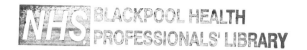
Obstetric Anesthesia

Principles and Practice

Third Edition

Obstetric Anesthesia

Principles and Practice

Third Edition

David H. Chestnut, M.D.
Alfred Habeeb Professor and Chair of Anesthesiology
Professor of Obstetrics and Gynecology
University of Alabama at Birmingham School of Medicine
Birmingham, Alabama

with 272 illustrations

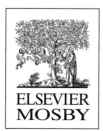

ELSEVIER
MOSBY

ELSEVIER
MOSBY

The Curtis Center
170 S Independence Mall W 300E
Philadelphia, Pennsylvania 19106

OBSTETRIC ANESTHESIA: PRINCIPLES AND PRACTICE

Previous editions copyrighted 1999, 1994

Obstetric anesthesia / [edited by] David H. Chestnut.—3rd ed.
    p. ; cm.
    Includes bibliographical references and index.
    ISBN 0-323-02357-6
    1. Anesthesia in obstetrics. I. Chestnut, David H.
    [DNLM: 1. Anesthesia, Obstetrical—methods. 2. Anesthetics. 3. Labor Complications.
WO 450 O141 2004]
RG732.O265 2004
617.9′682—dc22

2003061404

Acquisitions Editor: Natasha Andjelkovic
Developmental Editor: Donna Morrissey
Publishing Services Manager: Joan Sinclair
Project Manager: Mary Stermel

Printed in the United States of America

Last digit is the print number: 9 8 7 6 5 4 3 2 1

Contributors

Susan W. Aucott, M.D.
Assistant Professor of Pediatrics
Director, Neonatal Intensive Care Unit
The Johns Hopkins University School of Medicine
Baltimore, Maryland

Chakib M. Ayoub, M.D.
Assistant Professor of Anesthesiology
Beirut Medical Center
Beirut, Lebanon
Clinical Assistant Professor of Anesthesiology
Yale University School of Medicine
New Haven, Connecticut

Angela M. Bader, M.D.
Associate Professor of Anaesthesia
Harvard Medical School
Director, Center for Preoperative Evaluation
Brigham and Women's Hospital
Boston, Massachusetts

B. Wycke Baker, M.D.
Director of Obstetric Anesthesia
St. Luke's Episcopal Hospital
Houston, Texas

Elizabeth A. Bell, M.D., M.P.H.
Associate Professor of Anesthesiology
University of North Carolina School of Medicine
Chapel Hill, North Carolina

Jonathan L. Benumof, M.D.
Professor of Anesthesiology
University of California, San Diego, School of Medicine
San Diego, California

David J. Birnbach, M.D.
Professor of Anesthesiology and Obstetrics
  and Gynecology
Chief, Women's Anesthesia
Associate Director, Institute for Women's Health
University of Miami School of Medicine
Miami, Florida

Lisa Vincler Brock, J.D.
Assistant Attorney General, State of Washington
Faculty Associate, Department of Medical History and Ethics
University of Washington School of Medicine
Seattle, Washington

Philip R. Bromage, M.B., B.S., FRCA, FRCPC
Professor of Anaesthesia (retirement status)
McGill University
Montreal, Quebec, Canada

David L. Brown, M.D.
Professor and Head, Department of Anesthesia
University of Iowa Carver College of Medicine
Iowa City, Iowa

William R. Camann, M.D.
Associate Professor of Anaesthesia
Harvard Medical School
Brigham and Women's Hospital
Boston, Massachusetts

Harvey Carp, M.D., Ph.D.
Staff Anesthesiologist
Columbia Anesthesia Group
Southwest Washington Medical Center
Vancouver, Washington

Donald Caton, M.D.
Professor of Anesthesiology and Obstetrics and Gynecology
University of Florida College of Medicine
Gainesville, Florida

H.S. Chadwick, M.D.
Associate Professor of Anesthesiology
University of Washington School of Medicine
Seattle, Washington

Anita Backus Chang, M.D.
Associate Clinical Professor of Anesthesiology
David Geffen School of Medicine at UCLA
Director of Obstetric Anesthesia
UCLA Medical Center
Los Angeles, California

Paula D. M. Chantigian, M.D., FACOG
Obstetrician and Gynecologist
Byron, Minnesota

Robert C. Chantigian, M.D.
Associate Professor of Anesthesiology
Mayo Clinic College of Medicine
Rochester, Minnesota

David H. Chestnut, M.D.
Alfred Habeeb Professor and Chair of Anesthesiology
Professor of Obstetrics and Gynecology
University of Alabama at Birmingham School of Medicine
Birmingham, Alabama

Sheila E. Cohen, M.B., Ch.B., FRCA
Professor of Anesthesia and Obstetrics and Gynecology
Stanford University School of Medicine
Stanford, California

Edward T. Crosby, M.D., FRCPC
Professor of Anesthesiology
University of Ottawa
The Ottawa Hospital—General Campus
Ottawa, Ontario, Canada

Robert D'Angelo, M.D.
Associate Professor of Anesthesiology
Vice Chair and Section Head of Obstetric Anesthesia
Wake Forest University School of Medicine
Winston-Salem, North Carolina

David D. Dewan, M.D.
Professor of Anesthesiology (retirement status)
Wake Forest University School of Medicine
Winston-Salem, North Carolina

M. Joanne Douglas, M.D., FRCPC
Clinical Professor of Anesthesia
University of British Columbia Faculty of Medicine
British Columbia Women's Hospital and Health Centre
Vancouver, British Columbia, Canada

James C. Eisenach, M.D.
F.M. James, III, Professor of Anesthesiology
Wake Forest University School of Medicine
Winston-Salem, North Carolina

Mieczyslaw Finster, M.D.
Professor of Anesthesiology
College of Physicians and Surgeons
Columbia University
New York, New York

David R. Gambling, M.B., B.S., FRCPC
Clinical Associate Professor
University of California, San Diego, School of Medicine
Staff Anesthesiologist
Sharp Mary Birch Hospital for Women
San Diego, California

Beth Glosten, M.D.
Anesthesiologist (retirement status)
Redmond, Washington

Vijaya Gottumukkala, M.B.B.S., M.D., FRCA
Associate Professor and Director of Resident Education
Department of Anesthesia
University of Iowa Carver College of Medicine
Iowa City, Iowa

Thomas S. Guyton, M.D.
Medical Anesthesia Group
Methodist Hospitals of Memphis
Memphis, Tennessee

Miriam Harnett, M.B., FFARCSI
Instructor in Anaesthesia
Harvard Medical School
Brigham and Women's Hospital
Boston, Massachusetts

Andrew P. Harris, M.D., M.H.S.
Associate Professor of Anesthesiology and Critical
    Care Medicine
The Johns Hopkins University School of Medicine
Baltimore, Maryland

Joy L. Hawkins, M.D.
Professor of Anesthesiology
Director of Obstetric Anesthesia
University of Colorado School of Medicine
Denver, Colorado

Norman L. Herman, M.D., Ph.D.
Assistant Professor of Anesthesiology (retirement status)
Cornell University Medical College
New York, New York

BettyLou Koffel, M.D.
Chief of Anesthesiology
Northwest Permanente, P.C.
Director of Obstetric Anesthesia Services
Providence St. Vincent Medical Center
Portland, Oregon

Krzysztof M. Kuczkowski, M.D.
Assistant Clinical Professor of Anesthesiology
    and Reproductive Medicine
Director of Obstetric Anesthesia
University of California, San Diego, School of Medicine
San Diego, California

Robert B. Lechner, M.D., Ph.D.
Staff Anesthesiologist
Fauquier Hospital
Warrenton, Virginia

Dennis Lin, M.D.
Staff Anesthesiologist
Quincy Hospital
Quincy, Massachusetts

Karen S. Lindeman, M.D.
Associate Professor of Anesthesiology and Critical Care
    Medicine
The Johns Hopkins University School of Medicine
Baltimore, Maryland

Elizabeth G. Livingston, M.D.
Associate Professor of Obstetrics and Gynecology
Duke University Medical Center
Durham, North Carolina

Andrew M. Malinow, M.D.
Professor of Anesthesiology
Professor of Obstetrics, Gynecology, and Reproductive
  Sciences
Director of Obstetric Anesthesia
University of Maryland School of Medicine
Baltimore, Maryland

David C. Mayer, M.D.
Associate Professor of Anesthesiology and Obstetrics
  and Gynecology
University of North Carolina School of Medicine
Chapel Hill, North Carolina

Marie E. Minnich, M.D., M.M.M.
Division of Anesthesiology
Geisinger Health System
Danville, Pennsylvania

Philip S. Mushlin, M.D.
Associate Professor of Anaesthesia
Harvard Medical School
Brigham and Women's Hospital
Boston, Massachusetts

Holly A. Muir, M.D.
Assistant Professor of Anesthesiology
Chief, Division of Women's Anesthesia
Duke University Medical Center
Durham, North Carolina

Norah N. Naughton, M.D.
Clinical Associate Professor of Anesthesiology
University of Michigan School of Medicine
Director of Obstetric Anesthesia
University of Michigan Health System
Ann Arbor, Michigan

Jennifer R. Niebyl, M.D.
Professor and Head
Department of Obstetrics and Gynecology
University of Iowa Carver College of Medicine
Iowa City, Iowa

Geraldine M. O'Sullivan, M.D.
Anaesthetic Department
St. Thomas' Hospital
London, United Kingdom

Robert K. Parker, D.O.
Associate Professor of Anesthesiology and Obstetrics
  and Gynecology
Tufts University School of Medicine
Boston, Massachusetts
Chief of Obstetric Anesthesia
Baystate Medical Center
Springfield, Massachusetts

Donald H. Penning, M.D., M.Sc., FRCP
Associate Professor of Anesthesiology and Obstetrics
  and Gynecology
Chief, Division of Obstetric Anesthesia
The Johns Hopkins University School of Medicine
Baltimore, Maryland

Linda S. Polley, M.D.
Clinical Associate Professor of Anesthesiology
University of Michigan School of Medicine
Ann Arbor, Michigan

Robert W. Reid, M.D.
International Children's Heart Foundation
Overland Park, Kansas

Laurence S. Reisner, M.D.
Professor Emeritus of Clinical Anesthesiology
  and Reproductive Medicine
University of California, San Diego, School of Medicine
San Diego, California

**Felicity Reynolds, M.B.,B.S., M.D., FRCA, FRCOG *ad
eundem***
Emeritus Professor of Obstetric Anaesthesia
Anaesthetic Department
St. Thomas' Hospital
London, United Kingdom

Edward T. Riley, M.D.
Associate Professor of Anesthesia
Director of Obstetric Anesthesia
Stanford University School of Medicine
Stanford, California

Mark A. Rosen, M.D.
Professor and Vice Chair of Anesthesia and Perioperative Care
Professor of Obstetrics, Gynecology, and Reproductive
  Sciences
Director of Obstetric Anesthesia
University of California, San Francisco, School of Medicine
San Francisco, California

Brian K. Ross, M.D., Ph.D.
Professor of Anesthesiology
University of Washington School of Medicine
Seattle, Washington

Dwight J. Rouse, M.D., M.S.P.H.
Professor of Obstetrics and Gynecology
University of Alabama at Birmingham School of Medicine
Birmingham, Alabama

Alan C. Santos, M.D., M.P.H.
Professor of Anesthesiology
St. Luke's–Roosevelt Hospital Center
Columbia University
New York, New York

Scott Segal, M.D.
Associate Professor of Anaesthesia
Harvard Medical School
Brigham and Women's Hospital
Boston, Massachusetts

Shiv K. Sharma, M.D., FRCA
Professor of Anesthesiology and Obstetrics
  and Gynecology
University of Texas Southwestern Medical Center at Dallas
Dallas, Texas

Raymond S. Sinatra, M.D., Ph.D.
Professor of Anesthesiology
Director, Pain Management Service
Yale University School of Medicine
New Haven, Connecticut

Fred J. Spielman, M.D.
Professor of Anesthesiology and Obstetrics and Gynecology
University of North Carolina School of Medicine
Chapel Hill, North Carolina

Lawrence C. Tsen, M.D.
Assistant Professor of Anaesthesia
Harvard Medical School
Director, Anesthesia for Assisted Reproductive Technologies
Brigham and Women's Hospital
Boston, Massachusetts

Robert D. Vincent, Jr., M.D.
Associate Professor of Anesthesiology
University of Alabama at Birmingham School of Medicine
Birmingham, Alabama

Marsha L. Wakefield, M.D.
Associate Professor of Anesthesiology
University of Alabama at Birmingham School of Medicine
Birmingham, Alabama

Sally K. Weeks, M.B., B.S., FRCA
Associate Professor of Anesthesia and Obstetrics
    and Gynecology
McGill University
Director of Obstetric Anesthesia
Royal Victoria Hospital
Montreal, Quebec, Canada

Carl P. Weiner, M.D., M.B.A., FACOG
Professor of Obstetrics, Gynecology, and Reproductive
    Sciences
Professor of Physiology
University of Maryland School of Medicine
Baltimore, Maryland

Katharine D. Wenstrom, M.D.
Professor of Obstetrics and Gynecology and Human Genetics
Director, Division of Maternal-Fetal Medicine
    and Reproductive Genetics
University of Alabama at Birmingham School of Medicine
Birmingham, Alabama

Mark S. Williams, M.D., M.B.A., J.D.
Clinical Associate Professor
University of Alabama at Birmingham School of Medicine
Chair of Anesthesiology
Carraway Methodist Medical Center
Birmingham, Alabama

Richard N. Wissler, M.D., PhD.
Associate Professor of Anesthesiology and Obstetrics
    and Gynecology
Director of Obstetric Anesthesia
University of Rochester School of Medicine and Dentistry
Rochester, New York

David J. Wlody, M.D.
Vice Chair for Clinical Affairs in Anesthesiology
Director of Obstetric Anesthesia
State University of New York
Downstate Medical Center
Brooklyn, New York

Jerome Yankowitz, M.D.
Professor of Obstetrics and Gynecology
Director, Division of Maternal-Fetal Medicine
University of Iowa Carver College of Medicine
Iowa City, Iowa

Mark I. Zakowski, M.D.
Chief of Obstetric Anesthesia
Cedars-Sinai Medical Center
Los Angeles, California

Frank J. Zlatnick, M.D.
William C. Keettel Professor of Obstetrics and Gynecology
University of Iowa Carver College of Medicine
Iowa City, Iowa

Rhonda L. Zuckerman, M.D.
Assistant Professor of Anesthesiology and Critical Care
Assistant Professor of Gynecology and Obstetrics
The Johns Hopkins University School of Medicine
Baltimore, Maryland

To
my wife, **Janet,**
and
our children, **John Mark, Michael, Mary Beth, Annie,** *and* **Stephen**

Preface to the Third Edition

Sometimes less is more.

As we planned the third edition of this text, we sought the advice of our contributors and readers. We asked whether we should add chapters on this or that subject. The responses were clear and uniform: "Revise . . . update . . . amplify a few subjects . . . but do not lengthen or enlarge."

For the third edition, we solicited the services of 15 new contributors while retaining most of the outstanding contributors to the second edition. Some chapters were rewritten in their entirety. Others were revised extensively. New subjects were added. Some chapters were shortened. All chapters (except Chapter 1) were updated. Further, the publisher has used a tighter publication style. Altogether, the third edition is comprehensive and up-to-date, but it has *fewer* pages than the second edition. In my judgment, this is the best of the three editions that we have published.

I should like to express my gratitude to my extraordinary secretaries, Vickie Ray and Cindy Louderback, who provided invaluable assistance during the preparation of this third edition.

David H. Chestnut, M.D.

Preface to the Second Edition

Five years have elapsed since the publication of the first edition of this text. With pride and gratitude, 68 contributing authors and I offer this second edition to anesthesiologists, obstetricians and other clinicians who provide care for pregnant women. We welcome nine new contributors to the second edition, including new authors for six chapters. I am grateful for the hard work and selfless commitment of all these contributors. Each chapter (except chapter 1) has been thoroughly updated and revised. Dr. Don Caton introduces each part of the text with a relevant historical vignette. The Appendix includes the new Practice Guidelines for Obstetrical Anesthesia, recently approved by the House of Delegates of the American Society of Anesthesiologists. Together, our goal was to create a thorough, scholarly, and practical text for all clinicians who provide care for obstetric patients.

Two controversies in obstetric anesthesia have received substantial attention during the last five years. The first controversy—the relationship between epidural analgesia and the risk of cesarean section for dystocia—first waxed and (thankfully) has now waned. For several years, some obstetricians and third-party payers attributed the cesarean section "epidemic" to the increased use of epidural analgesia. Some third-party payers even denied reimbursement for epidural analgesia administered before 5 cm cervical dilation. This controversy has subsided for at least three reasons. First, several randomized clinical trials have demonstrated that the contemporary use of epidural analgesia does *not* increase the overall incidence of cesarean section. Second, the cesarean section rate in the United States has steadily declined during the last decade, despite the increased use of epidural analgesia. Third, most anesthesiologists currently use more dilute solutions of local anesthetic when providing epidural analgesia for laboring women. Even some critics of epidural analgesia have modified their earlier assessment. They currently contend—and I would agree—that dense epidural anesthesia, using a concentrated solution of local anesthetic, may increase the incidence of cesarean section for dystocia, but the use of a more dilute solution of local anesthetic is less likely to affect the progress of labor and the method of delivery (i.e., "that was then, and this is now"). Despite these highly publicized criticisms, the intrapartum use of epidural analgesia has continued to increase, and recent clinical studies have demonstrated that the contemporary use of epidural analgesia is compatible with an acceptable cesarean section rate. Maternal-fetal factors and obstetric management—*not* epidural analgesia—are the most important determinants of the cesarean section rate.

More recently, another controversy has threatened to divide our own specialty. This controversy results from some highly publicized cases of alleged denial of epidural analgesia for indigent parturients. Some anesthesiologists defend the practice of withholding epidural analgesia for indigent patients, claiming that epidural analgesia during labor is an elective procedure. In contrast, others argue that all women should have ready access to effective pain relief—including epidural analgesia—during labor.

This controversy highlights the dilemma that challenges many anesthesiologists. I understand this dilemma well. Obstetric anesthesia is the love of my professional career. I helped write the ASA-ACOG opinion, "Pain Relief During Labor," which includes the following observations:

> Labor results in severe pain for many women. There is no other circumstance where it is considered acceptable for a person to experience severe pain, amenable to safe intervention, while under a physician's care.

However, I am also chair of a university department of anesthesiology that provides anesthesia care for over 3500 obstetric patients per year. Medicaid is the payer for most of our patients. In some states, our obstetric colleagues have successfully lobbied their state governments for equitable reimbursement for their services, but the reimbursement for obstetric anesthesia services continues to lag.

Despite inequities in reimbursement, we offer epidural analgesia to *all* our obstetric patients, regardless of their ability to pay. Heretofore we and other anesthesiologists subsidized this service by cost-shifting. We do this willingly—one colleague says it is our "joyful burden"—but we worry whether we can continue to provide the same quality of service unless some third-party payers place greater economic value on our services. As is often stated, "no margin, no mission."

Herein lies the dilemma. If we agree to provide a service at *any* price, we lose all leverage in negotiations with third-party payers. Also, our ability to attract the best and brightest medical students to our specialty is jeopardized. On the other hand, we should not allow a dispute between ourselves and a third-party payer to cause a patient to suffer. The prophet Micah declared: "He has showed you, O man, what is good. And what does the Lord require of you? To act justly and to love mercy and to walk humbly with your God." *(Micah 6:8)*

I understand the frustration of my colleagues, but I also remain grateful for the privilege of providing care to all our patients, rich and poor.

What controversies can we expect during the next five years? I am not a futurist, but I suspect that intrathecal opioid analgesia—and combined spinal-epidural (CSE) analgesia—will undergo continued scrutiny. Use of the CSE technique has exploded during the last five years. The CSE technique allows the anesthesiologist to provide analgesia that is almost instantaneous, and the patient retains the ability to ambulate. However, several questions remain unanswered. Does ambulation provide a benefit clinically? Does CSE analgesia increase the risk of emergency cesarean section for fetal bradycardia? What is the incidence of maternal respiratory depression? Does CSE analgesia result in an increased risk of neuraxial infection? The CSE technique is more "invasive" than epidural analgesia alone, and in Chapter 33, Dr. Philip Bromage calls attention to several case reports of meningitis after administration of CSE analgesia in laboring women. Do these case reports signal an increased risk of meningitis? Does the indwelling epidural catheter serve as a conduit for pathogens to enter the subarachnoid space through the dural puncture site? Or, as suggested by Dr. Jim Eisenach, do these reports reflect the ease of publishing a case report of a complication resulting from a new technique? Answers to these questions likely will affect decisions regarding the possible reintroduction of spinal microcatheters—and the administration of continuous spinal analgesia—in obstetric anesthesia practice.

Notwithstanding existing economic pressures, more anesthesiologists are involved in the practice of obstetric anesthesia than at any time in the history of our specialty. Our journals are publishing an increasing number of quality papers related to obstetric anesthesia, and I am confident that these and other questions will be answered with care and clarity.

Finally, I express my gratitude to my extraordinary secretaries, Margaret Dodd and Cindy Louderback, who provided invaluable assistance during the preparation of this second edition. Likewise, I thank the production staff at Mosby for their support and attention to detail. Together, their competence, enthusiasm, and patience (with me) allowed this project to proceed smoothly and successfully.

David H. Chestnut, M.D.

Preface to the First Edition

Several years ago, I could not decide whether I wanted to be an anesthesiologist or an obstetrician. I obtained training in both specialties largely because of my love of perinatal medicine. This text is the result of my long-standing desire to prepare a truly comprehensive obstetric anesthesia text. In this book, I attempted to fulfill two goals: (1) to collate the most important information that anesthesiologists should know about obstetrics and (2) to prepare a thorough review of anesthesia care for obstetric patients. I asked each contributor to prepare a comprehensive, scholarly discussion of the subject and also to provide clear, practical recommendations for clinical management. Hopefully, this book will provide the necessary foundation for anesthesiology and obstetric residents, be a user-friendly resource for both experienced and occasional practitioners, and serve as a complete reference text for subspecialists in obstetric anesthesia.

This book would not have seen the light of day without the effort of 62 other contributors. I am grateful for their selfless commitment and hard work. I should like to thank several colleagues—David Murray, Alan Ross, and Carl Weiner—who reviewed chapters related to their areas of expertise. I should also like to thank my chairman, John Tinker, a true friend who provided encouragement and support. Finally, I should like to express my deepest gratitude to my extraordinary secretary, Teresa Block, who tirelessly revised the manuscript for each chapter. Her competence, attention to detail, and enthusiasm allowed this project to proceed smoothly.

David H. Chestnut, M.D.

Contents

Part I
Introduction

Chapter 1
The History of Obstetric Anesthesia

Donald Caton, M.D.

For I heard a cry as of a woman in travail, anguish as of one bringing forth her first child, the cry of the daughter of Zion gasping for breath, stretching out her hands, "Woe is me!"

Jeremiah 4:31

"The position of woman in any civilization is an index of the advancement of that civilization; the position of woman is gauged best by the care given her at the birth of her child." So wrote Haggard[1] in 1929. If his thesis is true, Western civilization made a giant leap on January 19, 1847, when James Young Simpson used diethyl ether to anesthetize a woman with a deformed pelvis for delivery. This first use of a modern anesthetic for childbirth occurred a scant 3 months after Morton's historic demonstration of the anesthetic properties of ether at the Massachusetts General Hospital in Boston. Strangely enough, Simpson's innovation evoked strong criticism from contemporary obstetricians, who questioned its safety, and from many segments of the lay public, who questioned its wisdom. The debate over these issues lasted more than 5 years and influenced the future of obstetric anesthesia.[2]

JAMES YOUNG SIMPSON

Few people were better equipped than Simpson to deal with controversy. Just 36 years old, Simpson already had 7 years' tenure as Professor of Midwifery at the University of Edinburgh, one of the most prestigious medical schools of its day (Figure 1-1). By that time, he had established a reputation as one of the foremost obstetricians in Great Britain, if not the world. On the day he first used ether for childbirth, he also received a letter of appointment as Queen's Physician in Scotland. Etherization for childbirth was only one of Simpson's contributions. He also designed obstetric forceps (which still bear his name), discovered the anesthetic properties of chloroform, made important innovations in hospital architecture, and wrote a textbook on the practice of witchcraft in Scotland, which was used by several generations of anthropologists.[3]

An imposing man, Simpson had a large head, a massive mane of hair, and the pudgy body of an adolescent. Contemporaries described his voice as "commanding," with a wide range of volume and intonation. Clearly Simpson had "presence" and "charisma." These attributes were indispensable to someone in his profession, because in the mid-nineteenth century the role of science in the development of medical theory and practice was minimal; rhetoric resolved more issues than facts. The medical climate in Edinburgh was particularly contentious and vituperative. In this milieu, Simpson had trained, competed for advancement and recognition, and succeeded. The rigor of this preparation served him well.

Initially, virtually every prominent obstetrician, including Montgomery of Dublin, Ramsbotham of London, Dubois of Paris, and Meigs of Philadelphia, opposed etherization for childbirth. Simpson called on all of his professional and personal finesse to sway opinion in the ensuing controversy.

MEDICAL OBJECTIONS TO THE USE OF ETHER FOR CHILDBIRTH

Shortly after Simpson administered the first obstetric anesthetic he wrote the following[4]:

It will be necessary to ascertain anesthesia's precise effect, both upon the action of the uterus and on the assistant abdominal muscles; its influence, if any, upon the child; whether it has a tendency to hemorrhage or other complications.

With this statement he identified the issues that would most concern obstetricians who succeeded him and thus shape the subsequent development of the specialty.

Simpson's most articulate, persistent, and persuasive critic was Charles D. Meigs, Professor of Midwifery at Jefferson Medical College in Philadelphia (Figure 1-2). In character and stature, Meigs equaled Simpson. Born to a prominent New England family, Meigs' forebears included heroes of the American revolutionary war, the first governor of the state of Ohio, and the founder of the University of Georgia. His descendants included a prominent pediatrician, an obstetrician, and one son who served the Union Army as Quartermaster General during the Civil War.[5]

At the heart of the dispute between Meigs and Simpson was a difference in their interpretation of the nature of labor and the significance of labor pain. Simpson maintained that all pain, labor pain included, is without physiologic value. He said that pain only degrades and destroys those who experience it. In contrast, Meigs argued that labor pain has purpose, that uterine pain is inseparable from contractions, and that any drug that abolishes pain will alter contractions. Meigs also believed that pregnancy and labor are normal processes that usually end quite well. He said that physicians should therefore not intervene with powerful, potentially disruptive drugs (Figure 1-3). We must accept the statements of both men as expressions of natural philosophy because neither had facts to buttress his position. Indeed, in 1847, physicians had little information of any sort about uterine function, pain, or the relationship between them. Studies of the anatomy and physiology of pain had just begun. It was only during the preceding 20 years that investigators had recognized that specific nerves and areas of the brain have different functions and that specialized peripheral receptors for painful stimuli exist.[2]

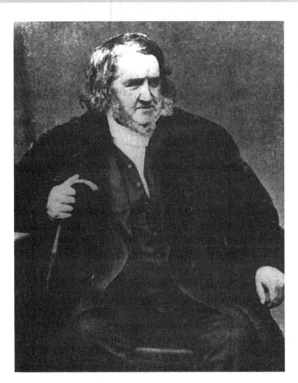

FIGURE 1-1. James Young Simpson, the obstetrician who first administered a modern anesthetic for childbirth. He also discovered the anesthetic properties of chloroform. Many believe that he was the most prominent and influential physician of his day. (Courtesy Yale Medical History Library.)

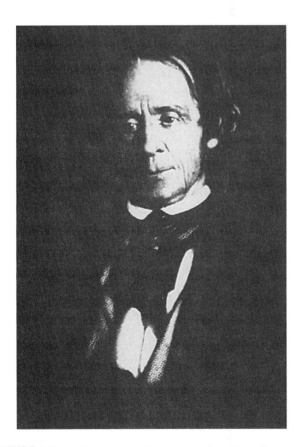

FIGURE 1-2. Charles D. Meigs, the American obstetrician who opposed the use of anesthesia for obstetrics. He questioned the safety of anesthesia and said that there was no demonstrated need for it during a normal delivery. (Courtesy Wood Library Museum.)

OBSTETRICS:

THE

SCIENCE AND THE ART.

BY

CHARLES D. MEIGS, M.D.,

PROFESSOR OF MIDWIFERY AND THE DISEASES OF WOMEN AND CHILDREN IN JEFFERSON MEDICAL COLLEGE AT PHILADELPHIA; LATELY ONE OF THE PHYSICIANS TO THE LYING-IN DEPARTMENT OF THE PENNSYLVANIA HOSPITAL; MEMBER OF THE SOCIETY OF SWEDISH PHYSICIANS AT STOCKHOLM; CORRESPONDING MEMBER OF THE HUNTERIAN SOCIETY OF LONDON; MEMBER OF THE AMERICAN PHILOSOPHICAL SOCIETY; OF THE ACADEMY OF NATURAL SCIENCES OF PHILADELPHIA; OF THE AMERICAN MEDICAL ASSOCIATION, ETC. ETC.

THIRD EDITION. REVISED.

WITH ONE HUNDRED AND TWENTY-NINE ILLUSTRATIONS.

PHILADELPHIA:
BLANCHARD AND LEA.
1856.

FIGURE 1-3. Frontispiece from Meigs' textbook of obstetrics.

In 1850, more physicians expressed support for Meigs' views than for Simpson's. For example, Baron Paul Dubois[6] of the Faculty of Paris wondered whether ether, "after having exerted a stupefying action over the cerebro-spinal nerves, could not induce paralysis of the muscular element of the uterus?" Similarly, Ramsbotham[7] of London Hospital said that he believed the "treatment of rendering a patient in labor completely insensible through the agency of anesthetic remedies . . . is fraught with extreme danger." These physicians' fears gained credence from the report by a special committee of the Royal Medical and Surgical Society documenting 123 deaths that "could be positively assigned to the inhalation of chloroform."[8] Although none involved obstetric patients, safety was on the minds of obstetricians.

The reaction to the delivery of Queen Victoria's eighth child in 1853 illustrated the aversion of the medical community to obstetric anesthesia. According to private records, John Snow anesthetized the Queen for the delivery of Prince Leopold at the request of her personal physicians. Although no one made a formal announcement of this fact, rumors surfaced and provoked strong public criticism. Thomas Wakley, the irascible founding editor of *The Lancet*, was particularly incensed. He "could not imagine that anyone had incurred the awful responsibility of advising the administration of chloroform to her Majesty during a perfectly natural labour with a seventh child."[9] (It was her eighth child, but Wakley had apparently lost count—a forgivable error considering the propensity of the Queen to bear children.) Court physicians did not defend their decision to use ether. Perhaps not wanting a public confrontation, they simply denied that the Queen had received an anesthetic. In fact, they first acknowledged a royal anesthetic 4 years later when the Queen delivered her ninth and last child, Princess Beatrice. By that time, however, the issue was no longer controversial.[9]

PUBLIC REACTION TO ETHERIZATION FOR CHILDBIRTH

The controversy surrounding obstetric anesthesia was not resolved by the medical community. Physicians remained skeptical, but public opinion changed. Women lost their reservations, decided they wanted anesthesia, and virtually forced physicians to offer it to them. The change in the public's attitude in favor of obstetric anesthesia marked the culmination of a more general change in social attitudes that had been developing over several centuries.

Before the nineteenth century, pain meant something quite different from what it does today. Since antiquity, people believed that all manner of calamities—disease, drought, poverty, and pain—signified divine retribution inflicted as punishment for sin. According to Scripture, childbirth pain originated when God punished Eve and her descendants for Eve's disobedience in the Garden of Eden. Many believed that it was wrong to avoid the pain of divine punishment. This belief was sufficiently prevalent and strong to retard acceptance of even the idea of anesthesia, especially for obstetric patients. Only when this tradition weakened did people seek ways to free themselves from disease and pain. In most Western countries, the transition occurred during the nineteenth century. Disease and pain lost their theologic connotations and became biologic processes subject to study and control by new methods of science and technology. This evolution of thought facilitated the development of modern medicine and stimulated public acceptance of obstetric anesthesia.[10]

The reluctance that physicians felt toward the administration of anesthesia for childbirth pain stands in stark contrast to the enthusiasm expressed by early obstetric patients. In 1847, Fanny Longfellow, wife of the American poet Henry Wadsworth Longfellow and the first woman in the United States anesthetized for childbirth, wrote the following[11]:

> I am very sorry you all thought me so rash and naughty in trying the ether. Henry's faith gave me courage, and I had heard such a thing had succeeded abroad, where the surgeons extend this great blessing more boldly and universally than our timid doctors. . . . This is certainly the greatest blessing of this age.

Queen Victoria, responding to news of the birth of her first grandchild in 1860 and perhaps remembering her own recent confinement, wrote: "What a blessing she [Victoria, her oldest daughter] had chloroform. Perhaps without it her strength would have suffered very much."[9] The new understanding of pain as a controllable biologic process left no room for Meigs' idea that pain might have physiologic value. The eminent nineteenth-century social philosopher John Stuart Mill stated that the "hurtful agencies of nature" promote good only by "inciting rational creatures to rise up and struggle against them."[12]

Simpson prophesied the role of public opinion in the acceptance of obstetric anesthesia, a fact not lost on his adversaries. Early in the controversy he wrote: "Medical men may oppose for a time the superinduction of anaesthesia in parturition but they will oppose it in vain; for certainly our patients themselves will force use of it upon the profession. The whole question is, even now, one merely of time."[13] By 1860, Simpson's prophecy came true; anesthesia for childbirth became part of medical practice by public acclaim.

OPIOIDS AND OBSTETRICS

The next major innovation in obstetric anesthesia came approximately 50 years later. *Dämmerschlaff*, which means "twilight sleep," was a technique developed by von Steinbüchel[14] of Graz and popularized by Gauss[15] of Freiberg. It combined opioids with scopolamine to make women amnestic and somewhat comfortable during labor (Figure 1-4). Until that time, opioids had been used sparingly for obstetrics. Although opium had been part of the medical armamentarium since the Roman Empire, it was not used extensively, in part because of the difficulty of obtaining consistent results with the crude extracts available at that time. Therapeutics made a substantial advance in 1809 when Sertürner, a German pharmacologist, isolated codeine and morphine from a crude extract of the poppy seed. Methods for administering the drugs remained unsophisticated, however. Physicians gave morphine orally or by a method resembling vaccination, in which they placed a drop of solution on the skin and then made multiple small puncture holes with a sharp instrument to facilitate absorption. In 1853, the year Queen Victoria delivered her eighth child, the syringe and hollow metal needle were developed. This technical advance simplified the administration of opioids and facilitated the development of twilight sleep approximately 50 years later.[16]

Although reports of labor pain relief with hypodermic morphine appeared as early as 1868, few physicians favored its use. For example, in an article published in *Transactions of the Obstetrical Society of London*, Sansom[17] listed four agents for relief of labor pain: (1) carbon tetrachloride, the use of which he favored; (2) bichloride of methylene, which was under evaluation; (3) nitrous oxide, which had been introduced recently by Klikgowich of Russia; and (4) chloroform. He did not mention opioids, but neither did he mention diethyl ether, which many physicians still favored. Similarly, Gusserow,[18] a prominent German obstetrician, wrote about salicylic acid but not morphine for labor pain. (Von Beyer did not introduce acetylsalicylic acid to medical practice until 1899.) In retrospect, von Steinbüchel's and Gauss' description of twilight sleep in the first decade of the century may have

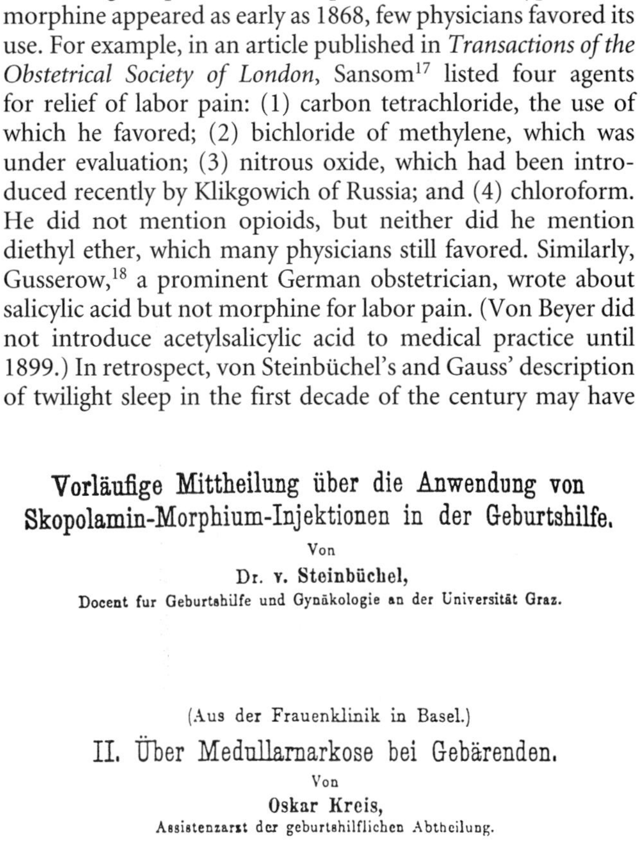

Vorläufige Mittheilung über die Anwendung von Skopolamin-Morphium-Injektionen in der Geburtshilfe.

Von

Dr. v. Steinbüchel,
Docent fur Geburtshilfe und Gynäkologie an der Universität Graz.

(Aus der Frauenklinik in Basel.)

II. Über Medullarnarkose bei Gebärenden.

Von

Oskar Kreis,
Assistenzarzt der geburtshilflichen Abtheilung.

FIGURE 1-4. Title pages from two important papers published in the first years of the twentieth century. The paper by von Steinbüchel introduced twilight sleep. The paper by Kreis described the first use of spinal anesthesia for obstetrics.

been important more for popularizing morphine than for suggesting that scopolamine be given with morphine.

Physicians reacted to twilight sleep as they had reacted to diethyl ether several years earlier. They resisted it, questioning whether the benefits justified the risks. Patients also reacted as they had before. Not aware of, or perhaps not concerned with, the technical considerations that confronted physicians, patients harbored few doubts and persuaded physicians to use it, sometimes against the physicians' better judgment. The confrontation between physicians and patients was particularly strident in the United States. Champions of twilight sleep lectured throughout the country and published articles in popular magazines. Public enthusiasm for the therapy subsided slightly after 1920 when a prominent advocate of the method died during childbirth. She was given twilight sleep, but her physicians said that her death was unrelated to any complication from its use. Whatever anxiety this incident may have created in the minds of patients, it did not seriously diminish their resolve. Confronted by such firm insistence, physicians acquiesced and used twilight sleep with increasing frequency.[19,20]

Although the reaction of physicians to twilight sleep resembled their reaction to etherization, the medical milieu in which the debate over twilight sleep developed was quite different from that in which etherization was deliberated. Between 1850 and 1900, medicine had changed, particularly in Europe. Physiology, chemistry, anatomy, and bacteriology became part of medical theory and practice. Bright students from America traveled to leading clinics in Germany, England, and France. They returned with new facts and methods that they used to examine problems and critique ideas. These developments became the basis for the revolution in American medical education and practice launched by the Flexner report published in 1914.[21]

Obstetrics also changed. During the years preceding World War I, it had earned a reputation as one of the most exciting and scientifically advanced specialties. Obstetricians experimented with new drugs and techniques. They recognized that change entails risk, and they examined each innovation more critically. In addition, they turned to science for information and methods to help them solve problems of medical management. Developments in obstetric anesthesia reflected this change in strategy. New methods introduced during this time stimulated physicians to reexamine two important but unresolved issues, the effects of drugs on the child, and the relationship between pain and labor.

THE EFFECTS OF ANESTHESIA ON THE NEWBORN

Many physicians, Simpson included, worried that anesthetic drugs might cross the placenta and harm the newborn. Available information justified their concern. The idea that gases cross the placenta appeared long before the discovery of oxygen and carbon dioxide. In the sixteenth century, English physiologist John Mayow[22] suggested that "nitro aerial" particles from the mother nourish the fetus. By 1847, physiologists had corroborative evidence. Clinical experience gave more support. John Snow observed depressed neonatal breathing and motor activity and smelled ether on the breath of neonates delivered from mothers who had been given ether. In an early paper, he surmised that anesthetic gases cross the placenta.[23] Regardless, some advocates of obstetric anesthesia discounted the possibility. For example, Harvard professor Walter Channing denied that ether crossed the placenta because he could not detect its odor in the cut ends of the

umbilical cord. Oddly enough, he did not attempt to smell ether on the child's exhalations as John Snow had done.[24]

In 1874, Swiss obstetrician Paul Zweifel[25] published an account of work that finally resolved the debate about the placental transfer of drugs (Figure 1-5). He used a chemical reaction to demonstrate the presence of chloroform in the umbilical blood of neonates. In a separate paper, Zweifel[26] used a light-absorption technique to demonstrate a difference in oxygen content between umbilical arterial and venous blood, thereby establishing the placental transfer of oxygen. Although clinicians recognized the importance of these data, they accepted the implications slowly. Some clinicians pointed to several decades of clinical use "without problems." For example, Otto Spiegelberg,[27] Professor of Obstetrics at the University of Breslau, wrote in 1887: "As far as the fetus is concerned, no unimpeachable clinical observation has yet been published in which a fetus was injured by chloroform administered to its mother." Experience lulled them into complacency, which may explain their failure to appreciate the threat posed by twilight sleep.

Dangers from twilight sleep probably developed insidiously. The originators of the method, von Steinbüchel and Gauss, recommended conservative doses of drugs. They suggested that 0.3 mg of scopolamine be given every 2 to 3 hours to induce amnesia and that no more than 10 mg of morphine be administered subcutaneously for the whole labor. Gauss, who was especially meticulous, even advised physicians to administer a "memory test" to women in labor to evaluate the need for additional scopolamine.[28] However, as other physicians used the technique, they changed it. Some gave larger doses of opioid—as much as 40 or 50 mg of morphine during labor. Others gave additional drugs (e.g., as much as 600 mg

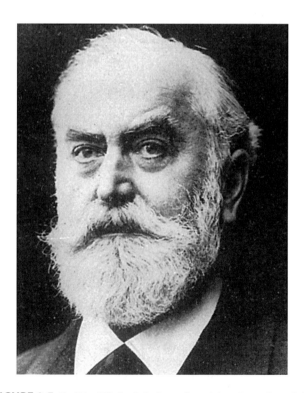

FIGURE 1-5. Paul Zweifel, the Swiss-born obstetrician who performed the first experiments that demonstrated chemically the presence of chloroform in the umbilical blood and urine of infants delivered of women who had been anesthetized during labor. (Courtesy J.F. Bergmann-Verlag, München, Germany.)

of pentobarbital during labor and inhalation agents for delivery). Despite administering these large doses to their patients, some physicians said they had seen no adverse effects on the infant. They probably spoke the truth, but this says more about their powers of observation than the safety of the method.

Two situations eventually made physicians confront problems associated with placental transmission of anesthetic drugs. The first was the changing use of morphine.[29] In the latter part of the nineteenth century (before the enactment of laws governing the use of addictive drugs), morphine was a popular ingredient of patent medicines and a drug frequently prescribed by physicians. As addiction became more common, obstetricians saw many pregnant women who were taking large amounts of morphine daily. When they tried to decrease their patients' opioid use, several obstetricians noted unexpected problems (e.g., violent fetal movements, sudden fetal death), which they correctly identified as signs of withdrawal. Second, physiologists and anatomists began extensive studies of placental structure and function. By the turn of the century, they had identified many of the physical and chemical factors that affect rates of drug transfer. Thus even before twilight sleep became popular, physicians had clinical and laboratory evidence to justify caution. As early as 1877, Gillette[30] described 15 instances of neonatal depression that he attributed to morphine given during labor. Similarly, in a review article published in 1914, Knipe[31] identified stillbirths and neonatal oligopnea and asphyxia as complications of twilight sleep and gave the incidence of each problem as reported by other authors.

When the studies of obstetric anesthesia published between 1880 and 1950 are considered, four characteristics stand out. First, few of them described effects of anesthesia on the newborn. Second, those that did report newborn apnea, oligopnea, or asphyxia seldom defined these words. Third, few used controls or compared one mode of treatment with another. Finally, few authors used their data to evaluate the safety of the practice that they described. In other words, by today's standards, even the best of these papers lacked substance. They did, however, demonstrate an increasing concern among physicians about the effects of anesthetic drugs on neonates. Perhaps even more important, their work prepared clinicians for the work of Virginia Apgar (Figure 1-6).

Apgar became an anesthesiologist when the chairman of the Department of Surgery at the Columbia University College of Physicians and Surgeons dissuaded her from becoming a surgeon. After training in anesthesia with Ralph Waters at the University of Wisconsin and with E. A. Rovenstine at Bellevue Hospital, she returned to Columbia Presbyterian Hospital as Director of the Division of Anesthesia. In 1949, she was appointed professor, the first woman to attain that rank at Columbia.[32]

In 1953, Apgar[33] described a simple, reliable system for evaluating newborns and showed that it was sufficiently sensitive to detect differences among neonates whose mothers had been anesthetized for cesarean section by different techniques (Figure 1-7). Infants delivered of women with spinal anesthesia had higher scores than those delivered with general anesthesia. The Apgar score had three important effects. First, it replaced simple observation of neonates with a reproducible measurement—that is, it substituted a numerical score for the ambiguities of words such as *oligopnea* and *asphyxia*. Thus it established the possibility of the systematic comparison of different treatments. Second, it provided objective criteria for the initiation of neonatal resuscitation. Third, and most important, it helped change the focus of obstetric care. Until that time the primary criterion for success or failure had been the survival and well-being of the mother, a natural goal considering the maternal risks of childbirth until that time. After 1900, as maternal risks diminished, the well-being of the mother no longer served as a sensitive measure of outcome. The Apgar score called attention to the child and made its condition the new standard for evaluating obstetric management.

THE EFFECTS OF ANESTHESIA ON LABOR

The effects of anesthesia on labor also worried physicians. Again their fears were well founded. Diethyl ether and chloroform depress uterine contractions. If given in sufficient amounts, they also abolish reflex pushing with the abdominal muscles during the second stage of labor. These effects are not difficult to detect, even with moderate doses of either inhalation agent.

Simpson's method of obstetric anesthesia used significant amounts of drugs. He started the anesthetic early, and

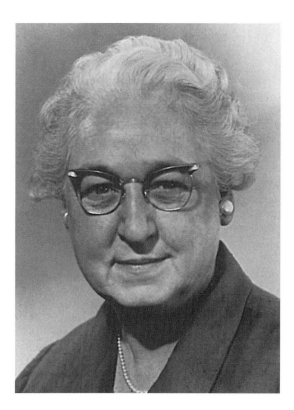

FIGURE 1-6. Virginia Apgar, whose scoring system revolutionized the practice of obstetrics and anesthesia. Her work made the well-being of the infant the major criterion for the evaluation of medical management of pregnant women. (Courtesy Wood Library Museum.)

Current Researches in Anesthesia and Analgesia—July-August, 1953

A Proposal for a New Method of Evaluation of the
Newborn Infant.*
Virginia Apgar, M.D., New York, N. Y.
*Department of Anesthesiology, Columbia University, College of Physicians and
Surgeons and the Anesthesia Service, The Presbyterian Hospital*

FIGURE 1-7. Title page from the paper in which Virginia Apgar described her new scoring system for evaluating the well-being of a newborn.

sometimes he rendered patients unconscious during the first stage of labor. In addition, he increased the depth of anesthesia for the delivery.[34] As many people copied his technique, they presumably had ample opportunity to observe uterine atony and postpartum hemorrhage.

Some physicians noticed the effects of anesthetics on uterine function. For example, Meigs[35] said unequivocally that etherization suppressed uterine function, and he described occasions in which he had had to suspend etherization to allow labor to resume. Other physicians waffled, however. For example, Walter Channing,[36] Professor of Midwifery and Jurisprudence at Harvard (seemingly a strange combination of disciplines, but at that time neither of the two was thought sufficiently important to warrant a separate chair), published a book about the use of ether for obstetrics. He endorsed etherization and influenced many others to use it. However, his book contained blatant contradictions (Figure 1-8). On different pages Channing contended that ether had no effect, that it increased uterine contractility, and that it suspended contractions entirely. Then, in a pronouncement smacking more of panache than reason, Channing swept aside his inconsistencies and said that whatever effect ether may have on the uterus he "welcomes it." Noting similar contradictions among other writers, W. F. H. Montgomery,[37] Professor of Midwifery at the King and Queen's College of Physicians in Ireland, wrote: "By one writer we are told that, if uterine action is excessive, chloroform will abate it; by another that

if feeble, it will strengthen it and add new vigor to each parturient effort."

John Snow[38] gave a more balanced review of the effects of anesthesia on labor. Originally a surgeon, Snow became the first physician to restrict his practice to anesthesia. He experimented with ether and chloroform and wrote many insightful papers and books describing his work (Figure 1-9). Snow's technique differed from Simpson's. Snow withheld anesthesia until the second stage of labor, limited administration to brief periods during contractions, and attempted to keep his patients comfortable but responsive. To achieve better control over the depth of anesthesia, he recommended using the vaporizing apparatus that he had developed for surgical cases. Snow[38] spoke disparagingly of Simpson's technique and the tendency of people to use it simply because of Simpson's reputation:

> The high position of Dr. Simpson and his previous services in this department, more particularly in being the first to administer ether in labour, gave his recommendations very great influence; the consequence of which is that the practice of anesthesia is presently probably in a much less satisfactory state than it would have been if chloroform had never been introduced.

Snow's method, which was the same one he had used to anesthetize Queen Victoria, eventually prevailed over Simpson's. Physicians became more cautious with anesthesia, reserving it for special problems such as cephalic version, the application of forceps, abnormal presentation, or eclampsia. They also became more conservative with dosage, often giving anesthesia only during the second stage of labor. Snow's methods were applied to each new inhalation agent—including

A TREATISE

ON

ETHERIZATION IN CHILDBIRTH.

ILLUSTRATED BY

FIVE HUNDRED AND EIGHTY-ONE CASES.

BY WALTER CHANNING, M.D.

PROFESSOR OF MIDWIFERY AND MEDICAL JURISPRUDENCE IN THE UNIVERSITY
AT CAMBRIDGE.

―――――――

" Give me the facts, said my Lord Judge: your reasonings are the mere guess-
work of the imagination." — OLD PLAY.

―――――――

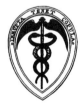

BOSTON:

WILLIAM D. TICKNOR AND COMPANY,
CORNER OF WASHINGTON AND SCHOOL STREETS.

M.DCCC.XL.VIII.

FIGURE 1-8. Frontispiece from Walter Channing's book on the use of etherization for childbirth. Channing favored the use of etherization, and he convinced others to use it, although evidence ensuring its safety was scant.

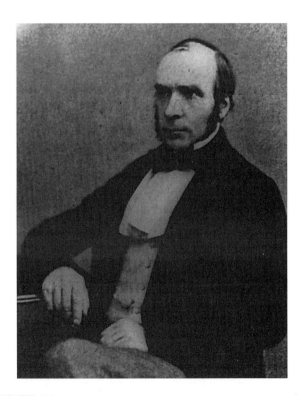

FIGURE 1-9. John Snow, a London surgeon who gave up his surgical practice to become the first physician to devote all his time to anesthesia. He wrote many monographs and papers, some of which accurately describe the effects of anesthesia on infant and mother. (Courtesy Wood Library Museum.)

nitrous oxide, ethylene, cyclopropane, trichloroethylene, and methoxyflurane—as it was introduced to obstetric anesthesia.

Early physicians modified their use of anesthesia from experience, not from study of normal labor or from learning more about the pharmacology of the drugs. Moreover, they still had not defined the relationship between uterine pain and contractions. As physicians turned more to science during the latter part of the century, however, their strategies began to change. For example, in 1893 the English physiologist Henry Head[39] published his classic studies of the innervation of abdominal viscera. His work stimulated others to investigate the role of the nervous system in the control of labor. Subsequently, clinical and laboratory studies of pregnancy after spinal cord transection established the independence of labor from nervous control.[40] When regional anesthesia appeared during the first decades of the twentieth century, physicians therefore had a conceptual basis from which to explore its effects on labor.

Carl Koller[41] introduced regional anesthesia when he used cocaine for eye surgery in 1884. Recognizing the potential of Koller's innovation, surgeons developed techniques for other procedures. Obstetricians quickly adopted many of these techniques for their own use. The first papers describing obstetric applications of spinal, lumbar epidural, caudal, paravertebral, parasacral, and pudendal nerve block appeared between 1900 and 1930 (see Figure 1-4).[42-44] Recognition of the potential effects of regional anesthesia on labor developed more slowly, primarily because obstetricians seldom used it. They continued to rely on inhalation agents and opioids, partly because there were few drugs and materials available for regional anesthesia at that time, but also because obstetricians did not appreciate the chief advantage of regional over general anesthesia—the relative absence of drug effects on the infant. Moreover, they rarely used regional anesthesia except for delivery, and then they often used elective forceps anyway. This set of circumstances limited their opportunity and motivation to study the effects of regional anesthesia on labor.

Among early papers dealing with regional anesthesia, one written by Cleland[45] stands out. Cleland described his experience with paravertebral anesthesia, but he also wrote a thoughtful analysis of the nerve pathways mediating labor pain, an analysis he based on information he had gleaned from clinical and laboratory studies. Few investigators were as meticulous or insightful as Cleland. Most of those who studied the effects of anesthesia simply timed the length of the first and second stages of labor. Some timed the duration of individual contractions or estimated changes in the strength of contractions by palpation. None of the investigators measured the intrauterine pressures, even though a German physician had described such a method in 1898 and had used it to evaluate the effects of morphine and ether on the contractions of laboring women.[46]

More detailed and accurate studies of the effects of anesthesia started to appear after 1944. Part of the stimulus was a method for continuous caudal anesthesia, introduced by Hingson and Edwards,[47] in which a malleable needle remained in the sacral canal throughout labor. Small, flexible plastic catheters eventually replaced malleable needles and made continuous epidural anesthesia even more popular. With the help of these innovations, obstetricians began using anesthesia earlier in labor. Ensuing problems, real and imagined, stimulated more studies. Although good studies were scarce, the strong interest in the problem represented a marked change from the early days of obstetric anesthesia.

Ironically, "natural childbirth" appeared just as regional anesthesia started to become popular and as clinicians began to understand how to use it without disrupting labor. Dick-Read,[48] the originator of the natural method, recognized "no physiological function in the body which gives rise to pain in the normal course of health." He attributed pain in an otherwise uncomplicated labor to an "activation of the sympathetic nervous system by the emotion of fear." He argued that fear made the uterus contract and become ischemic and therefore painful. He said that women could avoid the pain if they simply learned to abolish their fear of labor. Dick-Read never explained why uterine ischemia that results from fear causes pain, whereas ischemia that results from a normal contraction does not. In other words, Dick-Read, like Simpson a century earlier, claimed no necessary or physiologic relationship between labor pain and contractions. Dick-Read's book, written more for the public than for the medical profession, represented a regression of almost a century in medical thought and practice. It is important to note that contemporary methods of childbirth preparation do not maintain that fear alone causes labor pain. However, they do attempt to reduce fear by education and to help patients manage pain by teaching techniques of self-control. This represents a significant difference and an important advance from Dick-Read's original theory.

SOME LESSONS

History is important in proportion to the lessons it teaches. With respect to obstetric anesthesia, three lessons stand out. First, every new drug and method entails risks. Physicians who first used obstetric anesthesia seemed reluctant to accept this fact, perhaps because of their inexperience with potent drugs (pharmacology was in its infancy) or because they acceded too quickly to patients who wanted relief from pain and who had little understanding of the technical issues confronting physicians. Whatever the reason, this period of denial lasted almost half a century, until 1900. Almost another half-century passed before obstetricians learned to modify their practice to limit the effects of anesthetics on the child and the labor process.

Second, new drugs or therapies often cause problems in completely unexpected ways. For example, in 1900, physicians noted a rising rate of puerperal fever.[49] The timing was odd. Several decades had passed since Robert Koch had suggested the germ theory of disease and since Semmelweis had recognized that physicians often transmit infection from one woman to the next with their unclean hands. With the adoption of aseptic methods, deaths from puerperal fever had diminished dramatically. During the waning years of the nineteenth century, however, they increased again. Some physicians attributed this resurgence of puerperal fever to anesthesia. In a presidential address to the Obstetrical Society of Edinburgh in 1900, Murray[50] stated the following:

> I feel sure that an explanation of much of the increase of maternal mortality from 1847 onwards will be found in, first the misuse of anaesthesia and second in the ridiculous parody which, in many hands, stands for the use of antiseptics.... Before the days of anaesthesia, interference was limited and obstetric operations were at a minimum because interference of all kinds increased the conscious suffering of the patient.... When anaesthesia became possible, and interference became more frequent because it involved no additional suffering, operations were undertaken when really unnecessary...and so complications arose and the dangers of the labor increased.

Although it was not a direct complication of the use of anesthesia in obstetric practice, puerperal fever appeared to be an indirect consequence of it.

Changes in obstetric practice also had unexpected effects on anesthetic complications. During the first decades of the twentieth century, when cesarean sections were rare and obstetricians used only inhalation analgesia for delivery, few women were exposed to the risk of aspiration during deep anesthesia. As obstetric practice changed and cesarean sections became more common, this risk increased. The syndrome of aspiration was not identified and labeled until 1946, when obstetrician Curtis Mendelson[51] described and named it. The pathophysiology of the syndrome had already been described by Winternitz et al.,[52] who instilled hydrochloric acid into the lungs of dogs to simulate the lesions found in veterans poisoned by gas during the trench warfare of World War I. Unfortunately, the reports of these studies, although excellent, did not initiate any change in practice. Change occurred only after several deaths of obstetric patients were highly publicized in lay, legal, and medical publications. Of course, rapid-sequence induction, now recommended to reduce the risk of aspiration, creates another set of risks—those associated with a failed intubation.

The third—and perhaps most important—lesson offered by the history of obstetric anesthesia concerns the role of basic science. Modern medicine developed during the nineteenth century after physicians learned to apply principles of anatomy, physiology, and chemistry to the study and treatment of disease. Obstetric anesthesia underwent a similar pattern of development. Studies of placental structure and function called physicians' attention to the transmission of drugs and the potential effects of drugs on the infant. Similarly, studies of the physiology and anatomy of the uterus helped elucidate potential effects of anesthesia on labor. In each instance, lessons from basic science helped improve patient care.

During the past 50 years, scientists have accumulated a wealth of information about many processes integral to normal labor: the processes that initiate and control lactation; neuroendocrine events that initiate and maintain labor; the biochemical maturation of the fetal lung and liver; the metabolic requirements of the normal fetus and the protective mechanisms that it may invoke in times of stress; and the normal mechanisms that regulate the amount and distribution of blood flow to the uterus and placenta. At this point, we have only the most rudimentary understanding of the interaction of anesthesia with any of these processes. Only a fraction of the information available from basic science has been used to improve obstetric anesthesia care. Realizing the rewards from the clinical use of such information may be the most important lesson from the past and the greatest challenge for the future of obstetric anesthesia.

KEY POINTS

- Physicians have debated the safety of obstetric anesthesia since 1847, when James Young Simpson first administered anesthesia for delivery.
- Two issues have dominated the debate: the effects of anesthesia on labor and the effects of anesthesia on the newborn.
- Despite controversy, physicians quickly incorporated anesthesia into clinical practice, largely because of their patients' desire to avoid childbirth pain.
- Only after obstetric anesthesia was in use for many years did problems become apparent.
- Important milestones in obstetric anesthesia include the introduction of inhalation agents in 1847, the expanded use of opioids in the early decades of the twentieth century, and the refinement of regional anesthesia starting in the mid-twentieth century.
- Outstanding conceptual developments included (1) Zweifel's idea that drugs given to the mother cross the placenta and affect the fetus and (2) Apgar's idea that the condition of the newborn is the most sensitive assay of the quality of anesthetic care of the mother.
- The history of obstetric anesthesia suggests that the major improvements in patient care have followed the application of principles of basic science.

REFERENCES

1. Haggard HW. Devils, Drugs and Doctors: The Theory of the Science of Healing from Medicine Man to Doctor. New York, Harper & Brothers, 1929.
2. Caton D. Obstetric anesthesia: The first ten years. Anesthesiology 1970; 33:102-9.
3. Shepherd JA. Simpson and Syme of Edinburgh. Edinburgh, London, E & S Livingstone, 1969.
4. Simpson WG, editor. The Works of Sir JY Simpson, Vol II: Anaesthesia. Edinburgh, Adam and Charles Black, 1871: 199-200.
5. Levinson A. The three Meigs and their contribution to pediatrics. Ann Med Hist 1928; 10:138.
6. Dubois P. On the inhalation of ether applied to cases of midwifery. Lancet 1847; I:246-9.
7. Ramsbotham FH. The Principles and Practice of Obstetric Medicine and Surgery in Reference to the Process of Parturition. Philadelphia, Blanchard and Lea, 1855.
8. Report of the Committee Appointed by the Royal Medical and Surgical Society to Inquire into the Uses and the Physiological, Therapeutical and Toxical Effects of Chloroform. London, JR Adlarto, 1864.
9. Sykes WS. Essays on the First Hundred Years of Anaesthesia, Vol I. Park Ridge, Ill, Wood Library Museum of Anesthesiology, 1982.
10. Caton D. The secularization of pain. Anesthesiology 1985; 62:493-501.
11. Wagenknecht E, editor. Mrs. Longfellow. Selected Letters and Journals of Fanny Appleton Longfellow (1817-1861). New York, Longmans, Green, 1956.
12. Cohen M, editor. Nature: The Philosophy of John Stuart Mill. New York, Modern Library, 1961: 463-7.
13. Simpson WG, editor. The Works of Sir JY Simpson, Vol II: Anaesthesia. Edinburgh, Adam and Charles Black, 1871: 177.
14. von Steinbüchel R. Vorläufige Mittheilung über die Anwendung von Skopolamin-Morphium-Injektionen in der Geburtshilfe. Centralblatt Gyn 1902; 30:1304-6.
15. Gauss CJ. Die Anwendung des Skopolamin-Morphium-Dämmerschlafes in der Geburtshilfe. Medizinische Klinik 1906; 2:136-8.
16. Macht DI. History of opium and some of its preparations and alkaloids. JAMA 1915; 6:477-81.
17. Sansom AE. On the pain of parturition, and anaesthetics in obstetric practice. Trans Obstetr Soc Lond 1868; 10:121-40.
18. Gusserow A. Zur Lehre vom Stoffwechsel des Foetus. Arch Gyn 1871; III:241.
19. Wertz RW, Wertz DC. Lying In: A History of Childbirth in America. New York, Schocken Books, 1979.
20. Leavitt JW. Brought to Bed—Child Bearing in America 1750-1958. New York, Oxford University Press, 1986.
21. Kaufman M. American Medical Education: The Formative Years, 1765-1910. Westport, Conn, Greenwood Press, 1976.
22. Mayow J: Tractutus quinque medico-physici. Quoted by J Needham, Chemical Embryology, New York, Hafner Publishing, 1963.

23. Snow J. On the administration of chloroform during parturition. Assoc Med J 1853; 1:500-2.
24. Caton D. Obstetric anesthesia and concepts of placental transport: A historical review of the nineteenth century. Anesthesiology 1977; 46:132-7.
25. Zweifel P. Einfluss der Chloroformnarcose Kreissender auf den Fötus. Klinische Wochenschrift 1874; 21:1-2.
26. Zweifel P. Die Respiration des Fötus. Arch Gyn 1876; 9:291-305.
27. Speigelberg O. A Textbook of Midwifery. Translated by JB Hurry. London, The New Sydenham Society, 1887.
28. Gwathmey JT. A further study, based on more than twenty thousand cases. Surg Gynecol Obstet 1930; 51:190-5.
29. Terry CE, Pellens M. The Opium Problem. Camden, NJ, Bureau of Social Hygiene, 1928.
30. Gillette WR. The narcotic effect of morphia on the new-born child, when administered to the mother in labor. Am J Obstet Gynecol 1877; 10:612-23.
31. Knipe WHW. The Freiburg method of Däammerschlaf or twilight sleep. Am J Obstet Gynecol 1914; 70:884.
32. Calmes SH. Virginia Apgar: A woman physician's career in a developing specialty. J Am Med Wom Assoc 1984; 39:184-8.
33. Apgar V. A proposal for a new method of evaluation of the newborn infant. Curr Res Anesth Analg 1953; 32:260-7.
34. Thoms H. Anesthesia á la Reine—a chapter in the history of anesthesia. Am J Obstet Gynecol 1940; 40:340-6.
35. Meigs CD. Obstetrics, the Science and the Art. Philadelphia, Blanchard and Lea, 1865: 364-76.
36. Channing W. A Treatise on Etherization in Childbirth. Boston, William D. Ticknor, 1848.
37. Montgomery WFH. Objections to the Indiscriminate Administration of Anaesthetic Agents in Midwifery. Dublin, Hodges and Smith, 1849.
38. Snow J. On the administration of chloroform during parturition. Assoc Med J 1853; 1:500-2.
39. Head H. On disturbances of sensation with especial reference to the pain of visceral disease. Brain 1893; 16:1-132.
40. Gertsman NM. Über Uterusinnervation an Hand des Falles einer Geburt bei Quersnittslähmung. Monatsschrift Gebürtshüfle Gynäkologie 1926; 73:253-7.
41. Koller C. On the use of cocaine for producing anaesthesia on the eye. Lancet 1884; 2:990-2.
42. Kreis O. Über Medullarnarkose bei Gebärenden. Centralblatt Gynäkologie 1900; 28:724-7.
43. Bonar BE, Meeker WR. The value of sacral nerve block anesthesia in obstetrics. JAMA 1923; 81:1079-83.
44. Schlimpert H. Concerning sacral anaesthesia. Surg Gynecol Obstet 1913; 16:488-92.
45. Cleland JGP. Paravertebral anaesthesia in obstetrics. Surg Gynecol Obstet 1933; 57:51-62.
46. Hensen H. Ueber den Einfluss des Morphiums und des Aethers auf die Wehenthätigkeit des Uterus. Arch Gyn 1898; 53:129-77.
47. Hingson RA, Edwards WB. Continuous caudal analgesia: An analysis of the first ten thousand confinements thus managed with the report of the authors' first thousand cases. JAMA 1943; 123:538-46.
48. Dick-Read G. Childbirth Without Fear: The Principles and Practice of Natural Childbirth. New York, Harper & Row, 1970.
49. Lea AWW. Puerperal Infection. London, Henry Frowdie, 1910.
50. Murray M. Presidential address to the Obstetrical Society of Edinburgh, 1900. Quoted in Oliver Wendell Holmes and Puerperal Fever. London, MJ Glaisher, 1906.
51. Mendelson CL. The aspiration of stomach contents into the lungs during obstetric anesthesia. Am J Obstet Gynecol 1946; 52:191-205.
52. Winternitz MC, Smith GH, McNamara FP. Effect of intrabronchial insufflation of acid. J Exper Med 1920; 32:199-209.

Part II

Maternal and Fetal Physiology

Metabolism was among the first areas of physiology to influence clinical practice. By the beginning of the twentieth century, physiologists had established many of the principles that we recognize today, including normal rates of oxygen consumption and carbon dioxide production, the relationship between oxygen consumption and heat production, and the relationship between metabolic rate and body weight and surface area among individuals and species. Almost simultaneously, clinicians began to apply these principles to their studies of patients in different states of health and disease.

In one early study, physiologist Magnus Levy[1] found an exception to the rule that basal metabolic rate varied in proportion to body surface area. As he measured a woman's oxygen consumption during pregnancy, he observed that her metabolic rate increased out of proportion to increments in her body weight and surface area. Subsequent studies by other investigators established the basis of this phenomenon. Per unit of weight, the fetus, placenta, and uterus together consumed oxygen (and released carbon dioxide and heat) at a higher rate than the mother. In effect, the metabolism of a pregnant woman represented the sum of two independent organisms, each metabolizing at its own rate in proportion to its own surface area. Thus, each kg of maternal tissue consumed oxygen at a rate of approximately 4 mL/min, whereas the average rate for the fetus, placenta, and uterus was approximately 12 mL/min, although it could increase to rates as high as 20 mL/min. Therefore, during pregnancy, the mother's metabolism was the sum of her metabolic rate plus that of the fetus, placenta, and uterus.[1-4] Subsequent studies established that the highest rates of fetal metabolism occurred during the periods of most rapid growth, thereby reaffirming another physiologic principle—the high metabolic cost of synthesizing new tissue.[5]

The aforementioned studies gave clinicians estimates of the stress imposed by pregnancy. To maintain homeostasis during pregnancy, a pregnant woman had to make an appropriate adjustment in each of the physiologic mechanisms involved in the delivery of substrates to the fetal placental unit and in the excretion of metabolic wastes. Thus, for every increment in fetal weight, clinicians could expect to find a proportional change in all the mechanisms involved in the delivery of substrate to the fetus and in the excretion of all byproducts. In fact, subsequent clinical studies established predictable changes in uterine blood flow, cardiac output, blood volume, minute ventilation, the dissipation of body heat, and the renal excretion of nitrogenous waste and other materials.

Donald Caton, M.D.

REFERENCES

1. Magnus-Levy. Stoffwechsel und Nahrungbedarf in der Schwangerschaft, A. Geburtsh. u. Gynaek, lii:116-84.
2. Carpenter TM, Murlin JR. The energy metabolism of mother and child just before and just after birth. AMA Arch Intern Med 1911; 7:184-222.
3. Root H, Root HK. The basal metabolism during pregnancy and the puerperium. Arch Intern Med 1923; 32:411-24.
4. Sandiford I, Wheeler T. The basal metabolism before, during, and after pregnancy. J Bio Chem. lxii:329-52.
5. Caton D, Henderson DJ, Wilcox CJ, Barron DH. Oxygen consumption of the uterus and its contents and weight at birth of lambs. In Longo LD, Reneau DD, editors: Fetal and Newborn Cardiovascular Physiology, vol 2. New York, Garland STPM Press, 1978:123-34.

Chapter 2
Physiologic Changes of Pregnancy

Anita Backus Chang, M.D.

Marked anatomic and physiologic changes occur in women during pregnancy. Many of these adaptations dictate alterations of anesthetic technique from that appropriate for nonpregnant individuals. This chapter reviews the physiologic alterations of normal pregnancy and their anesthetic implications.

BODY WEIGHT AND COMPOSITION

The mean weight increase during pregnancy is 17% of the prepregnant weight, or approximately 12 kg.[1] Weight gain results from an increase in the size of the uterus and its contents (uterus, 1 kg; amniotic fluid, 1 kg; fetus and placenta, 4 kg), increases in blood volume and interstitial fluid (approximately 2 kg each), and deposition of new fat and protein (approximately 4 kg). Normal weight gain during the first trimester is 1 to 2 kg, and there is a 5 to 6 kg gain in each of the last two trimesters.

METABOLISM AND RESPIRATION

Oxygen Consumption

Several authors have reported that oxygen consumption increases by 30% to 40% during pregnancy, although use of

relatively early postpartum values for the control in most of these studies underestimates the increase. Spätling et al.,[1] using the value at 8 to 12 months postpartum as the control, reported that oxygen consumption increases by 60% during pregnancy. The progressive rise is caused primarily by the metabolic needs of the fetus, uterus, and placenta and secondarily by increased cardiac and respiratory work. Carbon dioxide production shows changes similar to those of oxygen consumption.[1]

Anatomy

The thoracic cage increases in circumference by 5 to 7 cm during pregnancy because of increases in both the anteroposterior and transverse diameters.[2,3] Flaring of the ribs, which begins at the end of the first trimester, results in an increase in the subcostal angle from 68.5 to 103.5 degrees at term.[3] The vertical measurement of the chest decreases by as much as 4 cm, which results from the elevated position of the diaphragm.[3]

Capillary engorgement of the nasal and oropharyngeal mucosae and larynx begins early in the first trimester and increases progressively throughout pregnancy.[2] Voice changes frequently result from involvement of the false vocal cords and the arytenoid region of the larynx.[2] Nasal breathing commonly becomes difficult, and epistaxis may occur because of nasal mucosal engorgement.[2]

Airway conductance increases, indicating a dilation of the larger airways below the larynx.[4] Factors contributing to airway dilation include the direct effects of progesterone, cortisone, and relaxin[4] and possibly enhanced beta-adrenergic activity induced by progesterone.[5]

Radiographs of the lungs have shown no characteristic changes of the parenchyma or pulmonary vasculature during gestation.

Mechanics

Inspiration in nonpregnant individuals results from the descent (i.e., contraction) of the diaphragm and expansion of the thoracic cage by the external intercostal muscles. Inspiration in the term pregnant woman is almost totally attributable to diaphragmatic excursion.[6] This is caused by a greater descent of the diaphragm from its elevated resting position and limitation of thoracic cage expansion because of its expanded resting position (Table 2-1).

Functioning of the large airways is unimpaired during pregnancy, as shown by the unaltered flow-volume loop[7] and the lack of change in maximum expiratory flow rate, forced expiratory volume in 1 second (FEV$_1$), and ratio of FEV$_1$ to forced vital capacity.[5,7-9] Thus dilation of the large airways compensates for the expected increase in airway resistance, which results from hypocapnia and reduction of the resting lung volume during pregnancy.[5] The unaltered flow-volume loop[7] and lack of change in closing capacity[10] indicate that small airway function is unaffected by pregnancy.

Lung Volumes and Capacities

Tidal volume increases by 45% during pregnancy, with approximately half of the change occurring during the first trimester (Figure 2-1).[8,11] The early change in tidal volume is associated with a reduction in inspiratory reserve volume. The changes during the latter half of pregnancy are accompanied by a decline in functional residual capacity (FRC) and an increase in inspiratory reserve volume.

FRC begins to decrease by the fifth month of pregnancy. This is caused by elevation of the relaxed diaphragm, which occurs as the enlarging uterus enters the abdominal cavity. FRC is reduced to 80% of the nonpregnant volume by term gestation.[4,8,10] A 25% reduction in expiratory reserve volume[4,7,8] and

a 15% reduction in residual volume[8] account for the change (Table 2-2). The FRC of the *supine* parturient is 70% of the volume measured in the upright position.[10]

Inspiratory capacity increases by 15% during the third trimester because of increases in tidal volume and inspiratory reserve volume.[4,8] There is a corresponding decrease in expiratory reserve volume, and vital capacity is unchanged.[3,4,7,8] Total lung capacity is slightly reduced during pregnancy.[4,7,8]

Ventilation

Minute ventilation increases by 45% during pregnancy, with an increase evident early in the first trimester (Table 2-2).[8,11] This change results from the increase in tidal volume.

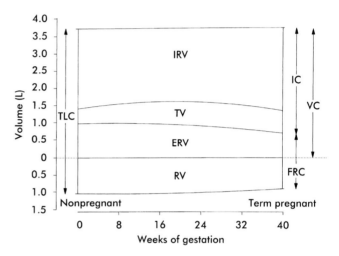

FIGURE 2-1. Lung volumes and capacities during pregnancy. *ERV,* Expiratory reserve volume; *FRC,* functional residual capacity; *IC,* inspiratory capacity; *IRV,* inspiratory reserve volume; *RV,* residual volume; *TLC,* total lung capacity; *TV,* tidal volume; *VC,* vital capacity.

TABLE 2-1	EFFECTS OF PREGNANCY ON RESPIRATORY MECHANICS
Parameter	**Change***
Diaphragm excursion	Increased
Chest wall excursion	Decreased
Pulmonary resistance	Decreased 50%
FEV$_1$	No change
FEV$_1$/FVC	No change
Flow volume loop	No change
Closing capacity	No change

FEV$_1$, Forced expiratory volume in 1 second; *FVC,* forced vital capacity.
*Relative to nonpregnant women.
Adapted from Conklin KA. Maternal physiological adaptations during gestation, labor, and the puerperium. Semin Anesth 1991; 10:221–34.

TABLE 2-2	CHANGES IN RESPIRATORY PHYSIOLOGY AT TERM GESTATION
Parameter	**Change***
Lung volumes	
Inspiratory reserve volume	+5%
Tidal volume	+45%
Expiratory reserve volume	−25%
Residual volume	−15%
Lung capacities	
Inspiratory capacity	+15%
Functional residual capacity	−20%
Vital capacity	No change
Total lung capacity	−5%
Dead space	+45%
Respiratory rate	No change
Ventilation	
Minute ventilation	+45%
Alveolar ventilation	+45%

*Relative to nonpregnant women.
From Conklin KA. Maternal physiological adaptations during gestation, labor, and the puerperium. Semin Anesth 1991; 10:221–34.

Although the respiratory rate declines slightly during mid-gestation, it is essentially unaltered during pregnancy.[8,11] Some investigators have reported that alveolar ventilation increases to a greater degree than minute ventilation,[1] but others have found that dead space increases (from dilation of the large airways[4]) in parallel with the increase in tidal volume.[11] The latter studies suggest that the ratio of dead space to tidal volume does not change during pregnancy and that the increase in alveolar ventilation is equivalent to the increase in minute ventilation throughout gestation.

The increased ventilation during pregnancy results from hormonal changes and increased carbon dioxide production.[1] The arterial partial pressure of carbon dioxide ($PaCO_2$) is closely related to the blood level of progesterone.[12] This hormone increases the sensitivity of the central respiratory center to carbon dioxide and acts as a direct respiratory stimulant. Estrogens also may contribute to increased ventilation. Because increased ventilation[8,11] and maternal hypocapnia[11] precede the increase in carbon dioxide production, early changes in ventilation result from elevated hormone levels, whereas later changes are the result of both factors.

Blood Gases

The $PaCO_2$ declines to approximately 30 mm Hg by 12 weeks' gestation but does not change further during the remainder of pregnancy (Table 2-3).[11,12] Although in nonpregnant individuals a gradient exists between the end-tidal carbon dioxide tension and $PaCO_2$, the two measurements are equivalent during early pregnancy,[13] at term gestation,[14] and in the early postpartum period.[15] This is attributed to a reduction in alveolar dead space (i.e., unperfused alveoli), which results from a marked increase in cardiac output during pregnancy. The mixed venous PCO_2 is 6 to 8 mm Hg below the nonpregnant level from the late first trimester until term.[1]

The arterial partial pressure of oxygen (PaO_2) of *erect* pregnant women increases to approximately 107 mm Hg by the end of the first trimester and falls by 2 mm Hg during each of the following trimesters (see Table 2-3).[11] The increased PaO_2 results from the decline in $PaCO_2$ and a reduced arteriovenous oxygen difference, which reduces the impact of the venous admixture on the PaO_2.[16,17] An increase in the arteriovenous oxygen difference during the second and third trimesters accounts for the small, progressive decline in PaO_2.[16] The decreased arteriovenous oxygen difference during early pregnancy results from an increase in cardiac output that is proportionately greater than the increase in oxygen consumption. As pregnancy progresses, oxygen consumption continues to increase while cardiac output increases to a lesser degree, resulting in decreased mixed venous oxygen content and increased arteriovenous oxygen difference.

After mid-gestation, pregnant women frequently exhibit a PaO_2 below 100 mm Hg when in the supine position. This occurs because FRC is less than closing capacity in as many as 50% of these individuals,[10] which results in the closure of small airways during normal tidal ventilation. A decline in cardiac output as a result of aortocaval compression also contributes to hypoxemia because it results in a decreased mixed venous oxygen content and an increased arteriovenous oxygen difference. Thus moving a pregnant woman from the supine to the erect[18] or lateral decubitus[19] position improves arterial oxygenation and decreases the alveolar-to-arterial oxygen gradient.

Acid-Base Status

Metabolic compensation for the respiratory alkalosis of pregnancy reduces the serum bicarbonate concentration to approximately 20 mEq/L, the base excess by 2 to 3 mEq/L, and the total buffer base by approximately 5 mEq/L.[20] This compensation is incomplete, as demonstrated by the elevation of venous,[21] capillary,[22] and arterial[11] blood pH by 0.02 to 0.06 units (see Table 2-3).

Metabolism and Respiration During Labor

Minute ventilation of the unmedicated parturient increases by 70% to 140% and by 120% to 200% in the first and second stages of labor, respectively, compared with prepregnant values.[1,23] The $PaCO_2$ may fall to measurements as low as 10 to 15 mm Hg. Oxygen consumption increases above the prelabor value by 40% in the first stage and by 75% in the second stage.[23] The changes in oxygen consumption result from the increased metabolic demands of hyperventilation (a doubling of ventilation by the parturient increases oxygen consumption by 50%), uterine activity, and maternal expulsive efforts during the second stage. The maternal aerobic requirement for oxygen exceeds oxygen consumption during labor, as is evident from the progressive rise of the blood lactate concentration, which is an index of anaerobic metabolism.[24-26]

Parenteral opioid analgesia reduces maternal hyperventilation, although the $PaCO_2$ values measured during the first and second stages of labor (21 to 28 mm Hg and 16 to 24 mm Hg, respectively) are still below normal for pregnancy.[24,25] When epidural analgesia is administered during the first stage of labor, minute ventilation, oxygen consumption, lactate concentration, and $PaCO_2$ remain at levels comparable with those measured before the onset of labor.[23-26] During the second stage of labor, maternal expulsive efforts result in increased minute ventilation, oxygen consumption, and lactate concentration, and a decreased $PaCO_2$, even when epidural analgesia is used.[23,25,26]

Metabolism and Respiration During the Puerperium

FRC increases after delivery but remains below the prepregnant value for 1 to 2 weeks. Oxygen consumption, tidal volume, and minute ventilation remain elevated until at least 6 to 8 weeks after delivery.[1] The alveolar and mixed venous PCO_2 increase slowly after delivery and are still slightly below prepregnant levels at 6 to 8 weeks postpartum.[1]

| TABLE 2-3 | BLOOD GASES DURING PREGNANCY |

		Trimester		
	Nonpregnant	First	Second	Third
$PaCO_2$ (mm Hg)	40	30	30	30
PaO_2 (mm Hg)	100	107	105	103
pH	7.40	7.44	7.44	7.44
$[HCO_3^-]$ (mEq/L)	24	21	20	20

THE HEART AND CIRCULATION

Examination of the Heart

The elevation of the diaphragm shifts the heart anteriorly and to the left during pregnancy. The apical impulse moves cephalad to the fourth intercostal space and laterally to at least the midclavicular line.

Auscultation and phonocardiography reveal several changes during pregnancy.[27] An accentuation of the first heart sound occurs with exaggerated splitting of the mitral and tricuspid components, both of which move closer to the Q wave. The second heart sound changes little, although the aortic-pulmonic interval tends to vary less with respiration during the third trimester. The third heart sound is easily heard during the latter half of pregnancy. A fourth heart sound is identified in up to 16% of pregnant women, although it typically disappears by term in healthy individuals. A grade I or II early- to mid-systolic murmur is commonly heard at the left sternal border and is attributable to cardiac enlargement, which results in a dilation of the tricuspid annulus that causes regurgitation.

Electrocardiography (ECG) reveals sinus tachycardia with a shortening of the P-R and uncorrected Q-T intervals during pregnancy. The QRS axis shifts to the right during the first trimester but may shift to the left during the third trimester. The T-wave axis shifts to the left.[28] Depressed S-T segments and isoelectric or low-voltage T waves in the left-sided precordial and limb leads are commonly observed during pregnancy.[29]

Echocardiography reveals left ventricular hypertrophy by 12 weeks' gestation, with a 50% increase in mass at term.[30] A significant increase in the annular diameters of the mitral, tricuspid, and pulmonic valves occurs; 94% of term pregnant women exhibit tricuspid and pulmonic regurgitation, and 27% exhibit mitral regurgitation.[31] The aortic annulus is not dilated.

Central Hemodynamics

Prerequisites for the accurate determination of hemodynamic changes during pregnancy require that measurements be made with subjects in the resting state and in a position that minimizes compression of the aorta and inferior vena cava by the gravid uterus. Further, comparisons must be made using an appropriate control, such as the same women before pregnancy or a matched group of nonpregnant women. If control measurements are made during the postpartum period, a sufficient interval of time must elapse so that hemodynamic parameters return to prepregnant values, which for some measurements may take 24 weeks or more.[32]

Studies meeting these criteria have demonstrated a significant increase in cardiac output by 5 weeks after the last menstrual period and a 35% to 40% increase by the end of the first trimester of pregnancy (Figure 2-2).[30,33] Cardiac output continues to rise throughout the second trimester until it reaches a level that is approximately 50% greater than that of nonpregnant women.[30,32,34-37] It does not change from this level during the remainder of pregnancy (Table 2-4). An apparent decline in cardiac output during late pregnancy, which has been reported by some investigators, has resulted from measurements taken with pregnant women in the supine position.

The earliest change in cardiac output is attributed to an increase in heart rate, which occurs by the fourth to fifth week of pregnancy.[30] Heart rate increases by approximately 15% to 25% above the nonpregnant level by the end of the first and second trimesters, respectively, and undergoes no further

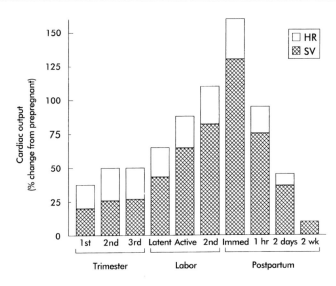

FIGURE 2-2. Cardiac output during pregnancy, labor, and the puerperium. Values during pregnancy are measured at the end of the first, second, and third trimesters. Values during labor are measured between contractions. For each measurement the relative contribution of heart rate (HR) and stroke volume (SV) to the change in cardiac output is illustrated.

TABLE 2-4	CENTRAL HEMODYNAMICS AT TERM GESTATION
Parameter	**Change***
Cardiac output	+50%
Stroke volume	+25%
Heart rate	+25%
Left ventricular end-diastolic volume	Increased
Left ventricular end-systolic volume	No change
Ejection fraction	Increased
Left ventricular stroke-work index	No change
Pulmonary capillary wedge pressure	No change
Pulmonary artery diastolic pressure	No change
Central venous pressure	No change
Systemic vascular resistance	−20%

*Relative to nonpregnant women.
Adapted from Conklin KA. Maternal physiological adaptations during gestation, labor, and the puerperium. Semin Anesth 1991; 10:221–34.

change during the third trimester.[30,32-37] Stroke volume increases by approximately 20% between the fifth and eighth week of gestation, increases by 25% to 30% by the end of the second trimester, and remains at that level until term.[30,32,33,36]

Left ventricular end-diastolic volume increases during gestation, whereas end-systolic volume remains unchanged, resulting in an increase in ejection fraction.[30,32-36] This occurs without a change in myocardial contractility because the left ventricular stroke-work index is unaffected by pregnancy (Figure 2-3).[37] Although enhanced myocardial contractility is suggested by the increased velocity of left ventricular circumferential fiber shortening,[30,34,36] this observation can be explained by changes in heart rate and afterload.

Central venous, pulmonary artery diastolic, and pulmonary capillary wedge pressures during pregnancy are within the normal range for nonpregnant individuals. Thus increased end-diastolic volume occurs without a change in cardiac filling pressures (see Table 2-4).[16,37] The apparent discrepancy between left ventricular filling pressure and end-diastolic volume is explained by hypertrophy and dilation,

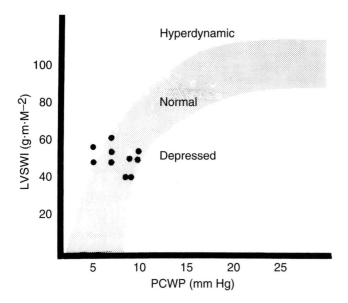

FIGURE 2-3. Left ventricular function in late phase of third-trimester normotensive pregnant patients. *LVSWI*, left ventricular stroke work index; *PCWP*, pulmonary capillary wedge pressure. (From Clark SL, Cotton DB, Lee W, et al. Central hemodynamic assessment of cardiac function. Am J Obstet Gynecol 1989; 161:1439-42.)

with the dilated ventricle accommodating a greater volume without an increase in pressure.

Organ Perfusion

The uterus, kidneys, and extremities (i.e., skin and skeletal muscle) benefit from the more than 2 L/min increase in cardiac output during pregnancy. Uterine blood flow, estimated to be from 50 to 190 mL/min before conception,[38,39] increases to 700 to 900 mL/min at term gestation.[39-43] Approximately 90% of this flow perfuses the intervillous space, with the balance perfusing the myometrium.[40,41]

Renal plasma flow is increased by 80% at 16 to 26 weeks' gestation, but declines to 50% above the nonpregnant level at term.[44] Skin perfusion begins to increase at approximately 15 weeks' gestation, reaching a value that is three to four times the nonpregnant level at term.[45] Increased skin perfusion results in an increase in skin temperature. Blood flow to other major organs, including the brain and liver, does not change.

Blood Pressure

Position, age, and parity affect blood pressure measurements in pregnant women. Brachial sphygmomanometry yields pressures that are highest in the supine position, somewhat lower in the sitting or standing positions, and lowest in the lateral position.[35,46,47] Blood pressure increases with advancing maternal age, and for a given age, nulliparous women have a higher mean blood pressure than parous women.[48]

Systolic blood pressure is minimally affected by pregnancy, with a maximum decline of approximately 8% during early- to mid-gestation and a return to the prepregnant level at term.[1,46,47,49,50] Systolic blood pressure is determined primarily by stroke volume and the distensibility of large arterial vessels. Because stroke volume increases during pregnancy, the decline in systolic blood pressure is explained by increased aortic size and compliance.[51]

Diastolic blood pressure falls to a greater degree than does systolic blood pressure, with early- to mid-gestational decreases of approximately 20%.[1,46,47,49,50] It also returns to the prepregnant level at term. The decreased diastolic blood pressure is consistent with changes in systemic vascular resistance, which falls during early gestation, reaches its nadir (i.e., a 35% decline) at 20 weeks' gestation, and rises during late gestation. However, systemic vascular resistance remains approximately 20% below the nonpregnant level at term.[30,37] The decreased systemic vascular resistance results from the development of a low resistance vascular bed (i.e., the intervillous space) as well as vasodilation caused by prostacyclin, estrogens, and progesterone. Compression of the aorta by the gravid uterus may partly account for the greater systemic vascular resistance during the third trimester.

Aortocaval Compression

The degree of compression of the aorta and inferior vena cava by the term gravid uterus depends on the position of the pregnant woman. In the lateral decubitus position, angiographic studies reveal partial caval obstruction.[52] This is consistent with the 75% elevation—above nonpregnant levels—of femoral venous[53] and lower inferior vena caval[54] pressures. Despite caval compression, collateral circulation maintains venous return, as reflected by the right ventricular filling pressure, which is unaltered in the lateral position.[37]

In the supine position, radiographic studies and magnetic resonance imaging reveal complete or nearly complete obstruction of the inferior vena cava in a high proportion of term pregnant women.[52,54,55] Venous return occurs primarily by diversion of blood through the intraosseous vertebral veins, paravertebral veins, and epidural venous plexus. The ovarian veins, which partially drain the uteroplacental vascular bed, also serve to bypass the caval obstruction.[56] Despite collateral circulation, right atrial pressure falls,[54,57] which indicates that venous return is not maintained in the supine position. Compression of the inferior vena cava occurs as early as 13 to 16 weeks' gestation and is evident from the 50% increase in femoral venous pressure that occurs when a woman assumes the supine position at this stage of pregnancy.[58] By term, femoral venous (Figure 2-4)[53,58] and lower inferior vena cava[54] pressures are approximately 2.5 times the nonpregnant values in the supine position.

Angiographic studies show that the aorta is little affected by the uterus when the term gravid woman is in the lateral position.[59] This finding is consistent with the observation that blood pressure is higher in the femoral artery than in the brachial artery in this position.[60] In the lateral tilt position, 40% of term pregnant women experience a fall in femoral arterial pressure, which is consistent with compression of the aorta.[60,61] In the supine position, femoral arterial pressure falls to an even greater degree,[60-62] with the fall being inversely proportional to the maternal arterial pressure.[62] These findings are consistent with angiographic studies in supine pregnant women that reveal partial obstruction of the aorta at the level of the lumbar lordosis (i.e., L_3 to L_5) and enhanced compression during periods of maternal hypotension.[59,63]

In late pregnancy (i.e., 30 to 38 weeks' gestation) the left lateral decubitus position results in less enhancement of cardiac sympathetic activity and less suppression of cardiac vagal activity, when compared with the supine or right lateral decubitus position; this is attributed to minimization of infe-

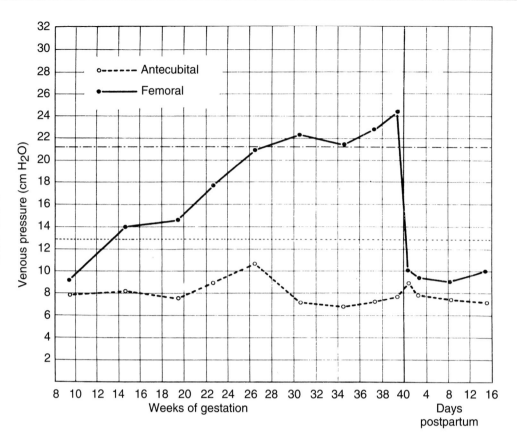

FIGURE 2-4. Femoral and antecubital venous pressure in the supine position throughout normal pregnancy and the puerperium. (From McLennan CE. Antecubital and femoral venous pressure in normal and toxemic pregnancy. Am J Obstet Gynecol 1943; 45:568-91.)

rior vena caval compression in the left lateral decubitus position. In contrast, in *nonpregnant* controls, the *right* lateral decubitus position results in greater enhancement of cardiac vagal activity, presumably because of the advantageous gravitational effect of left ventricular pumping from the "superior" position and better venous drainage into the "inferior" right atrium.[64]

Women who assume the supine position at term gestation experience a 10% to 20% decline in stroke volume and cardiac output.[36,57,65,66] These effects are consistent with the fall in right atrial filling pressure.[54,57] Heart rate changes minimally.[36,54,65,66] Blood flow in the upper extremities is unchanged,[67] whereas uterine blood flow decreases by 20%[42,68] and lower extremity blood flow falls by 50%.[67] Perfusion of the uterus is less affected than that of the lower extremities because caval compression does not obstruct uterine venous outflow by means of the ovarian veins.[56] Although aortic compression results in an equal reduction of arterial pressure in both circuits, perfusion pressure of the uterus is better maintained because uterine venous pressure is lower than femoral venous pressure. The adverse hemodynamic effects of aortocaval compression are reduced once the fetal head is engaged.[54,57,60,61]

Most term pregnant women exhibit an increase in brachial artery pressure when they assume the supine position.[35,46,47,65] This is caused by a higher systemic vascular resistance,[65] which is attributed to compression of the aorta. Approximately 8% of women at term experience bradycardia and a substantial drop in blood pressure when they assume the supine position.[69] It may take several minutes for the bradycardia and hypotension to develop, and the bradycardia usually is preceded by a period of tachycardia. This **supine hypotensive syndrome** results from a profound drop in venous return for which the cardiovascular system cannot compensate.

Hemodynamics During Labor

Cardiac output during labor (between uterine contractions) increases from prelabor values by approximately 10% in the early first stage, 25% in the late first stage, and 40% in the second stage (see Figure 2-2).[70-72] These changes result from increases in stroke volume with minimal changes in heart rate. Systolic and diastolic blood pressures also are elevated during the late first stage and second stage of labor. A progressive elevation of sympathetic nervous system activity, which peaks at the time of delivery,[73-75] accounts for these changes by increasing myocardial contractility, systemic vascular resistance, and venous return. Central venous pressure also increases.[71,72] Suppression of sympathetic nervous system activity with epidural analgesia[74,75] reduces the increase in cardiac output during labor.[71]

Cardiac output and stroke volume are augmented by an additional 15% to 25% during uterine contractions, with lesser increases of 10% to 15% when parturients receive effective analgesia.[70-72,76] The change in stroke volume results from increased venous return, reflected by the elevation of central venous pressure.[72,77] This occurs in response to increased sympathetic nervous system activity (which is reduced by maternal analgesia) and the displacement of 300 to 500 mL of blood from the intervillous space (i.e., autotransfusion).[76,77] Heart rate changes are variable. Among patients who have received analgesia, heart rate tends to decrease during uterine contractions; otherwise, heart rate increases during uterine contractions.

Autotransfusion is explained by an alteration of uterine hemodynamics. Compression of the aorta occurs (or increases) when the uterus contracts, as shown by angiography[59,63] and by a fall in femoral arterial pressure[62]; this reduces blood flow to the intervillous space because the uterine arteries originate below the site of compression.

Simultaneously, increased intrauterine pressure forces blood from the intervillous space through the relatively unimpeded ovarian venous outflow[56] into the central circulation of the parturient. The enhanced stroke volume and increased cardiac afterload result in an increase in brachial artery blood pressure during contractions.[72,76,77]

Hemodynamics During the Puerperium

A state of relative hypervolemia and increased venous return follows a vaginal delivery. This results from relief of caval compression, reduced lower extremity venous pressure (which enhances transcapillary refill), and a reduction of maternal vascular capacitance (i.e., elimination of the intervillous space) by a volume that exceeds blood loss (i.e., an autotransfusion). Central venous pressure rises,[72] and stroke volume and cardiac output increase to as much as 75% above predelivery values immediately postpartum.[71] During the next hour, cardiac output decreases to approximately 30% above prelabor levels because of a decline in both stroke volume and heart rate.[71,72]

Cardiac output falls to just below prelabor values at 48 hours postpartum.[78] It subsequently decreases to 10% above the prepregnant level after 2 weeks and then gradually returns to the prepregnant level between 12 and 24 weeks postpartum (see Figure 2-2).[32] Heart rate falls rapidly after delivery, reaches the prepregnant rate by 2 weeks postpartum, and is slightly below the prepregnant rate for the next several months.[32,78] Stroke volume remains above prelabor values at 48 hours and slowly declines postpartum for 24 weeks, at which time it is still 10% above the prepregnant level.[32,78] Left ventricular wall thickness and mass remain above prepregnant values at 24 weeks postpartum.[32]

In multiparous women (having had a minimum of four term pregnancies) who were studied an average of 12.7 years after their last pregnancy, cardiac chamber dimensions, left ventricular mass, systolic and diastolic function, valvular incompetence, and heart rate were similar to an age-matched control group of nulliparous women.[79] These studies demonstrate that the anatomic and functional changes of the heart during pregnancy are fully reversible.

HEMATOLOGY AND COAGULATION

Blood Volume

Plasma volume increases by 15% during the first trimester (becoming detectable by 6 to 12 weeks' gestation[80]), rises rapidly during the second trimester to 50% to 55% above the prepregnant level, and changes little during the remainder of pregnancy.[81-83] Red blood cell volume falls during the first 8 weeks of pregnancy, increases to the prepregnant level by 16 weeks, and undergoes a further rise to 30% above the prepregnant volume at term.[81,83,84] These changes result in 10%, 30%, and 45% increases in total blood volume by the end of the first, second, and third trimesters, respectively (Figure 2-5). Expressed in milliliters per kilogram (mL/kg), pregnancy results in an increase in plasma volume from 49 to 67 mL/kg, an increase in total blood volume from 76 to 94 mL/kg, and no change in red blood cell volume (27 mL/kg).[81] Although considerable variation occurs among individuals, these changes in blood volume tend to be repeated for the same woman in successive pregnancies.[81,84] Furthermore, greater increases in blood volumes occur with twins than with singleton pregnan-

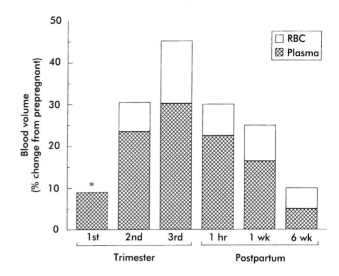

FIGURE 2-5. Blood volume during pregnancy and the puerperium. Values during pregnancy are measured at the end of the first, second, and third trimesters. Postpartum values are measured after a vaginal delivery. The values for red blood cell *(RBC)* mass and plasma volume *(Plasma)* do not represent the actual percentage of change in these parameters but instead reflect the relative contribution of each to the change in blood volume. The asterisk indicates that RBC volume is below the prepregnant volume at the end of the first trimester.

cies,[84] and volumes are positively correlated with the size of the fetus in singleton pregnancies.[82]

The increase in plasma volume results from fetal and maternal hormone production. The maternal concentrations of estrogens and progesterone increase nearly 100-fold during pregnancy.[1] Estrogens increase plasma renin activity, which enhances renal sodium reabsorption and water retention by means of the renin-angiotensin-aldosterone system. Fetal adrenal production of the estrogen precursor dehydroepiandrosterone may be the underlying control mechanism. Progesterone also enhances aldosterone production. These changes result in a marked increase in plasma renin activity and aldosterone level[85] and in retention of approximately 900 mEq of sodium and 7000 mL of total body water during pregnancy.

Red blood cell volume increases in response to the elevated erythropoietin concentration[86] and the erythropoietic effects of progesterone, prolactin, and placental lactogen. The delay in enhanced erythrocyte production during early pregnancy is consistent with the lack of change in erythropoietin concentration until 8 to 12 weeks' gestation.[86]

The hemoglobin concentration and hematocrit fall after conception until they are approximately 11.2 g/dL and 34%, respectively, by mid-gestation.[1,83,84,87-89] This represents a 15% decrease from prepregnant levels. The hemoglobin concentration and hematocrit increase during late gestation to approximately 11.6 g/dL and 35.5%, respectively, because of a greater increase in red blood cell mass than in plasma volume after mid-gestation (Table 2-5). Patients who do not receive iron supplementation during pregnancy experience greater decreases in their hemoglobin concentration and hematocrit.[83]

The hemodilution that occurs during pregnancy may be essential for maintaining the patency of the uteroplacental vascular bed. Because increased blood viscosity is associated with thrombosis, hemodilution and decreased viscosity may decrease the risk of intervillous thrombosis and infarction. This contention is supported by the observation that placental infarcts are positively correlated with the maternal hemoglobin concentration and hematocrit.[90]

Plasma Proteins

Plasma albumin concentration decreases from 4.5 to 3.9 g/dL during the first trimester and to 3.3 g/dL by term pregnancy (Table 2-6).[91,92] Globulins decline by 10% in the first trimester and then rise throughout the remainder of pregnancy to 10% above the prepregnant level at term.[91] The albumin to globulin ratio falls during pregnancy from a prepregnant value of 1.4 to 0.9,[91] and total protein falls from approximately 7.8 to 7.0 g/dL.[91] Maternal colloid osmotic pressure decreases by approximately 5 mm Hg during pregnancy.[37,87,93] The plasma cholinesterase concentration falls by approximately 25% during the first trimester and remains at that level until the end of pregnancy.[94,95]

Coagulation

Pregnancy is associated with enhanced platelet turnover, clotting, and fibrinolysis (Box 2-1). Thus pregnancy represents a state of accelerated but compensated intravascular coagulation.

Increases in platelet factor 4 and beta-thromboglobulin signal elevated platelet activation,[96] and the progressive increase in platelet width[97] and volume[98] are consistent with increased platelet consumption during pregnancy. Platelet aggregation in response to collagen, epinephrine, adenosine diphosphate, and arachidonic acid is increased.[99] Although an increase in platelet consumption might be expected to result in a decline in platelet count, as noted by some investigators,[98,100-102] others have found no change in platelet count, suggesting that increased production compensates for increased platelet activation.[96,97] However, 7.6% of otherwise normal parturients have a platelet count of less than 150,000/mm³, and 0.9% have a platelet count of less than 100,000/mm³.[103] Despite changes in platelet count and/or function, the bleeding time measurement is not altered during normal gestation.[104]

The concentrations of most coagulation factors, including fibrinogen (factor I), proconvertin (factor VII), antihemophilic factor (factor VIII), Christmas factor (factor IX), Stuart-Prower factor (factor X), and Hageman factor (factor XII), increase during pregnancy. The concentrations of some factors increase by more than 100%.[96,97,101,105,106] Prothrombin (factor II) and proaccelerin (factor V) concentrations do not change, whereas the concentrations of thromboplastin antecedent (factor XI) and fibrin-stabilizing factor (factor XIII) decrease.[100,101,105-107] A shortening of the prothrombin and partial thromboplastin times[101] is consistent with an elevation of most factor concentrations. An increase in most factor concentrations, an increase in fibrinopeptide A (formed during fibrin generation), and a decrease in antithrombin III concentration suggest an activation of the clotting system.[96] Changes in thromboelastography also suggest that pregnancy is a hypercoagulable state.[108]

The increased concentration of fibrin degradation products signals increased fibrinolytic activity during gestation.[96,107] The marked increase in the plasminogen concentration also is consistent with enhanced fibrinolysis.[100]

Hematology and Coagulation During the Puerperium

Blood loss during vaginal delivery and the early puerperium is approximately 600 mL.[109] Blood volume falls to 125% of the

TABLE 2-5	HEMATOLOGIC PARAMETERS AT TERM GESTATION
Parameter	**Change* or actual measurement**
Blood volume	+45%*
Plasma volume	+55%*
Red blood cell volume	+30%*
Hemoglobin	11.6 g/dL
Hematocrit	35.5%

*Relative to nonpregnant women.
From Conklin KA. Maternal physiological adaptations during gestation, labor, and the puerperium. Semin Anesth 1991; 10:221–34.

TABLE 2-6	PLASMA PROTEINS DURING PREGNANCY			
		Trimester		
	Nonpregnant	**First**	**Second**	**Third**
Total protein (g%)	7.8	6.9	6.9	7.0
Albumin (g%)	4.5	3.9	3.6	3.3
Globulin (g%)	3.3	3.0	3.3	3.7
Albumin/globulin ratio	1.4	1.3	1.1	0.9
Plasma cholinesterase	—	−25%	−25%	−25%
Colloid osmotic pressure (mm Hg)	27	25	23	22

Box 2-1   CHANGES IN COAGULATION AND FIBRINOLYTIC PARAMETERS AT TERM GESTATION*
INCREASED FACTOR CONCENTRATIONS Factor I (fibrinogen) Factor VII (proconvertin) Factor VIII (antihemophilic factor) Factor IX (Christmas factor) Factor X (Stuart-Prower factor) Factor XII (Hageman factor) **UNCHANGED FACTOR CONCENTRATIONS** Factor II (prothrombin) Factor V (proaccelerin) **DECREASED FACTOR CONCENTRATIONS** Factor XI (thromboplastin antecedent) Factor XIII (fibrin-stabilizing factor) Prothrombin time: shortened 20% Partial thromboplastin time: shortened 20% Thromboelastography: hypercoagulable Fibrinopeptide A: increased Antithrombin III: decreased Platelet count: no change or decreased Bleeding time: no change Fibrin degradation products: increased Plasminogen: increased

*Relative to nonpregnant women.

prepregnant level during the first week postpartum,[81,109] followed by a more gradual decline to 110% of the prepregnant level at 6 to 9 weeks postpartum.[81] The hemoglobin concentration and hematocrit fall during the first 3 postpartum days, rise rapidly during the next 3 days (because of a relatively greater reduction in plasma than in red blood cell volume), and continue to rise to prepregnant levels by 6 weeks postpartum.[110]

Cesarean section results in a blood loss of approximately 1000 mL within the first few hours of delivery.[109] General anesthesia using approximately 0.6 MAC (minimum alveolar concentration) of a volatile halogenated agent results in a somewhat greater blood loss than use of a nitrous oxide/opioid (i.e., balanced) technique or regional anesthesia.[111,112] The blood volume change after cesarean section is similar to that after vaginal delivery, although the hematocrit is lower because of the greater blood loss during cesarean delivery.[109]

Albumin and total protein concentrations and colloid osmotic pressure decline after delivery and gradually rise to prepregnant levels by 6 weeks postpartum.[87,91] Plasma cholinesterase falls below the predelivery level by 1 day postpartum and remains at that level during the next week.[94,95] Globulins are elevated throughout the first postpartum week.[91]

Beginning with delivery and during the first postpartum day, a rapid fall in the platelet count and in the concentrations of fibrinogen, factor VIII, and plasminogen occurs, as does an increase in antifibrinolytic activity.[113] Clotting tests remain shortened during the first postpartum day,[114] and thromboelastography remains consistent with a hypercoagulable state.[108] During the first 3 to 5 postpartum days the fibrinogen concentration and platelet count rise, which may account for the increased incidence of thrombotic complications during the puerperium.[114] The coagulation profile returns to that of the nonpregnant state by 2 weeks postpartum.[113]

THE IMMUNE SYSTEM
The blood leukocyte count rises progressively during pregnancy from the prepregnant level of approximately 6000/mm^3 to 9000 to 11,000/mm^3.[89,102] This increase reflects a rise in polymorphonuclear cells,[88,89,102] with the appearance of immature granulocytic forms (i.e., myelocytes and metamyelocytes) in most pregnant women.[88] The proportion of immature forms falls during the last 2 months of pregnancy.[88] The lymphocyte, eosinophil, and basophil counts fall, whereas the monocyte count does not change during pregnancy.[88,89,102] During labor the leukocyte count rises to approximately 13,000/mm^3,[89] and it increases further to an average of 15,000/mm^3 on the first postpartum day.[110] The leukocyte count falls during the puerperium to an average of 9250/mm^3 by the sixth postpartum day, although at 6 weeks postpartum it is still elevated above the prepregnant level.[110]

Polymorphonuclear leukocyte function is impaired during pregnancy, as shown by depressed neutrophil chemotaxis and adherence.[115] This may account for the increased incidence of infection during pregnancy and the decreased incidence of symptoms in some pregnant women with autoimmune diseases (e.g., rheumatoid arthritis). However, pregnancy does not appear to be associated with suppression of autoantibody production.[116] Although the serum concentrations of immunoglobulins A, G, and M are unchanged during gestation,[92] humoral antibody titers to certain viruses (e.g., herpes simplex, measles, influenza A) are decreased.[117]

THE GASTROINTESTINAL SYSTEM
Anatomy, Barrier Pressure, and Pyrosis
The stomach is displaced upward toward the left side of the diaphragm during pregnancy, and its axis is rotated approximately 45 degrees to the right from its normal vertical position. The altered position of the stomach displaces the intraabdominal segment of the esophagus into the thorax in most pregnant women. This causes a reduction in tone of the lower esophageal high-pressure zone (LEHPZ), which normally prevents the reflux of gastric contents. This displacement of the esophagus also prevents the rise in lower esophageal tone that normally accompanies an increase in intragastric pressure (IGP).[118-120] Progestins also may contribute to a relaxation of the LEHPZ.[121] IGP is elevated during the last trimester in all pregnant women.[118-120] Thus pyrosis (heartburn) occurs frequently in pregnant women as a result of the reduced barrier pressure (LEHPZ minus IGP). The incidence of pyrosis increases with gestational age, from 22% in the first trimester to 39% in the second trimester and 72% in the third trimester.[122] It is positively correlated with parity and inversely correlated with maternal age, but not influenced by race, body mass index before pregnancy, or weight gain during pregnancy.[122]

Gastrointestinal Motility and Secretions
The gastric emptying of liquid and solid materials is not altered at any time during pregnancy (Table 2-7). This has been demonstrated in studies that measured the absorption of orally

TABLE 2-7   CHANGES IN GASTROINTESTINAL PHYSIOLOGY DURING PREGNANCY*

Parameter	Trimester			Labor	Postpartum (18 hr)
	First	Second	Third		
Barrier pressure[†]	Decreased	Decreased	Decreased	Decreased	?
Gastric emptying	No change	No change	No change	Delayed	No change
Gastric acid secretion	No change or decreased	No change or decreased	No change	?	?
Proportion of women with gastric volume > 25 mL	No change	No change	No change	Increased	No change
Proportion of women with gastric pH < 2.5	No change	No change	No change	Decreased	No change

*Relative to nonpregnant women.
†Difference between intragastric pressure and tone of the lower esophageal high-pressure zone.

administered paracetamol[123,124] and in studies that assessed the emptying of a test meal by radiographic,[125] ultrasonographic,[126] and dye-dilution techniques[127]; epigastric impedance[128]; and applied potential tomography.[129] Measurements in studies that showed delayed gastric emptying during the first trimester[130,131] may have been affected by the stress associated with the upcoming surgical procedure for termination of pregnancy.

Esophageal peristalsis and intestinal transit time are slowed during pregnancy.[126,132,133] These effects on motility have been attributed to the inhibition of gastrointestinal contractile activity by progesterone. However, this may be an indirect action that results from a negative effect of progesterone on the plasma concentration of motilin, which declines during pregnancy.[126]

Studies of gastric acid secretion during pregnancy have demonstrated conflicting results. Early work suggested that both basal and maximal gastric acid secretion fell in midgestation, reaching a nadir at 20 to 30 weeks' gestation.[134] However, Van Thiel et al.[135] demonstrated no difference in basal or peak gastric acid secretion in four pregnant women studied in each trimester and at 1 to 4 weeks postpartum, although a significantly reduced plasma gastrin level was observed during the first trimester compared with postpartum.[135] A study of 11 women who had symptoms of mild dyspepsia showed no change in plasma gastrin levels in the first and third trimesters and at 4 to 6 months postpartum.[126] No difference in gastric acidity (measured using a radiotelemetry technique) was seen in pregnant women in the third trimester, when compared with nonpregnant women.[136]

It is most likely that differences in plasma gastrin levels and gastric acid secretion during pregnancy are small, if they exist at all. Peptic ulcer disease appears to be less common in pregnant women than in nonpregnant women, but this may be true for reasons unrelated to changes in gastric acidity, such as (1) increased plasma histaminase, (2) a decreased immune/inflammatory response to *Helicobacter pylori* colonization, and/or (3) avoidance of exposure to ulcerogenic factors such as smoking, alcohol, and nonsteroidal antiinflammatory drugs during pregnancy.[137]

Several investigators have reported results of nasogastric aspiration of gastric contents in nonpregnant patients undergoing elective surgery[138-142] and in pregnant women undergoing elective cesarean section.[143-148] Among those patients who received no preoperative medication that would alter gastric volume or pH, approximately 80% of individuals in *each* group (pregnant and nonpregnant) had a gastric pH of 2.5 or less, approximately 50% had gastric volumes of 25 mL or greater, and 40% to 50% exhibited both a low pH and a volume of at least 25 mL. An investigation of women with a mean gestational age of 15 weeks revealed similar results.[142]

Gastric Function During Labor

Gastric emptying is slowed during labor, as shown by sonographic imaging,[149] emptying of a test meal,[125,127,128] and the rate of absorption of oral paracetamol.[150] Direct measurements show that the mean gastric volume increases.[143] However, postpartum gastric volume was not different in parturients who consumed water in labor compared with those who consumed an isotonic "sports drink" composed of mixed carbohydrates and electrolytes.[151] Gastric acid secretion may decrease during labor because only 25% of laboring parturients have a gastric pH of 2.5 or less.[152]

Effects of Analgesia on Gastric Function During Labor

When compared with parturients who do not receive analgesia, women who receive intramuscular opioids during labor exhibit impaired gastric emptying.[125,128,150,153] Intramuscular opioids also reduce the tone of the LEHPZ.[154]

Epidural analgesia using local anesthetics does not delay gastric emptying during labor,[153] a result that is consistent with results from studies in postoperative patients and nonpregnant volunteers. Epidural fentanyl, administered in a bolus dose of 100 μg, significantly delays gastric emptying during labor[155-157] and after cesarean section,[158] although a 50-μg bolus may be without effect.[159] A 25-μg dose of intrathecal fentanyl also inhibits gastric emptying during labor.[159] An epidural fentanyl infusion (2.5 μg/mL with 0.0625% bupivacaine), without a preceding fentanyl bolus, does not alter gastric emptying during labor.[160] A 4-mg dose of epidural morphine administered to nonpregnant volunteers has also been shown to inhibit gastric emptying and to have a greater inhibitory effect than the same dose given intramuscularly.[161]

Gastric Function During the Puerperium

Gastric emptying is delayed during the early postpartum period,[162] but beyond 18 hours postpartum it is comparable to that of nonpregnant women (see Table 2-7).[124,129,163] Gastric volume and pH are similar in fasting women who are more than 18 hours postpartum and in nonpregnant individuals who have been without oral intake before elective surgery.[139,164,165]

THE LIVER AND GALLBLADDER

Liver size, morphology, and blood flow do not change during pregnancy, although the liver is displaced upward, posterior, and to the right during late pregnancy.

Serum bilirubin, alanine aminotransferase (ALT, SGPT), aspartate aminotransferase (AST, SGOT), and lactic dehydrogenase increase to the upper limits of the normal range during pregnancy.[166,167] The total alkaline phosphatase activity increases twofold to fourfold, mostly from production by the placenta with only a small increase from hepatic sources.[166] Excretion of sulfobromophthalein into bile decreases, whereas hepatic extraction and retention of this compound increases.[168]

The fasting and residual volumes of the gallbladder increase markedly during the second and third trimesters, and the rate of gallbladder emptying slows.[169] The bile tends to concentrate; thus pregnancy predisposes to gallstone formation.

THE KIDNEYS

The kidneys enlarge during pregnancy and return to prepregnant size by 6 months postpartum. The ureters and renal pelves dilate by the end of the first trimester as a result of hormonal changes (primarily increased progesterone) and, as gestation progresses, the obstructive effect of the uterus.

Renal plasma flow increases by approximately 75% to 85% during pregnancy, although it falls slightly as term approaches.[44] Because the glomerular filtration rate (GFR) increases by 50%, the filtration fraction decreases. Creatinine clearance increases early in pregnancy, is maximum by the end of the first trimester, falls slightly near term, and returns to the prepregnant level by 8 to 12 weeks postpartum.[170]

The increased GFR results in decreased blood concentrations of nitrogenous metabolites. The blood urea nitrogen concentration falls to 8 to 9 mg/dL by the end of the first trimester and remains at that level until term.[171] The serum creatinine concentration falls progressively to 0.5 to 0.6 mg/dL by the end of pregnancy.[171] The serum urate concentration falls during the first two trimesters to 2 to 3 mg/dL, after which it returns to the nonpregnant level at term.[172] Tubular reabsorption of urate accounts for the rise during the third trimester.

Pregnancy imposes a change in the glucose resorptive capacity of the proximal tubules so that all pregnant women exhibit an elevation of glucose excretion over the normal nonpregnant level. In pregnant women who have normal glucose tolerance to an oral load and normal glucose excretion when not pregnant, approximately half exhibit a doubling of glucose excretion, most of the remainder have increases of 3 to 10 times the nonpregnant amount, and a small proportion (less than 10%) excrete as much as 20 times the nonpregnant amount.[173] The normal nonpregnant pattern of glucose excretion is reestablished within a week of delivery.

NONPLACENTAL ENDOCRINOLOGY

Thyroid Function

The thyroid gland enlarges during pregnancy because of follicular hyperplasia and increased vascularity. The estrogen-induced increase in thyroid-binding globulin results in a 50% increase in total T_3 and T_4 concentrations during the first trimester, and these concentrations are maintained until term.[174] The concentrations of free T_3 and T_4 are unchanged during pregnancy.[174] The concentration of thyroid-stimulating hormone falls during the first trimester but returns to the nonpregnant level shortly thereafter and undergoes no further change during the remainder of pregnancy.[174]

Adrenal Cortical Function

The concentration of corticosteroid-binding globulin (CBG) doubles during gestation as a result of estrogen-induced enhanced hepatic synthesis. The elevated CBG results in a 100% increase in the plasma cortisol concentration at the end of the first trimester and a 200% increase at term.[175] The concentration of unbound, metabolically active cortisol at the end of the third trimester is 2.5 times the nonpregnant level. The increase in free cortisol results from increased production (which is consistent with hypertrophy of the zona fasciculata producing the hormone) and decreased clearance.

Pancreas and Glucose Metabolism

Pregnancy is characterized by reduced tissue sensitivity to insulin.[176] This diabetogenic effect is caused by hormones secreted by the placenta, primarily placental lactogen. Thus the blood glucose levels after a carbohydrate load are greater in pregnant than in nonpregnant women, despite a hyperinsulinemic response in pregnant women. These alterations resolve within 24 hours of delivery.

The *fasting* blood glucose level of women during the third trimester is significantly lower than that of nonpregnant individuals.[177] The altered response to fasting during pregnancy is explained by the high glucose use of the fetoplacental unit. The relative hypoglycemic state results in fasting hypoinsulinemia. Pregnant women also exhibit an exaggerated starvation ketosis.[177]

THE MUSCULOSKELETAL SYSTEM

As the uterus enlarges during pregnancy, the lumbar lordosis is enhanced, thus maintaining the woman's center of gravity over the lower extremities (Figure 2-6). The exaggerated lumbar lordosis tends to stretch the lateral femoral cutaneous

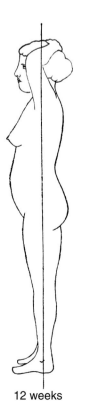
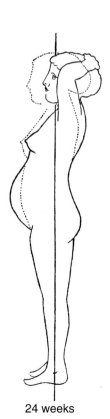
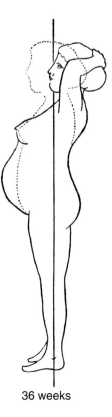

12 weeks   24 weeks   36 weeks

FIGURE 2-6. Changes in posture during pregnancy. The first figure and the subsequent dotted-line figures represent a woman's posture before growth of the uterus and its contents have affected the center of gravity. As the uterus enlarges and the abdomen protrudes, the lumbar lordosis is enhanced and the shoulders slump and move posteriorly. (From Beck AC, Rosenthal AH. Obstetrical Practice. Baltimore, Williams and Wilkins, 1955:146.)

nerve and can result in meralgia paresthetica, a mild sensory loss over the antero-lateral thigh. Anterior flexion of the neck and slumping of the shoulders usually accompany the enhanced lordosis; this can result in a brachial plexus neuropathy with aching, numbness, and weakness of the upper extremities from traction on the brachial plexus.

The mobility of the sacroiliac, sacrococcygeal, and pubic joints increases during pregnancy in preparation for passage of the fetus. A widening of the pubic symphysis is evident by 30 weeks' gestation. These changes are attributable to the hormone relaxin and the biomechanical strain of pregnancy on the ligaments and skeleton, and they are the leading cause of low back pain and pelvic discomfort, which occur in about 50% of pregnant women.[178] Relaxin also may contribute to the increased incidence of carpal tunnel syndrome during pregnancy by changing the nature of the connective tissue so that more fluid is absorbed.[179]

THE NERVOUS SYSTEM

Pregnancy-Induced Analgesia

Women experience an elevation in the threshold to pain and discomfort near the end of pregnancy and during labor.[180] Evidence that this pregnancy-induced analgesia is caused by endogenous analgesic neuropeptides, such as endorphins, enkephalins, and others, includes: (1) elevation of plasma and cerebrospinal fluid (CSF) concentrations of these compounds in pregnant women[181]; (2) elevation in brain levels of these compounds in pregnant experimental animals[182]; and (3) abolition of this phenomenon by systemic and intrathecal administration of opioid antagonists in experimental animals.[183,184]

Sympathetic Nervous System

Dependence on the sympathetic nervous system for maintenance of hemodynamic stability increases progressively throughout pregnancy and reaches a peak at term.[185-187] The effect is primarily on the venous capacitance system of the lower extremities,[187] which counteracts the adverse effects of uterine compression of the inferior vena cava on venous return. Thus pharmacologic sympathectomy in term pregnant women results in a marked decrease in blood pressure, whereas nonpregnant women experience a minimal decline (Figure 2-7).[185] The dependence on sympathetic nervous system activity returns to that of the nonpregnant state by 36 to 48 hours postpartum.[185]

The Vertebral Column

The epidural space is contained within boundaries formed superiorly by the dura, which adheres firmly to the periosteum around the foramen magnum; inferiorly by the sacrococcygeal membrane; and circumferentially by the vertebral lamina and pedicles, the posterior longitudinal ligament, and the ligamentum flavum. Thus the epidural space can be regarded as a rigid tube that contains two fluid-filled distensible tubes, the dural sac and the epidural veins. When the

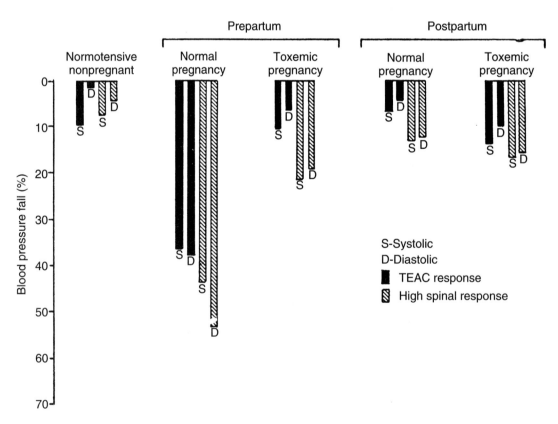

FIGURE 2-7. Blood pressure response of normotensive nonpregnant, normal term pregnant, severely preeclamptic, and postpartum women to pharmacologic sympathectomy. High spinal anesthesia (sensory level between T_2 and C_3) or ganglionic blockade with tetraethylammonium chloride (TEAC, a ganglionic blocker) was used to produce extensive sympathetic blockade. Intravenous fluids were not administered during the study period. (From Assali NS, Prystowsky H. Studies on autonomic blockade. I. Comparison between the effects of tetraethylammonium chloride (TEAC) and high selective spinal anesthesia on blood pressure of normal and toxemic pregnancy. J Clin Invest 1950; 29:1354-66.)

volume within one distensible tube increases, a compensatory loss of fluid from the other occurs. During pregnancy, compression of the inferior vena cava by the gravid uterus increases venous pressure below the obstruction[53,54,58] and diverts venous blood through the vertebral plexus within the epidural space. This diversion distends the epidural veins[52,54] and reduces the spinal CSF volume.

Fiberoptic epiduroscopy has revealed (1) a reduction in the size of the epidural pneumatic space following injection of 5 mL of air in the third trimester of pregnancy, (2) an increase in the density of the epidural vascular network in the third trimester of pregnancy, and (3) an increase in the amount of engorged blood vessels in the first and third trimesters, when compared with nonpregnant women.[188]

In the lateral position, lumbar epidural pressure is positive in term pregnant women but negative in greater than 90% of nonpregnant women.[189] Turning a parturient from the lateral to the supine position increases the epidural pressure.[189] Epidural pressure also increases during labor.[189] The increased pressure results from increased diversion of venous blood through the vertebral plexus. Specifically, it results from either enhanced compression of the inferior vena cava in the supine position or increased intraabdominal pressure during pain and/or pushing. The epidural pressure returns to the nonpregnant level by 6 to 12 hours postpartum.[189]

Despite compression of the dural sac by the epidural veins, the CSF pressure of parturients—between contractions in the lateral position—is the same as in nonpregnant women.[190] The result of uterine contractions and pushing is an increase in CSF pressure that is secondary to acute increases in epidural vein distention.[190]

ANESTHETIC IMPLICATIONS

Positioning the Pregnant Patient

Objective parameters of fetal well-being deteriorate when parturients labor in the supine position compared with the lateral or tilted position. Such evidence includes decreased fetal scalp capillary blood pH, decreased fetal transcutaneous Po_2, and an increased incidence of late decelerations of the fetal heart rate.[191,192] Neonatal outcome, assessed by umbilical cord pH and Apgar scores, also is compromised when parturients are positioned supine instead of tilted during labor or cesarean section.[193] These adverse effects are explained by aortocaval compression and impairment of uteroplacental blood flow when the pregnant woman is in the supine position.[42]

Aortocaval compression should be minimized in all pregnant women. This can be accomplished by placing a cushion or wedge under the parturient's right hip (Figure 2-8) or by placing her in the lateral decubitus position. Because the supine position impairs maternal hemodynamics as early as 20 weeks of pregnancy, such measures should be used from mid-term to term gestation. When identifying the epidural or subarachnoid space, the lateral flexed position may be more likely to cause concealed aortocaval compression than the sitting position. Andrews et al.[194] observed that laboring women who assumed the left lateral decubitus position with "maximal" lumbar flexion were more likely to experience a decrease in cardiac output than similar patients who assumed the sitting position during identification of the epidural space.

Blood Replacement

At delivery, maternal vascular capacitance is reduced by the volume of the intervillous space (by at least 500 mL).[76,77] Thus during vaginal delivery or cesarean section, this volume of blood does not need to be replaced for hemodynamic stability, nor should it be considered when estimating blood loss for the purpose of replacing red blood cells. Hemoconcentration occurs as maternal blood volume declines from 94 mL/kg at term gestation to 76 mL/kg during the postpartum period[81]; this should be considered when making a decision as to whether a parturient should receive crystalloid, colloid, or blood for volume replacement.

General Anesthesia

ENDOTRACHEAL INTUBATION

The internal diameter of the trachea is reduced during pregnancy because of capillary engorgement of the mucosa.[2] Therefore small-caliber endotracheal tubes should be used to facilitate endotracheal intubation and to prevent mucosal trauma in pregnant women (Box 2-2). A 6.5-mm endotracheal tube is a good choice for most pregnant women. Nasotracheal intubation should be avoided in pregnant women because mucosal engorgement increases the risk of nasopharyngeal trauma,[2] which may lead to severe epistaxis.

Engorgement of the oropharyngeal mucosa[2] most likely accounts for the increase in Mallampati score during gestation and its further increase during labor[195,196] and contributes to intubation difficulties during pregnancy. Samsoon and Young[197] found the incidence of failed endotracheal intubation in obstetric patients to be 1:280 (i.e., 7 of 1980 cases),

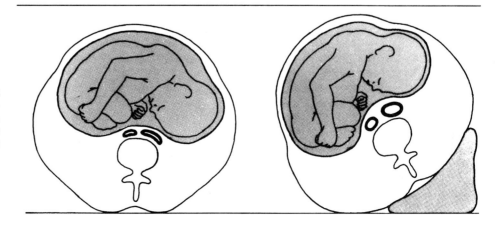

FIGURE 2-8. Compression of the aorta and inferior vena cava in the supine and lateral tilt position. (From Camann WR, Ostheimer GW. Physiological adaptations during pregnancy. Int Anesth Clin 1990; 28:2-10.)

whereas in nonpregnant patients it was 1:2230 (i.e., 6 of 13,380 cases). None of the obstetric patients who had a failed intubation presented with externally apparent anatomic features usually associated with difficult endotracheal intubation, but 6 of 7 women had a class-IV assessment of oropharyngeal structures (i.e., the soft palate was not visible).

Rocke et al.[198] reported that failed endotracheal intubation occurred in 2 of 1500 parturients receiving general anesthesia for cesarean section and that intubation was *very difficult* in another 30 (2%) of these cases. They also found a correlation between diminished visualization of oropharyngeal structures and difficulty at intubation. Further, they observed a significant association between difficult/failed intubation and short neck, receding mandible, and protruding maxillary incisors.

MATERNAL OXYGENATION

Pregnant women become hypoxemic more rapidly than nonpregnant women during episodes of apnea (see Box 2-2). This is caused by the reduced FRC and the higher oxygen consumption of pregnant women. Moreover, FRC is less than closing capacity in as many as 50% of supine pregnant women.[10] Therefore during the apnea associated with rapid-sequence induction of general anesthesia, the PaO_2 of parturients falls at more than twice the rate in nonpregnant women (139 mm Hg/min versus 58 mm Hg/min).[199] Because oxygenation before induction of anesthesia results in a PaO_2 of approximately 500 mm Hg,[199] parturients become hypoxemic after about 3 minutes of apnea, whereas nonpregnant women maintain a PaO_2 above 100 mm Hg for approximately 7 minutes.

Denitrogenation is achieved more rapidly in pregnant than in nonpregnant women. This is attributed to the elevated minute ventilation and decreased FRC seen in pregnancy.

MATERNAL VENTILATION

Ventilation during general anesthesia should be adjusted so that the $PaCO_2$ of the parturient is maintained at 30 mm Hg. Allowing the $PaCO_2$ to increase to the normal level for nonpregnant women (40 mm Hg) results in acute respiratory acidosis. Because the $PaCO_2$ reaches 30 mm Hg during the first trimester, this consideration applies equally to women who receive anesthesia during early pregnancy. A $PaCO_2$ of 30 mm Hg during cesarean section can be achieved by maintaining minute ventilation at 121 mL/kg/min, which is greater than the 77 mL/kg/min required to maintain a comparable $PaCO_2$ in nonpregnant women (see Box 2-2).[200]

INHALATION ANESTHETICS

The MAC of volatile halogenated anesthetic agents is reduced by 15% to 40% during pregnancy in animals (Box 2-3).[201-203] In human pregnancy MAC is reduced by 30% during early gestation,[204] and in postpartum women MAC returns to that of the nonpregnant state within 3 days of delivery.[205] Several factors have been proposed to account for this change: (1) the elevated level of progesterone, which has a sedative effect and can produce unconsciousness in humans, and reduces MAC in experimental animals,[203,206] (2) increased central nervous system (CNS) serotonergic activity,[207] and (3) activation of the endorphin system.[183-185]

The rate of rise of the alveolar anesthetic concentration compared with that of inspired gas (i.e., the rate of anesthetic induction) increases during pregnancy as a result of the increased minute ventilation and the reduced FRC. This occurs despite increased cardiac output, which slows the rate of induction.

INTRAVENOUS ANESTHETICS

Christensen et al.[208] found that the average induction dose of thiopental in parturients was reduced by 35% compared with that in nonpregnant women. This change in sensitivity to thiopental is similar to that for inhalation anesthetic agents (see Box 2-3). In early gestation (7 to 14 weeks), sensitivity to thiopental is increased by 18%.[209]

Pharmacokinetic analysis of thiopental in healthy parturients demonstrates a prolongation of the elimination half-life to 26.1 hours, compared with 11.5 hours for nonpregnant women.[210] The longer half-life is explained by a marked increase in the volume of distribution of thiopental, despite an

---

Box 2-2 GENERAL ANESTHESIA: ANESTHETIC IMPLICATIONS OF MATERNAL PHYSIOLOGIC CHANGES

ENDOTRACHEAL INTUBATION

- Smaller endotracheal tube required
- Increased risk of trauma with nasotracheal intubation
- Increased risk of failed intubation
- Increased risk of pulmonary aspiration of gastric contents

MATERNAL OXYGENATION

- Increased physiologic shunt when supine
- Increased rate of denitrogenation
- Increased rate of decline of PaO_2 during apnea
  - Decreased FRC (store of oxygen)
  - Increased oxygen consumption

MATERNAL VENTILATION

- Increased minute ventilation required

Adapted from Conklin KA. Maternal physiological adaptations during gestation, labor, and the puerperium. Semin Anesth 1991; 10:221-34.

Box 2-3 GENERAL ANESTHESIA: PHARMACOLOGY DURING PREGNANCY*

INHALATION ANESTHETICS

- Minimum alveolar concentration reduced 15% to 40%
- Rate of induction increased

INDUCTION AGENTS

- ED_{50} of thiopental reduced 35% (term pregnancy)
- Elimination half-life of thiopental prolonged
- Elimination half-life of propofol unaltered

MEPERIDINE

- Elimination half-life unaltered

SUCCINYLCHOLINE

- Duration of blockade unaltered (or decreased)
- Sensitivity reduced

NONDEPOLARIZING MUSCLE RELAXANTS

- Increased sensitivity to vecuronium and rocuronium
- Elimination half-life of vecuronium and pancuronium shortened
- Atracurium pharmacodynamics and pharmacokinetics unaltered

CHRONOTROPIC AGENTS

- Response diminished

*Changes relative to nonpregnant women.

increase in thiopental clearance. The shorter elimination half-life measured by some observers was likely caused by a shorter sampling time (1 day versus 3 to 4 days), which underestimates this parameter.[208] Plasma protein binding of thiopental is similar in term pregnant and nonpregnant women.[210]

There is scant information on the sensitivity to propofol in pregnancy, although clinical experience suggests that it is an effective induction agent. One study showed that the C_{50} for loss of consciousness with propofol is not reduced in early pregnancy (i.e., 8 weeks' gestation).[211] Maternal recovery from anesthesia occurs more rapidly when propofol is used for induction than when thiopental is used.[212] In contrast to thiopental, the elimination half-life of propofol is unaffected by pregnancy, although clearance of the drug may increase.[213] Propofol pharmacokinetics are similar in term pregnant and postpartum (2 to 3 days) women.

Pregnant and nonpregnant women metabolize and excrete meperidine and produce and eliminate normeperidine (an active metabolite of meperidine) in a similar manner.[214]

SUCCINYLCHOLINE

Pregnant women exhibit a 25% decrease in plasma cholinesterase activity.[94,95] In individuals with a genotypically normal enzyme, this reduction of enzyme activity does not significantly alter the elimination half-life or clinical duration of action of succinylcholine because it is eliminated by first-order kinetics.[215] Only a marked reduction in enzyme activity, which allows first-order kinetics to approach zero-order kinetics, results in a prolonged duration of the action of succinylcholine.[215]

These considerations explain why twitch height recovery after administration of succinylcholine does not differ significantly between normal pregnant and nonpregnant women who receive the same dose (mg/kg or mg/m^2).[95] Recovery may be even faster in pregnant women.[95] Faster recovery is explained by the increased volume of distribution of succinylcholine during gestation, which results in a lower initial drug concentration and a shorter time before the threshold for recovery is attained. Pregnant women may be less sensitive than nonpregnant women to comparable plasma concentrations of succinylcholine, which also would contribute to more rapid recovery during pregnancy (see Box 2-3).

After delivery the decrease in plasma cholinesterase activity (to less than 60% of the nonpregnant value[95]) and plasma volume alters succinylcholine pharmacokinetics. This is illustrated by a longer recovery time in women 1 to 2 days postpartum compared with term pregnant or nonpregnant women receiving the same dose of relaxant.[95] Postpartum women also require a reduced dose of succinylcholine to achieve an 80% depression of twitch height.[216] Although the postpartum changes are statistically significant, their magnitude is small and has minimal impact on anesthetic management.

NONDEPOLARIZING MUSCLE RELAXANTS

Pregnant and postpartum women exhibit enhanced sensitivity to the aminosteroid muscle relaxants vecuronium and rocuronium.[217-219] The ED_{50} of vecuronium in pregnant rabbits is reduced by more than 50%.[220] The increase in sensitivity to vecuronium is not explained by altered pharmacokinetics because the drug exhibits increased clearance and a shortened elimination half-life in pregnant women (see Box 2-3).[221] The pharmacokinetics of pancuronium undergo changes during pregnancy that are similar to those of vecuronium.[221,222]

In contrast to the aminosteroid relaxants, the pharmacodynamics and pharmacokinetics of atracurium, a bisquaternary ammonium benzylisoquinoline compound, are unaltered during pregnancy.[217,223]

CHRONOTROPIC AGENTS

Pregnancy reduces the chronotropic response to isoproterenol and epinephrine, possibly as a result of the downregulation of beta-adrenergic receptors.[224] Thus these agents are less sensitive markers of intravascular injection during administration of regional anesthesia in pregnant patients than in nonpregnant patients.

PRESSORS

The effect of pregnancy on the magnitude of the pressor response has not been established, although several pregnancy-induced alterations of vascular reactivity to adrenergic agonists have been demonstrated. Nisell et al.[225] found that the pressor response in *nonpregnant* women was caused by increased systemic vascular resistance (i.e., arterial vasoconstriction), whereas in *pregnant* women it was caused by an increase in stroke volume resulting from venoconstriction and increased venous return. Both systemic and uterine vascular resistance increase less during the infusion of norepinephrine and phenylephrine in pregnant ewes than in nonpregnant ewes.[226] Pregnancy is associated with a marked increase in the sensitivity of mesenteric veins to exogenous norepinephrine stimulation in rats.[227] However, pregnancy is associated with a reduced response to constriction of systemic arteries by the alpha$_1$-agonist phenylephrine in rats; this reduced response is mediated by increased production of nitric oxide.[228] The endothelium-dependent and endothelium-independent responses to vasodilators and overall nitric oxide synthase activity in systemic arteries are not affected by pregnancy in rats.[228] Altogether, these results suggest that pregnancy induces a refractoriness to arterial vasoconstriction by alpha-adrenergic agonists, but that it increases venous sensitivity to these agents. Enhanced venous sensitivity is consistent with the increased dependence of maternal venous return on sympathetic nervous system activity.[185-187]

In a preparation of rat *uterine* arterioles, pregnancy increased the contractile response to alpha$_1$-agonist (phenylephrine) stimulation, increased the relaxation response to the alpha$_2$-agonist clonidine, and attenuated the vasodilation elicited by the beta-agonist isoproterenol.[229] These observations suggest that pregnancy enhances alpha$_2$-agonist-mediated uterine arteriolar dilation by an increase in the release of nitric oxide.[229] This evidence supports the continued preferential use of ephedrine (which has alpha$_1$-, alpha$_2$-, and beta-agonist activity) over phenylephrine to treat hypotension in obstetric patients, given that ephedrine seems to protect uterine blood flow better than does phenylephrine.

Regional Analgesia and Anesthesia

TECHNICAL CONSIDERATIONS

The enhancement of lumbar lordosis during pregnancy may reduce the vertebral interspinous gap, thus creating technical difficulty when regional anesthesia is administered (Figure 2-9, Box 2-4). Widening of the pelvis results in a head-down tilt when a parturient is in the lateral position (Figure 2-10). This may increase the rostral subarachnoid spread of local anesthetic solution—especially hyperbaric solution—when an injection is made with the patient in this position.

The flow of CSF from a spinal needle should be unchanged throughout gestation because pregnancy does not alter CSF pressure.[190] However, the rate of flow may increase during a uterine contraction because the CSF pressure is increased at this time.[190]

HYPOTENSION DURING REGIONAL ANESTHESIA

Pregnancy increases dependence on the sympathetic nervous system for the maintenance of venous return.[185-187] This has been illustrated best by Assali et al.,[185] who produced complete sympathectomy with either high spinal anesthesia or ganglionic blockade, without a fluid preload, in pregnant and nonpregnant women in the supine position. Pregnant women exhibited a 50% fall in blood pressure, whereas the fall in

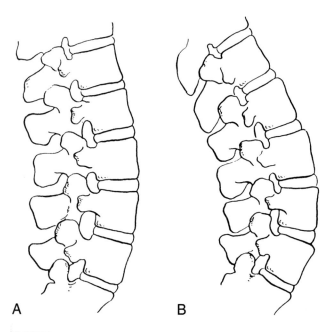

A   B

FIGURE 2-9. Effects of pregnancy on the lumbar spine. **A,** Nonpregnant. **B,** Pregnant. There is a marked increase in lumbar lordosis and a narrowing of the interspinous space during pregnancy. (From Bonica JJ. Principles and Practice of Obstetric Analgesia and Anesthesia, Volume 1. Philadelphia, FA Davis Company, 1967:35.)

Box 2-4 REGIONAL ANESTHESIA: ANESTHETIC IMPLICATIONS OF MATERNAL PHYSIOLOGIC CHANGES

TECHNICAL CONSIDERATIONS

- Lumbar lordosis increased
- Apex of thoracic kyphosis at higher level
- Head-down tilt when in lateral position
- CSF return unaltered
- Reduced sensitivity of "hanging drop" technique

PREVENTION OF HYPOTENSION

- Increased need for fluids and/or vasopressors*

LOCAL ANESTHETIC DOSE REQUIREMENTS†

- Subarachnoid dose reduced 25%
- Epidural dose (large dose) unaltered
- Epidural dose (small dose) reduced

*Relative to that required by nonpregnant women.
†Change in the segmental dose requirement relative to nonpregnant women.
Adapted from Conklin KA. Maternal physiological adaptations during gestation, labor, and the puerperium. Semin Anesth 1991; 10:221-34.

nonpregnant women was less than 10% (see Figure 2-7). Thus pregnant women require more medical intervention (i.e., intravenous fluids and/or pressors) than nonpregnant patients to maintain hemodynamic stability during the administration of regional anesthesia (see Box 2-4). By 48 hours postpartum the blood pressure response to regional anesthesia returns to that of the nonpregnant state.[185]

The ideal method for augmenting central blood volume to prevent hypotension—and the ideal pharmacologic regimen to prevent and/or treat hypotension—during administration of regional anesthesia in pregnant women is currently a matter of some dispute.[230] A recent metaanalysis concluded that colloid infusion is more uniformly effective than crystalloid in reducing the incidence of hypotension; leg wrapping or use of thromboembolic stockings was also found to be effective in decreasing the occurrence of hypotension.[231] Some investigators have recently challenged the long-standing dogma that ephedrine is the vasopressor of choice for treatment of hypotension in pregnant women receiving regional anesthesia. Recent studies suggest that phenylephrine and ephedrine have similar efficacy in the treatment of hypotension, and that use of phenylephrine is associated with a slightly higher umbilical arterial blood pH, although the incidence of frank fetal acidemia (pH < 7.2) is not reduced when compared with babies of mothers treated with ephedrine.[232]

PHARMACODYNAMICS OF LOCAL ANESTHETICS

Pregnancy enhances the neural sensitivity of peripheral nerves to local anesthetics (i.e., a given degree of neural blockade occurs at a lower intraneuronal local anesthetic concentration in the axons of pregnant animals).[233,234] Pregnant women exhibit a more rapid onset and a longer duration of spinal anesthesia than nonpregnant women who receive the same dose of local anesthetic.[235] This is consistent with enhanced neural sensitivity, although the pregnancy-associated reduction in CSF protein[236] (which may reduce protein binding of local anesthetics) and elevated CSF pH[237] (which increases the proportion of unionized local anesthetic) may contribute to these effects.

SPINAL ANESTHETIC DOSE REQUIREMENTS

Pregnancy enhances the spread of hyperbaric local anesthetic solution in the subarachnoid space, resulting in a 25% reduction in the segmental dose requirement (i.e., milligrams of drug necessary to block one spinal segment) in term pregnant women.[235,238-241] This enhanced spread occurs during the second and third trimesters, but not during the first.[241] The decreased segmental dose requirement (see Box 2-4) can be attributed to the following: (1) reduction of the spinal CSF volume, which accompanies distention of the vertebral venous plexus,[52,54,55] (2) enhanced neural susceptibility to local anesthetics, (3) increased rostral spread, caused by the widening of the pelvis, when injections are made with patients in the lateral position, (4) inward displacement of intervertebral foraminal soft tissue, resulting from increased abdominal pressure,[242] and (5) a higher level of the apex of the thoracic kyphosis (the lowest point of the thoracic spinal canal in the supine position) during late pregnancy.[243]

Spinal dose requirements change rapidly in the postpartum period, with segmental dose requirements returning to that of nonpregnant women within 24 to 48 hours.[185,240] The postpartum change can be explained by an expansion of the spinal CSF volume that accompanies the relief of vena caval compression.

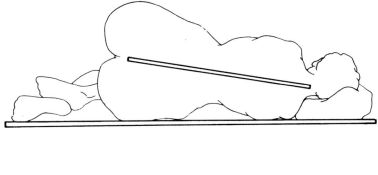

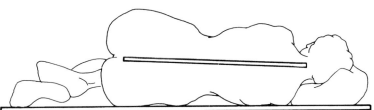

FIGURE 2-10. Pelvic widening and resultant head-down tilt in the lateral position during pregnancy. Upper panel: pregnant; lower panel: nonpregnant. (From Camann WR, Ostheimer GW. Physiological adaptations during pregnancy. Int Anesth Clin 1990; 28:2-10.)

EPIDURAL ANALGESIC/ANESTHETIC DOSE REQUIREMENTS

The local anesthetic dose requirement for epidural anesthesia is widely reported as reduced in term pregnant women. This has been attributed to enhanced neural susceptibility to local anesthetics and distention of the epidural veins, which results in a reduced volume of the epidural space. However, the distention of the veins results in a compensatory decrease in the spinal CSF volume[52,54,55] because of the rigid boundaries of the epidural space. Thus, the extravascular epidural space volume does not change, and mechanical factors should not affect the spread of local anesthetic solutions. Results show that uterine contractions, which increase venous distention and epidural space pressure, do not affect the epidural spread of local anesthetics.[244]

Despite enhanced neural susceptibility during pregnancy, the administration of *large* doses of local anesthetics results in the same spread of epidural anesthesia in term pregnant and in nonpregnant women (see Box 2-4). Grundy et al.[245] observed a similar spread of epidural anesthesia after the administration of 112.5 to 150 mg of bupivacaine for elective surgery in pregnant and nonpregnant women. Sharrock and Greenidge[246] also found no difference in the segmental dose requirement between pregnant and nonpregnant women when bupivacaine was administered in doses above 127.5 mg. (These results are consistent with the following clinical observation: after epidural administration of a large dose of local anesthetic to *any* patient, it may be difficult to achieve a higher sensory level by giving additional incremental doses of local anesthetic.)

The epidural segmental dose requirement decreases in both pregnant and nonpregnant women as the dose of local anesthetic is reduced, but pregnant women exhibit a greater decrease in segmental dose requirement.[246] Therefore, although epidural administration of large doses of bupivacaine produces the same anesthetic spread in pregnant and nonpregnant women,[245,246] *the spread of smaller doses is greater in pregnant women.*[246] Similarly, a small dose of lidocaine (e.g., 140 mg) has a greater spread in parturients than in nonpregnant women.[247]

PHARMACOKINETICS OF LOCAL ANESTHETICS

The rate of absorption of bupivacaine from the epidural space and the time required for peak plasma concentration is unaltered during pregnancy.[248] Earlier work demonstrated a reduced protein binding of bupivacaine in term pregnant women compared with nonpregnant women.[249] However, a more recent study has shown that this is true at higher (toxic) levels of bupivacaine (5 µg/ml), but that there is no change in bupivacaine protein binding at low (therapeutic) levels (1 µg/ml) in pregnancy.[250] Bupivacaine is bound by two proteins, both of which decline during pregnancy: (1) alpha-1-acid glycoprotein, a high-affinity, low-capacity site, and (2) albumin, a low-affinity, high-capacity site. The lack of reduction in the bound fraction of bupivacaine at low bupivacaine concentrations in pregnancy has been attributed to the fact that the alpha-1-acid glycoprotein is not fully saturated at this concentration.[250] Although the primary metabolites of bupivacaine are different in pregnant and nonpregnant women, the elimination half-life does not differ between the two groups.[248]

The pharmacokinetics of lidocaine during pregnancy have not been investigated thoroughly, although protein binding of lidocaine progressively decreases throughout gestation.[251] Ropivacaine pharmacokinetics are little affected by pregnancy.[252]

SYSTEMIC TOXICITY OF LOCAL ANESTHETICS

Morishima et al.[253] reported that the intravenous dose and plasma concentration of lidocaine that result in seizures, respiratory arrest, hypotension, and cardiovascular collapse are the same in pregnant and nonpregnant ewes. Bucklin et al.[254] found that the intravenous dose and the plasma and brain concentrations of lidocaine at the onset of electroencephalographic seizure activity are similar in male, nonpregnant, and pregnant rats. These results suggest that pregnancy does not alter the systemic toxicity of lidocaine. Similarly, pregnancy does not alter the intravenous dose or plasma concentration of mepivacaine[255] necessary to produce CNS and cardiovascular toxicity in sheep.

In humans, most cardiac deaths that result from intravascular injection of large doses of bupivacaine have occurred in pregnant women.[256] This has been ascribed to enhanced bupivacaine toxicity during pregnancy, but it might simply be a result of the fact that more pregnant women have received large doses of bupivacaine intended for epidural anesthesia. Older work had shown that pregnant ewes manifested cardiovascular collapse at a lower bupivacaine dose and plasma concentration, with a tendency toward enhanced CNS toxicity (although the latter trend was not statistically significant) than in nonpregnant ewes.[257] More recent, larger studies (using improved study design, including randomization and blinding) have revealed that pregnancy does *not* enhance susceptibility of ewes to the serious toxic effects (e.g., hypotension, apnea, circulatory collapse) of bupivacaine, levobupivacaine, or ropivacaine.[258,259] The seizure threshold is slightly lower (10% to 15%) for all three drugs during ovine pregnancy.[259] At equimolar doses the risk of systemic toxicity is greatest with bupivacaine, intermediate with levobupivacaine, and lowest with ropivacaine.[259]

Although in vitro studies suggested that elevated levels of progesterone during pregnancy enhanced the sensitivity of the rabbit myocardium to bupivacaine,[260,261] the two large in vivo studies by Santos et al.[258,259] showed no increase in the incidence of lethal ventricular arrhythmias in pregnant versus nonpregnant sheep treated with bupivacaine, ropivacaine, or levobupivacaine.

EFFECTS OF REGIONAL ANESTHESIA ON RESPIRATORY FUNCTION

FRC decreases during regional anesthesia.[262] This results in an increase in respiratory dead space and a ventilation-perfusion mismatch. Because pregnancy alone is associated with a decreased FRC,[4,8,10] which is further reduced in the supine position,[10] the parturient is at greater risk than the nonpregnant patient for developing airway closure and hypoxemia during major regional anesthesia.

During high spinal or epidural anesthesia, paralysis of the external intercostal muscles, which are muscles of inspiration, does not affect resting minute ventilation or arterial $Paco_2$ in pregnant[263] or nonpregnant[262,264] subjects. Abdominal muscles are important for forced expiration and coughing, and paralysis of these muscles during regional anesthesia decreases the peak expiratory flow rate, the maximum expiratory pressure, and the ability to increase intraabdominal and intrathoracic pressures during coughing.[264-267] The greater decrease of the peak expiratory flow rate in pregnant[266,267] versus nonpregnant[264] individuals suggests that the ability to cough effectively may be impaired to a greater degree during regional anesthesia in pregnant women.

KEY POINTS

- Increased minute ventilation and reduced functional residual capacity are the respiratory changes that have the greatest impact on anesthetic management during pregnancy.
- Compression of the inferior vena cava by the gravid uterus occurs in all patient positions, but vena caval compression is greatest in the supine position.
- Gastric volume and pH are unaltered during pregnancy, but lower esophageal tone is reduced in 80% of pregnant women.
- Pregnancy increases dependence on the sympathetic nervous system for maintenance of venous return.
- Parturients can tolerate greater blood loss than nonpregnant women undergoing surgery because maternal vascular capacitance is reduced at the time of delivery.

REFERENCES

1. Spätling L, Fallenstein F, Huch A, et al. The variability of cardiopulmonary adaptation to pregnancy at rest and during exercise. Br J Obstet Gynaecol 1992; 99(Suppl 8):1-40.
2. Leontic EA. Respiratory disease in pregnancy. Med Clin North Am 1977; 61:111-28.
3. Thomson KJ, Cohen ME. Studies on the circulation in pregnancy. II. Vital capacity observations in normal pregnant women. Surg Gynecol Obstet 1938; 66:591-603.
4. Gee JBL, Packer BS, Millen JE, Robin ED. Pulmonary mechanics during pregnancy. J Clin Invest 1967; 46:945-52.
5. Milne JA, Mills RJ, Howie AD, Pack AI. Large airways function during normal pregnancy. Br J Obstet Gynaecol 1977; 84:448-51.
6. Grenville-Mathers R, Trenchard HJ. The diaphragm in the puerperium. J Obstet Gynaecol Br Emp 1953; 60:825-33.
7. Baldwin GR, Moorthi DS, Whelton JA, MacDonnell KF. New lung functions and pregnancy. Am J Obstet Gynecol 1977; 127:235-9.
8. Alaily AB, Carrol KB. Pulmonary ventilation in pregnancy. Br J Obstet Gynaecol 1978; 85:518-24.
9. Brancazio LR, Laifer SA, Schwartz T. Peak expiratory flow rate in normal pregnancy. Obstet Gynecol 1997; 89:383-6.
10. Russell IF, Chambers WA. Closing volume in normal pregnancy. Br J Anaesth 1981; 53:1043-7.
11. Templeton A, Kelman GR. Maternal blood-gases (PAO_2-Pao_2), physiological shunt and V_D/V_T in normal pregnancy. Br J Anaesth 1976; 48:1001-4.
12. Machida H. Influence of progesterone on arterial blood and CSF acid-base balance in women. J Appl Physiol 1981; 51:1433-6.
13. Shankar KB, Moseley H, Vemula V, et al. Arterial to end-tidal carbon dioxide tension difference during anaesthesia in early pregnancy. Can J Anaesth 1989; 36:124-7.
14. Shankar KB, Moseley H, Kumar Y, Vemula V. Arterial to end tidal carbon dioxide tension difference during caesarean section anaesthesia. Anaesthesia 1986; 41:698-702.
15. Shankar KB, Moseley H, Kumar Y, et al. Arterial to end-tidal carbon dioxide tension difference during anaesthesia for tubal ligation. Anaesthesia 1987; 42:482-6.
16. Bader RA, Bader ME, Rose DJ, Braunwald E. Hemodynamics at rest and during exercise in normal pregnancy as studied by cardiac catheterization. J Clin Invest 1955; 34:1524-36.
17. Sady MA, Haydon BB, Sady SP, et al. Cardiovascular response to maximal cycle exercise during pregnancy and at two and seven months post partum. Am J Obstet Gynecol 1990; 162:1181-5.
18. Ang CK, Tan TH, Walters WAW, Wood C. Postural influence on maternal capillary oxygen and carbon dioxide tension. Br Med J 1969; 4:201-3.
19. Calvin S, Jones OW III, Knieriem K, Weinstein L. Oxygen saturation in the supine hypotensive syndrome. Obstet Gynecol 1988; 71:872-7.
20. Dayal P, Murata Y, Takamura H. Antepartum and postpartum acid-base changes in maternal blood in normal and complicated pregnancies. J Obstet Gynaecol Br Commonw 1972; 79:612-24.
21. Seeds AE, Battaglia FC, Hellegers AE. Effects of pregnancy on the pH, Pco_2, and bicarbonate concentrations of peripheral venous blood. Am J Obstet Gynecol 1964; 88:1086-9.
22. Lim VS, Katz AI, Lindheimer MD. Acid-base regulation in pregnancy. Am J Physiol 1976; 231:1764-70.
23. Hägerdal M, Morgan CW, Sumner AE, Gutsche BB. Minute ventilation and oxygen consumption during labor with epidural analgesia. Anesthesiology 1983; 59:425-7.
24. Pearson JF, Davies P. The effect of continuous lumbar epidural analgesia on the acid-base status of maternal arterial blood during the first stage of labour. J Obstet Gynaecol Br Commonw 1973; 80:218-24.
25. Jouppila R, Hollmén A. The effect of segmental epidural analgesia on maternal and foetal acid-base balance, lactate, serum potassium and creatine phosphokinase during labour. Acta Anaesth Scand 1976; 20:259-68.
26. Thalme B, Raabe N, Belfrage P. Lumbar epidural analgesia in labour. II. Effects on glucose, lactate, sodium, chloride, total protein, haematocrit and haemoglobin in maternal, fetal and neonatal blood. Acta Obstet Gynecol Scand 1974; 53:113-9.
27. Cutforth R, MacDonald CB. Heart sounds and murmurs in pregnancy. Am Heart J 1966; 71:741-7.
28. Carruth JE, Mirvis SB, Brogan DR, Wenger NK. The electrocardiogram in normal pregnancy. Am Heart J 1981; 102:1075-8.
29. Oram S, Holt M. Innocent depression of the S-T segment and flattening of the T-wave during pregnancy. J Obstet Gynaecol Br Commonw 1961; 68:765-70.

30. Robson SC, Hunter S, Boys RJ, Dunlop W. Serial study of factors influencing changes in cardiac output during human pregnancy. Am J Physiol 1989; 256:H1060-5.

31. Campos O, Andrade JL, Bocanegra J, et al. Physiologic multivalvular regurgitation during pregnancy: A longitudinal Doppler echocardiographic study. Int J Cardiol 1993; 40:265-272.

32. Robson SC, Hunter S, Moore M, Dunlop W. Haemodynamic changes during the puerperium: A Doppler and M-mode echocardiographic study. Br J Obstet Gynaecol 1987; 94:1028-39.

33. Capeless EL, Clapp JF. Cardiovascular changes in early phase of pregnancy. Am J Obstet Gynecol 1989; 161:1449-53.

34. Laird-Meeter K, Van de Ley G, Bom TH, et al. Cardiocirculatory adjustments during pregnancy: An echocardiographic study. Clin Cardiol 1979; 2:328-32.

35. Katz R, Karliner JS, Resnik R. Effects of a natural volume overload state (pregnancy) on left ventricular performance in normal human subjects. Circulation 1978; 58:434-41.

36. Rubler S, Damani PM, Pinto ER. Cardiac size and performance during pregnancy estimated with echocardiography. Am J Cardiol 1977; 40:534-40.

37. Clark SL, Cotton DB, Lee W, et al. Central hemodynamic assessment of normal term pregnancy. Am J Obstet Gynecol 1989; 161:1439-42.

38. Assali NS, Rauramo L, Peltonen T. Measurement of uterine blood flow and uterine metabolism. VIII. Uterine and fetal blood flow and oxygen consumption in early human pregnancy. Am J Obstet Gynecol 1960; 79:86-98.

39. Thaler I, Manor D, Itskovitz J, et al. Changes in uterine blood flow during human pregnancy. Am J Obstet Gynecol 1990; 162:121-5.

40. Assali NS, Douglass RA Jr, Baird WW, et al. Measurement of uterine blood flow and uterine metabolism. IV. Results in normal pregnancy. Am J Obstet Gynecol 1953; 66:248-53.

41. Rekonen A, Luotola H, Pitkänen M, et al. Measurement of intervillous and myometrial blood flow by an intravenous ^{133}Xe method. Br J Obstet Gynaecol 1976; 83:723-8.

42. Kauppila A, Koskinen M, Puolakka J, et al. Decreased intervillous and unchanged myometrial blood flow in supine recumbency. Obstet Gynecol 1980; 55:203-5.

43. Palmer SK, Zamudio S, Coffin C, et al. Quantitative estimation of human uterine artery blood flow and pelvic blood flow redistribution in pregnancy. Obstet Gynecol 1992; 80:1000-6.

44. Dunlop W. Serial changes in renal haemodynamics during normal human pregnancy. Br J Obstet Gynaecol 1981; 88:1-9.

45. Katz M, Sokal MM. Skin perfusion in pregnancy. Am J Obstet Gynecol 1980; 137:30-3.

46. Wilson M, Morganti AA, Zervoudakis I, et al. Blood pressure, the renin-aldosterone system and sex steroids throughout normal pregnancy. Am J Med 1980; 68:97-104.

47. MacGillivray I, Rose GA, Rowe B. Blood pressure survey in pregnancy. Clin Sci 1969; 37:395-407.

48. Christianson RE. Studies on blood pressure during pregnancy. 1. Influence of parity and age. Am J Obstet Gynecol 1976; 125:509-13.

49. Pyörälä T. Cardiovascular response to the upright position during pregnancy. Acta Obstet Gynecol Scand 1966; 45(Suppl 5):1-116.

50. Villar MA, Sibai BM. Clinical significance of elevated mean arterial blood pressure in second trimester and threshold increase in systolic or diastolic blood pressure during third trimester. Am J Obstet Gynecol 1989; 160:419-23.

51. Hart MV, Morton MJ, Hosenpud JD, Metcalfe J. Aortic function during normal human pregnancy. Am J Obstet Gynecol 1986; 154:887-91.

52. Kerr MG, Scott DB, Samuel E. Studies of the inferior vena cava in late pregnancy. Br Med J 1964; 1:532-3.

53. Howard BK, Goodson JH, Mengert WF. Supine hypotensive syndrome in late pregnancy. Obstet Gynecol 1953; 1:371-7.

54. Kerr MG. The mechanical effects of the gravid uterus in late pregnancy. J Obstet Gynaecol Br Commonw 1965; 72:513-29.

55. Hirabayashi Y, Shimizu R, Fukuda H, et al. Soft tissue anatomy within the vertebral canal in pregnant women. Br J Anaesth 1996; 77:153-6.

56. Bieniarz J, Yoshida T, Romero-Salinas G, et al. Aortocaval compression by the uterus in late human pregnancy. IV. Circulatory homeostasis by preferential perfusion of the placenta. Am J Obstet Gynecol 1969; 103:19-31.

57. Lees MM, Scott DB, Kerr MG, Taylor SH. The circulatory effects of recumbent postural change in late pregnancy. Clin Sci 1967; 32:453-65.

58. McLennan CE. Antecubital and femoral venous pressure in normal and toxemic pregnancy. Am J Obstet Gynecol 1943; 45:568-91.

59. Abitbol MM. Aortic compression by pregnant uterus. NY State J Med 1976; 76:1470-5.

60. Eckstein KL, Marx GF. Aortocaval compression and uterine displacement. Anesthesiology 1974; 40:92-6.

61. Kinsella SM, Whitwam JG, Spencer JAD. Aortic compression by the uterus: Identification with the Finapres digital arterial pressure instrument. Br J Obstet Gynaecol 1990; 97:700-5.

62. Bieniarz J, Maqueda E, Caldeyro-Barcia R. Compression of aorta by the uterus in late human pregnancy. I. Variations between femoral and brachial artery pressure with changes from hypertension to hypotension. Am J Obstet Gynecol 1966; 95:795-808.

63. Bieniarz J, Crottogini JJ, Curuchet E, et al. Aortocaval compression by the uterus in late human pregnancy. II. An arteriographic study. Am J Obstet Gynecol 1968; 100:203-17.

64. Kuo C-D, Chen G-Y, Yang M-J, Tsai Y-S. The effect of position on autonomic nervous activity in late pregnancy. Anaesthesia 1997; 52:1161-5.

65. Milsom I, Forssman L. Factors influencing aortocaval compression in late pregnancy. Am J Obstet Gynecol 1984; 148:764-71.

66. Clark SL, Cotton DB, Pivarnik JM, et al. Position change and central hemodynamic profile during normal third-trimester pregnancy and post partum. Am J Obstet Gynecol 1991; 164:883-7.

67. Drummond GB, Scott SEM, Lees MM, Scott DB. Effects of posture on limb blood flow in late pregnancy. Br Med J 1974; 2:587-8.

68. Suonio S, Simpanen AL, Olkkonen H, Haring P. Effect of the left lateral recumbent position compared with the supine and upright positions on placental blood flow in normal late pregnancy. Ann Clin Res 1976; 8:22-6.

69. Kinsella SM, Lohmann G. Supine hypotensive syndrome. Obstet Gynecol 1994; 83:774-88.

70. Robson SC, Dunlop W, Boys RJ, Hunter S. Cardiac output during labour. Br Med J 1987; 295:1169-72.

71. Ueland K, Hansen JM. Maternal cardiovascular dynamics. III. Labor and delivery under local and caudal analgesia. Am J Obstet Gynecol 1969; 103:8-18.

72. Kjeldsen J. Hemodynamic investigations during labour and delivery. Acta Obstet Gynecol Scand 1979; 89(Suppl):1-252.

73. Lederman RP, Lederman E, Work B Jr, McCann DS. Anxiety and epinephrine in multiparous women in labor: Relationship to duration of labor and fetal heart rate pattern. Am J Obstet Gynecol 1985; 153:870-7.

74. Grenman S, Erkkola R, Kanto J, et al. Epidural and paracervical blockades in obstetrics: Catecholamines, arginine vasopressin and analgesic effect. Acta Obstet Gynecol Scand 1986; 65:699-704.

75. Falconer AD, Powles AB. Plasma noradrenaline levels during labour: Influence of elective lumbar epidural blockade. Anaesthesia 1982; 37:416-20.

76. Adams JQ, Alexander AM Jr. Alterations in cardiovascular physiology during labor. Obstet Gynecol 1958; 12:542-9.

77. Hendricks CH. The hemodynamics of a uterine contraction. Am J Obstet Gynecol 1958; 76:969-82.

78. Robson SC, Dunlop W, Hunter S. Haemodynamic changes during the early puerperium. Br Med J 1987; 294:1065.

79. Sadaniantz A, Laurent LS, Parisi AF. Long-term effects of multiple pregnancies on cardiac dimensions and systolic and diastolic function. Am J Obstet Gynecol 1996; 174:1061-4.

80. Bernstein IM, Zeigler W, Badger GJ. Plasma volume expansion in early pregnancy. Obstet Gynecol 2001; 97:669-72.

81. Lund CJ, Donovan JC. Blood volume during pregnancy: Significance of plasma and red cell volumes. Am J Obstet Gynecol 1967; 98:393-403.

82. Hytten FE, Paintin DB. Increase in plasma volume during normal pregnancy. J Obstet Gynaecol Br Commonw 1963; 70:402-7.

83. Taylor DJ, Lind T. Red cell mass during and after normal pregnancy. Br J Obstet Gynaecol 1979; 86:364-70.

84. Pritchard JA. Changes in the blood volume during pregnancy and delivery. Anesthesiology 1965; 26:393-9.

85. Barron WM, Mujais SK, Zinaman M, et al. Plasma catecholamine responses to physiologic stimuli in normal human pregnancy. Am J Obstet Gynecol 1986; 154:80-4.

86. Cotes PM, Canning CE, Lind T. Changes in serum immunoreactive erythropoietin during the menstrual cycle and normal pregnancy. Br J Obstet Gynaecol 1983; 90:304-11.

87. Robertson EG, Cheyne GA. Plasma biochemistry in relation to oedema of pregnancy. J Obstet Gynaecol Br Commonw 1972; 79:769-76.

88. Efrati P, Presentey B, Margalith M, Rozenszajn L. Leukocytes of normal pregnant women. Obstet Gynecol 1964; 23:429-32.

89. Rath CE, Caton W, Reid DE, et al. Hematological changes and iron metabolism of normal pregnancy. Surg Gynecol Obstet 1950; 90:320-6.

90. Naeye RL. Placental infarction leading to fetal or neonatal death. A prospective study. Obstet Gynecol 1977; 50:583-8.

91. Coryell MN, Beach EF, Robinson AR, et al. Metabolism of women during the reproductive cycle. XVII. Changes in electrophoretic patterns of

plasma proteins throughout the cycle and following delivery. J Clin Invest 1950; 29:1559-67.

92. Mendenhal HW. Serum protein concentrations in pregnancy. I. Concentrations in maternal serum. Am J Obstet Gynecol 1970; 106:388-99.

93. Wu PYK, Udani V, Chan L, et al. Colloid osmotic pressure: Variations in normal pregnancy. J Perinat Med 1983; 11:193-9.

94. Evans RT, Wroe JM. Plasma cholinesterase changes during pregnancy: Their interpretation as a cause of suxamethonium-induced apnoea. Anaesthesia 1980; 35:651-4.

95. Leighton BL, Cheek TG, Gross JB, et al. Succinylcholine pharmacodynamics in peripartum patients. Anesthesiology 1986; 64:202-5.

96. Gerbasi FR, Buttoms S, Farag A, Mammen E. Increased intravascular coagulation associated with pregnancy. Obstet Gynecol 1990; 75:385-9.

97. Tygart SG, McRoyan DK, Spinnato JA, et al. Longitudinal study of platelet indices during normal pregnancy. Am J Obstet Gynecol 1986; 154:883-7.

98. Fay RA, Hughes AO, Farron NT. Platelets in pregnancy: Hyperdestruction in pregnancy. Obstet Gynecol 1983; 61:238-40.

99. Norris LA, Sheppard BL, Bonnar J. Increased whole blood platelet aggregation in normal pregnancy can be prevented in vitro by aspirin and dazmegrel (UK38485). Br J Obstet Gynaecol 1992; 99:253-7.

100. Hellgren M, Blömback M. Studies on blood coagulation and fibrinolysis in pregnancy, during delivery and in the puerperium. I. Normal conditions. Gynecol Obstet Invest 1981; 12:141-54.

101. Talbert LM, Langdell RD. Normal values of certain factors in the blood clotting mechanism in pregnancy. Am J Obstet Gynecol 1964; 90:44-50.

102. Pitkin RM, Witte DL. Platelet and leukocyte counts in pregnancy. JAMA 1979; 242:2696-8.

103. Burrows RF, Kelton JG. Thrombocytopenia at delivery: A prospective survey of 6715 deliveries. Am J Obstet Gynecol 1990; 162:731-4.

104. Berge LN, Lyngmo V, Svensson B, Nordoy A. The bleeding time in women: An influence of the sex hormones? Acta Obstet Gynecol Scand 1993; 72:423-7.

105. Kasper CK, Hoag MS, Aggeler PM, Stone S. Blood clotting factors in pregnancy: Factor VIII concentrations in normal and AHF-deficient women. Obstet Gynecol 1964; 24:242-7.

106. Stirling Y, Woolf L, North WR, et al. Haemostasis in normal pregnancy. Thromb Haemost 1984; 52:176-82.

107. Coopland A, Alkjaersig N, Fletcher AP. Reduction in plasma factor XIII (fibrin stabilizing factor) concentration during pregnancy. J Lab Clin Med 1969; 73:144-53.

108. Sharma SK, Philip J, Wiley J. Thromboelastographic changes in healthy parturients and postpartum women. Anesth Analg 1997; 85:94-8.

109. Ueland K. Maternal cardiovascular dynamics. VII. Intrapartum blood volume changes. Am J Obstet Gynecol 1976; 126:671-7.

110. Taylor DJ, Lind T. Puerperal haematological indices. Br J Obstet Gynaecol 1981; 88:601-6.

111. Gilstrap III LC, Hauth JC, Hankins GDV, Patterson AR. Effect of type of anesthesia on blood loss at cesarean section. Obstet Gynecol 1987; 69:328-32.

112. Andrews WW, Ramin SM, Maberry MC, et al. Effect of type of anesthesia on blood loss at elective repeat cesarean section. Am J Perinatol 1992; 9:197-200.

113. Ygge J. Changes in blood coagulation and fibrinolysis during the puerperium. Am J Obstet Gynecol 1969; 104:2-12.

114. Bonnar J, McNicol GP, Douglas AS. Coagulation and fibrinolytic mechanisms during and after normal childbirth. Br Med J 1970; 2:200-3.

115. Krause PJ, Ingardia CJ, Pontius LT, et al. Host defense during pregnancy: Neutrophil chemotaxis and adherence. Am J Obstet Gynecol 1987; 157:274-80.

116. Patton PE, Coulam CB, Bergstrahl E. The prevalence of autoantibodies in pregnant and nonpregnant women. Am J Obstet Gynecol 1987; 157:1345-50.

117. Baboonian C, Griffiths P. Is pregnancy immunosuppressive? Humoral immunity against viruses. Br J Obstet Gynaecol 1983; 90:1168-75.

118. Brock-Utne JG, Downing JW, Dimopoulos GE, et al. Effect of domperidone on lower esophageal sphincter tone in late pregnancy. Anesthesiology 1980; 52:321-3.

119. Dow TGB, Brock-Utne JG, Rubin J, et al. The effect of atropine on the lower esophageal sphincter in late pregnancy. Obstet Gynecol 1978; 51:426-30.

120. Ulmsten U, Sundström G. Esophageal manometry in pregnant and nonpregnant women. Am J Obstet Gynecol 1978; 132:260-4.

121. Van Thiel DH, Gavaler JS, Stremple J. Lower esophageal sphincter pressure in women using sequential oral contraceptives. Gastroenterology 1976; 71:232-4.

122. Marrero JM, Goggin PM, de Caestecker JS, et al. Determinants of pregnancy heartburn. Br J Obstet Gynaecol 1992; 99:731-4.

123. Macfie AG, Magides AD, Richmond MN, Reilly CS. Gastric emptying in pregnancy. Br J Anaesth 1991; 67:54-7.

124. Whitehead EM, Smith M, Dean Y, O'Sullivan G. An evaluation of gastric emptying times in pregnancy and the puerperium. Anaesthesia 1993; 48:53-7.

125. La Salvia LA, Steffen EA. Delayed gastric emptying time in labor. Am J Obstet Gynecol 1950; 59:1075-81.

126. Chiloiro M, Darconza G, Piccioli E, et al. Gastric emptying and orocecal transit time in pregnancy. J Gastroenterol 2001; 36:538-43.

127. Davison JS, Davison MC, Hay DM. Gastric emptying time in late pregnancy and labour. J Obstet Gynaecol Br Commonw 1970; 77:37-41.

128. O'Sullivan GM, Sutton AJ, Thompson SA, et al. Noninvasive measurement of gastric emptying in obstetric patients. Anesth Analg 1987; 66:505-11.

129. Sandhar BK, Elliott RH, Windram I, Rowbotham DJ. Peripartum changes in gastric emptying. Anaesthesia 1992; 47:196-8.

130. Simpson KH, Stakes AF, Miller M. Pregnancy delays paracetamol absorption and gastric emptying in patients undergoing surgery. Br J Anaesth 1988; 60:24-7.

131. Levy DM, Williams OA, Magides AD, Reilly CS. Gastric emptying is delayed at 8-12 weeks' gestation. Br J Anaesth 1994; 73:237-8.

132. Parry E, Shields R, Turnbull AC. Transit time in the small intestine in pregnancy. J Obstet Gynaecol Br Commonw 1970; 77:900-1.

133. Wald A, Van Thiel DH, Hoechstetter L, et al. Effect of pregnancy on gastrointestinal transit. Digest Dis Sci 1982; 27:1015-8.

134. Murray FA, Erskine JP, Fielding J. Gastric secretion in pregnancy. J Obstet Gynaecol Br Emp 1957; 64:373-81.

135. Van Thiel DH, Gavaler JS, Joshi SN, et al. Heartburn of pregnancy. Gastroenterology 1977; 72:666-8.

136. O'Sullivan GM, Bullingham RE. The assessment of gastric acidity and antacid effect in pregnant women by a non-invasive radiotelemetry technique. Br J Obstet Gynaecol 1984; 91:973-8.

137. Cappell MS, Garcia A. Gastric and duodenal ulcers during pregnancy. Gastroenterol Clin N Am 1998; 27:169-95.

138. Gryboski WA, Spiro HM. The effect of pregnancy on gastric secretion. New Engl J Med 1956; 255:1131-4.

139. James CF, Gibbs CP, Banner T. Postpartum perioperative risk of aspiration pneumonia. Anesthesiology 1984; 61:756-9.

140. Manchikanti L, Grow JB, Colliver JA, et al. Bicitra (sodium citrate) and metoclopramide in outpatient anesthesia for prophylaxis against aspiration pneumonitis. Anesthesiology 1985; 63:378-84.

141. Detmer MD, Pandit SK, Cohen PJ. Prophylactic single-dose oral antacid therapy in the preoperative period: Comparison of cimetidine and Maalox. Anesthesiology 1979; 51:270-3.

142. Wyner J, Cohen SE. Gastric volume in early pregnancy: Effect of metoclopramide. Anesthesiology 1982; 57:209-12.

143. Roberts RB, Shirley MA. Reducing the risk of acid aspiration during cesarean section. Anesth Analg 1974; 53:859-68.

144. Baraka A, Saab M, Salem MR, Winnie AP. Control of gastric acidity by glycopyrrolate premedication in the parturient. Anesth Analg 1977; 56:642-5.

145. McCaughey W, Howe JP, Moore J, Dundee JW. Cimetidine in elective caesarean section. Effect on gastric acidity. Anaesthesia 1981; 36:167-72.

146. Cohen SE, Jasson J, Talafre ML, et al. Does metoclopramide decrease the volume of gastric contents in patients undergoing cesarean section? Anesthesiology 1984; 61:604-7.

147. Boschi S, Di Marco MG, Pigna A, Rossi R. The effect of ranitidine on gastric pH and volume in patients undergoing cesarean section: Possible relationship to Mendelson's syndrome. Curr Ther Res 1984; 35:654-62.

148. Dewan DM, Floyd HM, Thistlewood JM, et al. Sodium citrate pretreatment in elective cesarean section patients. Anesth Analg 1985; 64:34-7.

149. Carp H, Jayaram A, Stoll M. Ultrasound examination of the stomach contents of parturients. Anesth Analg 1992; 74:683-7.

150. Murphy DF, Nally B, Gardiner J, Unwin A. Effect of metoclopramide on gastric emptying before elective and emergency caesarean section. Br J Anaesth 1984; 56:1113-6.

151. Kubli M, Scrutton MJ, Seed PT, O'Sullivan G. An evaluation of isotonic "sports drinks" during labor. Anesth Anal 2002; 94:404-8.

152. Lahiri SK, Thomas TA, Hodgson RMH. Single-dose antacid therapy for the prevention of Mendelson's syndrome. Br J Anaesth 1973; 45:1143-6.

153. O'Sullivan GM, Bullingham RE. Noninvasive assessment by radiotelemetry of antacid effect during labor. Anesth Analg 1985; 64:95-100.

154. Hall AW, Moossa AR, Clark J, et al. The effects of premedication drugs on the lower oesophageal high pressure zone and reflux status of Rhesus monkeys and man. Gut 1975; 16:347-52.

155. Wright PMC, Allen RW, Moore J, Donnelly JP. Gastric emptying during lumbar extradural analgesia in labour: Effect of fentanyl supplementation. Br J Anaesth 1992; 68:248-51.

156. Ewah B, Yau K, King M, et al. Effect of epidural opioids on gastric emptying in labour. Int J Obstet Anesth 1993; 2:125-8.

157. Wright PMC, Allen RW, Moore J, Donnelly JP. Gastric emptying during lumbar extradural analgesia in labour: Effect of fentanyl supplementation. Br J Anaesth 1992; 68:248-51.

158. Geddes SM, Thorburn J, Logan RW. Gastric emptying following caesarean section and the effect of epidural fentanyl. Anaesthesia 1991; 46:1016-8.

159. Kelly MC, Carabine UA, Hill DA, Mirakhur RK. A comparison of the effect of intrathecal and extradural fentanyl on gastric emptying in laboring women. Anesth Analg 1997; 85:834-8.

160. Porter J, Bonello E, Reynolds F. The influence of epidural fentanyl infusion on gastric emptying in labour. Int J Obstet Anesth 1995; 4:261.

161. Thorén T, Wattwil M. Effects on gastric emptying of thoracic epidural analgesia with morphine or bupivacaine. Anesth Analg 1988; 67:687-94.

162. Bowen M, Jayaram A, Carp H. Ultrasound examination of the stomach contents of post partum patients (abstract). Anesthesiology 1995; 83:A956.

163. Gin T, Cho AMW, Lew JKL, et al. Gastric emptying in the postpartum period. Anaesth Intens Care 1991; 19:521-4.

164. Blouw R, Scatliff J, Craig DB, Palahniuk RJ. Gastric volume and pH in postpartum patients. Anesthesiology 1976; 45:456-7.

165. Lam KK, So HY, Gin T. Gastric pH and volume after oral fluids in the postpartum patient. Can J Anaesth 1993; 40:218-21.

166. McNair RD, Jaynes RV. Alterations in liver function during normal pregnancy. Am J Obstet Gynecol 1960; 80:500-5.

167. Romalis G, Claman AD. Serum enzymes in pregnancy. Am J Obstet Gynecol 1962; 84:1104-10.

168. Combes B, Shibata H, Adams R, et al. Alterations in sulfobromophthalein sodium-removal mechanisms from blood during normal pregnancy. J Clin Invest 1963; 42:1431-42.

169. Braverman DZ, Johnson ML, Kern F Jr. Effects of pregnancy and contraceptive steroids on gallbladder function. New Engl J Med 1980; 302:362-4.

170. Davison JM, Hytten FE. Glomerular filtration during and after pregnancy. J Obstet Gynaecol Br Commonw 1974; 81:588-95.

171. Sims EAH, Krantz KE. Serial studies of renal function during pregnancy and the puerperium in normal women. J Clin Invest 1958; 37:1764-74.

172. Lind T, Godfrey KA, Otun H. Changes in serum uric acid concentrations during normal pregnancy. Br J Obstet Gynaecol 1984; 91:128-32.

173. Davison JM, Hytten FE. The effect of pregnancy on the renal handling of glucose. Br J Obstet Gynaecol 1975; 82:374-81.

174. Harada A, Hershman JM, Reed AW, et al. Comparison of thyroid stimulators and thyroid hormone concentrations in the sera of pregnant women. J Clin Endocrinol Metab 1979; 48:793-7.

175. Rosenthal HE, Slaunwhite WR Jr, Sandberg AA. Transcortin: A corticosteroid-binding protein of plasma. X. Cortisol and progesterone interplay and unbound levels of these steroids in pregnancy. J Clin Endocrinol Metab 1969; 29:352-67.

176. Fisher PM, Sutherland HW, Bewsher PD. The insulin response to glucose infusion in normal human pregnancy. Diabetologia 1980; 19:15-20.

177. Felig P, Lynch V. Starvation in human pregnancy: Hypoglycemia, hypoinsulinemia, and hyperketonemia. Science 1970; 170:990-2.

178. Berg G, Hammar M, Moller-Nielsen J, et al. Low back pain during pregnancy. Obstet Gynecol 1988; 71:71-5.

179. Wilkinson M. The carpal-tunnel syndrome in pregnancy. Lancet 1960; 1:453-4.

180. Cogan R, Spinnato JA. Pain and discomfort thresholds in late pregnancy. Pain 1986; 27:63-8.

181. Abboud TK, Sarkis F, Hung TT, et al. Effects of epidural anesthesia during labor on maternal plasma beta-endorphin levels. Anesthesiology 1983; 59:1-5.

182. Wardlaw SL, Frantz AG. Brain beta-endorphin during pregnancy, parturition, and the postpartum period. Endocrinology 1983; 113:1664-8.

183. Iwasaki H, Collins JG, Saito Y, Kerman-Hinds A. Naloxone-sensitive, pregnancy-induced changes in behavioral responses to colorectal distention: Pregnancy-induced analgesia to visceral stimulation. Anesthesiology 1991; 74:927-33.

184. Sander HW, Gintzler AR. Spinal cord mediation of the opioid analgesia of pregnancy. Brain Res 1987; 408:389-93.

185. Assali NS, Prystowsky H. Studies on autonomic blockade. I. Comparison between the effects of tetraethylammonium chloride (TEAC) and high selective spinal anesthesia on blood pressure of normal and toxemic pregnancy. J Clin Invest 1950; 29:1354-66.

186. Tabsh K, Rudelstorfer R, Nuwayhid B, Assali NS. Circulatory responses to hypovolemia in the pregnant and nonpregnant sheep after pharmacologic sympathectomy. Am J Obstet Gynecol 1986; 154:411-9.

187. Goodlin RC. Venous reactivity and pregnancy abnormalities. Acta Obstet Gynecol Scand 1986; 65:345-8.

188. Igarashi T, Hirabayashi Y, Shimizu R, et al. The fiberscopic findings of the epidural space in pregnant women. Anesthesiology 2000; 92:1631-6.

189. Messih MNA. Epidural space pressures during pregnancy. Anaesthesia 1981; 36:775-82.

190. Marx GF, Zemaitis MT, Orkin LR. Cerebrospinal fluid pressures during labor and obstetrical anesthesia. Anesthesiology 1961; 22:348-54.

191. Abitbol MM. Supine position in labor and associated fetal heart rate changes. Obstet Gynecol 1985; 65:481-6.

192. Huch A, Huch R, Schneider H, Rooth G. Continuous transcutaneous monitoring of fetal oxygen tension during labour. Br J Obstet Gynaecol 1977; 84 (Suppl 1):1-39.

193. Crawford JS, Burton M, Davies P. Time and lateral tilt at caesarean section. Br J Anaesth 1972; 44:477-84.

194. Andrews PJD, Ackerman III WE, Juneja MM. Aortocaval compression in the sitting and lateral decubitus positions during extradural catheter placement in the parturient. Can J Anaesth 1993; 40:320-4.

195. Pilkington S, Carli F, Dakin MJ, et al. Increase in Mallampati score during pregnancy. Br J Anaesth 1995; 74:638-42.

196. Dresner M, Lyons G. Increase in Mallampati score during labour (abstract). Int J Obstet Anesth 1996; 5:214.

197. Samsoon GLT, Young JRB. Difficult tracheal intubation: A retrospective study. Anaesthesia 1987; 42:487-90.

198. Rocke DA, Murray WB, Rout CC, Gouws E. Relative risk analysis of factors associated with difficult intubation in obstetric anesthesia. Anesthesiology 1992; 77:67-73.

199. Archer GW Jr, Marx GF. Arterial oxygen tension during apnoea in parturient women. Br J Anaesth 1974; 46:358-60.

200. Rampton AJ, Mallaiah S, Garrett CPO. Increased ventilation requirements during obstetric general anaesthesia. Br J Anaesth 1988; 61:730-7.

201. Palahniuk RJ, Shnider SM, Eger EI II. Pregnancy decreases the requirement for inhaled anesthetic agents. Anesthesiology 1974; 41:82-3.

202. Strout CD, Nahrwold ML. Halothane requirement during pregnancy and lactation in rats. Anesthesiology 1981; 55:322-3.

203. Thomas BA, Anzalone TA, Rosinia FA. Progesterone decreases the MAC of desflurane in the nonpregnant ewe (abstract). Anesthesiology 1995; 83:A952.

204. Chan MTV, Mainland P, Gin T. Minimum alveolar concentration of halothane and enflurane are decreased in early pregnancy. Anesthesiology 1996; 85:782-6.

205. Chan MTV, Gin T. Postpartum changes in the minimum alveolar concentration of isoflurane. Anesthesiology 1995; 82:1360-3.

206. Datta S, Migliozzi RP, Flanagan HL, Krieger NR. Chronically administered progesterone decreases halothane requirements in rabbits. Anesth Analg 1989; 68:46-50.

207. Spielman FJ, Mueller RA, Corke BC. Cerebrospinal fluid concentration of 5-hydroxyindoleacetic acid in pregnancy. Anesthesiology 1985; 62:193-5.

208. Christensen JH, Andreasen F, Jansen JA. Pharmacokinetics of thiopental in caesarian section. Acta Anaesth Scand 1981; 25:174-9.

209. Gin T, Mainland P, Chan MTV, Short TG. Decreased thiopental requirements in early pregnancy. Anesthesiology 1997; 86:73-8.

210. Morgan DJ, Blackman GL, Paull JD, Wolf LJ. Pharmacokinetics and plasma binding of thiopental. II. Studies at cesarean section. Anesthesiology 1981; 54:474-80.

211. Higuchi H, Adachi Y, Arimura S, et al. Early pregnancy does not reduce the C_{50} of propofol for loss of consciousness. Anesth Analg 2001; 93:1565-9.

212. Kanto J, Rosenberg P. Propofol in cesarean section. A pharmacokinetic and pharmacodynamic study. Methods Find Exp Clin Pharmacol 1990; 12:707-11.

213. Gin T, Gregory MA, Chan K, et al. Pharmacokinetics of propofol in women undergoing elective caesarean section. Br J Anaesth 1990; 64:148-53.

214. Kuhnert BR, Kuhnert PM, Prochaska AL, Sokol RJ. Meperidine disposition in mother, neonate, and nonpregnant females. Clin Pharmacol Ther 1980; 27:486-91.

215. Ritter DM, Rettke SR, Ilstrup DM, Burritt MF. Effect of plasma cholinesterase activity on the duration of action of succinylcholine in patients with genotypically normal enzyme. Anesth Analg 1988; 67:1123-6.

216. Ganga CC, Heyduk JV, Marx GF, Sklar GS. A comparison of the response to suxamethonium in post-partum and gynaecological patients. Anaesthesia 1982; 37:903-6.

217. Khuenl-Brady KS, Koeller J, Mair P, et al. Comparison of vecuronium- and atracurium-induced neuromuscular blockade in postpartum and nonpregnant patients. Anesth Analg 1991; 72:110-3.

218. Baraka A, Tabboush Z, Bijjani A, Karam K. Onset of vecuronium neuromuscular block is more rapid in patients undergoing caesarean section. Can J Anaesth 1992; 39:135-8.

219. Puhringer FK, Sparr HJ, Mitterschiffthaler G, et al. Extended duration of action of rocuronium in postpartum patients. Anesth Analg 1997; 84:352-4.

220. Rodrigue R, Durant NN, Nguyen N, et al. Comparison of vecuronium-induced neuromuscular blockade in pregnant and nonpregnant female rabbits (abstract). Anesthesiology 1986; 65:A401.

221. Dailey PA, Fisher DM, Shnider SM, et al. Pharmacokinetics, placental transfer, and neonatal effects of vecuronium and pancuronium administered during cesarean section. Anesthesiology 1984; 60:569-74.

222. Duvaldestin P, Demetriou M, Henzel D, Desmonts JM. The placental transfer of pancuronium and its pharmacokinetics during caesarian section. Acta Anaesth Scand 1978; 22:327-33.

223. Guay J, Crochetiere C, Gaudreault P, et al. Pharmacokinetics of atracurium in pregnant women (abstract). Abstracts, scientific papers, Society for Obstetric Anesthesia and Perinatology, 25th Annual Meeting, Indian Wells, CA, 1993.

224. DeSimone CA, Leighton BL, Norris MC, et al. The chronotropic effect of isoproterenol is reduced in term pregnant women. Anesthesiology 1988; 69:626-8.

225. Nisell H, Hjemdahl P, Linde B. Cardiovascular responses to circulating catecholamines in normal pregnancy and in pregnancy-induced hypertension. Clin Physiol 1985; 4:479-93.

226. Magness RR, Rosenfeld CR. Systemic and uterine responses to alpha-adrenergic stimulation in pregnant and nonpregnant ewes. Am J Obstet Gynecol 1986; 155:897-904.

227. Hohmann M, Keve TM, Osol G, McLaughlin MK. Norepinephrine sensitivity of mesenteric veins in pregnant rats. Am J Physiol 1990; 259:R753-9.

228. Ballego G, Barbosa TA, Coelho EB, et al. Pregnancy-associated increase in rat systemic arteries endothelial nitric oxide production diminishes vasoconstrictor but does not enhance vasodilator responses. Life Sci 2002; 70:3131-42.

229. Wang SY, Datta S, Segal S. Pregnancy alters adrenergic mechanisms in uterine arterioles of rats. Anesth Analg 2002; 94:1304-9.

230. McKinlay J, Lyons G. Obstetric neuraxial anaesthesia: which pressor agents should we be using? Internat J Obstet Anesth 2002; 11:117-21.

231. Morgan PJ, Halpern SH, Tarshis J. The effects of an increase of central blood volume before spinal anesthesia for cesarean delivery: a qualitative systematic review. Anesth Analg 2001; 92:997-1005.

232. Lee A, Ngan Kee WD, Gin T. A quantitative, systematic review of randomized controlled trials of ephedrine versus phenylephrine for the management of hypotension during spinal anesthesia for cesarean delivery. Anesth Anal 2002; 94:920-6.

233. Popitz-Bergez FA, Leeson S, Thalhammer JG, Strichartz GR. Intraneural lidocaine uptake compared with analgesic differences between pregnant and nonpregnant rats. Regional Anesth 1997; 22:363-71.

234. Flanagan HL, Datta S, Lambert DH, et al. Effect of pregnancy on bupivacaine-induced conduction blockade in the isolated rabbit vagus nerve. Anesth Analg 1987; 66:123-6.

235. Marx GF, Orkin LR. Physiology of Obstetric Anesthesia. Springfield, Mass, Charles C Thomas, 1969: 83-114.

236. Sheth AP, Dautenhahn DL, Fagraeus L. Decreased CSF protein during pregnancy as a mechanism facilitating the spread of spinal anesthesia (abstract). Anesth Analg 1985; 64:280.

237. Hirabayashi Y, Shimizu R, Saitoh K, et al. Acid-base state of cerebrospinal fluid during pregnancy and its effect on spread of spinal anaesthesia. Br J Anaesth 1996; 77:352-5.

238. Barclay DL, Renegar OJ, Nelson EW Jr. The influence of inferior vena cava compression on the level of spinal anesthesia. Am J Obstet Gynecol 1968; 101:792-800.

239. Datta S, Hurley RJ, Naulty JS, et al. Plasma and cerebrospinal fluid progesterone concentrations in pregnant and nonpregnant women. Anesth Analg 1986; 65:950-4.

240. Abouleish EI. Postpartum tubal ligation requires more bupivacaine for spinal anesthesia than does cesarean section. Anesth Analg 1986; 65:897-900.

241. Hirabayashi Y, Shimizu R, Saitoh K, Fukuda H. Spread of subarachnoid hyperbaric amethocaine in pregnant women. Br J Anaesth 1995; 74:384-6.

242. Hogan QH, Prost R, Kulier A, et al. Magnetic resonance imaging of cerebrospinal fluid volume and the influence of body habitus and abdominal pressure. Anesthesiology 1996; 84:1341-9.

243. Hirabayashi Y, Shimizu R, Fukuda H, et al. Anatomical configuration of the spinal column in the supine position. II. Comparison of pregnant and non-pregnant women. Br J Anaesth 1995; 75:6-8.

244. Sivakumaran C, Ramanathan S, Chalon J, Turndorf H. Uterine contractions and the spread of local anesthetics in the epidural space. Anesth Analg 1982; 61:127-9.

245. Grundy EM, Zamora AM, Winnie AP. Comparison of spread of epidural anesthesia in pregnant and nonpregnant women. Anesth Analg 1978; 57:544-6.

246. Sharrock NE, Greenidge J. Epidural dose responses in pregnant and non pregnant patients (abstract). Anesthesiology 1979; 51:S298.

247. Kalas DB, Senfield RM, Hehre FW. Continuous lumbar peridural anesthesia in obstetrics. IV: Comparison of the number of segments blocked in pregnant and nonpregnant subjects. Anesth Analg 1966; 45:848-51.

248. Pihlajamäki K, Kanto J, Lindberg R, et al. Extradural administration of bupivacaine: Pharmacokinetics and metabolism in pregnant and nonpregnant women. Br J Anaesth 1990; 64:556-62.

249. Denson DD, Coyle DE, Thompson GA, et al. Bupivacaine protein binding in the term parturient: Effects of lactic acidosis. Clin Pharmacol Ther 1984; 35:702-9.

250. Tsen LC, Tarshis J, Denson DD, et al. Measurements of maternal protein binding of bupivacaine throughout pregnancy. Anesth Analg 1999; 89:965-8.

251. Fragneto RY, Bader AM, Rosinia F, et al. Measurements of protein binding of lidocaine throughout pregnancy. Anesth Analg 1994; 79:295-7.

252. Arthur GR, Santos A, Finster M. Comparative pharmacokinetics of ropivacaine and bupivacaine in pregnant and non-pregnant sheep (abstract). Anesthesiology 1994; 81:A1178.

253. Morishima HO, Finster M, Arthur R, Covino BG. Pregnancy does not alter lidocaine toxicity. Am J Obstet Gynecol 1990; 162:320-4.

254. Bucklin BA, Warner DS, Choi WW, et al. Pregnancy does not alter the threshold for lidocaine-induced seizures in the rat. Anesth Analg 1992; 74:57-61.

255. Santos AC, Pedersen H, Harmon TW, et al. Does pregnancy alter the systemic toxicity of local anesthetics? Anesthesiology 1989; 70:991-5.

256. Albright GA. Clinical aspects of bupivacaine toxicity. Presentation to the Food and Drug Administration, Anesthetic and Life Support Drugs Advisory Committee, Oct 4, 1983.

257. Morishima HO, Pedersen H, Finster M, et al. Bupivacaine toxicity in pregnant and nonpregnant ewes. Anesthesiology 1985; 63:134-9.

258. Santos AC, Arthur GR, Wlody D, et al. Comparative systemic toxicity of ropivacaine and bupivacaine in nonpregnant and pregnant ewes. Anesthesiology 1995; 82:734-40.

259. Santos AC, DeArmas PI. Systemic Toxicity of levobupivacaine, bupivacaine, and ropivacaine during continuous intravenous infusion to nonpregnant and pregnant ewes. Anesthesiology 2001; 95:1256-64.

260. Moller RA, Datta S, Fox J, et al. Effects of progesterone on the cardiac electrophysiologic action of bupivacaine and lidocaine. Anesthesiology 1992; 76:604-8.

261. Moller RA, Covino BG. Effect of progesterone on the cardiac electrophysiological alterations produced by ropivacaine and bupivacaine. Anesthesiology 1992; 77:735-41.

262. Askrog VF, Smith TC, Eckenhoff JE. Changes in pulmonary ventilation during spinal anesthesia. Surg Gynecol Obstet 1964; 119:563-7.

263. Moya F, Smith B. Spinal anesthesia for cesarean section. Clinical and biochemical studies of effects on maternal physiology. JAMA 1962; 179:609-14.

264. Moir DD. Ventilatory function during epidural analgesia. Br J Anaesth 1963; 35:3-7.

265. Egbert LD, Tamersoy K, Deas TC. Pulmonary function during spinal anesthesia: The mechanism of cough depression. Anesthesiology 1961; 22:882-5.

266. Gamil M. Serial peak expiratory flow rates in mothers during caesarean section under extradural anaesthesia. Br J Anaesth 1989; 62:415-8.

267. Harrop-Griffiths AW, Ravalia A, Browne DA, Robinson PN. Regional anaesthesia and cough effectiveness. A study in patients undergoing caesarean section. Anaesthesia 1991; 46:11-3.

Chapter 3
Uteroplacental Blood Flow

Carl P. Weiner, M.D., M.B.A., FACOG · James C. Eisenach, M.D.

Uteroplacental blood flow is the major determinant of oxygen and nutrient transport to the fetus. There is a direct correlation between uterine blood flow and fetal P_{O_2} in both sheep (Figure 3-1) and humans.[1,2] In the latter, there is a direct correlation between uterine blood flow (determined by Doppler) and fetal umbilical venous P_{O_2} (determined by percutaneous umbilical cord blood sampling in utero).

An understanding of the regulation of uteroplacental blood flow is an essential foundation for optimal obstetric anesthesia practice. The measurement of a drug's effect on uteroplacental blood flow is a cornerstone for the assessment of the safety of any new drug in obstetric anesthesia practice. In addition, studies of the underlying mechanisms of changes in systemic and uterine vascular resistance during pregnancy may lead to novel treatments for diseases of pregnancy.

ANATOMY

Uteroplacental perfusion originates from the uterine and ovarian arteries. Although the fractional contribution of *ovarian* arterial blood flow to total human uteroplacental perfusion is unknown, it approximates one sixth of total uteroplacental flow in monkeys.[3] Maternal blood enters the disc-shaped basal plate of the placenta, spurting like a fountain into the intervillous space, where exchange occurs with the fetal blood that courses through the villi. Maternal blood then passes into the veins of the basal plate and exits the uterus. Normally, the two circulations are separate, and there is no mixing.

CHANGES DURING PREGNANCY

Uterine blood flow increases dramatically during pregnancy, from 50 to 100 mL/min *before* pregnancy to 700 to 900 mL/min at term. Using transvaginal ultrasound probes, Thaler et al.[4] observed a progressive increase in the diameter of the parametrial branch of the ascending uterine artery and a decrease in flow velocity with advancing pregnancy. By contrast, Palmer et al.[5] observed an increase in both diameter and flow velocity during pregnancy upstream from the main uterine artery close to the internal iliac-uterine artery bifurcation.

Not only does absolute uterine blood flow increase during pregnancy, but also the distribution of cardiac output changes. Uterine blood flow increases from less than 5% of cardiac output before pregnancy to approximately 12% of cardiac output at term. The proportion of common iliac artery blood distributed to the uterus increases progressively during pregnancy. Indeed, absolute blood flow to the external iliac artery actually *decreases* during pregnancy, which constitutes a "steal" phenomenon (Figure 3-2). Approximately 90% of uterine blood flow is distributed to the intervillous space.

Altered Response to Vasoactive Agents

A generalized reduction in maternal sensitivity to vasoconstrictors occurs during pregnancy. The pressor response to intravenous epinephrine, norepinephrine, phenylephrine, serotonin, thromboxane, and angiotensin II is diminished during pregnancy in many species, including humans. Women destined to develop preeclampsia fail to mount a normal adaptive response to pregnancy, and this failure is exploited for screening tests. For example, women who are more likely to develop preeclampsia never develop refractoriness to angiotensin II that is infused intravenously.

Uterine vascular responsiveness to endogenous vasoconstrictors also changes during pregnancy, although it often does so in a way that is different from that of the systemic vessels. For example, the uterine vasculature is less responsive than the systemic vasculature to the peptide vasoconstrictors (i.e., angiotensin II, endothelin)[6] and to a thromboxane analog.[7] Circulating concentrations of angiotensin II increase during pregnancy, and some investigators have proposed that the reduced sensitivity of uterine vessels to angiotensin II (as compared with systemic vessels) may be in part responsible for the redistribution of cardiac output and the increase in uterine blood flow during pregnancy.

Maternal sensitivity to alpha-adrenergic agonists also declines during pregnancy. Although uterine vessels are less sensitive to angiotensin II and endothelin than are systemic vessels, the uterine vessels in sheep are *more* sensitive to constriction from alpha-adrenergic agonists than are the systemic vessels.[8] Infusions of phenylephrine, epinephrine, and norepinephrine all decrease uterine blood flow in pregnant sheep[9,10] and produce parallel decreases in myometrial and placental blood flow.[11] However, placental flow declines less than myometrial flow at any given infusion rate. Whether this increased response to infused norepinephrine in the uterine as compared with the systemic vasculature reflects a uterine sympathetic denervation and supersensitivity[12] or some other factor is unknown. Powerful uterine artery vasoconstriction from alpha-adrenergic agonists has important clinical implications.

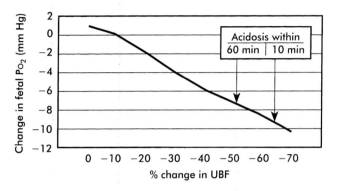

FIGURE 3-1. Effect of uterine blood flow *(UBF)* on fetal arterial P_{O_2} in sheep. With sustained reductions of UBF of 55%, fetal acidosis occurs within 60 minutes. With sustained reductions of UBF of 65%, fetal acidosis occurs within 10 minutes. (Adapted from Skillman CA, Plessinger MA, Woods JR, Clark KE. Effect of graded reductions in uteroplacental blood flow on the fetal lamb. Am J Physiol 1985; 149:1098-105.)

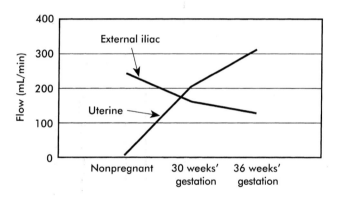

FIGURE 3-2. Steal of blood flow from the external iliac to the uterine artery in humans. Unilateral blood flows determined by Doppler in nonpregnant women and during pregnancy at 30 and 36 weeks' gestation. (Adapted from Palmer SK, Zamudio S, Coffin C, et al. Quantitative estimation of human uterine artery blood flow and pelvic blood flow redistribution in pregnancy. Obstet Gynecol 1992; 80:1000-6.)

Mechanisms of Changes

Global and regional changes in vascular reactivity during pregnancy may be caused by the following: (1) changes in receptor number or function[13]; (2) changes in metabolism and clearance of drugs[14]; (3) altered *release* of endogenous vasodilators or constrictors; and/or (4) altered *sensitivity* to endogenous vasodilators or constrictors. Much recent work has focused on the role of endogenous vasodilators—especially prostaglandins and nitric oxide—in pregnancy-induced changes in vascular tone and responsiveness and in the pathophysiology of preeclampsia.

Prostacyclin (PGI_2) production is increased during pregnancy, and this is evidenced by increased circulating and urinary concentrations of its stable metabolites.[15] Angiotensin II stimulates the release of both PGI_2 and nitric oxide from human uterine arteries, and this response is increased during pregnancy.[16] PGI_2 production is greater in uterine than systemic vessels, which may explain the diminished contraction of uterine as compared with systemic vessels in response to angiotensin II (Figure 3-3, left panel). Most PGI_2 is produced by vascular endothelium rather than smooth muscle, and increased PGI_2 is associated with increased cAMP concentrations in vascular smooth muscle. Together these studies support the hypothesis that increased uterine arterial endothelial release of PGI_2 during pregnancy results in increased cAMP concentrations, which contribute to the relaxation of uterine arterial smooth muscle and the resulting decrease in uterine vascular resistance.

This PGI_2 hypothesis predicts that prostaglandin synthetase inhibitors such as indomethacin and aspirin should reduce uterine blood flow; however, these drugs do not cause a clinically significant reduction in uterine blood flow. Although indomethacin reduces PGI_2 production by uterine arteries exposed to thromboxane and angiotensin II in vitro[7] and also increases blood pressure in response to infused angiotensin II,[16] indomethacin alone causes only a transient reduction in uterine blood flow.[17] This suggests that either the release of other vasodilating substances compensates for the decreased PGI_2 production after indomethacin administration or, alternatively, PGI_2 is less important during pregnancy than previously thought. The truth is probably somewhere in between. It has also been suggested that angiotensin-converting enzyme (ACE) inhibitors may decrease uterine perfusion

FIGURE 3-3. Vascular response to angiotensin II during pregnancy. During normal pregnancy *(left panel)*, there is an increase in uterine artery endothelial cell mass, which responds to angiotensin II *(Ang II)* by releasing prostacyclin *(PGI_2)*. This results in a vasodilator (−) response that counteracts the vasoconstricting (+) effect of Ang II on the smooth muscle. Collectively, these responses result in a minimal change in uterine artery diameter. However, Ang II constricts peripheral arteries. In contrast with normal pregnancy, endothelial cell dysfunction occurs in preeclampsia, and less PGI_2 is released in response to Ang II *(right panel)*. This leads to decreased uterine blood flow *(UBF)*.

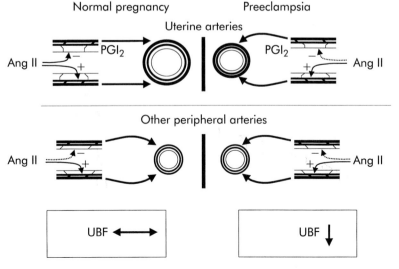

in pregnancy by producing a "steal" phenomenon that results from reduced vasoconstriction in peripheral vascular beds.[18]

The PGI$_2$ hypothesis is also consistent with several observations in preeclamptic women. PGI$_2$ excretion is decreased in women who have preeclampsia as compared with women who experience normal pregnancies.[19] Uterine arteries of women who have preeclampsia do not produce PGI$_2$ in response to angiotensin II, as do uterine arteries of women with normal pregnancies. Roberts et al.[20] have provided significant evidence that preeclampsia is characterized by a sequence of events consistent with endothelial dysfunction. Serum from preeclamptic women reportedly contains a factor that damages the endothelium, which could explain the decreased production of PGI$_2$ and many of the cardiovascular hallmarks of the disease. Thus, endogenous angiotensin II or exogenously infused angiotensin II could produce a reduction in uterine blood flow in preeclamptic women (Figure 3-3, right panel). Similar maladaptive responses are also seen in normotensive women whose pregnancies are complicated by intrauterine growth restriction (IUGR).

More recently, the role of endothelium-derived relaxing factors (e.g., nitric oxide [NO]) in uterine vascular regulation has been examined. Nitric oxide is synthesized from arginine in vascular endothelial cells. It diffuses to the smooth muscle cell, where it stimulates soluble guanylate cyclase, which increases cGMP and causes vascular smooth muscle relaxation. Several observations support a role of an estrogen-induced increase in nitric oxide production by vascular endothelium in the changes in systemic and uterine vascular resistance during pregnancy (Figure 3-4). First, Weiner et al.[7,21-23] demonstrated the proliferation of endothelial cells during pregnancy and an enhanced release of nitric oxide in vitro. Second, the urinary excretion of cGMP is increased during pregnancy,[23] which is consistent with increased stimulation of soluble guanylate cyclase by nitric oxide. This declines rapidly after delivery, suggesting that the placenta has an important role in this activity. Third, the removal of the endothelium diminishes or eliminates the refractoriness of the uterine artery to vasoconstrictor agents in vitro.[7] Fourth, the inhibition of nitric oxide synthesis by an infusion of N-monomethyl-L-arginine increases blood pressure and reverses the pregnancy-induced refractoriness to many vasopressor agents.[22,23] Finally, the application of acetylcholine (which stimulates nitric oxide

synthesis) or nitroglycerin (which directly stimulates guanylate cyclase) to isolated uterine arteries from pregnant guinea pigs results in nitric oxide-mediated smooth muscle relaxation.[21] This nitric oxide mechanism may underlie the phenomenon of preserved uterine perfusion after administration of ephedrine.

In addition to endothelium-derived relaxing factors (e.g., PGI$_2$, nitric oxide), there is strong evidence that atrial natriuretic peptide (ANP) and protein kinase C play a role in controlling uterine vascular tone. ANP diminishes the in vitro vasoconstriction of human placental cotyledons to angiotensin II,[24] and the intravenous infusion of ANP reduces blood pressure while increasing uterine blood flow in preeclamptic women.[25] Intravenous estrogen infusion increases uterine blood flow in animals, and steroids may also have a specific local effect on the uterine vasculature during pregnancy. For example, protein kinase C activity, which may mediate vasoconstriction, is decreased in uterine arteries but not in systemic arteries.[26] Although circulating estrogen concentrations increase during pregnancy, the ovarian lymphatic drainage (which runs through the broad ligament) may bathe uterine vessels selectively with higher concentrations of estrogen, and these high concentrations of estrogen may cause decreased protein kinase C activity, decreased uterine vascular resistance, and increased uteroplacental blood flow.[26]

Recent evidence suggests that estrogen and pregnancy may alter receptor-mediated G-protein coupling so that a functional decrease in GTPase activity occurs.[27,28] As a result, the effect of receptor activation is magnified. This would explain the observations that almost all pregnancy-mediated effects on the vasculature are receptor-coupled, the contractile responses to some agonists are actually enhanced during pregnancy, and receptor stimulation results in an increased release of both PGI$_2$ and nitric oxide.[27,28]

In summary, advances in our understanding of the mechanisms underlying the normal adaptation of the cardiovascular system to pregnancy focus on local hormonal actions and the activity of vascular endothelium. Selective uterine artery relaxation may be the result of the following: (1) enhanced release of vasodilators, such as PGI$_2$ and nitric oxide, by the vascular endothelium; (2) high local estrogen concentrations, which lead to the diminished activity of key intracellular enzymes that mediate vasoconstriction; and (3) altered recep-

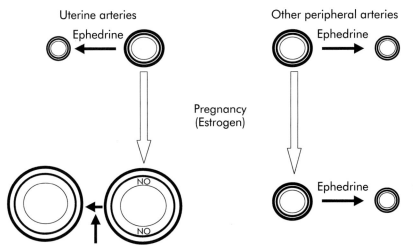

FIGURE 3-4. Vascular response to ephedrine. Ephedrine constricts nonpregnant uterine and other peripheral arteries in a similar manner *(upper circles)*. During pregnancy, estrogen produces an increase in uterine artery vessel diameter, endothelial cell mass, and the endothelium's ability to synthesize the vasodilator nitric oxide *(NO)*; this does not occur in peripheral vessels. Under these circumstances *(lower circles)*, ephedrine stimulates nitric oxide synthase *(NOS)* in uterine arterial endothelium, thereby counterbalancing its direct vasoconstriction. Because this does not occur in other peripheral vessels, ephedrine increases blood pressure while sparing the uterine circulation.

tor-mediated G-protein coupling. Disruption of normal endothelial cell function may be partly responsible for the increased blood pressure and uteroplacental insufficiency of preeclampsia. Not only do these concepts hold promise for a better understanding and treatment of preeclampsia, but they also help explain the rationale for the choice of analgesic, anesthetic, and vasopressor drugs that are used in contemporary obstetric anesthesia practice.

DETERMINANTS OF UTERINE BLOOD FLOW

The previous discussion describes the adaptive changes in uteroplacental perfusion that occur during normal pregnancy, many of the proposed mechanisms for those changes, and how preeclampsia and IUGR are associated with maladaptation. Other factors affect uterine blood flow in the acute setting. In general, uterine blood flow is related to perfusion pressure and vascular resistance according to the following formula:

$$UBF = \frac{\text{Uterine arterial} - \text{Uterine venous pressure}}{\text{Uterine vascular resistance}}$$

As a result, uterine blood flow decreases whenever perfusion pressure decreases or uterine vascular resistance increases (Box 3-1).

First, uterine blood flow may decline when the perfusion pressure decreases because of decreased uterine arterial pressure, which occurs during systemic hypotension. For example, the supine hypotension syndrome results from compression of the inferior vena cava, which leads to decreased venous return, decreased cardiac output, and systemic hypotension. As with other causes of hypotension, not only does uterine blood flow decrease because of the decline in perfusion pressure, but uterine vascular resistance increases because of increased concentrations of vasopressin

and angiotensin II, which are secreted in an attempt to maintain systemic blood pressure.

Second, uterine blood flow may decline when perfusion pressure decreases because of increased uterine venous pressure. This typically occurs in the following situations: (1) with vena caval compression; (2) during each uterine contraction; and (3) during the Valsalva maneuver that accompanies pushing during the second stage of labor. Drug-induced uterine hypertonus (which may occur during intravenous administration of oxytocin or with cocaine abuse) is another example of decreased uterine blood flow as a result of increased uterine venous pressure.

Third, uterine blood flow may decline because of increased uterine vascular resistance. The effect of vasoconstrictors on uterine blood flow depends on their relative potency for the constriction of systemic versus uterine arteries. These differences in potency often reflect modulating effects of the vascular endothelium. For example, the diminished potency of epinephrine in the causation of constriction of the pregnant guinea pig uterine artery in vitro parallels this vessel's increased secretion of nitric oxide,[22] which "protects" the uterine circulation from the constricting effects of this agent. This is not to say that high circulating concentrations of epinephrine or other vasoconstrictors do not decrease uterine blood flow; however, their detrimental effect on uterine blood flow is somewhat diminished by endothelial modulation. Further, that detrimental effect can be much more evident and profound when endothelium is dysfunctional, as it is in women with preeclampsia or IUGR.

The observation that the failure of an intravenous infusion of a vasodilator to increase uterine blood flow at rest has been interpreted to mean that the uterine vasculature is maximally dilated at rest and passively depends on perfusion pressure. However, there are alternative explanations. Just as with vasoconstrictors, the net effect of vasodilators on uterine blood flow depends on the balance of effects on systemic and uterine vessels and on myometrial versus placental vessels. Direct uterine arterial injection of a vasodilator such as acetylcholine or nitroglycerin increases uterine blood flow in pregnant animals. Systemic injection of the vasodilator nitroglycerin diminishes the decrease in uterine blood flow that occurs during a systemic infusion of norepinephrine in pregnant animals.[10] These observations suggest that the resting uterine vasculature is quite capable of vasodilation but that systemically administered vasodilators do not selectively dilate the uterine vasculature. Thus, the intravenous administration of a vasodilator may increase uterine blood flow, depending on the clinical circumstances (e.g., high circulating concentrations of catecholamines). It is important to remember that, just because total uterine blood flow increases, it does not necessarily mean that placental perfusion is enhanced. For example, the intravenous infusion of adenosine into pregnant ewes also receiving angiotensin II results in an increase in total uterine blood flow but no change in placental blood flow.[29]

It is unclear when a systemically administered vasodilator might improve uteroplacental perfusion in clinical practice. For example, hydralazine does not improve uterine blood flow in cocaine-intoxicated pregnant sheep, but it does cause a marked maternal tachycardia.[30] Nitroglycerin and sodium nitroprusside diminish the hypertensive response to endotracheal intubation in women with severe preeclampsia. These agents are nitric oxide donors, and nitric oxide directly stimulates soluble guanylate cyclase. Recent studies reveal that nitroglycerin (given intravenously at a dose that does not

---

Box 3-1 CAUSES OF DECREASED UTERINE BLOOD FLOW

DECREASED PERFUSION PRESSURE

DECREASED UTERINE ARTERIAL PRESSURE

- Supine position (aortocaval compression)
- Hemorrhage/hypovolemia
- Drug-induced hypotension
- Hypotension during sympathetic blockade

INCREASED UTERINE VENOUS PRESSURE

- Vena caval compression
- Uterine contractions
- Drug-induced uterine hypertonus (oxytocin, local anesthetics)
- Skeletal muscle hypertonus (seizures, Valsalva)

INCREASED UTERINE VASCULAR RESISTANCE

ENDOGENOUS VASOCONSTRICTORS

- Catecholamines (stress)
- Vasopressin (in response to hypovolemia)

EXOGENOUS VASOCONSTRICTORS

- Epinephrine
- Vasopressors (phenylephrine > ephedrine)
- Local anesthetics (in high concentrations)

affect blood pressure) can increase uterine blood flow during normal early pregnancy[31] and in women with preeclampsia (after transdermal application of a dose that reduces blood pressure by only 5%).[32] Magnesium sulfate increases resting uterine blood flow in pregnant sheep,[33] but the mechanisms by which it does this and its usefulness as a uterine artery vasodilator in clinical practice have not been examined in detail.

In summary, systemic blood pressure, uterine venous pressure, and uterine vascular resistance are the determinants of an acute change in uterine blood flow. Uterine blood flow is often reduced, especially in the third trimester, by maternal position, drugs, uterine contractions, pushing efforts, and endogenous and exogenous vasoconstrictors. The fact that intravenous administration of a vasodilator does not increase uterine blood flow at rest does not mean that the uterine vasculature is incapable of further dilation or that an intravenously administered vasodilator will not improve uterine blood flow in certain circumstances.

METHODS OF UTERINE BLOOD FLOW MEASUREMENT

Unfortunately, many of the available methods for the measurement of uterine blood flow have large inherent errors, or they measure something other than the variable of primary interest. Technologic advances have improved accuracy, but they have also generated reasons to question the validity of older methods.

From a clinical perspective, the parameter of central interest is placental perfusion. The ideal technique would measure the perfusion of *functional placenta*, which is the area where maternal-fetal exchange occurs. (In a way that is analogous to the lung, there may be areas of the placenta that receive maternal but not fetal blood flow.) No technique exclusively measures functional placental perfusion. However, in most circumstances, the measurement of intervillous blood flow provides a close approximation of functional placental blood flow. The measurement of total uterine artery blood flow—the most commonly used technique—may not always reflect placental perfusion.[30] For example, blood flow may be redistributed from the placenta to the myometrium (i.e., "steal") without a change in total uterine artery blood flow. Thus, placental blood flow might increase or decrease without any change in total uterine artery blood flow. Conversely, placental blood flow may stay constant despite an increase or decrease in total uterine artery blood flow. Moreover, studies typically measure the flow through only one uterine artery, and authors often do not note or discuss the relationship of that artery to the placenta; this is an important omission. When the placenta is located laterally rather than midline, the uterine artery on the side of the placenta usually has greater flow than the contralateral uterine artery and often responds differently to vasoactive substances. Finally, ovarian arterial blood flow is generally not measured, but it may contribute as much as one sixth of placental perfusion.[3]

Placental perfusion can be measured in animals with the injection of radioactive microspheres. This method allows for the separate calculation of placental and myometrial blood flows, but it only provides single-point-in-time information. More commonly, total uterine arterial blood flow is measured using electromagnetic or Doppler flow probes. These probes are surgically implanted around one or both uterine arteries or, in sheep, around the common uterine artery at the aortic trifurcation.

Placental perfusion can also be measured in humans by the injection of trace amounts of a radioactive-labeled substance, typically ^{133}Xe.[34] During the washout phase, the rapid decrease in measured radioactivity over the placenta is calculated as a biexponential or triexponential process. The most rapid decay constant is ascribed to intervillous perfusion. Alternatively, radioactive-tagged proteins (e.g., albumin) can be injected; scintigraphy is then performed over the placenta for the analysis of blood flow.[35] Because of the many assumptions inherent in both techniques, their accuracy for the determination of absolute flow is limited, but they are probably adequate for the measurement of relative change over time. Ethical concerns have precluded their use during pregnancy in the United States.

Clinically, uterine artery blood flow is typically assessed with noninvasive Doppler ultrasound techniques. Briefly, a probe sends an ultrasound signal, and the phase shift in reflected ultrasound energy is measured and interpreted as velocity of blood flow (i.e., red blood cell movement). Mean flow velocities and the ratio of systolic-to-diastolic velocity (the SD ratio) are reported; changes in either the mean velocity or the SD ratio are interpreted as changes in resistance to flow.

There are several significant sources of error when working with noninvasive Doppler measurements (Figure 3-5). First, the reproducibility of the measurement depends greatly on the examination of the same portion of the same artery each time. Second, in many circumstances, a change in the SD ratio is a poor reflection of a change in resistance. The SD ratio can be affected by both "upstream" variables (e.g., cardiac output) and "downstream" variables (e.g., changes in the number and site of capillaries recruited and open at one time); thus, this variable should never be used in isolation. It was not possible to obtain accurate mean velocity measurements until a decade ago, and reports of such measurements before 1992 should be questioned. Third, the variable of interest—blood flow—is not directly measured with Doppler ultrasound. The calculation of blood flow requires the precise determination of mean velocity, vessel diameter, and angle of insonation (Figure 3-5). Accurate measurement of vessel diameter is difficult with small vessels or vessels that are distant from the probe. Small errors in the estimation of the angle of insonation can result in blood flow measurement errors as large as 30%.[5] Therefore, the methods used in any clinical study that employs Doppler to measure uterine artery blood flow should be examined critically. This is especially important if no difference was

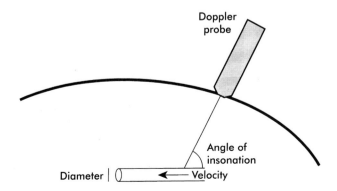

FIGURE 3-5. Sources of error in the determination of blood flow by Doppler ultrasound. Calculation of flow requires the precise determination of the velocity of blood flow, the diameter of the vessel, and the angle of insonation between the Doppler beam and the axis of blood flow of the vessel.

observed with experimental treatment (e.g., epidural anesthesia), because the margin of error is likely large and the power to detect clinically significant differences small.

Finally, uterine artery responses to vasoactive substances can be measured in arteries from humans or animals in vitro. This approach is particularly suited for investigations of the vascular endothelium or intracellular mechanisms of vasomotor activity and the changes that occur during pregnancy. Indeed, much of our understanding of these mechanisms comes from such studies. Unfortunately, the integrated response cannot be examined in studies of isolated vessels because of the following: (1) the direct effects of drugs, (2) sympathetic reflexes, and (3) the complex interactions among neurohormones secreted to maintain cardiovascular homeostasis. This may explain the discrepancy noted earlier, in which uterine blood vessels were less sensitive than systemic vessels to constriction from epinephrine in vitro,[24] but uterine vascular resistance increased more than systemic vascular resistance when epinephrine was infused in vivo.[8] In summary, it is difficult to extrapolate from in vitro vascular responses to the clinical response, which includes a complex interaction among neurohumoral controls, the determinants of perfusion pressure, and systemic versus uterine vascular responses.

REGIONAL ANESTHESIA

Epidural and spinal anesthesia can each affect uterine blood flow by several mechanisms, some of which may oppose one another (Box 3-2). Pain relief is the core mechanism by which epidural anesthesia may *increase* uterine blood flow. Pain and stress lead to the activation of the sympathetic nervous system, which causes decreased uterine blood flow by release of norepinephrine and epinephrine. Shnider et al.[36] observed that acute stress increased plasma norepinephrine by 25% and decreased uterine blood flow by 50% in gravid ewes. Pain and stress are associated with increased plasma epinephrine and an increased prevalence of abnormal fetal heart rate patterns in laboring women.[37] Effective pain relief using epidural analgesia is associated with a decrease in circulating catecholamines. In addition, women hyperventilate during painful uterine contractions. Not only do the subsequent periods of hypoventilation *between* contractions cause transient maternal and fetal hypoxemia, but hyperventilation itself may reduce uterine blood flow. Therefore, pain relief by epidural analgesia can increase uterine blood flow by decreasing circulating catecholamines and preventing periods of hyperventilation during painful contractions.

During epidural and spinal anesthesia, it is unclear whether the sympathetic blockade per se alters uterine blood flow. In the absence of hypotension, epidural anesthesia does not alter uterine blood flow in pregnant sheep,[38] laboring women,[39] or women undergoing cesarean section.[40] It is possible that sympathetic blockade alters the uterine and systemic vascular tone of the normal parturient in similar ways, with no net effect on uterine blood flow. In women with severe preeclampsia, epidural anesthesia using a plain local anesthetic may increase intervillous blood flow,[41] perhaps because of the heightened sympathomimetic activity associated with this disease.

Both epidural and spinal anesthesia may *decrease* uterine blood flow as a result of maternal hypotension. Hypotension decreases uterine blood flow by at least two mechanisms: (1) decreased perfusion pressure; and (2) stimulation of the

---

Box 3-2 EFFECTS OF REGIONAL ANESTHESIA ON UTERINE BLOOD FLOW

INCREASED UTERINE BLOOD FLOW AS A RESULT OF THE FOLLOWING:

- Pain relief
- Decreased sympathetic activity
- Decreased maternal hyperventilation

DECREASED UTERINE BLOOD FLOW AS A RESULT OF THE FOLLOWING:

- Hypotension
- Unintentional intravenous injection of local anesthetic and/or epinephrine
- Absorbed local anesthetic (little effect)

---

release of endogenous vasoconstrictors (e.g., vasopressin, angiotensin II). Indeed, epidural anesthesia (with its associated sympathetic blockade) causes increased vasopressin concentrations in dogs, even in the absence of hypotension.[42] However, Carp et al.[43] concluded that endogenous vasopressin does not play an important role in the maintenance of blood pressure during the administration of spinal and epidural anesthesia in nonpregnant patients and volunteers.

Unintentional intravenous injection of solutions intended for the epidural space may also decrease uterine blood flow. Small doses of epinephrine, which are commonly included in the epidural test dose, reduce uterine blood flow by more than 40% in pregnant sheep when given intravenously.[44] However, this reduction is short-lived (i.e., lasting less than 3 minutes) if the epinephrine is given as a single intravenous bolus (e.g., as might occur with a positive test dose clinically). Some anesthesiologists give a test dose of a local anesthetic alone (e.g., 40 mg of 2-chloroprocaine or lidocaine as an intrathecal test dose followed by 100 mg of the same local anesthetic as an intravenous test dose). The intravenous injection of small doses of 2-chloroprocaine or lidocaine has little effect on uterine blood flow as compared with epinephrine.[45]

Local anesthetics can decrease uterine blood flow. Unintentional intravenous injection of 25 mg of bupivacaine is associated with transient uterine hypertonus and fetal bradycardia in humans. Fishburne et al.[46] found that bupivacaine is more potent than either lidocaine or 2-chloroprocaine for increasing myometrial tone and decreasing uterine blood flow in gravid ewes (Figure 3-6).[46] These ovine studies may be relevant to humans, as evidenced by the pressor response to intravenous bupivacaine in volunteers.[47] In vitro, local anesthetics constrict arteries directly and inhibit endothelium-mediated vasodilation,[48] which may help explain these observations. Ropivacaine, which is a bupivacaine congener, produces more peripheral vasoconstriction than bupivacaine in pigs[49]; this initially raised some concern over its use in pregnancy. However, one study concluded that epidural injection of 115 to 140 mg of 0.5% ropivacaine has no effect on uterine blood flow in women undergoing cesarean section.[50]

Aside from unintentional intravenous injection or paracervical block, local anesthetics used for epidural anesthesia are unlikely to produce uterine vasoconstriction. The calculation of plasma concentrations achieved during epidural bupivacaine anesthesia for cesarean section suggests that, at most,

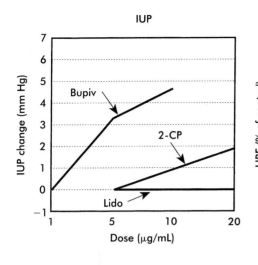

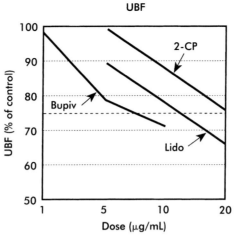

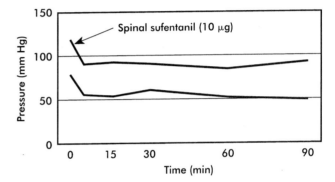

FIGURE 3-6. Effects of injection of local anesthetics into the common uterine artery at the aortic trifurcation in pregnant sheep. Bupivacaine *(Bupiv)* is more potent than lidocaine *(Lido)* or 2-chloroprocaine *(2-CP)* with regard to increasing intrauterine pressure *(IUP)* and decreasing uterine blood flow *(UBF)*. (Adapted from Fishburne JI Jr, Greiss FC Jr, Hopkinson R, Rhyne AL. Responses of the gravid uterine vasculature to arterial levels of local anesthetic agents. Am J Obstet Gynecol 1979; 133:753-61.)

the absorbed bupivacaine would decrease uterine blood flow by less than 5%.

Adjuvant Drugs

Three classes of adjuvant drugs are commonly used in the provision of regional anesthesia in obstetric patients: (1) opioids, (2) alpha$_2$-adrenergic agonists, and (3) vasopressors. Opioids or alpha$_2$-adrenergic agonists are combined with local anesthetics for epidural administration, and vasopressors are administered intravenously for the treatment of hypotension. Each of these three classes of adjuvant drugs can affect uterine blood flow.

OPIOIDS

Lipid-soluble opioids such as fentanyl and sufentanil often are combined with local anesthetics for epidural analgesia during labor. Craft et al.[51] observed that epidural fentanyl had no effect on uterine blood flow in gravid ewes. Likewise, they noted that epidural morphine, which is more often used for postoperative analgesia, also had no effect on uterine blood flow in gravid ewes.[52] Alahuhta et al.[53] reported that epidural sufentanil (50 µg) decreased the maternal mean arterial pressure—but did not alter uterine blood velocity waveform indices—in laboring women.

Lipid-soluble opioids are also administered intrathecally during labor, either as a single injection or repetitively through an intrathecal catheter. Intrathecal meperidine is associated with a higher prevalence of hypotension[54]; this is ascribed to its local anesthetic properties, and it could decrease uterine blood flow by this mechanism. Intrathecal sufentanil (10 µg) provides analgesia for 90 to 120 minutes in laboring women. It too is associated with a significant risk of hypotension,[55] which could decrease uterine blood flow. Figure 3-7 illustrates a clinical example; this patient had hypotension and extensive sensory blockade after intrathecal injection of sufentanil (10 µg).

The mechanism underlying the decrease in blood pressure after intrathecal sufentanil is unclear, but it may be a result of sympathetic blockade. (However, this proposed mechanism is a matter of debate.[56]) There is a high density of opioid receptors on the preganglionic sympathetic neurons in the spinal cord,[57] and the intrathecal injection of opioids decreases blood pressure in animals.[58] Early clinical studies may not have observed hypotension for at least two reasons. First, most studies evaluated the use of small doses of lipid-soluble

FIGURE 3-7. Effect of spinal injection of sufentanil (10 µg) on systolic *(upper line)* and diastolic *(lower line)* blood pressure in a laboring woman. The sensory level to pin testing was at the second thoracic dermatome by 5 minutes and at the fifth cervical dermatome by 10 minutes after injection.

opioids, which would result in cerebrospinal fluid concentrations much lower than those that occur following intrathecal administration. Second, morphine—the most common intrathecally administered opioid—may have inadequate lipid solubility to penetrate deep into the spinal cord, where the preganglionic sympathetic neurons are located.

ALPHA$_2$-ADRENERGIC AGONISTS

Epinephrine is a mixed adrenergic agonist that is often combined with local anesthetics for spinal and epidural anesthesia in obstetric patients. Among alpha-adrenoceptors, epinephrine has a greater affinity for the alpha$_2$-subtype. The effect of an intravenous injection of epinephrine on uterine blood flow was described previously. Wallis et al.[38] found that the epidural injection of an epinephrine-containing local anesthetic produced a small, brief reduction in uterine blood flow in pregnant sheep. By contrast, Alahuhta et al.[59] reported that epidural bupivacaine with epinephrine had no effect on intervillous blood flow in women undergoing cesarean section. Bonica et al.[60] observed that an epidural injection of epinephrine alone in human volunteers increased heart rate and cardiac output and decreased systemic vascular resistance to a degree similar to that observed after intravenous administration of low-dose epinephrine; these changes are consistent with a predominance of beta-adrenoceptor activation. Although there is no evidence for decreased uterine blood flow from absorbed epinephrine in epidural solutions given to healthy women during labor, some anesthesiologists avoid epinephrine in women with preeclampsia, because they fear an exaggerated uterine vasoconstrictive response to low concentrations of epinephrine. This practice, at least for cesarean section, is supported by the observation that the addition of 85 to 100 µg of epinephrine to epidural bupivacaine reduced uterine blood flow in hypertensive parturients with chronic fetal asphyxia.[61]

Epidural and intrathecal administration of more selective alpha$_2$-adrenergic agonists (e.g., clonidine, dexmedetomidine) has been a subject of recent clinical investigation. Both epidural and intrathecal injection of these drugs produce analgesia by a spinal mechanism; these drugs also enhance the action of opioids and local anesthetics. Clonidine has been used as an antihypertensive agent for preeclampsia, and its potential use as an epidural analgesic was examined in animals.[62] The intravenous administration of clonidine decreases uterine blood flow in gravid ewes,[63] possibly as a result of direct uterine artery vasoconstriction. By contrast, epidural clonidine does not alter uterine blood flow in pregnant sheep.[62] Clonidine-induced hypotension is more common and severe in humans than in sheep, and such hypotension would be expected to decrease uterine blood flow. Although epidural administration of clonidine in obstetric patients has been studied extensively in Europe, the United States package insert contains a warning against such use.[64]

VASOPRESSORS

Most anesthesiologists consider ephedrine the vasopressor of choice for the treatment of hypotension during regional anesthesia in obstetric patients. Ephedrine is more effective than alpha-adrenergic agonists in either the restoration or protection of uterine blood flow in pregnant sheep[65] and baboons.[66] As compared with alpha-adrenergic agonists, ephedrine is more likely to increase blood pressure by increasing cardiac output with less direct vasoconstriction.

Proponents of alpha-adrenergic agonists challenge these concepts. They argue that earlier studies were flawed by the use of excessively large doses of alpha-adrenergic agonists rather than small doses of drug carefully titrated to effect. Ramanathan and Grant[67] showed that both ephedrine and phenylephrine increase maternal preload and cardiac output when given for the treatment of hypotension during epidural anesthesia for cesarean section. Further, both phenylephrine[67,68] and methoxamine[69] are associated with favorable neonatal outcomes when used to treat hypotension during epidural or spinal anesthesia for cesarean section. Doppler ultrasound evaluation of uterine artery blood flow has yielded conflicting results. One study found no difference between phenylephrine and ephedrine,[70] whereas another noted increased uterine vascular resistance after the administration of phenylephrine but not ephedrine.[71] In vitro, uterine but not systemic arteries become less responsive to both ephedrine and methoxamine during pregnancy, and the maximal constriction in uterine arteries is reduced more in response to ephedrine than in response to metaraminol, which is an alpha-adrenergic agonist.[72] In other words, "ephedrine may spare uterine perfusion during pregnancy due to more selective constriction of systemic vessels than that caused by metaraminol."[72] Of interest, endothelium removal (which may mimic endothelial dysfunction in preeclampsia) accentuates the difference between the effects of ephedrine and metaraminol on uterine artery constriction in vitro.[72] The enhanced release of nitric oxide from uterine artery endothelium may be the main mechanism underlying ephedrine's

protection of uterine perfusion (Figure 3-4).[73] In summary, although there is some evidence that small doses of an alpha-adrenergic agonist can be used safely and effectively to treat regional anesthesia-induced hypotension in healthy women, most clinicians prefer ephedrine because of its apparent protective effect on uterine blood flow, its history of safety, and its ease of administration.

Finally, given the potential advantages of angiotensin II as a vasopressor without major effects on uterine blood flow, some investigators have examined its use for the treatment of hypotension during regional anesthesia. Although the initial results in healthy women receiving spinal anesthesia for cesarean section were promising,[74] this agent remains experimental. Of particular concern is the possibility that angiotensin II could be a potent uterine vasoconstrictor in women with preeclampsia or IUGR (recognized or unrecognized) and endothelial cell dysfunction (Figure 3-3, right panel).

GENERAL ANESTHESIA

Induction Agents

Barbiturates seem to have minimal direct effect on uterine blood flow; however, there are two indirect mechanisms by which they might reduce uterine blood flow. They may reduce systemic arterial pressure, which results in decreased uterine perfusion pressure. With typical doses of short-acting barbiturates (e.g., thiopental 4 mg/kg), this is a brief effect that is followed by a surge in circulating catecholamines during laryngoscopy and tracheal intubation. This surge in catecholamines directly produces uterine vasoconstriction and decreases uterine blood flow. In one study, uterine blood flow decreased 20% to 35% in pregnant women during thiopental induction and endotracheal intubation.[75] It seems reasonable to speculate that the sympathetic nervous system response to laryngoscopy and its effect on uterine blood flow might be reduced by increasing the dose of the induction agent and that this sympathetic response may produce an even more dramatic decrease in uterine blood flow in women with preeclampsia. However, neither of these hypotheses has been critically tested.

The effect of propofol or etomidate on uterine blood flow has not been tested in humans, but their pharmacology suggests that their direct and indirect actions should be similar to the barbiturates. Alon et al.[76] found that uterine blood flow does not significantly change during propofol administration for the induction of anesthesia, laryngoscopy and intubation, and maintenance of anesthesia in gravid ewes. By contrast, uterine blood flow decreased significantly during the induction of anesthesia and intubation in animals given thiopental. Unfortunately, the combined administration of propofol and succinylcholine produced a transient but severe maternal bradycardia, and one animal experienced sinus arrest.

Ketamine differs from other intravenous induction agents in terms of its actions on sympathetic nervous system activity and uterine tone. The effect of ketamine on uterine blood flow has been tested only in animals. In doses of 0.7 to 5.0 mg/kg, ketamine produces minor increases in both blood pressure and heart rate in gravid ewes.[77] Ketamine also increases uterine tone, which could decrease uterine blood flow, but this effect was not significant with doses used clinically.[78] Overall, the effects of anesthetic induction with ketamine on uterine blood flow appear similar to the effects of barbiturates—namely, a small effect of the drug itself and reduced uterine blood flow during the sympathetic response to tracheal intubation. However, in the setting of decreased intravascular volume, ketamine's effect would be expected to differ markedly from that of other induction agents by virtue of its ability to maintain systemic blood pressure near normal.

Inhalation Agents

Usual clinical doses (i.e., 0.5 to 1.5 minimum alveolar concentration [MAC]) of halothane, isoflurane, enflurane, desflurane, and sevoflurane have little or no effect on uterine blood flow, although deeper planes of anesthesia are associated with decreased maternal blood pressure, cardiac output, and uterine blood flow.[79,80] Thus, there is little reason to choose one of these agents over the other on the basis of their effect on uterine blood flow. Although some controversy persists regarding their impact on blood loss during cesarean section, the preponderance of evidence suggests that blood loss is not increased by the administration of a low concentration (i.e., less than 0.5 MAC) of one of these agents. Inhalation agents produce a dose-dependent reduction in uterine tone and would be expected to increase uterine blood flow in circumstances in which tone is increased (e.g., hyperstimulation with oxytocin, cocaine overdose, placental abruption).

Ventilation

Uterine blood flow is affected by the management of ventilation during general anesthesia. Although hypoxemia and hypercapnia per se do not alter uterine blood flow directly,[81,82] marked hypoxemia or hypercapnia may reduce uterine blood flow by activating the sympathetic nervous system. The effect of hypocapnia on uterine blood flow is controversial. Some authors have noted small (i.e., 10% to 20%) decreases in uterine blood flow,[83] whereas others have found no effect.[84] Levinson et al.[85] observed that positive-pressure hyperventilation decreases uterine blood flow in gravid ewes; the addition of CO_2 did not improve uterine blood flow. They concluded that mechanical hyperventilation itself—rather than hypocapnia—caused the decreased uterine blood flow. Although it is conceivable that a reduction in venous return, cardiac output, and uterine perfusion pressure may have caused the decreased uterine blood flow, it is also possible that noxious stimulation of these conscious sheep resulted in the release of catecholamines, which in turn decreased uterine perfusion. Nonetheless, most authors recommend that anesthesiologists avoid hyperventilation, in part because of concern for uterine blood flow.

EFFECTS OF OBSTETRIC DRUGS

Magnesium sulfate increases uterine blood flow in pregnant ewes at rest[33] and results in a modest decrease in uterine vascular resistance, as determined by Doppler, in women in preterm labor.[86] In addition, infusion of magnesium sulfate increases the release of prostacyclin in women in preterm labor.[87] Although hypermagnesemia exacerbates maternal hypotension during epidural anesthesia in gravid ewes, it does not decrease uterine blood flow under such conditions.[33] (In other words, hypermagnesemia seems to protect uterine blood flow during modest hypotension in pregnant sheep.) Surprisingly, hypermagnesemia significantly worsens maternal hypotension in gravid ewes subjected to progressive hem-

orrhage.[88] These results provide important clues to the regulation and reflex control of uterine blood flow, and suggest that the administration of magnesium sulfate may be one of the few available methods of causing a selective decrease in uterine vascular resistance.

In addition to magnesium sulfate, beta-adrenergic agonists, calcium-entry blocking drugs, prostaglandin synthetase inhibitors, and nitroglycerin are administered for tocolysis. Ritodrine has no significant effect on uterine blood flow in gravid ewes, and it does not significantly alter the maternal hemodynamic response to hemorrhage.[87] Murad et al.[89] observed that verapamil (0.2 mg/kg) decreased maternal blood pressure and increased pulmonary artery pressure while decreasing uterine blood flow by 25% in pregnant sheep. Lindow et al.[90] observed that sublingual nifedipine decreased blood pressure but not uterine blood flow in women with preeclampsia. Many obstetricians now consider nifedipine the tocolytic agent of choice. Indomethacin produces only a transient reduction in uterine blood flow.[17]

Beta-adrenergic receptor antagonists, methyldopa, and vasodilators are commonly employed for the treatment of hypertension in pregnancy. Esmolol does not affect uterine blood flow, but one study noted that prolonged maternal infusion caused beta-adrenergic receptor blockade and hypoxemia in fetal lambs.[91,92] The maternal administration of labetalol, a mixed alpha- and beta-adrenergic receptor antagonist, produces little beta blockade in fetal lambs[93] and does not decrease uterine blood flow in humans.[94] Methyldopa is often used for the treatment of chronic hypertension during pregnancy, and it does not decrease uterine blood flow in pregnant women.[95] Hydralazine increases total uterine blood flow more than nitroprusside does during phenylephrine infusion, and it maintains placental perfusion during angiotensin II infusion in gravid ewes.[96,97] Hydralazine either improves or does not decrease intervillous blood flow when used to decrease blood pressure in hypertensive women; for these reasons, it remains a preferred vasodilator for the initial treatment of severe hypertension in most pregnant women. One exception may be the patient who is hypertensive due to cocaine intoxication. Vertommen et al.[30] found that hydralazine did not restore uterine blood flow and caused a marked maternal tachycardia when given to treat cocaine-induced hypertension in gravid ewes. Labetalol also fails to restore uterine blood flow, but it is not associated with maternal tachycardia.[98]

Both nitroglycerin and nitroprusside are clinically useful for the acute control of severe hypertension, and evidence in animals suggests that nitroglycerin is more likely to improve uterine blood flow.[99] However, these data are based on animals infused with a vasoconstrictor, an action that does not mimic the clinical situation. We suggest that clinicians choose a potent vasodilator on the basis of other considerations (e.g., availability, efficacy, toxicity) rather than on the basis of small differences in uterine blood flow in laboratory animals.

Finally, positive inotropic drugs rarely are indicated in obstetric patients. On the basis of studies of normal pregnant sheep, milrinone and amrinone can be expected to increase uterine blood flow, whereas dopamine and epinephrine can be expected to decrease it.[100,101] However, any direct but negative effect of these agents on the uterine vasculature may be blunted by improved cardiac function and arterial oxygenation and decreased sympathetic outflow. The choice of an inotropic agent should be based primarily on the desired efficacy (i.e., maternal considerations) rather than on the potential direct effects on uterine blood flow.

KEY POINTS

- Uteroplacental blood flow increases during pregnancy (beginning in the first trimester) and constitutes approximately 12% of maternal cardiac output at term.

- Substances released by vascular endothelium (e.g., prostacyclin, nitric oxide) help maintain uteroplacental perfusion and protect the uteroplacental circulation from endogenous vasoconstrictors. Preeclampsia is characterized by endothelial injury or dysfunction and a deficiency of these substances.

- Uteroplacental blood flow is reduced by a decrease in uterine arterial pressure, an increase in uterine venous pressure, and an increase in uterine vascular resistance.

- Doppler ultrasonography is the method most commonly used to estimate uterine blood flow in humans, but it is fraught with methodologic errors in a quantitative sense.

- Regional anesthesia can *increase* uterine blood flow by decreasing pain and stress. Regional anesthesia can *decrease* uterine blood flow by causing hypotension.

- Unintentional intravenous injection of epinephrine or a local anesthetic may cause a transient decrease in uterine blood flow.

- Intrathecal administration of sufentanil can cause hypotension and decreased uterine blood flow. Likewise, alpha$_2$-adrenergic agonists can cause hypotension and thereby would be expected to reduce uterine blood flow.

- Ephedrine is the vasopressor that is most likely to restore or protect uterine blood flow, and it remains the preferred vasopressor for most cases of hypotension in obstetric anesthesia practice. (Recent studies suggest that the enhanced release of nitric oxide in uterine blood vessels represents the primary mechanism of ephedrine's protection of uterine perfusion during pregnancy.) Alternatively, phenylephrine seems to be a safe choice when given in small doses titrated to effect. Phenylephrine may be preferred when clinical conditions (e.g., maternal tachycardia) dictate the use of an alpha-adrenergic agonist.

- The doses of general anesthetic agents used clinically have minimal direct effects on uterine blood flow. General anesthesia may decrease uterine blood flow by causing hypotension. Conversely, noxious stimulation during light anesthesia may precipitate the release of catecholamines, which results in decreased uterine blood flow.

- Magnesium sulfate appears to increase uterine blood flow.

- For cardiovascular emergencies, the choice of drug should depend primarily on drug efficacy rather than minor differences in the direct effects on uterine blood flow.

REFERENCES

1. Skillman CA, Plessinger MA, Woods JR, Clark KE. Effect of graded reductions in uteroplacental blood flow on the fetal lamb. Am J Physiol 1985; 149:1098-105.
2. Bilardo CM, Nicolaides KH, Campbell S. Doppler measurements of fetal and uteroplacental circulations: Relationship with umbilical venous blood gases measured at cordocentesis. Am J Obstet Gynecol 1990; 162:115-20.
3. Wehrenberg WB, Chaichareon DP, Dierschke DJ, et al. Vascular dynamics of the reproductive tract in the female rhesus monkey: Relative contributions of ovarian and uterine arteries. Biol Reprod 1977; 17:148-53.
4. Thaler I, Manor D, Itskovitz J, et al. Changes in uterine blood flow during human pregnancy. Am J Obstet Gynecol 1990; 162:121-5.
5. Palmer SK, Zamudio S, Coffin C, et al. Quantitative estimation of human uterine artery blood flow and pelvic blood flow redistribution in pregnancy. Obstet Gynecol 1992; 80:1000-6.
6. Yang D, Clark KE. Effect of endothelin-1 on the uterine vasculature of the pregnant and estrogen-treated nonpregnant sheep. Am J Obstet Gynecol 1992; 167:1642-50.
7. Weiner CP, Thompson LP, Liu K-Z, Herrig JE. Endothelium-derived relaxing factor and indomethacin-sensitive contracting factor alter arterial contractile responses to thromboxane during pregnancy. Am J Obstet Gynecol 1992; 166:1171-81.
8. Magness RR, Rosenfeld CR. Systemic and uterine responses to α-adrenergic stimulation in pregnant and nonpregnant ewes. Am J Obstet Gynecol 1986; 155:897-904.
9. Rosenfeld CR. Circulatory response to systemic infusion of norepinephrine in the pregnant ewe. Am J Obstet Gynecol 1977; 127:376-83.
10. Wheeler AS, James FM III, Meis PJ, et al. Effects of nitroglycerin and nitroprusside on the uterine vasculature of gravid ewes. Anesthesiology 1980; 52:390-4.
11. Anderson SG, Still JG, Greiss FC Jr. Differential reactivity of the gravid uterine vasculatures: Effects of norepinephrine. Am J Obstet Gynecol 1977; 129:293-7.
12. Ekesbo R, Alm P, Ekström P, et al. Innervation of the human uterine artery and contractile responses to neuropeptides. Gynecol Obstet Invest 1991; 31:30-6.
13. Shaul PW, Magness RR, Muntz KH, et al. α_1-Adrenergic receptors in pulmonary and systemic vascular smooth muscle: Alterations with development and pregnancy. Circ Res 1990; 67:1193-200.
14. Friedman SA. Preeclampsia: A review of the role of prostaglandins. Obstet Gynecol 1988; 71:122-37.
15. Magness RR, Rosenfeld CR, Faucher DJ, Mitchell MD. Uterine prostaglandin production in ovine pregnancy: Effects of angiotensin II and indomethacin. Am J Physiol Heart Circ Physiol 1992; 263:H188-97.
16. Magness RR, Rosenfeld CR, Hassan A, Shaul PW. Endothelial vasodilator production by uterine and systemic arteries. I. Effects of ANG II on PGI$_2$ and NO in pregnancy. Am J Physiol Heart Circ Physiol 1996; 270:H1914-23.
17. Sibai BM, Caritis SN, Thom E, et al: Prevention of preeclampsia with low-dose aspirin in healthy, nulliparous pregnant women. N Engl J Med 1993; 329:1213-8.
18. Lumbers ER. Effects of drugs on uteroplacental blood flow and the health of the foetus. Clin Exp Pharmacol Physiol 1997; 24:864-8.
19. Minuz P, Covi G, Paluani F, et al. Altered excretion of prostaglandin and thromboxane metabolites in pregnancy-induced hypertension. Hypertension 1988; 11(suppl 6):550-6.
20. Roberts JM, Taylor RN, Goldfien A. Clinical and biochemical evidence of endothelial cell dysfunction in the pregnancy syndrome preeclampsia. Am J Hypertens 1991; 4:700-8.
21. Weiner C, Martinez E, Zhu LK, et al. In vitro release of endothelium-derived relaxing factor by acetylcholine is increased during the guinea pig pregnancy. Am J Obstet Gynecol 1989; 161:1599-605.
22. Weiner C, Liu KZ, Thompson L, et al. Effect of pregnancy on endothelium and smooth muscle: Their role in reduced adrenergic sensitivity. Am J Physiol Heart Circ Physiol 1991; 261:H1275-83.
23. Weiner CP, Thompson LP. Nitric oxide and pregnancy. Semin Perinatol 1997; 21:367-80.
24. Holcberg G, Kossenjans W, Brewer A, et al. Selective vasodilator effects of atrial natriuretic peptide in the human placental vasculature. J Soc Gynecol Invest 1995; 2:1-5.
25. Grunewald C, Nisell H, Jansson T, et al. Possible improvement in uteroplacental blood flow during atrial natriuretic peptide infusion in preeclampsia. Obstet Gynecol 1994; 84:235-9.
26. Magness RR, Rosenfeld CR, Carr BR. Protein kinase C in uterine and systemic arteries during ovarian cycle and pregnancy. Am J Physiol Endocrinol Metab 1991; 260:E464-70.

27. Buhimschi IA, Hall G, Thompson LP, Weiner CP. Pregnancy and estradiol decrease GTPase activity in the guinea pig uterine artery. Am J Physiol Heart Circ Physiol 2001; 281:H2168-75.

28. Thompson LP, Weiner CP. Pregnancy enhances G protein activation and nitric oxide release from uterine arteries. Am J Physiol Heart Circ Physiol 2001; 280:H2069-75.

29. Landauer M, Phernetton TM, Rankin JHG. Maternal ovine placental vascular responses to adenosine. Am J Obstet Gynecol 1986; 154:1152-5.

30. Vertommen JD, Hughes SC, Rosen MA, et al. Hydralazine does not restore uterine blood flow during cocaine-induced hypertension in the pregnant ewe. Anesthesiology 1992; 76:580-7.

31. Ramsay B, De Belder A, Campbell S, et al. A nitric oxide donor improves uterine artery diastolic blood flow in normal early pregnancy and in women at high risk for preeclampsia. Eur J Clin Invest 1994; 24:76-8.

32. Cacciatore B, Halmesmäki E, Kaaja R, et al. Effect of transdermal nitroglycerin on impedance to flow in the uterine, umbilical, and fetal middle cerebral arteries in pregnancies complicated by preeclampsia and intrauterine growth retardation. Am J Obstet Gynecol 1998; 179:140-5.

33. Vincent RD Jr, Chestnut DH, Sipes SL, et al. Magnesium sulfate decreases maternal blood pressure but not uterine blood flow during epidural anesthesia in gravid ewes. Anesthesiology 1991; 74:77-82.

34. Jouppila R, Jouppila P, Hollmen A, Kuikka J. Effect of segmental extradural analgesia on placental blood flow during normal labour. Br J Anaesth 1978; 50:563-7.

35. Skjolderbrand A, Eklund J, Johansson H, et al. Uteroplacental blood flow measured by placental scintigraphy during epidural anaesthesia for caesarean section. Acta Anaesthesiol Scand 1990; 34:79-84.

36. Shnider SM, Wright RG, Levinson G, et al. Uterine blood flow and plasma norepinephrine changes during maternal stress in the pregnant ewe. Anesthesiology 1979; 50:524-7.

37. Lederman RP, Lederman E, Work B, McCann DS. Anxiety and epinephrine in multiparous labor: Relationship to duration of labor and fetal heart rate pattern. Am J Obstet Gynecol 1985; 153:870-7.

38. Wallis KL, Shnider SM, Hicks JS, Spivey HT. Epidural anesthesia in the normotensive pregnant ewe: Effects on uterine blood flow and fetal acid-base status. Anesthesiology 1976; 44:481-7.

39. Hollmen A, Jouppila R, Jouppila P, et al. Effect of extradural analgesia using bupivacaine and 2-chloroprocaine on intervillous blood flow during normal labour. Br J Anaesth 1982; 54:837-42.

40. Alahuhta S, Räsänen J, Jouppila R, et al. Uteroplacental and fetal haemodynamics during extradural anaesthesia for caesarean section. Br J Anaesth 1991; 66:319-23.

41. Jouppila P, Jouppila R, Hollmen A, Koivula A. Lumbar epidural analgesia to improve intervillous blood flow during labor in severe preeclampsia. Obstet Gynecol 1982; 59:158-61.

42. Peters J, Schlaghecke R, Thouet H, Arndt JO. Endogenous vasopressin supports blood pressure and prevents severe hypotension during epidural anesthesia in conscious dogs. Anesthesiology 1990; 73:694-702.

43. Carp H, Vadhera R, Jayaram A, Garvey D. Endogenous vasopressin and renin-angiotensin systems support blood pressure after epidural block in humans. Anesthesiology 1994; 80:1000-7.

44. Hood DD, Dewan DM, James FM III. Maternal and fetal effects of epinephrine in gravid ewes. Anesthesiology 1986; 64:610-3.

45. Chestnut DH, Weiner CP, Herrig JE. The effect of intravenously administered 2-chloroprocaine upon uterine artery blood flow velocity in gravid guinea pigs. Anesthesiology 1989; 70:305-8.

46. Fishburne JI Jr, Greiss FC Jr, Hopkinson R, Rhyne AL. Responses of the gravid uterine vasculature to arterial levels of local anesthetic agents. Am J Obstet Gynecol 1979; 133:753-61.

47. Hasselstrom LJ, Mogensen T, Kehlet H, Christensen NJ. Effects of intravenous bupivacaine on cardiovascular function and plasma catecholamine levels in humans. Anesth Analg 1984; 63:1053-8.

48. Johns RA. Local anesthetics inhibit endothelium-dependent vasodilation. Anesthesiology 1989; 70:805-11.

49. Kopacz DJ, Carpenter RL, Mackey DC. Effect of ropivacaine on cutaneous capillary blood flow in pigs. Anesthesiology 1989; 71:69-74.

50. Alahuhta S, Räsänen J, Jouppila P, et al. The effects of epidural ropivacaine and bupivacaine for cesarean section on uteroplacental and fetal circulation. Anesthesiology 1995; 83:23-32.

51. Craft JB, Coaldrake LA, Bolan JC, et al. Placental passage and uterine effects of fentanyl. Anesth Analg 1983; 62:894-8.

52. Craft JB, Bolan JC, Coaldrake LA, et al. The maternal and fetal cardiovascular effects of epidural morphine in the sheep model. Am J Obstet Gynecol 1982; 142:835-9.

53. Alahuhta S, Räsänen J, Jouppila P, et al. Epidural sufentanil and bupivacaine for labor analgesia and Doppler velocimetry of the umbilical and uterine arteries. Anesthesiology 1993; 78:231-6.

54. Honet JE, Arkoosh VA, Norris MC, et al. Comparison among intrathecal fentanyl, meperidine, and sufentanil for labor analgesia. Anesth Analg 1992; 75:734-9.

55. D'Angelo R, Anderson MT, Philip J, Eisenach JC. Intrathecal sufentanil compared to epidural bupivacaine for labor analgesia. Anesthesiology 1994; 80:1209-15.

56. Riley ET, Walker D, Hamilton CL, Cohen SE. Intrathecal sufentanil for labor analgesia does not cause a sympathectomy. Anesthesiology 1997; 87:874-8.

57. Romagnano MA, Hamill RW. Spinal sympathetic pathway: An enkephalin ladder. Science 1984; 225:737-9.

58. Li SJ, Han JS. Depressor and bradycardic effect following intrathecal injection of [NMePhe3,D-Pro4]morphiceptin in rats. Eur J Pharmacol 1984; 99:91-5.

59. Alahuhta S, Räsänen J, Jouppila R, et al. Effects of extradural bupivacaine with adrenaline for caesarean section on uteroplacental and fetal circulation. Br J Anaesth 1991; 67:678-2.

60. Bonica JJ, AkAmatsu TJ, Berges PU, et al. Circulatory effects of peridural block. II. Effects of epinephrine. Anesthesiology 1971; 34:514-22.

61. Alahuhta S, Räsänen J, Jouppila P, et al. Uteroplacental and fetal circulation during extradural bupivacaine-adrenaline and bupivacaine for caesarean section in hypertensive pregnancies with chronic fetal asphyxia. Br J Anaesth 1993; 71:348-53.

62. Eisenach JC, Castro MI, Dewan DM, Rose JC. Epidural clonidine analgesia in obstetrics: Sheep studies. Anesthesiology 1989; 70:51-6.

63. Eisenach JC, Castro MI, Dewan DM, Rose JC, et al. Intravenous clonidine hydrochloride toxicity in pregnant ewes. Am J Obstet Gynecol 1989; 160:471-6.

64. Eisenach JC, De Kock M, Klimscha W. α_2-Adrenergic agonists for regional anesthesia: A clinical review of clonidine (1984-1995). Anesthesiology 1996; 85:655-74.

65. James FM III, Greiss FC Jr, Kemp RA. An evaluation of vasopressor therapy for maternal hypotension during spinal anesthesia. Anesthesiology 1970; 33:25-34.

66. Eng M, Berges PU, Ueland K, et al. The effects of methoxamine and ephedrine in normotensive pregnant primates. Anesthesiology 1971; 35:354-60.

67. Lee A, Ngan Kee WD, Gin T. A quantitative, systematic review of randomized controlled trials of ephedrine versus phenylephrine for the management of hypotension during spinal anesthesia for cesarean delivery. Anesth Analg 2002; 94:920-6.

68. Cooper DW, Carpenter M, Mowbray P, et al. Fetal and maternal effects of phenylephrine and ephedrine during spinal anesthesia for cesarean delivery. Anesthesiology 2002; 97:1582-90.

69. Wright PMC, Iftikhar M, Fitzpatrick KT, et al. Vasopressor therapy for hypotension during epidural anesthesia for cesarean section: Effects on maternal and fetal flow velocity ratios. Anesth Analg 1992; 75:56-63.

70. Thomas DG, Robson SC, Redfern N, et al. Randomized trial of bolus phenylephrine or ephedrine for maintenance of arterial pressure during spinal anesthesia for caesarean section. Br J Anaesth 1996; 76:61-5.

71. Alahuhta S, Rasanen J, Jouppila P, et al. Ephedrine and phenylephrine for avoiding maternal hypotension due to spinal anesthesia for ceasarean section: Effects on uteroplacental and fetal haemodynamics. Int J Obstet Anesth 1992; 1:129-34.

72. Tong C, Eisenach JC. The vascular mechanism of ephedrine's beneficial effect on uterine perfusion during pregnancy. Anesthesiology 1992; 76:792-8.

73. Li P, Tong C, Eisenach JC. Pregnancy and ephedrine increase the release of nitric oxide in ovine uterine arteries. Anesth Analg 1996; 82:288-93.

74. Vincent RD Jr, Werhan CF, Norman PF, et al. Prophylactic angiotensin II infusion during spinal anesthesia for elective cesarean delivery. Anesthesiology 1998; 88:1475-9.

75. Jouppila P, Kuikka J, Jouppila R, Hollmen A. Effect of induction of general anesthesia for cesarean section on intervillous blood flow. Acta Obstet Gynecol Scand 1979; 58:249-53.

76. Alon E, Ball RH, Gillie MH, et al. Effects of propofol and thiopental on maternal and fetal cardiovascular and acid-base variables in the pregnant ewe. Anesthesiology 1993; 78:562-76.

77. Craft JB, Coaldrake LA, Yonekura JL, et al. Ketamine, catecholamines, and uterine tone in pregnant ewes. Am J Obstet Gynecol 1983; 146:429-34.

78. Galloon S. Ketamine for obstetric delivery. Anesthesiology 1976; 44:522-4.

79. Palahniuk RJ, Shnider SM. Maternal and fetal cardiovascular and acid-base changes during halothane and isoflurane anesthesia in the pregnant ewe. Anesthesiology 1974; 41:462-72.

80. Stein D, Masaoka T, Wlody D, et al. The effects of sevoflurane and isoflurane in pregnant sheep: Uterine blood flow and fetal well-being (abstract). Anesthesiology 1991; 75:A851.

81. Greiss FC Jr, Anderson SG, King LC. Uterine vascular bed: Effects of acute hypoxia. Am J Obstet Gynecol 1972; 113:1057-64.

82. Makowski EL, Hertz RH, Meschia G. Effect of acute maternal hypoxia and hyperoxia on the blood flow to the pregnant uterus. Am J Obstet Gynecol 1973; 115:624-9.

83. Morishima HO, Daniel SS, Adamsons K Jr, James LS. Effects of positive pressure ventilation of the mother upon the acid-base state of the fetus. Am J Obstet Gynecol 1965; 93:269-73.

84. Parer JT, Eng M, Aoba H, Ueland K. Uterine blood flow and oxygen uptake during maternal hyperventilation in monkeys at cesarean section. Anesthesiology 1970; 32:130-5.

85. Levinson G, Shnider SM, deLorimier AA, Steffenson JL. Effects of maternal hyperventilation on uterine blood flow and fetal oxygenation and acid-base status. Anesthesiology 1974; 40:340-7.

86. Keeley MM, Wade RV, Laurent SL, Hamann VD. Alterations in maternal-fetal Doppler flow velocity waveforms in preterm labor patients undergoing magnesium sulfate tocolysis. Obstet Gynecol 1993; 81: 191-4.

87. Sipes SL, Weiner CP, Gellhaus TM, Goodspeed JD. The plasma renin-angiotensin system in preeclampsia: Effects of magnesium sulfate. Obstet Gynecol 1989; 73:934-7.

88. Chestnut DH, Thompson CS, McLaughlin GL, Weiner CP. Does the intravenous infusion of ritodrine or magnesium sulfate alter the hemodynamic response to hemorrhage in gravid ewes? Am J Obstet Gynecol 1988; 159:1467-73.

89. Murad SHN, Tabsh KMA, Shilyanski G, et al. Effects of verapamil on uterine blood flow and maternal cardiovascular function in the awake pregnant ewe. Anesth Analg 1985; 64:7-10.

90. Lindow SW, Davies N, Davey DA, Smith JA. The effect of sublingual nifedipine on uteroplacental blood flow in hypertensive pregnancy. Br J Obstet Gynaecol 1988; 95:1276-81.

91. Östman PL, Chestnut DH, Robillard JE, et al. Transplacental passage and hemodynamic effects of esmolol in the gravid ewe. Anesthesiology 1988; 69:738-41.

92. Eisenach JC, Castro MI. Maternally administered esmolol produces fetal β-adrenergic blockade and hypoxemia in sheep. Anesthesiology 1989; 71:718-22.

93. Eisenach JC, Mandell G, Dewan DM. Maternal and fetal effects of labetalol in pregnant ewes. Anesthesiology 1991; 74:292-7.

94. Joupilla P, Kirkinen P, Koivula A, Ylikorkala O. Labetalol does not alter the placental and fetal blood flow or maternal prostanoids in preeclampsia. Br J Obstet Gynaecol 1986; 93:543-7.

95. Rey E. Effects of methyldopa on umbilical and placental artery blood flow velocity waveforms. Obstet Gynecol 1992; 80:783-7.

96. Ring G, Krames E, Shnider SM, et al. Comparison of nitroprusside and hydralazine in hypertensive pregnant ewes. Obstet Gynecol 1977; 50:598-602.

97. Pedron SL, Reid DL, Barnard JM, et al. Differential effects of intravenous hydralazine on myoendometrial and placental blood flow in hypertensive pregnant ewes. Am J Obstet Gynecol 1992; 167:1672-8.

98. Hughes SC, Vertommen JD, Rosen MA, et al. Cocaine induced hypertension in the ewe and response to treatment with labetalol (abstract). Anesthesiology 1991; 75:A1075.

99. Craft JB Jr, Co EG, Yonekura ML, Gilman RM. Nitroglycerin therapy for phenylephrine-induced hypertension in pregnant ewes. Anesth Analg 1980; 59:494-9.

100. Fishburne JI Jr, Dormer KJ, Payne GG, et al. Effects of amrinone and dopamine on uterine blood flow and vascular responses in the gravid baboon. Am J Obstet Gynecol 1988; 158:829-37.

101. Santos AC, Baumann AL, Wlody D, et al. The maternal and fetal effects of milrinone and dopamine in normotensive pregnant ewes. Am J Obstet Gynecol 1992; 166:257-62.

Chapter 4

The Placenta: Anatomy, Physiology, and Transfer of Drugs

Mark I. Zakowski, M.D. · Norman L. Herman, M.D., Ph.D.

The placenta presents unceremoniously after delivery of the neonate, and it has been given the undignified name *afterbirth*. This often-ignored structure is, in fact, a critical organ that should not be an afterthought in the study of obstetric anesthesia.

Revered by ancient cultures as the seat of the external soul or the bundle of life, the placenta has been held in high esteem by many peoples, and it has been the subject of many cultural rituals.[1] However, a true understanding of the indispensable role of the placenta in the development of the fetus did not begin to evolve until the seventeenth century. Much of the placenta's function remained a mystery until the development of microanatomic, biochemical, and molecular biologic techniques during the past 50 years. The concept of the placenta as a passive sieve (which does little more than serve as a conduit for oxygen, nutrients, and waste) has been dispelled. Rather, the placenta is a complex, dynamic organ.

The placenta brings the maternal and fetal circulations into close apposition for physiologic exchange across an immense area.[2] Massive exchange of materials occurs at this interface, without substantial interchange of maternal and fetal blood. This important function is accomplished within a complex structure that is almost entirely of fetal origin.

ANATOMY

Embryology

At implantation, the developing blastocyst erodes the surrounding decidua, leaving a sludge of cellular debris on which it survives. The placenta develops as the needs of the embryo outstrip its ability to gain oxygen and nutrients by simple diffusion. The syncytiotrophoblasts (invasive cells located at the margin of the growing conceptus) continue to erode the surrounding deciduas and the associated capillaries and arterioles of the spiral arteries until the blastocyst is surrounded by a sea of circulating maternal blood (trophoblastic lacunae).

The vitelline vein system develops in the yoke sac of the embryo to enhance the transport of nutrients, which diffuse from maternal blood through the trophoblast layer and the chorionic plate and into the chorionic cavity. The embryo exponentially accelerates its growth as its dependence on simple diffusion diminishes.[3]

At 2 weeks of development, the primitive extraembryonic mesoderm (cytotrophoblast layer) begins to proliferate and extend cellular fingers into the syncytiotrophoblast. These cytotrophoblast cell columns and their syncytiotrophoblast covering, which extend into the lacunae of maternal blood, are **primary villi**. Further mesodermal invasion into the core of the primary villi marks the progression of the primary villi into the **secondary villi**. Cellular differentiation of the villus mesoderm results in the formation of blood cells and vessels, which compose the villous vascular network. The presence of vessels within the villi changes their classification to **tertiary villi**. The vascular components of each villus develop connections within the chorionic plate and into the connecting stalk that connects the developing embryo and primitive placenta. Penetration of the cytotrophoblast continues through the syncytiotrophoblastic layer until many of the villi reach the decidua and form anchoring villi (Figure 4-1).[3]

With continued development, these initial villi branch extensively into treelike structures; the numerous branches extend into the lacunar (or intervillous) spaces, thereby increasing the surface area for transport. Further maturation of the villi results in a marked reduction in the cytotrophoblastic component and a decrease in the diffusional distance between the fetal villi and maternal intervillous blood.[3]

The growing embryo within the blastocyst connects to the chorion through a connecting or body stalk. Mesodermal components of this stalk coalesce to form the allantoic (or rudimentary umbilical) vessels (Figure 4-2). As the embryo continues its exponential growth phase, the connecting stalk shifts ventrally from its initial posterior attachment. The expansive open region at the ventral surface of the embryo constricts as the body wall grows and closes. By so doing, the body wall surrounds the yoke stalk, allantois, and developing vessels within the connecting stalk to form the primitive umbilicus. As the expanding amnion surrounds and applies itself over the connecting stalk and yoke sac, the cylindrical umbilical cord takes on its mature form.[3]

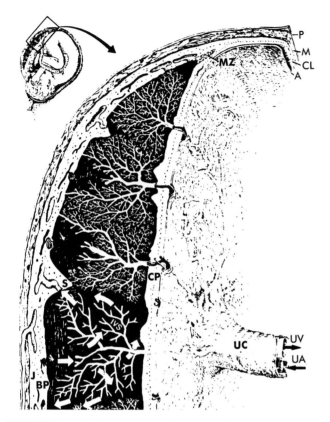

FIGURE 4-1. The placenta is a complex structure that brings the maternal and fetal circulations into close apposition for exchange of substances. *A,* Amnion; *BP,* basal plate; *CL,* chorionic laeve; *CP,* chorionic plate; *IVS,* intervillous space; *J,* junctional zone; *M,* myometrium; *MZ,* marginal zone; *P,* perimetrium; *S,* septum; *UA,* umbilical artery; *UC,* umbilical cord; *UV,* umbilical vein. (From Kaufmann P, Scheffen I. Placental development. In Polin RA, Fox WW, editors. Fetal and Neonatal Physiology, 2nd ed. Philadelphia, WB Saunders, 1998:59-70.)

The placenta grows dramatically from the third month of gestation until term. A direct correlation exists between the growth of the placenta and the growth of the fetus. By term, the mature placenta is oval and flat, with an average diameter of 18.5 cm, an average weight of 500 g, and an average thickness of 23 mm.[4] Wide variations in size and shape are within the range of normal and make little difference in function.

Comparative Anatomy

Great variation exists among the placentas of different species. The varieties of placental attachment (i.e., implantation) include adhesion, interdigitation, and fusion. In addition, there are differences in the number of tissue layers between the maternal and fetal circulations at their point of apposition. The most commonly used placental categorization system—the Grossner classification—uses the number of tissue layers of the placental barrier to classify the differences among species (Figure 4-3).[5] This system is imperfect and has been modified, but it remains a useful means of placental classification.

Animal studies have noted differences in placental function among species. The sheep is the most frequently used animal model of placental transfer because of its availability and the relatively easy access to the placenta. The sheep placenta has a markedly thicker epitheliochorial placenta, with all three maternal layers (epithelium, connective tissues, and endothelium) separating maternal blood from fetal blood. By contrast, the human hemochorial placenta lacks these maternal layers, and maternal blood directly bathes fetal tissues (Figure 4-3). For example, fatty acids do not cross the sheep placenta as they do in humans.[6] This wide diversity of placental structure and function among species makes extrapolation from animal experiments to clinical medicine tenuous.

Vascular Architecture

MATERNAL

Under the initial hormonal influences of the corpus luteum, the spiral arteries of the uterus become elongated and more extensively coiled. In the area beneath the developing conceptus, the compression and erosion of the decidua induces

FIGURE 4-2. The embryo at 19 days' gestation, showing the connecting stalk (the rudimentary umbilical cord) that connects the embryo and chorion with the developing placenta. The vascular system develops from the extraembryonic mesoderm of the yolk sac and chorion. (From Sadler TW. Langman's Medical Embryology, 7th ed. Baltimore, Williams and Wilkins, 1995:72.)

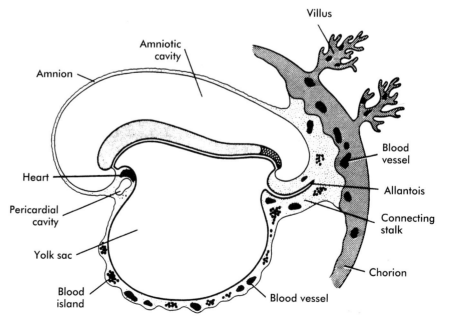

lateral looping of the already convoluted spiral arteries.[7] These vessels under the placenta gain access to the intervillous spaces. In late pregnancy, the increasing demands of the developing fetus require the 200 spiral arteries that directly feed the placenta to handle a blood flow of approximately 600 mL/min.[7] The vasodilation required to accommodate this flow is the result of the replacement of the elastic and muscle components of the artery, initially by cytotrophoblast cells and later by fibroid cells. This replacement reduces the vasoconstrictor activity of these arteries and exposes the vessels to the dilating forces of the increased blood volume of pregnancy, especially at the terminal segments, where they form funnel-shaped sacs as they enter the intervillous space.[7] The increased diameter of the vessels slows blood flow and reduces blood pressure.

The intervillous space is a large cavernous expanse into which the villous trees reach. It develops from the fusion of the trophoblastic lacunae of maternal blood, and it increases in size as the decidua is eroded by the expanding development of the blastocyst. This huge blood sinus is bounded by the chorionic plate and the decidua basalis (i.e., the maternal or basal plate). Folds in the basal plate form septae that separate the space into 13 to 30 anatomic compartments known as *lobules*. Each lobule contains numerous villous trees that are also known as *cotyledons* or *placentones*. Although it is packed with highly branched villous trees, the intervillous space of the mature placenta can accommodate approximately 350 mL of maternal blood.[8]

Maternal arterial blood leaves the funnel-shaped spiral arteries and enters the intervillous space. The blood first moves into the nearly hollow, low-resistance area, where villi are very loosely packed (the intercotyledonary space) (Figure 4-4).[9] Maternal blood then moves fairly homogeneously into the region of the densely packed intermittent and terminal villi. The densely packed zone of terminal villi represents the area

in which placental exchange predominates. After passing through this dense region, maternal venous blood collects between neighboring villous trees in an area called the *perilobular zone*.[10] Collecting veins penetrate the maternal plate at the periphery of the villous trees to drain perilobular blood from the intervillous space.

As the trophoblasts of the early blastocyst invade the decidua to form the trophoblastic lacunae that ultimately coalesce into the intervillous space, they invade the walls of existing endometrial venous channels. Blood from the intervillous space is drained through these fenestrations in decidual veins created by the trophoblasts. Initially the space is drained by masses of veins; however, as pregnancy progresses, increasing pressure on the uterine wall from intrauterine contents drastically reduces the number of these draining veins. In addition, these veins exhibit the same changes (i.e., atrophy of the tunica media and replacement with fibroid cells) that are seen in the spiral arteries.[4,10] The remaining venous channels dilate to accommodate the increasing venous return from the placenta.[7]

FETAL

Two coiled umbilical arteries conduct fetal blood within the umbilical cord to the placenta. These two arteries separate and course along the chorionic surface, where they further divide into the chorionic arteries that feed the multiple placental lobules. Chorionic arteries plunge beneath the chorionic plate to further subdivide and feed the villous trees (Figure 4-5).[4,11]

The arterial supply to the approximately 50 villous trees in the normal human placenta is complex. After an artery perforates the chorionic plate, it becomes the main villous stem or truncal artery at the base of the villous tree (first-order vessel). After a short distance, it branches into four to eight ramal or cotyledonary arteries (second-order vessels), which course

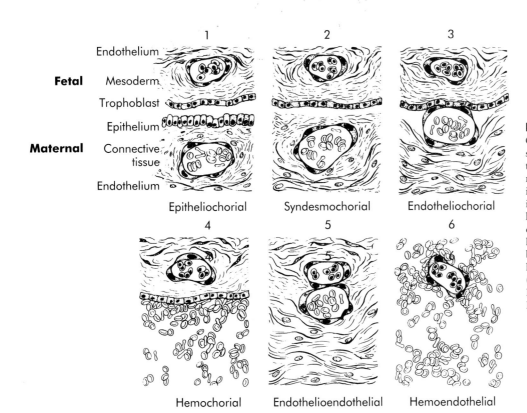

Fetal
Endothelium
Mesoderm
Trophoblast

Maternal
Epithelium
Connective tissue
Endothelium

1   2   3

Epitheliochorial   Syndesmochorial   Endotheliochorial

4   5   6

Hemochorial   Endothelioendothelial   Hemoendothelial

FIGURE 4-3. Modification of Grossner's original classification scheme, showing the number and types of tissue layers between the fetal and maternal circulations. Examples of each include the following: *(1)* epitheliochorial, sheep; *(2)* syndesmochorial, no known examples; *(3)* endotheliochorial, dogs and cats; *(4)* hemochorial, man and hamster; *(5)* endothelioendothelial, bandicoot (Australian opossum); and *(6)* hemoendothelial, Rocky Mountain pika. (From Ramsey EM. The Placenta: Human and Animal. New York, Praeger Publishers, 1982.)

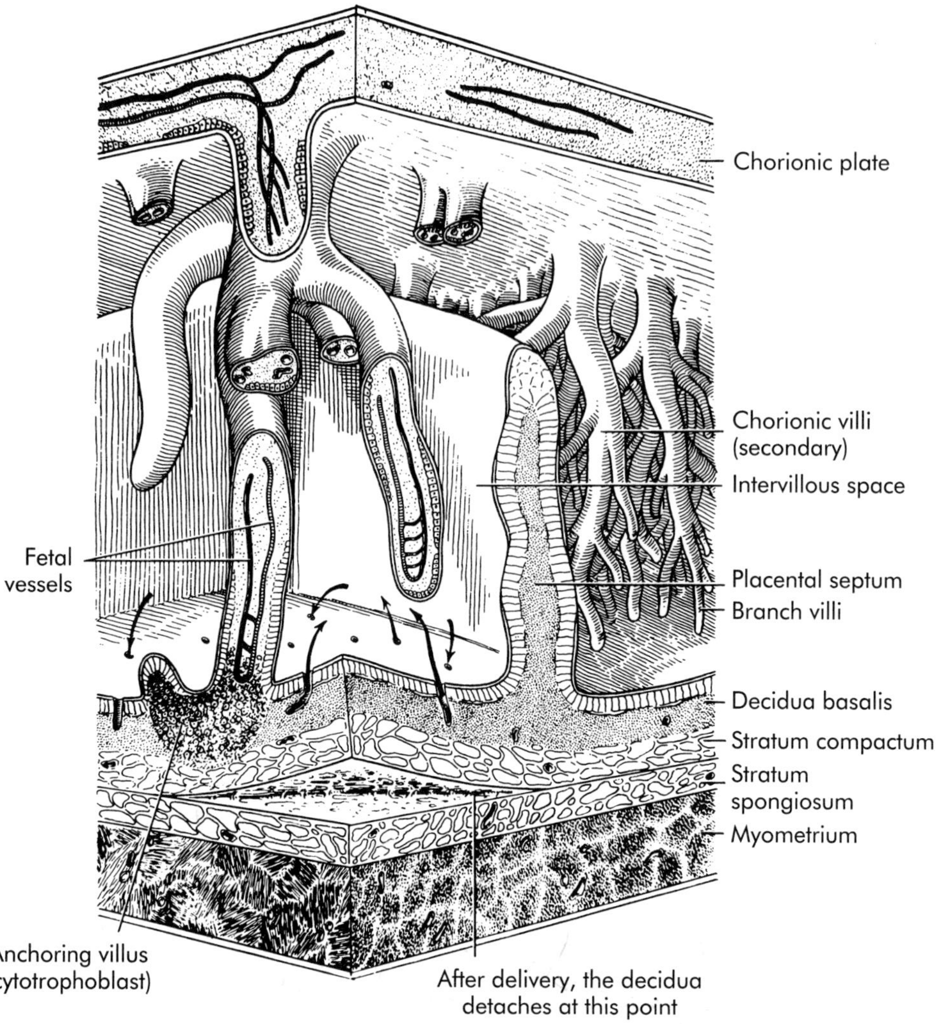

FIGURE 4-4. The relationship between the villous tree and maternal blood flow. The arrows indicate the maternal blood flow from the spiral arteries into the intervillous space and back out through the spiral veins. (From Tuchmann-Duplessis H, David G, Haegel P. Illustrated Human Embryology. Vol 1: Embryogenesis. New York, Springer Verlag, 1972: 73.)

Chorionic plate

Chorionic villi (secondary)

Intervillous space

Placental septum

Branch villi

Decidua basalis

Stratum compactum

Stratum spongiosum

Myometrium

Fetal vessels

Anchoring villus (cytotrophoblast)

After delivery, the decidua detaches at this point

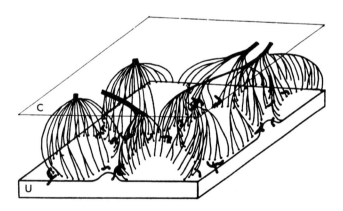

FIGURE 4-5. The dispersal of chorionic arteries through the chorionic plate *(C)* and into the villous trees (or placentones or cotyledons) of the human placenta. *U,* Basal plate of the uterus. (From Gruenwald P. Lobular architecture of primate placentas. In Gruenwald P, editor. The Placenta and Its Maternal Supply Line: Effects of Insufficiency on the Fetus. Baltimore, University Park Press, 1975:35-55.)

parallel to the chorionic plate for a variable length and then curve toward the maternal plate. As they pass toward the maternal plate, they further subdivide into third-order vessels (ramulus chorii).[4]

The third-order vessels course along the branches of the tree (intermediate villi) out toward the terminal villi, where they form the terminal arterioles. The terminal arterioles lead through a neck region to form two to four narrow capillaries within convolutions (or bulbous enlargements) of the terminal villi. The capillary loops within these convolutions dilate to form the fetal sinusoids (Figure 4-6). This massive increase in endothelial surface area—in conjunction with the near absence of connective tissue—makes these the optimal regions for maternal-fetal exchange (Figure 4-7).[10,12]

The venous ends of the capillary coils narrow and return through the neck region to collecting venules, which coalesce to form larger veins as they course toward the stems of the villous tree. Each villous tree drains into a large vein that perforates the chorionic plate to become a chorionic vein. All of the venous tributaries course toward the umbilical cord attachment site, where they empty into one umbilical vein that returns blood to the fetus.

PHYSIOLOGY

Barrier Function

Much has been made of the concept of the placental barrier. However, it is an imperfect barrier: occasionally even red blood cells cross the placenta, and we now understand that almost all substances cross the placenta. Placental transfer varies according to the degree of permeability; however, some mechanisms may restrict fetal exposure. First, a vast array of

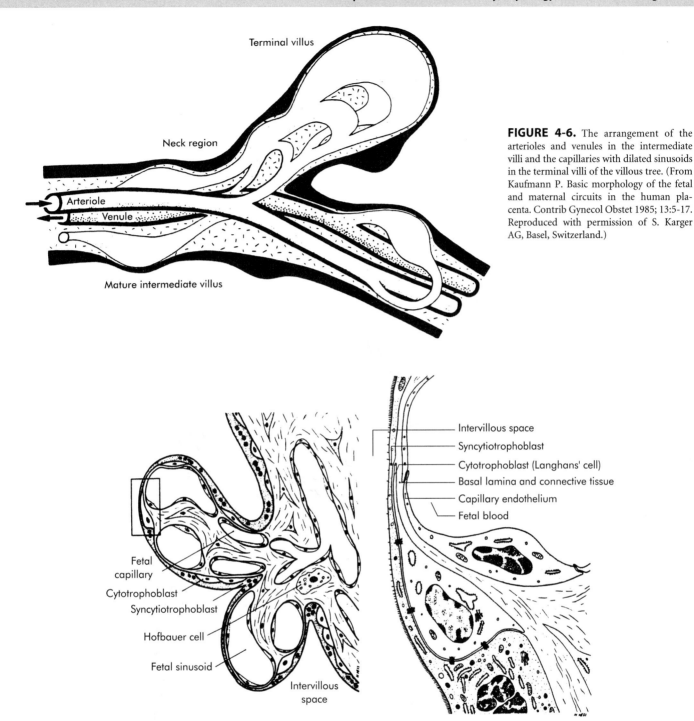

FIGURE 4-6. The arrangement of the arterioles and venules in the intermediate villi and the capillaries with dilated sinusoids in the terminal villi of the villous tree. (From Kaufmann P. Basic morphology of the fetal and maternal circuits in the human placenta. Contrib Gynecol Obstet 1985; 13:5-17. Reproduced with permission of S. Karger AG, Basel, Switzerland.)

FIGURE 4-7. Two terminal villi showing their cellular morphology at lower magnification *(left)*. The higher magnification (of the boxed region in the left diagram) exhibits the placental barrier between fetal and maternal blood *(right)*. (From Kaufmann P. Basic morphology of the fetal and maternal circuits in the human placenta. Contrib Gynecol Obstet 1985; 13:5-17. Reproduced with permission of S. Karger AG, Basel, Switzerland.)

cytochrome P-450 isoenzymes are found within the placenta; some of these are inducible, whereas others are constitutive.[13] The inducible enzymes are mainly of the 3-methylcholanthrene-inducible type rather than the phenobarbital-inducing variety found in the liver. The role these oxidative enzymes may play in reducing fetal exposure is poorly understood. Second, some substances may be bound (by specific or nonspecific binding) within placental tissue, and this binding may minimize fetal exposure and accumulation.[14] Third, diffusion may be influenced by membrane thickness. The thickness of the placental barrier decreases as gestation progresses, which

should increase the rate of diffusion.[15] However, the rate of transfer of some substances (e.g., glucose, water) differs very little among species, even though the placental thickness varies greatly.[16] Therefore, placental barrier thickness cannot be the only determinant of the ease of placental transfer.

Hormonal Function

Through a sophisticated transfer of precursor and intermediate compounds in the maternal-fetal-placental unit, placental enzymes convert steroid precursors into estrogens and progesterone. This steroidogenic function of the placenta begins very early during pregnancy; however, it is not until 35 to 47 days postovulation that the placental production of estrogen and progesterone exceeds that of the corpus luteum (i.e., the ovarian-placental shift).[17]

The placenta is also a vast protein synthetic factory that produces a wide array of enzymes, binding proteins, and polypeptide hormones. For example, the placenta produces human chorionic gonadotropin, human placental lactogen (a growth hormone also known as *human chorionic somatomammotropin*), all of the hypothalamic release and inhibitory factors, and a myriad of other control proteins.[17] These protein and steroid hormones produced by the placenta allow it to influence and control the environment in which it and the fetus exist.

Regulation of Placental Blood Flow

MATERNAL BLOOD FLOW
In addition to the trophoblastic invasion of the musculoelastic lining of the spiral arteries, a functional denervation of these arteries also occurs; this is demonstrated by a decrease in perivascular concentrations of dopamine and norepinephrine.[18] This denervation may represent an adaptive mechanism that decreases vascular reactivity.[19] Both pregnancy-induced adaptations keep the spiral arteries vasodilated by as much as 10 times their normal diameters.[20] These low-resistance pathways shunt blood to the intervillous spaces to ensure adequate perfusion.

Maternal blood (at a pressure of 70 to 80 mm Hg) enters the intervillous space within the center of a cotyledon (a zone relatively free of villi).[7] The pressure of this arterial jet of blood rapidly diminishes to approximately 10 mm Hg, and the velocity of blood flow decreases as it passes from the basal plate into the high-resistance, densely packed villi of the placentone.[15]

FETAL BLOOD FLOW
Effective exchange also requires adequate fetoplacental blood flow. Fetoplacental blood flow increases gradually during pregnancy; however, unlike maternoplacental blood flow, this increase probably reflects vascular growth of the villous beds to a greater extent than vasodilation.[21] Fetoplacental blood flow is autoregulated and is independent of catecholamines or angiotensin for the maintenance of basal arteriolar tone.[22] The mechanism of this autoregulatory process is not well defined. Maternal hyperglycemia[23] and hypoxemia[24] are examples of

derangements that cause alterations in regional fetal blood flow, probably through vascular mediators of vasodilation or vasoconstriction. There is increasing evidence of the role of endothelium-derived relaxing factors—especially prostacyclin[25] and nitric oxide[26]—in the control of fetoplacental circulation. Recent evidence suggests that hypoxia-induced fetoplacental vasoconstriction is mediated by a reduction in basal release of nitric oxide.[27]

The placenta's functional similarities to the lung are reflected in the hypoxia-induced vasoconstrictor activity of the perfused human placenta.[24] By this mechanism, the placenta may be able to optimize fetal oxygenation through the redistribution of fetal blood flow from lobules in hypoxic regions to lobules in better perfused zones.

Transport Mechanisms
Substances are transferred across the placenta by one of several mechanisms. These processes have been reviewed extensively elsewhere.[28-31]

PASSIVE TRANSPORT
The passive transfer of molecules across a membrane depends on the following: (1) concentration and electrochemical differences across the membrane; (2) molecular weight; (3) lipid solubility; (4) degree of ionization; and (5) membrane surface area and thickness. This process requires no expenditure of cellular energy. Transfer is driven solely by the concentration and potential differences across a membrane. Simple transmembrane diffusion can occur either through the lipid membrane (e.g., lipophilic molecules and water) or within protein channels that traverse the lipid bilayer (e.g., charged substances such as ions) (Figure 4-8).[30,32]

FACILITATED TRANSPORT
Carrier-mediated transport of relatively lipid-insoluble molecules down their concentration gradient is called *facilitated diffusion*.[32] Facilitated diffusion differs from simple diffusion in several ways. Specifically, this mode of transfer exhibits the following: (1) saturation kinetics; (2) competitive and noncompetitive inhibition; (3) stereospecificity; and (4) temperature influences (e.g., an increased temperature results in increased transfer).[29] With simple diffusion, the net rate of diffusion is proportional to the difference in

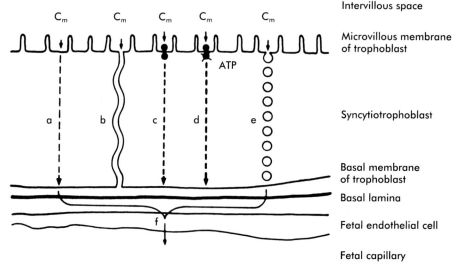

FIGURE 4-8. The transfer mechanisms used for the transfer of substances across the placental barrier: *a*, simple diffusion; *b*, simple diffusion through channels; *c*, facilitated diffusion; *d*, active transport; *e*, endocytosis. C_m, Intervillous concentration at the trophoblastic membrane. (From Morriss FH Jr, Boyd RDH, Mahendran D. Placental transport. In: Knobil E, Neill JD, editors. The Physiology of Reproduction, 2nd ed. New York, Raven Press, 1994; 2:813-61.)

concentrations between the two sides of the membrane. This is the case for facilitated diffusion only when transmembrane concentration differences are small. At higher concentration gradients, a maximum rate of transfer (V_{max}) is reached; thereafter, a further increase in the concentration gradient does not affect the rate of transfer. Intramembrane protein carrier molecules assist in transmembrane transport. The rate of transfer is determined by the number of membranous carrier complexes and the degree of interaction between the carrier and the substance that is undergoing transport.[30] An example of facilitated diffusion is the transplacental transfer of glucose.

A special type of facilitated diffusion involves the "uphill" transport of molecules, which is not directly driven by cellular energy expenditure. Transfer by this mechanism involves the uphill transport of a substance linked to another substance traveling down its own concentration gradient. In most cases, sodium is the molecule that facilitates transport. For the membrane-bound carrier to transfer these molecules, both molecules must be bound to the carrier. This hybrid system is called **secondary active transport** or **co-transport**.[29,30] Much of the transplacental transport of amino acids appears to occur by means of secondary active transport.

ACTIVE TRANSPORT

When the movement of any substance across a cell membrane is linked to the metabolic activity of that cell, the movement is called *active transport*. In general, net transport occurs against a concentration, electrical, or pressure gradient; however, not all active transport need be uphill.[29] Active transport requires cellular energy. If this energy supply is blocked, active transport ceases.

Like facilitated diffusion, active transport requires a protein membrane carrier that exhibits saturation kinetics and competitive inhibition (Figure 4-8).[32] However, unlike secondary active transport, this movement of a substance against its concentration gradient is directly linked to the hydrolysis of high-energy phosphate bonds of adenosine triphosphate (ATP). The best known example of primary active transport is the translocation of sodium and potassium through the Na^+/K^+ ATPase pump.

PINOCYTOSIS

Large macromolecules (e.g., proteins that exhibit negligible diffusion properties) still find their way across cell membranes. By the process of pinocytosis (a type of endocytosis), the cell membrane invaginates around the macromolecule to surround it with a membrane vesicle; this process usually requires energy. Many pinocytotic vesicles are subject to intracellular digestion; however, electron microscopic studies have demonstrated that some vesicles move across the cytoplasm and fuse with the membrane at the opposite pole.[33] This appears to be the mechanism by which immunoglobulin G is transferred from the maternal to the fetal circulation.[32,34]

OTHER FACTORS THAT INFLUENCE PLACENTAL TRANSPORT

Other factors that affect maternal-fetal exchange include the following: (1) changes in maternal and fetal blood flow[35]; (2) placental binding[14]; (3) placental metabolism[13,36]; (4) diffusion capacity[15]; (5) degree of maternal and fetal plasma protein binding[28]; and (6) gestational age (i.e., the placenta is more permeable during early pregnancy than at term).[37]

Transfer of Respiratory Gases and Nutrients

OXYGEN

As the "lung" for the fetus, the placenta allows the transfer of adequate oxygen for fetal growth and development. The placenta must supply approximately 8 mL O_2/min/kg fetal body weight[38] with only one fifth of the oxygen transfer efficiency of the adult lung.[39] It is necessary to determine changes in oxygen tension on both sides of the diffusional surface (i.e., within the placenta itself) to determine the transplacental diffusion capacity for oxygen. However, this is not practical. Therefore, blood must be obtained from the uterine and umbilical vessels. One study in sheep revealed a transplacental pressure gradient of 37 to 42 mm Hg,[40] which suggests a poor diffusion capacity for oxygen. Subsequently, other researchers have determined that these measurements are inaccurate; they do not represent true end-capillary O_2 tensions for at least three reasons. First, approximately 16% of uterine blood flow and 6% of umbilical blood flow are shunted around diffusional areas of the placenta, which results in an admixture.[15] Second, unlike the lung, the placenta uses a significant amount of the oxygen that is transferred; this accounts for 20% to 30% of the oxygen consumed by the fetal-placental unit.[41,42] Third, the uterus uses oxygen, which also contributes to the inaccuracy of using umbilical and uterine venous P_{O_2} to calculate the placental diffusion capacity for respiratory gases.

By contrast, carbon monoxide is not used by any organ; therefore it is not affected by shunt or consumption. When placental diffusion capacity was estimated using carbon monoxide, it was found to be four times greater than that obtained with calculations made from arterial-venous P_{O_2} differences.[43] Because oxygen and carbon monoxide have similar coefficients of diffusion, the placental diffusion capacity for oxygen must be essentially the same as that for carbon monoxide. Therefore, as with carbon monoxide, the transfer of oxygen is limited by flow and not by diffusion.[15]

The force that drives oxygen across the placenta is the difference in P_{O_2} between maternal and fetal blood. As physically dissolved oxygen diffuses across the villous membranes, bound oxygen is released by maternal hemoglobin in the intervillous space, and it too diffuses across the placenta. Several factors affect the fetal blood P_{O_2} at the completion of end-capillary equilibration within the villus. The geometry of the relationship between maternal and fetal blood flow plays a key role. Both concurrent and countercurrent arrangements of maternal and fetal blood flow have been identified in the placenta of various species. Studies that have demonstrated an almost complete equilibration of maternal and fetal P_{O_2} suggest that a concurrent (or parallel) relationship between maternal and fetal blood exists within the human placenta (Figure 4-9).[15,44] One study demonstrated that umbilical venous P_{O_2} was slightly higher than intervillous P_{O_2}, which would suggest a more complex, multivillous pool relationship.[45] In addition, the differences between the oxyhemoglobin dissociation curves of maternal and fetal blood may influence transplacental oxygen transfer to the fetus,[46] although this is a matter of some dispute.[15] The fetal oxyhemoglobin dissociation curve is positioned to the left of the maternal oxyhemoglobin dissociation curve because of the lower P_{50} for fetal blood in vivo (see Figure 5-3). In theory, this enhances oxygen uptake by fetal red blood cells and promotes the transfer of additional oxygen across the placenta. The **Bohr effect** may also augment the transfer of oxygen

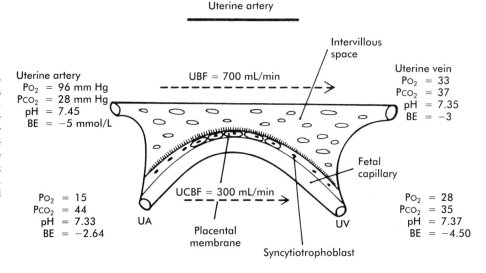

FIGURE 4-9. The concurrent relationship between the maternal and fetal circulations within the placenta and the way this arrangement affects gas transfer. These values were obtained from patients breathing room air during elective cesarean section. *BE,* Base excess; *UA,* umbilical artery; *UBF,* uterine blood flow; *UCBF,* umbilical cord blood flow; *UV,* umbilical vein. (From Ramanathan S. Obstetric Anesthesia. Philadelphia, Lea and Febiger, 1988:27.)

across the placenta. Specifically, concomitant fetal-to-maternal transfer of carbon dioxide makes maternal blood more acidic and fetal blood more alkalotic, which causes a right shift in the maternal oxyhemoglobin dissociation curve and a left shift in the fetal oxyhemoglobin dissociation curve. Both changes enhance the transfer of oxygen from mother to fetus. This "double" Bohr effect accounts for 2% to 8% of the transplacental transfer of oxygen.[47]

The maximum fetal arterial Po_2 is never greater than 50 to 60 mm Hg (even when maternal fractional inspired oxygen concentration [Fio_2] is 1.0), for several reasons. First, the placenta tends to function as a venous rather than an arterial equilibrator. Because of the shape of the maternal oxyhemoglobin dissociation curve, an increase in maternal Pao_2 above 100 mm Hg does not result in a substantial increase in maternal arterial oxygen content. Therefore, under conditions of constant uterine and umbilical blood flow and fetal oxygen consumption, fetal Pao_2 increases only slightly when maternal Fio_2 is increased. Although this increase in Pao_2 is of limited significance at normal levels of fetal Pao_2, it may be more important at decreased levels of fetal Pao_2 that are closer to the P_{50} of fetal blood (approximately 21 mm Hg in humans), because the fetal oxyhemoglobin dissociation curve is rather steep in that range. Second, the placenta itself has a relatively high rate of oxygen consumption, which lowers the amount of oxygen transferred to the umbilical circulation (see Chapter 5). Third, fetal arterial blood is a mixture of oxygenated umbilical venous blood and deoxygenated inferior vena cava blood (which returns centrally from the fetal lower extremities).

CARBON DIOXIDE

An understanding of the transfer of carbon dioxide is complicated by the number of different forms it takes in the blood. It is present as dissolved CO_2, carbonic acid (H_2CO_3), bicarbonate ion (HCO_3^-), carbonate ion (CO_3^{2-}), and carbaminohemoglobin. Dissolved CO_2 (8%) and HCO_3^- (62%) are the predominant forms involved in the transplacental transfer of carbon dioxide, because the concentrations of H_2CO_3 and CO_3^{2-} are almost negligible, and carbaminohemoglobin (30%) is present only within red blood cells.[15,39] The equilibrium between CO_2 and HCO_3^- is maintained by a reaction that is catalyzed by carbonic anhydrase in red blood cells.

A difference in Pco_2 normally exists between fetal and maternal blood (i.e., 40 mm Hg versus 34 mm Hg, respectively); this gradient favors fetal-to-maternal transfer. Carbon dioxide readily crosses the placenta; it is 20 times more diffusible than oxygen.[39] However, dissolved CO_2 is the form of carbon dioxide that actually crosses the placenta. As CO_2 rapidly moves from fetal capillary blood to maternal blood, the principle of La Chatelier causes a shift in the equilibrium of the carbonic anhydrase reaction, which produces more CO_2 for diffusion. The transfer of CO_2 is augmented further by the **Haldane effect** within the maternal blood. The maternal-to-fetal transfer of oxygen produces deoxyhemoglobin in the maternal blood, which has a greater affinity for CO_2 than does oxyhemoglobin. The Haldane effect may account for as much as 46% of the transplacental transfer of carbon dioxide.[47] Although a sizable fetal-maternal concentration gradient exists for HCO_3^-, its charged nature impedes its transfer, and therefore it is not a major contributor to carbon dioxide transport except as a source for the production of more CO_2 through the carbonic anhydrase reaction.[48]

GLUCOSE

Simple diffusion alone cannot explain the transfer of concentrations of glucose that are adequate for meeting the demands of the placenta and the fetus. Studies have demonstrated a stereospecific facilitated diffusion system for the movement of glucose down its concentration gradient, which does not depend on insulin, a sodium gradient, or cellular energy.[49,50] A D-glucose transport protein has been identified within the various components of the trophoblast membrane.[51] The placenta, which must maintain its own metabolic processes, competes with the fetus for maternal glucose. At term, only 28% of the glucose absorbed from the maternal surface is transferred to the umbilical vein.[32]

AMINO ACIDS

Concentrations of amino acids in umbilical venous blood exceed those found in maternal blood, and the concentrations in the placenta are higher than both of these.[52] The maternal-fetal transplacental transfer of amino acids is an active process that is inhibited by metabolic inhibitors; the energy required for this transfer apparently comes from the large gradient for sodium established by the Na+/K+ ATPase pump.[53] Much of the transplacental transport of amino acids appears to occur by way of linked carriers for both amino acids and sodium. The binding of sodium and amino acids allows for their translocation across the placenta. The transport of sodium down its concentration gradient "drags" amino acids into the cell. This results in increased intracellular concentrations of amino acids, which then "leak" down their gradients into the fetal circulation. However, this may not be the case for all amino acids. For example, histidine does not exhibit an elevated intracellular concentration.[15]

FATTY ACIDS

Free fatty acids cross the human placenta—but not the ovine placenta—in significant amounts.[6,54,55] Radiolabeled palmitic and linoleic acids readily cross the perfused human placenta.[56] A concentration gradient from mother to fetus exists for most fatty acids (with arachidonic acid being the most notable exception[57]), and evidence suggests that the rate of transfer depends on the magnitude of this gradient.[55] These findings imply that fatty acids cross the placenta by means of simple diffusion, although the actual mechanism remains unclear.

DRUG TRANSFER

Placental permeability and pharmacokinetics help determine the fetal exposure to a maternal drug. Animal models (e.g., pregnant ewes, in situ perfusion of the guinea pig placenta) have been used to assess the placental transport of drugs. Interspecies differences in anatomy and function limit the application of these data to humans.[58] Investigations of transport within the human placenta have been performed on placental slices, isolated villi, membrane vesicles, homogenates, and tissue culture cells. However, the direct application of these data is also in question, because these models do not account for the dual (i.e., maternal and fetal) perfusion of the intact placenta in situ.[58]

The inaccessibility of the placenta in situ and concerns for maternal and fetal safety have limited direct studies of the placenta in humans. Only one published study has reported the real-time pharmacokinetics of the transfer of an anesthetic drug across the human placenta in vivo.[59] This type of direct human testing would not be allowed in the present medicolegal environment. Data about the transplacental transfer of anesthetic agents have been extrapolated primarily from single measurements of drug concentrations in maternal and umbilical cord blood samples obtained at delivery. Most studies have reported fetal:maternal (F/M) ratios of the drug concentration. (In these studies, the umbilical vein blood concentrations represent the fetal blood concentrations of the drug.)

Single-measurement studies obtain only one set of measurements for each parturient. Maternal and fetal concentrations of a drug are influenced by drug metabolism in the mother, the placenta, and the fetus and also by changes at delivery (e.g., altered uteroplacental blood flow).[58,60] Unless a study includes a large number of patients with variable durations of exposure, it is difficult to reach conclusions about the type and time course of transplacental transfer of an individual drug. In addition, single-measurement studies only provide information on the **net transfer** of a drug across the maternal-placental-fetal unit and do not allow for the determination of unidirectional fluxes at any point (i.e., maternal-to-fetal or fetal-to-maternal). Nonetheless, these studies have provided the best data available for most anesthetic agents.

Investigators have developed a dual-perfused, in vitro human placental model that allows for the independent perfusion of the maternal and fetal sides of the placenta and thereby permits the investigation of maternal-to-fetal (or fetal-to-maternal) transport. The validity of this method for the study of placental transfer has been well established.[58] Equilibration studies (i.e., recirculating maternal and fetal perfusates) using this model probably are not directly applicable to the placenta in vivo.[61] However, when a non-recirculating scheme is used, steady-state clearance of a drug can be determined for either direction (maternal-to-fetal or fetal-to-maternal) and may have direct application to the actual clinical situation. A number of studies have used this method to assess the placental transfer of a variety of anesthetic agents (e.g., thiopental,[62] methohexital,[63] propofol,[64] bupivacaine,[65] ropivacaine,[66] alfentanil,[67] sufentanil[68,69]). Transfer across the placenta may be reported as drug clearance or as a ratio that is also referred to as the *transfer index* (i.e., drug clearance/reference compound clearance). The use of a transfer index improves interplacental comparisons by accounting for differences between placentas (e.g., lobule sizes). The transfer of commonly used reference compounds is either flow-limited (e.g., antipyrine, tritiated water) or membrane-limited (e.g., creatinine). These studies have enhanced our understanding of the placental transfer of anesthetic drugs.

Pharmacokinetic Principles

Factors affecting drug transfer across the human placenta include lipid solubility, protein binding, tissue binding, pKa of the drug, pH of the fetal blood, and blood flow. High lipid solubility may allow a drug to penetrate the cell membrane (a lipid bilayer) easily, but it also may allow the drug (e.g., sufentanil) to be trapped in the placental tissue.[69] Transfer of a drug that is highly protein bound is affected by the concentration of both maternal and fetal plasma proteins, which varies with gestational age and disease. Some drugs (e.g., diazepam) bind to albumin, whereas others (e.g., sufentanil, cocaine) bind predominantly to alpha$_1$-glycoprotein (AGP). Although the free, unbound fraction of drug equilibrates across the placenta, the total drug concentration is greatly affected by both the degree of protein binding and the quantity of protein in both the maternal and fetal blood. For example, fetal blood typically contains less than half the AGP contained in maternal blood.[70] One in vitro study of placental transfer of sufentanil noted different results when fresh frozen plasma—rather than albumin—was used as a perfusate.

The pKa of a drug determines the fraction of drug that is nonionized at physiologic pH. Thus, fetal acidemia will greatly enhance the maternal-to-fetal transfer (i.e., "ion trapping") of many *basic* drugs, such as local anesthetics and opioids (Figure 4-10).[71] Most anesthetic drugs are passively transferred, with blood flow rates (hence drug delivery) affecting the amount of drug that crosses the placenta.[72] One of the authors (M.I.Z.) has used the in vitro perfused human placenta model to perform a number of studies of the placental transfer of opioids; Table 4-1 summarizes some of the results of those studies.

Inhalation Anesthetic Agents

When general anesthesia is necessary in the pregnant patient, it is common practice to maintain anesthesia with an inhalation agent or agents. The lipid solubility and low molecular weight of these agents facilitates rapid transfer across the placenta. A prolonged induction-to-delivery interval results in lower Apgar scores in infants exposed to general anesthesia.[73]

Placental transfer of **halothane** is brisk. When administered during cesarean section, it is detectable in both umbilical venous and arterial blood within 1 minute. Even with relatively short induction-to-delivery times, an F/M ratio of between 0.71 and 0.87 is established.[74,75] **Enflurane** also exhibits unrestricted transfer across the placenta. Even brief exposure results in an F/M ratio of approximately 0.6.[76] **Isoflurane** distributes rapidly across the placenta during cesarean section, resulting in an F/M ratio of approximately 0.71.[75] To our knowledge, there are no published data regarding the placental transfer of either **desflurane** or **sevoflurane**.

Nitrous oxide also rapidly crosses the placenta. An F/M ratio of 0.83 is expected within 3 minutes.[77] Maternal administration of nitrous oxide decreases fetal central vascular resistance by 30%,[78] and a prolonged induction-to-delivery interval may cause neonatal depression.[79] Diffusion hypoxia may occur during the rapid elimination of nitrous oxide from the neonate; therefore, it seems prudent to administer supplemental oxygen to any neonate who has been exposed to nitrous oxide immediately before delivery.[80]

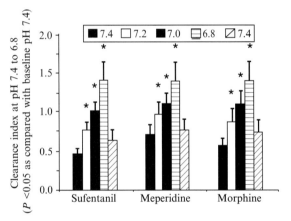

FIGURE 4-10.   The effects of changes in fetal pH on the transfer of opioids during in vitro perfusion of the human placenta. This figure demonstrates the "ion trapping" of opioids, which is similar to that of local anesthetics. Clearance index = clearance drug/clearance creatinine (a reference compound). (From Zakowski MI, Krishna R, Grant GJ, Turndorf H. Effect of pH on transfer of narcotics in human placenta during in vitro perfusion (abstract). Anesthesiology 1995; 85:A890.)

Induction Agents

The same lipophilic characteristics that make these agents ideal for the induction of anesthesia also enhance their transfer across the placenta. Our understanding of the transplacental transfer of these drugs is better than for any other group of anesthetic agents.

BARBITURATES

Thiopental is the most popular agent used for the induction of general anesthesia, and it is the most extensively studied member of this drug class. This extremely short-acting barbiturate quickly appears in umbilical venous blood after maternal injection.[81,82] Studies have reported mean F/M ratios between 0.4 and 1.1.[83,84] Studies with high F/M ratios suggest that thiopental is freely diffusible; however, factors other than simple diffusion must play a role in thiopental transfer, because studies have also demonstrated a wide intersubject variability in umbilical cord blood concentrations at delivery. Studies of the perfused human placenta have verified the rapid maternal-fetal transfer of thiopental. Both maternal-to-fetal and fetal-to-maternal transfer of thiopental are strongly influenced by maternal and fetal perfusate protein concentrations.[62]

Some anesthesiologists use the oxybarbiturate **methohexital** rather than thiopental for the induction of general anesthesia. Marshall[59] assessed the transfer of methohexital across the human placenta in vivo; he noted a rapid transfer of methohexital into the fetal circulation and simultaneous peak concentrations in maternal and fetal blood. Evidence from studies of in vitro perfusion of the human placenta suggests that methohexital rapidly crosses the placenta in both maternal-to-fetal and fetal-to-maternal directions, with transfer indices of 0.83 and 0.61, respectively,[63] when the albumin concentration is equal in both perfusates. This transfer asymmetry disappears when the albumin concentrations are altered to approximate physiologic levels of protein binding in maternal and fetal blood (8 g/100 mL and 4 g/100 mL, respectively). These conditions significantly increase fetal-to-maternal transfer so that it approximates maternal-to-fetal transfer.[63]

KETAMINE

Some anesthesiologists prefer to give ketamine during the induction of general anesthesia for cesarean section, especially to patients with hypovolemia or asthma. This phencyclidine

TABLE 4-1	OPIOID TRANSFER DURING IN VITRO PERFUSION OF THE HUMAN PLACENTA				
	Morphine	**Meperidine**	**Alfentanil**	**Fentanyl**	**Sufentanil**
Lipid solubility	1.4	39	129	816	1727
Percent nonionized at pH 7.4	23%	7.4%	89%	8.5%	20%
Percent protein binding	30%	70%	93%	84%	93%
Placenta drug ratio	0.1	0.7	0.53	3.4	7.2
F/M ratio, MTF	0.08	0.27	0.22	0.19	0.14
F/M ratio, FTM	0.08	0.13	0.11	0.08	0.18
Minutes to steady state	30	20	20	40-60	40-60
Clearance index MTF	0.4	0.95	0.75	0.76	0.41
Clearance index FTM	0.5	0.91	0.78	0.61	0.76

Data from non-recirculated experiments, using perfusate Media 199 without protein, with maternal flow 12 mL/min and fetal flow 6 mL/min.[67,69,104,107,113]
Clearance index, clearance drug/clearance antipyrine (a flow-limited reference compound); *FTM,* fetal-to-maternal; *MTF,* maternal-to-fetal; *Placenta drug ratio,* placenta drug concentration/g placental tissue/maternal drug concentration.

derivative rapidly crosses the placenta. Although it is less lipid soluble than thiopental, a mean F/M ratio of 1.26 was achieved in as little as 1 minute and 37 seconds after maternal administration of 2 mg/kg before vaginal delivery.[85]

PROPOFOL

Some anesthesiologists now give propofol to obstetric patients, although its exact role in obstetric anesthesia practice remains unclear.[86] Studies have noted that maternal administration of a bolus dose of 2.0 to 2.5 mg/kg results in a mean F/M ratio between 0.65 and 0.85.[87–89] Gin et al.[90] noted that bolus administration of 2.0 mg/kg followed by a continuous infusion of propofol (either 6 mg/kg/hr or 9 mg/kg/hr) resulted in mean F/M ratios of 0.50 and 0.54, respectively. Another study demonstrated that the F/M ratio was approximately 0.5 in early (i.e., 12 to 18 weeks) gestation and was independent of time over 5 to 20 minutes of study.[91] Celleno et al.[86] observed that the administration of propofol 2.8 mg/kg resulted in lower 1- and 5-minute Apgar scores than administration of thiopental 5 mg/kg during the induction of general anesthesia for elective cesarean section. In another study, administration of propofol was associated with an Apgar score of 5 or less in 3 of 10 neonates, with an average umbilical vein propofol concentration of 0.32 µg/mL.[92]

He et al.[93-95] have studied the factors that affect propofol transfer during in vitro human placental perfusion. Increased maternal blood flow increases both placental tissue uptake and transplacental transfer of propofol.[93] Propofol is highly protein bound; thus placental transfer is affected by changes in plasma protein concentrations. Increasing the fetal albumin concentration increases the total—but not the free—concentration of propofol in umbilical venous blood.[94] In addition, the umbilical venous blood concentration of propofol decreases by approximately two thirds when the maternal albumin concentration is doubled.[95]

ETOMIDATE

In 1979, Downing et al.[96] first described the use of etomidate, a carboxylated imidazole, for the induction of general anesthesia in obstetric patients. A dose of 0.3 to 0.4 mg/kg administered before cesarean section results in an F/M ratio of approximately 0.5.[97]

BENZODIAZEPINES

Diazepam is highly unionized and very lipophilic. Fetal-maternal ratios of 1.0 are attained within minutes of maternal injection[98] and increase to nearly 2.0 after 1 hour.[99] **Lorazepam** is less lipophilic, and as would be predicted, it takes almost 3 hours after its administration for the F/M ratio to reach unity.[100] **Midazolam** is even more polar, and its F/M ratio is approximately 0.76 at 20 minutes after administration. However, unlike those of the other benzodiazepines, its ratio falls quickly; by 200 minutes, it is only 0.3.[101]

Opioids

Opioids have long been the mainstay for systemic pain relief in obstetric patients. Safety associated with their use has increased because of a better understanding of their pharmacokinetics, improved monitoring, and the ability to reverse adverse effects with the antagonist naloxone.

Meperidine remains a commonly used opioid in obstetrics, even though it has been associated with neonatal central nervous system (CNS) and respiratory depression. Intravenous administration of meperidine is followed by a rapid transfer of the drug across the human placenta; the drug can be detected in umbilical venous blood as soon as 90 seconds after maternal administration.[102] F/M ratios for meperidine may exceed 1.0 after 2 to 3 hours; maternal levels fall more rapidly than do fetal levels because of the greater capacity for maternal metabolism of the drug.[103] In vitro perfusion of the human placenta has shown that meperidine is transferred rapidly across the placenta in both maternal-to-fetal and fetal-to-maternal directions, with equal clearances, little placental tissue binding, and no metabolism of the drug.[104]

Morphine also rapidly crosses the placenta. Morphine is often used to "rest" patients during early labor, although one study suggested that it caused a significant decrease in the biophysical profile score, with a mean umbilical cord concentration of 25 ng/mL and a mean F/M plasma ratio of 0.61.[105] Intrathecal administration of morphine results in a high F/M ratio (approximately 0.92), although the absolute fetal concentrations are less than those that cause fetal and neonatal complications.[106] In vitro perfusion of the human placenta showed that morphine, which is a hydrophilic compound, exhibits membrane-limited transfer with a low placental tissue content and a fast washout.[107] Concurrent naloxone administration apparently does not affect the placental transfer of morphine.[108]

Fentanyl and its analogs currently are used extensively as intrapartum analgesics. These drugs are administered by the epidural, intrathecal, and intravenous routes. Fentanyl has a high degree of lipophilicity and albumin binding (74%).[109] Maternal epidural administration of fentanyl results in an F/M ratio between 0.37 and 0.57.[110,111] During early pregnancy, fentanyl is rapidly transferred and may be detected not only in the placenta but also in the fetal brain.[112] In vitro perfusion of the human placenta has revealed rapid transfer in both maternal-to-fetal and fetal-to-maternal directions, with the placenta acting as a moderate drug depot.[113]

Maternal administration of **alfentanil** results in an F/M ratio of approximately 0.30,[114] but it is associated with a reduction of 1-minute Apgar scores.[115] In vitro perfusion of the human placenta reveals rapid and symmetric maternal-to-fetal and fetal-to-maternal transfer of alfentanil, with low placental drug uptake and rapid washout.[67]

Maternal administration of **sufentanil** results in a very high F/M ratio of 0.81. However, its greater lipid solubility and more rapid uptake by the CNS (as compared with fentanyl) results in less systemic absorption from the epidural space, which reduces maternal and umbilical vein concentrations and subsequent fetal exposure (and perhaps reduces the risk of neonatal respiratory depression).[110] Studies of in vitro perfusion of the human placenta have confirmed the rapid transplacental transfer of sufentanil. The placental transfer of sufentanil is influenced by differences in maternal and fetal plasma protein binding and fetal pH. High placental tissue uptake suggests that the placenta serves as a drug depot.[68,69]

Kan et al.[116] demonstrated that maternal intravenous administration of the new ultrashort-acting opioid **remifentanil** is followed by rapid placental transfer. Maternal intravenous administration of remifentanil (0.1 µg/kg/min), combined with epidural anesthesia for nonemergent cesarean section, resulted in an average F/M ratio of 0.88. In some cases, administration of remifentanil has resulted in excessive maternal sedation, but no adverse neonatal effects have been observed.[116,117]

Some physicians favor systemic administration of an opioid agonist/antagonist during labor, because some studies have suggested that these agents result in fewer maternal, fetal, and neonatal side effects. Both **butorphanol** and **nalbuphine** rapidly cross the placenta; studies have noted mean F/M ratios of 0.84 and 0.74 to 0.97, respectively.[118-120] In one study, maternal administration of nalbuphine resulted in "flattening" of the fetal heart rate tracing in 54% of cases.[120]

Local Anesthetics

Local anesthetic agents readily cross the placenta. See Chapter 12 for a discussion of the placental transfer of these agents.

Muscle Relaxants

Muscle relaxants are quaternary ammonium salts. These drugs are fully ionized, and they do not readily cross the placenta. Maternal administration of a single clinical dose of a muscle relaxant results in a detectable concentration in fetal blood. However, during induction of general anesthesia for cesarean section, maternal administration of a muscle relaxant rarely affects neonatal muscle tone at delivery.

When a single dose of **succinylcholine** is administered to facilitate intubation, it is not detected in umbilical venous blood at delivery.[121] Maternal doses of more than 300 mg are required before the drug can be detected in umbilical venous blood.[122] Neonatal neuromuscular blockade can occur when high doses are given repeatedly or when the fetus has a pseudocholinesterase deficiency.[123,124] Hinkle and Dorsch[125] reported a case of maternal masseter muscle rigidity and neonatal fasciculations after administration of succinylcholine before emergency cesarean section; both the mother and the newborn were diagnosed with central core myopathy and malignant hyperthermia susceptibility.

The administration of a nondepolarizing muscle relaxant also results in a low F/M ratio. The mean F/M ratios for the most commonly used nondepolarizing muscle relaxants are as follows: 0.12 for **d-tubocurare**[126]; 0.19 to 0.26 for pancuronium[127-129]; 0.06 to 0.11 for **vecuronium**[129,130]; and 0.07 for **atracurium**.[131] In one study, the F/M ratio of vecuronium nearly doubled as the induction-to-delivery interval increased from 180 to 420 seconds.[130] To our knowledge, no published study has investigated the placental transfer of the atracurium isomer **cisatracurium**. In one study, administration of **rapacuronium**, which is a short-acting analog of vecuronium, increased maternal heart rate and produced an F/M ratio of 0.09.[132] Although no published reports have documented problems with rapacuronium in parturients or neonates, reports of bronchospasm have resulted in the withdrawal of rapacuronium from the market. Some anesthesiologists have advocated the use of **rocuronium** as an alternative to succinylcholine during rapid-sequence induction of general anesthesia for cesarean section.[133,134] Published studies have not demonstrated any evidence of adverse neonatal effects after rocuronium administration; however, these studies did not determine umbilical cord blood concentrations of the drug.

Nondepolarizing muscle relaxants typically are administered in a bolus; although the transfer rates are low, the fetal blood concentrations increase over time.[130] Fetal blood concentrations of nondepolarizing muscle relaxants can be minimized by giving succinylcholine to facilitate intubation followed by the administration of small doses of either succinylcholine or a nondepolarizing muscle relaxant to maintain paralysis.[128]

Anticholinergic Agents

The placental transfer rate of anticholinergic agents correlates directly with their ability to cross the blood-brain barrier. **Atropine** is detected in the umbilical circulation within 1 to 2 minutes of maternal administration, and an F/M ratio of approximately 0.93 is attained at 5 minutes.[1] **Scopolamine**, which is the other commonly used tertiary amine, also crosses the placenta easily. Intramuscular administration of scopolamine results in an F/M ratio of almost unity within 55 minutes.[136] By contrast, **glycopyrrolate** is poorly transferred across the placenta; maternal intramuscular administration results in low absolute fetal blood concentrations, with a mean F/M ratio of only 0.22.[137] Maternal intravenous administration of glycopyrrolate does not result in a detectable fetal hemodynamic response.[138]

Anticholinesterase Agents

Neostigmine, **pyridostigmine**, and **edrophonium** are quaternary ammonium compounds that are ionized at physiologic pH; thus they undergo limited transplacental transfer.[139] For example, maternal administration of neostigmine does not reverse atropine-induced fetal tachycardia. However, small amounts of these agents do cross the placenta to the fetus. Clark et al.[140] reported a case of fetal bradycardia after maternal administration of neostigmine and glycopyrrolate at the completion of surgery in a 22-year-old pregnant woman. The authors speculated that the neostigmine crossed the placenta to a greater extent than the glycopyrrolate. They suggested that "neostigmine and atropine, rather than neostigmine and glycopyrrolate, be used to reverse nondepolarizing muscle relaxants in pregnant patients."[140]

Antihypertensive Agents

Beta-adrenergic receptor antagonists are used as antihypertensive agents in pregnancy. Early studies suggested that these agents were associated with intrauterine growth restriction and neonatal bradycardia, hypoglycemia, and respiratory depression.[141,142] Erkkola et al.[143] noted an F/M ratio of 0.26 after a single dose of **propranolol** administered 3 hours before cesarean section. Chronic administration of propranolol during pregnancy may result in F/M ratios greater than 1.0.[141] Other studies have noted that maternal administration of **atenolol** and **metoprolol** results in mean F/M ratios of 0.94 and 1.0, respectively.[144,145]

Some obstetricians and anesthesiologists now favor the maternal administration of **labetalol** for the treatment of either chronic or acute hypertension in pregnant women. At least one study observed mild neonatal bradycardia after maternal administration of labetalol.[146] Another study noted that chronic oral administration of labetalol resulted in an F/M ratio of 0.38.[147]

Some anesthesiologists favor maternal administration of the extremely short-acting beta-adrenergic receptor antagonist **esmolol** to attenuate the hypertensive response to laryngoscopy and intubation. Östman et al.[148] noted a mean F/M ratio of 0.2 after maternal administration of esmolol in gravid ewes. However, Ducey and Knape[149] reported a case of fetal bradycardia that required the performance of an emergency cesarean section after maternal administration of esmolol.

Clonidine and **methyldopa** are antihypertensive agents that act through the central stimulation of alpha₂-adrenergic receptors. Human studies have noted a mean F/M ratio of

0.89 for clonidine[150] and 1.17 for methyldopa.[151] In concentrations likely to be present in maternal blood when the drugs are used therapeutically, magnesium and nifedipine—but *not* clonidine—produced fetal vasodilation during in vitro perfusion of the human placenta.[152] **Dexmedetomidine** is a new alpha$_2$-adrenergic agonist. During in vitro perfusion of the human placenta, one study demonstrated an F/M ratio of 0.12, with evidence of high placental tissue content due to dexmedetomidine's high lipophilicity.[153] **Phenoxybenzamine**, an alpha-adrenergic receptor antagonist, is commonly used to treat hypertension in patients with pheochromocytoma. Chronic maternal administration results in an F/M ratio of 1.6.[154]

Direct-acting vasodilators are used for short-term treatment of severe hypertension in pregnant women. **Hydralazine** is frequently used to treat severe hypertension in preeclamptic women. Fetal and maternal concentrations are similar, so the F/M ratio approximates unity.[155] In vitro administration of hydralazine into the maternal side of a human placenta produces fetal vasodilation.[156] **Sodium nitroprusside** is lipid soluble and rapidly crosses the placenta.[157] Nitroprusside breakdown produces cyanide. One study in gravid ewes demonstrated that sodium thiosulfate, which is the agent used to treat cyanide toxicity, did not cross the placenta in the maternal-to-fetal direction but instead treated fetal cyanide toxicity via enhanced fetal-to-maternal transfer of cyanide. (An increased gradient occurred with the lowering of maternal cyanide levels.[158])

Glyceryl trinitrate (nitroglycerin) also crosses the placenta, with an F/M ratio of 0.18 observed during a study using in vitro perfusion of the human placenta. No change in fetal perfusion pressure was noted. The presence of dinitrate metabolites in both the maternal and fetal venous samples indicates the capacity for placental biotransformation of glyceryl trinitrate.[159] Administration of nitroglycerin resulted in no changes in fetal umbilical blood flow, blood pressure, heart rate, or blood gas measurements in gravid ewes.[160] Indeed, placental tissue production of nitric oxide may be an important factor that enhances the uterine relaxation caused by nitroglycerin in vivo.[161] In an in vitro study of nitrovasodilator compounds, perfusion of the maternal intervillous space produced fetal vasodilation (in the presence of fetal vasoconstriction caused by prostaglandin $F_{2\alpha}$), with the order of potency being as follows: glyceryl trinitrate $\geq$ sodium nitroprusside $\geq$ NaNO$_2$ $\geq$ S-nitroso-N-acetylpenicillamine (SNAP) = S-nitroso-N-glutathione (SNG).[162] SNG and NaNO$_2$ were significantly more potent under conditions of low oxygen tension. The antioxidants cysteine, glutathione, and superoxide dismutase significantly enhanced the vasodilatory effects of NaNO$_2$ only.[162] The nitric oxide donors and even vitamins and antioxidants affect fetal vascular tone and require further study.

Placental transfer of angiotensin-converting enzyme (ACE) inhibitors may adversely affect fetal renal function. **Enalaprilat** rapidly crosses the placenta; maternal administration of high doses lowered fetal arterial pressure by 20% in rhesus monkeys.[163]

Vasopressor Agents

Vasopressor agents are often administered to prevent or treat hypotension during the administration of regional anesthesia in obstetric patients; however, few studies have evaluated the transplacental transfer of these agents. Hughes et al.[164] observed that **ephedrine** easily crosses the placenta and results in an F/M ratio of approximately 0.7.

Cocaine, a common drug of abuse during pregnancy, has a potent vasoconstrictor activity. During in vitro perfusion of the human placenta, cocaine was rapidly transferred (without metabolism) in both maternal-to-fetal and fetal-to-maternal directions; transfer was constant over a wide range of concentrations.[165] Cocaine and its active metabolites norcocaine and cocaethylene—but not the inactive metabolite benzoylecgonine—are rapidly transferred across the placenta.[166,167] Chronic maternal administration results in higher cocaine levels in the fetal circulation.[168]

Anticoagulants

Patients with prosthetic heart valves or thromboembolic disease require anticoagulation therapy during pregnancy. However, anticoagulation therapy has been associated with maternal and fetal morbidity. Maternal administration of **warfarin** results in an increased rate of fetal loss and congenital anomalies[169]; these findings confirm the transplacental transfer of warfarin, although no study has directly measured the F/M ratio of this drug. By contrast, studies have confirmed that heparin does *not* cross the placenta; this was determined by coagulation studies in the newborn[170] and the measurement of radiolabeled heparin in fetal lambs.[171] Warfarin is contraindicated during the first trimester, and most physicians prefer the administration of heparin rather than warfarin throughout pregnancy. An increasing number of patients are receiving **low molecular weight heparin (LMWH)**. Maternal administration of **enoxaparin** does not alter fetal anti-IIa or anti-Xa activity.[172] Even at concentrations used for the acute treatment of thromboembolism, studies using in vitro perfusion of the human placenta demonstrated no placental transfer of enoxaparin or **fondaparinux** (a new pentasaccharide that selectively inhibits factor Xa).[173]

Drug Delivery Systems

New drug delivery systems may influence drug transfer and distribution across the human placenta. Liposome encapsulation of valproic acid significantly reduces drug transfer and placental uptake.[174] The type and charge of the liposomes affect transfer across the placenta. Anionic and neutral liposomes increase placental transfer, whereas cationic liposomes decrease placental transfer and placental tissue uptake.[175] New drug delivery vehicles should be evaluated for effects on placental uptake and transfer.

PLACENTAL PATHOLOGY

There has been a growing interest in the clinical-pathologic correlation between placental abnormalities and adverse obstetric outcomes.[176,177] In some cases, a skilled and systematic examination of the umbilical cord, fetal membranes, and placenta may provide insight into antepartum pathophysiology; in most of these cases, examination of the placenta will confirm the clinical diagnosis (e.g., chorioamnionitis). In other cases of adverse outcome, "a disorder that was not suspected clinically may be revealed by placental pathology" (e.g., microabscesses of listeriosis; amnion nodosum, which suggests long-standing oligohydramnios).[176] Drugs may produce placental abnormalities (e.g., cocaine produces chorionic villus hemorrhage and villus edema).[178] However, the significance of most findings (e.g., villous edema, hemorrhagic endovasculitis, chronic villitis) is unclear.

Several factors limit the assessment of placental pathology: (1) "the paucity of properly designed studies of adequate size with appropriate outcome parameters,"[176] which limits attempts to correlate placental abnormalities with adverse clinical outcome; (2) the limited number of pathologists with expertise in the recognition and interpretation of subtle abnormalities of the placenta; and (3) the cost of the routine assessment of placental pathology. The American College of Obstetricians and Gynecologists Committee on Obstetrics has concluded the following[176]:

> An examination of the umbilical cord, membranes, and placenta may assist the obstetric care provider in clinical-pathologic correlation when there is an adverse perinatal outcome. However, the scientific basis for clinical correlation with placenta pathology is still evolving, and the benefit of securing specimens on a routine basis is as yet unproven.

KEY POINTS

- The placenta is a dynamic organ with a complex structure. It brings two circulations close together for the exchange of blood gases, nutrients, and other substances (e.g., drugs).
- During pregnancy, anatomic adaptations result in substantial (near maximal) vasodilation of the uterine spiral arteries; this results in a low-resistance pathway for the delivery of blood to the placenta. Therefore, adequate uteroplacental blood flow depends on the maintenance of a normal maternal perfusion pressure.
- A marked diversity in placental structure and function exists among various animal species; this limits our ability to extrapolate the results of animal investigations to human pregnancy and clinical practice.
- Placental transfer involves all of the physiologic transport mechanisms that exist in other organ systems.
- Physical factors (e.g., molecular weight, lipid solubility, degree of ionization) affect the placental transfer of drugs and other substances. In addition, other factors affect maternal-fetal exchange, including changes in maternal and fetal blood flow, placental binding, placental metabolism, diffusion capacity, and degree of maternal and fetal plasma protein binding.
- Lipophilicity, which enhances the central nervous system uptake of general anesthetic agents, also heightens the transfer of these drugs across the placenta. However, the placenta itself may take up highly lipophilic drugs, thereby creating a placental drug depot that limits the initial transfer of drug.
- Fetal acidemia can result in the so-called "ion trapping" of both local anesthetics and opioids.
- Vasoactive drugs cross the placenta and may affect the fetal circulation.

REFERENCES

1. Haynes DM. The human placenta: Historical considerations. In: Lavery JP, editor. The Human Placenta: Clinical Perspectives. Rockville, Md, Aspen Publishers, 1987:1-10.
2. Kaufmann P, Scheffen I. Placental development. In: Polin RA, Fox WW, editors. Fetal and Neonatal Physiology, 2nd ed. Philadelphia, WB Saunders, 1998:59-70.
3. Sadler TW. Langman's Medical Embryology, 7th ed. Baltimore, Williams and Wilkins, 1995.
4. Boyd JD, Hamilton WJ. The Human Placenta. Cambridge, W. Heffer and Sons Ltd., 1970.
5. Flexner LB, Gellhorn A. The comparative physiology of placental transfer. Am J Obstet Gynecol 1942; 43:965-74.
6. James E, Meschia G, Battaglia FC. A-V differences of free fatty acids and glycerol in the ovine umbilical circulation. Proc Soc Exp Biol Med 1971; 138:823-6.
7. Ramsey EM, Donner MW. Placental Vasculature and Circulation: Anatomy, Physiology, Radiology, Clinical Aspects. Atlas and Textbook. Philadelphia, WB Saunders, 1980.
8. Arey LB. Developmental Anatomy: A Textbook and Laboratory Manual of Embryology. Philadelphia, WB Saunders, 1974.
9. Freese UE. The fetal-maternal circulation of the placenta. I: Histomorphological, plastoid injection, and x-ray cinematographic studies on human placentas. Am J Obstet Gynecol 1966; 94:354-60.
10. Leiser R, Kosanke G, Kaufmann P. Human placental vascularization: Structural and quantitative aspects. In: Soma H, editor. Placenta: Basic Research for Clinical Application. Basel, Switzerland, Karger, 1991:32-45.
11. Gruenwald P. Lobular architecture of primate placentas. In: Gruenwald P, editor. The Placenta and Its Maternal Supply Line: Effects of Insufficiency on the Fetus. Baltimore, University Park Press, 1975:35-55.
12. Kaufmann P. Basic morphology of the fetal and maternal circuits in the human placenta. Contrib Gynecol Obstet 1985; 13:5-17.
13. Juchau MR, Namkung MJ, Rettie AE. P-450 cytochromes in the human placenta: Oxidation of xenobiotics and endogenous steroids—A review. Trophoblast Res 1987; 2:235-63.
14. Wier PJ, Miller RK. The pharmacokinetics of cadmium in the dually perfused human placenta. Trophoblast Res 1987; 2:357-66.
15. Faber JJ, Thornburg KL. Placental Physiology: Structure and Function of Fetomaternal Exchange. New York, Raven Press, 1983.
16. Russo P. Maternal-fetal exchange of nutrients. In Nutrition and Metabolism in Pregnancy: Mother and Fetus. New York, Oxford University Press, 1990:133-67.
17. Siler-Khodr TM. Endocrine and paracrine function of the human placenta. In: Polin RA, Fox WW, editors. Fetal and Neonatal Physiology, 2nd ed. Philadelphia, WB Saunders, 1998:89-102.
18. O'Shaughnessy RW, O'Toole R, Tuttle S, Zuspan FP. Uterine catecholamines in normal and hypertensive human pregnancy. Clin Exp Hypertens 1983; 82:447-57.
19. Thorbert G, Alm P, Björklund AB, et al. Adrenergic innervation of the human uterus. Disappearance of the transmitter and transmitter-forming enzymes during pregnancy. Am J Obstet Gynecol 1979; 135:223-6.
20. Greiss FC, Jr. Uterine blood flow in pregnancy: An overview. In: Moawad AH, Lindheimer MD, editors. Uterine and Placental Blood Flow. New York, Masson Publishing, 1982:19-26.
21. Rosenfeld CR. Regulation of placental circulation. In: Polin RA, Fox WW, editors. Fetal and Neonatal Physiology, 2nd ed. Philadelphia, WB Saunders, 1998:70-7.
22. Rankin JHG, McLaughlin MK. The regulation of the placental blood flows. J Dev Physiol 1979; 1:3-30.
23. Roth JB, Thorp JA, Palmer SM, et al. Response of placental vasculature to high glucose levels in the isolated human placental cotyledon. Am J Obstet Gynecol 1990; 163:1828-30.
24. Howard RB, Hosokawa T, Maguire MH. Hypoxia-induced fetoplacental vasoconstriction in perfused human placental cotyledons. Am J Obstet Gynecol 1987; 157:1261-6.
25. Kuhn DC, Stuart MJ. Cyclooxygenase inhibition reduces placental transfer: Reverse by carbacyclin. Am J Obstet Gynecol 1987; 157:194-8.
26. Myatt L, Brewer A, Brockman DE. The action of nitric oxide in the perfused human fetal-placental circulation. Am J Obstet Gynecol 1991; 164:687-92.
27. Byrne BM, Howard RB, Morrow RJ, et al. Role of the L-arginine nitric oxide pathway in hypoxic fetoplacental vasoconstriction. Placenta 1997;18:627-34.
28. Miller RK, Koszalka TR, Brent RL. The transport of molecules across the placental membranes. In: Poste G, Nicolson GL, editors. The Cell Surface in Animal Embryogenesis and Development. Amsterdam, The Netherlands, Elsevier/North-Holland Biomedical Press, 1976:145-223.

29. Schuster VL. Properties and functions of cell membranes. In: West JB, editor. Best and Taylor's Physiological Basis of Medical Practice, 12th ed. Baltimore, Williams and Wilkins, 1991:14-30.

30. Guyton AC, Hall JE. Transport of ions and molecules through the cell membrane. Textbook of Medical Physiology, 9th ed. Philadelphia, WB Saunders, 1996:43-55.

31. van Kreel BK. Basic mechanisms of placental transfer. Int J Biol Res Pregnancy 1981; 2:28-36.

32. Morriss FH Jr, Boyd RDH, Mahendran D. Placental transport. In: Knobil E, Neill JD, editors. The Physiology of Reproduction, 2nd ed. New York, Raven Press, 1994:813-61.

33. Casley-Smith JR, Chin JC. The passage of cytoplasmic vesicles across endothelial and mesothelial cells. J Microsc 1971; 93:167-89.

34. Griffiths GD, Kershaw D, Booth AG. Rabbit peroxidase-antiperoxidase complex (PAP) as a model for the uptake of immunoglobulin G by the human placenta. Histochem J 1985; 17:867-81.

35. Illsley NP, Hall S, Stacey TE. The modulation of glucose transfer across the human placenta by intervillous flow rates: An in vitro perfusion study. Trophoblast Res 1987; 2:535-44.

36. Battaglia FC, Meschia G. Foetal and placental metabolism: Their interrelationship and impact upon maternal metabolism. Proc Nutr Soc 1981; 40:99-113.

37. Jauniaux F, Gulbis B. In vivo investigation of placental transfer early in human pregnancy. Eur J Obstet Gynecol Reprod Biol 2000; 92:45-9.

38. Longo LD. Respiration in the fetal-placental unit. In: Cowett RM, editor. Principles of Perinatal-Neonatal Metabolism. New York, Springer-Verlag, 1991:304-15.

39. Dancis J, Schneider H. Physiology: Transfer and barrier function. In: Gruenwald P, editor. The Placenta and Its Maternal Supply Line: Effects of Insufficiency on the Fetus. Baltimore, University Park Press, 1975:98-124.

40. Barron DH, Alexander G. Supplementary observations on the oxygen pressure gradient between the maternal and fetal blood of sheep. Yale J Biol Med 1952; 25:61-6.

41. Faber JJ, Hart FM. The rabbit placenta as an organ of diffusional exchange: Comparison with other species by dimensional analysis. Circ Res 1966; 19:816-33.

42. Campbell AGM, Dawes GS, Fishman AP, et al. The oxygen consumption of the placenta and foetal membranes in the sheep. J Physiol 1966; 182:439-64.

43. Longo LD, Power GG, Forster RE II. Respiratory function of the placenta as determined with carbon monoxide in sheep and dogs. J Clin Invest 1967; 46:812-28.

44. Wilkening RB, Meschia G. Current topic: Comparative physiology of placental oxygen transport. Placenta 1992; 13:1-15.

45. Nicolaides KH, Soothill PW, Rodeck CH, Campbell S. Ultrasound-guided sampling of umbilical cord and placental blood to assess fetal well-being. Lancet 1986; 1:1065-7.

46. Longo LD, Hill EP, Power GG. Theoretical analysis of factors affecting placental O_2 transfer. Am J Physiol 1972; 222:730-9.

47. Hill EP, Power GG, Longo LD. A mathematical model of carbon dioxide transfer in the placenta and its interaction with oxygen. Am J Physiol 1973; 224:283-99.

48. Longo LD, Delivoria-Papadopoulos M, Forster RE II. Placental CO_2 transfer after fetal carbonic anhydrase inhibition. Am J Physiol 1974; 226:703-10.

49. Rice PA, Rourke JE, Nesbitt REL Jr. In vitro perfusion studies of the human placenta. VI. Evidence against active glucose transport. Am J Obstet Gynecol 1979; 133:649-55.

50. Challier JC, Nandakumaran M, Mondon F. Placental transport of hexoses: A comparative study with antipyrine and amino acids. Placenta 1985; 6:497-504.

51. Johnson LW, Smith CH. Glucose transport across the basal plasma membrane of human placental syncytiotrophoblast. Biochim Biophys Acta 1985; 815:44-50.

52. Reynolds ML, Young M. The transfer of free a-amino nitrogen across the placental membrane in the guinea-pig. J Physiol 1971; 214:583-97.

53. Yudilevich DL, Sweiry JH. Transport of amino acids in the placenta. Biochim Biophys Acta 1985; 822:169-201.

54. Leat WMF, Harrison FA. Transfer of long-chain fatty acids to the fetal and neonatal lamb. J Dev Physiol 1980; 2:257-74.

55. Elphick MC, Hull D, Sanders RR. Concentrations of free fatty acids in maternal and umbilical cord blood during elective caesarean section. Br J Obstet Gynaecol 1976; 83:539-44.

56. Booth C, Elphick MC, Hendrickse W, Hull D. Investigation of [^{14}C]linoleic acid conversion into [^{14}C]arachidonic acid and placental transfer of linoleic and palmitic acids across the perfused human placenta. J Dev Physiol 1981; 3:177-89.

57. Filshie GM, Anstey MD. The distribution of arachidonic acid in plasma and tissues of patients near term undergoing elective or emergency caesarean section. Br J Obstet Gynaecol 1978; 85:119-23.

58. Dancis J. Why perfuse the human placenta? Contrib Gynecol Obstet 1985; 13:1-4.

59. Marshall JR. Human antepartum placental passage of methohexital sodium. Obstet Gynecol 1964; 23:589-92.

60. Tropper PJ, Petrie RH. Placental exchange. In: Lavery JP, editor. The Human Placenta: Clinical Perspectives. Rockville, Md, Aspen Publishers, 1987:199-206.

61. Reynolds F, Knott C. Pharmacokinetics in pregnancy and placental drug transfer. Oxf Rev Reprod Biol 1989; 11:389-449.

62. Herman NL, Li A-T, Bjoraker R, et al. The effects of maternal-fetal perfusate protein differences on the bidirectional transfer of thiopental across the human placenta (abstract). Anesthesiology 1998; 89:A1046.

63. Herman NL, Li AT, Van Decar TK, et al. Transfer of methohexital across the perfused human placenta. J Clin Anesth 2000; 12:25-30.

64. Herman N, Van Decar TK, Lanza M, et al. Distribution of propofol across the perfused human placenta (abstract). Anesthesiology 1994; 81:A1140.

65. Johnson RF, Herman N, Johnson HV, et al. Bupivacaine transfer across the human term placenta: A study using the dual human placental model. Anesthesiology 1995; 82:459-68.

66. Johnson RF, Cahana A, Olenick M, et al. A comparison of the placental transfer of ropivacaine versus bupivacaine. Anesth Analg 1999; 89:703-8.

67. Zakowski MI, Ham AA, Grant GJ. Transfer and uptake of alfentanil in the human placenta during in vitro perfusion. Anesth Analg 1994; 79:1089-93.

68. Johnson RF, Herman N, Arney TL, et al. The placental transfer of sufentanil: Effects of fetal pH, protein binding, and sufentanil concentration. Anesth Analg 1997; 84:1262-8.

69. Krishna BR, Zakowski MI, Grant GJ. Sufentanil transfer in the human placenta during in vitro perfusion. Can J Anaesth 1997; 44:996-1001.

70. Yang Y, Schenker S. Effects of binding on human transplacental transfer of cocaine (letter). Am J Obstet Gynecol 1995; 172:720-2.

71. Zakowski MI, Krishna R, Grant GJ, Turndorf H. Effect of pH on transfer of narcotics in human placenta during in vitro perfusion (abstract). Anesthesiology 1995; 85:A890.

72. Giroux M, Teixera MG, Dumas JC, et al. Influence of maternal blood flow on the placental transfer of three opioids—fentanyl, alfentanil, sufentanil. Biol Neonate 1997; 72:133-41.

73. Lumley J, Walker A, Marum J, Wood C. Time: An important variable at Caesarean section. J Obstet Gynaecol Br Commonw 1970; 77:10-23.

74. Kangas L, Erkkola R, Kanto J, Mansikka M. Halothane anaesthesia in caesarean section. Acta Anaesthesiol Scand 1976; 20:189-94.

75. Dwyer R, Fee JP, Moore J. Uptake of halothane and isoflurane by mother and baby during caesarean section. Br J Anaesth 1995; 74:379-83.

76. Dick W, Knoche E, Traub E. Clinical investigations concerning the use of Ethrane for caesarean section. J Perinat Med 1979; 7:125-33.

77. Marx GF, Joshi CW, Orkin LR. Placental transmission of nitrous oxide. Anesthesiology 1970; 32:429-32.

78. Polvi HJ, Pirhonen JP, Erkkola RU. Nitrous oxide inhalation: Effects on maternal and fetal circulations at term. Obstet Gynecol 1996; 87:1045-8.

79. Stenger VG, Blechner JN, Prystowsky H. A study of prolongation of obstetric anesthesia. Am J Obstet Gynecol 1969; 103:901-7.

80. Mankowitz E, Brock-Utne JG, Downing JW. Nitrous oxide elimination by the newborn. Anaesthesia 1981; 36:1014-6.

81. Flowers CE Jr. The placental transmission of barbiturates and thiobarbiturates and their pharmacological action on the mother and the infant. Am J Obstet Gynecol 1959; 78:730-42.

82. Finster M, Mark LC, Morishima HO, et al. Plasma thiopental concentrations in the newborn following delivery under thiopental-nitrous oxide anesthesia. Am J Obstet Gynecol 1966; 95:621-9.

83. Morgan DJ, Blackman GL, Paull JD, Wolf LJ. Pharmacokinetics and plasma protein binding of thiopental. II. Studies at cesarean section. Anesthesiology 1981; 54:474-80.

84. Levy CJ, Owen G. Thiopentone transmission through the placenta. Anaesthesia 1964; 19:511-23.

85. Ellingson A, Haram K, Sagen N, Solheim E. Transplacental passage of ketamine after intravenous administration. Acta Anaesthesiol Scand 1977; 21:41-4.

86. Celleno D, Capogna G, Tomassetti M, et al. Neurobehavioural effects of propofol on the neonate following elective caesarean section. Br J Anaesth 1989; 62:649-54.

87. Dailland P, Cockshott ID, Lirzin JD, et al. Intravenous propofol during cesarean section: Placental transfer, concentration in breast milk, and neonatal effects. A preliminary study. Anesthesiology 1989; 71:827-34.

88. Valtonen M, Kanto J, Rosenberg P. Comparison of propofol and thiopentone for induction of anaesthesia for elective caesarean section. Anaesthesia 1989; 44:758-62.

89. Gin T, Gregory MA, Chan K, Oh TE. Maternal and fetal levels of propofol at caesarean section. Anaesth Intensive Care 1990; 18:180-4.

90. Gin T, Yau G, Chan K, et al. Disposition of propofol infusions for caesarean section. Can J Anaesth 1991; 38:31-6.

91. Jauniaux E, Gulbis B, Shannon C, et al. Placental propofol transfer and fetal sedation during maternal general anaesthesia in early pregnancy. Lancet 1998;352:290-1.

92. Sanchez-Alcaraz A, Quintana MB, Laguarda M. Placental transfer and neonatal effects of propofol in caesarean section. J Clinical Phar Ther 1998; 23:19-23.

93. He YL, Seno H, Tsujimoto S, Tashiro C. The effects of uterine and umbilical blood flows on the transfer of propofol across the human placenta during in vitro perfusion. Anesth Analg 2001; 93:151-6.

94. He YL, Tsujimoto S, Tanimoto M, et al. Effects of protein binding on the placental transfer of propofol in the human dually perfused cotyledon in vitro. Br J Anaesth 2000; 85:281-6.

95. He YL, Seno H, Sasaki K, Tashior C. The influences of maternal albumin concentrations on the placental transfer of propofol in the human dually perfused cotyledon in vitro. Anesth Analg 2002; 94:1312-4.

96. Downing JW, Buley RJR, Brock-Utne JG, Houlton PC. Etomidate for induction of anaesthesia at caesarean section: Comparison with thiopentone. Br J Anaesth 1979; 51:135-40.

97. Gregory MA, Davidson DG. Plasma etomidate levels in mother and fetus. Anaesthesia 1991; 46:716-8.

98. Mandelli M, Morselli PL, Nordio S, et al. Placental transfer to diazepam and its disposition in the newborn. Clin Pharmacol Ther 1975; 17:564-72.

99. Erkkola R, Kangas L, Pekkarinen A. The transfer of diazepam across the placenta during labour. Acta Obstet Gynecol Scand 1973; 52:167-70.

100. McBride RJ, Dundee JW, Moore J, et al. A study of the plasma concentrations of lorazepam in mother and neonate. Br J Anaesth 1979; 51:971-8.

101. Wilson CM, Dundee JW, Moore J, et al. A comparison of the early pharmacokinetics of midazolam in pregnant and nonpregnant women. Anaesthesia 1987; 42:1057-62.

102. Shnider SM, Way EL, Lord MJ. Rate of appearance and disappearance of meperidine in fetal blood after administration of narcotics to the mother (abstract). Anesthesiology 1966; 27:227-8.

103. Caldwell J, Wakile LA, Notarianni LJ, et al. Transplacental passage and neonatal elimination of pethidine given to mothers in childbirth (abstract). Br J Clin Pharmacol 1977; 4:715P-6P.

104. Zakowski MI, Krishna BR, Wang SM, et al. Uptake and transfer of meperidine in human placenta during in vitro perfusion (abstract). Annual Meeting of the Society for Obstetric Anesthesia and Perinatology, Vancouver, 1997:104.

105. Kopecky EA, Ryan ML, Barrett JFR, et al. Fetal response to maternally administered morphine. Am J Obstet Gynecol 2000; 183:424-30.

106. Hée P, Sørensen SS, Bock JE, et al. Intrathecal administration of morphine for the relief of pains in labour and estimation of maternal and fetal plasma concentration of morphine. Eur J Obstet Gynecol Reprod Biol 1987; 25:195-201.

107. Bui T, Zakowski MI, Grant GJ, Turndorf H. Uptake and transfer of morphine in human placenta during in vitro perfusion (abstract). Anesthesiology 1995; 83:A932.

108. Kopecky EA, Simone C, Knie B, Koren G. Transfer of morphine across the human placenta and its interaction with naloxone. Life Sci 1999; 65:2359-71.

109. Bower S. Plasma protein binding of fentanyl. J Pharm Pharmacol 1981; 33:507-14.

110. Loftus JR, Hill H, Cohen SE. Placental transfer and neonatal effects of epidural sufentanil and fentanyl administered with bupivacaine during labor. Anesthesiology 1995; 83:300-8.

111. Bang U, Helbo-Hansen HS, Lindholm P, Klitgaard NA. Placental transfer and neonatal effects of epidural fentanyl-bupivacaine for cesarean section (abstract). Anesthesiology 1991; 75:A847.

112. Cooper J, Jauniaux E, Gulbis B, et al. Placental transfer of fentanyl in early human pregnancy and its detection in fetal brain. Br J Anaesth 1999; 82:929-31.

113. Zakowski M, Schlesinger J, Dumbroff S, et al. In vitro human placental uptake and transfer of fentanyl (abstract). Anesthesiology 1993; 79:A1006.

114. Gepts E, Heytens L, Camu F. Pharmacokinetics and placental transfer of intravenous and epidural alfentanil in parturient women. Anesth Analg 1986; 65:1155-60.

115. Gin T, Ngan-Kee WD, Siu YK, et al. Alfentanil given immediately before the induction of anesthesia for elective cesarean delivery. Anesth Analg 2000; 90:1167-72.

116. Kan RE, Hughes SC, Rosen MA, et al. Intravenous remifentanil: Placental transfer, maternal and neonatal effects. Anesthesiology 1998; 88:1467-74.

117. Santos Iglesias LJ, Sanchez LJ, Reboso Morales JA, et al. General anesthesia with remifentanil in two cases of emergency cesarean section [Spanish]. Rev Esp Anestesiol Reanim 2001; 48:244-7.

118. Pittman KA, Smyth RD, Losada M, et al. Human perinatal distribution of butorphanol. Am J Obstet Gynecol 1980; 138:797-800.

119. Wilson SJ, Errick JK, Balkon J. Pharmacokinetics of nalbuphine during parturition. Am J Obstet Gynecol 1986; 155:340-4.

120. Nicolle E, Devillier P, Delanoy B, et al. Therapeutic monitoring of nalbuphine: Transplacental transfer and estimated pharmacokinetics in the neonate. Eur J Clin Pharmacol 1996; 49:485-9.

121. Moya F, Kvisselgaard N. The placental transmission of succinylcholine. Anesthesiology 1961; 22:1-6.

122. Kvisselgaard N, Moya F. Investigation of placental thresholds to succinylcholine. Anesthesiology 1961; 22:7-10.

123. Owens WD, Zeitlin GL. Hypoventilation in a newborn following administration of succinylcholine to the mother: A case report. Anesth Analg 1975; 54:38-40.

124. Baraka A, Haroun S, Dassili M, Abu-Haider G. Response of the newborn to succinylcholine injection in homozygotic atypical mothers. Anesthesiology 1975; 43:115-6.

125. Hinkle AJ, Dorsch JA. Maternal masseter muscle rigidity and neonatal fasciculations after induction for emergency cesarean section. Anesthesiology 1993; 79:175-7.

126. Kivalo I, Saarikoski S. Placental transfer of ^{14}C-dimethyltubocurarine during Caesarean section. Br J Anaesth 1976; 48:239-42.

127. Duvaldestin P, Demetriou M, Henzel D, Desmonts JM. The placental transfer of pancuronium and its pharmacokinetics during caesarian section. Acta Anaesthesiol Scand 1978; 22:327-33.

128. Abouleish E, Wingard LB Jr, de la Vega S, Uy N. Pancuronium in caesarean section and its placental transfer. Br J Anaesth 1980; 52:531-6.

129. Dailey PA, Fisher DM, Shnider SM, et al. Pharmacokinetics, placental transfer, and neonatal effects of vecuronium and pancuronium administered during cesarean section. Anesthesiology 1984; 60:569-74.

130. Iwama H, Kaneko T, Tobishima S, et al. Time dependency of the ratio of umbilical vein/maternal artery concentration of vecuronium in caesarean section. Acta Anaesthesiol Scand 1999; 43:9-12.

131. Shearer ES, Fahy LT, O'Sullivan EP, Hunter JM. Transplacental distribution of atracurium, laudanosine and monoquaternary alcohol during elective caesarean section. Br J Anaesth 1991; 66:551-6.

132. Abouleish EI, Abboud TS, Bikhazi G, et al. Rapacuronium for modified rapid sequence induction in elective caesarean section: neuromuscular blocking effects and safety compared with succinylcholine, and placental transfer. Br J Anaesth 1999; 83:862-7.

133. Abouleish E, Abboud T, Lechevalier T, et al. Rocuronium (Org 9426) for caesarean section. Br J Anaesth 1994; 73:336-41.

134. Baraka AS, Sayyid SS, Assaf BA. Thiopental-rocuronium versus ketamine-rocuronium for rapid-sequence intubation in parturients undergoing cesarean section. Anesth Analg 1997; 84:1104-7.

135. Kivalo I, Saarikoski S. Placental transmission of atropine at full-term pregnancy. Br J Anaesth 1977; 49:1017-21.

136. Kanto J, Kentala E, Kaila T, Pihlajamäki K. Pharmacokinetics of scopolamine during caesarean section: Relationship between serum concentration and effect. Acta Anaesthesiol Scand 1989; 33:482-6.

137. Ali-Melkkilä T, Kaila T, Kanto J, Iisalo E. Pharmacokinetics of glycopyrronium in parturients. Anaesthesia 1990; 45:634-7.

138. Abboud TK, Read J, Miller F, et al. Use of glycopyrrolate of the parturient: Effect on the maternal and fetal heart and uterine activity. Obstet Gynecol 1981; 57:224-7.

139. Briggs GG, Freeman RK, Yaffee SJ. Drugs in Pregnancy and Lactation: A Reference Guide to Fetal and Neonatal Risk, 4th ed. Baltimore, Williams and Wilkins, 1994.

140. Clark RB, Brown MA, Lattin DL. Neostigmine, atropine, and glycopyrrolate: Does neostigmine cross the placenta? Anesthesiology 1996; 84:450-2.

141. Cottrill CM, McAllister RGJ, Gettes L, Noonan JA. Propranolol therapy during pregnancy, labor, and delivery: Evidence for transplacental drug transfer and impaired neonatal drug disposition. J Pediatr 1977; 91:812-4.

142. Witter FR, King TM, Blake DA. Adverse effects of cardiovascular drug therapy on the fetus and neonate. Obstet Gynecol 1981; 58:100S-5S.

143. Erkkola R, Lammintausta R, Liukko P, Anttila M. Transfer of propranolol and sotalol across the human placenta. Their effect on maternal and fetal plasma renin activity. Acta Obstet Gynecol Scand 1982; 61:31-4.

144. Melander A, Niklasson B, Ingemarsson I, et al. Transplacental passage of atenolol in man. Eur J Clin Pharmacol 1978; 14:93-4.

145. Lindeberg S, Sandström B, Lundborg P, Regårdh C-G. Disposition of the adrenergic blocker metoprolol in the late-pregnant woman, the amniotic fluid, the cord blood and the neonate. Acta Obstet Gynecol Scand Suppl 1984; 118:61-4.
146. Macpherson M, Broughton-Pipkin F, Rutter N. The effect of maternal labetalol on the newborn infant. Br J Obstet Gynaecol 1986; 93:539-42.
147. Michael CA. Use of labetalol in the treatment of severe hypertension during pregnancy. Br J Clin Pharmacol 1979; 8:211S-5S.
148. Östman PL, Chestnut DH, Robillard JE, et al. Transplacental passage and hemodynamic effects of esmolol in the gravid ewe. Anesthesiology 1988; 69:738-41.
149. Ducey JP, Knape KG. Maternal esmolol administration resulting in fetal distress and cesarean section in a term pregnancy. Anesthesiology 1992; 77:829-32.
150. Hartikainen-Sorri A-L, Heikkinen JE, Koivisto M. Pharmacokinetics of clonidine during pregnancy and nursing. Obstet Gynecol 1987; 69:598-600.
151. Jones HMR, Cummings AJ, Setchell KD, Lawson AM. A study of the disposition of α-methyldopa in newborn infants following its administration to the mother for the treatment of hypertension during pregnancy. Br J Clin Pharmacol 1979; 8:433-40.
152. David R, Leitch IM, Read MA, et al. Actions of magnesium, nifedipine and clonidine on the fetal vasculature of the human placenta. Aust NZ J Obstet Gynaecol 1996;36:267-71.
153. Ala-Kokko TI, Pienimaki P, Lampela E, et al. Transfer of clonidine and dexmedetomidine across the isolated perfused human placenta. Acta Anaesth Scand 1997; 41:313-9.
154. Santeiro ML, Stromquist C, Wyble L. Phenoxybenzamine placental transfer during the third trimester. Ann Pharmacother 1996; 30:1249-51.
155. Liedholm H, Wahlin-Boll E, Hanson A, et al. Transplacental passage and breast milk concentrations of hydralazine. Eur J Clin Pharmacol 1982; 21:417-9.
156. Magee KP, Bawdon RE. Ex vivo human placental transfer and the vasoactive properties of hydralazine. Am J Obstet Gynecol 2000; 182:167-9.
157. Naulty J, Cefalo RC, Lewis PE. Fetal toxicity of nitroprusside in the pregnant ewe. Am J Obstet Gynecol 1981; 139:708-11.
158. Gracine KA, Curry SC, Bikin DS, et al. The lack of transplacental movement of the cyanide antidote thiosulfate in gravid ewes. Anesth Analg 1999; 89:1448-52.
159. Bustard MA, Farley AE, Smith GN. The pharmacokinetics of glyceryl trinitrate with the use of the in vitro term human placental perfusion setup. Am J Obstet Gynecol 2002; 187:187-90.
160. Bootstaylor BS, Roman C, Parer JT, Heymann MA. Fetal and maternal hemodynamic and metabolic effects of maternal nitroglycerin infusion in sheep. Am J Obstet Gynecol 1997; 176:644-50.
161. Segal S, Csavoy AN, Datta S. Placental tissue enhances uterine relaxation by nitroglycerin. Anesth Analg 1998; 86:304-9.
162. Zhang XQ, Kwek K, Read MA, et al. Effects of nitrovasodilators on the human fetal-placental circulation in vitro. Placenta 2001; 22: 337-46.
163. Ducsay CA, Umezaki H, Kanshal KM, et al. Pharmacokinetic and fetal cardiovascular effects of enalaprilat administration to maternal rhesus macaques. Am J Obstet Gynecol 1996; 175:50-5.
164. Hughes SC, Ward MG, Levinson G, et al. Placental transfer of ephedrine does not affect neonatal outcome. Anesthesiology 1985; 63:217-9.
165. Krishna RB, Levitz M, Dancis J. Transfer of cocaine by the perfused human placenta: the effect of binding to serum proteins. Am J Obstet Gynecol 1995; 172:720-2.
166. Schenker S, Yang Y, Johnson RF, et al. The transfer of cocaine and its metabolites across the term human placenta. Clin Pharmacol Ther 1993; 53:329-39.
167. Simone C, Derewlany LO, Oskamp M, et al. Transfer of cocaine and benzoylecgonine across the perfused human placental cotyledon. Am J Obstet Gynecol 1994; 170:1404-10.
168. Zhou M, Song ZM, Lidow MS. Pharmacokinetics of cocaine in maternal and fetal rhesus monkeys at mid-gestation. J Pharmacol Exper Ther 2001; 297:556-62.
169. Hall JG, Pauli RM, Wilson KM. Maternal and fetal sequelae of anticoagulation during pregnancy. Am J Med 1980; 68:122-40.
170. Flessa HC, Kapstrom AB, Glueck HI, Will JJ. Placental transport of heparin. Am J Obstet Gynecol 1965; 93:570-3.
171. Andrew M, Boneu B, Cade J, et al. Placental transport of low molecular weight heparin in the pregnant sheep. Br J Haematol 1985; 59:103-8.
172. Dimitrakakis C, Papageorgiou P, Papageorgiou I, et al. Absence of transplacental passage of the low molecular weight heparin enoxaparin. Haemostasis 2000; 30:243-8.
173. Lagrange F, Vergnes C, Brun JL, et al. Absence of placental transfer of pentasaccharide (fondaparinux, Arixtra^R) in the dually perfused human cotyledon in vitro. Thromb Haemost 2002; 87:831-5.
174. Barzago MM, Bortolotti A, Stellari FF, et al. Placental transfer of valproic acid after liposome encapsulation during in vitro human placenta perfusion. J Pharmacol Exper Ther 1996; 277:79-86.
175. Bajoria R, Contractor SF. Effect of surface change on small unilamellar liposome on uptake and transfer of carboxyfluorescein across the perfused human term placenta. Pediatric Research 1997; 42:520-7.
176. American College of Obstetricians and Gynecologists Committee on Obstetrics: Maternal and Fetal Medicine. Placental pathology. ACOG Committee Opinion No. 125, 1993.
177. College of American Pathologists Conference XIX. The examination of the placenta: Patient care and risk management. Arch Pathol Lab Med 1991; 115:641-732.
178. Mooney EE, Boggess KA, Herbert WN, Layfield LJ. Placental pathology in patients using cocaine: An observational study. Obstet Gynecol 1998; 91:925-9.

Chapter 5
Fetal Physiology

Andrew P. Harris, M.D., M.H.S.

Because the fetus depends completely on maternal sources of metabolic substrate to maintain viability, special physiology patterns are present in the fetus that are different from those in postnatal animals. The fetus also must be prepared to undergo an abrupt transition to a state of physiologic independence: the process known as birth. This process necessarily involves adaptive mechanisms that attempt to ameliorate the stress that occurs during the transition from in utero to postnatal life.

FETAL OXIDATIVE METABOLISM

Oxygen Uptake and Substrate Use

Like postnatal animals, the fetus depends on the metabolism of oxygen to provide the energy necessary to maintain life. Unlike postnatal animals, the fetus has almost no oxygen reservoir in its body. Therefore, the fetal oxidative metabolic requirement is totally dependent on the ongoing transplacental transfer of oxygen from the mother to the fetus. When this transfer is hindered significantly, the fetal response is directed toward the preservation of oxygen transport to vital organ systems for as long as possible (vide infra).

Oxygen is transferred from the uterine circulation to the umbilical circulation by passive diffusion (see Chapter 4). Fetal arterial Po_2 is much lower than that in postnatal animals. However, under chronic basal conditions, the fetus is not "hypoxemic" despite this low Pao_2, primarily because of an increased hemoglobin concentration. Despite a lower Sao_2, oxygen content is normal by postnatal standards. Evidence supporting a normoxemic state includes the following: (1) a net lactate uptake (not production) by the fetus occurs, (2) only small amounts of hydrogen ion are transferred from fetus to mother, (3) no increase in oxygen consumption ($\dot{V}O_2$) occurs when increased oxygen is made available to the fetus, and (4) the healthy fetus has a normal basal pH.[1]

Total uterine oxygen uptake can be divided into two components: placental consumption and umbilical oxygen uptake (i.e., uptake by the fetus as opposed to the placenta). At term gestation, placental oxygen consumption accounts for approximately 40% of total uterine oxygen uptake,[2] but it is even higher at mid-gestation.[3] The placenta is metabolically active and plays an important role in carbohydrate and amino acid metabolism and substrate transport; all of these functions depend on oxidative metabolism as an energy source.

Umbilical $\dot{V}O_2$ is fairly constant and varies little among different mammalian species when it is corrected for fetal weight.[4] Human fetal $\dot{V}O_2$ is estimated to be approximately 6.8 to 8.0 mL O_2/kg/min.[5,6] By contrast, there is a clear inverse relationship between weight and metabolic rate in adult mammals.

Factors that influence fetal $\dot{V}O_2$ include the following: (1) fetal growth, (2) fetal activity (e.g., breathing movements, limb movements, cardiac activity), (3) substrate availability, (4) fetal organ metabolism, and (5) fetal hormonal status. Growth and activity account for a significant portion of $\dot{V}O_2$[7,8]; however, the use of oxygen for growth and activity is not necessary for survival and can be eliminated in times of stress.

Studies of sheep suggest that approximately 15% of total $\dot{V}O_2$ is used for striated muscle activity. In fact, skeletal muscle paralysis results in a 10% to 15% decrease in $\dot{V}O_2$ in fetal lambs.[7] The fetal brain accounts for approximately 8% to 9% of total $\dot{V}O_2$, and liver, intestines, and kidneys together account for approximately 29% (Figure 5-1).[9-14]

Fetal $\dot{V}O_2$ is increased above normal levels in utero in at least three circumstances: (1) during increased fetal activity; (2) during increased glucose uptake; and (3) during increased secretion of various hormones. Maternal hyperglycemia results in excessive maternal-fetal glucose transfer; the resulting hyperinsulinemia can cause as much as a 30% increase in fetal $\dot{V}O_2$.[15] Although such large increases in fetal $\dot{V}O_2$ can result in acidosis and even death in fetal lambs, the same does not consistently occur in humans.[16] Excessive secretion of catecholamines or thyroid hormones also can result in a 20% to 30% increase in $\dot{V}O_2$ in fetal lambs; thus the increased fetal catecholamine concentrations that may occur normally during labor and delivery may adversely affect fetal oxygenation, especially if oxygen transport is decreased and the fetal response to decreased oxygen transport is impaired.

Fetal $\dot{V}O_2$ does not change during fetal hypoglycemia, because hypoglycemia stimulates glycogenolysis and gluconeogenesis. By contrast, during severe fetal hypoxemia, $\dot{V}O_2$ may be depressed by as much as 40% in fetal lambs.[17] Potential causes of fetal hypoxemia include maternal hypoxemia, abnormal uterine or placental blood flow, placental

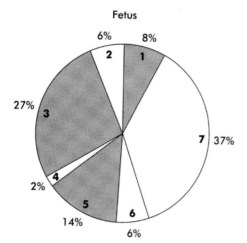

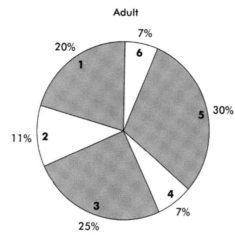

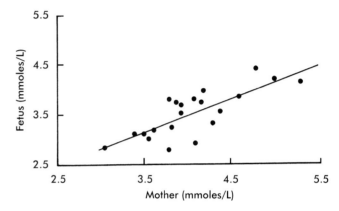

FIGURE 5-1. Tissue-specific oxygen consumption in chronically instrumented fetal lambs and resting adult humans.[12,13] *1*, Brain; *2*, heart; *3*, liver and intestines; *4*, kidney; *5*, muscle; *6*, other; *7*, growth (fetus only).

abnormalities, and fetal disorders. During fetal hypoxemia, the decreased fetal $\dot{V}O_2$ is associated with decreased metabolism in the fetal liver, intestines, and kidney[11,17,18]; cerebral and myocardial oxygen uptake are unchanged. If bradycardia occurs, myocardial oxygen uptake decreases. Fetal skeletal muscle activity (including fetal breathing movements) also decreases. Glycogenolysis occurs, resulting in an increased availability of substrate for both the brain and myocardium, which are the two organ systems that are essential for survival.

Glucose/Lactate Metabolism

Under normal conditions, gluconeogenesis does not occur to any significant extent in mammalian fetuses. Under normal fasting conditions at term gestation, maternal glucose transferred across the placenta is the sole source of glucose for the human fetus.[19] Fetal glucose concentrations are linearly related to maternal concentrations over the range of 3 to 5 mmol/L (Figure 5-2). Isolated placental studies suggest that the relationship remains linear up to a glucose concentration of 20 mmol/L.[20] Glucose is transferred across the placenta by facilitated, carrier-mediated diffusion. An analysis of total uterine glucose uptake reveals that the majority of the glucose is used by the placenta and that the remainder is transferred to the umbilical circulation. Glucose is used by the placenta for oxidation, glycogen storage, and conversion to lactate. Interestingly, when ovine uterine blood flow is reduced by 50%, there is no corresponding effect on fetal glucose uptake or fetal arterial glucose concentration.[21] However, when uterine blood flow is decreased further or when umbilical arterial flow is reduced by ligation of one of the umbilical arteries, fetal glucose uptake decreases.[21,22]

The umbilical glucose uptake is approximately 5 mg/kg/min at normal maternal arterial plasma glucose concentrations.[23] Because the umbilical glucose/oxygen quotient varies from approximately 0.5 in sheep[24] to 0.8 in human fetuses during labor,[25] it must be assumed that substrates other than glucose (e.g., lactate, amino acids) fuel a significant amount of fetal oxidative metabolism. Lactate and amino acids may each account for approximately 25% of total fetal $\dot{V}O_2$.[26,27]

Lactate is produced even in well-oxygenated fetal lambs. Total lactate production is approximately 4 mg/kg/min.[28] Although the exact origin of fetal lactate is unclear, the skeletal muscle and bone are definite sources of lactate production under resting conditions in fetal lambs. This lactate produc-

FIGURE 5-2. The linear relationship between maternal and fetal blood glucose concentrations during the third trimester. Fetal blood was obtained by percutaneous umbilical cord blood sampling. (From Kalhan SC. Metabolism of glucose and methods of investigation in the fetus and newborn. In: Polin RA, Fox WW, editors. Fetal and Neonatal Physiology, vol. I. Philadelphia, WB Saunders, 1992:477-88.)

tion becomes even greater during episodes of acute hypoxemia, although the increase may be blunted in fetuses previously exposed to oxidative stress.[29] Other organs are probably net producers as well. In terms of lactate use, the fetal myocardium is a net consumer of lactate, and the fetal liver also is a likely site of lactate utilization.[30] Exogenous lactate infusion in fetal lambs (sufficient to lower the pH to 7.20) results in transient fetal bradycardia and increased fetal breathing movements but no adverse effects.[31]

Amino Acid and Lipid Metabolism

Amino acids are taken up by the fetus for protein synthesis, growth, and oxidation. Most maternal-to-fetal amino acid transfer occurs against a concentration gradient and involves energy-dependent transfer mechanisms. Under conditions in which fetal aerobic metabolism is decreased, amino acid uptake by the placenta and fetus may be reduced because it involves an expenditure of energy. Hypoxia results in a large reduction in nitrogen uptake in fetal lambs.[32] During a maternal fast, fetal amino acid uptake does not change; however, evidence suggests that it may cause enhanced fetal proteolysis, which could result in amino acid oxidation or gluconeogenesis.

Lipid products also are transferred from the mother to the fetus. The fetus requires free fatty acids for growth, brain development, and the deposition of body fat for postnatal life. Fatty acids are transferred across the placenta by simple diffusion. Ketones also are transferred by simple diffusion; in humans, the maternal:fetal ratio is approximately 2.0.[33] The fetus can use ketones as energy or as lipogenic substrates.[34] Fetal tissues that can oxidize ketones include the brain, kidney, heart, liver, and placenta. Beta-hydroxybutyrate metabolism can replace glucose metabolism deficits in the placenta, brain, and liver during episodes of fetal hypoglycemia that result from maternal fasting.[34] Cholesterol synthesis or free cholesterol diffusion does not appear to occur in the placenta.[35] However, there is a significant correlation between maternal and fetal concentrations of lipoprotein(a), which implies that diffusion of lipoprotein(a) may occur.[35]

GENERAL GROWTH AND DEVELOPMENT

Normal growth and development occur when the fetus has an adequate supply of metabolic substrate and is able to use it. Conversely, growth and development are abnormal when adequate supplies are not available or when the fetus is unable to use the substrate that is available. Fetal measurements allow not only a dynamic assessment of fetal growth but also a static indication of fetal well-being. Normal fetal growth curves have been constructed using birth weights in a large series of newborns at varying weeks of gestation; these curves indicate a normal rate of human fetal growth of approximately 1.45% per day.

Such growth curves are useful when defining static categorizations of infant size. For example, infants who are appropriate for gestational age (AGA) are those with a weight between the 10th and 90th percentile for their gestational age. Infants who are large for gestational age (LGA) are those with a weight greater than the 90th percentile for their gestational age; infants who are small for gestational age (SGA) are those with a weight below the 10th percentile. However, evidence suggests that the 15th percentile would be a more useful threshold, because fetuses between the 10th and 15th percentile also are at increased risk for fetal death.[36] These terms (AGA, LGA, and SGA) should not be confused with terms used to describe birth weight independent of gestational age. Specifically, low birth weight (LBW) infants are those who weigh less than 2500 g, regardless of gestational age. Very low birth weight (VLBW) infants are those who weigh less than 1500 g, and extremely low birth weight (ELBW) infants are those who weigh less than 1000 g, regardless of gestational age. These last terms may not indicate abnormal growth. For example, although it would be normal for a newborn at 25 weeks' gestation to be an ELBW infant, it would not be normal at term. Babies who are SGA or LGA may not have suffered from pathophysiologic processes. Infants may be SGA for a variety of reasons, including genetic predetermination of small size.[37] Likewise, an LGA infant may represent a normal genetic expression.

However, the diagnosis of intrauterine growth restriction (IUGR)* signals an ongoing process of subnormal fetal growth over time. IUGR is more likely than birth weight to represent an underlying physiologic abnormality. Any process that results in a chronically inadequate availability of substrate or that impedes the fetus' ability to use substrate will cause the fetus to grow at a less-than-normal rate. For example, the plasma concentrations of a number of amino acids (but not glucose) are decreased in cases of IUGR, possibly as a result of decreased placental transport. In cases of IUGR, the activity of the placental microvillous transport system A is reduced in vitro.[38] Fetuses who suffer intrauterine oxidative stress also have a reduction in oxygen consumption, even after the stress is removed.[29] Of course, if an affected fetus remains in utero long enough, it is likely that it will be SGA at birth. Most cases of IUGR result in the delivery of an infant who is SGA.

IUGR may be **asymmetric** or **symmetric**. In cases of asymmetric IUGR, fetal brain growth is relatively preserved, but growth of the remainder of the body is diminished, which results in an asymmetry between head growth and body growth. An asymmetric growth pattern may be the consequence of a chronically decreased supply of substrate, which may occur for a variety of reasons. In cases of symmetric IUGR, head circumference and body length are reduced proportionately to overall weight. In some instances, this may be a normal growth pattern (e.g., genetic predisposition); in other cases, it may signal an insult that began early in gestation (e.g., genetic abnormality, congenital infection, prolonged uteroplacental insufficiency). Either category of IUGR makes the fetus less tolerant of a superimposed acute substrate deprivation, which may occur in a variety of circumstances, including labor and delivery. The diagnosis of IUGR is associated with an increased risk of fetal death.[39]

The diagnosis of IUGR, although more useful than static measurements, is also more difficult to ascertain. Various diagnostic techniques are used to assess intrauterine fetal growth. Physical examination (e.g., serial measurement of fundal height) is an inexpensive means of assessment, but it is neither sensitive nor specific for the diagnosis of IUGR. Serial sonographic examinations represent the most reliable method for the diagnosis of IUGR. During early gestation, a sonographic examination includes the measurement of crown-rump length. Subsequently, serial sonographic examinations include measurements of head size, abdominal circumference, and femur length. These measurements may be used to provide an estimate of fetal weight.

Other methods may be used to study fetuses in whom abnormalities of growth are suspected. Doppler ultrasonography can be used to study both the uteroplacental and umbilical vessels. However, these techniques do not measure fetal size or growth alone. A correlation exists between abnormal flow patterns[40,41] or pulse waveforms[42] and adverse fetal outcome. Growth-restricted fetuses may have an increased resistance in the umbilical arteries and descending aorta, with relatively normal internal carotid[43] or middle cerebral[44] (especially the subcortical segment[45]) artery flow; these findings are consistent with the brain sparing that occurs with asymmetric IUGR. In SGA infants, abnormality of both umbilical and middle cerebral artery velocimetry predicts adverse fetal outcome.[46] Abnormal Doppler flow studies of the fetal aorta are associated with poor perinatal outcome, especially if associated with abnormal umbilical artery flow studies.[47]

---

*Editor's note: Throughout this text, I have substituted the word *restriction* for the word *retardation*. This reflects my preference—and the preference of a growing number of obstetricians—for the use of the word *restriction* to describe abnormal somatic growth.

FETAL HEAT PRODUCTION AND THERMOREGULATION

At term, the human fetus consumes oxygen at the rate of approximately 6.8 to 8.0 mL/kg/min; this is approximately twice the rate of adult oxygen consumption, which is 3 to 4 mL/kg/min. Therefore, fetal heat production is large relative to that of the adult. Assuming that approximately 5 cal of heat are produced for each milliliter of oxygen consumed, a 4-kg human fetus produces approximately 136 cal/min, which is approximately 10 watts. This heat accumulates until a relatively constant temperature gradient is established, which causes heat to be dissipated into the mother. At steady state, this gradient is approximately 0.5° C. Because the gradient remains relatively constant, fetal temperature parallels maternal temperature. This temperature relationship, in which fetal temperature depends on maternal temperature, is sometimes referred to as a *heat clamp*, which prevents independent fetal thermoregulation in utero.

Heat dissipates from the fetus by means of two possible avenues: (1) the umbilical circulation (and therefore the placenta), and (2) fetal skin (by means of the amniotic fluid). Of these two, experimental evidence suggests that the umbilical circulation is the major source of fetal heat loss. In both baboons[48] and sheep,[49] fetal temperature increases shortly after umbilical cord occlusion, which may result in part from the activation of normal postnatal thermogenic mechanisms.[50] A decrease in uterine blood flow likewise would be expected to increase fetal temperature, but this has not been studied directly. However, the maternal-fetal temperature gradient does increase during uterine contractions in humans,[51] which indirectly confirms the importance of the placenta as a heat exchanger for the fetus. Heat loss through the skin and amniotic fluid represents only a small portion (15%) of fetal-maternal heat exchange.[50] Epidural anesthesia during labor may result in increased fetal temperature,[52] possibly because epidural anesthesia "alters the [maternal] thermoregulatory response to warming by increasing the threshold for thermoregulatory sweating and in some cases, [by] preventing leg sweating"[53] (see Chapter 36).

FETAL CIRCULATION

The fetal circulation allows the fetus to match the local supply of metabolic substrate to local demand. An understanding of fetal circulation requires an understanding of the following: (1) fetal oxygen transport, (2) the regulation of fetal blood volume, (3) the unique fetal circulatory pattern, and (4) the various factors that control the distribution of blood flow. These factors become critically important when substrate demand exceeds substrate supply during periods of fetal stress.

Fetal Oxygen Transport

Oxygen delivery to a fetal organ is the product of blood flow to that organ times the oxygen content of fetal arterial blood. The oxygen content of fetal blood is largely determined by the product of the concentration of hemoglobin (the predominant vehicle of oxygen transport in blood), the percent of hemoglobin that is bound to oxygen, and a constant of approximately 1.39 mL O_2/g Hgb (the oxygen-carrying capacity of hemoglobin). In adults, as the P_{O_2} is increased toward 1 atm, the oxygen content of arterial blood is augmented significantly by the presence of oxygen dissolved in plasma. Plasma oxygen content increases by approximately 0.003 mL O_2/dL

blood per mm Hg increase in Pa_{O_2}. In theory, an increased Pa_{O_2} allows adult animals to augment their total blood oxygen content by 1.5 to 1.8 mL O_2/dL (i.e., by approximately one third of adult oxygen consumption). By contrast, fetal umbilical venous P_{O_2} does not increase by more than 50 to 60 mm Hg, even when maternal oxygenation is optimized under isobaric oxygen conditions. The amount of oxygen dissolved in fetal plasma is insignificant relative to fetal oxygen demand or fetal hemoglobin oxygen-carrying capacity. The normal fetal hemoglobin concentration is approximately 18 g/dL. The oxygen-carrying capacity of fetal blood should be approximately 25 mL O_2/dL, a capacity that is greater than that of adults. However, this is only a theoretical capacity, because fetal hemoglobin never approaches complete saturation at the relatively low levels of P_{O_2} in utero.

At the low P_{O_2} of the intervillous space, a higher affinity of fetal blood for oxygen would augment the transfer of oxygen from the mother to the fetus. In fact, fetal blood has a higher affinity for oxygen than does maternal blood in vivo. The P_{50} of human fetal blood is approximately 19 to 21 mm Hg, which is in contrast with the 27 mm Hg found in adult blood (Figure 5-3). This observed difference in affinity for oxygen is largely a result of the relatively high concentration of hemoglobin F in fetal blood (i.e., approximately 75% to 84% of total hemoglobin at term).[54] The tetramer for hemoglobin F consists of two alpha chains and two gamma chains, whereas the tetramer for adult hemoglobin A includes two alpha chains and two beta chains. This change in globin composition does not result in a change in the absorption spectra of oxygenated and reduced hemoglobin[55] or in a change in oxygen affinity outside of the erythrocyte in vitro.[56] Instead, the shift in fetal blood oxygen affinity in vivo can be explained by a decreased interaction between hemoglobin F and intraerythrocyte 2,3-diphosphoglycerate (DPG), which normally acts to lower oxygen affinity by binding to and stabilizing the

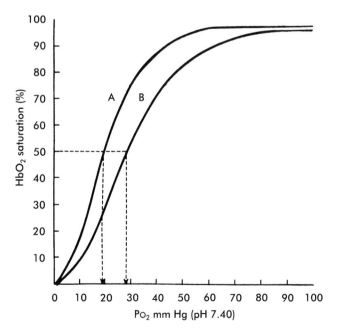

FIGURE 5-3. Oxyhemoglobin saturation curves for fetal *(A)* and adult *(B)* human blood. The P_{50} is indicated by the dashed vertical line. (Modified from Delivoria-Papadopoulos M, DiGiacomo JE. Oxygen transport. In: Polin RA, Fox WW, editors. Fetal and Neonatal Physiology, vol. 1. Philadelphia, WB Saunders, 1992:807.)

deoxygenated hemoglobin tetramer. The gamma chains of hemoglobin F do not bind as readily to 2,3-DPG. The net effect is that 2,3-DPG does not decrease the oxygen affinity of hemoglobin F as much as it decreases the oxygen affinity of hemoglobin A. Thus, although fetuses and adults have similar intraerythrocyte 2,3-DPG concentrations, fetal blood exhibits a lower P_{50} than adult blood. In utero, this increased affinity of fetal blood for oxygen results in a 6% to 8% higher saturation of hemoglobin on the fetal side of the intervillous membrane.

Hemoglobin A levels begin to increase and 2,3-DPG concentrations transiently increase above fetal and adult levels during the first few months of life. Therefore, the affinity of neonatal blood for oxygen is equivalent to that of the adult within 3 to 4 months of birth, despite the persistence of approximately 25% hemoglobin F.

The Regulation of Extracellular Fluid Volume

Extracellular fluid volume includes both interstitial fluid and intravascular volume. The distribution between these two compartments is determined predominantly by the colloid osmotic pressure in the intravascular compartment, the capillary hydrostatic pressure, and the capillary membrane permeability according to the Starling equation:

$$Q = K_f [(P_c - P_t) - \delta (\pi_c - \pi_t)]$$

where

Q = Fluid flux
K_f = Filtration coefficient (which expresses the membrane permeability to water flux)
P_c and P_t = Capillary and tissue hydrostatic pressures, respectively
δ = Reflection coefficient (which expresses the membrane's permeability to protein)
π_c and π_t = Capillary and tissue oncotic pressures, respectively

The intravascular volume of the term human fetus is approximately 100 to 110 mL/kg. This is larger than the blood volume in either the newborn or the adult, but approximately one third of fetal blood volume is contained outside of the fetal body in the umbilical cord and placenta.

Blood volume is regulated by the balance between interstitial volume and intravascular volume and is determined by plasma fluid loss across the capillaries. Given the relative stability of colloid osmotic pressure and capillary permeability, changes in hydrostatic pressure predominantly affect fetal blood volume. For example, blood volume decreases when hydrostatic pressure is transiently increased; such transient increases in hydrostatic pressure can occur during uterine contractions as blood is transferred from the placental vascular bed into the fetal body. Another etiology of decreased blood volume is an increase in capillary pressure as a result of the release of vasoconstrictive hormones, which occurs during periods of stress. Both factors may account for the observed decrease in circulating blood volume during labor and delivery.[57]

The maternal infusion of water or crystalloid also results in a change in fetal extracellular fluid volume. Under these conditions, transient changes in colloid osmotic pressure lead to transplacental osmotic gradients, and rapid equilibration occurs across the placenta. When this fluid is transferred to the fetus, its disposition differs from that found in adults. Specifically, adults who receive an intravenous infusion of crystalloid retain a significant amount of the infused volume in the intravascular space. In unanesthetized fetal lambs, a crystalloid infusion increases blood volume by only 6% to 7%; the remainder of the infusion rapidly enters the interstitial space.[58] This difference can be explained by the relatively high interstitial space compliance in the fetus and an apparently higher capillary filtration coefficient.[59] Thus, maternal infusion of crystalloid ultimately may result in a significant increase in fetal extracellular fluid volume. Anesthesiologists should consider this potential effect when giving a large volume of crystalloid to the mother.

Circulatory Pattern in Utero

The most striking difference between the fetal and postnatal circulations is that fetal systemic and pulmonary circulations are parallel, whereas postnatal circulations are in series. Blood flowing through the fetal right atrium is directed either through the foramen ovale into the left atrium or through the right ventricle into the pulmonary artery. Most pulmonary artery blood flow crosses the ductus arteriosus into the descending aorta and the left side of the circulation; only a small percentage travels through the lungs into the left atrium. The reason the fetal systemic and pulmonary circulations are parallel is obvious: the fetal lungs do not participate in blood oxygenation (a role that is met by the umbilical circulation, which is a component of the systemic circulation). Therefore, any pulmonary artery blood flow would be wasted and would gain no metabolic substrate in return for right ventricular work expended.

To maximize the efficiency of cardiac work and transplacental oxygen transfer, almost all deoxygenated blood from the fetal head and upper extremities enters the right atrium by means of the superior vena cava, moves into the right ventricle, and then moves through the ductus arteriosus into the distal aorta, from which a large percentage of flow goes to the placenta to be reoxygenated. By contrast, the oxygenated umbilical venous blood returns from the placenta, enters the right atrium by means of the inferior vena cava, and preferentially flows across the foramen ovale into the left atrium. From there it enters the left ventricle and the preductal circulation, which includes the brain and myocardium, the two organs with the highest oxygen requirements. This circulatory pattern facilitates the delivery of highly oxygenated blood to areas of high oxygen consumption and allows for the delivery of deoxygenated blood to the placenta, where oxygen uptake occurs. At birth, the circulatory pattern changes dramatically (see Chapter 9).

Cardiac Output

In postnatal mammals, the right ventricular output is approximately equal to the left ventricular output. Therefore, *cardiac output* is defined as the output of either the **right ventricle** (commonly measured with a thermodilution technique using a pulmonary artery catheter) or the **left ventricle** (measured with a green dye technique). By contrast, the fetus has an almost complete right-to-left shunt at the level of the ductus arteriosus. Therefore, fetal systemic flow consists of the sum of right and left ventricular output. Fetal cardiac output to the systemic circulation actually is **biventricular output**, which is also called **combined ventricular output (CVO)**. The CVO is approximately 500 mL/min/kg in near-term fetal lambs.[60-62] Right ventricular output is greater than left ventricular output, and right ventricular coronary blood flow is 50% greater than left ventricular coronary blood flow.[63] In fetal lambs, approximately two thirds of CVO originates from the right ventricle.[64] The primary function of the right ventricle (both in utero as well as after delivery) is to deliver blood for oxygen uptake. The purpose of the left ventricle is to deliver oxygenated blood.

CVO in utero is approximately equal to the output of each individual ventricle after birth.[65] Although total ventricular output doubles immediately after birth, it appears that the fetus is unable to increase CVO in utero, even during periods of stress. To understand the reason that cardiac output cannot be augmented in utero, we should consider the four major determinants of ventricular function: **preload, afterload, contractility,** and **heart rate**. The fetal response to changes in each of these factors differs from that of postnatal mammals.

VENTRICULAR RESPONSE TO CHANGES IN PRELOAD
According to the Frank-Starling curve, increased distention of the ventricles normally results in increased diastolic fiber length and an augmentation of contractility. Although fetal hemorrhage leads to an immediate decrease in fetal cardiac output, an increase in preload does not necessarily result in an increase in ventricular output. Volume infusions in normovolemic fetuses do not consistently result in increased ventricular output, for reasons that are not clear.[66-69]

Several factors may help explain this finding. First, isolated fibers of fetal myocardium demonstrate diminished tension development (as compared with mature myocardium) at all muscle lengths examined.[70] This finding may be explained by the significantly greater proportion of noncontractile proteins in fetal myocytes relative to adult myocytes. Further, at any given level of developed tension, myocardial shortening velocity and the extent of shortening are decreased in the fetus relative to the adult.[70] The velocity of force development is primarily determined by adenosine triphosphatase (ATPase) activity that is present in the myosin heavy chain. The myosin heavy chain isoform is different in fetuses and adults, and this may explain the difference in myocardial shortening.

Second, the highly compliant umbilical-placental circulation prevents a large increase in intracardiac volume, which prevents a significant increase in end-diastolic fiber length. The placental vascular bed can accommodate a large increase in intravascular volume, which typically prevents increased filling pressures in the relatively stiff fetal myocardium. However, even when end-diastolic pressures are increased as a result of intravascular transfusion, cardiac output does not increase.[71]

Third, volume infusion in the fetus typically results in a simultaneous increase in afterload, and the fetal heart is quite sensitive to an increase in afterload.[72] Fourth, the presence of a large interatrial shunt allows right and left ventricular end-diastolic pressures to increase equally during volume infusion, which impedes filling of the opposite ventricle. This diastolic ventricular interaction is a possible impediment to increasing ventricular volume in the relatively stiff fetal ventricles during volume infusion.

VENTRICULAR RESPONSE TO AFTERLOAD CHANGES
The second determinant of ventricular systolic function is afterload, which commonly is approximated by the calculation of systemic vascular resistance (SVR). In normal adults, an increase in afterload results in little if any decrease in cardiac output. In adults, a decrease in afterload typically results in an increase in cardiac output. By contrast, in fetal animals, the right ventricle responds to an increase in afterload with a decrease in cardiac output.[66] Conversely, the fetal right ventricle responds to a decrease in afterload with little change in right ventricular output.[66] The fetal left ventricle responds similarly.[67]

FETAL CARDIAC CONTRACTILITY
The third determinant of ventricular function is contractility. At all muscle lengths, a significant decrease in active tension is generated by fetal myocardium as compared with the mature heart. The sarcoplasmic reticulum is relatively immature in both structure and function. In addition, myofibrils are structurally and functionally immature in the fetus.[73,74] Finally, the beta-adrenergic receptor may be relatively unresponsive. Isoproterenol infusion does not result in an increase in cardiac output in fetal lambs.[75]

VENTRICULAR RESPONSE TO ALTERED HEART RATES
The fourth determinant of ventricular function is heart rate. In adult mammals, significant changes in heart rate do not result in proportional changes in cardiac output. As heart rate decreases, an increased diastolic filling time results in increased end-diastolic volume and increased end-diastolic fiber length. This results in an increase in stroke volume, which compensates for the decreased heart rate and helps keep cardiac output constant. An increased heart rate is accompanied by an increase in intrinsic myocardial contractility, but decreased diastolic filling time results in decreased end-diastolic and stroke volumes. The net result is no change or a slight increase in cardiac output. At either extreme of heart rate, cardiac output decreases.

By contrast, fetal ventricular output appears to be more sensitive to changes in heart rate. As heart rate increases, cardiac output increases.[76-78] As heart rate decreases, stroke volume increases only slightly, most likely because of the decreased compliance of the fetal myocardium and the ventricular diastolic interaction described previously. Although fetal bradycardia results in an increased diastolic filling time, the stiff, interactive ventricles are limited in their ability to distend. Therefore, fetal bradycardia is associated with a marked decrease in cardiac output.

Distribution of Cardiac Output
Figure 5-4 shows the distribution of CVO in near-term fetal lambs and resting adult humans. Approximately 41% of fetal CVO perfuses the placenta, and another 38% perfuses the skeletal muscle and bone. Renal, gastrointestinal, myocardial, and cerebral blood flow account for 2%, 6%, 4%, and 3% of CVO, respectively. The fetal systemic circulation is considered a low-resistance circulation, because a large fraction of CVO perfuses the relatively compliant placental circulation. In both fetal and adult animals, approximately equal volumes of blood proceed to the oxygen-uptake organ (i.e., the placenta before delivery, the lungs after delivery) and to the oxygen-consuming organs (i.e., the remainder of the body before delivery, the systemic circulation after delivery).

Control of the Systemic Circulation and the Fetal Response to Stress
Fetal cardiovascular function adapts to varying metabolic and environmental conditions through neuroregulation and endocrine regulation. The predominant form of neuroregulation occurs by means of the autonomic nervous system in

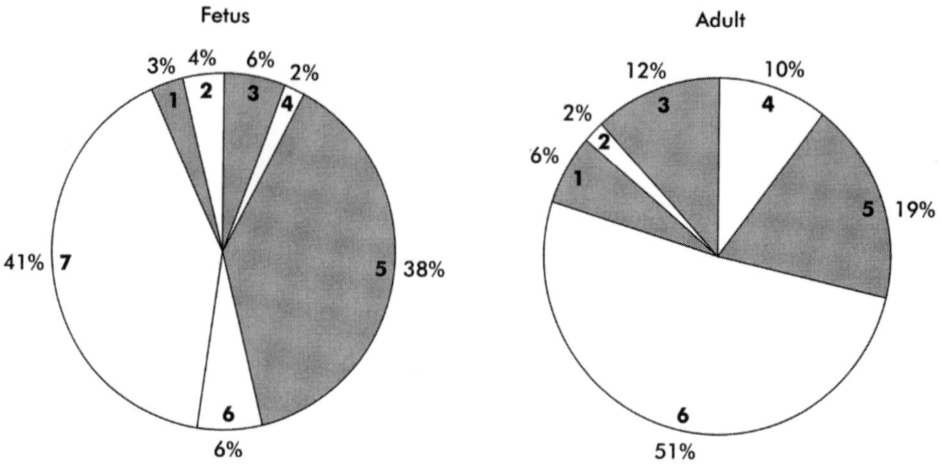

FIGURE 5-4. Regional distribution of the combined ventricular output in fetal lambs[51] and resting adult humans.[13] 1, Brain; 2, heart; 3, liver and intestines; 4, kidney; 5, muscles and other; 6, lungs; 7, placenta.

response to baroreceptor and chemoreceptor afferent input and through modulation of adrenergic receptor activity on the myocardium. In this capacity, the autonomic nervous system functions to reversibly redirect blood flow and oxygen delivery where and when required.

Arterial baroreceptor function has been demonstrated in several different fetal animal models. The predominant baroreceptors are located in the aortic arch and at the bifurcation of the common carotid arteries. These receptors project signals to the vasomotor center in the medulla, from which autonomic responses emanate. These baroreceptors begin to function relatively early in gestation. Resetting of the baroreceptors occurs as blood pressure increases during normal gestation.[79] An acute increase in fetal mean arterial pressure (MAP)—as occurs with partial or complete occlusion of the umbilical arteries—results in cholinergic stimulation, which causes fetal bradycardia.

Chemoreceptor activity is also present in many species of animals. Peripheral chemoreceptors are present in at least two locations: (1) between the aortic arch and the main pulmonary artery, and (2) at the bifurcation of the common carotid arteries. In addition, a peripheral chemoreceptor appears to be present in the adrenal gland in some species, but it disappears after birth.[80] The fetal aortic chemoreceptors are quite active and respond to small changes in arterial oxygenation.[81,82] Fetal carotid chemoreceptors are also active, but to a lesser extent. Dawes et al.[83] concluded that carotid chemoreceptors are more important for postnatal respiratory control, whereas aortic chemoreceptors are important in cardiovascular control and the regulation of oxygen delivery. Central chemoreceptors appear to play little if any role in the fetal chemoreceptor response.

Hypoxemia is the most common form of fetal stress that occurs during labor and delivery. Many studies have assessed the fetal circulatory response to hypoxemia in chronically instrumented pregnant sheep. Investigators have produced fetal hypoxemia by a variety of methods (e.g., administration of a hypoxic gas mixture to the mother, partial occlusion of the umbilical cord, partial occlusion of the uterine artery). Fetal hypoxemia results in a redistribution of blood flow away from the kidneys, spleen, carcass, and skin and toward the heart, brain, placenta, and adrenal glands. Nitric oxide appears to be an important mediator in the response of the coronary[84] and cerebral[85-87] circulations to hypoxia. Prostaglandins also play a prominent role.[85]

To a large extent, the increase in myocardial and cerebral blood flow can completely compensate for the decreased oxygen content of the blood and can help maintain myocardial and cerebral oxygen delivery, even during episodes of severe hypoxemia. At modest levels of hypoxemia, CVO is not affected, and blood pressure and heart rate are unchanged. However, extreme hypoxemia results in a decrease in cardiac output as a result of the bradycardic response to chemoreceptor stimulation. This decrease in CVO may be exacerbated by the presence of acidemia[88] and increased afterload resulting from umbilical cord occlusion. Combined blood flow to the heart and brain, which accounts for 7% to 8% of cardiac output under baseline conditions, increases to approximately 25% of cardiac output when oxygen content is reduced by 80% (Figure 5-5).[89] The absolute placental blood flow does not change during hypoxemia; however, when CVO decreases, the fraction of CVO distributed to the placenta increases. Animal studies suggest that fetal placental vascular resistance increases slightly during acute hypoxemia[88,89]; this response can be reversed by fetal alpha-adrenergic blockade.[90] Chronic hypoxemia in utero may lead to vascular remodeling that maintains the ability of the fetal coronary circulation to dilate in response to superimposed acute hypoxemia, even in the presence of a preexisting increase in flow that has occurred in response to the chronic hypoxemia.[84]

Sympathetic and Parasympathetic Development

Autonomic regulation of the peripheral circulation occurs predominantly through adrenergic mechanisms. The contractile response to norepinephrine is present in the fetal vasculature, although it is somewhat immature relative to the adult response.[91,92] Administration of alpha-adrenergic agonists results in the redistribution of fetal blood flow away from the kidneys, skin, and splanchnic organs and toward the heart, brain, placenta, and adrenal glands.[93]

Parasympathetic tone also affects the circulation, predominantly through an effect on heart rate. Parasympathetic activity first appears at approximately 16 weeks' gestation, when fetal administration of atropine results in fetal tachycardia. Sympathetic innervation of the heart becomes significant at the end of the second trimester. At this time, the fetal administration of a beta-adrenergic antagonist results in fetal bradycardia. Inotropic and chronotropic responses to adrenergic agents are present much earlier in gestation and have been measured as early as 4 to 5 weeks' gestation.[94] Likewise, the fetal myocardial pacemaker can be inhibited by the cholinergic agonists carbamylcholine and acetylcholine as early as 4 weeks' gestation.[95]

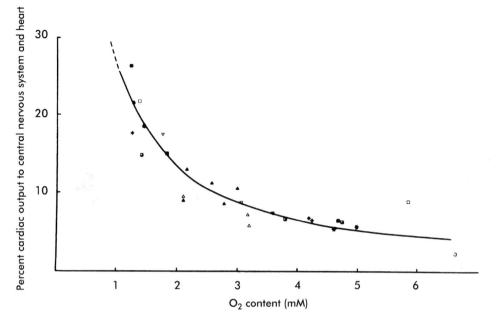

FIGURE 5-5. The redistribution of cardiac output to the heart and central nervous system during hypoxemia in fetal lambs. (Modified from Sheldon RE, Peeters LLH, Jones MD Jr, et al. Redistribution of cardiac output and oxygen delivery in the hypoxic fetal lamb. Am J Obstet Gynecol 1979; 135:1071.)

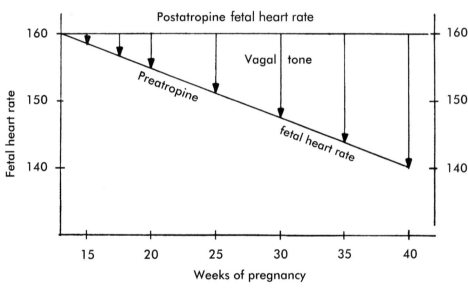

FIGURE 5-6. The increasing influence of the parasympathetic nervous system on fetal heart rate as gestation progresses. (From Schifferli P, Caldeyro-Barcia R. Effects of atropine and beta-adrenergic drugs on the heart rate of the human fetus. In: Broeus L, editor. Fetal Pharmacology. New York, Raven Press, 1973:264.)

Therefore, it is clear that autonomic receptor function appears much earlier than functional autonomic tone. Autonomic function is delayed even though nerve cells have been found in the human heart at 5 to 6 weeks' gestation,[96] parasympathetic cholinergic nerves have been identified in the human heart by 8 weeks' gestation,[97,98] and sympathetic adrenergic nerves are present by 9 to 10 weeks' gestation.[94]

Most studies have confirmed that parasympathetic innervation occurs earlier than sympathetic innervation and is present to a more complete extent at birth. As pregnancy progresses, parasympathetic activity becomes more dominant; thus the baseline fetal heart rate (FHR) at 40 weeks' gestation is less than the baseline FHR at 26 weeks' gestation. This decrease in FHR is reversible with atropine (Figure 5-6). Adrenergic innervation is relatively incomplete at birth.

Endocrine Control and the Response to Stress
Epinephrine released by the adrenal medulla is present in fetal plasma but at much lower concentrations than norepineph-

rine. Stress (e.g., hypoxemia, hemorrhage) may result in the release of epinephrine.

Arginine vasopressin (AVP) is detectable as early as 11 weeks' gestation in the posterior pituitary of human fetuses.[99] Even before mid-gestation, hemorrhage is a potent stimulus of vasopressin release in fetal lambs.[100,101] Under normal conditions, however, vasopressin is not an important regulator of fetal circulation. Fetal administration of a vasopressin-receptor antagonist has little or no effect on fetal arterial blood pressure in fetal lambs.[102] Vasopressin is released during episodes of acute fetal hypoxia,[103] and fetal infusion of vasopressin results in fetal hypertension. Vasopressin levels also increase dramatically during hypotension in fetal lambs,[104] and at vasopressin concentrations similar to those seen during stress responses, splanchnic and skin blood flow decrease. These changes are accompanied by a proportionate increase in cerebral, myocardial, and placental blood flow.[105] As a result, fetal Po_2 increases significantly, which implies that vasopressin may be an important mediator of the fetal response to acute hypoxemia.[88]

The renin-angiotensin system appears to be active under basal conditions in fetal animals.[106,107] Renin activity is present, and circulating angiotensin II concentrations can be measured in fetal lambs by 0.6 of the gestational period (i.e., just after mid-gestation). Various stresses result in increased renin-angiotensin system activity in fetal lambs. The renin response to hypotension[104] is greater than that seen in response to hypoxemia.[103] Interestingly, angiotensin II constricts the umbilical circulation when it is infused to achieve plasma concentrations similar to those observed during hemorrhage.[108] Basal concentrations of angiotensin II maintain chronic vasoconstriction of the peripheral circulation, which helps maintain arterial blood pressure and umbilical-placental blood flow. When angiotensin II receptors are blocked under basal conditions, blood pressure decreases, and umbilical-placental blood flow falls.[109]

Circulatory Responses to Increased Intracranial Pressure

As the fetal head descends into the maternal pelvis during normal labor, fetal intracranial pressure (ICP) increases out of proportion to the increases in intrauterine pressure. Pressures measured at the equator of the fetal head far exceed intraamniotic pressure.[110] These observations were confirmed in a study that used an intracranial catheter to measure ICP in two hydrocephalic fetuses during labor.[111] Outside of the range of cerebral autoregulation, cerebral perfusion pressure (defined as the MAP minus the greater of either cerebral venous pressure or ICP) is the determining factor in cerebral perfusion. Large increases in ICP in postnatal animals cause a transient decrease in cerebral perfusion pressure; this results in a Cushing response (i.e., vasoconstriction, increased MAP, increased cardiac output, decreased heart rate), which acts to return cerebral perfusion pressure toward normal. During labor, the fetal response to increased ICP may be important in preserving cerebral viability.

In fetal lambs, increased ICP results in a dramatic redistribution of the circulation. During gradual increases in ICP, MAP increases to maintain a cerebral perfusion pressure of approximately 26 mm Hg. Under these conditions, the redistribution of circulation includes the following: (1) decreased perfusion of the splanchnic organs, kidneys, and skin, (2) preservation of blood flow to the skeletal muscle and bone, and (3) augmented blood flow to the heart, brain, placenta, and adrenal glands.[112] Cardiac output does not change. Over time, fetal pH decreases as a result of these compensatory mechanisms. Nonetheless, cerebral oxygen delivery and uptake are maintained. In a similar model, when ICP is periodically increased to the level of MAP (using an oscillatory pattern), similar redistributions of blood flow occur over time. Cardiac output does not change.[113] Experiments involving alpha-adrenergic blockade indicate that the alpha-adrenergic system is primarily responsible for mediating this redistribution of the circulation,[102] which appears effective in preserving cerebral oxygen uptake, despite increased ICP.

Postnatal Effects of Intrauterine Stress

Investigators have expressed an interest in the postnatal effect of intrauterine stress on the autonomic nervous system. In one study, the postnatal sympathetic nervous system response to postural change (tilt) stress was enhanced, and the parasympathetic response to odor was blunted in infants who had chronic intrauterine stress (CIUSTR) from causes such as maternal smoking or maternal hypertension.[114] In a similar study,[115] a painful stimulus elicited a greater sympathetic response (i.e., increase in heart rate and blood pressure) in CIUSTR neonates than in a control group. In this study, an altered response to ocular compression indicated an enhanced parasympathetic response in the CIUSTR neonates. Thus, it appears that intrauterine stress affects the maturation and activity of the autonomic nervous system in the neonate.

KEY POINTS

- Unlike postnatal animals, the fetus has no effective oxygen reservoir.
- The basal rate of oxygen uptake in the fetus is approximately twice that of the adult, but it may decrease significantly during episodes of hypoxemia.
- Lactate is produced and consumed even in well-oxygenated fetuses.
- The diagnosis of intrauterine growth restriction signals an increased fetal susceptibility to physiologic stress.
- Although the level of fetal Pao_2 is low in utero, the fetus is neither hypoxemic nor hypoxic under basal conditions.
- The P_{50} of fetal blood is significantly lower than the P_{50} of adult blood.
- Fluid moves readily between the maternal intravascular and fetal interstitial spaces.
- The fetal circulation directs oxygenated blood toward the brain and heart and directs deoxygenated blood to the umbilical circulation and placenta.
- The fetus cannot significantly increase its combined ventricular output above basal values.
- Hypoxemia results in chemoreceptor stimulation, which results in significant redistribution of cardiac output toward the heart, brain, placenta, and adrenal glands.
- The fetal autonomic nervous system is relatively immature, even in term fetuses.
- As pregnancy progresses, tonic parasympathetic activity increases; thus the baseline fetal heart rate at 40 weeks' gestation is less than the baseline fetal heart rate at 26 weeks' gestation.
- Increased fetal intracranial pressure can significantly alter the fetal circulatory pattern.
- Intrauterine stress affects the maturation and activity of the autonomic nervous system in the neonate.

REFERENCES

1. Philipps AF. Carbohydrate metabolism of the fetus. In: Polin RA, Fox WW, editors. Fetal and Neonatal Physiology, vol. 1. Philadelphia, WB Saunders, 1992:373-84.
2. Meschia G, Battaglia FC, Hay WW Jr, Sparks JW. Utilization of substrates by the ovine placenta in vivo. Fed Proc 1980; 39:245-9.
3. Molina RD, Meschia G, Wilkening RB. Uterine blood flow, oxygen and glucose uptakes at mid-gestation in the sheep. Proc Soc Exp Biol Med 1990; 195:379-85.

4. Battaglia FC, Meschia G. An Introduction to Fetal Physiology. Orlando, Fla, Academic Press, 1986:65.

5. Sandiford I, Wheeler T. The basal metabolism before, during and after pregnancy. J Biol Chem 1924; 62:329-50.

6. Bonds DR, Crosby LD, Cheek TG, et al. Estimation of human fetal-placental unit metabolic rate by application of the Bohr principle. J Dev Physiol 1986; 8:49-54.

7. Brooke OG. Energy expenditure in the fetus and neonate: Sources of variability. Acta Paediatr Scand (suppl) 1985; 319:128-34.

8. Rurak DW, Gruber NC. The effect of neuromuscular blockage on oxygen consumption and blood gases in the fetal lamb. Am J Obstet Gynecol 1983; 145:258-62.

9. Jones MD Jr, Traystman RJ. Cerebral oxygenation of the fetus, newborn, and adult. Semin Perinatol 1984; 8:205-16.

10. Battaglia FC, Meschia G. An Introduction to Fetal Physiology. New York, Academic Press, 1986:136-53.

11. Bristow J, Rudolph AM, Itskovitz J. A preparation for studying liver blood flow, oxygen consumption, and metabolism in the fetal lamb in utero. J Dev Physiol 1981; 3:255-66.

12. Edelstone DI, Holzman IR. Fetal intestinal oxygen consumption at various levels of oxygenation. Am J Physiol 1982; 242:H50-4.

13. Philipps AF. Carbohydrate metabolism of the fetus. In: Polin RA, Fox WW, editors. Fetal and Neonatal Physiology. Philadelphia, WB Saunders, 1992:375.

14. Milnor WR. Normal circulatory function. In: Mountcastle VB, editor. Medical Physiology, 13th ed. St Louis, Mosby, 1974:934.

15. Philipps AF, Porte PJ, Stabinsky S, et al. Effects of chronic fetal hyperglycemia upon oxygen consumption in the ovine uterus and conceptus. J Clin Invest 1984; 74:279-86.

16. Philipson EH, Kalhan SC, Riha MM, Pimentel R. Effects of maternal glucose infusion on fetal acid-base status in human pregnancy. Am J Obstet Gynecol 1987; 157:866-73.

17. Edelstone DI. Fetal compensatory responses to reduced oxygen delivery. Semin Perinatol 1984; 8:184-91.

18. Peeters LL, Sheldon RE, Jones MD Jr, et al. Blood flow to fetal organs as a function of arterial oxygen content. Am J Obstet Gynecol 1979; 135:637-46.

19. Kalhan SC, D'Angelo LJ, Savin S, Adam PAJ. Glucose production in pregnant women at term gestation: Sources of glucose for the human fetus. J Clin Invest 1979; 63:388-94.

20. Haugel S, Desmaizieres V, Challier JC. Glucose uptake, utilization, and transfer by the human placenta as functions of maternal glucose concentration. Pediatr Res 1986; 20:269-73.

21. Wilkening RB, Battaglia FC, Meschia G. The relationship of umbilical glucose uptake to uterine blood flow. J Develop Physiol 1985; 7:313-9.

22. Oh W, Omori K, Hobel CJ, et al. Umbilical blood flow and glucose uptake in lamb fetus following single umbilical artery ligation. Biol Neonate 1975; 26:291-9.

23. Hay WW Jr, Sparks JW, Wilkening RB, et al. Fetal glucose uptake and utilization as functions of maternal glucose concentration. Am J Physiol 1984; 246:E237-42.

24. Boyd RDH, Morriss FH Jr, Meschia G, et al. Growth of glucose and oxygen uptakes by fetuses of fed and starved ewes. Am J Physiol 1973; 225:897-907.

25. Morriss FH Jr, Makowski EL, Meschia G, Battalga FC. The glucose/oxygen quotient of the term human fetus. Biol Neonate 1975; 25:44-52.

26. Burd LI, Jones MD Jr, Simmons MA, et al. Placental production and foetal utilization of lactate and pyruvate. Nature 1975; 254:710-1.

27. Gresham EL, James EJ, Raye JR, et al. Production and excretion of urea by the fetal lamb. Pediatrics 1972; 50:372-9.

28. Battaglia FC, Meschia G. An Introduction to Fetal Physiology. Orlando, Fla, Academic Press, 1986:91.

29. Gardner DS, Giussani DA, Fowden AL. Hindlimb glucose and lactate metabolism during umbilical cord compression and acute hypoxemia in the late-gestation ovine fetus. Am J Physiol Regul Integr Comp Physiol 2003; 284:R954-964.

30. Sparks JW, Hay WW Jr, Bonds D, et al. Simultaneous measurements of lactate turnover rate and umbilical lactate uptake in the fetal lamb. J Clin Invest 1982; 70:179-92.

31. Bocking AD, Challis JR, White SE. Effect of acutely-induced lactic acidemia on fetal breathing movements, heart rate, blood pressure, ACTH and cortisol in sheep. J Dev Physiol 1991; 16:45-50.

32. Milley JR. Protein synthesis during hypoxia in fetal lambs. Am J Physiol 1987; 252:E519-24.

33. Palacin M, Lasuncion MA, Herrara E. Lactate production and absence of gluconeogenesis from placental transferred substrates in fetuses from fed and 48-h starved rats. Pediatr Res 1987; 22:6-10.

34. Shambaugh GE III, Mrozak SC, Freinkel N. Fetal fuels. I. Utilization of ketones by isolated tissues at various stages of maturation and maternal nutrition during late gestation. Metabolism 1977; 26:623-35.

35. Neary RH, Kilby MD, Kumpatula P, et al. Fetal and maternal lipoprotein metabolism in human pregnancy. Clin Sci 1995; 88:311-8.

36. Seeds JW, Peng T. Impaired growth and risk of fetal death: Is the tenth percentile the appropriate standard? Am J Obstet Gynecol 1998; 178:658-69.

37. Klebanoff MA, Schulsinger C, Mednick BR, Secher NJ. Preterm and small-for-gestational-age birth across generations. Am J Obstet Gynecol 1997; 176:521-6.

38. Jansson T, Ylven K, Wennergren M, et al. Glucose transport and system A activity in syncytiotrophoblast microvillous and basal plasma membranes in intrauterine growth restriction. Placenta 2002; 23:392-9.

39. Ferguson R, Myers SA. Population study of the risk of fetal death and its relationship to birth weight, gestational age, and race. Am J Perinatol 1994; 11:267-72.

40. Zelop CM, Richardson DK, Heffner LJ. Outcomes of severely abnormal umbilical artery Doppler velocimetry in structurally normal singleton fetuses. Obstet Gynecol 1996; 87:434-8.

41. Poulain P, Palaric JUC, Paris-Liado J, Jacquemart F, and the Doppler Study Group. Fetal umbilical Doppler in a population of 541 high-risk pregnancies: Prediction of perinatal mortality and morbidity. Doppler Study Group. Eur J Obstet Gynecol Reprod Biol 1994; 54:191-6.

42. Madazli C, Sen S, Uludag V, et al. Doppler dynamics: their clinical significance and relationship with fetal blood gases and pH measurements. J Obstet Gynaecol 2001; 21:448-52.

43. Wladimiroff JW, Wijngaard JAGW, Degani S, et al. Cerebral and umbilical arterial blood flow velocity waveforms in normal and growth retarded pregnancies. Obstet Gynecol 1987; 69:705-9.

44. Yoshimura S, Masuzaki H, Miura K, et al. Fetal blood flow redistribution in term intrauterine growth retardation (IUGR) and post-natal growth. Int J Gynaecol Obstet 1998; 60:3-8.

45. Luzi G, Coata G, Caserta G, et al. Doppler velocimetry of different sections of the fetal middle cerebral artery in relation to perinatal outcome. J Perinat Med 1996; 24:327-34.

46. Strigini FA, De Luca G, Lencioni G, et al. Middle cerebral artery velocimetry: Different clinical relevance depending on umbilical velocimetry. Obstet Gynecol 1997; 90:953-7.

47. Madazli R, Uludag S, Ocak V. Doppler assessment of umbilical artery, thoracic aorta and middle cerebral artery in the management of pregnancies with growth restriction. Acta Obstet Gynecol Scand 2001; 80:702-7.

48. Morishima HO, Yeh M-N, Niemann WH, James LS. Temperature gradient between fetus and mother as an index for assessing intrauterine fetal condition. Am J Obstet Gynecol 1977; 129:443-8.

49. Power GG, Kawamura T, Dale PS, et al. Temperature responses following ventilation of the fetal sheep in utero. J Dev Physiol 1986; 8:477-84.

50. Schroder HJ, Power GG. Engine and radiator: Fetal and placental interactions for heat dissipation. Exp Physiol 1997; 82:403-14.

51. Peltonen R. The difference between fetal and maternal temperatures during delivery (abstract). Fifth European Congress of Perinatal Medicine, Uppsala, Sweden, June 1976:188.

52. Camann WR, Hortvet LA, Hughes N, et al. Maternal temperature regulation during extradural analgesia for labour. Br J Anaesth 1991; 67:565-8.

53. Glosten B, Savage M, Rooke GA, Brengelmann GL. Epidural anesthesia and the thermoregulatory responses to hyperthermia: Preliminary observations in the volunteer subjects. Acta Anaesthesiol Scand 1998; 42:442-6.

54. Kirschbaum TH. Fetal hemoglobin composition as a parameter of the oxyhemoglobin dissociation curve of fetal blood. Am J Obstet Gynecol 1962; 84:477-85.

55. Harris AP, Sendak MJ, Donham RT, et al. Absorption characteristics of human fetal hemoglobin at wavelengths used in pulse oximetry. J Clin Monit 1988; 4:175-7.

56. Allen DW. The oxygen equilibrium of fetal and adult human hemoglobin. J Br Chem 1953; 203:81-7.

57. Comline RS, Silver M. The composition of foetal and maternal blood during parturition in the ewe. J Physiol 1972; 222:233-56.

58. Brace RA. Fetal blood volume responses to intravenous saline solution and dextran. Am J Obstet Gynecol 1983; 147:777-81.

59. Brace RA, Gold PS. Fetal whole-body interstitial compliance, vascular compliance, and capillary filtration coefficient. Am J Physiol 1984; 247:R800-5.

60. Anderson DF, Bissonette JM, Faber JJ, Thornburg KL. Central shunt flows and pressures in the mature fetal lamb. Am J Physiol 1981; 241:H60-6.

61. Gilbert RD. Control of fetal cardiac output during changes in blood volume. Am J Physiol 1980; 238:H80-6.
62. Rudolph AM, Heymann MA. Circulatory changes during growth in the fetal lamb. Circ Res 1970; 26:289-99.
63. Thornburg KL, Reller MD. Coronary flow regulation in the fetal sheep. Am J Physiol 1999; 277:R1249-60.
64. Rasanen J, Wood DC, Weiner S, et al. Role of the pulmonary circulation in the distribution of human fetal cardiac output during the second half of pregnancy. Circulation 1196; 94:1068-73.
65. Klopfenstein HS, Rudolph AM. Postnatal changes in the circulation and the responses to volume loading in sheep. Circ Res 1978; 42:839-45.
66. Thornburg KL, Morton MJ. Filling and arterial pressures as determinants of RV stroke volume in the sheep fetus. Am J Physiol 1983; 244:H656-63.
67. Gilbert RD. Effects of afterload and baroreceptors on cardiac function in fetal sheep. J Dev Physiol 1982; 4:299-309.
68. Heymann MA, Rudolph AM. Effects of increasing preload on right ventricular output in fetal lambs in utero (abstract). Circulation 1973; 48(Suppl 4):37.
69. Kirkpatrick SE, Pitlick PT, Naliboff J, Friedmon WF. Frank-Starling relationship as an important determinant of fetal cardiac output. Am J Physiol 1976; 231:495-500.
70. Friedman WF. The intrinsic physiologic properties of the developing heart. Prog Cardiovasc Dis 1982; 15:87-111.
71. Kilby MD, Szware RS, Benson LN, Morrow RJ. Left ventricular hemodynamic effects of rapid, in utero intravascular transfusion in anemic fetal lambs. J Matern Fetal Med 1998; 7:51-8.
72. Hawkins JA, Van Hare GF, Rudolph AM. The effect of preload and afterload on left ventricular output in the fetal lamb. Pediatr Res 1988; 23:244A.
73. Friedman WF, Pool PE, Jacobowitz D, et al. Sympathetic innervation of the developing rabbit heart. Circ Res 1968; 23:25-32.
74. Nassar R, Reedy MC, Anderson PAW. Developmental changes in the ultrastructure and sarcomere shortening of the isolated rabbit ventricular myocyte. Circ Res 1987; 61:465-83.
75. Picardo S, Li C, Tyndall M, Rudolph AM. Fetal cardiovascular response to beta adrenoreceptor (BAR) stimulation. Pediatr Res 1986; 20:371A.
76. Anderson PAW, Glick KL, Killam AP, Mainwaring RD. The effect of heart rate on in utero left ventricular output in the fetal sheep. J Physiol 1986; 372:557-73.
77. Anderson PAW, Killam AP, Mainwaring RD, Oakeley AE. In utero right ventricular output in the fetal lamb: The effect of heart rate. J Physiol 1987; 387:297-316.
78. Rudolph AM, Heymann MA. Cardiac output in the fetal lamb: The effects of spontaneous and induced changes of heart rate on right and left ventricular output. Am J Obstet Gynecol 1976; 124:183-92.
79. Blanco CE, Dawes GS, Hanson MA, McCooke HB. Studies of carotid baroreceptor afferents in fetal and newborn lambs. In: Jones CT, Nathaniels PW, editors. The Physiological Development of the Fetus and Newborn. Orlando, Fla, Academic Press, 1985:595-8.
80. Long WA. Developmental pulmonary circulatory physiology. In: Long WA, editor. Fetal and Neonatal Cardiology. Philadelphia, WB Saunders, 1990:76-96.
81. Walker AM. Physiological control of the fetal cardiovascular system. In: Beard RW, Nathanielsz PW, editors. Fetal Physiology and Medicine. New York, Marcel Dekker, 1984:287-316.
82. Boekkooi PF, Baan J Jr, Teitel D, Rudolph AM. Chemoreceptor responsiveness in fetal sheep. Am J Physiol 1992; 263:H162-7.
83. Dawes GS, Duncan SLD, Lewis BV, et al. Cyanide stimulation of the systemic arterial chemoreceptors in foetal lambs. J Physiol (Lond) 1969; 201:117-28.
84. Thornburg KL, Jonker S, Reller MD. Nitric oxide and fetal coronary regulation. J Card Surg 2002; 17:307-16.
85. van Bel F, Sola A, Roman C, et al. Perinatal regulation of the cerebral circulation: Role of nitric oxide and prostaglandins. Pediatr Res 1997; 42:299-304.
86. Gardner DS, Fowden AL, Giussani DA. Adverse intrauterine conditions diminish the fetal defense against acute hypoxia by increasing nitric oxide activity. Circulation 2002; 106:2278-83.
87. van Bel F, Sola A, Roman C, et al. Role of nitric oxide in the regulation of the cerebral circulation in the lamb fetus during normoxemia and hypoxemia. Biol Neonate 1995; 68:200-10.
88. Cohn HE, Sacks EJ, Heymann MA, Rudolph AM. Cardiovascular responses to hypoxemia and acidemia in fetal lambs. Am J Obstet Gynecol 1974; 120:817-24.
89. Sheldon RE, Peeters LLH, Jones MD Jr, et al. Redistribution of cardiac output and oxygen delivery in the hypoxemic fetal lamb. Am J Obstet Gynecol 1979; 135:1071-8.
90. Reuss ML, Parer JT, Harris JL, Krueger TR. Hemodynamic effects of alpha-adrenergic blockade during hypoxia in fetal sheep. Am J Obstet Gynecol 1982; 142:410-5.
91. Assali NS, Brinkman CR III, Wood R Jr, et al. Ontogenesis of the autonomic control of cardiovascular functions in the sheep. In: Longo LD, Reneau DD, editors. Fetal and Newborn Cardiovascular Physiology 1. New York, Garland, 1978:47-91.
92. Van Petten GR, Harris WH, Mears GJ. Development of fetal cardiovascular responses to alpha-adrenergic agonists. In: Longo LD, Reneau DD, editors. Fetal and Newborn Cardiovascular Physiology 1. New York, Garland, 1978:158-66.
93. Lorijn RHW, Longo LD. Norepinephrine elevation in the fetal lamb: Oxygen consumption and cardiac output. Am J Physiol 1980; 239: R115-22.
94. Papp JG. Autonomic responses and neurohumoral control in the human early antenatal heart. Basic Res Cardiol 1988; 83:2-9.
95. Long WA, Henry GW. Autonomic and central neuroregulation of fetal cardiovascular function. In: Polin RA, Fox WW, editors. Fetal and Neonatal Physiology, vol. 1. Philadelphia, WB Saunders, 1992: 629-45.
96. Walls EW. The development of the specialized conducting tissue of the human heart. J Anat 1947; 81:93-107.
97. Smith RB. The development of the intrinsic innervation of the human heart between the 10 and 70 mm stages. J Anat 1970; 107:271-9.
98. Taylor IM, Smith RB. Cholinesterase activity in the human fetal heart rate between the 35 and 160 mm crown rump length stages. J Histochem Cytochem 1971; 19:498-503.
99. Levina SE. Endocrine features in development of human hypothalamus, hypophysis, and placenta. Gen Comp Endocrinol 1968; 11:151-9.
100. Drummond WH, Rudolph AM, Keil LC, et al. Arginine vasopressin and prolactin after hemorrhage in the fetal lamb. Am J Physiol 1980; 238: E214-9.
101. Rurak DW. Plasma vasopressin levels during haemorrhage in mature and immature fetal sheep. J Dev Physiol 1979; 1:91-101.
102. Harris AP, Takahashi H, Koehler RC, et al. Circulatory response to increased intracranial pressure after α-adrenergic and vasopressin blockade in fetal sheep (abstract). Proceedings of the Annual Meeting of the Society for Obstetric Anesthesia and Perinatology, Charleston, SC, 1991.
103. Raff H, Wood CE. Effect of age and blood pressure on the heart rate, vasopressin, and rennin response to hypoxia in fetal sheep. Am J Physiol Regul Integr Comp Physiol 1992; 263:R880-4.
104. Wood CE, Tong H. Central nervous system regulation of reflex responses to hypotension during fetal life. Am J Physiol 1999; 277:R1541-52.
105. Iwamoto HS, Rudolph AM, Keil LC, Heymann MA. Hemodynamic responses of the sheep fetus to vasopressin infusion. Circ Res 1979; 44:430-6.
106. Mott JC. The kidneys and arterial pressure in immature and adult rabbits. J Physiol 1969; 202:25-44.
107. Robillard JE, Gomez RA, Meernik JG, et al. Role of angiotensin II on the adrenal and vascular responses to hemorrhage during development in fetal lambs. Circ Res 1982; 50:645-50.
108. Iwamoto HS, Rudolph AM. Effects of angiotensin II on the blood flow and its distribution in fetal lambs. Circ Res 1981; 48:183-9.
109. Iwamoto HS, Rudolph AM. Effects of endogenous angiotensin II on the fetal circulation. J Dev Physiol 1979; 1:283-93.
110. Schwarcz RL, Strada-Saenz G, Althabe O, et al. Pressure exerted by uterine contractions on the head of the human fetus during labor. In Perinatal Factors Affecting Human Development. Washington, DC, Pan Am Health Organ (Sci Publ 185) 1969:115-26.
111. Mocsary P, Gaal J, Komaromy B, et al. Relationship between fetal intracranial pressure and fetal heart rate during labor. Am J Obstet Gynecol 1970; 106:407-11.
112. Harris AP, Koehler RC, Gleason CA, et al. Cerebral and peripheral circulatory responses to intracranial hypertension in fetal sheep. Circ Res 1989; 64:991-1000.
113. Harris AP, Koehler RC, Nishijima MK, et al. Circulatory dynamics during periodic intracranial hypertension in fetal sheep. Am J Physiol 1992; 263:R95-102.
114. Van Reempts PJ, Wouters A, De Cock W, Van Acker KJ. Stress responses to tilting and odor stimulus in preterm neonates after intrauterine conditions associated with chronic stress. Physiol Behav 1997; 61:419-24.
115. Van Reempts PJ, Wouters A, De Cock W, Van Acker KJ. Stress responses in preterm neonates after normal and at-risk pregnancies. J Paediatr Child Health 1996; 32:450-6.

Part III
Fetal and Neonatal Assessment and Therapy

Ostensibly, concern for the neonate began in 1861 when London physician W.J. Little published a paper entitled "On the influence of abnormal parturition, difficult labors, premature birth, and asphyxia neonatorum, on the mental and physical condition of the child, especially in relation to deformities."[1] Hailed as "an original field of observation," Little's paper was among the first to identify antepartum asphyxia as the cause of problems in the neonate.

Almost half a century passed, however, before clinicians developed a sustained interest in fetal oxygenation. This came through the influence of Sir Joseph Barcroft and his book, "Researches on Prenatal Life."[2] A professor of physiology at Cambridge University, Barcroft was already highly respected for his studies of respiration when his book was published.

From his laboratory studies, Barcroft discovered a progressive decrease in fetal oxygen saturation during the last half of pregnancy. He attributed this to the fetal demands for oxygen, which slowly increased until the capacity of the placenta was exhausted. Barcroft compared the fetus to a mountaineer climbing Mt. Everest, in that the oxygen environment of the fetus became progressively less dense. He suggested that the term fetus faced either asphyxia in utero or escape, through the initiation of labor. Barcroft's depiction of the fetal environment disturbed clinicians who were already well aware of the additional stress imposed by labor.

Ironically, one of Barcroft's own students proved him wrong. D. H. Barron, Professor of Physiology at Yale, suggested that Barcroft's data had been skewed by the conditions of his experiments, all of which had been conducted on animals anesthetized for acute surgery. Barron and his colleagues developed methods to sample fetal blood in awake, unstressed animals. Under these circumstances, they observed no deterioration in the fetal environment until the onset of labor. Oxygen saturation, hemoglobin concentration, and pH remained stable and normal.[3]

Barcroft's data have had the most impact on clinical practice. Virtually all current methods of fetal monitoring grew out of the belief that oxygen availability is the single most important factor influencing the well-being of the newborn. However, Barron's studies impacted physiologists, who began to study the mechanisms that maintained the stability of the intrauterine environment in the face of increasing fetal demands.

Donald Caton, M.D.

REFERENCES

1. Little WJ. On the influence of abnormal parturition, difficult labors, premature birth, and asphyxia neonatorum, on the mental and physical condition of the child, especially in relation to deformities. Trans Obstet Soc Lond, 1861; 293-344.
2. Barcroft J. Researches on prenatal life. Springfield, Charles C Thomas, 1947.
3. Barron DH. The environment in which the fetus lives: Lessons learned since Barcroft. In Mack HC, editor: Prenatal Life: Biological and Clinical Perspectives. Wayne State University Press, Detroit, 1970:109-128.

Chapter 6
Antepartum Fetal Assessment and Therapy

Katharine D. Wenstrom, M.D.

Advances in technology and increased knowledge of maternal-fetal physiology have led to the introduction, application, and widespread use of a variety of methods of antepartum fetal assessment and therapy. Many "new" technologies (e.g., ultrasonography and fetal chromosomal analysis) are now fully integrated into routine prenatal care, but others (e.g., fetal bladder shunt placement) are used only rarely.

ROUTINE PRENATAL CARE

Antenatal fetal assessment begins with an **estimate of gestational age**. Evaluation of fetal growth, efficient use of screening and diagnostic tests, appropriate initiation of fetal surveillance, and optimal timing of delivery all depend on accurate dating of the pregnancy. If the last menstrual period (LMP) is known with certainty, Nägele's rule can be used to determine the estimated date of confinement (EDC):

$$EDC = [LMP + 1 \text{ week}] - 3 \text{ months}$$

In many cases, however, patient recall of the LMP is inaccurate. By using LMP dates alone, one study estimated that one fourth of infants believed to be preterm and one eighth of infants thought to be postmature were neither preterm nor postmature, respectively.[1] Factors that contribute to confusion regarding the LMP include (1) a history of irregular menstrual periods, (2) irregular bleeding, (3) conception after oral contraceptive use, and (4) conception in the postpartum period.

Other historical data and physical findings may help the obstetrician determine the EDC. These include (1) the date of the first positive pregnancy test, (2) uterine size during the first examination, (3) the date that fetal heart sounds are first audible, and (4) the date of quickening. The first unamplified fetal heart sounds (20 to 22 weeks' gestation) and the date of quickening (18 to 19 weeks' gestation) improve the accuracy of the estimated gestational age to approximately 90%.[2] However, the methods of pregnancy-dating most often used in current practice are the date of the first positive pregnancy test and performance of an early ultrasound examination.

Most pregnancy tests involve the identification and quantitation of human chorionic gonadotropin (hCG) in maternal serum or urine.[3,4] Produced by the fetal trophoblast, hCG levels in maternal blood increase exponentially between implantation and 60 to 70 days' gestation, at which time a gradual decline occurs. Commercially available hCG test kits typically use an anti-hCG antibody to identify hCG and can detect concentrations as low as 50 mIU/mL (using the International Reference Preparation standard), by 8 or 9 days after ovulation, in serum or urine. Comparison of the date of the first positive pregnancy test with the date of the LMP is one way to assess the accuracy of the gestational age estimate.

Coincident ultrasound examination allows more accurate pregnancy dating as well as the identification of abnormal pregnancies. By using the transabdominal technique, an intrauterine sac is identified in 94% of normal pregnancies with a serum hCG concentration of 6000 to 6500 mIU/mL.[5] When transvaginal sonography is used, an intrauterine sac is visible with a serum hCG concentration between 1000 and 2000 mIU/mL.[6] Failure to see an intrauterine sac with these hCG levels indicates an abnormal pregnancy (e.g., ectopic pregnancy, missed abortion) and should prompt further evaluation. A fetal pole should be visible at $5\frac{1}{2}$ to 6 weeks of gestation, with a corresponding serum hCG concentration of approximately 17,000 mIU/mL. Between 8 and 14 weeks' gestation, the fetal crown-rump length correlates well with actual gestational age ($\pm$ 3 to 5 days).

Patients with early pregnancy complications (e.g., bleeding) and those who are actively attempting conception are likely to undergo early evaluation (i.e., physical examination, determination of serum hCG concentration, and sonographic fetal measurements). Unfortunately, many patients do not present for obstetric care during early pregnancy. For such patients, ultrasound dating criteria may be used exclusively to establish the EDC. The biparietal diameter (BPD) and femur length are the sonographic measurements that are most important for the determination of fetal age in the second trimester. Between 14 and 26 weeks' gestation, the BPD is a very accurate reflection of gestational age, with a variation of only 7 to 10 days.[7] Two large studies, which together included nearly 50,000 pregnancies, demonstrated that when a second-trimester BPD measurement was used to establish the EDC, there was a significant increase in the number of women who delivered within 7 days of their EDC, as well as a 60% to 70%

reduction in the number of pregnancies considered postterm.[8,9] Moreover, the BPD is unchanged by fetal Down syndrome,[10] making this an especially useful measurement for timing maternal serum alpha-fetoprotein (MSAFP) testing. After 26 weeks' gestation, the variation in the BPD measurement is greater (i.e., ± 14 to 21 days); thus, it becomes a less reliable indicator of fetal age.[7]

Fetal long-bone measurements are useful in pregnancy dating. Both femur and humerus lengths correlate strongly with the BPD and gestational age.[11] Abdominal circumference is less accurate than either BPD or femur length, in part because this measurement reflects fetal nutritional status and growth as well as age. Because all fetal measurements individually entail some degree of inaccuracy, an algorithm that employs multiple sonographic predictors is frequently used. Several age estimates may be averaged, or ratios of various measurements (e.g., femur length/BPD) may be calculated. When ultrasound evaluation occurs late in gestation, serial examinations that document appropriate interval growth provide support for the estimate of fetal age.

The utility of performing a routine, second-trimester ultrasound examination on all pregnant women remains a subject of debate. Early studies provided conflicting data regarding the efficacy of routine ultrasound screening, but in general they were limited by small sample size and relatively primitive ultrasound technology.[12-15] In one prospective, randomized trial conducted in Helsinki, Finland, 9310 women were assigned to receive either a screening ultrasound examination at 16 to 20 weeks' gestation or an ultrasound examination for obstetric indications only.[16] Perinatal mortality was significantly lower in the screening ultrasound group (4.6/1000) than in the control group (9.0/1000), largely because of early detection of fetal malformations (which prompted elective abortion) and early detection and appropriate care of twin pregnancies. Routine ultrasound examination resulted in improved pregnancy dating and a reduced rate of postmaturity at the onset of spontaneous labor.

In contrast, a large, multicenter, randomized trial involving 15,151 low-risk American women (the RADIUS study) concluded that screening ultrasonography did not improve perinatal or maternal outcomes and had no impact on the management of anomalous fetuses.[17-19] Although this was a well-designed clinical trial of adequate size, this study has been criticized because of its highly selective entry criteria (by one estimate, less than 1% of pregnant women in the United States were eligible[20]) and the selection of primary outcomes (perinatal morbidity and mortality) that were inappropriate for the low-risk population studied. In addition, only 17% of major congenital anomalies were detected before 24 weeks' gestation in the routine ultrasound examination group, and the rate of pregnancy termination after the detection of a major anomaly was lower than that in the Helsinki study. A similar trial conducted in one tertiary care center, in which all ultrasound examinations were performed by maternal-fetal medicine specialists using state-of-the-art equipment, identified only half of all fetal anomalies in the women who received routine ultrasound examination.[21] The results of both of these trials illustrate that the value of a routine obstetric ultrasound examination is directly related to the skill and experience of the operator and the sophistication of the sonographic equipment used, and that ultrasound examination has limitations even in the best of hands. Whether a routine mid-trimester ultrasound examination should be offered to all pregnant women remains controversial.

Evaluation of Fetal Growth

After an initial evaluation, all gravid women should be examined serially to monitor maternal and fetal condition and to assess fetal growth. Most women should have a weight gain of approximately 10 to 12 kg during pregnancy; pregnant teenagers should gain more and obese women may gain less. Weight gain should be accompanied by an increase in fundal height of approximately 1 cm per week. Between 20 and 31 weeks' gestation, the fundal height (in centimeters) equals the gestational age in weeks in most healthy women of average weight with an appropriately grown fetus. Although fundal-height measurements are frequently decreased in patients whose fetuses are growth restricted, the range of normal fundal heights at each gestational age is wide; on average, there is a 6-cm difference between the 10th and 90th percentiles at each week after 20 weeks' gestation.[22] As a result, serial fundal height measurements can reflect fetal growth with a sensitivity as high as 86%,[22] but isolated measurements may be difficult to interpret.

A skilled clinician is able to evaluate fetal size and growth by examining the gravid uterus in a systematic way. Leopold's maneuvers include four basic steps that allow determination of (1) the number of fetuses, (2) the fetal lie, and (3) the position of the presenting part. The obstetrician also can estimate fetal size with a degree of accuracy that improves with experience.

A thorough ultrasound evaluation augments the assessment of fetal size and growth. If the gestational age is known, an alteration in fetal growth can be verified in 80% of cases and excluded in 90% of cases.[23] Sonographic estimates of fetal weight commonly are derived from formulas that use a combination of fetal measurements. A fairly accurate estimate, in which the estimated weight varies from the actual weight by only ± 7.5%, is derived from a combination of measurements of the fetal head, abdomen, and femur.[24] When such a formula is used, the absolute error is smaller in the lower weight range (i.e., ± 7.5% = ± 75 g in a 1000-g fetus) and larger in the upper weight range (i.e., ± 7.5% = ± 300 g in a 4000-g fetus). Thus, sonographic estimates of fetal weight in grams seem more accurate in preterm or growth-restricted fetuses than in term or macrosomic fetuses. Accordingly, sonographic estimates of fetal weight must be evaluated in the context of the clinical situation and balanced against the clinical estimate of fetal weight. Serial sonographic evaluations at 3- to 4-week intervals improve the assessment of fetal size.

Intrauterine growth restriction (IUGR) is commonly defined as an estimated fetal weight that is less than the 10th percentile for gestational age. (The word *restriction* has replaced the word *retardation,* because the latter term has other implications and may be upsetting for the parents of the child.) This definition is not ideal, because the short but appropriately grown fetus may be inappropriately classified as having IUGR, whereas the long but abnormally thin fetus may have an estimated weight above the 10th percentile. If IUGR is defined as an estimated fetal weight that is less than the third percentile, severely growth-restricted fetuses will be identified, but more mildly affected fetuses will be missed. In addition, selecting an inappropriate growth curve to which the fetus will be compared can introduce error. For example, a growth curve derived from a population that lives at high altitude (e.g., Denver) includes generally lower weights than a growth curve derived from patients who live at sea level (e.g., Iowa).

IUGR can also be described as symmetric or asymmetric. In cases of **asymmetric IUGR**, head growth is normal but body growth lags, which suggests relatively recent pathologic stressors that may be reversible. Asymmetric IUGR usually develops in the third trimester and occurs when a normal fetus matures in an unfavorable intrauterine environment (e.g., uteroplacental insufficiency and maternal illness). In cases of **symmetric IUGR**, both cephalic size and body weight are small, indicating a global insult that occurred early in gestation. Symmetric IUGR may reflect an inherent fetal abnormality (e.g., genetic disease, early congenital infection), or it may provide evidence that the placenta was severely dysfunctional throughout pregnancy (e.g., severe maternal hypertension, longstanding insulin-dependent diabetes, collagen vascular disease). Antepartum recognition of IUGR is important because the condition is associated with a significantly increased risk of perinatal morbidity and mortality.

If ultrasonography and clinical data suggest that the estimated fetal weight is less than the 10th percentile on the appropriate growth curve, the patient and fetus should be evaluated thoroughly. In some cases, the etiology of the IUGR can be determined and contributing factors can be modified or eliminated. Up to 20% of cases of severe IUGR are associated with fetal chromosome abnormalities or congenital malformations, 25% to 30% are related to maternal conditions characterized by vascular disease, and a portion are the result of abnormal placentation. In a substantial number of cases the etiology of IUGR is unknown.[25] Discovery of severe, symmetric IUGR warrants referral to a maternal-fetal medicine specialist.

Assessment of Fetal Well-Being

One of the most important components of routine antepartum care is the assessment of fetal well-being. Although fetal health is generally reflected by fetal size and pattern of growth, more immediate indicators of fetal status are required to verify that the fetus is in good condition at any given time. In low-risk pregnancies, the patient may be instructed in fetal assessment techniques. In high-risk pregnancies, more specific tests are used.

Fetal movement counting is the most basic method for assessment of fetal well-being, and is ideal for monitoring low-risk pregnancies. The normal fetus exhibits 20 to 50 gross body movements per hour (range, 0 to 130). Fewer movements occur during the day, and increasing activity occurs between 9:00 PM and 1:00 AM.[26] The mother perceives approximately 80% of sonographically visualized fetal movements.[27] Thus, patient involvement in antenatal fetal assessment is both logical and practical. Several different schemes for routine daily assessment of fetal activity have been proposed and tested. All of these schemes consider the marked variation in activity patterns between fetuses, as well as the variation in maternal perception of fetal movement. With one commonly used method, a patient at 28 weeks' gestation or more is instructed to rest quietly on her left side once each day in the evening (e.g., sometime between 7:00 PM and 11:00 PM) and to record the time interval required to appreciate 10 fetal movements. Most patients with a healthy fetus will feel 10 movements in approximately 20 minutes; 99.5% of women with a healthy fetus will feel 10 fetal movements within 90 minutes.[28] If 10 movements are not perceived within 2 hours, the patient is instructed to call her physician and/or to report to the hospital for further fetal testing. In one large study, use of this scheme resulted in a reduc-

tion of fetal mortality from 44.5 to 10.3 per 1000 births.[28] Patient perception of decreased fetal movement prompted further evaluation and resulted in a significant increase in both the number of labor inductions and the number of cesarean sections for fetal intolerance of labor. This outcome suggests that fetal movement counting helps identify stressed fetuses in an otherwise low-risk population.

Patients at high risk for fetal compromise generally undergo more sophisticated antenatal testing. Commonly used tests include the **nonstress test (NST)**, the **biophysical profile (BPP)**, and the **contraction stress test (CST)** or **oxytocin challenge test (OCT)**. Although several different criteria for evaluation of these tests have been described, standard definitions for fetal heart rate (FHR) interpretation have recently been established by the National Institute of Child Health and Human Development Research Planning Workshop.[29]

NONSTRESS TEST

During an NST, the FHR is recorded for a period and evaluated for the presence or absence of specific, periodic changes. During antepartum testing, the FHR is determined externally by use of Doppler ultrasound. With Doppler ultrasound, sound waves emitted from the transducer are deflected by the movement of any fetal cardiac structure; the shift in the frequency of these deflected sound waves is detected by a sensor and then converted into a heart rate by computer software. If the membranes are ruptured (e.g., during labor), the FHR can be recorded directly using a fetal scalp electrode, which records the R-to-R interval of the fetal electrocardiogram (ECG). With either method, each successive signal received by the monitor and the interval between signals is rapidly transformed into a rate (e.g., the number of heart beats or signals per 60 seconds, if that rate were to continue for a full 60 seconds). The FHR is recorded on a strip-chart recorder.

Evaluation of an FHR tracing includes several components. First, the **baseline FHR** is noted. A normal FHR is between 110 and 160 beats per minute. Persistent fetal **tachycardia** may be associated with fetal hypoxia, but it also may reflect maternal fever, chorioamnionitis, administration of an anticholinergic or beta-adrenergic agent, or fetal anemia or heart failure. Persistent fetal **bradycardia** may be a result of congenital heart block, administration of a beta-adrenergic receptor antagonist, or hypothermia. Most often, fetal bradycardia reflects acute fetal hypoxia.[30] Both tachyarrhythmias and bradyarrhythmias require immediate evaluation and therapy.

Second, short- and long-term variability are evaluated. The FHR is determined on a beat-to-beat basis by the competing influences of the sympathetic and parasympathetic nervous systems on the fetal sinoatrial node. A variable heart rate, characterized by fluctuations that are irregular in both amplitude and frequency,[29] indicates that the autonomic nervous system is functioning and that the fetus has normal acid-base status. Although traditionally each type of variability has had its own definition and has been evaluated separately, both components of variability are closely interrelated, and in practice most clinicians consider them together.[29] **Short-term** or **beat-to-beat variability** is defined as the difference in heart rate noted between successive beats. Short-term FHR reactivity can be confirmed only by recording the fetal R-to-R intervals with a fetal scalp electrode; hence, membranes must be ruptured. Doppler ultrasound (external) monitoring cannot be used to assess short-term variability. Because the sensor detects the movement of any fetal cardiac structure, Doppler monitoring may overestimate the true short-term variability. Conversely, if Doppler monitoring indicates that short-term variability is absent, it is likely that no short-term variability will be detected with a fetal scalp electrode. **Long-term variability** describes the presence of crude sine waves that appear in cycles of three to six per minute. Long-term variability can be detected with either Doppler ultrasound or a fetal scalp electrode. Long-term variability is described as **normal** (i.e., amplitude of variability is greater than 6 beats per minute), **decreased** (i.e., amplitude of 2 to 6 beats per minute), or **absent** (i.e., amplitude of less than 2 beats per minute) (Figure 6-1).[29] Both long- and short-term variability result from normal, intact interaction between the sympathetic and parasympathetic control of FHR. Normal variability indicates the absence of cerebral hypoxia. With **acute hypoxia**, variability may increase (i.e., a saltatory pattern with an amplitude greater than 25 beats per minute). **Persistent or chronic hypoxia** results in a loss of variability. Reduced variability also may be the result of other factors, including maternal opioid administration, vagal blockade (e.g., administration of atropine), fetal arrhythmia, or neurologic abnormality (e.g., anencephaly).[29-31]

An NST is performed when formal documentation of the fetal condition is necessary. In a normal fetus, the FHR accelerates in response to fetal movement; these accelerations usually indicate fetal health and adequate oxygenation.[31,32] Several different definitions of a reactive or normal NST have been used, and most have been evaluated in (largely nonrandomized) clinical trials. All definitions require a normal baseline heart rate, normal long-term variability, and between one and three FHR accelerations (defined as an increase from baseline of 10 to 15 beats per minute for 10 to 30 seconds) within a 15- to 60-minute period (Figure 6-2).[31] Because most healthy fetuses move within a 75-minute period, the testing period for an NST should not exceed 80 minutes.[33] The NST is a direct indicator of the fetal condition but provides only an indirect assessment of uteroplacental function. It is best applied to cases in which uteroplacental insufficiency is not the prime concern (e.g., gestational diabetes, multiple gestation, preterm labor).

BIOPHYSICAL PROFILE

In some cases, an NST alone may not be interpretable or may be insufficient. In these cases, a BPP may be performed. The BPP is a simple test that can be completed relatively rapidly, but requires the use of both an FHR monitor and an ultrasound machine. It consists of the sonographic assessment of four variables, all of which must be present within one 30-minute period, and an NST. The ultrasound variables are: (1) fetal breathing movements, (2) gross fetal body movements, (3) fetal tone (i.e., flexion and extension of limbs), and (4) amniotic fluid volume (Table 6-1). These characteristics develop in the normal fetus in a predictable sequence (fetal tone appears at 7.5 to 8.5 weeks' gestation, fetal movement at 9 weeks, fetal breathing at 20 to 21 weeks, and FHR reactivity at 24 to 28 weeks' gestation). In the presence of hypoxia, these characteristics typically disappear in the reverse order in which they appeared (i.e., reactivity is lost first and then fetal breathing) (Figure 6-3).[34] The amniotic fluid volume, which is composed almost entirely of fetal urine in the second and third trimesters, is not influenced by acute fetal hypoxia or acute fetal central nervous system (CNS) function. Rather, it reflects the chronic fetal condition.

The BPP can be scored in several ways. Usually, the presence of one characteristic results in a score of 2; the absence of that characteristic yields a score of 0. Thus 10 is a perfect score, a score of 8 to 10 is generally reassuring, a score of 4 to 6 is suspicious and requires reevaluation, and a score of 0 to 2 signals fetal stress.[35,36] However, in order to make the BPP result most meaningful, the clinician must evaluate the individual criteria that determined the score in addition to the score itself. For example, a score of 8 for a patient with anhydramnios would be ominous rather than reassuring, whereas a score of 4 for a patient with a reactive NST and adequate amniotic fluid volume would suggest fetal health rather than stress.[34,37] Some clinicians do not assess all five variables. If all of the sonographic variables are normal (i.e., a score of 8/10), some clinicians do not perform the NST.[38] Alternatively, in the presence of a reactive NST with normal amniotic fluid volume, some do not assess the three additional sonographic variables.[39] Prospective evaluation of the BPP in thousands of high-risk pregnancies has suggested that it is relatively easy to perform and has a low false-negative rate.[36]

CONTRACTION STRESS TEST/OXYTOCIN CHALLENGE TEST

The CST and OST are traditional tests of uteroplacental function. Because they require the induction of uterine contractions by either oxytocin administration (OCT) or nipple stimulation (CST), many clinicians consider them cumbersome and relatively unsafe for outpatient testing. However, because they allow the indirect evaluation of fetal oxygenation during periods of placental stress, they may provide a better assessment of uteroplacental function than either the NST or BPP. Both tests require the occurrence of three mild-to-moderate contractions within 10 minutes. A healthy, well-oxygenated fetus exhibits normal FHR reactivity without

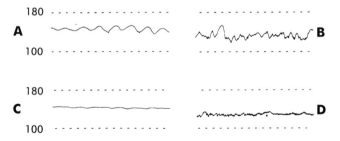

FIGURE 6-1. Components of heart rate variability from internal monitor. **A,** Long-term variability without short-term variability. **B,** Long- and short-term variability. **C,** No long- or short-term variability. **D,** Short-term variability without long-term variability. (From Zanini B, Paul RH, Huey JR. Intrapartum fetal heart rate: correlation with scalp pH in the preterm fetus. Am J Obstet Gynecol 1980; 136:43-4.)

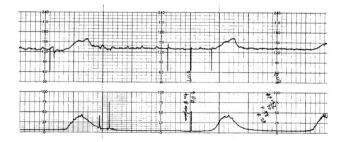

FIGURE 6-2. Reactive fetal heart rate tracing. (From Rabello YA, Lapidus MR, editors. Fundamentals of Electronic Fetal Monitoring. Corometric Medical Systems, 1991;45.)

TABLE 6-1	BIOPHYSICAL PROFILE SCORING: TECHNIQUE AND INTERPRETATION	
Biophysical variable	**Normal score (score = 2)**	**Abnormal score (score = 0)**
Fetal breathing movements (FBM)	At least one episode of FBM of at least 30 sec duration in 30 min of observation	Absent FBM or no episode of ≥ 30 sec duration in 30 min
Gross body movement	At least three discrete body/limb movements in 30 min (episodes of active continuous movement considered as a single movement)	Less than three episodes of body/limb movements in 30 min
Fetal tone	At least one episode of active extension with return to flexion of fetal limb(s) or trunk; opening and closing of hand considered normal tone	Slow extension with return to partial flexion, movement of limb in full extension, or absent fetal movement
Qualitative amniotic fluid (AF) volume	At least one pocket of AF that measures at least 1 cm in two perpendicular planes	No AF pockets or a pocket < 1 cm in two perpendicular planes
Reactive FHR	At least two episodes of an FHR acceleration of ≥ 15 bpm and of at least 15 sec duration associated with fetal movement in 30 min of observation	Less than two episodes of an acceleration of FHR or accelerations of < 15 bpm in 30 min

FHR, Fetal heart rate.
Modified from Manning FA. Fetal biophysical assessment by ultrasound. In Creasy RK, Resnik R, editors. Maternal-Fetal Medicine: Principles and Practice, 2nd ed. Philadelphia, WB Saunders, 1989;359.

periodic decelerations during this period; such a response is considered a negative test. A positive test is defined as the presence of late FHR decelerations after more than half of the uterine contractions (Figure 6-4). A **late deceleration** is a smooth reduction in FHR that begins just after the peak of the uterine contraction and returns to baseline only after the end of the contraction.[29] This pattern suggests impaired maternal-fetal oxygen exchange during uterine contractions and possible fetal jeopardy. The combination of a positive CST and absent FHR variability is especially ominous. A positive CST, with or without FHR variability, should prompt either further testing or delivery.

All three tests (NST, BPP, and OCT) are evaluated according to their ability to predict the absence of fetal death during the 1-week period following the test. The false-negative (a reassuring test with a bad outcome) and false-positive (an abnormal test with a normal outcome) rates for each test are listed in Table 6-2.[40] The false-negative rates for all three tests are fairly low. Because the NST has a high false-positive rate, some consider it a screening test for identifying fetuses that require further assessment with either a BPP or an OCT. No method of fetal assessment is perfect, and clinical judgment plays a large role in any management decision.

FETAL HEART RATE MONITORING DURING LABOR

The ideal method of FHR monitoring during labor is a subject of much debate at present. Many obstetricians employ con-tinuous electronic FHR monitoring, with attention to the baseline rate, short- and long-term variability, and the presence or absence of periodic decelerations. However, some obstetricians prefer intermittent auscultation: obtaining a FHR every 30 minutes during the first stage of labor and every 15 minutes during the second stage for low-risk patients, and every 15 minutes during the first stage and every 5 minutes during the second for high-risk patients. Although it was initially hoped that continuous fetal monitoring would result in a significant reduction in perinatal morbidity and mortality, randomized trials have failed to detect a difference between continuous monitoring and intermittent auscultation with respect to rates of intrapartum death, fetal acidosis, or long-term neurologic sequelae in the neonate.[41-45] Accordingly, the American College of Obstetricians and Gynecologists (ACOG) supports the use of either method for FHR monitoring during labor[46] (see Chapter 8). Continuous FHR monitoring was rapidly adopted nationwide and was in routine use in many labor and delivery units long before research determined that it offered no advantage over intermittent auscultation. To avoid a similar scenario in the future, many researchers advocate the thorough testing of any new fetal monitoring device or protocol *before* it is introduced into clinical practice. **Fetal pulse oximetry** is a new and potentially valuable method of intrapartum fetal monitoring. The pulse oximetry sensor is introduced through the cervix and rests against the fetal cheek or scalp. Fetal pulse oximetry allows a continuous, noninvasive assessment of fetal oxyhemoglobin saturation. Prospective trials, in which fetal pulse oximetry is compared to standard FHR monitoring, are currently in progress.

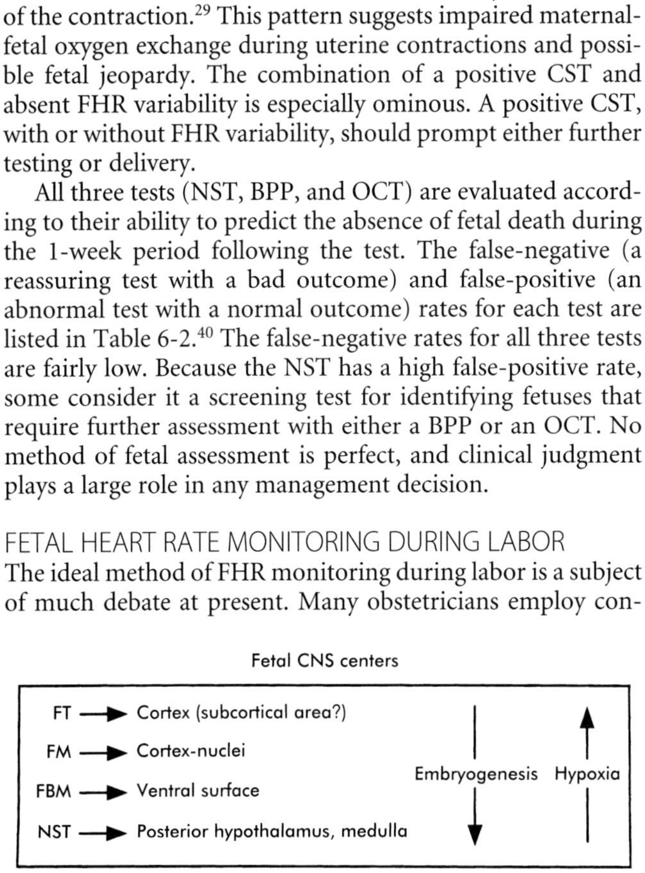

Fetal CNS centers

FT ⟶ Cortex (subcortical area?)

FM ⟶ Cortex-nuclei

FBM ⟶ Ventral surface

NST ⟶ Posterior hypothalamus, medulla

Embryogenesis   Hypoxia

FIGURE 6-3. Order of appearance and disappearance of biophysical profile parameters. *FT,* Fetal tone; *FM,* fetal movements; *FBM,* fetal breathing movements; *NST,* nonstress test. (From Vintzileos AM, Campbell WA, Ingardia CJ, Nochimson DJ. The fetal biophysical profile and its predictive value. Reprinted with permission from the American College of Obstetricians and Gynecologists. Obstet Gynecol 1983; 62:271-8.)

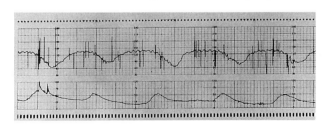

FIGURE 6-4. Positive oxytocin challenge test. Contractions occur every 3 minutes. The fetal heart rate has a baseline of 130 bpm and decelerates to 65 to 90 bpm after every contraction.

TABLE 6-2	FALSE-POSITIVE AND FALSE-NEGATIVE RATES FOR THE NONSTRESS TEST, OXYTOCIN CHALLENGE TEST, AND BIOPHYSICAL PROFILE		
		False-positive rate	False-negative rate
Nonstress test		58%	6.2/1000
Oxytocin challenge test		30%	1.2/1000
Biophysical profile		45%* to 0%†	0.68/1000

*With score = 6.
†With score = 0.
Adapted from Eden RD, Boehm FH, editors. Assessment and Care of the Fetus; Physiological, Clinical, and Medicolegal Principles. East Norwalk, CT, Appleton and Lange, 1990;351-96.

SPECIAL TECHNIQUES

Although they are not a substitute for sound clinical judgment and experience, special techniques may improve the accuracy of fetal diagnosis and facilitate fetal therapy.

Ultrasonography

Widespread clinical application of two-dimensional ultrasonography began in the 1960s after pioneering work by researchers in the United States and Britain.[47] Diagnostic ultrasonography uses high-frequency sound waves that are directed into the body by a transducer, reflected by maternal and fetal tissue, detected by a receiver, processed, and displayed on a screen. No deleterious biologic effects have been associated with obstetric sonography.

Three types of ultrasound evaluation currently are performed: the basic examination, the targeted (comprehensive) examination, and the limited examination. The **basic examination** includes determination of the following: (1) the number of fetuses, (2) fetal position, (3) fetal viability, (4) placental location, (5) amniotic fluid volume, (6) gestational age, (7) the presence or absence of a maternal pelvic mass, and (8) the presence of gross fetal malformations.[48] Most pregnancies can be evaluated adequately by this basic examination alone. If the patient's history, physical examination, or basic ultrasound examination suggest the presence of a fetal malformation, a **targeted** or **comprehensive examination** should be performed by a sonographer who is more skilled in fetal evaluation. During a targeted examination, all fetal structures are carefully examined in great detail to confirm or exclude the presence of a malformation. If a malformation is present, the targeted scan characterizes the abnormality more fully. In some situations, a **limited examination** may be appropriate. Rather than performing a complete examination, the sonographer evaluates only certain features (e.g., amniotic fluid volume, FHR for confirmation of fetal viability, fetal presentation, placental location), or provides sonographic guidance for an invasive procedure (e.g., amniocentesis).

Current debate centers on who should undergo sonographic examination and what type of evaluation these patients should have. Advocates of routine sonography cite several advantages of universal ultrasound evaluation. First, the accuracy of pregnancy dating can be improved; this makes evaluation of fetal growth and the diagnosis of prematurity and postdatism more accurate. Some studies suggest that a single BPD measurement between 13 and 24 weeks' gestation provides a more accurate assessment of gestational age than

does accurate recollection of the date of the LMP.[8] Second, routine sonography results in earlier diagnosis of multiple gestation, which leads to improved antepartum care and optimal delivery planning. Third, fetal malformations are detected earlier, which allows improved perinatal management of high-risk fetuses and leads to a reduction in perinatal mortality rates (largely as the result of early termination of affected pregnancies).[16] Fourth, routine sonography may facilitate screening for fetal Down syndrome (*vide infra*). Opponents of routine sonographic examination argue that the high cost of the procedure ($75 to $200 for a basic examination) makes it a very expensive screening test. They contend that the cost is not justified by published research.[17-19] (See the discussion of the RADIUS study earlier in this chapter.)

Although routine sonography for all pregnant women is controversial, few would disagree that the benefits far outweigh the costs for selected patients. A mid-trimester ultrasound examination can be of tremendous benefit for patients with (1) an uncertain LMP, (2) uterine size larger or smaller than expected for the estimated gestational age, (3) a medical disorder that can affect fetal development or well-being (e.g., diabetes, hypertension, collagen vascular disorder), (4) a family history of a genetic abnormality, or (5) a history that increases the possibility of a fetal malformation or growth disturbance.[48] Most patients undergo a basic screening examination before referral for a targeted examination.

Screening for Chromosomal Abnormalities

Chromosomal abnormalities are a major cause of morbidity and mortality, accounting for 50% of first-trimester abortions, 6% to 12% of all stillbirths and neonatal deaths, 10% to 15% of anomalies in live-born infants, and more than 60 different syndromes characterized by developmental delay and anatomic malformation. One type of aneuploidy, autosomal trisomy, is caused by meiotic nondysjunction. Meiotic nondysjunction usually results from an error in maternal meiosis I, a phenomenon that increases in frequency with greater maternal age. Women 35 years of age and older are considered to have a risk of fetal aneuploidy that is high enough to justify an invasive diagnostic procedure (i.e., amniocentesis or chorionic villus sampling). However, because only 8% to 12% of all births occur in women age 35 and older, only 20% to 25% of all cases of trisomy 21 (Down syndrome) will be identified if amniocentesis is offered only to older women.[49]

Screening methods have been developed to identify those younger women who are at greater risk of having a fetus with Down syndrome. These screening methods also can be used to modify the age-related risk in older women. The most commonly used screening test involves the measurement of three second-trimester maternal serum analytes (alpha-fetoprotein [AFP], hCG, and unconjugated estriol), and uses the results of these measurements to modify patients' age-related risk. Women whose final estimated risk exceeds a predetermined threshold (usually a risk of Down syndrome of ≥ 1:200 or 1:270) are offered amniocentesis to determine the fetal karyotype. If all screen-positive women undergo genetic amniocentesis, this screening and diagnostic protocol can identify 60% of Down syndrome cases at a screen-positive (amniocentesis) rate of 5% in women younger than 35 years of age; a separate algorithm allows the detection of 75% of fetuses with trisomy 18 at a screen-positive rate of 1% or less.[50] Because the maternal age-related Down syndrome risk is the basis of the test, older women are more likely to be screen-positive, but also benefit from a higher Down syndrome detection rate. Seventy-five percent or more of all Down syndrome cases are detected at a 25% screen-positive rate in women 35 years of age or older.[49,51]

Many variations of this screening algorithm exist. The sensitivity and specificity of the second-trimester test can be improved by adding measurement of dimeric inhibin A. Some centers now offer first-trimester screening with measurement of pregnancy-associated placental protein-A (PAPP-A) and free beta-hCG, combined with an ultrasonographic assessment of nuchal translucency.[52] The so-called "genetic sonogram" includes the second-trimester assessment of several sonographic markers of fetal aneuploidy, including nuchal translucency; long-bone measurements; and the presence or absence of the nasal bone, echodense bowel, renal pelvis dilation, a gap between the first and second toes, and major structural malformations. This genetic sonogram can be used as another type of screening test, in which the patient's age-related Down syndrome risk is modified by the risk indicated by the ultrasound examination.[53,54] Although many patients request this type of ultrasound examination, it must be emphasized that it is only a screening test, and it is not more sensitive than the second-trimester maternal serum screening test (50% Down syndrome detection with sonographic screening versus 60% with serum screening).[53] Although the results of any of these Down syndrome screening tests or the presence of sonographic abnormalities may signal an increased risk of Down syndrome and lead to invasive testing, it should be remembered that most women will receive a reassuring screening test result and have a fetus without obvious abnormalities, indicating decreased risk and enabling the avoidance of an invasive procedure.

Amniocentesis

For many patients, visual evaluation of fetal anatomy is insufficient to make a diagnosis or support a treatment plan. Amniotic fluid analysis may aid in fetal diagnosis and in the assessment of a variety of fetal conditions. Amniotic fluid is composed largely of fetal urine, lung fluid, skin transudate, and water filtered across the amniotic membranes, and it contains electrolytes, proteins, and desquamated fetal cells. Substances present in the fluid can be measured (e.g., lecithin and sphingomyelin to assess fetal lung maturity, and bacteria and white blood cells to diagnose intraamniotic infection), and fetal cells contained in the fluid can be cultured to obtain a fetal karyotype or DNA for other genetic tests. Because of recent advances in cytogenetic technology, a fetal karyotype with high-resolution banding usually can be performed on amniocytes within 9 days or less. Fluorescence in situ hybridization (FISH) allows the identification of fetal gender and common trisomies (X, Y, 13, 18, or 21) or specific chromosome deletions (e.g., the DiGeorge deletion) within just a few days.[55]

Amniocentesis typically involves the insertion of a 20- or 22-gauge spinal needle through the maternal abdominal wall and into the uterine cavity. Although amniocentesis was performed blindly in the past, the procedure currently is performed with sonographic guidance. Sonographic guidance permits the operator to choose the safest site, preferably in the fundus and away from the placenta and fetus, thus enhancing safety. Transient leakage of amniotic fluid occurs after 1% to 2% of amniocentesis procedures, and amnionitis complicates approximately 0.1% of cases.[56] The greatest risk associated with amniocentesis is spontaneous abortion after the premature rupture of membranes (PROM). Fortunately, this is an uncommon complication that occurs in 1 of 200 to 400 procedures at most major centers.

The most common indications for amniocentesis include (1) cytogenetic analysis of fetal cells, (2) amniotic fluid AFP and acetylcholinesterase measurement for the diagnosis of fetal neural tube defects, (3) determination of fetal pulmonary maturity, and (4) spectrophotometric analysis of amniotic fluid bilirubin and determination of fetal Rh type (by direct analysis of fetal DNA from amniocytes) in pregnant women with isoimmunization. For genetic assessment, most traditional amniocenteses are performed in the early part of the second trimester, after 14 weeks' gestation. Early amniocentesis, performed from 11 to 14 weeks' gestation, is now performed less frequently because several studies have shown that it entails a higher risk of spontaneous postprocedure pregnancy loss (2.2% versus 0.2% in one study[57]) and increases the incidence of positional fetal foot deformities (e.g., club foot) when compared with either traditional amniocentesis or chorionic villus sampling (CVS).[58] Because the safety of either traditional or early amniocentesis is directly related to operator skill, it should be performed only by a trained operator who is experienced in ultrasound-guided procedures.

During the third trimester, amniocentesis is less technically difficult and may be used for the assessment of pregnancy complications, including preterm labor, preterm PROM, and polyhydramnios. In these situations, fluid obtained by amniocentesis can be evaluated by means of culture and Gram staining to confirm or rule out infection, or it can be tested to document fetal pulmonary maturity. If PROM is suspected but unproven, the obstetrician can use the amniocentesis technique to instill indigo carmine into the amniotic cavity. If blue stains appear on a perineal pad worn by the patient, the diagnosis of PROM is confirmed. Amniocentesis can be therapeutic as well as diagnostic. In cases in which polyhydramnios results in an overdistention of the uterus and preterm labor, transabdominal removal of a large volume (e.g., 1000 mL) of amniotic fluid may decrease intrauterine pressure and allow effective tocolysis. Serial amniocenteses have been advocated for the treatment of stuck twin syndrome, a situation in which a monochorionic/diamnionic twin pregnancy is complicated by polyhydramnios in one sac and anhydramnios in the other sac.[59] Correction of the polyhydramnios by amniocentesis is believed to change the placental intravascular pressure differential, resulting in the restoration of relatively normal fluid volumes in each sac.

Chorionic Villus Sampling

The safest time for genetic amniocentesis is ≥ 14 weeks of gestation; early amniocentesis at 11 to 14 weeks is associated with a higher rate of complications (*vide supra*). Patients who desire earlier cytogenetic analysis may undergo CVS at 10 to 12 weeks of gestation. Because the chromosome content of the placenta and the fetus are identical in most cases, cytogenetic analysis of the placental villus obviates the need for analysis of fetal cells. In addition, certain genetic conditions (e.g., collagen diseases such as osteogenesis imperfecta) can be diagnosed only by analysis of placental tissue.

Chorionic villus sampling entails ultrasound-guided aspiration of chorionic villi by means of a 16-gauge catheter inserted transcervically or a 20-gauge spinal needle inserted transabdominally into the placenta. Approximately 15 to 30 mg of villus material is obtained and analyzed in one or both of two ways: by the **direct method**, in which overnight incubation followed by an arrest of cell division and chromosome band staining yields results in 2 to 3 days, and by the **long-term tissue-culture method**, in which cells are cultured for several days before analysis and results are available in 6 to 8 days.[60] In order to both provide a rapid result and confirm its accuracy, many centers report the results of both methods.

The main advantage of CVS compared to amniocentesis is that it allows cytogenetic analysis of the fetus to be performed in the first trimester. Chorionic villus sampling allows fetal diagnosis immediately after first-trimester Down-syndrome screening, and earlier termination of the pregnancy if an abnormality is detected. Transabdominal CVS can also be performed in the second or third trimester and is an alternative to cordocentesis *(vide infra)* for obtaining tissue for a rapid fetal karyotype.[61] The most common minor complication of the procedure is vaginal spotting, which occurs in 10% to 25% of patients. The incidence of amnionitis (0.3%) and rupture of membranes (0.3%) after CVS does not differ significantly from the incidence of these complications after traditional amniocentesis, and is lower than after early amniocentesis.[60] Some investigators have reported that women undergoing CVS have a greater number of postprocedure pregnancy losses (i.e., spontaneous losses up to 20 weeks' gestation, or elective abortions chosen because of a fetal abnormality) than women undergoing amniocentesis, but this may be a function of the early gestational age at the time of the procedure.[62,63] Because the rate of spontaneous abortion is highest during early gestation and decreases toward term, and because early diagnosis of fetal aneuploidy may lead to the termination of pregnancies that might otherwise have been lost spontaneously before amniocentesis could be performed, it is reasonable to expect that patients undergoing CVS at 10 to 12 weeks' gestation would have a higher rate of pregnancy loss than those who defer genetic testing until after 15 weeks' gestation. However, some investigators have not found an increased loss rate associated with CVS.

Another potential complication of CVS that received considerable media attention more than 10 years ago is **fetal limb reduction defects**. In 1991, a British group reported five cases of severe limb abnormalities among the infants of 289 women who had undergone CVS between 56 and 66 days' gestation.[64] In 1992, a group from Chicago reported four severe transverse limb reduction deformities among 391 surviving infants whose karyotypes had been evaluated with CVS at 9.5 to 11 weeks' gestation.[65] Because four of the five British infants also had a recognized genetic syndrome called **oromandibular hypogenesis** (which has nothing to do with CVS), and both reports involved a small series of patients who underwent CVS during the early clinical experience with this procedure, the significance of these cases was unclear. The World Health Organization (WHO) subsequently issued their report of nearly 139,000 CVS procedures, which confirmed that the incidence of fetal limb reduction defects in women who undergo CVS is not different from the background rate, especially if the procedure is performed after 66 days' gestation.[66] Most large centers currently do not perform CVS before 10 weeks' gestation.

A diagnostic problem affecting a small number of CVS procedures is **confined placental mosaicism (CPM)**. In this situation, the placental and fetal karyotypes are not identical.

The karyotype of the chorionic villus is mosaic (e.g., containing two or more populations of cells with two or more different karyotypes, usually one normal and one or more trisomic), although the karyotype of the fetus is actually normal. The incidence of CPM is as high as 1% to 2% with the direct method, but most cases are not confirmed by the long-term tissue-culture method[60]; this suggests that the majority of cases of CPM identified with use of the direct method are spurious and are related more to the method itself than to the actual placental karyotype. Accordingly, most centers report only the long-term culture results. The reverse situation (in which the CVS result is normal but the fetus actually has an aneuploidy) has been reported[67] but fortunately is quite rare. Because of the possibility of CPM, a patient undergoing CVS should be informed of the small chance that she will need to undergo a second procedure.

Fluorescence in situ hybridization (FISH) is an alternative for women who require a rapid fetal chromosome analysis or who are at increased risk of having a fetus with a specific chromosome deletion or duplication. Most FISH protocols utilize a spread of metaphase chromosomes obtained by the direct method, but each chromosome is then identified by FISH. Typically, probes for X, Y, 13, 18, and 21 are used; this combination allows determination of fetal gender and the presence or absence of the trisomies most compatible with fetal survival beyond the first trimester.[68] If the fetus is at risk of a specific translocation, deletion, or duplication for which FISH probes are available, the presence or absence of such an abnormality could also be determined by FISH.[69] This kind of analysis is reserved for those with a personal or family history of a specific chromosome abnormality and those whose fetus has structural abnormalities suggestive of a specific chromosome deletion or duplication (e.g., a fetus with a certain kind of heart defect might be tested by FISH for the DiGeorge deletion). Most standard FISH protocols do not routinely include testing for less common trisomies or for specific translocations, deletions, or duplications and will, therefore, miss these types of karyotypic abnormalities. Accordingly, the American College of Medical Genetics and the American Society of Human Genetics recommend that all FISH results be confirmed by a complete karyotype.[70]

Cordocentesis

In cases in which pregnancy complications or fetal abnormalities are discovered later in gestation, cordocentesis is an option for rapid evaluation of the fetus. Cordocentesis involves the insertion of a 22-gauge spinal needle through the maternal abdomen and uterine wall and into the umbilical vein, preferably at the umbilical cord origin on the placenta, using direct ultrasound guidance. The first report of this procedure was published in 1983,[71] and many subsequent studies have documented the safety and efficacy of cordocentesis for a variety of indications.

Complications associated with cordocentesis are infrequent in skilled hands and are similar to those incurred with amniocentesis. Specifically, there is a low risk of bleeding, infection, and PROM. The risk of losing the pregnancy as a result of the procedure is estimated to be 1.4%,[72] although this risk is not evenly distributed among all patients. The fetus with severe IUGR and/or severe anomalies (e.g., cordocentesis for rapid karyotype) has the highest risk, and the appropriately grown, structurally normal fetus (e.g., cordocentesis for fetal hematocrit) has the lowest risk. Transient fetal bradycardia may occur during the procedure, most often when the needle inadvertently enters the umbilical artery rather than the umbilical vein, stimulating a reactive vasospasm. Most perinatologists who perform this procedure on viable fetuses use facilities wherein cesarean section can be performed immediately after a procedure-related complication. Controversy exists regarding the need for prophylactic antibiotics, tocolysis, and maternal sedation. As with most invasive techniques, success rates and safety improve with experience. A skilled operator is the most important factor for a successful outcome.

Although cordocentesis was once considered superior to amniocentesis for a variety of diagnostic indications, recent advances in laboratory analysis currently allow much of the same information to be obtained with amniocentesis.[73] For example, one of the most common indications for diagnostic cordocentesis is the need for a rapid fetal karyotype, usually in cases where a structural fetal anomaly and/or severe symmetric IUGR is identified in the third trimester. Although a karyotype can be obtained within 24 to 48 hours using fetal blood, amniocytes isolated from the amniotic fluid or chorionic villi obtained by transabdominal CVS currently can be subjected to FISH analysis to confirm or exclude certain trisomies within a few days, with a complete karyotype usually available within a week. Many other diagnostic tests for a variety of genetic syndromes or pregnancy complications can now be performed on amniocytes or chorionic villi as well as on fetal blood. For example, the fetal Rh D and CE genes, the presence of certain other red cell antigens (e.g., Kell), and the platelet type can be determined by direct analysis of fetal amniocyte DNA, thus shortening the list of indications for fetal blood sampling.[74] Although cordocentesis has been used for the assessment of fetal oxygenation, acid-base status, and other parameters of fetal well-being in cases of severe IUGR and/or fetal compromise, it currently is rarely performed for this indication.

Cordocentesis, unlike amniocentesis, also can be used therapeutically. Fetal intravascular transfusion for severe fetal anemia (e.g., from isoimmunization, parvovirus infection, or fetal-maternal hemorrhage) can be performed safely using cordocentesis and is preferable to the older method of fetal intraperitoneal transfusion.[75] The maternal-fetal medicine specialist can use cordocentesis to monitor fetal drug concentrations and the fetal response to pharmacologic therapy.[76] It also is possible to give drugs directly to the fetus by means of cordocentesis.[76]

Doppler Ultrasound Velocimetry

Doppler ultrasound velocimetry uses the Doppler principle to detect blood flow in maternal and fetal vessels. Sound waves of a known frequency are focused on the target (e.g., blood moving in a vessel), reflected backward at a different frequency, recorded by a crystal probe, and converted to a visual display of blood velocity. The instrument must account for the angle of the ultrasound beam, the frequencies of the original and returning beams, and the velocity of ultrasound propagation in tissue. First used to assess the fetoplacental circulation in 1978,[77] this technique has been applied to the study of several high-risk obstetric conditions.

The umbilical artery is one of only a few arteries that normally has diastolic flow, and as a result is one of the most frequently targeted vessels during pregnancy. Doppler assessment of umbilical artery blood flow provides an indirect measure of fetal status; decreased diastolic flow, resulting in

an increased systolic-to-diastolic (SD) ratio, suggests increased placental vascular resistance and fetal compromise. An increased SD ratio is found most often in pregnancies complicated by maternal hypertension or IUGR.[78,79] Absent or reversed diastolic flow is an especially ominous finding. It suggests a fetal anomaly, severe fetal growth restriction, or severe uteroplacental insufficiency, and indicates the need for possible intervention (Figure 6-5).[80] However, as a test of fetal well-being, Doppler velocimetry has not been useful in the evaluation of a variety of high-risk pregnancies, including diabetic and postdates pregnancies, and generally has a high false-positive rate.[81,82] Accordingly, other tests of fetal well-being or a targeted ultrasound examination are usually performed after identifying abnormal diastolic flow, and management decisions are not usually made on the basis of Doppler studies alone. Nonetheless, new applications for Doppler technology are still being investigated. A potentially useful new application of Doppler velocimetry is the noninvasive evaluation of fetal anemia resulting from isoimmunization. When a fetus gradually becomes severely anemic, blood is preferentially shunted to vital organs, and middle cerebral artery blood flow increases significantly. Increased middle cerebral artery blood flow correlates well with fetal anemia and indicates the need to perform a cordocentesis to determine the fetal hematocrit and/or perform a fetal blood transfusion.[83] Doppler studies of other vessels (including the uterine artery, fetal aorta, and fetal carotid arteries) have contributed to our knowledge of maternal-fetal physiology but have resulted in few clinical applications. Doppler velocimetry initially was viewed with great enthusiasm, but currently its role in the clinical management of various high-risk conditions is unclear.

Other Techniques

In certain situations, two otherwise infrequently used procedures may add significantly to the diagnostic evaluation of an anomalous fetus or a maternal anatomic abnormality. **Radiographic imaging** of fetal and maternal bone structure is superior to that of sonography. In cases in which the fetus is believed to have a bony dystrophy, radiographic evaluation may prove invaluable. At least 25 different forms of osteochondrodysplasia are identifiable at birth, and 11 of these are

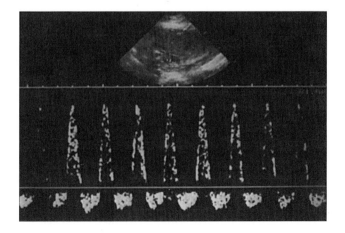

FIGURE 6-5. Doppler velocimetry demonstrating absent or reverse diastolic flow. (From Wenstrom KD, Weiner CP, Williamson RA. Diverse maternal and fetal pathology associated with absent diastolic flow in the umbilical artery of high risk fetuses. Reprinted with permission from the American College of Obstetricians and Gynecologists. Obstet Gynecol 1991; 77:374-8.)

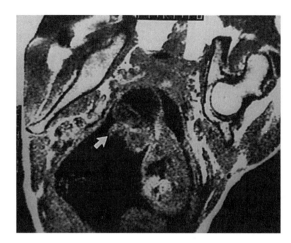

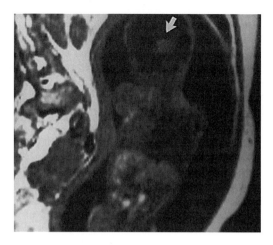

FIGURE 6-6. Sagittal MRI view of a fetus with holoprosencephaly, identifying a proboscis *(arrow)*. (From Wenstrom KD, Williamson RA, Weiner CP, et al. Magnetic resonance imaging of fetuses with intracranial defects. Reprinted with permission from the American College of Obstetricians and Gynecologists. Obstet Gynecol 1991; 77:529-32.)

FIGURE 6-7. Coronal MRI view of fetus with holoprosencephaly, showing a single ventricle and fused thalami *(arrow)*. (From Wenstrom KD, Williamson RA, Weiner CP, et al. Magnetic resonance imaging of fetuses with intracranial defects. Reprinted with permission from the American College of Obstetricians and Gynecologists. Obstet Gynecol 1991; 77:529-32.)

lethal in the peripartum period.[84] Although a few forms may be identified by a unique sonographic appearance (e.g., cloverleaf skull and small thorax in thanatophoric dysplasia), others may escape diagnosis when only routine sonography is used. The timely performance of a radiographic study may allow an experienced pediatric radiologist to more thoroughly evaluate the fetal skull, vertebrae, and long bones (including the epiphysis, metaphysis, and diaphysis) and thus identify the chondrodystrophy more precisely. A simple maternal abdominal radiographic examination that includes good views of the fetal skull, thorax, and spine is all that is required. If performed at or shortly before 20 weeks' gestation, ossification is sufficient to allow good visualization of the bones, and termination of the pregnancy remains an option.

With **magnetic resonance imaging (MRI)**, the interaction between an applied magnetic field and radio waves with the inherent nuclear magnetism of atomic nuclei in the patient's tissues is converted into an anatomic image by computer software. Because MRI does not involve ionizing radiation, it is ideal for maternal or fetal imaging of certain structures during pregnancy. Bone is visualized poorly, but soft tissues create bright images. Thus MRI is uniquely suited to the evaluation of fetal intracranial defects (Figures 6-6 and 6-7), other fetal organs, and soft tissues in the maternal pelvis.[85] Although fetal motion degraded the image obtained with older machines, new ultrafast technology allows such rapid image acquisition that fetal movement is no longer a problem. A knowledgeable radiologist with experience in obstetric imaging should evaluate fetal radiographic and MRI studies.

EVALUATION OF PREGNANCY COMPLICATIONS

All methods of fetal assessment can be applied, singly or in combination, to the management of various pregnancy complications. Obstetric complications can be categorized as acute or chronic (nonacute) and as primarily maternal or fetal.

Maternal Complications

Chronic maternal complications that can affect fetal status include maternal hypertension, diabetes, and collagen vascu-

lar disorders. Patients with one or more of these conditions are at increased risk of developing uteroplacental insufficiency, which can affect fetal growth and well-being. In addition, because drug therapy usually is required to control maternal symptoms, the developing fetus is exposed to various pharmacologic agents, some of which may affect embryogenesis and fetal growth. In these cases, fetal assessment usually begins with an early (first trimester) ultrasound examination to confirm gestational age. Often this is followed by a targeted sonographic examination to evaluate fetal anatomy at 20 to 22 weeks' gestation. If exposure to certain drugs makes a particular defect (e.g., cardiac) more likely, special imaging studies (e.g., fetal echocardiography) may be considered. More specific genetic evaluation also is possible, depending on the patient's age and past history.

In the late second or early third trimester, clinical assessment of fetal weight may prompt serial ultrasound examinations to document appropriate fetal growth. If interval growth is inadequate or if the fetus is growth restricted, a modification in maternal therapy may be considered. At some point, weekly fetal testing (NST, BPP, or OCT) is initiated. Some centers begin testing at a predetermined gestational age (usually 32 to 34 weeks' gestation), whereas others begin testing when the gestational age is compatible with intact survival should delivery be required (e.g., more than 28 weeks' gestation). Ultrasound evaluation of amniotic fluid volume often is included. The development of oligohydramnios in a fetus with apparently normal kidneys indicates placental dysfunction and usually prompts consideration of delivery.[86] In situations in which the mother is relatively stable but the fetus exhibits stress, delivery may be indicated after multiple factors are considered (e.g., gestational age, presence of pulmonary maturity, and degree of fetal compromise). If the maternal condition has deteriorated to the point where the mother's health or life is in jeopardy, delivery usually is planned, regardless of gestational age.

One nonacute maternal condition that requires attention is **postdatism**, defined as a gestation extending beyond 42 weeks' gestation (294 days). The proportion of postdates pregnancies is related in part to the method of initial pregnancy dating; postdatism complicates 3% to 12% of all pregnancies but is less frequent in pregnancies dated by ultrasound.[17] It occurs most often in young and elderly primigravidas and grand multiparas and is associated with a perinatal mortality rate that is two to three times higher than that of pregnancies that end earlier. Surviving postdates infants tend to be heavier, are more likely to be delivered by forceps or cesarean section, are more likely to experience shoulder dystocia, have lower Apgar scores, and have an increased incidence of meconium aspiration than infants delivered before 42 weeks' gestation.[87] Because of these risks, many clinicians perform a cervical examination between 41 and 42 weeks' gestation and induce labor in those patients with a favorable cervix.

The management of patients with an unfavorable cervix is strongly influenced by tests of fetal well-being. Debate continues regarding the optimal combination of tests, but most schemes include an ultrasound assessment of amniotic fluid volume. Amniotic fluid volume typically reaches a peak of 1000 to 1200 mL at 38 weeks' gestation and decreases rapidly to 300 mL at 42 weeks' gestation. A further reduction in volume occurs beyond 42 weeks' gestation. This decline indicates placental dysfunction and places the patient at increased risk of cord accident or another untoward event. In most centers, the discovery of oligohydramnios at or near term (i.e., at or beyond 37 weeks' gestation) prompts delivery. If amniotic fluid volume is normal, an NST, BPP, or OCT is performed to provide further assessment of the fetal-placental unit. Each test has a substantial false-positive rate (see Table 6-2). If amniotic fluid volume is normal and once- or twice-weekly NSTs, BPPs, or OCTs are reassuring, some clinicians choose expectant management and await the onset of labor. Others advocate the induction of labor in all patients at 41 weeks' gestation; they argue that fetal outcome is improved and maternal outcome (including the cesarean section rate) is unaffected. Hannah et al.[88] randomized 3407 low-risk Canadian women to either labor induction at 41 weeks' gestation or to expectant management. Women in the elective induction group had a decreased incidence of meconium-stained amniotic fluid and less frequent fetal intolerance of labor. They also underwent fewer cesarean sections, primarily because fewer cesarean sections were performed for fetal stress. Whatever the initial plan of management, few obstetricians allow a well-dated pregnancy to continue past 42 to 43 weeks' gestation.

Acute maternal complications require immediate maternal and fetal assessment and institution of therapy. The mother is evaluated first and stabilized. Fetal monitoring typically is performed while the maternal evaluation is conducted, but intervention on behalf of the fetus usually is not considered unless the mother's condition is known and believed to be secure. An exception to this dictum is the postmortem cesarean delivery of a viable fetus, a controversial procedure that is rarely successful.

One example of an acute complication is third-trimester bleeding. In this situation, the patient is likely to be hypovolemic, and the fetus may exhibit signs of acute stress (e.g., tachycardia and late FHR decelerations). Bleeding usually is caused by placenta previa, placental abruption, or rarely, vasa previa (i.e., the umbilical cord has a velamentous insertion, and vessels course unsupported over the cervical os). While the mother is resuscitated with intravenous fluid and possibly blood products, an ultrasound examination is performed to determine the source of bleeding. Placenta previa and placental abruption result in loss of **maternal blood**, which may lead to decreased uteroplacental perfusion and signs of fetal stress. Vasa previa, however, can result in an acute loss of **fetal blood**,

fetal stress, and a 50% chance of fetal death. Management is determined by maternal and fetal status and gestational age. If the mother is relatively stable, the fetus is viable and acutely stressed, and the condition is unlikely to resolve (e.g., ongoing abruption), immediate delivery usually is warranted. If the mother is unstable, if the fetus is pre-viable, or if the bleeding stops, efforts are made to optimize maternal and fetal condition and delivery is deferred (see Chapter 37).

Preterm labor is another acute maternal complication that requires prompt evaluation (see Chapter 34). Preterm labor is associated with infection, bleeding, rupture of membranes, uterine overdistention (e.g., multiple gestation, polyhydramnios), uterine malformations, illicit drug use (e.g., cocaine), trauma, and nutritional or socioeconomic factors. Assessment of the mother includes an attempt to confirm or exclude these potential causes. Fetal assessment begins with an ultrasound examination to determine fetal age, size, and position; amniotic fluid volume; and placental condition. FHR monitoring is used to verify fetal status. Therapeutic decisions are based on both maternal and fetal assessments. If both the mother and fetus appear stable, efforts are made to correct predisposing conditions. Examples of such therapy include the administration of antibiotics for bladder infection or therapeutic amniocentesis for hydramnios. Tocolytic agents may be administered if there are no maternal or fetal contraindications, but they generally do not prolong pregnancy for more than the 48 hours required to achieve optimal benefit from corticosteroid administration. Labor is allowed to continue and delivery is planned if cervical dilation is advanced, if labor is proceeding in the presence of ruptured membranes, or if either the mother or fetus exhibits signs of compromise that are unresponsive to therapy.

Fetal Complications

Certain pregnancy complications may be primarily fetal in origin. These include anatomic malformations, nonimmune hydrops, congenital infection, and IUGR resulting from a genetic abnormality. A maternal-fetal medicine specialist with expertise in fetal diagnosis and therapy should assess these conditions. Evaluation begins with a thorough targeted ultrasound examination. Further diagnostic testing (e.g., fetal echocardiography, fetal blood sampling for karyotype, evaluation for infection) may help delineate abnormalities precisely. Consultation with appropriate specialists (e.g., medical geneticist; pediatric neurosurgeon, urologist, or cardiologist; infectious disease specialist) may be necessary to determine the diagnosis and develop the best therapeutic plan. Depending on the fetal condition, gestational age, and prognosis, termination of the pregnancy may be considered. Patients who elect to continue the pregnancy should be counseled regarding the desirability of aggressive intervention, including cesarean section for fetal stress. Some patients who decline abortion may still decide against cesarean delivery or heroic therapy at the time of delivery. If the fetus has a nonlethal condition and the parents want to do everything possible for the fetus, fetal assessment should begin at the gestational age when intervention would be considered, and delivery conditions should be optimized; delivery in a tertiary care center with appropriate specialists close at hand may be beneficial.

INTRAUTERINE FETAL DEMISE

The most serious fetal complication is intrauterine fetal demise (IUFD). Multiple maternal, fetal, and placental factors can contribute to IUFD, including hypertensive disease, diabetes, autoimmune disorders, erythroblastosis fetalis, umbilical cord and placental abnormalities, congenital malformations, and antenatal infections.[89,90] Although older studies suggest that approximately 50% of such cases are unexplained, recent data indicate that an aggressive approach to autopsy, using a team of obstetricians, pediatricians, geneticists, and other professionals, can reduce the "etiology unknown" category to 10%.[90,91] Once fetal demise is suspected, confirmation usually is obtained by sonographic examination. The absence of fetal cardiac activity confirms the diagnosis. Other signs indicate the duration of the demise. Spalding's sign (overlapping of the cranial sutures), scalp edema, and soft tissue maceration develop in 10 to 14 days.

After fetal demise is confirmed, the mother should be evaluated to determine whether she is in labor and, if not, whether she is hemodynamically stable. Approximately 75% of patients begin labor spontaneously within 2 weeks of fetal demise, with a shorter demise-to-delivery interval near term.[89] If the patient remains undelivered, she should be evaluated for a consumptive coagulopathy, which can result from the release of fetal thromboplastic substances into the maternal circulation. Coagulopathy typically does not appear until 3 to 5 weeks after the death of the fetus. Useful laboratory tests include complete blood count, fibrinogen level, thrombin time, prothrombin time, activated partial thromboplastin time, and quantitation of fibrin degradation products; baseline measurements should be obtained and followed serially.

If a coagulopathy is confirmed, the patient should be resuscitated with crystalloid and packed red blood cells if necessary, and labor should be induced. The administration of coagulation factors usually is unnecessary and does not halt ongoing disseminated intravascular coagulation (DIC). Rather, such therapy "fuels the fire" of coagulopathy, and the transfused coagulation factors suffer the same fate as the patient's factors.[92] Delivery also should be effected if the demise is related to a medical complication that can be corrected by uterine evacuation (e.g., preeclampsia, chorioamnionitis).

If the laboratory evaluation is normal and no high-risk condition exists, management options include expectant management, induction of labor, or mechanical dilation and evacuation (if the uterus is small enough and an experienced and skilled operator is available). In general, expectant management is preferred because labor ensues spontaneously in the majority of patients. Elective induction of labor shortly after the occurrence of IUFD is associated with maternal risks, including hemorrhage, infection, and uterine rupture. Dorlman et al.[93] evaluated nine maternal deaths that occurred after IUFD; seven resulted from complications that occurred during elective induction or uterine evacuation.[93] Malpresentation or a large estimated fetal weight usually does not prevent vaginal delivery; soft tissue collapse and maceration allow even large fetuses to pass through the birth canal. Cesarean delivery should be avoided in cases of IUFD.

After adequate counseling and consideration, if the patient strongly desires immediate delivery, labor may be induced with prostaglandin E_2 vaginal suppositories or an intravenous infusion of a concentrated oxytocin solution. Chances for a successful induction are improved if the cervix is ripened with an osmotic cervical dilator (e.g., *Laminaria digitata*), prostaglandin gel, or extraamniotic saline infusion (EASI).[94]

After delivery, every effort should be made to determine the etiology of the loss. The fetus should be examined thoroughly and should undergo autopsy, if possible. Even when a full autopsy is declined, information can be gathered that may indicate the reason for the loss. Photographs can be taken for later reference, fetal blood or skin can be obtained for karyotype, and bacterial and viral cultures may be helpful. A Kleihauer-Betke stain of maternal blood for fetal cells will provide evidence of a fetal-maternal hemorrhage. Maternal evaluation should include determination of blood type, an antibody screen, and tests for the presence of antiphospholipid antibodies.

FETAL THERAPY

Because the physician caring for a pregnant woman has two patients, the mother and the fetus, fetal assessment is an integral part of obstetric care. For the majority of obstetric complications, fetal assessment is used primarily to help the obstetrician decide whether to deliver the fetus or to stop labor. In certain situations, however, fetal therapy is available and may improve or even correct the underlying problem. Therapy can range from general supportive measures to aggressive intervention. Therapy may be designed to alter a maternal factor that affects fetal development (e.g., maternal diet, blood pressure, or hemoglobin concentration), or therapy may primarily target the fetus. For example, fetal drug therapy can be initiated by administering drugs to the mother that will cross the placenta and have direct fetal effects. Occasionally, more aggressive intervention such as shunt placement or fetal transfusion may be indicated. Data proving the efficacy of such therapies have been acquired slowly, because cases amenable to therapy are rare and prospective randomized trials with strict outcome measures are difficult to perform. However, data supporting some therapies are now available, and as prenatal assessment and diagnostic techniques improve, suitable patients are being identified more frequently.

Noninvasive Therapies

The noninvasive therapy that has been most widely used and most thoroughly investigated is the antenatal maternal administration of corticosteroids to improve neonatal outcome after a preterm delivery. Infants delivered preterm are at increased risk of developing **respiratory distress syndrome (RDS)**, a condition characterized by insufficient surfactant and the formation of hyaline membranes in distal bronchioles and alveoli. The risk of developing RDS is inversely proportional to the gestational age at delivery. Antenatal maternal administration of a glucocorticoid accelerates the appearance of pulmonary surfactant in laboratory animals, and numerous clinical trials have confirmed the efficacy of antenatal steroid administration in reducing RDS in humans. A meta-analysis of 12 controlled trials (with over 3000 participants) concluded that antenatal administration of corticosteroids to women in preterm labor reduced the incidence of neonatal respiratory morbidity by 40% to 60%.[95] Although the greatest effect was observed in infants delivered at 30 to 32 weeks' gestation, some benefit was observed at all gestational ages at which RDS can occur. Corticosteroid administration has also resulted in a decreased incidence of neonatal periventricular hemorrhage and necrotizing enterocolitis.[95] Risks to patients and fetuses are minimal and are significantly outweighed by these obvious benefits. Although various protocols for corticosteroid administration exist, most clinicians administer two 12-mg doses of betamethasone intramuscularly, 12 to 24 hours apart. The infant receives maximum benefit if delivery is delayed until at least 24 hours after the last dose.

Sometimes maternal dietary alteration may be a form of fetal therapy. Women with **insulin-dependent diabetes** who adhere to a strict diabetic diet and maintain their blood glucose within the normal range before conception and throughout the first trimester can reduce their risk of having a fetus with a structural malformation from as high as 40% (without blood glucose control) to that of the general population (2% to 3%).[96] Initiation of a diabetic diet may also alter the course of **gestational diabetes** by preventing fetal macrosomia and neonatal metabolic instability. Initiation of a phenylalanine-free diet can prevent congenital anomalies in the offspring of women with **phenylketonuria (PKU)**, an autosomal recessive disease characterized by a deficiency of the enzyme phenylalanine hydroxylase. Untreated women with PKU have excessive levels of phenylalanine in their blood because they cannot metabolize it, and the excess phenylalanine readily crosses the placenta and is toxic to fetal tissues. Thus the otherwise-normal fetus may develop a cardiac malformation, microcephaly, growth restriction, and/or mental retardation. A diet low in phenylalanine can prevent this poor outcome. If such a diet is initiated before conception and phenylalanine levels are maintained at levels below 10 mg/dL throughout gestation, the chances of having a normal infant improve significantly.[97] Because chronic hyperphenylalaninemia is believed to cause continued cognitive and neuropsychological deterioration in adults, the patient should be advised to continue the diet even after delivery.

Other conditions amenable to noninvasive fetal therapy occur less frequently, with data regarding the natural history of each disease and the best antenatal treatment usually presented as case series from tertiary care centers. An example of such a condition is **alloimmune thrombocytopenia (ATP)**, the platelet analog of Rh disease. With ATP, a mother who is platelet-antigen negative makes IgG antibodies against her fetus' antigen-positive platelets. These antibodies readily cross the placenta and cause severe fetal thrombocytopenia. In untreated mothers, complications include fetal intracranial hemorrhage and fetal or neonatal demise. Similar to Rh disease, the fetal thrombocytopenia characteristic of ATP appears earlier and is more severe with each subsequent affected pregnancy. In contrast to Rh disease, however, even the first fetus affected by ATP can have a severe intracranial hemorrhage antepartum. Several large series have shown that weekly maternal infusion of gamma globulin can halt or reverse the fetal thrombocytopenia in most pregnancies complicated by ATP; even fetuses whose platelet response is suboptimal avoid antepartum intracranial hemorrhage with this treatment.[98] The addition of corticosteroids does not further improve the platelet count.[99]

Although the therapy of ATP initially required invasive evaluation of the fetus by cordocentesis, advances in genetic laboratory technology have now made it possible to evaluate the fetus less invasively. The likelihood that the fetus is platelet-antigen positive can be estimated by evaluating the father's platelets. If paternal testing indicates that the fetus has a 100% chance of being platelet-antigen positive, gamma globulin therapy can be initiated without invasive fetal testing; those fetuses with a 50% chance can have their platelet antigen status confirmed by testing amniocytes obtained by amniocentesis, and thus can avoid a cordocentesis for fetal blood sampling. At term, the treated patient can undergo a single cordocentesis to confirm that the fetal platelet count is high enough for safe vaginal delivery; alternatively, treated women may decline cordocentesis and instead opt for delivery by elective cesarean section. Vaginal delivery is preferred, since gamma globulin therapy raises the fetal platelet count sufficiently to allow term, vaginal delivery of an intact fetus in the majority of cases.[98,99]

The gamma globulin administered to the mother with ATP does not cross the placenta. Sometimes, however, drugs known to cross the placenta are deliberately given to the mother for the purpose of treating the fetus. An example of a condition for which such treatment is considered is **fetal hyperthyroidism**. Fetal hyperthyroidism occurs when a pregnant women has Graves' disease, an autoimmune disorder in which maternal IgG antibodies stimulate the maternal thyroid gland. These antibodies can cross the placenta and can also stimulate the fetal thyroid. Patients with this disease can be rendered asymptomatic by undergoing either surgical or ^{131}I thyroid ablation. However, because thyroid ablation does not diminish antibody production, 1.5% to 12% of fetuses born to such women exhibit signs of thyrotoxicosis.[100] If untreated, the fetal mortality rate approaches 15% to 25%. Survivors are likely to have serious morbidity, including high-output heart failure, growth restriction, neonatal Graves' disease, postnatal craniosynostosis, and persistent neurologic and developmental abnormalities.[101] Fortunately, fetal hyperthyroidism can be diagnosed by performing thyroid studies on blood obtained by cordocentesis, and affected fetuses can be treated with maternally administered propylthiouracil.[102] This antithyroid medication crosses the placenta and blocks the synthesis of thyroxine within the fetal thyroid gland. It also blocks the conversion of thyroxine to triiodothyronine in peripheral fetal tissues. Although the thyroid-ablated mother must take replacement thyroxine, this does not affect the fetus because thyroxine does not cross the placenta.

Another example of a condition that requires antenatal fetal drug therapy is **congenital adrenal hyperplasia**, an HLA-linked autosomal recessive disorder that results from 21-hydroxylase deficiency. Affected fetuses have elevated levels of cortisol, androgen precursors, and androgens that do not require 21-hydroxylase for their biosynthesis. An affected male fetus may undergo premature masculinization and accelerated development, whereas a female fetus may be virilized to the point of having ambiguous genitalia. Such virilization can be avoided by the antenatal administration of dexamethasone to the mother.[103] Dexamethasone readily crosses the placenta and suppresses fetal adrenal androgen production. Therapy is begun at 5 weeks' gestation in patients at high risk (i.e., those with a previously affected child). Subsequent genetic analysis of the fetus by CVS or amniocentesis then determines the gender and confirms the presence or absence of the affected gene. Therapy is continued only in patients with an affected female fetus. Amniotic fluid levels of 17-hydroxyprogesterone and androgens can be measured by amniocentesis at mid-gestation; if these levels are still elevated, the corticosteroid dose can be adjusted upward. Not all affected fetuses respond equally well to this regimen, but the degree of virilization is minimized in most cases.

Occasionally, drugs that fail to cross the placenta in therapeutic doses can be administered to the fetus directly. One report documented a fetus with **supraventricular tachycardia** who failed to respond to maternal digoxin therapy. An excellent response was achieved when the drug was administered directly to the fetus by serial, sonographically guided intramuscular injections.[75]

Unfortunately, other commonly used noninvasive therapies are not supported by research data. One of the therapies most widely prescribed for improving maternal and fetal status is **bed rest**. By one estimate, bed rest is recommended at some point in nearly 20% of all pregnancies.[104] It is used for a variety of pregnancy complications, including threatened miscarriage, vaginal bleeding, preterm labor, IUGR, pregnancy-induced hypertension, and preeclampsia. However, there are few data to support its effectiveness for any of these conditions.[104] Bed rest has been shown to improve outcomes only in cases of twin gestation; several studies have demonstrated that in-hospital bed rest results in significant fetal weight gain in twin fetuses,[105,106] although no studies have demonstrated a significant improvement in other outcome measures, such as the incidence of preterm birth, low birth weight, or perinatal death.

Another form of therapy that has been disappointing is maternal administration of **low-dose aspirin**. Because low-dose aspirin inhibits the formation of thromboxane (which is a vasoconstrictor) more than the formation of prostacyclin (which is a vasodilator),[107] it has been suggested that daily aspirin ingestion should result in dilation of the placental vessels and improved uteroplacental blood flow in a variety of obstetric conditions, including IUGR and preeclampsia. However, the largest prospective, randomized, double-blind, multicenter study performed to date (Collaborative Low-dose Aspirin Study in Pregnancy [CLASP]), which included 9364 women who had or were at risk for IUGR or preeclampsia, concluded that low-dose aspirin had no significant effect on either of these conditions[108,109] (see Chapter 44).

Invasive Therapies

The most commonly used and thoroughly tested invasive fetal therapy is **fetal intravascular transfusion for the treatment of fetal hemolytic disease**. Before the 1980s, fetuses who were anemic and/or hydropic as a result of Rh disease or other red cell antigen incompatibility were treated with intraperitoneal transfusion of packed red blood cells. The transfused blood presumably was absorbed by subdiaphragmatic lymphatic tissue and then transported into the fetal vasculature. However, severely compromised fetuses absorbed the blood poorly. After cordocentesis was introduced in 1983, several groups investigated the possibility of transfusing the compromised fetus directly through the umbilical vein. Several large series have demonstrated that fetal intravascular transfusion can be performed safely and can result in greatly improved neonatal outcome.[110] In addition, precise evaluation of fetal status is possible because pretransfusion and posttransfusion fetal hematocrits can be determined, and other parameters (e.g., venous blood pH and Po_2) can be measured directly. Certain fetal blood tests, including the reticulocyte count and direct Coombs test, can be used to predict the optimum time interval between serial transfusions.[111] This allows the maternal-fetal medicine specialist to optimize the efficacy and safety of each procedure.

Rarely, **fetal surgery** is performed to prevent progressive damage to a fetal structure or to restore normal anatomy so that development can proceed. Fetal surgery usually is considered only in cases in which a fetus with a normal karyotype has an isolated malformation that, if untreated, will result in fetal or neonatal demise. An understanding of the natural history of the untreated malformation is essential. Fetal surgery should not be attempted if the natural history is unknown or if the chances of survival without treatment are equal to or greater than the risks of the procedure. Before such procedures are considered, a thorough evaluation must be performed to (1) confirm a normal fetal karyotype, (2) exclude associated malformations, (3) characterize the malformation completely, and (4) eliminate the possibility of other contributing and/or treatable factors. Malformations for which surgical intervention is considered are rare.

Surgical intervention is sometimes considered in cases of **obstructive fetal uropathy**. A complete obstruction of urine output that occurs before 20 weeks' gestation results in anhydramnios and subsequent pulmonary hypoplasia. Complete obstruction also results in marked ureteral dilation and renal damage. Thus, this condition meets the criterion of lethality in the absence of treatment. If urine is diverted from the overdistended bladder into the amniotic cavity, urinary tract pressure is relieved and amniotic fluid volume is restored. Shunts designed for this purpose currently are available and have been placed in the fetal bladder under ultrasound guidance in many cases. The key to success in this situation is the accurate identification and selection for therapy of only those fetuses who have not already sustained severe irreversible renal damage, or who do not have intrinsic renal dysplasia. The most successful diagnostic approach reported to date includes a targeted ultrasound examination, determination of the fetal karyotype, exclusion of other genetic syndromes or structural defects, and serial evaluation of fetal urinary electrolytes and protein. In one series, the use of this approach resulted in the correct identification of all fetuses with a good prognosis and 100% survival in this group after antenatal shunting.[112]

Shunting may also improve the outcome of **fetal hydrothorax**, another entity that results in mortality in 57% to 100% of cases. Death usually is caused by pulmonary hypoplasia that occurs as a result of compression of the developing fetal lung; the intrathoracic fluid increases the pressure in the fetal chest and reduces the potential space required for pulmonary growth. Because the increased intrathoracic pressure also affects cardiac function and fetal swallowing, cardiac failure and nonimmune hydrops often are present. The most common cause appears to be congenital chylothorax. Placement of a thoracoamniotic shunt diverts intrathoracic fluid to the amniotic cavity, creating room within the thorax for pulmonary expansion and development, and preventing or reversing hydrops by restoring normal cardiac positioning.[113] However, shunt placement does not always fulfill these goals, and there is currently no test or algorithm with which to identify those fetuses most likely to have a favorable response to this therapy.

A **congenital cystic adenomatoid malformation (CCAM)** is a hamartoma characterized by overgrowth of the terminal pulmonary bronchioles. A CCAM can occupy a lot of space in the fetal thorax and thus inhibit normal pulmonary development in the affected lung. A CCAM can also cause (1) mediastinal shift and compression of the opposite lung,

(2) hydramnios as a result of reduced fetal swallowing, and (3) hydrops as a result of cardiac compromise. Pulmonary hypoplasia with or without associated heart failure is a frequent cause of early neonatal death. Although fetuses with this malformation that do not develop hydrops have a good chance of survival, virtually 100% of those with hydrops are stillborn or die in the neonatal period. For hydropic fetuses, antenatal resection of the mass can be life-saving.[114] Adzick et al.[115] reported a series of CCAM cases in which all 76 fetuses without hydrops survived without antenatal intervention, another 6 with large isolated cysts survived after thoracoamniotic shunt placement, and 8 of 13 hydropic fetuses survived after antenatal surgical resection of the mass. All 25 fetuses with hydrops who were not treated with antenatal surgery died.

Antenatal surgical intervention has been explored for other diagnoses but with little success. Attempts at intrauterine, intraventricular shunt placement for treatment of **fetal hydrocephalus** have been unsuccessful, in part because an accurate prognosis for intact survival cannot be obtained from prenatal studies, and it is impossible to predict antenatally who would benefit from this therapy.[116] A variety of fetal surgical techniques to correct **congenital diaphragmatic hernia** have been investigated, but so far have been disappointing. One problem is that a proportion of affected fetuses have a good outcome with postnatal repair and neonatal extracorporeal oxygenation, whereas those fetuses unlikely to survive with only postnatal surgery also frequently fail to respond to antenatal surgical repair.[117] Accordingly, substantial benefits from antenatal surgery have been difficult to detect.

Recently, fetal surgery to repair **open spina bifida** has been investigated. This surgery is controversial, because spina bifida is not a lethal malformation, and therefore does not meet the aforementioned criteria for fetal surgery, and because fetuses with lesions of the lower spine can have a good prognosis with only postnatal repair. Some proponents of antenatal surgical repair of this lesion feel that it is justified by the "two hit" hypothesis. Namely, the neurologic deficits associated with open spina bifida are believed to result from two "hits," with the first "hit" being the open spina bifida itself and the second "hit" being damage to the exposed neural tissues that presumably occurs sometime during fetal life. They hypothesize that antenatal surgical closure of the spina bifida will prevent the trauma associated with the second insult.[118] Although more than 200 intrauterine closures of fetal spina bifida have been performed to date in the United States, no obvious improvement in either bowel or bladder function or ambulatory ability as the result of the surgery has been demonstrated.[119,120] There does seem to be a reduction in hindbrain herniation after fetal surgery, and many of the children treated antenatally seem less likely to need a ventriculoperitoneal shunt after birth. However, none of the fetuses who underwent antenatal surgery were randomly assigned to this treatment, and there may have been bias in both assignment of the surgery and evaluation of its outcome. In order to evaluate this surgery objectively, the NIH is currently sponsoring a prospective randomized trial of antenatal surgical closure of open spina bifida. Until the results of this trial are known, there is a moratorium on such surgery performed outside this research study.

Fetal surgery is discussed in greater detail in Chapter 7.

KEY POINTS

- Accurate determination of the estimated gestational age is essential for the management of pregnancy complications and the effective use of various antepartum tests.
- Ultrasound examination can estimate gestational age, assess fetal growth, monitor amniotic fluid volume, and detect and characterize fetal anomalies.
- Appropriate fetal growth suggests fetal health and can be assessed clinically or by ultrasound examination. Inappropriate fetal growth requires maternal and fetal evaluation.
- Fetal well-being can be assessed in low-risk pregnancies by simple counting of fetal movements. High-risk pregnancies should be monitored with the nonstress test, the oxytocin challenge test, or the biophysical profile.
- A fetal karyotype can be obtained by chorionic villus sampling, early or traditional amniocentesis, and cordocentesis.
- Doppler velocimetry has advanced our understanding of maternal-fetal physiology, but its role in the management of various high-risk conditions is unclear.
- Radiographic and magnetic resonance imaging may be used to assess certain fetal malformations and can provide unique information that is unavailable by other methods.
- Various maternal and fetal therapies, including corticosteroid administration, fetal transfusion, pharmacologic treatment, and (rarely) fetal surgery may be used to improve fetal outcome.

REFERENCES

1. Kramer MS, Mclean FH, Boyd ME, Usher RH. The validity of gestational age estimation by menstrual dating in term, preterm, and post-term gestations. JAMA 1988; 260:3306-8.
2. Hertz RH, Sokol RJ, Knoke JD, et al. Clinical estimation of gestational age: Rules for avoiding preterm delivery. Am J Obstet Gynecol 1978; 131:395-402.
3. Rasor JL, Farber S, Braunstein GD. An evaluation of 10 kits for determination of human chorionic gonadotropin in serum. Clin Chem 1983; 29:1828-31.
4. American College of Obstetricians and Gynecologists. Medical Management of Tubal Pregnancy. ACOG Practice Bulletin No. 3, December 1998.
5. Kadar N, DeVore G, Romero R. Discriminating hCG zone: Its use in the sonographic evaluation for ectopic pregnancy. Obstet Gynecol 1981; 58:156-61.
6. Fossum GT, Davajan V, Kletzky OA. Early detection of pregnancy with transvaginal ultrasound. Fertil Steril 1988; 49:788-91.
7. Sabbaha RE, Hughey M. Standardization of sonar cephalometry and gestational age. Obstet Gynecol 1978; 52:402-6.
8. Mongelli M, Wilcox M, Gardosi J. Estimating the date of confinement: Ultrasonographic biometry versus certain menstrual dates. Am J Obstet Gynecol 1996; 174:278-81.
9. Tunon K, Eik-Nes SH, Grottum P. A comparison between ultrasound and a reliable last menstrual period as predictors of the day of delivery in 15,000 examinations. Ultrasound Obstet Gynecol 1996; 8:178-85.
10. Cuckle HS, Wald NJ. The effect of estimating gestational age by ultrasound cephalometry on the sensitivity of alpha feto-protein screening for Down's syndrome. Br J Obstet Gynaecol 1987; 94:274-6.

11. Seeds JW, Cefalo RC. Relationship of fetal limb lengths to both biparietal diameter and gestational age. Obstet Gynecol 1982; 60:680-5.

12. Persson PH, Kullander S. Long-term experience of general ultrasound screening in pregnancy. Am J Obstet Gynecol 1983; 146:942-7.

13. Belfrage P, Fernström I, Hallenberg G. Routine or selective ultrasound examinations in early pregnancy. Obstet Gynecol 1987; 69:747-50.

14. Waldenström U, Axelsson O, Nilsson S, et al. Effects of routine one stage ultrasound screening in pregnancy: A randomized controlled trial. Lancet 1988; ii:585-8.

15. Thacker SB. Quality of controlled clinical trials: The case of imaging ultrasound in obstetrics: A review. Br J Obstet Gynaecol 1985; 92:432-44.

16. Saari-Kemppainen A, Karjalainen O, Ylostalo P, Heinonen OP. Ultrasound screening and perinatal mortality: Controlled trial of systematic one-stage screening in pregnancy. Lancet 1990; 336:387-91.

17. Ewigman BG, Crane JP, Frigoletto FD, et al. Effect of prenatal ultrasound screening on perinatal outcome. N Engl J Med 1993; 329:821-7.

18. Crane JP, LeFevre ML, Winborn RC, et al. A randomized trial of prenatal ultrasonographic screening: Impact on the detection, management, and outcome of anomalous fetuses. Am J Obstet Gynecol 1994; 171: 392-9.

19. LeFevre ML, Bain RP, Ewigman BG. A randomized trial of prenatal ultrasonographic screening: Impact on maternal management and outcome. Am J Obstet Gynecol 1993; 169:483-9.

20. American Institute of Ultrasound in Medicine Bioeffects Committee. Review of the Radius Study. AIUM Reporter 1994; 10:2-4.

21. Van Dorsten JP, Hulsey TC, Newman RB, Menard MK. Fetal anomaly detection by second-trimester ultrasonography in a tertiary center. Am J Obstet Gynecol 1998; 178:742-9.

22. Belizan JM, Villar J, Nardin JC, et al. Diagnosis of intrauterine growth retardation by a simple clinical method: Measurement of fundal height. Am J Obstet Gynecol 1978; 1313:643-6.

23. Sabbagha RE. Intrauterine growth retardation. In Sabbagha RE, editor. Diagnostic Ultrasound Applied to Obstetrics and Gynecology, 2nd ed. Philadelphia, JB Lippincott, 1987:112.

24. Hadlock FP, Harris RB, Carpenter RJ, et al. Sonographic estimation of fetal weight. Radiology 1984; 150:535-40.

25. Resnik R. Intrauterine growth restriction. Obstet Gynecol 2002; 99:490-6.

26. Patrick J, Campbell K, Carmichael L, et al. Patterns of gross fetal body movements over 24-hour observation intervals during the last 10 weeks of pregnancy. Am J Obstet Gynecol 1982; 142:363-71.

27. Rayburn WF. Clinical significance of perceptible fetal motion. Am J Obstet Gynecol 1980; 138:210-2.

28. Moore TR, Piacquadio K. A prospective evaluation of fetal movement screening to reduce the incidence of antepartum fetal death. Am J Obstet Gynecol 1989; 160:1075-80.

29. National Institute of Child Health and Human Development Research Planning Workshop. Electronic fetal heart rate monitoring: Research guidelines for interpretation. Am J Obstet Gynecol 1997; 177:1385-90.

30. Parer JT. Fetal heart rate. In Creasy RK, Resnik R, editors. Maternal Fetal Medicine: Principles and Practice, 2nd ed. Philadelphia, WB Saunders, 1989:314-43.

31. American College of Obstetricians and Gynecologists. Antepartum Fetal Surveillance. ACOG Practice Bulletin No. 9, October 1999.

32. Lee CY, DiLoreto PC, Logrand B. Fetal activity acceleration determination for the evaluation of fetal reserve. Obstet Gynecol 1976; 48:19-26.

33. Brown R, Patrick J. The nonstress test: How long is enough? Am J Obstet Gynecol 1981; 141:646-51.

34. Vintzileos AM, Campbell WA, Nochimson DJ, Weinbaum PJ. The use and misuse of the fetal biophysical profile. Am J Obstet Gynecol 1987; 156:527-33.

35. Manning FA, Baskett TF, Morrison I, Lange I. Fetal biophysical profile scoring: A prospective study in 1,184 high-risk patients. Am J Obstet Gynecol 1981; 140:289-94.

36. Manning FA, Morrison I, Harmanck, et al. Fetal assessment based on fetal biophysical profile scoring: Experience in 19,221 referred high-risk pregnancies. Am J Obstet Gynecol 1987; 157:880-4.

37. Vintzileos AM, Gaffney SE, Salinger LM, et al. The relationships among the fetal biophysical profile, umbilical cord pH, and Apgar scores. Am J Obstet Gynecol 1987; 157:627-31.

38. Manning FA, Morrison I, Lagne IR, et al. Fetal assessment based on fetal biophysical profile scoring: Experience in 12,620 referred high-risk pregnancies. I. Perinatal mortality by frequency and etiology. Am J Obstet Gynecol 1985; 151:343-50.

39. Vintzileos AM, Campbell WA, Ingardia CJ, Nochimson DJ. The fetal biophysical profile and its predictive value. Obstet Gynecol 1983; 62:271-8.

40. Freeman RK, Lagrew DC. The contraction stress test. In Eden RD, Boehm FH, editors. Assessment and Care of the Fetus: Physiological, Clinical, and Medicolegal Principles. East Norwalk, CT, Appleton and Lange, 1990:351-84.

41. Leveno KJ, Cunningham FG, Nelson S, et al. A prospective comparison of selective and universal electronic fetal monitoring in 34,995 pregnancies. N Engl J Med 1986; 315:615-9.

42. Shy KK, Luthy DA, Bennett FC, et al. Effects of electronic fetal-heart-rate monitoring, as compared with periodic auscultation, on the neurologic development of premature infants. N Engl J Med 1990; 322:588-93.

43. Nelson JP. Electronic fetal heart rate monitoring during labor: Information from randomized trials. Birth 1994; 21:101-4.

44. Rosen MG, Dickinson JC. The paradox of electronic fetal monitoring: More data may not enable us to predict or prevent infant neurologic morbidity. Am J Obstet Gynecol 1993; 168:745-51.

45. Herbst A. Intermittent versus continuous electronic monitoring in labour: A randomized study. Br J Obstet Gynecol 1994; 101:663-8.

46. American College of Obstetricians and Gynecologists. Fetal heart rate patterns: Monitoring, interpretation, and management. ACOG Technical Bulletin No. 207, July 1995.

47. Donald I. On launching a new diagnostic science. Am J Obstet Gynecol 1969; 103:609-28.

48. American College of Obstetricians and Gynecologists. Ultrasonography in pregnancy. ACOG Technical Bulletin No. 187, 1993.

49. Haddow JE, Palomake GE, Knight GJ, et al. Prenatal screening for Down's syndrome with use of maternal serum markers. N Engl J Med 1992; 327:588-93.

50. Canick JA, Palomaki GE, Osathanondh R. Prenatal screening for trisomy 18 in the second trimester. Prenat Diag 1987; 7:623-30.

51. Haddow JE, Palomaki GE, Knight GJ, et al. Reducing the need for amniocentesis in women 35 years of age or older with serum markers for screening. N Engl J Med 1994; 330: 1114-8.

52. Wapner R for the BUN Study Group. First trimester aneuploid screening: Results of the NICHD multicenter study (abstract). Am J Obstet Gynecol 2002; 185:S70.

53. Drugan A, Johnson MP, Reichler A, et al. Second trimester minor ultrasound abnormalities: Impact on the risk of aneuploidy associated with advanced age. Obstet Gynecol 1996; 88:203-6.

54. Vintzeleos AM, Campbell WA, Rodis JF, et al. The use of second-trimester genetic sonogram in guiding clinical management of patients at increased risk for fetal trisomy 21. Obstet Gynecol 1996; 87:948-52.

55. D'Alton ME, Malone FD, Chelmow DM, et al. Defining the role of fluorescence in situ hybridization on uncultured amniocytes for prenatal diagnosis of aneuploidies. Am J Obstet Gynecol 1997; 176:769-74.

56. Daegan A, Johnson MP, Evans MI. Amniocentesis. In Eden RD, Boehm FH, editors. Assessment and Care of the Fetus: Physiological, Clinical, and Medicolegal Principles. East Norwalk, CT, Appleton and Lange, 1990:283-90.

57. The Canadian Early and Mid-Trimester Amniocentesis Trial (CEMAT) Group. Randomized trial to assess safety and fetal outcome of early and midtrimester amniocentesis. Lancet 1998; 351:242-7.

58. Farrell SA, Summers AM, Dallaire L, et al. Club foot, an adverse outcome of early amniocentesis: Disruption or deformation? J Med Genet 1999; 36:843-46.

59. Mahoney BS, Petty CN, Nyberg DA, et al. The "stuck twin" phenomenon: Ultrasonographic findings, pregnancy outcome, and management with serial amniocenteses. Am J Obstet Gynecol 1990; 163:1513-22.

60. Wapner RJ, Jackson L. Chorionic villus sampling. Clin Obstet Gynecol 1988; 31:328-44.

61. Carroll SGM, Davies T, Kyle PM, et al. Fetal karyotyping by chorionic villus sampling after the first trimester. Br J Obstet Gynaecol 1999; 106:1035-40.

62. MRC Working Party on the Evaluation of Chorion Villus Sampling. Medical Research Council European trial of chorion villus sampling. Lancet 1991; 337:1491-9.

63. Canadian Collaborative CVS-Amniocentesis Clinical Trial Group. Multicentre randomised clinical trial of chorion villus sampling and amniocentesis: First report. Lancet 1989; i:1-6.

64. Firth HV, Boyd PA, Chamberlain P, et al. Severe limb abnormalities after chorion villus sampling at 56-66 days' gestation. Lancet 1991; 337:762-3.

65. Burton BK, Schulz CJ, Burd LI. Limb anomalies associated with chorionic villus sampling. Obstet Gynecol 1992; 79:726-30.

66. Kuliev A, Jackson L, Froster U, et al. Chorionic villus sampling safety. Report of World Health Organization/EURO meeting in association with the Seventh International Conference on Early Prenatal Diagnosis

of Genetic Diseases, Tel-Aviv, Israel, May 21, 1994. Am J Obstet Gynecol 1996; 174:807-11.

67. Martion AO, Elias S, Rosinsky B, et al. False negative findings on chorion villus sampling. Lancet 1986; 2:391-2.

68. D'Alton ME, Malone FD, Chelmow D, et al. Defining the role of fluorescence in situ hybridization on uncultured amniocytes for prenatal diagnosis of aneuploidies. Am J Obstet Gynecol 1997; 176:769-76.

69. Oh DC, Min JY, Lee MH, et al. Prenatal diagnosis of tetralogy of Fallot associated with chromosome 22q11 deletion. J Korean Med Science 2002; 17:125-8.

70. ACMG/ASHG Test and Technology Transfer Committee. Technical and clinical assessment of fluorescence in situ hybridization: An ACMG/ASHG position statement. I. Technical considerations. Genet Med 2000; 2:356-61.

71. Daffos F, Capella-Bilovsky M, Forestier F. A new procedure for fetal blood sampling in utero: Preliminary results of fifty three cases. Am J Obstet Gynecol 1983; 146:985-7.

72. Ghidini A, Sepulveda W, Lockwood C, Romero R. Complications of fetal blood sampling. Am J Obstet Gynecol 1993; 168:1339-44.

73. Fisk N, Bower S. Fetal blood sampling in retreat. BMJ 1993; 307:143-4.

74. Van den Veyver IB, Moise KJ. Fetal RhD typing by polymerase chain reaction in pregnancies complicated by rhesus alloimmunization. Obstet Gynecol 1996; 88:1061-7.

75. Harman CR, Bowman JM, Manning FA, Menticoglou SM. Intrauterine transfusion–intraperitoneal versus intravascular approach: A case-control comparison. Am J Obstet Gynecol 1990; 162:1053-9.

76. Weiner CP, Thompson MIB. Direct treatment of fetal supraventricular tachycardia after failed transplacental therapy. Am J Obstet Gynecol 1988; 158:570-3.

77. McCallum WD, Williams CS, Nagel S, Daigle RE. Fetal blood velocity waveforms and intrauterine growth retardation. Am J Obstet Gynecol 1978; 132:425-9.

78. Rochelson B, Schulman H, Fleischer A, et al. The clinical significance of Doppler umbilical artery velocimetry in the small for gestational age fetus. Am J Obstet Gynecol 1987; 156:1223-6.

79. Ducey J, Schulman H, Farmalcaides G, et al. A classification of hypertension in pregnancy based on Doppler velocimetry. Am J Obstet Gynecol 1987; 157:680-5.

80. Wenstrom KD, Weiner CP, Williamson RA. Diverse maternal and fetal pathology associated with absent diastolic flow in the umbilical artery of high risk fetuses. Obstet Gynecol 1991; 77:374-8.

81. Farmakides G, Schulman H, Ducey J, et al. Uterine and umbilical artery Doppler velocimetry in postterm pregnancy. J Reprod Med 1988; 33:259-61.

82. Landon MB, Gable SG, Bruner JP, Ludmir J. Doppler umbilical artery velocimetry in pregnancy complicated by insulin-dependent diabetes mellitus. Obstet Gynecol 1989; 73:961-5.

83. Mari G, Adrignolo A, Abuhamad AZ, et al. Diagnosis of fetal anemia with Doppler ultrasound in the pregnancy complicated by maternal blood group immunization. Ultrasound Obstet Gynecol 1995; 5:400-5.

84. Rimoin DL, Lachman RS. The chondrodysplasias. In Emergy AE, Rimoin DL, editors. Principles and Practice of Medical Genetics, 2nd ed. New York, Churchill Livingston, 1990:895-932.

85. Levine D, Barnes PD, Edelman RR. Obstetric MR imaging. Radiology 1999; 211:609-17.

86. Queenan JT. Polyhydramnios and oligohydramnios. Contemp Obstet Gynecol 1991; 30:60-81.

87. Eden RD, Seifert LS, Winegar A, Spellacy WN. Perinatal characteristics of uncomplicated postdate pregnancies. Obstet Gynecol 1987; 69:296-9.

88. Hannah ME, Hannah WJ, Hellman J, et al. Induction of labor as compared with serial antenatal monitoring in post-term pregnancy: A randomized controlled trial. N Engl J Med 1992; 326:1587-92.

89. Pitkin RM. Fetal death: Diagnosis and management. Am J Obstet Gynecol 1987; 157:583-9.

90. Faye-Petersen OM, Guinn DA, Wenstrom KD. The value of perinatal autopsy. Obstet Gynecol 1999; 96:915-20.

91. Craven CM, Demsey S, Carey JC, Kochenour NK. Evaluation of perinatal autopsy protocol: Influence of the prenatal diagnosis conference team. Obstet Gynecol 1990; 76:684-8.

92. Green JR. Placenta previa and abrupto placentae. In Maternal-Fetal Medicine: Principles and Practice, 2nd ed. Philadelphia, WB Saunders, 1989:610.

93. Dorlman SF, Grimes DA, Cates W. Maternal deaths associated with antepartum fetal death in utero, United States, 1972 to 1978. South Med J 1983; 76:838-43.

94. Owen J, Hauth JC, Winkler CL, Gray SE. Midtrimester pregnancy termination: A randomized trial of prostaglandin E_2 versus concentrated oxytocin. Am J Obstet Gynecol 1992; 167:1112-6.

95. Crowley PA, Chalmers I, Kirse MJNC, et al. The effects of corticosteroid administration before preterm delivery: An overview of the evidence from controlled trials. Br J Obstet Gynaecol 1990; 97:11-25.

96. Greene MF, Hare JW, Cloherty JP, et al. First-trimester hemoglobin A_1 and risk for major malformation and spontaneous abortion in diabetic pregnancy. Teratology 1989; 39:225-31.

97. Leuke RR, Levy HL. Maternal phenylketonuria and hyperphenylalaninemia. N Engl J Med 1980; 303:1202-8.

98. Bussel JB, Berkowitz RL, McFarland JG, et al. Antenatal treatment of neonatal alloimmune thrombocytopenia. N Engl J Med 1988; 319:1374-8.

99. Bussel JB, Berkowitz RL, Lynch L, et al. Antenatal management of alloimmune thrombocytopenia with intravenous gammaglobulin: A randomized trial of the addition of low dose steroid to intravenous gammaglobulin. Am J Obstet Gynecol 1996; 174:1414-23.

100. Bruinse HW, Vermeulen-Meiners C, Wit JM. Fetal treatment for thyrotoxicosis in non-thyrotoxic pregnant women. Fetal Ther 1988; 3:152-7.

101. Hollingsworth DR. Graves disease. Clin Obstet Gynecol 1983; 26:615-34.

102. Wenstrom KD, Weiner CP, Williamson RA, Grant SS. Prenatal diagnosis of fetal hyperthyroidism using funipuncture. Obstet Gynecol 1990; 76:513-7.

103. Pang S, Pollack MS, Marshall RN, Immken L. Prenatal treatment of congenital adrenal hyperplasia due to 21-hydroxylase deficiency. N Engl J Med 1990; 322:111-5.

104. Goldenberg RL, Cliver S, Bronstein J, et al. Bed rest in pregnancy. Obstet Gynecol 1994; 84:131-6.

105. Komaromy B, Lampe L. Value of bed rest in twin pregnancies. Int J Gynaecol Obstet 1977; 14:262-6.

106. Jeffrey RL, Bowes WA, Delaney JJ. Role of bed rest in twin gestation. Obstet Gynecol 1974; 43:822-6.

107. Benigni A, Gregorini G, Frusca T. Effect of low-dose aspirin on fetal and maternal generation of thromboxane by platelets in women at risk for pregnancy induced hypertension. N Engl J Med 1989; 321:357-62.

108. CLASP (Collaborative Low-dose Aspirin Study in Pregnancy) Collaborative Group. CLASP: a randomized trial of low-dose aspirin for the prevention and treatment of pre-eclampsia among 9364 pregnant women. Lancet 1994; 343:619-29.

109. CLASP Collaborative Group. Low dose aspirin in pregnancy and early childhood development: Follow up of the collaborative low dose aspirin study in pregnancy. Br J Obstet Gynecol 1995; 102:861-8.

110. Weiner CP, Williamson RA, Wenstrom KD, et al. Management of hemolytic disease by cordocentesis. II. Outcome of treatment. Am J Obstet Gynecol 1991; 165:1303-7.

111. Weiner CP, Williamson RA, Wenstrom KD, et al. Management of hemolytic disease by cordocentesis. I. Prediction of fetal anemia. Am J Obstet Gynecol 1991; 165:546-53.

112. Johnson MP, Bukowski TP, Reitleman C, et al. In utero surgical treatment of fetal obstructive uropathy: A new comprehensive approach to identify candidates for vesicamniotic shunt therapy. Am J Obstet Gynecol 1994; 170:1770-9.

113. Rodeck CH, Fisk NM, Fraser DI, Nicolini U. Long term in utero drainage of fetal hydrothorax. N Engl J Med 1988; 319:1135-8.

114. Romero R, Pilu G, Jeanty P, et al. Congenital cystic adenomatoid malformation of the lung. In Prenatal Diagnosis of Congenital Anomalies. Norwalk, CT, Appleton Lange, 1988:198-201.

115. Adzick NS, Harrison MR, Crombleholme TM, et al. Fetal lung lesions: Management and outcome. Am J Obstet Gynecol 1998; 179:884-9.

116. Manning FA, Harrison MR, Rodeck CR, et al. Catheter shunts for fetal hydronephrosis and hydrocephalus: Report of the international fetal surgery registry. N Engl J Med 1986; 315:336-40.

117. Dommergues M, Louis-Sylvestre C, Mandelbrot L, et al. Congenital diaphragmatic hernia: Can prenatal ultrasonography predict outcome? Am J Obstet Gynecol 1996; 174:1377-81.

118. Meuli M, Meuli-Simmen C, Hutchins GM, et al. The spinal cord lesion in fetuses with meningomyelocele: Implications for fetal surgery. J Ped Surgery 1997; 32:448-52.

119. Holzbeierlein J, Pope JC, Adams MC, et al. The urodynamic profile of myelodysplasia in children with spinal closure during gestation. J Urology 2000; 164:1336-9.

120. Hirose S, Farmer DL, Albanese CT. Fetal surgery for meningomyelocele. Curr Opin Obstet Gynecol 2001; 13:215-22.

Chapter 7

Anesthesia for Fetal Surgery and Other Intrauterine Procedures

Mark A. Rosen, M.D.

In 1981, physicians at the University of California-San Francisco (UCSF) performed the first successful human fetal surgery to treat a fetus with bilateral hydronephrosis, and a new field of medicine was born.[1] Advances in prenatal diagnostic technology have contributed to an increasingly sophisticated capability of prenatal diagnosis of fetal disorders that are amenable to antenatal therapy. These advances have included biochemical and cytogenetic analysis of amniotic fluid and fetal blood, as well as imaging techniques such as ultrasonography, computed tomography, and magnetic resonance. Some of the identified disorders are amenable to antenatal therapy, including intrauterine surgery for fetal structural anomalies. Fetal therapy is not new; it originated with Liley's successful intraperitoneal blood transfusion to a fetus with erythroblastosis fetalis.[2] Subsequently, attempts were made to perform intrauterine exchange transfusion through a hysterotomy, but this procedure was abandoned owing to a high incidence of maternal morbidity.[3]

Fetal therapy is largely nonsurgical (e.g., administration of medications or blood) (see Chapter 6). Surgical correction of anatomic malformations in utero is more difficult technically. The potential for antenatal correction of anatomic defects led to the development of the Fetal Treatment Program at UCSF. The program's multidisciplinary team includes perinatologists, geneticists, radiologists, surgeons, anesthesiologists, neonatologists, specialized nurses, social workers, and other support personnel.[4] This program offers a full range of services, including fetal assessment and medical therapy, and continues to pioneer procedures in fetal therapy. These advances have included (1) fetal surgery performed through a maternal hysterotomy (i.e., "open" fetal surgery) for repair of malformations; (2) percutaneous needle insertion for administration of drugs or blood products, or for stent or shunt placement; and (3) endoscopic techniques for fetal tracheal occlusion to treat congenital diaphragmatic hernia, laser ablation of communicating placental vessels for treatment of twin-twin transfusion syndrome, and umbilical cord radiofrequency ablation for treatment of twin reversed arterial perfusion sequence.[5] Special attention to fetal monitoring and the management of anesthesia for *both* patients—mother and fetus—is required to ensure maternal and fetal welfare.

THERAPEUTIC ALTERNATIVES FOR FETAL MALFORMATIONS

Although there was rapid progress in prenatal diagnosis two to three decades ago, few invasive therapies were available or even considered other than blood transfusion. The only other alternatives included pregnancy termination, early delivery, or alteration of the delivery site to facilitate the availability of highly specialized care. Currently more alternatives are available. However, most malformations diagnosed in utero remain unsuitable for antenatal intervention. Antenatal diagnosis of a serious malformation (i.e., one that is neither correctable nor compatible with normal postnatal life) often prompts the early termination of pregnancy (Box 7-1).

Most correctable malformations are best managed by therapy *after* delivery at term gestation (Box 7-2). Some fetal malformations cause dystocia and require cesarean delivery (Box 7-3). When early correction or treatment of a malformation can minimize the progressive impairment associated with continued gestation, preterm delivery is considered; however, the risks of prematurity must be weighed against the risks of continued gestation.

Some defects, especially those that cause airway obstruction, can be treated by intrapartum intervention, in which the fetus undergoes repair of the defect and/or the airway is secured during birth, while the uteroplacental unit remains functional (Box 7-4). This technique of <u>ex</u> utero <u>in</u>trapartum <u>t</u>reatment (i.e., EXIT) was developed to allow the safe delivery of fetuses that had undergone intrauterine tracheal occlusion to treat congenital diaphragmatic hernia earlier in the pregnancy.[6]

Fetal surgery is a reasonable alternative for selected fetal anomalies that might result in fetal death, severe disability, or irreversible harm *before* the adequate development of fetal

Box 7-1 FETAL MALFORMATIONS OFTEN MANAGED BY ELECTIVE ABORTION

- Anencephaly, alobar holoprosencephaly
- Severe anomalies associated with chromosomal abnormalities (e.g., trisomy 13, trisomy 18)
- Bilateral renal agenesis or bilateral polycystic kidney disease
- Inherited, nontreatable chromosomal, metabolic, and hematologic abnormalities (e.g., Tay-Sachs disease)
- Lethal bone dysplasias (e.g., recessive osteogenesis imperfecta)

Box 7-2 FETAL MALFORMATIONS DETECTABLE IN UTERO BUT BEST CORRECTED AFTER DELIVERY AT TERM

- Esophageal, duodenal, jejunoileal, and anorectal atresias
- Meconium ileus (cystic fibrosis)
- Enteric cysts and duplications
- Small intact omphalocele
- Small intact meningocele, myelomeningocele, and spina bifida
- Unilateral hydronephrosis
- Craniofacial, extremity, and chest wall deformities
- Cystic hygroma
- Small sacrococcygeal teratoma
- Benign cysts (e.g., ovarian, mesenteric)

Box 7-3 FETAL MALFORMATIONS THAT MAY REQUIRE CESAREAN DELIVERY

- Conjoined twins
- Giant omphalocele or gastroschisis
- Large hydrocephalus, sacrococcygeal teratoma, cystic hygroma, or myelomeningocele

Box 7-4 DEFECTS THAT CAN BE MANAGED BY "EXIT" DELIVERY

- Cervical teratoma or large goiter causing airway compression
- Cervical cystic hygroma
- Cervical hemangioma
- Congenital high airway obstruction syndrome (laryngeal atresia)
- Lung mass preventing lung expansion
- Anticipated need for immediate extracorporeal membrane oxygenation (ECMO)

Box 7-5 ANATOMIC MALFORMATIONS THAT MAY BENEFIT FROM ANTENATAL SURGICAL CORRECTION

- Bilateral obstructive hydronephrosis
- Diaphragmatic hernia
- Cystic adenomatoid malformation
- Sacrococcygeal teratoma
- Obstructive hydrocephalus
- Cardiac abnormalities (e.g., ventricular outflow tract obstruction)
- Complete heart block
- Selected neural tube defects (myelomeningocele)
- Selected skeletal abnormalities (amniotic band syndrome, allogenic bone grafting)
- Craniofacial abnormalities
- Gastroschisis, omphalocele

and potential intrauterine therapeutic intervention, including fetal surgery.

INDICATIONS AND RATIONALE FOR FETAL SURGERY

Bilateral Hydronephrosis

Congenital bilateral hydronephrosis results from fetal urethral obstruction at the bladder outlet, most often by posterior urethral valves in male fetuses. It is easily detected by ultrasonography, which is often performed to investigate the associated oligohydramnios resulting from decreased fetal urine output. This lesion often has devastating developmental consequences, including renal dysplasia and pulmonary hypoplasia, which can prevent postnatal survival (Figure 7-1).[8] Delivery of the fetus preterm allows early urinary tract decompression ex utero, but fetal pulmonary immaturity limits the efficacy of this approach. Early intrauterine intervention allows drainage of urine from the fetal bladder into the amniotic cavity, which decompresses the urinary tract and allows fetal renal development. It can also restore normal amniotic fluid volume and prevent the sequelae of oligohydramnios (e.g., pulmonary hypoplasia and umbilical cord compression). Animal models of obstructive uropathy reveal changes in renal histology similar to those seen in kidneys of human neonates with congenital hydronephrosis. Relief of obstruction in utero ameliorates but does not eliminate the dysplastic changes in these animal models.[9] Restoration of normal urine flow and amniotic fluid volume allows the lungs to grow and prevents the development of pulmonary hypoplasia.

Two decades ago, the UCSF Fetal Treatment Program introduced the use of vesicoamniotic catheter shunts for the intrauterine treatment of bilateral hydronephrosis.[10] These

lung maturity necessary for extrauterine survival. Fetal surgery is reasonable only if (1) the lesion is diagnosed accurately; (2) the lesion's severity is assessed correctly; (3) associated anomalies that contraindicate intervention are excluded; (4) maternal risk is acceptably low; and (5) neonatal outcome is improved by fetal surgery when compared with surgery performed after preterm or term delivery. Emphasis is always placed on maternal welfare to guard against undue maternal risk.[7]

Examples of anatomic anomalies that are considered for invasive correction by the UCSF Fetal Treatment Program include obstructive hydronephrosis, diaphragmatic hernia, cystic adenomatoid malformation, large sacrococcygeal teratomas, myelomeningoceles, and valvular cardiac stenosis. These lesions result from failure of embryonic tissue closure, obstructive phenomena, or fetal tumor growth. If untreated, these lesions can interfere with fetal organ development or cause high-output fetal cardiac failure. Correction in utero may prevent irreversible organ damage. Some day, yet other malformations that interfere with organ development or that cause fetal cardiac failure, or other nonlethal defects such as craniofacial deformities, also may benefit from antenatal correction (Box 7-5). Although technically feasible, fetal surgery remains an innovative, investigational therapy, and controversy persists about its efficacy and expense, especially for nonlethal lesions such as myelomeningocele. Controlled clinical trials are needed to establish efficacy and substantiate the safety of fetal surgery for each lesion considered. We conduct weekly multidisciplinary meetings to discuss cases referred to the UCSF Fetal Treatment Program for evaluation

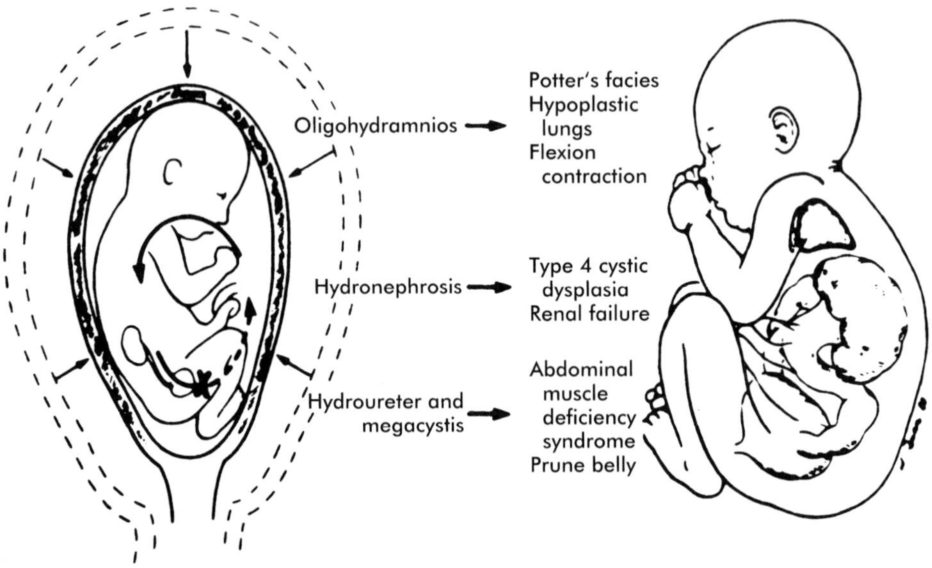

FIGURE 7-1. Developmental consequences of fetal urethral obstruction. Obstructed fetal urinary flow results in hydronephrosis, hydroureter, megacystis, oligohydramnios, and pulmonary hypoplasia. (From Harrison MR, Filly RA, Parer JT, et al. Management of the fetus with a urinary tract malformation. JAMA 1981; 246:635-9.)

valveless, double-coiled catheters are placed percutaneously with use of ultrasonographic guidance. By 1985, 73 human fetuses had undergone successful urinary tract decompression with vesicoamniotic catheters, but only 30 had successful clinical outcomes.[11] Frequent problems associated with use of these catheters include difficult placement, occlusion, and displacement. The first open surgical procedure, fetal vesicostomy, was performed as an alternative to catheter decompression of fetal obstructive uropathy.[12]

Preoperative assessment includes evaluation of fetal renal function (e.g., assessment of fetal urine volume, electrolytes, and beta$_2$-microglobulin levels; and ultrasonographic assessment of the renal parenchyma). Despite some early problems,[13] success has been reported with careful selection and the use of techniques including fetoscopic vesicostomy, cystoscopic laser ablation of valves, and placement of wire-mesh stents.[14] Clinical experience suggests that fetal surgery for the correction of obstructive uropathy is feasible, safe, and effective in the restoration of amniotic fluid volume and the prevention of pulmonary hypoplasia.[15] However, its potential for reversal of renal functional damage remains unclear.

Congenital Diaphragmatic Hernia and the EXIT Procedure

Approximately 1 in 2400 newborn infants has a congenital diaphragmatic hernia. This relatively simple anatomic defect can be corrected after birth in less severely affected babies by removing the herniated viscera from the chest and closing the diaphragm, and survival has improved by use of extra corporeal membrane oxygenation (ECMO). However, when correctable lesions diagnosed before 25 weeks' gestation are considered among fetuses without chromosomal or other life-threatening abnormalities, the mortality from pulmonary hypoplasia and insufficiency remains approximately 60% without fetal surgical intervention.[16] This high mortality rate occurs despite optimal postnatal management at a tertiary care medical center and the use of ECMO. Intrauterine correction of congenital diaphragmatic hernia can prevent pulmonary hypoplasia and allow the fetal lung to develop before delivery.[17]

Using a fetal lamb model, Harrison[17] demonstrated that the broad range of severity of congenital diaphragmatic her-

nia is explained by the timing and extent of visceral herniation and pulmonary compression, and that fatal pulmonary hypoplasia is caused by compression of the developing lung. Further studies demonstrated that parenchymal hypoplasia and associated pulmonary vascular changes may be reversed by correction in utero. The UCSF Fetal Treatment Program has performed primary repairs of fetal diaphragmatic hernia in utero with limited success, but with many lessons learned.[18-20] Enlargement of the fetal abdomen using an abdominal patch was necessary to accommodate the added abdominal contents without increasing intraabdominal pressure, which compromises ductus venosus blood flow.[18] The procedure is technically difficult and usually unsuccessful when the liver has herniated into the fetal chest. Reduction of the herniated liver compromises umbilical circulation with devastating consequences; many fetuses have died intraoperatively because of this problem. We have learned that more careful evaluation of the umbilical vein by color Doppler imaging allows more accurate preoperative assessment of the extent of liver herniation. Also, we have learned that the performance of *both* subcostal and thoracotomy incisions on the fetus improves surgical exposure, allows the reduction of viscera by pushing and pulling techniques, and facilitates the reconstruction of a diaphragm with a prosthetic patch.[21] Other lessons learned include (1) the advantages of opening the uterus with a stapling device to ensure effective hemostasis; (2) improved techniques of uterine closure; and (3) use of fibrin glue to help prevent amniotic fluid leaks. However, adequate control of intraoperative and postoperative uterine tone remains a substantial problem. In a prospective trial, open fetal surgery did not improve survival over standard postnatal treatment for fetuses without herniation of the liver into the thorax.[22]

Fetal tracheal occlusion impedes the normal egress of fetal lung fluid and results in expansion of the hypoplastic lung. This technique has replaced in utero primary repair for the correction of the pulmonary hypoplasia associated with congenital diaphragmatic hernia. It is a less extensive, palliative fetal surgical procedure, which allows postponement of the definitive repair until after birth.[23-25] Once the trachea is occluded, fetal pulmonary fluid slowly accumulates and expands the lung, pushing the viscera out of the thorax, a technique that we call "plug the lung until it grows" (i.e.,

PLUG).[25] In our first attempts at establishing reversible, controlled tracheal occlusion techniques, a foam plug was placed in the trachea during open fetal surgery, but this failed to completely occlude the trachea. Subsequently, an open procedure was used to place metallic hemoclips around the trachea after meticulous neck dissection to avoid injury to the recurrent laryngeal and vagus nerves. Subsequently, fetal endoscopic (i.e., FETENDO) surgical techniques replaced the open technique for placement of the clips.[26] Currently we place a small balloon in the trachea by endoscopic endotracheal intubation. The balloon, made for neuroangiographic occlusion of an intracranial aneurysm or arteriovenous malformation, is inflated and left in place until delivery. However, in a randomized trial, fetal tracheal occlusion for intrauterine treatment of severe congenital diaphragmatic hernia did not improve survival or reduce morbidity when compared with postnatal treatment with ECMO at a tertiary care center.[27]

Intrapartum management of the iatrogenic airway obstruction prompted the development of the EXIT procedure for these babies.[6] Adequate time and operating conditions are necessary for surgical removal of the tracheal balloon at delivery using the EXIT technique. During the EXIT procedure, the baby continues to exchange gases (including inhaled anesthetic agents) at the placenta rather than at the lungs. The EXIT procedure provides time to secure the airway while the infant remains on "placental bypass." In our experience, with appropriate anesthetic management to ensure uterine relaxation and avoid placental separation, normal uteroplacental gas exchange can be maintained for at least 2 hours. After inducing maternal and fetal anesthesia and ensuring uterine relaxation, a uterine incision is made with a stapling device to ensure hemostasis, and the baby is partially delivered. The surgeons then perform fetal bronchoscopy and pierce the balloon and retrieve it from the trachea. The trachea is then secured with an endotracheal tube, surfactant is administered if indicated, and the lungs are ventilated with oxygen. The cord is clamped after the baby's oxygen saturation increases, and the baby is delivered.

This technique is now widely used for a variety of other fetal problems (e.g., embryonic cervical tumors, laryngeal atresia) that compress the airway and/or render neonatal intubation unfeasible, and has generated numerous published case reports of success (see Box 7-4).[28-31] During the EXIT procedure for airway obstruction, either the fetal trachea is intubated directly using a laryngoscope or bronchoscope or a tracheostomy is performed. Following successful use of the EXIT procedure for management of airway compromise, the procedure has been used for a wide variety of problems, including (1) thoracotomy for cystic adenomatoid malformation; (2) transitioning from placental gas exchange to ECMO for anticipated pulmonary insufficiency; and (3) excision of a giant cervical teratoma.[32] We have performed several procedures lasting 1 to 2 hours or longer, without evidence of neonatal hypercarbia or acidosis at delivery.

Congenital Cystic Adenomatoid Malformation

Congenital cystic adenomatoid malformation is a pulmonary cystic tumor that can cause fetal hydrops and pulmonary hypoplasia. Small lesions detected in utero or in the newborn infant are treated after birth by surgical excision of the affected pulmonary lobe. Large lesions cause mediastinal shift and hydrops, which interfere with fetal survival. Large lesions also cause pulmonary hypoplasia, which may preclude neona-

tal survival.[33] In utero pulmonary lobectomy has been successful, allowing compensatory lung growth and resolution of hydrops. Macrocystic lesions have been decompressed in utero by the placement of shunt catheters between large cysts and the amniotic cavity, resulting in sustained decompression and resolution of hydrops; these procedures were followed by successful postnatal surgery.[34] However, not all lesions are decompressed successfully by thoracentesis because the cysts are not always contiguous (i.e., in communication with each other) and because they can refill rapidly. Refined selection criteria, as well as the potential for radiofrequency ablation of the tumor using a minimally invasive technique, hold promise for improved outcomes.[35]

Sacrococcygeal Teratoma

Some fetuses with a sacrococcygeal teratoma undergo massive tumor enlargement, develop hydrops and placentomegaly, and die in utero. These tumors function as large arteriovenous fistulae, and fetal demise results from high-output cardiac failure. Fetuses with large lesions are at risk for intrapartum dystocia or tumor rupture and hemorrhage; these fetuses may require delivery by cesarean section. Fetuses with lesions diagnosed before 30 weeks' gestation have a poor prognosis and may benefit from surgical excision in utero. However, fetal surgical techniques have not reached the necessary level of sophistication to allow resection of lesions that deeply invade the pelvis, where considerable fetal blood loss would be expected. In addition, the "maternal mirror syndrome," a hyperdynamic state (e.g., hypertension, peripheral and pulmonary edema) in which the maternal physiology mirrors the abnormal circulatory physiology of the hydropic fetus, does not resolve by rapid correction of the fetal pathophysiology.[36]

Successful operations for large sacrococcygeal teratomas have been performed with catheterization of a fetal hand or umbilical cord vein for blood and crystalloid transfusion during tumor resection.

Obstructive Hydrocephalus

In fetuses with obstructive hydrocephalus, perinatologists have performed cephalocentesis to relieve increased intracranial pressure and protect the development of the fetal brain. However, attempts at percutaneous placement of ventriculoamniotic shunts for obstructive ventriculomegaly have been disappointing and have not resulted in improved outcome. Selection of appropriate cases, development of an effective catheter with a one-way valve, and refinement of the procedure remain unsolved problems. By mid-1989, more than 40 cases of fetal ventriculomegaly treated by shunt catheter placement in utero had been reported to the International Fetal Medicine and Surgery Society Registry.[11] The poor outcomes prompted a de facto international moratorium on intrauterine therapy for ventriculomegaly.

Myelomeningocele

Although not lethal, a myelomeningocele (i.e., protrusion of meninges and spinal cord through a congenital defect in the vertebrae and overlying muscles and skin) can result in serious, lifelong morbidity and disability, including paraplegia, incontinence, hydrocephalus, and occasionally impaired cognition. Myelomeningocele is relatively common, with an incidence of about one in 2000 births, but it is becoming less common owing to folate supplementation of maternal diet and early detection of the lesion by alpha-fetoprotein screening of maternal blood, which allows the option of pregnancy termination. Recent experimental work has demonstrated that the associated neurologic damage may result from exposure of the spinal cord to amniotic fluid, suggesting that the spinal cord is not inherently defective. The purpose of in utero surgery for myelomeningocele is to cover the cord, preventing its further contact with amniotic fluid. Both endoscopic and open techniques have been employed to repair this lesion.[37,38] Preliminary results suggest successful reversal of the hindbrain herniation of the Arnold-Chiari malformation; however, it remains unclear what gestational age is optimal for intervention and what surgical technique should be employed. More important, it remains unclear whether in utero correction reverses the need for postnatal ventriculoperitoneal shunting and/or decreases the likelihood of paraplegia, and it is unclear whether the benefits (e.g., improved neurologic function) outweigh the complications and risks.[39] A multicenter, prospective trial is underway to determine the efficacy of in utero myelomeningocele repair.[40]

Twin-Twin Transfusion Syndrome

Abnormal connection of chorionic blood vessels in the placenta between two monochorionic twins results in a substantial incidence of mortality (i.e., as high as 75% for anatomically normal twins). The twin-twin transfusion syndrome usually presents in the second trimester of monochorionic twin gestation. Intertwin transfusion, common between monochorionic twins, is usually balanced through arterioarterial and venovenous connections but unidirectional and unbalanced through arteriovenous chorionic vessels. Unbalanced net intertwin transfusion results in the twin-twin transfusion syndrome, with one twin (the recipient) developing polycythemia, polyuria, and hypertrophic cardiomyopathy in a polyhydramniotic sac. This twin is at risk for hydrops and fetal death. The donor twin is typically hypovolemic, oliguric, growth-restricted, and stuck against the endometrium in an oligohydramniotic sac (hence the designation *stuck twin*) and often has a velamentous cord insertion. This twin is at risk for neonatal renal failure or renal tubular dysgenesis and dysfunction. For unclear reasons, the survivors are at risk for neurologic injury with white-matter lesions and long-term disability. A variety of therapeutic management techniques have been developed, including (1) amnioreduction to control polyhydramnios and reduce the risk of preterm labor; (2) surgical septostomy of the amnions to equalize amniotic pressures; (3) selective termination of one twin to allow the other to survive; and (4) laser photocoagulation of the vascular anastomoses between the two twins.[41] The photocoagulation technique has been effective. The laser can be inserted either percutaneously or through a maternal laparotomy or minilaparotomy incision. Depending on placental location, laparotomy and exteriorization of the uterus may be necessary to access the chorionic plate. Location of the placenta has a direct impact on choice of anesthesia. A variety of anesthetic techniques have been employed for management of fetoscopic surgery, ranging from local infiltration to general anesthesia.[42]

Twin Reversed Arterial Perfusion Sequence

In monozygotic twins, one twin can perfuse the other by retrograde blood flow though arterioarterial anastomoses. Twin reversed arterial perfusion sequence (i.e., TRAP) affects 1% of monozygotic twins and 1 in 30 triplets. Inadequate perfusion to the perfused twin via retrograde flow results in the development of a lethal set of anomalies that include acardia and acephalus. Cardiovascular failure in the normal twin is the indication for intervention. The goal of therapy is interruption of the vascular communication between the two twins. In contrast to the treatment of twin-twin transfusion syndrome, treatment results in the demise of the anomalous fetus. This is most readily achieved by percutaneous umbilical cord ligation with suture or by radiofrequency coagulation. Alternative therapy has included sectio parva or percutaneous thrombosis of the acardiac twin's umbilical cord. Without treatment, the normal fetus invariably will die in utero. Operative endoscopy for cord ligation by radiofrequency coagulation is relatively simple and effective. Anesthetic considerations are identical to those for twin-twin transfusion syndrome and other fetoscopic procedures.

Other Lesions

Placement of thoracoamniotic shunts has resulted in successful decompression of massive congenital pleural effusions caused by fetal chylothorax that otherwise would have resulted in hydrops, pulmonary compression, and fetal or neonatal death.[43] Other potentially correctable defects include certain cardiac abnormalities (e.g., ventricular outflow tract obstruction), refractory complete heart block, gastroschisis, cleft lip and palate, other craniofacial anomalies, and skeletal anomalies correctable by allogenic bone grafting (see Box 7-5). Techniques for extracorporeal circulation have undergone investigation in fetal lambs.[44]

Fetal surgery in utero has some unique advantages. The intrauterine environment supports rapid wound healing (i.e., without scarring before midgestation), and the umbilical circulation meets nutritional and respiratory needs without outside assistance. The poorly developed fetal immune surveillance system may facilitate certain invasive procedures. Intrauterine cleft palate or lip surgery may restore normal form without scarring, allow midfacial growth without restriction or scar formation, and prevent associated nasal deformities. However, continued refinement of surgical and anesthetic techniques and reduction of maternal and fetal risk must occur before we can perform fetal surgery on a more routine basis, or for less severe fetal anomalies.

ANESTHETIC MANAGEMENT

Fundamental considerations for anesthetic management of fetal surgery are similar to those for performance of nonobstetric surgery during pregnancy (see Chapter 16). Maternal safety is paramount. Women at increased risk are excluded following preoperative assessment by the anesthesiologist. To ensure both maternal and fetal safety, the anesthesiologist must understand the physiologic changes of pregnancy and their effects on anesthetic management, and he/she must take an active role in perioperative management.

Unlike other surgical procedures performed during pregnancy, fetal surgery requires both complete uterine relaxation (i.e., atony) and fetal anesthesia. Fetal surgery also entails a high risk of preterm labor, preterm rupture of membranes, and preterm delivery.

Minimally Invasive and Percutaneous Procedures

Local anesthetic infiltration of the abdominal wall is sufficient to reduce maternal discomfort for many percutaneous procedures (e.g., amniocentesis, cordocentesis, and intrauterine blood transfusion). Supplemental maternal analgesia and anxiolysis can be provided by administration of an opioid and/or a benzodiazepine. We routinely administer supplemental oxygen whenever conscious sedation is employed.

Cordocentesis occasionally results in prolonged fetal bradycardia, especially if the needle punctures the umbilical artery rather than the umbilical vein. The risk of fetal bradycardia secondary to cord trauma increases with gestational age. Persistent fetal bradycardia may prompt performance of emergency cesarean section if the gestational age is compatible with extrauterine viability. For patients with a viable fetus, we have the mother fast overnight and we establish intravenous access, administer medication for aspiration prophylaxis, and monitor as though general anesthesia may be required for emergency cesarean section. In some cases we administer "prophylactic" spinal or epidural anesthesia *before* cordocentesis, especially at later gestational ages (i.e., 30 weeks' gestation or later).

Some percutaneous techniques that do not require large ports to accommodate the endoscope (e.g., placement of vesicoamniotic catheter shunts, laser surgery on placental vessels) include procedures similar to those for cordocentesis. Adequate maternal anesthesia may be obtained with local anesthetic infiltration of the maternal abdomen, and some fetal sedation may be achieved by placental transfer of the opioid and benzodiazepine administered to the mother.[45] However, if larger needles and/or multiple attempts are necessary, maternal comfort can be difficult to achieve safely by local infiltration and/or sedation. In these circumstances we administer spinal or epidural anesthesia. We also use epidural anesthesia for percutaneous or minilaparotomy approaches for endoscopic surgery, when large or multiple access ports are required, provided the placenta is positioned so that access can be achieved without requiring uterine exteriorization. We find that general anesthesia is preferred when surgical exposure requires uterine exteriorization, both for maternal comfort and to block the uterine response to the increased manipulation that is required.

Unfortunately, fetal activity may render the procedure technically difficult or impossible. Placental transfer of the opioid and/or benzodiazepine does not ensure an immobile fetus. Fetal movement may be hazardous for the fetus because displacement of the needle or catheter may lead to trauma, bleeding, or compromise of the umbilical circulation. Fetal movement can be safely controlled by use of direct fetal intramuscular or umbilical venous administration of pancuronium or vecuronium (0.3 mg/kg intramuscularly or 0.05 to 0.1 mg/kg intravenously). The onset of fetal paralysis occurs in approximately 2 minutes, with a duration of 1 to 2 hours.[46]

Fetal paralysis has replaced reliance on placental transfer of agents used for maternal sedation to achieve fetal immobilization for many percutaneous procedures that do not involve noxious stimulation of the fetus. We have not found that fetal immobilization is necessary for laser surgery involving the chorionic plate, such as twin-twin transfusion syndrome. If cordocentesis results in fetal bradycardia and emergency cesarean section, the neonatologist must be informed if the infant is paralyzed.

Anesthesia for Open Fetal Surgery

When corrective fetal surgery or an in utero procedure requires surgical access through a hysterotomy, we administer a high concentration of a volatile halogenated agent to provide both maternal and fetal anesthesia and to provide the required uterine relaxation.[47]

Preoperatively, the mother receives medication for aspiration prophylaxis and rectal indomethacin for tocolysis, and an epidural catheter is placed. Minimal doses of preanesthetic medication and adjuvant anesthetic agents are given to supplement the volatile halogenated agent. This allows administration of maximum doses of a volatile halogenated agent to achieve uterine relaxation. With left uterine displacement—and following denitrogenation of the lungs—rapid-sequence induction of general anesthesia and tracheal intubation are performed. We maintain anesthesia with a low concentration of a volatile halogenated agent while further preparations for surgery are undertaken, including (1) obtaining additional vascular access; (2) prophylactic antibiotic administration; (3) urinary bladder catheterization; and (4) performance of ultrasonography to assess fetal presentation and placental location. During this time, we prepare additional medications for providing fetal anesthesia (fentanyl 25 µg/kg), immobility (vecuronium 0.2 mg/kg), and resuscitation (atropine 0.02 mg/kg, epinephrine 1 µg/kg, and crystalloid 10 mL/kg), and we deliver these drugs to the surgeon in a sterile fashion for subsequent administration, as per our direction.

In anticipation of maternal skin incision, the concentration of the volatile halogenated agent is increased to 2 to 3 minimum alveolar concentration (MAC). Any volatile halogenated agent can be used.[48] We support maternal blood pressure with ephedrine as necessary to maintain mean arterial pressure at >65 mm Hg. Before surgery begins, it is important to achieve an increased end-tidal concentration of the volatile halogenated agent to provide both fetal anesthesia and uterine relaxation. We assess fetal well-being primarily by fetal heart rate (FHR) monitoring using ultrasonography, fetal pulse oximetry, fetal echocardiography, and/or direct fetal ECG. We intermittently assess fetal ventricular size and contractility, and we monitor fetal oxygen saturation by oximetry when feasible. Prior to uterine incision, the uterus is assessed both visually and by palpation for contractions or increased tone. The inspired concentration of the volatile halogenated agent is increased if the uterus is not soft and flaccid, and we then wait for the desired uterine response. If a uterine contraction band is seen or increased uterine tone is palpated after the hysterotomy incision is made, we give boluses of nitroglycerin (50 to 200 µg intravenously) to provide supplemental tocolysis. By using ultrasonographic guidance, fentanyl and vecuronium are administered to the fetus intramuscularly prior to uterine incision. The uterine incision is made (remote from the location of the placenta) with a stapling device devised to prevent excessive bleeding and to seal the membranes to the endometrium. During surgery, the exposed fetus and uterus are bathed with warmed fluids.

When uterine closure is initiated at the conclusion of the procedure, a loading dose of magnesium sulfate is administered (4 to 6 g intravenously over 20 minutes), followed by an intravenous infusion of 2 g/hr. We discontinue the volatile halogenated agent when the magnesium sulfate bolus is given, and maternal anesthesia is maintained with fentanyl and nitrous oxide in oxygen, as well as activation of epidural anesthesia with a bolus dose of a local anesthetic agent and an opioid administered through the epidural catheter. This regimen

(1) allows time for elimination of the volatile halogenated agent; (2) facilitates tracheal extubation shortly after surgery is completed, with a fully awake patient who is capable of protecting her airway with minimal coughing or straining that might jeopardize the integrity of the water-tight uterine closure; and (3) allows the patient to awaken without pain.

Intraoperative maternal intravenous fluids are restricted to minimize the risk of the frequently seen problem of postoperative pulmonary edema, despite evidence that the pulmonary edema is not a result of volume overload.[20] Other postoperative concerns are maternal and fetal pain, preterm labor, rupture of membranes, infection, and a variety of potential fetal complications, including heart failure, intracranial hemorrhage, constriction of the ductus arteriosus from indomethacin, and fetal demise. We maintain analgesia with a continuous epidural infusion of a dilute solution of local anesthetic and opioid for the first 2 to 3 days. Effective analgesia may help prevent postoperative preterm labor.[49] Early postoperative uterine contractions are expected, and tocolysis is provided with an infusion of magnesium sulfate, which may be supplemented with indomethacin and occasionally terbutaline. Uterine activity and FHR are monitored continuously or very frequently during the first 2 to 3 postoperative days. The fetus is evaluated postoperatively by ultrasonography and magnetic resonance imaging.

We have also used an alternative anesthetic and tocolytic technique for open fetal surgery. With this technique, we administer nitrous oxide, fentanyl, and a low concentration of the volatile halogenated agent. Intravenous fluids are administered to maintain a normal central venous pressure. We achieve intraoperative uterine relaxation by administration of intravenous nitroglycerin in doses as large as 20 µg/kg/min, and we support blood pressure with ephedrine. Fetal anesthesia is achieved primarily by intramuscular administration of an opioid such as fentanyl. This technique has been successful, but it has no clear advantage and it may be associated with maternal and perhaps fetal morbidity. For example, postoperative administration of nitroglycerin for tocolysis can result in maternal nonhydrostatic pulmonary edema, possibly due to peroxynitrite, a nitroglycerin metabolite.[20] Fetal intraventricular and periventricular hemorrhage and cerebral ischemia can result from changes in fetal cerebral blood flow, and concern has been raised that tocolytic agents that affect vascular tone and cross the placenta may be harmful. We now reserve this technique for unusual circumstances, such as that for a recent patient who was at risk for malignant hyperthermia.[50]

Further studies are needed to determine the optimal anesthetic technique that ensures maternal cardiovascular stability, optimal uteroplacental perfusion, total uterine relaxation, adequate fetal anesthesia and immobility, minimal fetal myocardial depression, and blockade of the fetal stress response. Direct fetal administration of vasoactive agents may block the fetal autonomic response to stress, which may redistribute blood flow away from the placenta.[51] Total fetal spinal anesthesia would block the fetal autonomic response to noxious stimuli, but it does not seem feasible technically at this time.

Anesthesia for the EXIT Procedure

For the EXIT procedure, we modify our usual anesthetic technique for cesarean section and administer a combined epidural and general anesthetic technique. Unlike general anesthesia for cesarean section, sufficient time must be allowed after induction of anesthesia—before surgery commences—to achieve the high end-tidal concentration of volatile halogenated agent needed to ensure uterine relaxation. Anesthesia is supplemented by fetal intramuscular administration of an opioid and a paralytic agent to provide sufficient fetal anesthesia and immobility. After ensuring that uterine relaxation has been achieved, a uterine incision is made with the stapling device, and the fetal head and shoulders are delivered in preparation for tracheal intubation. For more extensive procedures such as fetal thoracotomy, or when there is fetal bradycardia suggestive of umbilical cord compression, the fetus is completely delivered and placed on the maternal chest and abdomen. The umbilical cord is not manipulated; it is kept wet with warmed fluids, and the fetoplacental circulation is maintained. The fetus is monitored with (1) a pulse oximeter probe placed on the fetal hand; (2) periodic ultrasonography; and (3) direct visualization. Once the fetal surgery is completed, the baby's lungs are ventilated. When the baby's oxygen saturation increases (typically above 90%), the umbilical cord is cut and the (already intubated) newborn infant is transferred to the neonatologist for further resuscitation. At this point the maternal anesthetic technique is changed: (1) the inspired concentration of the volatile halogenated agent is substantially reduced or discontinued; (2) nitrous oxide 70% and an opioid are administered; and (3) epidural anesthesia is activated with a bolus dose of a local anesthetic agent and an opioid administered through the epidural catheter. Oxytocin is administered in the usual fashion, and hyperventilation is achieved to rapidly decrease the end-tidal concentration of the volatile halogenated agent. When using this technique we have not encountered postpartum uterine atony or excessive blood loss, and to date, we have not needed to give methylergonovine or a prostaglandin to achieve adequate uterine tone.[52]

Fetal Response to Surgical Stimulation

The subjective phenomenon of pain has not been assessed adequately in human fetuses. Studies of preterm neonates undergoing surgery with minimal anesthesia have noted circulatory, sympathoadrenal, and pituitary adrenal responses characteristic of stress (e.g., increased release of catecholamines, growth hormone, glucagon, cortisol, aldosterone, and other corticosteroids; decreased secretion of insulin).[53-56] Administration of adequate anesthesia abolishes the neonatal stress response,[57] and in preterm neonates, attenuation of the stress response with opioids improves outcome.[58]

Surgical needling of the human fetus during intrahepatic vein blood transfusion increases plasma beta-endorphin and cortisol concentrations and causes a decrease in the Doppler-determined middle cerebral artery pulsatility index, which is consistent with redistribution of blood flow to vital organs, including the brain.[59] Human fetuses elaborate pituitary-adrenal, sympathoadrenal, and circulatory stress responses to noxious stimuli as early as 18 weeks' gestation.[60-63] Administration of fentanyl, 10 µg/kg, blocks the increase in plasma endorphins and the Doppler-determined arterial resistance changes, but not the plasma cortisol changes.[64] Possibly this dose of fentanyl is insufficient or the cortisol response is too fast. (The fentanyl was administered immediately *after* needling.) During late gestation, fetuses respond to environmental stimuli such as noises, light, music, pressure, touch, and cold.[65]

However, these physiologic responses are not necessarily equivalent to the multidimensional, subjective phenomenon that we call *pain*.[66] When is the fetus adequately developed to *feel* pain? Thalamocortical axons reach the somatosensory cortex at 24 to 26 weeks' gestation, but nociceptive information may be transmitted earlier through a complete neurologic connection from the peripheral tissue through the brainstem and the thalamus to the cerebral cortex via transient thalamocortical fibers.[67] Can the fetus experience pain before development of this final anatomic link from periphery to cortex? Even if not, given that descending inhibitory pathways are formed much later, is it possible that the fetus is *more* sensitive to noxious stimuli? Can the neonate or fetus feel pain if not sentient? If a neonate can feel pain, does the fetus feel pain at the same gestational age, or is there something about birth that initiates this capability? Even if noxious stimulation does not affect consciousness, can it influence development, given that circumcision in a nonanesthetized neonate increases the infant's pain response to injections 6 months later[68] and that fetal stress affects hormonal activity in young monkeys?[69]

Clearly, many questions remain unanswered. However, it is possible that pain can have adverse long-term neurodevelopmental consequences that could be attenuated or blocked by anesthesia. Further, it seems doubtful that fetal exposure to general anesthesia for fetal surgery would be more harmful to the fetus than similar exposure to anesthesia in neonates, older children, or the fetuses of mothers who undergo nonobstetric surgery during pregnancy (see Chapter 16).[70,71] It seems best to err on the side of adequate fetal anesthesia administration.[72]

Altogether, clinical observations of fetal and neonatal behavior, information about the development of mechanisms of pain perception, and studies of fetal and neonatal responses to noxious stimuli provide a compelling physiologic and philosophic rationale for the provision of adequate fetal anesthesia, especially after 24 to 26 weeks' gestation. This has been my practice since the inception of fetal surgery at UCSF more than two decades ago. I have emphasized the importance of fetal immobility, cardiovascular homeostasis, analgesia, and perhaps amnesia.

Effects of Anesthesia on Fetal Circulation

In fetal lambs, the concentration of halothane required to prevent movement in response to painful stimuli is lower than that for adult sheep or newborn lambs (Table 7-1).[73] Despite rapid placental transfer of volatile halogenated agents, fetal concentrations of volatile halogenated agents remain lower than maternal concentrations for significant periods after maternal administration (Figures 7-2 and 7-3).[74,75]

TABLE 7-1	FETAL ANESTHETIC REQUIREMENT (MAC) FOR HALOTHANE IN SHEEP (MEAN ± SE)	
	Blood concentration at MAC* (mg/L)	**Theoretical (calculated) end-tidal concentration* (%)**
Mothers	133 ± 5	0.69 ± 0.25
Fetuses	49 ± 28	0.33 ± 0.29

*Maternal and fetal values are significantly different (P <0.001).
Modified from Gregory GA, Wade JG, Biehl DR, et al. Fetal anesthetic requirement (MAC) for halothane. Anesth Analg 1983; 62:9-14.

Experimental studies of the fetal effects of maternal administration of a volatile halogenated agent have not produced uniform results.[74-77] Maternal administration of 0.7% halothane or 1.0% isoflurane (i.e., 1.0 MAC for sheep) caused a modest decrease in fetal blood pressure with no change in fetal heart rate, oxygen saturation, or acid-base status. However, maternal administration of 1.5% halothane or 2.0% isoflurane caused decreased fetal blood pressure, heart rate, oxygen saturation, and base excess, with development of progressive fetal acidosis.[76] Other studies of maternal administration of 1.5% halothane demonstrated decreased fetal arterial pressure caused by decreased peripheral vascular resistance, with no change in fetal heart rate, cardiac output, oxygenation, acid-base status, or blood flow to the fetal brain or other major fetal organs (Figures 7-4 through 7-6).[74,77] Another

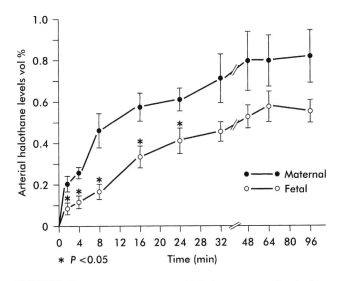

FIGURE 7-2. Maternal and fetal arterial halothane concentrations in sheep during maternal administration of 1.5% halothane (mean ± SE). (From Biehl DR, Cote J, Wade JG, et al. Uptake of halothane by the foetal lamb in utero. Can Anaesth Soc J 1983; 30:24-7.)

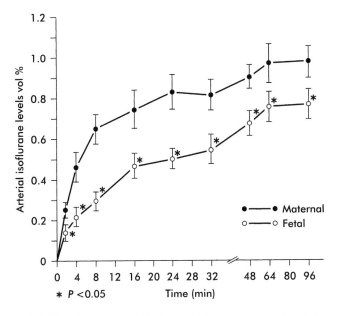

FIGURE 7-3. Maternal and fetal arterial isoflurane concentrations in sheep during maternal administration of 2.0% isoflurane (mean ± SE). (From Biehl DR, Yarnell R, Wade JG, Sitar D. The uptake of isoflurane by the foetal lamb in utero: effect on regional blood flow. Can Anaesth Soc J 1983; 30:581-6.)

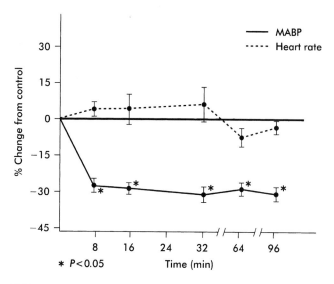

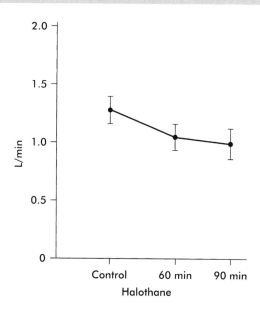

FIGURE 7-4. Changes in fetal sheep mean arterial blood pressure *(MABP)* and heart rate during maternal administration of 1.5% halothane, expressed as percentage change from control levels (mean ± SE). (From Biehl DR, Tweed WA, Cote J, et al. Effect of halothane on cardiac output and regional flow in the fetal lamb in utero. Anesth Analg 1983; 62:489-92.)

FIGURE 7-6. Fetal sheep cardiac output calculated using the labeled microsphere injection technique during maternal administration of 1.5% halothane (mean ± SE). Measurements were made at control and after 60 and 90 minutes of halothane anesthesia. (From Biehl DR, Tweed WA, Cote J, et al. Effect of halothane on cardiac output and regional flow in the fetal lamb in utero. Anesth Analg 1983; 62:489-92.)

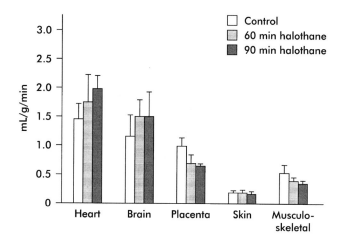

FIGURE 7-5. Fetal sheep regional blood flow during maternal administration of 1.5% halothane (mean ± SE). Measurements were made at control and after 60 and 90 minutes of halothane anesthesia using the labeled microsphere injection technique. (From Biehl DR, Tweed WA, Cote J, et al. Effect of halothane cardiac output and regional flow in the fetal lamb in utero. Anesth Analg 1983; 62:489-92.)

study noted decreased fetal cardiac output and placental blood flow and progressive fetal acidosis during maternal administration of 2% isoflurane for 90 minutes. Exposures lasting as long as 30 minutes did not significantly decrease fetal cardiac output or result in fetal acidosis.[75]

In the chronic maternal-fetal sheep model, with no surgical stimulus to either the mother or fetus, it appears that prolonged, deep maternal inhalation anesthesia (i.e., 2.0 MAC) results in progressive fetal acidosis and is unsafe. Whether this adverse response results from direct impairment of fetal myocardial contractility, adverse redistribution of fetal blood flow, or reduced maternal uterine blood flow remains unclear. Light maternal inhalation anesthesia (i.e., 1.0 MAC) may be undesirable because it does not block the fetal response to a painful stimulus (e.g., surgery), which includes increased fetal catecholamines, vasoconstriction, and redistri-

bution of fetal blood flow.[78] Fetal exposure to light maternal inhalation anesthesia (i.e., 1.0 MAC), *without* fetal stimulation, or *brief* fetal exposure to deep maternal inhalation anesthesia (i.e., 2.0 to 3.0 MAC) seems safe. Inhibition of the stress response using fetal spinal anesthesia in fetal sheep improves the fetal hemodynamic status during surgery and facilitates placental function after fetal cardiac bypass, compared to a technique of fetal ketamine administration.[79] However, the *combined* impact of adequate fetal anesthesia with a halogenated agent, intrauterine manipulation, and fetal stress on fetal cardiovascular stability and regional blood flow remains unknown. In our experience, long and deep maternal inhalation anesthesia has not caused fetal hypoxia, hypercarbia, or acidosis, even after exposures of 2 hours. However, others have seen acidosis after 45 minutes of fetal exposure to anesthesia.[80]

Fetal Monitoring

Maternal and fetal anesthesia, uterine incision, fetal manipulation, and surgical stress may adversely affect uteroplacental and fetoplacental circulation by several mechanisms. Maternal hypotension, increased uterine activity, and maternal hyperventilation and hypocarbia impair uteroplacental and/or umbilical blood flow. Fetal manipulation may affect fetal cardiac output, *regional distribution* of cardiac output, and/or umbilical blood flow. Direct compression of the umbilical cord, inferior vena cava, and/or mediastinum adversely affects fetal circulation.

Current methods of intraoperative fetal monitoring include FHR monitoring, pulse oximetry, ultrasonography, and blood gas and pH determinations. Initially we monitored FHR with a standard fetal electrocardiogram (ECG) electrode and a reference electrode on the maternal abdomen, with both connected to a maternal ground pad. The signal, processed by a standard FHR cardiotachometer, was of low amplitude and was very sensitive to movement artifact. Thus

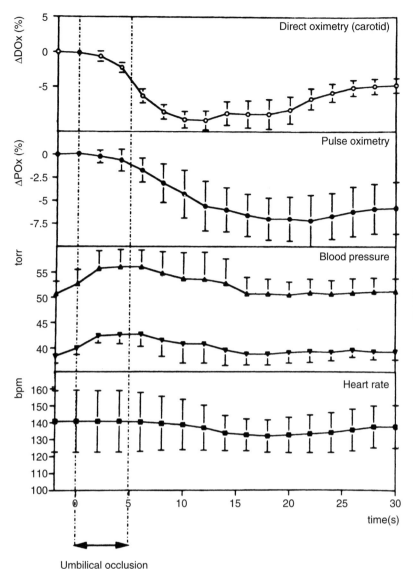

FIGURE 7-7. Response to 5 seconds of umbilical cord occlusion in the fetal lamb. Direct and pulse oximetry are expressed as delta saturation $(T_x - T_0)$. (From Luks FI, Johnson BD, Papadakis K, et al. Predictive value of monitoring parameters in fetal surgery. J Pediatr Surg 1998; 33:1297-1301.)

interpretation was unreliable. Direct fetal ECG monitoring using modified, insulated atrial pacing wires was more reliable. The distal end of the bare wire was sutured subcutaneously onto the fetal thorax. The proximal end of the insulated wire was attached to coaxial shielded cables, which connected the three leads to a cardiotachometer. We used a cardiotachometer that was modified with an increased gain to allow signal amplification. The cardiotachometer was modified further by the addition of a fixed low-pass frequency filter and a variable high-pass frequency filter, which substantially reduced motion artifact. These modifications allowed more reliable display of fetal ECG, with visible P waves and QRS complexes. Unfortunately, this technique did not eliminate motion artifact. Further, this technique allowed only intraoperative assessment of fetal ECG.

Plethysmography combined with spectrophotometric oximetry (pulse oximetry) has proven to be very useful, especially for the EXIT procedure. We currently use a noninvasive neonatal digital sensor wrapped around a fetal foot or palmar arch. We have experimented with a flat sensor placed over exposed fetal skin, which measures light by reflectance rather than transmission. In fact, we designed the flat sensor that

eventually led to the commercially available fetal oximeter and its probe (Nellcor, Hayward, CA), which we are comparing with commercially available finger sensors for use during myelomeningocele repairs. We have seen fetal oxygen saturations sustained at approximately 75% for more than an hour during fetal surgery, with maternal anesthesia comprising high-dose isoflurane (i.e., 2.0 to 3.0 MAC*) in oxygen, which suggests good fetal cardiac output, perfusion pressure, and oxygenation, despite the high concentration of isoflurane. The predictive value of pulse oximetry may be superior to FHR monitoring; bradycardia was found to be a late sign of fetal distress in fetal lambs subjected to umbilical cord compression (Figure 7-7).[82] However, we have seen bradycardia precede desaturation during human fetal surgery, and others have made similar observations during labor (Figures 7-8 through 7-10).[83]

---

*Gin and Chan[81] demonstrated that MAC for isoflurane is approximately 0.775% in pregnant woman at 8 to 12 weeks' gestation.

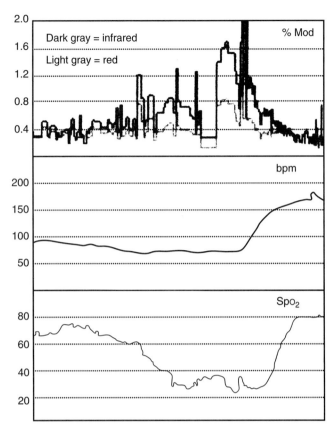

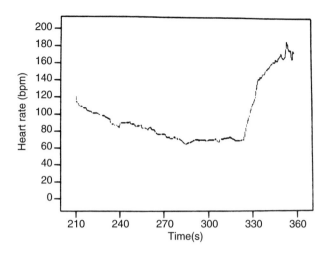

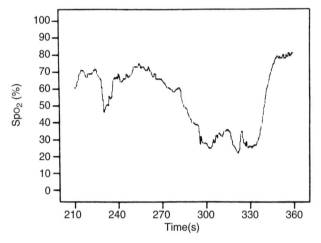

FIGURE 7-8. Two-minute tracing showing fetal heart rate (FHR) (beats per minute [bpm]; scale 0 to 250), oxygen saturation (SpO$_2$; scale 0% to 100%), and modulation of red and infrared light signals (light grey = red, dark grey = infrared; scale 0% to 2%) in a 24-week gestation fetus undergoing open diaphragmatic hernia repair. Note that the decrease in FHR from about 90 to 70 bpm precedes the decrease in oxygen saturation from about 70% to 22%, and recovery in FHR to about 160 bpm precedes the recovery in oxygen saturation. This may represent a transport delay in propagation of blood to the peripheral SpO$_2$ sensor. FHR may be a better monitor than SpO$_2$ for acute changes. (From Rosen MA. Anesthesia for fetal surgery. In Shnider and Levinson's Anesthesia for Obstetrics, 4th ed. Hughes SC, Levinson G, Rosen MA [eds]. Lippincott Williams, & Wilkins, Philadelphia, 2002.)

FIGURE 7-9. Graphic representation of the data in Figure 7-8 showing fetal heart rate (bpm) and oxygen saturation (SpO$_2$) more precisely detailed over the 120-second period. (From Rosen MA. Anesthesia for fetal surgery. In Shnider and Levinson's Anesthesia for Obstetrics, 4th ed. Hughes SC, Levinson G, Rosen MA [eds]. Lippincott Williams & Wilkins, Philadelphia, 2002.)

Intermittent ultrasonography also facilitates intraoperative fetal monitoring. The FHR can be determined by visualization of the heart or by Doppler assessment of umbilical cord blood flow. Fetal cardiac contractility and volume also can be assessed qualitatively. Unfortunately, the sterile transducer cannot be positioned continuously because it often interferes with surgery.

Invasive methods used in experimental fetal animal preparations require indwelling catheters that have not been used routinely for human fetal surgery to date. Capillary or umbilical venous blood samples have been obtained for blood gas, pH, electrolyte, and glucose determinations. Vascular access has been achieved by surgical cut-down on the internal jugular vein for fluid, blood, and/or drug administration during prolonged procedures (e.g., correction of a diaphragmatic hernia). On three occasions we have placed an intravenous catheter into a fetal arm vein, and twice we have administered blood to replace blood loss during a sacrococcygeal teratoma resection. In the future, placental vessels may be catheterized for continuous blood pressure monitoring and blood gas determinations, and more information may be obtained from waveform analysis of the fetal ECG. Intraosseous access has

been investigated in fetal sheep,[84] and chronic fetal vascular access has been achieved with use of laparoscopic techniques to cannulate chorionic vessels by an extraamniotic approach in rhesus monkey fetuses.[85] New devices may become available for monitoring the fetal EEG; for continuous monitoring of arterial blood oxygen saturation, Po$_2$, and Pco$_2$; and for monitoring cerebral oxygenation, blood volume, and blood flow by near-infrared spectroscopy.

Preterm Labor

The human uterus has a thick, muscular layer that is sensitive to stimulation or manipulation. Uterine incision and stimulation may result in strong uterine contractions, which have resulted in a high incidence of postoperative abortion in studies of primate fetuses. Therefore, fetal surgery entails a high risk of preterm labor. Uterine contractions also may impede uterine blood flow and/or induce partial placental separation. Management of postoperative preterm labor has been the "Achilles heel" of fetal surgery.[86] The size of the uterine incision appears to directly relate to the likelihood and intensity of preterm labor. We have seen less preterm labor (or more

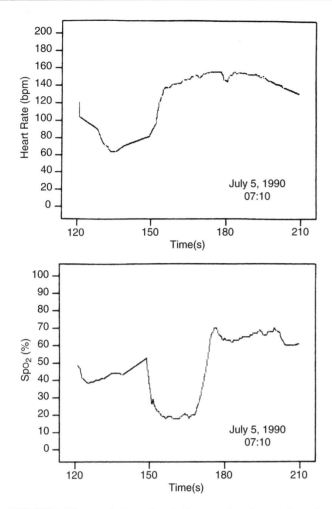

FIGURE 7-10. Data similar to those in Figure 7-9 from the same fetus a few minutes earlier, showing an acute decrease in fetal heart rate (FHR) with an associated decrease in fetal saturation. Note that the onset of the desaturation detected in the fetal hand is delayed relative to the onset of the bradycardia. Similarly, the recovery in FHR precedes the onset of the rapid increase in saturation. This most likely represents a transport delay of the blood from the heart to the fetal hand. (From Rosen MA. Anesthesia for fetal surgery. In Shnider and Levinson's Anesthesia for Obstetrics, 4th ed. Hughes SC, Levinson G, Rosen MA (eds), Philadelphia, Lippincott Williams & Wilkins, 2002.)

easily treated preterm labor) among women who have undergone minimally invasive surgery compared to those who have undergone open procedures involving a large hysterotomy.

Prevention of uterine contractions is ideal, and the treatment of uterine contractions is essential. Our tocolytic therapy has included a variety of agents, including preoperative indomethacin; intraoperative volatile halogenated agents; intraoperative and postoperative magnesium sulfate; and postoperative beta-adrenergic, indomethacin, and calcium-entry blockade therapies. A recent study suggests that volatile anesthetic agents may inhibit myometrial contractility by calcium-sensitive potassium channel modulation.[87] Magnesium probably competes with calcium at these voltage-operated calcium channels, indomethacin blocks the synthesis of prostaglandins, and beta-adrenergic agents have a direct action on the uterus, activating adenylate cyclase and thereby reducing intracellular calcium. The relative inefficacy of tocolytic agents and their potential adverse side effects have made this aspect of postoperative management frustrating. Use of nitric oxide donor agents has not been very beneficial. Perhaps the development of new tocolytic agents with increased efficacy and selectivity will substantially improve our ability to prevent preterm labor and delivery after fetal surgery.

Tocolysis typically is unnecessary after cordocentesis or intrauterine transfusion. For more invasive percutaneous procedures (e.g., shunt catheter placement, endoscopic techniques), we routinely administer magnesium sulfate.

THE FUTURE OF FETAL THERAPY

Although the rationale for fetal surgery seems straightforward, many issues remain problematic. Questions remain regarding maternal and fetal rights, safety, efficacy, cost effectiveness, and societal resource allocation. We must balance societal expectations and the availability of therapy with increased budgetary constraints in health care. In addition, there is concern regarding the sensitivity, specificity, and appropriate use of diagnostic testing. Fetal therapy raises complex social, ethical, and legal issues that go beyond those customary for therapeutic intervention. There is considerable controversy about fetal surgery, particularly for nonlethal lesions such as myelomeningocele.[88]

In some cases, distinguishing innovative therapy from experimentation is difficult. The ethical framework for the transition from innovation in fetal surgery to clinical trials to offering fetal surgery as a standard of care must be managed thoughtfully and responsibly.[89,90] Fetal therapy must be evaluated carefully in properly conducted trials and undertaken only with great caution and informed maternal consent. The UCSF Fetal Treatment Program founded the International Fetal Medicine and Surgery Society, which sets general and specific guidelines for fetal therapy and maintains a voluntary registry of fetal surgical procedures. This facilitates the moral obligation of researchers to report *all* results to allow peer-review of the merits and liabilities of fetal surgery.

Fetal surgical and anesthetic techniques and tocolytic therapy continue to evolve. Less invasive endoscopic techniques, which obviate the need for a large uterine incision and reduce risk by causing less uterine trauma and less preterm labor, are significant advances. More therapeutic procedures (e.g., stem cell transplantation, gene therapy) are likely to become available in the future. The future of fetal surgery depends on advances in the ability to control preterm labor and prevent preterm delivery. Technical advances will likely permit use of less invasive techniques. We must carefully distinguish fetuses that may benefit from invasive therapy from those that will not, and we should intervene only when there is a reasonable probability of benefit. Despite two decades of experience, we have much to study, a great deal to learn, and hopefully a lot to achieve.

KEY POINTS

- **Advances in antenatal diagnostic technology have resulted in the recognition and delineation of fetal disorders amenable to treatment in utero.**
- **Most malformations diagnosed in utero are not suitable for antenatal intervention. Fetal surgery is a reasonable option for anomalies that cause harm to the fetus before adequate development of fetal lung maturity necessary for extrauterine survival.**

- Currently, the conditions amenable to potential fetal surgical correction include bilateral hydronephrosis, diaphragmatic hernia, cystic adenomatoid malformation, large sacrococcygeal teratoma, twin-twin transfusion abnormalities, and perhaps myelomeningocele.
- Anesthetic considerations for intrauterine fetal surgery are similar to those for nonobstetric surgery in pregnant patients, with the following exceptions: (1) fetal surgery entails greater requirements for intraoperative fetal monitoring; (2) the fetus should be anesthetized and immobile; (3) intraoperative uterine relaxation is essential; and (4) the patient is at high risk for preterm labor during or after surgery.
- Many minimally invasive intrauterine procedures can be performed with use of local or regional anesthesia, but open surgery requires general anesthesia.
- There are many medical, social, ethical, and legal questions regarding the efficacy and safety of intrauterine fetal surgery. It is crucial that we continue to evaluate the risks and benefits of fetal surgical and anesthetic techniques.

REFERENCES

1. Harrison MR, Golbus MS, Filly RA, et al. Fetal surgery for congenital hydronephrosis. N Engl J Med 1982; 306:591-3.
2. Liley AW. Intrauterine transfusion of foetus in haemolytic disease. Br Med J 1963; 2:1107-9.
3. Adamsons K. Fetal surgery. N Engl J Med 1966; 275:204-6.
4. Howell LJ, Adzick NS, Harrison MR. The fetal treatment center. Semin Pediatr Surg 1993; 2:143-6.
5. Albanese CT, Harrison MR. Surgical treatment for fetal disease. The state of the art. Ann NY Acad Sci 1998; 847:74-85.
6. Mychaliska GB, Bealer JF, Rosen MA, et al. Operating on placental support: The ex utero intrapartum treatment procedure. J Pediatr Surg 1997; 32:227-31.
7. Longaker MT, Golbus MS, Filly RA, et al. Maternal outcome after open fetal surgery: A review of the first 17 human cases. JAMA 1991; 265: 737-41.
8. Harrison MR, Filly RA, Parer JT, et al. Management of the fetus with a urinary tract malformation. JAMA 1981; 246:635-9.
9. Glick PL, Harrison MR, Adzick NS, et al. Congenital hydronephrosis in utero. IV: In utero decompression prevents renal dysplasia. J Pediatr Surg 1984; 19:649-57.
10. Golbus MS, Harrison MR, Filly RA, et al. In utero treatment of urinary tract obstruction. Am J Obstet Gynecol 1982; 142:383-8.
11. Manning F, Harrison MR, Rodeck C, and the members of the International Fetal Medicine and Surgery Society. Report of the International Fetal Surgery Registry: Catheter shunts for fetal hydronephrosis and hydrocephalus. N Engl J Med 1986; 315:336-40.
12. Crombleholme TM, Harrison MR, Langer JC, et al. Early experience with open fetal surgery for congenital hydronephrosis. J Pediatr Surg 1988; 23:1114-21.
13. Johnson MD, Birnbach DJ, Burchman C, et al. Fetal surgery and general anesthesia: A case report and review. J Clin Anesth 1989; 1:363-7.
14. Quintero RA, Hume R, Smith C, et al. Percutaneous fetal cystoscopy and endoscopic fulguration of posterior urethral valves. Am J Obstet Gynecol 1995; 173:206-9.
15. Agarwal SK, Fisk NM. In utero therapy for lower urinary tract obstruction. Prenat Diagn 2001; 21:970-6
16. Harrison MR, Adzick NS, Estes JM, et al. A prospective study of the outcome for fetuses with diaphragmatic hernia. JAMA 1994; 271:382-4.
17. Harrison MR. The fetus with a diaphragmatic hernia[?]. In Harrison MR, Evans MI, Adzick NS, Holzgreve W, editors. The Unborn Patient: The Art and Science of Fetal Therapy, 3rd ed. Philadelphia, WB Saunders, 2001:297-314.
18. Harrison MR, Adzick NS, Longaker MT, et al. Successful repair in utero of a fetal diaphragmatic hernia after removal of herniated viscera from the left thorax. N Engl J Med 1990; 22:1582-4.
19. Harrison MR, Adzick NS, Flake AW, et al. Correction of congenital diaphragmatic hernia in utero. VI: Hard-earned lessons. J Pediatr Surg 1993; 28:1411-8.
20. DiFederico EM, Harrison MR, Matthay MA. Pulmonary edema in a woman following fetal surgery. Chest 1996; 109:1114-7.
21. Harrison MR, Adzick NS, Flake AW, et al. The CDH two-step: A dance of necessity. J Pediatr Surg 1993; 28:813-6.
22. Harrison MR, Adzick NS, Rosen MA, et al. Correction of congenital diaphragmatic hernia in utero. VII: A prospective trial. J Pediatr Surg 1997; 32:1637-42.
23. Wilson JM, Difore JW, Peters CA. Experimental fetal tracheal ligation prevents the pulmonary hypoplasia associated with fetal nephrectomy: Possible application for congenital diaphragmatic hernia. J Pediatr Surg 1993; 28:1433-40.
24. Difore JW, Fauza DO, Slavin R, et al. Experimental fetal tracheal ligation reverses the structural and physiological effects of pulmonary hypoplasia in congenital diaphragmatic hernia. J Pediatr Surg 1994; 29:248-57.
25. Bealer JF, Skarsgard ED, Hedrick MH, et al. The "PLUG" odyssey: Adventures in experimental fetal tracheal occlusion. J Pediatr Surg 1995; 30:361-4.
26. Harrison MR, Adzick NS, Rosen MA, et al. Correction of congenital diaphragmatic hernia in utero. VIII: Response of the hypoplastic lung to tracheal occlusion. J Pediatr Surg 1996; 31:1339-48.
27. Harrison MR, Keller RL, Hawgood SB, et al. A randomized trial of fetal endoscopic tracheal occlusion for severe fetal congenital diaphragmatic hernia. N Engl J Med 2003; 349:1916-24.
28. Schulman SR, Jones BR, Slotnick N, et al. Fetal tracheal intubation with intact uteroplacental circulation. Anesth Analg 1993; 76:197-9.
29. Gaiser RR, Cheek TG, Kurth CD. Anesthetic management of cesarean delivery complicated by ex utero intrapartum treatment of the fetus. Anesth Analg 1997; 84:1150-3.
30. Midrio P, Zadra N, Grismondi G et al. EXIT procedure in a twin gestation and review of the literature. Am J Perinat 2001; 18:357-62
31. Bouchard S, Johnson MP, Flake AW, et al. The EXIT procedure: Experience and outcome in 31 cases. J Pediatr Surg 2002; 37:418-26.
32. MacKenzie TC, Crombleholme TM, Flake AW. The ex-utero intrapartum treatment. Curr Opin Pediatr 2002; 14:453-8
33. Harrison MR, Adzick NS, Jennings RW, et al. Antenatal intervention for congenital cystic adenomatoid malformation. Lancet 1990; 336:965-7.
34. Clark SL, Vitale DJ, Minton SD, et al. Successful fetal therapy for cystic adenomatoid malformation associated with second trimester hydrops. Am J Obstet Gynecol 1987; 157:294-5.
35. Crombleholme TM, Coleman B, Hedrick H, et al. Cystic adenomatoid malformation volume ratio predicts outcome in prenatally diagnoses cystic adenomatoid malformation of the lung. J Pediatr Surg 2002; 37:331-8.
36. Langer JC, Harrison MR, Schmidt KG, et al. Fetal hydrops and death from sacrococcygeal teratoma: Rationale for fetal surgery. Am J Obstet Gynecol 1989; 160:1145-50.
37. Bruner JP, Tulipan N, Paschall RL, et al. Fetal surgery for myelomeningocele and the incidence of shunt-dependent hydrocephalus. JAMA 1999; 282:1819-25.
38. Sutton LN, Adzick NS, Bilaniuk LT et al. Improvement in hindbrain herniation demonstrated by serial fetal magnetic resonance imaging following fetal surgery for myelomeningocele. JAMA 1999; 282:1826-31.
39. Mazzola CA, Albright AL, Sutton LN, et al. Dermoid inclusion cysts and early spinal cord tethering after fetal surgery for myelomeningocele. N Engl J Med 2002; 347:256-9.
40. Jobe AH. Perspective: Fetal surgery for myelomeningocele. N Engl J Med 2002; 347:230-1.
41. Yves V, Hyett J, Hecher K, et al. Preliminary experience with endoscopic laser surgery for severe twin-twin transfusion syndrome. N Engl J Med 1995; 332:224-7.
42. Galinkin JL, Gaiser RR, Cohen DE, et al. Anesthesia for fetoscopic fetal surgery: Twin reverse arterial perfusion sequence and twin-twin transfusions syndrome. Anesth Analg 2000; 91:1394-7.
43. Rodeck CH, Fisk NM, Fraser DI, et al. Long-term in utero drainage of fetal hydrothorax. N Engl J Med 1988; 319:1135-8.
44. Fenton KN, Heinemann MK, Hickey PR, et al. Inhibition of the fetal stress response improves cardiac output and gas exchange after fetal cardiac bypass. J Thorac Cardiovasc Surg 1994; 107:1416-22.
45. Spielman FJ, Seeds JW, Corke BC. Anaesthesia for fetal surgery. Anaesthesia 1984; 39:756-9.
46. Leveque C, Murat I, Toubas F, et al. Fetal neuromuscular blockade with vecuronium bromide: Studies during intravascular intrauterine transfusion in isoimmunized pregnancies. Anesthesiology 1992; 76:642-4.

47. Harrison MR, Anderson J, Rosen MA, et al. Fetal surgery in the primate. I. Anesthetic, surgical, and tocolytic management to maximize fetal-neonatal survival. Pediatr Surg 1982; 17:115-22.

48. Sakawi Y, Boyd G, Shaw B, et al. Use of sevoflurane to provide uterine relaxation for the ex-utero intrapartum procedure. Am J Anesthesiol 2001; 28:195-8.

49. Tame JD, Abrams LM, Ding XY, et al. Level of postoperative analgesia is a critical factor in regulation of myometrial contractility after laparotomy in the pregnant baboon: Implications for human fetal surgery. Am J Obstet Gynecol 1999; 180:1196-1201.

50. Rosen MA, Andreae M, Cameron A. Nitroglycerin for fetal surgery: Fetoscopy and ex utero intrapartum treatment procedure with malignant hyperthermia precautions. Anesth Analg 2003; 96:698-700.

51. Bradley SM, Hanley FL, Duncan BW, et al. Fetal cardiac bypass alters regional blood flows, arterial blood gases, and hemodynamics in sheep. Am J Physiol 1992; 263:H919-28.

52. Noah MMS, Norton ME, Sandberg P, et al. Short-term maternal outcomes that are associated with the EXIT procedure, as compared to cesarean section. Am J Obstet Gynecol 2002; 186:773-7

53. Anand KJS. Hormonal and metabolic function of neonates and infants undergoing surgery. Curr Opin Cardiol 1986; 1:681-9.

54. Anand KJS, Brown MJ, Bloom SR, et al. Studies on the hormonal regulation of fuel metabolism in the human newborn infant undergoing anaesthesia and surgery. Horm Res 1985; 22:115-28.

55. Milne EMG, Elliott MJ, Pearson DT, et al. The effect on intermediary metabolism of open-heart surgery with deep hypothermia and circulatory arrest in infants of less than 10 kilograms body weight. Perfusion 1986; 1:29-40.

56. Anand KJS, Brownk MJ, Causon RC, et al. Can the human neonate mount an endocrine and metabolic response to surgery? J Pediatr Surg 1985; 20:41-8.

57. Anand KJS, Sippell WG, Aynsley-Green A. Randomized trial of fentanyl anaesthesia in preterm neonates undergoing surgery: Effects on the stress response. Lancet 1987; 1:243-8.

58. Anand KJS, Hickey PR. Pain and its effects in the human neonate and fetus. N Engl J Med 1987; 317:1321-9.

59. Giannakoulopoulos X, Sepulveda W, Kourtis P et al. Fetal plasma cortisol and beta-endorphin response to intrauterine needling. Lancet 1994; 344:77-81.

60. Teixeria J, Fogliani R, Giannakoulopoulos X, et al. Fetal haemodynamic stress response to invasive procedures. Lancet 1996; 347:624.

61. Giannakoulopoulos X, Teixeira J, Fisk N, Glover V. Human fetal and maternal noradrenaline responses to invasive procedures. Pediatr Res 1999; 45:494-9.

62. Teixeria JM, Glover V, Fisk NM. Acute cerebral redistribution in response to invasive procedures in the human fetus. Am J Obstet Gynecol 1999; 181:1018-25.

63. Gitau R, Fisk NM, Teixeira JM et al. Fetal hypothalamic-pituitary-adrenal stress responses to invasive procedures are independent of maternal responses. J Clin Endocrinol Metab 2001; 86:104-9.

64. Fisk NM, Gitau R, Teixeira JM, et al. Effect of direct fetal opioid analgesia on fetal hormonal and hemodynamic stress response to intrauterine needling. Anesthesiology 2001; 95:828-35.

65. Liley AW. The foetus as a personality. Aust N Z J Psych 1972; 6:99-105.

66. Derbyshire SWG. Locating the beginnings of pain. Bioethics 1999; 13:1-31.

67. Kostovic I, Rakic P. Developmental history of the transient subplate zone in the visual and somatosensory cortex of the macaque money and human brain. J Comp Neurol 1990; 297:441-470.

68. Taddio A, Katz J, Ilersich Al, et al. Effect of neonatal circumcision on pain response during subsequent routine vaccination. Lancet 1997; 349:599-603.

69. Carke AS, Wittwer DJ, Abbott DH, et al. Long-term effects of prenatal stress in HPA axis activity in juvenile rhesus monkeys. Dev Psychobiol 1994; 27:257-69.

70. Bhutta AT, Anand KJ. Vulnerability of the developing brain. Neuronal mechanisms. Clin Perinatol 2002; 29:357-72.

71. Lidow MS. Long-term effects of neonatal pain on nociceptive systems. Pain 2002; 99:377-83.

72. Glover V, Fisk NM. Do fetuses feel pain? We don't know: Better to err on the safe side from mid-gestation. Br Med J 1996: 313:796.

73. Gregory GA, Wade JG, Biehl DR, et al. Fetal anesthetic requirement (MAC) for halothane. Anesth Analg 1983; 62:9-14.

74. Biehl DR, Cote J, Wade JG, et al. Uptake of halothane by the foetal lamb in utero. Can Anaesth Soc J 1983; 30:24-7.

75. Biehl DR, Yarnell R, Wade JG, et al. The uptake of isoflurane by the foetal lamb in utero: Effect on regional blood flow. Can Anaesth Soc J 1983; 30:581-6.

76. Palahniuk RJ, Shnider SM. Maternal and fetal cardiovascular and acid-base changes during halothane and isoflurane anesthesia in the pregnant ewe. Anesthesiology 1974; 41:462-72.

77. Biehl DR, Tweed WA, Cote J, et al. Effect of halothane on cardiac output and regional flow in the fetal lamb in utero. Anesth Analg 1983; 62:489-92.

78. Sabik J, Assad RS, Hanley FL. Halothane as an anesthetic for fetal surgery. J Pediatr Surg 1993; 28:542-7.

79. Fenton KN, Zinn HE, Heinemann MK, et al. Long-term survivors of fetal cardiac bypass in lambs. J Thorac Cardiovasc Surg 1994; 107:1423-7.

80. Gaiser TT, Kurth CD, Cohen D, et al. The cesarean delivery of a twin gestation under 2 minimum alveolar anesthetic concentration of isoflurane: one normal and one with a large anesthetic neck mass. Anesth Analg 1999; 88:584-6.

81. Gin T, Chan MTV. Decreased minimum alveolar concentration of isoflurane in pregnant humans. Anesthesiology 1994; 81:829-32.

82. Luks FI, Johnson BD, Papadakis K, et al. Predictive value of monitoring parameters in fetal surgery. J Pediatr Surg 1998; 33:1297-301.

83. Izumi A, Minakami H, Sato I. Fetal heart rate decelerations precede a decrease in fetal oxygen content. Gynecol Obstet Invest 1997; 44: 26-31.

84. Jennings RW, Adzick NS, Longaker MT, et al. New techniques in fetal therapy. J Pediatr Surg 1992; 27:1329-33.

85. Hedrick MH, Jennings RW, MacGillivray TE, et al. Chronic fetal vascular access. Lancet 1993; 342:1086-7.

86. Harrison MR. Fetal surgery. Am J Obstet Gynecol 1996; 174:1255-64.

87. Kafali H, Kaya T, Gursoy S, et al. The role of K+ channels on the inhibitor effect of sevoflurane in pregnant rat myometrium. Anesth Analg 2002; 94:174-8.

88. Lyerly AD, Cefalo RC, Socol M, et al. Attitudes of maternal-fetal specialists concerning maternal-fetal surgery. Am J Obstet Gynecol 2001; 185:1052-8.

89. Lyerly D, Gates EA, Cefalo RC, et al. Toward the ethical evaluation and use of maternal-fetal surgery. Obstet Gynecol 2001; 98:689-97.

90. Chervenak FA, McCullough LB. A comprehensive ethical framework for fetal research and its application to fetal surgery for spina bifida. Am J Obstet Gynecol 2002; 187:10-14.

Chapter 8

Intrapartum Fetal Assessment and Therapy

Elizabeth G. Livingston, M.D.

Both professional journals and the lay press have scrutinized the value of obstetric interventions during labor and delivery. Obstetricians have reassessed old technologies and introduced new ones. An increased cesarean section rate, persistent cases of fetal/neonatal neurologic injury, and excessive malpractice litigation have prompted an ongoing search for optimal intrapartum fetal assessment and therapy.

FETAL RISK DURING LABOR

Epidemiologic data suggest that the fetus is at increased risk for morbidity and mortality during labor and delivery. In 1970, one report suggested that one third of intrauterine fetal deaths occur intrapartum.[1] In 1963, the British Perinatal Mortality Survey reviewed autopsy data for 1400 stillborn infants and concluded that slightly more than 30% of these losses resulted from intrapartum asphyxia.[2] At the same time, the United States Perinatal Collaborative Project (conducted between 1959 and 1966) revealed that the risk of neonatal death or neurologic impairment (as a result of late pregnancy events) was approximately 2% for infants with a birth weight greater than 2500 g.[3] A recent report from Latvia revealed that intrapartum asphyxia accounts for 12% of perinatal deaths.[4] Further, in 1989, birth certificates in the United States attributed 720 infant deaths (17.6/100,000 live births) to intrauterine hypoxia and birth asphyxia.[5]

Experimental models lend support to the hypothesis that intrapartum events can lead to long-term neurologic sequelae. Fetal monkeys subjected to hypoxia in utero have suffered neurologic injury similar to that seen in children who presumably suffered asphyxia in utero.[6] Epidemiologic and experimental data suggest that the fetus is at significant jeopardy during labor and delivery.

Studies suggest that some fetuses are at greater risk for adverse intrapartum events than others. Older studies suggest that high-risk mothers constitute 20% of the pregnant population, but their offspring represent 50% of the cases of perinatal morbidity and mortality.[7] Various schemes for identification of high-risk pregnancies have been published (Box 8-1).[8] High-risk pregnancies include but are not limited to women with (1) **medical complications** (e.g., hypertension, preeclampsia, diabetes, autoimmune disease, hemoglobinopathy), (2) **fetal complications** (e.g., intrauterine growth restriction, nonlethal anomalies, prematurity, multiple gestation, postdatism, hydrops), and (3) **intrapartum complications** (e.g., abnormal vaginal bleeding, maternal fever, meconium-stained amniotic fluid, oxytocin augmentation of labor). The identification of high-risk pregnancies predicts perinatal morbidity and mortality with a high incidence of false-positive and false-negative results.[9] A study of intrapartum stillbirths in Australia was unable to identify antenatal risk factors among the mothers of stillborn infants when compared with a group of matched controls.[10]

The magnitude of risk for intrapartum fetal neurologic injury has been a matter of some dispute. In 2003 the American College of Obstetricians and Gynecologists (ACOG) Task Force on Neonatal Encephalopathy and Cerebral Palsy concluded that 70% of these types of fetal neurologic injuries result from events that occur *before* the onset of labor.[11] Examples of antepartum events that may cause fetal neurologic injury include congenital anomalies, chemical exposure, infection, and fetal thrombosis/coagulopathy. Only 4% of cases of neonatal encephalopathy result solely from intrapartum hypoxia—an incidence of approximately 1.6/1000.[11] Approximately 25% of fetuses may have antepartum and intrapartum risk factors for neurologic injury. Box 8-2 lists the criteria required to define an acute intrapartum hypoxic event as sufficient to cause cerebral palsy.[11,12]

The ability of contemporary obstetricians to recognize and treat pregnancies at risk during labor is an evolving science. With our current understanding of pathophysiology and the contemporary technology used clinically, the extent to which obstetricians can prevent intrapartum injury is unclear. It is hoped that a clearer definition of intrapartum injury will lead to more precise identification of fetuses that are at risk and help us develop strategies and interventions that may correct reversible pathophysiology.

Efforts to understand placental physiology and pathophysiology are central to our efforts to support the health of the pregnant woman and her fetus, both antepartum and intrapartum. The fetus depends on the placenta for the diffusion of nutrients and for respiratory gas exchange. Many factors affect placental transfer, including concentration gradients, villus surface area, placental permeability, and placental metabolism. Maternal hypertensive disease, congenital anomalies, and intrauterine infection are examples of conditions that may impair placental transfer. One of the most important determinants of placental function is uterine blood flow.[13] A uterine contraction results in a transient decrease in uteroplacental blood flow. Thus a placenta with borderline function before labor may be unable to maintain adequate gas exchange to prevent fetal asphyxia during labor. The healthy fetus may compensate for the effects of hypoxia during labor.[14,15] The compensatory response includes (1) decreased oxygen consumption, (2) vasoconstriction of nonessential vascular beds, and (3) redistribution of blood flow to the vital organs (e.g., brain, heart, adrenal glands, placenta).[16,17] Humoral responses (e.g., release of epinephrine from the adrenal medulla, release of vasopressin and endogenous opioids) may enhance fetal cardiac function during hypoxia.[13] Prolonged or severe hypoxia overwhelms these compensatory mechanisms and results in fetal injury or death.

INTRAPARTUM FETAL ASSESSMENT

Electronic Fetal Heart Rate Monitoring

The optimal practical method for assessing fetal health during labor and delivery has not been determined.[18] Most contemporary methods include assessment of the fetal heart rate (FHR). The FHR can be monitored intermittently using a simple DeLee stethoscope. Alternatively, either Doppler ultrasound or a fetal electrocardiographic (ECG) electrode can be used to monitor the FHR intermittently or continuously.

Experimental models have provided insight into the regulation of the FHR. Both neuronal and humoral factors affect the intrinsic FHR. Parasympathetic outflow by means of the vagus nerve decreases the FHR, whereas sympathetic activity increases FHR and cardiac output.[13] Baroreceptors respond to increased blood pressure and chemoreceptors respond to decreased PaO_2 and increased $PaCO_2$ to modulate the FHR through the autonomic nervous system. Cerebral cortical activity and hypothalamic activity affect the FHR through their effects on integrative centers in the medulla oblongata (Figure 8-1).[13] Both animal studies and clinical observations have helped establish a correlation between FHR and perinatal outcomes.

An electronic fetal monitor simultaneously records the FHR and uterine contractions. Use of an electronic monitor allows determination of the **baseline rate** and **patterns** of the FHR and their relationship to uterine contractions. External or internal techniques can assess the FHR and uterine contractions (Figure 8-2). Doppler ultrasonography detects the changes in ventricular wall motion and blood flow in major vessels during each cardiac cycle. The monitor calculates the FHR by measuring the interval between each fetal myocardial contraction. Alternatively, an ECG lead attached to the fetal scalp allows the cardiotachometer to calculate the FHR by measuring each successive R-R interval. Both external and internal methods allow continuous assessment of the FHR.

The FHR is superimposed over the uterine contraction pattern. Uterine contractions can be monitored externally with a tocodynamometer or internally with an intrauterine pressure catheter. The tocodynamometer allows determination of the approximate onset, duration, and offset of each uterine contraction. An intrauterine pressure catheter must be used to determine the strength of uterine contractions. In some cases, an intrauterine pressure catheter is needed to determine the precise onset and offset of uterine contractions. Such information may be needed to distinguish among early, variable, and late FHR decelerations.

Several features of the FHR pattern can be assessed: (1) **baseline** FHR, (2) FHR **variability** (the degree to which

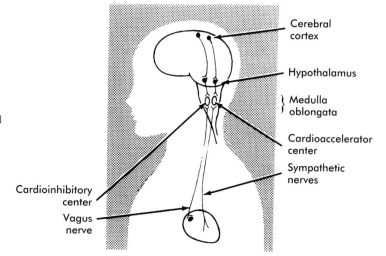

FIGURE 8-1. Regulation of FHR. (From Parer JT. Physiological regulation of fetal heart rate. JOGN 1976; 5:26S-9S.)

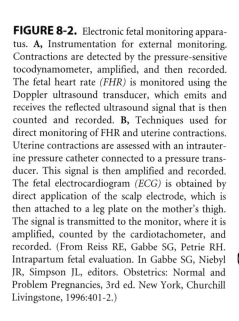

FIGURE 8-2. Electronic fetal monitoring apparatus. A, Instrumentation for external monitoring. Contractions are detected by the pressure-sensitive tocodynamometer, amplified, and then recorded. The fetal heart rate *(FHR)* is monitored using the Doppler ultrasound transducer, which emits and receives the reflected ultrasound signal that is then counted and recorded. B, Techniques used for direct monitoring of FHR and uterine contractions. Uterine contractions are assessed with an intrauterine pressure catheter connected to a pressure transducer. This signal is then amplified and recorded. The fetal electrocardiogram *(ECG)* is obtained by direct application of the scalp electrode, which is then attached to a leg plate on the mother's thigh. The signal is transmitted to the monitor, where it is amplified, counted by the cardiotachometer, and recorded. (From Reiss RE, Gabbe SG, Petrie RH. Intrapartum fetal evaluation. In Gabbe SG, Niebyl JR, Simpson JL, editors. Obstetrics: Normal and Problem Pregnancies, 3rd ed. New York, Churchill Livingstone, 1996:401-2.)

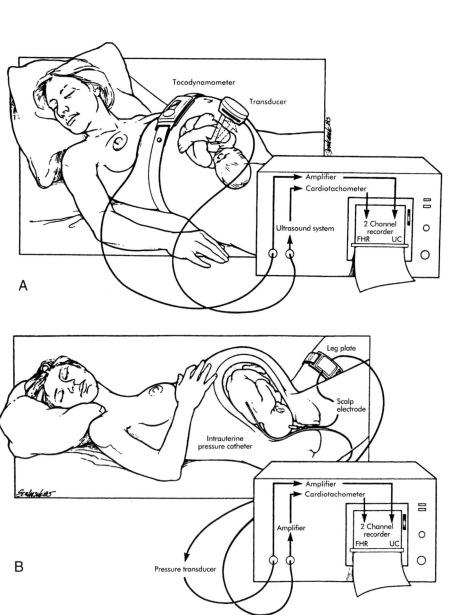

the rate varies both instantaneously and over longer periods), and (3) **periodic changes** (i.e., patterns of acceleration or deceleration) and their association with uterine contractions.

BASELINE FHR

A normal baseline FHR often is defined as 120 to 160 beats per minute (bpm). However, many obstetricians currently extend the lower limit of normal to 110 bpm. In general, term fetuses have a lower baseline FHR than preterm fetuses because of increased parasympathetic nervous system activity near term. Laboratory studies suggest that bradycardia (caused by increased vagal activity) is the initial fetal response to acute hypoxemia. After prolonged hypoxemia, the fetus may develop tachycardia as a result of catecholamine secretion and sympathetic nervous system activity.[14] Other causes of a change in baseline FHR include maternal fever and/or intrauterine infection. Medications, such as the beta-adrener-

gic receptor agonist terbutaline (given to treat preterm labor) or the anticholinergic agent atropine, may increase both maternal heart rate and FHR. A fetal tachyrhythmia or bradyrhythmia (caused by an anatomic or functional etiology) also may cause abnormalities in the baseline FHR.

FHR VARIABILITY

FHR variability includes short- (beat-to-beat) and long-term variability (Figure 8-3). **Short-term variability** is the difference between two or three adjacent beats. Doppler ultrasonography may not always detect short-term variability accurately. In some cases, it may overestimate FHR variability because the signal (i.e., cardiac movement) is not as discrete as the R wave of the electrocardiogram. A fetal ECG electrode should be used to obtain the most reliable estimate of short-term variability. However, the newer Doppler monitors that use auto-correlation techniques seem to provide a close

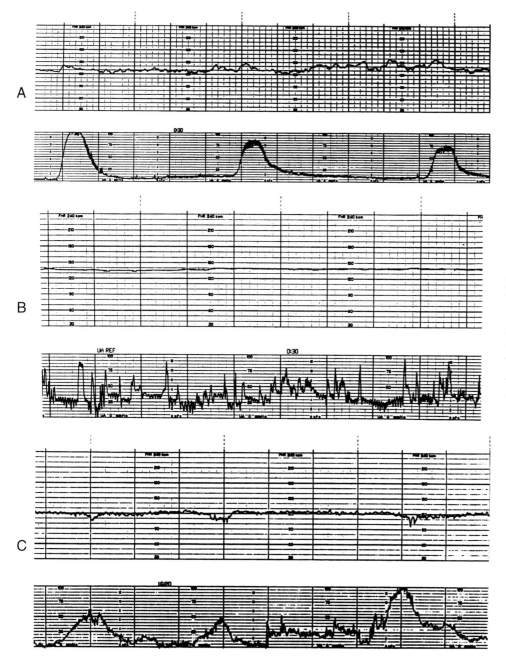

FIGURE 8-3. **A,** Normal intrapartum fetal heart rate (FHR) tracing. The infant had Apgar scores of 8 and 8 at 1 and 5 minutes, respectively. **B,** Absent variability in a FHR tracing. Placental abruption was noted at cesarean section. The infant had an umbilical arterial blood pH of 6.75 and Apgar scores of 1 and 4. **C,** Early FHR decelerations. After a normal spontaneous vaginal delivery, the infant had Apgar scores of 8 and 8.

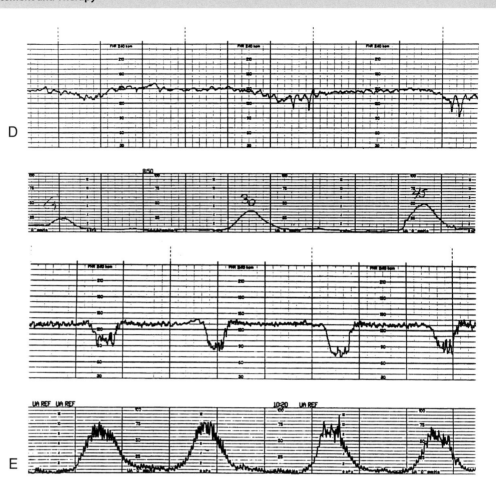

FIGURE 8-3, cont'd. **D,** Late FHR decelerations. This fetus had meconium-stained amniotic fluid. Despite the late FHR decelerations, the variability remained acceptable. The infant was delivered by cesarean section and had an umbilical venous blood pH of 7.30. Apgar scores were 9 and 9. **E,** Variable FHR decelerations. A tight nuchal cord was noted at low forceps vaginal delivery. The infant had Apgar scores of 6 and 9.

approximation of short-term variability. **Long-term variability** denotes the rough sine waves that occur three to six times per minute, with variation of at least 6 bpm.

The presence of normal FHR variability reflects the presence of normal, intact pathways from (and within) the fetal cerebral cortex, midbrain, vagus nerve, and cardiac conduction system (see Figure 8-1).[13] Short-term variability most likely results from the influence of parasympathetic tone (by means of the vagus nerve) on the intrinsic FHR. Maternal administration of atropine (which readily crosses the placenta) eliminates short-term FHR variability. In humans, the sympathetic nervous system appears to have a lesser role in the origin of short-term variability.[13] Maternal administration of the beta-adrenergic receptor antagonist propranolol has little effect on FHR variability.[13]

During hypoxemia, myocardial and cerebral blood flow increase to maintain oxygen delivery.[19,20] With severe hypoxemia, blood flow cannot increase sufficiently to maintain oxygen delivery. The decompensation of cerebral blood flow and oxygen delivery results in a loss of FHR variability.[13] The absence of variability in an anencephalic fetus also suggests that FHR variability reflects the integrity of the central nervous system (CNS). In animal models, perfusion of the CNS with calcium results in depolarization of EEG activity, which abolishes FHR variability.

Clinically, the presence of normal FHR variability predicts early neonatal health, as defined by an Apgar score of greater than 7 at 5 minutes.[21,22] In a case series of monitored fetal deaths, no fetus had normal short-term or long-term variability immediately before demise.[13] The differential diagnosis of decreased variability includes fetal hypoxia, fetal sleep state,

fetal neurologic abnormality, and decreased CNS activity that results from exposure to drugs such as opioids.

PERIODIC CHANGES

Periodic changes include accelerations and early, late, or variable FHR decelerations. **Early decelerations** occur simultaneously with uterine contractions and usually are less than 20 bpm below baseline. The onset and offset of each deceleration coincides with the onset and offset of the uterine contraction (see Figure 8-3). In animal models, head compression can precipitate early decelerations.[14] In humans, early decelerations are believed to result from reflex vagal activity secondary to mild hypoxia. Early decelerations are not ominous.

Late decelerations begin 10 to 30 seconds after the beginning of a uterine contraction, and likewise, they end 10 to 30 seconds after the end of the uterine contraction. Late decelerations are smooth and repetitive (i.e., they occur with each uterine contraction). Animal studies suggest that late decelerations represent a response to hypoxemia. The delayed onset of the deceleration reflects the time needed for the chemoreceptors to detect decreased oxygen tension and mediate the change in FHR by means of the vagus nerve.[14] Late decelerations also may result from decompensation of the myocardial circulation and myocardial failure. Unfortunately, clinical and animal studies suggest that late decelerations may be an oversensitive test of fetal asphyxia.[14] However, the combination of late decelerations and decreased/absent FHR variability is an accurate, ominous signal of fetal distress.[15]

Variable decelerations vary in depth, shape, and/or duration. They often are abrupt in onset and offset. Variable decelerations result from baroreceptor- or chemoreceptor-mediated vagal activity. Experimental models and clinical studies suggest that **umbilical cord occlusion,** either partial or complete, results in variable decelerations. During the second stage of labor, variable decelerations may result from compression of the fetal head. In this situation, dural stimulation leads to increased vagal discharge.[23] The healthy fetus typically can tolerate mild-to-moderate variable decelerations (not below 80 bpm) without decompensation. With prolonged, severe variable decelerations (less than 60 bpm) or persistent fetal bradycardia, it is difficult for the fetus to maintain cardiac output and umbilical blood flow.[23]

During the antepartum period, the heart rate of the healthy fetus accelerates in response to fetal movement. Antepartum FHR **accelerations** signal fetal health, and the presence of FHR accelerations represent a reactive nonstress test. During the intrapartum period, the significance of FHR accelerations is less clear.[14,21] In some cases, accelerations may signal the presence of a vulnerable umbilical cord. However, the presence of intrapartum FHR accelerations most likely precludes the presence of significant fetal metabolic acidosis.

The sinusoidal pattern and the saltatory pattern are two unusual FHR patterns that may indicate fetal compromise. The **sinusoidal** FHR pattern is a regular, smooth, wavelike pattern with absent short-term variability; this pattern may signal fetal anemia.[13] Occasionally, maternal administration of an opioid may result in a sinusoidal FHR pattern. The **saltatory** pattern includes excessive swings in variability (more than 25 bpm). Some obstetricians contend that a saltatory pattern signals the occurrence of acute fetal hypoxia. There is a weak association between this pattern and low Apgar scores.[13]

Limitations of Electronic Fetal Heart Rate Monitoring

Despite laboratory and clinical data suggesting that FHR monitoring accurately reflects fetal health, controversy exists over the ability of this measure to improve fetal/neonatal outcome when it is applied to large obstetric populations. Continuous electronic FHR monitoring was first described 35 years ago, and it became more widespread during the decades that followed. Retrospective reports suggested that continuous FHR monitoring was associated with a decrease in the incidence of intrauterine fetal demise, neonatal seizures, and neonatal death.[24-27]

At least 12 prospective, randomized trials of electronic FHR monitoring have been performed, with the control arms including some type of intermittent FHR auscultation.[28,29] Electronic FHR monitoring is consistently associated with an increased rate of operative delivery.[28,29] Other findings have been mixed, although the majority of studies have demonstrated no clear benefit associated with electronic FHR monitoring. A meta-analysis of these trials, which included over 50,000 women from several continents, suggested that electronic FHR monitoring results in a decreased incidence of 1-minute Apgar scores less than 4 and a decreased incidence of neonatal seizures.[28] The long-term clinical significance of these findings is unclear. This meta-analysis[28] did not confirm the conclusion of an earlier meta-analysis, namely that electronic FHR monitoring is associated with decreased perinatal mortality from fetal hypoxia.[29]

It is unclear why prospective studies have not confirmed greater benefit to the use of continuous electronic FHR monitoring during labor. In these prospective randomized trials, women who were randomized to receive intermittent FHR auscultation were monitored by dedicated nursing staff that provided intensive intrapartum care. In contrast, the historical cohorts (whose outcome was compared to patients who received continuous electronic FHR monitoring) had intermittent FHR auscultation with *non*intensive nursing care. There are no published studies in which patients were randomized to receive no FHR monitoring. Consistent with the results of the prospective trials, the ACOG endorses the use of either intermittent auscultation or continuous electronic FHR monitoring during labor. In high-risk patients, ACOG guidelines recommend that the obstetrician or nurse monitor the FHR every 15 minutes during the first stage of labor and every 5 minutes during the second stage. For low-risk patients, the time intervals may be lengthened to 30 minutes for the first stage and 15 minutes for the second stage.[18]

Freeman[30] recently proposed several hypotheses for the apparent failure of intrapartum FHR monitoring to reduce the incidence of cerebral palsy: (1) a large proportion of the asphyxial damage begins before the onset of labor; (2) catastrophic events (e.g., cord prolapse, placental abruption, uterine rupture) may not allow sufficient time for intervention before neurologic damage occurs; (3) "a larger proportion of surviving very low birth weight [VLBW] infants undoubtedly contributes to the current pool of children with cerebral palsy"; (4) infection is associated with abnormal FHR patterns and subsequent development of cerebral palsy, and it is unclear that early intervention offers any benefit in such cases; and (5) "the amount of asphyxia required to cause permanent neurologic damage is very near the amount that causes fetal death," leaving a narrow window for intervention. Freeman[30] concluded that "the number of patients who develop cerebral palsy caused by intrapartum asphyxia is probably quite small."

Another limitation is that an abnormal FHR tracing has a poor positive predictive value for abnormal outcome. Because of this imprecision, ACOG has recommended that the term *nonreassuring fetal status* be used to describe an abnormal FHR tracing, rather than the terms *fetal distress* or *birth asphyxia*.[31] In one population-based study of California children with cerebral palsy, the authors retrospectively reviewed their FHR tracings and compared them with those of neurologically normal children. A markedly higher incidence of tracings with late decelerations and decreased short-term variability occurred in children with cerebral palsy than in controls. However, of the estimated 10,791 monitored infants weighing 2500 g or more who had these FHR abnormalities, only 21 (0.19%) had cerebral palsy. Thus the authors calculated the false-positive rate to be 99.8%.[32]

In addition to a greater incidence of operative delivery, other possible limitations of continuous FHR monitoring include (1) poor intraobserver and interobserver agreement,[33,34] (2) the need for a nurse or physician to assess the FHR tracing continually, (3) inconvenience for the patient (e.g., confinement to bed and application of monitor belts or a scalp electrode), and (4) the need to maintain the FHR tracing as a legal document.

With its value so questionable, why does FHR monitoring remain in widespread use after 35 years? Parer and King[35] have noted that, despite little evidence for its efficacy, obstetricians continue to heavily rely on FHR monitoring for at least three reasons: (1) professional obstetric organizations (e.g., ACOG) advise some form of monitoring during labor, (2) electronic FHR monitoring is logistically easier and less expensive than one-on-one nursing care during labor, and (3) individual (often anecdotal) experience causes "many obstetricians [to] believe that in their own hands FHR monitoring is . . . efficacious." In an effort to improve the utility of FHR monitoring, a 1997 National Institutes of Health workshop recommended standardization of nomenclature regarding the FHR interpretation, followed by research into the validity of electronic FHR monitoring as a predictor of fetal health. Such research should include quantitation of abnormal patterns, correlation with short- and long-term outcomes, and evaluation of the role of ancillary techniques of fetal health evaluation.[36]

Methods for Improving the Efficacy of Electronic Fetal Heart Rate Monitoring

Several technologies have been suggested to overcome limitations in the use of electronic FHR monitoring. To facilitate continual assessment of FHR, many labor-and-delivery units transmit the FHR tracing from the bedside to the nurses' station. Presumably, this facilitates a rapid response to worrisome FHR tracings.

Several computer systems may assist with interpretation of the FHR. Computerized analysis may be more accurate than traditional methods of analysis in the identification of those pregnancies with a pathologic neonatal outcome.[37,38] However, none of these methods has achieved widespread use.

Another strategy involves transmitting the FHR tracing by telephone to a central station for expert consultation. A review of the University of Connecticut's experience with this system revealed that half of the strips considered worrisome by outside inquirers were compatible with fetal well-being, and that the consulting obstetricians were encouraged to manage the labors expectantly. Such a service may reduce unnecessary intervention.[39]

Continuous FHR monitoring requires the patient to wear FHR and uterine contraction monitoring devices. The patient also must remain within several feet of the monitor, which precludes ambulation. One alternative is the use of telemetry, which transmits the FHR from the ambulating patient to the monitor. Of course, the low-risk patient who wishes to ambulate probably does not require continuous electronic FHR monitoring.

Electronic archiving allows electronic storage of FHR tracings and eliminates the need for long-term storage of the paper record. The electronic record also may allow for more efficient retrieval of strips. The FHR tracing is a medicolegal document, and if it is lost, the plaintiff's lawyer may allege that the tracing was discarded intentionally because it was detrimental to the defendant.[40]

Supplemental Methods of Fetal Assessment

Electronic FHR monitoring is very accurate in the identification of a healthy fetus and in the prediction of the birth of a healthy infant. It is more than 99% accurate in predicting a 5-minute Apgar score greater than 7. Unfortunately, electronic FHR monitoring suffers from a lack of specificity. The prediction of fetal compromise has a 35% to 50% false-positive rate.[41,42] **Fetal scalp blood pH determination** is one method that is used to confirm or exclude the presence of fetal acidosis when FHR monitoring suggests the presence of fetal compromise. Suggested indications include decreased or absent FHR variability or persistent late or variable FHR

decelerations.[13] The obstetrician inserts an endoscope into the vagina, makes a small laceration in the fetal scalp (or buttock), and uses a capillary tube to collect a sample of fetal capillary blood (Figure 8-4). Obviously, the obstetrician cannot perform this procedure if there is minimal cervical dilation. Relative contraindications include (1) the presence of intact membranes and an unengaged vertex; (2) fetal coagulopathy (which entails the potential for fetal exsanguination); (3) infection, such as chorioamnionitis, human immunodeficiency virus (HIV), or herpes simplex virus (disruption of the fetal scalp allows a portal of entry for infection); and (4) an anticipated need for many samples, which might result in significant fetal trauma.[13] Further, some small hospitals do not have the laboratory facilities necessary to perform a blood gas analysis of a microsample of blood.

In general, a fetal scalp blood pH of more than 7.25 is acceptable and indicates that the patient may continue to labor. If the FHR tracing abnormalities continue, repeated sampling is recommended approximately every 30 minutes. A pH of less than 7.20 is considered abnormal, and delivery should be expedited if the value is confirmed by a second pH determination. A pH between 7.20 and 7.25 usually warrants a second scalp pH determination. Interpretation of the fetal scalp blood pH requires consideration of conditions that may give a false-positive result (e.g., abnormalities of the maternal pH, an inadequate sample, contamination with amniotic fluid, sampling from the caput succedaneum). Although early studies suggested that fetal scalp sampling may decrease the cesarean delivery rate,[43] a 1994 report showed no change in the rate of cesarean delivery or perinatal asphyxia when the technique was essentially abandoned at that institution.[44]

An alternative to fetal scalp blood sampling is **fetal scalp stimulation**. The fetal scalp can be digitally stimulated during vaginal examination or it can be squeezed with an Allis clamp. (Of course, fetal scalp blood sampling also results in fetal scalp stimulation.) The heart rate of a healthy, nonacidotic fetus accelerates in response to scalp stimulation. In these circumstances, FHR acceleration is associated with a fetal pH of at least 7.19.[45,46]

Vibroacoustic stimulation is another method for assessing a worrisome FHR tracing. Advocates of this technique contend that the application of an artificial larynx to the

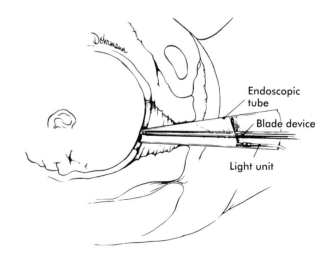

FIGURE 8-4. Technique of obtaining fetal scalp blood during labor. (From Creasy RK, Parer JT. Perinatal care and diagnosis. In Rudolph AM, editor. Pediatrics, 16th ed. New York, Appleton-Century-Crofts, 1977:121.)

maternal abdomen results in an FHR acceleration in a healthy fetus and improves the specificity of FHR monitoring.[47] The use of the scalp stimulation test and vibroacoustic stimulation has resulted in a marked decline in the use of fetal scalp blood pH determination in some centers. A meta-analysis of intrapartum stimulation tests (i.e., fetal scalp blood pH determination, Allis clamp scalp stimulation, vibroacoustic stimulation, and digital fetal scalp stimulation) found the tests to be equivalent at predicting fetal acidemia, with digital fetal scalp stimulation having the greatest ease of use.[48] The authors recommended fetal scalp pH assessment in the presence of a positive test (i.e., lack of FHR accelerations) to improve accuracy.

The intrapartum use of **umbilical artery velocimetry** and the **biophysical profile** have been used as adjuncts to FHR monitoring with mixed results[49,50] (see Chapter 6).

The presence of **meconium-stained amniotic fluid** has long been associated with an increased risk for depression at birth. Moderate-to-thick meconium is associated with lower Apgar scores, lower umbilical arterial blood pH, an increased incidence of neonatal seizures, and higher rates of cesarean section and admission to intensive care nurseries.[51,52] Although approximately 10% to 20% of all deliveries are complicated by meconium-stained amniotic fluid, not all of these infants experience neonatal depression. In one series, the false-positive rate for prediction of neonatal acidemia was 95%, and the sensitivity was only 32%.[53] Our understanding of the physiology of the passage of meconium is incomplete. Ultrasonographic imaging suggests that the fetus may regularly pass rectal contents into the amniotic fluid throughout gestation.[54] Meconium-stained amniotic fluid is more common in pregnancies complicated by postdatism or intrauterine growth restriction (IUGR). Potential triggers for the passage of meconium include umbilical cord compression and hypoxia. The combination of the presence of meconium and an abnormal FHR tracing or another risk factor (e.g., IUGR, postdatism) is associated with an increased likelihood of neonatal depression.[51,52]

Thick meconium probably reflects defecation into a reduced volume of amniotic fluid, whereas light meconium suggests a normal amniotic fluid volume. Meis et al.[55] observed that the presence of early, heavy meconium-stained amniotic fluid was associated with increased fetal and neonatal morbidity and mortality. The passage of meconium during late labor also was associated with an increased incidence of neonatal morbidity. In contrast, the presence of light meconium-stained amniotic fluid during early labor was not associated with an increased incidence of fetal or neonatal morbidity or death.[55]

Aside from its association with neonatal depression, the aspiration of meconium also may result in the **meconium aspiration syndrome,** which may cause neonatal morbidity or mortality. Thorough suction of the airway at the time of delivery may decrease the incidence of meconium aspiration syndrome, although this is controversial (see Chapter 9). The fact that suctioning of the infant's airway at the time of delivery does not prevent all cases of meconium aspiration syndrome suggests that some cases of meconium aspiration occur antepartum. Alternatively, the lung injury may result from intrapartum fetal hypoxia in some cases.[56]

New Technologies for Fetal Assessment

FHR monitoring is an indirect assessment of fetal oxygenation and acid-base status. Alternative technologies may provide a more direct assessment of fetal oxygenation. Transcutaneous PO_2, PCO_2, and pH monitors have been described.[57-59] These techniques are limited by technical difficulty in application of the probe(s), drift of the baseline, and a slow response time.

The technique of reflectance pulse oximetry has been adapted for assessment of fetal oxygenation. The U.S. Food and Drug Administration (FDA) has approved the Nellcor N-400 fetal pulse oximeter (Nellcor, Puritan Bennett, Pleasanton, CA) for use in the setting of a term, singleton fetus at *greater than* 36 weeks' gestation, with a vertex presentation and a nonreassuring heart rate pattern after rupture of membranes.[60] The most commonly used probes are held in place against the fetal head or cheek with pressure from the cervix. A reliable pulse oximetry signal can be obtained in 60% to 70% of cases; however, environmental factors and/or physiologic events (e.g., fetal scalp congestion, thick fetal hair, vernix caseosa, uterine activity, movement artifacts) may affect the accuracy of fetal pulse oximetry.[60] The saturation measurements are averaged every 45 seconds.[61] The human fetus typically has a oxygen saturation of 35% to 65%. Animal and human data suggest that metabolic acidosis does not occur until the oxygen saturation has fallen below 30% for at least 10 minutes, as measured with this device.[62,63] Two recent studies have challenged the accuracy of fetal pulse oximetry in human fetuses when the measurements are less than 30%.[61,64] A clinical trial of fetal pulse oximetry used in conjunction with FHR monitoring demonstrated a reduction in the rate of cesarean section for a nonreassuring FHR tracing. However, more cesarean sections were performed for dystocia, resulting in no overall reduction in the rate of cesarean delivery.[65] The lack of overall reduction in cesarean delivery prompted the ACOG to withhold endorsement of the clinical use of fetal pulse oximetry, pending further investigation of its utility.[60]

Fetal electrocardiography with **ST waveform analysis** is another proposed adjunctive technique of fetal assessment. Fetal hypoxia induces changes in the morphology of the ST segment and the T wave of the fetal ECG. A randomized controlled trial in Sweden of the STAN S21 system (Neoventa Medical, Goteborg, Sweden), which performs automatic ST waveform analysis, showed that a combination of FHR monitoring and analysis of the ST waveform of the fetal ECG reduced the risk of fetal exposure to significant hypoxia that leads to metabolic acidosis at birth, and reduced the incidence of newborn infants with marked neurologic symptoms.[66] The FDA is currently reviewing the potential use of this assessment tool in the United States.

Near-infrared spectroscopy offers promise as a tool to measure fetal cerebral oxygenation directly.[67] Near-infrared spectroscopy can detect changes in the ratio of reduced versus oxygenated cytochrome-c oxidase in the brain and in the ratio of oxygenated versus deoxygenated hemoglobin in the blood perfusing the brain. It also measures the total amount of hemoglobin in the tissue, which provides an estimate of tissue blood perfusion.[67] In theory, this may offer the opportunity to determine whether neurons are at risk for hypoxic damage. Currently this technology is being correlated with other measures of fetal well-being, such as periodic changes of the FHR and umbilical cord blood pH at delivery.[68,69] Like fetal pulse oximetry, current near-infrared spectroscopy technology is limited by frequent (i.e., 20%) inability to obtain an interpretable reading.[68] A correlation with long-term neurodevelopmental outcome remains to be determined.

Proton magnetic resonance spectroscopy (^{1}H MRS) is a new technique for obtaining metabolic information from human and animal brains. Investigations are underway to assess its ability to assess fetal brain oxygenation.[70] It has proven useful in the evaluation of hypoxic-ischemic encephalopathy and metabolic disorders in pediatric patients. ^{1}H MRS can measure levels of the metabolites N-acetylaspartate, creatine, choline, and inositol in fetal and neonatal neural tissue. These measurements can be correlated to the level of tissue oxygenation. The clinical utility of this technique as a means of fetal assessment remains unclear.

INTRAPARTUM FETAL THERAPY

Once intrapartum fetal compromise has been identified, physicians should make a careful assessment of maternal, placental, and fetal factors that may contribute to this compromise. Clinical history, physical examination, laboratory findings, and fetal monitoring (e.g., FHR, ultrasonography) should be used to identify the etiology.

Correctable **maternal factors** that may contribute to fetal compromise include pathologic states that result in hypoxemia or decreased oxygen delivery to the placenta (Table 8-1). **Respiratory failure** caused by long-standing disease (e.g., asthma) should be suggested by history and physical examination. Physical examination and laboratory measurements may suggest pneumonia or pulmonary edema as the underlying cause. **Decreased oxygen delivery** to the placenta may result from **chronic disease.** Decreased uteroplacental perfusion may result from decreased maternal cardiac output (e.g., cardiovascular disease) or chronic vascular disease (e.g., chronic hypertension and diabetes). Alternatively, decreased oxygen delivery may result from **acute causes** (e.g., sepsis, hypotension during maternal hemorrhage, or regional anes-thesia). Dehydration from prolonged labor may be a more subtle cause of decreased uteroplacental perfusion.

The treatment of maternal causes of fetal hypoxemia includes treatment of the underlying maternal disease (e.g., bronchospasm). Administration of supplemental oxygen may enhance fetal oxygenation, even in the previously normoxemic mother.[18,71] Whether maternal oxygen therapy improves fetal outcome remains unclear.[72,73]

Uterine tetany or **frequent uterine contractions** also may result in decreased uteroplacental perfusion. Uterine tetany is one of the hazards of the use of oxytocin or prostaglandin compounds for the induction of labor. Uterine contractions constrict the uterine spiral arteries and cause decreased oxygen delivery to the placenta. A rare cause of fetal distress is **uterine rupture**, which may be a result of uterine hyperstimulation and/or an old uterine scar. **Placental abruption** may result in a partial or complete cessation of oxygen transfer to the fetus. Placental abruption may result from chronic or acute disease. For example, it is associated with long-standing vascular disease that is associated with chronic hypertension or smoking. Acute factors such as cocaine abuse and abdominal trauma also may precipitate abruption.

The treatment of uteroplacental causes of fetal compromise includes correction of uterine tetany by cessation of oxytocin infusion (see Table 8-1). Oxytocin has a plasma half-life of 1 to 6 minutes. Therefore, it may take several minutes for the tetany to be relieved. Another option is administration of a tocolytic agent (e.g., terbutaline, nitroglycerin) to relieve the tetanic contraction.[18,74] Normal maternal circulation should be maintained by avoiding aortocaval compression, expanding intravascular volume, and giving a vasopressor (e.g., ephedrine) if indicated.[75]

TABLE 8-1	INTRAUTERINE TREATMENT FOR ABNORMAL FETAL HEART RATE (FHR) PATTERNS			
Causes	**Resulting FHR patterns**	**Corrective maneuver**	**Mechanism**
Hypotension (e.g., supine hypotension, regional anesthesia)	Bradycardia, late decelerations	Intravenous fluids, position change, ephedrine	Return of uterine blood flow toward normal
Excessive uterine activity	Bradycardia, late decelerations	Decrease in oxytocin, lateral position, tocolysis (e.g., terbutaline, nitroglycerin)	Return of uterine blood flow toward normal
Transient umbilical cord compression	Variable decelerations	Change in maternal position (e.g., left or right lateral or Trendelenburg), amnioinfusion	Return of umbilical blood flow toward normal
Head compression, usually during the second stage	Variable decelerations	Pushing only with alternate contractions	Return of umbilical blood flow toward normal
Decreased uterine blood flow associated with uterine contractions, below limits of fetal basal O$_2$ needs	Late decelerations	Change in maternal position (e.g., left lateral), administration of supplemental oxygen	Return of uterine blood flow toward normal, increase in maternal-fetal O$_2$ gradient
		Tocolysis (e.g., terbutaline, nitroglycerin)	Decrease in contractions or uterine tone, thus abolishing the associated decrease in uterine blood flow
Prolonged asphyxia	Decreased FHR variability*	Change in maternal position (e.g., left lateral or Trendelenburg), administration of supplemental oxygen	Return of uterine blood flow toward normal, increase in maternal-fetal O$_2$ gradient

FHR, Fetal heart rate.
*During labor, this is always preceded by a heart rate pattern that signals asphyxial stress (e.g., late decelerations or a prolonged bradycardia). This is not necessarily so in the antepartum period, *before* the onset of uterine contractions.
Modified from Parer JT. Fetal heart rate. In Creasy RK, Resnik R, editors. Maternal-Fetal Medicine. Philadelphia, WB Saunders, 1989:332.

Fetal factors may contribute to fetal hypoxemia and acidosis. Umbilical cord compression is a frequent cause of fetal compromise. **Umbilical cord prolapse** through the cervix represents an obvious cause of cord compression. Cord prolapse often results in sudden fetal bradycardia. Treatment of a prolapsed cord consists of fetal head elevation until operative delivery can be accomplished. Katz et al.[76] reported the installation of 500 to 700 mL of 0.9% saline into the maternal bladder to accomplish head elevation and cord decompression. Manual reduction of the prolapsed cord also has been reported.[77]

Variable decelerations or bradycardia may signal **intrauterine cord compression**. Oligohydramnios is a risk factor for cord compression. In some cases of cord compression a change in maternal position may alleviate the cord compression and correct fetal compromise. Another alternative is **saline amnioinfusion** to alleviate cord compression. Presumably, restoration of the natural cushion of amniotic fluid alleviates cord compression. Controlled studies suggest that amnioinfusion results in a decreased frequency of severe variable decelerations, a decreased incidence of cesarean section, and increased umbilical cord blood pH in patients with preterm premature rupture of membranes (PROM), oligohydramnios, and/or variable decelerations during labor.[78-81]

Saline amnioinfusion requires a dilated cervix, ruptured membranes, and placement of an intrauterine catheter. Equipment that allows simultaneous saline amnioinfusion and measurement of intrauterine pressure is preferred. Either normal saline or Ringer's lactate may be infused as a bolus or as a continuous infusion.[18] The ideal rate of infusion has not been determined, but a commonly used regimen includes a bolus of as much as 800 mL (infused at a rate of 10 to 15 mL/min) followed by either a continuous infusion at a rate of 3 mL/min or repeated boluses of 250 mL, as needed.[18] The necessity of either an infusion pump or a fluid warmer has not been demonstrated.[18] Alleviation of abnormal FHR patterns generally requires 20 to 30 minutes.[18] A meta-analysis suggested that prophylactic intrapartum amnioinfusion in patients with oligohydramnios (rather than therapeutic amnioinfusion in the setting of FHR abnormalities) may improve neonatal outcomes and decrease the rate of cesarean delivery without an increase in the incidence of endometritis.[82] Nevertheless, most centers reserve amnioinfusion for patients with oligohydramnios only in the setting of FHR abnormalities.

The presence of thick, meconium-stained amniotic fluid is another indication for the use of amnioinfusion during labor. By definition, the presence of thick meconium signals the presence of decreased amniotic fluid volume. In these cases, amnioinfusion may dilute the meconium and ameliorate the consequences of meconium aspiration in utero. Increased amniotic fluid volume also should decrease the likelihood of umbilical cord compression and perhaps prevent the passage of additional meconium. Some studies have suggested that in patients with thick, meconium-stained amniotic fluid, amnioinfusion results in a decreased incidence of meconium aspiration syndrome and fetal acidosis.[83,84] However, these benefits have not been demonstrated in all studies.[85,86] A meta-analysis suggested that amnioinfusion in patients with meconium staining improves neonatal outcomes and lowers the cesarean section rate without resulting in an increased rate of endometritis.[87]

Although most studies suggest that amnioinfusion is safe for the mother and fetus, some complications have been reported. Overdistention of the uterus has occurred; thus care should be taken to note the amount of fluid loss from the uterus during infusion.[18] Ultrasonography may be used to evaluate fluid volume in the amniotic cavity. At least one study noted an increased rate of maternal infection with use of prophylactic amnioinfusion.[86] Cases of respiratory distress, including two cases of fatal amniotic fluid embolism, have occurred during saline amnioinfusion.[88,89] This association is troubling, although a cause-and-effect relationship has not been determined. Maher et al.[89] have altered their amnioinfusion protocol so that the infusion occurs by gravity rather than by means of a mechanical infusion pump, and they also take care to prevent uterine overdistention.

Maternal fever may increase fetal oxygen consumption. Obstetricians should treat maternal fever with acetaminophen, a cooling blanket, and antibiotics as indicated to maintain maternal and fetal euthermia. **Hyperglycemia** also increases fetal oxygen consumption. Thus administration of a large bolus of a glucose-containing solution is contraindicated.

Fetal cardiac failure results in inadequate umbilical blood flow and fetal hypoxemia and acidosis. **Fetal anemia** caused by maternal isoimmunization, fetal hemoglobinopathy, or fetal hemorrhage results in decreased fetal oxygen-carrying capacity. There are few options for the treatment of fetal cardiac failure or anemia during labor.

If intrapartum assessment suggests the presence of fetal compromise and fetal therapy is unsuccessful, the obstetrician should effect an expeditious, atraumatic delivery.

KEY POINTS

- A normal FHR tracing accurately predicts fetal well-being. An abnormal tracing is not very specific in the prediction of fetal compromise. Exceptions include the fetus with a prolonged bradycardia or the fetus with late FHR decelerations and absent variability. Both suggest a high likelihood of fetal distress.
- Large prospective, randomized studies have not confirmed that continuous electronic FHR monitoring confers substantial clinical benefit over intermittent FHR auscultation, as performed by dedicated labor nurses.
- The specificity of FHR monitoring may be augmented by use of fetal scalp stimulation, fetal vibroacoustic stimulation, and fetal scalp blood sampling.
- When possible, FHR resuscitation in utero is preferable to emergency delivery of an acidotic fetus.
- Saline amnioinfusion effectively prevents or relieves variable decelerations caused by umbilical cord compression, and it may improve perinatal outcome in patients with oligohydramnios and/or thick, meconium-stained amniotic fluid.

REFERENCES

1. Lilien AA. Term intrapartum fetal death. Am J Obstet Gynecol 1970; 107:595-603.
2. Butler NR, Bonham DG. Perinatal Mortality. The First Report on the British Perinatal Mortality Survey. Edinburgh, E & S Livingstone, 1963.

3. Nelson KB, Ellenberg JH. Obstetric complications as risk factors for cerebral palsy or seizure disorders. JAMA 1984; 251:1843-8.

4. Jansome M, Lazdane G. Perinatal problems and quality assurance in Latvia–a country in economic transition. Acta Obstet Gynecol Scand 1997; Suppl 164; 76:31-3.

5. United States Preventive Services Task Force. Screening for fetal distress with intrapartum electronic fetal monitoring. Guide to clinical preventive services: An assessment of 169 interventions. Baltimore, Williams & Wilkins, 1989; 233-8.

6. Brann AW, Myers RE. Central nervous system findings in the newborn monkey following severe in utero partial asphyxia. Neurology 1975; 25:327-8.

7. Nesbitt RE, Aubry RH. High-risk obstetrics. II. Value of semi-objective grading system in identifying the vulnerable group. Am J Obstet Gynecol 1969; 103:972-85.

8. Knox AJ, Sadler L, Pattison NS, et al. An obstetric scoring system: Its development and application in obstetric management. Obstet Gynecol 1993; 81:195-9.

9. Low JA, Simpson MD, Tonni G, et al. Limitations in the clinical prediction of intrapartum fetal asphyxia. Am J Obstet Gynecol 1995; 172:801-4.

10. Alessandri LM, Stanley FJ, Read AW. A case-control study of intrapartum stillbirths. Br J Obstet Gynaecol 1992; 99:719-23.

11. American College of Obstetricians and Gynecologists Task Force on Neonatal Encephalopathy and Cerebral Palsy. Neonatal Encephalopathy and Cerebral Palsy: Defining the Pathogenesis and Pathophysiology. The American College of Obstetricians and Gynecologists and the American Academy of Pediatrics, Washington, D.C., January 2003.

12. MacLennan A. A template for defining a causal relation between acute intrapartum events and cerebral palsy: International consensus statement. BMJ 1999; 319:1054-9.

13. Parer JT. Handbook of Fetal Heart Rate Monitoring, 2nd ed. Philadelphia, WB Saunders, 1997:1-14.

14. Court DJ, Parer JT. Experimental studies of fetal asphyxia and fetal heart rate interpretation. In Nathanielsz PW, Parer JT, eds. Research in Perinatal Medicine, Vol 1. New York, Perinatology Press, 1984:113-69.

15. Parer JT, Livingston EG. What is fetal distress? Am J Obstet Gynecol 1990; 162:1421-7.

16. Cohn HE, Sacks EJ, Heymann MA, et al. Cardiovascular responses to hypoxemia and acidemia in fetal lambs. Am J Obstet Gynecol 1974; 120:817-24.

17. Peeters LL, Shellen RE, Jones MD, et al. Blood flow to fetal organs as a function of arterial oxygen content. Am J Obstet Gynecol 1979; 135:637-46.

18. American College of Obstetricians and Gynecologists. Fetal Heart Rate Patterns: Monitoring, Interpretation and Management. ACOG Technical Bulletin No 207, July 1995.

19. Fisher DJ, Heymann MA, Rudolph AM. Myocardial oxygen and carbohydrate consumption during acutely induced hypoxia. Am J Physiol 1982; 242:H657-61.

20. Jones MD, Sheldon RE, Peeters LL, et al. Fetal cerebral oxygen consumption at different levels of oxygenation. J Appl Physiol 1977; 43:1080.

21. Krebs HB, Petres RE, Dunn LJ, et al. Intrapartum fetal rate monitoring. I. Classification and prognosis of fetal heart rate patterns. Am J Obstet Gynecol 1979; 133:762-72.

22. Hammacher K, Herter KA, Bokelmann J, et al. Foetal heart frequency and perinatal condition of the foetus and newborn. Gynaecologia 1968; 166:349-60.

23. Ball RH, Parer JT. The physiologic mechanisms of variable decelerations. Am J Obstet Gynecol 1992; 166:1683-9.

24. Yeh SY, Diaz F, Paul RH. Ten year experience in intrapartum fetal monitoring in Los Angeles County. University of Southern California Medical Center. Am J Obstet Gynecol 1982; 143:496-500.

25. Paul RH, Huey JR, Yaeger CF. Clinical fetal monitoring: Its effect on cesarean section rate and perinatal mortality–5 year trends. Postgrad Med 1977; 61:160-6.

26. Quirk JG, Miller FC. Fetal heart rate tracing characteristics that jeopardize the diagnosis of fetal well being. Clin Obstet Gynecol 1986; 29:12-22.

27. Renou P, Chang A, Anderson I, et al. Controlled trial of fetal intensive care. Am J Obstet Gynecol 1976; 126:470-6.

28. Thacker SB, Stroup DF, Peterson HB. Efficacy and safety of intrapartum electronic fetal monitoring: An update. Obstet Gynecol 1995; 86:613-20.

29. Vintzileos AM, Nochimson DJ, Guzman ER, et al. Intrapartum electronic fetal heart rate monitoring versus intermittent auscultation: A meta-analysis. Obstet Gynecol 1995; 85:149-55.

30. Freeman RK. Problems with intrapartum fetal heart rate monitoring interpretation and patient management. Obstet Gynecol 2002; 100:813-26.

31. American College of Obstetricians and Gynecologists. Inappropriate use of the terms fetal distress and birth asphyxia. ACOG Committee Opinion No. 197, Feb 1998.

32. Nelson KB, Danbrosia JM, Ting TY, et al. Uncertain value of electronic fetal monitoring in predicting cerebral palsy. N Engl J Med 1996; 334:613-8.

33. Lotgering FK, Wallenburg HC, Schouten HJ. Interobserver and intraobserver variation in the assessment of antepartum cardiotocograph. Am J Obstet Gynecol 1982; 144:701-5.

34. Grant JM. The fetal heart rate trace is normal, isn't it? Observer agreement of categorical assessments. Lancet 1991; 337:215-8.

35. Parer JT, King T. Fetal heart rate monitoring: Is it salvageable? Am J Obstet Gynecol 2000; 182:982-7.

36. National Institutes of Child Health and Human Development Research Planning Workshop. Electronic fetal heart rate monitoring: Research guidelines for interpretation. Am J Obstet Gynecol 1997; 177:1385-90.

37. Mantel R, van Geijn HP, Ververs IA, et al. Automated analysis of near-term antepartum fetal heart rate in relation to fetal behavioral states: The Sonicaid System 8000. Am J Obstet Gynecol 1991; 165:57-65.

38. Scibilia MR, Borri P, Di Tommaso M, et al. Cardiotocographic monitoring of fetal health: Comparative evaluation of traditional and computerized methods. Minerva Ginecol 1991; 43:269-72.

39. Vintzileos AM, Montgomery JT, Nochimson DJ, et al. Telephone transmission of fetal heart rate monitor data: The experience at the University of Connecticut Health Center. Am J Obstet Gynecol 1986; 155:630-4.

40. Phelan JP. Confronting medical liability. Contemp Obstet Gynecol 1991; 36:70-81.

41. Tejani N, Mann L, Bhakthanathsalan A. Correlation of fetal heart rate patterns and fetal pH with neonatal outcome. Obstet Gynecol 1976; 48:460-3.

42. Schifrin BS, Dame L. Fetal heart rate patterns: Prediction of Apgar scores. JAMA 1972;219:1322-5.

43. Young DC, Gray JH, Luther ER, et al. Fetal scalp blood pH sampling: Its value in active obstetric unit. Am J Obstet Gynecol 1980; 136:276-81.

44. Goodwin TM, Milner-Masterson L, Paul RH. Elimination of fetal scalp blood sampling on a large clinical service. Obstet Gynecol 1994; 83:971-4.

45. Clark SL, Gimovsky ML, Miller FC. The scalp stimulation test: A clinical alternative to fetal scalp blood sampling. Am J Obstet Gynecol 1984; 148:274-7.

46. Rice PE, Benedetti TJ. Fetal heart rate acceleration with fetal blood sampling. Obstet Gynecol 1986; 68:469-72.

47. Smith CV, Ngeyeu HN, Phelan JP, et al. Intrapartum assessment of fetal well being: A comparison of fetal acoustic stimulation with acid-base determination. Am J Obstet Gynecol 1986; 155:726-8.

48. Skupski DW, Rosenberg CR, Eglinton GS. Intrapartum fetal stimulation tests: A meta-analysis. Obstet Gynecol 2002; 99:129-34.

49. Ogunyemi D, Stanley R, Lynch C, et al. Umbilical artery velocimetry in predicting perinatal outcome with intrapartum fetal distress. Obstet Gynecol 1992; 80:377-80.

50. Dawes GS, Moulden M, Redman KW. Short term fetal heart rate variations, decelerations, and umbilical flow velocity waveforms before labor. Obstet Gynecol 1992; 80:673-8.

51. Nathan L, Leveno KJ, Carmody TJ, et al. Meconium: A 1990's perspective on an old obstetric hazard. Obstet Gynecol 1994; 83:39-42.

52. Berkus MD, Langer O, Samueloff A, et al. Meconium-stained amniotic fluid: Increased risk for adverse neonatal outcome. Obstet Gynecol 1994; 84:115-20.

53. Low JA. The role of blood gas and acid base assessment in the diagnosis of intrapartum fetal asphyxia. Am J Obstet Gynecol 1988; 159:1235-40.

54. Cajal CLR, Martinez RO. Defecation in utero: A physiologic function. Am J Obstet Gynecol 2003;188:153-6.

55. Meis PJ, Hall M, Marshall JR, et al. Meconium passage: A new classification for risk assessment in labor. Am J Obstet Gynecol 1978; 131:509-13.

56. Katz VL, Bowes WA. Meconium aspiration syndrome: Reflections on a murky subject. Am J Obstet Gynecol 1992; 166:171-83.

57. Stamm O, Latscha U, Janecek P, et al. Development of a special electrode for continuous subcutaneous pH measurement in the infant scalp. Am J Obstet Gynecol 1976; 124:193-5.

58. Mueller-Heubach E, Caritis SN, Echelstone DI, et al. Comparison of continuous transcutaneous Po_2 measurement with intermittent arterial Po_2 determinations in fetal levels. Obstet Gynecol 1981; 57:248-52.

59. Nickelsen C, Thomsen SG, Weber T. Continuous acid-base assessment of the human fetus during labor by tissue pH and transcutaneous carbon dioxide monitoring. Br J Obstet Gynaecol 1985; 92:220-5.

60. American College of Obstetricians and Gynecologists. Fetal Pulse Oximetry. ACOG Committee Opinion No 258. Obstet Gynecol 2001; 98:523-4.

61. Stiller R, Mering R, Konig V, et al. How well does reflectance pulse oximetry reflect intrapartum fetal acidosis? Am J Obstet Gynecol 2002; 186:1351-7.

62. Nijland R, Jongsma HW, Nijhuis JG, et al. Arterial saturation in relation to metabolic acidosis in fetal lambs. Am J Obstet Gynecol 1995; 172:810-9.

63. Kuhnert M, Seelbach-Gobel B, Butterwegge M. Predictive agreement between the fetal arterial oxygen saturation and fetal scalp pH: Results of the German multicenter study. Am J Obstet Gynecol 1998; 178:330-5.

64. Luttkus AK Lubke M, Buscher U, et al. Accuracy of fetal pulse oximetry. Acta Obstet Gynecol Scand 2002;81:417-23.

65. Garite TJ Dildy GA, McNamara H, et al . A multicenter control trial of fetal pulse oximetry in the intrapartum management of nonreassuring fetal heart rate patterns. Am J Obstet Gynecol 2000;183:1049-58.

66. Noren H, Amer-Wahlin I, Hagberg H, et al. Fetal electrocardiography in labor and neonatal outcome: Data from the Swedish randomized controlled trial on intrapartum fetal monitoring. Am J Obstet Gynecol 2003;188:183-92.

67. Brazy JF. Near infrared spectroscopy. Clin Perinatol 1991; 18:519-34.

68. Aldrich CJ, D'antonia D, Wyatt JS, et al. Fetal cerebral oxygenation measured by near infrared spectroscopy shortly before birth and acid-base status at birth. Obstet Gynecol 1994; 84:861-6.

69. Aldrich CJ, D'Antonia D, Spencer JA, et al. Late fetal heart decelerations and changes in cerebral oxygenation during the first stage of labor. Br J Obstet Gynecol 1995; 102:9-13.

70. Kok RD, van den Bergh AJ, Heerschap A, et al. Metabolic information from the human fetal brain obtained with proton magnetic resonance spectroscopy. Am J Obstet Gynecol 2001; 185:1011-5.

71. McNamara H, Johnson N, Lilford R. The effect on fetal arteriolar oxygen saturation resulting from giving oxygen to the mother measured by pulse oximetry. Br J Obstet Gynaecol 1993; 100:446-9.

72. Dildy GA, Clark SL, Loucks CA. Intrapartum, fetal pulse oximetry: The effect of maternal hyperoxia on fetal arterial oxygen saturation. Am J Obstet Gynecol 1994; 171:1120-4.

73. Thorp JA, Trobough T, Evans R, et al. The effect of maternal oxygen administration during the second stage of labor on umbilical cord blood gas values: A randomized controlled prospective trial. Am J Obstet Gynecol 1995; 172:465-74.

74. Magann EF, Cleveland RS, Dockery JR, et al. Acute tocolysis for fetal distress: Terbutaline versus magnesium sulphate. Aust NZ J Obstet Gynecol 1993; 33:362-4.

75. Thurlow JA, Kinsella SM. Intrauterine resuscitation: Active management of fetal distress. Int J Obstet Anesth 2002;11:105-16.

76. Katz Z, Shoham Z, Lancet M, et al. Management of labor with umbilical cord prolapse: A 5-year study. Obstet Gynecol 1988; 72:278-81.

77. Barrett JM. Funic reduction for the management of umbilical cord prolapse. Am J Obstet Gynecol 1991; 165:654-7.

78. Nageotte MP, Freeman RK, Garite TJ, et al. Prophylactic intrapartum amnioinfusion in patients with preterm premature rupture of membranes. Am J Obstet Gynecol 1985; 153:557-62.

79. Strong TH, Hetzler G, Sarno AP, et al. Prophylactic intrapartum amnioinfusion: A randomized clinical trial. Am J Obstet Gynecol 1990; 162:1370-5.

80. Miyazaki FS, Nevarez F. Saline amnioinfusion for relief of repetitive variable decelerations: A prospective randomized study. Am J Obstet Gynecol 1985; 153:301-6.

81. Owen J, Henson BV, Hauth JC. A prospective randomized study of saline solution amnioinfusion. Am J Obstet Gynecol 1990; 162:1146-9.

82. Pitt C, Sanchez-Ramos L , Kaunitz AM , et al. Prophylactic amnioinfusion for intrapartum oligohydramnios: A meta-analysis of randomized control trials. Obstet Gynecol 2000; 96:861-6.

83. Cialone PR, Sherer DM, Ryan RM, et al. Amnioinfusion during labor complicated by particulate meconium-stained amniotic fluid decreases neonatal morbidity. Am J Obstet Gynecol 1994; 170:842-9.

84. Eriksen NL, Hostetter M, Parisi VM. Prophylactic amnioinfusion in pregnancies complicated by thick meconium. Am J Obstet Gynecol 1994; 171:1026-30.

85. Usta IM, Mercer BM, Aswad NK, et al. The impact of a policy of amnioinfusion for meconium-stained amniotic fluid. Obstet Gynecol 1995; 85:237-41.

86. Spong CY, Ogundipe OA, Ross MG. Prophylactic amnioinfusion for meconium-stained amniotic fluid. Am J Obstet Gynecol 1994; 171:931-5.

87. Pierce J, Gaudier FL, Sanchez-Ramos L. Intrapartum amnioinfusion for meconium-stained fluid: Meta-analysis of prospective clinical trials. Obstet Gynecol 2000; 95:1051-6.

88. Dragich DA, Ross AF, Chestnut DH, et al. Respiratory failure associated with amnioinfusion during labor. Anesth Analg 1991; 72:549-51.

89. Maher JE, Wenstrom KD, Hauth JC, et al. Amniotic fluid embolism after saline amnioinfusion: Two cases and review of the literature. Obstet Gynecol 1994; 83:851-4.

Chapter 9
Neonatal Assessment and Resuscitation

Susan W. Aucott, M.D. · Rhonda L. Zuckerman, M.D.

The transition from intrauterine to extrauterine life represents the most important adjustment that the newborn will make in its life. It is remarkable that this transition occurs uneventfully after most deliveries. Satisfactory transition depends on the following: (1) the anatomic and physiologic condition of the fetus at delivery; (2) the ease or difficulty of the delivery itself; and (3) the extrauterine environment. When transition is unsuccessful, prompt assessment and supportive care must be initiated immediately.

At least one person skilled in neonatal resuscitation should be present at every delivery. Available individuals may include personnel from the pediatrics, anesthesiology, obstetrics, respiratory therapy, and nursing services. The composition of the resuscitation team will vary from place to place, but some type of in-house, 24-hour coverage is essential for all hospitals that have labor and delivery services.[1] The departments of pediatrics, anesthesiology, and obstetrics should participate in the process of ensuring that appropriate personnel and equipment are available for neonatal resuscitation.[2]

All personnel working in the delivery area should receive training in neonatal resuscitation to facilitate the prompt initiation of neonatal resuscitation when the appointed resuscitation team has not arrived in time for the delivery. The International Guidelines 2000 Conference on Cardiopulmonary Resuscitation and Emergency Cardiovascular Care resulted in the publication of revised guidelines for neonatal resuscitation.[3] Changes in these guidelines reflect the careful review of scientific evidence by members of the American Academy of Pediatrics (AAP), the American Heart Association (AHA), and the International Liaison Committee on Resuscitation. In October 2000, the revised *Textbook of Neonatal Resuscitation* and *Instructor's Manual for Neonatal Resuscitation* were published by the AAP and the AHA.[4] The new guidelines have been included in the Neonatal Resuscitation Program (NRP), which is the standardized training and certification program administered by the AAP. The NRP, which was originally sponsored by the AAP and the AHA in 1987, is designed to be appropriate for all personnel who attend deliveries. To ensure the implementation of current guidelines for neonatal resuscitation, the AAP recommends that at least one NRP-certified practitioner attend every delivery.[5]

Both the American Society of Anesthesiologists (ASA) and the American College of Obstetricians and Gynecologists (ACOG) have published specific goals and guidelines regarding neonatal resuscitation (Box 9-1).[6] The ASA has emphasized that a single anesthesiologist should not be expected to assume responsibility for the concurrent care of *both* the mother and her child. Rather, a second anesthesia care provider or a qualified individual from another service should assume responsibility for the care of the newborn, except in unforeseen emergency conditions.

In clinical practice, anesthesiologists often are involved in resuscitation of the newborn.[7-9] In 1991, Heyman et al.[7] noted that anesthesia personnel were involved in newborn resuscitation in 99 (31%) of 320 selected Midwestern community hospitals. The individual who administered anesthesia to the mother was also responsible for the care of the newborn in 13.4% of these hospitals. In 6.8% of these institutions, a second anesthesia care provider routinely assumed primary responsibility for the infant. In a survey of the obstetric anesthesia workforce in the United States, Hawkins et al.[9] found that fewer anesthesiologists were involved in neonatal resuscitation in 1992 than in 1981, although anesthesiologists still provided neonatal resuscitation in 10% of cesarean deliveries.

Even when the anesthesiologist is not primarily responsible for neonatal resuscitation, he or she is often asked to provide assistance in cases of difficult airway management or in emergency cases, when members of the neonatal resuscitation team have not arrived. The anesthesiologist should be prepared to offer assistance to those in charge of neonatal resuscitation, provided such care does not compromise the care of the mother. A recent study of University of Pennsylvania residency graduates from 1989 to 1999 revealed that most anesthesiologists are not certified in neonatal resuscitation, although they would like to be.[10] Hopefully opportunities for anesthesiologists to become NRP-certified will increase; the NRP course is now offered at the annual meeting of the Society for Obstetric Anesthesiology and Perinatology (SOAP).[11]

In the ASA Closed-Claims Database, 13% of malpractice claims for obstetric anesthesia were related to neonatal resuscitation.[12] Of the five cases listed, three involved delayed or failed tracheal intubation, and one involved an unrecognized esophageal intubation. A review of obstetric anesthesia-related lawsuits from 1985 to 1993 revealed that 12 (17%) of the 69 obstetric anesthesia cases involved claims of inadequate neonatal resuscitation by anesthesia personnel[13]; 10 of these 12 cases resulted in payment to the plaintiff. It is clear that written hospital policies should identify the personnel responsible for neonatal resuscitation and that obstetric anesthesia care providers should maintain a high level of skill in neonatal resuscitation.

Box 9-1 OPTIMAL GOALS FOR ANESTHESIA CARE IN OBSTETRICS: NEONATAL RESUSCITATION

Personnel other than the surgical team should be immediately available to assume responsibility for resuscitation of the depressed newborn.

The surgeon and anesthesiologist are responsible for the mother and may not be able to leave her care for the newborn, even when a regional anesthetic is functioning adequately. Individuals qualified to perform neonatal resuscitation should demonstrate the following:

A. Proficiency in rapid and accurate evaluation of the newborn's condition, including Apgar scoring;
B. Knowledge of the pathogenesis of a depressed newborn (acidosis, drugs, hypovolemia, trauma, anomalies, and infection), as well as specific indications for resuscitation; and
C. Proficiency in newborn airway management, laryngoscopy, endotracheal intubations, suctioning of airways, artificial ventilation, cardiac massage, and maintenance of thermal stability.

In larger maternity units and those functioning as high-risk centers, 24-hour in-house anesthesia, obstetric, and neonatal specialists are usually necessary.

From the American College of Obstetrics and Gynecologists Committee on Obstetric Practice and the American Society of Anesthesiologists Committee on Obstetric Anesthesia. ACOG Committee Opinion No. 256, May 2001.

TRANSITION FROM INTRAUTERINE TO EXTRAUTERINE LIFE

Circulation

At birth, the circulatory system changes from fetal circulation (which is in parallel), through a transitional circulation, to adult circulation (which is in series) (Figure 9-1).[14,15] In the fetus, blood from the placenta travels through the umbilical vein and the ductus venosus to the inferior vena cava and the right side of the heart. The anatomic orientation of the inferior vena caval–right atrial junction favors the shunting (i.e., streaming) of this well-oxygenated blood through the foramen ovale to the left side of the heart. This well-oxygenated blood is pumped through the ascending aorta, where branches that perfuse the upper part of the body (e.g., heart, brain) exit proximal to the entrance of the ductus arteriosus.[16] Desaturated blood returns to the heart from the upper part of the body by means of the superior vena cava. The anatomic orientation of the superior vena caval–right atrial junction favors the streaming of blood into the right ventricle. Because fetal pulmonary vascular resistance is higher than systemic vascular resistance (SVR), approximately 90% of the right ventricular output passes through the ductus arteriosus and enters the aorta distal to the branches of the ascending aorta and aortic arch; therefore, less well-oxygenated blood perfuses the lower body, which consumes less oxygen than the heart and brain.

At the time of birth and during the resulting circulatory transition, the amount of blood that shunts through the foramen ovale and ductus arteriosus diminishes, and the flow becomes bidirectional. Clamping the umbilical cord (or exposing the umbilical cord to room air) results in increased SVR. Meanwhile, expansion of the lungs and increased alveolar oxygen tension and pH result in decreased pulmonary vascular resistance.[17,18] Decreased pulmonary vascular resistance allows an increased flow of pulmonary artery blood through the lungs. Increased pulmonary artery blood flow results in

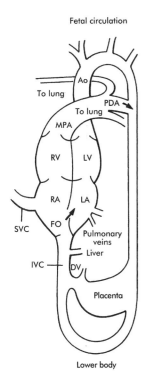

Fetal circulation

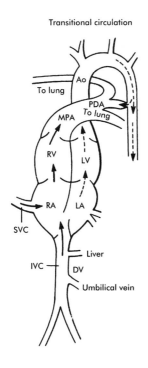

Transitional circulation

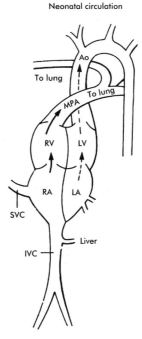

Neonatal circulation

FIGURE 9-1. Transition of the circulation from the fetal to the normal postnatal flow patterns. During the normally short-lived transitional period, the patent ductus arteriosus *(PDA)* and foramen ovale *(FO)* may be significant conduits. *RV,* Right ventricle; *RA,* right atrium; *DV,* ductus venosus; *LV,* left ventricle; *LA,* left atrium; *Ao,* aorta; *MPA,* main pulmonary artery; *SVC* and *IVC,* superior and inferior vena cava, respectively. (Adapted from Polin RA, Burg FD. Workbook in Practical Neonatology. Philadelphia, WB Saunders, 1983:156-7.)

improved oxygenation and increased left atrial pressure; the latter results in a decreased shunt across the foramen ovale. Increased PaO_2 and SVR and decreased pulmonary vascular resistance result in a constriction of the ductus arteriosus.[19,20] Together, these changes in vascular resistance result in functional closure of the foramen ovale and the ductus arteriosus. This process does not occur instantaneously, and SaO_2 remains higher in the right upper extremity (which is preductal) than in the left upper extremity and the lower extremities until blood flow through the ductus arteriosus is minimal.[21] Differences in SaO_2 are usually minimal by 10 minutes and absent by 24 hours after birth. Provided that there is no interference with the normal fall in pulmonary vascular resistance, both the foramen ovale and the ductus arteriosus close functionally, and the infant develops an adult circulation (which is in series).

Persistent fetal circulation—more correctly called *persistent pulmonary hypertension of the newborn* (PPHN)—can occur when the pulmonary vascular resistance remains elevated at the time of birth. Factors that may contribute to this problem include hypoxia, acidosis, hypovolemia, and hypothermia.[17,22,23] Maternal use of nonsteriodal antiinflammatory agents may also be problematic, because these agents may cause premature constriction of the ductus arteriosus in the fetus and thus predispose it to PPHN.

Respiration

Fetal breathing movements have been observed in utero as early as 11 weeks' gestation. These movements increase with advancing gestational age, but they are markedly reduced within days of the onset of labor. They are stimulated by hypercapnia and maternal smoking and are inhibited by hypoxia and central nervous system (CNS) depressants (e.g., barbiturates). Under normal conditions, this fetal breathing activity results only in the movement of pulmonary dead space.[24] The fetal lung contains a liquid that is composed of an ultrafiltrate of plasma, which is secreted by the lungs in utero[25,26]; the volume of this lung liquid is approximately 30 mL/kg. Partial reabsorption of this liquid occurs during labor and delivery, and approximately two thirds is expelled from the lungs of the term newborn by the time of delivery.[27] Small preterm babies and those delivered by cesarean section may have increased residual lung liquid after delivery. These infants experience decreased chest compression at delivery as compared with larger infants or those who are delivered vaginally; this can lead to difficulty in the initiation and maintenance of a normal breathing pattern. Retained fetal lung liquid is the presumed cause of **transient tachypnea of the newborn (TTN)**.[28]

The first breath occurs approximately 9 seconds after delivery. Air enters the lungs as soon as the intrathoracic pressure begins to fall. This air movement during the first breath is important, because it establishes the newborn's functional residual capacity (IRC) (Figure 9-2).

Lung inflation is a major physiologic stimulus for the release of lung surfactant into the alveoli.[29] Surfactant, which is necessary for normal breathing, is present within the alveolar lining cells by 20 weeks' gestation,[30] and it is present within the lumen of the airways by 28 to 32 weeks' gestation. However, significant amounts of surfactant do not appear in terminal airways until 34 to 38 weeks' gestation unless surfactant production has been stimulated by chronic stress or maternal steroid administration.[31]

Stress during labor and delivery can lead to gasping efforts by the fetus, which may result in the inhalation of amniotic fluid into the lungs.[32] This can produce problems if the stress caused the fetus to pass meconium into the amniotic fluid before gasping.

Catecholamines

Transition to extrauterine life is associated with a catecholamine surge. Catecholamines may be necessary for the transition process to be successful. In chronically catheterized sheep, catecholamine levels begin to increase a few hours before delivery. At the time of delivery, the catecholamine levels may be higher than at any other time during life.[33]

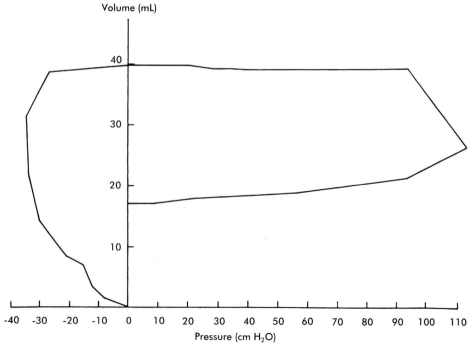

FIGURE 9-2. Typical pressure-volume loop of the first breath. The intrathoracic pressure falls to −30 to −40 cm H_2O, drawing air into the lungs. The expiratory pressure is much greater than the inspiratory pressure. (From Milner AD, Vyas H. Lung expansion at birth. J Pediatr 1982; 101:881.)

Catecholamines have an important role in the following areas: (1) the production and release of surfactant; (2) the mediation of preferential blood flow to vital organs during the period of stress that occurs during every delivery; and (3) the thermoregulation of the newborn.

Thermal Regulation

Thermal stress challenges the newborn in the extrauterine environment. Newborns increase their metabolic rates and release norepinephrine in response to cold; this facilitates the oxidation of brown fat, which contains numerous mitochondria. This oxidation results in **nonshivering thermogenesis,** which is the major mechanism for newborn heat regulation.[34] This process may result in significant oxygen consumption, especially if the newborn has not been dried off and kept in an appropriate thermoneutral environment, such as a radiant warmer. Thermal stress is an even greater problem in infants with low fat stores, such as preterm infants or infants who are small for gestational age. It is important to maintain a neutral thermal environment (i.e., 34° to 35° C) for newborns. Recent studies of perinatal brain injury suggest that mild hypothermia may be neuroprotective in the setting of hypoxia-ischemia. Hyperthermia, which may worsen neurologic outcome, should be avoided.[3,35]

Administration of epidural analgesia during labor is associated with an increase in maternal and fetal temperature.[36] Concern has been expressed regarding whether the temperature elevation associated with epidural analgesia results in an increased frequency of neonatal sepsis evaluations.[36,37] In one study, such an increase was observed only when the mother developed fever (>38° C).[36] In another study, an increased frequency of neonatal sepsis evaluations was observed in women who received epidural analgesia, even if the mother did not have fever.[37] A recent retrospective study evaluated other variables besides epidural analgesia, such as preeclampsia/hypertension, gestational age, birth weight, meconium aspiration and respiratory distress at birth, hypothermia at birth, and group B beta-hemolytic streptococcal colonization of the maternal birth canal. These other factors were strong predictors of the performance of neonatal sepsis evaluations, whereas maternal fever and epidural analgesia were not.[38] Many confounding variables may influence results; patients who receive epidural analgesia are inherently different than those who do not receive epidural analgesia. The incidence of actual neonatal sepsis is not higher in term infants whose mothers receive epidural analgesia than in infants whose mothers do not receive epidural analgesia. At this time, there is no evidence to suggest that parturients should hesitate to receive epidural analgesia because of concerns regarding an epidural analgesia-associated increase in maternal temperature.

ANTENATAL ASSESSMENT

Approximately 14% of newborns require some level of resuscitation.[39] The need for resuscitation can be predicted *before* labor and delivery with approximately 80% accuracy on the basis of a number of antepartum factors (Box 9-2).

Preterm delivery increases the likelihood that the newborn will require resuscitation. When a mother is admitted with either preterm labor or premature rupture of membranes (PROM), plans should be made for neonatal care in the event of delivery. The antenatal assessment of gestational age is based on the presumed date of the last menstrual period, the fundal height, and ultrasonographic measurements of the fetus. Unfortunately, it may be difficult to assess gestational age accurately, because menstrual dates may be unknown or incorrect, the fundal height may be affected by abnormalities of fetal growth or amniotic fluid volume, and ultrasonographic assessment of fetal age is less precise after mid-pregnancy. The assessment of gestational age is most accurate in patients who receive prenatal care early in pregnancy. An accurate approximation of gestational age enables the health care team to plan for the needs of the newborn and to counsel the parents regarding neonatal morbidity and mortality. These plans and expectations must be formulated with caution and flexibility, because the antenatal assessment may not accurately predict the size, maturity, and/or condition of the newborn at delivery.

Box 9-2 RISK FACTORS SUGGESTING AN INCREASED NEED FOR NEONATAL RESUSCITATION

ANTEPARTUM RISK FACTORS

Maternal diabetes
Pregnancy-induced hypertension
Chronic hypertension
Chronic maternal illness (e.g., cardiovascular, thyroid, neurologic, pulmonary, renal)
Anemia or isoimmunization
Previous fetal or neonatal death
Bleeding in second or third trimester
Maternal infection
Polyhydramnios
Oligohydramnios
Premature rupture of membranes
Post-term gestation
Multiple gestation
Size/dates discrepancy
Drug therapy (e.g., lithium carbonate, magnesium, adrenergic-blocking drugs)
Maternal substance abuse
Fetal malformation
Diminished fetal activity
No prenatal care
Age <16 or >35 years

INTRAPARTUM RISK FACTORS

Emergency cesarean section
Forceps or vacuum-assisted delivery
Breech or other abnormal presentation
Preterm labor
Precipitous labor
Chorioamnionitis
Prolonged rupture of membranes (>18 hours before delivery)
Prolonged labor (>24 hours)
Prolonged second stage of labor (>2 hours)
Fetal bradycardia
Nonreassuring fetal heart rate patterns
Use of general anesthesia
Uterine tetany
Opioids administered to mother within 4 hours of delivery
Meconium-stained amniotic fluid
Prolapsed cord
Placental abruption
Placenta previa

Adapted from Niermeyer S (ed), Kattwinkel J, Van Reempts P, et al. International Guidelines for Neonatal Resuscitation: An excerpt from the Guidelines 2000 for Cardiopulmonary Resuscitation and Emergency Cardiovascular Care: International Consensus on Science. Pediatrics 2000; 106:E29:1-16.

A variety of **intrauterine insults** can impair the fetal transition from intrauterine to extrauterine life. For example, neonatal depression at birth can result from acute or chronic uteroplacental insufficiency or acute umbilical cord compression. Chronic uteroplacental insufficiency, regardless of its etiology, may result in fetal growth restriction. Fetal hemorrhage, viral or bacterial infection, meconium aspiration, and exposure to opioids or other CNS depressants also can result in neonatal depression. Although randomized trials have not confirmed that fetal heart rate (FHR) monitoring improves neonatal outcome, a nonreassuring FHR tracing is considered to be a predictor of the need for neonatal resuscitation.[40]

Infants with **congenital anomalies** (e.g., tracheoesophageal fistula, diaphragmatic hernia, CNS and cardiac malformations) may need resuscitation and cardiorespiratory support. Improved ultrasonography allows for the antenatal diagnosis of many congenital anomalies and other fetal abnormalities (e.g., nonimmune hydrops). Obstetricians should communicate knowledge or suspicions regarding these entities to those who will provide care for the newborn in the delivery room; this allows the resuscitation team to make specific resuscitation plans.

In the past, infants delivered by either elective or emergency cesarean section were considered more likely to require resuscitation than infants delivered vaginally. More recent evidence suggests that repeat cesarean sections and cesarean sections performed for dystocia—in patients without FHR abnormalities—result in the delivery of infants at low risk for neonatal resuscitation, especially when those cesarean deliveries are performed with regional anesthesia.[41] However, infants delivered by elective repeat cesarean section are at increased risk for subsequent respiratory problems (e.g., transient tachypnea of the newborn) as compared with similar infants whose mothers had a trial of labor before cesarean section.[42] Emergency cesarean section is considered a risk factor for the need for neonatal resuscitation.

ASSESSMENT OF THE NEWBORN

Apgar Score

Resuscitative efforts typically precede the performance of a thorough physical examination of the newborn. Because new NRP instructions require simultaneous assessment and treatment, it is important that assessment of the newborn be both simple and sensitive.[43] In 1953, Dr. Virginia Apgar, an anesthesiologist, described a simple method for the assessment of the newborn that could be performed while care was being delivered.[44] She developed this system to provide a standardized and relatively objective method of assessing the newborn's clinical status. Dr. Apgar suggested that this scoring system would differentiate between infants who require resuscitation and those who need only routine care.[45]

The Apgar score is based on five parameters that are assessed at 1 and 5 minutes after birth. Further scoring at 5- or 10-minute intervals may be done if initial scores are low. The parameters include heart rate, respiratory effort, muscle tone, reflex irritability, and color. A score of 0, 1, or 2 is assigned for each of these five entities (Table 9-1). A total score of 8 to 10 is normal; a score of 4 to 7 indicates moderate impairment; and a score of 0 to 3 signals the need for immediate resuscitation. Dr. Apgar emphasized that this system does not replace a complete physical examination and serial observation of the newborn for several hours after birth.[46]

The Apgar score is widely used to assess newborns, although its value has been questioned repeatedly. The scoring system may help predict mortality and neurologic morbidity in *populations* of infants, but Dr. Apgar cautioned against the use of the Apgar score to make these predictions in an *individual* infant. Dr. Apgar[46] noted that the risk of neonatal mortality was inversely proportional to the 1-minute score. In addition, the 1-minute Apgar score was a better predictor of mortality within the first 2 days of life than within 2 to 28 days of life.

Several studies have challenged the notion that a low Apgar score signals perinatal asphyxia. In a prospective study of 1210 deliveries, Sykes et al.[47] noted a poor correlation between the Apgar score and the umbilical cord blood pH. Several studies, including those of low birth weight (LBW) infants, have found that a low Apgar score is a poor predictor of neonatal acidosis, although a high score is reasonably specific for the exclusion of the presence of severe acidosis.[48-54] By contrast, the fetal biophysical profile has a good correlation with the acid-base status of the fetus and the newborn[55] (see Chapter 6). The biophysical profile includes performance of a nonstress test (NST) and ultrasonographic evaluation of fetal tone, fetal movement, fetal breathing movements, and amniotic fluid volume.[55]

Other studies that have evaluated the relationship between Apgar scores and neurologic outcome suggest that Apgar

---

TABLE 9-1	APGAR SCORING SYSTEM		
	Score		
Parameter	**0**	**1**	**2**
Heart rate	Absent	< 100	> 100
Respiratory effort	Absent	Irregular, slow, shallow, or gasping respirations	Robust, crying
Muscle tone	Absent, limp	Some flexion of extremities	Active movement
Reflex irritability (nasal catheter, oropharyngeal suctioning)	No response	Grimace	Active coughing and sneezing
Color	Cyanotic	Acrocyanotic (trunk pink, extremities blue)	Pink

Adapted from Tabata BK. Neonatal resuscitation. In: Rogers MC, editor. Current Practice in Anesthesiology. 2nd ed. St. Louis, Mosby, 1990:368.

scores are poor predictors of long-term neurologic impairment.[56,57] The Apgar score is more likely to predict a poor neurologic outcome when the score remains 3 or less at 10, 15, and 20 minutes. However, when a child develops cerebral palsy, low Apgar scores alone are not adequate proof that perinatal hypoxia was responsible for the neurologic injury.

The ACOG Task Force on Neonatal Encephalopathy and Cerebral Palsy recently published criteria for defining an intrapartum event sufficient to cause cerebral palsy.[58] An Apgar score of 0 to 3 beyond 5 minutes of age is not included in the list of "essential criteria"; rather, it is one of five criteria that "collectively suggest an intrapartum timing (within close proximity to labor and delivery . . .) but are nonspecific to asphyxial insults."[58-62]

In a retrospective analysis of 151,891 singleton infants born at 26 weeks' gestation or later between 1988 and 1998, Casey et al.[63] examined the relationship between Apgar scores and neonatal death rates during the first 28 days of life. The highest relative risk for neonatal death was observed in infants with an Apgar score of 3 or less at 5 minutes of age. The 5-minute Apgar score was a better predictor of neonatal death than the umbilical artery pH. In term infants, the relative risk was eight times higher in infants with a 5-minute Apgar score of 3 or less than in those with an umbilical artery pH of 7.0 or less.[63,64] In preterm infants, lower 5-minute Apgar scores were associated with younger gestational age (i.e., mean score 6.6 ± 2.1 for infants born at 26 to 27 weeks' and 8.7 ± 0.8 for infants born at 34 to 36 weeks' gestation).[63] Similarly, earlier studies found that preterm infants are more likely than term infants to have low 1- and 5-minute Apgar scores, independent of neonatal oxygenation and acid-base status. Respiratory effort, muscle tone, and reflex irritability are the components of the score that are most influenced by gestational age.[65]

The earlier the gestational age, the greater the likelihood of a low Apgar score, even in the presence of a normal umbilical cord blood pH. Preterm infants often require active resuscitation efforts immediately after delivery, and these manipulations may affect the components of the Apgar score. For example, pharyngeal and tracheal stimulation may cause a reflex bradycardia, which affects the heart rate score.[50] In addition, it is difficult to judge respiratory effort during suctioning and/or endotracheal intubation. Likewise, it is difficult to assess respiratory effort in infants (either preterm or term) who require laryngoscopy for the removal of meconium.

During cases of active neonatal resuscitation, the Apgar scores often are not assigned at the appropriate times; rather, these scores may be assigned retrospectively. In these situations, the individual must rely on recall of the infant's condition at earlier times, which introduces inaccuracy. Even if the scores are assigned at the appropriate times, there may be disagreement among the several individuals who are providing care for the infant. To avoid bias, Dr. Apgar recommended that the score be assigned by someone not involved in the care of the mother.

Noninvasive monitoring of newborn heart rate and SaO_2 (the latter a more objective criterion than assessment of color) can be accomplished with a pulse oximeter. These measurements, coupled with the other components of the Apgar score (i.e., muscle tone, reflex irritability, respiratory effort) may strengthen the correlations between Apgar scores and other outcome predictors, such as umbilical cord blood pH measurements.[66] Although there is some appeal to the use of objective measurements (e.g., SaO_2, heart rate) rather than subjective observations, it should not be inferred that the subjective components of the Apgar score (e.g., muscle tone) are less important than the objective measurements. Also, there are some practical limitations to the usefulness of pulse oximetry in the delivery room (e.g., movement artifact).[21] However, newer-generation pulse oximeters provide more accurate estimations of SaO_2 (vide infra).[67]

In summary, the usefulness of the Apgar score is still being debated some 50 years after its inception.[63,64,68] The Apgar scoring system is used throughout the world, but its limitations must be kept in mind. Low Apgar scores alone do not provide sufficient evidence of perinatal asphyxia; rather, Apgar scores can be low for a variety of reasons. Preterm delivery, congenital anomalies, neuromuscular diseases, antenatal drug exposure, manipulation at delivery, and subjectivity and error may influence the Apgar score.

Umbilical Cord Blood Gas and pH Analysis

Some obstetricians routinely assess umbilical cord blood gas and pH measurements immediately after delivery. Others obtain these measurements only in cases of neonatal depression. Umbilical cord blood gas and pH measurements reflect the fetal condition immediately before delivery and may be a more objective indication of a newborn's condition than the Apgar score. However, there is a lag between the time that the samples are obtained and the time that analysis is complete; during this interval, decisions must be made on the basis of clinical assessment.

Acids produced by the fetus include carbonic acid (produced during oxidative metabolism) and lactic and beta-hydroxybutyric acids (which result primarily from anaerobic metabolism). Carbonic acid, which is often called **respiratory acid,** is cleared rapidly by the placenta as carbon dioxide, provided that placental blood flow is normal. However, metabolic clearance of lactic and beta-hydroxybutyric acids requires hours; thus these acids are called **metabolic** or **fixed acids.** In the fetus, the presence of metabolic acidemia is more ominous than respiratory acidemia, because it reflects a significant amount of anaerobic metabolism.

The measured components of umbilical cord blood gas analysis include pH, PCO_2, PO_2, and HCO_3^-. Bicarbonate (HCO_3^-) is a major buffer in fetal blood. The measure of change in the buffering capacity of umbilical cord blood is reflected in the delta base, which is also known as the base excess or deficit. This value can be calculated from the pH, PCO_2, and HCO_3^-. Ideally, blood samples from both the umbilical artery and vein are collected. Umbilical artery blood gas measurements represent the fetal condition, whereas umbilical vein measurements reflect the maternal condition and uteroplacental gas exchange. Unfortunately, it may be difficult to obtain blood from the umbilical artery, especially when it is small, as it is in very low birth weight (VLBW) infants. Caution should be used when interpreting an isolated umbilical venous blood pH, which can be normal despite the presence of arterial acidemia.

The blood samples should be drawn and handled properly to obtain accurate measurements. The measurements should be accurate, provided that the following are true: (1) the umbilical cord is doubly clamped immediately after delivery[69-71]; (2) the samples are drawn, within 15 minutes of delivery,[72] into a syringe containing the proper amount of heparin[73]; and (3) the samples are analyzed within 30 to 60 minutes.[74-76] The PO_2 measurement is more accurate if residual air bubbles are removed from the syringe.

TABLE 9-2	STUDIES REPORTING UMBILICAL CORD ARTERIAL BLOOD GAS VALUES					
Study	**pH**	**Pco$_2$**	**Bicarbonate**	**Base deficit**	**Po$_2$**
Huisjes and Aarnoudse (1979)[85] (n = 852)	7.20 ± 0.09 (7.02-7.38)				
Sykes et al. (1982)[47] (n = 899)	7.20 ± 0.08 (7.04-7.36)			8.3 ± 4.0 (0.3-16.3)	
Eskes et al. (1983)[86] (n = 4667)	7.23 ± 0.07 7.09-7.37				
Yeomans et al. (1985)[82] (n = 146)	7.28 ± 0.05 (7.18-7.38)	49.2 ± 8.4 (32.4-66.0)	22.3 ± 2.5 (17.3-27.3)		
Low (1988)[87] (n = 4500)	7.26 ± 0.07 (7.12-7.40)	54.9 ± 9.9 (35.1-74.7)			15.1 ± 4.9 (5.3-24.9)
Ruth and Raivio (1988)[91] (n = 106)	7.29 ± 0.07 (7.15-7.43)			4.7 ± 4.0 (−3.3-12.7)	
Thorp et al. (1989)[88] (n = 1694)	7.24 ± 0.07 (7.10-7.38)	56.3 ± 8.6 (39.1-73.5)	24.1 ± 2.2 (19.7-28.5)	3.6 ± 2.7 (−1.8-9.0)	17.9 ± 6.9 (4.1-31.7)
Ramin et al. (1989)[83] (n = 1292)	7.28 ± 0.07 (7.14-7.42)	49.9 ± 14.2 (21.5-78.3)	23.1 ± 2.8 (17.5-28.7)	3.6 ± 2.8 (−2.0-9.4)	23.7 ± 10.0 (3.7-43.7)
Riley and Johnson (1993)[89] (n = 3522)	7.27 ± 0.07 (7.13-7.41)	50.3 ± 11.1 (28.1-72.5)	22.0 ± 3.6 (14.8-29.2)	2.7 ± 2.8 (−2.9-8.3)	18.4 ± 8.2 (2.0-34.8)
Nagel et al. (1995)[90] (n = 1614)	7.21 ± 0.09 (7.03-7.39)				

Data are presented as mean ± 1 SD and (−2 to +2 SD). Sample size pertains to cord arterial pH and not necessarily to other parameters. Some studies report selected low-risk populations with normal vaginal deliveries only,[82,83] unselected patients with vaginal deliveries,[89] and unselected nulliparous patients,[88] and others report all deliveries at one hospital.[47,87,90,91]

From Thorp JA, Dildy BA, Yeomans ER, et al. Umbilical cord blood gas analysis at delivery. Am J Obstet Gynecol 1996; 175:517-22.

Historically, the normal umbilical cord blood pH was thought to be 7.2 or higher[77,78]; however, investigators have challenged the validity of this number. The assumption that 7.2 was the lower limit of normal made no distinction between umbilical arterial and venous blood, although there are clear differences between the normal measurements for the two.[79] One study noted that the median umbilical arterial pH in vigorous infants (those with 5-minute Apgar scores greater than or equal to 7) was 7.26, with a 2.5th percentile value of 7.10.[80] Published studies suggest that the lower limit of normal umbilical arterial pH may range from 7.02 to 7.18 (Table 9-2).[47,81-91] Other factors may also influence the umbilical arterial blood pH measurement. A fetus subjected to the stress of labor will have lower pH measurements than one delivered by cesarean section without labor.[92] Offspring of nulliparous women tend to have a lower pH than offspring of parous women, which is likely related to the difference in the duration of labor.[88]

Some studies have suggested that preterm infants have an increased incidence of acidemia. More recent studies suggest that term and preterm infants have similar umbilical cord blood gas and pH measurements.[83,84,92] Preterm infants often receive low Apgar scores, despite the presence of normal umbilical cord blood gas and pH measurements; therefore, assessment of umbilical cord blood is especially helpful in the evaluation of preterm neonates.

Physicians should use strict definitions when interpreting umbilical cord blood gas and pH measurements. Terms such as *birth asphyxia* should be avoided in most cases.[58] Acidemia refers to an increase in the hydrogen ion concentration in the blood. Acidosis occurs when there is an increased hydrogen ion concentration in tissue. Asphyxia is a clinical situation that includes hypoxia (i.e., a decreased level of oxygen in tissue), damaging acidemia, and metabolic acidosis.

When acidemia is present, it is important to identify the type: respiratory, metabolic, or mixed (Table 9-3). Metabolic acidemia is more likely to be associated with acidosis than respiratory acidemia and is more significant clinically. Similarly, mixed acidemia with a high Pco$_2$, an extremely low HCO$_3^-$, and a high base deficit is more ominous than a mixed acidemia with a high Pco$_2$ but only a slightly reduced HCO$_3^-$ and a low base deficit. Mixed or metabolic acidemia (but not respiratory acidemia) is associated with an increased incidence of neonatal complications and death.[92] Goldaber et al.[93] noted that an umbilical arterial blood pH of less than 7.00 was associated with a significant increase in the incidence of neonatal death. All neonatal seizures occurred in infants with an umbilical arterial blood pH of less than 7.05. By contrast, a short-term outcome study failed to show a good correlation between arterial pH and the subsequent health of an infant.[54] Casey et al.[63] found that an umbilical artery pH of 7.0 or less was a poorer predictor of the relative risk of neonatal death during the first 28 days of life than was a 5-minute Apgar score of 3 or less.[63] However, 6264 infants were excluded from the study because umbilical arterial blood gas measurements could not be obtained, and these infants had a higher incidence of neonatal death than those for whom blood gas measurements were available (4.5 per 1000 versus 1.2 per 1000).

According to the ACOG Task Force, an umbilical artery pH of less than 7.0 and a base deficit greater than or equal to 12 mmol/L at delivery are considered one part of the definition of an acute intrapartum hypoxic event sufficient to cause cerebral palsy.[58] The base deficit and bicarbonate (the metabolic component) are the most significant factors associated with neonatal morbidity in newborns with an umbilical artery pH of less than 7.0.

There is a lack of consistent correlation between abnormal FHR patterns and umbilical cord blood gas measurements

TABLE 9-3	CRITERIA USED TO DEFINE TYPES OF ACIDEMIA IN NEWBORNS WITH AN UMBILICAL ARTERIAL PH LESS THAN 7.20		
Classification	**P_{CO_2} (mm Hg)**	**HCO_3^- (mEq/L)**	**Base deficit (mEq/L)***
Respiratory	High (> 65)	Normal (≥ 22)	Normal (−6.4 ± 1.9)
Metabolic	Normal (< 65)	Low (≤ 17)	High (−15.9 ± 2.8)
Mixed	High (≥ 65)	Low (≤ 17)	High (−9.6 ± 2.5)

*Means ± SD are included in parentheses.
From the American College of Obstetricians and Gynecologists. Assessment of fetal and newborn acid-base status. Technical Bulletin No. 127. Washington, DC, April 1989.

and newborn outcome.[40] Because the correlation is poor, it is important to remember that a newborn may suffer multi-organ system damage, including neurologic injury, even in the absence of a low pH and a low Apgar score.

As Dr. Apgar emphasized in 1962, the most important components of newborn assessment are a careful physical examination and continued observation for several hours.[46] Additional information can be gained from the antenatal history, Apgar scores, and umbilical cord blood gas and pH measurements, provided clinicians are aware of the proper methods of interpretation and the limitations of these methods of assessment.

Respiration and Circulation

There are some similarities between the initial assessment of the newborn and the initial assessment of an adult who requires resuscitation. In both situations, the physician should give immediate attention to the ABCs of resuscitation (i.e., airway, breathing, circulation).

The normal respiratory rate of the newborn is between 30 and 60 breaths per minute. Breathing should begin by 30 seconds and be regular by 90 seconds of age. The newborn who is not breathing by 90 seconds of age has either primary or secondary apnea. These two distinct apneic states have been observed in a neonatal rhesus monkey model.[14] During intrauterine surgery, a plastic bag was placed over the fetal head and intravascular catheters were placed for postdelivery monitoring and blood sampling. After surgery, the fetus was delivered vaginally. Immediately after delivery, gasping motions were observed for approximately 1 minute; this was followed by a 1-minute period of apnea, then 5 minutes of gasping motions, and a final period of apnea. The two periods of apnea have been called *primary* and *secondary* (or *terminal*) *apnea.* During **primary apnea,** tactile stimulation of the newborn monkey initiated breathing efforts. This was not the case during **secondary apnea.** The heart rate was low during both periods of apnea; however, blood pressure decreased only during secondary apnea. By the time of the onset of secondary apnea (approximately 8 minutes after birth), the pH was 6.8 and the Pa_{O_2} and Pa_{CO_2} were less than 2 and 150 mm Hg, respectively. This experimental model illustrates two important points. First, distinguishing primary from secondary apnea is not possible without measuring blood pressure and/or blood gases and pH. Second, by the time secondary

apnea has begun, blood gas measurements have deteriorated significantly. Therefore, during evaluation of the apneic newborn, aggressive resuscitation must be initiated promptly if tactile stimulation does not result in the initiation of spontaneous breathing.

Assessment of the adequacy of respiratory function requires comprehensive observation for signs of newborn respiratory distress. These signs include cyanosis, grunting, flaring of the nares, retracting chest motions, and unequal breath sounds. The adequacy of respiratory function can also be assessed by the estimation of Sa_{O_2}. The reliability of pulse oximetry for the assessment of newborn Sa_{O_2} was questioned initially because of concerns regarding the accuracy of spectrophotometric assessments of fetal hemoglobin and the difficult signal detection caused by the rapidity of the newborn's heart rate.[94-96] Newer-generation pulse oximeters employ signal extraction and averaging techniques, and they provide more reliable measurements than conventional oximeters, especially when poor perfusion, patient movement, and ambient light artifacts are present.[67,97]

Pulse oximetry provides accurate estimates of Sa_{O_2} during periods of stability, but it may overshoot during periods of a rapid decrease in saturation.[98] The Sa_{O_2} (Sp_{O_2}) measurements may fluctuate in the delivery room as a result of the ongoing transition from the fetal to the adult circulation. Overall, the newer-generation pulse oximeters reliably provide continuous noninvasive Sa_{O_2} measurements and are useful for monitoring the newborn.[99]

The pulse oximeter sensor should be applied to the newborn's right upper extremity. This extremity receives preductal blood flow *(vide supra);* therefore, right upper extremity Sa_{O_2} measurements provide a more accurate assessment of CNS oxygenation, because CNS blood flow also is preductal.[21] Sensor placement can be difficult on skin that is wet and that may be covered with vernix caseosa. It may be easier to place the sensor over the right radial artery rather than on a finger, especially in preterm infants.[97]

It is technically difficult to obtain an arterial blood sample from a newborn; thus neonatal arterial blood samples are rarely obtained in the delivery room. It is helpful to cannulate the umbilical artery in infants who will require frequent blood sampling. This procedure often requires the use of microinstruments (especially in preterm and VLBW infants) and the ability to monitor an infant's condition while the infant is obscured from view by surgical drapes; thus this procedure is usually performed in the neonatal intensive care unit.

The normal heart rate in the newborn is 120 to 160 beats per minute (bpm). The heart rate may be greater than 160 bpm in the tiny preterm newborn, but it should be within the range of 120 to 160 bpm by 28 weeks' gestational age. The heart rate can be determined in several ways. The clinician can lightly grasp the base of the umbilical cord to feel the arterial pulsations. (This method cannot be used in situations in which the pulsations become difficult to feel, such as with an infant with a low cardiac output.) Alternatively, the clinician can listen to the apical heartbeat. When either of these two methods is used, the evaluator should tap a hand with each heartbeat so that other members of the resuscitation team are aware of the rate. A third method involves the use of a cardiotachometer, which is a monitor that detects the heart rate by means of electrodes taped to the chest and emits a sound for each beat. Use of this monitor—unlike the use of the first two methods—eliminates the need for an additional team member.

Measurement of arterial blood pressure is not a priority during the initial assessment and resuscitation of the newborn.[4] However, observation for signs of abnormal circulatory function is considered essential. These signs include cyanosis, pallor, mottled coloring, prolonged capillary refill time, and weak or absent pulses in the extremities. One of the causes of abnormal circulatory function is hypovolemia. Hypovolemia should be anticipated in cases of bleeding from the umbilical cord or the fetal side of the placenta or whenever a newborn does not respond appropriately to resuscitation. The hypovolemic newborn may exhibit not only signs of abnormal circulatory function but also tachycardia and tachypnea. (Neonatal hypovolemia usually does not accompany placental abruption, which may cause maternal bleeding or other conditions associated with fetal asphyxia.)

Neurologic Status

The initial neurologic assessment of the newborn requires only simple observation. The newborn should demonstrate evidence of vigorous activity, including crying and active flexion of the extremities. Signs of possible neurologic abnormality include apnea, seizures, hypotonia, and unresponsiveness. Newborns should be assessed for physical signs of hypoxic-ischemic encephalopathy (HIE) (Table 9-4). The different stages of HIE are associated with different outcomes: stage I, good; stage II, moderate; and stage III, poor.[100] While detailed neurologic assessment is performed after the newborn is transferred to the neonatal intensive care unit, assessment of tone, baseline heart rate, respirations, and reflex activity are part of both the Apgar scoring system and the HIE assessment and are done initially in the delivery room.

Gestational Age

When evaluating a very small newborn whose gestational age appears to be lower than that of viability, the evaluator must consider whether it is appropriate to initiate and maintain resuscitation efforts. The neonatal gestational age often is assessed by use of the scoring systems described by Dubowitz et al.[101] and Ballard et al.[102] The **Dubowitz system** makes use of an external score based on physical characteristics described earlier by Farr et al.[103,104] and a neurologic score. The **Ballard system** uses simplified scoring criteria to assess gestational age. Ballard et al.[102] eliminated certain physical criteria such as edema and skin color because of the unreliability of these criteria in some clinical conditions. In addition, they abbreviated the neurologic criteria, based on the observations of Amiel-Tison.[105]

Both the Dubowitz and Ballard scores are most accurate when they are used to estimate gestational age at 30 to 42 hours after delivery rather than during the first several minutes after birth[102]; therefore these scores are of limited value in determining the gestational age immediately after delivery.

These scoring systems are also less accurate in very small, preterm infants. In one study of 100 preterm babies with birth weights less than 1500 g, agreement among antenatal measures of gestational age (e.g., last menstrual period, ultrasonography determination) and postnatal measures (e.g., Dubowitz and Ballard scores) was poor.[106] Both scoring systems overestimated gestational age in this subset of VLBW babies. Ballard et al.[107] refined the Ballard score to provide a more accurate estimate of gestational age in preterm babies (Figure 9-3). The new Ballard score assesses **physical**

TABLE 9-4	STAGES OF NEONATAL HYPOXIC-ISCHEMIC ENCEPHALOPATHY	
Stage I HIE	**Stage II HIE**	**Stage III HIE**
Irritable	Lethargic/obtunded	Coma
Normal respirations	Depressed respirations	Apnea
Hypertonic	Hypotonic	Flaccid
Increased reflexes	Decreased reflexes	Absent reflexes
No seizures	Occasional seizures	Status epilepticus or nearly isoelectric electroencephalogram
Good outcome	**Moderate outcome**	**Poor outcome**

HIE, Hypoxic-ischemic encephalopathy.
Adapted from Eicher DJ, Wagner C. Update on neonatal resuscitation. J South Car Med Assoc 2002; 98:115.

criteria such as eyelid fusion, breast tissue, lanugo hair, and genitalia and **neurologic criteria** such as wrist "square window." (The square window assessment is performed by flexing the infant's wrist on the forearm and noting the angle between the hypothenar eminence and the ventral aspect of the forearm [Figure 9-3]). Although the new Ballard score may be more accurate than the older score for the assessment of preterm infants, inconsistencies occur with all of these methods. Of particular interest is the observation that fetuses of different racial origin mature at different rates (i.e., black fetuses mature faster than white fetuses); this suggests that gestational-age scoring systems should be race specific.[108]

Another commonly used criterion for the estimation of gestational age is birth weight. Normal values for birth weight are published and readily available.[109] Although birth weight may help physicians estimate the gestational age of an otherwise healthy preterm baby, physicians cannot rely on birth weight to provide an accurate estimate of gestational age in a baby who suffered from intrauterine growth restriction or who is large for gestational age.

Because of the potential for inaccurate gestational age estimation in the delivery room, it is best not to use these scoring systems to guide decisions regarding the initiation or continuation of neonatal resuscitation immediately after delivery. In most circumstances, the newborn's response to resuscitative efforts is the best indicator of whether further intervention is warranted.

NEONATAL RESUSCITATION

The equipment and medications needed for neonatal resuscitation are listed in Box 9-3. Equipment, supplies, and medications should be checked regularly to ensure that all components are available and functional.

Care of the newborn ideally begins as soon as the head is delivered, before the baby takes its first breath. First the mouth and then the nose should be suctioned gently with a bulb syringe to remove residual amniotic fluid, mucus, blood, and meconium. (The management of the newborn who has expelled meconium into the amniotic fluid is discussed separately.)

After delivery is complete, the newborn is transferred to the resuscitation area. The availability of sterile blankets allows the individual performing the delivery to remain ster-

Neuromuscular maturity

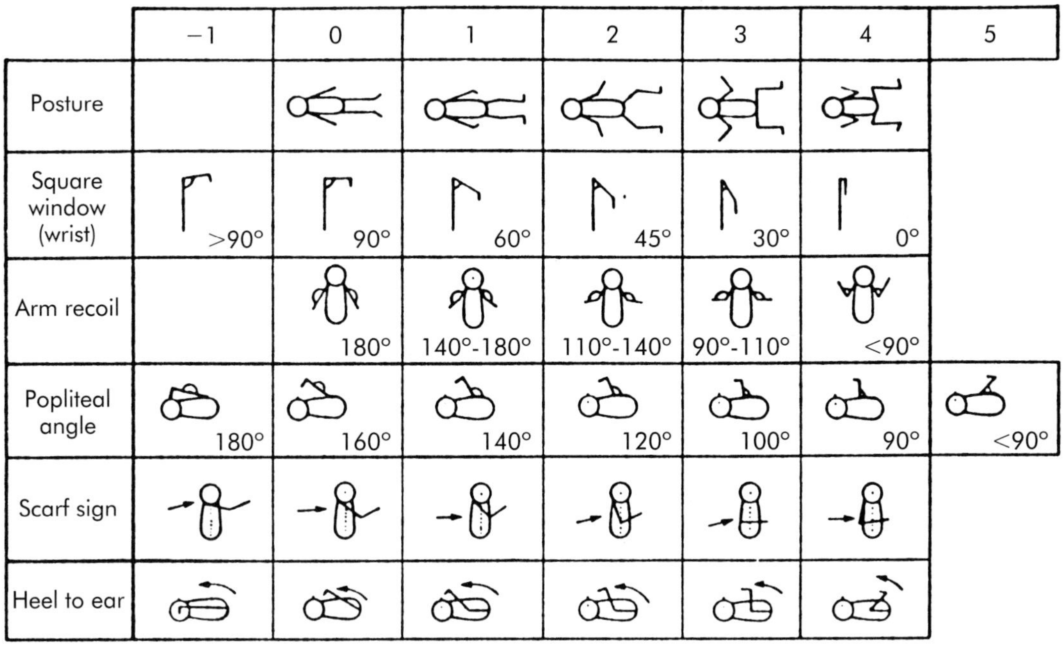

	−1	0	1	2	3	4	5
Posture		⬚	⬚	⬚	⬚	⬚	
Square window (wrist)	>90°	90°	60°	45°	30°	0°	
Arm recoil		180°	140°-180°	110°-140°	90°-110°	<90°	
Popliteal angle	180°	160°	140°	120°	100°	90°	<90°
Scarf sign	⬚	⬚	⬚	⬚	⬚	⬚	
Heel to ear	⬚	⬚	⬚	⬚	⬚	⬚	

Physical maturity

								Maturity rating
Skin	Sticky, friable, transparent	Gelatinous, red, translucent	Smooth, pink, visible veins	Superficial peeling and/or rash, few veins	Cracking, pale areas, rare veins	Parchment, deep cracking, no vessels	Leathery, cracked, wrinkled	
Lanugo	None	Sparse	Abundant	Thinning	Bald areas	Mostly bald		
Plantar surface	Heel-toe 40 to 50 mm: −1 <40 mm: −2	>50 mm no crease	Faint red marks	Anterior transverse crease only	Creases anterior two thirds	Creases over entire sole		
Breast	Imperceptible	Barely perceptible	Flat areola, no bud	Stippled areola, 1 to 2-mm bud	Raised areola, 3 to 4-mm bud	Full areola, 5 to 10-mm bud		
Eye/ear	Lids fused loosely: −1 tightly: −2	Lids open, pinna flat, stays folded	Slightly curved pinna, soft, slow recoil	Well-curved pinna, soft but ready recoil	Formed and firm, instant recoil	Thick cartilage, ear stiff		
Genitals —male	Scrotum flat, smooth	Scrotum empty, faint rugae	Testes in upper canal, rare rugae	Testes descending, few rugae	Testes down, good rugae	Testes pendulous, deep rugae		
Genitals —female	Clitoris prominent, labia flat	Prominent clitoris, small labia minora	Prominent clitoris, enlarging minora	Majora and minora equally prominent	Majora large, minora small	Majora cover clitoris and minora		

Maturity rating

Score	Weeks
−10	20
−5	22
0	24
5	26
10	28
15	30
20	32
25	34
30	36
35	38
40	40
45	42
50	44

FIGURE 9-3. New Ballard scoring system for clinical assessment of maturation in newborns. This scoring system has been expanded to include extremely preterm infants, and it has been refined to improve the accuracy of assessment of more mature infants. (Adapted from Ballard JL, Khoury JC, Wedig K, et al. New Ballard score, expanded to include extremely premature infants. J Pediatr 1991; 119:418.)

ile while transferring the newborn; this is especially important during cesarean deliveries. The timing of delivery should be noted, assessment and appropriate resuscitative measures should continue, and Apgar scores should be assigned at the appropriate intervals (Figure 9-4).

The examination table should be adjustable to allow for 30-degree Trendelenburg and reverse Trendelenburg positioning. The former favors the drainage of secretions, and the latter may increase PaO_2 during spontaneous ventilation.[110] In healthy, vigorous infants delivered at term gestation, the physician or nurse should promptly dry the skin and wrap the baby in a warm, dry blanket. Babies who are delivered preterm or who are depressed should also be placed beneath an overhead radiant warmer, which maintains body temperature while allowing access to the baby during resuscitation. Hypothermia can result in increased oxygen consumption

Box 9-3 EQUIPMENT AND DRUGS NEEDED FOR NEONATAL RESUSCITATION

SUCTION EQUIPMENT

Bulb syringe
Mechanical suction and tubing
Suction catheters, 5-F or 6-F, 8-F, and 10-F or 12-F
8-F feeding tube and 20-mL syringe
Meconium aspiration device

BAG-AND-MASK EQUIPMENT

Neonatal resuscitation bag with a pressure-release valve or pressure manometer (the bag must be capable of delivering 90% to 100% oxygen)
Face masks, newborn and preterm sizes (masks with cushioned rim preferred)
Oxygen with flowmeter (flow rate up to 10 L/min) and tubing (including portable oxygen cylinders)

INTUBATION EQUIPMENT

Laryngoscope with straight blades, No. 0 (preterm) and No. 1 (term)
Extra bulbs and batteries for laryngoscope
Tracheal tubes, 2.5, 3.0, 3.5, and 4.0 mm ID
Stylet (optional)
Scissors
Tape or securing device for tracheal tube
Alcohol sponges
CO_2 detector (optional)
Laryngeal mask airway (optional)

MEDICATIONS

Epinephrine 1:10,000 (0.1 mg/mL): 3- or 10-mL ampules
Isotonic crystalloid (normal saline or Ringer's lactate) for volume expansion: 100 or 250 mL
Sodium bicarbonate 4.2% (5 mEq/10 mL): 10-mL ampules
Naloxone hydrochloride 0.4 mg/mL: 1-mL ampules (or 1.0 mg/mL: 2-mL ampules)
Normal saline, 30 mL
Dextrose 10%, 250 mL
Normal saline "fish" or "bullet" (optional)
Feeding tube, 5-F (optional)
Umbilical vessel catheterization supplies
    Sterile gloves
    Scalpel or scissors
    Povidone-iodine solution
    Umbilical tape
    Umbilical catheters, 3.5-F, 5-F
    Three-way stopcock
Syringes, 1, 3, 5, 10, 20, and 50 mL
Needles, 25-, 21-, and 18-gauge, or puncture device for needleless system

MISCELLANEOUS

Gloves and appropriate personal protection
Radiant warmer or other heat source
Firm, padded resuscitation surface
Clock (timer optional)
Warmed linens
Stethoscope
Tape, $1/2$- or $3/4$-inch
Cardiac monitor and electrodes and/or pulse oximeter with probe (optional for delivery room)
Oropharyngeal airways

Adapted from Niermeyer S (ed), Kattwinkel J, Van Reempts P, et al. International Guidelines for Neonatal Resuscitation: An excerpt from the Guidelines 2000 for Cardiopulmonary Resuscitation and Emergency Cardiovascular Care: International Consensus on Science. Pediatrics 2000; 106:E29:1-16.

and metabolic acidosis,[111,112] and it results in a significant increase in mortality among preterm infants.[113]

Recent studies suggest that selective cerebral hypothermia may protect against brain injury in the asphyxiated infant. This treatment is not yet included in the neonatal resuscitation guidelines, because results of controlled human studies have not been reported.[3,35] However, the current guidelines recommend avoidance of *hyper*thermia.[7] In fact, avoidance of hyperthermia is one of the primary recommendations relevant to the prevention of neonatal encephalopathy in term infants.

The newborn should be positioned in a way that allows the airway to remain open and that favors the drainage of secretions. For example, the lateral decubitus/slight Trendelenburg position meets these criteria. Additional suctioning of the mouth and nose with a bulb syringe may be necessary if secretions accumulate.

The newborn with a normal respiratory pattern, heart rate, and color requires no further intervention. However, evaluation for choanal atresia can be performed at this time. This is accomplished by gently inserting a small suction catheter through each nostril into the nasopharynx. Vigorous nasal suctioning should be avoided, because it can cause trauma to the nasal mucosa and result in progressive edema and airway obstruction. The newborn is an obligate nasal breather; thus choanal atresia is a potentially lethal anomaly that requires immediate attention. If this anomaly is present (as evidenced by failure to pass the catheter nasally), an oral airway or endotracheal tube should be inserted, and the newborn should be evaluated for repair of the obstruction. The classic clinical presentation is an infant with cyanosis and respiratory distress at rest who becomes pink when crying.

Often the newborn has a normal respiratory pattern and heart rate but may not be pink. Acrocyanosis often persists for several minutes after delivery. If the newborn is breathing but not vigorous (i.e., Apgar score less than 8), the administration of supplemental oxygen may be beneficial. It is preferable to use a flow-through system, which does not require positive pressure for the delivery of oxygen. Indeed, administration of "blow-by" oxygen, without positive pressure, is adequate for most newborns.

Tactile stimulation should be used if the newborn does not breathe immediately; this consists of rubbing the back and flicking the soles of the feet. Tactile stimulation does not trigger respiratory efforts during secondary apnea in the newborn. Therefore, if the newborn does not begin to breathe spontaneously after tactile stimulation, the evaluator should begin positive-pressure mask ventilation with 100% oxygen. Overzealous tactile stimulation (e.g., slapping the back) is not useful; it provides no advantage over the more moderate methods and can result in traumatic injury.

If the newborn has a normal respiratory pattern but an abnormally slow heart rate (i.e., less than 100 bpm), positive-pressure ventilation with 100% oxygen should be performed until the heart rate increases to the normal range. If supplemental oxygen is not available, positive-pressure ventilation should be initiated with room air.[3]

High concentrations of oxygen (as opposed to ambient air) can result in an increased production of oxygen free radicals, which have been linked to hypoxia-reoxygenation injury. Because of this concern, recent studies have evaluated the use of room air versus 100% oxygen for neonatal resuscitation.[114,115] In a randomized trial of 609 term infants, no major outcome difference was found between the infants who received 100% oxygen and those who received room air for

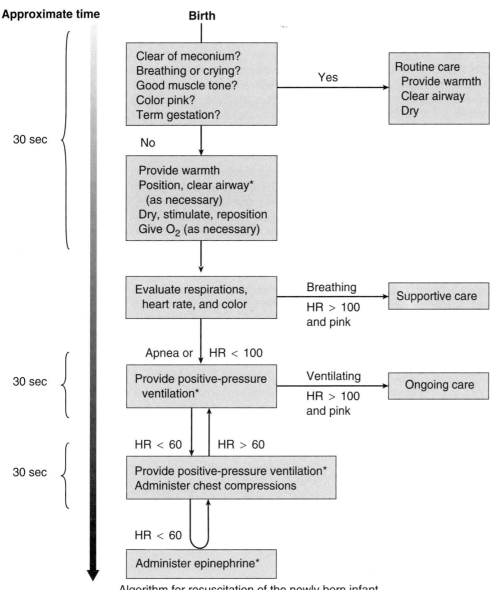

Approximate time

Birth

Clear of meconium?
Breathing or crying?
Good muscle tone?
Color pink?
Term gestation?

Yes → Routine care
Provide warmth
Clear airway
Dry

No

Provide warmth
Position, clear airway*
(as necessary)
Dry, stimulate, reposition
Give O_2 (as necessary)

30 sec

Evaluate respirations,
heart rate, and color

Breathing
HR > 100
and pink → Supportive care

Apnea or | HR < 100

30 sec

Provide positive-pressure
ventilation*

Ventilating
HR > 100
and pink → Ongoing care

HR < 60 | HR > 60

30 sec

Provide positive-pressure ventilation*
Administer chest compressions

HR < 60

Administer epinephrine*

Algorithm for resuscitation of the newly born infant.
*Endotracheal intubation may be considered at several steps

FIGURE 9-4. Algorithm for resuscitation of the newly born infant. (Adapted from Niermeyer S [ed], Kattwinkel J, Van Reempts P, et al. International Guidelines for Neonatal Resuscitation: An excerpt from the Guidelines 2000 for Cardiopulmonary Resuscitation and Emergency Cardiovascular Care: International Consensus on Science. Pediatrics 2000; 106:E29:7.)

resuscitation.[114] Use of a concentration of oxygen of less than 100% for resuscitation of some newborns may be incorporated into future guidelines for neonatal resuscitation. However, current guidelines continue to recommend the use of 100% oxygen for assisted ventilation during neonatal resuscitation. In preterm and/or asphyxiated newborns, it is believed that the benefits of 100% oxygen (including its pulmonary vasodilating effect, which aids in the prevention of PPHN) outweigh the risk.[116] Of course, the inspired oxygen concentration should be decreased as soon as possible—especially in preterm newborns—to decrease the risk of retinopathy of prematurity and pulmonary toxicity.[117] Oxygen saturations of 92% to 95% are thought to be adequate and appropriate for newborns of less than 34 weeks' gestation.[114,115]

Positive-pressure ventilation must be performed correctly to ensure that it is effective and does not cause barotrauma. A ventilation bag with a volume of 250 to 500 mL should be used. The circuit must contain a safety pop-off pressure valve (e.g., 35 cm H_2O) and/or a visible pressure gauge. An oxygen flow rate of 5 to 10 L/min is adequate. The mask must be of appropriate size and shape to ensure a good seal around the

nose and mouth. A variety of masks should be available to accommodate infants of all sizes and gestational ages. For infants with excessive occipital scalp edema (e.g., caput succedaneum), it may be helpful to place a small roll under the baby's shoulders to alleviate hyperflexion of its neck.

During the first assisted breath, positive pressure at 30 to 40 cm H_2O should be maintained for 4 to 5 seconds at the end of inspiration to overcome the surface tension of the lungs and open the alveoli.[118] The neonatal response to a large, rapid inflation of the lungs is a sharp inspiration of its own (Head's paradoxical reflex).[2] Subsequent breaths should be delivered at a rate of 40 to 60 per minute, with intermittent inspiratory pauses to prevent the development of atelectasis. The maximum pressure generated should range between 20 and 30 cm H_2O, with an inspiration-to-expiration ratio of approximately 1:1. If mask ventilation is needed for longer than 2 to 3 minutes, the stomach should be emptied with an orogastric catheter. Distention of the stomach with oxygen or air can compromise respiratory function in the newborn. This maneuver should be performed with care, because pharyngeal stimulation can result in arrhythmias and apnea.[119]

The adequacy of respiratory resuscitation can be monitored by its effect on heart rate: an increase in heart rate is the first reliable sign of effective oxygenation. By contrast, changes in color occur slowly and are a relatively poor index of successful resuscitation. Color also is difficult to assess in many newborns.

When the newborn's heart rate is greater than 100 bpm, positive-pressure ventilation can be stopped, and the newborn can be reevaluated for spontaneous respiratory effort. If the newborn does not begin to breathe and if an opioid effect is the suspected etiology, administration of **naloxone** (0.1 mg/kg) should be considered. Naloxone may be given intravenously, endotracheally, or, if perfusion is adequate, intramuscularly or subcutaneously.[3] Naloxone should be given only if it is indicated and with caution, because it can worsen the neurologic damage caused by asphyxia.[120,121] The duration of action of naloxone is shorter than that of many opioids. A newborn who responds to naloxone may require observation for as long as 24 hours, especially if the infant was exposed to a relatively long-acting opioid and/or a large dose of opioid in utero. Signs of recurrent respiratory depression may be noted. Use of naloxone is contraindicated in cases of maternal opioid abuse. Naloxone can precipitate acute neonatal opioid withdrawal, which may include seizures.

If positive-pressure mask ventilation does not improve oxygenation (as reflected by an increase in heart rate), prompt endotracheal intubation is indicated. Endotracheal intubation must be performed gently to avoid damage to the delicate newborn neck and airway. The size of the newborn's head is large relative to that of its body; therefore the newborn is in the "sniffing position" when it lies supine. In most cases, it is not necessary to elevate or hyperextend the newborn's head during laryngoscopy. The neonatal larynx is more anterior than that of the adult, and visualization often is easier when cricoid pressure is applied. The practitioner should hold the laryngoscope and apply cricoid pressure with the same hand. The thumb and first two fingers hold the base of the laryngoscope, the third finger rests on the mandible, and the fourth finger applies cricoid pressure. This technique promotes gentleness during airway manipulation. The distance from the gums to the larynx often is surprisingly short. A common mistake is to advance the laryngoscope blade too deeply—past the larynx and into the esophagus. When this occurs, the larynx falls into view if the laryngoscope blade is withdrawn slowly.

The diameter of the endotracheal tube should be large enough to allow adequate ventilation and insertion of a suction catheter (if needed) but small enough to avoid causing trauma and subsequent subglottic stenosis. The internal diameter/gestational age ratio should be less than 0.1 (e.g., 3.0 mm tube/35 weeks' gestation = 0.09).[122,123]

After endotracheal intubation, positive-pressure ventilation should be resumed with 100% oxygen using an appropriate circuit as described for mask ventilation. Assessment of proper tube placement is accomplished by listening for breath sounds in both axillae. The revised neonatal resuscitation guidelines suggest that exhaled CO_2 can be useful to confirm placement of the tube in the trachea.[3] As noted above, the fractional inspired oxygen concentration (FiO_2) should be reduced as soon as possible, especially in the preterm neonate. In practice, changes in FiO_2 often are made after the newborn has been stabilized and transferred to the neonatal intensive care unit. If the endotracheal tube will remain in the newborn, a chest radiographic study should be done to confirm the exact position of the tube.

Because endotracheal intubation and/or effective bag-and-mask ventilation may be difficult for those who are inexperienced with neonatal resuscitation, some investigators have evaluated the use of the laryngeal mask airway (LMA) for neonatal resuscitation.[124,125] The LMA is blindly inserted into the pharynx, and a cuff is inflated to provide a low-pressure seal around the larynx. This allows for more effective ventilation than bag-and-mask ventilation but does not require the skill and experience needed for endotracheal intubation. When evaluated in term infants requiring resuscitation at delivery, use of the LMA was found to be highly successful and without complications.[108,109] A recent report described the successful use of a size 1 LMA in a preterm newborn (35 weeks' gestation). Endotracheal intubation via direct laryngoscopy was unsuccessful, but intubation was accomplished successfully with fiberoptic bronchoscopy performed through the LMA.[126] The revised guidelines state that the LMA is an acceptable alternative means of establishing an airway that can be used by appropriately trained providers, especially when bag-and-mask ventilation is ineffective or attempts at endotracheal intubation have been unsuccessful.[3]

One cause of unequal breath sounds and eventual circulatory collapse is tension pneumothorax. Some physicians have recommended that providers of neonatal resuscitation should be skilled in needle aspiration of a tension pneumothorax.[2] This is accomplished by placing a 22- or 25-gauge needle in the second intercostal space in the mid-clavicular line (on the side where no breath or heart sounds are heard). Air will rush out of the needle hub, thereby reducing the tension pneumothorax.

Given the emphasis on ventilatory support, the need for chest compressions often is forgotten during neonatal resuscitation. Chest compressions are needed in only 0.03% of deliveries.[112] Moreover, the guidelines regarding chest compressions have changed.[3] In the past, chest compressions were indicated when the heart rate was less than 60 bpm or when the heart rate was between 60 and 80 bpm and was not increasing after 30 seconds of adequate ventilation with 100% oxygen. Review of scientific evidence prompted the International Liaison Committee on Resuscitation (ILCOR) to recommend the performance of chest compressions only when the heart rate is less than 60 bpm. The revised guidelines recommend that providers concentrate on improving ventilation when the heart rate is between 60 and 80 bpm; the rationale is that the performance of chest compressions can interfere with the ability to provide adequate ventilatory support, and adequate ventilation is the most important aspect of neonatal resuscitation.

Chest compressions can be done either with the first two fingers of one hand or with the thumbs of both hands; the latter method generates a better cardiac output and is preferred.[3,127] Pressure is applied over the sternum just below an imaginary line drawn between the nipples; pressure applied over the lower part of the sternum or xiphoid can result in abdominal injury. The sternum should be compressed to approximately one third to one half the anterior-posterior dimension of the chest, and the compression depth must be adequate to produce a palpable pulse.[3,128-130] The compression time should be slightly shorter than the release time; this may be the best timing for improving blood flow in the very young infant.[131] Ventilation will be compromised if the chest is compressed simultaneously with the administration of positive-pressure ventilation. The recommended ratio of compressions to breaths is 3:1.[132,133] The chest is compressed three times in

1½ seconds, leaving a ½ second for ventilation (thus 90 chest compressions and 30 breaths should be administered per minute). After 30 seconds of compressions and ventilations, the heart rate should be rechecked. Compressions should be resumed until the heart rate is greater than or equal to 60 bpm. Positive-pressure ventilation with 100% oxygen should be continued until the heart rate is greater than 100 bpm.

Medications are rarely required during neonatal resuscitation, because most newborns that require resuscitative measures respond well to satisfactory oxygenation and ventilation alone.[134] However, a variety of pharmacologic agents should be available in the delivery room (Box 9-3). **Epinephrine** is the drug recommended for use during neonatal resuscitation.[3] The current recommended practice is to administer epinephrine (0.01 to 0.03 mg/kg or 0.1 to 0.3 mL/kg of a 1:10,000 solution) if the heart rate remains less than 60 bpm after 30 seconds of adequate ventilation and chest compressions. (In the past, epinephrine administration was recommended if the heart rate remained less than 80 bpm after 30 seconds of chest compressions.) Administration of epinephrine is especially important if the heart rate is zero. Epinephrine increases the heart rate (the major determinant of newborn cardiac output), and it restores coronary and cerebral blood flow.[135]

Sodium bicarbonate is used infrequently during resuscitation. Because of its high osmolarity, it can cause hepatic injury at any gestational age, and it can cause cerebral hemorrhage in the preterm newborn[136]; it may also compromise myocardial and cerebral function.[137-139] It should be given only during prolonged resuscitation and only when adequate ventilation and circulation have been established. Arterial blood gas measurements and serum chemistry determinations should guide the use of sodium bicarbonate. The current recommended dose is 1 to 2 mEq/kg of a 0.5 mEq/mL solution given over at least 2 minutes by slow intravenous push.

Atropine is no longer recommended for use during the resuscitation of the newborn. Epinephrine is considered the drug of choice for the treatment of bradycardia.

Calcium administration is no longer recommended for neonatal resuscitation, unless it is given specifically to reverse the effect of magnesium (which may have crossed the placenta from the mother to the fetus). Evidence suggests that calcium administration causes cerebral calcification and decreases survival in stressed newborns.[140]

During neonatal resuscitation, the easiest way to administer epinephrine is by means of an endotracheal tube. Agents that may be given to the newborn using this route include lidocaine, atropine, naloxone, and epinephrine (**l-a-n-e**).[141-145] In the past, it was recommended that intratracheal doses be higher than intravenous doses to ensure absorption and delivery of an adequate amount of drug. However, current guidelines do *not* recommend a higher dose for intratracheal administration. For example, current guidelines recommend a uniform dose of epinephrine (i.e., 0.01 to 0.03 mg/kg) when it is given *either* intravenously or by means of an endotracheal tube. Dilution with normal saline to a volume of 1 to 2 mL is recommended.

Volume expanders must be given strictly according to the recommended dose. A continuous infusion is dangerous in the newborn, because it can easily result in the administration of an excessive fluid volume. Fluid overload can cause hepatic capsular rupture, brain swelling in the asphyxiated infant, or intracranial hemorrhage in the preterm infant. Fluids and medications can be administered either intravenously (most commonly through the umbilical vein) or, if necessary, intraosseously.

There are at least two ways to cannulate the umbilical vein (Figure 9-5). The first requires that an ample length of umbilical cord be left attached to the newborn at delivery; this should be discussed with the obstetrician before delivery, especially if resuscitation is anticipated. A 20- or 22-gauge catheter can be inserted into the umbilical vein using the same technique that is used to cannulate a peripheral vein. The standard intravenous catheter is relatively stiff; therefore, it must be inserted into the *distal* cord so that the tip does not extend into the abdomen, where it can cause trauma. The second method uses a soft catheter that is inserted into the cut end of the vein. It is advanced until blood return is noted but no more than 2 cm past the abdominal surface. If central

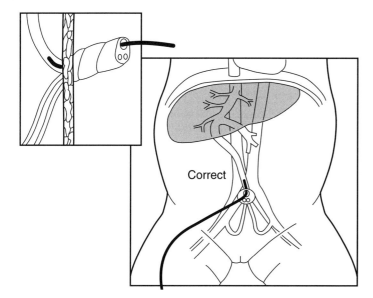
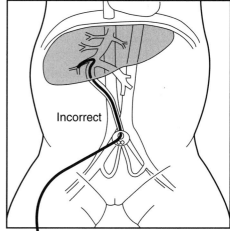

FIGURE 9-5. Cannulation of the umbilical vein. A 3.5-F or 5-F umbilical catheter with a single end hole nend a radiopaque marker should be used. For emergency use, the catheter should be inserted into the vein of the umbilical stump until the tip of the catheter is just below the skin level but free flow of blood is present. If the catheter is inserted farther, there is a risk of infusing solutions into the liver and possibly causing damage. (Adapted from Kattwinkel J, editor. Textbook of Neonatal Resuscitation. 4th ed. American Heart Association and American Academy of Pediatrics, Elk Grove Village, IL, 2000:6-6.)

venous pressure (CVP) monitoring is required during the newborn's hospital course, the soft umbilical catheter can be advanced through the ductus venosus into the inferior vena cava. Care must be taken to avoid leaving the tip in an intermediate location because of possible hepatic damage if a high-osmolarity substance (e.g., improperly diluted sodium bicarbonate) is injected. Other complications of umbilical venous catheterization are hemorrhage and sepsis.

Intraosseous access is accomplished by inserting a 20-gauge needle into the proximal tibia approximately 1 cm below the tibial tuberosity.[146] This technique may be easier to perform than umbilical venous cannulation for individuals who have little experience with intravenous catheterization in the newborn. Absorption from the newborn bone marrow into the general circulation occurs almost immediately.[147-150] This rapid absorption results from the preponderance of red bone marrow rather than yellow bone marrow, which is less vascular and is the dominant form of marrow after age 5. Complications related to this technique are rare and include tibial fracture (which occurs more often in older children)[151] and osteomyelitis. The risk of infection is proportional to the duration of intraosseous infusion[152-154]; therefore, the needle should be removed after 1 to 2 hours, and, if necessary, a more conventional route of access should be established. Current guidelines state that intraosseous access should be used for medication administration or volume expansion when venous access is difficult to achieve.[3]

The current guidelines for use of volume expanders have changed somewhat from previous recommendations. Normal saline or Ringer's lactate are the preferred volume expanders, given initially at 10 mL/kg over 5 to 10 minutes and repeated as necessary following reassessment for ongoing hypovolemia. Intravascular volume should be assessed by evaluating heart rate, capillary refill time, and color. If heavy blood loss is suspected, O-negative packed red blood cells may be used according to the same dosage regimen.[3] Red blood cells replete the oxygen-carrying capacity as well as the intravascular volume. O-negative blood should be available at all times for emergency use during neonatal resuscitation. If time permits, this blood should be cross-matched with a maternal sample before it is given to the newborn. Placental blood can be used for newborn volume expansion,[155] but this practice is discouraged in many institutions because of the risk of infection and/or transfusion of clots. Albumin administration is no longer recommended, because it carries a risk of infectious disease and has been associated with higher mortality.[156]

SPECIAL RESUSCITATION CIRCUMSTANCES

Meconium Aspiration

A great deal of interest has centered on the management of the newborn whose airway has been exposed to meconium-containing amniotic fluid. Meconium is present in the intestinal tract of the fetus after approximately 31 weeks' gestation. Meconium-stained amniotic fluid is present in approximately 10% to 15% of all pregnancies; the incidence is higher in postterm pregnancies. Intrapartum passage of meconium may be associated with fetal stress and hypoxia.[157,158] Among newborns exposed to meconium in the amniotic fluid, as many as 60% have meconium in the trachea.

Meconium aspiration syndrome (MAS) is defined as respiratory distress in a newborn whose airway was exposed to meconium and whose chest radiographic study exhibits char-

acteristic findings, including pulmonary consolidation and atelectasis.[159] Treatment of MAS often involves the use of positive-pressure ventilation and is associated with a 5% to 20% incidence of pneumothorax from pulmonary air leaks.[160] Extracorporeal membrane oxygenation (ECMO) and inhaled nitric oxide have been used for the treatment of MAS.[161-163] In one study of 176,790 infants born between 1973 and 1987, the annual death rate from MAS was as high as 6 per 10,000 live infants.[164]

Prevention of MAS is preferable to treatment, and preventive measures should be taken both before and after delivery. FHR monitoring and fetal scalp blood pH determination (when indicated) help detect fetal stress that can lead to the passage of meconium.[165] When moderate or thick meconium-stained amniotic fluid is noted during labor, transcervical amnioinfusion often is performed in an attempt to decrease the incidence and severity of MAS.[166,167]

Since 1974, neonatologists have attempted to determine whether peripartum suctioning of the newborn's airway decreases the risk of developing MAS. Gregory et al.[164] published the original study of 80 meconium-exposed newborns who were delivered either vaginally or by cesarean section. All of these infants underwent endotracheal intubation and suctioning after delivery. In 34 infants, no meconium was observed below the vocal cords; none of these infants developed MAS. Meconium was noted below the cords in the remaining 46 infants, and a total of 16 (35%) of these infants developed MAS. The authors concluded that "all infants born through thick, particulate, or 'pea soup' meconium should have the trachea aspirated immediately after birth."[164]

Another study conducted soon thereafter reviewed the delivery room airway management of newborns who required intensive care unit admission for the treatment of MAS.[168] The authors observed that 37% of infants who developed MAS had undergone endotracheal suctioning, whereas 85% of those who did *not* develop MAS had undergone endotracheal suctioning. Almost 20% of the infants with MAS died; most of those that died had not undergone endotracheal suctioning. The authors concluded that immediate endotracheal suctioning is indicated for infants exposed to meconium.[168]

A third study, which was published in 1976, investigated the effect of pharyngeal suctioning (immediately after delivery of the fetal head) on the incidence of MAS.[169] The purpose of this early suctioning (before delivery of the thorax) was to remove the meconium from the pharynx before the newborn took the first breath; this would prevent meconium passage into the distal areas of the lung and therefore prevent MAS. In this study, 273 meconium-exposed infants underwent early pharyngeal suctioning. Afterward, all underwent laryngoscopy, but only those who had visible meconium below the cords (two of 273 infants) underwent endotracheal intubation and suctioning. Only one of these two infants developed MAS, whereas none of the 271 who received only pharyngeal suctioning developed MAS. None of the infants died.[169]

There has been controversy regarding whether severe MAS is caused by meconium aspiration or whether the pathophysiologic changes in the lung may be caused by intrauterine stress such as asphyxia or sepsis. Two schools of thought have emerged. One school believes that the development of MAS is primarily an intrauterine event caused by fetal stress. Hypoxia induces pathologic changes in the pulmonary vasculature, which results in pulmonary hypertension and respiratory distress after birth. The pulmonary damage is independent of meconium aspiration; therefore, it is not prevented by the suctioning of meconium. The other school believes that MAS is the direct result of meconium aspiration and that the suctioning of meconium is indicated in selected high-risk cases of meconium-stained amniotic fluid.

Murphy et al.[170] examined the lungs of 11 newborns who had MAS and died within 4 days of birth. Of the 11 newborns, 10 also had a diagnosis of persistent pulmonary hypertension, and these 10 had evidence of excessive muscularization of the intraacinar arteries. Previous studies[171,172] had shown that muscularization of these arteries is not a normal finding in the fetus or neonate. Meyrick and Reid[173] had earlier shown that chronic hypoxia (i.e., at least 4 weeks' duration) but not acute hypoxia results in pulmonary vascular muscularization in an animal model. Murphy et al.[170] concluded that the observed changes in the 1- to 4-day-old human lung could not be explained by the postdelivery effects of meconium aspiration; rather, they concluded that the pathologic findings in MAS must result from intrauterine maldevelopment of the pulmonary vasculature. They suggested a potential link between increased intestinal motility, passage of meconium, and precocious muscularization of the intraacinar arteries.

Perlman et al.[174] have challenged the belief that muscularization of the intraacinar arteries is an abnormal event in the newborn. They examined lung tissue from 62 newborns; 24 had meconium aspiration, 20 had meconium staining but no aspiration, and 18 had placental abruption without meconium aspiration or staining. The newborns with meconium aspiration or staining died within 48 hours of birth. Meconium was found in the lungs of all newborns with meconium aspiration. Newborns with either meconium aspiration or staining showed a greater inflammatory response than those with placental abruption. The authors identified muscularized intraacinar arteries in *all* newborns except for one infant in the group with meconium staining. They observed no difference in the degree of muscularization among these three groups. The authors stated that this increased muscularization is not an abnormal finding indicative of intrauterine stress. They also noted that muscularization of these arteries normally occurs in the fetus,[175-177] but its degree is underestimated when the pulmonary vessels are injected and distended before examination.[178,179] They concluded that the etiology of pulmonary hypertension in newborns with MAS lies in the pathophysiology of meconium aspiration and its associated events and *not* in pulmonary vascular structural changes.

Some investigators have not confirmed that airway suctioning at birth prevents MAS and its associated mortality. One retrospective study examined the outcome of 1420 meconium-exposed live-born infants between 1977 and 1981.[180] The airway management included early pharyngeal suctioning followed by endotracheal intubation and suctioning if meconium was present in the pharynx. If it was necessary, repetitive intubations were performed until no meconium was seen during endotracheal suctioning. Meconium aspiration syndrome occurred in 30 (2.1%) of the meconium-exposed newborns; approximately 40% of those newborns died. The authors compared these results with those from studies in which combined obstetric and pediatric suctioning was not used. The authors concluded that vigorous airway management does not always prevent either MAS or death from MAS but that the incidence of symptomatic

MAS is reduced by early pharyngeal suctioning followed by endotracheal intubation and suctioning.

Falciglia et al.[181] compared the incidence of MAS in newborns who underwent early pharyngeal suctioning versus the incidence among those who underwent delayed suctioning after delivery of the thorax and the onset of breathing. Both groups of patients received subsequent endotracheal inspection and suctioning. There was no difference between the two groups in the incidence of MAS. The authors concluded that, because early suctioning did not decrease the incidence of MAS, it is likely that MAS is primarily the result of intrauterine events.

Linder et al.[182] performed a prospective study to assess the efficacy of routine endotracheal suctioning of meconium to prevent MAS. The authors randomized 572 meconium-exposed newborns into two groups. All infants were delivered vaginally and had 1-minute Apgar scores of greater than 8. All newborns received early pharyngeal suctioning. Infants in one group also underwent endotracheal suctioning, whereas those in a second group did not. Among the infants in the first group, four developed MAS, and two had laryngeal stridor. None of the infants in the second group had complications. The authors cautioned practitioners about the hazards of endotracheal intubation and suction. They suggested that vigorous newborns who have begun breathing before transfer to the resuscitation table derive little or no benefit from endotracheal suctioning and in fact may suffer some harm.

Ghidini and Spong[183] reviewed studies published between 1980 and 1999 to determine whether a causal relationship exists between meconium aspiration and MAS. They found that most cases of severe MAS were not causally related to meconium aspiration but rather resulted from intrauterine stress. They concluded that severe MAS is a misnomer because, in most cases, much more than meconium aspiration has contributed to the damage to the lung. The implication is that, when severe MAS occurs, inadequate suctioning at delivery or during resuscitation should not be considered the cause, and so other causes of intrauterine lung damage should be investigated.

The revised neonatal resuscitation guidelines include revised recommendations with regard to the suctioning of meconium at birth. In the past, determination of the consistency of the meconium (i.e., thin versus thick or particulate) guided the decision as to whether endotracheal suctioning was indicated. The current recommendations do not depend on the consistency of the meconium. When meconium is noted in the amniotic fluid, the infant's head should be delivered, and the hypopharynx should be suctioned. If the infant is not vigorous at birth (i.e., if the infant has absent or depressed respirations, a heart rate of less than 100 bpm, or poor muscle tone), direct tracheal suctioning should be performed to remove meconium from the airway.[3] If the infant is vigorous at birth, it is not necessary to perform endotracheal suctioning. Because of the potential harm of endotracheal intubation, this practice is no longer recommended for the vigorous infant, regardless of the presence of thick or particulate meconium. In this situation, meconium should be cleared from the mouth and then the nose using a bulb syringe or a large suction catheter (e.g., 12-F to 14-F).[184]

The preferred method of applying suction to the endotracheal tube has changed since the early 1970s. Originally, meconium was removed by means of oral suctioning with the resuscitator. A face mask and a DeLee trap were often used to prevent the transmission of newborn secretions into the resuscitator's mouth, but this was not always successful.[185] Conversely, secretions apparently can be transmitted from the resuscitator to the newborn, as noted in a case report of a newborn who contracted herpes simplex virus infection from the resuscitating physician.[186] In contemporary practice, endotracheal suctioning is performed by connecting the endotracheal tube to a meconium aspirator that has been connected to a regulated suction source.[187] Suction is then applied as the endotracheal tube is withdrawn. Repeated endotracheal suctioning is performed until little additional meconium is recovered or until the heart rate indicates that other resuscitative measures (e.g., oxygenation, ventilation) should be begun.[3] If a vigorous meconium-stained newborn subsequently develops apnea or respiratory distress, endotracheal suctioning of meconium should be performed before the administration of positive-pressure ventilation.

Because the passage of meconium has been associated with fetal stress and hypoxia, the liberal administration of supplemental oxygen to meconium-exposed newborns is recommended (after suctioning). Once the newborn has a normal heart rate, the resuscitator should gently pass a soft nasogastric or orogastric catheter to remove gastric meconium that may have been swallowed and could later be regurgitated and aspirated.

Preterm Infant

The preterm newborn, especially the VLBW infant, is at increased risk for problems with multiple organ systems simply because of immaturity. During resuscitation, the physician should give special attention to the effect of prematurity on the lungs and the brain. Before the addition of surfactant and high-frequency ventilation to the therapeutic armamentarium of the neonatologist, pulmonary hyaline membrane disease (also known as *neonatal respiratory distress syndrome* [NRDS]) was the overwhelming obstacle in the attempted salvage of the very preterm newborn.

Between 1970 and 2000, the proportion of infants weighing less than 1500 g at delivery increased from 1.17% to 1.45%.[188] The survival rate of these 500 to 1500 g infants has increased to approximately 85%.[189] Of these, approximately 5% to 10% develop what is characterized as cerebral palsy, and 25% to 50% exhibit behavioral and cognitive deficits that result in important school problems[189-191] (see Chapter 10). These VLBW infants comprise a tiny proportion of the birth population, but they are at the highest risk for developing cerebral palsy; infants weighing less than 1500 g at birth account for 25% of cases.[58]

Markers for brain injury affecting preterm infants are germinal matrix intraventricular hemorrhage (IVH) and periventricular leukomalacia. The brain injury may occur either as a consequence of the IVH and its sequelae or as an associated finding.[188] The incidence of germinal matrix IVH in preterm infants has declined from 35% to 50% in the late 1970s and early 1980s to approximately 15% in the mid-1990s.[192] Volpe[188,192] has stated that this decrease in the incidence of IVH does not mean that the problem is becoming less important given that the incidence is directly related to degree of prematurity,[193] and survival rates for very preterm infants continue to increase. Periventricular leukomalacia, which is the classic neuropathology associated with hypoxic-ischemic cerebral injury in the preterm infant, frequently accompanies IVH.[194]

The fragility of the immature subependymal germinal matrix predisposes the preterm newborn to the development of IVH. The hemorrhage originates from the endothelial cell-lined vessels that course through the germinal matrix in free communication with the venous circulation (i.e., the capillary-venule junction). The mechanism of damage to these endothelial cells and to the integrity of these capillaries has been investigated in the fetal lamb[195] and beagle puppy[196] models and in newborn humans by means of Doppler velocimetry.[197]

Volpe[198-200] has reviewed the theories of the pathogenesis of germinal matrix IVH. He has concluded that the pathogenesis of IVH is multifactorial; different combinations of factors are relevant in different patients. The three major categories in the pathogenesis of IVH are intravascular, vascular, and extravascular. **Intravascular factors** include fluctuating cerebral blood flow (CBF), which can result from respiratory disturbances in the ventilated preterm infant with neonatal respiratory distress syndrome[197,201]; increases in CBF[202]; increases in cerebral venous pressure[203]; decreases in CBF followed by reperfusion; and platelet and coagulation disturbances.[204] **Vascular factors** include the tenuousness of the capillary integrity of the germinal matrix and the vulnerability of the matrix capillaries to hypoxic-ischemic injury.[205] **Extravascular factors** include deficient vascular support, excessive fibrinolytic activity, and a possible postnatal decrease in extravascular tissue pressure.[206]

Of special interest in the discussion of antepartum and intrapartum care and neonatal resuscitation are the possible interventions that may prevent or lessen the severity of IVH. The surest way to prevent germinal matrix IVH is the prevention of preterm birth. Infection and inflammation are the most common identified causes of preterm birth at the lowest relevant gestational age.[207] Antenatal treatment of infections has not been proven to prevent preterm labor or PROM.[58] Prevention of infection, if possible, may be an important way to decrease the risk of IVH. Another intervention that decreases the incidence of IVH is the transportation of the preterm mother while the fetus is still in utero to a center that specializes in the care of high-risk newborns.[188]

Various antenatal pharmacologic interventions have been tried for the prevention of IVH. Clinical trials of antenatal maternal administration of phenobarbital[208,209] and vitamin K[210,211] have yielded conflicting results, and their routine use is not currently recommended.[58]

Glucocorticoids are currently the most clearly beneficial antenatal pharmacologic intervention for the prevention of IVH. This was first noticed when obstetricians began giving betamethasone and dexamethasone to pregnant women to help accelerate fetal lung maturity. The mechanism behind this protection is thought to be improved neonatal cardiovascular stability, which results in less hypotension and less need for blood pressure treatment in these infants.[212] Antenatal betamethasone administration leads to decreased placental vascular resistance and increased placental blood flow.[213] This improvement in placental blood flow may decrease impairment of the preterm infant's cerebral autoregulation. In addition, glucocorticoids may stimulate the maturation of the germinal matrix.[188] There is consensus regarding the efficacy of a single course of corticosteroids in patients at risk for preterm delivery, but there remains controversy regarding the risks and benefits of *multiple* courses of steroids for women who remain undelivered 7 days after the initial dose. Obstetricians must balance the possible benefits versus the potentially deleterious effects on neuronal and organ growth (see Chapter 34).

Some studies have noted a lower incidence of cerebral palsy in infants of mothers given magnesium sulfate for the treatment of preeclampsia or for tocolysis.[214,215] However, most evidence does not suggest that maternal magnesium sulfate administration results in a decreased incidence of IVH, although the incidence of high-grade (III or IV) lesions may be decreased.[216] At least one group of investigators has suggested that antenatal exposure to magnesium sulfate results in an increased risk of adverse neonatal outcome (see Chapter 34).[217]

Volpe[188] has also noted that the avoidance of prolonged labor and/or vaginal breech delivery may help prevent IVH. Some investigators have suggested that early cesarean delivery—performed before the onset of the active phase of labor—may help prevent IVH in preterm infants. Data are needed to confirm this hypothesis before this practice can be recommended.[218]

Postnatal interventions that may prevent IVH include the avoidance of the overly rapid infusion of volume expanders or hypertonic solutions such as sodium bicarbonate.[136,188] The establishment of adequate ventilation is the most beneficial immediate intervention that helps preserve cerebrovascular autoregulation in the preterm infant. The prevention of hypoxemia and hypercarbia is essential, because they are both linked to pressure-passive cerebral circulation, which in turn leads to the development of IVH.[188]

Among infants who exhibit fluctuating cerebral blood flow velocity, Volpe's group has found that treatment with pancuronium bromide, which corrects this fluctuation, decreases the incidence and severity of IVH.[219] Volpe[188] has emphasized that the future direction of IVH prevention should involve trials of other pharmacologic agents for correcting fluctuating hemodynamic disturbances. Studies with meperidine[220] and fentanyl[221] have shown some benefit.

If the use of antepartum and intrapartum pharmacologic prophylaxis against IVH becomes part of preterm delivery management, the practice of obstetric anesthesia for preterm patients will be affected directly. For example, the conventional wisdom is that preterm infants are more sensitive than term infants to the effects of maternally administered agents such as analgesics[222] and that this effect is inherently deleterious. However, if this effect is found to protect the preterm infant brain from factors that may lead to IVH (e.g., hemodynamic instability), perhaps obstetric anesthesiologists will no longer attempt to avoid the placental transfer of pharmacologic agents but will deliberately administer these agents to the mother, with the intent that they reach the fetus.

Congenital Anomalies

Occasionally resuscitation of the newborn is complicated by congenital anomalies of the airway or diaphragm. These anomalies may manifest as respiratory distress, which resolves only when appropriate resuscitation techniques are used. For example, newborns are obligatory nose breathers. The diagnosis and management of choanal stenosis and atresia include placement of an oral airway or endotracheal intubation until a definitive surgical procedure can be performed.

Other congenital anomalies that cause upper airway obstruction include the following: (1) micrognathia, as in Pierre Robin syndrome; (2) macroglossia, as in Beckwith-Wiedeman syndrome; (3) glycogen storage disease type II;

(4) laryngeal webs; (5) laryngeal atresia; (6) stenosis or paralysis at the level of the vocal cords; (7) subglottic stenosis; (8) subglottic webs; (9) tracheal agenesis; and (10) tracheal rings. Obstruction also can occur as a result of tumors such as subglottic hemangiomas. The presence of a cleft palate may result in difficult manual ventilation. In an infant with micrognathia or macroglossia, airway patency may be maintained if the newborn is kept in the prone position; this position reduces posterior movement of the tongue into the pharynx. If macroglossia is extreme, use of an oral airway or a small nasogastric or orogastric suction catheter may be necessary to prevent complete obstruction of the pharynx by the tongue.

When respiratory distress and difficulty with bag-and-mask ventilation are encountered, laryngoscopy should be performed. The cause of the obstruction may be evident if it is supraglottic. Some supraglottic entities (e.g., laryngeal webs) may be treated successfully by forcing an endotracheal tube through the obstruction and into the trachea. Subglottic lesions may require tracheostomy. The help of an otolaryngologist may be invaluable during resuscitation of a newborn with congenital airway obstruction. If evidence of such a condition (e.g., laryngeal stenosis)[223] exists antepartum, it is best to have an otolaryngologist present at the time of delivery. If obstruction is first noted after delivery, the resuscitator should not hesitate to call for surgical assistance.

Fetal neck masses such as cervical teratoma and lymphangioma can lead to extrinsic airway compression. The resulting distortion of the airway can result in airway obstruction, and it may be difficult—if not impossible—to secure an airway in a timely fashion at the time of delivery. These masses often are diagnosed before delivery because of the associated occurrence of polyhydramnios resulting from esophageal compression. In these rare cases, a multidisciplinary team should be assembled to assist in securing the airway. Leichty et al.[224] have described a method to provide time to secure an airway; this method is known as the **ex utero intrapartum treatment (EXIT) procedure**. The procedure was used initially for the delivery of fetuses with a diaphragmatic hernia who had undergone intrauterine tracheal clip application for the induction of fetal lung growth (see Chapter 7).

The following summarizes the EXIT procedure used by Leichty et al.[224] in the management of five fetuses with life-threatening neck masses. The multidisciplinary team consisted of two or three pediatric surgeons, an obstetrician, a neonatologist, and an anesthesiologist. Following rapid-sequence induction and endotracheal intubation, maternal anesthesia was maintained with 50% nitrous oxide and isoflurane at 0.3% to 1.9% expired. Maternal muscle relaxation was maintained with vecuronium. The isoflurane concentration was titrated to achieve and maintain uterine relaxation to preserve uteroplacental circulation and fetal gas exchange. At the time of hysterotomy, nitrous oxide administration was discontinued. The fetal head and shoulders were delivered while the umbilical cord and lower torso remained in the uterus. The fetus was given additional agents intramuscularly (fentanyl, vecuronium, and atropine) to provide fetal analgesia and to prevent movement and breathing. The FHR and SaO_2 were monitored continuously by a pulse oximeter probe attached to the fetal hand. The surgeon performed direct laryngoscopy in an attempt to secure the airway with a 2.5- to 3.5-mm endotracheal tube. If the airway was not visualized adequately, a rigid bronchoscope was used. If an endotracheal tube still could not be passed, tracheostomy was performed.

After establishment of the airway, the infant was completely delivered. Maternal isoflurane was decreased to 0.3% expired, and oxytocin was administered to prevent uterine atony and excessive maternal bleeding.

Since its initial description, the EXIT procedure has been considered an option for fetuses with other congenital anomalies.[225] A common indication for the EXIT procedure is intrinsic airway obstruction. Intrinsic high airway obstruction from defects such as laryngeal webs, subglottic cysts, or tracheal atresias is classified as the **congenital high airway obstruction syndrome (CHAOS)**.[225] Use of the EXIT procedure has resulted in the first long-term surviving child with CHAOS.[226]

The EXIT procedure may also be useful in conditions such as severe congenital heart disease, when the need for emergent ECMO at birth is anticipated. The EXIT procedure allows for the placement of arterial and venous cannulas before umbilical cord clamping, thereby avoiding an unstable period between the termination of placental perfusion and the institution of ECMO.[225]

Other possible indications for the EXIT procedure include the resection of congenital cystic adenomatoid malformations and a first step in separation procedures for conjoined twins with cardiovascular involvement.

Noah et al.[227] have reviewed maternal outcomes associated with the EXIT procedure. In 34 patients who underwent the EXIT procedure between 1994 and 1999, short-term outcomes were compared with a control group who underwent non-emergent primary cesarean delivery. The EXIT procedure patients had higher estimated blood loss, but there was no difference in postoperative hematocrit or duration of hospital stay. The EXIT procedure patients had a higher rate of superficial wound infection (15% versus 2%), but there was no difference between the two groups in the incidence of endometritis.

Anesthetic considerations for the mother during the EXIT procedure include those relevant to general anesthesia for the mother undergoing cesarean delivery or other surgical procedures during pregnancy (see Chapters 16 and 25). Several volatile halogenated agents have been used for the EXIT procedure, including isoflurane, desflurane, and seroflurane.[225] Sevoflurane has the advantage of providing uterine relaxation similar to that achieved with isoflurane without the resulting tachycardia associated with isoflurane and desflurane. Sevoflurane also has the advantage of being eliminated quickly once the procedure is completed so that the uterus can readily contract in response to oxytocin.[228]

Esophageal atresia and **tracheoesophageal fistula** occur in 1 out of every 3000 births.[229] There are many variations of these anomalies, the most common being esophageal atresia with a distal tracheoesophageal fistula (80% to 90%). Newborns with a tracheoesophageal fistula are at increased risk for the pulmonary aspiration of gastric contents through the fistula into the lung. If the presence of a tracheoesophageal fistula is not known antepartum, it should be suspected if bubbling secretions are noted during spontaneous or bag-and-mask ventilation. Once a tracheoesophageal fistula is suspected, bag-and-mask ventilation should be discontinued, because its use may contribute to overdistention of the gastrointestinal tract with air; this can lead to difficulty in ventilation from impingement of the enlarged stomach on the diaphragm. The newborn should be kept in the reverse Trendelenburg position, and a suction catheter should be placed in the esophageal pouch to facilitate the removal of oral secretions. If mechanical ventilation is necessary, an endotracheal tube should be inserted, and the tip should be distal to the entrance of the fistula. This usually can be accomplished by the performance of a right mainstem bronchial intubation followed by a slow withdrawal of the tube until breath sounds are auscultated on the left; a lack of breath sounds over the stomach should then be confirmed. Percutaneous gastrostomy placement may be necessary during resuscitation to facilitate decompression of the gastrointestinal tract.

Congenital diaphragmatic hernia (CDH) occurs in approximately 1 in 4000 live births.[230] The mortality rate from CDH is 30% to 60%. Approximately 80% to 90% of cases occur on the left side and are the result of herniation of the gut through the posteriolateral defect of Bochdalek. During formation of the lung, herniation of the gut into the thoracic cavity results in hypoplasia of the lung tissue and pulmonary vasculature. This hypoplasia may be unilateral, but often it is bilateral because of the shift of mediastinal structures to the contralateral side. CDH should be suspected when a newborn has respiratory difficulty and a scaphoid abdomen; this abnormal abdominal shape results from the presence of abdominal contents in the thorax.

During resuscitation of the newborn with CDH, bag-and-mask ventilation is contraindicated, because it allows further distention of the gut, which will further impinge on the lung. If mechanical ventilation is required, endotracheal intubation should be performed and followed by the placement of a nasogastric or orogastric tube to ensure decompression of the gastrointestinal tract. Ventilation should consist of low-positive-pressure breaths (e.g., less than 15 cm H_2O, if possible) delivered at a rapid rate (e.g., 60 to 100 per minute). This low-pressure ventilation may decrease the risk of causing a pneumothorax on the side contralateral to the CDH. If a pneumothorax does occur, it must be evacuated promptly. In the newborn, this is accomplished initially by placing a 22-gauge needle into the second intercostal space in the midclavicular line and aspirating air with an attached stopcock and syringe.

Severe pulmonary hypertension often accompanies CDH. Maintenance of euthermia, normoxia, and hypocapnia ($Paco_2$ = 25 to 35 mm Hg) promote pulmonary artery blood flow.

Whenever congenital anomalies of the respiratory tract are noted, the presence of other anomalies should be suspected. It is important to evaluate the newborn promptly for cardiac malformations, especially if appropriate resuscitative efforts are not successful. Echocardiography is used for the investigation of cardiac structures and function.

ETHICAL CONSIDERATIONS

The current neonatal resuscitation guidelines address the ethical considerations of noninitiation or discontinuation of resuscitation in the delivery room.[3] Extremes of prematurity (<23 weeks' confirmed gestation) and severe congenital anomalies (e.g., anencephaly, confirmed trisomy 13 or 18) are examples of circumstances when noninitiation of resuscitation is considered appropriate. Because intrapartum confirmation of pertinent information may not be possible, it is recognized that initiation of resuscitation may occur and that discontinuation may then be appropriate after further information has been obtained and discussion with family has occurred. In some cases, a trial of therapy may be appropriate, and this does not always mandate continued support.

Discontinuation of resuscitation of an infant with cardiopulmonary arrest may be appropriate if spontaneous circulation has not occurred in 15 minutes. After 10 minutes of asystole, survival or survival without severe disabilities is very unlikely.[231-234]

NEUROBEHAVIORAL TESTING

It is difficult to detect subtle neurobehavioral differences among newborns during the assignment of Apgar scores or the performance of the initial neurologic examination; therefore, investigators have developed and studied methods of documenting newborn neurobehavioral status. In the past, the newborn was considered incapable of exhibiting higher cortical function. However, investigators have noted that the term newborn is able to sense and respond to a variety of stimuli in a well-organized fashion.[235-237]

In 1973, Brazelton[238] described the Neonatal Behavioral Assessment Scale (NBAS). Brazelton listed four variables as key determinants of newborn neurobehavior: (1) various prenatal influences (e.g., infection); (2) the degree of maturity of the infant, especially its CNS; (3) the effects of analgesics and anesthetics administered to the mother before and during delivery; and (4) the effects of difficulties encountered during delivery (e.g., trauma).[239] The NBAS was developed as a tool to detect neurobehavioral abnormalities that resulted from any of these four variables.

The NBAS consists of 47 individual tests; 27 tests evaluate behavior, and the remaining 20 evaluate elicited or provoked responses. The 47 tests can be completed in approximately 45 minutes. The NBAS evaluates the ability of the newborn to perform complex motor behaviors, to alter the state of arousal, and to suppress meaningless stimuli. The goal is to provide an extensive evaluation of newborn cortical function and to detect subtle differences among groups of infants. Habituation (i.e., the ability to suppress the response to meaningless, repetitive stimuli) is considered an excellent indicator of normal early cortical function.[240]

In 1974, Scanlon et al.[240] described the Early Neonatal Behavioral Scale (ENNS). The ENNS is based on descriptions of newborn neurobehavioral activity by Prechtal and Beintema,[241] Beintema,[242] and Brazelton.[239] The researchers selected tests that are easy to perform and score quantitatively during the neonatal period. The ENNS was developed primarily for the evaluation of the effects of maternal medications (e.g., analgesic and anesthetic agents) on newborn neurobehavior. The ENNS includes the following: (1) 15 observations of muscle tone and power, reflexes (e.g., rooting, sucking, Moro), and response to stimuli (e.g., light, sound, pinprick); (2) 11 observations of the infant's state of wakefulness; (3) an assessment of the ability of the newborn to habituate to repetitive stimuli; and (4) an overall general assessment of neurobehavioral status. The ENNS can be performed in 6 to 10 minutes.

In 1982, Amiel-Tison et al.[243] described the Neurologic and Adaptive Capacity Score (NACS). It was intended to differentiate drug-induced depression from depression resulting from asphyxia, birth trauma, or neurologic disease. The ENNS concentrates on the infant's habituation ability, but the NACS emphasizes motor tone as a key indicator of drug-induced abnormal neurobehavior. The basis for this emphasis on newborn motor tone is explained as follows: unilateral or upper body hypotonus may occur as a result of either birth trauma or anoxia, but global motor depression is more likely a result of anesthetic- or analgesic-induced depression. A total of 20 criteria are tested in the areas of adaptive capacity, passive tone (e.g., scarf sign), active tone (e.g., assessment of the flexor and extensor muscles of the neck), primary reflexes (e.g., Moro), and alertness. The total possible score is 40, and a score of 35 to 40 is considered normal. The NACS can be performed in 3 to 4 minutes.

Amiel-Tison et al.[243] examined interobserver reliability, and they assessed the correlation of results between the NACS and ENNS. A total of 61 infants underwent 183 NACS and 122 ENNS examinations; this yielded 3660 joint observations for the NACS examinations and 2074 joint observations for the ENNS examinations. The interobserver reliability was 93% for the NACS and 88% for the ENNS. Approximately 92% of infants with high scores on the ENNS scored equally well on the NACS. Brockhurst et al.[244,245] reviewed studies that have relied on the NACS, and they have questioned its reliability. Halpern et al.[246] examined 200 healthy term infants and found poor interrater reliability. Amiel-Tison[247] has reported her ongoing experience with the NACS, and she has documented good interrater reliability.

Anesthesiologists have used neurobehavioral testing primarily to document the effects of analgesic and anesthetic agents and techniques on newborn neurobehavior; the AAP[248] and the Food and Drug Administration[249,250] have recommended that these investigations be performed. Investigators have evaluated the effects of maternally administered systemic agents (e.g., meperidine, diazepam) on newborn neurobehavior, and many of these studies have demonstrated a transient serum concentration-dependent depression of newborn neurobehavior.[251-254] However, one study that controlled for differences in patient and labor and delivery characteristics noted only decreased habituation during NBAS examination after systemic administration of meperidine to the mother.[255] Similarly, maternal systemic administration of fentanyl minimally affects performance on the NACS.[256]

As is the case with many studies of systemic agents, studies of epidural anesthesia are often confounded by variables that are difficult to control, such as different patient populations, varied durations of labor, and multiple drug administrations. Scanlon et al.[240] introduced the ENNS in a study of the effect of maternal epidural anesthesia on newborn neurobehavior. The authors concluded that epidural anesthesia was associated with lower ENNS scores because of decreased muscle strength and tone. In this study, all patients who had received epidural anesthesia were considered part of one group, although 9 patients had received lidocaine and 19 had received mepivacaine. Further investigation revealed that epidural lidocaine, even when administered in larger doses for cesarean delivery, does not affect ENNS scores.[257] The difference in ENNS scores between the epidural and nonepidural groups, noted in the earlier study,[240] was most likely related to the use of mepivacaine rather than lidocaine.[258] As was observed with lidocaine, epidural bupivacaine, 2-chloroprocaine, and etidocaine—when administered for cesarean delivery—do not affect ENNS scores.[257,259] Kuhnert et al.[260] assessed performance on the NBAS in a group of infants exposed to either epidural lidocaine or 2-chloroprocaine. Although the authors observed subtle changes in neurobehavior in the group of infants whose mothers had received lidocaine, they concluded that other variables (e.g., mode of delivery) are more likely to affect neurobehavioral examination performance.

Sepkoski et al.[261] compared NBAS scores between two groups of vaginally delivered infants. In one group, the mothers had received epidural bupivacaine, and in the other group, the mothers had received no anesthesia or analgesia. The infants in the epidural group showed less alertness, less orientation ability, and less motor function maturity than the infants in the control group. However, variables such as duration of labor, incidence of oxytocin administration, and incidence of instrumental delivery were not similar between the two groups. Earlier, Abboud et al.[262] performed ENNS examinations on vaginally delivered infants whose mothers had received epidural bupivacaine. In this study, epidural administration of bupivacaine did not affect the ENNS scores. The maternal doses of epidural bupivacaine and the maternal venous and umbilical cord blood bupivacaine concentrations were similar to those noted by Sepkoski et al.[261] Abboud et al.[262] also noted normal ENNS scores for infants whose mothers had received epidural lidocaine or 2-chloroprocaine.

Critics of the ENNS and the NACS claim that these examinations fail to show subtle differences in neurobehavior that would be detected by the more comprehensive NBAS.[263] However, although some investigators have observed differences in NBAS performance among groups of infants exposed or not exposed to local anesthetics, confounding variables have prevented clear conclusions of cause and effect.

Hodgkinson et al.[264] observed that the subarachnoid administration of tetracaine for cesarean section did not adversely affect ENNS performance. Other studies have used the NACS to evaluate the effects of maternal epidural opioids[265-271] and epinephrine (in combination with a local anesthetic).[272-275] These drugs did not significantly affect NACS performance in these studies.

Other studies have used the ENNS and NACS to study the effects of general anesthetic agents on newborn neurobehavior. In a prospective, randomized study, Abboud et al.[276] assessed NACS performance at 15 minutes, 2 hours, and 24 hours of age in infants whose mothers received general, epidural, or spinal anesthesia for cesarean delivery. Women who received general anesthesia received thiopental 4 mg/kg followed by enflurane 0.5% with nitrous oxide 50% in oxygen. Although the NACS was lower at both 15 minutes and 2 hours of age in the infants in the general anesthesia group than in the infants in either regional anesthesia group, no difference in the NACS was noted at 24 hours of age.

Hodgkinson et al.[264] used the ENNS to evaluate outcomes among three groups of infants, all of which were delivered by elective cesarean section. One group of women received general anesthesia with thiopental 4 mg/kg followed by 50% nitrous oxide. A second group received general anesthesia with ketamine 1 mg/kg followed by 50% nitrous oxide. A third group received spinal anesthesia with 6 to 8 mg of tetracaine. The ENNS evaluations were conducted at 4 to 8 hours of age and again 24 hours later. During the 4- to 8-hour examination, infants in the spinal anesthesia group scored significantly higher on multiple components of the ENNS than did infants in either of the general anesthesia groups. At 24 hours, infants in the spinal anesthesia group scored significantly higher than those in the thiopental group in alertness, total decrement score, and overall assessment. Similarly, infants in the spinal anesthesia group scored higher than those in the ketamine group in alertness and overall assessment. No significant differences existed between the scores of the thiopental group infants and the ketamine group infants.[264] Palahniuk et al.[277] observed similar results in a study that compared groups of infants whose mothers received either epidural anesthesia or general anesthesia for elective cesarean section. Infants whose mothers had received thiopental and nitrous oxide scored significantly lower in the alertness component of the ENNS than infants whose mothers had received epidural lidocaine with epinephrine.

Stefani et al.[278] observed that subanesthetic maternal doses of enflurane or nitrous oxide did not affect newborn neurobehavior (as assessed by ENNS and NACS) at 15 minutes, 2 hours, and 24 hours of age. Abboud et al.[279] obtained similar results from NACS examinations of infants whose mothers had received subanesthetic doses of isoflurane.

In summary, subtle changes in newborn neurobehavior may result from factors such as antepartum maternal drug exposure. Parent-infant bonding and the ability of the infant to breast-feed may be adversely affected by these neurobehavioral changes.[239] These transient effects may seem trivial to some observers but important to others. With regard to the long-term neurologic outcome of individual infants, performance during neurobehavioral assessment may aid the observer in the formulation of a prognosis. However, as demonstrated with Apgar scores, the prognostic value of an isolated test score is likely to be lower than the prognostic value of multiple factors considered together during the overall assessment of an individual infant.

KEY POINTS

- The anesthesia care provider attending the mother should not be responsible for resuscitation of the newborn. However, all anesthesia care providers should be prepared to provide assistance during neonatal resuscitation when it is needed.
- Adverse conditions at birth (e.g., hypoxia, acidosis, profound hypovolemia, hypothermia) may impair the transition from intrauterine to extrauterine life. Impaired transition may manifest as persistent pulmonary hypertension of the newborn (PPHN).
- The Apgar scoring system provides the practitioner with a standard guide for assessing the need for newborn resuscitation.
- No single factor should be considered prognostic of poor neurologic outcome. A combination of factors, including severe metabolic acidemia and Apgar scores of 3 or less beyond 5 minutes, are included among the criteria that suggest the occurrence of intrapartum hypoxia of sufficient severity to cause long-term neurologic impairment. However, not all infants who fulfill these criteria suffer permanent neurologic injury.
- Severe mixed or metabolic acidemia—but not respiratory acidemia alone—is associated with an increased incidence of neonatal complications and death.
- During evaluation of the apneic newborn, assisted ventilation should be initiated promptly if tactile stimulation does not result in the initiation of spontaneous breathing.

- In most circumstances, decisions regarding the initiation or continuation of resuscitation in the delivery room should be based on the newborn's response to resuscitative efforts rather than an estimation of gestational age.
- During the first assisted breath, positive pressure (30 to 40 cm H_2O) should be maintained for 4 to 5 seconds at the end of inspiration to overcome the surface tension of the lungs and open the alveoli. Thereafter, the maximum pressure generated for all assisted breaths should range between 20 and 30 cm H_2O.
- All meconium-exposed newborns should undergo nasopharyngeal and oropharyngeal suctioning before delivery of the thorax. Further suctioning (by means of endotracheal intubation) may be necessary, especially for those meconium-exposed newborns believed to be at highest risk for developing meconium aspiration syndrome (i.e., those who are depressed).

REFERENCES

1. Nogami WM. Neonatal resuscitation: Who should respond? SOAP Newsletter. 1997; Summer:5-6.
2. Ostheimer GW. Resuscitation of the newborn. In: Stanley TH and Schafer PG, editors. Pediatric and Obstetrical Anesthesia. Dordrecht, Netherlands, Kluwer Academic Publishers, 1995:159-86.
3. Niermeyer S (editor), Kattwinkel J, Van Reempts P, et al. International Guidelines for Neonatal Resuscitation: An excerpt from the Guidelines 2000 for Cardiopulmonary Resuscitation and Emergency Cardiovascular Care: International Consensus on Science. Pediatrics 2000; 106:E29.
4. Kattwinkel, J, editor. Textbook of Neonatal Resuscitation. 4th edition. American Heart Association and American Academy of Pediatrics, Elk Grove Village, IL, 2000.
5. Eicher DJ, Wagner CL. Update on neonatal resuscitation. J South Car Med Assoc 2002; 98:114-20.
6. American College of Obstetrics and Gynecologists Committee on Obstetric Practice and American Society of Anesthesiologists Committee on Obstetric Anesthesia. ACOG Committee Opinion No. 256, May 2001.
7. Heyman HJ, Joseph NJ, Salem MR, Heyman K. Anesthesia personnel, neonatal resuscitation, and the courts (abstract). Anesthesiology 1991; 75:A1074.
8. Gibbs CP, Krischer J, Peckham BM, et al. Obstetric anesthesia: A national survey. Anesthesiology 1986; 65:298-306.
9. Hawkins JL, Gibbs CP, Orleans M, et al. Obstetric anesthesia workforce survey, 1981 versus 1992. Anesthesiology 1997; 87:135-43.
10. Gaiser RR, Lewis SB, Cheek TG, Gutsche BB. Neonatal resuscitation and the anesthesiologist (abstract). Anesthesiology 2001; 94:A80.
11. Gaiser RR, Lewin SB, Cheek TG, Gutsche BB. Anesthesiologists' interest in neonatal resuscitation certification. J Clin Anesth 2001; 13:374-6.
12. Chadwick HS, Posner K, Caplan RA, Ward RJ, Cheney FW. A comparison of obstetric and nonobstetric anesthesia malpractice claims. Anesthesiology 1991; 74:242-9.
13. Heyman HJ. Neonatal resuscitation and anesthesiologist liability. Anesthesiology 1994; 81:783.
14. Dawes GS. Foetal and Neonatal Physiology. Chicago, Mosby, 1968: 160-76.
15. Rudolph AM, Heymann MA. Fetal and neonatal circulation and respiration. Annu Rev Physiol 1974; 36:187-207.
16. Rudolph AM. The changes in the circulation after birth. Circulation 1970; 41:343.
17. Rudolph AM, Yuen S. Response of the pulmonary vasculature to hypoxia and H^+ ion concentration changes. J Clin Invest 1966; 45:399-411.
18. Cassen S, Dawes GS, Mott JC, et al. The vascular resistance of the foetal and newly ventilated lung of the lamb. J Physiol (Lond) 1964; 171: 61-79.
19. Assali NS, Morris JA, Smith EW, Manson WA. Studies on ductus arteriosus circulation. Circ Res 1963; 13:478-89.
20. Boreus LO, Malmfors T, McMurphy DM, Olson L. Demonstration of adrenergic receptor function and innervation in the ductus arteriosus of the human fetus. Acta Physiol Scand 1969; 77:316-21.
21. Dimich I, Singh PP, Adell A, et al. Evaluation of oxygen saturation monitoring by pulse oximetry in neonates in the delivery system. Can J Anaesth 1991; 38:985-8.
22. Brady JP, Rigatto H. Pulmonary capillary flow in infants. Circulation (suppl) 1969; 3:50.
23. Walsh-Sukys MC. Persistent pulmonary hypertension of the newborn. Clin Perinatol 1993; 20:127-43.
24. Alano MA, Ngougmna E, Ostrea EM Jr, Konduri GG. Analysis of nonsteroidal antiinflammatory drugs in meconium and its relation to persistent pulmonary hypertension of the newborn. Pediatrics 2001; 107:519-23.
25. Adams FH, Moss AJ, Fagan L. The tracheal fluid of the foetal lamb. Biol Neonate 1963; 5:151-8.
26. Ross BB. Comparison of foetal pulmonary fluid with foetal plasma and amniotic fluid. Nature 1963; 199:1100-1.
27. Karlberg P. The adaptive changes in the immediate postnatal period, with particular reference to respiration. J Pediatr 1960; 56:585-604.
28. Usher RH, Allen AC, McLean FH. Risk of respiratory distress syndrome related to gestational age, route of delivery, and maternal diabetes. Am J Obstet Gynecol 1971; 111:826-32.
29. Lawson EW, Birdwell RL, Huang PS, et al. Augmentation of pulmonary surfactant secretion by lung expansion at birth. Pediatr Res 1979; 13:611-4.
30. Platzker ACG, Kitterman JA, Mescher EJ, et al. Surfactant in the lung and tracheal fluid of the fetal lamb and acceleration of its appearance by dexamethasone. Pediatrics 1975; 56:544-9.
31. Platzker ACG, Kitterman JA, Clements JA, et al. Surfactant appearance and secretion in the fetal lamb lung in response to dexamethasone. Pediatr Res 1972; 6:406.
32. Tuberville DF, McCaffree MA, Block MF, Krous HF. In utero distal pulmonary meconium aspiration. South Med J 1979; 72:535-6.
33. Lagercrantz H, Bistoletti P. Catecholamine release in the newborn infant at birth. Pediatr Res 1973; 11:889-93.
34. Dahm LS, James LS. Newborn temperature and calculated heat loss in the delivery room. Pediatrics 1972; 49:504-13.
35. Volpe JJ. Perinatal brain injury: From pathogenesis to neuroprotection. Ment Retard Dev Disabil Res Rev 2001; 7:56-64.
36. Philip J, Alexander JM, Sharma SK, et al. Epidural analgesia during labor and maternal fever. Anesthesiology 1999; 90:1271-5.
37. Lieberman E, Lang JM, Frigoletto F Jr, et al. Epidural analgesia, intrapartum fever, and neonatal sepsis evaluation. Pediatrics 1997; 99:415-9.
38. Kaul B, Vallejo M, Ramanathan S, Mandell G. Epidural labor analgesia and neonatal sepsis evaluation rate: A quality improvement study. Anesth Analg 2001; 93:986-90.
39. Wimmer JE. Neonatal resuscitation. Pediatr Rev 1994; 15:255-65.
40. Huddleston JF. Intrapartum fetal assessment: A review. Clin Perinatol 1999; 26:549-68.
41. Jacob J, Pfenninger J. Cesarean deliveries: When is a pediatrician necessary? Obstet Gynecol 1997; 89:217-20.
42. Hook B, Kiwi R, Amini S, et al. Neonatal morbidity after elective repeat cesarean section and trial of labor. Pediatrics 1997; 100:348-53.
43. Zaichkin J. Introduction to the revised neonatal resuscitation program guidelines: Questions and answers to get you started. Neonatal Network 2000; 19:49-54.
44. Apgar V. A proposal for a new method of evaluation of the newborn infant. Curr Res Anesth Analg 1953; 32:260-7.
45. Apgar V. The newborn Apgar scoring system: Reflections and advice. Pediatr Clin North Am 1966; 13:645-50.
46. Apgar V, James LS. Further observations on the newborn scoring system. Am J Dis Child 1962; 104:419-28.
47. Sykes GS, Johnson P, Ashworth F, et al. Do Apgar scores indicate asphyxia? Lancet 1982; 1:494-6.
48. Lauener PA, Calame A, Janecek P, et al. Systematic pH-measurements in the umbilical artery: Causes and predictive value of neonatal acidosis. J Perinat Med 1983; 11:278-85.
49. Suidan JS, Young BK. Outcome of fetuses with lactic acidemia. Am J Obstet Gynecol 1984; 150:33-7.
50. Fields LM, Entman SS, Boehm FH. Correlation of the one-minute Apgar score and the pH value of umbilical arterial blood. South Med J 1983; 76:1477-9.
51. Boehm FH, Field L, Entman S, et al. Correlation of the one minute Apgar score and umbilical cord acid-base status. South Med J 1986; 79:429-31.
52. Page FO, Martin J, Palmer S, et al. Correlation of neonatal acid base status with Apgar scores and fetal heart rate tracings. Am J Obstet Gynecol 1986; 154:1306-11.

53. Luthy DA, Kirkwood KS, Strickland D, et al. Status of infants at birth and risk for adverse neonatal events and long-term sequelae: A study in low birth weight infants. Am J Obstet Gynecol 1987; 157:676-9.

54. Josten BE, Johnson TRB, Nelson JP. Umbilical cord blood pH and Apgar scores as an index of neonatal health. Am J Obstet Gynecol 1987; 157:843-8.

55. Vintzileos AM, Gaffney SE, Salinger LM, et al. The relationships among the fetal biophysical profile, umbilical cord pH, and Apgar scores. Am J Obstet Gynecol 1987; 157:627-31.

56. Drage JS, Kennedy C, Berendes H, et al. The Apgar score as an index of infant morbidity. Dev Med Child Neurol 1966; 8:141-8.

57. Drage JS, Kennedy C, Schwarz BK. The Apgar score as an index of neonatal mortality: A report from the collaborative study of cerebral palsy. Obstet Gynecol 1964; 24:222-30.

58. American College of Obstetricians and Gynecologists and American Academy of Pediatrics. Neonatal Encephalopathy and Cerebral Palsy: Defining the Pathogenesis and Pathophysiology. Washington, DC, American College of Obstetricians and Gynecologists, 2003.

59. Freeman JM, Nelson KB. Intrapartum asphyxia and cerebral palsy. Pediatrics 1988; 82:240-9.

60. Gilstrap LC, Leveno KJ, Burris J, et al. Diagnosis of birth asphyxia on the basis of fetal pH, Apgar score and newborn cerebral dysfunction. Am J Obstet Gynecol 1989; 161:825-30.

61. Nelson KB, Ellenberg JH. Antecedents of cerebral palsy: Multivariate analysis of risk. N Engl J Med 1986; 315:81-6.

62. American College of Obstetricians and Gynecologists. Use and abuse of the Apgar score. Pediatrics 1996; 98:141-2.

63. Casey BM, McIntire DD, Leveno KJ. The continuing value of the Apgar score for the assessment of newborn infants. N Engl J Med 2001; 344:467-71.

64. Papile L. The Apgar score in the 21st century (editorial). N Engl J Med 2001; 344:519.

65. Catlin EA, Carpenter MW, Brann IV, et al. The Apgar revisited: Influence of gestational age. J Pediatr 1986; 109:865-8.

66. Helmy SAK, Ebeid AM. Modified Apgar score using pulse oximetry (abstract). Anesth Analg 1995; 80:S179.

67. Urschitz MS, Von Einem V, Seyfang A, Poets CF. Use of pulse oximetry in automated oxygen delivery to ventilated infants. Anesth Analg 2002; 94:537-540.

68. Halpern S. Obstetrical and pediatric anesthesia. Best evidence in anesthetic practice. Prognosis: the Apgar score predicts 28-day neonatal mortality (editorial). Can J Anesth 2002; 49:46-8.

69. Lievaart M, deJong PA. Acid-base equilibrium in umbilical cord blood and time of cord clamping. Obstet Gynecol 1984; 63:44-7.

70. Ackerman BD, Sosna MM, Ullrich JR. A technique for serial sampling of umbilical artery blood at birth. Biol Neonate 1972; 20:458-65.

71. Chou PJ, Ullrich JR, Ackerman BD. Time of onset of effective ventilation at birth. Biol Neonate 1974; 24:74-81.

72. Santos DJ. Discussion of: Page FO, Martin JN, Palmer SM, et al. Correlation of neonatal acid-base status with Apgar scores and fetal heart rate tracings. Am J Obstet Gynecol 1986; 154:1309-10.

73. Kirshon B, Moise KJ. Effect of heparin on umbilical arterial blood gases. J Reprod Med 1989; 34:267-9.

74. Strickland DM, Gilstrap LC, Hauth JC, Widmer K. Umbilical cord pH and Pco_2: Effects of interval from delivery to determination. Am J Obstet Gynecol 1984; 148:191-4.

75. Hilger JS, Holzman IR, Brown DR. Sequential changes in placental blood gases and pH during the hour following delivery. J Reprod Med 1981; 26:305-7.

76. Sato I, Saling E. Changes of pH value during storage of fetal blood samples. J Perinatal Med 1975; 3:211-4.

77. Gilstrap LC, Hauth JC, Hankins GDV, et al. Second-stage fetal heart rate abnormalities and type of neonatal acidemia. Obstet Gynecol 1987; 70:191-5.

78. Wible JL, Petrie RH, Koons A, et al. The clinical use of umbilical cord acid-base determinations in perinatal surveillance and management. Clin Perinatol 1982; 9:387-97.

79. Miller JM, Bernard M, Brown HL, et al. Umbilical cord blood gases for term healthy newborns. Am J Perinatol 1990; 7:157-9.

80. Helwig JT, Paker JT, Kilpatrick SJ, Laros RK. Umbilical cord blood acid-base state: What is normal? Am J Obstet Gynecol 1996; 174:1807-14.

81. American College of Obstetricians and Gynecologists. Assessment of Fetal and Newborn Acid-Base Status. ACOG Technical Bulletin No. 127, 1989.

82. Yeomans ER, Hauth JC, Gilstrap LC, et al. Umbilical cord pH, Pco_2 and bicarbonate following uncomplicated term vaginal deliveries. Am J Obstet Gynecol 1985; 151:798-800.

83. Ramin SM, Gilstrap LC, Leveno KJ, et al. Umbilical artery acid-base status in the preterm infant. Obstet Gynecol 1989; 74:256-8.

84. Thorp JA, Dildy GA, Yeomans ER, et al. Umbilical cord blood gas analysis at delivery. Am J Obstet Gynecol 1996; 175:517-22.

85. Huisjes HJ, Aarnoudse JG. Arterial or venous umbilical pH as a measure of neonatal morbidity? Early Hum Dev 1979; 3:155-61.

86. Eskes TKAB, Jongsma HW, Houx PCW. Percentiles for cord gas values in human umbilical cord blood. Eur J Obstet Gynecol Reprod Biol 1983; 14:341-6.

87. Low JA. The role of blood gas and acid base assessment in the diagnosis of intrapartum fetal asphyxia. Am J Obstet Gynecol 1988; 159:1235-40.

88. Thorp JA, Sampson JE, Parisi VM, Creasy RK. Routine umbilical cord blood gas determinations? Am J Obstet Gynecol 1989; 161:600-5.

89. Riley RJ, Johnson JWC. Collecting and analyzing cord blood gases. Clin Obstet Gynecol 1993; 36:13-23.

90. Nagel HTC, Vandenbussche FPHA, Oekes D, et al. Follow-up of children born with an umbilical arterial blood pH <7. Am J Obstet Gynecol 1995; 173:1758-64.

91. Ruth VJ, Raivio K. Perinatal brain damage: Predictive value of metabolic acidosis and the Apgar score. BMJ 1988; 297:24-7.

92. Vintzileos AM, Egan JFX, Campbell WA, et al. Asphyxia at birth as determined by cord blood pH measurements in preterm and term gestations: Correlation with neonatal outcome. J Matern Fetal Med 1992; 1:7-13.

93. Goldaber KG, Gilstrap LC, Leveno KJ, et al. Pathologic fetal acidemia. Obstet Gynecol 1991; 78:1103-7.

94. Zwart A, Buursma A, Oeseburg B, et al. Determination of hemoglobin derivatives with the IL 282 CO-Oximeter as compared with a manual spectrophotometric five-wavelength method. Clin Chem 1981; 27:1903-7.

95. Huch R, Huch A, Tuchschmid P, et al. Carboxyhemoglobin concentration in fetal cord blood (letter). Pediatrics 1983; 71:461-2.

96. Zijlstra WG, Buursma A, Koek JN, et al. Problems in the spectrophotometric determination of HbO_2 and HbCO in fetal blood. In: Maas AHJ, Kofstad J, Siggard-Andersen O, et al, editors. Proceeding of the Ninth Meeting of the IFCC Expert Panel on pH and Blood Gases. Oslo, Norway, Private Press, 1984:44-55.

97. Kopotic RJ, Lindner W. Assessing high-risk infants in the delivery room with pulse oximetry. Anesth Analg 2002; 94:S31-6.

98. Jennis MS, Peabody JL. Pulse oximetry: An alternative method for the assessment of oxygenation in newborn infants. Pediatrics 1987; 79:524-8.

99. Severinghaus JW, Noifeh KH. Accuracy of response of six pulse oximeters to profound hypoxia. Anesthesiology 1987; 67:551-8.

100. Sarnat HB, Sarnat MS. Neonatal encephalopathy following fetal distress. A clinical and electroencephalographic study. Arch Neurol 1976; 33:696-705.

101. Dubowitz LMS, Dubowitz V, Goldberg C. Clinical assessment of gestational age in the newborn infant. J Pediatr 1970; 77:1-10.

102. Ballard JL, Novak KK, Driver M. A simplified score for assessment of fetal maturation of newly born infants. J Pediatr 1979; 95:769-74.

103. Farr V, Mitchell RG, Neligan GA, Parkin JM. The definition of some external characteristics used in the assessment of gestational age in the newborn infant. Dev Med Child Neurol 1966; 8:507-11.

104. Farr V, Kerridge DF, Mitchell RG. The value of some external characteristics in the assessment of gestational age at birth. Dev Med Child Neurol 1966; 8:657.

105. Amiel-Tison C. Neurological evaluation of the maturity of newborn infants. Arch Dis Child 1968; 43:89-93.

106. Sanders M, Allen M, Alexander GR, et al. Gestational age assessment in preterm neonates weighing less than 1500 grams. Pediatrics 1991; 88:542-6.

107. Ballard JL, Khoury JC, Wedig K, et al. New Ballard score, expanded to include extremely premature infants. J Pediatr 1991; 119:417-23.

108. Alexander GR, deCaunes F, Hulsey TC, et al. Ethnic variation in postnatal assessments of gestational age: A reappraisal. Paediatr Perinat Epidemiol 1992; 6:423-33.

109. Battaglia FC, Lubchenco LO. A practical classification of newborn infants by weight and gestational age. J Pediatr 1967; 71:159-163.

110. Thoresen M, Cowan F, Whitelaw A. Effect of tilting on oxygenation in newborn infants. Arch Dis Child 1988; 63:315-7.

111. Schubring C. Temperature regulation in healthy and resuscitated newborns immediately after birth. J Perinatol 1986; 14:27-33

112. Leuthner SR, Jansen RD, Hageman JR. Cardiopulmonary resuscitation of the newborn. Pediatr Clin N Am 1994; 41:893-907.

113. Hazan J, Maag V, Chessex P. Association between hypothermia and mortality rate of premature infants: Revisited. Am J Obstet Gynecol 1991; 164:111-2.

114. Saugstaad OD, Rootwelt T, Aalen O. Resuscitation of asphyxiated newborn infants with room air or oxygen: an international controlled trial: The Resair 2 study. Pediatrics 1998; 102:E1.

115. Vento M, Arseni M, Sastre J, et al. Resuscitation with room air instead of 100% oxygen prevents oxidative stress in moderately asphyxiated term neonates. Pediatrics 2001; 107:642-7.

116. Perlman JM. Resuscitation: Air versus 100% oxygen (letter). Pediatrics 2002; 109:347-9

117. Weinberger B, Laskin DL, Heck DE, Laskin JD. Review oxygen toxicity in premature infants. Toxicol Appl Pharmacol 2002; 181:60-7.

118. Vyas H, Milner AD, Hopkin IE, Boon AW. Physiologic responses to prolonged and slow-rise inflation in the resuscitation of the asphyxiated newborn infant. J Pediatr 1981; 99:635-9.

119. Cordero L, Hon EH. Neonatal bradycardia following nasopharyngeal stimulation. J Pediatr 1971; 78:441-7.

120. Young RS, Hessert TR, Pritchard GA, Yagel SK. Naloxone exacerbates hypoxic-ischemic brain injury in the neonatal rat. Am J Obstet Gynecol 1984; 150:52-6.

121. Chernick V, Manfreda J, DeBooy V, et al. Clinical trial of naloxone in birth asphyxia. J Pediatr 1988; 113:519-25.

122. Sherman JM, Lowitt S, Stephenson C, Ironson JM. Factors influencing acquired subglottic stenosis in infants. J Pediatr 1986; 109:322-7.

123. Laing IA, Cowan DL, Ballantine GM, Hume R. Prevention of subglottic stenosis in neonatal ventilation. Int J Pediatr Otorhinolaryngol 1986; 11:61-6.

124. Paterson SJ, Byrne PJ, Molesky MG, et al. Neonatal resuscitation using the laryngeal mask airway. Anesthesiology 1994; 80:1248-53.

125. Brimacombe J, Berry A. The laryngeal mask airway for obstetric anaesthesia and neonatal resuscitation. Int J Obstet Anesth 1994; 3:211-8.

126. Fernandez-Jurado MI, Fernandez-Baena M. Use of laryngeal mask airway for prolonged ventilatory support in a preterm newborn. Paediatr Anaesth 2002; 12:369-70.

127. David R. Closed chest cardiac massage in the newborn infant. Pediatrics 1988; 81:552-4.

128. Orlowski JP. Optimum position for external cardiac compression in infants and young children. Ann Emerg Med 1986; 15:667-73.

129. Phillips GWL, Zideman DA. Relation of infant heart to sternum: Its significance in cardiopulmonary resuscitation. Lancet 1986; 1:1024-5.

130. Finholt DA, Kettrick RG, Wagner R, Swedlow DB. The heart is under the lower third of the sternum: Implications for external cardiac massage. Am J Dis Child 1986; 140:646-9.

131. Dean JM, Koehler RC, Schleien CL, et al. Age-related effects of compression rate and duration in cardiopulmonary resuscitation. J Appl Physiol 1990; 68:554-60.

132. Fitzgerald KR, Babbs CF, Frissora HA, et al. Cardiac output during cardiopulmonary resuscitation at various compression rates and durations. Am J Physiol 1981; 241:H442-8.

133. Babbs CF, Tacker WA, Paris RL, et al. CPR with simultaneous compression and ventilation at high airway pressure in four animal models. Crit Care Med 1982; 10:501-4.

134. Burchfield DJ. Medication use in neonatal resuscitation. Clin Perinatol 1999; 26:683-691.

135. Schlein CL, Dean JM, Koehler RC, et al. Effect of epinephrine on cerebral and myocardial perfusion in an infant animal preparation of cardiopulmonary resuscitation. Circulation 1986; 73:809-17.

136. Simmons MA, Adcock EW, Bard H, Battagia FC. Hypernatremia and intracranial hemorrhage in neonates. N Engl J Med 1974; 291:6-10.

137. Kette F, Weil MH, von Planta M, Gazmuri RJ, Rackow EC. Buffer agents do not reverse intramyocardial acidosis during cardiac resuscitation. Circulation 1990; 81:1660-6.

138. Kette F, Weil MH, Gazmuri RJ. Buffer solutions may compromise cardiac resuscitation by reducing coronary perfusion pressure. JAMA 1991; 266:2121-6 (published correction appears in JAMA 1991; 266:3286).

139. Papile LA, Burstein J, Burstein R, Koffler H, Koops B, Relationship of intravenous sodium bicarbonate infusions and cerebral intraventricular hemorrhage. J Pediatr 1978; 93:834-6.

140. Changaris DG, Purohit DM, Balentine JD, et al. Brain calcification in severely stressed neonates receiving parenteral calcium. J Pediatr 1984; 104:941-6.

141. Lindemann R. Resuscitation of the newborn: Endotracheal administration of epinephrine. Acta Paediatr Scand 1984; 73:210-2.

142. Quinton DN, O'Byrne G, Aitkenhead AR. Comparison of endotracheal and peripheral intravenous adrenaline in cardiac arrest. Lancet 1987; 1:828-9.

143. Greenberg M, Mayeda DV, Chrzanowski R, et al. Endotracheal administration of atropine sulfate. Ann Emerg Med 1982; 11:546-8.

144. Greenberg M, Roberts JR, Baskin SI. Endotracheal naloxone. Ann Emerg Med 1980; 9:289-92.

145. McDonald JL. Serum lidocaine levels during cardiopulmonary resuscitation after intravenous and endotracheal administration. Crit Care Med 1985; 13:914-5.

146. Fiser DH. Intraosseous infusions. N Engl J Med 1990; 322:1579-81.

147. Tocantins LM. Rapid absorption of substance injected into the bone marrow. Proc Soc Exp Biol Med 1940; 45:292-6.

148. Papper EM. The bone marrow route for injecting fluids and drugs into the general circulation. Anesthesiology 1942; 3:307-13.

149. Hodge D III, Delgado-Paredes C, Fleisher G. Intraosseous infusion flow rates in hypovolemic "pediatric" dogs. Ann Emerg Med 1987; 16:305-7.

150. Redmond AD, Plunkett PK. Intraosseous infusion. Arch Emerg Med 1986; 3:231-3.

151. La Fleche R, Slepin MJ, Vargas J, et al. Iatrogenic bilateral tibial fractures after intraosseous infusion attempts in a 3 month old infant. Ann Emerg Med 1989; 18:1099-101.

152. Rosetti VA, Thompson BM, Miller J, et al. Intraosseous infusion: An alternative route of pediatric intravascular access. Ann Emerg Med 1985; 14:885-8.

153. Quilligan JJ Jr, Turkel H. Bone marrow infusion and its complications. Am J Dis Child 1946; 71:457-65.

154. Heinild S, Sndergaard T, Tudvad F. Bone marrow infusion in childhood: Experiences from a thousand infusions. J Paediatr 1947; 30:400-12.

155. Golden SM, O'Brien EW, Metz SA. Anticoagulation of autologous cord blood for neonatal resuscitation. Am J Obstet Gynecol 1982; 144:103-4.

156. Cochrane Injuries Group Albumin Reviewers. Human albumin administration in critically ill patients: Systematic review of randomised controlled trials. BMJ 1998; 317:235-40.

157. Desmond MM, Moore J, Lindley JE, Brown CA. Meconium staining of the amniotic fluid: A marker of fetal hypoxia. Obstet Gynecol 1957; 9:91.

158. Matthews TG, Warshaw JB. Relevance of the gestational age distribution of meconium passage in utero. Pediatrics 1979; 64:30-1.

159. Yeh TF, Harris V, Srinivasan G, et al. Roentgenographic findings in infants with meconium aspiration syndrome. JAMA 1979; 242:60-3.

160. Wiswell TE, Tuggle JM, Turner BS. Meconium aspiration syndrome: Have we made a difference? Pediatrics 1990; 85:715-21.

161. Short BL, Miller MK, Anderson KO. ECMO in the management of respiratory failure in the newborn. Clin Perinatol 1987; 14:737-48.

162. Truog WE. Inhaled nitric oxide: A tenth anniversary observation. Pediatrics 1998; 101:696-7.

163. Wessel DL, Adatia I, Van Marter LJ, et al. Improved oxygenation in a randomized trial of inhaled nitric oxide for persistent pulmonary hypertension of the newborn. Pediatrics 1997; 100:E7.

164. Gregory GA, Gooding CA, Phibbs RH, Tooley WN. Meconium aspiration in infants: A prospective study. J Pediatr 1974; 85:848-52.

165. Gadzinowski J. Contemporary treatment options for meconium aspiration syndrome. Croat Med J 1998; 39:158-64.

166. Hofmeyr GJ, Gulmezoglu AM, Buchmann E, et al. The Collaborative Randomised Amnioinfusion for Meconium Project (CRAMP): 1. South Africa. Br J Obstet Gynaecol 1998; 105:304-8.

167. Mahomed K, Mulambo T, Woelk G, et al. The Collaborative Randomised Amnioinfusion for Meconium Project (CRAMP): 2. Zimbabwe. Br J Obstet Gynaecol 1998; 105:309-13.

168. Ting P, Brady JP. Tracheal suction in meconium aspiration. Am J Obstet Gynecol 1975; 122:767-71.

169. Carson BS, Losey RW, Bowes Jr WA, Simmons MA. Combined obstetric and pediatric approach to prevent meconium aspiration syndrome. Am J Obstet Gynecol 1976; 126:712-5.

170. Murphy JD, Vawter GF, Reid LM. Pulmonary vascular disease in fatal meconium aspiration. J Pediatr 1984; 104:758-62.

171. Hislop A, Reid LM. Intrapulmonary arterial development during fetal life: Branching pattern and structure. J Anat 1972; 113:35-48.

172. Hislop A, Reid LM. Pulmonary arterial development during childhood. Thorax 1973; 28:129-35.

173. Meyrick B, Reid LM. Effect of continued hypoxia on rat pulmonary arterial circulation. Lab Invest 1978; 38:188-200.

174. Perlman EJ, Moore GW, Hutchins GM. The pulmonary vasculature in meconium aspiration. Hum Pathol 1989; 20:701-6.

175. O'Neal RM, Ahlvin RC, Bauer WC, Thomas WA. Development of fetal pulmonary arterioles. AMA Arch Pathol 1957; 63:309-15.

176. Naeye RL. Arterial changes during the perinatal period. Arch Pathol 1961; 71:121-8.

177. Davies G, Reid L. Growth of the alveoli and pulmonary arteries in childhood. Thorax 1970; 25:669-81.

178. Haworth SG, Hislop AA. Pulmonary vascular development: Normal values of peripheral vascular structure. Am J Cardiol 1983; 52:578-83.

179. Wagenvoort CA, Dingemans KP. Pulmonary vascular smooth muscle and its interaction with endothelium. Chest 1985; 88:200S-2S.

180. Davis RO, Philips JB, Harris BA, et al. Fatal meconium aspiration syndrome occurring despite airway management considered appropriate. Am J Obstet Gynecol 1985; 151:731-6.

181. Falciglia HS, Henderschott C, Potter P, Helmchen R. Does DeLee suction at the perineum prevent meconium aspiration syndrome? Am J Obstet Gynecol 1992; 167:1243-9.

182. Linder N, Aranda JV, Tsur M, et al. Need for endotracheal intubation and suction in meconium-stained neonates. J Pediatr 1988; 112:613-5.

183. Ghidini A, Spong CY. Severe meconium aspiration syndrome is not caused by aspiration of meconium. Am J Obstet Gynecol 2001; 185:931-8.

184. Locus P, Yeomans E, Crosby U. Efficacy of bulb versus DeLee suction at deliveries complicated by meconium stained amniotic fluid. Am J Perinatol 1990; 7:87-91.

185. Ballard JL, Musial MJ, Myers MG. Hazards of delivery room resuscitation using oral methods of endotracheal suctioning. Pediatr Infect Dis 1986; 5:198-200.

186. Van Dyke RB, Spector SA. Transmission of herpes simplex virus type 1 to a newborn infant during endotracheal suctioning for meconium aspiration. Pediatr Infect Dis 1984; 3:153-6.

187. Oriol NE. Aspiration of meconium from the trachea of neonates. Anesthesiology 1990; 73:1294.

188. Volpe JJ. Neurology of the Newborn. 4th edition. Philadelphia, WB Saunders, 2001.

189. MacDorman MF, Minino AM, Stobino DM, Guyer B. Annual summary of vital statistics: 2001. Pediatrics 2002; 110:1037-52.

190. Wolke D, Meyer R: Cognitive status, language attainment, and prereading longitudinal study. Dev Med Child Neurol 1999; 41:94-109.

191. Paneth N. Classifying brain damage in preterm infants. J Pediatr 1999; 134:527-9.

192. Volpe JJ. Brain injury in the premature infant: Overview of clinical aspects, neuropathology, and pathogenesis. Semin Pediatr Neurol 1998; 5:135-51.

193. Vohr BR, Wright LL, Dusick AM, et al. Neurodevelopmental and functional outcomes of extremely low birth weight infants in the national institute of child health and human development neonatal research network, 1993-1994. Pediatrics 2000; 105:1216-26.

194. Chen CH, Shen WC, Wang TM, Chi CS. Cerebral magnetic resonance imaging of preterm infants after corrected age of one year. Acta Paed Sin 1995; 36:261-5.

195. Reynolds ML, Evans CAN, Reynolds EDR, et al. Intracranial hemorrhage in the preterm sheep fetus. Early Hum Dev 1979; 3:163-86.

196. Goddard J, Lewis RM, Armstrong DL, Zeller RS. Moderate, rapidly induced hypertension as a cause of intraventricular hemorrhage in the newborn beagle model. J Pediatr 1980; 96:1057-60.

197. Perlman JM, McMenamin JB, Volpe JJ. Fluctuating cerebral blood-flow velocity in respiratory-distress syndrome. N Engl J Med 1983; 309:204-9.

198. Volpe JJ. Intraventricular hemorrhage in the premature infant—current concepts. Part I. Ann Neurol 1989; 25:3-11.

199. Volpe JJ. Neurologic outcome of prematurity. Arch Neurol 1998; 55:297-300.

200. Volpe JJ. Brain injury in the premature infant. Clin Perinatol 1997; 24:567-87.

201. Perlman JM, Volpe JJ. Are venous circulatory abnormalities important in the pathogenesis of hemorrhagic and/or ischemic cerebral injury? Pediatrics 1987; 80:705-11.

202. Goldberg RN, Chung D, Goldman SL, et al. The association of rapid volume expansion and intraventricular hemorrhage in the preterm infant. J Pediatr 1980; 96:1060-3.

203. Nakamura Y, Okudera T, Fukuda S, et al. Germinal matrix hemorrhage of venous origin in preterm neonates. Hum Pathol 1990; 21:1059-62.

204. van de Bor M, Briet E, Van Bel F, et al. Hemostasis and periventricular-intraventricular hemorrhage of the newborn. Am J Dis Child 1986; 140:1131-4.

205. Goldstein GW. Pathogenesis of brain edema and hemorrhage: role of the brain capillary. Pediatrics 1979; 64:357-60.

206. Gould SJ, Howard S. An immunohistochemical study of the germinal layer in the late gestation human fetal brain. Neuropathol Appl Neurobiol 1987; 13:421-37.

207. Goldenberg RL, Hauth JC, Andrews WW. Intrauterine infection and preterm delivery. N Engl J Med 2000; 342:1500-7.

208. Shankaran S, Cepeda E, Muran G, et al. Antenatal phenobarbital therapy and neonatal outcome. I. Effect on intracranial hemorrhage. Pediatrics 1996; 97:644-8.

209. Shankaran S, Woldt E, Nelson J, et al. Antenatal phenobarbital therapy and neonatal outcome. II. Neurodevelopmental outcome at 36 months. Pediatrics 1996; 97:649-52.

210. Morales WJ, Angel JL, O'Brien WF, et al. The use of antenatal vitamin K in the prevention of early neonatal intraventricular hemorrhage. Am J Obstet Gynecol 1988; 159:774-9.

211. Thorp JA, Parriott J, Ferrettesmith D, et al. Antepartum vitamin K and phenobarbital for preventing intraventricular hemorrhage in the premature newborn: A randomized, double-blind, placebo-controlled trial. Obstet Gynecol 1994; 83:70-6.

212. Moise AA, Wearden ME, Kozinetz CA, et al. Antenatal steroids are associated with less need for blood pressure support in extremely premature infants. Pediatrics 1995; 95:845-50.

213. Wallace EM, Baker LS. Effect of antenatal betamethasone administration on placental vascular resistance. Lancet 1999; 353:1404-7.

214. Nelson KG, Grether JK. Can magnesium sulfate reduce the risk of cerebral palsy in very low birth weight infants? Pediatrics 1995; 95:263-9.

215. Paneth N, Jetton J, Pinto-Martin J, Susser M. Magnesium sulfate in labor and risk of neonatal brain lesions and cerebral palsy in low birth weight infants. Pediatrics 1997; 99:1-10.

216. Hirtz DG, Nelson K. Magnesium sulfate and cerebral palsy in premature infants. Curr Opin Pediatr 1998; 10:131-137.

217. Mittendorf R, Dambrosia J, Pryde PG, et al. Association between the use of antenatal magnesium sulfate in preterm labor and adverse health outcomes in infants. Am J Obstet Gynecol 2002; 186:1111-8.

218. Anderson GD, Bada HS, Shaver DC, et al. The effect of cesarean section on intraventricular hemorrhage in the preterm infant. Am J Obstet Gynecol 1992; 166:1091-1101.

219. Perlman JM, Goodman S, Kreusser KL, Volpe JJ. Reduction in intraventricular hemorrhage by elimination of fluctuating cerebral blood-flow velocity in preterm infants with respiratory distress syndrome. N Engl J Med 1985; 312:1353-7.

220. Miall-Allen VM, Whitelaw AG. Effect of pancuronium and pethidine on heart rate and blood pressure in ventilated infants. Arch Dis Child 1987; 62:1179-80.

221. Saarenmaa E, Hultunen P, Leppaluoto J, et al. Advantages of fentanyl over morphine in analgesia for ventilated newborn infants after birth: A randomized trial. J Pediatr 1999; 134:144-50.

222. Myers RE, Myers SE. Use of sedative, analgesic, and anesthetic drugs during labor and delivery: Bane or boon? Am J Obstet Gynecol 1979; 133:83-104.

223. Richards DS, Yancey MK, Duff P, Stieg FH. The perinatal management of severe laryngeal stenosis. Obstet Gynecol 1992; 80:537-40.

224. Leichty KW, Crombleholme TM, Flake AW, et al. Intrapartum airway management for giant fetal neck masses: The EXIT (ex utero intrapartum treatment) procedure. Am J Obstet Gynecol 1997; 177:870-4.

225. MacKenzie TC, Crombleholme TM, Flake AW. The ex-utero intrapartum treatment. Curr Opin Pediatr 2002; 14:453-8.

226. Crombleholme TM, Sylvester K, Flake AW, et al. Salvage of a fetus with congenital high airway obstruction syndrome by ex utero intrapartum treatment (EXIT) procedure. Fetal Diagn Ther 2000; 15:280-2.

227. Noah MMS, Norton ME, Sandberg P, Esakoff T, Farrell J, Albanese CT. Short-term maternal outcomes that are associated with the EXIT procedure, as compared with cesarean delivery. Am J Obstet Gynecol 2002; 186:773-7.

228. Sakawi Y, Boyd G, Shaw B, Rouse D, Philips JB. Use of sevoflurane to provide uterine relaxation for the ex-utero intrapartum procedure. Am J Anesthesiol 2001; 28:195-8.

229. Gregory GA. Esophageal atresia and tracheoesophageal fistula. In: Rogers MCR, editor. Current Practice in Anesthesiology. 2nd ed. St. Louis, Mosby, 1990:218-22.

230. Haberkern CM, Crone RK. Congenital diaphragmatic hernia. In: Rogers MCR, editor. Current Practice in Anesthesiology. 2nd ed. St. Louis, Mosby, 1990:211-7.

231. Davis DJ. How aggressive should delivery room cardiopulmonary resuscitation be for extremely low birth weight neonates? Pediatrics 1993; 92:447-50.

232. Jain L, Ferre C, Vidyasagar D, Nath S, Sheftel D. Cardiopulmonary resuscitation of apparently stillborn infants: survival and long-term outcome. J Pediatr 1991; 118:778-82.

233. Yeo CL, Tudehope DI. Outcome of resuscitated apparently stillborn infants: A ten year review. J Paediatr Child Health 1994; 30:129-33.

234. Casalaz DM, Marlow N, Speidel BD. Outcome of resuscitation following unexpected apparent stillbirth. Arch Dis Child Fetal Neonatal Ed 1998; 78:F112-5.

235. Brazelton TB, Scholl ML, Robey J. Visual behavior in the neonate. Pediatrics 1966; 37:284-90.

236. Ball W, Tronick E. Infant response to impending collision: Optical and real. Science 1971; 171:818-20.

237. Kearsley RB. The newborn's response to auditory stimulation: A demonstration of orienting and defensive behavior. Child Dev 1973; 44:582-90.

238. Brazelton TB. Neonatal behavioral assessment scale. Clinics in Developmental Medicine, No. 50. Spastics International Medical Publications. London, William Heinemann Medical Books, 1973.

239. Brazelton TB. Psychophysiologic reactions in the neonate. II. Effect of maternal medication on the neonate and his behavior. J Pediatr 1961; 58:513-8.

240. Scanlon JW, Brown WU Jr, Weiss JB, et al. Neurobehavioral responses of newborn infants after maternal epidural anesthesia. Anesthesiology 1974; 40:121-8.

241. Prechtal HFR, Beintema D. The neurological examination of the full term infant. Clinics in Developmental Medicine, No. 12. Lavenham, England, Spastics International Medical Publications, 1964.

242. Beintema DJ. A neurological study of newborn infants. Clinics in Developmental Medicine, No. 28. Lavenham, England, Spastics International Medical Publications, 1968.

243. Amiel-Tison C, Barrier G, Shnider SM, et al. A new neurologic and adaptive capacity scoring system for evaluating obstetric medications in full-term newborns. Anesthesiology 1982; 56:340-50.

244. Brockhurst NJ, Littleford JA, Halpern SH. The neurologic and adaptive capacity score. Anesthesiology 2000; 92:3-5.

245. Camann W, Brazelton TB. Use and abuse of neonatal neurobehavioral testing (editorial). Anesthesiology; 2000; 92:237-46.

246. Halpern SH, Littleford JA, Brockhurst NJ, Youngs PJ, Malik N, Owen HC. The neurologic and adaptive capacity score is not a reliable method of newborn evaluation. Anesthesiology 2001; 94:958-62.

247. Amiel-Tison C. Update of the Amiel-Tison neurologic assessment for the term neonate or at 40 weeks corrected age. Pediatr Neurol 2002; 27:196-212.

248. American Academy of Pediatrics Committee on Drugs. Effects of medication during labor and delivery on infant outcome. Pediatrics 1978; 62:402-3.

249. US Department of Health, Education, and Welfare; Public Health Service; and the Food and Drug Administration. Guidelines for the Clinical Evaluation of Local Anesthetics. HEW (FDA) 78-3053. Rockville, Md, 1977:78-3053.

250. US Department of Health, Education, and Welfare; Public Health Service; and the Food and Drug Administration. Guidelines for the Clinical Evaluation of General Anesthetics. HEW (FDA) 78-3052. Rockville, Md, 1977:78-3052.

251. Brackbill Y, Kane J, Manniello RL, Abramson D. Obstetric meperidine usage and assessment of neonatal status. Anesthesiology 1974; 40: 116-20.

252. Rolbin SH, Wright RG, Shnider SM, et al. Diazepam during cesarean section: Effects on neonatal Apgar scores, acid-base status, neurobehavioral assessment and maternal and fetal plasma norepinephrine levels. In: Abstracts of Scientific Papers. New Orleans, American Society of Anesthesiologists, 1977:449.

253. Dailey PA, Baysinger CL, Levinson G, Shnider SM. Neurobehavioral testing of the newborn infant: Effects of obstetric anesthesia. Clin Perinatol 1982; 9:191-214.

254. Hodgkinson R, Bhatt M, Wang CN. Double-blind comparison of the neurobehavior of neonates following administration of different doses of meperidine to the mother. Can Anaesth Soc J 1978; 25:405-11.

255. Lieberman BA, Rosenblatt DB, Belsey E, et al. The effects of maternally administered pethidine or epidural bupivacaine on the fetus and newborn. Br J Obstet Gynaecol 1979; 86:598-606.

256. Rayburn WF, Smith CV, Leuschen MP, Hoffman K. Comparison of patient-controlled and nurse-administered analgesia using intravenous fentanyl during labor. Anesth Rev 1991; 18:31-3.

257. Kileff ME, James FM, Dewan DM, Floyd HM. Neonatal neurobehavioral responses after epidural anesthesia for cesarean section using lidocaine and bupivacaine. Anesth Analg 1984; 63:413-7.

258. Brown WU Jr, Bell GC, Lurie AO, et al. Newborn blood levels of lidocaine and mepivacaine in the first postnatal day following maternal epidural anesthesia. Anesthesiology 1975; 42:698-706.

259. Datta S, Corke BC, Alper MH, et al. Epidural anesthesia for cesarean section: A comparison of bupivacaine, chloroprocaine, and etidocaine. Anesthesiology 1980; 52:48-51.

260. Kuhnert BR, Harrison MJ, Linn PL, Kuhnert PM. Effects of maternal epidural anesthesia on neonatal behavior. Anesth Analg 1984; 63:301-8.

261. Sepkoski CM, Lester BM, Ostheimer GW, Brazelton TB. The effects of maternal epidural anesthesia on neonatal behavior during the first month. Dev Med Child Neurol 1992; 34:1072-80.

262. Abboud TK, Khoo SS, Miller F, et al. Maternal, fetal, and neonatal responses after epidural anesthesia with bupivacaine, 2-chloroprocaine, or lidocaine. Anesth Analg 1982; 61:638-44.

263. Tronick E. A critique of the neonatal neurologic and adaptive capacity score (NACS). Anesthesiology 1982; 56:338-9.

264. Hodgkinson R, Bhatt M, Kim SS, et al. Neonatal neurobehavioral tests following cesarean section under general and spinal anesthesia. Am J Obstet Gynecol 1978; 132:670-4.

265. Hughes SC, Rosen MA, Shnider SM, et al. Maternal and neonatal effects of epidural morphine for labor and delivery. Anesth Analg 1984; 63: 319-24.

266. Preston P, Rosen M, Hughes SC, et al. Epidural anesthesia with fentanyl and lidocaine for cesarean section: Maternal effects and neonatal outcome. Anesthesiology 1988; 68:938-43.

267. Murakawa K, Abboud TK, Yanagi T, et al. Clinical experience of epidural fentanyl for labor pain. J Anesth (Jap) 1987; 1:93-5.

268. Cohen SE, Tan S, Albright GA, Halpern J. Epidural fentanyl/bupivacaine mixtures for obstetric analgesia. Anesthesiology 1987; 67:403-7.

269. Abboud TK, Afrasiabi A, Zhu J, et al. Epidural morphine or butorphanol augments bupivacaine analgesia during labor. Reg Anesth 1989; 14:115-20.

270. Zhu J, Abboud TK, Afrasiabi A, et al. Epidural butorphanol augments lidocaine sensory analgesia during labor. Reg Anesth 1991; 16:265-7.

271. Little MS, McNitt JD, Choi HJ, Tremper KK. A pilot study of low dose epidural sufentanil and bupivacaine for labor anesthesia (abstract). Anesthesiology 1987; 67:A444.

272. Abboud TK, David S, Nagappala S, et al. Maternal, fetal and neonatal effects of lidocaine with and without epinephrine for epidural anesthesia in obstetrics. Anesth Analg 1984; 63:973-9.

273. Abboud TK, Sheik-Ol-Eslam A, Yanagi T, et al. Safety and efficacy of epinephrine added to bupivacaine for lumbar epidural analgesia in obstetrics. Anesth Analg 1985; 64:585-91.

274. Abboud TK, DerSarkissian L, Terrasi J, et al. Comparative maternal, fetal and neonatal effects of chloroprocaine with and without epinephrine for epidural anesthesia in obstetrics. Anesth Analg 1987; 66:71-5.

275. Abboud TK, Afrasiabi A, Zhu J, et al. Bupivacaine/butorphanol/epinephrine for epidural anesthesia in obstetrics: Maternal and neonatal effects. Reg Anesth 1989; 14:219-24.

276. Abboud TK, Nagappala S, Murakawa K, et al. Comparison of the effects of general and regional anesthesia for cesarean section on neonatal neurologic and adaptive capacity scores. Anesth Analg 1985; 64: 996-1000.

277. Palahniuk RJ, Scatliff J, Biehl D, et al. Maternal and neonatal effects of methoxyflurane, nitrous oxide and lumbar epidural anaesthesia for caesarean section. Can Anaesth Soc J 1977; 24:586-96.

278. Stefani SJ, Hughes SC, Shnider SM, et al. Neonatal neurobehavioral effects of inhalation analgesia for vaginal delivery. Anesthesiology 1982; 56:351-5.

279. Abboud TK, Gangolly J, Mosaad P, Crowell D. Isoflurane in obstetrics. Anesth Analg 1989; 68:388-91.

Chapter 10
Fetal and Neonatal Neurologic Injury

Donald H. Penning, M.D., M.Sc., FRCP

Our understanding of fetal brain injury has increased substantially during the last several years. Advances in imaging and the identification of potential biochemical markers have made the detection and diagnosis of fetal and newborn brain injury easier. We also have a greater knowledge of the pathophysiology of fetal brain injury, including responsible factors and clinical associations. The role of overt and subclinical chorioamnionitis in the etiology and pathophysiology of both preterm labor and fetal brain injury remains an area of active investigation. Inflammatory mediators clearly play a role in the pathophysiology of neurologic injury. Studies have demonstrated the efficacy of magnesium sulfate therapy for seizure prophylaxis in preeclamptic women, but there remains controversy regarding its efficacy for tocolysis and its effect on fetal neurologic outcome.

Notwithstanding our increased understanding of the pathophysiology, it is frustrating that little progress has been made to reduce the incidence of fetal brain injury. However, there is reason to hope that significant strides may soon be made.

HISTORY, DEFINITIONS, AND SIGNIFICANCE

In 1861, John Little, an orthopedic surgeon, first described cerebral palsy in a report to the Obstetrical Society of London. He drew attention to a newborn neurologic disorder that was associated with difficult labor or birth trauma, and it was known as Little's disease until William Osler coined the term *cerebral palsy* in 1888.[1] Today, **cerebral palsy** can be defined as a nonprogressive disorder of the central nervous system (CNS) that has been present since birth and that includes some impairment of motor function or posture.[2] Mental retardation may or may not be present and is not an essential diagnostic criterion. Various forms of cerebral palsy exist, and differences also exist with regard to pathology, pathophysiology, and potential relationships with intrapartum events.

It is difficult to review and understand the literature on the subject of cerebral palsy. Terms such as *hypoxic-ischemic encephalopathy (HIE) of the newborn, newborn asphyxia, birth asphyxia,* and *asphyxia neonatorum* can be difficult to distinguish. Some obstetricians and anesthesiologists have requested that physicians abandon the term **birth asphyxia.**[3] The American College of Obstetricians and Gynecologists prefers the use of the terms **hypercarbia, hypoxia, metabolic acidemia,** and **respiratory** or **lactic acidosis.**[4,5] Although these terms are more descriptive and less pejorative than the term *birth asphyxia,* it is naive to believe that the term *birth asphyxia* will soon disappear.[6] In this chapter, the term *asphyxia*—although imprecise—has been retained, because it reflects our incomplete knowledge of the factors responsible for neurologic injury.

Intrapartum misadventures continue to receive blame for many cases of cerebral palsy. It is a logical and widely held theory that an intrapartum reduction in fetal oxygen delivery causes some forms of cerebral palsy, and early reports linked perinatal events to poor neurologic outcome in the newborn. Years ago, studies in primates demonstrated that perinatal asphyxia could cause brain injury.[7] It is widely believed that electronic fetal heart rate (FHR) monitoring should detect the vast majority of these episodes. Electronic FHR monitoring has largely replaced intermittent auscultation during labor, although many studies have failed to demonstrate its clear superiority. Use of electronic FHR monitoring has prompted many cesarean deliveries for nonreassuring FHR tracings. Despite the increased incidence of cesarean section for this indication, there has been no reduction in the incidence of cerebral palsy. Indeed, it is estimated that, among patients with new-onset late FHR decelerations, there is a 99% probability that the tracing is a false positive "if used as an indicator for subsequent development of cerebral palsy."[8] This is probably a surprise to many laypersons and trial lawyers, but it is also poorly appreciated among obstetricians. A recent survey of maternal-fetal medicine fellows showed that they, too, greatly overestimated the diagnostic accuracy of FHR monitoring.[8]

Lest we be too hard on our obstetric colleagues, let us remember that great medicolegal pressure exists, and it is understandable that many cesarean sections are performed in an effort to avoid the astronomic jury awards against obstetricians for fetal/neonatal neurologic injury. These awards are not limited to the United States; in the United Kingdom, payments to plaintiffs "regularly exceed £3 million and in some cases lawyers' fees exceed the award."[1] Many attorneys and physicians contend that most cases of cerebral palsy are a direct result of a perinatal complication or misadventure.[9] One plaintiff's attorney stated, "If the doctor does not know or is not apprised of the possibility of a depressed fetus and does not remove the fetus by cesarean section so that the baby can survive the birth process, then that doctor has committed malpractice."[10] Clearly this represents an extreme view. Intrapartum events are likely responsible for some cases of cerebral palsy[11]; however, these cases are few in number. Peripartum events probably account for only 8% to 10% of the cases of cerebral palsy.[12,13] Indeed, when one excludes significant congenital anomalies, it is estimated that only 6% of cases of cerebral palsy result from intrapartum asphyxial insults.[8] Templates exist to help define abnormalities that are *potentially* a result of intrapartum events; these templates also describe proper behavior and credentials for expert witnesses in this arena.[14]

Until recently it had been hoped that greater fetal surveillance would lead to the identification and prompt delivery of the fetus at risk, which would result in lower rates of cerebral palsy. Although such surveillance has been largely responsible for increasing the cesarean section rate, it has made little impact on the incidence of cerebral palsy.[15,16] Large randomized trials have failed to demonstrate improved fetal and neonatal outcome when continuous electronic FHR monitoring was compared with intermittent FHR auscultation.[17,18] In an editorial, Friedman[19] cited observations made by Schifrin and Dame[20] and opined, "the absence of either suggestive or overtly ominous fetal heart rate patterns is reliably reassuring." Unfortunately, there is also little objective evidence that reassuring FHR tracings exclude the subsequent occurrence of cerebral palsy. Rosen and Dickinson[21] reviewed published studies of FHR monitoring and were unable to identify FHR patterns that were consistently associated with neurologic injuries. When they examined a subset of 55 brain-damaged infants, they observed no consistent FHR pattern. The authors stated, "We do not advocate the abandonment of the use of electronic fetal monitoring, but we do believe that it is yet to be proved to be of value in predicting or preventing neurologic morbidity." Perhaps the more focused use of FHR monitoring may prove useful. For example, fetal inflammatory changes—which can be associated with neurologic injury—may have characteristic FHR findings.[22]

EPIDEMIOLOGY OF CEREBRAL PALSY

Rosen and Dickinson[23] reviewed studies from Europe, Australia, and the United States that were published between 1985 and 1990 and that included data from the years 1959 to 1982 (Table 10-1). The rate of cerebral palsy ranged from 1.8 to 4.9 cases per 1000 live births, with a composite rate of 2.7 cases per 1000 live births. Approximately 36% of these cases of cerebral palsy occurred among infants with a birth weight of less than 2500 g. Composite data revealed that the incidences of certain conditions were as follows: diplegia, 34%; hemiplegia, 30%; quadriplegia, 20%; and extra-pyramidal forms, 16%.[24-34] It is difficult to compare data among these studies. For example, the studies varied in the duration of follow-up evaluation. One study excluded all congenital abnormalities, one study excluded deaths before the age of 2 years, and one failed to state whether deaths were included. Some studies did not group patients by birth weight, and those studies that grouped patients by birth weight did not use the same birth weight groups. Diagnostic accuracy is very important. Various registries of cerebral palsy are used to compare trends and prevalence rates between populations and to identify subjects for collaborative studies. The use of accurate and precise diagnostic criteria is essential. In the past, cerebral palsy has been used as an umbrella diagnosis for a number of separate conditions. With the refinement of diagnostic accuracy, some forms of neurologic injury may be omitted from these registries. This may suggest that a lower rate of cerebral palsy exists, when in fact the apparent decrease resulted from a reclassification of neurologic injuries.[35]

An older but large study from Western Australia examined trends in the epidemiology of cerebral palsy between 1968 and 1981.[30] The authors concluded that the increased survival of

---

TABLE 10-1 CUMULATIVE INCIDENCE OF CEREBRAL PALSY PER 1000 LIVE BIRTHS

Study	Year published	Birth years	Country	Length of follow-up (years)	Rate, excluding acquired (per 1000)
Jarvis et al.[24]	1995	1972-1975	England	5	1.8
Nelson and Ellenberg[25]	1986	1959-1966	United States*	7	4.6
Emond et al.[26]	1989	1970	England	7	2.5
Hagberg et al.[27†]	1989	1979-1982	Sweden	4	2.2
Holst et al.[28]	1989	1978	Denmark	4	4.9
Dowding and Barry[29‡]	1988	1979-1981	Ireland	4	1.9
Stanley and Watson[30]	1988	1979-1981	West Australia	5	2.3
Riikonen et al.[31]	1989	1978-1982	Finland	5	2.5
Torfs et al.[32]	1990	1959-1966	United States	5	2.0§
Pharoah et al.[33]	1990	1984	England	5	1.9
Meberg[34]	1990	1980-1984	Norway	4	2.1
Composite Rate					2.7

*Collaborative Perinatal Project.
†Excluded deaths before age 2.
‡Excluded all congenital anomalies.
§Did not indicate whether deaths were included.
From Rosen MG, Dickinson JC. The incidence of cerebral palsy. Am J Obstet Gynecol 1992; 167:417-23.

low birth weight (LBW) infants probably has resulted in an increased number of patients with cerebral palsy but that "most cerebral palsy syndromes still occur in normal birth weight infants."[30]

ETIOLOGY OF CEREBRAL PALSY

The cause(s) of cerebral palsy is/are not known, but the varying forms suggest a multifactorial etiology. The Collaborative Perinatal Project presents older data but still represents one of the largest studies of the antecedent factors associated with cerebral palsy. The investigators evaluated the outcomes of 54,000 pregnancies among patients who delivered at 12 university hospitals between 1959 and 1966. The investigators subjected more than 400 variables to univariate analysis[36]; variables identified as potential risk factors were then subjected to a more rigorous multivariate analysis.[25] The univariate analysis did not suggest that maternal age, parity, socioeconomic status, smoking history, maternal diabetes, duration of labor, or use of anesthesia was associated with cerebral palsy. Using multivariate analysis, the investigators determined that the leading factors associated with cerebral palsy were as follows: (1) maternal mental retardation; (2) birth weight of 2000 g or less; and (3) fetal malformations. Other factors associated with cerebral palsy included the following: (1) breech presentation (but not vaginal breech delivery); (2) severe proteinuria (more than 5 g/24 hr) during the second half of pregnancy; (3) third-trimester bleeding; and (4) a gestational age of 32 weeks or less. There was a slight association between cerebral palsy and fetal bradycardia, chorioamnionitis, and low placental weight. However, only 34% of the cases of cerebral palsy occurred among the 5% of the population deemed to be at highest risk before pregnancy; this proportion increased slightly (to 37%) when the investigators included factors identified during pregnancy or after delivery. These data suggest that most cases of cerebral palsy cannot be predicted and that the identification of pregnancy-related conditions contributes minimally to the identification of patients at risk for having a child with cerebral palsy. A recent large epidemiologic study noted an incidence of neonatal encephalopathy of 3.8 per 1000 term births.[37] The authors identified certain preconception and antepartum factors that were associated with neonatal encephalopathy (Box 10-1). It is estimated that intrapartum factors alone are associated with neonatal encephalopathy in less than 5% of cases.[37,38]

In 2000, the American College of Obstetrics and Gynecology and the American Academy of Pediatrics convened the Neonatal Encephalopathy and Cerebral Palsy Task Force. The final, landmark report,[38] which was released in January 2003, was reviewed and endorsed by such groups as the United States Department of Health, the Child Neurology Society, the March of Dimes Birth Defects Foundation, the National Institutes of Health, the Royal Australian and New Zealand College of Obstetricians and Gynaecologists, the Society for Maternal-Fetal Medicine, and the Society of Obstetricians and Gynaecologists of Canada. The Task Force extended the initial international consensus regarding what is required to establish a potential relationship between intrapartum events and cerebral palsy.[14] The most important results are summarized in Box 10-2. This leads to several medicolegal conclusions: (1) the only types of cerebral palsy associated with intrapartum hypoxia are spastic quadriplegia, and less commonly, dyskinesia; (2) mental retardation, epilepsy, and learning disorders should not be ascribed to birth asphyxia unless accompanied by spastic

---

Box 10-1 WESTERN AUSTRALIAN RISK FACTORS FOR NEWBORN ENCEPHALOPATHY

PRECONCEPTION FACTORS*

Increasing maternal age
Unemployed, unskilled laborer or housewife
No private health insurance
Family history of seizures
Family history of neurologic disorders
Infertility treatment

ANTEPARTUM FACTORS*

Maternal thyroid disease
Severe preeclampsia
Bleeding in pregnancy
Viral illness in pregnancy
Postdates pregnancy
Growth restriction in the fetus
Placental abnormalities

---

*Significantly and independently associated with newborn encephalopathy in multiple logistic regression analysis.
Information compiled from Badawi N, Kurinczuk JJ, Keogh JM, et al. Antepartum risk factors for neonatal encephalopathy: The Western Australia case-control study. BMJ 1998; 317:1549-53.

Box 10-2 CRITERIA TO DEFINE AN ACUTE INTRAPARTUM HYPOXIC EVENT AS SUFFICIENT TO CAUSE CEREBRAL PALSY

ESSENTIAL CRITERIA (MUST MEET ALL FOUR)

1. Evidence of a metabolic acidosis in fetal umbilical cord arterial blood obtained at delivery (pH < 7 and base deficit ≥ 12 mmol/L)
2. Early onset of severe or moderate neonatal encephalopathy in infants born at 34 or more weeks' gestation
3. Cerebral palsy of the spastic quadriplegic or dyskinetic type*
4. Exclusion of other identifiable etiologies such as trauma, coagulation disorders, infectious conditions, or genetic disorders

CRITERIA THAT COLLECTIVELY SUGGEST AN INTRAPARTUM TIMING (WITHIN CLOSE PROXIMITY TO LABOR AND DELIVERY [E.G., 0 TO 48 HOURS]) BUT ARE NONSPECIFIC TO ASPHYXIAL INSULTS

1. A sentinel (signal) hypoxic event occurring immediately before or during labor
2. A sudden and sustained fetal bradycardia or the absence of fetal heart rate variability in the presence of persistent, late, or variable decelerations, usually after an hypoxic sentinel event when the pattern was previously normal
3. Apgar scores of 0 to 3 beyond 5 minutes
4. Onset of multisystem involvement within 72 hours of birth
5. Early imaging study showing evidence of acute nonfocal cerebral abnormality

---

*Spastic quadriplegia and, less commonly, dyskinetic cerebral palsy are the only types of cerebral palsy associated with acute hypoxic intrapartum events. Spastic quadriplegia is not specific to intrapartum hypoxia. Hemiparetic cerebral palsy, hemiplegic cerebral palsy, spastic diplegia, and ataxia are unlikely to result from acute intrapartum hypoxia. (Nelson KB, Grether JK. Potentially asphyxiating conditions and spastic cerebral palsy in infants of normal birth weight. Am J Obstet Gynecol 1998; 179:507-13.)
From the American College of Obstetricians and Gynecologists Taskforce on Neonatal Encephalopathy and Cerebral Palsy. Neonatal Encephalopathy and Cerebral Palsy: Defining the Pathogenesis and Pathophysiology. Washington, DC, American College of Obstetricians and Gynecologists, 2003. Modified from MacLennan A. A template for defining a causal relation between acute intrapartum events and cerebral palsy: International consensus statement. BMJ 1999; 319: 1054-9.

quadriplegia; (3) no statements of severity should be made before 3 to 4 years of age, because mild cases may improve and dyskinesia may not be evident until then; and (4) intrapartum hypoxia sufficient to cause cerebral palsy is always accompanied by neonatal encephalopathy and seizures.[14,38]

Peripartum Asphyxia and Cerebral Palsy

In 1953, Dr. Virginia Apgar, an anesthesiologist, introduced her scoring system to help identify those newborn infants who require resuscitation and to facilitate assessment of the adequacy of subsequent resuscitation efforts.[39] Physicians hoped that the Apgar score would help identify those infants at risk for cerebral palsy.[40,41] At best, there is a weak association between low Apgar scores and cerebral palsy. In the Collaborative Perinatal Project, only 1.7% of children with a 1-minute Apgar score of 3 or less developed cerebral palsy.[2] Among infants who weighed more than 2500 g at delivery, the incidence of cerebral palsy was 4.7% if the 5-minute Apgar score was 0 to 3, but the incidence was only 0.2% if the 5-minute Apgar score was at least 7; among infants who weighed less than 2500 g, the incidence of cerebral palsy was 6.7% and 0.8%, respectively. Among all infants, there was an increased incidence of cerebral palsy if the Apgar score remained 3 or less for longer than 5 minutes. Likewise, the incidence of early neonatal death increased among those infants with prolonged neonatal depression.

Most infants who subsequently manifest evidence of cerebral palsy have a normal 5-minute Apgar score. In the Collaborative Perinatal Project, only 15% of the infants who later developed cerebral palsy had a 5-minute Apgar score of 3 or less. Approximately 12% had a 5-minute Apgar score of 4 to 6, and the remaining 73% had a 5-minute Apgar score of at least 7.[2]

The Apgar scoring system should be modified when it is used to assess preterm newborns. Even under ideal circumstances, preterm neonates are more likely to have hypotonia and peripheral cyanosis and typically are less responsive than infants delivered at term; thus it is unusual for a healthy preterm infant to have an Apgar score of more than 7.[42] Current guidelines for neonatal resuscitation (for both term and preterm newborns) delineate assessment on the basis of the triad of heart rate, respiration, and color.[43,44]

Although most cases of cerebral palsy result from insults that predate the intrapartum period, we should understand that intrapartum asphyxia does occur and can have serious consequences. The degree of intrapartum asphyxia that will produce irreversible CNS injury is unclear. In some cases, an intrapartum insult may be superimposed on subclinical chronic fetal compromise; in these cases, an insult that might otherwise be innocuous may result in permanent injury to the fetus.

The definition of *asphyxia* may be reduced to "insufficient exchange of respiratory gases."[45] This definition, although accurate, does not include any index of severity and does not have any predictive value. Unfortunately, most studies have not used a uniform definition of birth asphyxia.[46-48] As recently as 1996, one study defined "normal" umbilical cord blood gas and pH measurements.[45] In that study, the authors limited their assessment to vigorous neonates, whom they arbitrarily defined as having a 5-minute Apgar score of 7 or more. Data were available for 16,060 (61%) of 26,249 newborn infants during the study period of 1977 to 1993. Of these newborns, 15,073 (94%) satisfied the inclusion criteria. The

median umbilical artery measurements (with the 2.5th percentile in parentheses) were pH 7.26 (7.10), Po_2 17 (6) mm Hg, Pco_2 52 (74) mm Hg, and base excess −4 (−11) mEq/L. Only small differences in median pH were present when infants were grouped according to gestational age. The effects of gestational age on other cord blood measurements were not reported, but the authors stated that these results were similar to those for pH measurements. It would have been useful if the authors had reported data for all newborns, including those with Apgar scores of less than 7. It should be remembered that Apgar scores are not good predictors of the eventual development of cerebral palsy; thus the inclusion of only "vigorous" infants in this study may be misleading if the data are used to predict the risk of cerebral palsy.

Although events in the intrapartum period likely cause a minority of the cases of cerebral palsy, these events remain important and have been studied extensively. Clinical studies have attempted to define the degree and duration of perinatal asphyxia that is associated with this subset of cases. Fee et al.[49] defined asphyxia as an umbilical artery pH of less than 7.05 with a base deficit greater than 10 mEq/L; they found that this was a poor predictor of adverse neurologic outcome. Goodwin et al.[50] defined asphyxia as an umbilical artery pH of less than 7.00; they found that morbidity "occurred with greater frequency as the degree of acidemia increased." Goldaber et al.[51] also observed increased neonatal morbidity and mortality among term infants (birth weight greater than 2500 g) with an umbilical artery pH of less than 7.00. In summary, asphyxia—by definition—represents an insufficient exchange of respiratory gases; however, the magnitude of impairment that is clinically significant remains unclear.

Low et al.[52,53] have attempted to further define the role of perinatal asphyxia in cases of neurologic injury. They have described a unique (but not universally accepted) definition of asphyxia. At their institution, a buffer base* of less than 36 mmol/L is more than two standard deviations below the mean for "clinically normal" term fetuses at delivery.[54] Lactic acid contributes to the metabolic acidosis produced by asphyxia. It was reasoned that, because a proportion (approximately one third) of lactate may be derived normally from pyruvate, the buffer base threshold should be adjusted down to be less than 34 mmol/L to "serve as a measure of metabolic acidosis due to hypoxia."[55] Using this definition, the authors demonstrated that the incidence of asphyxia in term newborns was approximately 2%; however, in a much smaller cohort of preterm fetuses (less than 2000 g at birth), the incidence was approximately 6%.[55,56] The authors performed neurodevelopmental studies of the term infants at 1 year of age, and they found an increased incidence of neurologic deficits among those infants who had an umbilical artery buffer base of less than 34 mmol/L at birth; the relationship was especially strong when the umbilical artery buffer base was less than 20 mmol/L at birth.[57] These investigators demonstrated a similar relationship in a study of preterm newborns.[58]

Continuing their investigations, Low et al.[59,60] studied complications in newborns after intrapartum asphyxia in term and preterm fetuses. From these studies, they developed a complication score that expressed the magnitude of neona-

---

Buffer base is defined as the amount of buffer in blood available to combine with nonvolatile acids. A buffer base of 34 mmol/L is equivalent to a whole blood base deficit of 12 mmol/L.

tal complications. Among the term fetuses, newborn complications increased in frequency and severity with increased severity and duration of metabolic acidosis at birth. A low Apgar score at 1 minute was a better predictor of neonatal complications than a low Apgar score at 5 minutes. Of interest, respiratory acidosis at birth did not predict complications in newborns. Similar results were noted for preterm fetuses delivered between 32 and 36 weeks' gestation. For fetuses delivered before 32 weeks' gestation, complications were similar in the control and asphyxia groups. Using this scoring system in term fetuses, the investigators predicted that the threshold for moderate or severe newborn complications was an umbilical artery base deficit of 12 mmol/L.[61]

Some investigators do not accept Low's definition of asphyxia, but few have performed follow-up neurodevelopment examinations. Nagel et al.[62] performed such examinations in children who had an umbilical arterial blood pH of less than 7.00 at delivery. Thirty children qualified for the study, and 28 of them survived the neonatal period. Evaluation at 1 to 3 years of age detected three children who had experienced an episode of hypertonia. Only one child displayed a mild motor developmental delay, and the majority of children exhibited no major problems. Another study examined neonatal complications in babies with an umbilical arterial blood pH of less than 7.00 at delivery.[63] Only three of 35 affected newborns died during the neonatal period. These investigators did not perform any follow-up neurologic examinations after the neonatal period.[63]

Because Low and others have placed an emphasis on the importance of metabolic acidosis as a predictor of complications in newborns, it would be helpful if the severity of acidosis could be anticipated intrapartum. Gull et al.[64] studied a small cohort of 27 patients with "terminal bradycardia" who were delivered vaginally. Not surprisingly, the umbilical arterial blood base deficit was greater in infants with end-stage bradycardia than in controls. Although this was a very small study, the authors suggested a correlation between the loss of short-term FHR variability for more than 4 minutes during end-stage bradycardia and the development of metabolic acidosis.

The relationship between the umbilical artery base excess and the timing of hypoxic injury has been estimated on the basis of data from human and animal studies.[65] Unfortunately, this relationship alone cannot accurately time the injury, because it does not consider the role of previous or repetitive hypoxic episodes before the episode in question. The human fetus is very robust. Most babies born after an episode of in utero asphyxia will be normal, whereas a smaller number will die in utero. Blumenthal[1] concluded that "there is a fine threshold between normality and death from asphyxia."

Some investigators have suggested that the presence of increased numbers of nucleated red blood cells in the umbilical circulation at delivery is a marker of intrauterine asphyxia.[66-68] These investigators have also suggested that the nucleated red blood cell count might be used to time an asphyxial event. Their data showed considerable variability; thus the predictive value of the test in an individual case may be limited. In addition, results varied according to birth weight and gestational age.[69] Furthermore, it may be more difficult to time the occurrence of an injury if the fetus suffered multiple episodes of asphyxia, including some that were remote from delivery. In such cases, the nucleated red blood cell count may reflect only the most recent and possibly least important event and thus falsely implicate the recent event as the cause of an injury. Both nucleated red blood cell and lymphocyte counts seem to be elevated longer in cases of antepartum asphyxia than in intrapartum asphyxia.[38]

Chorioamnionitis, Fever, and Cerebral Palsy

Recent studies have demonstrated an association between cerebral palsy and chorioamnionitis, both in preterm infants and in term infants of normal birth weight.[70,71] An elevated maternal temperature is one sign of chorioamnionitis, but fever alone is insufficient for the diagnosis. Other signs include—but are not limited to—the following: maternal and fetal tachycardia, foul-smelling amniotic fluid, uterine tenderness, and maternal leukocytosis. A Gram-stain examination of amniotic fluid may be useful. Often the diagnosis is presumed but remains unproved unless it is confirmed by culture or histologic examination of the placenta. The mechanism by which chorioamnionitis may be associated with cerebral palsy is unclear. Some investigators have suggested that inflammatory cytokines are a potential cause of perinatal brain injury.[72-74]

Several studies have demonstrated a tendency for maternal temperature to increase after administration of epidural analgesia during labor.[75,76] The relationship between epidural analgesia and maternal fever remains a matter of dispute. Furthermore, it would be erroneous to conclude that epidural analgesia-associated maternal pyrexia indicates chorioamnionitis and therefore increases the risk of cerebral palsy.[77] It is common practice for obstetricians to give antibiotics to mothers with fever and no other evidence of chorioamnionitis; this may lead to unnecessary neonatal sepsis evaluations and antibiotic exposure for which epidural analgesia has been blamed.[78] Mayer et al.[79] correctly stated that "rather than treating all women with temperature elevations and epidurals for presumed chorioamnionitis," physicians should make an effort to differentiate true chorioamnionitis from incidental maternal fever. These investigators found that additional signs of chorioamnionitis were present in all cases in which the diagnosis was later confirmed by culture or pathologic examination. The influence of epidural analgesia-associated maternal fever on the incidence of cerebral palsy has not been studied directly. However, it should be emphasized that the largest univariate analysis did *not* identify regional anesthesia as a risk factor for cerebral palsy.[36]

The mode of delivery has been examined as an independent risk factor for periventricular leukomalacia in preterm deliveries (25 to 32 weeks' gestation) complicated by chorioamnionitis.[80] The authors identified 99 cases that met the criteria for chorioamnionitis, and these infants were serially examined for evidence of periventricular leukomalacia. The investigators identified a significant association between vaginal birth and periventricular leukomalacia. Given that the cesarean section group likely included a substantial number of infants with a non-reassuring FHR tracing, it is striking that the infants delivered by cesarean section had better outcomes. The authors correctly cautioned that a prospective trial is needed to confirm the observations from this retrospective study.

Advances in the Radiologic Diagnosis of Cerebral Injury

Great strides have been made in the diagnosis of neonatal brain injury with magnetic resonance imaging (MRI).[81-83]

MRI has been used most often during the neonatal period, but it has also been used for the intrauterine diagnosis of fetal brain injury.[84] Younkin[85] reviewed the use of MRI in the diagnosis of HIE in newborn infants. Three-dimensional MRI can be used to determine the volume of gray matter and the degree of white matter myelination and thus can provide valuable insights into normal and abnormal brain development in humans.[86] Although it is far from an exact science, MRI can be used in some cases to estimate the timing of the brain injury in patients with cerebral palsy.[87] There is a strong correlation between anatomic brain lesions detected on MRI and specific types of cerebral palsy.[88] MRI is particularly sensitive in the detection of periventricular leukomalacia, but it is important to stress that many children with this MRI abnormality will have clinically normal neurologic development.[89] The presence of cerebral edema confirms that the brain injury is of recent onset (i.e., develops in 6 to 12 hours and clears in 4 days).[1] Unfortunately, the changes may be subtle. Also, this time frame typically exceeds the duration of the intrapartum period. Nonetheless, this information can be quite helpful, and early imaging should be sought. Cerebral ultrasonography remains a useful technique in the early neurologic assessment of the newborn.[90] This is especially true for the critically ill infant who would be unsuitable for transport to an MRI facility.

PATHOPHYSIOLOGY OF FETAL ASPHYXIA

Much of our knowledge regarding the fetal response to asphyxia has been gained through the use of animal models; however, the limitations of these models must be acknowledged. Raju[91] has reviewed the various animal models of fetal brain injury. One advantage of the chronically instrumented fetal lamb is that it is similar in size to the human fetus; this facilitates the placement of electrodes and vascular catheters in both the fetus and the mother. Investigators may obtain measurements while the mother (and fetus) remain anesthetized, or they may obtain measurements from animals who have recovered from surgery. Studies of chronically instrumented animals allow the assessment of fetal breathing movements, gross body movements, the electroencephalogram, and blood gas and pH measurements. Blood concentrations of glucose, lactate, and various hormones also can be determined.[92-94] Recent studies have used microdialysis techniques to evaluate neurotransmitter release within the fetal brain in vivo in acute, exteriorized, and chronic preparations.[95-97] Other studies have measured fetal cerebral blood flow in vivo during episodes of hypoxemia[98] and during maternal infusion of ethanol.[99] Together, these studies have enhanced our understanding of the fetal brain response to pathophysiologic insults in utero. Ultimately, these new insights may lead to improved diagnoses, treatment, and/or prevention of fetal brain injury.

Studies have used a variety of methods to produce fetal hypoxemia and acidemia in fetal lambs. Each method may mimic one or more clinically relevant situations. These methods involve the following: (1) decreasing the concentration of maternal-inspired oxygen for several hours[92] or days[93]; (2) decreasing uterine blood flow, which may be accomplished by placing an adjustable clamp on the common iliac artery[100]; (3) decreasing umbilical blood flow, either by total obstruction[101] or by means of a slow, progressive obstruction[102,103]; (4) uteroplacental embolization[104]; (5) maternal hemorrhage[105]; and (6) a combination of two insults, such as hypoxemia plus hypotension.[106]

Care must be exercised when applying knowledge gained from hypoxia/ischemia studies conducted on nonfetal models (e.g., rat pups) to the problem of asphyxia in utero. The fetus and the fetal brain exist in a relatively hypoxemic environment. Despite preferential streaming of the most highly oxygenated blood to the brain and heart, the average Po_2 measured in the carotid artery of fetal lambs at term is approximately 22 mm Hg.[107] Furthermore, unlike adult conditions in which global anoxia (i.e., cardiac arrest) or focal ischemia (i.e., stroke) is the clinical correlate, fetal asphyxia typically involves diminished—but not absent—delivery of oxygen, with variable degrees of respiratory or metabolic acidosis. A complete loss of cerebral blood flow rarely occurs, except as a terminal event. Of course, prolonged hypoxemia and decreased oxygen delivery will result in acidemia and myocardial failure, followed by ischemia and rapid fetal demise. Fetal hypoxemia may result from the compromise of any or all of the steps involved in maternal-fetal oxygen transport (Box 10-3).[108] The impact of repeated hypoxic-ischemic insults should not be underestimated, and numerous clinical scenarios can be envisioned whereby this might occur (e.g., repetitive cord occlusion). Moreover, brief insults that might of themselves be harmless could cause damage if repeated; this has been demonstrated in adult rats[109] and in fetal lambs.[110]

The fetus takes advantage of several adaptive responses that help it survive and grow in the relatively hypoxemic intrauterine environment. These responses may be categorized as those that involve altered fetal metabolism and those that maximize fetal oxygen transport (Box 10-4).[108] Richardson[111] has defined the *oxygen margin of safety* as the degree to which fractional oxygen extraction can increase and fetal arterial Po_2 can decrease before tissue oxygen supplies are inadequate. Regardless of the etiology of decreased oxygen delivery to the fetus, fetal oxygen consumption is maintained by increasing oxygen extraction until oxygen delivery is approximately 50% of normal.[112] Lower levels of tissue oxygen tension result in progressive metabolic acidemia and a terminal decrease in oxygen consumption.[111]

Box 10-3 FACTORS DECREASING O_2 TRANSFER TO THE FETUS

ENVIRONMENTAL PO_2

High altitude

MATERNAL CARDIOPUL-MONARY FUNCTION

Cyanotic heart disease

O_2 TRANSPORT BY MATERNAL BLOOD

Anemia
Cigarette smoking

PLACENTAL BLOOD FLOW

Hypertension
Diabetes
Placental abruption
Uterine contractions

PLACENTAL O_2 TRANSFER

Placental abruption
Placental infarcts

UMBILICAL BLOOD FLOW AND FETAL CIRCULATION

Umbilical cord occlusion
Heart disease

O_2 TRANSPORT BY FETAL BLOOD

Anemia
Hemorrhage

From Richardson B. The fetal brain: Metabolic and circulatory responses to asphyxia. Clin Invest Med 1993; 16:103-14.

Alterations in substrate use may affect the fetal response to asphyxia. Unlike the adult brain, the fetal brain can use ketone bodies and lactate as alternative energy sources.[38] In gravid ewes, decreased uterine blood flow results in decreased fetal glucose consumption.[113] In the adult, current opinion holds that hyperglycemia should be avoided in patients at risk for ischemia.[114] Hyperglycemia may exacerbate metabolic acidosis by providing substrate for anaerobic metabolism, which results in an increased production of lactic acid. Vannucci and Mujsce,[115] citing experiments in neonatal rat pups, suggested that the immature brain may respond differently and that glucose administration may reduce hypoxic-ischemic brain injury. These authors did not consider earlier work by Blomstrand et al.,[116] who studied the effects of hypoxia in the anesthetized, exteriorized fetal lamb. In that study, hyperglycemia accelerated the loss of somatosensory evoked potentials, the onset of metabolic acidosis, and the reduction of cerebral oxygen consumption. Until these different observations are reconciled, it seems prudent to maintain normoglycemia in utero.

During chronic hypoxemia, the fetus may also restrict the use of energy derived from oxidative metabolism to maintain essential cellular processes; this may lead to decreased somatic growth and intrauterine growth restriction. Using an ovine model of asphyxia, Hooper et al.[117] detected a decreased incorporation of tritiated [3H]-thymidine (which reflects decreased DNA turnover and presumably decreased cell division) in fetal tissue. However, the decreased incorporation of tritiated [3H]-thymidine was not uniform in all tissues. Rates of DNA synthesis were maintained in most fetal tissues (including the fetal brain) but were greatly reduced in the lung, the skeletal muscle, and the thymus gland.

The fetus can conserve additional energy by decreasing breathing and gross body movements. Rurak and Gruber[118] demonstrated a 17% decrease in fetal oxygen consumption in fetal lambs that were paralyzed by a neuromuscular blocking agent. Perceptible fetal movements represent an index of fetal health. Many obstetricians instruct their patients to count episodes of fetal activity at specified periods and to consult them immediately if fetal movements are decreased or absent. Fetal hypoxemia results in decreased activity and decreased rapid eye movement (REM) sleep in fetal lambs. REM sleep states are associated with an increased cerebral metabolic rate for oxygen ($CMRO_2$).[98] Thus, during periods of fetal stress, a reduction in fetal body movements or REM sleep results in a significant decrease in fetal energy expenditure.

Oxygen deprivation typically results in a change and/or redistribution of fetal cardiac output[119]; the magnitude of these changes depends on the mechanism and severity of oxygen deprivation. Sheldon et al.[120] demonstrated that experimental fetal hypoxemia (produced by the administration of a decreased maternal-inspired concentration of oxygen) resulted in *increased* blood flow to the brain, myocardium, and adrenal glands. In fetal lambs, a brief (4-minute) complete arrest of uterine and ovarian blood flow resulted in a decrease in blood flow to all organs (including the brain) except the myocardium and adrenal glands.[121]

Adaptive changes to intrauterine hypoxemia vary between the immature and the mature fetus. The neuropathology of intrauterine asphyxia depends, to some extent, on gestational age. The neuropathologic response to sustained hypoxia with developing acidemia was studied in mid-gestation and near-term fetal lambs.[122] In this study, it was demonstrated that immature fetuses had predominantly periventricular

---

Box 10-4 FETAL CEREBRAL RESPONSES TO ASPHYXIA

FETAL CEREBRAL METABOLISM

Oxygen margin of safety
Substrate alterations
Decreased growth
Behavioral state alterations

FETAL CEREBRAL O$_2$ TRANSPORT

Cerebral blood flow redistribution

From Richardson B. The fetal brain: Metabolic and circulatory responses to asphyxia. Clin Invest Med 1993; 16:103-14.

---

injury and that mature fetuses had primarily cortical injury, although there was some overlap (Figure 10-1). This is consistent with injury patterns in humans. It is not surprising that the biophysical and biochemical responses to hypoxemia vary between preterm and term fetuses. Matsuda et al.[92] observed that the development of metabolic acidemia, decreased fetal breathing and body movements, and an altered sleep state were much less pronounced in mid-gestation fetal lambs subjected to hypoxemia as compared with fetal lambs at term.

Studies of fetal lambs are valuable and have provided data that cannot be obtained from human fetuses. However, one should understand this model's limitations before extrapolating the experimental findings to the human fetus. At birth, both the sheep and the guinea pig brain are much closer to maturity than the human brain. In this regard, the rat pup is more similar to the human; both the rat pup brain and the human brain undergo significant extrauterine development (Figure 10-2).[123] Unfortunately, no animal model exactly duplicates human fetal development.

Placentation also varies among animal species, and the type of placentation affects the extent of transplacental transfer of various substances. Moreover, the relationship of maternal and fetal blood flow varies among species. Among animals used for studies of fetal physiology, the morphology of the placenta may be either hemochorial or epitheliochorial. In **hemochorial** forms, the fetal chorion invades the uterine stroma, thereby destroying the maternal endothelium and coming in direct contact with maternal blood. By contrast, **epitheliochorial** placentas have an intact maternal vascular epithelium.[124]

Maternal and fetal blood can flow past each other in an efficient countercurrent pattern, or the exchange can be less well coordinated—and hence less efficient—as occurs in the concurrent (or venous equilibration) pattern.[124]

Magnesium Sulfate and Cerebral Palsy

Controversy continues regarding the role of magnesium sulfate in preventing or possibly exacerbating fetal brain injury. Two reports documented a decreased incidence of cerebral palsy in surviving very low birth weight (VLBW) infants who were exposed to magnesium sulfate in utero.[125,126] In a retrospective study, Nelson and Grether[126] reviewed the outcomes of a cohort of San Francisco-area VLBW children born between 1983 and 1985 who had survived to at least 3 years of age. There were 155,636 live births during this period, and 881 VLBW survivors met the study criteria. Of these, 42 children had moderate to severe cerebral palsy. These children were matched with 75 randomly selected VLBW controls. Magnesium sulfate had been administered to 7% of the chil-

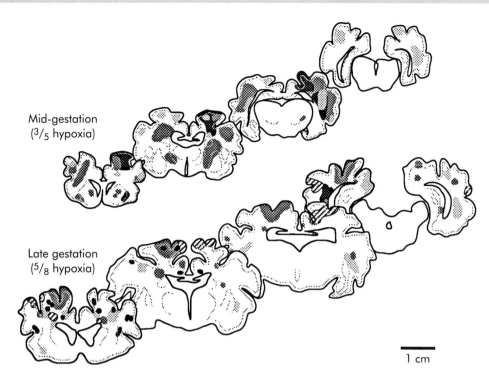

Mid-gestation
($^3/_5$ hypoxia)

Late gestation
($^5/_8$ hypoxia)

1 cm

FIGURE 10-1. Composite diagram showing distribution of hypoxic injury in mid-gestation *(top)* and near-term *(bottom)* fetal lambs 3 days after 8 hours of arterial hypoxemia. Hypoxemia was produced by placing the pregnant ewe in a chamber with reduced ambient oxygen. Each shading pattern represents an individual animal. The severity of injury is not indicated in this diagram. (From Penning DH, Grafe MR, Hammond R, et al. Neuropathology of the near-term and midgestation ovine fetal brain after sustained in utero hypoxemia. Am J Obstet Gynecol 1994; 170:1425-32.)

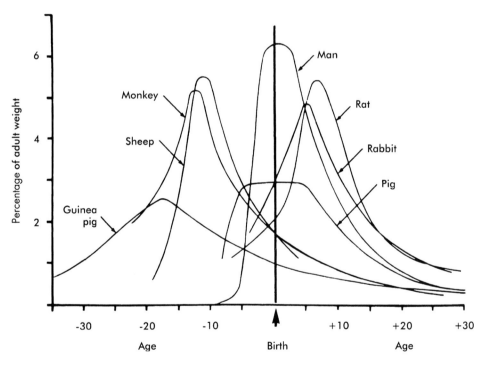

FIGURE 10-2. Brain growth spurts of seven mammalian species expressed as first-order velocity curves of the increase in weight with age. The units of time for each species are as follows: guinea pig (days); rhesus monkey (4 days); sheep (5 days); pig (weeks); man (months); rabbit (2 days); rat (days). Rates are expressed as a percentage of adult weight for each unit of time. (From Dobbing J, Sands S. Comparative aspects of the brain growth spurt. Early Hum Dev 1979; 3:79-83.)

dren in the cerebral palsy group and to 36% of the controls (odds ratio [OR], 0.14; 95% confidence interval [CI], 0.05 to 0.51), which suggested that magnesium sulfate had a protective effect. In the majority of cases, magnesium sulfate was administered for seizure prophylaxis in preeclamptic patients; thus an alternative explanation is that preeclampsia confers a protective effect. Indeed the hypothesis that preeclampsia alone is protective to the fetus has been entertained, and this issue is far from settled.[127]

The number of subjects was too small to separate the effect of preeclampsia from the proposed protective action of magnesium sulfate. However, further analysis supported the conclusion that magnesium sulfate had a protective effect.

In a subset of patients who received magnesium sulfate for tocolysis during preterm labor, the apparent protective effect of magnesium sulfate was maintained. Furthermore, when a covariate analysis was performed to assess the potential contribution of antenatal steroids administered to accelerate fetal lung maturity, the protective effect of magnesium continued to be maintained.

In a study that has received international attention,[128] Schendel et al.[125] evaluated a cohort of children in Georgia to examine the relationship between prenatal exposure to magnesium sulfate and the risk of developing cerebral palsy or mental retardation among VLBW survivors. These investigators studied all VLBW infants born in Atlanta and surrounding counties during a 2-year period. Among the children who were alive at 3 to 5 years of age, they determined the presence or absence of cerebral palsy, mental retardation, and intrauterine exposure to magnesium sulfate. Among Atlanta-born survivors, the incidence of cerebral palsy for the magnesium sulfate-treated group was 0.9% versus 7.7% for the group that was not exposed to magnesium sulfate (OR, 0.11; 95% CI, 0.02 to 0.81). The incidence of mental retardation for the magnesium sulfate-treated group was 1.8% versus 5.8% for the group that was not exposed to magnesium sulfate (OR, 0.3; 95% CI, 0.07 to 1.29). The authors performed a multivariate analysis to assess the contribution of risk factors, including preeclampsia/eclampsia; antihypertensive therapy; maternal administration of other drugs (i.e., antibiotics, other tocolytic agents, corticosteroids); maternal age, education, and race; neonatal birth weight; gender; and gestational age at delivery. All of these factors had a negligible effect on the relative risk for either cerebral palsy or mental retardation. Because the selective mortality of magnesium sulfate-exposed children could have created bias in favor of a protective effect of magnesium sulfate, the authors determined whether there was any difference in mortality between magnesium sulfate-exposed and unexposed children; they found no association between prenatal magnesium sulfate exposure and infant mortality.

In an accompanying editorial, Nelson[129] delineated several possible interpretations of these data, including the possibility that magnesium protects against fetal neurologic injury. Alternatively, because magnesium sulfate often is administered for seizure prophylaxis in preeclamptic patients, it is possible that preeclampsia itself is protective. The small sample size in this study precluded a definite conclusion, but the results suggested that magnesium exerted an independent protective effect. Nelson[129] discussed the potential contribution of concurrent corticosteroid therapy, which is most often combined with magnesium sulfate when the latter is used for tocolysis. However, Nelson[129] noted that other studies have failed to demonstrate a protective effect of corticosteroids.

The question of a potential fetal therapeutic role for magnesium sulfate in *term* pregnancy is unresolved. It is difficult to separate the effect of magnesium sulfate from the possible effects of preeclampsia per se. Preeclampsia/eclampsia is essentially the only indication for the use of magnesium sulfate at term; only randomized clinical trials or animal studies that specifically test for a neuroprotective effect of magnesium sulfate will resolve this issue. It has been estimated that a clinical trial to investigate the possible benefit of magnesium sulfate for the prevention of cerebral palsy would require the enrollment of 900,000 to 1,500,000 patients.[130]

These studies[126,127] have also prompted interest in the potential of magnesium sulfate to protect the fetal brain during a pathophysiologic insult such as hypoxia. The neuroprotective effects of magnesium sulfate appear to result primarily from the magnesium ion's interaction with the glutamate neuronal system. When present in the synapse at a high concentration, glutamate can produce excitotoxic neuronal cell death by means of excessive calcium ion influx, primarily because of N-methyl-D-aspartate (NMDA) receptor overactivation. The developing CNS also is vulnerable to the excitotoxic actions of glutamate. In fact, areas such as the cerebral cortex are much more susceptible to glutamate/NMDA receptor-induced excitotoxic injury during the period of rapid fetal brain growth and development than in adulthood.[131]

The fetus reacts to decreased arterial oxygen content by centralizing blood flow to the vital organs, including the brain.[119] Reynolds et al.[105] performed a study of the effect of fetal hypermagnesemia on this compensatory mechanism during an episode of hypoxia in fetal lambs. The results were disturbing; the administration of magnesium sulfate caused an increase in the proportion of fetal deaths produced by maternal hemorrhage. Furthermore, among surviving fetuses, hypermagnesemia inhibited the compensatory increase in fetal cerebral blood flow that was observed in the saline-treated animals. Although caution must be used in extrapolating these data to humans, the results suggest that the effects of magnesium sulfate may not be entirely beneficial (or benign).

By contrast, de Haan et al.[132] did not observe any effect (either positive or negative) of magnesium sulfate on fetal survival or compensatory cerebral blood flow in fetal lambs subjected to umbilical cord occlusion. However, these investigators used a different method of producing fetal hypoxemia, and they also used a different method of measuring changes in blood flow (i.e., Doppler measurements of carotid artery flow instead of radioactive microspheres). Moon et al.[133] also found that magnesium sulfate did not impair the redistribution of cardiac output or cause fetal death in response to maternal hemorrhage in gravid ewes. A study in rats found that magnesium sulfate was protective if given *before* an hypoxic-ischemic insult but that it increased neuronal injury if given *after* the insult.[134] This again raises the possibility that magnesium has intrinsic neuroprotective properties at the cellular and molecular level but that it may impair important compensatory responses at the whole-organism level.

In a controversial randomized controlled trial, Mittendorf et al.[135] observed that women randomized to receive magnesium sulfate for tocolysis had worse perinatal outcomes and that this effect was dose-related. It seems intuitive that women having refractory preterm labor would have higher magnesium sulfate requirements and possibly also worse outcomes. This was a small study, but it gives pause in view of the conflicting data regarding the efficacy of magnesium sulfate for tocolysis.[136]

In summary, the best studies support the continued use of magnesium sulfate for seizure prophylaxis in preeclampsia. Clinical evidence suggests that the antenatal use of magnesium sulfate confers some protection against neonatal demise.[137] However, in certain situations that may produce fetal hypoxemia (e.g., maternal hemorrhage), magnesium sulfate may inhibit the expected compensatory increase in fetal cerebral blood flow.

NEUROPATHOLOGY OF PERINATAL ASPHYXIA

The mechanism and timing of an asphyxial insult affects the pattern of pathology that is seen in the fetus and neonate. Acute complete asphyxia must be distinguished from incomplete, brief, or intermittent asphyxia or chronic hypoxemia. **Complete asphyxia** may occur in the setting of a total placental abruption or umbilical cord occlusion. If unrecognized and untreated, it rapidly leads to fetal demise. **Incomplete asphyxia** may occur in any setting in which oxygen delivery to the fetus is inadequate to meet all of its needs (e.g., brief and/or repeated episodes of umbilical cord occlusion, placental embolization, or incomplete placental abruption). This latter category of incomplete or intermittent asphyxia most likely contributes to the largest proportion of cases of cerebral palsy. In these cases, the insult is not severe enough to lead to immediate fetal demise, but it can profoundly affect fetal brain growth and development. Ongoing studies are attempting to determine whether there is a period of time in utero when the fetus is especially vulnerable to neurologic injury.

Myers[7] used a primate model to perform seminal research on the subject of perinatal brain injury. He identified two patterns of injury, depending on whether the fetus suffered complete or partial asphyxia. First, fetal monkeys at term were subjected to varying lengths (0 to 25 minutes) of **complete asphyxia.** These fetuses were resuscitated when possible, which often required the use of cardiac massage and epinephrine. Postmortem examination revealed extensive pathology in brainstem areas. In humans, it is unlikely that such a severe intrauterine insult would be compatible with extrauterine survival. If survival could follow such a severe insult, the infant would show obvious encephalopathy and multiorgan system dysfunction at birth. More relevant to our discussion of cerebral palsy were the findings in the fetal monkeys subjected to **partial asphyxia;** a number of these animals demonstrated cortical necrosis and damage to subcortical white matter and the basal ganglia.[138] Although these two studies form the core of our knowledge of perinatal brain injury in primates, it should be noted that there were relatively few animals in each experimental group and that the animals demonstrated considerable variability in their responses. Some animals suffered no injury, and others could not be resuscitated.

Several authors have attempted to summarize the neuropathology of fetal and newborn asphyxia.[138-140] Volpe[141] has emphasized the fact that intrauterine asphyxia results in varying neuropathology that depends on the gestational age of the fetus. Volpe also has described a framework of major neuropathologic variations. White matter (especially the periventricular white matter) and the basal ganglia are the principal sites of injury in preterm fetuses. In older fetuses, injury occurs primarily (but not exclusively) in the gray matter of the cortex and cerebellum.

Two pathologic entities deserve additional discussion: periventricular leukomalacia and selective neuronal injury. **Periventricular leukomalacia** is the most common pathologic finding in preterm infants with brain injury.[142] This lesion is characterized by coagulative necrosis of the white matter adjacent to the lateral ventricles and around the foramen of Monro, especially at the external angle of the lateral ventricles and optic radiation.[143] With long-term survival, the lesion may progress to a widening of the ventricles and hydrocephalus ex vacuo. Clinically, periventricular leukomalacia may not be apparent at birth.[139] Developing hydrocephalus may be detected by computed tomography or ultrasound examination. In more subtle cases, MRI may detect decreased myelination (vide supra).[144]

The pathophysiology of periventricular leukomalacia is unclear. Conventional wisdom has held that periventricular leukomalacia is an ischemic lesion unique to preterm infants.[145] The insult is thought to occur in an arterial border zone perfused by end-arterial branches of the middle and posterior cerebral arteries. This border zone has been identified by DeReuck,[145] who demonstrated periventricular arborizations between vessels penetrating to the ventricles (i.e., ventriculopedal vessels) and between vessels arising from the ventriculochoroidal arteries (i.e., ventriculofugal vessels). Others have challenged DeReuck's anatomic findings and have questioned whether periventricular leukomalacia is a purely ischemic lesion.[146,147]

Box 10-5 MAJOR SITES FOR SELECTIVE NEURONAL NECROSIS IN NEONATAL HYPOXIC-ISCHEMIC ENCEPHALOPATHY

Cerebral cortex: Hippocampus more than supralimbic cortex
Diencephalon: Thalamus, hypothalamus, and lateral geniculate body
Basal ganglia: Caudate, putamen, and globus pallidus
Midbrain: Inferior colliculus, oculomotor and trochlear nuclei, red nucleus, substantia nigra, and reticular formation
Pons: Motor nuclei of trigeminal and facial nerves, dorsal more than ventral cochlear nuclei, reticular formation, and pontine nuclei
Medulla: Dorsal motor nucleus of vagus nerve nucleus ambiguus, inferior olivery nuclei, and cuneate and gracilis nuclei
Cerebellum: Purkinje cells, dentate, and other roof nuclei

From Volpe JJ. Hypoxic-ischemic encephalopathy: Neuropathology and pathogenesis. In Volpe JJ. Neurology of the Newborn. 2nd ed. Philadelphia, WB Saunders, 1987:209-35.

White matter in the immature fetal brain may be at increased risk for hypoxic-ischemic injury, because its vessels may have a limited ability to vasodilate.[142] If this is true, autoregulation would be precluded in situations of hypotension. However, at least one study has shown that blood flow to white matter actually may increase (relative to gray matter) during fetal asphyxia.[148] Fetal white matter may be more metabolically active than gray matter because of large numbers of actively myelinating cells.[142] In situations of marginal oxygen supply, this would place glia at risk for injury. One study has suggested that immature astrocytes are more susceptible to ischemic death than mature astrocytes.[149] Studies in fetal lambs have successfully produced pathologic changes similar to those that are present in infants with periventricular leukomalacia[122]; these models may help clarify the mechanism of this common pathologic correlate of cerebral palsy in the preterm infant.

Selective neuronal injury also may occur during the perinatal period. Selective neuronal injury refers to neuronal death without infarction (i.e., without any obvious disturbance of the associated glia or vascular elements). This is the entity most often associated with glutamate-induced neuronal death (vide infra).[150,151] It is difficult to identify the brain sites that are the most vulnerable in humans, because this injury often occurs in infants with severe HIE, multiorgan system failure, and a prolonged intensive care unit stay, which may confound the eventual findings at autopsy. Box 10-5 lists the brain sites that are known to exhibit selective neuronal necrosis.[141]

GLUTAMATE-INDUCED NEURONAL INJURY

Glutamate is the most prevalent neurotransmitter in the CNS. Its action on postsynaptic neurons is excitatory (i.e., depolarizing).[152] (An example of an inhibitory neurotransmitter is gamma-aminobutyric acid.) In an in vitro preparation, hypoxia has been shown to be associated with an increase in extracellular glutamate and a cessation of synaptic activity.[153] Some investigators have reviewed the role of glutamate in ischemic neuronal injury.[150,151,154-157] Figures 10-3 and 10-4 depict the pathogenesis of hypoxic-ischemic injury and the function of excitatory amino acid (EAA) receptors.[158,159] Figure 10-5 gives an overview of the cascade of events that result from the pathologic activation of EAA receptors.

More than 60 years ago, it was observed that the immature animal is more likely to withstand asphyxia than the adult animal.[160-162] The evidence for the role of excitatory amino acids in the pathophysiology of hypoxic-ischemic brain injury in adults has stimulated research on the development (ontogeny) of these neurotransmitter systems in the fetus. It is known from experiments using rat pups that asphyxia causes a disruption in EAA receptors, which suggests that they are susceptible to hypoxic-ischemic injury.[163] Hypoxia-ischemia is known to decrease glutamate reuptake, thus inhibiting the normal process that terminates glutamate's action at the synapse.[164]

The ontogeny of EAA systems has been studied in many species, including the fetal sheep.[165] Anatomically distinct binding patterns exist for each of the major glutamate receptor subtypes (Box 10-6).[158,166] These receptors are commonly referred to as **NMDA type** or **non-NMDA type.** Non-NMDA types include kainate, alpha-amino-3-hydroxy-5-methyl-4-isoxazole-propionic acid (AMPA), and metabotropic subtypes. The metabotropic subtype is unique; activation of the other receptors is linked to ion flow across the postsynaptic membrane, but metabotropic receptor activation is linked to turnover of phosphoinositol (an intracellular second messenger) in the postsynaptic cell. The metabotropic subclass of glutamate receptor also shows developmental alterations.[167] The changing pattern of the glutamate receptor profile may explain, in part, why some neuronal populations are more sensitive to injury at different stages of brain development. Cells with EAA receptors may have an enhanced susceptibility to ischemic injury during specific periods of development[168]; this underlines the importance of determining the developmental profile of these neurotransmitter systems in the fetus.

The chronic in utero microdialysis technique has been used to document the accumulation of glutamate in the fetal brain after a pathophysiologic insult. Increased cortical glutamate concentrations have been noted after acute fetal hypoxemia caused by severe maternal hemorrhage[96] and during chronic hypoxemia produced by restricting uterine artery blood flow for 24 hours.[100] Presumably the released glutamate is free to participate in processes that ultimately lead to fetal brain injury.

Lee and Choi[169] have identified the density and distribution of EAA receptors in the developing human brain. There are clear gestational age-dependent changes in glutamate receptor subtype binding in the fetal brain; for example, a sharp increase in receptor density occurs at mid-gestation. The investigators suggested that these changes may be related to the role of EAA pathways in synaptogenesis. They also suggested that the changing density and distribution of these receptors may be responsible for the age-dependent selective vulnerability in the developing human fetal brain.[169] Greenamyre et al.[170] have shown that there is virtually no glutamatergic innervation of the adult human globus pallidus (a portion of the basal ganglia) but that this area has a high concentration of glutamate receptors in fetuses. The authors

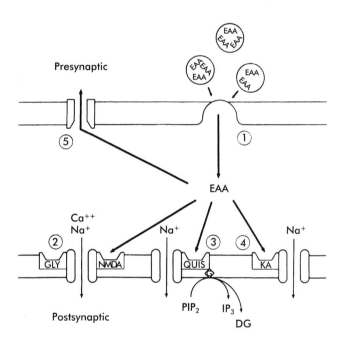

FIGURE 10-4. Excitatory amino acid *(EAA)* synaptic components that contribute to synaptic transmission, second messenger generation, and cessation of these responses are shown. *1,* Glutamate and related excitatory amino acids are released from presynaptic neuronal terminals in a calcium-dependent process by depolarization of the presynaptic neuron. *2 to 4,* Once released into the synaptic cleft, glutamate can depolarize the postsynaptic neuronal membrane by binding to at least three subsets of excitatory amino acid receptors. Activation of the NMDA receptor channel complex *(2),* quisqualate *(QUIS)* receptors *(3)* or kainate *(KA)* receptors *(4)* can produce cationic fluxes through receptor-associated ionophores. Alternatively, a subset of quisqualate receptors are linked with phospholipase C, which activates phosphoinositol hydrolysis and generates the second messengers inositol triphosphate *(IP₃)* and diacylglycerol *(DG).* The distribution of these subtypes of excitatory amino acid receptors in brain can be examined with radiolabeled ligands specific to each receptor subtype. *5,* The excitatory action of glutamate on postsynaptic membranes is inactivated by a presynaptic, high-affinity, energy-dependent transport process. *GLY,* Glycine; *NMDA,* N-methyl-D-aspartate. (From McDonald JW, Johnston MV. Physiological and pathophysiologic roles of excitatory amino acids during central nervous system development. Brain Res Rev 1990; 15:41-70.)

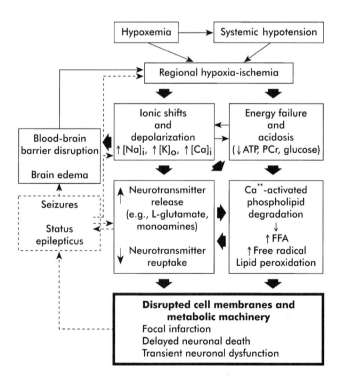

FIGURE 10-3. Pathogenesis of events that may mediate hypoxic-ischemic injury to neurons and other tissues in the brain in the hours following asphyxia. *ATP,* Adenosine triphosphate; *FFA,* Free fatty acid; *PC,* phosphocreatine. (From Nelson N, editor. Current Therapy in Neonatal-Perinatal Medicine, volume 2. Toronto, B.C. Decker, 1990:276.)

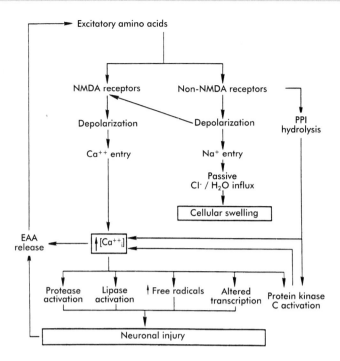

FIGURE 10-5. Some of the mechanisms that may contribute to excitatory amino acid (EAA) neurotoxicity are shown. Experiments in vitro suggest that EAA neurotoxicity may have two components. The first component, mediated by excessive activation of non-NMDA receptors, is characterized by an influx of Na$^+$ followed by passive influx of Cl$^-$ and H$_2$O, which may produce osmotic neuronal swelling. These are acute events occurring within hours of the exposure to EAA agonists. The second, more prominent component is produced by overactivation of NMDA receptors, which leads to a rise in the intracellular concentration of Ca^{2+}. A sustained rise in intracellular Ca^{2+} may trigger a biochemical cascade of events that lead to neuronal injury and death. Furthermore, activation of a subset of non-NMDA receptors coupled with polyphosphoinositide hydrolysis also may elevate intracellular Ca^{2+}. Excitatory amino acids released from synaptic terminals would further propagate neuronal injury. *NMDA,* N-methyl-D-aspartate. (From McDonald JW, Johnston MV. Physiological and pathophysiological roles of excitatory amino acids during central nervous system development. Brain Res Rev 1990; 15:41-70.)

suggested that a glutamate pathway may transiently exist in the globus pallidus during development and may play a role in the basal ganglia damage seen in some forms of cerebral palsy after intrauterine hypoxic-ischemic injury.

In addition to variations in EAA receptor distribution and density, some data suggest that the fetal brain responds differently to anoxia than the adult brain. An increase in intracellular calcium seems to be one component of the final common pathway that leads to irreversible neuronal injury.[171,172] Both the glutamate receptor subtypes and their functions are undoubtedly important in the susceptibility of the fetal brain to glutamate-induced hypoxic-ischemic injury. For example, although kainate is a potent neurotoxin in the adult brain, it is relatively nontoxic in the immature brain, where its receptors lag in appearance behind NMDA and AMPA receptors (Figure 10-6). These receptors also serve a different function in the immature brain than in the mature brain. For example, in the neocortex, striatum, and cerebellum of the rat, the rise in intracellular calcium that results from kainate/AMPA receptor activation is highest in the immature brain and markedly declines with age.[173]

The activation of EAA receptors can also lead to the intracellular production of nitric oxide, which can exacerbate the neurotoxic process (Figure 10-7). This is an area of active research.[174,175]

Box 10-6 CLASSIFICATION OF GLUTAMATE RECEPTORS

NMDA-TYPE RECEPTORS

Ionotropic receptor/channel complex

NON-NMDA–TYPE RECEPTORS

AMPA ionotropic receptors
Kainate ionotropic receptors
Metabotropic receptors

From Johnston MV. Cellular alterations associated with perinatal asphyxia. Clin Invest Med 1993; 16:122-32.

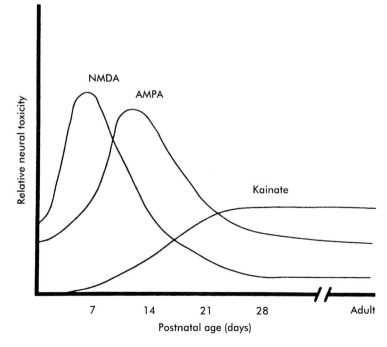

FIGURE 10-6. Relative neurotoxicity of three analogues of glutamate injected into the brain at different ages. Lines represent trends based on experimental work. *AMPA,* Alpha-amino-3-hydroxy-5-methyl-4-isoxazole propionate; *NMDA,* N-methyl-D-aspartate. (From Johnston MV. Cellular alterations associated with perinatal asphyxia. Clin Invest Med 1993;122-32.)

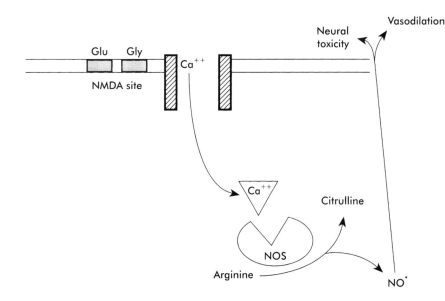

FIGURE 10-7. Proposed mechanism by which calcium entering neurons through excitatory amino acid channels stimulates production of the free-radical second messenger nitric oxide *(NO)*. Nitric oxide can diffuse through membranes to cause vasodilation and neuronal toxicity. *NOS,* Nitric oxide synthase. (From Johnston MV. Cellular alterations associated with perinatal asphyxia. Clin Invest Med 1993; 16:122-32.)

ENDOGENOUS FETAL NEUROPROTECTION

The fetus lives, moves, and grows in a low-oxygen environment; indeed, very high concentrations of oxygen may be toxic to fetal neurons. Nevertheless, immediately after birth, the neonate experiences a rapid increase in oxygen requirement that does not seem to be explained purely on the basis of increased metabolic needs. It is possible that some maternal influence works in utero to suppress oxygen requirements. Progesterone is present in high concentrations in utero, has anesthetic and neuroprotective properties, and is therefore a candidate substance. This hypothesis was tested in neuronal cell cultures mimicking the developing brain.[176] In this study, allopregnanolone, which is the endogenous metabolite of progesterone, protected neurons against NMDA-induced cell necrosis and apoptosis. Perhaps one day these naturally occurring compounds may have a therapeutic role in perinatology and neonatology.

OTHER CAUSES OF FETAL AND NEONATAL BRAIN INJURY

Drugs

Although most drugs cross the placenta and may affect the fetus, discussion in this chapter is limited to two commonly used and abused drugs: alcohol and cocaine. The **fetal alcohol syndrome** is characterized by the triad of intrauterine growth restriction, craniofacial anomalies, and CNS abnormalities[177]; the heart, kidney, and musculoskeletal system may also be affected. The most common craniofacial abnormalities are microcephaly, short palpebral fissures, and midfacial hypoplasia. CNS effects include intellectual impairment and behavioral manifestations. During the early neonatal period, a withdrawal syndrome may occur that may include tremors, hypertonia, abdominal distention, irritability, and seizures. This syndrome may be difficult to distinguish from that of opioid withdrawal. Useful clinical signs include abdominal distention (which occurs more often in cases of alcohol withdrawal) and yawning and diaphoresis (which occur more often in cases of opioid withdrawal).[178]

Smith et al.[179] have reviewed the pathophysiologic effects of ethanol on the fetus. In rats, prenatal ethanol exposure results in a permanent reduction in hippocampal neurons in offspring.[180] Chronic ethanol ingestion also affects glutamate receptor composition.[181] These receptors are known to be important in the normal process of synaptogenesis in the brain; thus it seems reasonable to assume that fetal exposure to ethanol at crucial periods may disrupt normal development. Using chronic in utero microdialysis, Reynolds et al.[97] demonstrated that doses of ethanol that mimic binge ingestion are associated with paroxysmal increases in cortical glutamate concentrations.

Maternal cocaine abuse has increased dramatically and is associated with numerous deleterious effects[182] (see Chapter 52). Cocaine may cause uteroplacental vasoconstriction and decreased uteroplacental perfusion. Cocaine abuse also is associated with preterm labor and placental abruption. In addition, cocaine may affect the fetal brain directly by causing cerebral vasoconstriction, which may result in neuronal injury (Figure 10-8). Various teratogenic and developmental disturbances in infants and children have been reported after exposure to cocaine in utero (Table 10-2). In addition to direct neuronal injury, there is a much higher incidence of subarachnoid and intraventricular hemorrhage in infants exposed to cocaine in utero. Neurobehavioral abnormalities also have been detected in babies exposed to cocaine in utero.[183-185]

Maternal Trauma

Maternal trauma is an uncommon cause of fetal neurologic injury. It is the leading cause of nonobstetric maternal mortality and accounts for approximately 20% of maternal deaths[186] (see Chapter 53). A study from Western Australia noted an incidence of cerebral palsy of 2.6 per 1000 pregnant women who required hospitalization for trauma versus only 1.8 per 1000 who were hospitalized for another reason; however, this difference was not statistically significant.[187]

Mechanisms of injury vary, but placental abruption, uterine rupture, and placental hypoperfusion as a result of maternal hypovolemia are more common than direct fetal injury. Fetal injury that results from placental abruption or fetal-maternal hemorrhage may be delayed; therefore serial examinations may be necessary. It is possible for the fetal head to be

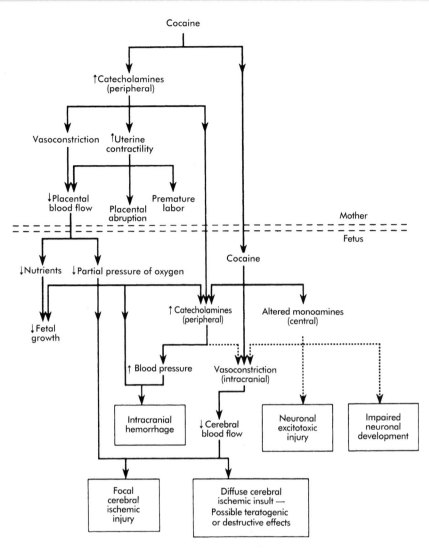

FIGURE 10-8. Deleterious effects of maternal cocaine use on fetuses. Effects that appear plausible on the basis of current information but whose confirmation require more supporting evidence are indicated by dotted lines. ↑, Increased; ↓, decreased. (From Volpe JJ. Effect of cocaine use on the fetus. N Engl J Med 1992; 327:399-407.)

| TABLE 10-2 | DISTURBANCES IN HUMAN BRAIN DEVELOPMENT REPORTED AFTER INTRAUTERINE EXPOSURE TO COCAINE |

Event	Peak gestational period	Abnormality reported after cocaine exposure
Neural tube formation	3-4 weeks	Myelomeningocele, encephalocele
Prosencephalic development	2-3 months	Agenesis of corpus callosum, agenesis of septum pellucidum, septo-optic dysplasia
Neuronal proliferation	3-4 months	Microcephaly
Neuronal migration	3-5 months	Schizencephaly, neuronal heterotopias
Neuronal differentiation	5 months (postnatal)	Abnormal cortical neuronal cytodifferentiation (preliminary)
Myelination	After birth	None

From Volpe JJ. Effect of cocaine use on the fetus. N Engl J Med 1992; 327:399-407.

crushed between the mother's seat belt and the maternal sacral promontory.[188] However, fetal survival depends on maternal survival, which is more likely when the mother is wearing both a lap and a shoulder belt. Thus, seat belts should be worn (appropriately) during pregnancy (see Chapter 53).

Severe trauma does not necessarily mandate the performance of cesarean section. Late FHR decelerations may result from maternal hypovolemia, which may be relieved by volume replacement. The physiologic changes of pregnancy (e.g., uterine enlargement) may compromise cardiopulmonary resuscitation.[189] Aortocaval compression should be avoided at all times.

Fetal Trauma

Some obstetricians favor the elective performance of an episiotomy and the use of outlet forceps to protect the preterm fetal head during vaginal delivery,[190,191] but this is a matter of some dispute.[192] Other factors may affect delivery outcome, including operator skill, maternal anatomy and parity, gestational age, and the station of the fetal head.

Vacuum-assisted delivery has waxed and waned in popularity. The availability of Silastic cups has resulted in more frequent use of this method of delivery.[193] Some obstetricians argue that vacuum extraction is contraindicated in the delivery of preterm infants because of the increased risk of neonatal jaundice associated with the use of this technique.[194] Of course, preterm infants are at increased risk for intracranial hemorrhage, and it is unclear whether vacuum extraction increases the risk of this complication.

Brachial plexus injuries (e.g., Erb's palsy) most often result from fetal macrosomia and shoulder dystocia (see Chapter 17). To avoid these injuries, the anesthesiologist may be asked to provide anesthesia and relaxation of the pelvic floor to facilitate delivery. In some cases, emergency cesarean section is required.

ANESTHESIA AND BRAIN INJURY

Anesthetic agents can have profound effects on brain metabolism and synaptic transmission.[195-199] Anesthetic agents are known to decrease neuronal metabolism and therefore may increase the "oxygen margin of safety."[111] There is abundant rationale to support the use of anesthetic agents as cerebral protective agents; however, experimental and clinical evidence is controversial. Barbiturates prolong the time that neurons can withstand anoxia and regain synaptic activity in vitro.[200] Studies in vivo are much more difficult to interpret, because the systemic effects of anesthetic agents also must be considered. This is especially relevant in pregnant animal models, because profound fetal effects may result from manipulations that the mother tolerates easily.[92] Furthermore, there are subtle differences in the various animal models of cerebral hypoxia-ischemia.[201] Warner et al.[202] demonstrated that volatile anesthetic agents reduce focal ischemic brain damage in nonpregnant rats as compared with awake controls. Previously the apparent protective effects of some drugs have been explained on the basis of drug-induced hypothermia.[203] Even mild hypothermia (2 to 3° C) may be neuroprotective,[204] and this strategy is used effectively in cardiac surgery.

It is unlikely that any protective effect of anesthetic agents can be explained purely on the basis of cerebral metabolic depression. More likely, protective effects result from a complex combination of factors, including alterations in the release or activity of EAA neurotransmitters such as glutamate.[205] In experimental preparations, anesthetic agents such as thiopental, ketamine, isoflurane, halothane, diethyl ether, and chloroform have been shown to inhibit glutamate-induced responses.[206] It also may be possible that hyperpolarizing GABA-receptor agonist drugs (e.g., benzodiazepines) may antagonize the depolarizing effects of glutamate and provide neuroprotection.[207,208]

There is little information on the effects of anesthetic agents on the fetal brain. Myers and Myers[209] have suggested that maternal administration of sedative or anesthetic drugs may prevent or ameliorate the effects of fetal asphyxia at the time of delivery. Suggested mechanisms for this effect include the following: (1) decreased fetal brain metabolism; (2) a decreased maternal stress response, which would tend to improve uteroplacental perfusion; (3) decreased uterine contractility, which would increase uteroplacental perfusion; and (4) a limited increase in fetal glucose concentration. (Fetal hyperglycemia predisposes the fetus to brain lactic acidosis as a result of increased glycolysis.) However, there are no published data that suggest that any anesthetic drug or technique is more likely to protect the fetal brain (provided the chosen technique is administered according to the recommended guidelines for good clinical practice).

The blockade of EAA receptors may help prevent hypoxic-ischemic neuronal injury during episodes of hypoxia in the fetus and neonate.[210-212] However, before unbridled enthusiasm results in the premature clinical use of these drugs, we also must recognize that EAAs have profound trophic effects on normal brain development[213,214]; thus we must exercise caution before we intervene in this process.[215]

Future Directions

A new concept in neurobiology is that of **apoptosis,** which is also known as programmed cell death.[216,217] This naturally occurring process is responsible for the purposeful killing of specific cells in the developing CNS. Apoptosis ensures that the number of surviving cells is appropriate and optimal. Glutamate receptor-mediated neuronal death is closely associated with this process and may represent an inappropriate activation of apoptosis. Although the regulation of this process appears to be very complex and is incompletely understood, it is apparent that further knowledge of apoptosis will be fundamental to any significant progress in the therapy of cerebral palsy.

The underappreciated role of white matter in the attenuation of hypoxic-ischemic brain damage (e.g., by uptake of EAAs or sequestration of K^+ and H^+) will likely receive more attention as we learn more about the unique metabolism of that brain component.[218-220] In addition to EAA receptor antagonists, drugs that inhibit EAA release may be of benefit.[221] Future studies will evaluate the use of multiple strategies to inhibit the deleterious cascades initiated by brain ischemia and hypoxia.[222] Oxygen free-radical scavengers and calcium-entry blocking agents have been given together for the treatment of postasphyxial injury in newborn sheep.[223] In previous editions of this text, I speculated that the day may arrive when a "brain cocktail" consisting of free-radical scavengers, modifiers of nitric oxide activity, metabolic inhibitors, calcium and iron chelators, and drugs that affect the EAA systems will be administered to fetuses and neonates at risk for brain injury. Today the list of possible therapeutic agents has grown. One day we might add drugs that affect or interrupt the inflammatory cascade; these compounds have the potential to reduce the processes that lead to unplanned CNS necrosis or apoptosis. In addition, the role of progesterone and other steroids in relation to brain development is under investigation, and therapeutic opportunities exist for manipulating these systems, not only in utero, but perhaps also during the neonatal period.

Meanwhile, we must redouble our efforts to identify the most vulnerable periods of fetal development, and we need to develop noninvasive techniques for identifying the fetus at risk. We still lack the tools to specifically and sensitively identify these babies in utero; only then can we design effective treatment regimens and clinical trials that interfere as little as possible with the normal trophic activities in the developing brain.

KEY POINTS

- Cerebral palsy is a nonprogressive disorder of the central nervous system that is present (but not always obvious) at birth and that involves some impairment of motor function or posture. Mental retardation may or may not be present.

- The term *birth asphyxia* should be used sparingly, if at all, in medical records. More descriptive terms that describe the newborn's tone, color, respiratory effort, and metabolic status should be used when possible.

- The incidence of cerebral palsy is approximately two per 1000 live births and has not decreased despite the widespread use of intrapartum FHR monitoring and an increased cesarean section rate.

- The false-positive rate for new-onset, persistent, late FHR decelerations as a predictor for the development of cerebral palsy is 99%.

- The Apgar score is a poor predictor of cerebral palsy.

- Spastic quadriplegia and, less commonly, dyskinesia are the only types of cerebral palsy associated with acute intrapartum hypoxic events.

- Intrapartum hypoxia sufficient to cause cerebral palsy is always accompanied by neonatal encephalopathy and seizures.

- Fetal compensatory responses to hypoxemia in utero include the following: (1) a redistribution of fetal cardiac output, with increased blood flow to the brain, myocardium, and adrenal glands; (2) decreased fetal energy consumption as a result of decreased fetal breathing and body movements; and (3) maintenance of essential cellular processes at the expense of intrauterine fetal growth.

- Chorioamnionitis is associated with an increased risk of cerebral palsy. Epidural analgesia during labor is associated with an increased maternal temperature (but not chorioamnionitis). More accurate diagnosis of chorioamnionitis may prevent unnecessary evaluations for sepsis in newborns of mothers with a small increase in temperature during labor.

- EAA neurotransmitters (e.g., glutamate) likely play an important role in hypoxic-ischemic brain injury in utero, and the intrauterine maturation of these transmitter systems may result in periods of susceptibility to hypoxic injury.

- The high levels of progesterone to which the fetus is exposed in utero may afford some endogenous fetal neuroprotection.

- No published data suggest that a given anesthetic drug or technique is more likely to protect fetal neurologic function (provided that the anesthetic technique is administered according to the recommended guidelines for good anesthesia practice).

- There is no scientific basis for the "30-minute rule" for emergency cesarean delivery; it merely represents a realistic standard for many community hospitals.

- Improved knowledge of the process and regulation of apoptosis (programmed neuronal cell death) may lead to the development of strategies to prevent irreversible fetal neurologic injury.

REFERENCES

1. Blumenthal I. Cerebral palsy: Medicolegal aspects. J Royal Soc Med 2001; 94:624-7.
2. Nelson KB, Ellenberg JH. Apgar scores as predictors of chronic neurologic disability. Pediatrics 1981; 68:36-44.
3. Clark RB, Quirk JG. What is birth asphyxia? (letter). Am J Obstet Gynecol 1990; 163:1367-8.
4. American College of Obstetricians and Gynecologists Committee on Obstetrics: Maternal and Fetal Medicine. Utility of Umbilical Cord Blood Acid-Base Assessment. ACOG Committee Opinion No. 91. February, 1991.
5. American College of Obstetricians and Gynecologists Committee on Obstetric Practice. Inappropriate Use of the Terms Fetal Distress and Birth Asphyxia. ACOG Committee Opinion No. 197. February, 1998.
6. Thorp JA. Letter to the editor. Am J Obstet Gynecol 1990; 163:1368-9.
7. Myers RE. Two patterns of perinatal brain damage and their conditions of occurrence. Am J Obstet Gynecol 1972; 112:246-76.
8. Hankins GDV, Erickson K, Zinberg S, et al. Neonatal encephalopathy and cerebral palsy: A knowledge survey of fellows of the American College of Obstetricians and Gynecologists. Obstet Gynecol 2003; 101:11-7.
9. Towbin A. Obstetric malpractice litigation: The pathologist's view. Am J Obstet Gynecol 1986; 155:927-35.
10. American College of Obstetricians and Gynecologists. Shifting strategies in neurologic injury cases. ACOG Newsletter, November 1991:5.
11. Bakketeig LS. Only a minor part of cerebral palsy cases begin in labour. BMJ 1999; 319:1016-7.
12. Blair E, Stanley FJ. Intrapartum asphyxia: A rare cause of cerebral palsy. J Pediatrics 1988; 112:515-9.
13. Espinosa MI, Parer JT. Mechanisms of asphyxial brain damage, and possible pharmacological interventions, in the fetus. Am J Obstet Gynecol 1991; 164:1582-91.
14. MacLennan A. A template for defining a causal relation between acute intrapartum events and cerebral palsy: International consensus statement. BMJ 1999; 319:1054-9.
15. Grant A, Joy M, O'Brien N, et al. Cerebral palsy among children born during the Dublin randomized trial of intrapartum monitoring. Lancet 1989; 2:1233-6.
16. Freeman R. Intrapartum fetal monitoring: A disappointing story. N Engl J Med 1990; 322:624-6.
17. MacDonald D, Grant A, Sheridan-Pereira M, et al. The Dublin randomized controlled trial of intrapartum fetal heart rate monitoring. Am J Obstet Gynecol 1985; 152:524-39.
18. Leveno KJ, Cunningham FG, Nelson S, et al. A prospective comparison of selective and universal electronic fetal monitoring in 34,995 pregnancies. N Engl J Med 1986; 315:615-9.
19. Friedman EA. The obstetrician's dilemma: How much fetal monitoring and cesarean section is enough? N Engl J Med 1986; 315:641-3.
20. Schifrin BS, Dame L. Fetal heart rate patterns: Prediction of Apgar score. JAMA 1972; 219:1322-5.
21. Rosen MG, Dickinson JC. The paradox of electronic fetal monitoring: More data may not enable us to predict or prevent infant neurologic morbidity. Am J Obstet Gynecol 1993; 168:745-51.
22. Freeman RK. Problems with intrapartum fetal heart rate monitoring interpretation and patient management. Obstet Gynecol 2002; 100:813-26.
23. Rosen MG, Dickinson JC. The incidence of cerebral palsy. Am J Obstet Gynecol 1992; 167:417-23.
24. Jarvis SN, Holloway JS, Hey EN. Increase in cerebral palsy in normal birth weight babies. Arch Disease Child 1985; 60:1113-21.
25. Nelson KB, Ellenberg JH. Antecedents of cerebral palsy. N Engl J Med 1986; 315:81-6.
26. Emond A, Golding J, Pecklam C. Cerebral palsy in two national cohort studies. Arch Dis Child 1989; 64:848-52.
27. Hagberg B, Hagberg G, Olow I, Von Wendt L. The changing panorama of cerebral palsy in Sweden. V. The birth year period 1979-82. Acta Pediatr Scand 1989; 78:283-90.
28. Holst K, Anderson E, Philip J, Henningsen I. Antenatal and perinatal conditions correlated to handicap among 4-year-old children. Am J Perinatol 1989; 6:258-67.
29. Dowding VM, Barry C. Cerebral palsy: Changing patterns of birth weight and gestational age (1976/81). Irish Med J 1988; 81:25-8.
30. Stanley FJ, Watson L. The cerebral palsies in Western Australia: Trends, 1968 to 1981. Am J Obstet Gynecol 1988; 158:89-93.
31. Riikonen R, Raumavirta S, Sinivuori E, Seppala T. Changing pattern of cerebral palsy in the southwest region of Finland. Acta Pediatr Scand 1989; 78:581-7.

32. Torfs CP, Van den Berg BJ, Oechsli FW, Cummins S. Prenatal and perinatal factors in the etiology of cerebral palsy. J Pediatrics 1990; 116:615-9.

33. Pharoah POD, Cooke T, Cooke RW, Rosenbloom L. Birth weight specific trends in cerebral palsy. Arch Dis Child 1990; 65:602-6.

34. Meberg A. Declining incidence of low birth weight: Impact on perinatal mortality and incidence of cerebral palsy. J Perinatal Med 1990; 18:195-200.

35. Badawi N, Watson L, Petterson B, et al. What constitutes cerebral palsy? Dev Med Child Neurol 1998; 40:520-7.

36. Nelson KB, Ellenberg JH. Antecedents of cerebral palsy. I. Univariate analysis of risks. Am J Dis Child 1985; 139:1031-8.

37. Badawi N, Kurinczuk JJ, Keogh JM, et al. Intrapartum risk factors for neonatal encephalopathy: The Western Australia case-control study. BMJ 1998; 317:1554-8.

38. American College of Obstetricians and Gynecologists Taskforce on Neonatal Encephalopathy and Cerebral Palsy. Neonatal Encephalopathy and Cerebral Palsy: Defining the Pathogenesis and Pathophysiology. American College of Obstetricians and Gynecologists. Washington, DC, 2003.

39. Apgar V. A proposal for a new method of evaluation of the newborn infant. Anesth Analg 1953; 32:260-7.

40. Sykes GS, Johnson P, Ashworth F, et al. Do Apgar scores indicate asphyxia? Lancet 1982; 1:494-6.

41. Marrin M, Paes BA. Birth asphyxia: Does the Apgar score have diagnostic value? Obstet Gynecol 1988; 72:120-3.

42. Catlin EA, Carpenter MW, Brann BS. The Apgar score revisited: Influence of gestational age. J Pediatrics 1986; 109:865-8.

43. Williams TJ, Carlo WA. Neonatal resuscitation guidelines 2000: A framework for practice. J Matern-Fetal Neonatal Med 2002; 11:4-10.

44. Niermeyer S, Kattwinkel J, Van Reempts P, et al. International Guidelines for Neonatal Resuscitation: An excerpt from the Guidelines 2000 for Cardiopulmonary Resuscitation and Emergency Cardiovascular Care: International Consensus on Science. Contributors and Reviewers for the Neonatal Resuscitation Guidelines. Pediatrics 2000; 106:E29.

45. Helwig JT, Parer JT, Kilpatrick SJ, Laros RK. Umbilical cord blood acid-base state: What is normal? Am J Obstet Gynecol 1996; 174:1807-12.

46. Chiswick ML. Birth asphyxia and cerebral palsy. Int J Obstet Anesth 1992; 1:178-9.

47. Gilstrap LC III, Leveno KJ, Burris J, et al. Diagnosis of birth asphyxia on the basis of fetal pH, Apgar score, and newborn cerebral dysfunction. Am J Obstet Gynecol 1989; 161:825-30.

48. Hull J, Dodd K. What is birth asphyxia? Br J Obstet Gynaecol 1991; 98:953-5.

49. Fee SC, Malee K, Deddish R, et al. Severe acidosis and subsequent neurological status. Am J Obstet Gynecol 1990; 162:802-6.

50. Goodwin TM, Belai I, Hernandez P, et al. Asphyxial complications in the term newborn with severe umbilical acidemia. Am J Obstet Gynecol 1992; 167:1506-12.

51. Goldaber KG, Gilstrap LC, Leveno KJ, et al. Pathologic fetal acidemia. Obstet Gynecol 1991; 78:1103-7.

52. Low JA, Simpson LL, Ramsey DA. The clinical diagnosis of asphyxia responsible for brain damage in the human fetus. Am J Obstet Gynecol 1992; 167:11-5.

53. Low JA. Relationship of fetal asphyxia to neuropathology and deficits in children. Clin Invest Med 1993; 16:133-40.

54. Low JA, Pancham SR, Worthington D, Boston RW. Acid-base, lactate, and pyruvate characteristics of the normal obstetric patient and fetus during the intrapartum period. Am J Obstet Gynecol 1974; 120:862-7.

55. Low JA. The role of blood gas and acid-base assessment in the diagnosis of intrapartum fetal asphyxia. Am J Obstet Gynecol 1988; 159:1235-40.

56. Low JA, Wood SL, Killen HL, et al. Intrapartum asphyxia in the preterm fetus < 2000 gm. Am J Obstet Gynecol 1990; 162:378-82.

57. Low JA, Galbraith RS, Muir DW, et al. Motor and cognitive deficits after intrapartum asphyxia in the mature fetus. Am J Obstet Gynecol 1988; 158:356-61.

58. Low JA, Galbraith RS, Muir DW, et al. Mortality and morbidity after intrapartum asphyxia in the preterm fetus. Obstet Gynecol 1992; 80:57-61.

59. Low JA, Panagiotopoulos C, Derrick EJ. Newborn complications after intrapartum asphyxia with metabolic acidosis in the term fetus. Am J Obstet Gynecol 1994; 170:1081-7.

60. Low JA, Panagiotopoulos C, Derrick EJ. Newborn complications after intrapartum asphyxia with metabolic acidosis in the preterm fetus. Am J Obstet Gynecol 1995; 172:805-10.

61. Low JA, Lindsay BG, Derrick EJ. Threshold of metabolic acidosis associated with newborn complications. Am J Obstet Gynecol 1997; 177:1391-4.

62. Nagel HTC, Vandenbussche FPHA, Oepkes D, et al. Follow-up of children born with an umbilical arterial blood pH < 7. Am J Obstet Gynecol 1995; 173:1758-64.

63. Sehdev HM, Stamilio DM, Macones GA, et al. Predictive factors for neonatal morbidity in neonates with an umbilical arterial cord pH less than 7.00. Am J Obstet Gynecol 1997; 177:1030-4.

64. Gull I, Jaffa AJ, Oren M, et al. Acid accumulation during end-stage bradycardia in term fetuses: How long is too long? Br J Obstet Gynaecol 1996; 103:1096-101.

65. Ross MG, Gala R. Use of umbilical artery base excess: Algorithm for the timing of hypoxic injury. Am J Obstet Gynecol 2002; 187:1-9.

66. Phelan JP, Korst LM, Ahn MO, Martin GI. Neonatal nucleated red blood cell and lymphocyte counts in fetal brain injury. Obstet Gynecol 1998; 91:485-9.

67. Phelan JP, Ahn MO, Korst LM, Martin GI. Nucleated red blood cells: A marker for fetal asphyxia? Am J Obstet Gynecol 1995; 173:1380-4.

68. Korst LM, Phelan JP, Ahn MO, Martin GI. Nucleated red blood cells: An update on the marker for fetal asphyxia. Am J Obstet Gynecol 1996; 175:843-6.

69. Leikin E, Verma U, Klein S, Tejani N. Relationship between neonatal nucleated red blood cell counts and hypoxic-ischemic injury. Obstet Gynecol 1996; 87:439-43.

70. Murphy DJ. Placental infection and risk of cerebral palsy in very low birth weight infants. J Pediatr 1996; 129:776-7.

71. Grether JK, Nelson KB. Maternal infection and cerebral palsy in infants of normal birth weight. JAMA 1997; 278:207-11.

72. Silverstein F, Barks J, Hagan P, et al. Cytokines and perinatal brain injury. Neurochem Int 1997; 30:375-83.

73. Dammann O, Leviton A. Intrauterine infection, cytokines, and brain damage in the preterm newborn. Pediatr Res 1997; 42:1-8.

74. Dammann O, Leviton A. Does prepregnancy bacterial vaginosis increase a mother's risk of having a preterm infant with cerebral palsy? Develop Med Child Neurol 1997; 39:836-40.

75. Camann WR, Hortvet LA, Hughes N, et al. Maternal temperature regulation during extradural analgesia for labour. Br J Anaesth 1991; 67:565-8.

76. Fusi L, Steer PJ, Maresh MJA, Beard RW. Maternal pyrexia associated with the use of epidural analgesia in labour. Lancet 1989; 1:1250-2.

77. Gray D, Finucane BT. Epidurals and fever: Association or cause? Can Med Assoc J 1997; 157:511-2.

78. Lieberman E, Lang JM, Frigoletto F, et al. Epidural analgesia, intrapartum fever, and neonatal sepsis evaluation. Pediatrics 1997; 99:415-9.

79. Mayer DC, Chescheir NC, Spielman FJ. Increased intrapartum antibiotic administration associated with epidural analgesia in labor. Am J Perinatol 1997; 14:83-6.

80. Baud O, Ville Y, Zupan V, et al. Are neonatal brain lesions due to intrauterine infection related to mode of delivery? Br J Obstet Gynaecol 1998; 105:121-4.

81. Barkovich AJ, Sargent SK. Profound asphyxia in the premature infant: Imaging findings. Am J Neuroradiol 1995; 16:1837-46.

82. Barkovich AJ, Westmark K, Partridge C, et al. Perinatal asphyxia: MR findings in the first 10 days. Am J Neuroradiol 1995; 16:427-38.

83. Martin E, Barkovich AJ. Magnetic resonance imaging in perinatal asphyxia. Arch Dis Child 1995; 72:F62-70.

84. Sibony O, Stempfle N, Luton D, et al. In utero fetal cerebral intraparenchymal ischemia diagnosed by nuclear magnetic resonance. Develop Med Child Neurol 1998; 40:122-3.

85. Younkin DP. Magnetic resonance spectroscopy in hypoxic-ischemic encephalopathy. Clin Invest Med 1993; 16:115-21.

86. Huppi PS, Warfield S, Kikinis R, et al. Quantitative magnetic resonance imaging of brain development in premature and mature newborns. Ann Neurol 1998; 43:224-35.

87. Sugimoto T, Woo M, Nishida N, et al. When do brain abnormalities in cerebral palsy occur? An MRI study. Dev Med Child Neurol 1995; 37:285-92.

88. Okumura A, Kato T, Kuno K, et al. MRI findings in patients with spastic cerebral palsy. 2: Correlation with type of cerebral palsy. Dev Med Child Neurol 1997; 39:369-72.

89. Olsen P, Paakko E, Vainionpaa L, et al. Magnetic resonance imaging of periventricular leukomalacia and its clinical correlation in children. Ann Neurol 1997; 41:754-61.

90. Eken P, Jansen GH, Groenendaal F, et al. Intracranial lesions in the full-term infant with hypoxic ischaemic encephalopathy: Ultrasound and autopsy correlation. Neuropediatrics 1994; 25:301-7.

91. Raju TNK. Some animal models for the study of perinatal asphyxia. Biol Neonate 1992; 62:202-14.

92. Matsuda Y, Patrick J, Carmichael L, et al. Effects of sustained hypoxemia on the sheep fetus at midgestation: Endocrine, cardiovascular, and biophysical responses. Am J Obstet Gynecol 1992; 167:531-40.

93. Richardson BS, Carmichael L, Homan J, Patrick JE. Electrocortical activity, electroocular activity, and breathing movements in fetal sheep with prolonged and graded hypoxemia. Am J Obstet Gynecol 1992; 167:553-8.

94. Richardson BS, Patrick JE, Bousquet J, et al. Cerebral metabolism in fetal lamb after maternal infusion of ethanol. Am J Physiol 1985; 249:R505-9.

95. Hagberg H, Andersson P, Kjellmer I, et al. Extracellular overflow of glutamate, aspartate, GABA and taurine in the cortex and basal ganglia of fetal lambs during hypoxia-ischemia. Neurosci Lett 1987; 78:311-7.

96. Penning DH, Chestnut DH, Dexter F, et al. Glutamate release from the ovine fetal brain during maternal hemorrhage: A study using chronic in utero cerebral microdialysis. Anesthesiology 1995; 82:521-30.

97. Reynolds JD, Penning DH, Dexter F, et al. Dose-dependent effects of acute in vivo ethanol exposure on extracellular glutamate concentration in the cerebral cortex of the near-term fetal sheep. Alcohol Clin Exp Res 1995; 19:1447-53.

98. Richardson BS, Patrick JE, Abduljabbar H. Cerebral oxidative metabolism in the fetal lamb: Relationship to electrocortical state. Am J Obstet Gynecol 1985; 153:426-31.

99. Richardson B, Patrick J, Homan J, et al. Cerebral oxidative metabolism in fetal sheep with multiple-dose ethanol infusion. Am J Obstet Gynecol 1987; 157:1496-502.

100. Henderson JL, Reynolds JD, Dexter F, et al. Chronic hypoxemia causes extracellular glutamate concentration to increase in the cerebral cortex of the near-term fetal sheep. Develop Brain Res 1998; 105:287-93.

101. Mallard EC, Gunn AJ, Williams CE, et al. Transient umbilical cord occlusion causes hippocampal damage in the fetal sheep. Am J Obstet Gynecol 1992; 167:1423-30.

102. Johnson G, Palahniuk R, Tweed W, et al. Regional cerebral blood flow changes during severe fetal asphyxia produced by slow partial umbilical cord compression. Am J Obstet Gynecol 1979; 135:48-52.

103. Clapp JF, Peress NS, Wesley M, Mann LI. Brain damage after intermittent partial cord occlusion in the chronically instrumented fetal lamb. Am J Obstet Gynecol 1988; 159:504-9.

104. Clapp JF, Mann LI, Peress NS, Szeto HH. Neuropathology in the chronic fetal lamb preparation: Structure-function correlates under different environmental conditions. Am J Obstet Gynecol 1981; 141:973-86.

105. Reynolds JD, Chestnut DH, Dexter F, et al. Magnesium sulfate adversely affects fetal lamb survival and blocks fetal cerebral blood flow response during maternal hemorrhage. Anesth Analg 1996; 83:493-9.

106. Hohimer AR, Chao CR, Bissonnette JM. The effect of combined hypoxemia and cephalic hypotension on fetal cerebral blood flow and metabolism. J Cerebral Blood Flow Metabol 1991; 11:99-105.

107. Robillard JE, Weitzman RE, Burmeister L, Smith FG. Developmental aspects of the renal response to hypoxemia in the lamb fetus. Circ Res 1981; 48:128-38.

108. Richardson BS. The fetal brain: Metabolic and circulatory responses to asphyxia. Clin Invest Med 1993; 16:103-14.

109. Lin BW, Globus MYT, Dietrich WD, et al. Differing neurochemical and morphological sequelae of global ischemia: Comparison of single-multiple and multiple-insult paradigms. J Neurochem 1992; 59:2213-23.

110. Mallard EC, Williams CE, Gunn AJ, et al. Frequent episodes of brief ischemia sensitize the fetal sheep brain to neuronal loss and induce striatal injury. Pediatr Res 1993; 33:61-5.

111. Richardson BS. Fetal adaptive responses to asphyxia. Clin Perinatol 1989; 16:595-611.

112. Edelstone DI. Fetal compensatory responses to reduced oxygen delivery. Semin Perinatol 1984; 8:184-91.

113. Gu W, Jones CT, Parer JT. Metabolic and cardiovascular effects on fetal sheep of sustained reduction of uterine blood flow. J Physiol 1985; 368:109-29.

114. Sieber FE, Smith DS, Traystman RJ, Wollman H. Glucose: A reevaluation of its intraoperative use. Anesthesiology 1987; 67:72-81.

115. Vannucci RC, Mujsce DJ. Effect of glucose on perinatal hypoxic-ischemic brain damage. Biol Neonate 1992; 62:215-24.

116. Blomstrand SB, Hrbek A, Karlsson K, et al. Does glucose administration affect the cerebral response to fetal asphyxia? Acta Obstet Gynecol Scand 1984; 63:345-53.

117. Hooper S. DNA synthesis is reduced in selected fetal tissue during prolonged hypoxemia. Am J Physiol 1991; 261:R508-14.

118. Rurak DW, Gruber NC. The effect of neuromuscular blockade on oxygen consumption and blood gases in the fetal lamb. Am J Obstet Gynecol 1983; 145:258-62.

119. Jensen A, Berger R. Fetal circulatory responses to oxygen lack. Develop Brain Res 1991; 16:181-207.

120. Sheldon RE, Peeters LLH, Jones MD, et al. Redistribution of cardiac output and oxygen delivery in the hypoxic fetal lamb. Am J Obstet Gynecol 1979; 135:1071-8.

121. Jensen A, Hohmann M, Kunzel W. Dynamic changes in organ blood flow and oxygen consumption during acute asphyxia in fetal sheep. J Develop Physiol 1987; 9:543-59.

122. Penning DH, Grafe MR, Hammond R, et al. Neuropathology of the near-term and midgestation ovine fetal brain after sustained in utero hypoxemia. Am J Obstet Gynecol 1994; 170:1425-32.

123. Dobbing J, Sands J. Comparative aspects of the brain growth spurt. Early Hum Dev 1979; 3:79-83.

124. Battaglia FC, Meschia G. An Introduction to Fetal Physiology. Orlando, FL, Academic Press, 1986:257.

125. Schendel DE, Berg CJ, Yearginallsopp M, et al. Prenatal magnesium sulfate exposure and the risk for cerebral palsy or mental retardation among very low-birth-weight children aged 3 to 5 years. JAMA 1996; 276:1805-10.

126. Nelson KB, Grether JK. Can magnesium sulfate reduce the risk of cerebral palsy in very low birth weight infants? Pediatrics 1995; 95:263-9.

127. Collins M, Paneth N. Preeclampsia and cerebral palsy: Are they related? Dev Med Child Neurol 1998; 40:207-11.

128. Mayor S. Prenatal magnesium sulphate cuts risk of cerebral palsy. Br Med J 1996; 313:1505.

129. Nelson KB. Magnesium sulfate and risk of cerebral palsy in very low-birth-weight infants (editorial). JAMA 1996; 276:1843-4.

130. Rouse DJ, Hauth JC, Nelson KG, Goldenberg RL. The feasibility of a randomized clinical perinatal trial: Maternal magnesium sulfate for the prevention of cerebral palsy. Am J Obstet Gynecol 1996; 175:701-5.

131. Johnston MV. Neurotransmitters and vulnerability of the developing brain. Brain Dev 1995; 17:301-6.

132. de Haan HH, Alistair AJ, Williams CE, et al. Magnesium sulfate therapy during asphyxia in near-term fetal lambs does not compromise the fetus but does not reduce cerebral injury. Am J Obstet Gynecol 1997; 176:18-27.

133. Moon PF, Ramsay MM, Nathanielsz PW. Intravenous infusion of magnesium sulfate and regional redistribution of fetal blood flow during maternal hemorrhage in late gestation gravid ewes. Am J Obstet Gynecol 1999; 181:1486-94.

134. Sameshima H, Ota A, Ikenoue T. Pretreatment with magnesium sulfate protects against hypoxic-ischemic brain injury but postasphyxial treatment worsens brain damage in seven-day-old rats. Am J Obstet Gynecol 1999; 180:725-30.

135. Mittendorf R, Dambrosia J, Pryde PG, et al. Association between the use of antenatal magnesium sulfate in preterm labor and adverse health outcomes in infants. Am J Obstet Gynecol 2002; 186:1111-8.

136. Kirschbaum TH. Magnesium sulfate and prematurity. J Soc Gynecol Investig 2002; 9:58-9.

137. Farkouh LJ, Thorp JA, Jones PG, et al. Antenatal magnesium exposure and neonatal demise. Am J Obstet Gynecol 2001; 185:869-72.

138. Brann AW, Myers RE. Central nervous system findings in the newborn monkey following severe in utero partial asphyxia. Neurology 1975; 25:327-38.

139. Larroche JC. Fetal and perinatal brain damage. In: Wigglesworth JS, Singer DB, editors. Textbook of Fetal and Perinatal Pathology. Boston, Blackwell Scientific Publications, 1991:807-38.

140. Allan WC, Riviello JJ. Perinatal cerebrovascular disease in the neonate: Parenchymal ischemic lesions in term and preterm infants. Pediatr Clin North Am 1992; 39:621-50.

141. Volpe JJ. Hypoxic-ischemic encephalopathy: Neuropathology and pathogenesis. In: Volpe JJ, editor. Neurology of the Newborn. 2nd ed. Philadelphia, W.B. Saunders, 1987:209-35.

142. Volpe JJ. Brain injury in the premature infant: Current concepts of pathogenesis and prevention. Biol Neonate 1992; 62:231-42.

143. Banker BQ, Larroche LJC. Periventricular leukomalacia of infancy: A form of neonatal anoxic encephalopathy. Arch Neurol 1962; 7:386-410.

144. Dubowitz LMS, Bydder GM, Mushin J. Developmental sequence of periventricular leukomalacia. Arch Dis Child 1985; 60:349-55.

145. DeReuck J. The human periventricular arterial blood supply and the anatomy of cerebral infarctions. Eur Neurol 1971; 5:321-34.

146. Nelson MDJ, Gonzalez-Gomez I, Gilles FH. The search for human telencephalic ventriculofugal arteries. Am J Neuroradiol 1991; 12: 215-22.

147. Mayer PL, Kier EL. The controversy of the periventricular white matter circulation: A review of the anatomic literature. Am J Neuroradiol 1991; 12:223-8.

148. Ashwal S, Dale PS, Longo LD. Regional cerebral blood flow: Studies in the fetal lamb during hypoxia, hypercapnia, acidosis, and hypotension. Pediatr Res 1984; 18:1309-16.

149. Juurlink BHJ, Hertz L, Yager JY. Astrocyte maturation and susceptibility to ischaemia or substrate deprivation. Neuroreport 1992; 3:1135-7.

150. Choi DW. Excitotoxic cell death. J Neurobiol 1992; 23:1261-76.

151. Rothman SM, Olney JW. Glutamate and the pathophysiology of hypoxic-ischemic brain damage. Ann Neurol 1986; 19:105-11.

152. Fonnum F. Glutamate: A neurotransmitter in mammalian brain. J Neurochem 1984; 42:1-11.

153. Penning DH, Goh JW, Elbeheiry H, Brien JF. Effect of hypoxia on glutamate efflux and synaptic transmission in the guinea pig hippocampus. Brain Res 1993; 620:301-4.

154. Choi D. Glutamate neurotoxicity and diseases of the nervous system. Neuron 1988; 1:623-34.

155. Choi D. Cerebral hypoxia: Some new approaches and unanswered questions. J Neurosci 1990; 10:2493.

156. Choi D, Rothman S. The role of glutamate neurotoxicity in hypoxic-ischemic neuronal death. Ann Rev Neurosc 1990; 13:171-82.

157. Benveniste H. The excitotoxin hypothesis in relation to cerebral ischemia. Cerebrovasc Brain Metab Review 1991; 3:213-45.

158. Nelson N, editor. Current Therapy in Neonatal-Perinatal Medicine. Toronto, B.C. Decker, 1990:276.

159. McDonald JW, Johnston MV. Physiological and pathophysiological roles of excitatory amino acids during central nervous system development. Brain Res Rev 1990; 15:41-70.

160. Fazekas JF, Alexander FAD, Himwich HE. Tolerance of the newborn to anoxia. Am J Physiol 1941; 134:281-7.

161. Kabat H. The greater resistance of very young animals to arrest of the brain circulation. Am J Physiol 1940; 130:588-99.

162. Glass HG, Snyder FF, Webster E. The rate of decline in resistance to anoxia of rabbits, dogs and guinea pigs from the onset of viability to adult life. Am J Physiol 1944; 140:609-15.

163. Silverstein FS, Torke L, Barks J, Johnston MV. Hypoxia-ischemia produces focal disruption of glutamate receptors in developing brain. Dev Brain Res 1987; 34:33-9.

164. Silverstein FS, Buchanan K, Johnston MV. Perinatal hypoxia-ischemia disrupts striatal high-affinity [3H]glutamate uptake into synaptosomes. J Neurochem 1986; 47:1614-9.

165. Penning DH, Patrick J, Jimmo S, Brien JF. Release of glutamate and gamma-aminobutyric acid in the ovine fetal hippocampus: Ontogeny and effect of hypoxia. J Develop Physiol 1991; 16:301-7.

166. Johnston MV. Cellular alterations associated with perinatal asphyxia. Clin Invest Med 1993; 16:122-32.

167. Gombos G, Levy O, Debarry J. Developmental changes of EAA metabotropic receptor activity in rat cerebellum. Neuroreport 1992; 3:877-80.

168. Ikonomidou C, Mosinger JL, Salles KS, et al. Sensitivity of the developing rat brain to hypobaric/ischemic damage parallels sensitivity to N-methyl-aspartate neurotoxicity. J Neuroscience 1989; 9:2809-18.

169. Lee HS, Choi BH. Density and distribution of excitatory amino acid receptors in the developing human fetal brain: A quantitative autoradiographic study. Exp Neurol 1992; 118:284-90.

170. Greenamyre T, Penney JB, Young AB, et al. Evidence for transient perinatal glutamatergic innervation of globus pallidus. J Neuroscience 1987; 7:1022-30.

171. Siesjo BK. Pathophysiology and treatment of focal cerebral ischemia: 2. Mechanisms of damage and treatment. J Neurosurg 1992; 77:337-54.

172. Siesjo BK. Pathophysiology and treatment of focal cerebral ischemia: 1. Pathophysiology. J Neurosurg 1992; 77:169-84.

173. Pellegrini-Giampietro DE, Bennett MVL, Zukin RS. Are Ca^{2+}-permeable kainate/AMPA receptors more abundant in immature brain? Neurosci Lett 1992; 144:65-9.

174. Dawson VL, Dawson TM. Nitric oxide in neuronal degeneration. Proc Soc Exp Biol Med 1996; 211:33-40.

175. Dawson DA. Nitric oxide and focal cerebral ischemia: Multiplicity of actions and diverse outcome. Cerebrovasc Brain Metab Rev 1994; 6:299-324.

176. Lockhart EM, Warner DS, Pearlstein RD, et al. Allopregnanolone attenuates N-methyl-D-aspartate-induced excitotoxicity and apoptosis in the human NT2 cell line in culture. Neurosci Lett 2002; 328:33-6.

177. Clarren SK, Smith DW. The fetal alcohol syndrome. N Engl J Med 1978; 298:1063-7.

178. Cohen RS, Benitz WE, Stevenson DK. Fetal injury from drug abuse in pregnancy: Alcohol, narcotic, cocaine and phencyclidine. In: Stevenson DK, Sunshine P, editors. Fetal and Neonatal Brain Injury: Mechanisms, Management, and the Risks of Practice. Philadelphia, B.C. Decker, 1989:57-64.

179. Smith GN, Patrick J, Sinervo KR, Brien JF. Effects of ethanol exposure on the embryo-fetus: Experimental considerations, mechanisms, and the role of prostaglandins. Canad J Physiol Pharmacol 1990; 69: 550-69.

180. Barnes DE, Walker DW. Prenatal ethanol exposure permanently reduces the number of pyramidal neurons in rat hippocampus. Dev Brain Res 1981; 1:333-40.

181. Snell LD, Tabakoff B, Hoffman PL. Radioligand binding to the N-methyl-D-aspartate receptor/ionophore complex: Alterations by ethanol in vitro and by chronic in vivo ethanol ingestion. Brain Res 1993; 602:91-8.

182. Volpe JJ. Effect of cocaine use on the fetus. N Engl J Med 1992; 327: 399-407.

183. Cutler AR, Wilkerson AE, Gingras JL, Levin ED. Prenatal cocaine and/or nicotine exposure in rats: Preliminary findings on long-term cognitive outcome and genital development at birth. Neurotoxicol Teratol 1996; 18:635-43.

184. Richardson GA, Conroy ML, Day NL. Prenatal cocaine exposure: Effects on the development of school-age children. Neurotoxicol Teratol 1996; 18:627-34.

185. Martin JC, Barr HM, Martin DC, Streissguth AP. Neonatal neurobehavioral outcome following prenatal exposure to cocaine. Neurotoxicol Teratol 1996; 18:617-25.

186. Smith CV, Phelan JP. Trauma in Pregnancy. In: Clark SL, Cotton DB, Hankins GDV, Phelan JP, editors. Critical Care Obstetrics. 2nd ed. Boston, Blackwell Scientific Publications, 1991.

187. Gilles MT, Blair E, Watson L, et al. Trauma in pregnancy and cerebral palsy: Is there a link? Med J Aust 1996; 164:500-1.

188. Chetcuti P, Levene M. Seat belts: A potential hazard to the fetus. J Perinat Med 1987; 15:207.

189. Lee RV, Rodgers BD, White LM, Harvey RC. Cardiopulmonary resuscitation of pregnant women. Am J Med 1986; 81:311-8.

190. Bishop EH, Israel SL, Briscoe CC. Obstetric influences on the premature infant's first year of development: A report from the collaborative study of cerebral palsy. Obstet Gynecol 1965; 26:628.

191. Huff DL, Thurnau GR, Sheldon R. The outcome of protective forceps deliveries of 26-33 week infants (abstract). Proceedings of the Annual Meeting of the Society of Perinatal Obstetricians. Orlando, FL, 1987.

192. Barrett JM, Boehm FH, Vaughn WK. The effect of type of delivery on neonatal outcome in singleton infants of birth weight of 1,000 g or less. JAMA 1983; 250:625.

193. Thomas RL, Ferguson JE, Repke JT. Complications of labor and delivery: Selected medical and surgical considerations. In: Stevenson DK, Sunshine P, editors. Fetal and Neonatal Brain Injury: Mechanisms, Management, and the Risks of Practice. 1st ed. Philadelphia, B.C. Decker, 1989:34-45.

194. Broekhuizen FF, Washington JM, Johnson F. Vacuum extraction versus forceps delivery: Indications and complications, 1979 to 1984. Obstet Gynecol 1987; 69:338.

195. El-Beheiry H, Puil E. Anesthetic depression of excitatory synaptic transmission in neocortex. Exper Brain Res 1989; 77:87-93.

196. Puil E, El-Beheiry H. Anaesthetic suppression of transmitter actions in neocortex. Br J Pharmacol 1990; 101:61-6.

197. Charlesworth P, Pocock G, Richards CD. The action of anaesthetics on stimulus-secretion coupling and synaptic activity. Gen Pharmacol 1992; 23:977-84.

198. Elliott JR, Elliott AA, Harper AA, Winpenny JP. Effects of general anaesthetics on neuronal sodium and potassium channels. Gen Pharmacol 1992; 23:1005-11.

199. Krnjevic K. Cellular and synaptic actions of general anaesthetics. Gen Pharmacol 1992; 23:965-75.

200. Aitken PG, Schiff SJ. Barbiturate protection against hypoxic neuronal damage in vitro. J Neurosurg 1986; 65:230-2.

201. Ginsberg M, Busto R. Rodent models of cerebral ischemia. Stroke 1989; 20:1627-42.

202. Warner DS, Todd MM, Ludwig P, et al. Volatile anesthetics reduce focal ischemic brain damage in the rat. J Cereb Blood Flow Metab 1993; 13:S684.

203. Buchan A, Pulsinelli W. Hypothermia but not the N-methyl-D-aspartate antagonist, MK-801, attenuates neuronal damage in gerbils subjected to transient global ischemia. J Neurosci 1990; 10:311-6.

204. Ginsberg MD, Sternau LL, Globus MYT, et al. Therapeutic modulation of brain temperature: Relevance to ischemic brain injury. Cerebrovasc Brain Metab Rev 1992; 4:189-225.

205. Todd M, Warner D. A comfortable hypothesis reevaluated: Cerebral metabolic depression and brain protection during ischemia. Anesthesiology 1992; 76:161-4.

206. Carla V, Moroni F. General anaesthetics inhibit the responses induced by glutamate receptor agonists in the mouse cortex. Neurosci Lett 1992; 146:21-4.

207. Lyden PD, Hedges B. Protective effect of synaptic inhibition during cerebral ischemia in rats and rabbits. Stroke 1992; 23:1463-9.
208. Yatsu FM, Grotta JC. Protective effect of synaptic inhibition during cerebral ischemia in rats and rabbits (editorial comment). Stroke 1992; 23:1469-70.
209. Myers RE, Myers SE. Use of sedative, analgesic, and anesthetic drugs during labor and delivery: Bane or boon? Am J Obstet Gynecol 1979; 133:83-104.
210. Olney JW, Ikonomidou C, Mosinger JL, Frierdich G. MK-801 prevents hypobaric-ischemic neuronal degeneration in infant rat brain. J Neurosci 1989; 9:1701-4.
211. McDonald JW, Silverstein FS, Johnston MV. MK-801 protects the neonatal brain from hypoxic-ischemic damage. Eur J Pharmacol 1987; 140:359-61.
212. Tan WKM, Williams CE, Gunn AJ, et al. Suppression of postischemic epileptiform activity with MK-801 improves neural outcome in fetal sheep. Ann Neurol 1992; 32:677-82.
213. Komuro H, Rakic P. Modulation of neuronal migration by NMDA receptors. Science 1993; 260:95-7.
214. Emerit MB, Riad M, Hamon M. Trophic effects of neurotransmitters during brain maturation. Biol Neonate 1992; 62:193-201.
215. Gluckman PD, Williams CE. Is the cure worse than the disease? Caveats in the move from laboratory to clinic. Dev Med Child Neurol 1992; 34:1015-8.
216. Choi DW, Lobner D, Dugan LL. Glutamate receptor-mediated neuronal death in the ischemic brain. In: Hsu CY, editor. Ischemic Stroke: From Basic Mechanisms to New Drug Development. Basel, Switzerland, Karger, 1998:2-13.
217. Choi DW. At the scene of ischemic brain injury: Is PARP a perp? Nature Med 1997; 3:1073-4.
218. Swanson RA, Choi DW. Glial glycogen stores affect neuronal survival during glucose deprivation in vitro. J Cereb Blood Flow Metab 1993; 13:162-9.
219. Swanson RA. Astrocyte glutamate uptake during chemical hypoxia in vitro. Neurosci Lett 1992; 147:143-6.
220. Ransom BR. The pathophysiology of anoxic injury in central nervous system white matter. Stroke 1990; 21(Suppl III):III52-7.
221. Graham SH, Chen J, Sharp FR, Simon RP. Limiting ischemic injury by inhibition of excitatory amino acid release. J Cereb Blood Flow Metab 1993; 13:88-97.
222. Volpe JJ. Brain injury in the premature infant: From pathogenesis to prevention. Brain Dev 1997; 19:519-34.
223. Thiringer K, Hrbek A, Karlsson K, et al. Postasphyxial cerebral survival in newborn sheep after treatment with oxygen free radical scavengers and a calcium antagonist. Pediatr Res 1987; 22:62-66.

Part IV
Foundations in Obstetric Anesthesia

Simpson was right. As he predicted, physicians used obstetric anesthesia sparingly until patients themselves forced the issue. The major impetus for the incorporation of anesthesia into obstetric practice came from nineteenth century feminists. Although suffrage was their primary goal, feminists recognized that women could participate fully in the economic and political life of the country only if they were healthy and had the physical stamina to compete. For this reason they made obstetric care, including anesthesia, part of their campaign for political parity.

Early feminists had good reason to be concerned about obstetric care. Despite many improvements in medicine, the morbidity and mortality associated with childbirth hardly changed between 1830 and 1930. Women were debilitated by the physical sequelae of poorly managed deliveries by untrained physicians and midwives, and they were exhausted by frequent pregnancies and the care of large families. As part of their campaign, feminists sought care by obstetricians rather than by midwives, obstetric care in hospitals rather than at home, and adequate time for recuperation from childbirth before they returned to their normal responsibilities. Other initiatives included the construction of special maternity units or hospitals, better instruction in obstetrics in medical schools, and the training of an increased number of obstetricians.

Anesthesia was also part of the feminist campaign for better obstetric care. Feminists and physicians alike believed that the pain of childbirth, in and of itself, contributed to the disability of women later in life. To increase the quality and availability of obstetric anesthesia, feminists founded two organizations. The National Twilight Sleep Association began in the United States just before the beginning of World War I and the National Birthday Trust Fund started in Great Britain in 1928.

Both organizations influenced the practice of obstetric anesthesia. Physicians began exploring new ways to manage the pain of childbirth. Between 1900 and 1940 a large number of papers were published describing the use of new methods and drugs for obstetric anesthesia, among them rectal ether and intravenous opioids. They also performed many important studies on the use of regional anesthesia.

For obstetricians, regional anesthesia had several advantages. First, it appeared to be safe and easy to administer. Ease of administration was especially important because qualified anesthesiologists were in short supply. Second, the use of regional anesthesia allowed obstetricians to make more liberal use of operative techniques for vaginal delivery (e.g., episiotomy, use of forceps), which were just coming into vogue. No less important, regional anesthesia appeared to satisfy the desires of women who wanted safer and more comfortable deliveries. Similar motives prompted the use of other blocks, including presacral, paravertebral, spinal, lumbar epidural, and caudal epidural anesthesia. In conjunction with this clinical work, scientists studied the anatomy and physiology of uterine function and childbirth pain, including the neurologic pathways involved in the perception of childbirth pain. Our current practices of obstetric anesthesia, particularly the emphasis on regional anesthesia, are a direct outgrowth of scientific studies and clinical trials that began during this period.[1-3]

Donald Caton, M.D.

REFERENCES

1. Loudon I. Death in Childbirth: An International Study of Maternal Care and Maternal Mortality 1800-1950. Oxford, Clarendon Press, 1992:187, 220-3, 172-233, 216-32.
2. Claye AM. Anaesthesia and analgesia in normal labour cases; one year's experience at a maternity hospital. Lancet 1932; 223:180-2.
3. Lewis J. Mothers and maternal policies in the twentieth century, in Garcia J, Kilpatrick R, Richards M, editors: The Politics of Maternity Care: Services for Childbearing Women in Twentieth-Century Britain. Oxford, Clarendon Paperbacks, 1990:15-29.

Chapter 11

Spinal, Epidural, and Caudal Anesthesia: Anatomy, Physiology, and Technique

David L. Brown, M.D. · Vijaya Gottumukkala, M.B.B.S., M.D., FRCA

Regional anesthesia is used extensively for obstetric patients. Of the estimated 3,700,000 women that go through childbirth in the United States each year, approximately 50% receive regional anesthesia. Of these, the overwhelming majority receives spinal or epidural anesthesia.[1,2] The purpose of this chapter is to review the anatomy, physiology, and techniques relevant to the administration of major regional anesthesia in obstetric patients. Technical features represent only one element of the successful use of spinal or epidural anesthesia. Conversely, sound medical judgment is of little benefit if a physician uses inadequate technique.

ANATOMY

Obstetric Pain Pathways

Pain during the first stage of labor results primarily from uterine contractions and dilation of the cervix. Pain is transmitted by visceral afferent nerve fibers that accompany the sympathetic nerves and enter the spinal cord at the T10 to T12 and L1 segments.

During the late first stage and second stage of labor, pain results from distention of the pelvic floor, vagina, and perineum. Pain is transmitted by somatic nerve fibers, which enter the spinal cord at the S2 to S4 segments (Figure 11-1).

During cesarean section, additional nociceptive pathways are involved in the transmission of pain. Most cesarean sections are performed with a horizontal (e.g., Pfannenstiel) skin incision, which involves the infraumbilical T11 to T12 dermatomes; during surgery, stretching of the skin may involve dermatomes two to four levels higher. Intraperitoneal manipulation and dissection involve poorly localized visceral pain pathways. Visceral pain may be transmitted by pathways as high as the celiac plexus. Additional somatic pain impulses may occur as a result of diaphragmatic stimulation, because the intercostal nerves innervate a portion of the peripheral diaphragm.

Anatomic Changes of Pregnancy

The normal anatomic changes of pregnancy affect the use of regional anesthesia techniques. Uterine enlargement and vena caval compression result in engorgement of the epidural veins. Unintentional intravascular cannulation and injection of local anesthetic are more common in pregnant patients than in nonpregnant patients. In addition, the vertebral foraminal veins, which are contiguous with the epidural veins, are enlarged and obstruct one of the pathways for local anesthetic to exit the epidural space during administration of epidural anesthesia. The enlarged epidural veins also may displace cerebrospinal fluid (CSF) from the thoracolumbar region of the subarachnoid space, as does the increased intraabdominal pressure of pregnancy; this partly explains the lowered dose requirement for spinal anesthesia in pregnant women.[3] Subarachnoid dose requirements are also affected by the lower specific gravity of CSF in pregnant patients as compared with nonpregnant patients.[4]

The hormonal changes of pregnancy affect the perivertebral ligamentous structures,[5] including the ligamentum flavum. The ligamentum flavum may feel less dense and "softer" in pregnant women than in nonpregnant patients; thus it may be more difficult to feel the movement of the epidural needle through the ligamentum flavum. It is difficult for trainees to provide successful epidural anesthesia consistently unless they are able to identify the ligamentum flavum.

It is more difficult for a pregnant woman to achieve flexion of the lumbar spine. Progressive accentuation of lumbar lordosis alters the relationship of surface anatomy to the vertebral column (Figure 11-2). At least three changes may occur. First, a pregnant woman's pelvis rotates on the long axis of the spinal column; thus the line joining the iliac crests assumes a more cephalad relationship to the vertebral column. (For example, this imaginary line might cross the vertebral column at the L3 to L4 interspace rather than the L4 to L5 interspace.) Second, less space exists between adjacent lumbar spinous processes during pregnancy. It may be more difficult to use the midline approach to identify the epidural or subarachnoid space in pregnant women. (Thus the often-heard comment, "She has a narrow interspace.") In addition, labor pain makes it more difficult for some women to assume and maintain an ideal position while the anesthesiologist performs regional anesthesia. Third, magnetic resonance imaging (MRI) has shown that the apex of the lumbar lordosis is shifted caudad during pregnancy, and the typical thoracic kyphosis in women is reduced in pregnant women.[6]

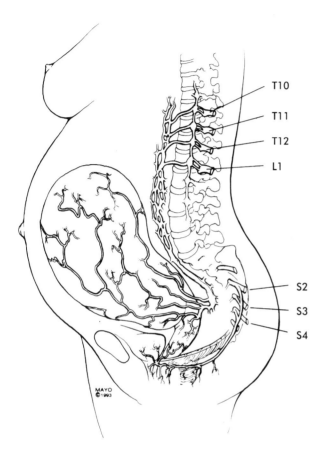

FIGURE 11-1. Pain pathways during labor and delivery. The afferent pain pathways from the cervix and uterus involve nerves that accompany sympathetic fibers and enter the neuraxis at T10 to L1. The pain pathways for the pelvic floor and perineum include the pudendal nerve fibers, which enter the neuraxis at S2 to S4.

Vertebral Anatomy

The administration of regional anesthesia requires a complete understanding of the lumbar and sacral vertebral and perivertebral anatomy.[7] Local anesthetics ultimately produce anesthesia through their effects on the spinal cord and nerve roots. The spinal cord is continuous cephalad with the brainstem through the foramen magnum. In women of childbearing age, the spinal cord terminates as the conus medullaris at the level of the lower border of the first lumbar vertebral body. The conus medullaris is attached to the coccyx by means of a neural-fibrous band called the *filum terminale,* which is surrounded by the nerves of the lower lumbar and sacral roots, known as the *cauda equina* (Figure 11-3). Within the bony vertebral column are three membranes: the pia mater, the arachnoid mater, and the dura mater. The pia mater is a highly vascular membrane that closely invests the spinal cord and distally forms the filum terminale. The arachnoid mater is a delicate nonvascular membrane closely attached to the outermost layer, which is the dura. The subarachnoid space is located between the pia and arachnoid mater. The subarachnoid space includes the following: (1) CSF; (2) spinal nerves; (3) a trabecular network between the two membranes; (4) blood vessels that supply the spinal cord; and (5) lateral extensions of the pia mater—the dentate ligaments (these ligaments supply lateral support from the spinal cord to the dura mater). Although the spinal cord ends at the lower border of L1 in obstetric patients, the subarachnoid space continues to the S2 level. At the end of the spinal cord the cauda equina begins and continues to the level of S2. The cauda equina nerves are surrounded by CSF, and the structure is affected by gravity; it assumes a dependent position in the spinal canal in both the supine and prone positions (Figure 11-4).

The third and outermost membrane in the spinal canal is a longitudinally organized fibroelastic membrane called the *dura mater.* This layer is a direct extension of the cranial dura mater and extends from the foramen magnum to S2, where the filum terminale blends with the periosteum of the coccyx. A potential space (e.g., the subdural space) exists between the dura and the arachnoid mater. The subdural space contains only small amounts of serous fluid, which allow the dura and arachnoid to move easily over one another. This space is not used intentionally by anesthesiologists. Unintentional subdural injection may explain some cases of failed spinal anesthesia; it may also explain the rare, slow-to-develop cases of high spinal anesthesia after a negative epidural test dose and injection of additional local anesthetic.

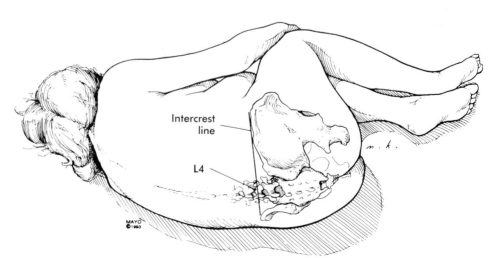

FIGURE 11-2. The surface anatomy used to estimate the lumbar vertebral level. In pregnant women, the interiliac crest line (Tuffier's line) may be slightly higher in relation to the lumbar vertebral axis because of the difficulty in flexing the lumbar spine.

Immediately peripheral to the dura mater is the epidural space. The spinal epidural space extends from the foramen magnum to the sacral hiatus. The posterior longitudinal ligaments form the anterior boundary of this space. The pedicles and intervertebral foramina form the lateral boundaries, and the ligamentum flavum forms the posterior boundary. The contents of the epidural space include nerve roots, fat, areolar tissue, lymphatics, and blood vessels, including the well-organized venous plexus of Batson. The epidural space is segmented; it is not the uniform cylindrical space many authors have described. As shown in Figure 11-5, its segmentation often assumes vertebral level division.[8,9]

Epiduroscopy and epidurography suggest the presence of a dorsal median connective tissue band in some individuals. Anatomic dissection and computerized tomographic epidurography also have suggested the presence of epidural space septa. This band (or these septa) may explain one etiology of unilateral or incomplete epidural anesthesia.[10,11] However, some investigators have suggested that the dorsal median band is an artifact of epidural space distention, and it may be an anatomic manifestation of the previously unappreciated epidural space segmentation.[12]

Posterior to the epidural space lies the ligamentum flavum, which also extends from the foramen magnum to the sacral hiatus. Historically some physicians have described the ligamentum flavum as a single ligament. In actuality, however, it is composed of two curvilinear ligaments that join in the middle and form an acute angle with a ventral opening (Figure 11-6).[12,13] The ligamentum flavum is not uniform from skull to sacrum; indeed, it is not uniform even within a single intervertebral space.[7] The thickness of the ligamentum flavum varies with vertebral column level, as does the distance between the skin and the epidural space (Tables 11-1 and 11-2).[14-17] Hormonal changes may cause the ligamentum flavum to feel "softer" in pregnant women than in nonpregnant patients. The lamina, the spinous processes of the vertebral bodies, and the interspinous ligaments lie posterior to the ligamentum flavum. Posterior to these structures are the supraspinous ligament (which extends from the external occipital protuberance to the coccyx), subcutaneous tissue, and skin (Figure 11-7).

Successful administration of caudal epidural anesthesia is complicated by frequent variations in sacral anatomy.

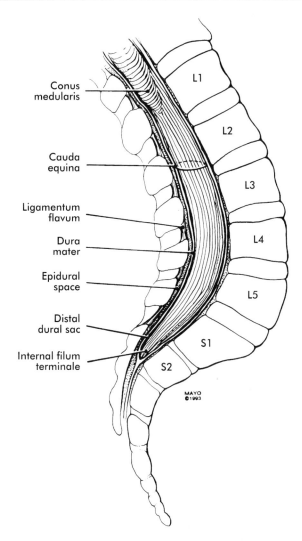

FIGURE 11-3. Distal centroneuraxis anatomy. In pregnant women, the spinal cord ends at the lower border of the first lumbar vertebral body. The subarachnoid space continues to the second sacral vertebral level.

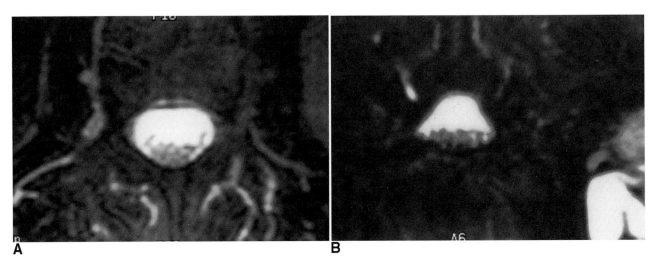

A   **B**

FIGURE 11-4. Cross-sectional magnetic resonance images of low lumbar vertebral anatomy, including the cauda equina. **A,** Supine cross-sectional image showing the cauda equina in a posterior location in the subarachnoid space. **B,** Prone cross-sectional image showing the cauda equina in an anterior location in the subarachnoid space.

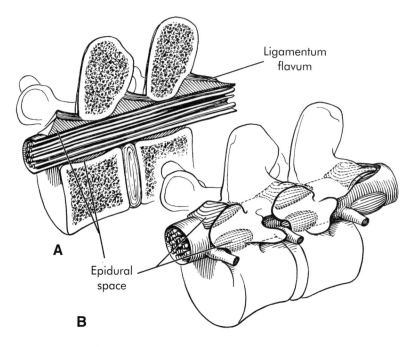

FIGURE 11-5. **A,** Sagittal section of the epidural space demonstrates that the contents of the epidural space depend on the level of the section. **B,** Three-dimensional drawing of the epidural space shows the discontinuity of the epidural contents. However, this potential space can be dilated by the injection of fluid into the epidural space. (Reprinted with permission from the Mayo Foundation. From Stevens RA. Neuraxial blocks. In: Brown DL, editor. Regional Anesthesia and Analgesia. Philadelphia, WB Saunders, 1976:323.)

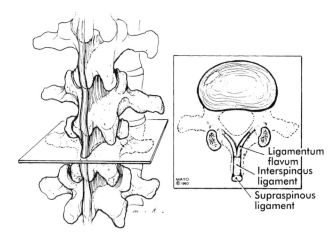

FIGURE 11-6. A horizontal section of the ligamentum flavum and associated neuraxis structures is shown next to an oblique parasagittal section of the lumbar vertebral neuraxis. The horizontal section illustrates the posterior ligamentous structures of the spinal column. The ligamentum flavum is composed of two leaves that meet in the midline at 90 degrees. The interspinous and supraspinous ligaments lie external to the posterior portion of the ligamentum flavum.

TABLE 11-1	DISTANCE FROM THE SKIN TO THE EPIDURAL SPACE IN 1000 PARTURIENTS		
	Distance from skin to epidural space (cm)		
		Percentile	
Lumbar interspace	**Median**	**5th**	**95th**
L1-2	4.23	3.12	6.33
L2-3	4.86	3.29	7.32
L3-4	4.93	3.57	7.44
L4-5	4.78	3.25	6.75

From Harrison GR, Clowes, NWB. The depth of the lumbar epidural space from the skin. Anaesthesia 1985; 40:685-7.

TABLE 11-2	CHARACTERISTICS OF THE LIGAMENTUM FLAVUM AT DIFFERENT VERTEBRAL LEVELS[15-17]	
Site	**Skin to ligament (cm)**	**Average thickness of ligament (mm)**
Lumbar	3.0-8.0*	5.0-6.0†
Caudal	Variable	2.0-6.0

*Distance is ≤ 4 cm for 50% of patients and ≤ 6 cm for 80% of patients.
†Within each interlaminar space, the epidural space varies in depth from cephalad to caudad; near the rostral lamina, 1.3 to 1.6 mm; near the caudad lamina, 6.9 to 9.1 mm.

Developmentally, the five sacral vertebrae fuse to form the sacrum. The sacral hiatus results from the failure of the laminae of S5 and usually part of S4 to fuse in the midline. The sacral hiatus is covered posteriorly by the posterior sacrococcygeal ligament, which is the functional counterpart to the ligamentum flavum. The shape of the bony defect varies from a narrow, slit-like opening to a wide-based, inverted V. The sacral hiatus is absent in as many as 5% of all adult patients, and such an absence precludes the administration of caudal anesthesia.[18,19] The sacral hiatus is less likely to be absent in obstetric patients than in nonobstetric patients, because ossification of this opening seems to increase with age.

The interior of the sacrum contains the sacral canal, which contains the terminal portion of the dural sac. The dural sac terminates cephalad to a line joining the posterior superior iliac spines at the level of the second sacral segment. The sacral canal also contains a venous plexus, which is part of the valveless internal vertebral venous plexus.

PHYSIOLOGY

Safe, successful administration of regional anesthesia in pregnant women requires an understanding of the normal physiologic changes of pregnancy (see Chapter 2). Anesthesiologists, obstetricians, and nurses must appreciate the potential for

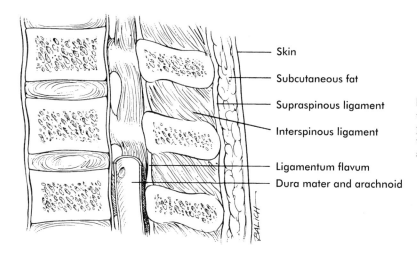

FIGURE 11-7. Midline sagittal anatomy of the vertebral column. When a needle is placed into the cerebrospinal fluid, it must pass through skin, subcutaneous fat, the supraspinous ligament, the interspinous ligament, the ligamentum flavum, the epidural space, and finally the dura.

Skin

Subcutaneous fat

Supraspinous ligament

Interspinous ligament

Ligamentum flavum

Dura mater and arachnoid

aortocaval compression during spinal and epidural anesthesia. Only 10% of *unanesthetized* pregnant women manifest clinical evidence of the supine hypotension syndrome.[20,21] The sympathectomy and vasodilation that accompany neuraxial anesthesia cause pregnant women to be more susceptible to the effects of aortocaval compression. These undesirable hemodynamic changes can be mitigated by hydration with crystalloid and avoidance of aortocaval compression. Pregnant women should not lie supine during the maintenance of spinal or epidural anesthesia. Physicians and nurses should maintain left uterine displacement during labor, the performance of a vaginal examination, and the placement of a fetal scalp electrocardiogram (ECG) electrode or urethral catheter.

The increased oxygen consumption and decreased functional residual capacity associated with pregnancy result in a faster onset of hypoxemia during maternal apnea. Aortocaval compression hastens the onset of cardiovascular collapse during high/total spinal anesthesia. In addition, laboratory evidence suggests that pregnancy increases susceptibility to cardiac toxicity caused by intravenous injection (or overdose) of bupivacaine (but not lidocaine), although this is a matter of some dispute (see Chapter 12).[22] Anesthesiologists should administer spinal or epidural anesthesia only in a physical setting in which complications such as unintentional intravenous or subarachnoid injection of local anesthetic can be rapidly and efficiently managed. In cases of cardiovascular collapse, endotracheal intubation may be necessary to facilitate mechanical ventilation and oxygenation and to protect the lungs from aspiration of gastric contents. Equipment and supplies necessary for laryngoscopy, intubation, and mechanical ventilation should be immediately available.

Physiology of Neural Blockade

Hormonal changes and accompanying decreases in CSF specific gravity likely are responsible for the decreased local anesthetic dose requirements during spinal anesthesia in pregnant women.[4,23] Local anesthetics produce conduction block primarily by blocking sodium channels in nerve membranes, thereby preventing the propagation of neural impulses. For many years, anesthesiologists have known that the zone of differential block of motor-sensory-sympathetic function is wider with spinal than with epidural anesthesia.[24] During spinal anesthesia, local anesthetics act directly on neural tissue in the subarachnoid space. Regression of anesthesia can be explained by the simple vascular uptake of local anesthetic from the subarachnoid space.[25]

Epidural anesthesia has a much smaller zone of differential motor-sensory-sympathetic block; this suggests that the mechanism of epidural anesthesia must involve more than simple diffusion across the dura. For many years, nerve fiber size was presumed to be the primary determinant of susceptibility to local anesthetic blockade (i.e., smaller fibers are blocked more readily than larger fibers). However, recent studies have shown that the length of nerve fiber exposed to local anesthetic is as important as the size of the nerve fiber. Fink[26] hypothesized that the length of nerve fiber exposed to local anesthetic affects the extent of the differential zone of motor and sensory blockade. With spinal anesthesia, the local anesthetic concentration required to block sufficient sodium channels to affect motor, sensory, and sympathetic function is less than that needed for the better protected nerves found in the epidural space; thus a wider band of differential block occurs during spinal anesthesia than during epidural anesthesia (Figure 11-8).

Our understanding of the mechanisms of spinal and epidural anesthesia likely remains oversimplified. Nonetheless, it seems clear that spinal anesthesia results primarily from the effects of local anesthetic on the spinal cord, whereas epidural anesthesia results from the effects of local anesthetic within both the epidural and subarachnoid spaces.

TECHNIQUE

Contraindications for these techniques include the following: (1) patient refusal or inability to cooperate; (2) increased intracranial pressure as a result of a mass lesion, which may predispose the patient to brainstem herniation after dural puncture; (3) skin or soft tissue infection at the site of needle puncture; (4) frank coagulopathy; (5) uncorrected maternal hypovolemia; and (6) inadequate training or experience in the technique. Whether mild or isolated abnormalities in tests of blood coagulation preclude the use of regional anesthesia is controversial. However, it is clear that the prophylactic administration of low molecular weight heparin is a clinical risk factor that mandates caution in the administration of neuraxial anesthesia.[27] The anesthesiologist should weigh the risks and benefits of regional anesthesia for each patient.

Patient Position

Pregnant women have an exaggerated lumbar lordosis, and it is more difficult for them to flex the lumbar spine. However, most pregnant women are young, and youth usually allows

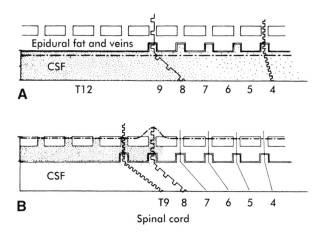

FIGURE 11-8. The mechanism of differential block in the thoracic spinal cord. The two crenated lines represent long and short internode myelinated fibers, respectively, and are intersected by a dashed line at the critical bathed lengths. **A,** Subarachnoid conduction blockade. The concentration gradient of anesthetic in the cerebrospinal fluid (CSF) is symbolized by the density of stippling. The security of conduction has decreased to the same degree in the short-internode fibers of segmental nerve T4 as in the long-internode fibers of segment T8, because the product of node number and anesthetic concentration is the same. Only the short-internode fibers will be blocked at T8. **B,** Epidural conduction blockade. The epidural concentration of anesthetic is approximately the same throughout the affected portion of the epidural space, except at the edges of the bathed area. For clarity, long- and short-internode fibers are represented in different segments but may be discussed as if present in the same segment, because the length of axon between the end of the dural cuff and the exit from the intervertebral foramen is approximately the same and measures only a few millimeters in all thoracic segments. The number of nodes bathed in the intervertebral canal is not sufficient to establish conduction block in the long-internode fiber but does suffice in the short-internode fiber. The spread of epidural anesthetic beyond the intervertebral foramina can abolish the differential block, as may diffusion in sufficient concentration through the dura into the CSF and nerve roots. (From Fink BR. Mechanisms of differential axial blockade in epidural and subarachnoid anesthesia. Anesthesiology 1989; 70:851-8.)

sufficient flexibility to facilitate the insertion of a needle into the epidural or subarachnoid space. Most obstetric patients may assume the lateral decubitus position comfortably during the administration of spinal or epidural anesthesia; this position likely has less adverse effect on venous return and cardiac output than the sitting position. Some anesthesiologists have debated whether the lateral decubitus position or the sitting position is more comfortable for the patient. Vincent and Chestnut[28] performed a study in which they observed that neither position was consistently superior with regard to patient comfort. However, pregnant women who preferred the left lateral decubitus position weighed less and had lower body mass indices than women who preferred the sitting position.

When spinal or epidural anesthesia is performed with the patient in a lateral position, the patient's back should lie parallel with the edge of the bed for at least two reasons. First, the edge is the most firm section of the mattress. (If the patient lies away from the edge of the bed, the patient's weight will depress the mattress, and the anesthesiologist must work in a "downhill" direction.) Second, this position allows anesthesiologists to keep their elbows flexed, which facilitates control of fine hand and wrist muscle movements. This is especially important when using the loss-of-resistance technique for performing epidural anesthesia.

The sitting position is likely associated with an increased incidence of orthostatic hypotension and syncope, and an

assistant is often required during use of the sitting position. The sitting position is preferred—and may be required—in obese parturients. In obese patients, the sitting position facilitates identification of the spinous processes. Further, morbidly obese women may develop hypoxemia when placed in the lateral decubitus position. It seems intuitive that the sitting position might compromise venous return, cardiac output, and uteroplacental perfusion. However, one study demonstrated a greater reduction in maternal cardiac output with *maximal* lumbar flexion in the lateral decubitus position than in the sitting position during identification of the epidural space. The authors speculated that maximal lumbar flexion in the lateral decubitus position results in concealed aortocaval compression.[29] (Editor's note: Notwithstanding this study, I have observed more fetal heart rate abnormalities when giving epidural anesthesia in the sitting position than in the lateral decubitus position. When possible, I prefer to monitor the fetal heart rate continuously when performing epidural or spinal anesthesia in a parturient in the sitting position.) Finally, Bamberger and Birnbach[30] reported the administration of epidural anesthesia in a patient who remained in the knee-chest position because that was the only position that relieved and prevented fetal bradycardia.

It is preferred that spinal anesthesia for cesarean section be performed with the patient in the right lateral decubitus position for two reasons. First, use of the lateral position facilitates the establishment of a T4 sensory level, which is preferable for an intra-abdominal procedure. Second, the patient will be tilted leftward during surgery. When giving a hyperbaric local anesthetic solution, it makes sense to inject the local anesthetic with the patient lying on her right side, knowing that she will be tilted leftward thereafter. If the local anesthetic is injected with the patient lying on her left side and the leftward tilt is maintained thereafter, an asymmetric and inadequate block may result (i.e., a higher level may result on the left side than on the right side). By contrast, when giving spinal anesthesia for instrumental vaginal delivery, it often makes sense to perform the procedure with the patient sitting to ensure the rapid onset of sacral anesthesia.

Posture has less influence on the spread of epidural anesthesia.[31-33] During epidural anesthesia, a unilateral block more likely results from the malposition of the catheter (or perhaps an anatomic barrier within the epidural space) than from the prolonged use of one position. Norris et al.[33] observed that gravity did not augment the spread of anesthesia in patients receiving epidural anesthesia for cesarean section, and they concluded that posture does not need to be manipulated to ensure adequate bilateral epidural anesthesia for cesarean section. At least two studies have noted that the use of the sitting position is not necessary for the development of good sacral anesthesia when giving large volumes of local anesthetic epidurally for cesarean section.[31,33] However, Reid and Thorburn[33] observed that use of the sitting position appeared to delay the spread of anesthesia to the midthoracic dermatomes.

Caudal anesthesia is used infrequently in modern obstetric anesthesia practice. However, there remain some circumstances in which a caudal technique is useful and/or advantageous. Caudal anesthesia is a good choice for the second stage of labor in selected patients in whom the lumbar epidural approach is hazardous or contraindicated. In most cases, caudal anesthesia can be successfully performed with the patient in a lateral decubitus position. Anatomic variation may require use of the knee-chest position in some patients.

Choice of Drug*

SPINAL ANESTHESIA

Anesthesiologists may give spinal anesthesia for cerclage, nonobstetric surgery, forceps delivery, cesarean section, or the removal of a retained placenta. Cesarean section represents the most frequent indication for spinal anesthesia in pregnant women. Most anesthesiologists give a hyperbaric solution of local anesthetic for spinal anesthesia in obstetric patients. Use of a hyperbaric solution results in a faster onset of block and a higher maximum sensory level with a shorter duration of nerve block.[34] The urgency and anticipated duration of surgery dictate the choice of local anesthetic agent. The drug choices for spinal anesthesia in the United States include lidocaine (Xylocaine), tetracaine (Pontocaine), ropivacaine (Naropin), S(−)-levobupivacaine (Chirocaine), and bupivacaine (Marcaine or Sensorcaine). **Lidocaine** provides a short-to-intermediate duration of action. Although some physicians are limiting their use of spinal lidocaine because of concerns about the development of neurotoxicity, many anesthesiologists continue to use the drug successfully.[35] Tetracaine, bupivacaine, levobupivacaine, and ropivacaine provide intermediate-to-long durations of action.

It was previously thought that epinephrine did not prolong the duration of spinal anesthesia with lidocaine. However, earlier studies defined duration as time to high thoracic two-segment regression. Moore et al.[36] observed that epinephrine prolonged the duration of spinal anesthesia for lower thoracic two-segment regression and lower abdominal incision. Some anesthesiologists also contend that epinephrine improves the *quality* of spinal anesthesia. At least one study has suggested that the addition of epinephrine may increase the incidence of nausea and vomiting during spinal anesthesia.[37]

Tetracaine is packaged as niphanoid crystals (20 mg) and as a 1% solution (20 mg/2 mL). Niphanoid crystals should be diluted with preservative-free sterile water immediately before subarachnoid injection. Either the crystal-diluted or pre-mixed solution is mixed with an equal volume of 10% dextrose to create a solution of 0.5% tetracaine in 5% dextrose. The addition of epinephrine prolongs the duration of spinal anesthesia with tetracaine.[38] Epinephrine also improves the quality of tetracaine spinal anesthesia. The addition of 0.1 to 0.2 mg of epinephrine does not adversely affect uteroplacental or spinal cord blood flow.[39,40]

Bupivacaine 0.75% is prepackaged with 8.5% dextrose. Hyperbaric 0.75% bupivacaine is the most widely used agent for spinal anesthesia in obstetric anesthesia practice in the United States. (Bupivacaine is prepared and distributed as a hyperbaric 0.5% solution in some countries, but not in the United States.) Some anesthesiologists contend that epinephrine improves the quality of spinal anesthesia with bupivacaine[41]; others have found that it is unnecessary to add epinephrine to bupivacaine when giving spinal anesthesia for cesarean section.

Ropivacaine is attractive because of experimental evidence that it is less likely to cause cardiac toxicity. With spinal anesthesia, this difference seems insignificant because such small doses of drugs are administered. Ropivacaine is not as potent as bupivacaine when administered for spinal anesthesia, and it may be necessary to give a dose of ropivacaine as large as twice that of bupivacaine to achieve the same effect.[42] Ropivacaine is associated with earlier recovery of motor function and shorter discharge times, although many believe it to be indistinguishable from bupivacaine when equipotent doses are used.[43]

Levobupivacaine is the isolated S-enantiomer of bupivacaine and is now available for spinal anesthesia. Clinical data suggest that this drug is indistinguishable from racemic bupivacaine when used for spinal anesthesia. The spinal dose for levobupivacaine is the same as that for bupivacaine. In clinical situations in which systemic toxicity is not an issue, the advantage of levobupivacaine over bupivacaine seems more theoretic than real.[44]

Anesthesiologists often add an opioid to the local anesthetic to improve the quality of anesthesia and to provide postoperative analgesia. It was hoped that other adjuncts (e.g., clonidine, neostigmine) might allow for the administration of a smaller dose of local anesthetic and thereby minimize the sympatholytic side effects and perhaps hasten recovery. Side effects from these other adjuncts have precluded their wide use in obstetric anesthesia practice (see Chapters 25 and 28).

EPIDURAL ANESTHESIA

Local anesthetic agents available for epidural administration in obstetric patients include 2-chloroprocaine (Nesacaine), lidocaine (Xylocaine), mepivacaine (Carbocaine), bupivacaine (Marcaine or Sensorcaine), ropivacaine (Naropin), levobupivacaine (Chirocaine), and etidocaine (Duranest). Mepivacaine and etidocaine are used infrequently in obstetric anesthesia practice.

Bupivacaine remains the most popular local anesthetic for analgesia during labor and vaginal delivery because of its differential sensory blockade, long duration of action, and low frequency of tachyphylaxis (see Chapters 12 and 22). Anesthesiologists currently administer bupivacaine for cesarean section less frequently than they did two decades ago because of several cases of cardiac toxicity and maternal mortality following unintentional intravascular injection of the drug. With the introduction of local anesthetic agents with safer cardiotoxic profiles (e.g., ropivacaine, levobupivacaine), long-acting alternatives to bupivacaine are now available.

Ropivacaine has gained popularity as an agent for epidural analgesia because of evidence that it results in less cardiac toxicity and greater differential sensory blockade than bupivacaine.[45] Some studies have suggested that epidural ropivacaine is only 60% as potent as epidural bupivacaine on the basis of the median effective dose (ED_{50}) determined using an up-down sequential allocation study design.[46] However, Chua et al.[47] observed "clinically indistinguishable" pain relief when either 0.125% ropivacaine or 0.125% bupivacaine was used for initiation and maintenance of patient-controlled epidural analgesia in laboring women. The addition of an opioid allows for the administration of a more dilute solution of ropivacaine. One study suggested that 0.075% ropivacaine with 2 μg/mL of fentanyl provides satisfactory analgesia with minimal motor blockade and excellent hemodynamic stability.[48]

Levobupivacaine has recently been introduced into clinical practice because of its apparent favorable safety profile as compared with bupivacaine. Clinical trials have shown it to have similar potency and analgesic qualities as bupivacaine with the probable exception of less motor block.[48,49] Bupivacaine, ropivacaine, and levobupivacaine all have a slower onset than lidocaine, and they may be preferred over shorter-acting agents when a slow onset of anesthesia is desirable.

Despite some variation among the reports, published studies suggest no more than slight differences in onset and

---

*Chapter 12 includes a detailed discussion of local anesthetic agents.

potency and no differences in quality or duration of neuronal block between ropivacaine, levobupivacaine and bupivacaine. However, bupivacaine is more cardiotoxic than these other agents in vitro and perhaps when unintentionally administered intravascularly.[50] No clinical studies have confirmed the decreased toxicity of these newer agents in humans. Whether the decreased cardiac toxicity profile and enhanced sensorimotor differentiation of these new agents are sufficient advantages to displace bupivacaine as the "standard" for epidural anesthesia remains to be determined.

The most popular choice of local anesthetic when giving epidural anesthesia for cesarean section is 2% **lidocaine with epinephrine**. The addition of epinephrine causes a modest prolongation of the block. However, epinephrine's major advantage is that it improves the *quality* of epidural lidocaine anesthesia. Clinically, the addition of 1 mL of 8.4% sodium bicarbonate for every 10 mL of 2% lidocaine with 1:200,000 epinephrine produces a significantly faster onset of anesthesia and a more rapid spread of sensory block.[51] The quality of the block can be further enhanced by the addition of 50 to 100 μg of fentanyl or 10 to 20 μg of sufentanyl. Lam et al.[52] have shown that surgical anesthesia for cesarean section can be achieved in 5.2 ± 1.5 minutes with the addition of bicarbonate and fentanyl to 2% lidocaine with epinephrine.

Many anesthesiologists reserve **2-chloroprocaine** for cases in which they need the rapid extension of epidural anesthesia for vaginal delivery or urgent cesarean section. A disadvantage of 2-chloroprocaine is its apparent antagonism of subsequently injected epidural opioids[53] and amide local anesthetics.[54] 2-Chloroprocaine was earlier associated with arachnoiditis following unintentional subarachnoid injection of the drug.[55] Replacement of bisulfite (an antioxidant that was added to stabilize the formulation) by ethylenediaminetetraacetic acid exchanged the associated danger of arachnoiditis with the less-serious side effect of backache.[56] It remains to be seen whether preservative-free 2-chloroprocaine will be associated with back pain in clinically used doses. With the luxury of fast-onset blockade resulting from alkalinized lidocaine with epinephrine and an opioid, some anesthesiologists question the clinical relevance of 2-chloroprocaine in contemporary obstetric anesthesia practice.

For cesarean section, anesthesiologists typically need to give at least 15 to 20 mL of local anesthetic in 5-mL increments, regardless of the choice of drug. 2-Chloroprocaine, lidocaine with epinephrine, ropivacaine, and bupivacaine provide anesthesia for durations of approximately 40 minutes, 75 to 90 minutes, 100 to 130 minutes, and 120 to 150 minutes, respectively.

CAUDAL ANESTHESIA

The drugs used for caudal epidural anesthesia are identical to those used for lumbar epidural block. The major difference is that a much larger volume (e.g., 25 to 35 mL) of local anesthetic solution must be administered to extend a caudal block for cesarean section. Such large volumes entail an increased risk for systemic local anesthetic toxicity, and perhaps with this technique ropivacaine and levobupivacaine will prove to be better choices than racemic bupivacaine. However, there are few indications for the use of caudal anesthesia for cesarean section in contemporary practice.

Needle Placement

SPINAL ANESTHESIA

The first equipment decision involves determining whether to perform a single-shot or continuous technique. Continuous spinal anesthesia is not a new technique; indeed, some physicians gave continuous spinal anesthesia 50 years ago. Early techniques required the use of large needles and catheters, which resulted in a high incidence of postdural puncture headache. The development of small-bore microcatheters resulted in renewed interest in the use of continuous spinal anesthesia. In 1992, the Food and Drug Administration rescinded approval for the use of these small-bore catheters.[57] Currently a large-bore epidural needle and catheter must be used for continuous spinal anesthesia. Thus a single-shot technique is used for most spinal anesthetics in obstetric patients.

The primary decision the anesthesiologist must make is whether to use a cutting-bevel or a non-cutting-bevel needle. It seems clear that the non-cutting needles (e.g., Whitacre, Sprotte, Greene) result in a lower incidence of postdural puncture headache than the cutting needles (e.g., Quincke) of similar size (Figure 11-9).[58-60] Some anesthesiologists refer to the Whitacre and Sprotte needles as *pencil-point* needles. It is now believed that these pencil-point needles result in more trauma to the dura, which then results in a more intense inflammatory response than occurs with cutting-bevel

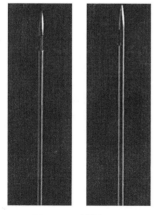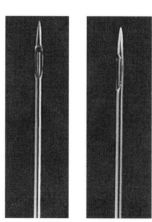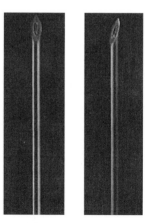

25–gauge Whitacre   24–gauge Sprotte   25–gauge Quincke

FIGURE 11-9. Spinal needle assortment often used in parturients. The needles are shown in an open-bevel view and an oblique orientation. The Whitacre and Sprotte needles have cone-shaped bevels, whereas the Quincke has a cutting bevel. (Other sizes are available in some of these needle designs.)

needles. Presumably the inflammation results in edematous closure of the dural defect.[61]

Needle size also must be determined. In general, there are "ease-of-use" advantages associated with larger needles that must be balanced against a decreased incidence of postdural puncture headache with smaller needles. For most anesthesiologists, the two curves cross at the use of a 25-gauge needle (i.e., with needles smaller than 25-gauge, the technical difficulties increase enough to offset the small decrease in the incidence of postdural puncture headache). However, anesthesiologists should make individual decisions based on their own skills and practice setting. The urgency of the procedure may also influence the choice of needle size. For example, a 27-gauge needle might be chosen for spinal anesthesia for an elective procedure and a larger (e.g., 22-gauge) needle might be chosen when the subarachnoid space must be entered quickly in cases of severe fetal distress.

When using a small-gauge needle, use of an introducer needle is preferable. The introducer needle allows for more accurate introduction of the spinal needle than is possible with use of a small-gauge spinal needle alone.

Either the midline or paramedian approach can be used to enter the subarachnoid space. The **midline** approach requires the patient to reduce her lumbar lordosis to allow access to the subarachnoid space between adjacent spinous processes (usually L3 to L4, or sometimes L4 to L5). Two fingers (usually the index and middle finger) identify the interspinous space by palpating the caudad border of the more cephalad spine. The two fingers identify the midline by rolling the fingers in a medial-to-lateral direction (Figure 11-10). Next, the anesthesiologist injects local anesthetic intradermally and subcutaneously (it is important to raise a skin wheal; otherwise introduction of the introducer will be painful). The anesthesiologist then inserts the introducer into the substance of the interspinous ligament. At this time, it is useful to make certain that the introducer is directed midline. The introducer is then grasped with the palpating fingers and steadied while the other hand is used to hold the spinal needle like a dart. The fifth finger is used as a tripod against the patient's back to prevent patient movement from causing unintentional needle insertion to a level deeper than intended. If a cutting-bevel needle is chosen, the needle should be inserted with the bevel parallel to the longitudinal-directed dural fibers. When a non-cutting-bevel needle is chosen, the needle may be inserted without attention to fiber direction. As the needle passes through the ligamentum flavum and the dura, characteristic changes in resistance are noted. The stylet is removed, and CSF should appear in the needle hub. If it does not, the needle is rotated in 90-degree increments until CSF appears. If CSF does not appear in any quadrant, the stylet is replaced, the needle is advanced a few millimeters, and then it is again checked for CSF flow. If CSF does not appear at this point and the needle is at an appropriate depth for the patient, the needle and introducer are withdrawn, and the process is repeated.

The most common reason for lack of CSF flow is insertion of the needle away from the midline. If the anesthesiologist achieves good anesthesia of the skin and subcutaneous tissues,

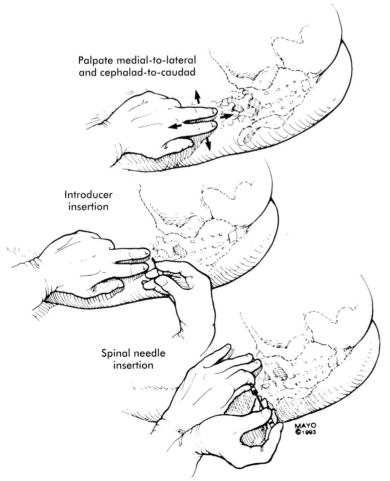

Palpate medial-to-lateral and cephalad-to-caudad

Introducer insertion

Spinal needle insertion

MAYO ©1993

FIGURE 11-10. The midline approach for spinal needle insertion requires accurate identification of a lumbar interspinous space. The palpating fingers are rolled in a medial-to-lateral and cephalad-to-caudad direction; an introducer is then inserted through the interspinous space almost perpendicular to the lumbar spinous process. Once the introducer is seated in the interspinous ligament, the spinal needle is inserted; the needle is stabilized in a tripod fashion during insertion (similar to a dart being thrown).

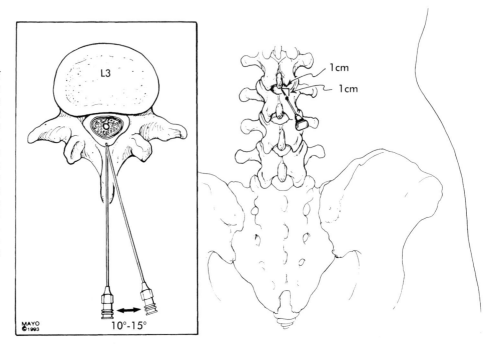

FIGURE 11-11. Vertebral anatomy of midline and paramedian approaches for spinal and epidural anesthesia. The midline approach requires anatomic projection in only two planes: sagittal and horizontal. The paramedian approach also requires consideration of the oblique plane. However, the paramedian approach requires less patient cooperation in reducing lumbar lordosis to allow for successful needle insertion. The paramedian needle insertion site is made 1 cm lateral and 1 cm caudad to the caudad edge of the more cephalad spinous process. The paramedian needle is inserted approximately 10 to 15 degrees off the sagittal plane (inset).

correct use of the midline approach is almost painless. Significant pain suggests that the needle is directed away from the midline; indeed, a patient often indicates that the pain is located on either the left or right side of the back. In such cases, correct direction of the needle should be confirmed. Redirection of the needle often eliminates the patient's pain and results in the successful identification of the subarachnoid space.

Once CSF is freely dripping from the needle hub, the dorsum of the anesthesiologist's nondominant hand steadies the introducer and spinal needle against the patient's back while the syringe with local anesthetic is attached to the needle. After aspirating to ensure the free flow of CSF, the anesthesiologist injects the dose at a rate of approximately 0.2 mL per second. After completion of the injection, the anesthesiologist again aspirates approximately 0.2 mL of CSF and reinjects that CSF into the subarachnoid space. This last step reconfirms the needle location and clears the needle of the remaining local anesthetic. The patient is then positioned as appropriate.

For most patients, the midline approach is faster and less painful than the paramedian approach. The midline approach is also easier to teach than the paramedian approach, because it requires mental projection of the anatomy in only two planes, whereas the paramedian approach requires appreciation of a third plane (Figure 11-11). Nevertheless, the **paramedian** approach is a useful technique that allows for the successful identification of the subarachnoid or epidural space in difficult cases. The paramedian approach does not require that the patient fully reduce her lumbar lordosis. This approach exploits the larger target that is available when the needle is inserted slightly off the midline.

A common error that is made with the paramedian approach is the insertion of the needle too far off the midline; the vertebral lamina then becomes a barrier to needle insertion. With the paramedian approach, the palpating fingers should again identify the caudad edge of the more cephalad spinous process. A skin wheal is raised 1 cm lateral and 1 cm caudad to this point; a longer needle is then used to infiltrate the deeper tissues in a cephalomedial plane. (This contrasts

with the midline approach, in which the local anesthetic is not injected beyond the subcutaneous tissue.) The spinal introducer is then inserted 10 to 15 degrees off the sagittal plane in a cephalomedial direction, and the spinal needle is advanced by means of the introducer toward the subarachnoid space. Another common error is to use an excessive cephalad angle with initial needle insertion. When the needle is inserted correctly and contacts bone, it is redirected slightly cephalad. If bone is again encountered but at a deeper level, the slight stepwise increase in cephalad angulation is continued, and the needle is "walked" up and off the lamina. As with the midline approach, the characteristic feel of the ligamentum flavum and dura can be appreciated. However, use of the paramedian approach requires insertion of a greater length of needle. Once CSF is obtained, the block is performed as it is with the midline approach.

The **Taylor** approach is a variation of the paramedian approach. It uses the L5 to S1 space, which has the largest interlaminar space in the lumbosacral region. A 5-inch spinal needle is inserted in a cephalomedial plane from a site 1 cm medial and 1 cm caudad to the lowermost prominence of the posterior superior iliac spine (Figure 11-12). If bone is encountered on the first needle insertion, the needle is redirected in small steps cephalad to walk off the sacrum and into the subarachnoid space.

EPIDURAL ANESTHESIA

When choosing equipment, anesthesiologists must decide whether to use a continuous or a single-shot technique. With a continuous technique, a needle with a lateral-faced opening should be used. (Figure 11-13). With a single-shot technique, *any* epidural needle—including a Crawford needle—may be used.

Some anesthesiologists use the hanging-drop method to identify the epidural space. However, most use a loss-of-resistance technique (Figure 11-14). With the latter technique, the type of syringe and the syringe content must be chosen. The ideal syringe is a finely ground glass syringe with a Luer-lock connector. We prefer that the syringe contain both saline and

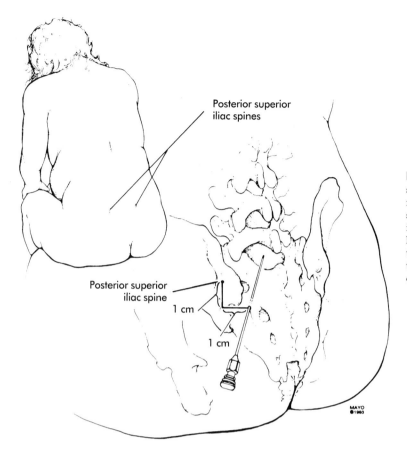

Posterior superior
iliac spines

Posterior superior
iliac spine

1 cm

1 cm

MAYO
©1993

FIGURE 11-12. Anatomy of Taylor's approach to spinal anesthesia. This is a true paramedian approach at the L5 to S1 level. A skin mark is made 1 cm caudad and 1 cm medial to one of the posterior superior iliac spines. Through this skin mark, the spinal needle is inserted cephalad and medially (to walk off the sacrum) and into the largest interspinous space, the L5 to S1 intervertebral space. The posterior superior iliac spines typically are located immediately anterior to the skin dimples that often are found overlying the superior aspect of the sacrum.

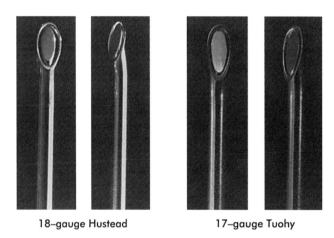

18–gauge Hustead   17–gauge Tuohy

FIGURE 11-13. Epidural needles often used in parturients. The needles are shown in an open-bevel view and oblique orientation. The 18-gauge Hustead and 17-gauge Tuohy needles have lateral-faced openings, which direct epidural catheters to enter the epidural space more easily than if a single-shot Crawford needle design is used. (Other sizes and needle designs are available for obstetric epidural anesthesia.)

a small (e.g., 0.25 mL) compressible bubble of air. (Editor's note: Saline causes some syringe plungers to stick, and in the past I used a dry syringe that contained air only.[62] However, there is controversy regarding the use of air for detecting the point of loss of resistance.[63-65] The authors of a recently published review concluded that better analgesia and decreased morbidity result from the use of saline as the medium for determining the loss of resistance.[65] I now use saline with a small bubble of air, as recommended by Drs. Brown and Gottumukkala.)

Regardless of the technique that is used, success depends on the correct placement of the needle tip within the ligamentum flavum. It is helpful to advance the needle into the ligmentum flavum before attaching the syringe or before placing the hanging drop of solution into the needle hub. This has at least three advantages. First, it encourages the anesthesiologist to use proprioception while directing and advancing the needle. Second, it decreases the time required for successful identification of the epidural space. Third, it decreases the likelihood of having a false-positive loss of resistance. (Undoubtedly, this false-positive identification of the epidural space is responsible for many cases of unsuccessful epidural anesthesia; it is even possible to insert a catheter between the interspinous ligament and the ligamentum flavum.)

During advancement of the needle-syringe assembly, the needle should be advanced toward the epidural space by the nondominant hand while the thumb of the dominant hand applies pressure on the syringe plunger. We prefer to apply constant pressure on the syringe plunger. (Anesthesiologists who use an air-filled syringe typically employ an intermittent, oscillating technique.) When the needle enters the epidural space, the pressure applied to the syringe plunger causes the solution to flow easily into the epidural space (Figure 11-14).

When the hanging-drop technique is used, a drop of solution is placed into the needle hub once the needle tip is placed into the ligamentum flavum. When the needle tip enters the epidural space, the drop of solution is "sucked in." Historically, anesthesiologists have believed that this technique depends on the presence of true subatmospheric pressure within the epidural space. However, it is more likely that artifactual subatmospheric pressure occurs as a result of expansion of the epidural space as the needle pushes the dura away from the ligamentum flavum.[66]

FIGURE 11-14. Techniques of epidural needle insertion most often used in locating the epidural space. **A,** Loss-of-resistance technique. The needle is first inserted into the ligamentum flavum, and a syringe containing an air bubble in saline is attached to the hub. After compression of the air bubble by pressure to the syringe-plunger, the needle is carefully advanced until a loss of resistance to syringe-plunger pressure is noted as the needle enters the epidural space. **B,** Hanging-drop technique. Here the needle is again inserted into the ligamentum flavum, and a drop of saline or local anesthetic is placed in the hub. The needle is carefully advanced until the entry of the needle into the epidural space is signaled by the drop of solution being "sucked" into the epidural space.

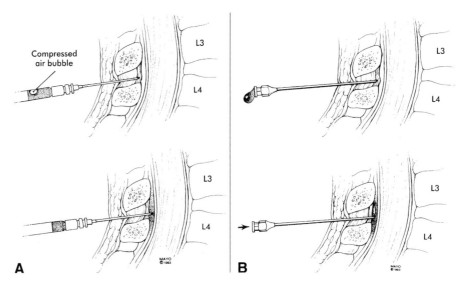

In most obstetric cases, anesthesiologists insert a catheter and use a continuous technique. Anesthesiologists must decide whether to insert the catheter before or after the test and the therapeutic doses of local anesthetic. Most anesthesiologists insert the catheter before injecting local anesthetic; they contend that this method allows for a more controlled development of epidural anesthesia. However, there is little evidence that the incremental injection of local anesthetic through the catheter results in less significant hemodynamic change than incremental injection through the needle (followed by insertion of the catheter). Nonetheless, if the principal reason for using an epidural technique is the provision of continuous analgesia, it seems most practical to insert the catheter before injecting the therapeutic dose of local anesthetic so that correct catheter placement can be verified promptly. If a catheter technique is chosen, it may be helpful to advance the epidural needle another 1 to 2 mm before threading the catheter.

If the catheter is placed before the test and therapeutic doses of local anesthetic, it may be helpful to inject 10 mL of saline before threading the catheter. Some anesthesiologists contend that this expands the epidural space and decreases the likelihood of unintentional intravenous cannulation of the catheter.[67-69] Some studies have noted that injection of 5 mL[68] or 10 mL[67,69] of 0.9% saline[69] or bupivacaine[67,68] through the epidural needle significantly reduces the incidence of cannulation of an epidural vein. By contrast, Rolbin et al.[70] noted that there was no advantage to the injection of 3 mL of fluid into the epidural space before insertion of the epidural catheter.

The anesthesiologist must decide whether to use a single-orifice or multi-orifice catheter.[71-76] The proposed advantage of single orifice, open-end catheters is that the injection of drugs is restricted to a single anatomic site. In theory, this should facilitate the detection of intravenous or subarachnoid placement of the catheter. Likewise, the purported disadvantage of multi-orifice, closed-end catheters is that local anesthetic may be injected into more than one anatomic site (e.g., both the epidural and subarachnoid spaces). However, increasing evidence suggests that multi-orifice, closed-end catheters result in a more even distribution of local anesthetic and a greater likelihood of successful epidural anesthesia.[76] Although many anesthesiologists have their personal prefer-

ences, there are no compelling reasons to favor one catheter over the other, provided the anesthesiologist gives careful attention to detail during the injection of a local anesthetic. Regardless of the choice of catheter, aspiration should be performed before each dose of local anesthetic. A catheter initially placed in the epidural space can migrate into a vein or the subdural or subarachnoid space.

Many techniques are available for securing the catheter at the skin entry site; institutional tradition often is the determining factor. If a catheter will be used for prolonged intrapartum or postoperative analgesia, the anesthesiologist should be able to assess the skin surrounding the catheter. Many find that a clear, sterile adhesive dressing applied over the catheter works well. (The periphery of the dressing can be reinforced with tape.) Others have developed methods of placing gauze or a commercially designed sponge at the skin entry site before taping the catheter in place, believing that this lessens the chance of catheter kinking. One study demonstrated that the position of the epidural catheter may change significantly with patient movement from the sitting flexed to the sitting upright or lateral decubitus position. To minimize the risk of catheter displacement, especially in obese patients, the authors recommended that multi-orifice catheters be inserted at least 4 cm into the epidural space and that patients assume the sitting upright or lateral position *before* the anesthesiologist secures the catheter to the skin.[77]

The potential for the contamination of local anesthetic solutions has prompted some anesthesiologists to use a micropore filter during the administration of continuous epidural anesthesia for labor. However, Abouleish et al.[78,79] concluded that micropore filters are unnecessary during the administration of epidural anesthesia in obstetric patients. Micropore filters may also decrease the reliability of aspiration.[80] We believe that micropore filters have little utility in clinical practice.

CAUDAL ANESTHESIA

Equipment for caudal anesthesia is similar to that used for lumbar epidural techniques except that a needle with a lateral-faced opening is not needed. A blunt-tipped needle is satisfactory even when a catheter is used, because the angle of needle insertion allows insertion of the catheter. Successful administration of caudal anesthesia requires the accurate identifica-

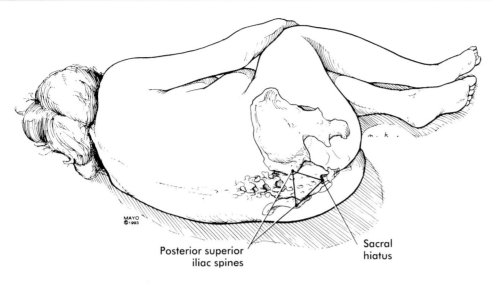

FIGURE 11-15. The location of the sacral hiatus for caudal anesthesia is facilitated by the identification of the posterior superior iliac spines. The posterior superior spines are marked, and a line is drawn between them that forms one edge of an equilateral triangle. If the triangle is completed as illustrated, the sacral hiatus should underlie the caudad tip of the equilateral triangle.

Posterior superior
iliac spines

Sacral
hiatus

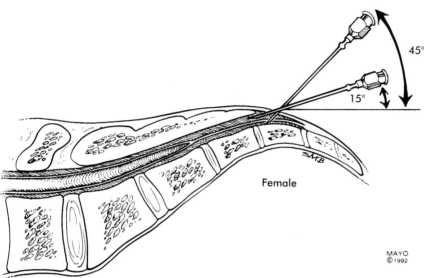

FIGURE 11-16. Once the sacral hiatus is identified, the needle is inserted by insertion and withdrawal in a stepwise fashion from an initial 45-degree angle off the coronal plane. In pregnant women, the needle eventually enters the caudal canal at an angle approximately 15 degrees off the coronal plane. If the needle is placed properly, no subcutaneous "lump" develops after the injection of the local anesthetic solution.

tion of the sacral hiatus. The sacrococcygeal ligament (an extension of the ligamentum flavum) overlies the sacral hiatus between the sacral cornu. Identification of the posterior superior iliac spines facilitates the identification of the sacral cornu; the location of the sacral hiatus is approximated by using the line between them as one side of an equilateral triangle (Figure 11-15). Once the sacral hiatus is identified, the palpating fingers are placed on the cornu, and the caudal needle is inserted with the hub at an angle approximately 45 degrees from the skin (Figure 11-16). A decrease in resistance is noted when the needle enters the caudal canal. The needle is advanced until it contacts bone (i.e., the dorsal aspect of the ventral plate of the sacrum); next, the needle is withdrawn slightly and redirected so that the angle of insertion relative to the skin surface is decreased. In pregnant women, the final angle is approximately 15 degrees from a plane parallel to the sacrum.

Accurate placement of the caudal needle is verified primarily by the "feel" of the needle passing through the sacrococcygeal ligament. There is a maneuver that may help those with less experience to verify correct needle placement. Once the needle is believed to be within the caudal canal, a 5-mL dose of saline is rapidly injected through the needle while the anesthesiologist's other hand is placed over the dorsum of the sacrum. If the needle is placed correctly, no mass or pressure wave is detected over the midline of the sacrum. Conversely, if the needle is malpositioned (often posterior to the caudal canal), a fluid mass or pressure wave is felt by the anesthesiologist's palpating hand. If the needle is malpositioned, the anesthesiologist should reassess the patient's anatomy, and the technique should be repeated.

The needle should be advanced only 1 to 2 cm into the caudal canal. Dural puncture and/or unintentional intravascular cannulation are more likely to occur with deeper insertion. A test dose similar to that used during administration of lumbar epidural anesthesia should be given first.

Combined Spinal and Epidural Technique

In 1981, Brownridge[81] first described his experience with a combined spinal-epidural (CSE) technique in 200 patients undergoing cesarean section. He placed an epidural catheter at L1 to L2 to provide postoperative analgesia, and he placed a small-gauge spinal needle at L3 to L4 to provide intraoperative anesthesia. He cited the advantages of a rapid onset of spinal anesthesia for surgery and continuous epidural analgesia postoperatively. His original technique used separate interspaces for the epidural and spinal techniques.

Subsequently, many have used this technique by placing both needles at the same interspace.[82-84] With this method, an epidural needle is first used to identify the epidural space. A smaller needle is inserted into the subarachnoid space either by directing the spinal needle through the lumen of the epidural needle or through a side lumen. The CSE technique allows flexibility in a number of clinical settings and has become a common anesthetic technique for both labor and cesarean section (Box 11-1).[85]

CSE anesthesia allows one to minimize the intrathecal dose of local anesthetic, thereby reducing the impact on maternal blood pressure. As compared with conventional epidural anesthesia for cesarean section, CSE anesthesia is associated with a more rapid onset of surgical anesthesia, less intraoperative pain and discomfort, better muscle relaxation, less shivering, and less vomiting.[86]

During labor, CSE analgesia is associated with a faster onset of pain relief, fewer requests for supplementation of analgesia, less motor blockade, and increased maternal satisfaction than conventional epidural analgesia.[87] Some studies suggest that CSE analgesia results in a decreased incidence of instrumental vaginal delivery, although this is a matter of some dispute (see Chapter 21, Section III).[88,89]

Potential problems of the CSE technique include the inability to reliably test the epidural catheter for proper placement and the enhanced spread of previously injected spinal drug following the epidural injection of local anesthetic.[90]

Inadequate Anesthesia

During labor, inadequate epidural anesthesia usually results from failure to identify the epidural space correctly or from malposition of the catheter within the epidural space. A unilateral block may occur despite the use of good technique. Sometimes the anesthesiologist can correct the problem by withdrawing the catheter 1 to 2 cm, thereby changing the position of the catheter tip within the epidural space. Unilateral block can often be prevented by limiting the length of catheter within the epidural space to 3 cm or less. The problem with limited insertion of the catheter is that, in some patients, the catheter tends to migrate outward over time (patients undergoing surgery remain still; by contrast, laboring women change position frequently). Obese women seem to be at increased risk for outward migration of the catheter tip. Prospective studies suggest that 4 to 6 cm is the optimal depth of epidural catheter insertion in laboring women.[91-93]

In some cases, partial withdrawal of the catheter does not solve the problem of unilateral block. Gielen et al.[94] performed a radiologic study in which they observed no consistent relationship between catheter position and the asymmetric onset of sympathetic blockade. Sometimes the unilateral block may result from midline obstruction in the epidural space (e.g., dorsomedian connective tissue band).[95] In these cases, it seems preferable to place another catheter at another interspace.

The management of inadequate anesthesia is more problematic during cesarean section. If inadequate *spinal* anesthesia is noted *before* incision, the anesthesiologist may perform a second spinal anesthetic procedure and give additional local anesthetic. Recently some investigators have suggested that failed spinal anesthesia results from the maldistribution of local anesthetic within the subarachnoid space.[96,97] Drasner and Rigler[97] noted that, within the American Society of Anesthesiologists Closed-Claim Database, three cases of cauda equina syndrome complicated spinal anesthesia. In two cases, a "failed spinal" had occurred, followed by a repeat injection of local anesthetic. The authors recommended that anesthesiologists determine the presence of anesthesia in the sacral dermatomes before giving additional local anesthetic into the subarachnoid space. They stated the following[77]:

> If CSF [was] aspirated following anesthetic injection, it should be assumed that the local anesthetic [was] delivered into the subarachnoid space; total anesthetic dosage should be limited to the maximum dose a clinician would consider reasonable to administer in a single injection. If an injection is repeated, the technique should be modified to avoid reinforcing the same restricted distribution (e.g., alter the patient's position, use an anesthetic with a different baricity, or straighten the lumbosacral curvature).

If the patient complains of pain *after* incision, the anesthesiologist must decide between the administration of inhalation or intravenous analgesia versus general anesthesia. Supplemental analgesia may be provided by giving 40% nitrous oxide in oxygen or small incremental boluses of ketamine (0.1 to 0.25 mg/kg). Supplemental infiltration with local anesthetic is sometimes helpful, especially when spinal anesthesia regresses near the end of an unexpectedly long operation. The anesthesiologist must ensure that the patient remains sufficiently alert to protect the airway. In most cases, severe pain unrelieved by modest doses of analgesia requires rapid-sequence induction of general anesthesia, followed by endotracheal intubation.

In some cases, inadequate *epidural* anesthesia results from failure to give a sufficient dose of local anesthetic or failure to wait a sufficient length of time after administration. For example, if 0.5% bupivacaine is given epidurally, approximately 20 minutes must pass to achieve an adequate *level* of anesthesia, and additional local anesthetic may be needed to achieve an adequate *density* of blockade. In urgent cases or in cases with a "missed" segment, local infiltration with a local anesthetic often results in satisfactory anesthe-

---

Box 11-1 POSSIBLE ADVANTAGES OF THE COMBINED SPINAL AND EPIDURAL ANESTHETIC TECHNIQUE

- Initial epidural needle placement allows the spinal needle to be guided near the dura, thereby minimizing the number of times the spinal needle tip hits bone, which dulls the needle.
- The combined technique results in lower maternal, fetal, and neonatal blood concentrations of local anesthetic than does epidural anesthesia alone.
- The rapid onset of spinal anesthesia allows surgical anesthesia to be established more rapidly than does epidural anesthesia alone.
- The combined technique is less likely to result in inadequate anesthesia than either technique alone. If the initial subarachnoid dose is inadequate, a higher sensory level can be achieved by giving additional local anesthetic through the epidural catheter. This allows the anesthesiologist to give a conservative subarachnoid dose of local anesthetic, and it may decrease the incidence of high spinal anesthesia.
- A small dose of opioid—with or without a small dose of local anesthetic—can be given to establish analgesia during early labor. Subsequently, local anesthetic—with or without an opioid—can be administered through the epidural catheter.
- For cases in which the obstetrician plans a trial of forceps, low spinal anesthesia can be established for forceps delivery. If the trial of forceps fails, additional local anesthetic can be administered through the epidural catheter, and anesthesia can be extended for cesarean section.

sia. Sometimes it is difficult to separate the beneficial effect of the local infiltration from the beneficial effect of waiting for the obstetrician to obtain, prepare, and inject the local anesthetic solution. Finally, the anesthesiologist should exercise caution when giving spinal anesthesia after failed epidural anesthesia because of an apparent increase in the incidence of high spinal anesthesia in this circumstance. Presumably the large volume of local anesthetic within the epidural space results in decreased volume in the lumbar subarachnoid space, which predisposes the patient to high spinal anesthesia.

COMPLICATIONS OF NEEDLE OR CATHETER PLACEMENT

During planned spinal anesthesia, Mihic[98] demonstrated that splitting rather than cutting the longitudinally directed dural fibers results in a lower incidence of postdural puncture headache (Figure 11-17). The author did not specify the type of needle he used, but it is likely that he used a cutting-bevel needle. It now seems clear that the use of a non-cutting-bevel needle decreases the incidence of postdural puncture headache.[58,59] Some anesthesiologists have also suggested that the paramedian approach results in a decreased incidence of this complication as compared with the midline approach.[99,100]

Enforced bed rest does not decrease the incidence or severity of postdural puncture headache.[81] At least one study has suggested that early ambulation decreases the severity of headache as compared with 24 hours of bed rest after the procedure.[101]

Unfortunately, postdural puncture headache remains a problem after unintentional dural puncture during planned epidural anesthesia. In residency training programs, the incidence of unintentional dural puncture is approximately 2% to 3%. Given the popularity of non-cutting needles for spinal anesthesia, the incidence of postdural puncture headache may be greater with planned epidural anesthesia than with spinal anesthesia. When a 17- or 18-gauge epidural needle results in unintentional dural puncture, the subsequent incidence of postdural puncture headache is as great as 70% to 80%. Techniques to minimize the incidence of unintentional dural puncture include the following: (1) identification of the liga-

mentum flavum before seeking the loss of resistance; (2) understanding the likely depth of the epidural space in an individual patient; (3) advancement of the needle between contractions when unexpected patient movement is less likely; and (4) adequate control of the needle-syringe assembly during advancement of the needle. Norris et al.[102] observed that unintentional dural puncture is less likely to result in headache if the epidural needle bevel is parallel to the longitudinal direction of the dural fibers. With this technique, the needle bevel must be rotated 90 degrees before catheter insertion. Some anesthesiologists prefer to avoid rotation of the needle within the epidural space; they fear that rotation of the sharp epidural needle will "core" a hole in the dura. Meiklejohn[103] performed a study using postmortem dura mater and demonstrated that "rotation of the epidural needle significantly decreased the force required to puncture the dura." By contrast, Huffnagle et al.[104] noted that careful cephalad rotation of the epidural needle bevel does not increase the risk of dural puncture. Nonetheless, we prefer to insert the epidural needle with the bevel oriented in a cephalad direction so that there is no need to rotate the needle bevel within the epidural space. (Insertion of the epidural catheter through a needle oriented in the cephalad direction increases the likelihood of success of epidural anesthesia.[104])

The management of unintentional dural puncture depends on the clinical setting. One option is to place the epidural catheter within the subarachnoid space and use a continuous spinal anesthetic technique. Norris and Leighton[105] have shown that insertion of a subarachnoid catheter and administration of continuous spinal anesthesia do not result in an increased incidence of headache as compared with withdrawal of the needle and administration of epidural anesthesia using an adjacent interspace.

Another option is to withdraw the epidural needle and identify the epidural space at another interspace. In such cases, anesthesiologists must be wary of an unexpected high level of anesthesia after administration of usual doses of local anesthetic.[106,107] Leach and Smith[107] reported a patient who had extensive block after unintentional dural puncture and subsequent epidural injection of bupivacaine. They presented radiologic evidence of the spread of local anesthetic from the epidural to the subarachnoid space, and they stated the following[107]:

> That such transarachnoid spread can occur at first seems unlikely because of the pressure gradient which causes CSF to leak outward into the epidural space.... In patients with low compliance, epidural pressure during injection, especially when large volumes of solution are used and during regular uterine contractions, may briefly exceed CSF pressure and allow such transarachnoid flow to occur.

Epidural Test Dose

The purpose of the test dose is to help recognize unintentional cannulation of a vein or the subarachnoid space. Pregnant women are at increased risk for unintentional intravenous cannulation. The test dose should contain a dose of local anesthetic and/or another marker sufficient to allow the recognition of intravenous or subarachnoid injection but not so large as to cause systemic toxicity or total spinal anesthesia.[108,109] Most anesthesiologists give a test dose that includes 15 μg of epinephrine, as recommended by Moore and Batra.[110] Those authors observed that the intravenous injection of 15 μg of epinephrine consistently causes a transient increase in heart

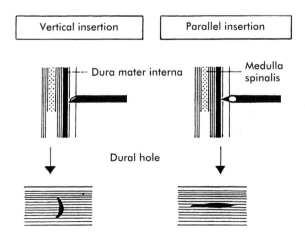

FIGURE 11-17. Types of needle insertion. The bevel of the spinal needle is inserted through the dura perpendicular (*left*) instead of parallel to the long axis of the vertebral column. (From Mihic DN. Postspinal headache and the relationship of the needle bevel to the longitudinal dural fibers. Reg Anesth 1985; 10:76-81.)

rate during the first minute after injection in nonpregnant subjects. Some anesthesiologists fear that intravenous injection of epinephrine may decrease uteroplacental perfusion and precipitate fetal distress.[111-113] Others have noted that a cyclic change in maternal heart rate during labor complicates interpretation of the test dose.[114,115] For this reason, the test dose should be given immediately after a uterine contraction so that there is no need to distinguish between tachycardia as a result of pain versus tachycardia as a result of the intravenous injection of epinephrine.[116]

Rebuttal of criticisms of the epinephrine-containing test dose includes the following arguments. First, the changes in uterine blood flow after intravenous injection of epinephrine in pregnant laboratory animals were transient[111,112]; similar transient declines in perfusion undoubtedly occur during normal uterine contractions. Second, the adverse maternal and fetal consequences of intravenous injection of a large therapeutic dose of local anesthetic would likely be more severe. Third, there has been no report of adverse neonatal outcome after intravenous injection of an epinephrine-containing test dose. Mulroy and Glosten[117] wrote a detailed review of the epinephrine-containing test dose in obstetric patients. (Box 11-2 lists test-dose options for the recognition of intravenous injection of a local anesthetic.)

Chadwick et al.[133] searched the American Society of Anesthesiologists Closed-Claim Database and identified that convulsions are a more common reason for malpractice litigation in obstetric anesthesia than in other types of anesthesia. Among the claims involving obstetric patients, 83% of convulsions during regional anesthesia resulted in neurologic injury or death to the mother, newborn, or both. There was no evidence that an epinephrine-containing test dose was given in any of these cases (see Chapter 29).

Some anesthesiologists do not give adequate attention to the exclusion of unintentional subarachnoid injection of local anesthetic. Subarachnoid injection of 30 to 45 mg of lidocaine or 12.5 to 15 mg of bupivacaine is likely to produce objective evidence of spinal anesthesia within 5 minutes.[108,109,134] However, the anesthesiologist must take the time to look for evidence of spinal anesthesia. Clinicians often do not wait a sufficient length of time or perform the necessary assessment to exclude unintentional subarachnoid injection. It is inadequate to ask the patient whether she can wiggle her toes.

Rather, anesthesiologists should wait at least 3—if not 5—minutes before excluding objective evidence of either sensory or motor blockade.

Finally, every anesthesiologist should remember that no test-dose regimen will exclude every case of unintentional intravenous or subarachnoid injection.[117,135] (Editor's note: Box 11-3 summarizes the editor's approach to avoiding complications of intravenous or subarachnoid injection of local anesthetic.)

Resuscitation of the Obstetric Patient

Intravenous, spinal, or epidural injection of local anesthetic may rarely precipitate maternal cardiac arrest. If this event occurs before delivery, left uterine displacement must be maintained and aortocaval compression avoided during maternal resuscitation. Initially, the ABCs of resuscitation are important. These include the following: (1) the establishment and protection of the patient's airway; (2) the provision of adequate ventilation; and (3) the restoration and maintenance of circulation. The American Heart Association (AHA)[136] has reviewed cardiopulmonary resuscitation in pregnant women. The AHA noted that, if ventricular fibrillation is present, it should be treated with defibrillation according to the standard algorithm. The AHA also noted that standard pharmacologic therapy (e.g., epinephrine, norepinephrine, dopamine) should be used without modification. If initial resuscitative efforts are unsuccessful, the obstetrician should deliver the infant immediately (i.e., within 4 to 5 minutes of the cardiac arrest). Rapid delivery may save the infant's life, and evacuation of the uterus may facilitate resuscitation of the mother.[136-138] According to the AHA, "While the optimum interval from arrest to delivery is within 5 minutes, there are case reports of intact infant survival after more than 20 minutes of complete maternal arrest."[136,137,139]

Equipment Problems

The frequency of major equipment malfunction is very low during the administration of regional anesthesia. Most anesthesiologists in the United States use disposable needles, and the plastic needle hubs are attached to the needles' shafts with epoxy. However, some disposable needles have a metal hub, and, rarely, the needle may break at the hub-shaft junction.[140] If the needle should break, the portion of the needle that remains in the patient should be removed, because it may migrate and cause injury.[141]

Box 11-2 TEST-DOSE REGIMENS DESIGNED TO RECOGNIZE UNINTENTIONAL INTRAVASCULAR INJECTION OF LOCAL ANESTHETIC

CHANGE IN HEART RATE AND/OR BLOOD PRESSURE

Epinephrine[108-110,116-118]
Isoproterenol[119-122]
Ephedrine[123,124]

SUBJECTIVE SYMPTOMS

Local anesthetic alone
    2-Chloroprocaine[125-127]
    Lidocaine[128]
    Bupivacaine[126]
Fentanyl[129,130]

DOPPLER CHANGES

Air[131,132]

Box 11-3 STEPS TO AVOID COMPLICATIONS OF UNINTENTIONAL INTRAVENOUS OR SUBARACHNOID INJECTION OF LOCAL ANESTHETIC

1. Lower the catheter below the site of insertion and observe for the passive return of blood or cerebrospinal fluid through the catheter.
2. Aspirate before injecting each dose of local anesthetic.
3. Give the test dose *after* a uterine contraction.
4. Use dilute solutions of local anesthetic during labor.
5. Do not inject more than 5 mL of local anesthetic as a single bolus.
6. Maintain verbal contact with the patient.
7. If little or no block is produced after the injection of an appropriate dose of local anesthetic, assume that the local anesthetic was injected intravenously, and remove the catheter.

It is possible to shear off an epidural or spinal catheter any time that it is withdrawn through a needle; thus an epidural or spinal catheter should never be withdrawn in this manner. It is also possible to break a catheter during attempted removal. The 18- and 20-gauge catheters used for epidural anesthesia rarely break. If resistance to catheter removal is encountered, the patient should assume a position that reduces lumbar lordosis, because this often lessens the kinking of the catheter between perivertebral structures. Once the catheter has been removed successfully, it should be examined to ensure that it has been removed completely. The anesthesiologist should document in the medical record that the catheter was removed intact.

Some problems with the breakage of spinal microcatheters have occurred.[142] These catheters most often break during attempts at removal. The tensile strength of many of the small-bore microcatheters is one third to one half of that found in a typical epidural catheter.[143] We favor aggressive attempts to remove broken *spinal* catheters. However, it may be unnecessary to remove broken *epidural* catheters; rather, in these circumstances, the patient can be informed of the complication and observed over time. The incidence of catheter migration or other delayed sequelae appears to be low. Computed tomography may help identify the precise location of a broken catheter, if necessary.[144]

KEY POINTS

- Accentuation of lumbar lordosis during pregnancy may complicate attempts to use the midline approach to identify the epidural or subarachnoid space in pregnant women.
- The midline approach is faster and less painful than the paramedian approach to the epidural or subarachnoid space. However, the paramedian approach allows for the successful identification of the subarachnoid or epidural space in difficult cases.
- Anesthesiologists must identify the ligamentum flavum if they want to identify the epidural space quickly and consistently.
- When using the loss-of-resistance technique, the anesthesiologist must ensure that the syringe plunger does not stick.
- Use of a non-cutting-bevel spinal needle reduces the incidence of postdural puncture headache.
- No epidural test dose will exclude every case of unintentional intravenous or subarachnoid injection. However, appropriate use of the epinephrine-containing test dose is safe and likely excludes most cases of unintentional intravenous cannulation. Anesthesiologists should give equal attention to the exclusion of the unintentional subarachnoid injection of local anesthetic.
- Aortocaval compression hastens the onset of cardiovascular collapse during high/total spinal anesthesia. Evacuation of the uterus (i.e., delivery of the infant) may facilitate resuscitation of the mother.

REFERENCES

1. Hawkins JL, Gibbs CP, Orleans M, et al. Obstetric anesthesia work force survey, 1981 versus 1992. Anesthesiology 1997; 8:135-43.
2. Buckin BA, Hawkins JL, Anderson JR. Obstetric anesthesia workforce survey: Preliminary work (abstract). Proceedings of the Annual Meeting of the American Society of Anesthesiologists. San Francisco, October, 2003: A-1182.
3. Hogan QH, Prost R, Kulier A, et al. Magnetic resonance imaging of cerebrospinal fluid volume and the influence of body habitus and abdominal pressure. Anesthesiology 1996; 84:1341-9.
4. Richardson MG, Thakur R, Abramowicz JS, Wissler RN. Maternal posture influences the extent of sensory block produced by intrathecal dextrose-free bupivacaine with fentanyl for labor analgesia. Anesth Analg 1996; 83:1229-33.
5. Cunningham FG, MacDonald PC, Gant NF. Williams Obstetrics. 18th ed. Norwalk, Conn, Appleton & Lange, 1989:157.
6. Hirabayashi Y, Shimizu R, Fukuda H, et al. Anatomical configuration of the spinal column in the supine position. II. Comparison of pregnant and non-pregnant women. Br J Anaesth 1995; 75:6-8.
7. Brown DL. Spinal, epidural, and caudal anesthesia. In: Miller RD, editor. Anesthesia. 4th ed. New York, Churchill Livingstone, 1994:1505-33.
8. Hogan QH. Reexamination of anatomy in regional anesthesia. In: Brown DL, editor. Regional Anesthesia and Analgesia. Philadelphia, W.B. Saunders, 1996:50-83.
9. Hogan QH. Epidural anatomy examined by cryomicrotome section. Reg Anesth 1996; 21:395-406.
10. Savolaine ER, Pandya JB, Greenblatt SH, Conover SR. Anatomy of the human lumbar epidural space: New insights using CT-epidurography. Anesthesiology 1988; 68:217-20.
11. Santos DJ, Bridenbaugh PO, Heins S, Pai U. Unilateral epidural analgesia for labor. Regional Anesth 1985; 10:41A.
12. Hogan QH. Lumbar epidural anatomy: A new look by cryomicrotome section. Anesthesiology 1991; 75:767-75.
13. Zarzur E. Anatomic studies of the human lumbar ligamentum flavum. Anesth Analg 1984; 63:499-502.
14. Harrison GR, Clowes NWB. The depth of the lumbar epidural space from the skin. Anaesthesia 1985; 40:685-7.
15. Bromage PR. Epidural Analgesia. Philadelphia, W.B. Saunders, 1978.
16. Reynolds AF, Roberts PA, Pollay M, Stratemeier PH. Quantitative anatomy of the thoracolumbar epidural space. Neurosurgery 1985; 17:905-7.
17. Cousins MJ, Bromage PR. Epidural neural blockade. In: Cousins MJ, Bridenbaugh PO, editors. Neural Blockade in Clinical Anesthesia and Management of Pain. Philadelphia, J.B. Lippincott, 1988:255.
18. Thompson JE. An anatomical and experimental study of sacral anesthesia. Ann Surg 1917; 66:718-27.
19. Trotter M. Variations of the sacral canal: Their significance in the administration of caudal anesthesia. Anesth Analg 1947; 26:192-202.
20. Marx GF. Aortocaval compression: Incidence and prevention. Bull NY Acad Med 1974; 50:443-6.
21. Bieniarz J, Crottogini JJ, Curuchet E, et al. Aortocaval compression by the uterus in late human pregnancy. Am J Obstet Gynecol 1978; 100:203-17.
22. Moller RA, Datta S, Fox J, et al. Effects of progesterone on the cardiac electrophysiologic action of bupivacaine and lidocaine. Anesthesiology 1992; 76:604-8.
23. Datta S, Hurley RJ, Naulty JS, et al. Plasma and cerebrospinal fluid progesterone concentrations in pregnant and nonpregnant women. Anesth Analg 1986; 65:950-4.
24. Greene NM. Physiology of Spinal Anesthesia. 3rd ed. Baltimore, Williams & Wilkins, 1981.
25. Burm AGL, van Kleef JW, Gladines MPRR, et al. Spinal anesthesia with hyperbaric lidocaine and bupivacaine: Effects of epinephrine on the plasma concentration profiles. Anesth Analg 1987; 66:1104-8.
26. Fink BR. Mechanisms of differential axial blockade in epidural and subarachnoid anesthesia. Anesthesiology 1989; 70:851-8.
27. Heit JA, Horlocker TT, editors. Neuraxial Anesthesia and Anticoagulation. Reg Anesth Pain Med 1998; 23(Suppl 2):129-93.
28. Vincent RD, Chestnut DH. Which position is more comfortable for the parturient during identification of the epidural space? Int J Obstet Anesth 1991; 1:9-11.
29. Andrews PJD, Ackerman WE, Juneja MM. Aortocaval compression in the sitting and lateral decubitus positions during extradural catheter placement in the parturient. Can J Anaesth 1993; 40:320-4.
30. Bamberger PD, Birnbach DJ. Lumbar epidural anesthesia initiated in the knee-chest position. Regional Anesth 1991; 16:240-1.
31. Norris MC, Dewan DM. Effect of gravity on the spread of extradural anaesthesia for caesarean section. Br J Anaesth 1987; 59:338-41.

32. Norris MC, Leighton BL, DeSimone CA, Larijani GE. Lateral position and epidural anesthesia for cesarean section. Anesth Analg 1988; 67: 788-90.

33. Reid JA, Thorburn J. Extradural bupivacaine or lignocaine anaesthesia for elective caesarean section: The role of maternal posture. Br J Anaesth 1988; 61:149-53.

34. Khaw KS, Kee WDN, Wong M, et al. Spinal ropivacaine for cesarean delivery: A comparison of hyperbaric and plain solutions. Anesth Analg 2002; 94:680-5.

35. Pollock J, Neal J, Stephenson C, et al. Prospective study of the incidence of transient radicular irritation in patients undergoing spinal anesthesia. Anesthesiology 1996; 84:1361-7.

36. Moore DC, Chadwick HS, Ready LB. Epinephrine prolongs lidocaine spinal: Pain in the operative site the most accurate method of determining local anesthetic duration. Anesthesiology 1987; 67:416-8.

37. Carpenter RL, Caplan RA, Brown DL, et al. Incidence and risk factors for side effects of spinal anesthesia. Anesthesiology 1992; 76:906-16.

38. Caldwell C, Neilsen C, Baltz T, et al. Comparison of high-dose epinephrine and phenylephrine in spinal anesthesia with tetracaine. Anesthesiology 1985; 62:804-7.

39. Kennedy WF Jr, Bonica JJ, Ward RJ, et al. Cardiorespiratory effects of epinephrine when used in regional anesthesia. Acta Anaesth Scand (Suppl) 1966; 23:320-33.

40. Bahar M, Cole G, Rosen M, Vickers MD. Histopathology of the spinal cord after intrathecal cocaine, bupivacaine, lignocaine, and adrenaline in the rat. Eur J Anesthesiol 1984; 1:293-7.

41. Abouleish EI. Epinephrine improves quality of spinal anesthesia of bupivacaine (abstract). Anesthesiology 1986; 65:A375.

42. McDonald SB, Lui SS, Kopacs DJ, Stephensen CA. Hyperbaric spinal ropivacaine: A comparison to bupivacaine in volunteers. Anesthesiology 1999; 90:971-7.

43. Gauthier P, DeKock M, Van Steenberge AM, et al. Intrathecal ropivacaine for ambulatory surgery: A comparison between intrathecal bupivacaine and intrathecal ropivacaine for knee arthroscopy. Anesthesiology 1999; 91:1239-45.

44. Alley EA, Kopacz DJ, McDonald SB, Liu SS. Hyperbaric spinal levobupivacaine: A comparison to racemic bupivacaine in volunteers. Anesth Analg 2002; 94:188-93.

45. Lyons G, Reynolds F. Toxicity and safety of epidural local anesthetics. Int J Obstet Anesth 2001; 10:259-62.

46. Polley LS, Columb MO, Naughton NN, et al. Relative analgesic potencies of ropivacaine and bupivacaine for epidural analgesia in labor: Implications for therapeutic indexes. Anesthesiology 1999; 90:944-50.

47. Chua NP, Sia AT, Ocampo CE. Parturient controlled epidural analgesia during labour: Bupivacaine vs ropivacaine. Anaesthesia 2001; 56:1169-73.

48. Owen MD, Thomas JA, Smith T et al. Ropivacaine 0.075% and bupivacaine 0.075% with fentanyl 2 µg/ml are equivalent for labor analgesia. Anesth Analg 2002; 94:179-83.

49. Vercauteren MP, Hans G, De Decker K, Adriaensen HA. Levobupivacaine combined with sufentanil and epinephrine for intrathecal labor analgesia: A comparison with racemic bupivacaine. Anesth Analg 2001; 93:996-1000.

50. Brown DL, Ransom DM, Hall JA, et al. Regional anesthesia and local anesthetic-induced systemic toxicity: Seizure frequency and accompanying cardiovascular changes. Anesth Analg 1995; 81:321-8.

51. Di Fazio CA, Carron HO, Grosslight KR, et al. Comparison of pH adjusted lidocaine solutions for epidural anesthesia. Anesth Analg 1986; 65:760

52. Lam DTC, Ngan Kee WD, Khaw KS. Extension of epidural blockade in labour for emergency cesarean section using 2% lidocaine with ephedrine and fentanyl, with or without alkalinisation. Anesthesia 2001; 56:777-98.

53. Camann WR, Hartigan PM, Gilbertson LI, et al. Chloroprocaine antagonism of epidural opioid analgesia: A receptor specific phenomenon. Anesthesiology 1990; 73:860.

54. Corke BC, Carlson CG, Dettbarn WD. The influence of 2-chloroprocaine on the subsequent analgesic potency of bupivacaine. Anesthesiology 1984; 60:25.

55. Reisner LS, Hochman BN, Plumer MH. Persistent neurologic deficit and adhesive arachnoiditis following intrathecal 2-chloroprocaine injection. Anesth Analg 1980; 59:452.

56. Fibuch EE, Opper SE. Back pain following epidurally administered Nesacaine-MPF. Anesth Analg 1989; 69:113.

57. Benson JS. FDA Safety Alert: Cauda equina syndrome associated with use of small-bore catheters in continuous spinal anesthesia. Rockville, Md, Food and Drug Administration, May 29, 1992.

58. Snyder GE, Person DL, Flor CE, Wilden RT. Headache in obstetrical patients: Comparison of Whitacre needle versus Quincke needle (abstract). Anesthesiology 1989; 71:A860.

59. Ross BK, Chadwick HS, Mancuso JJ, Benedetti C. Sprotte needle for obstetric anesthesia: Decreased incidence of post dural puncture headache. Reg Anesth 1992; 17:29-33.

60. Shutt LE, Valentine SJ, Wee MYK, et al. Spinal anaesthesia for caesarean section: Comparison of 22-gauge and 25-gauge Whitacre needles with 26-gauge Quincke needles. Br J Anaesth 1992; 69:589-94.

61. Reina MA, de Leon-Casasola OA, Lopez A, et al. An in vitro study of dural lesions produced by 25-gauge Quincke and Whitacre needles evaluated by scanning electron microscopy. Reg Anesth 2000; 25: 393-402.

62. Leiman BC, Katz J, Salzarulo H, et al. A comparison of different methods of lubrication of glass syringes used to identify the epidural space. Anaesthesia 1988; 43:397-8.

63. Saberski LR, Kondamuri S, Osinubi OYO. Identification of the epidural space: Is loss of resistance to air a safe technique? Reg Anesth 1997; 22:3-15.

64. Scott DB: Identification of epidural space: Loss of resistance to air or saline? (editorial). Reg Anesth 1997; 22:1-2.

65. Shenouda PE, Cunningham BJ. Assessing the superiority of saline versus air for use in the epidural loss of resistance technique: A literature review. Reg Anesth Pain Med 2003; 28:48-53.

66. Zarzur E. Genesis of "true" negative pressure in the lumbar epidural space: A new hypothesis. Anaesthesia 1984; 39:1101-4.

67. Verniquet AJW. Vessel puncture with epidural catheters. Anaesthesia 1980; 35:660-2.

68. Ahn NN, Ung DA, DeFay S, et al. Blood vessel puncture with epidural catheters (abstract). Anesthesiology 1989; 71:A916.

69. Mannion D, Walker R, Clayton K. Extradural vein puncture: An avoidable complication. Anaesthesia 1991; 46:585-7.

70. Rolbin SH, Halpern SH, Braude BM, et al. Fluid through the epidural needle does not reduce complications of epidural catheter insertion. Can J Anaesth 1990; 37:337-40.

71. Ward CF, Osborne R, Benumof JL, Saidman LJ. A hazard of double-orifice epidural catheters. Anesthesiology 1978; 48:362-4.

72. Beck H, Brassow F, Doehn M, et al. Epidural catheters of the multi-orifice type: Dangers and complications. Acta Anaesthesiol Scand 1986; 30:549-55.

73. Power I, Thorburn J. Differential flow from multihole epidural catheters. Anaesthesia 1988; 43:876-8.

74. Michael S, Richmond MN, Birks RJS. A comparison between open-end (single hole) and closed-end (three lateral holes) epidural catheters: Complications and quality of sensory blockade. Anaesthesia 1989; 44:578-80.

75. Morrison LMM, Buchan AS. Comparison of complications associated with single-holed and multi-holed extradural catheters. Br J Anaesth 1990; 64:183-5.

76. D'Angelo R, Foss ML, Livesay CH. A comparison of multiport and uniport epidural catheters in laboring patients. Anesth Analg 1997; 84:1276-9.

77. Hamilton CL, Riley ET, Cohen SE. Changes in the position of epidural catheters associated with patient movement. Anesthesiology 1997; 86:778-84.

78. Abouleish E, Amortegui AJ, Taylor FH. Are bacterial filters needed in continuous epidural analgesia for obstetrics? Anesthesiology 1977; 46:351-4.

79. Abouleish E, Amortegui AJ. Millipore filters are not necessary for epidural block. Anesthesiology 1981; 55:604.

80. Charlton GA, Lawes EG. The effect of micropore filters on the aspiration test in epidural analgesia. Anaesthesia 1991; 46:573-5.

81. Brownridge P. Epidural and subarachnoid analgesia for elective caesarean section (letter). Anesthesia 1981; 36:70.

82. Dennsion B. Combined subarachnoid and epidural block for caesarean section. Can Anaesth Soc J 1987; 34:105-7.

83. Rawal N, Schollin J, Wesström G. Epidural versus combined spinal epidural block for cesarean section. Acta Anaesth Scand 1988; 32:61-6.

84. Carrie LES. Epidural versus combined spinal epidural block for caesarean section. Acta Anaesth Scand 1988; 32:595-6.

85. Eisenach JC. Combined spinal-epidural analgesia in obstetrics. Anesthesiology 1999; 91:299-302.

86. Choi DH, Kim JA, Chung IS. Comparison of combined spinal epidural anesthesia and epidural anesthesia for cesarean section. Acta Anesthesiol Scand 2000; 44:214-9.

87. Collis RE, Davies DW, Aveling W. Randomised comparison of combined spinal-epidural and standard epidural analgesia in labour. Lancet 1995; 345:1413-6.

88. Nageotte MP, Larson D, Rumney PJ, Sidhu M, Hollenbach K. Epidural analgesia compared with combined spinal epidural analgesia during labor in nulliparous women. N Engl J Med 1997; 337:1715-9.

89. Comparative Obstetric Mobile Epidural Trial (COMET) Study Group UK. Effect of low dose mobile versus traditional techniques on mode of delivery. Lancet 2001; 358:19-23.

90. Blumgart CH, Ryall D, Dennison B, et al. Mechanism of extension of spinal anesthesia by extradural injection of local anesthetic. Br J Anesth 1992; 69:457.

91. Beilin Y, Bernstein HH, Zucker-Pinchoff B. The optimal distance that a multiorifice epidural catheter should be threaded into the epidural space. Anesth Analg 1995; 81:301-4.

92. D'Angelo R, Berkebile BL, Gernacher JC. Prospective examination of epidural catheter insertion. Anesthesiology 1996; 84:88-93.

93. Hamilton CL, Riley ET, Cohen SE. Changes in the position of epidural catheters associated with patient movement. Anesthesiology 1997; 86:778-84.

94. Gielen MJM, Slappendel R, Merx JL. Asymmetric onset of sympathetic blockade in epidural anaesthesia shows no relation to epidural catheter position. Acta Anaesthesiol Scand 1991; 35:81-4.

95. Narang VPS, Linter SPK. Failure of extradural blockade in obstetrics. Br J Anaesth 1988; 60:402-4.

96. Rigler ML, Drasner K. Distribution of catheter-injected local anesthetic in a model of the subarachnoid space. Anesthesiology 1991; 75:684-92.

97. Drasner K, Rigler ML. Repeat injection after a "failed spinal": At times, a potentially unsafe practice (letter). Anesthesiology 1991; 75:713-4.

98. Mihic DN. Postspinal headache and the relationship of the needle bevel to the longitudinal dural fibers. Reg Anesth 1985; 10:76-81.

99. Hatfalvi BI. The dynamics of postspinal headache. Headache 1977; 17:64-7.

100. Ready LB, Cuplin S, Haschke RH, Nessley M. Spinal needle determinants of rate of transdural fluid leak. Anesth Analg 1989; 69:457-60.

101. Thornberry EA, Thomas TA. Posture and post-spinal headache. Br J Anaesth 1988; 60:195-7.

102. Norris MC, Leighton BC, DeSimone CA. Needle bevel direction and headache after inadvertent dural puncture. Anesthesiology 1989; 70:729-31.

103. Meiklejohn BH. The effect of rotation of an epidural needle: An in vitro study. Anaesthesia 1987; 42:1180-2.

104. Huffnagle SL, Norris MC, Arkoosh VA, et al. The influence of epidural needle bevel orientation on spread of sensory blockade in the laboring parturient. Anesth Analg 1998; 87:326-30.

105. Norris MC, Leighton BL. Continuous spinal anesthesia after unintentional dural puncture in parturients. Reg Anesth 1990; 15:285-7.

106. Hodgkinson R. Total spinal block after epidural injection into an interspace adjacent to an inadvertent dural perforation. Anesthesiology 1981; 55:593-5.

107. Leach A, Smith GB. Subarachnoid spread of epidural local anaesthetic following dural puncture. Anaesthesia 1988; 43:671-4.

108. Abraham RA, Harris AP, Maxwell LG, Kaplow S. The efficacy of 1.5% lidocaine with 7.5% dextrose and epinephrine as an epidural test dose for obstetrics. Anesthesiology 1986; 64:116-9.

109. Van Zundert AA, Vaes LE, Soetens M, et al. Every dose given in epidural analgesia for vaginal anesthesia can be a test dose. Anesthesiology 1987; 67:436-40.

110. Moore DC, Batra MS. The components of an effective dose prior to epidural block. Anesthesiology 1981; 55:693-6.

111. Hood DD, Dewan DM, James FM. Maternal and fetal effects of epinephrine in gravid ewes. Anesthesiology 1986; 64:610-3.

112. Chestnut DH, Weiner CP, Martin JG, et al. Effect of intravenous epinephrine upon uterine artery blood flow velocity in the pregnant guinea pig. Anesthesiology 1986; 65:633-6.

113. Leighton BL, Norris MC, Sosis M, et al. Limitations of epinephrine as a marker of intravascular injection in laboring women. Anesthesiology 1987; 66:688-91.

114. Cartwright PD, McCarroll SM, Antzaka C. Maternal heart rate changes with a plain epidural test dose. Anesthesiology 1986; 65:226-8.

115. Chestnut DH, Owen CL, Brown CK, et al. Does labor affect the variability of maternal heart rate during induction of epidural anesthesia? Anesthesiology 1988; 68:622-5.

116. Chadwick HS, Benedetti C, Ready LB, Williams V. Epinephrine-containing test doses: Don't throw the baby out with the bath water (letter). Anesthesiology 1987; 66:571.

117. Mulroy M, Glosten B. The epinephrine test dose in obstetrics: Note the limitations (editorial). Anesth Analg 1998; 86:923-5.

118. Colonna-Romano P, Nagaraj L. Tests to evaluate intravenous placement of epidural catheters in laboring women: A prospective clinical study. Anesth Analg 1998; 86:985-8.

119. Leighton BL, DeSimone CA, Norris MC, Chayen B. Isoproterenol is an effective marker of intravenous injection in laboring women. Anesthesiology 1989; 71:206-9.

120. Marcus MAE, Vertommen JD, Van Aken H, Wouters PF. Hemodynamic effects of intravenous isoproterenol versus epinephrine in the chronic maternal-fetal sheep preparation. Anesth Analg 1996; 82:1023-6.

121. Marcus MAE, Vertommen JD, Van Aken H, et al. Hemodynamic effects of intravenous isoproterenol versus saline in the parturient. Anesth Analg 1997; 84:1113-6.

122. Marcus MAE, Vertommen JD, Van Aken H, et al. The effects of adding isoproterenol to 0.125% bupivacaine on the quality and duration of epidural analgesia in laboring patients. Anesth Analg 1998; 86:749-52.

123. Fong J, Gadalla F, Fiamengo SA, et al. Ephedrine sulfate as the intravenous component of the epidural analgesia test dose in laboring parturients (abstract). Anesthesiology 1988; 69:A706.

124. Cherala SR, Greene R, Mehta D. Ephedrine as a marker of intravascular injection in laboring parturients. Reg Anesth 1990; 15:15-8.

125. Grice SC, Eisenach JC, Dewan DM, Mandell G. Evaluation of 2-chloroprocaine as an effective intravenous test dose for epidural analgesia (abstract). Anesthesiology 1987; 67:A627.

126. Harrington BE, Neal JM, Mackey DC, Mulroy MF. 2-Chloroprocaine and bupivacaine as indicators of intravascular injection (abstract). Anesthesiology 1988; 69:A357.

127. Rathmell JP, Viscomi CM, Ashikaga T. Detection of intravascular epidural catheters using 2-chloroprocaine. Reg Anesth 1997; 22:113-8.

128. Roetman KJ, Eisenach JC. Evaluation of lidocaine as an intravenous test dose for epidural anesthesia (abstract). Anesthesiology 1988; 69:A669.

129. Freeman AB, Hicks L. Epidural fentanyl as a test dose (letter). Anesth Analg 1989; 68:187-8.

130. Rottman RL, Miller M, Yoshii WY, et al. Fentanyl as an epidural intravascular test dose in obstetrics (abstract). Anesth Analg 1990; 70:S336.

131. Leighton BL, Gross JB. Air: An effective indicator of intravenously located epidural catheters. Anesthesiology 1989; 71:848-51.

132. Leighton BL, Norris MC, DeSimone CA, et al. The air test as a clinically useful indicator of intravenously placed epidural catheters. Anesthesiology 1990; 73:610-3.

133. Chadwick HS, Posner K, Caplan RA, et al. A comparison of obstetric and non-obstetric anesthesia malpractice claims. Anesthesiology 1991; 74:242-9.

134. Prince G, McGregor D. Obstetric epidural test doses: A reappraisal. Anaesthesia 1986; 41:1240-50.

135. McLean BY, Rottman RL, Kotelko DM. Failure of multiple test doses and techniques to detect intravascular migration of an epidural catheter. Anesth Analg 1992; 74:454-6.

136. American Heart Association. Guidelines for cardiopulmonary resuscitation and emergency cardiac care: Special resuscitation situations. JAMA 1992; 268:2242-50.

137. Katz VL, Dotters DJ, Droegemueller W. Perimortem cesarean delivery. Obstet Gynecol 1986; 68:571-6.

138. Strong TH, Lowe RA. Perimortem cesarean section. Am J Emerg Med 1989; 7:489-94.

139. Lopez-Zeno JA, Carlo WA, O'Grady JP, Fanaroff AA. Infant survival following delayed postmortem cesarean delivery. Obstet Gynecol 1990; 76:991-2.

140. Schlake PT, Peleman RR, Winnie AP. Separation of the hub from the shaft of a disposable epidural needle. Anesthesiology 1988; 68:611-3.

141. Moore DC. Complications of Regional Anesthesia. Springfield, Ill, CC Thomas, 1955:242-6.

142. DeVera HV, Ries M. Complication of continuous spinal microcatheters: Should we seek their removal if sheared? (letter). Anesthesiology 1991; 74:794.

143. Ley SJ, Jones BR. Strength of continuous spinal catheters. Anesth Analg 1991; 73:394-6.

144. Moore DC, Artru AA, Kelley WA, Jenkins D. Use of computed tomography to locate a sheared epidural catheter. Anesth Analg 1987; 66:795-6.

Chapter 12
Local Anesthetics

Alan C. Santos, M.D., M.P.H. · Mieczyslaw Finster, M.D.

Local anesthetics are the agents most often used for pain relief in obstetric patients. In the early 1880s, cocaine was the first local anesthetic introduced into clinical practice and it was used for spinal analgesia during labor by 1900. However, the toxicity of the drug was soon apparent, and the potential usefulness of local anesthetics was not appreciated until the early 1900s when procaine, a derivative of para-aminobenzoic acid, was synthesized. The introduction of procaine led the way for the synthesis of other substituted amino-esters, such as tetracaine and 2-chloroprocaine.

In the early 1950s, a new class of drugs became available—amide derivatives of diethylaminoacetic acid. In contrast to the ester-type agents, the formulations of these compounds were more stable and less allergenic. Lidocaine was the first amide local anesthetic introduced into clinical practice. Mepivacaine, prilocaine, bupivacaine, and etidocaine followed.

MOLECULAR STRUCTURE

With the exception of cocaine, all local anesthetic molecules contain a desaturated carbon ring (aromatic portion) and a tertiary amine connected by an intermediate alkyl chain (Figure 12-1). The intermediate alkyl chain, by virtue of its ester or amide linkage, is the basis for the classification of local anesthetics as **amino-esters** (which are hydrolyzed by pseudocholinesterase) and **amino-amides** (which undergo hepatic microsomal metabolism) (Table 12-1). For the **ester-linked** agents, the aromatic ring, which renders the molecule lipid soluble, is a derivative of benzoic acid. For the **amide-linked** agents, the aromatic ring is a homolog of aniline. The tertiary-amine portion acts as a proton acceptor, which makes local anesthetics behave as weak bases. In its quaternary (i.e., "protonated") form, the terminal amine also is the water-soluble portion. The Henderson-Hasselbalch equation predicts the relative proportions of local anesthetic that exist in the ionized versus the unionized form. The higher the pK_B relative to physiologic pH, the smaller the proportion of drug that exists in an unionized form. All amide local anesthetics (with the exception of lidocaine) exist as stereoisomers because of the presence of an asymmetric carbon adjacent to the terminal amine.

Clinical formulations of local anesthetics are prepared as hydrochloride salts to increase their solubility in water. These solutions usually are acidic (i.e., they have a pH of 4 to 6) to enhance formation of the water-soluble quaternary amine.[1] A low pH also prevents oxidation of the epinephrine present in epinephrine-containing solutions.

MODE OF ACTION

At rest, the interior of a nerve cell is negatively charged in relation to its exterior. This resting potential of 60 to 90 mV exists because the concentration of sodium in the extracellular space greatly exceeds that in the intracellular space. The converse is true for potassium. Excitation results in the opening of membrane channels, which allows sodium ions to flow freely down their concentration gradient into the cell interior. Thus the electrical potential within the nerve cell becomes less negative until, at the critical threshold, rapid depolarization occurs. This is necessary for initiating the same sequence of events in adjacent membrane segments and for propagation of the action potential. Thereafter, sodium channels close and the membrane once again becomes impermeable to the influx of sodium. Rather, sodium is removed from the cell by active transport. At the same time, potassium passively accumulates within the resting cell.

Interference with sodium-ion conductance appears to be the mechanism by which local anesthetics reversibly inhibit the propagation of the action potential. Four major theories attempt to explain this effect. The most prominent hypothesis is that the local anesthetic interacts with receptors in the nerve cell membrane, which control channels involved in sodium conductance.[2] There may be more than one site at which local anesthetics bind to sodium-channel receptors (Figure 12-2).[3]

The Meyer-Overton theory offers a second explanation for local anesthetic action. This hypothesis suggests that the lipid-soluble portion of the local anesthetic molecule expands the cell membrane and interferes with rapid sodium conductance. Third, local anesthetics may alter the membrane surface charge, which would inhibit propagation of the action

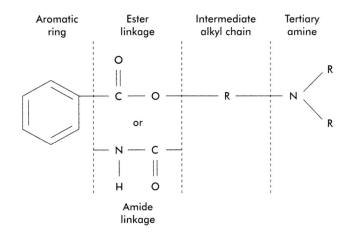

FIGURE 12-1. Structure of a local anesthetic molecule. *R*, Alkyl group. (Modified from Santos AC, Pedersen H. Local anesthetics in obstetrics. In Petrie RH, editor. Perinatal Pharmacology. Cambridge, Mass, Blackwell Scientific Publishing, 1989:373.)

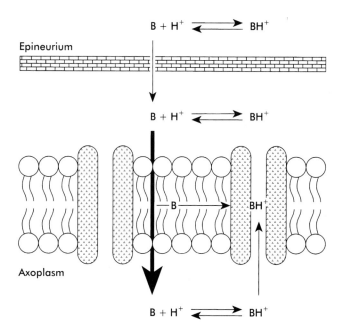

FIGURE 12-2. Local anesthetic access to the sodium channel. The uncharged molecule *(B)* diffuses most easily across the lipid membrane and interacts with the sodium channel at an intramembranous site. The charged molecule *(BH⁺)* gains access to a specific receptor on the sodium channel in the intracellular space. (Modified from Carpenter RL, Mackey DC. Local anesthetics. In Barash PG, Cullen BF, Stoelting RK, editors. Clinical Anesthesia, Philadelphia, Lippincott, 1992:510.)

TABLE 12-1	PHYSICOCHEMICAL CHARACTERISTICS AND FETAL-MATERNAL (F/M) BLOOD CONCENTRATION RATIOS AT DELIVERY FOR COMMONLY USED LOCAL ANESTHETIC AGENTS				
	Molecular weight (base)	pK_B	Lipid solubility*	% Protein bound	F/M
Esters					
2-Chloroprocaine	271	8.9	0.14	—	—
Tetracaine	264	8.6	4.1	—	—
Amides					
Lidocaine	234	7.9	2.9	64	0.5-0.7
Mepivacaine	246	7.8	0.8	78	0.7
Etidocaine	276	7.7	141	94	0.2-0.3
Bupivacaine	288	8.2	28	96	0.2-0.4
Ropivacaine	274	8.0	3	90-95	0.2

*N-heptane/pH = 7.4 buffer.
Modified from Santos AC, Pederson H. Local anesthetics in obstetrics. In Petrie RH, editor. Perinatal Pharmacology. Cambridge, Mass, Blackwell Scientific Publishing, 1989:375.

potential. Fourth, local anesthetics may displace calcium from sites that control sodium conductance.

Both the unionized and ionized forms of a local anesthetic are involved in pharmacologic activity. The base, which is lipid soluble, diffuses through the cell membrane, whereas the charged form is much more active in blocking the sodium channel.

EFFECTS OF PREGNANCY ON THE PHARMACODYNAMICS AND PHARMACOKINETICS OF LOCAL ANESTHETICS

Pharmacodynamics

During administration of spinal or epidural anesthesia, pregnant women typically require smaller doses of local anesthetic than do nonpregnant patients.[4] In the past, this was attributed to an enhanced spread of local anesthetic caused by epidural venous engorgement. However, mechanical effects alone do not account for the observation that the spread of epidural analgesia in early pregnancy is similar to that in pregnant women at term.[4,5] More recent observations support the hypothesis that pregnancy may enhance neuronal sensitivity to local anesthetics. For example, pregnancy increases median nerve susceptibility to lidocaine.[6] In vitro studies demonstrated that the onset of neural blockade was faster and that lower concentrations of bupivacaine were required to block vagal nerve fibers in pregnant rabbits than in nonpregnant rabbits.[7]

Hormonal and biochemical changes may be responsible for the increased susceptibility to neural blockade during pregnancy. For example, one study demonstrated an enhanced effect of bupivacaine in isolated vagus nerve fibers from nonpregnant, ovariectomized rabbits who had received chronic (4 days) but not acute exposure to progesterone.[8] A higher pH, as well as decreased bicarbonate and total carbon dioxide content, have been demonstrated in cerebrospinal fluid (CSF) in patients undergoing elective cesarean section when compared with CSF from age-matched nonpregnant controls. A higher pH increases the proportion of local anesthetic that exists in the base form and facilitates diffusion of the drug across nerve membranes.[5,9]

Pharmacokinetics

Pregnancy is associated with progressive physiologic adaptations that may influence drug disposition (see Chapter 2). However, it is difficult to predict with certainty the effects of pregnancy on the pharmacokinetics of an individual drug.

2-CHLOROPROCAINE

Of the ester-type local anesthetics, only 2-chloroprocaine is used in large doses that may be affected by pregnancy-induced changes in pharmacokinetics. 2-Chloroprocaine is hydrolyzed very rapidly by plasma pseudocholinesterase to chloroaminobenzoic acid and H_2O. The in vitro half-life of 2-chloroprocaine incubated with sera from male volunteers is less than 15 seconds.[10] Although pregnancy is associated with a 30% to 40% decrease in pseudocholinesterase activity, the half-life of 2-chloroprocaine in maternal plasma in vitro is 11 to 21 seconds.[10] After epidural injection, the half-life of 2-chloroprocaine in the mother ranges from 1.5 to 6.4 minutes.[11] The longer half-life observed after epidural administra-

tion results from continued absorption of the drug from the injection site. Administration of 2-chloroprocaine to patients with low pseudocholinesterase activity may result in prolonged local anesthetic effect and an increased potential for systemic toxicity.[12]

LIDOCAINE

In sheep, the volume of the central compartment and the volume of distribution are greater in pregnant than in nonpregnant animals.[13,14] Bloedow et al.[13] observed that the total body clearance of lidocaine was similar in the two groups of animals. Therefore, the elimination half-life of lidocaine, which depends on the balance between volume of distribution and clearance, was longer in pregnant ewes.[13] Subsequently, we observed that the elimination half-life of lidocaine was similar in the two groups of sheep because the total body clearance of the drug was greater in pregnant animals than in nonpregnant animals.[14] The discrepancy between these results could be a result of differences in the complexity of the surgical preparation and the recovery period allowed.[15] In pregnant women, the elimination half-life of lidocaine after epidural injection is approximately 114 minutes.[16]

Lidocaine is metabolized to two active compounds, monoethylglycinexylidide (MEGX) and glycinexylidide (GX). MEGX can be detected in maternal plasma within 10 to 20 minutes after subarachnoid or epidural injection of the parent compound, whereas GX can be detected within 1 hour of epidural injection but rarely after subarachnoid injection.[17,18] Urinary excretion of unchanged lidocaine is negligible in sheep (i.e., less than 2% of the administered dose) and is not affected by pregnancy.[14]

The physiologic changes that occur during pregnancy are progressive. However, little information is available concerning the pharmacokinetics of local anesthetics before term. In one study, total clearance of lidocaine was similar at 119 and 138 days' gestation in gravid ewes (term is 148 days).[19]

Lidocaine is predominantly bound to alpha-1-acid glycoprotein (AAG) in plasma.[20] Pregnancy results in a decreased concentration of AAG, and as a result, the free fraction of lidocaine is higher in plasma obtained from term pregnant women compared with plasma obtained from nonpregnant controls.[20] The increase in the free fraction of lidocaine occurs early in gestation and is progressive.[21]

BUPIVACAINE

Bupivacaine is perhaps the most commonly used local anesthetic in obstetric anesthesia practice because it tends to preserve motor function and is compatible with intraspinal opioids. At least two studies compared the pharmacokinetics of bupivacaine after epidural administration in pregnant and nonpregnant women.[22,23] The absorption rate, the area under the concentration-time curve, and the elimination half-life (12 to 13 hours) were similar in the two groups.[22,23] As is the case with other local anesthetics, the elimination half-life of bupivacaine after epidural administration is much longer than that reported after intravenous injection, largely because the drug is continuously absorbed over time.[22,23]

After intravenous injection, the volume of distribution of bupivacaine is lower in pregnant sheep than in nonpregnant sheep.[24] In contrast, ovine pregnancy is associated with a greater volume of distribution of lidocaine.[13,14] The differences in gestational effects on the volume of distribution of the two local anesthetics may result from the greater binding of bupivacaine to plasma proteins during gestation (whereas pregnancy is associated with decreased protein binding of lidocaine).[24] One study noted that urinary excretion of unchanged bupivacaine was not affected by pregnancy and was less than 1% of the administered dose.[22] Nonetheless, low concentrations of bupivacaine may be detected in the urine of pregnant women for as long as 3 days after delivery.[25]

Bupivacaine undergoes dealkylation in the liver to 2,6-pipecolyxylidide (PPX). After epidural injection of bupivacaine for cesarean section, PPX was detected in maternal plasma within 5 minutes and remained detectable for as long as 24 hours.[25] With the lower drug dose required for labor analgesia, PPX was found only if the block was maintained with multiple reinjections during a period that exceeded 4 hours.[26] Pregnancy may affect metabolic pathways involved in bupivacaine degradation.[22] For example, pregnant women have higher serum PPX concentrations, but the unconjugated 4-hydroxy metabolite is not produced in significant amounts. The reason for this is unclear but may be related to the effects of hormonal changes on hepatic enzyme systems. Both progesterone and estradiol are competitive *inhibitors* of microsomal oxidases, whereas reductive enzymes are *induced* by progesterone.[24]

Bupivacaine is bound extensively to AAG and albumin.[27] This protein binding is reduced during late pregnancy in humans.[28]

Effect of H₂-Receptor Antagonists

H₂-receptor antagonists (e.g., cimetidine, ranitidine) are administered to increase gastric pH and reduce the parturient's risk of aspiration. Both may affect drug disposition by binding to hepatic cytochrome P450, thereby reducing hepatic blood flow and renal clearance; however, this effect is more pronounced for cimetidine than for ranitidine.[29,30] Indeed, altered drug disposition has been documented in surgical patients who had received chronic treatment with cimetidine.[31]

Short-term administration of either cimetidine or ranitidine, however, does not alter the pharmacokinetics of amide local anesthetics in pregnant women.[32,33]

Effects of Preeclampsia

Pathophysiologic changes associated with preeclampsia (e.g., reduced hepatic blood flow, abnormal liver function, decreased intravascular volume) also may affect maternal blood concentrations of local anesthetics (see Chapter 44). For example, total body clearance of lidocaine after epidural injection was significantly decreased in women with preeclampsia when compared with normotensive women.[34] However, the elimination half-life of lidocaine was similar in the two groups. Nonetheless, a decreased clearance may result in greater drug accumulation with repeated injections of lidocaine in women with preeclampsia. In contrast, bupivacaine has a low hepatic extraction, and changes in liver blood flow with preeclampsia may have less effect on the metabolic clearance of bupivacaine.

Effect of Diurnal Variation

Local anesthetic activity may be affected by the time of day that the drug is administered. For example, in one study, the duration of action of epidural bupivacaine was approximately 25% longer when given between 7:00 AM and 7:00 PM when compared to epidural administration between 7:00 PM and 7:00 AM.[35]

TOXICITY OF LOCAL ANESTHETICS

Systemic absorption or intravascular injection of a local anesthetic may result in systemic toxicity. Toxicity most often involves the central nervous system (CNS), but cardiovascular toxicity also may occur. Less common complications include tissue toxicity and hypersensitivity reactions.

CNS Toxicity

The severity of CNS effects is directly proportional to the blood concentration of a local anesthetic. This relationship is well described for lidocaine (Figure 12-3). Initially, the patient may complain of numbness of the tongue, tinnitus, or lightheadedness. At high plasma concentrations, convulsions occur because of a selective blockade of central inhibitory neurons, which results in increased CNS excitation.[36] At still higher concentrations, generalized CNS depression or coma may result from reversible blockade of both inhibitory and excitatory neuronal pathways. Finally, depression of the brainstem and cardiorespiratory centers may occur.

The relative toxicity of a local anesthetic correlates with its potency. For lidocaine, etidocaine, and bupivacaine, the ratio of the mean cumulative doses that cause convulsions in dogs is approximately 4:2:1, which is similar to their relative anesthetic potencies.[37] The same relative toxicity was demonstrated in human volunteers.[38] Local anesthetics may be ranked in order of decreasing CNS toxicity as follows: bupivacaine, tetracaine, etidocaine, lidocaine, mepivacaine, and 2-chloroprocaine.[39]

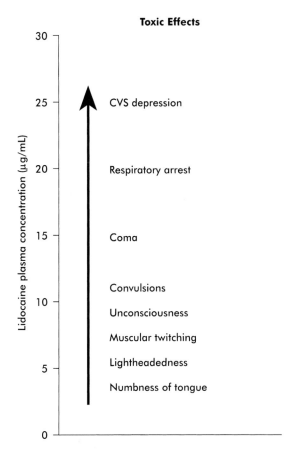

FIGURE 12-3. Signs and symptoms of systemic toxicity with increasing lidocaine concentrations. *CVS,* Cardiovascular system. (Modified from Carpenter RL, Mackey DC. Local anesthetics. In Barash PG, Cullen BF, Stoelting RK, editors. Clinical Anesthesia. Philadelphia, Lippincott, 1992:527.)

Other factors (e.g., the speed of injection) may affect CNS toxicity. In humans, the mean dose of etidocaine that elicited signs of CNS toxicity was substantially smaller during a 20 mg/min infusion than during a 10 mg/min infusion.[38] The seizure threshold also may be affected by metabolic factors. For example, in cats, an increase in $Paco_2$ or a decrease in pH results in a reduction in the seizure-dose threshold for several local anesthetics. Respiratory acidosis may result in increased drug delivery to the brain. Alternatively, respiratory acidosis may result in "ion trapping" of the local anesthetic and/or an increase in the unbound fraction of drug available for pharmacologic effect.[40-42]

Cardiovascular Toxicity

The cardiovascular system is much more resistant to the toxic effects of local anesthetics than the CNS. Severe, direct cardiovascular depression is rare, especially in association with the use of lidocaine and mepivacaine. Prompt oxygenation, ventilation, and, if necessary, circulatory support usually prevents cardiac arrest after unintentional intravenous injection of clinical doses of these drugs.[43] Progressive depression of myocardial function and profound vasodilation occur only at extremely high plasma concentrations of lidocaine or mepivacaine.[43] In contrast, the more potent amide local anesthetics, bupivacaine and etidocaine, have a more narrow margin of safety, expressed as the ratio between the dose (or plasma concentration) required to produce cardiovascular collapse and the dose (or plasma concentration) required to produce convulsions.[43] This results in part from the fact that supraconvulsant doses of bupivacaine (but not lidocaine or mepivacaine) precipitate lethal ventricular arrhythmias.[44-46] These arrhythmias may be caused by exaggerated electrophysiologic effects (e.g., depression of ventricular conduction) out of proportion to bupivacaine's anesthetic potency.[47]

Two theories have been proposed to explain why malignant ventricular arrhythmias occur with bupivacaine but not with lidocaine. Both bupivacaine and lidocaine rapidly block cardiac sodium channels during systole, but bupivacaine dissociates from these channels during diastole at a much slower rate than lidocaine.[47] Thus, at physiologic heart rates, the diastolic period is of sufficient duration for lidocaine to dissociate from sodium channels, whereas a bupivacaine block becomes intensified. This makes bupivacaine much more potent than lidocaine in depressing conduction and inducing reentrant-type ventricular arrhythmias. Alternatively, others have suggested that high concentrations of local anesthetic in the brainstem may result in systemic hypotension, bradycardia, and ventricular arrhythmias.[48] This may occur more frequently with bupivacaine because of its high lipid solubility, which facilitates transfer across the blood-brain barrier. An echocardiographic study in dogs suggested that bolus intravenous injection of bupivacaine results in systolic dysfunction, especially involving the right ventricle, which precedes the occurrence of arrhythmias.[49] Unfortunately, this study is difficult to interpret because the dogs were anesthetized with pentobarbital, a myocardial depressant.

Effects of Pregnancy on Systemic Toxicity

CNS TOXICITY

It is unclear whether pregnancy reduces the seizure threshold for amide local anesthetic agents. In a recent study, seizures occurred at lower doses of bupivacaine, levobupivacaine, and ropivacaine in pregnant ewes than in nonpregnant ewes.[50] However, the difference was small (10% to 15%) and probably of negligible clinical significance. In other studies in sheep and rats, pregnancy did *not* reduce the doses required to cause convulsions after intravenous administration of mepivacaine, bupivacaine, or lidocaine.[46,51] Magnesium sulfate, which is frequently used in obstetrics, does not affect the seizure-dose threshold of lidocaine.[52]

CARDIOVASCULAR TOXICITY

In 1979, Albright[53] alerted anesthesiologists to several cases of sudden cardiovascular collapse after unintentional intravascular injection of clinical doses of bupivacaine ($n = 5$) and etidocaine ($n = 1$) in pregnant women. The fact that cardiac arrest occurred concurrently with or shortly after the onset of convulsions in otherwise healthy parturients was especially disconcerting.[53,54] Most of these cases were fatal, and subsequent controversy centered on whether resuscitation was instituted promptly and effectively. Nonetheless, in response to the apparent epidemic, the U.S. Food and Drug Administration (FDA) restricted the use of the highest concentration (0.75%) of bupivacaine in pregnant women.

Several physiologic changes that occur during pregnancy place the parturient at increased risk for refractory cardiac arrest. First, reduced functional residual capacity and increased metabolic rate increase the risk and hasten the onset of hypoxemia during periods of hypoventilation or apnea. Second, aortocaval compression decreases the efficacy of closed-chest cardiac massage in the supine position.[55] Third, a large bolus of drug injected into an epidural vein might reach the heart rapidly through a dilated azygous system. However, none of these factors adequately explain the reason why cardiac arrest and difficult resuscitation are very rare in parturients intoxicated with lidocaine or mepivacaine.[53,54]

Laboratory studies of the effects of pregnancy on bupivacaine cardiotoxicity have been contradictory. Pregnancy-related hormones enhance the cardiotoxicity and arrhythmogenicity of bupivacaine in vitro.[56,57] For example, the magnitude and severity of bupivacaine-induced electrophysiologic changes were greater in myocardium obtained from nonpregnant rabbits treated with progesterone or beta-estradiol when compared with untreated controls.[56,57] The electrophysiologic effects of lidocaine were less pronounced than those resulting from bupivacaine even in hormonally treated animals. Studies in vivo have been less conclusive. In earlier investigations, significantly lower doses and plasma concentrations of bupivacaine, but not of mepivacaine or lidocaine, were required to produce circulatory collapse in pregnant sheep than in nonpregnant sheep.[44-46] However, a recent study, involving a larger number of sheep and more rigorous methods (e.g., randomization, blinding), failed to confirm that pregnancy enhances the cardiotoxicity of bupivacaine.[50]

Extrapolation of animal toxicity studies to clinical obstetric anesthesia is difficult for several reasons. First, in the aforementioned sheep studies, the drug was administered by constant-rate intravenous infusion. In contrast, in pregnant women intoxicated with bupivacaine, cardiac arrest occurred after unintended, rapid intravascular injection of a large bolus of drug. Second, a potential for bias existed because randomization and blinding were not used in all studies and some relied on historical controls.[44-46] Third, it is unclear whether resuscitation in the reported clinical cases was accompanied by prompt and effective relief of aortocaval compression.[55] Nonetheless, bupivacaine remains the most popular local anesthetic for obstetric anesthesia. In current practice, heightened vigilance, use of an appropriate test dose, and fractionation of the therapeutic dose have made epidural anesthesia a safe technique for use in obstetric patients. In a recent study of anesthesia-related maternal mortality, Hawkins et al.[58] noted that the number of maternal deaths resulting from local anesthetic toxicity decreased after 1984, which was the year that the FDA withdrew approval for the epidural administration of 0.75% bupivacaine in obstetric patients. In our judgment, adherence to the aforementioned clinical precautions—rather than the proscription against the epidural administration of 0.75% bupivacaine—has been responsible for the decreased number of maternal deaths resulting from local anesthetic toxicity. Anesthesiologists should be aware that intravenous injection of 0.5% bupivacaine also can cause systemic local anesthetic toxicity.

Treatment of Systemic Toxicity

Meticulous attention to good technique and strict adherence to maximum-recommended-dose guidelines are mandatory. (The use of a test dose to identify misplaced injections is discussed in Chapters 11, 21, and 25.) Incremental injection of the therapeutic dose, careful observation of the patient, and monitoring of vital signs usually provides early warning of an impending reaction. In mild cases, discontinuation of the administration of drug, administration of supplemental oxygen, and maintenance of normal ventilation often limit the severity of the reaction. In patients who show signs of CNS excitation, a small dose of thiopental (50 mg) or diazepam (2.5 to 5 mg) may prevent convulsions. Prophylactic administration of a benzodiazepine reduced the incidence of convulsions and decreased the incidence of mortality in mice intoxicated with amide local anesthetics.[59]

If convulsions should occur, oxygenation and ventilation must be maintained to prevent hypoxemia, hypercarbia, and acidosis.[40,41,60] Patency of the airway must be restored. (It may be necessary to suction the airway first in some patients.) Management should include administration of 100% oxygen, application of cricoid pressure, and endotracheal intubation, if required. Convulsions may be terminated quickly with a small dose of thiopental or diazepam. Maternal circulation should be supported by maintaining left uterine displacement and by administration of a vasopressor as needed. Because a high plasma concentration of local anesthetic may cause myocardial depression and vasodilation, a mixed alpha and beta agonist (e.g., ephedrine) may be preferable to a pure alpha agonist. Fortunately, convulsions induced by intravenous injection of a relatively small dose of local anesthetic are self-limited because of rapid redistribution of the drug.

Cardiac arrest should be treated with closed-chest cardiac massage, positive-pressure ventilation with 100% oxygen, administration of appropriate cardiotonic drugs, and defibrillation if necessary. In addition, the pelvis should be tilted leftward to prevent aortocaval compression, which would render cardiac massage ineffective. Prompt delivery of the infant may be necessary to restore maternal circulation.[61]

Persistent hypotension and bradycardia after bupivacaine intoxication may require administration of high doses of epinephrine and atropine.[62] A study in dogs suggested that amrinone may be superior to epinephrine in improving cardiac contractility depressed by bupivacaine.[63] However, amrinone may worsen ventricular arrhythmias.[64] Bupivacaine-induced ventricular arrhythmias should *not* be treated with lidocaine, because local anesthetic toxicity is additive.[65]

In the past, bretylium was recommended for the treatment of bupivacaine-induced ventricular arrhythmias.[65] However, the world's natural supply of bretylium is nearly exhausted, and the drug is no longer available. Bretylium has been deleted from the Advanced Cardiovascular Life Support (ACLS) algorithm for ventricular fibrillation/pulseless ventricular tachycardia. Currently there are no specific guidelines for the pharmacologic treatment of bupivacaine cardiotoxicity in parturients. Amiodarone is listed as the preferred antiarrhythmic agent in the most current ACLS algorithm. However, there may be some limitations to the utility of amiodarone in the treatment of bupivacaine-induced ventricular arrhythmias. Amiodarone may block the same ion channels that are affected by bupivacaine. Further, amiodarone has a relatively slower onset of action than bretylium and lidocaine, and it can cause hypotension. Nonetheless, amiodarone has been successfully used to resuscitate laboratory animals intoxicated with bupivacaine,[66] and it now seems to be the drug of choice for treatment of bupivacaine-induced ventricular arrhythmias. Bupivacaine toxicity may result in a *torsade de pointes*-like arrhythmia, which may require rapid atrial pacing and administration of isoproterenol.[67] Prolonged resuscitation may be needed until myocardial washout of bupivacaine has occurred.[47]

After maternal recovery, fetal condition should be assessed promptly. In theory, a delay in delivery may allow back-diffusion of local anesthetic from the fetus to the mother, which may be of benefit to the neonate. Laboratory studies have demonstrated this phenomenon after the administration of bupivacaine[68] but not lidocaine.[69]

Tissue Toxicity

Neurologic complications of regional anesthesia are rare (see Chapter 33). Most have resulted from direct neural trauma, infection, injection of toxic doses of local anesthetic, or, more likely, the presence of trace contaminants or detergents used to sterilize reusable equipment.

2-Chloroprocaine has resulted in prolonged or permanent sensory and motor deficits after subarachnoid injection of a large dose intended for epidural block.[70] Laboratory studies comparing the neurotoxicity of 2-chloroprocaine with that of other local anesthetics have yielded conflicting results, most likely related to the use of different methodologies and different species.[71,72] It has been suggested that neurotoxicity was caused by sodium meta-bisulfite, an antioxidant present in the commercial formulation (Nesacaine-CE) used in the reported cases.[73] The pH of Nesacaine-CE was between 2.7 and 4.0. In CSF rendered more acidic by 2-chloroprocaine, meta-bisulfite generates sulfur dioxide, which is lipid soluble and can diffuse into the nerve cell interior (Figure 12-4).[73] Intracellular hydration of sulfur dioxide generates sulfurous acid, which may cause profound intracellular acidosis and irreversible damage.

Subsequently, the manufacturer released another preparation of 2-chloroprocaine (i.e., Nesacaine-MPF, Astra Pharmaceutical Products), which was free of bisulfite but contained ethylenediamine-tetraacetic acid (EDTA). This was followed by several reports of severe, incapacitating paralumbar pain and spasm associated with epidural injection of large volumes of this new formulation.[74] The etiology is unclear, although some physicians have suggested that chelation of calcium by disodium EDTA may result in a decreased tissue calcium concentration and local tetany of the affected muscles.[74]

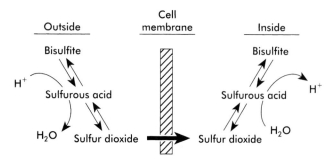

FIGURE 12-4. Effect of extracellular bisulfite in reducing intracellular pH by sulfur dioxide migration into the nerve cell interior. (Modified from Gissen AJ, Datta S, Lambert D. The chloroprocaine controversy. II. Is chloroprocaine neurotoxic? Reg Anesth 1984; 9:140.)

A rececent study[75] suggested that sodium bisulfite was the "scapegoat" for 2-chloroprocaine neurotoxicity. The authors concluded that neurologic deficits associated with unintentional intrathecal injection of 2-chloroprocaine likely resulted from a direct effect of the 2-chloroprocaine, *not* the sodium bisulfite.[75]

The current preparation of 2-chloroprocaine that is marketed for epidural administration (which is also called Nesacaine-MPF) does not contain EDTA or other preservatives. It is packaged in colored vials to reduce the oxidation of the 2-chloroprocaine.

Lidocaine has been used for spinal anesthesia for more than 50 years—in thousands upon thousands of patients—with apparent safety. However, during the past decade there have been reports of cauda equina syndrome, sacral nerve root deficits, or transient neurologic toxicity following subarachnoid injection of hyperbaric 5% lidocaine.[76-78] Neurotoxicity of local anesthetics is concentration-dependent[79,80] and is not unique to lidocaine.[81,82] Some investigators have speculated that slow injection of local anesthetic through a spinal microcatheter results in maldistribution and pooling of high concentrations of hyperbaric lidocaine in the cauda equina area.[76,77]

Milder manifestations of neurotoxicity also may occur. As early as 1954, mild, transient neurologic symptoms were reported after spinal anesthesia with lidocaine.[83] Transient neurologic symptoms (TNS) (dysesthesia or low back pain radiating to the buttocks, thighs, and calves) have been observed in surgical patients even after conventional (i.e., single shot) spinal anesthesia with hyperbaric 5% lidocaine.[78] In June 1994, in response to concerns that intrathecal injection of hyberbaric 5% lidocaine might be associated with TNS, the FDA Advisory Committee on Anesthetic Drugs recommended that the injected drug concentration be reduced by dilution with an equal volume of either preservative-free saline or CSF. To our knowledge, no prospective study has demonstrated the efficacy of this approach. Further, prospective randomized trials have demonstrated that, even with the use of 2% lidocaine, the incidence of TNS after spinal anesthesia (22% to 30%) is higher than that with mepivacaine (0%), prilocaine (3%), or bupivacaine (0%).[84,85]

The efficacy and safety of spinal lidocaine in concentrations of less than 2% can be determined only by prospective, randomized clinical trials. Interestingly, the exposure of frog sciatic nerve to lidocaine results in a progressive, irreversible loss of impulse activity beginning at a concentration of 1%.[80] These investigators noted that "the range of lidocaine that produces such changes in mammalian nerve awaits determination." Meanwhile, it seems prudent to take the following precautions: (1) dilute the commercial 5% lidocaine for intrathecal injection as recommended by the FDA, (2) administer the lowest possible dose, and (3) avoid the use of hyperbaric lidocaine in clinical conditions (e.g., obesity) or situations (e.g., the lithotomy position) that may be associated with an increased incidence of TNS.[78,86] If pencil-point, side-hole spinal needles are used, the injection port should be directed cephalad. However, a recent epidemiologic survey failed to implicate dose and needle bevel direction as factors that affect the risk of TNS.[86] Recent studies suggest that prilocaine, mepivacaine, and procaine may be suitable alternatives to lidocaine for spinal anesthesia.[84,85] However, larger studies of safety and efficacy are required before these drugs can be embraced for spinal anesthesia.

Pregnancy may be associated with a reduced risk of TNS. Recent studies suggest that the incidence of TNS following spinal anesthesia with lidocaine or bupivacaine is equally low (<3%) in women having cesarean delivery or postpartum tubal ligation.[87,88] However, the use of the lithotomy position seems to increase the risk of TNS with spinal lidocaine but not spinal bupivacaine in women undergoing cervical cerclage.[86]

Allergic Reactions

True allergy to a local anesthetic is rare.[89] Further, anaphylactic and anaphylactoid reactions may be the result of additives such as methylparaben or meta-bisulfite.[90] Clinical criteria are important in the diagnosis of allergic reactions because a delay in obtaining confirmatory laboratory data often occurs.[89] However, the alleged allergy to a local anesthetic can be substantiated in only 15% of patients by a history of urticaria, bronchospasm, facial edema, and/or cardiovascular instability.[91] Adverse reactions (e.g., CNS and cardiovascular symptoms) may mimic hypersensitivity, but they often do not result from hypersensitivity. These symptoms may be caused by hyperventilation or vasovagal syncope during injection of the drug, sympathetic stimulation (e.g., palpitations, tachycardia) from epinephrine, or edema related to the injection itself.

Some pregnant women claim to be allergic to "Novocain" or to "the caine" drugs. Obstetricians should refer such patients to an allergist and an anesthesiologist for appropriate evaluation well before the expected date of delivery. In many cases, a carefully obtained history excludes true hypersensitivity.[91] Otherwise, it may be necessary for an allergist to determine the type of reaction and the offending agent. The allergist may perform skin tests, drug-specific basophil degranulation, and/or the radioallergosorbent test (RAST). The last two tests, although highly specific, are costly and time consuming and may not be available for all anesthetic agents. Intradermal skin testing, although less costly and easy to perform, is associated with a false-positive rate of 8% to 15%.[92]

Alternatively, subcutaneous provocative dose testing is a useful method for rapid identification of a safe local anesthetic for an individual patient.[91,92] It can be performed by any physician qualified to manage hypersensitivity reactions. Appropriate emergency equipment and drugs (e.g., epinephrine, diphenhydramine) should be immediately available for resuscitation. Although not mentioned in many protocols, it seems prudent to establish intravenous access before testing.[93]

The back and the ventral aspect of the forearm are the preferred sites for testing. Areas with abnormal skin coloration or dermographia should be avoided. A history of recent treatment with antihistamines, salicylates, or steroids should be noted because these drugs may alter the test results.[94]

The following protocol has been proposed by Chandler et al.[92] (Table 12-2) and has been used successfully in at least one

TABLE 12-2	A PROTOCOL FOR PROVOCATIVE DOSE TESTING WITH LOCAL ANESTHETICS*			
Step	Route	Volume	Dilution
1	Skin prick		Undiluted
2	Subcutaneous	0.1 mL	Undiluted
3	Subcutaneous	0.5 mL	Undiluted
4	Subcutaneous	1.0 mL	Undiluted
5	Subcutaneous	2.0 mL	Undiluted

*See text for initial dilutions in patients with a severe history of allergy.
From Chandler MJ, Grammer LC, Patterson R. Provocative challenge with local anesthetics in patients with a prior history of reaction. J Allergy Clin Immunol 1987; 79:885.

published case.[93] After a negative needle-prick test, increasing volumes of undiluted local anesthetic (typically 1% concentration) are injected subcutaneously at 15-minute intervals. In patients with an especially strong history of a severe reaction, the series may be preceded by injection of diluted solutions (e.g., a 1:100 solution, followed by a 1:10 solution). A fresh syringe and a 30-gauge needle should be used for each injection. Additional refinements may include the use of a negative control (e.g., normal saline) and a positive control of diluted histamine. A local anesthetic that is not in the same class as the drug in question should be tested. (If an ester is suspected as the offending agent, testing should be performed with an amide agent, and vice versa.) If possible, the drug tested should be suitable for local infiltration and for epidural and subarachnoid block.

The test is considered positive if there is a change in the patient's clinical status or if a skin wheal greater than 10 mm in diameter, with or without a flare, arises within 10 minutes of injection and persists for at least 30 minutes.[94] If provocative dose testing is completed without a reaction, the local anesthetic used and the final dose given should be recorded and the patient (and the referring physician) should be informed that the risk of an adverse reaction to subsequent administration of that drug is no greater than that for the general population.[91-93]

MANAGEMENT OF AN ALLERGIC REACTION

Pharmacologic therapy of a severe allergic reaction includes (1) inhibition of mediator synthesis and release, (2) reversal of the effects of these mediators on target organs, and (3) prevention of the recruitment of other inflammatory processes. In general, catecholamines, phosphodiesterase inhibitors, antihistamines, and corticosteroids have been used for this purpose (Box 12-1).[95] Higher doses of catecholamines may be required in a patient with sympathetic blockade. In addition, pregnancy itself decreases responsiveness to catecholamines.[96] Despite its potential adverse effect on uterine blood flow, epinephrine remains the cornerstone of therapy for allergic reactions.[97] In one reported case, a mother was treated successfully with epinephrine 100 µg without any apparent adverse effects on the newborn.[97]

EFFECTS OF LOCAL ANESTHETICS ON THE UTERUS AND PLACENTA

Uterine Blood Flow

Much of the interest in this subject was generated by the association of paracervical block anesthesia with fetal bradycardia,

Box 12-1 MANAGEMENT OF ANAPHYLAXIS

INITIAL THERAPY

1. Stop administration of antigen
2. Maintain airway with 100% oxygen
3. Discontinue all anesthetic agents
4. Start intravascular volume expansion (2-4 L of crystalloid/colloid [25-50 mL/kg] to treat hypotension)
5. Give epinephrine:
   - 5-10 µg intravenously for treatment of hypotension; titrate as needed
   - 0.5-1.0 mg intravenously for treatment of cardiovascular collapse

SECONDARY TREATMENT

1. Catecholamine infusions (starting doses):
   - Epinephrine 4-8 µg/min (0.05-0.1 µg/kg/min)
   - Norepinephrine 4-8 µg/min (0.05-0.1 µg/kg/min)
   - Isoproterenol 0.05-0.1 µg/min
2. Antihistamines (0.5-1.0 mg/kg of diphenhydramine)
3. Corticosteroids (0.25-1.0 g of hydrocortisone; alternatively 1-2 g [25 mg/kg] of methylprednisolone)
4. Bicarbonate (0.5-1.0 mEq/kg) in patients with persistent hypotension or acidosis
5. Airway evaluation (before extubation)

From Levy JH. Anaphylactic Reactions in Anesthesia and Intensive Care. Stoneham, Mass, Butterworth-Heinemann, 1992:162.

which some investigators attributed to the high concentration of local anesthetic deposited in the vicinity of the uterine arteries.[98] Human uterine artery segments obtained at the time of cesarean hysterectomy constrict when exposed to high concentrations of lidocaine,[99] mepivacaine,[99] or bupivacaine.[100]

These findings also have been confirmed in laboratory animals.[101] Fishburne et al.[101] observed a dose-related decrease in uterine blood flow during uterine arterial infusion of 2-chloroprocaine, lidocaine, or bupivacaine in gravid ewes. A 25% reduction in uterine blood flow occurred at the following calculated plasma concentrations of local anesthetic: bupivacaine, 7 µg/mL; 2-chloroprocaine, 11.5 µg/mL; and lidocaine, 19.5 µg/mL.[101] However, when plasma local anesthetic concentrations mimic those that occur in ordinary clinical practice, local anesthetics have no adverse effect on uterine blood flow.[102-104] In pregnant ewes, uterine blood flow remained unchanged during an intravenous infusion of lidocaine or bupivacaine that resulted in plasma concentrations of 0.81 to 4.60 and 1.5 to 2.0 µg/mL, respectively.[102,103] Likewise, intravenous injection of 2-chloroprocaine, 0.67 and 1.34 mg/kg, did not reduce uterine blood flow velocity in pregnant guinea pigs.[104]

Pregnancy may enhance uterine vascular reactivity to local anesthetic agents. Studies have observed that isolated human uterine artery segments obtained from term parturients constrict at a lower lidocaine concentration than uterine artery segments from nonpregnant patients.[99,105] Uterine artery sensitivity to local anesthetics increases as early as the second trimester of pregnancy and may be related to an increase in estrogen concentrations.[99,101] However, these studies were performed before we recognized the importance of intact vascular endothelium in the in vitro assessment of vascular tone.

The exact mechanism by which high concentrations of local anesthetics cause uterine artery vasoconstriction (while causing dilation in other vascular beds) is unclear. This vaso-constriction may result from modulation of calcium-channel regulatory mechanisms because verapamil and nifedipine ablate the response.[105] Alternatively, local anesthetics may affect cyclic nucleotides and alter the ionic content and contractility of uterine vascular smooth muscle.[106] Clinical experience with the use of local anesthetics during labor and delivery supports the view that clinical concentrations of these drugs do not adversely affect the uterine vasculature.[107-113]

Umbilical Blood Flow

Fetal well-being also depends on the adequacy of fetal perfusion of the placenta. The regulatory mechanisms that control flow through the umbilical vessels are poorly understood. Lidocaine does not affect spiral strips obtained from human umbilical artery segments at concentrations of 1 to 5 μg/mL, but it produces relaxation in concentrations that range from 30 to 900 μg/mL.[114] Bupivacaine also does not constrict umbilical artery segments at clinically relevant concentrations of 0.3 and 1 μg/mL.[114] At higher concentrations, the effect of bupivacaine appears to be biphasic. Specifically, constriction occurs at concentrations of 5 to 25 μg/mL, and relaxation occurs at concentrations that exceed 125 μg/mL.[114,115] Hypercarbia but not hypoxia lessens the contractile response of umbilical vessels to bupivacaine in vitro.[116]

Decreases in umbilical blood flow of as much as 43% accompany intravenous administration of lidocaine 4 mg/kg in pregnant sheep.[117] However, plasma concentrations of the drug were high and all ewes exhibited signs of CNS toxicity, which may reduce umbilical blood flow.

Recent advances in noninvasive Doppler imaging have facilitated clinical assessment of umbilical cord blood flow velocity. The ratio of the systolic (S) peak to the diastolic (D) trough of the umbilical artery waveform is used as a measure of vascular resistance. The S/D ratio in the umbilical artery decreases during normal pregnancy, and high ratios usually are associated with fetal compromise.[118] Local anesthetics administered for epidural anesthesia do not seem to adversely affect the umbilical artery S/D ratio.[119,120] In fact, during labor, epidural analgesia with lidocaine 1.5% or 2-chloroprocaine 2% resulted in a decrease in the S/D ratio.[119,120] This favorable change may have resulted from pain relief. Others have noted no appreciable change or a slight decrease in the S/D ratio after the epidural administration of amide local anesthetics for elective cesarean section.[110,113,121]

Uterine Tone and Contractility

Changes in uterine tone and contractility also may affect uteroplacental perfusion. Local anesthetics exert direct effects on uterine smooth muscle. Exposure to high concentrations of lidocaine, procaine, or 2-chloroprocaine in vitro resulted in contraction of human myometrial segments obtained at the time of cesarean section.[122] These findings have been corroborated in laboratory animals.[101,123] Further, Belitzky et al.[124] observed that direct intramyometrial injection of 1% procaine resulted in uterine hyperstimulation and fetal distress in pregnant women. In all these reports, the myometrium was exposed to higher than normal concentrations of the drug. In contrast, intravenous infusion of lidocaine or bupivacaine, which resulted in clinically relevant plasma concentrations, did not affect uterine tone or uterine activity in pregnant ewes.[102,103]

ADJUVANTS

Epinephrine

Epinephrine often is added to local anesthetic solutions to reduce peak blood levels of the drug and to intensify and prolong neural blockade. Epinephrine itself exerts an antinociceptive effect mediated by an alpha$_2$-receptor stimulation.[125] For example, the addition of epinephrine 1:600,000 results in a 30% reduction in the minimum effective local analgesic concentration (MLAC) for epidural bupivacaine in laboring women.[126] The efficacy of epinephrine varies with the particular drug and concentration used as well as the site of injection. (The influence of epinephrine on the maternal blood concentration of local anesthetic is considered in the discussion of placental transfer.)

The routine use of epinephrine in obstetric anesthesia practice is not universally accepted because of its potential effects on uterine blood flow and labor. Intravenous administration of epinephrine causes a dose-related decrease in uterine blood flow in pregnant sheep and guinea pigs.[127,128] However, it is doubtful whether the drug, when absorbed from the epidural space, attains blood levels sufficiently high to cause a clinically significant reduction in uterine blood flow. Studies that used Doppler velocimetry and radioactive xenon have shown that the addition of epinephrine to local anesthetic solutions does not alter uteroplacental perfusion during administration of epidural anesthesia for labor or cesarean section.[110,121,129-131]

The effects of epinephrine on uterine contractility also may be dose dependent. Several studies demonstrated that epidural administration of a local anesthetic with epinephrine (1:200,000) was associated with a transient decrease in uterine activity[132-135] and a prolonged first stage of labor.[132,133,135] These effects were not observed after the epidural administration of a decreased concentration of epinephrine (e.g., 1:300,000).[136-138]

Epidural administration of epinephrine does not affect umbilical cord blood flow in healthy fetuses.[119,139,140] However, Marx et al.[119] observed an increase in the umbilical artery S/D ratio after the epidural administration of epinephrine in women whose fetuses had abnormally high umbilical vascular resistance. On the basis of this finding, it would seem prudent to avoid the routine use of epinephrine in conditions associated with fetal compromise.

Epinephrine also may affect the maternal cardiovascular system. Grant et al.[141] noted that epidural administration of bupivacaine with epinephrine (a total epinephrine dose of as much as 110 μg) was associated with mild vasodilation and a slightly greater incidence of hypotension when compared with the epidural administration of bupivacaine alone for cesarean section. In this study, the addition of epinephrine did not affect maternal cardiac output or heart rate.

Bicarbonate

Alkalinization of local anesthetics (which are weak bases) favors formation of the uncharged base and facilitates the penetration of neuronal membranes. The effects of alkalinization are most dramatic with commercially prepared, epinephrine-containing formulations of local anesthetic that have been adjusted to a pH of less than 6.0.[142] Several studies have suggested that the addition of 8.4% sodium bicarbonate (1.0 mEq of bicarbonate/10 mL of local anesthetic) to lidocaine, mepivacaine, or 2-chloroprocaine shortens the latent period of epidural analgesia.[143-147] This effect is least pronounced with 2-chloroprocaine.[146,147] In contrast, Gaggero et al.[148] recently found that alkalinization of 2% lidocaine did not shorten latency or improve the quality of epidural anesthesia for cesarean section.

Data regarding bupivacaine are conflicting. Bupivacaine is more difficult to alkalinize because of its tendency to precipitate. Some have noted a faster onset time and more intense motor blockade with the addition of 0.1 mL of 8.4% sodium bicarbonate to 20 mL of bupivacaine,[149,150] but others have failed to detect any effect of alkalinization.[151] Commercially prepared, epinephrine-containing bupivacaine may require more bicarbonate (e.g., 0.15 mL of bicarbonate/10 mL of solution) because of the lower pH of the epinephrine-containing solution.[150]

Care must be exercised when using an alkalinized solution of local anesthetic because hypotension, not unlike that observed with spinal anesthesia, occurs more frequently than with use of an unbuffered solution.[152] Presumably this is a result of an accelerated onset of sympathetic blockade.

Opioids

The addition of an opioid to the solution of local anesthetic has become widespread in obstetric anesthesia practice. Indeed, recent studies have demonstrated that the addition of a lipid-soluble opioid (e.g., fentanyl, sufentanil) decreases the MLAC for epidural bupivacaine,[153] predominantly by a spinal site of action.[154] Administration of a reduced concentration of local anesthetic results in less maternal motor block, which is especially important during the second stage of labor.

DRUG INTERACTIONS
WITH 2-CHLOROPROCAINE

Epidural 2-chloroprocaine may affect the efficacy of other drugs administered in the neuraxis. Previous use of 2-chloroprocaine (even a test dose) may reduce the quality and duration of analgesia produced by subsequent injection of morphine or fentanyl epidurally.[155,156] Several hypotheses have been proposed for this antagonism. The low pH of the 2-chloroprocaine solution may result in acidification of the epidural space, and it favors formation of the poorly diffusible, charged form of the opioid. However, administration of a buffered 2-chloroprocaine solution does not prevent the antagonism with epidural fentanyl.[157] Second, it has been suggested that 2-chloroprocaine (or its metabolite, chloroaminobenzoic acid) may act as a specific mu-receptor antagonist because a kappa-receptor agonist (e.g., butorphanol) is not antagonized by 2-chloroprocaine.[155] Third, Hughes et al.[158] proposed that there may be a "window" caused by the rapid regression of 2-chloroprocaine before the onset of analgesia with epidural morphine.

2-Chloroprocaine also reduces the subsequent efficacy of epidural bupivacaine.[159] Corke et al.[160] suggested that chloroaminobenzoic acid is responsible for this effect. Administration of buffered 2-chloroprocaine does not prevent the antagonism of epidural bupivacaine.[146]

PLACENTAL TRANSFER

Most drugs, including local anesthetics, readily cross the placenta. The factors that influence the placental transfer of a drug include (1) the physicochemical characteristics of the local anesthetic itself, (2) the concentration of free drug in the mater-

nal blood, (3) the permeability of the placenta, and (4) the hemodynamic events occurring within the fetal-maternal unit.

Local anesthetics cross placental membranes by a process of simple (i.e., passive) diffusion. The rate of transfer is described by the Fick equation:

$$Q/t = \frac{K \times A \, (Cm - Cf)}{D}$$

where:
Q/t = The rate of diffusion
K = A diffusion constant for a particular drug
A = The surface area available for transfer
Cm = The free drug concentration in the maternal blood
Cf = The free drug concentration in the fetal blood
D = The thickness of the trophoblastic epithelium

In general, K is affected by molecular size, lipid solubility, and the degree of ionization.

Molecular Size

Compounds with a molecular weight of less than 500 daltons typically cross the placenta easily, whereas drugs like digoxin, which have a molecular weight of greater than 500 daltons, have a slower rate of diffusion.[161] Commonly used local anesthetics have molecular weights that range from 234 to 288 daltons (see Table 12-1). These small differences in molecular weight should not affect the rate of placental transfer because K is inversely proportional to the square root of the molecular weight.[162]

Ionization and Lipid Solubility

The degree of ionization affects the rate of placental diffusion because the unionized molecule is more lipid soluble than the ionized moiety. Local anesthetics are weak bases; they have a relatively low degree of ionization and considerable lipid solubility at physiologic pH.

The relationship between pH and pK_B may affect drug accumulation in the fetus. For the amide local anesthetics in particular, pK_B values are sufficiently close to physiologic pH that changes in fetal acid-base status may significantly alter the balance between ionized and unionized drug. In the acidotic fetus, a greater proportion of drug in the ionized form results in a larger total amount of local anesthetic in fetal plasma. This is because of "ion trapping" (Figure 12-5).[163-165] Elimination of lidocaine from fetal blood is slower in the asphyxiated fetus than in the nonasphyxiated fetus.[117] Accumulation of lidocaine may be greater in the fetal tissues, where the pH is even lower than that of fetal blood.[165]

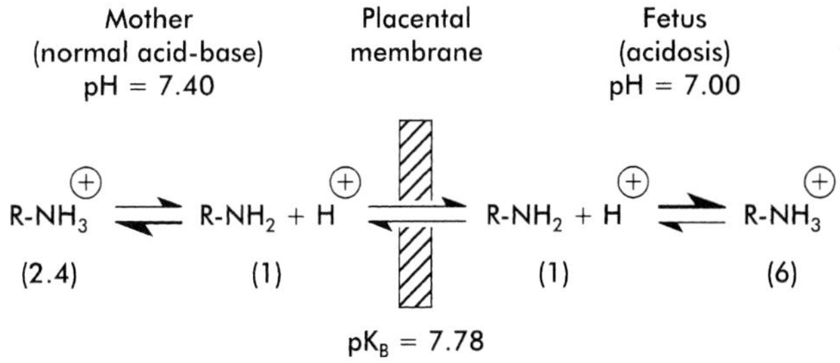

FIGURE 12-5. "Ion trapping" of a local anesthetic. (From the American College of Obstetricians and Gynecologists. Obstet Gynecol 1976; 48:29.)

Protein Binding

Perhaps most confusing and least understood are the effects of protein binding on the placental transfer of local anesthetic agents. Amide local anesthetics are predominantly bound to AAG and, to a much lesser degree, to albumin.[20] The extent of protein binding varies among the local anesthetic agents (see Table 12-1). For a given local anesthetic, the proportion of free drug increases as blood concentration increases because of the saturation of binding sites. Protein binding of local anesthetics in the fetal plasma is approximately half that in the mother.[68,69]

The fetal-maternal (F/M) blood concentration ratios of amide local anesthetic agents are listed in Table 12-1. The lower F/M blood concentration ratios of highly protein-bound drugs (e.g., bupivacaine, etidocaine) have been attributed to more restricted placental transfer compared with less protein-bound drugs (e.g., lidocaine, mepivacaine). Indeed the rate of bupivacaine transfer across rabbit placenta perfused in situ was lower than that for lidocaine.[166,167] Some investigators have suggested that protein binding in the maternal plasma should not affect the diffusion of drugs across the placenta because the dissociation from plasma proteins is essentially instantaneous.[168] This has been demonstrated for fentanyl but not for bupivacaine.[169] More recently, the relatively low umbilical vein/maternal vein blood concentration ratio for bupivacaine has been attributed to differences in protein binding between maternal and fetal plasma (Figure 12-6).[68,69,170,171] Let us assume that the total concentration of lidocaine or bupivacaine in the maternal plasma is 2 mg/L. Lidocaine and bupivacaine are approximately 50% and 90% bound to maternal plasma proteins, respectively. Thus the free concentration of drug available for placental transfer is 1.0 and 0.2 mg/L, respectively. At equilibrium, the concentration of free drug is equal on both sides of the placenta. However, in the fetus, lidocaine and bupivacaine are approximately 25% and 50% bound to fetal plasma proteins, respectively. Thus the total lidocaine concentration in fetal plasma is 1.33 mg/L, resulting in an F/M ratio of 0.67. For bupivacaine, the corresponding values are 0.4 mg/L and an F/M ratio of 0.2.

Kuhnert et al.[25] observed that substantial accumulation of bupivacaine occurred in human fetuses whose mothers received the drug for epidural anesthesia. After delivery, measurable plasma and urine concentrations persisted for as long as 3 days.

Maternal Blood Concentration of Drug

The maternal blood concentration of local anesthetic is determined by (1) the dose, (2) the site of administration, (3) metabolism and excretion, and (4) the effects of adjuvants such as epinephrine. For a given local anesthetic, the maternal blood concentration determines fetal drug exposure and is the only variable of the Fick equation that may be influenced by the clinician.

DOSE

In general, higher doses result in higher maternal and fetal blood concentrations. For example, a study in humans demonstrated that doubling the dose of epidural lidocaine from 300 ± 195 mg to 595 ± 127 mg almost doubled the lidocaine concentrations in umbilical cord blood.[17] The elimination half-life of amide local anesthetics is relatively long; thus repeated epidural injection or continuous infusion of the drug may lead to accumulation in the maternal plasma. This does not apply to 2-chloroprocaine, which is rapidly hydrolyzed by pseudocholinesterase.[11]

SITE OF ADMINISTRATION

The rates of absorption and peak plasma concentrations depend on the vascularity of the tissues at the site of administration. The peak plasma concentration of lidocaine is achieved within 9 to 10 minutes after paracervical block. In contrast, absorption from the lumbar epidural space, which is less vascular, occurs at a slower rate; the peak plasma concentration is not achieved until 25 to 40 minutes after epidural administration.[17,172] Injection of local anesthetic into the caudal rather than the lumbar epidural space may result in higher blood levels.[173]

In the past, it was thought that subarachnoid administration of a local anesthetic resulted in less systemic absorption of the drug than epidural administration. However, one study detected similar peak blood concentrations of lidocaine after either subarachnoid or epidural administration of 75 mg of lidocaine to nonpregnant patients.[174] In another study, subarachnoid administration of lidocaine 75 mg for cesarean section resulted in low but measurable fetal plasma concentrations of the drug.[18]

EPINEPHRINE

Epinephrine frequently is administered with a local anesthetic to enhance analgesia and delay the uptake of the drug from

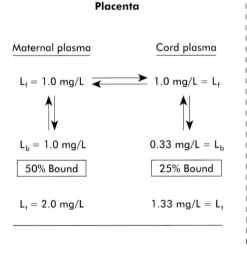
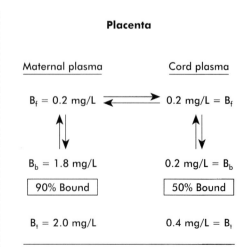

FIGURE 12-6. Demonstration of how distribution of local anesthetics across the placenta may be predicted from differences in drug protein binding in maternal and fetal plasma. *L*, Lidocaine; *B*, bupivacaine; *f*, *b*, *t*, free, bound, and total drug concentrations, respectively. Lidocaine U/M = 0.67; bupivacaine U/M = 0.20. (From Tucker GT, Mather LE, Properties, absorption, and disposition of local anesthetic agents. In Cousins MJ, Bridenbaugh PO, editors. Neural Blockade in Clinical Anesthesia and Management of Pain, 2nd ed. Philadelphia, Lippincott, 1988:95.)

the site of administration.[125] The latter action of epinephrine varies with the choice and concentration of local anesthetic as well as the concentration of epinephrine. The effect of epinephrine is greater when combined with lidocaine than when combined with mepivacaine or bupivacaine.[175,176] Even concentrations of epinephrine as low as 1:300,000 (i.e., 3.3 µg/mL) have been shown to be effective in reducing the plasma concentrations of lidocaine.[136]

In contrast, the addition of epinephrine to bupivacaine has transient effects. Reynolds and Taylor[177] observed that the addition of epinephrine 1:200,000 (i.e., 5 µg/mL) to bupivacaine resulted in decreased maternal plasma concentrations of drug only at 20 minutes after the first epidural injection and at 40 minutes after the second epidural injection in laboring women.[177] The addition of epinephrine 1:300,000 to 0.5% bupivacaine had no effect on maternal venous plasma concentrations of drug in laboring women.[137] Likewise, Reynolds et al.[178] observed no effect when they added epinephrine 1:200,000 to bupivacaine during administration of epidural anesthesia for cesarean section.

The site of administration also may influence the effect of epinephrine on the absorption of individual drugs. For example, the addition of epinephrine to bupivacaine resulted in a 50% decrease in maternal plasma concentrations of bupivacaine after paracervical block.[179] In contrast, Denson et al.[180] observed that epinephrine did not alter absorption of lidocaine after subarachnoid injection.

Studies of the effects of epinephrine on the placental transfer of local anesthetics have yielded contradictory results. In rabbits, epinephrine did not affect the F/M ratio of bupivacaine.[181] In pregnant women, the F/M ratio for bupivacaine was increased[177] or unchanged.[137,138,179] For mepivacaine, the F/M ratio was increased,[175] whereas for lidocaine it was increased,[175,182] decreased,[136] or unchanged.[183]

Placenta

The maturation of the placenta itself may affect the rate of drug transfer. In pregnant mice, diazepam and its metabolites cross the placenta more rapidly in late pregnancy.[184] Uptake and metabolism of drugs by the placenta would be expected to decrease transfer to the fetus. However, placental drug uptake of local anesthetics is limited, and it is unlikely that this organ metabolizes the amide local anesthetic agents.[185] This may not be true for the ester local anesthetics. Evidence suggests that cocaine is biotransformed when incubated with human placental microsomal fraction, presumably because of cholinesterase activity within the placenta.[186] Placental metabolism of para-aminobenzoic acid also has been demonstrated.[187]

Hemodynamic events within the placental unit also may affect the rate of transfer. For example, maternal hypoxia resulted in a decreased F/M ratio of lidocaine and decreased transfer of the drug as a result of stagnant circulation within the placenta.[188]

TERATOGENICITY

The teratogenicity of anesthetic agents is not an issue during parturition, but local anesthetics often are used for procedures during the first trimester of pregnancy. In vitro studies have suggested that local anesthetics have some adverse developmental effects. Even at low concentrations, these agents have caused reversible reduction of cell division in tissue culture.[189-194]

In contrast, structural anomalies have not been observed in intact animals.[195-197] Mid-pregnancy administration of lidocaine or mepivacaine in rats has been associated with behavioral changes only in the offspring.[198,199]

Extrapolation of laboratory findings to humans is tenuous for a number of reasons. First, a drug may be teratogenic in one species but not in others.[200] Second, a 1-hour drug exposure in a pregnant rat (with a gestation of 21 days) is excessive and not analogous to several hours of clinical anesthesia during human pregnancy. Third, the doses of local anesthetics used in animal studies greatly exceed those administered for clinical anesthesia. A large, multicenter study demonstrated that the risk of congenital anomalies in humans was not increased by the administration of benzocaine, procaine, tetracaine, or lidocaine during early pregnancy.[201] However, a twofold increase in the incidence of congenital anomalies was noted in infants whose mothers had received mepivacaine. The small number of patients who received mepivacaine ($n = 82$) and the fact that no adverse effects occurred with the use of other amide agents have raised doubts about the validity of this observation.[202]

FETUS AND NEWBORN

Pharmacokinetics

Local anesthetics, once transferred across the placenta, are distributed in the fetus. Factors that influence tissue uptake of the drug include (1) fetal plasma protein binding, (2) lipid solubility, (3) the degree of ionization of the drug, and (4) hemodynamic changes that affect the distribution of fetal cardiac output. As previously mentioned, the fetal plasma protein-binding capacity of local anesthetics is approximately 50% less than that of maternal plasma.[68,69] Thus at any given total plasma concentration of local anesthetic, there is greater availability of free drug in the fetus than in the mother.[68,69,203,204] Studies have examined the distribution of lidocaine in fetal tissues after an intravenous injection of the drug in pregnant sheep and guinea pigs.[19,205] The higher concentration of lidocaine in the liver, myocardium, and brain (when compared with other fetal tissues) probably reflects rapid distribution of the drug to highly perfused tissues. The only organ in which lidocaine concentrations in the fetus exceeded those in the mother was the liver. This is not surprising, given the high lipid content of the fetal liver and the fact that it receives most of the blood returning from the placenta by means of the umbilical vein.[205] Fetal acidosis and hypoxemia result in circulatory adaptations that increase blood flow to vital organs (e.g., brain, heart, adrenal glands).[206] The concentration of lidocaine in these organs is higher in asphyxiated fetuses than in healthy fetuses.[165,206]

Any drug that reaches the fetus undergoes metabolism and excretion. The term newborn has the hepatic enzymes necessary for the biotransformation of amide local anesthetics.[17,18,207-211] Nonetheless, the elimination half-life of these drugs is longer in the neonate compared with the adult.[209,211] The use of mepivacaine in obstetric epidural analgesia fell into disfavor after a report indicated that the elimination half-life of the drug in the newborn was approximately 9 hours, or three times as long as the neonatal half-life for lidocaine.[175] It is ironic that it later became known that the neonatal elimination half-life for bupivacaine may be as long as 14 hours.[212]

The pharmacokinetics of lidocaine have been compared among adult ewes and fetal and neonatal lambs.[211] The metabolic (hepatic) clearance in the newborn was similar to that in the adult, and renal clearance was greater than that in the adult. Nonetheless, the elimination half-life was more prolonged in the newborn. This has been attributed to a greater volume of distribution in the newborn. Thus at any given time, a smaller fraction of lidocaine accumulated in the body is available for clearance by hepatic metabolism. The greater renal clearance noted in neonates is a result of decreased protein binding, which increases the proportion of drug available to the kidneys for excretion.

The elimination half-life of local anesthetics in the fetus is similar to that of the adult because, unlike the newborn, the fetus can excrete drug across the placenta back to the mother.[68,211] With bupivacaine, this may occur even though the total plasma drug concentration in the mother may exceed that in the fetus.[68]

Systemic Toxicity

In general, the newborn is more sensitive than the adult to the depressant effects of drugs. This may not be the case for local anesthetics. The seizure threshold for local anesthetics in the newborn appears to be similar to that in the adult.[213]

The relative CNS and cardiovascular toxicity of lidocaine have been compared in adult ewes and fetal and neonatal lambs.[214] For both drugs, greater doses (when calculated on a milligram-per-kilogram basis) were required to elicit toxic manifestations in the fetus and newborn when compared with the adult. However, the plasma concentrations of the drug associated with toxic manifestations were similar among the three groups of animals. The greater dose tolerated by the fetus compared with the newborn and the adult was attributed to placental clearance of drug back to the mother and better maintenance of blood gas tensions during convulsions. In the newborn, a large volume of distribution most likely is responsible for the high doses of local anesthetic required to produce toxic effects.

Studies of bupivacaine cardiotoxicity are inconsistent. In vitro, the sinoatrial node of newborn guinea pigs was more sensitive than that of the adult to the cardiodepressant effect of bupivacaine.[215] In contrast, newborn piglets (2 days old) demonstrated greater resistance to the arrhythmogenic and CNS effects of bupivacaine than did older animals.[216]

Fetal Heart Rate

Changes in fetal heart rate (FHR) after administration of local anesthetics most often are related to indirect effects such as maternal hypotension and uterine hyperstimulation. Local anesthetics likely have little direct effect on FHR, except perhaps after paracervical block. Rather, labor itself may be the single most important factor that alters FHR patterns.[217] Transient changes in beat-to-beat FHR variability and an increase in the incidence of periodic decelerations have been observed during administration of epidural analgesia in laboring women.[218-222] In contrast, in the absence of labor, FHR patterns are not affected by the larger doses of local anesthetics required during administration of epidural anesthesia for cesarean delivery.[217] The FHR changes noted in laboring women were transient and did not affect the condition of the newborn.[218-222]

Neurobehavioral Tests

Neurobehavioral tests have been developed to detect subtle changes in organized behavior in the newborn. These tests include the Brazelton Neonatal Behavioral Assessment Scale (NBAS), the Early Neonatal Neurobehavioral Scale (ENNS), and the Neurologic and Adaptive Capacity Score (NACS). All are subjective and complex and lack specificity.

In 1974, Scanlon et al.[223] found that babies born to mothers who received epidural lidocaine or mepivacaine scored lower on tests of muscle strength and tone in the first 8 hours of life than babies who were not exposed to these local anesthetics. This report has been criticized for its lack of appropriate controls, inadequate sample size, and concomitant administration of opioids and barbiturates. In subsequent studies, all commonly used local anesthetics (e.g., lidocaine, mepivacaine, 2-chloroprocaine, bupivacaine) had minor transient effects on neonatal neurobehavior.[221,222,224-227] Other perinatal factors appear to have a more important effect on neonatal test performance than the choice of local anesthetic.[228]

Preterm Fetus and Newborn

It has become axiomatic that the preterm infant is more vulnerable than the term infant to the effects of drugs used in obstetric analgesia and anesthesia. There are several postulated causes of enhanced drug sensitivity in the preterm newborn: (1) less protein is available for drug binding; (2) higher levels of bilirubin are present and may compete with the drug for protein binding; (3) greater drug access to the CNS occurs because of a poorly developed blood-brain barrier; (4) the preterm infant has greater total body water and less fat content; and (5) the preterm infant has a decreased ability to metabolize and excrete drugs. Unfortunately, few systematic studies have determined the maternal and fetal pharmacokinetics and pharmacodynamics of drugs throughout gestation, but these deficiencies of the preterm infant may not be as serious as we have been led to believe. Although the plasma albumin and AAG concentrations are lower in the preterm fetus, this primarily affects drugs that are highly bound to these proteins. However, most local anesthetics exhibit only low-to-moderate degrees of binding in fetal plasma.[68,69]

The placenta efficiently eliminates fetal bilirubin. Thus the hyperbilirubinemia of prematurity normally occurs in the postpartum period. Bupivacaine has been implicated as a possible cause of neonatal jaundice.[229,230] High affinity of the drug for fetal erythrocyte membranes may lead to a decrease in filterability and deformability, which may render red blood cells more prone to hemolysis.[230] However, increased bilirubin production has not been demonstrated in newborns whose mothers received bupivacaine for epidural anesthesia during labor and delivery.[231]

Greater total body water in the preterm fetus results in a greater volume of distribution for drugs. Thus, to achieve equal blood concentrations, the immature fetus must receive a greater amount of drug transplacentally than the mature fetus.

The decreased ability to metabolize or excrete drugs associated with prematurity is certainly not a universal phenomenon. One study of the pharmacokinetics of lidocaine in preterm newborns noted that plasma clearance was similar to that in the adult.[209]

During anesthesia for preterm labor, concerns about drug effects on the newborn are far less important than the prevention of asphyxia and trauma to the fetus. Indeed, *healthy* preterm fetal lambs tolerated clinically relevant plasma concentrations of lidocaine (e.g., approximately 1.5 μg/mL) as well as mature ones.[19,232]

Asphyxia

Circulatory adaptations important for fetal survival during asphyxia result in increased blood flow and oxygen delivery to vital organs (e.g., heart, brain, adrenal glands).[206] Little information about the effects of local anesthetics on these fetal responses exists. In one study, adaptation to asphyxia was unaffected in mature fetal lambs exposed to lidocaine.[206] In contrast, lidocaine adversely affected asphyxiated preterm fetal lambs, who experienced a further deterioration of acid-base status and a reduction in cardiac output and blood flow to the brain and heart (Figure 12-7).[233] In asphyxiated preterm fetal lambs, exposure to bupivacaine reduced blood flow to vital organs; however, fetal heart rate, blood pressure, and acid-base measurements did not change.[234]

After performing an in vitro study using perfused human placentae, Johnson et al.[235] suggested that bupivacaine might be preferable to lidocaine in the presence of fetal acidosis because the greater maternal protein binding of bupivacaine may limit its placental transfer. However, this methodology does not consider the potential for greater fetal tissue uptake of bupivacaine (compared with lidocaine) because of the fact that bupivacaine is more lipid-soluble and protein-bound than lidocaine.

Although the effects of bupivacaine appear less severe than those of lidocaine in asphyxiated preterm fetal lambs, limitations are inherent in a historical comparison of two studies performed 8 years apart.[233,234] Further, it is unclear whether these findings are applicable to humans. Both lidocaine and bupivacaine have enjoyed a long history of safe use in obstetric anesthesia, and prospective clinical studies are required before recommending one drug over the other.

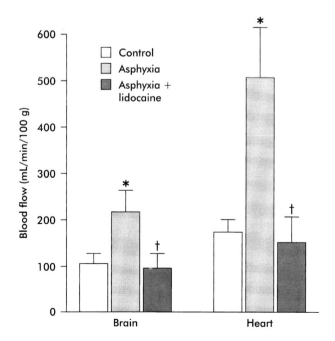

FIGURE 12-7. Blood flow to brain and heart in the preterm fetal lamb before and during asphyxia and during exposure to lidocaine while asphyxiated (mean ± SEM). *Significantly different from control. †Significantly different from asphyxia. (Modified from Morishima HO, Pedersen H, Santos AC, et al. Adverse effects of maternally administered lidocaine on the asphyxiated preterm fetal lamb. Anesthesiology 1989; 71:110-5.)

NEWER AMIDE LOCAL ANESTHETICS

In 1984, the FDA proscribed the use of the highest concentration of bupivacaine (0.75%) in pregnant women because of concerns regarding bupivacaine cardiotoxicity *(vide supra)*. Subsequently, many anesthesiologists have perceived a need for an alternative amide local anesthetic with the beneficial blocking properties of bupivacaine but a greater margin of safety. Two drugs may satisfy these requirements. Ropivacaine (Naropin, Astra) was approved for clinical use in 1994, and levobupivacaine (Chirocaine, Zeneca) was approved in 1999.

Chirality

With the exception of lidocaine, the commonly used amide local anesthetics are known as chiral compounds because they have a single asymmetric carbon adjacent to the amino group and thus exist in isomeric forms that are mirror images of each other. The direction in which the isomers rotate polarized light distinguishes them as either dextrorotary (D) or levorotary (L) isomers. This is important because individual isomers of the same drug may have different biologic effects. As a rule, the levorotary isomer has greater vasoconstrictor activity and a longer duration of action but less potential for systemic toxicity than the dextrorotary form of the same drug.[236] The reduction in systemic toxicity observed with administration of the levorotary isomers may be both drug- and concentration-dependent. For example, one study in isolated guinea pig hearts noted that bupivacaine isomers increased atrioventricular conduction time more than ropivacaine isomers did. In contrast to other measured variables, "atrioventricular conduction time showed evident stereoselectivity" for bupivacaine at the lowest concentration studied (0.5 uM) but only at much higher concentrations for ropivacaine (> 30 uM).[237]

In the past, single-isomer formulations have been costly to produce, and for that reason, local anesthetics used clinically have contained a racemic mixture of both the dextrorotary and levorotary forms of the drug. However, with improved techniques of selective extraction, commercially available single-isomer formulations of local anesthetic are now a reality.

Ropivacaine

Ropivacaine is a homolog of mepivacaine and bupivacaine, but unlike these other local anesthetics, it is formulated as a single levorotary isomer rather than as a racemic mixture. A propyl group on the pipechol ring distinguishes ropivacaine from bupivacaine (which has a butyl group) and mepivacaine (which has a methyl group).[238] Thus it is not surprising that the physicochemical characteristics of ropivacaine are intermediate between those of mepivacaine and bupivacaine. Ropivacaine is approximately 10 times less lipid soluble (N-heptane/buffer) than bupivacaine. This characteristic is important for two reasons.[238] First, it may result in slower penetration of ropivacaine into the large, heavily myelinated motor neurons, which may then result in less motor block than occurs with bupivacaine. Second, it raises questions as to whether ropivacaine truly is equipotent to bupivacaine. Indeed, a higher dose of ropivacaine is required to produce a sensory and motor block comparable to that produced by bupivacaine after spinal injection.[239,240] Similarly, the MLAC of epidural ropivacaine is almost twice as great as that of epidural bupivacaine in laboring women.[241] Critics of the use of MLAC argue that it provides no information on the shape and slope of the dose-effect relationship, which can vary with drug concentration, and further, that it provides no information on the effective clinical dose (ED_{95}).[242] Nonetheless, in clinical practice, ropivacaine appears to be less potent than bupivacaine during provision of epidural analgesia in laboring women.

PHARMACOKINETICS

In a recent study in sheep, we noted that pregnancy was associated with a smaller volume of distribution and a slower clearance of ropivacaine than occurs in nonpregnant animals.[24] However, the relationship between volume of distribution and clearance was such that the elimination half-life was similar in pregnant and nonpregnant animals.[24]

After intravenous injection in laboratory animals, the elimination half-life of ropivacaine is shorter than that of bupivacaine.[24,243] Similar findings have been described after intravenous injection in nonpregnant human volunteers.[244] The shorter elimination half-life of ropivacaine has been attributed to a faster clearance and a shorter mean residence time than that for bupivacaine.[24]

A clinical study demonstrated that the peak plasma concentration (C_{max}) after epidural administration of 0.5% ropivacaine or 0.5% bupivacaine for cesarean section was similar for the two drugs (1.3 µg/mL and 1.1 µg/mL, respectively).[245] The elimination half-life of ropivacaine was 5.2 ± 0.6 hours, which was shorter than that for bupivacaine (10.9 ± 1.1 hours).[245] No difference in clearance between the two drugs was noted.

Like bupivacaine, ropivacaine is metabolized by hepatic microsomal cytochrome P450. The major metabolite is 2,6 pipecolyxylidide and minor metabolites are 3′ and 4′ hydroxy-ropivacaine.[246]

Ropivacaine is highly bound (approximately 92%) to serum proteins but less so than bupivacaine (96%).[244] Indeed, at plasma concentrations occurring during epidural analgesia for cesarean section, the free fraction of ropivacaine is almost twice that of bupivacaine.[245] To our knowledge, no studies have compared the effects of pregnancy on the protein binding of ropivacaine in humans. However, in sheep, pregnancy is associated with a greater binding of ropivacaine (and bupivacaine) to serum proteins.[24]

SYSTEMIC TOXICITY

In perfused preparations of myocardium, ropivacaine is intermediate between bupivacaine and lidocaine in its depressant effect on cardiac excitation and conduction, as well as in its potential to induce reentrant type ventricular arrhythmias.[247] In dogs, the margin of safety between convulsive or lethal doses and plasma concentrations of drug is greater for ropivacaine than for bupivacaine but less than that for lidocaine.[248] The arrhythmogenicity of ropivacaine in pigs also is intermediate between that of lidocaine and bupivacaine.[249] In sheep, the ratio among fatal doses of bupivacaine, ropivacaine, and lidocaine is 1:2:9.[250]

Scott et al[251] administered intravenous infusions of ropivacaine and bupivacaine to human volunteers. Ropivacaine caused fewer CNS symptoms and was 25% less toxic than bupivacaine (as defined by the doses and plasma concentrations that were tolerated).

Progesterone does not increase myocardial sensitivity to ropivacaine.[252] Likewise, pregnancy does not enhance the systemic toxicity of ropivacaine in sheep.[50]

Most studies that have compared the systemic toxicity of ropivacaine and bupivacaine have used equal doses of each,

and, therefore, cannot resolve the controversy as to whether ropivacaine truly is less cardiotoxic or merely less potent than bupivacaine. This would be of concern only if greater doses of ropivacaine than bupivacaine were required to produce comparable regional blocks. Indeed, a recent study suggested that the MLAC of ropivacaine in women having epidural analgesia during labor is almost twice that for bupivacaine (vide supra).[241] If this is true, the need for a larger dose of ropivacaine could negate the expected benefits from its apparently wider margin of safety. Currently, this controversy remains unresolved. However, results of a recently published laboratory study demonstrated that ropivacaine produces less cardiotoxicity than bupivacaine, even when given at equipotent doses.[253]

UTERINE BLOOD FLOW

All local anesthetics can reduce uterine blood flow at plasma concentrations that greatly exceed those occurring during the routine practice of obstetric anesthesia.[101] There has been an added concern that the levorotary isomers of local anesthetics, which produce vasoconstriction at clinical doses,[254] may reduce uteroplacental perfusion and adversely affect fetal well-being. It is reassuring to note that ropivacaine, even at serum concentrations that are almost two times greater than would be expected to occur during clinical use, does not reduce uterine blood flow or affect fetal heart rate, blood pressure, or acid-base measurements in pregnant sheep.[103] In humans, Doppler velocimetry studies have shown that ropivacaine has little effect on the uteroplacental or fetal circulation when it is administered to provide epidural anesthesia for cesarean delivery.[113]

PLACENTAL TRANSFER

In vitro studies using perfused human placentae have found that the placental transfer of ropivacaine is similar to that for bupivacaine.[255] Intravenous infusion of ropivacaine or bupivacaine to pregnant sheep results in steady-state maternal plasma concentrations of 1.5 to 1.6 µg/mL and fetal concentrations of approximately 0.28 µg/mL.[103] Tissue concentrations of ropivacaine in fetal heart, brain, liver, lung, kidneys, and adrenals were similar to those for bupivacaine.[103] Datta et al[245] noted that the free fraction of ropivacaine at delivery was approximately twice that of bupivacaine in neonates whose mothers received the drug for epidural anesthesia during labor or cesarean delivery.

NEUROBEHAVIORAL EFFECTS

Some authors have reported that a greater proportion of neonates exposed to ropivacaine have a higher neonatal NACS than do similar infants exposed to bupivacaine administered epidurally during labor.[256] A meta-analysis of five published studies comparing ropivacaine and bupivacaine for epidural analgesia during labor also concluded that NACSs were better after the use of ropivacaine than after the use of bupivacaine.[257] In contrast, a recent prospective, randomized trial (which used a double-blind study design) found that NACSs were similar among infants exposed to ropivacaine or bupivacaine administered epidurally during labor.[258]

Levobupivacaine

Levobupivacaine also is a single levorotary isomer formulate of a local anesthetic. Preliminary evidence suggests that levobupivacaine causes fewer arrhythmias than the racemate. Valenzuela et al.[259] demonstrated that levobupivacaine caused less inhibition of inactivated sodium channels than either the dextrorotary or racemic drug. In comparison with dextrorotary and racemic bupivacaine, levobupivacaine resulted in less QRS widening and a lower frequency of malignant ventricular arrhythmias in isolated, perfused rabbit hearts.[260] Similarly, levobupivacaine produced less second-degree heart block and atrioventricular conduction delay than the other two forms of the drug in isolated perfused guinea pig hearts.[237]

In laboratory animals, the systemic toxicity of levobupivacaine is intermediate between that of bupivacaine and ropivacaine.[50] Unlike ropivacaine,[241] the MLAC of epidural levobupivacaine during labor is similar to that of bupivacaine.[261] Unfortunately, there is no single study that compares the MLAC of all three drugs. Altogether, published data and clinical experience suggest that any benefits from reduced risk of systemic toxicity with levobupivacaine are not obtained at the expense of efficacy. Pregnancy does not enhance the cardiotoxicity of levobupivacaine in sheep.[50] Clinically relevant serum concentrations of levobupivacaine had no adverse effect on uterine blood flow or fetal blood pressure, heart rate, or acid-base measurements in pregnant sheep.[103] Placental transfer[103] and fetal tissue uptake[103] of levobupivacaine were similar to those for bupivacaine and ropivacaine.

In obstetric practice, the clinical effects of epidural levobupivacaine are indistinguishable from epidural bupivacaine. Epidural administration of levobupivacaine 0.25% in laboring women results in sensory and motor block similar to that produced by epidural bupivacaine 0.25%.[262] The choice between bupivacaine and levobupivacaine does not affect the method of delivery or neonatal condition. For cesarean section, epidural levobupivacaine 0.5% is virtually identical to epidural bupivacaine 0.5%.[263]

The combined spinal-epidural (CSE) technique has become popular for analgesia during labor. Levobupivacaine may have a greater motor-sparing effect than bupivacaine when given for the initial intrathecal injection. For example, in one study, none of 37 women who received intrathecal levobupivacaine 2.5 mg (with sufentanil and epinephrine) had evidence of motor block. In contrast, 13 of 38 (34%) women given intrathecal bupivacaine 2.5 mg developed a Bromage-1 motor block.[264]

Conclusions

The availability of single levorotary isomers of a local anesthetic may be advantageous because these drugs have a greater margin of safety and blocking properties similar to bupivacaine, although at a higher cost. However, even before the introduction of these drugs, modifications in our clinical practice, such as appropriate use of an epidural test dose and fractionation of the therapeutic dose of local anesthetic, have made epidural anesthesia a very safe procedure.[58] Thus, it is difficult to predict with certainty the role that single isomers will assume in obstetric anesthesia practice. From the standpoint of systemic toxicity, their use may be more beneficial in parturients having a cesarean delivery, who require higher doses than those administered for analgesia during labor. Nonetheless, a greater margin of safety with these new drugs should be no substitute for proper technique.

KEY POINTS

- Pregnancy enhances the effect of local anesthetic agents.
- Appropriate administration of epidural anesthesia does not adversely affect uterine tone or uterine or umbilical blood flow.
- Repeated epidural injections of lidocaine may result in a greater accumulation of drug in women with preeclampsia than in healthy pregnant women.
- Bupivacaine has greater cardiotoxicity than lidocaine because of its greater electrophysiologic effects, which predispose to ventricular arrhythmias.
- Alkalinization of a local anesthetic solution shortens the latency of neural blockade but increases the risk of hypotension during administration of epidural anesthesia.
- Fetal acidosis results in a greater accumulation of amide local anesthetic in the fetus.
- Local anesthetics, as used clinically, are not teratogenic.
- The elimination half-life of amide local anesthetics is longer in the newborn than in the adult because the former has a greater volume of distribution.
- The fetus and newborn seem to be no more vulnerable to the toxic effects of local anesthetics than the adult.
- Neonatal neurobehavior depends on many factors other than the choice of local anesthetic.
- Single (levorotary) isomer formulations of amide local anesthetics, such as ropivacaine and levobupivacaine, have a lower potential for cardiotoxicity than racemic bupivacaine.

REFERENCES

1. Moore DC. The pH of local anesthetic solutions. Anesth Analg 1981; 60:833-4.
2. Strichartz GR. The inhibition of sodium currents in myelinated nerve by quaternary derivatives of lidocaine. J Gen Physiol 1973; 62:37-57.
3. Strichartz GR, Ritchie JM. The action of local anesthetics on ion channels of excitable tissues. In Strichartz GR, editor. Local Anesthetics, Handbook of Experimental Pharmacology. Berlin, Springer-Verlag, 1987:21.
4. Bromage PR. Continuous lumbar epidural analgesia for obstetrics. Can Med Assoc J 1961; 85:1136-40.
5. Fagraeus L, Urban BJ, Bromage PR. Spread of epidural analgesia in early pregnancy. Anesthesiology 1983; 58:184-7.
6. Butterworth JF, Walker FO, Lyzak SZ. Pregnancy increases median nerve susceptibility to lidocaine. Anesthesiology 1990; 72:962-5.
7. Datta S, Lambert DH, Gregus J, et al. Differential sensitivities of mammalian nerve fibers during pregnancy. Anesth Analg 1983; 62:1070-2.
8. Bader AM, Datta S, Moller RA, Covino BG. Acute progesterone treatment has no effect on bupivacaine-induced conduction blockade in the isolated rabbit vagus nerve. Anesth Analg 1990; 71:545-8.
9. Dautenhahn DL, Fagraeus L. Acid-base changes of spinal fluid during pregnancy (abstract). Anesth Analg 1984; 63:204.
10. O'Brien JE, Abbey V, Hinsvark O, et al. Metabolism and measurement of chloroprocaine, an ester-type local anesthetic. J Pharm Sci 1979; 68:75-8.
11. Kuhnert BR, Kuhnert PM, Philipson EH, et al. The half-life of 2-chloroprocaine. Anesth Analg 1986; 65:273-8.
12. Monedero P, Hess P. High epidural block with chloroprocaine in a parturient with low pseudocholinesterase. Can J Anaesth 2001; 48:318-20.

13. Bloedow DC, Ralston DH, Hargrove JC. Lidocaine pharmacokinetics in pregnant and nonpregnant sheep. J Pharm Sci 1980; 69:32-7.

14. Santos AC, Pedersen H, Morishima HO, et al. Pharmacokinetics of lidocaine in nonpregnant and pregnant ewes. Anesth Analg 1988; 67:1154-8.

15. Rutten AJ, Mather LE, Plummer JL, Henning EC. Postoperative course of plasma protein binding of lignocaine, ropivacaine, and bupivacaine in sheep. J Pharm Pharmacol 1992; 44:355-8.

16. Downing JW, Johnson HV, Gonzalez HP, et al. The pharmacokinetics of epidural lidocaine and bupivacaine during cesarean section. Anesth Analg 1997; 84:527-32.

17. Kuhnert BR, Knapp DR, Kuhnert PM, Prochaska AL. Maternal, fetal, and neonatal metabolism of lidocaine. Clin Pharmacol Ther 1979; 26:213-30.

18. Kuhnert BR, Philipson EH, Pimental R, et al. Lidocaine disposition in mother, fetus, and neonate after spinal anesthesia. Anesth Analg 1986; 65:139-44.

19. Pedersen H, Santos AC, Morishima HO, et al. Does gestational age affect the pharmacokinetics and pharmacodynamics of lidocaine in mother and fetus? Anesthesiology 1988; 68:367-72.

20. Wood M, Wood AJJ. Changes in plasma drug binding and alpha$_1$-acid glycoprotein in mother and newborn infant. Clin Pharmacol Ther 1981; 29:522-6.

21. Fragneto RY, Bader AM, Rosinia F, et al. Measurements of protein binding of lidocaine throughout pregnancy. Anesth Analg 1994; 79: 295-7.

22. Pihlajamäki K, Kanto J, Lindberg R, et al. Extradural administration of bupivacaine: Pharmacokinetics and metabolism in pregnant and nonpregnant women. Br J Anaesth 1990; 64:556-62.

23. Tucker GT, Mather LE. Clinical pharmacokinetics of local anesthetics. Clin Pharmacokinet 1979; 4:241-78.

24. Santos AC, Arthur GR, Lehning EJ, Finster M. Comparative pharmacokinetics of ropivacaine and bupivacaine in nonpregnant and pregnant ewes. Anesth Analg 1997; 85:87-93.

25. Kuhnert PM, Kuhnert BR, Stitts JM, Gross TL. The use of a selected ion monitoring technique to study the disposition of bupivacaine in mother, fetus and neonate following epidural anesthesia for cesarean section. Anesthesiology 1981; 55:611-7.

26. Reynolds F, Taylor G. Maternal and neonatal blood concentrations of bupivacaine: A comparison with lignocaine during continuous extradural analgesia. Anaesthesia 1970; 25:14-23.

27. Mather LE, Thomas J. Bupivacaine binding to plasma protein fractions. J Pharmacol Pharm 1978; 30:653.

28. Wulf H, Münstedt P, Maier C. Plasma protein binding of bupivacaine in pregnant women at term. Acta Anaesth Scand 1991; 35:129-33.

29. Pelkonen O, Puurunen J. The effect of cimetidine on in vitro and in vivo microsomal drug metabolism in the rat. Biochem Pharmacol 1980; 29:3075-80.

30. Abernethy DR, Greenblatt DJ, Eshelman FN, Shader RI. Ranitidine does not impair oxidative or conjugative metabolism: Noninteraction with antipyrine, diazepam, and lorazepam. Clin Pharmacol Ther 1984; 35:188-92.

31. Reimann IW, Klotz U, Frolich JC. Effects of cimetidine and ranitidine on steady-state propanolol kinetics and dynamics. Clin Pharmacol Ther 1982; 32:749-57.

32. Dailey PA, Hughes SC, Rosen MA, et al. Effect of cimetidine and ranitidine on lidocaine concentrations during epidural anesthesia for cesarean section. Anesthesiology 1988; 69:1013-7.

33. Brashear WT, Zuspan KJ, Lazebnik N, et al. Effect of ranitidine on bupivacaine disposition. Anesth Analg 1991; 72:369-76.

34. Ramanathan J, Bottorff M, Jeter JN, et al. The pharmacokinetics and maternal and neonatal effects of epidural lidocaine in preeclampsia. Anesth Analg 1986; 65:120-6.

35. Debon R, Chassard D, Duflo F, et al. Chronobiology of epidural ropivacaine. Variation in the duration of action related to the hour of administration. Anesthesiology 2002; 96:542-5.

36. de Jong RH, Robles R, Corbin RW. Central actions of lidocaine-synaptic transmission. Anesthesiology 1969; 30:19-23.

37. Liu PL, Feldman HS, Giasi R, et al. Comparative CNS toxicity of lidocaine, etidocaine, bupivacaine, and tetracaine in awake dogs following rapid intravenous administration. Anesth Analg 1983; 62:375-9.

38. Scott DB. Evaluation of the toxicity of local anaesthetic agents in man. Br J Anaesth 1975; 47:56-60.

39. Covino BG, Vassallo HG. Local Anesthetics: Mechanisms of Action and Clinical Use. New York, Grune & Stratton, 1976:126.

40. Englesson S. The influence of acid-base changes on central nervous system toxicity of local anaesthetic agents. I. Acta Anaesthesiol Scand 1974; 18:79-87.

41. Englesson S, Grevsten S. The influence of acid-base changes on central nervous system toxicity of local anaesthetic agents. II. Acta Anaesthesiol Scand 1974; 18:88-103.

42. Burney RG, Di Fazio CA, Foster JA. Effects of pH on protein binding of lidocaine. Anesth Analg 1978; 57:478-80.

43. De Jong RH, Ronfeld RA, De Rosa RA. Cardiovascular effects of convulsant and supraconvulsant doses of amide local anesthetics. Anesth Analg 1982; 61:3-9.

44. Morishima HO, Finster M, Arthur GR, Covino BG. Pregnancy does not alter lidocaine toxicity. Am J Obstet Gynecol 1990; 162:1320-4.

45. Santos AC, Pedersen H, Harmon TW, et al. Does pregnancy alter the systemic toxicity of local anesthetics? Anesthesiology 1989; 70:991-5.

46. Morishima HO, Pedersen H, Finster M, et al. Bupivacaine toxicity in pregnant and nonpregnant ewes. Anesthesiology 1985; 63:134-9.

47. Clarkson CW, Hondeghem LM. Mechanism for bupivacaine depression of cardiac conduction: Fast block of sodium channels during the action potential with slow recovery from block during diastole. Anesthesiology 1985; 62:396-405.

48. Thomas RD, Behbehani MM, Coyle DE, Denson DD. Cardiovascular toxicity of local anesthetics: An alternative hypothesis. Anesth Analg 1986; 65:444-50.

49. Coyle DE, Porembka DT, Sehlhorst CS, et al. Echocardiographic evaluation of bupivacaine cardiotoxicity. Anesth Analg 1994; 79:335-9.

50. Santos AC, DeArmas P. Systemic toxicity of levobupivacaine, bupivacaine and ropivacaine during continuous intravenous infusion to nonpregnant and pregnant ewes. Anesthesiology 2001; 95:1256-64.

51. Bucklin BA, Warner DS, Choi WW, et al. Pregnancy does not alter the threshold for lidocaine-induced seizures in the rat. Anesth Analg 1992; 74:57-61.

52. Kim YJ, McFarlane C, Warner DS, et al. The effect of plasma and brain magnesium concentrations on lidocaine-induced seizures in the rat. Anesth Analg 1996; 83:1223-8.

53. Albright GA. Cardiac arrest following regional anesthesia with etidocaine and bupivacaine. Anesthesiology 1979; 51:285-7.

54. Marx GF. Cardiotoxicity of local anesthetics: The plot thickens (editorial). Anesthesiology 1984; 60:3-5.

55. Kasten GW, Martin ST. Resuscitation from bupivacaine-induced cardiovascular toxicity during partial inferior vena cava occlusion. Anesth Analg 1986; 65:341-4.

56. Moller RA, Datta S, Fox J, et al. Effects of progesterone on the cardiac electrophysiologic action of bupivacaine and lidocaine. Anesthesiology 1992; 76:604-8.

57. Moller R, Datta S, Strichartz GR. Beta-estradiol acutely potentiates the depression of cardiac excitability by lidocaine and bupivacaine. J Cardiovasc Pharmacol 1999; 34:718-27.

58. Hawkins JL, Koonin LM, Palmer SK, et al. Anesthesia-related deaths during obstetric delivery in the United States, 1979-1990. Anesthesiology 1997; 86:277-84.

59. De Jong RH, Bonin JD. Benzodiazepines protect mice from local anesthetic convulsions and deaths. Anesth Analg 1981; 60:385-9.

60. Rosen MA, Thigpen JW, Shnider SM, et al. Bupivacaine-induced cardiotoxicity in hypoxic and acidotic sheep. Anesth Analg 1985; 64:1089-96.

61. Marx GF. Cardiopulmonary resuscitation of late-pregnant women. Anesthesiology 1982; 56:156.

62. Feldman HS, Arthur GR, Pitkanen M, et al. Treatment of acute systemic toxicity after the rapid intravenous injection of ropivacaine and bupivacaine in the conscious dog. Anesth Analg 1991; 73:373-84.

63. Saitoh K, Hirabayashi Y, Shimizu R, Fukuda H. Amrinone is superior to epinephrine in reversing bupivacaine-induced cardiovascular depression in sevoflurane-anesthetized dogs. Anesthesiology 1995; 83:127-33.

64. Lindgren L, Randell T, Suzuki N, et al. The effect of amrinone on recovery from severe bupivacaine intoxication in pigs. Anesthesiology 1992; 77:309-15.

65. Kasten GW, Martin ST. Bupivacaine cardiovascular toxicity: Comparison of treatment with bretylium and lidocaine. Anesth Analg 1985; 64:911-6.

66. Haasio J, Pitkanen MT, Kytta J, Rosenberg PH. Treatment of bupivacaine-induced cardiac arrhythmias in hypoxic and hypercarbic pigs with amiodarone or bretylium. Reg Anesth 1990; 15:174-9.

67. Smith WM, Gallagher JJ. "Les torsades de pointes": An unusual ventricular arrhythmia. Ann Intern Med 1980; 93:578-84.

68. Kennedy RL, Miller RP, Bell JU, et al. Uptake and distribution of bupivacaine in fetal lambs. Anesthesiology 1986; 65:247-53.

69. Kennedy RL, Bell JU, Miller RP, et al. Uptake and distribution of lidocaine in fetal lambs. Anesthesiology 1990; 72:483-9.

70. Covino BG, Marx GF, Finster M, Zsigmond EK. Prolonged sensory/motor deficits following inadvertent spinal anesthesia. Anesth Analg 1980; 59:399-400.

71. Barsa J, Batra M, Fink BR, Sumi SM. A comparative in vivo study of local neurotoxicity of lidocaine, bupivacaine, 2-chloroprocaine, and a mixture of 2-chloroprocaine and bupivacaine. Anesth Analg 1982; 61:961-7.

72. Ready LB, Plumer MH, Haschke RH, et al. Neurotoxicity of intrathecal local anesthetics in rabbits. Anesthesiology 1985; 63:364-70.

73. Gissen AJ, Datta S, Lambert D. The chloroprocaine controversy. II. Is chloroprocaine neurotoxic? Reg Anesth 1984; 9:135-45.

74. Fibuch EE, Opper SE. Back pain following epidurally administered Nesacaine-MPF. Anesth Analg 1989; 69:113-5.

75. Taniguchi M, Bollen AW, Drasner K. Sodium bisulfite: Scapegoat for chloroprocaine neurotoxicity? Anesthesiology 2004; 100: 85-91.

76. Rigler ML, Drasner K, Krejcie TC, et al. Cauda equina syndrome after continuous spinal anesthesia. Anesth Analg 1991; 72:275-81.

77. Schell RM, Braner FS, Cole DJ, Applegate RL II. Persistent sacral nerve root deficits after continuous spinal anaesthesia. Can J Anesth 1991; 38:908-11.

78. Schneider M, Ettlin T, Kaufman M, et al. Transient neurologic toxicity after hyperbaric subarachnoid anesthesia with 5% lidocaine. Anesth Analg 1993; 76:1154-7.

79. Lundy JS, Essex HE, Kernohan JW. Experiments with anesthetics: IV lesions produced in the spinal cord of dogs by a dose of procaine hydrochloride sufficient to cause permanent and fatal paralysis. JAMA 1933; 101:1546-50.

80. Bainton CR, Strichartz GR. Concentration dependence of lidocaine-induced irreversible conduction loss in frog sciatic nerve. Anesthesiology 1994; 81:657-67.

81. Lambert LA, Lambert DH, Strichartz GR. Irreversible conduction block in isolated nerve by high concentrations of local anesthetics. Anesthesiology 1994; 80:1082-93.

82. Li DF, Bahar M, Cole G, Rosen M. Neurological toxicity of the subarachnoid infusion of bupivacaine, lignocaine or 2-chloroprocaine in the rat. Br J Anaesth 1985; 57:424-9.

83. Dripps RD, Vandam LD. Long-term follow-up of patients who received 10,098 spinal anesthetics: Failure to discover major neurological sequelae. JAMA 1954; 156:1486-91.

84. Liguori GA, Zayas VM, Chisholm MF. Transient neurologic symptoms after spinal anesthesia with mepivacaine and lidocaine. Anesthesiology 1998; 88:619-23.

85. Hampl KF, Heinzmann-Wiedmer S, Luginbuehl I, et al. Transient neurologic symptoms after spinal anesthesia: A lower incidence with prilocaine and bupivacaine than with lidocaine. Anesthesiology 1998; 88:629-33.

86. Freedman JM, DeKun L, Drasner K, et al. Transient neurologic symptoms after spinal anesthesia. An epidemiologic survey. Anesthesiology 1998; 89:633-41.

87. Aouad MT, Siddik SS, Jalbout MI, Baraka AS. Does pregnancy protect against intrathecal lidocaine-induced transient neurologic symptoms? Anesthesiology 2001; 92:401-4.

88. Philip J, Sharma SK, Gottumukkala VNR, et al. Transient neurologic symptoms after spinal anesthesia with lidocaine in obstetric patients. Anesth Analg 2001; 92:405-9.

89. Brown DT, Beamish D, Wildsmith JAW. Allergic reactions to an amide local anaesthetic. Br J Anaesth 1981; 53:435-7.

90. Simon RA. Adverse reactions to drug additives. J Allergy Clin Immunol 1984; 74:623-30.

91. Incaudo G, Shatz M, Patterson R. Administration of local anesthetics to patients with a history of prior adverse reaction. J Allergy Clin Immunol 1978; 6l:339-45.

92. Chandler MJ, Grammer LC, Patterson R. Provocative challenge with local anesthetics in patients with a prior history of reaction. J Allergy Clin Immunol 1987; 79:883-6.

93. Palmer CM, Voulgaropoulos D. Management of the parturient with a history of local anesthetic allergy. Anesth Analg 1993; 77:625-8.

94. Fisher M. Intradermal testing after anaphylactoid reaction to anaesthetic drugs: Practical aspects of performance and interpretation. Anaesth Intens Care 1984; 12:115-20.

95. Levy JH. Anaphylactic Reactions in Anesthesia and Intensive Care. Stoneham, Mass, Butterworth-Heineman, 1992:115.

96. Magness RR, Rosenfeld CR. Mechanisms for attenuated pressor responses to α-agonists in ovine pregnancy. Am J Obstet Gynecol 1988; 159:252-61.

97. Zucker-Pinchoff B, Ramanathan S. Anaphylactic reaction to epidural fentanyl. Anesthesiology 1989; 71:599-601.

98. Teramo K. Effects of obstetrical paracervical blockade on the fetus. Acta Obstet Gynecol Scand 1971; 51(suppl 16):6-55.

99. Cibils LA. Response of human uterine arteries to local anesthetics. Am J Obstet Gynecol 1976; 126:202-10.

100. Norén H, Lindblom B, Källfelt B. Effects of bupivacaine and calcium antagonists on human uterine arteries in pregnant and non-pregnant women. Acta Anaesthesiol Scand 1991; 35:488-91.

101. Fishburne JI, Greiss FC, Hopkinson R, Rhyne AL. Responses of the gravid uterine vasculature to arterial levels of local anesthetic agents. Am J Obstet Gynecol 1979; 133:753-61.

102. Biehl D, Shnider SM, Levinson G, Callender K. The direct effects of circulating lidocaine on uterine blood flow and foetal well-being in the pregnant ewe. Can Anaesth Soc J 1977; 24:445-51.

103. Santos AC, Karpel B, Noble G. The placental transfer and fetal effects of levobupivacaine, racemic bupivacaine and ropivacaine. Anesthesiology 1999; 90:1698-703.

104. Chestnut DH, Weiner CP, Herrig JE. The effect of intravenously administered 2-chloroprocaine upon uterine artery blood flow velocity in gravid guinea pigs. Anesthesiology 1989; 70:305-8.

105. Gintautas J, Kraynack B, Havasi G, et al. Responses of isolated uterine arteries to local anesthetic agents. Proc West Pharmacol Soc 1981; 24:191-2.

106. Gintautas J, Kraynack BJ, Warren PR, et al. Effects of adenine nucleotides on lidocaine induced contractions in isolated uterine artery. Proc West Pharmacol Soc 1980; 23:299-300.

107. Hollmén AI, Jouppila R, Jouppila P, et al. Effect of extradural analgesia using bupivacaine and 2-chloroprocaine on intervillous blood flow during normal labour. Br J Anaesth 1982; 54:837-41.

108. Husemeyer RP, Crawley JCW. Placental intervillous blood flow measured by inhaled ^{133}Xe clearance in relation to induction of epidural analgesia. Br J Obstet Gynaecol 1979; 86:426-31.

109. Huovinen K, Lehtovirta P, Forss M, et al. Changes in placental intervillous blood flow measured by the ^{133}Xenon method during lumbar epidural block for elective caesarean section. Acta Anaesthesiol Scand 1979; 23:529-33.

110. Giles WB, Lah FX, Trudinger BJ. The effect of epidural anaesthesia for caesarean section on maternal uterine and fetal umbilical artery blood flow velocity waveforms. Br J Obstet Gynaecol 1987; 94:55-9.

111. Morrow RJ, Rolbin SH, Ritchie JWK, Haley S. Epidural anaesthesia and blood flow velocity in mother and fetus. Can J Anaesth 1989; 36:519-22.

112. Alahuhta S, Räsänen J, Jouppila P, et al. Effects of extradural bupivacaine with adrenaline for caesarean section on uteroplacental and fetal circulation. Br J Anaesth 1991; 67:678-82.

113. Alahuhta S, Räsänen J, Jouppila P, et al. The effects of epidural ropivacaine and bupivacaine for cesarean section on uteroplacental and fetal circulation. Anesthesiology 1995; 83:23-32.

114. Tuvemo T, Willdeck-Lund G. Smooth muscle effects of lidocaine, prilocaine, bupivacaine and etidocaine on the human umbilical artery. Acta Anaesthesiol Scand 1982; 26:104-7.

115. Norén H, Källfelt B, Lindblom B. Influence of bupivacaine and morphine on human umbilical arteries and veins in vitro. Acta Obstet Gynecol Scand 1990; 69:87-91.

116. Halevy S, Monuszko E, Freese KJ, Altura BM. Local anesthetics interaction with hypoxia, hypercarbia-induced acidosis and histamine on umbilical vascular reactivity (abstract). Anesthesiology 1988; 69:A673.

117. Morishima HO, Heymann MA, Rudolph AM, et al. Transfer of lidocaine across the sheep placenta to the fetus: Hemodynamic and acid-base responses of the fetal lamb. Am J Obstet Gynecol 1975; 122:581-8.

118. Trudinger BJ, Giles WB, Cook CM. Uteroplacental blood flow velocity: Time waveforms in normal and complicated pregnancy. Br J Obstet Gynaecol 1985; 92:39-45.

119. Marx GF, Elstein ID, Schuss M, et al. Effects of epidural block with lignocaine and lignocaine-adrenaline on umbilical artery velocity waveform ratios. Br J Obstet Gynaecol 1990; 97:517-20.

120. Marx GF, Patel S, Berman JA, et al. Umbilical blood flow velocity waveforms in different maternal positions and with epidural analgesia. Obstet Gynecol 1986; 68:61-4.

121. Lindlad A, Marsál K, Vernersson E, Renck H. Fetal circulation during epidural analgesia for caesarean section. Br Med J 1984; 288:1329-30.

122. McGaughey HS, Corey EL, Eastwood D, Thornton WN. Effect of synthetic anesthetics on the spontaneous motility of human uterine muscle in vitro. Obstet Gynecol 1962; 19:233-40.

123. Morishima HO, Covino BG, Yeh MN, et al. Bradycardia in the fetal baboon following paracervical block anesthesia. Am J Obstet Gynecol 198l; 140:775-80.

124. Belitzky R, Delrad LG, Novick LM. Oxytocic effect of intramyometrial injection of procaine in a prcgnant woman. Am J Obstet Gynecol 1970; 107:973-5.

125. Collins JG, Kitahata LM, Matsumoto M, et al. Spinally administered epinephrine suppresses noxiously evoked activity of WDR neurons in the dorsal horn of the spinal cord. Anesthesiology 1984; 60:269-75.

126. Polley LS, Columb MO, Naughton NN, et al. Effect of epidural epinephrine on minimum local analgesic concentration of epidural bupivacaine in labor. Anesthesiology 2002; 96:1123-8.

127. Hood DD, Dewan DM, James FM. Maternal and fetal effects of epinephrine in gravid ewes. Anesthesiology 1986; 64:610-3.

128. Chestnut DH, Weiner CP, Martin JG, et al. Effect of intravenous epinephrine upon uterine artery blood flow velocity in the pregnant guinea pig. Anesthesiology 1986; 65:633-6.

129. Jouppila R, Jouppila P, Hollmén A, Kuikka J. Effect of segmental extradural analgesia on placental blood flow during normal labour. Br J Anaesth 1978; 50:563-7.

130. Albright GA, Jouppila R, Hollmén AI, et al. Epinephrine does not alter human intervillous blood flow during epidural anesthesia. Anesthesiology 1981; 54:131-5.

131. Morrow RJ, Rolbin SH, Ritchie JWK, Haley S. Epidural anaesthesia and blood flow velocity in mother and fetus. Can J Anaesth 1989; 36:519-22.

132. Gunther RE, Bauman J. Obstetrical caudal anesthesia. I. A randomized study comparing 1% mepivacaine with 1% lidocaine plus epinephrine. Anesthesiology 1969; 31:5-19.

133. Gunther RE, Bellville JW. Obstetrical caudal anesthesia. II. A randomized study comparing 1 percent mepivacaine with 1 percent mepivacaine plus epinephrine. Anesthesiology 1972; 37:288-98.

134. Craft JB, Epstein BS, Coakley CS. Effect of lidocaine with epinephrine versus lidocaine (plain) on induced labor. Anesth Analg 1972; 51:243-6.

135. Matadial L, Cibils LA. The effect of epidural anesthesia on uterine activity and blood pressure. Am J Obstet Gynecol 1976; 125:846-54.

136. Abboud TK, David S, Nagappala S, et al. Maternal, fetal, and neonatal effects of lidocaine with and without epinephrine for epidural anesthesia in obstetrics. Anesth Analg 1984; 63:973-9.

137. Abboud TK, Sheik-ol-Eslam A, Yanagi T, et al. Safety and efficacy of epinephrine added to bupivacaine for lumbar epidural analgesia in obstetrics. Anesth Analg 1985; 64:585-91.

138. Abboud TK, Reyes A, Steffens Z, et al. Bupivacaine/butorphanol/epinephrine for epidural anesthesia in obstetrics: Maternal and neonatal effects. Reg Anesth 1989; 14:219-24.

139. Veille JC, Youngstrom P, Kanaan C, Wilson B. Human umbilical artery flow velocity waveforms before and after regional anesthesia for cesarean section. Obstet Gynecol 1988; 72:890-3.

140. McLintic AJ, Danskin FH, Reid JA, Thorburn J. Effect of adrenaline on extradural anaesthesia, plasma lignocaine concentrations and the fetoplacental unit during elective caesarean section. Br J Anaesth 1991; 67:683-9.

141. Grant GJ, Ramanathan S, Turndorf H. The maternal hemodynamic effects of bupivacaine-epinephrine mixture used for obstetrical anesthesia. Acta Anaesthesiol Scand 1990; 34:543-7.

142. Berrada R, Chassard D, Bryssine S, et al. Effects in vitro de l'alcalinisation de la bupivacaine, 0.25%, et de la lidocaine, 2%. Ann Fr Anesth Reanim 1994; 13:165-8.

143. Di Fazio CA, Carron H, Grosslight KR, et al. Comparison of pH-adjusted lidocaine solutions for epidural anesthesia. Anesth Analg 1986; 65:760-4.

144. Capogna G, Celleno D, Varrassi G, et al. Epidural mepivacaine for cesarean section: Effects of a pH-adjusted solution. J Clin Anesth 1991; 3:211-5.

145. Ackerman WE, Juneja MM, Denson DD, et al. The effect of pH and PCO_2 on epidural analgesia with 2% 2-chloroprocaine. Anesth Analg 1989; 68:593-8.

146. Chestnut DH, Geiger M, Bates JN, Choi WW. The influence of pH-adjusted 2-chloroprocaine on the quality and duration of subsequent epidural bupivacaine during labor: A randomized, double-blind study. Anesthesiology 1989; 70:437-41.

147. Ackerman WE, Denson DD, Juneja MM, et al. Alkalinization of chloroprocaine for epidural anesthesia: Effects of PCO_2 at constant pH. Reg Anesth 1990; 15:89-93.

148. Gaggero G, Meyer O, VanGessel E, Rifal K. Alkalinization of lidocaine 2% does not influence the quality of epidural anaesthesia for elective caesarean section. Can J Anaesth 1995; 42:1080-4.

149. McMorland GH, Douglas MJ, Jeffrey WK, et al. Effect of pH-adjustment of bupivacaine on onset and duration of epidural analgesia in parturients. Can Anaesth Soc J 1986; 33:537-41.

150. Tackley RM, Coe AJ. Alkalinized bupivacaine and adrenaline for epidural caesarean section: A comparison with 0.5% bupivacaine. Anaesthesia 1988; 43:1019-21.

151. Benhamou D, Labaille T, Bonhomme L, Perrachon N. Alkalinization of epidural 0.5% bupivacaine for cesarean section. Reg Anesth 1989; 14:240-3.

152. Parnass SM, Curran MJA, Becker GL. Incidence of hypotension associated with epidural anesthesia using alkalinized and nonalkalinized lidocaine for cesarean section. Anesth Analg 1987; 66:1148-50.

153. Polley LS, Columb MO, Wagner DS, Naughton NN. Dose-dependent reduction of the minimum local analgesic concentration of bupivacaine by sufentanil for epidural analgesia in labor. Anesthesiology 1998; 89:626-32.

154. Polley LS, Columb MO, Naughton NN, et al. Effect of intravenous versus epidural fentanyl on the minimum local analgesic concentration of epidural bupivacaine in labor. Anesthesiology 2000; 93:122-8.

155. Camann WR, Hartigan PM, Gilbertson LI, et al. Chloroprocaine antagonism of epidural opioid analgesia: A receptor-specific phenomenon? Anesthesiology 1990; 73:860-3.

156. Grice SG, Eisenach JC, Dewan DM. Labor analgesia with epidural bupivacaine plus fentanyl: Enhancement with epinephrine and inhibition with 2-chloroprocaine. Anesthesiology 1990; 72:623-8.

157. Malinow AM, Mokriski BLK, Wakefield ML, et al. Does pH adjustment reverse Nesacaine antagonism of post cesarean epidural fentanyl analgesia (abstract)? Anesth Analg 1988; 67:S137.

158. Hughes SC, Wright RG, Murphy D, et al. The effect of pH adjusting 3% 2-chloroprocaine on the quality of post-cesarean section analgesia with epidural morphine (abstract). Anesthesiology 1988; 69:A689.

159. Cohen SE, Thurlow A. Comparison of a chloroprocaine-bupivacaine mixture with chloroprocaine and bupivacaine used individually for obstetric epidural analgesia. Anesthesiology 1979; 51:288-92.

160. Corke BC, Carlson CG, Dettbarn WD. The influence of 2-chloroprocaine on the subsequent analgesic potency of bupivacaine. Anesthesiology 1984; 60:25-7.

161. Mirkin BL. Maternal and fetal distribution of drugs in pregnancy. Clin Pharmacol Ther 1973; 14:643-7.

162. Tucker GT, Mather LE. Properties, absorption, and disposition of local anesthetic agents. In Cousins MJ, Bridenbaugh PO, editors. Neural Blockade in Clinical Anesthesia and Management of Pain, 2nd ed. Philadelphia, Lippincott, 1988:49.

163. Brown WU, Bell GC, Alper MH. Acidosis, local anesthetics and the newborn. Obstet Gynecol 1976; 48:27-30.

164. Biehl D, Shnider SM, Levinson G, Callender K. Placental transfer of lidocaine: Effects of fetal acidosis. Anesthesiology 1978; 48:409-12.

165. Morishima HO, Covino BG. Toxicity and distribution of lidocaine in nonasphyxiated and asphyxiated baboon fetuses. Anesthesiology 1981; 54:182-6.

166. Hamshaw-Thomas A, Rogerson N, Reynolds F. Transfer of bupivacaine, lignocaine and pethidine across the rabbit placenta: Influence of maternal protein binding and fetal flow. Placenta 1984; 5:61-70.

167. Hamshaw-Thomas A, Reynolds F. Placental transfer of bupivacaine, pethidine and lignocaine in the rabbit: Effect of umbilical flow rate and protein content. Br J Obstet Gynaecol 1985; 92:706-13.

168. Tucker GT. Plasma binding and disposition of local anesthetics. Int Anesth Clin 1975; 13:33-59.

169. Vella ML, Knott C, Reynolds F. Transfer of fentanyl across the rabbit placenta. Br J Anaesth 1986; 58:49-54.

170. Petersen MC, Moore RG, Nation RL, McMeniman W. Relationship between the transplacental gradients of bupivacaine and alpha$_1$-acid glycoprotein. Br J Clin Pharmacol 1981; 12:859-62.

171. Thomas J, Long G, Moore G, Morgan D. Plasma protein binding and placental transfer of bupivacaine. Clin Pharmacol Ther 1976; 19:426-34.

172. Petrie RH, Paul WL, Miller FC, et al. Placental transfer of lidocaine following paracervical block. Am J Obstet Gynecol 1974; 120:791-801.

173. Mazze RI, Dunbar RW. Plasma lidocaine concentrations after caudal, lumbar epidural, axillary block and intravenous regional anesthesia. Anesthesiology 1966; 27:574-9.

174. Giasi RM, D'Agostino E, Covino BG. Absorption of lidocaine following subarachnoid and epidural administration. Anesth Analg 1979; 58:360-3.

175. Brown WU, Bell GC, Lurie AO, et al. Newborn levels of lidocaine and mepivacaine in the first postnatal day following maternal epidural anesthesia. Anesthesiology 1975; 42:698-702.

176. Tucker GT, Mather LE. Properties, absorption, and disposition of local anesthetic agents. In Cousins MJ, Bridenbaugh PO, editors. Neural Blockade in Clinical Anesthesia and Management of Pain, 2nd ed. Philadelphia, Lippincott, 1988:74.

177. Reynolds F, Taylor G. Plasma concentrations of bupivacaine during continuous epidural analgesia in labour: The effect of adrenaline. Br J Anaesth 1971; 43:436-9.

178. Reynolds F, Laishley R, Morgan B, Lee A. Effect of time and adrenaline on the feto-maternal distribution of bupivacaine. Br J Anaesth 1989; 62:509-14.

179. Beazley JM, Taylor G, Reynolds F. Placental transfer of bupivacaine after paracervical block. Obstet Gynecol 1972; 39:2-6.

180. Denson DD, Bridenbaugh PO, Turner PA, et al. Neural blockade and pharmacokinetics following subarachnoid lidocaine in the Rhesus monkey. I. Effects of epinephrine. Anesth Analg 1982; 61:746-50.

181. Laishley RS, Carson RJ, Reynolds F. Effect of adrenaline on placental transfer of bupivacaine in the perfused in situ rabbit placenta. Br J Anaesth 1989; 63:439-43.

182. Abboud TK, Kim KC, Noueihed R, et al. Epidural bupivacaine, chloro-procaine, or lidocaine for cesarean section: Maternal and neonatal effects. Anesth Analg 1983; 62:914-9.

183. Thomas J, Climie CR, Long G, Nighjoy LE. The influence of adrena-line on the maternal plasma levels and placental transfer of ligno-caine following lumbar epidural administration. Br J Anaesth 1969; 41:1029-34.

184. Idanpaan-Heikkila JE, Tasha RJ, Allen HA, Schoolar JC. Placental trans-fer of diazepam-^{14}C in mice, hamsters, and monkeys. J Pharmacol Exp Ther 1971; 176:752-7.

185. Shnider SM, Way EL. The kinetics of transfer of lidocaine (Xylocaine) across the human placenta. Anesthesiology 1968; 29:944-50.

186. Roe DA, Little BB, Bawdon RE, Gilstrap L. Metabolism of cocaine by human placentas: Implication for fetal exposure. Am J Obstet Gynecol 1990; 163:715-8.

187. Van Petten GR, Hirsch GH, Cherrington AD. Drug-metabolizing activ-ity of the human placenta. Can J Biochem 1968; 46:1057-61.

188. Waters JJ, Ramanathan S. Placental transfer of lidocaine during mater-nal hypoxia (abstract). Anesthesiology 1991; 75:A828.

189. Sturrock JE, Nunn JF. Cytotoxic effects of procaine, lignocaine and bupivacaine. Br J Anaesth 1979; 51:273-80.

190. Lee H, Nagele RG. Neural tube defects caused by local anesthetics in early chick embryos. Teratology 1985; 31:119-27.

191. Lee H, Bush KT, Nagele RG. Time-lapse photographic study of neural tube closure defects caused by Xylocaine in the chick. Teratology 1988; 37:263-9.

192. Anderson PL, Bamburg JR. Effects of local anesthetics on nerve growth in culture. Dev Neurosci 1981; 4:273-90.

193. O'Shea KS, Kaufman MH. Neural tube closure defects following in vitro exposure of mouse embryos to Xylocaine. J Exp Zool 1980; 214:235-8.

194. Stygall K, Mirsky R, Mowbray J. The effect of local anaesthetics and bar-biturates on myogenesis and myotube integrity in rat skeletal muscle cultures. J Cell Sci 1979; 37:231-41.

195. Ramazzotto LJ, Curro FA, Patterson JA, et al. Toxicological assessment of lidocaine in the pregnant rat. J Dent Res 1985; 64:1214-8.

196. Fujinaga M, Mazze RI. Reproductive and teratogenic effects of lidocaine in Sprague-Dawley rats. Anesthesiology 1986; 65:626-32.

197. Martin LVH, Jurand A. The absence of teratogenic effects of some anal-gesics used in anaesthesia: Additional evidence from a mouse model. Anaesthesia 1992; 47:473-6.

198. Smith RF, Wharton GG, Kurtz SL, et al. Behavioral effects of mid-pregnancy administration of lidocaine and mepivacaine in the rat. Neurobehav Toxicol Teratol 1986; 8:61-8.

199. Smith RF, Kurkjian MF, Mattran KM, Kurtz SL. Behavioral effects of prenatal exposure to lidocaine in the rat: Effects of dosage and of gesta-tional age at administration. Neurotoxicol Teratol 1989; 11:395-403.

200. Tuckermann-Duplessis H. Influence of certain drugs on the prenatal development. Int J Gynaecol Obstet 1970; 8:777-97.

201. Heinonen OP, Slone D, Shapiro S. Birth defects and drugs in pregnancy. Littleton, Mass, Publishing Sciences Group, 1977:357-65.

202. Friedman JM. Teratogen update: Anesthetic agents. Teratology 1988; 37:69-77.

203. Tucker GT, Boyes RN, Bridenbaugh PO, Moore DC. Binding of anilide-type local anesthetics in human plasma. II. Implications in vivo, with special reference to transplacental distribution. Anesthesiology 1970; 33:304-14.

204. Ehrnebo M, Agurell S, Jalling B, Boreus LO. Age differences in drug binding by plasma proteins: Studies on human foetuses, neonates and adult. Eur J Clin Pharmacol 1971; 3:189-93.

205. Finster M, Morishima HO, Boyes RN, Covino BG. The placental trans-fer of lidocaine and its uptake by fetal tissues. Anesthesiology 1972; 36:159-63.

206. Morishima HO, Santos AC, Pedersen H, et al. Effect of lidocaine on the asphyxial responses in the mature fetal lamb. Anesthesiology 1987; 66:502-7.

207. Meffin P, Long GJ, Thomas J. Clearance and metabolism of mepivacaine in the human neonate. Clin Pharmacol Ther 1973; 14:218-25.

208. Blankenbaker WL, Di Fazio CA, Berry FA. Lidocaine and its metabolites in the newborn. Anesthesiology 1975; 42:325-30.

209. Mihaly GW, Moore RG, Thomas J, et al. The pharmacokinetics and metabolism of the anilide local anaesthetics in neonates. 1. Lignocaine. Eur J Clin Pharmacol 1978; 13:143-52.

210. Morgan D, McQuillan D, Thomas J. Pharmacokinetics and metabolism of the anilide local anaesthetics in neonates. II. Etidocaine. Eur J Clin Pharmacol 1978; 13:365-71.

211. Morishima HO, Finster M, Pedersen H, et al. Pharmacokinetics of lido-caine in fetal and neonatal lambs and adult sheep. Anesthesiology 1979; 50:431-6.

212. Lieberman BA, Rosenblatt DB, Belsey E, et al. The effects of maternally administered pethidine or epidural bupivacaine on the fetus and new-born. Br J Obstet Gynaecol 1979; 86:598-606.

213. Finster M, Poppers PJ, Sinclair JC, et al. Accidental intoxication of the fetus with local anesthetic drug during caudal anesthesia. Am J Obstet Gynecol 1965; 92:922-4.

214. Morishima HO, Pedersen H, Finster M, et al. Toxicity of lidocaine in adult, newborn, and fetal sheep. Anesthesiology 1981; 55:57-61.

215. Bosnjak ZJ, Stowe DF, Kampine JP. Comparison of lidocaine and bupivacaine depression of sinoatrial nodal activity during hypoxia and acidosis in adult and neonatal guinea pigs. Anesth Analg 1986; 65:911-7.

216. Badgwell JM, Heavner JE, Kytta J. Bupivacaine toxicity in young pigs is age-dependent and is affected by volatile anesthetics. Anesthesiology 1990; 73:297-303.

217. Loftus JR, Holbrook RH, Cohen SE. Fetal heart rate after epidural lido-caine and bupivacaine for elective cesarean section. Anesthesiology 1991; 75:406-12.

218. Boehm FH, Woodruff LF, Growdon JH. The effect of lumbar epidural anesthesia on fetal heart rate variability. Anesth Analg 1975; 54:779-82.

219. Hehre FW, Hook R, Hon EH. Continuous lumbar peridural anesthesia in obstetrics. VI. The fetal effects of transplacental passage of local anes-thetic agents. Anesth Analg 1969; 48:909-13.

220. Lavin JP, Samuels SV, Miodovnik M, et al. The effects of bupiva-caine and chloroprocaine as local anesthetics for epidural anesthesia on fetal heart rate monitoring parameters. Am J Obstet Gynecol 1981; 141:717-22.

221. Abboud TK, Khoo SS, Miller F, et al. Maternal, fetal and neonatal responses after epidural anesthesia with bupivacaine, 2-chloroprocaine or lidocaine. Anesth Analg 1982; 61:638-44.

222. Abboud TK, Afrasiabi A, Sarkis F, et al. Continuous infusion epidural analgesia in parturients receiving bupivacaine, chloroprocaine or lido-caine: Maternal, fetal, and neonatal effects. Anesth Analg 1984; 63: 421-8.

223. Scanlon JW, Brown WU, Weiss JB, Alper MH. Neurobehavioral response of newborn infants after maternal epidural anesthesia. Anesthesiology 1974; 40:121-8.

224. Scanlon JW, Ostheimer GW, Lurie AO, et al. Neurobehavioral responses and drug concentrations in newborns after maternal epidural anesthesia with bupivacaine. Anesthesiology 1976; 45:400-5.

225. Kileff ME, James FM, Dewan DM, Floyd HM. Neonatal neurobehav-ioral responses after epidural anesthesia for cesarean section using lido-caine and bupivacaine. Anesth Analg 1984; 63:413-7.

226. Abboud TK, Kern S, Jacobs J, et al. The neonatal neurobehavioral effects of mepivacaine for epidural anesthesia during labor. Reg Anesth 1986; 11:143-6.

227. Abboud TK, Moore MJ, Jacobs J, et al. Epidural mepivacaine for cesarean section: Maternal and neonatal effects. Reg Anesth 1987; 12: 76-9.

228. Kuhnert BR, Harrison MJ, Linn PL, Kuhnert PM. Effects of maternal epidural anesthesia on neonatal behavior. Anesth Analg 1984; 63:301-8.

229. Campbell N, Harvey D, Norman AP. Increased frequency of neonatal jaundice in a maternity hospital. Br Med J 1975; 2:548-52.

230. Clark DA, Landaw SA. Bupivacaine alters red blood cell properties: A possible explanation for neonatal jaundice associated with maternal anesthesia. Pediatr Res 1985; 19:341-3.

231. Gale R, Ferguson JE II, Stevenson D. Effect of epidural analgesia with bupivacaine hydrochloride on neonatal bilirubin production. Obstet Gynecol 1987; 70:692-5.

232. Smedstad KG, Morison DH, Harris WH, Pascoe P. Placental transfer of local anaesthetics in the premature sheep fetus. Int J Obstet Anesth 1993; 2:34-8.

233. Morishima HO, Pedersen H, Santos AC, et al. Adverse effects of mater-nally administered lidocaine on the asphyxiated preterm fetal lamb. Anesthesiology 1989; 71:110-5.

234. Santos AC, Yun EM, Bobby PD, et al. The effects of bupivacaine, l-nitro-l-arginine-methyl ester, and phenylephrine on cardiovascular adapta-tion to asphyxia in the preterm fetal lamb. Anesth Analg 1997; 85:1299-306.

235. Johnson RF, Herman NL, Johnson HV, et al. Effects of fetal pH on local anesthetic transfer across the human placenta. Anesthesiology 1996; 85:608-15.

236. Aberg G. Toxicological and local anesthetic effects of optically active iso-mers of two local anaesthetic compounds. Acta Pharmacologica et Toxicologica 1972; 31:273-286.

237. Graf BM, Abraham I, Eberbach N, et al. Differences in cardiotoxicity of bupivacaine and ropivacaine are the result of physiochemical and stereoselective properties. Anesthesiology 2002; 96:1427-34.

238. McClure JH. Ropivacaine. Br J Anaesth 1996; 76:300-7.

239. Van Kleef JW, Veering BT, Burm AGL. Spinal anesthesia with ropivacaine: A double-blind study on the efficacy and safety of 0.5% and 0.75% solutions on patients undergoing minor lower limb surgery. Anesth Analg 1994; 78:1125-30.

240. Lacassie HJ, Columb MO, Lacassie HP, Lantadilla RA. The relative motor-blocking potencies of epidural bupivacaine and ropivacaine in labor. Anesth Analg 2002; 95:204-8.

241. Polley LS, Columb MO, Naughton NN, et al. Relative analgesic potencies of ropivacaine and bupivacaine for epidural analgesia in labor. Anesthesiology 1999; 90:944-50.

242. D'Angelo R, James RL. Is ropivacine less potent than bupivacaine. Anesthesiology 1999; 90:941-3.

243. Arthur R, Feldman HS, Covino BG. Comparative pharmacokinetics of bupivacaine and ropivacaine, a new amide local anesthetic. Anesth Analg 1988; 67:1053-8.

244. Lee A, Fagan D, Lamont M, et al. Disposition kinetics of ropivacaine in humans. Anesth Analg 1989; 69:736-38.

245. Datta S, Camann W, Bader A, et al. Clinical effects of maternal and fetal plasma concentrations of epidural ropivacaine versus bupivacaine for cesarean section. Anesthesiology 1995; 82:1346-52.

246. Oda Y, Furuichi K, Tanaka K, et al. Metabolism of a new local anesthetic, ropivacaine, by human hepatic cytochrome P450. Anesthesiology 1995; 82:214-20.

247. Moller R, Covino BG. Cardiac electrophysiologic properties of bupivacaine and lidocaine compared with those of ropivacaine, a new amide local anesthetic. Anesthesiology 1990; 72:322-9.

248. Feldman HS, Arthur GR, Covino BG. Comparative systemic toxicity of convulsant and supraconvulsant doses of intravenous ropivacaine, bupivacaine, and lidocaine in the conscious dog. Anesth Analg 1989; 69:794-801.

249. Reiz S, Häggmark S, Johanson G, Nath S. Cardiotoxicity of ropivacaine: A new amide local anaesthetic. Acta Anaesthesiol Scand 1989; 33:93-8.

250. Nancarrow C, Rutten AJ, Runciman WB, et al. Myocardial and cerebral drug concentrations and the mechanisms of death after fatal intravenous doses of lidocaine, bupivacaine, and ropivacaine in the sheep. Anesth Analg 1989; 69:276-83.

251. Scott DB, Lee A, Fagan D, et al. Acute toxicity of ropivacaine compared with that of bupivacaine. Anesth Analg 1989; 69:563-9.

252. Moller RA, Covino BG. Effects of progesterone on cardiac electrophysiologic alterations produced by ropivacaine and bupivacaine. Anesthesiology 1992; 77:735-41.

253. Dony P, Dewinde V, Vandereck B, et al. The comparative toxicity of ropivacaine and bupivacaine at equipotent doses in rats. Anesth Analg 2000; 91:1189-92

254. Kopacz DJ, Carpenter RL, MacKey DC. Effect of ropivacaine on cutaneous capillary blood flow in pigs. Anesthesiology 1989; 71:69-74.

255. Johnson RF, Cahana A, Olenick M, et al. A comparison of the placental transfer of ropivacaine versus bupivacaine: Effect of maternal protein binding. Anesth Analg 1999; 89:703-8.

256. Stienstra R, Jonker TV, Bourdez P, et al. Ropivacaine 0.25% versus bupivacaine 0.25% for continuous epidural analgesia in labor: A double blind comparison. Anesth Analg 1995; 80:285-9.

257. Writer WD, Stienstra R, Eddleston JM, et al. Neonatal outcome and mode of delivery after epidural analgesia for labor with ropivacaine and bupivacaine Br J Anaesth 1998; 81:713-7.

258. Muir HA, Write D, Douglas J, et al. Double-blind comparison of epidural ropivacaine 0.25% and bupivacaine 0.25% for the relief of childbirth pain. Can J Anaesth 1997; 44:599-04.

259. Valenzuela C, Snyders DJ, Bennett PB, et al. Stereoselective block of cardiac sodium channels by bupivacaine in guinea-pig ventricular myocytes. Circulation 1995; 92:3014-24.

260. Mazoit JX, Boico O, Samii K. Myocardial uptake of bupivacaine. II. Pharmacokinetics and pharmacodynamics of bupivacaine enantiomers in the isolated perfused rabbit heart. Anesth Analg 1993; 77:477-482.

261. Lyons G, Columb MO, Wilson RC, Johnson RV. Epidural pain relief in labour: Potencies of levobupivacaine and racemic bupivacaine. Br J Anaesth 1998; 81:899-901.

262. Burke D, Henderson DJ, Simpson AM, et al. Comparison of 0.25% S(-)-bupivacaine with 0.25% RS-bupivacaine for epidural analgesia in labor. Br J Anaesth 1999; 83:750-5.

263. Bader AM, Tsen LC, Camann WR, et al. Clinical effects and maternal and fetal plasma concentrations of 0.5% epidural levobupivacaine versus bupivacaine for cesarean delivery. Anesthesiology 1999; 90:1596-601.

264. Vercauteren MP, Hans G, De Decker K, Adriaesen HA. Levobupivacaine combined with sufentanil and epinephrine for intrathecal labor analgesia: a comparison with racemic bupivacaine. Anesth Analg 2001; 93:996-1000.

Part V
Anesthesia Before and During Pregnancy

During the early years of obstetric anesthesia, physicians were primarily concerned with its effect on neonatal respiration. Almost 25 years passed before some investigators began to suspect that anesthesia might cause other problems. In fact, it was suspected that chloroform caused icterus neonatorum and it was this suspicion that originally stimulated Paul Zweifel to study placental transmission.

Icterus neonatorum was not Zweifel's original interest. Under the guidance of Adolf Gusserow, one of the preeminent obstetricians in Europe, Zweifel had been studying glucose metabolism during pregnancy. In the course of his work, Zweifel unexpectedly found a reducing compound in the urine of infants whose mothers had received chloroform during labor. At first he suspected that the compound might be glucose, thinking that the metabolism of this compound had somehow been altered by chloroform. After further testing, however, he learned that the reducing substance was not glucose but chloroform itself.

Zweifel thought that chloroform, transmitted to the fetus during labor, might explain some cases of neonatal jaundice. By 1876 physicians already knew that chloroform affected the liver. To cause icterus neonatorum, sufficient quantities of the drug would have to traverse the placenta during the course of a normal labor; the rapidity of transfer was a point of contention among clinicians. To establish the possibility, Zweifel performed experiments that identified chloroform in fetal blood and urine.[1,2]

Zweifel later discounted chloroform as a cause of icterus neonatorum, and the issue was dropped. Another 75 years passed before physicians began to appreciate that drug exposure during pregnancy might have deleterious effects. Events that called attention to the problem included (1) sequelae from radiation exposure after the first use of the atomic bomb, (2) the skeletal deformities associated with the use of thalidomide, a drug once used to treat the nausea of early pregnancy, and (3) the high incidence of genital tumors among daughters of women who had been given diethylstilbestrol during pregnancy. By then the public had also been alerted through the publication of Rachel Carson's Silent Spring, *which gave such graphic descriptions of the environmental effects of the indiscriminate use of insecticides. Physicians also knew more about embryology and toxicology, better techniques for testing drugs were available, procedures for collecting information were standardized, and information about complications was disseminated. Undoubtedly, increased public awareness of these developments contributed to the resurgence of natural childbirth that began after 1950.*

Donald Caton, M.D.

REFERENCES

1. Zweifel P. Der Uebergang von Chloroformnarcose Kreissender auf den Fötus. Arch Gynaekol 1876; 9:291-305.

2. Zweifel P. Der Uebergang von Chloroform und Salicysaüre in die Placenta, nebst Bemerkungen über den Icterus Neonatorum. Arch Gynaekol 1877; 12:235-7.

Chapter 13
Nonanesthetic Drugs During Pregnancy and Lactation

Jerome Yankowitz, M.D. · Jennifer R. Niebyl, M.D.

GENERAL TERATOLOGY

The term *placental barrier* is a misnomer. The placenta allows many drugs and dietary substances to cross from mother to fetus. Several factors (e.g., lipid solubility, molecular weight, protein binding) affect the passage of drugs across the placenta. Lipid-soluble substances readily cross the placenta. Virtually all drugs cross the placenta to some degree, with the exception of large organic ions such as heparin and insulin.

Patients should be educated about nonpharmacologic techniques to cope with tension, aches and pains, and viral illnesses during pregnancy. Drugs should be used only when necessary. The risk:benefit ratio should justify the use of any drug, and the minimum effective dose should be employed. Long-term effects of fetal drug exposure may not become apparent for many years. Therefore, physicians and patients should exercise caution in the use of any drug during pregnancy. On the other hand, the physician should ask: What would be the appropriate treatment in the nonpregnant patient with the same condition? In most cases, the answer is the same for women who are pregnant.[1]

Sensitive serum pregnancy tests can diagnose pregnancy as early as 1 week after conception. Before drug therapy is started, a sensitive test should be used if there is any question with regard to drug safety during a potential pregnancy.

In the United States, major malformations affect 2% to 3% of neonates,[2] but account for approximately 20% of infant mortality.[3] Exogenous causes of birth defects (e.g., radiation, infections, maternal metabolic disorders, drugs, environmental chemicals) account for almost 10% of all birth defects, and therefore affect only 0.2% to 0.3% of all births. Drug exposure explains only 2% to 3% of birth defects. Thus the majority of birth defects are of unknown etiology.

A major malformation is defined as one that is incompatible with survival (e.g., anencephaly), one that requires major surgery for correction (e.g., cleft palate or congenital heart disease), or causes mental retardation. If all minor malformations (e.g., ear tags and extra digits) are included, the incidence of congenital anomalies may be as high as 7% to 10%.

Drug teratogenicity is affected by species specificity, timing of exposure, dose, maternal physiology, embryology, and genetics. Drug teratogenicity is markedly species specific. For example, thalidomide produces phocomelia in primates but not rodents. The timing of exposure is important. When administered between 35 and 37 days' gestation, thalidomide produces ear malformations; when administered between 41 and 44 days' gestation, it produces amelia or phocomelia. The dose of drug is also important. In most cases, administration of a low dose will result in no effect, whereas malformations may occur at intermediate doses and death may occur at higher doses. Fetal death may cause organ-specific teratogenic activity to go unnoticed. The route and/or timing of drug administration may also affect outcome. Small doses administered over several days may have an effect different from that observed with the same total dose given at once. Sequential drug administration may induce the production of an enzyme that metabolizes the drug and thus results in less exposure. Constant exposure may destroy cells that would have catabolized the drug if it had been administered in periodic doses. Pregnancy-associated changes in maternal physiology may affect absorption, distribution, metabolism, and excretion. Placental transfer must also be considered. For example, warfarin derivatives easily cross the placenta and have teratogenic potential; in contrast, heparin does not cross the placenta.

Teratogen exposure in the first 2½ weeks after conception is generally thought to have no effect or to result in spontaneous loss (i.e., all-or-nothing phenomenon). Among women with a 28-day menstrual cycle, the classic period of susceptibility to teratogenic agents is during the period of organogenesis, which occurs primarily at 2½ to 8 weeks' postconception (31 to 71 days–or 4½ to 10 weeks–after the first day of the last menstrual period or LMP) (Figure 13-1). After this period, embryonic development is characterized primarily by increasing organ size; thus, the principal effect of exposure will be growth restriction and/or effects on the nervous system and gonadal tissue. For example, diethylstilbestrol (DES) exposure during the second trimester results in uterine anomalies that do not become apparent until after puberty. Fetal alcohol syndrome may occur with chronic exposure to alcohol during pregnancy. During organogenesis each organ system will have different critical periods of sensitivity. A teratogen can act by causing cell death, altering tissue growth (e.g., hyperplasia, hypoplasia, asynchronous growth), or interfering with cellular differentiation or other basic morphogenic processes.

The genotype of the mother and fetus can affect individual susceptibility to an agent. For example, fetuses with low levels of the enzyme epoxide hydrolase are more likely to manifest the fetal hydantoin syndrome than those with normal levels of this enzyme.[4] Combinations of agents may produce different degrees of malformation and/or growth restriction than drugs given individually. For example, fetuses whose mothers receive combination anticonvulsant therapy are at the highest risk for malformations, including neural tube defects and facial dysmorphic features.

U.S. Food and Drug Administration Categories

In 1979, the U.S. Food and Drug Administration (FDA) introduced a drug classification system to discourage nonessential use of medications during pregnancy[5]:

1. **Category A:** Controlled studies have shown no risk. Adequate, well-controlled studies in pregnant women have failed to demonstrate a risk to the fetus in the first trimester (and there is no evidence of a risk in later trimesters), and the possibility of fetal harm appears remote.

2. **Category B:** No evidence of human fetal risk exists. Either animal reproduction studies have not demonstrated fetal risk but no controlled studies in pregnant women have been reported, or animal reproduction studies have shown an adverse effect (other than a decrease in fertility) that was not confirmed in controlled studies in women in the first trimester (and there is no evidence of risk in later trimesters).

3. **Category C:** Risk cannot be ruled out. Either studies in animals have revealed adverse effects on the fetus (teratogenic, embryocidal, or other) but no controlled studies in women have been reported, or studies in women and animals are not available. Drugs should be given only if the potential benefit justifies the potential risk to the fetus.

4. **Category D:** Positive evidence of human fetal risk exists. However, the benefits from use in pregnant women may be acceptable despite the risk (e.g., if the drug is needed for a life-threatening condition or for a serious disease for which safer drugs cannot be used or are ineffective).

5. **Category X:** Contraindicated in pregnancy. Studies in animals or human beings have demonstrated fetal abnormalities, or evidence exists of fetal risk based on human experience, or both, and the risk in pregnant women clearly outweighs any possible benefit. The drug is contraindicated in women who are or may become pregnant.

Unfortunately, maternal anxiety related to medication use can lead to unnecessary pregnancy terminations. Several characteristics of the FDA drug classification system contribute to public perception—and *mis*perception—of the dangers of medication use during pregnancy. Although only 20 to 30 commonly used drugs are known teratogens, 7% of all the medications that are listed in the Physicians Desk Reference (PDR) are classified as category X.[5,6] All new medications are classified as category C, leading to an exaggerated impression of the danger of many medications.

The Teratology Society has suggested abandonment of the FDA classification scheme.[5] The FDA categories imply a progressive fetal risk from category A to X, whereas the drugs in different categories may pose similar risks, but be listed in different categories based on risk:benefit considerations. Second, the categories create the impression that drugs within a category present similar risks, whereas the category definition permits inclusion (in the same category) of drugs that vary in type, degree, and/or extent of risk. When counseling patients or responding to queries from physicians, we prefer to avoid referring to the PDR. Rather, we use specific descriptions in teratogen databases to provide the best information that is available.

In 1997, the FDA held a public meeting to discuss labeling of drugs. There was consensus that the current classification scheme probably is oversimplified and confusing, does not address the range of clinical situations and/or the range of possible effects, and should be replaced with narrative labeling. Subsequently a concept paper was presented, which outlined a new model for labeling and included sections such as "clinical management statement," "summary risk assessment," and "discussion of data" for both pregnant and breastfeeding women.[7] This proposal has not yet been implemented.

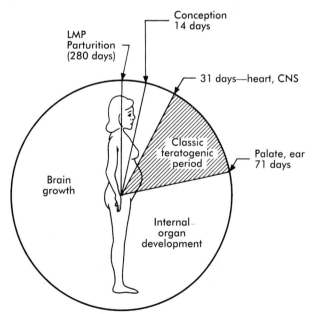

FIGURE 13-1. Gestational clock showing the classic teratogenic period. *CNS,* Central nervous system; *LMP,* last menstrual period. (From Niebyl JR. Drug Use in Pregnancy, 2nd ed. Philadelphia, Lea & Febiger, 1988:2.)

DRUG USE DURING PREGNANCY

Anticonvulsants

All anticonvulsants cross the placenta. Pregnant women with epilepsy who ingest anticonvulsant drugs have a fetal congenital anomaly rate of 4% to 8%, which is higher than the 2% to 3% background incidence quoted for the general population.[8,9] A twofold increase in the risk of minor malformations also exists in this population.[9] Cleft lip with or without cleft palate and congenital heart disease are especially common. Administration of valproic acid or carbamazepine entails a 1% risk of neural tube defects and other malformations; thus alpha-fetoprotein screening and targeted ultrasonography are appropriate for these patients. In addition, the offspring of epileptic women have a 2% to 3% incidence of epilepsy, which is five times that of the general population.

It has been proposed that the underlying maternal epilepsy is hereditary and that the inheritance of this genetic abnormality produces an increased frequency of birth defects.[10] Holmes et al.[11] attempted to refute this unproven theory. They studied children of women who had a history of seizures, but took no medications during pregnancy. There was no difference in physical features or cognitive function between these children and a group of matched controls. Unfortunately, this study was confounded by the fact that women in the seizure group were atypical (i.e., with mild disease), as evidenced by the fact that they had no need for anticonvulsant drugs.

More recently, Holmes et al.[12] screened 128,049 pregnant women at delivery to identify three groups of infants: those exposed to anticonvulsant drugs, those unexposed to anticonvulsant drugs but with a maternal history of seizures, and those unexposed to anticonvulsant drugs with no maternal history of seizures (control group). The combined frequency of anticonvulsant embryopathy was higher in 223 infants exposed to one anticonvulsant drug than in 508 control infants (20.6% versus 8.5%; odds ratio = 2.8; 95% confidence interval = 1.1 to 9.7). The frequency was also higher in 93 infants exposed to two or more anticonvulsant drugs than in the controls (28.0% versus 8.5%; odds ratio = 4.2; 95% confidence interval = 1.1 to 5.1). The 98 infants whose mothers had a history of epilepsy but took no anticonvulsant drugs during the pregnancy did *not* have a higher frequency of abnormalities than the control infants. The authors concluded that "a distinctive pattern of physical abnormalities in infants of mothers with epilepsy is associated with the use of anticonvulsant drugs during pregnancy, rather than with epilepsy itself."[12]

Possible causes of these congenital malformations include genetic differences in drug metabolism, the specific drugs themselves, and/or deficiency states (e.g., decreased serum folate) induced by the drugs. No congenital malformations appear to be unique to any one anticonvulsant. The characteristics of these syndromes are so similar that the term *fetal anticonvulsant syndrome* has been applied to almost every anticonvulsant drug. The fetal anticonvulsant syndrome primarily includes orofacial, cardiovascular, and digital malformations.[13]

Among women taking **phenytoin**, there is a 2% to 5% risk of major congenital anomalies, which primarily include midline heart defects, orofacial clefts, and urogenital defects.[8] The fetal hydantoin syndrome includes a constellation of minor anomalies, including craniofacial abnormalities (short nose, flat nasal bridge, wide lips, hypertelorism, ptosis, epicanthal folds, low-set ears, and low hairline), and limb anomalies (distal digital hypoplasia, absent nails, and altered palmar

crease). In addition, neonatal growth and performance delays have been documented. The risk of having the *fetal hydantoin syndrome* is approximately 10%.[12]

Phenytoin may act as a competitive inhibitor of the placental transport of vitamin K. This results in a decrease in the fetal coagulation factors II, VII, IX, and X. In addition, phenytoin may induce fetal hepatic metabolism of the coagulation factors. The resulting decrease in fetal coagulation factors is associated with an increased risk of hemorrhagic disease in the newborn.[14] To help prevent this coagulopathy, some physicians advocate oral vitamin K supplementation (10 mg daily) for pregnant epileptic patients during the last month of pregnancy, in addition to the parenteral administration of vitamin K to the neonate at birth.[15]

Several anticonvulsant medications have metabolites that typically are eliminated by the enzyme epoxide hydrolase. In one study, 19 women taking phenytoin underwent amniocentesis. Of four women with low enzyme activity in amniocytes, all four had affected fetuses. The 15 fetuses with normal amniocyte epoxide hydrolase activity did not have the characteristics of the fetal hydantoin syndrome.[4]

Carbamazepine (Tegretol) is used to treat all types of seizure disorders, with the exception of petit mal epilepsy. It is most commonly used in the treatment of psychomotor (temporal lobe) and grand mal epilepsy. In a prospective study involving 72 women with epilepsy taking carbamazepine, there was an increased incidence of congenital anomalies among the 35 fetuses exposed to the drug. There was an 11% incidence of craniofacial defects, a 26% incidence of fingernail hypoplasia, and a 20% incidence of developmental delay.[16] This constellation of fetal effects has been named the *fetal carbamazepine syndrome* and closely resembles the malformations seen in cases of fetal hydantoin syndrome. In addition, maternal carbamazepine exposure has been specifically associated with spina bifida. An analysis of all available data involving cohorts of pregnant women ingesting carbamazepine supports the conclusion that fetal exposure to this drug carries a 0.5% to 1% risk of spina bifida.[17]

Phenobarbital is used in the treatment of partial and generalized tonic-clonic seizures and status epilepticus.[18] Fetal exposure to phenobarbital has been associated with such major malformations as congenital heart defects and orofacial clefting. A *fetal phenobarbital syndrome* is characterized by minor dysmorphic features similar to those seen with the fetal hydantoin syndrome.[8] Fetal phenobarbital exposure has also been associated with decreased intellectual and cognitive development in neonates and children. Maternal phenobarbital use during pregnancy can result in hemorrhagic disease of the newborn and neonatal withdrawal symptoms following delivery. The withdrawal symptoms consist mostly of irritability, begin at approximately 7 days of life, and usually last for approximately 2 to 6 weeks.[18]

Valproic acid (Depakene, Depakote) is used to treat absence and generalized tonic-clonic seizures. Infants exposed to valproic acid have a 1% to 2% risk of spina bifida. The neural tube defect tends to be lumbosacral in location. Fetal valproic acid exposure has also been associated with cardiac defects, orofacial clefting, and genitourinary anomalies. A *fetal valproate syndrome* has been described, and is characterized by dysmorphic features, including epicanthal folds, shallow orbits, hypertelorism, low-set ears, flat nasal bridge, upturned nasal tip, microcephaly, thin vermillion borders, downturned mouth, thin overlapping fingers and toes, and hyperconvex fingernails.[8]

Among the new anticonvulsant drugs are felbamate, gabapentin, lamotrigine, oxcarbazepine, topiramate, tiagabine, and vigabatrin.[13] **Felbamate** was approved by the FDA for monotherapy, but later its use was severely restricted because of its association with aplastic anemia and hepatic failure. **Gabapentin** (Neurontin) was initially released in the United States as an adjunctive treatment for partial seizures and secondarily generated tonic-clonic seizures. Gabapentin inhibits dopamine release in the central nervous system (CNS). **Lamotrigine** (Lamictal) appears to have efficacy comparable to that of carbamazepine in the monotherapy of partial epilepsy. Lamotrigine is an inhibitor of dihydrofolate reductase and decreases embryonic folate levels in experimental animals. This raises the concern that human use of lamotrigine may result in developmental toxicity. The manufacturer has established a registry to evaluate this possibility.[19] A preliminary report from this registry has described a 6% congenital malformation rate in fetuses exposed to this drug; this does not represent a clear increase in the rate of malformations.[20] However, there have not been sufficient numbers of fetal exposures to draw any definite conclusions. Lamotrigine is not protein bound, has no effect on the cytochrome P450 system, and does not appear to result in significant accumulations of arene oxide metabolites.[20]

Many patients present to prenatal clinics already using these newer anticonvulsants. We counsel patients that there is no clear evidence of teratogenicity, but we acknowledge that little information is available. Some investigators have suggested avoiding the newer anticonvulsants until evidence of safety is accumulated.[18]

Some women may be taking anticonvulsant drugs without recent revaluation of the need to continue drug therapy. If a patient with idiopathic epilepsy has been seizure-free for 2 years and has a normal electroencephalogram (EEG), the neurologist may try to withdraw the drug before pregnancy.[21] If the patient has not been taking her drug regularly, a low blood level will confirm a lack of compliance. If she has not had recurrent seizures despite a low blood level of drug, she may not need to continue the drug.

If a patient first presents for care during pregnancy, most authorities agree that the benefits of anticonvulsant therapy during pregnancy outweigh the risks of discontinuing the drug. The blood level of the drug should be monitored to minimize the dose needed to ensure a therapeutic level of drug.

Isotretinoin (Accutane)

Isotretinoin is given for the treatment of cystic acne. Isotretinoin is highly teratogenic. Lammer et al.[22] reported 21 infants with birth defects, 12 spontaneous abortions, 95 elective abortions, and 26 normal infants in 154 women who were taking isotretinoin during early pregnancy. Characteristic features of this embryopathy include CNS malformations, microtia/anotia, micrognathia, cleft palate, cardiac and great vessel defects, thymic abnormalities, and eye anomalies. Prospective studies suggest that the risk of congenital anomalies is approximately 25%, and an additional 25% of the offspring have mental retardation.[23]

Unlike vitamin A, isotretinoin is not stored in tissue, and the drug is not detected in serum 5 days after ingestion. Therefore exposure *before* pregnancy does not seem to be hazardous. The package insert for isotretinoin explains the extreme risk of teratogenic effect and clearly states that, before

a woman capable of childbearing initiates isotretinoin treatment, she must have two negative pregnancy tests and commit to the use of two forms of contraception.

Topical **tretinoin** (Retin-A) has not been associated with any teratogenic risk.

Tranquilizers

Human epidemiologic studies regarding possible teratogenic effects of various tranquilizers, including **meprobamate** (Miltown) and **chlordiazepoxide** (Librium), are inconsistent. One report of nearly 400 patients found a 12% incidence of birth defects in the offspring of meprobamate users.[24] Another study of similar size failed to identify any increased risk of malformations.[25] Similar data are available for chlordiazepoxide.[24,25]

Some studies have suggested that first-trimester exposure to **diazepam** increases the risk of cleft lip, with or without cleft palate.[26] A calculated pooled risk of oral clefting after first-trimester exposure to **benzodiazepines** (i.e., diazepam or alprazolam) yielded an odds ratio of 2.4 (95% confidence interval = 1.40 to 4.03) for the development of oral clefts.[27] Although these data suggest an increased risk of an oral cleft after exposure to benzodiazepines, the baseline risk for this anomaly is only 0.06%.[27] Therefore, the absolute risk of oral clefting after intrauterine drug exposure is small.

Other reports have *not* suggested an increase in congenital abnormalities after fetal exposure to benzodiazepines. In a case-control study of 611 infants with cleft lip or cleft palate and 2498 controls with other birth defects, no association between diazepam and cleft palate was found; the odds ratios after adjustment for potential confounders were 0.8 for cleft lip with or without cleft plate (95% confidence interval = 0.4 to 1.7) and 0.8 for cleft palate alone (95% confidence interval = 0.2 to 2.5).[28] A study of 460 women exposed to benzodiazepines during pregnancy found no difference in the incidence of congenital anomalies, when compared to 424 control pregnancies (i.e., 3.1% versus 2.6%).[29] Nonetheless, in many clinical situations, the risk:benefit ratio does not justify the use of benzodiazepines during pregnancy. Perinatal use of diazepam has been associated with hypotonia, hypothermia, and respiratory depression.[30]

Lithium

In the International Registry of Lithium Babies, 25 (11.5%) of 217 infants exposed to lithium during the first trimester of pregnancy were malformed.[31] Eighteen infants had cardiovascular anomalies, and six had the rare Ebstein's anomaly, which occurs only once in 20,000 nonexposed pregnancies. Subsequent studies have suggested that ascertainment bias may have flawed the Registry; the reported risk of anomalies following lithium exposure is much less than that reported by the Registry.

In a cohort study linking the Swedish Birth Registry with the records of women with bipolar disorder, 59 infants were identified whose mothers were treated with lithium early in pregnancy.[32] Four (6.8%) of the 59 infants exposed to lithium had congenital heart disease compared to two (0.9%) infants of 228 bipolar women not exposed (relative risk = 7.7; 95% confidence interval = 1.5 to 41.2). None of the infants had Ebstein's anomaly. In a prospective cohort study of 148 women treated with lithium during the first trimester and 148 controls not exposed to any known teratogens, there was no significant difference between groups in the incidence of major congenital anomalies or cardiac malformations,[33] although one lithium-exposed infant did have Ebstein's anomaly. The authors concluded that lithium is not a major human teratogen, but they recommended that women exposed to lithium be offered ultrasonography and fetal echocardiography.[33] If the data are pooled, these two cohort studies do not suggest a statistically significant increase in risk of congenital malformations or cardiac malformations in women exposed to lithium during pregnancy. Although the risk for congenital malformations associated with intrauterine lithium exposure is likely to be lower than previously reported, an absence of risk cannot be assumed from the available data.

Two published cases associate polyhydramnios with maternal lithium treatment.[34,35] Nephrogenic diabetes insipidus has been reported in adults taking lithium; thus the presumed mechanism of polyhydramnios is fetal diabetes insipidus. Polyhydramnios may signal fetal lithium toxicity.

Pregnancy accelerates the excretion of lithium; thus serum lithium levels should be monitored in pregnant women.[36] Perinatal effects of lithium include hypotonia, lethargy, and poor feeding in the infant. In addition, complications (e.g., goiter, hypothyroidism) similar to those seen in adults taking lithium have been noted in newborns.

Some authorities recommend discontinuation of lithium and substitution with other medications during pregnancy. However, the discontinuation of lithium is associated with a 70% chance of relapse of the affective disorder in 1 year, as opposed to a 20% risk of relapse in those who continue taking lithium.[37]

Antidepressants

A summation of 14 studies assessing the effect of fetal exposure to **tricyclic antidepressants** evaluated 414 cases of first-trimester exposure.[27] When pooled or viewed individually, no significant association between fetal exposure to tricyclic antidepressants and congenital malformations was found.[27] In the Michigan Medicaid study, 467 newborns had been exposed to amitriptyline, and 75 newborns had been exposed to imipramine during the first trimester. There was no association between tricyclic antidepressant use and congenital anomalies.

The selective serotonin reuptake inhibitors include **sertraline** (Zoloft), **paroxetine** (Paxil), **fluoxetine** (Prozac), and **citalopram** (Celexa). No increased risk of major malformations or developmental (language and behavior) abnormalities has been identified.[38-40] However, in another report, infants who were exposed to fluoxetine in the third trimester were compared to those exposed only in the first trimester. Those exposed in the third trimester had a greater incidence of perinatal complications, including preterm delivery, admission to the special care nursery, poor neonatal adaptation, lower mean birth weight, and shorter length.[41] Although these results are concerning, their long-term clinical significance is unknown.

Anticoagulants

Warfarin (Coumadin) use in pregnancy can result in an embryopathy similar to the X-linked chondrodysplasia punctata (CDPX). The embryopathy can occur with fetal exposure between 6 and 12 weeks' gestation. This condition may result from inhibition of arylsulfatase E by warfarin. Deficiency of arylsulfatase E is responsible for CDPX. The period between 6 and 9 weeks' gestation is especially critical. The *fetal warfarin syndrome* consists of nasal hypoplasia, depressed nasal bridge (often with a deep groove between the alae and nasal tip), stippled epiphyses, nail hypoplasia, mental retardation, and growth restriction. Second- and third-trimester exposure can result in other adverse fetal effects, including microcephaly, blindness, deafness, and growth restriction.

Hall et al.[42] reviewed all published cases of warfarin embryopathy through 1980. They found 418 pregnancies complicated by warfarin use. One sixth of the liveborn had abnormalities, one sixth of the pregnancies ended in stillbirth or spontaneous abortion, and the remaining two thirds had a normal outcome. For the 45 pregnancies with only first-trimester exposure, 31 had some type of problem, including 22 abortions and 9 (20%) with a malformation. For those with isolated second- and/or third-trimester exposure, the overall problem rate was 20% to 30%, but this was not further subdivided between losses and malformations. At least one source[43] has stated that, based on three prospective studies of women exposed only in the second and third trimesters, the incidence of malformations in this group must be exceedingly low, as there was no evidence of fetal/neonatal CNS or eye abnormalities. There is some evidence that a lower dosage (≤ 5 mg daily) has less teratogenic potential.[44]

Heparin, the alternative drug, is a large, water-soluble molecule that does not cross the placenta. Maternal administration of heparin does not have an adverse effect on the fetus, and heparin is the drug of choice for most pregnant patients who require anticoagulation. Administration of 20,000 units per day for more than 20 weeks may be associated with maternal bone demineralization.[45] Heparin should be used for prolonged periods only when its use is clearly necessary.

An isolated history of deep vein thrombosis does not necessarily justify full anticoagulation during pregnancy. Conservative measures, such as the use of elastic stockings and the avoidance of prolonged sitting or standing, should be considered.

In contrast, full anticoagulation is necessary in pregnant women with cardiac valve prostheses. Unfortunately, there have been reports of catastrophic heparin failure and valve thrombosis leading to maternal and fetal morbidity and mortality. One report noted a 4.5-fold increase in valve thrombosis when heparin (rather than warfarin) was used, but in 8 of 12 cases there was evidence of suboptimal treatment.[46] Iturbe-Alessio et al.[47] studied 72 pregnant women with prosthetic heart valves. Among those who received warfarin, 25% to 30% had embryopathy, but there were cases of fatal prosthetic valve thrombosis in the patients who received low-dose heparin. The authors concluded that warfarin is a teratogen but that low-dose heparin is *not* appropriate for prophylaxis in patients with prosthetic heart valves. Similar results were found in a study of 92 pregnancies in 59 women.[48] In 31 women, oral anticoagulants were discontinued when pregnancy was diagnosed, and subcutaneous heparin was started with a goal of adjusting the activated partial thromboplastin time (aPTT) to 2 times the control. In 61 pregnancies, the oral anticoagulant was continued throughout the first trimester. However, there was one case of hydrocephalus in a pregnant woman who continued oral anticoagulation therapy. There were more embolic events in the group of women who received heparin.

Low-molecular-weight heparin (LMWH) has some advantages over standard unfractionated heparin.[49] Like standard heparin, LMWH does not cross the placenta. LMWH has a longer half-life, which allows once-daily dosing. However, during pregnancy, the increased volume of distribution and accelerated clearance may eliminate this benefit. In addition, LMWH has a much more predictable dose-response relationship, which obviates the need for monitoring. LMWH has a lower risk of heparin-induced thrombocytopenia and clinical bleeding at delivery, but studies that suggest a decreased risk of osteoporosis are preliminary. The cost of LMWH is substantially higher than that of standard heparin.

Thyroid and Antithyroid Drugs

Drugs used to treat hyperthyroidism include propylthiouracil and methimazole. **Propylthiouracil** has been the mainstay of treatment. It can cause fetal and neonatal hypothyroidism and rarely goiter. The rate of congenital malformations is not higher among the infants of women treated with propylthiouracil.[50] **Methimazole** (Tapazole, Carbimazole), like propylthiouracil, is given orally to treat hyperthyroidism. Aplasia cutis congenita of the scalp has been described among children whose mothers took methimazole during pregnancy.[51,52] On the other hand, the risk of a scalp defect appears to be small, as several large series found no cases of aplasia cutis.[50]

Radioactive iodine administered for thyroid ablation or diagnostic studies is not concentrated by the fetal thyroid until 10 to 12 weeks' gestation.[53] Thus inadvertent administration of ^{131}I or ^{125}I near conception causes no specific risk to the fetal thyroid.

Women with hypothyroidism may require a larger dose of **thyroxine** during pregnancy.[54] It is prudent to monitor thyroid function throughout pregnancy and to adjust the thyroxine dose to maintain a normal thyrotropin level, as there is some evidence of decreased intelligence in the offspring of women with subclinical thyroid deficiency during pregnancy.[55]

Inotropic Agents

The inotropic agents include dopamine, dobutamine, isoproterenol, and digoxin. There are no reports of teratogenicity related to use of dopamine or dobutamine during pregnancy. Among 31 women treated with isoproterenol during the first 4 months of pregnancy in the Collaborative Perinatal Project,[56] there was no increase in the incidence of malformations.

Digoxin is used to treat heart failure and cardiac arrhythmias. Physicians should monitor the maternal digoxin level to ensure a therapeutic level of drug during pregnancy. Among the infants of 142 women who were treated with digoxin during the first trimester, the frequency of congenital anomalies was no greater than expected.[57] The rate of anomalies was also not increased among the 52 women treated with cardiac glycosides in the first trimester or among the 129 women treated any time during pregnancy in the Collaborative Perinatal Project.[56]

Antihypertensive Drugs

Methyldopa is often used to treat mild chronic hypertension during pregnancy. The drugs commonly used for treatment of severe hypertension in pregnancy include hydralazine, labetalol, sodium nitroprusside, nitroglycerin, calcium-entry blocking agents (including nicardipine and nifedipine), and beta-adrenergic receptor antagonists (including propranolol and atenolol).

METHYLDOPA

Methyldopa (Aldomet) has been widely used for the treatment of chronic hypertension during pregnancy. Postural hypotension may occur, but there is no evidence of teratogenicity or other adverse fetal effects.

HYDRALAZINE

Hydralazine (Apresoline) is the preferred parenteral agent for treatment of severe hypertension during pregnancy. The frequency of congenital anomalies was not significantly increased among the children of 136 women treated with hydralazine during pregnancy in the Collaborative Perinatal Project.[56] However, only eight of these women were treated in the first trimester. There is no evidence that hydralazine is teratogenic.

BETA-ADRENERGIC RECEPTOR ANTAGONISTS

There is no evidence that **propranolol** (Inderal) is teratogenic. Maternal administration of propranolol within 2 hours of delivery may result in neonatal bradycardia.[58] There is some evidence that maternal administration of propranolol may result in modest intrauterine growth restriction (IUGR).[59] It seems prudent to use ultrasonography to assess intrauterine fetal growth.

Atenolol (Tenormin) is a cardioselective beta-adrenergic receptor antagonist. In a large analysis of published trials involving beta-adrenergic antagonist therapy, there was little or no information on teratogenicity for the multiple agents studied, including atenolol, labetalol, metoprolol, oxprenolol, pindolol, and propranolol.[60] Atenolol was associated with lower birth weight and a trend toward more frequent preterm delivery compared to other antihypertensive drugs or no therapy. These effects were more pronounced when the drug was given earlier in pregnancy and for a long duration.[61] In one study, treatment of hypertension (mostly with atenolol) reduced the risk of severe hypertension and preterm labor.[62] In a randomized clinical trial, the same group observed that atenolol prevented preeclampsia but resulted in the birth of infants who weighed 440 g less than those in the placebo group.[63]

LABETALOL

Labetalol (Normodyne, Trandate) is another commonly used agent for the treatment of severe hypertension. It is a nonselective beta-adrenergic receptor antagonist and a postsynaptic alpha$_1$-receptor antagonist. Labetalol slows heart rate and decreases systemic vascular resistance. There are few data about labetalol use and the risk of congenital malformations. In one randomized double-blind trial of 152 women with hypertension, there were no malformations in either the treatment group or the placebo group, although the exposure to labetalol occurred in the second and third trimesters.[64]

ANGIOTENSIN-CONVERTING ENZYME (ACE) INHIBITORS

These drugs do not appear to be teratogenic when given during the first trimester.[65] Later in pregnancy they can cause fetal renal failure and oligohydramnios, which may result in fetal limb contractures, craniofacial deformities, and pulmonary hypoplasia.[66] ACE inhibitors should be discontinued when pregnancy is diagnosed, and pregnant women should receive an alternative drug.

CALCIUM-ENTRY BLOCKING AGENTS

A recent report noted the occurrence of myocardial infarction in a pregnant woman who was receiving nifedipine for treatment of preterm labor.[67] However, the overall maternal risk of nifedipine seems low, and it does not seem to cause an increase in the rate of malformations among exposed fetuses.[68]

Antiarrhythmia Drugs

Amiodarone (Cordarone) is structurally similar to thyroxine and contains 37% iodine by weight.[69,70] In a review of the 64 reported pregnancies in which amiodarone was given to the mother, there was no clear increase in the incidence of malformations. However, 11 (17%) infants had evidence of hypothyroidism and two (3%) neonates had goiter. Evidence of transient hyperthyroidism occurred in two (3%) newborns. There was no clear effect on intelligence in the offspring, but there may be an association with a mild alteration of neurodevelopment.[70] This agent is most often used during pregnancy to treat fetal arrhythmias, so that first-trimester exposure is rare.

There are scant data on **quinidine** (Duraquin, Quinaglute, Quinalan, Cardioquin, and Quinidex), **procainamide** (Pronestyl), **flecainide** (Tambocor), or **sotalol** (Betapace), which are often used to treat fetal arrhythmias.

Antineoplastic and Immunosuppressant Drugs

Azathioprine (Imuran) has been used successfully in pregnant women with systemic lupus erythematosus and/or a renal transplant. There is no evidence of an increase in the incidence or distribution of anomalies among infants who are exposed to this drug in utero.[71,72]

Cyclosporine has been used for immunosuppression during pregnancy in renal transplant patients. No teratogenic effects have been reported.[73]

In human pregnancies, administration of **cyclophosphamide** during the first trimester has been associated with skeletal and palatal defects and with malformations of the limbs and eyes.[74] Administration of cyclophosphamide after the first trimester may be associated with low birth weight.

Chloroquine is safe in doses used as prophylaxis for malaria. One study noted no increased risk of birth defects in 169 infants exposed to 300 mg once weekly.[75] However, maternal administration of larger, therapeutic dosages (e.g., 250 to 500 mg/day) was associated with congenital abnormalities, including two cases of cochleovestibular paresis.[76]

Antiasthmatic Drugs

THEOPHYLLINE AND AMINOPHYLLINE

These drugs are safe for the treatment of asthma during pregnancy. No evidence of teratogenicity was found in 76 cases of fetal exposure in the Collaborative Perinatal Project,[77] although there was a slight increase over the expected rate of birth defects in the Michigan Medicaid study.[78]

EPINEPHRINE

Minor malformations have been reported after 3082 cases of exposure to a sympathomimetic amine in the first trimester.[77] The most common sources included a variety of over-the-counter preparations used to treat upper respiratory tract infections.

TERBUTALINE AND OTHER SHORT-ACTING BETA-SYMPATHOMIMETIC AGENTS

A Michigan Medicaid study with over 1000 first-trimester exposures to albuterol, and a smaller number of exposures to metaproterenol, terbutaline, and isoproterenol, did not demonstrate any significant teratogenic risk in humans.[78]

CORTICOSTEROIDS

Inhaled corticosteroids provide effective therapy, but some of the drug is absorbed systemically. All corticosteroids cross the placenta to some degree, but prednisone and prednisolone are inactivated by the placenta. After maternal administration of prednisone, the fetal concentration of active drug is less than 10% of that in the mother. Therefore, prednisone and prednisolone are the preferred systemic corticosteroids for treatment of maternal diseases such as asthma. Oral corticosteroid therapy has been reported to increase the relative risk of cleft lip and palate up to fivefold.[79,80]

CROMOLYN SODIUM

This mast cell stabilizer has been used for more than 25 years without a reported association with congenital defects.[78]

OTHER AGENTS

The 5-lipoxygenase (5-LO) inhibitors and leukotriene receptor antagonists are fairly new agents, and no data about teratogenic effect are available.

Antiemetics

Two randomized, placebo-controlled trials have confirmed that **vitamin B₆** is effective therapy for nausea and vomiting during early pregnancy.[81,82] Thus vitamin B₆ should be tried first for nausea and vomiting in pregnancy. **Doxylamine** is available over-the-counter as Unisom SleepTabs 25 mg. Thus patients can take a combination similar to the formerly marketed Bendectin. One 25-mg tablet of vitamin B₆ and one 25-mg tablet of doxylamine at bedtime, and half of each in the morning and again in the afternoon, is an effective combination. **Ginger** has also been shown to be an effective treatment for nausea and vomiting during pregnancy.[83,84]

TRIMETHOBENZAMIDE

Trimethobenzamide (Tigan) is an antinausea drug that is not classified as either an antihistamine or a phenothiazine. Data from a small number of patients are conflicting. In the Kaiser Health Plan study,[85] there was an increase in the incidence of congenital anomalies among 193 patients exposed to trimethobenzamide during pregnancy. However, the authors observed no pattern of specific anomalies in these children, and they noted that some of the mothers also took other drugs. There was no evidence of an association between this drug and congenital malformations in 340 patients in the Collaborative Perinatal Project.[86]

PHENOTHIAZINES

Chlorpromazine (Thorazine) and **promethazine** (Phenergan) effectively treat hyperemesis gravidarum. The most important side effect is drowsiness. Teratogenicity does not seem to be a problem with the phenothiazines as a group. Some 976 patients were treated in the Kaiser Health Plan study,[85] and 1309 patients were treated in the Collaborative Perinatal Project,[86] with no evidence of an association between these drugs and congenital malformations.

METOCLOPRAMIDE

Metoclopramide (Reglan) is an alternative agent for the treatment of nausea and vomiting in pregnancy. The frequency of malformations was no greater than expected among the infants of 190 women who had been given prescriptions for metoclopramide during the first trimester of pregnancy in a Danish record-linkage study.[87]

ONDANSETRON

Ondansetron (Zofran) has equal efficacy to promethazine in the treatment of hyperemesis gravidarum.[88] It is much more costly but less sedating than promethazine.

Antihistamines

Some patients will require treatment with antihistamines for allergies or other upper respiratory tract complaints such as the common cold. Patients should understand that these drugs represent symptomatic therapy for the common cold and have no influence on the course of the disease. Physicians should recommend other remedies, such as the use of a humidifier, rest, and fluids. If medication is necessary, patients should not use a combination of two drugs if one drug will suffice. If the patient has an allergy, an antihistamine alone may be all that is needed. If the patient needs a decongestant, a topical nasal spray will result in less fetal exposure than systemic medication. One study suggested an association between **pseudoephedrine** and gastroschisis.[89] Physicians should discourage the use of over-the-counter drugs for trivial indications because the long-term fetal effects of chronic maternal use of these drugs are unknown.

Most sedating antihistamines are not associated with an increased malformation rate. These include chlorpheniramine, diphenhydramine, methapyrilene, thonzylamine, pyrilamine, tripelennamine, phenyltoloxamine, and buclizine.

Although there have been some conflicting reports about **brompheniramine**, a meta-analysis found no evidence to implicate it as a teratogen.[90] In the Boston Collaborative Program,[57] none of the sedating antihistamines were associated with malformations. Two combination products: **triprolidine with pseudoephedrine** (Actifed), and **phenylpropanolamine with chlorpheniramine** (Ornade), were not associated with malformations. In a cohort of 1502 San Diego women, antihistamines were not associated with congenital malformations.[91] This study included 269 women exposed to **chlorpheniramine** (Chlor-Trimeton). **Azatadine** (Trinalin) was not found to be teratogenic among 127 Michigan Medicaid recipients.

Limited safety information is available for the newer nonsedating antihistamines. In a cohort study, 114 **astemizole** (Hismanal)-exposed women were matched with 114 women exposed to known nonteratogens (e.g., dental radiography, acetaminophen).[92] There were two major malformations in the astemizole group and two in the control group. In a study of 39 women exposed to **cetirizine** (Zyrtec), there was no increase in malformations compared with a control group.[93] There are no controlled human studies for **loratadine** (Claritin) or **fexofenadine** (Allegra).

Several antihistamines have primary indications not directly related to upper respiratory complaints. **Hydroxyzine** (Atarax and Vistaril) is used for treatment of pruritus, **meclizine** (Antivert) for dizziness, **diphenhydramine** (Benadryl) for sleep and pruritus, and **doxylamine** (a component of the former Bendectin) for treatment of nausea and vomiting of pregnancy. A metaanalysis of antihistamines, used mostly for nonrespiratory complaints, found a protective effect against malformations (odds ratio = 0.76; 95% confidence interval = 0.60 to 0.94).[94] This apparent benefit may have resulted from an association between maternal nausea and good fetal outcomes rather than from a direct effect of antihistamines.

Antibiotics

Pregnant women are especially susceptible to vaginal yeast infections, and an antifungal agent may be necessary after antibiotic therapy. Therefore, antibiotics should be used only when clearly indicated.

PENICILLINS AND CEPHALOSPORINS

Use of penicillin derivatives (e.g., amoxicillin, ampicillin) appears to be safe during pregnancy. Use of erythromycin and the cephalosporins also appears to be safe. In a large case-control study, Czeizel et al.[95] found no teratogenic risk from use of cephalosporins, primarily oral cephalexin.

ERYTHROMYCIN

Erythromycin is an alternative to penicillin for the treatment of many diseases in pregnancy, and it is used as a primary treatment for mycoplasma and chlamydial infections. No evidence of teratogenesis has been reported.[57]

SULFONAMIDES

Sulfonamides compete with bilirubin for albumin-binding sites, and they may cause an increased risk of hyperbilirubinemia in the newborn. Thus they are not the first choice during the third trimester, especially if the mother is at risk for preterm labor.

Sulfasalazine is poorly absorbed after oral administration. Thus it is used for treatment of ulcerative colitis and Crohn's disease. Sulfasalazine crosses the placenta. The fetal blood concentration approximates the maternal concentration, although both are low. Neither kernicterus nor severe neonatal jaundice has been reported after maternal use of sulfasalazine, even when the drug was administered until the time of delivery.[96]

TRIMETHOPRIM

Trimethoprim often is given with sulfa for the treatment of a urinary tract infection. In 2296 Michigan Medicaid recipients, first-trimester trimethoprim exposure was associated with a slightly increased risk of birth defects, particularly cardiovascular anomalies, and in a retrospective study the odds ratio was 2.3.[97] Folic acid antagonists, which include trimethoprim, may increase the risk not only of neural tube defects, but also of cardiovascular defects, oral clefts, and urinary tract defects.[98]

NITROFURANTOIN

No risk of birth defects has been noted after exposure to nitrofurantoin. However, it can induce hemolytic anemia in glucose 6-phosphate dehydrogenase-deficient patients. Because the newborn's red blood cells are deficient in reduced glutathione, the package insert warns against the use of this drug at term. However, there is no report of neonatal hemolytic anemia after intrauterine exposure.

TETRACYCLINES

There does not appear to be a teratogenic effect of first-trimester exposure to tetracycline or doxycycline.[99] However, tetracyclines bind to developing enamel and cause discoloration of the teeth. Tetracyclines affect deciduous teeth when given between approximately 26 weeks of pregnancy and

6 months of age in the infant. They affect the permanent teeth only if given to children between approximately 6 months and 5 years of age. In addition, tetracyclines deposit in developing osseous sites and cause an inhibition of bone growth beginning in the second trimester.[100] Physicians should give alternative drugs during pregnancy.

AMINOGLYCOSIDES

No teratogenic effect was observed in 135 infants exposed to **streptomycin** in the first trimester. Streptomycin crosses the placenta, and it has caused ototoxicity in 3% to 11% of children of mothers who received prolonged streptomycin treatment for tuberculosis during pregnancy.[101] Similar ototoxicity has been seen after prolonged intrauterine exposure to **kanamycin**.

Physicians should limit the duration of therapy with aminoglycosides and should monitor maternal serum levels to minimize fetal exposure. Once-daily dosing (4 mg/kg intravenously) of **gentamicin** increases efficacy and decreases toxicity and cost.[102] Aminoglycosides may also potentiate the neuromuscular weakness associated with the administration of magnesium sulfate or a nondepolarizing muscle relaxant.

QUINOLONES

The quinolones (e.g., ciprofloxacin, norfloxacin) have a high affinity for bone tissue and cartilage and may cause arthropathies in children. However, no malformations or musculoskeletal problems were noted in 38 infants exposed during the first trimester.[103] The manufacturer recommends against the use of this drug during pregnancy and in children.

METRONIDAZOLE

There is no apparent increase in the incidence of major congenital anomalies among the newborns of mothers treated with metronidazole (Flagyl) during early or late gestation. A recent meta-analysis confirmed no teratogenic risk.[104] It remains the most effective drug for trichomoniasis.

ACYCLOVIR AND OTHER ANTIVIRAL THERAPY

Administration of acyclovir (Zovirax) has resulted in no fetal abnormalities in 601 reported exposures.[105] The Centers for Disease Control and Prevention (CDC) recommends that pregnant women with disseminated infection (e.g., herpetic hepatitis, varicella pneumonia) be treated with acyclovir.

Zidovudine (AZT) has been studied because of its role in the treatment of AIDS. In a prospective cohort study, children exposed to AZT in the perinatal period through Pediatric AIDS Clinical Trials Group Protocol 076 (PACTG 076) were studied up to a median age of 4.2 years. No adverse effects were observed.[106] Combination antiretroviral therapy has not been associated with major infant toxicity, even when the therapy was initiated in the first trimester of pregnancy.[107]

The International Antiretroviral Registry was established in 1993 to detect any major teratogenic effect of the antiretroviral drugs. The registration process protects patient anonymity. The Registry depends on voluntary reporting of prenatal exposure to the antiretroviral drugs; therefore, drug-associated adverse events may not reflect true rates. Through July 1999, 916 pregnancies were enrolled in the study; of these, 403 were first-trimester exposures.[108] The Registry includes reports of prenatal exposure (in all three trimesters of pregnancy) to almost all of the antiretroviral drugs, alone or in combination, with the exception of zalcitabine and delavirdine. Exposure to the latter two drugs has been

reported in the first and second trimesters. The number of pregnancies exposed to the various drugs has been increasing, but in many cases an assessment of the effects of individual drugs on the fetus is not possible. No evidence of teratogenicity has been reported.[109]

Four drugs are currently approved for the control and prevention of influenza in the United States: amantadine, rimantadine, zanamivir, and oseltamivir. Amantadine and rimantadine are chemically related and demonstrate activity against influenza A but not influenza B viruses. Zanamivir and oseltamivir are neuraminidase inhibitors with activity against both influenza A and B viruses. In a surveillance study of 333,000 live-born infants, 64 pregnancies were exposed to amantadine.[110] Five of the children were diagnosed with congenital anomalies, while the expected number was 3.1. The CDC has stated that because of the unknown effects of influenza antiviral drugs on pregnant women and their fetuses, these four drugs should be used during pregnancy only if the potential benefit justifies the potential risk to the embryo or fetus.[111]

Mild Analgesics

Physicians should encourage patients to use nonpharmacologic remedies (e.g., locally applied heat, rest) for aches and pains during pregnancy.

ASPIRIN

There is no evidence of an overall increase in congenital malformations with maternal use of aspirin during the first trimester. One review suggested an increased risk of gastroschisis.[112]

Aspirin causes permanent inhibition of prostaglandin synthetase in platelets. Aspirin inhibits platelet aggregation, and platelet function returns to normal only after the production of new platelets in the bone marrow. Thus aspirin may increase the risk of peripartum hemorrhage. One study noted platelet dysfunction in the newborn as late as 5 days after maternal ingestion of aspirin.[113]

Prostaglandins help maintain the patency of the ductus arteriosus in utero. Areilla et al.[114] reported one case in which they suggested that the use of aspirin shortly before delivery caused closure of the ductus arteriosus in utero.

Low-dose aspirin may prevent fetal wastage associated with autoimmune disease. In patients with antiphospholipid antibody syndrome, treatment with low-dose aspirin may help prevent pregnancy loss.[115] Low-dose aspirin does not significantly prolong the bleeding time.[116]

ACETAMINOPHEN

There is no known teratogenic risk associated with the use of acetaminophen (Tylenol or Datril).[57] Acetaminophen does not cause permanent inhibition of prostaglandin synthesis, and it does not prolong the bleeding time. Moreover, the usual maternal doses of acetaminophen do not result in neonatal toxicity. Thus, if a mild analgesic or antipyretic is required during pregnancy, acetaminophen is preferred over aspirin.

PROPOXYPHENE

Propoxyphene (Darvon) has no known teratogenic risk, and it may be prescribed during pregnancy. Propoxyphene has the potential for addiction; thus it should not be used for trivial indications. There are case reports of neonatal opioid-withdrawal symptoms in infants whose mothers were addicted to propoxyphene.[117]

CODEINE

No increased risk of malformations was observed in the infants of 563 mothers who used codeine during pregnancy in the Collaborative Perinatal Project.[56] Excessive antepartum use of codeine can cause maternal addiction and neonatal opioid-withdrawal symptoms.

INDOMETHACIN

Indomethacin is a nonsteroidal antiinflammatory agent used in the treatment of disorders such as rheumatoid arthritis, ankylosing spondylitis, and osteoarthritis, as well as in the treatment of preterm labor. Unlike aspirin, which causes an irreversible inhibition of the cyclooxygenase enzyme necessary for prostaglandin synthesis, indomethacin results in a competitive and reversible inhibition of this enzyme.

Oral administration of indomethacin may result in intrauterine constriction of the ductus arteriosus, and this effect increases with advancing gestational age.[118] Use for longer than 48 hours may cause oligohydramnios. No increased risk of teratogenicity has been reported with first-trimester use.[57]

OTHER NONSTEROIDAL ANTIINFLAMMATORY AGENTS

No evidence of teratogenicity has been reported for other nonsteroidal antiinflammatory drugs, including **ibuprofen** (Motrin and Advil) and **naproxen**[119] (Naprosyn), but limited information is available. Chronic use may lead to oligohydramnios. Also, constriction of the fetal ductus arteriosus and/or neonatal pulmonary hypertension might occur.

Caffeine

No evidence suggests that caffeine has any teratogenic effect in humans. A national registry study from Finland evaluated over 700 malformations, including those of the CNS, cleft lip/palate, skeletal malformations, and congenital heart defects.[120] They found no association with coffee consumption. Two large U.S. studies also found no relationship between coffee intake and congenital malformations.[121,122] A Canadian study of 80,319 pregnancies found no increase in malformations related to coffee intake.[123]

Early uncontrolled studies suggested that heavy ingestion of caffeine was associated with an increased incidence of spontaneous abortion, low birth weight, preterm delivery, and stillbirth. However, these studies were not controlled for the use of tobacco and alcohol. In a subsequent study that was controlled for smoking, other habits, demographic characteristics, and medical history,[122] no relationship was found between heavy coffee consumption and low birth weight or preterm delivery. The retrospective data regarding caffeine and spontaneous abortion have not been widely accepted because of study bias.[124] Martin and Bracken[125] suggested that an increased incidence of growth-restricted infants may occur in women who consume more than 300 mg of caffeine daily. One study indicated that the ingestion of caffeine may increase the risk of an early spontaneous abortion among nonsmoking women carrying fetuses with normal karyotypes.[126] Ingestion of at least 300 mg per day was required to increase the risk. Concomitant consumption of caffeine and cigarette smoking may increase the risk of IUGR.[126] Maternal caffeine intake decreases iron absorption and may increase the risk of anemia.[127]

DRUG USE DURING LACTATION

Many drugs can be detected in breast milk at low concentrations that usually are not of clinical significance for the infant. The rate of drug transfer into milk depends on the lipid solubility, molecular weight, degree of ionization of the drug, degree of protein binding, and the presence or absence of active secretion. Nonionized molecules of small molecular weight (e.g., ethanol) cross easily.

The amount of a drug that is detected in breast milk is a variable fraction of the maternal blood level, which is proportional to the oral maternal dose. The resulting dose usually is subtherapeutic for the infant. The average fetal dose is 1% to 2% of the maternal dose. Usually, this amount is so trivial that no adverse effects are noted. Physicians and patients should be aware of the following disclaimers. First, in the case of toxic drugs, any exposure may be inappropriate. Second, the infant may be allergic to a drug consumed by the mother. Third, there may be unknown, long-term effects of even small doses of drugs. Fourth, if an increased dose of drug or decreased maternal renal function causes a high maternal blood concentration, a higher concentration of drug may be detected in breast milk. Finally, infants have immature enzyme systems and metabolic pathways, and some drugs are eliminated more slowly. The benefits of breast-feeding are well known, and the risk of drug exposure must be weighed against these benefits.

Lactation is not fully established during the first several days postpartum. The infant receives only a small volume of colostrum, and little drug is excreted through milk at this time. Thus it is unlikely that analgesics or other drugs administered after vaginal or cesarean delivery will adversely affect the infant.

When a mother requires a daily dose of a drug during lactation, knowledge of pharmacokinetics may minimize the dose for the infant. In general, medications should be taken *after* breast-feeding, and long-acting preparations should be avoided. If the infant nurses less frequently overnight, ingestion of a nighttime drug dose *after* nursing will decrease the infant's exposure.

The American Academy of Pediatrics[128] has reviewed the use of drugs during lactation and has categorized drugs as follows.

Cytotoxic Drugs that May Interfere with Cellular Metabolism of the Nursing Infant

Cytotoxic agents (e.g., cyclophosphamide, cyclosporine, doxorubicin, methotrexate) used for cancer chemotherapy may cause immunosuppression in the infant, although data are limited. There may also be an association with carcinogenesis. The potential risks of these drugs probably outweigh the benefits of continuing nursing.[128]

After oral administration to a lactating patient with choriocarcinoma, methotrexate was found in milk in low but detectable levels. Most mothers would elect to avoid any infant exposure to this drug, but in environments in which bottle feeding is rarely practiced and presents practical and cultural difficulties, therapy with this drug would not appear to constitute a contraindication to breast-feeding.[129]

Drugs of Abuse for which Adverse Effects on the Infant During Breast-Feeding Have Been Reported

Drugs of abuse such as amphetamines, cocaine, heroin, marijuana, and phencyclidine are all contraindicated during breast-feeding because they are hazardous to the nursing infant and to the health of the mother.[128]

Radioactive Compounds that Require Temporary Cessation of Breast-Feeding

The American Academy of Pediatrics[128] suggests that consultation with a nuclear medicine physician take place so that the radionuclide with the shortest excretion time in breast milk can be used. The mother can attempt to store breast milk prior to the study. She should continue to pump her breasts to maintain milk production, but she should discard the milk during therapy. Radiopharmaceuticals require variable intervals of interruption of nursing to ensure that no radioactivity is detectable in the milk. Recommended intervals are as follows:

1. Gallium-67: 2 weeks
2. ^{131}Iodine: 2 to 14 days
3. Radioactive sodium: 4 days
4. Technetium-99: 15 hours to 3 days

The physician may reassure the patient by counting the radioactivity of the milk before nursing is resumed.

Drugs for which the Effect on Nursing Infants is Unknown But May Be of Concern

This category includes several classes of psychotropic drugs, amiodarone (which might affect the infant's thyroid function), lamotrigine (due to the potential for therapeutic serum concentrations in the infant), metoclopramide (due to its antagonism of dopaminergic receptors, although no detrimental effects have been reported), and metronidazole.

PSYCHOTROPIC DRUGS

These drugs (e.g., antianxiety, antidepressant, and neuroleptic drugs) may be of concern when given to nursing mothers. Maternal ingestion of these drugs results in milk:plasma ratios of 0.5 to 1.0. Many of these medications often have a long half-life, and the effect of even small doses on the developing nervous system is not known. If these agents must be used in a lactating woman, it is recommended that relatively short-acting agents with inactive metabolites be selected, such as oxazepam, lorazepam, orazepam, alprazolam, or midazolam.[130] The infant should be monitored for sedation during use and for withdrawal symptoms after stopping the medication or after discontinuation of breast-feeding.[131]

METRONIDAZOLE

During maternal metronidazole therapy, a single dose is preferred, and the mother may interrupt nursing for 12 to 24 hours to allow elimination of the drug.

Drugs that Have Been Associated with Significant Effects on Some Nursing Infants and Should Be Given to Nursing Mothers with Caution

ATENOLOL

Atenolol been associated with cyanosis and bradycardia (vide infra).

BROMOCRIPTINE

Bromocriptine is an ergot alkaloid derivative. It has an inhibitory effect on lactation. Bromocriptine is no longer approved for postpartum lactation suppression, because of its association with puerperal seizures, stroke, and myocardial infarction.

ERGOTAMINE

Ergotamine, as used by patients with migraine headache, has been associated with vomiting, diarrhea, and convulsions in the infant. Therefore, ergotamine should be avoided during lactation. However, administration of an ergot alkaloid for the treatment of uterine atony does not contraindicate lactation.

LITHIUM

Breast milk levels of lithium are one third to one half maternal serum levels,[132,133] and the infant's serum levels while nursing are much lower than the fetal levels that occur when the mother takes lithium during pregnancy. The benefits of breast-feeding must be weighed against the theoretical effects of small amounts of the drug on the developing brain.

Drugs Usually Compatible with Breast-Feeding

ANALGESICS, OPIOIDS, SEDATIVES, AND ANTICONVULSANTS

There is little transfer of salicylates into breast milk because these acids exist primarily in the ionized form. Following single or repeated oral doses, peak milk levels occur at approximately 3 hours, with a milk:plasma ratio of 0.03 to 0.08.[134] Maternal ingestion of *high doses* (e.g., more than 16 tablets per day) may result in maternal and breast milk concentrations sufficiently high to affect platelet aggregation in the infant. The reduced clearance of salicylates by neonates may result in drug accumulation and toxic effects, even when repeated exposures are small.[135] Because of these concerns, the World Health Organization (WHO) Working Group on Human Lactation has classified the salicylates as unsafe for use by nursing women.[136] The American Academy of Pediatrics Committee on Drugs[128] has stated that aspirin is "associated with significant effects on some nursing infants and should be given to nursing mothers with caution," based on a single case report of a neonate who developed metabolic acidosis.

No harmful effects of acetaminophen or the classic nonsteroidal antiinflammatory agents (e.g., indomethacin, ibuprofen) have been noted. The breast milk concentration of propoxyphene was half that of the maternal serum level in one patient who took propoxyphene in a suicide attempt.[137] Theoretically, a breast-feeding infant could receive up to 1 mg of propoxyphene per day if the mother were to consume the maximum dose.

In general, opioid analgesics, sedatives, and anticonvulsants used by nursing mothers do not adversely affect their infants. Normal maternal doses of codeine, morphine, meperidine, carbamazepine, phenytoin, valproic acid, and magnesium sulfate do not cause obvious adverse effects in nursing infants.[8,128] The dose detectable in breast milk is approximately 1% to 2% of the mother's dose and is sufficiently low to have no significant pharmacologic activity.

Studies have detected only small amounts of phenytoin, phenobarbital, and diazepam in breast milk.[138,139] However, infants eliminate phenobarbital and diazepam slowly, and accumulation may occur. Women taking a barbiturate or a benzodiazepine should observe their infants for evidence of sedation and withdrawal.[9,128]

Cruikshank et al.[140] measured breast milk magnesium concentrations in 10 patients with preeclampsia who were receiving magnesium sulfate 1 g/hr intravenously for 24 hours after delivery. The mean breast-milk magnesium concentration was 6.4 ± 0.4 mg/dL, compared with 4.8 ± 0.5 mg/dL in controls. Breast-milk calcium concentrations were not affected by magnesium sulfate therapy.

ANTIBIOTICS AND OTHER ANTIMICROBIAL AGENTS

Penicillin and its derivatives are safe in nursing mothers. With the usual therapeutic doses of ampicillin, the milk:plasma ratio is 0.2 or less, and no adverse effects are noted in nursing infants.[141] Theoretically, infant diarrhea or candidiasis might occur with prolonged therapy.

Dicloxacillin is 98% protein bound.[141] If this drug is used to treat a breast infection, very little drug is transferred into the breast milk, and nursing may be continued.

Cephalosporins appear in trace amounts in breast milk. In one study, maternal administration of cefazolin (500 mg intramuscularly three times a day) resulted in nondetectable breast-milk concentrations of drug.[142] Intravenous injection of 2 g of cefazolin resulted in a milk-to-plasma ratio of 0.023. Thus the infant was exposed to only 0.075% of the maternal dose.[142]

Tooth staining and/or delayed bone growth have not been reported in offspring after ingestion of tetracycline by a breast-feeding mother. The breast-milk concentration of tetracycline is about half that in the mother's plasma. However, tetracycline has a high affinity for both calcium and protein. Thus the amount of free tetracycline available for systemic absorption is too small to be significant clinically.

Sulfonamides displace bilirubin from binding sites on albumin, and these drugs are best avoided during the first 5 days of life or in mothers of preterm infants with hyperbilirubinemia. Otherwise, sulfonamides are not contraindicated during nursing. Sulfonamides appear in breast milk in small amounts. One study of sulfapyridine noted that the infant receives less than 1% of the maternal dose.[143] In another study, sulfasalazine was not detected in the breast milk of a mother taking this drug.[144] Sulfasalazine should be used with caution, as it has been associated with a case of bloody diarrhea.[128]

Maternal administration of acyclovir does not contraindicate breast-feeding. If a mother takes 1 g/day, the infant probably receives less than 1 mg/day, a very low dose.[145] There are no reported adverse effects on the infant of isoniazid administered to nursing mothers, and its use is considered compatible with breast-feeding.[128]

Other specific agents listed as compatible with breast-feeding include amoxicillin, aztreonam, ciprofloxacin, clindamycin, erythromycin, fluconazole, gentamicin, ketoconazole, nitrofurantoin, ofloxacin, ticarcillin, and rifampin.

ANTIHISTAMINES AND PHENOTHIAZINES

No harmful effects have been noted with maternal use of antihistamines or phenothiazines.[146] These drugs do not appear to affect the milk supply. However, women who are having trouble with their milk supply should avoid decongestants (i.e., vasoconstrictive agents).

THEOPHYLLINE AND OTHER ANTIASTHMATIC DRUGS

Maximum milk concentrations of theophylline are achieved between 1 and 3 hours after an oral dose. It has been calculated that the nursing infant receives less than 1% of the maternal dose. Such exposure appears to cause no adverse effects.[128] Other asthma medications considered compatible with breast-feeding include terbutaline and metoprolol.[128]

ANTIHYPERTENSIVES

One study detected no chlorothiazide in breast milk after a single 500-mg oral dose.[147] Miller et al.[148] reported that daily ingestion of 50 mg of hydrochlorothiazide caused peak milk concentrations that were approximately 25% of maternal blood concentrations. They did not detect any drug in the infant's serum, and the infant's electrolytes were normal.

A single 40-mg dose of propranolol results in breast milk drug concentrations that are less than 40% of peak maternal plasma concentrations.[149] In one study, a 30-day regimen of propranolol (240 mg/day) resulted in predose and 3-hour postdose breast-milk concentrations of 26 ng/mL and 64 ng/mL, respectively. Thus, at a maternal dose of 240 mg/day, an infant ingesting 500 mL of milk per day would ingest a maximum dose of approximately 1% of the therapeutic dose for an infant; it is unlikely that this would cause any adverse effect.[150]

Atenolol is concentrated in breast milk at approximately three times the maternal plasma concentration.[151] However, after a peak-level feeding, the infant plasma concentration is less than 10 ng/mL, which is not associated with side effects in the infant. In addition, the total infant dose is only 1% of the maternal therapeutic dose. This agent should be used with caution when breast-feeding because of its association with neonatal cyanosis and bradycardia.[128]

Breast-milk clonidine concentrations are almost twice maternal serum concentrations. However, this exposure does not seem to have any adverse effects on the infant.[152]

ANTICOAGULANTS

Most mothers who require anticoagulation may continue to nurse their infants with no problems. Heparin does not cross into breast milk. Moreover, heparin is not active when given orally.

Warfarin is 98% protein bound. Orme et al.[153] studied seven women taking warfarin (Coumadin) 5 to 12 mg/day. They detected no warfarin in breast milk or infant plasma. deSwiet and Lewis[154] also confirmed that warfarin appears in breast milk in insignificant quantities.

CORTICOSTEROIDS

Katz and Duncan[155] obtained breast milk 2 hours after an oral dose of 10 mg of prednisone in one nursing mother. Breast-milk concentrations of prednisone and prednisolone were of an amount not likely to result in any deleterious effect. MacKenzie et al.[156] administered 5 mg of radioactive prednisolone to seven patients and found that 0.14% (a negligible quantity) of the radioactive label was secreted in the milk in the subsequent 60 hours. Thus breast-feeding is not contraindicated in mothers taking corticosteroids. Even at a maternal dosage of 80 mg/day, the nursing infant would ingest a dose equivalent to less than 10% of its endogenous cortisol production.[157]

DIGOXIN

After a maternal dose of 0.25 mg, peak breast-milk concentrations of 0.6 to 1.0 ng/mL occur, and the milk:plasma ratio at the 4-hour peak is 0.8 to 0.9. Maternal protein binding limits infant drug exposure. In 24 hours an infant might receive approximately 1% of the maternal dose,[158] and no adverse effects have been reported in nursing infants.

ORAL CONTRACEPTIVES

Some studies have suggested that the use of an estrogen-progestin oral contraceptive is associated with a decreased quantity of breast milk, a shorter duration of lactation, decreased infant weight gain, and decreased nitrogen and protein content in the milk.[159] However, most published studies evaluated the effect of the 50-μg estrogen preparations. Oral contraceptives cause less inhibition of lactation if the patient delays contraceptive therapy until 3 weeks postpartum.[160] Progestin-only contraceptives do not alter breast milk composition or volume. No long-term adverse effects on growth and development have been described in the children of mothers taking an oral contraceptive.[128,160]

PROPYLTHIOURACIL

Only small amounts of propylthiouracil are found in breast milk. One study noted no change in thyroid function (including levels of thyroid-stimulating hormone) through 5 months of age in an infant exposed to maternal propylthiouracil.[161]

H$_2$-RECEPTOR ANTAGONISTS

In theory, H$_2$-receptor antagonists (e.g., ranitidine, cimetidine) might suppress gastric acidity and/or cause CNS stimulation in the infant, but these effects have not been confirmed in published studies. The American Academy of Pediatrics considers cimetidine to be compatible with breast-feeding.[128] Famotidine, nizatidine, and roxatidine are less concentrated in breast milk and may be preferable in nursing mothers.[162]

CAFFEINE

Moderate maternal intake of caffeine does not adversely affect the infant. One study noted that breast milk contains only 1% of the total maternal dose of caffeine.[163] If a mother drinks excessive amounts of coffee, caffeine might accumulate in the infant, and the infant might show signs of caffeine stimulation (e.g., irritability, poor sleeping pattern). Nursing mothers should limit their intake to a moderate level of caffeinated beverages (e.g., 2 to 3 cups per day).[128]

KEY POINTS

- The critical period of organ development extends from approximately day 31 to day 71 after the first day of the LMP.
- Administration of anticonvulsants is associated with an increased risk of congenital anomalies, but monotherapy is associated with less risk than therapy with two or more drugs.
- Isotretinoin is highly teratogenic and should not be used during pregnancy.
- Heparin does not cross the placenta and is the anticoagulant of choice during pregnancy, except for women with prosthetic heart valves, who should receive warfarin.
- Angiotensin-converting enzyme inhibitors should be avoided during pregnancy because they cause fetal renal dysplasia and oligohydramnios.

- Only a small amount of prednisone crosses the placenta. Therefore, prednisone is the preferred corticosteroid for most maternal diseases. In contrast, betamethasone and dexamethasone readily cross the placenta and are preferred when the obstetrician wants to accelerate fetal lung maturity.
- Most antibiotics are safe during pregnancy. Tetracyclines should be avoided because they cause tooth discoloration and inhibit bone growth in the fetus. Quinolones are contraindicated during pregnancy. Trimethoprim most likely should be avoided during the first trimester.
- Analgesic doses of aspirin cause an increased risk of peripartum hemorrhage.
- Most drugs are safe for use during lactation. Typically only 1% to 2% of the maternal dose appears in breast milk. Lithium and ergotamine are best avoided during lactation.

REFERENCES

1. Yankowitz J. Use of medications in pregnancy: General principles, teratology, and current developments. In: Drug Therapy in Pregnancy. Yankowitz J, Niebyl JR, editors. Lippincott Williams & Wilkins, Baltimore, 2001.
2. American College of Obstetricians and Gynecologists. Teratology. ACOG Educational Bulletin No. 236, April 1997.
3. Sever LE, Mortensen ME. Teratology and the epidemiology of birth defects: Occupational and environmental perspectives. In: Gabbe SG, Niebyl JR, Simpson JL, editors. Obstetrics: Normal and Problem Pregnancies. 3rd edition. Churchill Livingston, New York, 1996.
4. Buehler BA, Delimont D, van Waes M, Finnell RH. Prenatal prediction of risk of the fetal hydantoin syndrome. N Engl J Med 1990; 322:1567-72.
5. Teratology Society Public Affairs Committee. FDA classification of drugs for teratogenic risk. Teratology 1994; 49:446-7.
6. Friedman JM. Report of the Teratology Society Public Affairs Committee Symposium on FDA Classification of Drugs. Teratology 1993; 48:5-6.
7. Doering PL, Boothby LA, Cheok M. Review of pregnancy labeling of prescription drugs: Is the current system adequate to inform of risks? Am J Obstet Gynecol 2002; 187:333-9.
8. Malone FD, D'Alton ME. Drugs in pregnancy: Anticonvulsants. Semin Perinatol 1997; 21:114-23.
9. Morrell MJ. Guidelines for the care of women with epilepsy. Neurology 1998; 51(suppl 4):S21-7.
10. Shapiro S, Hartz SC, Siskind V, et al. Anticonvulsants and parental epilepsy in the development of birth defects. Lancet 1976; i:272-5.
11. Holmes LB, Rosenberger PB, Harvey EA, et al. Intelligence and physical features of children of women with epilepsy. Teratology 2000; 61:196-202.
12. Holmes LB. Harvey EA, Cull BA, et al. The teratogenicity of anticonvulsant drugs. N Engl J Med 2001; 344:1132-8.
13. Morrell MJ. The new antiepileptic drugs and women: Efficacy, reproductive health, pregnancy and fetal outcome. Epilepsia 1996; 37 (suppl. 6): S34-4.
14. Cornelissen M, Steegers-Theunissen R, Kollee L, et al. Increased incidence of neonatal vitamin K deficiency resulting from maternal anticonvulsant therapy. Am J Obstet Gynecol 1993; 168:923-8.
15. Cornelissen M, Steegers-Theunissen R, Kollee L, et al. Supplementation of vitamin K in pregnant women receiving anticonvulsant therapy prevents neonatal vitamin K deficiency. Am J Obstet Gynecol 1993; 168:884-8.
16. Jones KL, Lacro RV, Johnson KA, Adams J. Patterns of malformations in the children of women treated with carbamazepine during pregnancy. N Engl J Med 1989; 320:1661-6.
17. Rosa FW. Spina bifida in infants of women treated with carbamazepine during pregnancy. N Engl J Med 1991; 324:674-7.
18. Levy RH, Yerby MS. Effects of pregnancy on antiepileptic drug utilization. Epilepsia 1985; 26 (suppl 1):S52-7.

19. Eldridge RR, White AD, Tennis PS, et. al. Three prospective registries to monitor prenatal maternal exposures: The acyclovir in pregnancy, the antiretroviral in pregnancy, and the lamotrigine in pregnancy registries (abstract). Reprod Toxicol 1993; 7:637.

20. Tennis P. Eldridge RR, and the International Lamotrigine Pregnancy Registry Scientific Advisory Committee. Preliminary results on pregnancy outcomes in women using lamotrigine. Epilepsia 2002; 43: 1161-7.

21. Callaghan N, Garrett A, Goggin T. Withdrawal of anticonvulsant drugs in patients free of seizures for two years. N Engl J Med 1988; 318:942-4.

22. Lammer EJ, Chen DT, Hoar RM, et al. Retinoic acid embryopathy. N Engl J Med 1985; 313:837-41.

23. Adams J. High incidence of intellectual deficits in 5 year old children exposed to isotretinoin "in utero." Teratology 1990; 41:614.

24. Milkovich L, van den Berg BJ. Effects of prenatal meprobamate and chlordiazepoxide hydrochloride on human embryonic and fetal development. N Engl J Med 1974; 291:1268-71.

25. Hartz SC, Heinonnen OP, Shapiro S, et al. Antenatal exposure to meprobamate and chlordiazepoxide in relation to malformations, mental development, and childhood mortality. N Engl J Med 1975; 292:726-8.

26. Safra MJ, Oakley GP. Association between cleft lip with or without cleft palate and prenatal exposure to diazepam. Lancet 1975; ii:478-80.

27. Altshuler LL, Cohen L, Szuba M, et al. Pharmacologic management of psychiatric illness during pregnancy: Dilemmas and guidelines. Am J Psychiatry 1996; 153:592-606.

28. Rosenberg L, Mitchell AA, Parsells JL, et al. Lack of relation of oral clefts to diazepam use during pregnancy. N Engl J Med 1983; 309:1282-5.

29. Ornoy A, Arnon J, Shectman S, et al. Is benzodiazepine use during pregnancy really teratogenic? Reprod Toxicol 1998; 12:511-5.

30. Gillberg C. "Floppy infant syndrome" and maternal diazepam. Lancet 1977; ii:244.

31. Linden S, Rich CL. The use of lithium during pregnancy and lactation. J Clin Psychiatr 1983; 44:358-61.

32. Kallen B, Tandberg A. Lithium and pregnancy: A cohort study on manic-depressive women. Acta Psychiatr Scand 1983; 68:134-9.

33. Jacobson SJ, Jones K, Johnson X, et al. Prospective multicenter study of pregnancy outcome after lithium exposure during the first trimester. Lancet 1992; 339:530-3.

34. Krause S, Ebbesen F, Lange AP. Polyhydramnios with maternal lithium treatment. Obstet Gynecol 1990; 75:504-6.

35. Ang MS, Thorp JA, Parisi VM. Maternal lithium therapy and polyhydramnios. Obstet Gynecol 1990; 76:517-9.

36. Schou M, Amdisen A, Streenstrup OP. Lithium and pregnancy. II. Hazards to women given lithium during pregnancy and delivery. Br Med J 1973; 2:137-8.

37. Linden S, Rich CL. The use of lithium during pregnancy and lactation. J Clin Psychiatr 1983; 44:358-361.

38. Goldstein DJ, Corbin LA, Sundell KL. Effects of first-trimester fluoxetine exposure on the newborn. N Engl J Med 1997; 89:713-8.

39. Nulman I, Rovet J, Stewart DE, et al. Child development following exposure to tricyclic antidepressants or fluoxetine throughout fetal life: A prospective, controlled study. Am J Psychiatr 2002; 159:1889-95.

40. Hendrick V, Smith LM, Suri R, et al. Birth outcomes after prenatal exposure to antidepressant medication. Am J Obstet Gynecol 2003; 188:812-5.

41. Chambers CD, Johnson KA, Dick LM, et al. Birth outcomes in pregnant women taking fluoxetine. N Engl J Med 1996; 335:1010-5.

42. Hall JG, Pauli RM, Wilson KM. Maternal and fetal sequelae of anticoagulation during pregnancy. Am J Med 1980; 68:122-40.

43. Jones KL. Smith's recognizable patterns of human malformation. 5th edition. WB Saunders, Philadelphia, 1997.

44. Vitale N, De Feo M, De Santo LS, et al. Dose-dependent fetal complications of warfarin in pregnant women with mechanical heart valves. J Am Coll Cardiol 1999; 33:1637-41.

45. Dahlman T, Lindvall N, Hellgren M. Osteopenia in pregnancy during long-term heparin treatment: A radiological study post-partum. Br J Obstet Gynaecol 1990; 97:221-8.

46. Frewin R, Chisholm M. Anticoagulation of women with prosthetic heart valves during pregnancy. Br J Obstet Gynaecol 1998; 105:683-6.

47. Iturbe-Alessio I, Fonseca MC, Mutchinik O, et al. Risks of anticoagulant therapy in pregnant women with artificial heart valves. N Engl J Med 1986; 315:1390-3.

48. Meschengieser SS, Fondevila CG, Santarelli MT, Lazzari MA. Anticoagulation in pregnant women with mechanical heart valve prostheses. Heart 1999; 82:23-6.

49. American College of Obstetricians and Gynecologists. Thromboembolism in pregnancy. ACOG Practice Bulletin No 19, August 2000.

50. Wing DA, Millar LK, Koonings PP, et al. A comparison of propylthiouracil versus methimazole in the treatment of hyperthyroidism in pregnancy. Am J Obstet Gynecol 1994; 170:90-5.

51. Martin-Denavit T, Edery P, Plauchu H, et al. Ectodermal abnormalities associated with methimazole intrauterine exposure. Am J Med Genet 2000; 94:338-40.

52. Vogt T, Stolz W, Landthaler M. Aplasia cutis congenita after exposure to methimazole: A causal relationship? Br J Dermatol 1995; 133:994-6.

53. Burrow GN. Thyroid diseases. In Burrow GN, Duffy TP, editors. Medical complications during pregnancy. Philadelphia, WB Saunders, 1999:135-61.

54. Mandel SJ, Larsen PR, Seely EW, et al. Increased need for thyroxine during pregnancy in women with primary hypothyroidism. N Engl J Med 1990; 323:91-6.

55. Haddow JE, Palomaki GE, Allan WC, et al. Maternal thyroid deficiency during pregnancy and subsequent neuropsychological development of the child. N Engl J Med 1999; 341:549-55.

56. Heinonen OP, Slone D, Shapiro S. Birth defects and drugs in pregnancy. Publishing Sciences Group, Massachusetts, 1977:441.

57. Aselton P, Jick H, Milunsky A, et al. First-trimester drug use and congenital disorders. Obstet Gynecol 1985; 65:451-5.

58. Pruyn SC, Phelan JP, Buchanan GC. Long-term propranolol therapy in pregnancy: Maternal and fetal outcome. Am J Obstet Gynecol 1979; 135:485-9.

59. Redmond GP. Propranolol and fetal growth retardation. Semin Perinatol 1982; 6:142-7.

60. Magee LA, Bull SB, Koren G, Logan A. The generalizability of trial data: A comparison of β-blocker trial participants with a prospective cohort of women taking β-blockers in pregnancy. Eur J Obstet Gynecol Reprod Biol 2001; 94:205-10.

61. Lydakis C, Lip GYH, Beevers M, Beevers DG. Atenolol and fetal growth in pregnancies complicated by hypertension. Am J Hypertens 1999; 12:541-7.

62. Easterling TR, Carr DB, Brateng D, et al. Treatment of hypertension in pregnancy: Effect of atenolol on maternal disease, preterm delivery, and fetal growth. Obstet Gynecol 2001; 98:427-33.

63. Easterling TR, Brateng D, Schmucker B, et al. Prevention of preeclampsia: A randomized trial of atenolol in hyperdynamic patients before onset of hypertension. Obstet Gynecol 1999; 93:725-33.

64. Pickles CJ, Symonds EM, Broughton PF. The fetal outcome in a randomized double-blind controlled trial of labetalol versus placebo in pregnancy-induced hypertension. Br J Obstet Gynecol 1989; 98: 38-43.

65. Burrows RF, Burrows EA. Assessing the teratogenic potential of angiotensin-converting enzyme inhibitors in pregnancy. Aust N Z J Obstet Gynecol 1998; 38:306-11.

66. Piper JM, Ray WA, Rosa FW. Pregnancy outcome following exposure to angiotensin-converting enzyme inhibitors. Obstet Gynecol 1992; 80:429-32.

67. Oei SG, Oei SK, Brolmann HA. Myocardial infarction during nifedipine therapy for preterm labor (letter). N Engl J Med 1999; 340:154.

68. Magee LA, Schick B, Donnenfeld AE, et al. The safety of calcium channel blockers in human pregnancy: A prospective, multicenter cohort study. Am J Obstet Gynecol 1996; 174:823-8.

69. Tan HL, Lie KI. Treatment of tachyarrhythmias during pregnancy and lactation. Eur Heart J 2001; 22:458-64.

70. Bartalena L, Bogazzi F, Braverman LE, Martino E. Effects of amiodarone administration during pregnancy on neonatal thyroid function and subsequent neurodevelopment. J Endocrinol Invest 2001; 24: 116-30.

71. Kallen B. Drug treatment of rheumatic diseases during pregnancy. The teratogenicity of antirheumatic drugs: What is the evidence? Scand J Rheumatol 1998; 27(suppl 107):119-24.

72. Polifka JE, Friedman JM. Teratogen update: Azathioprine and 6-mercaptopurine. Teratology 2002; 65:240-61.

73. Armenti VT, Moritz MJ, Davison JM. Drug safety issues in pregnancy following transplantation and immunosuppression. Effects and outcomes. Drug Saf 1998; 19:219-32.

74. Kirshon B, Wasserstram N, Willis R, et al. Teratogenic effects of first trimester cyclophosphamide therapy. Obstet Gynecol 1988; 72:462-7.

75. Wolfe MS, Cordero JF. Safety of chloroquine in chemosuppression of malaria during pregnancy. Br Med J 1985; 290:1466-7.

76. Hart CW, Naunton RF. The ototoxicity of chloroquine phosphate. Arch Otolaryngol 1964; 80:407-12.

77. Heinonen OP, Slone D, Shapiro S. Birth defects and drugs in pregnancy. Publishing Sciences Group, Massachusetts, 1977:367-70.

78. Rosa F. Databases in the assessment of the effect of drugs during pregnancy. J Allergy Clin Immunol 1999; 103:S360-1.

79. Park-Wyllie L, Mazzotta P, Pastuszak A, et al. Birth defects after maternal exposure to corticosteroids: Prospective cohort study and meta-analysis of epidemiological studies. Teratology 2000; 62:385-92.

80. Carmichael SL, Shaw GM. Maternal corticosteroid use and risk of selected congenital anomalies. Am J Med Genet 1999; 86:242-4.

81. Sahakian V, Rouse D, Sipes S, et al. Vitamin B6 is effective therapy for nausea and vomiting of pregnancy: A randomized, double-blind placebo-controlled study. Obstet Gynecol 1991; 78:33-6.

82. Vutyavanich T, Wongtra-Rjan S, Ruangsri R. Pyridoxine for nausea and vomiting of pregnancy: A randomized double-blind placebo-controlled trial. Am J Obstet Gynecol 1995; 173:881.

83. Vutyavanich T, Kraisarin T, Ruangsri R. Ginger for nausea and vomiting in pregnancy: Randomized, double-masked, placebo-controlled trial. Obstet Gynecol 2001; 97:577-82.

84. Fischer-Rasmussen W, Kjaer SK, Dahl C, Asping U. Ginger treatment of hyperemesis gravidarum. Eur J Obstet Gynecol Reprod Biol 1990; 38:19-24.

85. Milkovich L, Van Den Berg BJ. An evaluation of the teratogenicity of certain antinauseant drugs. Am J Obstet Gynecol 1976; 125:244-8.

86. Heinonen OP, Slove D, Shapiro S. Birth defects and drugs in pregnancy. Publishing Sciences Group, Massachusetts, 1977:324.

87. Sorensen HT, Nielsen GL, Christensen K, et al. Birth outcomes following maternal use of metoclopramide. Br J Clin Pharmacol 2000; 49:264-8.

88. Sullivan CA, Johnson CA, Roach H, et al. A pilot study of intravenous ondansetron for hyperemesis gravidarum. Am J Obstet Gynecol 1996; 174:1565-8.

89. Werler MM, Mitchell AA, Shapiro S. First trimester maternal medication use in relation to gastroschisis. Teratology 1992; 45:361-7.

90. Seto A, Einarson T, Koren G. Evaluation of brompheniramine safety in pregnancy. Reprod Toxicol 1993; 7:393-5.

91. Schatz M, Zeiger RS, Harden K, et al. The safety of asthma and allergy medications during pregnancy. J Allergy Clin Immunol 1997; 100: 301-6.

92. Pastuszak A, Schick B, D'Alimonte D, et al. The safety of astemizole in pregnancy. J Allergy Clin Immunol 1996; 98:748-50.

93. Einarson A, Bailey B, Jung G, et al. Prospective controlled study of hydroxyzine and cetirizine in pregnancy. Ann Allergy Asthma Immunol 1997; 78:183-6.

94. Seto A, Einarson T, Koren G. Pregnancy outcome following first trimester exposure to antihistamines: Meta-analysis. Am J Perinatol 1997; 14:119-24.

95. Czeizel AE, Rockenbauer M, Sorensen HT, Olsen J. Use of cephalosporins during pregnancy and in the presence of congenital abnormalities: A population-based, case-control study. Am J Obstet Gynecol 2001; 184:1289-96.

96. Jarnerot G, Into-Malmberg MB, Esbjorner E. Placental transfer of sulphasalazine and sulphapyridine and some of its metabolites. Scand J Gastroenterol 1981; 16:693-7.

97. Briggs GG, Freeman RK, Yaffe SJ. Drugs in pregnancy and lactation, 6th edition. Philadelphia, Lippincott Williams & Wilkins, 2002:1394.

98. Hernandez-Diaz S, Werler MM, Walker AM, Mitchell AA. Folic acid antagonists during pregnancy and the risk of birth defects. N Engl J Med 2002; 343:1608-14.

99. Czeizel AE, Rockenbauer M. Teratogenic study of doxycycline. Obstet Gynecol 1997; 89:524-8.

100. Totterman LE, Saxen L. Incorporation of tetracycline into human foetal bones after maternal drug administration. Acta Obstet Gynecol Scand 1969; 48:542-9.

101. Robinson GC, Cambon KG. Hearing loss in infants of tuberculous mothers treated with streptomycin during pregnancy. N Engl J Med 1964; 271:949-51.

102. Mitra AG, Whitten MK, Laurent SL, et al. A randomized, prospective study comparing once-daily gentamicin versus thrice-daily gentamicin in the treatment of puerperal infection. Am J Obstet Gynecol 1997; 177:786-92.

103. Berkovitch M, Pastuszak A, Gazarian M, et al. Safety of the new quinolones in pregnancy. Obstet Gynecol 1994; 84:535.

104. Bertin P, Taddio A, Ariburnu O, et al. Safety of metronidazole in pregnancy: A meta-analysis. Am J Obstet Gynecol 1995; 172:525.

105. Andrews EB, Yankaskas BC, Cordero JF, et al. Acyclovir in pregnancy registry: Six years' experience. Obstet Gynecol 1992; 79:7.

106. Culnane M, Fowler MG, Lee SS, et al. Lack of long-term effects of in utero exposure to zidovudine among uninfected children born to HIV-infected women. JAMA 1999; 281:151-7.

107. McGowan JP, Crane M, Wiznia AA, Blum S. Combination antiretroviral therapy in human immunodeficiency virus-infected pregnant women. Obstet Gynecol 1999; 94:641-46.

108. Antiretroviral Pregnancy Registry PharmaResearch Corporation, 1410 Commonwealth Drive, Wilmington, NC 28403 (Telephone: 1-800-258-4263 or 1-910-256-2955).

109. Watts, DH. Management of human immunodeficiency virus infection in pregnancy. N Engl J Med 2002; 346:1879-91.

110. Rosa F. Amantadine pregnancy experience. Reprod Toxicol 1994; 8:531.

111. Centers for Disease Control and Prevention. Prevention and Control of Influenza– Recommendations of the Advisory Committee on Immunization Practices. MMWR Morb Mortal Wkly Rep 2000; 49(RR03):1-38.

112. Kozer E, Nikfar S, Costei A, et al. Aspirin consumption during the first trimester of pregnancy and congenital anomalies: A meta-analysis. Am J Obstet Gynecol 2002; 187:1623-30.

113. Stuart JJ, Gross SJ, Elrad H, et al. Effects of acetylsalicylic acid ingestion on maternal and neonatal hemostasis. N Engl J Med 1982; 307:909-12.

114. Areilla RA, Thilenius OB, Ranniger K. Congestive heart failure from suspected ductal closure in utero. J Pediatr 1969; 75:74-8.

115. Farquharson RG, Quenby S, Greaves M. Antiphospholipid syndrome in pregnancy: A randomized, controlled trial of treatment. Obstet Gynecol 2002; 100:408-13.

116. Williams HD, Howard R, O'Donnell N, Findley I. The effect of low dose aspirin on bleeding times. Anaesthesia 1993; 48:331-3.

117. Tyson HK. Neonatal withdrawal symptoms associated with maternal use of propoxyphene hydrochloride (Darvon). J Pediatr 1974; 85:684-5.

118. Moise K. Effect of advancing gestational age on the frequency of fetal ductal constriction in association with maternal indomethacin use. Am J Obstet Gynecol 1993; 168:1350-3.

119. Briggs GG, Freeman RK, Yaffe SJ. Drugs in pregnancy and lactation. 6th edition. Baltimore, Lippincott Williams & Wilkins, 2002:973.

120. Kurpa K, Holmberg PC, Kuosma E, Saxen L. Coffee consumption during pregnancy and selected congenital malformations: A nationwide case-control study. Am J Public Health 1983; 73:1397-9.

121. Rosenberg L, Mitchell AA, Shapiro S, Slone D. Selected birth defects in relation to caffeine-containing beverages. JAMA 1982; 247:1429-32.

122. Linn S, Schoenbaum SC, Monson RR, Rosner B. No association between coffee consumption and adverse outcomes of pregnancy. N Engl J Med 1982; 306:141-5.

123. McDonald AD, Armstrong BG, Sloan M. Cigarette, alcohol and coffee consumption and congenital defects. Am J Public Health 1992; 82:91-3.

124. Infante-Rivard C, Fernandez A, Gauthier R, et al. Fetal loss associated with caffeine intake before and during pregnancy. JAMA 1993; 270:2940-3.

125. Martin TR, Bracken MB. The association between low birth weight and caffeine consumption during pregnancy. Am J Epidemiol 1987; 126:813-21.

126. Beaulac-Baillargeon L, Desrosiers C. Caffeine-cigarette interaction on fetal growth. Am J Obstet Gynecol 1987; 157:1236-40.

127. Munoz LM, Lonnerdal B, Keen CL, et al. Coffee consumption as a factor in iron deficiency anemia among pregnant women and their infants in Costa Rica. Am J Clin Nutr 1988; 48:645-51.

128. American Academy of Pediatrics. Committee on Drugs. The transfer of drugs and other chemicals into human milk. Pediatrics 2001; 108:776-89.

129. Johns BG, Rutherford CD, Laighton RC, et al. Secretion of methotrexate into human milk. Am J Obstet Gynecol 1972; 112:978.

130. Chisolm CA, Kuller JA. A guide to the safety of CNS-active agents during breastfeeding. Drug Saf 1997; 17:127-42.

131. Allaire AD, Kuller JA. Psychotropic drugs in pregnancy and lactation. In Yankowitz J, Niebyl JR, editors. Drug therapy in pregnancy, 3rd edition. Lippincott Williams & Wilkins, New York, 2001.

132. Sykes PA, Quarrie J, Alexander FW. Lithium carbonate and breastfeeding. Br Med J 1976; 2:1299.

133. Schou M, Amdisen A. Lithium and pregnancy. III: Lithium ingestion by children breast-fed by women in lithium treatment. Br Med J 1973; 2:138.

134. Findlay JWA, DeAngelis RL, Kearney MF, et al. Analgesic drugs in breast milk and plasma. Clin Pharmacol Ther 1981; 29:625-33.

135. McNamara PJ, Burgio D, Yoo SD. Pharmacokinetics of acetaminophen, antipyrine, and salicylic acid in the lactating and nursing rabbit, with model predictions of milk to serum concentration ratios and neonatal dose. Toxicol Appl Pharmacol 1991; 109:149-60.

136. The WHO Working Group, Bennet PN, editors. Drugs and human lactation. Elsevier, New York, 1988:335-40.

137. Catz C, Guiacoia G. Drugs and breast milk. Pediatr Clin North Am 1972; 19:155-66.

138. Cole AP, Hailey DM. Diazepam and active metabolite in breast milk and their transfer to the neonate. Arch Dis Child 1975; 50:741-2.

139. Nau H, Rating D, Hauser I, et al. Placental transfer and pharmacokinetics of primidone and its metabolites phenobarbital, PEMA and hydroxyphenobarbital in neonates and infants of epileptic mothers. Eur J Clin Pharmacol 1980; 18:31-42.

140. Cruikshank DP, Varner MW, Pitkin RM. Breast milk magnesium and calcium concentrations following magnesium sulfate treatment. Am J Obstet Gynecol 1982; 143:685-8.

141. Wilson J, Brown R, Cherek D, et al. Drug excretion in human breast milk: Principles, pharmacokinetics and projected consequences. Clin Pharmacol Ther 1980; 5:1-66.

142. Yoskioka H, Cho K, Takimoto M, et al. Transfer of cefazolin into human milk. J Pediatr 1979; 94:151-5.

143. Jarnerot G, Into-Malmberg MB. Sulfasalazine treatment during breast-feeding. Scand J Gastroenterol 1979; 14:869-71.

144. Berlin CM Jr, Yaffe SJ. Disposition of salicylazosulfapyridine (Azulfidine) and metabolites in human breast milk. Dev Pharmacol Ther 1980; 1:31-9.

145. Meyer LJ, deMiranda P, Sheth N, et al. Acyclovir in human breast milk. Am J Obstet Gynecol 1988; 158:586-8.

146. Lione A, Scialli AR. The developmental toxicity of the H1 histamine antagonists. Reprod Toxicol 1996; 10:247-55.

147. Weithmann MW, Krees SV. Excretion of chlorothiazide in human breast milk. J Pediatr 1972; 81:781-3.

148. Miller ME, Cohn RD, Burghart PH. Hydrochlorothiazide disposition in a mother and her breast-fed infant. J Pediatr 1982; 101:789-91.

149. Bauer JH, Pape B, Zajicek J, et al. Propranolol in human plasma and breast milk. Am J Cardiol 1979; 43:860-2.

150. Anderson PO, Slater FJ. Propranolol therapy during pregnancy and lactation. Am J Cardiol 1976; 37:325.

151. White WB, Andreoli JW, Wong SH, et al. Atenolol in human plasma and breast milk. Obstet Gynecol 1984; 63:S42-4.

152. Hartikainen-Sorri AL, Heikkinen JE, Koivisto M. Pharmacokinetics of clonidine during pregnancy and nursing. Obstet Gynecol 1987; 69:598-600.

153. Orme ME, Lewis PJ, deSwiet M, et al. May mothers given warfarin breast-feed their infants? Br Med J 1977; i:1564-5.

154. deSwiet M, Lewis PJ. Excretion of anticoagulants in human milk. N Engl J Med 1977; 297:1471.

155. Katz FH, Duncan BR. Entry of prednisone into human milk. N Engl J Med 1975; 293:1154.

156. MacKenzie SA, Seeley JA, Agnew JE. Secretion of prednisolone into breast milk. Arch Dis Child 1975; 50:894-6.

157. Ost L, Wettrell G, Bjorkhem I, et al. Prednisolone excretion in human milk. J Pediatr 1985; 106:1008-11.

158. Loughnan PM. Digoxin excretion in human breast milk. J Pediatr 1978; 92:1019-20.

159. Lonnerdal B, Forsum E, Hambraeus L. Effect of oral contraceptives on consumption and volume of breast milk. Am J Clin Nutr 1980; 33:816-24.

160. American Academy of Pediatrics. Committee on Drugs. Breast-feeding and contraception. Pediatrics 1981; 68:138-40.

161. Kampmann JP, Hansen JM, Johansen K, et al. Propylthiouracil in human milk. Lancet 1980; i:736-8.

162. Anderson PO. Drug use during breast-feeding. Clin Pharm 1991; 10:594-624.

163. Berlin CM Jr, Denson HM, Daniel CH, et al. Disposition of dietary caffeine in milk, saliva, and plasma of lactating women. Pediatrics 1984; 73:59-63.

Chapter 14

In Vitro Fertilization and Other Assisted Reproductive Techniques

Lawrence C. Tsen, M.D. · Robert D. Vincent, Jr., M.D.

In 1978, Steptoe and Edwards[1] reported the first live birth that occurred after in vitro fertilization (IVF) of a human oocyte. They described a case in which a single oocyte was recovered laparoscopically just before ovulation during a natural menstrual cycle. After insemination and fertilization in vitro, the resulting embryo was grown in culture media to the eight-cell stage and was transferred to the uterine cavity 2½ days after oocyte retrieval.

IVF was developed as a treatment for infertility secondary to chronic tubal disease. Indications for assisted reproductive techniques (ARTs) have now been extended to include women with inadequate oocyte quality or number (donor oocyte therapy), women with irreparable or absent uteri (surrogate uterus programs), women with significant comorbidities (embryo cryopreservation), men with sperm deficiencies, and couples with certain genetic aberrations.[2]

In 1981, Edwards[3] estimated that between 15 and 20 babies would be born worldwide in that year after IVF and embryo transfer (ET). Subsequently both the complexities and numbers of ART procedures performed have increased rapidly (Figure 14-1). For example, in 1999, 88,077 cycles of ART led to the birth of 39,967 neonates in the United States alone.[4]

Methodologic advances in ARTs have increased the probability of a live birth after a cycle of hormonal stimulation from 6% in 1985 to 30% in 1999.[4] These improved results have occurred, in part, because reproductive biologists have appreciated that even subtle differences in culture media and laboratory methods may affect outcomes with ARTs.[5] Given the limited insurance coverage of ART expenses (approximately $10,000 for each cycle that progresses to transfer) coupled with the reality that most cycles do not result in a live birth, it is prudent for the anesthesiologist to avoid (or minimize) patient exposure to anesthetic agents that have potential gamete or embryo toxicity.

ASSISTED REPRODUCTIVE TECHNIQUES (ARTs)

Hormonal Stimulation

Initially, IVF was performed after the collection of a *single* preovulatory oocyte during the natural ovarian menstrual cycle.[1] Later the institution of hormonal follicular stimulation allowed the harvesting of multiple oocytes for IVF and subsequent transfer. This advancement resulted in a dramatic increase in the number of mature oocytes harvested and the probability of a live birth for each hormonal stimulation cycle. A typical hormonal regimen begins with a gonadotropin-releasing hormone agonist (GnRH-a) to induce pituitary suppression. Follicle-stimulating hormone (FSH) and human menopausal gonadotropin (HMG) are then given to induce the stimulation and growth of multiple ovarian follicles. Later, human chorionic gonadotropin (HCG) is added to induce oocyte maturation before retrieval. Although the goal of this regimen is to generate 10 to 15 oocytes, superovulation may occur, resulting in the production of as many as 70 oocytes in some women. All visible ovarian follicles are aspirated (*vide infra*), with most follicles containing a single oocyte.

Following oocyte retrieval, pituitary function usually does not provide sufficient hormonal support to the growing corpus luteum. For this reason, parenteral progesterone is given daily until the results of a chemical pregnancy test are known. Should a chemical pregnancy occur, exogenous progesterone administration often is continued through the first trimester of pregnancy.

Oocyte Retrieval

Originally performed during pelvic laparoscopy to allow direct vision of the ovarian follicles,[1] oocyte retrieval is now performed principally through a transvaginal approach, using ultrasonographic guidance (Figure 14-2).[6] Laparoscopic oocyte retrieval is now usually reserved for situations in which immediate tubal transfer is planned (i.e., gamete intrafallopian transfer [GIFT] and zygote intrafallopian transfer [ZIFT]).

Typically oocyte retrieval is performed approximately 34 to 36 hours after HCG administration. Retrieval must be performed promptly, or spontaneous ovulation will reduce the number of mature oocytes available for harvesting. After visualization of the ovary with use of a transvaginal ultrasound probe, mature follicles are punctured and aspirated with a needle introduced through the vaginal fornix. Immediately after retrieval, oocytes are washed in culture media and examined microscopically to determine their stage of meiosis. Oocytes are classified as postmature metaphase II, mature

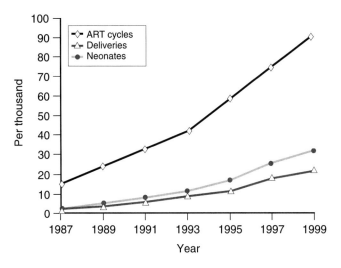

FIGURE 14-1. Numbers for all assisted reproductive cycles initiated, deliveries, and live births reported annually to the American Fertility Society/Society for Assisted Reproductive Technology Registry.[4,8-13]

metaphase II, metaphase I, or prophase I based on their nuclear, cytoplasmic, and extracellular composition.

In Vitro Fertilization (IVF)

Although the term *IVF* is often believed to be synonymous with all aspects of ART, it applies only to the process of oocyte fertilization with spermatozoa in culture media. After the oocytes are examined microscopically, they are incubated in culture media that resembles human tubal fluid and inseminated approximately 4 to 6 hours after retrieval. Some programs further delay insemination of immature oocytes (e.g., metaphase I) in an attempt to increase the probability of normal (i.e., monospermic) fertilization.

Approximately 16 to 20 hours after insemination, the oocytes are examined for evidence of fertilization (i.e., the presence of two pronuclei and two polar bodies in the perivitelline space) (Figure 14-3).[7] At this stage (i.e., pronuclear) the spermatozoon has penetrated the oocyte membrane, but fusion of the male and female pronuclei has not yet occurred. Advantages of IVF are the documentation of the process of fertilization and the implementation of techniques that improve sperm motility or penetration (e.g., intracytoplasmic sperm injection). Male factor infertility is present in approximately 37% of the couples seeking ART procedures, and intracytoplasmic sperm injection currently is used in more than 11,000 cases annually in the United States.[4]

Embryo Transfer (ET)

Embryos resulting from IVF may be transferred into the fallopian tubes (i.e., ZIFT) or the uterine cavity (IVF-ET). Usually performed 3 to 5 days following retrieval, most ET procedures are performed transcervically, with the embryos transferred via a catheter. Advantages of transcervical ET

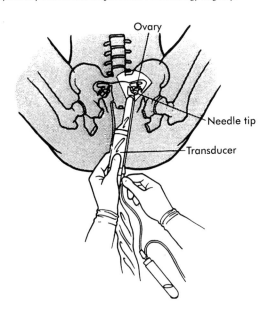

FIGURE 14-2. Transvaginal ultrasound-guided oocyte retrieval. The elasticity of the vagina and proximity of the ovaries to the posterolateral vaginal wall allow the aspiration needle to penetrate the ovary without traversing any vital structure. The transducer is placed in the vagina and advanced to the posterior fornix. The needle, previously inserted through the needle guide, is advanced through the vaginal wall and into the ovarian follicle. (From Wikland M, Enk L, Hammarberg K, Nilsson L. Use of a vaginal transducer for oocyte retrieval in an IVF/ET program. J Clin Ultrasound 1987; 15:245-51.)

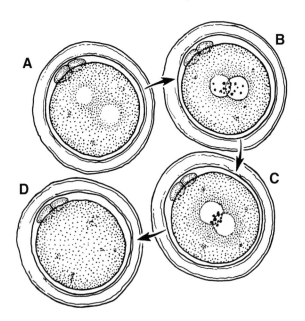

FIGURE 14-3. Pronuclear stage prezygote. **A,** 8 to 10 hours after insemination, pronuclei are barely visible and may be spaced slightly apart. **B,** After 12 hours, pronuclei migrate to the center of the cell and are clearly seen. **C,** At 20 to 22 hours, nuclear envelopes break down and pronuclei begin to fade from view. **D,** The one-cell zygote before the first cleavage. (From Veeck LL. Atlas of the Human Oocyte and Early Conceptus. Baltimore, Williams & Wilkins, 1991:43.)

include (1) simplicity—it does not require laparoscopy or anesthesia, (2) low cost when compared with laparoscopic intrafallopian transfer procedures, and (3) a patent fallopian tube is not essential. The primary disadvantage of transcervical ET is that the probability of successful pregnancy is slightly less than that with an ET performed directly into the fallopian tubes (i.e., ZIFT). Nevertheless, ET is the most common ART technique employed and its use continues to increase (Figure 14-4).[4,8-13] Embryos in excess of those required for transfer may be frozen in 1,2-propanediol or glycerol and stored for possible later transfer.

Gamete Intrafallopian Transfer (GIFT)

GIFT begins with the transabdominal or transvaginal collection of oocytes. Immediately after collection, the oocytes are inspected for quality and maturation under a microscope in a laboratory adjacent to the operating room. After examination, laboratory personnel load a transfer catheter with mature oocytes and washed husband or donor sperm. The surgeon places the transfer catheter through the fimbriated end of the fallopian tube, and the gametes are injected into the distal 3 to 6 cm of one or both fallopian tubes. Finally, the catheter is inspected microscopically to verify that no oocytes have been retained. Thus the GIFT procedure does not include IVF. Rather, fertilization occurs in vivo in the natural milieu of the fallopian tube.

Specific advantages of this procedure include (1) the greater convenience of a one-step procedure, (2) the necessity of IVF is eliminated, and (3) the embryos reach the uterine cavity at a more appropriate (i.e., later) stage of development than with IVF-ET.[14] The primary disadvantage of GIFT is that fertilization cannot be documented. This may be critical when fertilization capacity is questionable, as in couples with male or immunologic factors. Normally, 50% to 70% of inseminated oocytes will fertilize[15]; however, lower fertilization rates may be observed in couples with severe male factor infertility or in women with antisperm antibodies. Other disadvantages are that at least one patent fallopian tube is necessary and that laparoscopic surgery is required.

Zygote Intrafallopian Transfer (ZIFT)

ZIFT (also known as pronuclear stage transfer [PROST]) begins with oocyte retrieval followed by IVF. Approximately 16 to 20 hours after insemination, the oocytes are examined for the presence of two distinct pronuclei (i.e., the pronuclear stage). If fertilization is successful, pronuclear stage embryos (usually four or less) are loaded into a catheter in preparation for tubal transfer. The patient is anesthetized for laparoscopy and the pronuclear stage embryos are transferred into the distal portion of a fallopian tube (as described for GIFT). Advantages of ZIFT include (1) fertilization can be documented, (2) laparoscopy can be avoided if fertilization is not successful (approximately 13% of inseminations),[3] (3) exposure to the laboratory environment is shorter than with IVF-ET, and (4) embryos reach the uterine cavity at a more appropriate stage of development than with IVF-ET (i.e., approximately the fifth day after insemination). Disadvantages include (1) the added inconvenience and cost of a two-stage procedure, (2) laparoscopic surgery is required, and (3) there must be at least one patent fallopian tube.

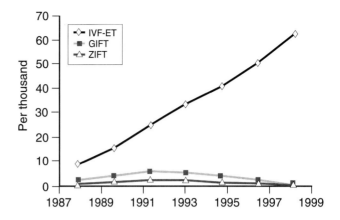

FIGURE 14-4. Numbers of IVF-ET, GIFT, and ZIFT procedures reported annually to the American Fertility Society/Society for Assisted Reproductive Technology Registry. A change in the configuration of the database led to underreporting in the number of ART procedures for 1994.[4,8-13]

SUCCESS OF ASSISTED REPRODUCTIVE TECHNIQUES

The Society for Assisted Reproductive Techniques (SART) and the American Society for Reproductive Medicine (ASRM) collaborate with the Centers for Disease Control and Prevention (CDC) to form a data registry and analyze the results of all ART cycles initiated within each calendar year in the United States.[4,8-13]

Maternal age is the dominant factor in determining the likelihood of successful pregnancy after an ART procedure. For example, in 1999, 36% of GIFT procedures led to the delivery of one or more infants among women less than 35 years of age.[4] In contrast, in the select group of women greater than 40 years of age meeting optimal fertility criteria, only 14% of these procedures resulted in a live birth.

Pregnancy and delivery rates are slightly higher for tubal transfers (i.e., GIFT, ZIFT) than for transcervical uterine transfers (IVF-ET), although the reasons for these differences remain unclear.[4,15] Some physicians believe that the early postovulatory uterine environment is unfavorable to early embryo growth.[15] After tubal transfer procedures, embryos may not reach the uterine cavity for 3 to 5 days, at which time the uterine environment may be more receptive to implantation. Other reasons that implantation rates are lower after transcervical ET may include (1) adverse uterine effects from the transfer procedure itself, (2) expulsion of transfer fluid from the uterine cavity by means of uterine contractions,[16] and (3) the absence of unknown tubal factors that may promote early embryo growth and enhance attachment to the endometrium.[15,17] Of interest, the difference in success rates between tubal and intrauterine transfers appears to have diminished in recent years (Figure 14-5). For this reason some physicians are beginning to reassess the role of tubal transfer procedures in programs that have consistent success with IVF-ET.

OBSTETRIC COMPLICATIONS

The hormonal stimulation associated with ARTs has been associated with increased coagulation and decreased fibrinolysis when evaluated by individual hemostatic markers and global assessment tools (i.e., thromboelastography).[18,19] These alterations may be associated with a phenomenon termed *ovarian hyperstimulation syndrome* (OHSS), which is the most common complication associated with iatrogenic

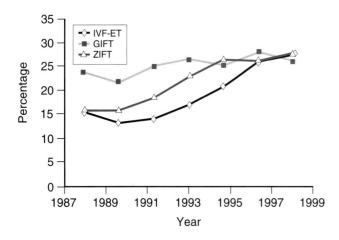

FIGURE 14-5. Delivery rates (per retrieval) over time for IVF-ET, GIFT, and ZIFT. Data were obtained from the American Fertility Society/Society for Assisted Reproductive Technology Registry.[4,8-13]

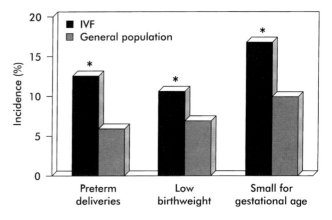

FIGURE 14-6. Incidence of preterm delivery, low birth weight, and small-for-gestational-age infants in IVF pregnancies and the general obstetric population. *$P < 0.05$ compared with the general population. (Modified from Doyle P, Beral V, Maconochie N. Preterm delivery, low birth weight and small-for-gestational age in liveborn singleton babies resulting from in-vitro fertilization. Hum Reprod 1992; 7:425-8.)

ovarian stimulation. Mild cases may present with abdominal discomfort, bilateral ovarian enlargement, and ascites. Severe cases of OHSS may result in follicular rupture and hemorrhage, pleural effusion, hemoconcentration, oliguria, and thromboembolic events.[20-22] OHSS is unlikely to complicate the anesthetic management of a patient undergoing oocyte retrieval or oocyte/embryo transfer because it presents after the transfer has occurred. Rarely these patients may require emergency laparoscopy/laparotomy for excision of a ruptured ovarian cyst or to prevent ovarian infarction caused by torsion of the ovarian pedicle.[22] Abdominal paracentesis and/or thoracentesis may be necessary before the induction of general anesthesia in patients with respiratory compromise caused by massive ascites or pleural effusion.

Multiple gestation pregnancies represented 37% of the deliveries that followed ART procedures in the United States in 1999.[4] Among these deliveries, 87% were twins and the remainder were a higher order. By transferring a greater number of embryos or oocytes, the probability of a live birth and the likelihood of a multifetal pregnancy increases. Although many infertile couples consider a twin or triplet pregnancy preferable to a singleton pregnancy, maternal and perinatal morbidity and mortality for multiple gestation pregnancies is at least double that of singleton gestation pregnancies.[23] Further, overall medical costs escalate with each additional fetus. Hidlebaugh et al.[24] noted that the mean obstetric and neonatal charges were approximately $9000, $20,000, and $153,000 for singleton, twin, and triplet deliveries, respectively, following IVF-ET. In an effort to reduce the incidence of multifetal pregnancies, many ART programs and some countries have mandated a limit on the number of oocytes/embryos that are transferred. In addition, some programs perform selective reductions if a triplet or higher order gestation occurs. Moral and ethical considerations prevent some patients and physicians from considering the option of selective reduction, even with the occurrence of a very high order multifetal pregnancy.

Ectopic pregnancies occur more often with ART pregnancies than with natural pregnancies.[25] This is largely a result of the increased prevalence of tubal disease among infertility patients. Surprisingly, the transfer site (uterine versus tubal) does not appear to be a predisposing factor in the development of ectopic pregnancies. Indeed, more ectopic pregnan-

cies occur after IVF-ET because women with bilateral tubal disease are not candidates for GIFT or ZIFT. Approximately 10% of ectopic pregnancies develop in conjunction with an ongoing intrauterine pregnancy.[25] In these instances it becomes necessary to surgically remove the ectopic pregnancy during the first trimester of an ongoing intrauterine pregnancy.

Preterm delivery, low birth weight (LBW), and small-for-gestational-age (SGA) babies are more common with IVF pregnancies than with natural pregnancies.[26] This phenomenon persists even when the analysis is restricted to singleton gestations (Figure 14-6). The difference appears to be a result of infertility per se rather than the IVF process because previously infertile women who conceive independent of IVF also are at greater risk for preterm delivery.[26]

EFFECTS OF ANESTHESIA ON REPRODUCTION

General Considerations

In 1987 Boyers et al.[27] reported that oocytes recovered by laparoscopic techniques in patients who had received general anesthesia (i.e., isoflurane or enflurane with 50% nitrous oxide and 50% oxygen) were less likely to fertilize if the case duration was prolonged. Specifically, fertilization rates for the first- and last-recovered oocytes were 69% and 57%, respectively, when the difference in exposure time exceeded 5 minutes. The authors advanced two plausible explanations for this difference: (1) the acidification of follicular fluid by intraperitoneal carbon dioxide and/or (2) the effects of general anesthesia. Regardless of the reason for the observed differences, this study encouraged scrutiny of all anesthetic techniques and agents used during ART procedures.

Ideally, anesthetic techniques and agents used for ART procedures should not interfere with oocyte fertilization or early embryo development and implantation. Although a number of studies have noted that anesthetic agents may interfere with some aspect of reproductive physiology in some species under certain conditions, the literature must be interpreted with caution. For example, one study concluded that general anesthesia significantly reduced oocyte cleavage rates when compared to epidural anesthesia.[28] However, a laparoscopic (instead of transvaginal) retrieval method was utilized

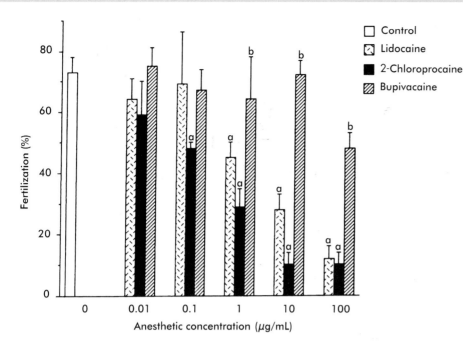

FIGURE 14-7. Fertilization of mouse oocytes at 48 hours (mean ± SD) for each anesthetic exposure group. *a*, $P < 0.05$ (anesthetics compared with control); *b*, $P < 0.05$ (lidocaine and 2-chloroprocaine compared with bupivacaine). (Reprinted from Schnell VL, Sacco AG, Savoy-Moore RT, et al. Effects of oocyte exposure to local anesthetics on in vitro fertilization and embryo development in the mouse. Reprod Toxicol 1992; 6:323-7 with kind permission from Elsevier Science, Ltd, The Boulevard, Langford Lane, Kidlington OX51GB, UK.)

in the general anesthesia group, and carbon dioxide pneumoperitoneum may significantly decrease both follicular fluid pH and oocyte fertilization rates. Another group of investigators suggested that it may be preferable to avoid general anesthesia, but the authors did not disclose the actual agents used in their study.[29] In addition, conclusions based on animal data may not reflect the human experience due to interspecies and assay method differences.[30]

Assessment of specific anesthetic drugs must also be interpreted in context to the techniques of administration, doses, and combinations of drugs, as well as the timing and duration of exposure. For example, a local anesthetic agent yields dissimilar pharmacokinetic profiles when given for paracervical, epidural, or intrathecal anesthesia. Anesthetic agents may also affect unfertilized oocytes and fertilized embryos differently; thus the same anesthetic technique and agents for a GIFT (prefertilization) procedure should not be directly compared with that for a ZIFT (postfertilization) procedure. Finally, a significantly higher free concentration of certain agents (e.g., bupivacaine) exists during ART stimulation due to a decrease in serum binding proteins.[31] Thus when selecting an anesthetic technique and agent(s) for an ART procedure, the clinician should weigh the known benefits (e.g., greater hemodynamic stability, less nausea, less psychomotor impairment) versus the hypothetical risks (e.g., lower delivery rates) for each anesthetic technique and drug.

Local Anesthetic Agents

In animal models, the effect of local anesthetic agents on reproductive physiology appears to be related to the agent, the timing, and the dose of exposure. By using mouse oocytes incubated for 30 minutes in culture media with known concentrations of lidocaine, bupivacaine, or 2-chloroprocaine, Schnell et al.[32] demonstrated that lidocaine and 2-chloroprocaine adversely affected both fertilization and embryo development at concentrations of 1.0 and 0.1 µg/mL, respectively (Figures 14-7 and 14-8). In contrast, bupivacaine produced adverse effects only at the highest concentration studied (100 µg/mL). Similarly, Del Valle et al.[33] demonstrated that after 48 hours of culture, 24% of mouse embryos exposed

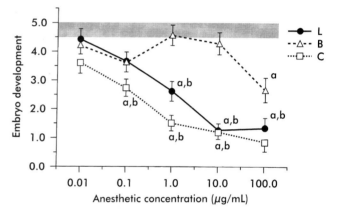

FIGURE 14-8. Embryo development scores (mean ± SD) at 72 hours as a function of anesthetic concentration. Shaded area represents embryo development score (4.75 ± 0.28) for the control mouse embryos. *a*, $P < 0.01$ (lidocaine, bupivacaine, and 2-chloroprocaine compared with control); *b*, $P < 0.01$ (bupivacaine compared with lidocaine and 2-chloroprocaine). (From Schnell VL, Sacco AG, Savoy-Moore RT, et al. Effects of oocyte exposure to local anesthetics on in vitro fertilization and embryo development in the mouse. Reprod Toxicol 1992; 6:323-7.)

to lidocaine, 10 µg/mL, versus none in the control group, showed evidence of degeneration. Finally, Ahuja[34] noted that hamster oocytes exposed to procaine or tetracaine demonstrated impaired zona reactions, potentially allowing additional sperm to enter the oocyte and create abnormal chromosomal numbers (polyploidy).

These in vitro findings may have limited relevance, however, given that much lower anesthetic concentrations occur clinically and that the oocytes are washed and screened prior to fertilization and transfer. More important, no data from human trials condemn the use of local anesthetic agents for oocyte retrieval, GIFT, or ZIFT. Wikland et al.[35] reported that the incidence of oocyte fertilization and clinical pregnancy was not decreased among women who received a modified paracervical block with lidocaine for transvaginal oocyte retrieval (Figure 14-9). Further, others have observed favorable pregnancy rates after GIFT performed during epidural lidocaine anesthesia.[28]

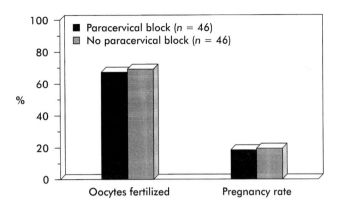

FIGURE 14-9. Fertilization and pregnancy rates after transvaginal oocyte retrieval with and without lidocaine paracervical block. Fertilization and cleavage rates did not differ between the two groups. (Modified from Wikland M, Evers H, Jakobsson AH, et al. The concentration of lidocaine in follicular fluid when used for paracervical block in a human IVF-ET programme. Hum Reprod 1990; 5:920-3.)

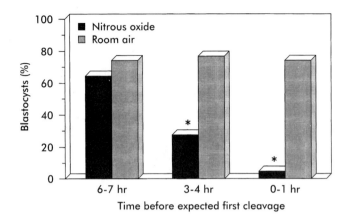

FIGURE 14-10. Developmental outcome of two-cell mouse embryos exposed to 60% nitrous oxide/40% oxygen for 30 minutes in vitro. Administration of nitrous oxide within 4 hours of anticipated cleavage decreased the percentage of embryos reaching the blastocyst stage. *$P < 0.05$ compared with the room air (i.e., control) group. (Modified from Warren JR, Shaw B, Steinkampf MP. Effects of nitrous oxide on preimplantation mouse embryo cleavage and development. Biol Reprod 1990; 43:158-61.)

Opioids, Benzodiazepines, and Ketamine

Fentanyl, alfentanil, remifentanil, and meperidine do not appear to interfere with either fertilization or preimplantation embryo development in animal and human trials.[36,37] When given during oocyte retrieval, fentanyl and alfentanil were detected in extremely low-to-nonexistent follicular fluid concentrations[38]; with alfentanil, a 10:1 ratio between serum and follicular fluid was observed 15 minutes following the initial bolus dose.[39] Morphine appears distinct in terms of adverse effects. When sea urchin eggs were incubated in morphine (equivalent to a human dose of 50 mg), more than one sperm entered approximately 30% of the oocytes.[40]

Midazolam administered systemically in preovulatory mice did not impair fertilization or embryo development in vivo or in vitro, even when given in doses up to 500 times that used clinically.[41] When used in small bolus or infusion doses for anxiolysis and sedation for ART in humans, midazolam has not been found in follicular fluid and does not appear to cause teratogenicity.[42,43]

Ketamine in a dose of 0.75 mg/kg, administered with midazolam, 0.06 mg/kg, has been noted to be an acceptable alternative to general anesthesia with isoflurane. Although the study had inadequate power, no differences in reproductive outcomes were observed.[44]

Propofol and Thiopental

The effect of propofol on reproductive outcomes has been a subject of controversy. Dichotomous alterations in fertilization and early embryo development have been observed in both animal and human trials.[45-49] Recent pharmacokinetic and pharmacodynamic studies have demonstrated a dose- and duration-dependent accumulation of propofol in the follicular fluid.[50,51] The threshold at which oocyte fertilization or early embryo development becomes impaired is unclear. However, in studies that correlated follicular fluid concentrations with reproductive outcome measures, no detrimental effects have been observed.[51,52] In addition, when general anesthesia with propofol and 50% oxygen in air was compared to paracervical block with mepivacaine, no differences in fertilization rates, embryo cleavage, or implantation rates were observed.[48] Moreover, a sensitive index of genotoxic effects (i.e., the sister chromatid

exchange assay) demonstrated no DNA damage—even through two metaphases—when hamster oocytes were exposed to very high concentrations of propofol (20 μg/mL).[53] Of interest, these concentrations are at least 40 times higher than those detected clinically in the follicular fluid of patients undergoing oocyte retrieval.[50,51] Studies of GIFT procedures performed using propofol for induction and/or maintenance of general anesthesia have demonstrated essentially no differences in outcomes, compared with other forms of anesthesia.[46] However, Vincent et al.[54] demonstrated that the incidence of ongoing pregnancies was lower among women given propofol-nitrous oxide anesthesia for ZIFT when compared with a similar group given thiopental-nitrous oxide-isoflurane anesthesia. Further investigation is necessary to elucidate the full effect of propofol on reproductive outcomes.

Both thiopental and thiamylal (5 mg/kg) can be detected in follicular fluid as early as 11 minutes after administration for induction of general anesthesia in patients undergoing GIFT procedures.[55] No adverse reproductive effects have been observed with these agents, and when compared specifically to propofol (2.7 mg/kg) for GIFT procedures, no differences in clinical pregnancy rates were noted.[47]

Nitrous Oxide

Nitrous oxide reduces methionine synthetase activity, concentrations of nonmethylated folate derivatives, and DNA synthesis in animals and humans.[56,57] Nitrous oxide also impairs function of the mitotic spindle in cell cultures.[58] Warren et al.[59] reported that two-cell mouse embryos exposed to nitrous oxide within 4 hours of the expected onset of cleavage were less likely to develop to the blastocyst stage (Figure 14-10). However, this difference resolved by later stages of embryo development.[60]

Clinical studies of anesthesia for laparoscopic ART procedures support the administration of nitrous oxide during GIFT and ZIFT.[46,54,61] In a multicenter study, Beilin et al.[46] observed a delivery rate of 35% among women given nitrous oxide for GIFT, compared with 30% among women who did not receive nitrous oxide.

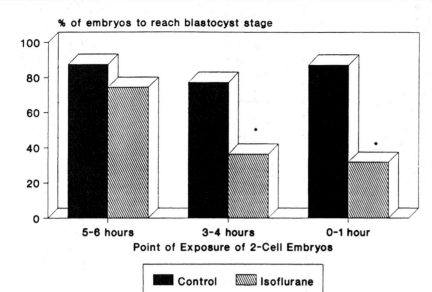

FIGURE 14-11. Developmental outcome of two-cell mouse embryos exposed in vitro to 3% isoflurane for 30 minutes at various times in relation to expected onset of the first cleavage in vitro. *$P < 0.01$ (From Warren JR, Shaw B, Steinkampf MP. Inhibition of preimplantation mouse embryo development by isoflurane. Am J Obstet Gynecol 1992; 166:693-8.)

Volatile Halogenated Agents

Volatile halogenated agents have been observed to depress DNA synthesis and mitosis in cell cultures.[62,63] Sturrock and Nunn[62] noted that volatile halogenated agents prevent cytoplasmic cleavage during mitosis, resulting in an increased number of abnormal mitotic figures (e.g., tripolar and tetrapolar nuclear phases). Isoflurane adversely affects embryo development in vitro.[60,64] Specifically, Warren et al.[64] reported that two-cell mouse embryos exposed to 3% (but not 1.5%) isoflurane for 1 hour were less likely to develop to the blastocyst stage (Figure 14-11). Similar to their earlier study of embryos exposed to nitrous oxide, the authors noted that the timing of anesthetic administration was critical. Developmental outcome was impaired only when isoflurane was given within 4 hours of the predicted onset of cleavage. It is questionable whether studies of two-cell mouse embryos are applicable to human oocytes and spermatozoa exposed during GIFT or to one-cell embryos that are exposed during ZIFT.

A possible mechanism by which volatile halogenated agents affect ART outcome is through an increase in prolactin levels. High prolactin levels have been associated with diminished oocyte development and uterine receptivity *(vide infra)*; whether volatile halogenated agents can affect mature oocytes in the process of being retrieved is questionable. Critchlow et al.[65] observed dramatic increases in plasma prolactin levels with an enflurane in nitrous oxide/oxygen technique for GIFT procedures. However, these changes did not occur until 4 to 10 minutes after induction and did not affect follicular fluid prolactin levels or fertilization rates.

Volatile anesthetic agents have been evaluated in clinical studies. Fishel et al.[66] reported that pregnancy rates were significantly lower among women given halothane anesthesia for ET when compared with a similar group of women given enflurane. (Anesthesia was administered in an effort to decrease uterine activity during ET). Similarly, Critchlow et al.[65] reported lower pregnancy and delivery rates among women who received halothane for GIFT, when compared with women who received enflurane (Figure 14-12). General anesthesia with volatile halogenated agents has also been compared to conscious sedation. In a retrospective study with a sequential study design, Wilhelm et al.[36] noted lower pregnancy rates in patients undergoing oocyte retrieval with general anesthesia (i.e., isoflurane or propofol in combination

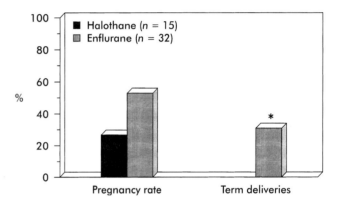

FIGURE 14-12. Pregnancy and term delivery rates after halothane and enflurane anesthesia for GIFT. The percentage of term pregnancies after GIFT was greater after enflurane-nitrous oxide anesthesia than after halothane-nitrous oxide anesthesia. *$P < 0.05$ compared with the halothane group. (Modified from Critchlow BM, Ibrahim Z, Pollard BJ. General anaesthesia for gamete intra-fallopian transfer. Eur J Anaesth 1991; 8:381-4.)

with 60% nitrous oxide in oxygen) than in subsequent patients who received a remifentanil-based MAC (monitored anesthesia care) technique. The authors acknowledged that "the success rates of ART programs . . . improve over time, [and] it is possible that physician-related factors also may have played a role in the improved success during the second (MAC) phase of [the] study."[36]

These data suggest that specific halogenated agents can affect ART outcomes. Of note, the metabolic byproduct of sevoflurane, compound A, has been associated with genotoxic ovarian cell effects, although reproductive outcome has not been assessed.[67] As such, caution is advised when selecting a volatile halogenated agent, especially when contemplating the use of new agents such as sevoflurane, desflurane, and isodesox (a combination of 1% desflurane, 0.25% isoflurane and 60% oxygen in nitrogen)[68] until further work has been done.

Antiemetic Agents

At least one study noted that droperidol and metoclopramide rapidly induce hyperprolactinemia with subsequent impairment of ovarian follicle maturation and corpus luteum function.[69] When given prior to oocyte retrieval, oocyte production may be diminished. After retrieval, uterine receptivity to the embryo could be affected. Forman et al.[70] demonstrated that low plasma prolactin concentrations during ART procedures were associated with a higher incidence of pregnancy.

ANESTHETIC MANAGEMENT

Most patients undergoing ART procedures are young and otherwise healthy, and as such, many institutions do not require preoperative laboratory studies, electrocardiograms, or chest radiographs. However, the application of ART procedures to patients with a growing spectrum of pathologies, such as morbid obesity, cancer (with oocyte retrieval performed prior to chemotherapy or radiation therapy), and severe cardiac, pulmonary, or renal morbidities (with oocyte retrieval performed for surrogate gestational carriers), has created special concerns that should be addressed individually.

All patients should follow the fasting guidelines typically used for other patients undergoing ambulatory surgery, and for patients with risk factors for aspiration, a nonparticulate antacid should be given prior to the procedure. On occasion, a patient may not adhere to strict fasting guidelines, and although delay or cancellation of the case is an option, this decision should be made with careful analysis of the potential risks and benefits. If the window for maximal oocyte retrieval (34 to 36 hours following HCG administration) is missed, spontaneous ovulation and loss of oocytes can occur, invalidating the considerable effort and expense leading to the retrieval procedure. Moreover, should follicle aspiration not be performed, the patient is at increased risk for ovarian hyperstimulation syndrome, with its potential for significant morbidity. In contrast, the magnitude of risk for aspiration is difficult to quantify.

As with other day surgery cases, the ideal anesthetic technique results in effective pain relief with minimal postoperative nausea, sedation, pain, and psychomotor impairment.

Ultrasonographic-Guided Transvaginal Oocyte Retrieval

Although transvaginal oocyte retrievals can be performed under paracervical, spinal, epidural, and general anesthetic techniques, conscious sedation is the most commonly utilized technique.[71,72] Although usually adequate for surgical analgesia, conscious sedation may need to progress to loss of consciousness (i.e., general anesthesia) to prevent patient movement at critical times. The need for additional pain relief should be anticipated when the needle penetrates the cul-de-sac and, later, each ovary. Of interest, one report noted a higher rate of admissions following oocyte retrieval, mostly secondary to intraabdominal bleeding, when conscious sedation was used rather than general anesthesia.[73] Self-administered inhalational analgesia with isodesox (*vide supra*) by face mask was associated with less effective analgesia and less patient satisfaction than with physician-administered intravenous analgesia.[68]

Because paracervical anesthesia incompletely blocks sensation from the vaginal and ovarian pain fibers, additional analgesia is required, even when increased doses of local anesthetic are utilized.[74] Epidural and spinal techniques provide excellent pain relief with minimal oocyte exposure to anesthetic agents. When compared to sedation with propofol and mask-assisted ventilation with nitrous oxide, epidural

bupivacaine anesthesia resulted in fewer complications, especially nausea and emesis.[75] Spinal anesthesia may be preferable to epidural anesthesia due to the reduced anesthetic failure rate, lower systemic and follicular concentrations of anesthetic agent, and a faster recovery profile.[76] Spinal administration of 1.5% hyperbaric lidocaine (60 mg) is associated with significantly shorter recovery times than spinal administration of 5% hyperbaric lidocaine in patients undergoing ART procedures.[77] The addition of intrathecal fentanyl (10 µg) to lidocaine 45 mg improves postoperative analgesia for the first 24 hours, with no increase in time to urination, ambulation, and discharge, when compared to lidocaine alone.[78] Low-dose spinal bupivacaine has been evaluated for use in these patients, given the apparent association between spinal lidocaine and postoperative transient neurologic symptoms. However, the prolonged time to urination and discharge may prevent it from becoming a commonly used alternative.[79]

General anesthesia can be provided by total intravenous anesthesia using propofol (titrated) and fentanyl (50 to 100 µg), with midazolam (1 to 2 mg) as an optional premedicant. By using this option, most patients can be managed with spontaneous ventilation via high-flow oxygen mask and the use of carbon dioxide analysis.[43] However, in individuals with multiple risk factors for aspiration, an endotracheal tube should be placed. Anesthetics managed in this fashion have higher patient acceptance than conscious sedation, due to improved pain relief and less awareness during the surgical procedure.[43] Alternatively, general anesthesia with intubation and maintenance with volatile halogenated agents has been utilized successfully; however, higher rates of nausea and emesis and more unplanned admissions have been observed when compared to use of a propofol, alfentanil, and an air/oxygen mixture.[80]

Novel analgesic measures have been investigated during oocyte retrieval. Electro-acupuncture has been suggested as an alternative to intravenous alfentanil, although both groups also received a paracervical block and the acupuncture group experienced higher degrees of preoperative stress and longer periods of discomfort during oocyte aspiration.[81]

Embryo Transfer

Described as relatively painless, transcervical embryo transfer is most commonly performed without analgesia or anesthesia; however, on rare occasion, intravenous sedation or regional or general anesthesia may be requested. In contrast, transabdominal gamete or embryo transfer (i.e., GIFT, ZIFT), are usually performed via laparoscopy with local, regional, or general anesthesia. The anesthetic management for these procedures, and the associated concerns of the laparoscopic technique and the Trendelenburg position, are described in subsequent text. Major intraoperative complications associated with laparoscopy are rare but include gastric or intestinal perforation, hemorrhage, pneumothorax, pneumopericardium, mediastinal emphysema, gas embolism, and cardiac arrest.[82,83]

PNEUMOPERITONEUM AND THE TRENDELENBURG POSITION

Carbon dioxide is the most common gas used to establish pneumoperitoneum. Its high solubility in blood facilitates absorption from the peritoneal cavity after laparoscopic surgery and may be life-saving in the rare but potentially catastrophic event of gas embolization. For example, rapid intravenous injection of 5 to 10 mL/kg of carbon dioxide produces only transient (less than 1 minute) hypotension in anesthetized dogs (Figure 14-13).[84] In contrast, intravascular administration of a similar volume of a less soluble gas (e.g., helium, oxygen, nitrogen) usually is fatal in laboratory animals.

Signs of embolization of large quantities of carbon dioxide (or any other gas) in anesthetized patients may include *hypo*capnia, hypotension, hypoxemia, S-T segment and T-wave changes, arrhythmias, and audible changes in the heart sounds.[85] Initial treatment of carbon dioxide embolism should include release of the pneumoperitoneum and pharmacologic support of the circulation. If initial resuscitation efforts are unsuccessful, aspiration of gas from the right atrium (using a multi-orifice central venous catheter) should be considered. Although the use of the left lateral recumbent position (Durant maneuver), with or without head-down positioning, has been suggested to facilitate removal of the postulated air lock from the right side of the heart,[86] laboratory evidence suggests that this maneuver may have a detrimental effect on cardiac function after venous gas embolism.[87]

Nearly as soluble in blood as carbon dioxide, nitrous oxide is associated with a reduction in peritoneal and diaphragmatic irritation,[88] and consequently some anesthesiologists advocate its use for the establishment of pneumoperitoneum in awake patients undergoing laparoscopy. A major disadvantage of nitrous oxide is the ability to support combustion, which could increase the possibility of an explosion should the surgeon elect to coagulate an area of endometriosis intraoperatively.

GIFT and ZIFT procedures are often performed with the patient in the Trendelenburg position to facilitate easier visualization of the fallopian tubes and other pelvic structures. Although their use is controversial, shoulder braces placed to prevent the patient from moving cephalad on the operating table should be positioned with padding against the acromioclavicular joints to prevent brachial plexus damage. Many anesthesiologists contend that adduction of the patient's arms against her trunk reduces the risk of a brachial plexus injury, but this is unproved.

Both pneumoperitoneum and the Trendelenburg position produce physiologic changes. Hemodynamic effects of moderate pneumoperitoneum (less than 20 mm Hg) in a patient in the Trendelenburg position include increased mean arterial and central venous pressures, increased systemic vascular resistance, and decreased stroke volume and cardiac output.[89] Heart rate usually does not change, but in some patients, pneumoperitoneum may elicit sinus bradycardia, heart block, or even cardiac arrest. Finally, pneumoperitoneum aggravates the respiratory effects of the Trendelenburg position (e.g., reduced chest wall compliance and increased venous admixture). Overall, most healthy patients easily tolerate the cardiovascular and pulmonary effects of intraabdominal pressures less than 20 mm Hg.

ANESTHESIA FOR LAPAROSCOPIC ART PROCEDURES

The anesthetic plan for GIFT typically is dictated by the method (i.e., transabdominal or transvaginal) of oocyte retrieval. Many ART programs harvest oocytes transabdominally during pelvic laparoscopy, with the principal advantage being that the patient is positioned and anesthetized once for both the retrieval and transfer portions of the procedure. The major disadvantage of this technique is that oocytes are exposed to both carbon dioxide pneumoperitoneum and anesthetic gases. Many anesthesiologists delay induction of general anesthesia for GIFT until just before the skin incision in an effort to minimize unnecessary exposure to these agents. Induction is usually performed with intravenous propofol, lidocaine, fentanyl, and succinylcholine. Following intubation, some advocate the decompressing of the patient's stomach with a suction catheter or Salem sump tube to potentially reduce the risk of gastric perforation during instrumentation. Subsequently, a volatile halogenated agent in oxygen and air, with or without a short-acting muscle relaxant (e.g., verocuronium, rocuronium) is given for the maintenance of anesthesia. A propofol/nitrous oxide technique has also been used, and has been noted to cause less postoperative sedation, lower pain scores, and less emesis when compared to an isoflurane/nitrous oxide technique.[54]

Alternatively, some reproductive endocrinologists prefer to harvest oocytes transvaginally and replace them laparoscopically. Of interest, this is the technique most commonly used with ZIFT procedures, where oocyte retrieval and IVF occur on the day before the ZIFT procedure under laparoscopy. Advantages to the combined transvaginal/

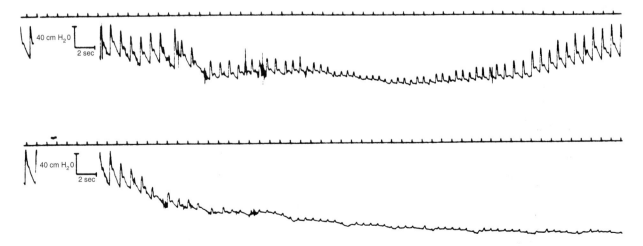

FIGURE 14-13. Arterial tracing after rapid intravenous injection of 7.5 mL/kg of carbon dioxide *(top)* and helium *(bottom)*. Recovery occurs within 1 min after the carbon dioxide injection, but complete cardiovascular collapse occurs after the helium injection. (From Wolf JS, Carrier S, Stoller ML. Gas embolism: Helium is more lethal than carbon dioxide. J Laparoendosc Surg 1994; 4:173-7.)

transabdominal approach include (1) laparoscopy is avoided in the 1% to 2% of cases where oocyte quality or number is inadequate to justify proceeding to tubal transfer[3] and (2) exposure of the oocytes to both carbon dioxide pneumoperitoneum and general anesthesia is eliminated. Disadvantages of this method include (1) the patient must be repositioned before laparoscopy and (2) operative time is prolonged.

A few patients prefer spinal or epidural anesthesia for GIFT procedures.[90,91] Obese women are not ideal candidates to receive regional anesthesia for laparoscopic surgery. However, studies have demonstrated that healthy, nonobese patients tolerate laparoscopic surgery in the Trendelenburg position during high thoracic (i.e., T-2 to T-4) spinal or epidural anesthesia.[90-93] Limiting intraperitoneal pressure to no more than 10 mm Hg may facilitate the use of regional anesthesia for these procedures.

A few investigators have reported adequate analgesia for laparoscopic ART procedures using local anesthesia supplemented with intravenous sedation.[94-97] Padilla et al.[94] reported that the quality of intraoperative analgesia is improved by limiting maximal intraabdominal pressure to 8 to 10 mm Hg, reducing the rate of carbon dioxide insufflation to 1 L/min, and minimizing ovarian manipulation. However, given the difficulty frequently encountered in cannulating the fallopian tubes and the pain resulting from this manipulation, local anesthesia may prove an unwise choice for laparoscopic ART procedures. Waterstone et al.[95] noted that all 21 patients undergoing local anesthesia for laparoscopy experienced some degree of discomfort when the fallopian tubes were mobilized. Moreover, use of this technique does not obviate the benefit of the continuous presence of an anesthesia care provider during the procedure. When rare but life-threatening complications (e.g., bradycardia, cardiac arrest) occur, the management and outcome is greatly assisted by individuals skilled in airway management and cardiopulmonary resuscitation.[98]

Postoperative Management

The incidence of anesthetic or surgical complications requiring hospital admission after ART procedures is low. Oskowitz et al.[73] reported admission rates after oocyte retrieval and GIFT of 0.16% and 0.18%, respectively. The most common indications for hospitalization included hemoperitoneum and syncope following oocyte retrieval, and nausea, vomiting, and bowel injury following laparoscopic GIFT. Incisional pain, diffuse abdominal pain, uterine cramping, and referred shoulder pain from diaphragmatic irritation occur frequently after laparoscopy. This pain results in part from retained intraperitoneal carbon dioxide. Although pain accompanied by nausea is usually a reasonable indication for the use of nonsteroidal antiinflammatory drugs, their use should be avoided, as changes in the prostaglandin milieu can affect embryo implantation.[99,100] Instead, small doses of intravenous fentanyl (25-50 μg) or oral acetaminophen with codeine can be used to allay this discomfort.

Nausea and emesis can also occur; however, exposure to droperidol and metoclopramide should be limited (*vide supra*); treatment with nondopaminergic agents can be considered. Prior to discharge, patients should be able to drink and retain oral liquids, ambulate, and void. Every patient undergoing anesthesia for ART should receive a follow-up call at 24 hours post procedure to respond to any questions or complications.

FUTURE CONSIDERATIONS

The use of ART procedures has been extended to include patients within a broader range of ages and comorbidities. Check et al.[101] reported the successful delivery of infants through the use of donor oocytes, IVF, and ET in two postmenopausal women who were 51 years old. Future studies should assess the maternal and perinatal outcomes following these techniques in these populations and the obstetric and anesthetic implications.

Technically, the improvement of ultrasonographic and fiberoptic methods of oocyte retrieval and fallopian tube cannulation could potentially make laparoscopic interventions unnecessary. For example, small-diameter laparoscopes with optical views comparable to conventional instruments have recently allowed "mini" laparoscopic procedures to be performed for GIFT procedures.[97] These alterations may allow for changes in anesthetic options.

The identification of agents and techniques that provide optimal analgesia or anesthesia with negligible impact on ART success is an important process to which anesthesiologists can and should contribute.

KEY POINTS

- Assisted reproductive techniques are procedures that are being applied to an increasingly diverse population of patients with a wide range of comorbidities.
- Assisted reproductive techniques usually include a regimen of hormonal stimulation and oocyte retrieval, followed by either in vitro fertilization and embryo transfer, or gamete intrafallopian transfer (GIFT).
- Hormonal stimulation creates a number of oocytes for retrieval. On occasion, ovarian hyperstimulation syndrome (OHSS) can occur, with severe cases being associated with ascites, pleural effusion, hemoconcentration, oliguria, and thromboembolic events.
- Oocyte retrieval must be performed promptly, or ovulation will reduce the number of mature oocytes available for harvesting. Embryo transfer usually occurs transcervically; however, laparoscopic techniques (ZIFT) can be utilized.
- Conscious sedation, regional anesthesia, and general anesthesia have all been used successfully to anesthetize women for ART procedures. Laboratory studies have suggested that local anesthetic agents, nitrous oxide, and the volatile halogenated agents interfere with some aspect of reproductive physiology in vitro. However, few clinical data suggest that brief administration of any contemporary anesthetic agent (except halothane) for an ART procedure adversely affects live-birth rates.
- The identification of agents and techniques that provide optimal analgesia or anesthesia with negligible impact on ART success is an important process to which anesthesiologists can and should contribute.

REFERENCES

1. Steptoe PC, Edwards RG. Birth after the reimplantation of a human embryo (letter). Lancet 1978; 2:366.
2. Toner JP. Progress we can be proud of: U.S. trends in assisted reproduction over the first 20 years. Fertil Steril 2002; 78:943-50.
3. Edwards RG. Test-tube babies. Nature 1981; 293:253-6.
4. Society for Assisted Reproductive Technology and the American Society for Reproductive Medicine. Assisted reproductive technology in the United States: 1999 Results generated from the American Society for Reproductive Medicine/Society for Assisted Reproductive Technology Registry. Fertil Steril 2002; 78:918-31.
5. Cooke S, Quinn P, Kime L, et al. Improvement in early human embryo development using new formulation sequential stage-specific culture media. Fertil Steril 2002;78:1254-60.
6. Wikland M, Enk L, Hammarberg K, Nilsson L. Use of a vaginal transducer for oocyte retrieval in an IVF/ET program. J Clin Ultrasound 1987; 15:245-51.
7. Veeck LL. Atlas of the human oocyte and early conceptus. Baltimore, Williams & Wilkins, 1991:43.
8. Medical Research International, et al. In vitro fertilization/embryo transfer in the United States: 1987 Results from the National IVF-ET Registry. Fertil Steril 1989; 51:13-9.
9. Medical Research International, et al. In vitro fertilization-embryo transfer (IVF-ET) in the United States: 1989 Results from the IVF-ET Registry. Fertil Steril 1991; 55:14-22.
10. Society for Assisted Reproductive Technology, The American Fertility Society. Assisted reproductive technology in the United States and Canada: 1991 Results from the Society for Assisted Reproductive Technology generated from the American Fertility Society Registry. Fertil Steril 1993; 59:956-62.
11. Society for Assisted Reproductive Technology, American Society for Reproductive Medicine. Assisted reproductive technology in the United States and Canada: 1993 Results generated from the American Society for Reproductive Medicine/Society for Assisted Reproductive Technology Registry. Fertil Steril 1995; 64:13-21.
12. Assisted reproductive technology in the United States and Canada: 1995 Results generated from the American Society for Reproductive Medicine/Society for Assisted Reproductive Technology Registry. Fertil Steril. 1998; 69:389-98.
13. Assisted reproductive technology in the United States: 1997 Results generated from the American Society for Reproductive Medicine/Society for Assisted Reproductive Technology Registry. Fertil Steril 2000;74: 641-53.
14. Corson SL, Batzer F, Eisenberg E, et al. Early experience with the GIFT procedure. J Reprod Med 1986; 31:219-23.
15. Yovich JL, Yovich JM, Edirisinghe WR. The relative chance of pregnancy following tubal or uterine transfer procedures. Fertil Steril 1988; 48:858-64.
16. Schulman JD. Delayed expulsion of transfer fluid after IVF/ET (letter). Lancet 1986;1:44.
17. Abyholm T, Tanbo T, Henriksen T, Magnus O. Preliminary experience with embryo intrafallopian transfer (EIFT). Int J Fertil 1990; 35: 339-42.
18. Magnani BJ, Tsen LC, Datta S, Bader AM. In-vitro fertilization: Do short-term changes in estrogen levels produce increased fibrinolysis? Am J Clin Path 1999; 112:485-91.
19. Harnett M, Bhavani-Shankar K, Datta S, Tsen LC. In-vitro fertilization induced alterations in coagulation and fibrinolysis as measured by thromboelastography. Anesth Analg 2002; 95:1063-6.
20. Dulitzky M, Cohen SB, Inbal A, et al. Increased prevalence of thrombophilia among women with severe ovarian hyperstimulation syndrome. Fertil Steril 2002; 77:463-7.
21. Bar-Hava I, Orvieto R, Dicker D, et al. A severe case of ovarian hyperstimulation: 65 Liters of ascites aspirated in an on-going IVF-ET twin pregnancy. Gynecol Endocrinol 1995; 9:295-8.
22. Pryor RA, Wiczyk HP, O'Shea DL. Adnexal infarction after conservative surgical management of torsion of a hyperstimulated ovary. Fertil Steril 1995; 63:1344-6.
23. Schenker JG, Ezra Y. Complications of assisted reproductive techniques. Fertil Steril 1994; 61:411-22.
24. Hidlebaugh DA, Thompson IE, Berger MJ. Cost of assisted reproductive technology for a health maintenance organization. J Reprod Med 1997; 42:570-4.
25. Cohen J. The efficiency and efficacy of IVF and GIFT. Hum Reprod 1991; 6:613-8.
26. Doyle P, Beral V, Maconochie N. Preterm delivery, low birth weight and small-for-gestational age in liveborn singleton babies resulting from in vitro fertilization. Hum Reprod 1992; 7:425-8.
27. Boyers SP, Lavy G, Russell JB, DeCherney AH. A paired analysis of in vitro fertilization and cleavage rates of first-and last-recovered pre-ovulatory human oocytes exposed to varying intervals of 100% CO_2 pneumoperitoneum and general anesthesia. Fertil Steril 1987; 48: 969-74.
28. Lefebvre G, Vauthier D, Seebacher J, et al.. In vitro fertilization: A comparative study of cleavage rates under epidural and general anesthesia–interest for gamete intrafallopian transfer (letter). J In Vitro Fert Embryo Transf 1988;5:305-6.
29. Lewin A, Margalioth EJ, Rabinowitz R, Schenker JG. Comparative study of ultrasonically guided percutaneous aspiration with local anesthesia and laparoscopic aspiration of follicles in an in vitro fertilization program. Am J Obstet Gynecol. 1985; 151:621-5.
30. Davidson A, Vermesh M, Lobo RA, Paulson RJ. Mouse embryo culture as quality control for human in vitro fertilization: the one-cell versus the two-cell model. Fertil Steril 1988; 49:516-21.
31. Tsen LC, Datta S, Bader AM. Estrogen induced changes in protein binding of bupivacaine during in-vitro fertilization. Anesthesiology 1997; 87:879-83.
32. Schnell VL, Sacco AG, Savoy-Moore RT, et al. Effects of oocyte exposure to local anesthetics on in vitro fertilization and embryo development in the mouse. Reprod Toxicol 1992; 6:323-7.
33. Del Valle LJ, Orihuela PA. Cleavage and development in cultured preimplantation mouse embryos exposed to lidocaine. Reprod Toxicol 1996; 10:491-6.
34. Ahuja KK. In-vitro inhibition of the block to polyspermy of hamster eggs by tertiary amine local anaesthetics. J Reprod Fertil 1982; 65: 15-22.
35. Wikland M, Evers H, Jakobsson AH, et al. The concentration of lidocaine in follicular fluid when used for paracervical block in a human IVF-ET programme. Hum Reprod 1990: 5:920-3.
36. Wilhelm W, Hammadeh ME, White PF, et al. General anesthesia versus monitored anesthesia care with remifentanil for assisted reproductive technologies: Effect on pregnancy rate. J Clin Anesth 2002; 14:1-5.
37. Chetkowski RJ, Nass TE. Isofluorane inhibits early mouse embryo development in vitro. Fertil Steril 1988; 49:171-3.
38. Bruce DL, Hinkley R, Norman PF. Fentanyl does not inhibit fertilization or early development of sea urchin eggs. Anesth Analg 1985; 64:498-500.
39. Shapira SC, Chrubasik S, Hoffmann A, et al. Use of alfentanil for in vitro fertilization oocyte retrieval. J Clin Anesth 1996; 8:282-5.
40. Cardasis C, Schuel H. The sea urchin egg as a model system to study the effects of narcotics on secretion. In: Ford DH, Clouet DH, eds. Tissue responses to addictive drugs. Spectrum, New York, 1976:631-40.
41. Swanson RF, Leavitt MG. Fertilization and mouse embryo development in the presence of midazolam. Anesth Analg 1992; 75:549-54.
42. Chopineau J, Bazin JE, Terrisse MP, et al. Assay for midazolam in liquor folliculi during in vitro fertilization under anesthesia. Clin Pharm 1993; 12:770-3.
43. Casati A, Valentini G, Zangrillo A, et al. Anaesthesia for ultrasound guided oocyte retrieval: Midazolam/remifentanil versus propofol/fentanyl regimens. Eur J Anaesthesiol 1999; 16:773-8.
44. Ben-Shlomo I, Moskovich R, Katz Y, Shalev E. Midazolam/ketamine sedative combination compared with fentanyl/propofol/isoflurane anaesthesia for oocyte retrieval.. Hum Reprod 1999; 14:1757-9.
45. Rosenblatt MA, Bradford CN, Bodian CA, Grunfeld L. The effect of propofol-based sedation technique on cumulative embryo scores, clinical pregnancy rates, and implantation rates in patients undergoing embryo transfers with donor oocytes. J Clin Anesth 1997; 9:614-7.
46. Beilin Y, Bodian CA, Mukherjee T, et al. The use of propofol, nitrous oxide, or isoflurane does not affect the reproductive success rate following gamete intrafallopian transfer (GIFT): A multicenter pilot trial/survey. Anesthesiology 1999; 90:36-41.
47. Pierce ET, Smalky M, Alper MM, et al. Comparison of pregnancy rates following gamete intrafallopian transfer (GIFT) under general anesthesia with thiopental sodium or propofol. J Clin Anesth 1992; 4:394-8.
48. Christiaens F, Janssenswillen C, Van Steirteghem AC, et al. Comparison of assisted reproductive technology performance after oocyte retrieval under general anaesthesia (propofol) versus paracervical local anaesthetic block: A case-controlled study. Hum Reprod 1998; 13:2456-60.
49. Hein HA, Putman JM. Is propofol a proper proposition for reproductive procedures? J Clin Anesth 1997; 9:611-3.
50. Christiaens F, Janssenswillen C, Verborgh C, et al. Propofol concentrations in follicular fluid during general anaesthesia for transvaginal oocyte retrieval. Hum Reprod 1999; 14:345-8.
51. Ben-Shlomo I, Moskovich R, Golan J, et al. The effect of propofol anaesthesia on oocyte fertilization and early embryo quality. Hum Reprod 2000; 15:2197-9.

52. Imoedemhe DA, Sigue AB, Abdul Ghani I, et al. An evaluation of the effect of the anesthetic agent profofol (Diprivan) on the outcome of human in vitro fertilization. J Assist Reprod Genet 1992; 9:488-91.

53. Tomioka S, Nakajo N. No genotoxic effect of propofol in chinese hamster ovary cells: Analysis by sister chromatid exchanges. Acta Anaesthesiol Scand 2000; 44:1261-5.

54. Vincent RD, Syrop CS, Van Voorhis BJ, et al. An evaluation of the effect of anesthetic technique on reproductive success after laparoscopic pronuclear stage transfer (PROST): Propofol-nitrous oxide versus isoflurane-nitrous oxide. Anesthesiology 1995; 82:352-8.

55. Endler GC, Stout M, Magyar DM, et al. Follicular fluid concentrations of thiopental and thiamylal during laparoscopy for oocyte retrieval. Fertil Steril 1987; 48:828-33.55.

56. Koblin DD, Waskell L, Watson JE, et al. Nitrous oxide inactivates methionine synthetase in human liver. Anesth Analg 1982; 61:75-8.

57. Baden JM, Serra M, Mazze RI. Inhibition of fetal methionine synthetase by nitrous oxide. Br J Anaesth 1984; 56:523-6.

58. Kieler J. The cytotoxic effect of nitrous oxide at different tensions. Acta Pharm Scand 1957; 13:301-8.

59. Warren JR, Shaw B, Steinkampf MP. Effects of nitrous oxide on preimplantation mouse embryo cleavage and development. Biol Reprod 1990; 43:158-61.

60. Chetkowski RJ, Nass TE. Isoflurane inhibits early mouse embryo development in vitro. Fertil Steril 1988; 49:171-3.

61. Rosen MA, Roizen MF, Eger EI, et al. The effect of nitrous oxide on in vitro fertilization success rate. Anesthesiology 1987; 67:42-4.

62. Sturrock JE, Nunn JF. Mitosis in mammalian cells during exposure to anesthetics. Anesthesiology 1975; 43:21-33.

63. Nunn JF, Lovis JD, Kimball KL. Arrest of mitosis by halothane. Br J Anaesth 1971; 43:524-30.

64. Warren JR, Shaw B, Steinkampf MP. Inhibition of preimplantation mouse embryo development by isoflurane. Am J Obstet Gynecol 1992; 166:693-8.

65. Critchlow BM, Ibrahim Z, Pollard BJ. General anaesthesia for gamete intrafallopian transfer. Eur J Anaesth 1991; 8:381-4.

66. Fishel S, Webster J, Faratian B, Jackson P. General anesthesia for intrauterine placement of human conceptuses after *in vitro* fertilization. J In Vitro Fertil Embryo Transf 1987; 4:260-4.

67. Eger EI 2nd, Laster MJ, Winegar R, et al. Compound A induces sister chromatid exchanges in Chinese hamster ovary cells. Anesthesiology. 1997; 86:918-22.

68. Thompson N, Murray S, MacLennan F, Ross JA, et al. A randomised controlled trial of intravenous versus inhalational analgesia during outpatient oocyte recovery. Anaesthesia 2000; 55:770-3.

69. Kauppila A, Leinonen P, Vihko R, Ylostalo P. Metoclopramide-induced hyperprolactinemia impairs ovarian follicle maturation and corpus luteum function in women. J Clin Endocrinol Metab 1982; 54:955-60.

70. Forman R, Fishel B, Edwards RG, Walters E. The influence of transient hyperprolactinemia on in vitro fertilization in humans. J Clin Endocrinol Metab 1984; 60:517-22.

71. Ditkoff ECX, Plumb J, Selick A, Sauer MV. Anesthesia practices in the United States common to in vitro fertilization (IVF) centers. J Assist Reprod Genet 1997; 14:145-7.

72. Bokhari A, Pollard BJ. Anaesthesia for assisted conception: a survey of UK practice. Eur J Anaesthesiol 1999; 16:225-30.

73. Oskowitz SP, Smalky M, Berger MJ, et al. Safety of a free standing surgical unit for the assisted reproductive technologies. Fertil Steril 1995; 63:874-9.

74. Ng EH, Tang OS, Chui DK, Ho PC. Comparison of two different doses of lignocaine used in paracervical block during oocyte collection in an IVF programme. Hum Reprod 2000; 15:2148-51.

75. Botta G, D'Angelo A, D'Ari G, et al. Epidural anesthesia in an in vitro fertilization and embryo transfer program. J Assist Reprod Genet 1995; 12:187-90.

76. Endler GC, Magyar DM, Hayes MF, Moghiosi KS. Use of spinal anesthesia in laparoscopy for IVF. Fert Steril 1985; 43:809.

77. Manica V, Bader AM, Fragneto G, et al. Anesthesia for in vitro fertilization: A comparison of 1.5% and 5% spinal lidocaine for ultrasonically guided oocyte retrieval. Anesth Analg 1993; 77:453-6.

78. Martin R, Tsen LC, Tseng G, Datta S. Comparison of 1.5% lidocaine with fentanyl with 1.5% lidocaine for in-vitro fertilization. Anesth Analg 1999; 88:523-6.

79. Tsen LC, Schultz R, Martin R, et al. Intrathecal low-dose bupivacaine vs. lidocaine for in-vitro fertilization procedures. Reg Anesth Pain Med 2001; 26:52-6.

80. Raftery S, Sherry E. Total intravenous anaesthesia with propofol and alfentanil protects against postoperative nausea and vomiting. Can J Anaesth 1992; 39:37-41.

81. Stener-Victorin E, Waldenstrom U, Nilsson L, et al. A prospective randomized study of electro-acupuncture versus alfentanil as anaesthesia during oocyte aspiration in in-vitro fertilization. Hum Reprod 1999; 14:2480-4.

82. Murphy AA. Diagnostic and operative laparoscopy. In Thompson JD, Rock JA, editors. TeLinde's operative gynecology. Philadelphia, JB Lippincott, 1992: 361-84.

83. Doctor NH, Hussain Z. Bilateral pneumothorax associated with laparoscopy: A case report of a rare hazard and review of literature. Anaesthesia 1973; 28:75-81.

84. Wolf JS, Carrier S, Stoller ML. Gas embolism: Helium is more lethal than carbon dioxide. J Laparoendosc Surg 1994; 4:173-7.

85. Couture P, Boudreault D, Derouin M, et al. Venous carbon dioxide embolism in pigs: An evaluation of end-tidal carbon dioxide, transesophageal echocardiography, pulmonary artery pressure, and precordial auscultation monitoring modalities. Anesth Analg 1994; 79:867-73.

86. Durant TM, Long J, Oppenheimer MJ. Pulmonary (venous) air embolism. Am Heart J 1947; 33:269-81.

87. Geissler HJ, Allen SJ, Mehlhorn U, et al. Effect of body positioning after venous air embolism. An echocardiographic study. Anesthesiology 1997; 86:710-7.

88. Brown DR, Fishburn JI, Roberson VO, Hulka JF. Ventilatory and blood gas changes during laparoscopy with local anesthesia. Am J Obstet Gynecol 1976; 124:741-5.

89. McKenzie R, Wadhwa R, Bedger RC. Noninvasive measurement of cardiac output during laparoscopy. J Reprod Med 1980; 24:247-50.

90. Silva PD, Kang SB, Sloane KA. Gamete intrafallopian transfer with spinal anesthesia. Fertil Steril 1993; 59:841-3.

91. Chung PH, Yeko TR, Mayer JC, et al. Gamete intrafallopian transfer: Comparison of epidural vs. general anesthesia. J Reprod Med 1998; 43:681-6.

92. Burke RK. Spinal anesthesia for laparoscopy: A review of 1063 cases. J Reprod Med 1978; 21:59-62.

93. Ciofolo MJ, Clergue F, Seebacher J, et al. Ventilatory effects of laparoscopy under epidural anesthesia. Anesth Analg 1990; 70:357-61.

94. Padilla SL, Smith RD, Dugan K, Zinder H. Laparoscopically assisted gamete intrafallopian transfer with local anesthesia. Fertil Steril 1996; 66:404-7.

95. Waterstone JJ, Bolton VN, Wren M, Parson JH. Laparoscopic zygote intrafallopian transfer using augmented local anesthesia. Fertil Steril 1992; 57:442-4.

96. Milki AA, Hardy RI, Danasouri IE, et al. Local anesthesia with conscious sedation for laparoscopic intrafallopian transfer. Fertil Steril 1992; 58:1240-2.

97. Pellicano M, Zullo F, Fiorentino A, et al. Conscious sedation versus general anaesthesia for minilaparoscopic gamete intra-Fallopian transfer: A prospective randomized study. Hum Reprod 2001; 16:2295-7

98. Ayestaran C, Matorras R, Gomez S, et al. Severe bradycardia and bradypnea following vaginal oocyte retrieval: A possible toxic effect of paracervical mepivacaine. Eur J Obstet Gynecol Reprod Biol 2000; 91:71-3.

99. von der Weiden RM, Helmerhorst FM, Keirse MJ. Influence of prostaglandins and platelet activating factor on implantation. Hum Reprod 1991; 6:436-42.

100. Marshburn PB, Shabanowitz RB, Clark MR. Immunohistochemical localization of prostaglandin H synthase in the embryo and uterus of the mouse from ovulation through implantation. Mol Reprod Dev 1990; 25:309-16.

101. Check JH, Nowroozi K, Barnea ER, et al. Successful delivery after age 50: A report of two cases as a result of oocyte donation. Obstet Gynecol 1993; 81:835-6.

Chapter 15
Problems of Early Pregnancy

Robert C. Chantigian, M.D. · Paula D. M. Chantigian, M.D., FACOG

PHYSIOLOGIC CHANGES OF EARLY PREGNANCY

Respiratory Changes

The respiratory system undergoes profound physiologic changes during early pregnancy.[1-3] Increased progesterone concentrations stimulate respiratory efforts by increasing the sensitivity of the respiratory center to carbon dioxide. The minute ventilation increases at least 15% by 12 weeks' gestation and 25% by 20 weeks' gestation. This increase in minute ventilation is due to an increase in tidal volume (respiratory rate is unchanged) and is in excess of the increase in oxygen consumption. The result is a respiratory alkalosis with maternal arterial partial pressure of carbon dioxide ($PaCO_2$) decreasing to 30 to 33 mm Hg by 10 to 12 weeks' gestation. Moreover, maternal arterial partial pressure of oxygen (PaO_2) increases to 106 to 108 mm Hg in the first trimester. A decreased bicarbonate concentration compensates for the modest respiratory alkalosis that results from the physiologic hyperventilation. The result is a maternal pH that is slightly above normal (e.g., approximately 7.44). There is little or no change in lung capacities during the first half of pregnancy.

Cardiovascular Changes

The cardiovascular system also undergoes profound changes early in pregnancy.[2-5] Cardiac output increases 20% to 25% by 8 weeks' gestation and 35% to 40% by 20 weeks' gestation. Systemic vascular resistance (SVR) decreases 30% by 8 weeks' gestation. Maternal mean arterial pressure (MAP) decreases approximately 6 mm Hg at 16 to 24 weeks' gestation and returns to normal near term. Aortocaval compression typically is not a problem until 18 to 20 weeks' gestation, when the uterus is large enough to compress the aorta and vena cava when the patient assumes the supine position.[6]

Blood volume increases throughout pregnancy; the average prepregnancy blood volume of 4350 mL (76 mL/kg) increases to 4700 mL (81 mL/kg) at 12 weeks' gestation, 5500 mL (89 mL/kg) at 20 weeks' gestation, and 6600 mL (97 mL/kg) at term. The increase in blood volume is primarily the result of increased plasma volume because the red blood cell (RBC) volume remains relatively constant at 27 mL/kg.[7] Because pregnant women have an expanded blood volume, they typically tolerate a blood loss of 500 to 1500 mL during the first half of pregnancy. A blood loss of 500 to 1500 mL rarely requires blood transfusion, provided the blood loss is replaced with an adequate volume of crystalloid or colloid.

Gastrointestinal Changes

During the first half of pregnancy, the physiologic changes of the gastrointestinal system are not clinically significant. Fasting gastric volume is approximately 30 mL in both nonpregnant women and women in early pregnancy (i.e., 15 weeks' gestation). Metoclopramide 10 mg, administered 15 to 30 minutes before anesthesia, can reduce this volume by 50%.[8] In a study of 100 pregnant women undergoing general anesthesia by mask at 6 to 22 weeks' gestation, a pH electrode revealed reflux of gastric contents into the esophagus in 17% of patients. (Most episodes of reflux occurred in patients who developed hiccups.) Only 2% had regurgitation of gastric contents into the pharynx, and no patient demonstrated clinical evidence of pulmonary aspiration.[9]

General anesthesia may be administered by means of a mask for selected extraabdominal procedures during early pregnancy, without complication. However, patients who receive general anesthesia during the first half of pregnancy should be intubated if they do not meet the criteria for an "empty stomach" (e.g., no oral intake for several hours). Likewise, intubation of patients with a difficult mask airway is recommended. Pharmacologic prophylaxis (e.g., sodium citrate, an H_2-receptor antagonist, and/or metoclopramide) is likely to further decrease the risk of aspiration pneumonia. Regional anesthesia is associated with a lower risk of aspiration than is general anesthesia.

Neurologic Changes

Pregnant women are more sensitive to both local anesthetics[10] and inhalation agents[11] during early pregnancy. The minimum alveolar concentration (MAC) is decreased approximately 30% with halothane, enflurane, and isoflurane. The exact mechanism for the increased sensitivity is unclear, but hormonal changes may play a role.

ECTOPIC PREGNANCY

Ectopic pregnancy results when the fertilized ovum implants outside the endometrial lining of the uterus. Death, infertility, and recurrent ectopic pregnancy are possible sequelae.

The frequency of ectopic pregnancy in the United States has increased almost fivefold, from 4.5 per 1000 pregnancies in 1970[12] to 19.7 per 1000 pregnancies in 1992.[13] Earlier diagnosis of previously unrecognized ectopic pregnancies, as well as an increased prevalence of associated risk factors, may account for the reported increase. Ruptured ectopic pregnancy is responsible for approximately 7% of all pregnancy-related maternal deaths in the United States[14] and is the leading cause of pregnancy-related maternal death during the first trimester.[12] Most (92%) ectopic pregnancy-related maternal deaths result from hemorrhage. Infection (3%), embolism (3%), and anesthetic complications (1%) are responsible for a minority of those deaths.[14] More than 30% of women who have had an ectopic pregnancy subsequently suffer from infertility, and 5% to 23% will have a recurrent ectopic pregnancy.[15]

Factors that increase the risk of an ectopic pregnancy involve alterations in the normal fallopian tube transport system for the fertilized ovum. These factors include (1) prior tubal surgery (e.g., tuboplasty, tubal ligation, previous ectopic pregnancy), (2) inflammation (e.g., prior pelvic inflammatory disease), (3) congenital anatomic distortion (e.g., exposure to diethylstilbestrol [DES] in utero), (4) previous pelvic or abdominal surgery (e.g., appendectomy), (5) concurrent use of an intrauterine contraceptive device, (6) delayed ovulation, (7) lifestyle choices (e.g., smoking, vaginal douching), (8) a history of infertility, (9) hormonal changes associated with ovulation induction, and (10) assisted reproductive technology (ART) procedures (e.g., zygote transfer into the fallopian tube or uterine cavity).[16-19] One third of patients with an ectopic pregnancy have no identifiable risk factors.[20]

The fertilized ovum may implant anywhere along the path of migration (Figure 15-1).[21] Some 98% of natural ectopic pregnancies are **tubal** (infundibular or fimbrial: 6%; ampullary: 78%; isthmic: 12%; interstitial or cornual: 2%). The remaining 2% implant on the **cervix**, **vagina**, **ovary**, or elsewhere within the **abdomen**.[16,22] With ART patients, most ectopic pregnancies are tubal; however, approximately 6% are ovarian, abdominal or cervical, and 12% to 15% are **heterotopic** (simultaneous intrauterine and extrauterine) pregnancies.[16,19]

Clinical Presentation

The clinical presentation of the patient with an ectopic pregnancy depends on the gestational age, the site of implantation, and the occurrence of significant hemorrhage. Classic clinical signs of impending rupture or a ruptured tubal pregnancy include abdominal or pelvic pain (90% to 100%), delayed menses (75% to 95%), and vaginal bleeding (50% to 80%).[18,20,22,23] Vaginal bleeding results from the breakdown and shedding of the decidual lining of the uterine wall, probably associated with decreased hormone production by the corpus luteum and inadequate human chorionic gonadotropin (hCG) production by the ectopic trophoblast. Pain often precedes vaginal bleeding. Patients with hemorrhage (with or

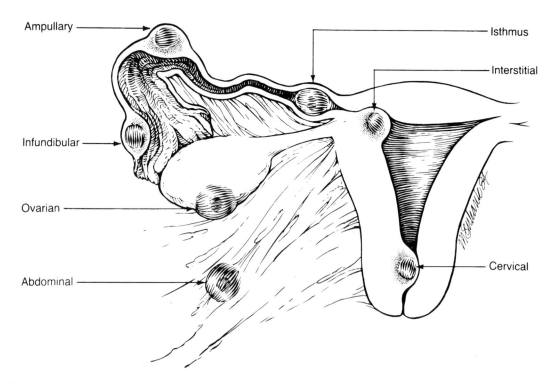

FIGURE 15-1. Potential location of ectopic pregnancies. The majority of ectopic pregnancies occur in the ampullary portion of the fallopian tube. (From DeCherney AH, Seifer DB. Ectopic pregnancy. In Gabbe SG, Niebyl JR, Simpson JL, editors. Obstetrics: Normal and Problem Pregnancies, 2nd ed. New York, Churchill Livingstone, 1991:811.)

without tubal rupture) may experience dizziness or syncope, or they may have the urge to defecate because of the presence of blood in the cul-de-sac.

Physical findings include abdominal tenderness with or without rebound (80% to 95%), a uterus that is smaller than expected for dates (30%), and a tender adnexal mass (30% to 50%). A bulging cul-de-sac suggests hemoperitoneum. With significant hemorrhage, orthostatic changes in blood pressure and heart rate or frank shock may occur. Some patients appear stable hemodynamically (e.g., normal blood pressure) despite a hemoperitoneum of 1000 to 1500 mL. Presumably, these patients have a slowly bleeding ectopic pregnancy, and they are able to compensate for the gradual blood loss.[22]

Diagnosis

In a woman of reproductive age, the symptoms of ectopic pregnancy must be differentiated from (1) a threatened, inevitable, or incomplete abortion, (2) infection after attempted abortion, (3) pelvic inflammatory disease, (4) a degenerating fibroid, (5) appendicitis or other gastrointestinal diseases, (6) ovarian torsion, (7) a ruptured or bleeding ovarian cyst, (8) a trapped retroverted pregnant uterus, and (9) nephrolithiasis.

For years, laparoscopy has been considered the gold standard for the diagnosis of an ectopic pregnancy in hemodynamically stable patients. Recent advances in diagnostic regimens (e.g., single measurement of the maternal serum progesterone concentration, serial beta-human chorionic gonadotropin [beta-hCG] levels, transvaginal ultrasonography, uterine curettage) allow early diagnosis of ectopic pregnancy.[15] Early diagnosis decreases morbidity and mortality and allows outpatient medical or conservative surgical (laparoscopic) treatment.[15] A positive pregnancy test and the absence of an intrauterine gestational sac during ultrasound examination indicate the diagnosis of ectopic pregnancy until proven otherwise.

Diagnostic algorithms include the following guidelines:
1. A serum progesterone concentration less than or equal to 5 ng/mL indicates a nonviable pregnancy with 100% sensitivity[24]; a concentration greater than 25 ng/mL usually is associated with a viable pregnancy.[25]
2. Serial beta-hCG concentrations that decrease, plateau, or show a subnormal rise (less than 66% over 48 hours) usually indicate a nonviable pregnancy—either an ectopic pregnancy or an impending abortion.[26] Beta-hCG concentrations greater than 100,000 mIU/mL usually are associated with viable intrauterine pregnancies.[24]
3. Ultrasonography can reliably confirm only the presence of an intrauterine pregnancy. The ectopic pregnancy itself may be difficult to visualize.[27] An intrauterine gestational sac is usually visible by **transabdominal ultrasonography** when serum beta-hCG concentrations are greater than 6000 to 6500 mIU/mL, using the International Reference Preparation (IRP) standard (i.e., approximately 42 days after the first day of the last menstrual period), or by **transvaginal ultrasonography** when beta-hCG concentrations are greater than 1400 mIU/mL IRP (i.e., approximately 35 days after the first day of the last menstrual period).[28]
4. Uterine curettage can be performed when nonviability is established. Identification of trophoblastic villi confirms miscarriage of an intrauterine pregnancy. Absence of villi signals either a complete spontaneous abortion (confirmed by rapidly decreasing beta-hCG concentrations) or an ectopic pregnancy.

When a diagnosis must be established and the serum progesterone concentration, beta-hCG testing, and ultrasonography are not available, culdocentesis can identify a hemoperitoneum and, with clinical signs, can establish the presumptive diagnosis of a ruptured ectopic pregnancy. Culdocentesis is considered positive when non-clotting bloody fluid or fragmented old clots are aspirated. Culdocentesis is positive in 80% to 95% of patients with a ruptured ectopic pregnancy; the false-positive rate is 5% to 10%.[18,20,23]

Obstetric Management

Management of an ectopic pregnancy may include expectant, medical, or surgical approaches. Management choice depends on the symptoms and findings.

Expectant management may be used for selected asymptomatic cases with early tubal ectopic pregnancies and stable or decreasing beta-hCG levels. Successful resolution has been reported in approximately 50% of these selected patients.[29] If expectant management is unsuccessful, a medical or surgical approach is required.

Methotrexate and citrovorum chemotherapy is the usual drug combination used for **medical management**. Methotrexate inhibits the growth of the trophoblastic cells of the placenta. Early tubal pregnancies (i.e., no cardiac activity, a diameter less than 4 cm, and no evidence of tubal rupture or hemoperitoneum) have been successfully treated with single-dose methotrexate and citrovorum chemotherapy in 67% to 100% of selected patients.[15,30] Side effects include abdominal pain, vomiting, stomatitis, severe neutropenia, and pneumonitis.[30] Unsuccessful resolution of the ectopic pregnancy requires surgical intervention.

Surgical management depends on the location of the pregnancy, the hemodynamic stability of the patient, the equipment available, and the surgeon's expertise. When a viable intrauterine pregnancy has been excluded, hemodynamically stable patients may first undergo a dilation and uterine evacuation (D and E) to eliminate the possibility of an incomplete abortion. Subsequently, diagnostic laparoscopy is performed to confirm the diagnosis and locate the ectopic pregnancy. For tubal ectopic pregnancies, a salpingostomy, salpingotomy, or salpingectomy (usually partial) is performed by means of laparoscopy or laparotomy. To aid hemostasis during laparoscopic removal of the ectopic pregnancy, some obstetricians inject dilute vasopressin into the surface of the fallopian tube. This causes marked blanching of the tube and results in a relatively bloodless surgical field. If the vasopressin is accidentally injected intravenously, a marked increase in maternal blood pressure may result.[31]

A laparotomy is indicated in cases in which the surgeon is not trained in operative laparoscopy, laparoscopic removal may be difficult (e.g., tube diameter greater than 6 cm or an interstitial location of the ectopic pregnancy), or there is uncontrollable bleeding.[31] Hemodynamic instability should prompt the immediate performance of a laparotomy. These cases often require a partial or total salpingectomy. If a partial salpingectomy is performed, tubal repair may be performed primarily or during a second operation.

Persistent ectopic pregnancy complicates laparoscopic salpingostomy in as many as 15% of cases. The performance of a salpingostomy during laparotomy results in an incidence of persistent ectopic pregnancy of 2% or less.[32]

Interstitial, cervical, and abdominal pregnancies present significant diagnostic and therapeutic challenges. **Interstitial** pregnancies often go unrecognized and may present with uterine wall rupture, massive hemorrhage, and shock. Conservative surgery (e.g., cornual resection) may be attempted, but hysterectomy may be required if uterine damage is severe.

Cervical pregnancies often result in massive hemorrhage because of the inability of the cervix to contract. In the past, most cervical pregnancies necessitated hysterectomy to control the hemorrhage. Other management regimens include (1) methotrexate therapy, (2) local excision, (3) cerclage and tamponade, (4) ligation of the hypogastric arteries or the cervical branches of the uterine arteries, and (5) angiographic embolization of the uterine arteries, followed by a D and E procedure.[33]

Abdominal pregnancies are associated with a high incidence of maternal morbidity and a maternal mortality rate of 0.5% to 4.5%.[34,35] Diagnosis is difficult and is missed in as many as 1 of 9 cases.[34] Abdominal pain, vaginal bleeding, symptoms consistent with partial bowel obstruction, shock, or death may be the first indication of this unusual type of pregnancy.[36] Ultrasonography may aid in diagnosis but may miss the diagnosis in more than 50% of cases. Magnetic resonance imaging (MRI) may prove to be a sensitive diagnostic tool.[36] Abdominal pregnancy is associated with decreased placental perfusion (which typically results in fetal growth restriction) and oligohydramnios (which often results in pulmonary hypoplasia and anatomic deformities). Stevens[35] reviewed published cases of abdominal pregnancy since 1809 and found that 63% of infants survived when born after 30 weeks' gestation. Delayed delivery places the mother at risk for massive hemorrhage from premature separation of the placenta.

Management of an abdominal pregnancy consists of laparotomy and delivery of the fetus. Once the fetus is delivered, management of the placenta is controversial and fraught with hazard. Removal of the placenta is associated with (1) massive hemorrhage, (2) prolonged, complicated surgery (e.g., bowel resection), and (3) increased maternal mortality. A decision to leave the placenta in situ results in an increased risk of infectious morbidity as well as a greater need for additional surgery.[23,35,36] The site of placental implantation and the ability to adequately ligate the blood supply often dictates the obstetrician's decision regarding management of the placenta.

Historically, **heterotopic** pregnancies were thought to occur in 1 in 30,000 natural pregnancies.[37-39] With the advent of ART, the overall incidence of heterotopic pregnancy may be as frequent as 1 in 2600.[37-39] In ART patients, 1% to 3% of pregnancies are heterotopic.[16] The difficulty in visualizing the entire fallopian tube by ultrasonography, combined with normal or slightly elevated beta-hCG measurements (i.e., low serum levels from the ectopic pregnancy combined with normal levels from the intrauterine pregnancy), make the early diagnosis of heterotopic pregnancy difficult.[40] A heterotopic pregnancy should be suspected in cases in which clinical signs of an ectopic pregnancy and a confirmed intrauterine pregnancy coexist. In most cases the ectopic pregnancy is removed surgically. (Alternatively, transvaginal ultrasound-guided injection of potassium chloride into the ectopic pregnancy has been performed successfully in a small number of cases.[41]) The patient usually sustains the normal intrauterine pregnancy to term.[38,40,42]

Patients who are Rh negative should receive Rh-immune globulin at the time of medical or surgical intervention.[30]

Anesthetic Management

Patients with an unruptured tubal pregnancy usually have a normal intravascular volume and little bleeding before and during surgery. These patients have low anesthetic and surgical risks. Laparoscopy or laparotomy can be performed safely with spinal, epidural, or general anesthesia (Box 15-1).[43] Most patients prefer general anesthesia.

Patients may have significant hemorrhage associated with a ruptured tubal pregnancy or an unruptured interstitial, cervical, or abdominal ectopic pregnancy. Young women often maintain a normal blood pressure despite a markedly reduced circulating blood volume. In one study of ruptured ectopic pregnancies, approximately 50% of patients had more than 500 mL, and 10% had greater than 1500 mL of blood in the peritoneal cavity.[23] General anesthesia is preferred for most patients with preoperative evidence of bleeding. Large-gauge intravenous catheters should be placed as soon as possible. Several units of packed RBCs should be immediately available. Intraoperative autologous blood transfusion can be used safely in women with a ruptured ectopic pregnancy.[44,45] Invasive monitoring may be required in patients with hemodynamic instability.

ABORTION AND INTRAUTERINE FETAL DEMISE

Abortion refers to a pregnancy loss or termination, either before 20 weeks' gestation or when the fetus weighs less than 500 g. It can occur spontaneously or can be performed electively for personal or medical reasons. Over 800,000 elective abortions (i.e., an abortion rate of approximately 250 abortions per 1000 live births) were performed in the United States in 1999. Almost all of these were surgical; over 98% were performed by curettage. Medical abortions (i.e., nonsurgical, usually performed at 8 or fewer weeks' gestation) have been performed since the mid-1990s and may become more common.[46]

Hutchon[47] has suggested that physicians substitute the word *miscarriage* for the word *abortion* in cases of spontaneous early pregnancy loss. Further, he suggested that the word *miscarriage* may be modified with descriptive adjectives such as *threatened, incomplete,* and *complete,* and that the term *delayed miscarriage* replace the term *missed abortion.* In our judgment, either set of terms is acceptable.

Five percent of all pregnancy-related maternal deaths in the United States are associated with an induced or spontaneous abortion.[14] Death results from sepsis in approximately 36% of cases, hemorrhage in approximately 20% of cases, and embolism in approximately 16% of cases.[14] Of the 21 abortion-related maternal deaths in the United States in 1998, 9 occurred with elective abortion, 11 occurred with spontaneous abortion, and 1 was not classified.[46]

Spontaneous abortion occurs in 10% to 15% of clinically recognized pregnancies; when subclinical pregnancies also are considered, the incidence of spontaneous pregnancy loss may be as high as 60%.[48,49] Although most spontaneous abortions manifest clinically at 8 to 14 weeks' gestation, ultrasonography suggests that fetal demise usually occurs before 8 weeks' gestation.[48,49] If the fetus is viable at 8 weeks' gestation, the incidence of subsequent fetal loss is only 3%.[50]

The etiology of spontaneous abortion varies among patients. Chromosomal abnormalities are responsible for at least 50% to 80% of all spontaneous abortions.[49,51,52] Other causes include (1) immunologic mechanisms, (2) maternal infections, (3) endocrine abnormalities (e.g., poorly con-

Box 15-1 ANESTHETIC TECHNIQUE FOR LAPAROSCOPY OR LAPAROTOMY FOR A PATIENT WITH AN ECTOPIC PREGNANCY

UNRUPTURED TUBAL ECTOPIC PREGNANCY WITH NO OR MINIMAL BLEEDING

- Type and screen
- Routine noninvasive monitors (electrocardiogram [ECG], blood pressure cuff, pulse oximeter, stethoscope, temperature probe)
- One intravenous catheter
- Foley catheter
- Spinal anesthesia
  1. Hydration with 1000 to 1500 mL of Ringer's lactate solution
  2. Single injection with a small-gauge spinal needle placed at the L2 to L3 or L3 to L4 interspace
  3. 12 to 15 mg of bupivacaine with 25 μg of fentanyl
  4. T2 to T4 level
- Epidural anesthesia
  1. Hydration with 1000 to 1500 mL of Ringer's lactate solution
  2. Placement of the epidural needle at the L2 to L3 or L3 to L4 interspace
  3. Approximately 20 to 25 mL of 2% lidocaine with 1:200,000 epinephrine and 100 μg of fentanyl, *injected incrementally*
  4. T2 to T4 level
- General anesthesia
  1. Rapid-sequence induction with cricoid pressure if patient has a full stomach
  2. Thiopental or propofol for induction
  3. Muscle relaxant for intubation and surgery (with the use of a nerve stimulator)
  4. Endotracheal intubation
  5. End-tidal carbon dioxide monitoring
  6. Maintenance of anesthesia with oxygen, nitrous oxide, a volatile halogenated agent, and an opioid

  7. Placement of oral gastric tube, performance of suctioning, and removal of tube
  8. Reversal of muscle relaxant and extubation when the patient is awake and responds to verbal commands

RUPTURED TUBAL PREGNANCY OR INTERSTITIAL, CERVICAL, OR ABDOMINAL PREGNANCY

- Type and cross for several units of blood
- Routine noninvasive monitors, consideration of invasive hemodynamic monitoring (e.g., arterial catheter, central venous pressure [CVP] catheter)
- Two large-gauge intravenous catheters with Ringer's lactate solution
- Foley catheter
- Consideration of intraoperative autologous blood transfusion
- General anesthesia
  1. Rapid-sequence induction with cricoid pressure
  2. Ketamine or etomidate for induction (thiopental or propofol can be used if the intravascular volume has been restored)
  3. Muscle relaxant for intubation and surgery (with the use of a nerve stimulator)
  4. Endotracheal intubation
  5. End-tidal carbon dioxide monitoring
  6. Maintenance with oxygen, nitrous oxide, an opioid, and a volatile halogenated agent as tolerated
  7. Placement of oral gastric tube, performance of suctioning, and removal of tube
  8. Reversal of muscle relaxant and extubation when the patient is awake and responds to verbal commands

trolled diabetes mellitus), (4) uterine anomalies, (5) incompetent cervix, (6) debilitating maternal disease, (7) trauma, and possibly (8) environmental exposures (e.g., irradiation, smoking, certain drugs).[49,53]

Although several studies (conducted before scavenging of anesthetic gases was routine) have suggested an increased incidence of spontaneous abortion among women who have been exposed to trace concentrations of anesthetic agents in the operating room,[54] reevaluation of those data demonstrated significant flaws in the study design, which casts doubt on the original conclusions.[55] Other studies have not shown an increased incidence of spontaneous abortion in women working in the operating room.[56,57]

Clinical Presentation and Obstetric Management

The clinical presentation and management of a patient undergoing a spontaneous abortion vary. A **threatened abortion** is defined as uterine bleeding *without* cervical dilation before 20 weeks' gestation. Bleeding may be accompanied by cramping or backache. Once the diagnosis is confirmed, activities are restricted until symptoms resolve. Approximately 25% of pregnancies are complicated by a threatened abortion; approximately half of these women will go on to have a spontaneous abortion.[58]

An **inevitable abortion** is defined as cervical dilation or rupture of membranes without expulsion of the fetus or placenta. Spontaneous expulsion of the uterine contents usually occurs, but infection can be a complication.

A **complete abortion** is defined as a complete, spontaneous expulsion of the fetus and placenta. Partial expulsion of

the uterine contents (i.e., an **incomplete abortion**) is more common after 8 weeks' gestation.[53] Persistent bleeding and cramping after expulsion of tissue are signs of an incomplete abortion. An incomplete abortion usually requires a D and E procedure to remove any remaining fetal or placental tissue. Oxytocin and/or an ergot alkaloid (e.g., methylergonovine) increases uterine tone and may be administered intraoperatively and/or postoperatively to decrease the amount of uterine bleeding.

In a patient with a **missed abortion**, fetal death goes unrecognized for several weeks. Occasionally, coagulation defects such as disseminated intravascular coagulopathy (DIC) may complicate an intrauterine fetal death (IUFD); this is more likely when the fetus dies at an advanced gestational age. If spontaneous expulsion of the uterine contents does not occur after a brief period of observation, evacuation of the uterus is indicated. Options include intravaginal or intracervical placement of a prostaglandin E_2 (PGE_2) preparation, or a D and E procedure after laminaria placement. Side effects of prostaglandins include nausea, vomiting, diarrhea, and fever. Intraamniotic instillation of hypertonic saline is not recommended in cases of IUFD because coagulation defects may be induced or enhanced.[59]

Recurrent or **habitual abortion** refers to the occurrence of three or more consecutive spontaneous abortions.

Obstetric Complications

Complications of a D and E include cervical laceration, uterine perforation, hemorrhage, retained products of conception, and infection. The risk of these complications is increased in pregnancies beyond the first trimester. Vasovagal events, postabortal syndrome (i.e., intrauterine blood clots with uterine atony, associated with lower abdominal pain, tachycardia, and diaphoresis), DIC, and unrecognized ectopic pregnancy also can occur.

Management of uterine perforation may include simple observation or immediate laparotomy with indicated repairs. Management depends on the suspected severity of injury to the uterus and adjacent structures.

Serious infection (e.g., **septic abortion**) complicates approximately 0.5 of 100,000 spontaneous abortions. Serious infection occurs more frequently after induced abortion, particularly illegal abortion.[58,60] Septic abortion causes significant morbidity and is life threatening. Blood cultures should be obtained, and broad-spectrum antibiotics are promptly administered intravenously. Some patients with hemodynamic instability require invasive hemodynamic monitoring to guide fluid, blood, and/or vasoactive drug therapy. Once the patient is stabilized and lower genital tract or bowel injury is excluded, the uterus is reevacuated. On occasion, hysterectomy is necessary and may be lifesaving.

If the mother who aborts is Rh-negative, Rh-immune globulin (e.g., anti-D immune globulin) is administered to prevent Rh-sensitization.[59] In the past, some obstetricians did not administer Rh-immune globulin to Rh-negative women with a threatened abortion. However, von Stein et al.[61] demonstrated a positive Kleihauer-Betke test (which indicates transplacental hemorrhage of fetal blood into the maternal circulation) in 11% of patients with a threatened abortion. Therefore Rh-negative women with a threatened abortion should receive Rh-immune globulin.

Women who suffer a spontaneous abortion are at increased risk for depressive disorders during the 6 months after miscarriage.[62]

Anesthetic Management

Anesthesiologists should consider whether the cervix is dilated, whether the patient has had significant blood loss or is septic, and whether the patient has a full stomach (Box 15-2). Dilation of the cervix is relatively painful, whereas the suction and/or curettage is less painful. If the cervix is dilated, sedation and a paracervical block may suffice. (Because spontaneous abortion is upsetting for many women, some women who have a dilated cervix prefer general anesthesia.) If the cervix is not dilated, anesthesia usually is needed for the surgical dilation. This may be accomplished with a paracervical block and sedation or with spinal, epidural, or general anesthesia.

The cervix is typically dilated in patients who have had significant preoperative bleeding. Rarely, a patient with a closed cervix has significant bleeding. With significant bleeding, it is first necessary to restore intravascular volume. A paracervical block and sedation may then provide adequate analgesia. If such a patient has significant discomfort despite receiving a paracervical block, general anesthesia is preferred. Substantial hemorrhage represents a relative contraindication to the use of spinal or epidural anesthesia. Likewise, it is probably best to avoid spinal or epidural anesthesia in patients with evidence of frank sepsis.

Thiopental, propofol, ketamine, or etomidate can be administered for the induction of general anesthesia. Ketamine may

---

Box 15-2 ANESTHETIC TECHNIQUE FOR DILATION AND EVACUATION FOR A SPONTANEOUS ABORTION

GENERAL CONSIDERATIONS

Performance of a type of screen in patients with a large blood loss or in those with advanced gestation

Oxytocin and/or an ergot alkaloid available

In all patients who have lost a significant amount of blood, observation of the patient on the operating table for evidence of hypotension for at least 5 minutes after the legs have been lowered from the lithotomy position

MONITORED ANESTHESIA CARE (WELL TOLERATED WHEN CERVIX IS DILATED)

Routine noninvasive monitors (ECG, blood pressure cuff, pulse oximeter, stethoscope)

One intravenous catheter with Ringer's lactate solution (two large-gauge intravenous catheters if the patient has had substantial hemorrhage)

Intravenous analgesia with fentanyl or alfentanil and sedation with midazolam or propofol

Paracervical block by the obstetrician

SPINAL ANESTHESIA (ONLY IF PATIENT HAS A NORMAL INTRAVASCULAR VOLUME AND IS NOT SEPTIC)

Routine noninvasive monitors

One intravenous catheter

Hydration with 1000 to 1500 mL of Ringer's lactate solution

Single injection using a small-gauge spinal needle placed at the L2 to L3 or L3 to L4 interspace

40 mg of lidocaine or 7.5 mg of bupivacaine, with 20 μg of fentanyl

T8 to T10 level

EPIDURAL ANESTHESIA (ONLY IF PATIENT HAS A NORMAL INTRAVASCULAR VOLUME AND IS NOT SEPTIC)

Routine noninvasive monitors

One intravenous catheter

Hydration with 1000 to 1500 mL of Ringer's lactate solution

Placement of the epidural needle at the L2 to L3 or L3 to L4 interspace

Approximately 12 to 15 mL of 2% lidocaine with epinephrine and 50 to 75 μg of fentanyl, *injected incrementally*

T8 to T10 level

GENERAL ANESTHESIA

Rapid-sequence induction with cricoid pressure if the patient has a full stomach

Routine noninvasive monitors (ECG, blood pressure cuff, pulse oximeter, stethoscope, temperature probe, nerve stimulator)

One intravenous catheter with Ringer's lactate solution (two intravenous catheters if the patient has had substantial hemorrhage)

Thiopental or propofol for induction (ketamine or etomidate in cases of severe hemorrhage)

Mask anesthesia during early pregnancy if there is no full stomach; otherwise endotracheal intubation with a muscle relaxant for intubation

End-tidal carbon dioxide monitoring

Maintenance with oxygen, nitrous oxide, an opioid, a benzodiazepine, and/or propofol; a low (< 0.5 MAC) concentration of a volatile halogenated agent may be added if there is little bleeding and no evidence of uterine atony

Placement of an oral gastric tube, performance of suctioning, and removal of tube if patient is intubated

Extubation when the patient is awake and responds to verbal commands be the ideal agent for induction of general anesthesia, especially in patients with significant bleeding. Large doses (1.5 to 2.0 mg/kg) of ketamine increase uterine tone,[63] which may be advantageous in patients who require evacuation of the uterus.

During general anesthesia, the drugs used may influence the amount of blood lost during the procedure. The volatile halogenated agents produce dose-dependent relaxation of uterine smooth muscle[64] and have been associated with increased uterine bleeding.[65-68] Two recent studies[67,68] assessed blood loss during elective first-trimester abortion. In all patients general anesthesia was induced with propofol and maintained with propofol infusion; nitrous oxide and oxygen; or isoflurane, nitrous oxide, and oxygen. In both studies blood loss was greater in the isoflurane group than in the propofol infusion group. However, these differences in blood loss may not be clinically significant in view of the expanded blood volume during pregnancy. Some obstetricians contend that relaxation of the uterus with a volatile halogenated agent increases the risk of uterine perforation. Because of this risk, these obstetricians prefer to avoid the administration of a volatile halogenated agent during a D and E procedure.

Anesthesia is maintained with oxygen, nitrous oxide, and an opioid (with or without a small dose of benzodiazepine). A propofol infusion or a low (less than 0.5 MAC) concentration of a volatile agent can be added. The volatile halogenated agent should be avoided or discontinued if there is any evidence of uterine atony. In most cases, oxytocin (20 units/L of crystalloid) is administered intravenously to increase uterine tone and decrease blood loss.

INCOMPETENT CERVIX

An inherent or traumatic deficiency in the structure or function of the uterine cervix results in an **incompetent cervix**, which is unable to sustain a pregnancy to full term. Typically, the woman with an incompetent cervix suffers recurrent second-trimester pregnancy losses that are characterized by (1) painless cervical dilation, (2) herniation followed by rupture of the fetal membranes, and (3) a short labor with delivery of a live, immature infant. The reported incidence of incompetent cervix varies from 0.001% to 1.84% of pregnant women.[69-72]

Cervical incompetence is caused by a spectrum of anatomic disorders, which include cervical deficiency or weakness at the level of the internal os. Cervical trauma, congenital abnormalities, a dysfunctional cervix, or hormonal abnormalities may cause the weakness.[73,74] Trauma appears to be a common cause of cervical incompetence. The trauma may have occurred during a previous vaginal delivery or during previous surgery (e.g., dilation and curettage, conization of the cervix, partial amputation or resection of the cervix, cervical cauterization). Congenital abnormalities (e.g., unicornuate or bicornuate uterus) of the reproductive tract may be present in as many as 2% of patients with cervical incompetence. Some anomalies may result from maternal exposure to DES in utero. Less often, a dysfunctional or muscular cervix may be present (i.e., more muscle than fibrous tissue weakens the cervix).

Diagnosis

Cervical incompetence remains a *clinical* diagnosis. A definitive diagnosis is made when herniating fetal membranes are visualized or palpated through a partially dilated cervix during the midtrimester of a current pregnancy. A characteristic history from a previous pregnancy allows the presumptive diagnosis of cervical incompetence, once other causes of recurrent pregnancy loss are excluded. Uterine contractions or vaginal bleeding during a previous pregnancy suggest that other mechanisms are responsible for pregnancy loss.

Physical examination may reveal cervical abnormalities or underlying congenital anomalies. Several tests suggestive of cervical incompetence (performed in the nonpregnant woman) have been described; unfortunately these tests may not reflect the condition of the pregnant cervix. These tests include the Hegar test, the traction test, and the compliance test.[73] Hysterosalpingography suggests a diagnosis of cervical incompetence when the internal os has a width of more than 1 cm[75] or when cervical funneling is observed.[76]

Symptoms of cervical incompetence may include increased vaginal discharge, lower abdominal or back pressure or discomfort, vaginal fullness, and/or urinary frequency.[77] During pregnancy, serial cervical and/or ultrasonographic examinations may be performed to evaluate cervical length and width.[73,78] MRI may prove to be a useful modality for the diagnosis of incompetent cervix.[79]

Obstetric Management

Despite the lack of prospective studies, most patients with a diagnosis of cervical incompetence undergo surgical reinforcement of the cervix or cervical cerclage. Cervical cerclage procedures have increased the fetal survival rate threefold to fourfold (from 20% to as high as 89%) when affected women are used as their own controls.[70-73,80]

The most commonly performed procedures are the modified **Shirodkar cerclage**[81] and the **McDonald cerclage**.[77] Both of these procedures are performed **transvaginally**. A ligature (e.g., Mersilene tape) is placed around the cervix at or near the level of the internal cervical os. In the more invasive modified Shirodkar procedure, the cervical mucosa is incised anteriorly and posteriorly, the bladder often is advanced, the ligature is placed submucosally and then tied, and the mucosal incisions are closed. The cervical mucosa is left intact with the McDonald cerclage. A purse-string ligature is placed around the cervix and then tied (Figure 15-2).[82] These two procedures result in comparable rates of fetal survival in patients with no history of prior cerclage.[70,83] In one study, better outcome (i.e., more advanced gestational age) was obtained when a Shirodkar cerclage was performed in patients who had a previous cerclage.[83] Advanced cervical dilation (i.e., 3 cm or greater) at the time of cerclage placement is associated with a decreased likelihood of successful outcome.[71,83]

Transvaginal cerclage can be performed in most patients with an incompetent cervix. However, if no substantial cervical tissue is present (e.g., severe cervical laceration, congenital or traumatic cervical shortening) or if a previous transvaginal cerclage has failed, a **transabdominal cerclage** may be performed.[84] The transabdominal cerclage can be performed before or during pregnancy. Although a posterior colpotomy and division of the transabdominal cerclage occasionally are performed in an attempt to allow vaginal delivery, most patients with transabdominal cerclage undergo cesarean section. The transabdominal cerclage can remain in situ if further pregnancies are desired, or it can be removed at the time of cesarean section.[80]

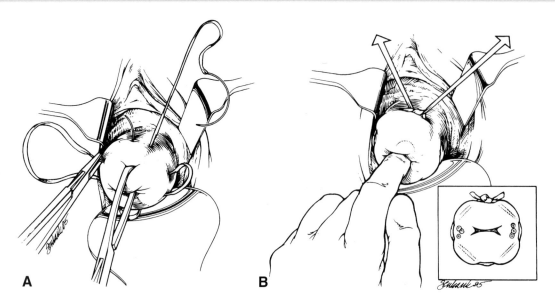

FIGURE 15-2. Placement of sutures for McDonald cervical cerclage. **A,** A double-headed Mersilene band with four "bites" is placed in the cervix, avoiding the vessels. **B,** The suture is placed high upon the cervix close to the cervical-vaginal junction, approximately at the level of the internal os. (From Iams JD. Preterm birth. In Gabbe SG, Niebyl JR, Simpson JL, editors. Obstetrics: Normal and Problem Pregnancies, 4th ed. New York, Churchill Livingstone, 2002: 803.)

The efficacy of perioperative antibiotics, tocolytic drugs, and/or progesterone drugs has not been confirmed; however, many obstetricians use one or more of these drugs empirically.[71,80,83]

Contraindications to a cerclage procedure include preterm labor, vaginal bleeding, fetal anomalies, fetal death, rupture of membranes, placental abruption, and chorioamnionitis. Some obstetricians obtain cervical cultures for gonorrhea, chlamydia, and group B streptococcus.

A cerclage can be performed either before (interval cerclage) or during pregnancy. An *interval* cerclage may increase the risk of infertility and may not allow easy evacuation of the uterus in the case of a first-trimester spontaneous abortion. *During* pregnancy, a cerclage can be performed prophylactically (before cervical dilation), or as an emergency procedure after the onset of cervical changes. Because prophylactic cerclage is more effective than emergency cerclage (fetal survival is 78% to 87% versus 42% to 68%, respectively),[70,71] most obstetricians perform prophylactic cerclage in the at-risk patient at 12 to 18 weeks' gestation, once fetal viability is established. A cervical dilation of 2 cm or more is associated with a greater risk of premature rupture of membranes and/or preterm delivery.[83]

The greatest risk during the performance of emergency cerclage is rupture of the membranes. Several techniques have been described to facilitate replacement of the bulging fetal membranes into the uterus. Uterine relaxation is essential. One option is to administer a volatile halogenated agent (e.g., isoflurane). Alternatively, a tocolytic drug (e.g., terbutaline, ritodrine) may be administered. Use of the steep Trendelenburg position allows for gravity assistance.

Some obstetricians insert a Foley catheter (with the tip removed) into the cervical canal and then inflate the balloon with 30 to 60 mL of saline. The balloon is deflated and the catheter is removed at the end of the procedure. Alternatively, some obstetricians fill the urinary bladder with sterile saline to assist in replacement of herniated membranes.

Immediate complications of cervical cerclage include rupture of the fetal membranes, hemorrhage, and stimulation of labor. Delayed complications include infection, cervical stenosis secondary to scarring, and cervical lacerations and uterine rupture if labor proceeds with the cerclage in place. Rarely, sepsis may result in maternal mortality. An increased need for cesarean section occurs in patients who have undergone cerclage. Patients who have undergone the Shirodkar procedure have an almost twofold increase in the incidence of cesarean section, compared with women who have had a McDonald cerclage (31% versus 17%).[83]

Anesthetic Management

Whether the cervix is dilated is of primary concern because this influences the type of anesthetic administered (Box 15-3). If the cervix is not dilated, spinal, epidural, or general anesthesia may be administered. (McCulloch et al.[85] described the use of pudendal nerve block for performance of McDonald cerclage, but pudendal block may not provide adequate anesthesia for many patients.) Either spinal or epidural anesthesia is an excellent choice for performance of prophylactic cerclage. Spinal anesthesia results in a rapid, predictable onset of sacral anesthesia, which is desirable for these procedures. In the past, administration of spinal anesthesia for cerclage resulted in a high incidence of postdural puncture headache.[86] Use of a small-gauge, non-cutting spinal needle (e.g., Whitacre, Sprotte) should reduce the incidence of postdural puncture headache in these patients.

If the cervix is dilated—and especially if the fetal membranes are bulging—the choice of anesthesia is more problematic. The advantages and disadvantages of each anesthetic technique must be weighed carefully. It is important to produce adequate analgesia for the mother and to prevent an increase in intraabdominal and intrauterine pressure that may lead to further bulging and possible rupture of the fetal membranes and subsequent fetal death. General anesthesia is preferred in patients with a dilated cervix and bulging fetal membranes. Administration of a volatile halogenated agent relaxes uterine smooth muscle and results in a decrease in intrauterine pressure. A decrease in intrauterine pressure facilitates replacement of the bulging membranes and placement of the cerclage. On occasion, an amniocentesis may

Box 15-3 ANESTHETIC TECHNIQUE FOR TRANSVAGINAL CERVICAL CERCLAGE

FETAL HEART RATE (FHR) MONITORING

Less than 20 weeks' gestation: FHR checked before and after cerclage procedure

Greater than 20 weeks' gestation: continuous FHR monitoring used during the procedure*

SPINAL ANESTHESIA

Routine noninvasive monitors

One intravenous catheter

Hydration with 1000 to 1500 mL of Ringer's lactate solution

Single injection with a small-gauge spinal needle placed at the L2 to L3 or L3 to L4 interspace

40 mg of lidocaine or 7.5 mg of bupivacaine, with 20 μg of fentanyl

T8 to T10 level

EPIDURAL ANESTHESIA

Routine noninvasive monitors

One intravenous catheter

Hydration with 1000 to 1500 mL of Ringer's lactate solution

Placement of the epidural needle at the L2 to L3 or L3 to L4 interspace

Approximately 12 to 15 mL of 2% lidocaine with epinephrine and 50 to 75 μg of fentanyl, *injected incrementally*

T8 to T10 level

GENERAL ANESTHESIA (IF CERVIX IS DILATED AND UTERINE RELAXATION IS NEEDED)

Routine noninvasive monitors

One intravenous catheter

Thiopental or propofol for induction

Intubation preferable in patients with a full stomach or patients who are greater than 18 to 20 weeks' gestation; mask anesthesia otherwise acceptable

End-tidal carbon dioxide monitoring

Maintenance with oxygen, nitrous oxide, and a volatile halogenated agent to provide uterine relaxation

*Use left uterine displacement if the patient is greater than 18 to 20 weeks' gestation.

be performed before or during a cerclage procedure in an attempt to decrease the intrauterine pressure and facilitate the reduction of the fetal membranes. During induction of general anesthesia, it is important to avoid coughing on the endotracheal tube, which may result in increased intrauterine pressure. A smooth induction of general anesthesia is preferred. Administration of regional anesthesia obviates the need for endotracheal intubation and the possibility of coughing on the endotracheal tube. However, some physicians worry that acute dorsiflexion during placement of the block may result in an increase in intrauterine pressure. In addition, vomiting results in a significant increase in intrauterine pressure.

Few clinical studies have assessed obstetric outcome after administration of regional versus general anesthesia for cerclage. One retrospective study observed no difference in fetal outcome after administration of either general anesthesia (375 cases) or epidural anesthesia (114 cases) for cerclage procedures.[87]

Fetal heart rate (FHR) monitoring should be performed during the procedure after 20 weeks' gestation. In theory, it is possible that replacement of bulging membranes and closure

of the cervix may lead to an increase in intrauterine pressure with a subsequent reduction in placental blood flow. In this case, it would be reasonable to give a tocolytic agent to help reduce intrauterine pressure.

The transvaginal cerclage is removed at 37 to 38 weeks' gestation. The suture is removed earlier if rupture of membranes occurs or if labor begins. Removal of a McDonald cerclage often requires no anesthesia. In the patient with a Shirodkar cerclage, anesthesia (e.g., paracervical block, spinal anesthesia, epidural anesthesia) usually is necessary. If the Shirodkar cerclage is epithelialized, some obstetricians leave the cerclage intact and perform an elective cesarean section.

Once the suture is removed, labor often begins within a few hours or days. If an epidural catheter was placed for cerclage removal, the epidural anesthetic can be allowed to regress while the patient is observed for evidence of cervical dilation and the onset of labor. If labor begins, the epidural catheter can be reinjected to provide analgesia for labor.

GESTATIONAL TROPHOBLASTIC DISEASE

In normal pregnancies, trophoblastic tissue forms the placenta. Abnormal trophoblastic proliferation of the human placenta results in gestational trophoblastic disease (GTD). The histologic spectrum of GTD includes (1) complete or partial **hydatidiform mole**, (2) **invasive mole** (i.e., chorioadenoma destruens), (3) **choriocarcinoma**, and (4) **placental site trophoblastic tumor (PSTT)**. Hydatidiform mole with spontaneous resolution and placental site trophoblastic tumors are considered as separate entities from the other gestational trophoblastic neoplasms (GTNs) when using current staging and risk-scoring systems.[88]

Gestational trophoblastic disease caused 0.5% of all pregnancy-related maternal deaths in the United States between 1991 and 1997.[14] There is marked geographic variation in the incidence of hydatidiform mole, with a rate of 1 in 82 pregnancies in Taiwan and a rate of 1 in 1300 to 1 in 2500 pregnancies in the United States.[89] Risk factors include advanced maternal age, very young maternal age, history of previous molar pregnancy, and possibly nutritional factors.[90]

Approximately 20% of patients with a complete molar pregnancy and 3% to 4% with a partial molar pregnancy will have persistent GTN (70% to 90%) or malignant GTN (10% to 30%) and require chemotherapy.[89-93] Because the histologic pattern does not always correlate with the clinical course and treatment response, the International Federation of Gynecology and Obstetrics (FIGO) updated the staging and risk-factor scoring systems for GTN in March, 2002 (Tables 15-1 and 15-2).[88] The identification of an individual patient's stage and risk-factor score is expressed by assigning a Roman numeral to the stage and an Arabic numeral to the risk-factor score, with the two numbers separated by a colon. Patients with a GTN risk factor score of 6 or less are considered low risk, and patients with a score of 7 or higher are considered high risk. Single-agent chemotherapy is used to treat patients with low-risk GTN, and combination chemotherapy is used for those with high-risk GTN.[91] The rate of cure is nearly 100% for nonmetastatic GTN and 65% to 94% for metastatic GTN.[88,90,91]

GTNs produce hCG in amounts proportional to the neoplastic volume.[94] Beta-hCG is a sensitive tumor marker, and serial measurements allow close follow-up for persistent and malignant disease. Placental site trophoblastic tumors are the exception. They produce little hCG because of their cytotrophoblastic cellular composition. However, some of these tumors produce human placental lactogen (HPL), and in these patients HPL may be used as a tumor marker.[90] Placental site trophoblastic tumors are less sensitive to chemotherapeutic agents, and hysterectomy often is required for treatment.[90]

Diagnosis

There are two types of hydatidiform mole: a complete or classic mole and a partial or incomplete mole. Partial moles often are focal and have associated fetal tissue. Patients with a partial mole usually have a preoperative diagnosis of incomplete or missed abortion. Only 5% of partial moles are diagnosed before evacuation.[95]

Approximately 90% of hydatidiform moles are complete and not associated with fetal tissue.[96] Complete molar pregnancies have a higher rate of associated complications and a higher rate of subsequent malignant GTN than do partial moles.[89-93]

Clinically, patients with a complete mole present with vaginal bleeding after delayed menses,[89,90,94] and they often spontaneously pass hydropic vesicles. The absence of an FHR, a uterus that is large for gestational age, and a markedly elevated concentration of beta-hCG strongly suggest the diagnosis of hydatidiform mole. Ultrasonography shows characteristic multiechogenic regions that represent hydropic villi or hemorrhagic foci.

Excessive uterine size occurs in one third to one half of patients with a complete molar pregnancy and is associated with a higher incidence of complications (Table 15-3).[89-94,97-100] Excessive uterine size is associated with a markedly elevated serum beta-hCG concentration (greater than 100,000 mIU/mL) secondary to an increased volume of the tumor.

Ovarian theca-lutein cysts occur primarily in patients with extremely high serum beta-hCG concentrations (greater than 100,000 mIU/mL).[94] These cysts typically regress over 2 to 3 months; however, torsion, rupture, or infarction may necessitate prompt oophorectomy.

Hyperemesis gravidarum can lead to significant electrolyte disturbances and volume depletion, which should be corrected before surgery.

Pregnancy-induced hypertension (PIH) occurs in 11% to 27% of women with a molar pregnancy. The syndrome of PIH includes hypertension with proteinuria, edema, and/or hyperreflexia. Although convulsions rarely occur in these patients,[94] magnesium sulfate is administered prophylactically. An antihypertensive agent (e.g., hydralazine, labetalol) is administered to reduce blood pressure. Most patients with PIH have an excessively large uterus.[93] Gestational trophoblastic neoplasia should be strongly suspected in any patient who presents with PIH during early pregnancy.

Anemia frequently complicates a complete molar pregnancy. The visible vaginal bleeding may lead to an underestimation of the total amount of hemorrhage. Occult bleeding

TABLE 15-1	INTERNATIONAL FEDERATION OF GYNECOLOGY AND OBSTETRICS (FIGO): STAGING OF GESTATIONAL TROPHOBLASTIC NEOPLASMS[88]

Stage	Description
I	Gestational trophoblastic tumors confined strictly to the uterine corpus
II	Gestational trophoblastic tumors extending to the adnexa or vagina but limited to the genital structures
III	Gestational trophoblastic tumors extending to the lungs, with or without genital tract involvement
IV	All other metastatic sites

TABLE 15-3	COMPLICATIONS OF COMPLETE MOLAR PREGNANCIES

Complication	Incidence (%)
Excessive uterine size	30-53
Ovarian theca-lutein cysts (> 6 cm)	4-50
Hyperemesis gravidarum	14-29
Pregnancy-induced hypertension	11-27
Anemia (hemoglobin < 10 g/dL)	10-54
Hyperthyroidism	1-7
Trophoblastic emboli	2-7
Acute cardiopulmonary distress	6-27
Malignant sequelae (metastasis)	4-36
Other (renal, DIC, infection)	Rare

References 89-94, 97-100.

TABLE 15-2	INTERNATIONAL FEDERATION OF GYNECOLOGY AND OBSTETRICS (FIGO): RISK-FACTOR SCORING FOR GESTATIONAL TROPHOBLASTIC NEOPLASMS[88]

Parameter	0	1	2	4
Age (yr)		≤ 39	>39	
Antecedent pregnancy	Hydatidiform mole	Abortion		Term pregnancy
Interval (mo) from index pregnancy	< 4	4-6	7-12	> 12
Pretreatment hCG (mIU/mL)	<10^3	10^3-10^4	10^4-10^5	> 10^5
Largest tumor size, including uterus (cm)		3-4	5	
Sites of metastasis		Spleen, kidney	GI tract	Brain, liver
Number of metastases identified	0	1-4	5-8	>8
Previously failed chemotherapy			1 drug	≥ 2 drugs

The identification of an individual patient's stage and risk-factor score is expressed by assigning a Roman numeral to the stage and an Arabic numeral to the risk score, with the two numbers separated by a colon.

into and around the tumor results in multiple hemorrhagic foci. Because blood loss may occur gradually, the patient may have a normal intravascular volume despite the presence of severe anemia. Transfusion is required in as many as 32% to 45% of patients.[89,92]

Although it occurs infrequently, **hyperthyroidism** may result from a marked elevation of hCG,[101,102] which may have a thyrotropin-like effect. Alternatively, hyperthyroidism may result from some other thyrotropic substance produced by the neoplasm.[103] Anesthesia or surgery can precipitate thyroid storm (e.g., sinus tachycardia, atrial fibrillation, hyperthermia, cardiovascular collapse). A beta-adrenergic antagonist is administered to treat the cardiovascular effects of thyroid storm.

Acute cardiopulmonary distress has been observed after evacuation of a molar pregnancy in as many as 27% of all patients.[94,97-99] An increased risk of cardiopulmonary complications occurs in patients with a uterine size of 16 weeks or greater.[99,100] Signs and symptoms include chest pain, cough, tachycardia, tachypnea, hypoxemia, diffuse rales, and bilateral pulmonary infiltrates on chest radiographic examination. When distress occurs, **trophoblastic embolization** is the proven etiology in more than half of the cases.[98,100] Other causes include (1) high-output cardiac failure from thyrotoxicosis, (2) pulmonary congestion from severe anemia, (3) PIH, (4) aspiration pneumonitis, and (5) iatrogenic fluid overload.[98,100] Symptoms usually develop within 12 hours of uterine evacuation.[98] Some patients require endotracheal intubation, mechanical ventilation, and invasive hemodynamic monitoring.[104] Symptoms usually subside within 72 hours; however, massive embolization[105] or adult respiratory distress syndrome[106] may result in death. If the patient survives trophoblastic embolization, **malignant sequelae** often develop.[90,98,106]

Other complications of GTD include **DIC** and **infection** (sepsis).

Obstetric Management

Thorough evaluation of the patient with GTD includes screening for evidence of metastasis (e.g., vaginal, liver, lung, brain) and other potential complications. Prompt treatment should be instituted. A delay in uterine evacuation may increase the risk of complications.

Once the patient is stabilized, suction curettage is performed to evacuate the uterus in patients who want to preserve fertility. Real-time ultrasonography may aid the obstetrician in performing a complete evacuation of the uterus in patients with excessive uterine size.[107] Hysterectomy is performed in patients who have completed childbearing.

The obstetrician should determine beta-hCG concentrations weekly or biweekly for several months postevacuation to detect persistent trophoblastic disease. Chest radiographic study and other tests may be indicated to screen for evidence of metastasis. Prevention of pregnancy is recommended for 6 to 12 months. Chemotherapy is indicated in patients with (1) histologic evidence of invasive mole or choriocarcinoma, (2) a rise in beta-hCG levels of 10% or greater in three or more samples taken over at least 2 weeks (days 1, 7, and 14), (3) a plateau of beta-hCG levels in four or more samples taken over 3 consecutive weeks (days 1, 7, 14, and 21), (4) persistence of measurable beta-hCG levels 6 months after molar evacuation, or (5) evidence of metastasis.[88] Some patients require a delayed hysterectomy, a thoracotomy for resection of pulmonary metastasis, and/or liver or brain irradiation.

Anesthetic Management

The anesthesiologist should evaluate the patient for specific complications of molar pregnancy, including hyperemesis gravidarum, PIH, anemia, and thyrotoxicosis. The presence of cardiopulmonary distress warrants the use of invasive hemodynamic monitoring before evacuation of the uterus.[90,98,100] Kohorn[100] recommended the preoperative determination of arterial blood gas measurements. If these are normal, a central venous or pulmonary artery catheter is *not* needed unless other conditions (e.g., severe anemia, hemorrhage) exist. If the PaO$_2$ is decreased, the anesthesiologist should consider the placement of an intraarterial catheter and a pulmonary artery catheter. The anesthesiologist also should consider the use of invasive hemodynamic monitoring in patients with PIH, severe anemia, hyperthyroidism, or a uterus of greater than 16 weeks' size.[108]

During evacuation of the uterus, blood loss may be substantial. Thus the anesthesiologist should establish adequate intravenous access (i.e., at least two large-gauge intravenous catheters), and blood should be immediately available.

General anesthesia is preferred because of the potential for rapid, substantial blood loss during evacuation of the uterus (Box 15-4). Thiopental and propofol may cause marked hypotension in hypovolemic patients, and ketamine may result in marked tachycardia in hyperthyroid patients.[109] Thus etomidate is an excellent choice for patients with preoperative bleeding or preoperative evidence of hyperthyroidism. Maintenance of anesthesia should include administration of oxygen, nitrous oxide, a benzodiazepine, and an opioid. It is best to avoid administration of a volatile halogenated agent in most patients with a molar pregnancy.[110]

> **Box 15-4 ANESTHETIC TECHNIQUE FOR PATIENTS WITH A GESTATIONAL TROPHOBLASTIC NEOPLASM**
>
> **PREOPERATIVE EVALUATION**
>
> Examination for complications of molar pregnancy
> Evaluation of baseline arterial blood gas measurements
>
> **GENERAL ANESTHESIA**
>
> Routine noninvasive monitors (ECG, blood pressure cuff, pulse oximeter, stethoscope, temperature probe, nerve stimulator)
> Consideration of invasive hemodynamic monitoring in patients with a decreased PaO$_2$, pregnancy-induced hypertension, severe anemia, hyperthyroidism, or a uterine size greater than 16 weeks' gestation
> Two large-gauge intravenous catheters
> Immediate availability of blood
> Etomidate for induction (avoidance of ketamine if patient is hyperthyroid)
> Muscle relaxant for intubation
> Endotracheal intubation
> End-tidal carbon dioxide monitoring
> Maintenance of anesthesia with oxygen, nitrous oxide and an opioid, with or without a small dose of midazolam; avoidance of volatile halogenated agents to decrease blood loss and the risk of uterine perforation
> Oxytocin infusion (20 units/L) after cervical dilation or after partial uterine evacuation

Spinal anesthesia has been performed for a D and E procedure in a hyperthyroid patient with a hydatidiform mole, but careful attention to blood loss and the ability to rapidly transfuse the patient is essential.[111]

An intravenous oxytocin infusion (20 units/L) is begun either before[94,99] or during[90] uterine evacuation. Oxytocin helps the uterus contract, which facilitates a safe curettage and decreases blood loss. Some obstetricians have speculated that oxytocin may decrease trophoblastic embolization by constricting the uterine veins.[99] Postoperatively, these patients should be monitored closely for any evidence of uterine hemorrhage or cardiopulmonary distress.

HYPEREMESIS GRAVIDARUM

As many as 70% of women experience nausea and vomiting during pregnancy. These symptoms often are worse during the morning hours; ergo the term *morning sickness*. Symptoms typically improve or resolve by the end of the first trimester.

On rare occasions, pregnant women experience a persistent severe form of nausea and vomiting called *hyperemesis gravidarum*. These women develop dehydration, ketonuria, nutritional compromise, weight loss, electrolyte abnormalities, and transient hepatic and renal dysfunction. Parenteral rehydration, correction of electrolyte abnormalities, pharmacologic antiemetic therapy, and, rarely, hyperalimentation are indicated.

Hyperemesis gravidarum may be associated with multiple gestation, thyrotoxicosis, and/or GTD. Other underlying diseases such as hepatitis, cholecystitis, pancreatitis, pyelonephritis, and partial bowel obstruction should be ruled out.[112]

CORPUS LUTEUM CYSTS

Symptomatic corpus luteum cysts occasionally occur during early pregnancy. Typically, they resolve over several weeks. In some cases, hemorrhage or ovarian torsion necessitates ovarian cystectomy or oophorectomy. After the cyst is removed, the fetus usually is not affected, provided that supplemental progesterone is administered until 10 to 12 weeks' gestation.

KEY POINTS

- Aortocaval compression is rare during the first half of pregnancy, except in patients with excessive uterine size (e.g., from hydatidiform mole or multiple gestation).
- General anesthesia may be administered by mask for selected extraabdominal procedures during the first 18 to 20 weeks of pregnancy, provided the patient fulfills the criteria for an empty stomach and there is no difficulty with mask ventilation. Some anesthesiologists prefer to limit the use of mask anesthesia to the first 12 to 14 weeks of pregnancy.
- Pregnant women are more sensitive to both local and general anesthetic agents during early pregnancy.
- Most ectopic pregnancies are located in one of the fallopian tubes. Ruptured tubal pregnancies and interstitial, abdominal, and cervical ectopic pregnancies may result in substantial hemorrhage.

- The most painful part of a D and E procedure is the dilation of the cervix. If the cervix is already dilated, sedation (with or without paracervical block) often will suffice. However, if the cervix is closed, a paracervical block with sedation or spinal, epidural, or general anesthesia often is necessary.
- Regional anesthesia is an excellent choice for the performance of prophylactic cervical cerclage.
- In a patient who requires emergency cervical cerclage, it is important to prevent a marked increase in intraabdominal and intrauterine pressures, which might cause the bulging fetal membranes to rupture.
- Patients with a molar pregnancy may have hyperemesis gravidarum, pregnancy-induced hypertension, severe anemia, and/or hyperthyroidism. These complications are more frequent in patients with excessive uterine size.
- Signs and symptoms of acute cardiopulmonary distress develop after uterine evacuation in as many as 27% of patients with a molar pregnancy.

REFERENCES

1. Elkus R, Popovich J Jr. Respiratory physiology in pregnancy. Clin Chest Med 1992; 13:555-65.
2. Spatling L, Fallenstein F, Huch A, et al. The variability of cardiopulmonary adaptation to pregnancy at rest and during exercise. Br J Obstet Gynaecol 1992; 99 Suppl 8:1-40.
3. Crapo RO. Normal cardiopulmonary physiology during pregnancy. Clin Obstet Gynecol 1996; 39:3-16.
4. van Oppen AC, Stigter RH, Bruinse HW. Cardiac output in normal pregnancy: A critical review. Obstet Gynecol 1996; 87:310-8.
5. Clapp JF III, Capeless E. Cardiovascular function before, during, and after the first and subsequent pregnancies. Am J Cardiol 1997; 80: 1469-73.
6. Marx GF. Aortocaval compression syndrome: Its 50 year history. Int J Obstet Anesth 1992; 1:60-4.
7. Lund CJ, Donovan JC. Blood volume during pregnancy: Significance of plasma and red cell volumes. Am J Obstet Gynecol 1967; 98:393-403.
8. Wyner J, Cohen SE. Gastric volume in early pregnancy: Effect of metoclopramide. Anesthesiology 1982; 57:209-12.
9. Vanner RG. Gastro-oesophageal reflux and regurgitation during general anesthesia for termination of pregnancy. Int J Obstet Anesth 1992; 1:123-8.
10. Butterworth JF IV, Walker FO, Lysak SZ. Pregnancy increases median nerve susceptibility to lidocaine. Anesthesiology 1990; 72:962-5.
11. Chan MTV, Mainland P, Gin T. Minimum alveolar concentration of halothane and enflurane are decreased in early pregnancy. Anesthesiology 1996; 85:782-6.
12. CDC. Ectopic pregnancy – United States, 1988-1989. MMWR 1992; 41:591-4.
13. CDC. Ectopic pregnancy – United States, 1990-1992. MMWR 1995; 44:46-8.
14. Berg CJ, Chang J, Callaghan WM, Whitehead SJ. Pregnancy-related mortality in the United States, 1991-1997. Obstet Gynecol 2003; 101:289-96.
15. Carson SA, Buster JE. Ectopic pregnancy. N Eng J Med 1993; 329: 1174-81.
16. Pisarska MD, Carson SA. Incidence and risk factors for ectopic pregnancy. Clin Obstet Gynecol 1999; 42:2-8.
17. Marchbanks PA, Annegers JF, Coulam CB, et al. Risk factors for ectopic pregnancy: A population-based study. JAMA 1988; 259:1823-7.
18. Weckstein LN. Clinical diagnosis of ectopic pregnancy. Clin Obstet Gynecol 1987; 30:236-46.
19. Marcus SF, Brinsden PR. Analysis of the incidence and risk factors associated with ectopic pregnancy following in-vitro fertilization and embryo transfer. Hum Reprod 1995; 10:199-203.
20. Green LK, Kott M. Ectopic pregnancy: Clinical and pathological review of 150 cases. Tex Med 1988; 84:30-5.

21. DeCherney AH, Seifer DB. Ectopic pregnancy. In Gabbe SG, Niebyl JR, Simpson JL, editors. Obstetrics: Normal and Problem Pregnancies, 2nd ed. New York, Churchill Livingstone, 1991:811.

22. Breen JL. A 21-year study of 654 ectopic pregnancies. Am J Obstet Gynecol 1970; 106:1004-19.

23. Brenner PF, Roy S, Mishell Jr DR. Ectopic pregnancy: A study of 300 consecutive surgically treated cases. JAMA 1980; 243:673-6.

24. Stovall TG, Ling FW, Carson SA, Buster JE. Serum progesterone and uterine curettage in differential diagnosis of ectopic pregnancy. Fertil Steril 1992; 57:456-8.

25. Stovall TG, Ling FW, Cope BJ, Buster JE. Preventing ruptured ectopic pregnancy with a single serum progesterone. Am J Obstet Gynecol 1989; 160:1425-31.

26. Kadar N, Caldwell BV, Romero R. A method of screening for ectopic pregnancy and its indications. Obstet Gynecol 1981; 58:162-6.

27. van Dam PA, Vanderheyden JS, Uyttenbroeck F. Application of ultrasound in the diagnosis of heterotopic pregnancy. A review of the literature. J Clin Ultrasound 1988; 16:159-65.

28. Fossum GT, Davajan V, Kletzky OA. Early detection of pregnancy with transvaginal ultrasound. Fertil Steril 1988; 49:788-91.

29. Shalev E, Peleg D, Tsabari A, et al. Spontaneous resolution of ectopic tubal pregnancy: Natural history. Fert Steril 1995; 63:15-9.

30. American College of Obstetricians and Gynecologists. Medical management of tubal pregnancy. ACOG Practice Bulletin No.3, December 1998.

31. Pouly JL, Mahnes H, Mage G, et al. Conservative laparoscopic treatment of 321 ectopic pregnancies. Fertil Steril 1986; 46:1093-7.

32. Seifer DB, Gutmann JN, Grant WD, et al. Comparison of persistent ectopic pregnancy after laparoscopic salpingostomy versus salpingostomy at laparotomy for ectopic pregnancy. Obstet Gynecol 1993; 81:378-82.

33. Meyerovitz MF, Lobel SM, Harrington DP, Bengtson JM. Preoperative uterine artery embolization in cervical pregnancy. J Vasc Intervent Rad 1991; 2:95-7.

34. Atrash HK, Friede A, Hogue CJR. Abdominal pregnancy in the United States: Frequency and maternal mortality. Obstet Gynecol 1987; 69: 333-7.

35. Stevens CA. Malformations and deformations in abdominal pregnancy. Am J Med Genet 1993, 47:1189-95.

36. Costa SD, Presley J, Bastert G. Advanced abdominal pregnancy. Obstet Gynecol Surv 1991; 46:515-25.

37. Bello GV, Schonholz D, Moshirpur J, et al. Combined pregnancy: The Mount Sinai experience. Obstet Gynecol Surv 1986; 41:603-13.

38. Reece EA, Petrie RH, Sirmans MF, et al. Combined intrauterine and extrauterine gestations: A review. Am J Obstet Gynecol 1983; 146: 323-30.

39. Lund PR, Sielaff GW, Aiman EJ. In vitro fertilization patient presenting in hemorrhagic shock caused by unsuspected heterotopic pregnancy. Am J Emerg Med 1989; 7:49-53.

40. Lewin A, Simon A, Rabinowitz R, Schenker JG. Second-trimester heterotopic pregnancy after in vitro fertilization and embryo transfer: A case report and review of the literature. Int J Fertil 1991; 36:227-30.

41. Fernandez H, Lelaidier C, Doumerc S, et al. Nonsurgical treatment of heterotopic pregnancy: A report of six cases. Fertil Steril 1993; 60: 428-32.

42. Goldman GA, Fisch B, Ovadia J, Tadir Y. Heterotopic pregnancy after assisted reproductive technologies. Obstet Gynecol Surv 1992; 47:217-21.

43. Chantigian RC, Chantigian PDM. Anesthesia for laparoscopy. In Corfman RS, Diamond MP, DeCherney A, editors. Complications of Laparoscopy and Hysteroscopy, 2nd ed. Boston, Blackwell Scientific Publications, 1997:5-13.

44. Silva PD, Beguin EA, Jr. Intraoperative rapid autologous blood transfusion. Am J Obstet Gynecol 1987; 160:1226-7.

45. Merrill BS, Mitts DL, Rogers W, Weinberg PC. Autotransfusion: Intraoperative use in ruptured ectopic pregnancy. J Reprod Med 1980; 24:14-6.

46. CDC. Abortion Surveillance – United States, 1999. MMWR 2002; 51: 1-28.

47. Hutchon DJR. Understanding miscarriage or insensitive abortion: Time for more defined terminology? Am J Obstet Gynecol 1998; 179:397-8.

48. Wilcox AJ, Weinberg CR, O'Connor JF, et al. Incidence of early loss of pregnancy. N Engl J Med 1988; 319:189-94.

49. Simpson JL. Fetal wastage. In Gabbe SG, Niebyl JR, Simpson JL, editors. Obstetrics: Normal and Problem Pregnancies, 4th ed. New York, Churchill Livingstone, 2002:729-53.

50. Simpson JL, Mills JL, Holmes LB, et al. Low fetal loss rates after ultrasound-proved viability in early pregnancy. JAMA 1987; 258:2555-7.

51. Strom CM, Ginsberg N, Applebaum M, et al. Analyses of 95 first-trimester spontaneous abortions by chorionic villus sampling and karyotype. J Assist Reprod Genetics 1992; 9:458-61.

52. Boué J, Boué A, Lazar P. Retrospective and prospective epidemiological studies of 1500 karyotyped spontaneous human abortions. Teratology 1975; 12:11-26.

53. McNeeley SG Jr. Early abortion. In Sciarra JJ, Dilts PV Jr, editors. Gynecology and Obstetrics, vol 2. Philadelphia, JB Lippincott, 1992; 23:1-6.

54. American Society of Anesthesiologists. Occupational disease among operating room personnel: A national study. Anesthesiology 1974; 41:321-40.

55. Tannenbaum TN, Goldberg RJ. Exposure to anesthetic gases and reproductive outcome: A review of the epidemiologic literature. J Occup Med 1985; 27:659-68.

56. Ericson HA, Kallen AJB. Hospitalization for miscarriage and delivery outcome among Swedish nurses working in operating rooms 1973-1978. Anesth Analg 1985; 64:981-8.

57. Hemminki K, Kyyronen P, Lindbohm M-L. Spontaneous abortions and malformations in the offspring of nurses exposed to anaesthetic gases, cytostatic drugs, and other potential hazards in hospitals, based on registered information of outcome. J Epidemiol Community Health 1985; 39:141-7.

58. Stabile I. Spontaneous abortion: A clinical perspective. Female Patient 1992; 17:14-30.

59. Stubblefield PG. Pregnancy termination. In Gabbe SG, Niebyl JR, Simpson JL, editors. Obstetrics: Normal and Problem Pregnancies, 3rd ed. New York, Churchill Livingstone, 1996:1249-78.

60. Grimes DA, Cates W Jr, Selik RM. Fatal septic abortion in the United States, 1975-1977. Obstet Gynecol 1981; 57:739-44.

61. von Stein GA, Munsick RA, Stiver K, Ryder K. Fetomaternal hemorrhage in threatened abortion. Obstet Gynecol 1992; 79:383-6.

62. Neugebauer R, Kline J, Strout P, et al. Major depressive disorder in the 6 months after miscarriage. JAMA 1997; 227:383-8.

63. Oats JN, Vasey DP, Waldron BA. Effects of ketamine on the pregnant uterus. Brit J Anaesth 1979; 51:1163-6.

64. Munson ES, Embro WJ. Enflurane, isoflurane, and halothane and isolated human uterine muscle. Anesthesiology 1977; 46:11-4.

65. Cullen BF, Margolis AJ, Eger EI II. The effects of anesthesia and pulmonary ventilation on blood loss during elective therapeutic abortion. Anesthesiology 1970; 32:108-13.

66. Dolan WM, Eger EI II, Margolis AJ. Forane increases bleeding in therapeutic suction abortion. Anesthesiology 1972; 36:96-7.

67. Hall JE, Ng WS, Smith S. Blood loss during first trimester termination of pregnancy: Comparison of two anaesthesic techniques. Br J Anaesth 1997; 78:172-4.

68. Kumarasinghe N, Harpin R, Stewart AW. Blood loss during suction termination of pregnancy with two different anesthetic techniques. Anaesth Intens Care 1997; 25:48-50.

69. Novy MJ. Managing reproductive failure by transabdominal isthmic cerclage. Contemp Obstet Gynecol 1977; 10:17-25.

70. Harger JH. Comparison of success and morbidity in cervical cerclage procedures. Obstet Gynecol 1980; 56:543-8.

71. Magrina JF, Kempers RD, Williams TJ. Cervical cerclage: 20 years' experience at the Mayo Clinic. Minnesota Med 1983; 66:599-602.

72. Barford DAG, Rosen MG. Cervical incompetence: Diagnosis and outcome. Obstet Gynecol 1984; 64:159-63.

73. Golan A, Barnan R, Wexler S, et al. Incompetence of the uterine cervix. Obstet Gynecol Surv 1989; 44:96-107.

74. McDonald IA. Incompetent cervix as a cause of recurrent abortion. J Obstet Gynaecol Br Commonw 1963; 70:105-9.

75. Maier DB, Hammond CB. Hysterosalpingography and hysteroscopy. Postgrad Obstet Gynecol 1984; 4:1-8.

76. American College of Obstetricians and Gynecologists. Cervical cerclage, prophylactic. ACOG Criteria Set, No. 17, October 1996.

77. McDonald IA. Suture of the cervix for inevitable miscarriage. J Obstet Gynaecol Br Commonw 1957; 64:346-50.

78. Andrews WW, Cooper R, Hauth JC, et al. Second-trimester cervical ultrasound: Associations with increased risk for recurrent early spontaneous delivery. Obstet Gynecol 2000; 95:222-6.

79. Maldjian C, Adam R, Pelosi M, Pelosi M III. MRI appearance of cervical incompetence in a pregnant patient. Magnetic Resonance Imaging 1999; 17:1399-402.

80. Craig S, Fliegner JRH. Treatment of cervical incompetence by transabdominal cervicoisthmic cerclage. Aust NZ J Obstet Gynaecol 1997; 37:407-11.

81. Shirodkar VN. A new method of operative treatment for habitual abortions in the second trimester of pregnancy. Antiseptic 1955; 52:229-30.

82. Iams JD. Preterm birth. In Gabbe SG, Niebyl JR, Simpson JL, editors. Obstetrics: Normal and Problem Pregnancies, 4th ed. New York, Churchill Livingstone, 2002:803.

83. Treadwell MC, Bronsteen RA, Bottoms SF. Prognostic factors and complication rates for cervical cerclage: A review of 482 cases. Am J Obstet Gynecol 1991; 165:555-8.

84. Zaveri V, Aghajafari F, Amankwah K, Hannah M. Abdominal versus vaginal cerclage after a failed transvaginal cerclage: A systematic review. Am J Obstet Gynecol 2002; 187:868-72.

85. McCulloch B, Bergen S, Pielet B, et al. McDonald cerclage under pudendal nerve block. Am J Obstet Gynecol 1993; 168:499-502.

86. Brownridge P. Spinal anaesthesia revised: An evaluation of subarachnoid block in obstetrics. Anaesth Intens Care 1984; 12:334-42.

87. Crawford JS, Lewis M. Nitrous oxide in early human pregnancy. Anaesthesia 1986; 41:900-5.

88. Kohorn EI. Negotiating a staging and risk factor scoring system for gestational trophoblastic neoplasia: A progress report. J Reprod Med 2002; 47:445-50.

89. Beischer NA, Bettinger HF, Fortune DW, Pepperell R. Hydatidiform mole and its complications in the state of Victoria. J Obstet Gynaecol Br Commonw 1970; 77:263-76.

90. Soper JT, Lewis JL Jr, Hammond CB. Gestational trophoblastic disease. In Hoskins WJ, Perez CA, Young RC, editors. Principles and Practice of Gynecologic Oncology, 2nd ed. Philadelphia, Lippincott-Raven Publishers, 1997:1039-77.

91. Kohorn EI. Gestational trophoblastic neoplasia and evidence-based medicine. J Reprod Med 2002; 47:427-32.

92. Schlaerth JB, Morrow CP, Montz FJ, d'Ablaing G. Initial management of hydatidiform mole. Am J Obstet Gynecol 1988; 158:1299-1306.

93. Curry SL, Hammond CB, Tyrey L, et al. Hydatidiform mole: Diagnosis, management, and long-term followup of 347 patients. Obstet Gynecol 1975; 45:1-8.

94. Berkowitz RS, Goldstein DP. Diagnosis and management of the primary hydatidiform mole. Obstet Gynecol Clin North Am 1988; 15:491-503.

95. Szulman AE, Surti U. The clinicopathologic profile of the partial hydatidiform mole. Obstet Gynecol 1982; 59:597-602.

96. Jones WB, Lauersen NH. Hydatidiform mole with coexistent fetus. Am J Obstet Gynecol 1975; 122:267-72.

97. Hammond CB: Diagnosis and management of hydatiform mole. Postgrad Obstet Gynecol 1982; 2:1-6.

98. Twiggs LB, Morrow CP, Schlaerth JB. Acute pulmonary complications of molar pregnancy. Am J Obstet Gynecol 1979; 135:189-94.

99. Cotton DB, Bernstein SG, Read JA, et al. Hemodynamic observations in evacuation of molar pregnancy. Am J Obstet Gynecol 1980; 138:6-10.

100. Kohorn EI. Clinical management and the neoplastic sequelae of trophoblastic embolization associated with hydatidiform mole. Obstet Gynecol Surv 1987; 42:484-8.

101. Kenimer JG, Hershman JM, Higgins HP. The thyrotropin in hydatidiform moles is human chorionic gonadotropin. J Clin Endocrinol Metab 1975; 40:482-91.

102. Higgins HP, Hershman JM, Kenimer JG, et al. The thyrotoxicosis of hydatidiform mole. Ann Intern Med 1975; 83:307-11.

103. Amir SM, Osathanondh R, Berkowitz RS, Goldstein DP. Human chorionic gonadotropin and thyroid function in patients with hydatidiform mole. Am J Obstet Gynecol 1984; 150:723-8.

104. Natonson R, Shapiro BA, Harrison RA, Stanhope RC. Massive trophoblastic embolization and PEEP therapy. Anesthesiology 1979; 51:469-71.

105. Lipp RG, Kindschi JD, Schmitz R. Death from pulmonary embolism associated with hydatidiform mole. Am J Obstet Gynecol 1962; 83:1644-7.

106. Orr JW Jr, Austin JM, Hatch KD, et al. Acute pulmonary edema associated with molar pregnancies: A high-risk factor for development of persistent trophoblastic disease. Am J Obstet Gynecol 1980; 136:412-4.

107. Evers JLH, Schijf CPT, Kenemans P, Martin CB Jr. Real-time ultrasound as an adjunct in the operative management of hydatidiform mole. Am J Obstet Gynecol 1981; 140:469-71.

108. Kim JM, Arakawa K, McCann V. Severe hyperthyroidism associated with hydatidiform mole. Anesthesiology 1976; 44:445-8.

109. Kaplan JA, Cooperman LH. Alarming reactions to ketamine in patients taking thyroid medication: Treatment with propranolol. Anesthesiology 1971; 35:229-30.

110. Ackerman WE III. Anesthetic considerations for complicated hydatidiform molar pregnancies. Anesth Rev 1984; 11:20-4.

111. Solak M, Aktürk G. Spinal anesthesia in a patient with hyperthyroidism due to hydatidiform mole. Anesth Analg 1993; 77:851-2.

112. Cruikshank DP, Wigton TR, Hays PM. Maternal physiology in pregnancy. In Gabbe SG, Niebyl JR, Simpson JL, editors. Obstetrics: Normal and Problem Pregnancies, 3rd ed. New York, Churchill Livingstone, 1996:91-109.

Chapter 16
Nonobstetric Surgery During Pregnancy
Norah N. Naughton, M.D. · Sheila E. Cohen, M.B., Ch.B., FRCA

Estimates of the frequency of nonobstetric surgery performed during pregnancy range from 0.75% to 2%.[1,2] Thus, in the United States, as many as 75,000 pregnant women may undergo anesthesia and surgery each year. These figures most likely are an underestimate, because pregnancy may be unrecognized at the time of operation. In two recent studies, 0.3% of 2056 female outpatients[3] and 1.2% of 412 adolescents[4] had positive pregnancy tests when they presented for surgery. Despite such data, universal pregnancy testing generally has not been recommended.[5,6] If a patient's history suggests that she may be pregnant, specific questions regarding the possibility of pregnancy should precede pregnancy testing.

Surgery may be necessary during any stage of pregnancy. Among 5405 Swedish women who had operations during pregnancy, 42% occurred during the first trimester, 35% during the second trimester, and 23% during the third trimester.[1] Laparoscopy was the most common first-trimester procedure (34% of 2252 operations), whereas appendectomy was the most frequent procedure during the remainder of pregnancy. Moreover, surgery often is performed for cervical incompetence, complications of ovarian cysts, trauma, gallbladder disease, bowel obstruction, and removal of breast tumors or other malignancies. Major surgery occasionally is necessary to alleviate life-threatening maternal cardiac or neurosurgical conditions.

Pregnancy-induced maternal changes pose hazards for the mother and fetus during surgery. Additional risks for the fetus include the following: (1) the effects of the disease process itself or of related therapy; (2) the possible teratogenicity of anesthetic agents; (3) intraoperative perturbations of uteroplacental perfusion and/or fetal oxygenation; and (4) the risk of abortion or preterm delivery. Although immediate delivery of the fetus usually is not planned, depressant effects of anesthetic drugs on the fetal central nervous system (CNS) or cardiovascular system may assume importance when high doses of these agents are administered during long procedures. (Anesthesia for fetal surgery involves special considerations and is discussed in detail in Chapter 7.)

MATERNAL SAFETY: ALTERED MATERNAL PHYSIOLOGY

During pregnancy, profound changes in maternal physiology result from increased concentrations of various hormones, mechanical effects of the gravid uterus, increased metabolic demand, and the hemodynamic consequences of the low-pressure placental circulation.[7,8] Hormonal changes most likely are responsible for most of the changes that occur during the first trimester. Mechanical effects become apparent when the uterus emerges from the pelvis, which occurs during the second half of gestation (see Chapter 2).

Respiratory System and Acid-Base Balance Changes

Alveolar ventilation increases 25% by the fourth month of gestation and 45% to 70% by term. This results in a chronic respiratory alkalosis, with a $PaCO_2$ of 28 to 32 mm Hg, a slightly alkaline pH (e.g., approximately 7.44), and decreased levels of bicarbonate and buffer base. Although oxygen consumption increases during gestation, PaO_2 usually increases slightly or remains within the normal range. Functional residual capacity (FRC) decreases by approximately 20% as the uterus expands, which results in decreased oxygen reserve and the potential for airway closure. When FRC is decreased further (e.g., from morbid obesity; perioperative intraabdominal distention; placement of the patient in the supine, Trendelenburg, or lithotomy positions), airway closure may be sufficient to cause hypoxemia.

Weight gain during pregnancy and capillary engorgement of the respiratory tract mucosa lead to more frequent problems with mask ventilation and endotracheal intubation. Failed intubation (which is the leading cause of maternal death from anesthesia) is as much a risk during nonobstetric surgery as it is during cesarean section.

Decreased FRC, increased oxygen consumption, and diminished buffering capacity result in the rapid development of hypoxemia and acidosis during periods of hypoventilation or apnea. Moreover, induction of general anesthesia occurs more rapidly during pregnancy, because alveolar hyperventilation and a decreased FRC allow faster equilibration of inhaled agents. An additional factor that accelerates the induction of anesthesia is the approximately 30% decrease in the minimum alveolar concentration (MAC) for volatile anesthetic agents that occurs even during early gestation.[9,10] The anesthesiologist must be especially vigilant when administering subanesthetic concentrations of analgesic and anesthetic agents to the parturient; unconsciousness can occur quickly and unexpectedly.

Cardiovascular System Changes

Cardiac output increases by 30% to 50% during pregnancy because of increases in heart rate and stroke volume; both systemic and pulmonary vascular resistance decrease. Serial measurements of cardiac output demonstrate striking alterations, even during the first trimester. By eight weeks' gestation, 57% of the increase in cardiac output, 78% of the increase in stroke volume, and 90% of the decrease in systemic vascular resistance that typically are achieved by 24 weeks' gestation have occurred (Figure 16-1).[11]

During the second half of gestation, the weight of the uterus compresses the inferior vena cava when the mother lies supine; this decreases venous return and cardiac output by approximately 25% to 30%. Although upper extremity blood pressure may be maintained by compensatory vasoconstriction and tachycardia, uteroplacental perfusion is jeopardized whenever the mother lies supine. Frank hypotension also can occur in the supine parturient, especially when regional or general anesthesia attenuates or abolishes normal compensatory mechanisms. For these reasons, it is essential to displace the uterus laterally during any operation performed after the twentieth week of pregnancy. Vena caval compression also results in distention of the epidural venous plexus, which increases the likelihood of intravascular injection of local anesthetic during the administration of epidural anesthesia. The decreased capacity of the epidural space most likely contributes to the enhanced spread of small doses of epidural local anesthetic that occurs during pregnancy.

Changes in Blood Volume and Blood Constituents

Blood volume expands in the first trimester and increases 30% to 45% by term. A smaller increase in red blood cell volume than in plasma volume results in a dilutional anemia. Although moderate blood loss is well tolerated during pregnancy, preexisting anemia decreases the patient's reserve when significant hemorrhage occurs. Pregnancy is associated with a benign leukocytosis, which makes the white blood cell count an unreliable indicator of infection. In general, pregnancy induces a hypercoagulable state, with increases in fibrinogen; factors VII, VIII, X, and XII; and fibrin degradation products. Pregnancy is associated with enhanced platelet turnover, clotting, and fibrinolysis, and there is a wide range in the normal platelet count; thus pregnancy represents a state of accelerated but compensated intravascular coagulation.[12] During the postoperative period, pregnant surgical patients are at high risk for thromboembolic complications.

Gastrointestinal System Changes

Incompetence of the lower esophageal sphincter and distortion of gastric and pyloric anatomy result in an increased risk of esophageal reflux; thus the pregnant woman is at risk for the regurgitation of gastric contents and aspiration pneumonitis. It is unclear at what stage during pregnancy this risk becomes significant. Although lower esophageal sphincter tone is impaired early in pregnancy (especially in patients with heartburn), the mechanically induced factors do not become relevant until later in pregnancy. It seems prudent to consider any pregnant patient at risk for aspiration after 18 to 20 weeks' gestation.

Altered Responses to Anesthesia

In addition to the decrease in MAC for inhaled anesthetic agents, thiopental requirements begin to decrease early in pregnancy.[13] In addition, more extensive neural blockade is obtained with epidural and spinal anesthesia in pregnant patients. Pregnancy also enhances the response to peripheral neural blockade.

Plasma cholinesterase levels decrease by approximately 25% from early in pregnancy until the seventh postpartum day. Fortunately, prolonged neuromuscular blockade with succinylcholine is uncommon, because the larger volume available for drug distribution offsets the impact of decreased drug hydrolysis.[14] Nevertheless, the dose of succinylcholine should be controlled carefully in the pregnant patient, and the anesthesiologist should monitor neuromuscular blockade with a nerve stimulator to ensure adequate reversal before extubation.

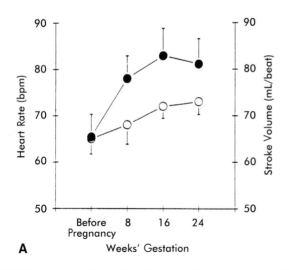

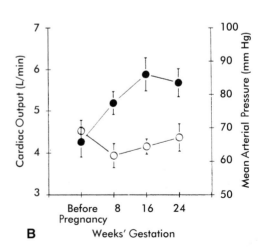

FIGURE 16-1. **A,** **Stroke volume (•) and heart rate** (○) components of cardiac output at four intervals during early pregnancy. **B,** Cardiac output (•) and mean arterial pressure (○) components of systemic vascular resistance at the same four intervals. (From Capeless EL, Clapp JF. Cardiovascular changes in early phase of pregnancy. Am J Obstet Gynecol 1989; 161:1449.)

Decreased protein binding associated with low albumin concentrations during pregnancy may result in a greater fraction of unbound drug, with the potential for greater drug toxicity during pregnancy. Pregnant surgical patients may also require drugs that are used infrequently in this population and about which little is known. Cautious administration of such agents is advisable, because their pharmacokinetic and pharmacodynamic profiles may differ from those in nonpregnant patients.

FETAL CONSIDERATIONS

Risk of Teratogenicity

Although maternal catastrophes that cause severe maternal hypoxia or hypotension pose the greatest risk to the fetus, considerable attention has focused on the role of anesthetic agents as abortifacients and teratogens. *Teratogenicity* has been defined as any significant postnatal change in function or form in an offspring after prenatal treatment. Concern about the potential harmful effects of anesthetic agents stems from their known effects on mammalian cells. These occur at clinical concentrations and include reversible decreases in cell motility, prolongation of DNA synthesis, and inhibition of cell division.[15-17] Despite these theoretical concerns, no data specifically link any of these cellular events with teratogenic changes. Unfortunately, prospective clinical studies of the teratogenic effects of anesthetic agents are impractical. To identify a teratogen that doubled the incidence of a congenital defect (e.g., anencephaly) with an incidence of 1 per 1000, 23,000 cases would be required in which the mother was exposed to the agent during the first trimester.[18] Therefore, investigations of anesthetic agents have followed three directions: (1) studies of the reproductive effects of anesthetic agents in small animals; (2) epidemiologic surveys of operating room personnel chronically exposed to subanesthetic concentrations of inhalation agents; and (3) studies of pregnancy outcome in women who have undergone surgery while pregnant.

PRINCIPLES OF TERATOGENICITY

A number of important factors influence the teratogenic potential of a substance, including species susceptibility, dose of the substance, duration and timing of exposure, and genetic predisposition. Like other toxicologic phenomena, the effects of teratogens are dose dependent (Figure 16-2).[19] Most teratologists accept the principle that any agent can be teratogenic in an animal provided enough is given at the right time. Thus, the finding of teratogenesis after either administration of a high dose or chronic administration of a low dose of an agent does not imply that a single, short exposure (e.g., during anesthesia) would incur similar risk. The interaction between dose and timing also is critical. A small dose of a teratogen may cause malformations or death in the susceptible early embryo, whereas much larger doses may prove harmless to the fetus,[19,20] as was shown with thalidomide. Most studies have used small animals (e.g., chick embryos, mice, rats), and their results cannot necessarily be extrapolated to other species, especially humans. Of the more than 2200 agents listed in Shepard's *Catalog of Teratogenic Agents*,[21] approximately 1200 are teratogenic in animals, but only about 30 of these are known to cause defects in humans.

Manifestations of teratogenicity include death, structural abnormality, growth restriction, and functional deficiency.[19] Depending on when it occurs, death is referred to as abortion, fetal death, or stillbirth in humans and fetal resorption in animals. Structural abnormalities can lead to death if they are severe, although death may occur in the absence of congenital anomalies. Growth restriction currently is considered a manifestation of teratogenesis and may relate to multiple factors, including placental insufficiency and genetic and environmental factors.[22] Functional deficiencies include a number of behavioral and learning abnormalities, the study of which is called *behavioral teratology*. The stage of gestation at which exposure occurs determines the target organs or tissues, the types of defects, and the severity of damage. Most structural abnormalities result from exposure during the period of organogenesis, which extends from approximately day 31 to day 71 after the first day of the last menstrual period. Figure 16-3 shows the critical stages of development and the related susceptibility of different organs to teratogens. Functional deficiencies are usually associated with exposure during late pregnancy or even after birth, because the CNS continues to mature during this period.

Consideration of the possible teratogenicity of anesthetic agents must be viewed against the naturally high occurrence of adverse pregnancy outcomes. Roberts and Lowe[23] estimated that as many as 80% of human conceptions ultimately are lost; many are lost even before pregnancy is recognized. Chromosomal abnormalities are present in half of these early abortions.[24] The incidence of congenital anomalies among humans is approximately 3%, and most of these are unexplained. Indeed, exposure to drugs and environmental toxins accounts for only 2% to 3% of such defects (Table 16-1).[19]

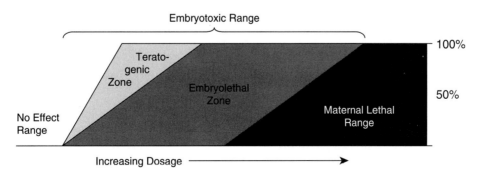

FIGURE 16-2. Toxic manifestations with increasing dosage of a teratogen. A no-effect range of dosage occurs below the threshold at which embryotoxic effects abruptly appear. Teratogenesis and embryolethality often have similar thresholds and may increase at roughly parallel rates as dosage increases to a point at which all conceptuses are affected. Increasing dosage causes increased embryolethality, but teratogenicity appears to decrease, because many defective embryos die before term. A further increase in dosage reaches the maternal lethal range. (From Wilson JG. Environment and Birth Defects. New York, Academic Press, 1973:31.)

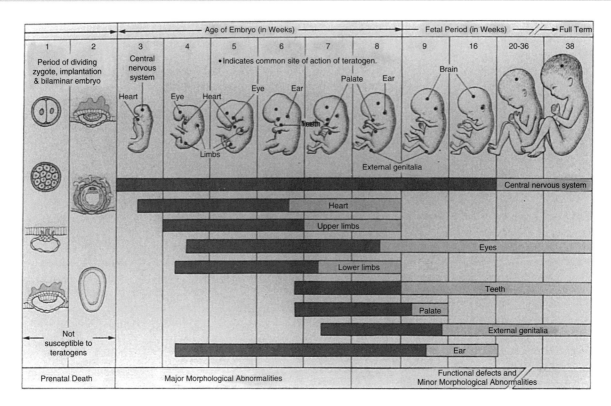

FIGURE 16-3. Critical periods in human development. During the first 2 weeks of development, the embryo typically is not susceptible to teratogens. During these predifferentiation stages, a substance either damages all or most cells of the embryo, resulting in its death, or it damages only a few cells, which allows the embryo to recover without developing defects. The dark shaded bars denote highly sensitive periods, whereas light bars indicate periods of lesser sensitivity. The ages refer to the actual ages of the embryo and fetus. *Clinical estimates* of gestational age represent intervals beginning with the first day of the last menstrual period. Because fertilization typically occurs 2 weeks after the first day of the last menstrual period, the reader should add 14 days to the ages shown here to convert to estimated gestational ages that are used clinically. (From Moore KL. The Developing Human. 4th ed. Philadelphia, WB Saunders, 1993:156.)

TABLE 16-1	ETIOLOGY OF HUMAN DEVELOPMENTAL ABNORMALITIES	
Causes of Developmental Defects in Humans		**Percent**
Genetic transmission		20
Chromosomal aberration		3-5
Environmental causes		
Radiation		<1
Infection		2-3
Maternal metabolic imbalance		1-2
Drugs and environmental chemicals		2-3
Unknown		65-70
TOTAL		100

Modified from Wilson JG. Environmental and Birth Defects. New York, Academic Press, 1973:49.

Shepard[21] has listed several criteria for determining that an agent is a human teratogen, including the following: (1) proven exposure to the agent at the critical time of development; (2) consistent findings in two or more high-quality epidemiologic studies; (3) careful delineation of the clinical cases, ideally with the identification of a specific defect or syndrome; and (4) an association that "makes biological sense." Documentation of teratogenicity in experimental animals is important but not essential. The list of agents or factors that are proven human teratogens does not include anesthetic agents (which are listed as "unlikely teratogens") or any drug routinely used during the course of anesthesia (Box 16-1).

NONDRUG FACTORS ENCOUNTERED IN THE PERIOPERATIVE PERIOD

Anesthesia and surgery can cause derangements of maternal physiology, which may result in hypoxia, hypercapnia, stress, and abnormalities of temperature and carbohydrate metabolism. These states may be teratogenic themselves, or they may enhance the teratogenicity of other agents.[21,25-28] Severe hypoglycemia and prolonged hypoxia and hypercarbia have caused congenital anomalies in laboratory animals,[21,25,26] but evidence is lacking to support teratogenicity after brief episodes in humans. The chronic hypoxemia experienced by mothers at high altitudes results in the delivery of infants with lower birth weights but with no increase in congenital defects.[21] Maternal stress and anxiety are teratogenic in animals[27] and have been implicated in clinical case reports[29]; however, their significance as human teratogens remains questionable, because supporting epidemiologic studies are lacking. Hypothermia is not teratogenic, whereas hyperthermia is both an animal and a human teratogen.[21] Congenital anomalies, especially involving the CNS, repeatedly have been associated with maternal fever (i.e., more than 38.9 ° C) during the first half of pregnancy. Ionizing radiation is also a known human teratogen; dose-related effects on reproduction range from an increased risk of childhood cancer in the offspring of exposed mothers to congenital anomalies or fetal death.[21,30,31] Animal and human data suggest that no increase in major anomalies or growth restriction results from exposures below 5 to 10 rads.[30,31] Fetal exposure from a chest radiograph is estimated to be 8 millirads and that from a barium enema 800 millirads.

Box 16-1   TERATOGENIC AGENTS IN HUMAN BEINGS

RADIATION

Atomic weapons, radioiodine, therapeutic uses

INFECTIONS

Cytomegalovirus, herpes virus hominis, parvovirus B-19, rubella virus, syphilis, toxoplasmosis, Venezualan equine encephalitis virus

MATERNAL METABOLIC IMBALANCE

Alcoholism, cretinism, diabetes, folic acid deficiency, hyperthermia, phenylketonuria, rheumatic disease and congenital heart block, virilizing tumors

DRUGS AND CHEMICALS

Aminopterin and methylaminopterin, androgenic hormones, busulphan, captopril, chlorobiphenyls, cocaine, coumarin anticoagulants, cyclophosphamide, diethylstilbestrol, diphenylhydantoin, enalapril, etretinate, iodides (goiter), lithium, mercury (organic), methimazole (scalp defects), penicillamine, 13-*cis*-retinoic acid (Accutane), tetracyclines, thalidomide, trimethadione, valproic acid

---

Modified from Shepard TH. Catalog of Teratogenic Agents. 7th ed. Baltimore, Johns Hopkins University Press, 1992.

SYSTEMIC AGENTS

Animal Studies

Early studies documented teratogenicity after a variety of neurotropic agents (e.g., opioids, tricyclic antidepressants, phenothiazines, benzodiazepines, butyrophenones) were administered in high doses to rodents.[32-36] The fetuses exhibited a characteristic group of CNS malformations as well as skeletal abnormalities and growth restriction. In one study, fetal abnormalities were dose related with diamorphine, methadone, pentazocine, phenazocine, and propoxyphene, whereas no further increase in anomalies occurred above a certain dose level with morphine, hydromorphone, and meperidine.[32] Whether these investigations really reflect the teratogenic potential of opioids is questionable, because the respiratory depression and impaired feeding that accompany large bolus injections of opioids may be teratogenic themselves. In a study designed to avoid such problems, Fujinaga and Mazze[37] maintained clinically relevant concentrations of morphine throughout most of pregnancy in rats by means of chronically implanted osmotic mini-pumps. Structural anomalies were not observed at any morphine dose, although fetal growth restriction was present, and mortality was increased among the offspring. Using the same methodology, these investigators found fentanyl, sufentanil, and alfentanil completely devoid of teratogenic effects.[38,39] Additional animal studies have confirmed the absence of teratogenicity with other opioids.[40]

The many tranquilizers and anxiolytics taken by pregnant women have been investigated less systematically than the opioids. Animal studies have demonstrated structural or behavioral teratogenesis after exposure to some of the barbiturate, phenothiazine, and tricyclic antidepressant agents.[41-44] The reader is referred to standard teratology reference sources for animal data related to specific drugs.[21,45,46] The package insert provided by a drug's manufacturer also typically describes unpublished in-house studies related to the drug's reproductive effects.

Human Studies

Teratogenesis has not been associated with the use of any of the commonly used induction agents—including the barbiturates, ketamine, and the benzodiazepines—when they are given in clinical doses during anesthesia.[21,22] Similarly, no evidence supports the teratogenicity of opioids in humans; this is evidenced by no increase in the incidence of congenital anomalies among the offspring of mothers who use morphine or methadone during pregnancy.[21,45,46]

Although human data relating to chronic tranquilizer therapy have raised questions about the possible teratogenicity of some agents, most studies have been retrospective and have suffered from a variety of methodologic flaws. In a review of 19,044 birth records, Milkovich and Van den Berg[47] reported an 11% to 12% incidence of severe birth anomalies when mothers took meprobamate or chlordiazepoxide during pregnancy as compared with rates of 4.6% when they took other anxiolytics and 2.6% when no drugs were taken. Other confounding factors were not controlled, the observed anomalies were unrelated, and the results reached statistical significance only when drug ingestion was confined to the first 6 weeks of pregnancy. By contrast, Hartz et al.[48] found no adverse effects in a follow-up study of 50,282 pregnancies in which 1870 children were exposed to meprobamate or chlordiazepoxide in utero.

Benzodiazepine therapy became controversial after several studies reported an association between maternal diazepam ingestion during the first trimester and infants with cleft palate, with or without cleft lip.[49,50] Safra and Oakley[49] interviewed 278 mothers whose infants had major malformations; they noted that diazepam ingestion was four times more common among mothers of infants with oral clefts than among mothers of infants with other defects. The authors commented that their results, even if confirmed, would predict only a 0.4% risk of cleft lip and a 0.2% risk for cleft palate. Another report described an association between maternal diazepam ingestion and oral clefts in 599 children with this anomaly among a large number of births examined in a Finnish registry study between 1967 and 1971.[50] Subsequently, a number of investigations,[51-53] including one prospective study of 854 women who ingested diazepam during the first trimester,[52] have failed to demonstrate increased risk associated with benzodiazepine therapy. Although the present consensus among teratologists is that diazepam is not a proven human teratogen,[21] it is appropriate to consider the risk/benefit ratio before initiating chronic benzodiazepine therapy during the first trimester. No evidence suggests that a single dose of a benzodiazepine (e.g., midazolam) during the course of anesthesia would prove harmful to the fetus.

LOCAL ANESTHETICS

Procaine, lidocaine, and bupivacaine cause reversible cytotoxic effects in cultures of hamster fibroblasts.[13] However, no evidence supports the morphologic or behavioral teratogenicity associated with lidocaine in rats,[54,55] and no evidence supports teratogenicity associated with any local anesthetic used clinically in humans.[21] Maternal cocaine abuse is associated with adverse reproductive outcomes, including abnormal neonatal behavior and, in some reports, an increased incidence of congenital defects of the genitourinary and gastrointestinal tracts.[21] The greatest risk to the fetus most likely results from the high incidence of placental abruption associated with maternal cocaine use (see Chapter 52).

MUSCLE RELAXANTS

Testing muscle relaxants for teratogenicity using standard in vivo animal studies is complicated by maternal respiratory depression and the need for mechanical ventilation (a complex undertaking in rats or mice), or it requires the administration of very low doses of a drug. Fujinaga et al.[56] avoided this problem by using the whole-embryo rat culture system to investigate the reproductive toxicity of high doses of d-tubocurarine, pancuronium, atracurium, and vecuronium. Although dose-dependent toxicity was manifested by decreased crown-rump length, a decreased number of somite pairs, and morphologic abnormalities, these effects occurred only at maternal concentrations thirty-fold greater than those encountered in clinical practice. These findings are consistent with earlier studies that failed to demonstrate toxicity with smaller doses of muscle relaxants.[57,58] Given that fetal blood concentrations of muscle relaxants are only 10% to 20% of maternal concentrations, these drugs appear to have a wide margin of safety when administered to the mother during organogenesis; whether their administration later in gestation results in adverse effects is uncertain. Prolonged disturbance of normal muscular activity by muscle relaxants has caused axial and limb deformities in the chick but has seldom been seen in other experimental animals. Although one case report described arthrogryposis (i.e., persistent joint flexure) in the infant of a woman with tetanus who received d-tubocurarine for 19 days beginning at 55 days' gestation, the patient also was hypoxic and received multiple other drugs.[59] Many women have received muscle relaxants for several days during late gestation without adverse effect on the neonate.

INHALATION ANESTHETICS

Animal Studies

Volatile Agents. Many studies have shown that, under certain conditions, the volatile halogenated anesthetic agents can produce teratogenic changes in chicks or small rodents. In 1968, Basford and Fink[60] observed skeletal abnormalities but no increase in fetal loss when rats were exposed in utero to 0.8% halothane for 12 hours on days 8 and 9 of pregnancy (i.e., the "critical period" in the 21-day rat gestation). Chronic exposure to subanesthetic concentrations of halothane caused fetal growth restriction in rats but no increase in the incidence of congenital anomalies,[61,62] whereas isoflurane had no adverse effects in similar studies of mice.[63] Reduced maternal food intake or other physiologic disturbances accompanying the halothane experiments were thought to be responsible for the delayed development.

More significant reproductive effects have occurred with greater exposures to anesthetic agents. Fetal skeletal abnormalities or death followed repeated or prolonged maternal exposure of mice to *anesthetic* concentrations of volatile anesthetic agents.[64-66] However, teratogenicity in these studies most likely was caused by the physiologic changes (e.g., profound hypothermia, hypoventilation) associated with anesthesia rather than by the anesthetic agent itself. Moreover, some strains of mice are especially likely to develop anomalies such as cleft palate. In a subsequent study, Mazze et al.[67] exposed rats to 0.75 MAC of halothane, isoflurane, or enflurane or 0.55 MAC of nitrous oxide for 6 hours daily on 3 consecutive days at various stages of pregnancy. The animals remained conscious throughout the study, and normal feeding and sleep patterns were preserved. Under these conditions, no teratogenic effects were associated with any of the

volatile agents. The only positive finding was a threefold increase in fetal resorptions with nitrous oxide. No evidence has suggested reproductive toxicity with either sevoflurane or desflurane in clinical concentrations.

Nitrous Oxide. In contrast with the volatile halogenated agents, nitrous oxide is a weak teratogen in rodents under certain conditions, even when normal homeostasis is maintained. In 1967, Fink et al.[68] found that rats continually exposed to 50% nitrous oxide for as long as 6 days (starting on day 8 of gestation) had an increased incidence of resorption and skeletal abnormalities. Shephard and Fink[69] also found that exposure to 70% nitrous oxide for 24 hours on days 8 or 9 of pregnancy consistently caused teratogenic effects; this finding was confirmed by other investigators.[61,67,70,71] To exclude the possibility that adverse effects were a consequence of the anesthetic state, Lane et al.[72] exposed rats to 70% nitrous oxide or to a similar concentration of xenon (a slightly more potent anesthetic devoid of biochemical effects) for 24 hours on day 9 of gestation. Again, abnormalities occurred only in the nitrous oxide group. With the exception of one study in which extremely prolonged exposure to a low concentration caused some minor effects,[73] at least 50% nitrous oxide has been required to consistently produce anomalies.[71] The threshold exposure time has not been determined accurately, although exposure for at least 24 hours typically has proved necessary.

In vivo and embryo culture studies in rats have confirmed that nitrous oxide produces several adverse reproductive effects, each of which results from exposure at a specific period of susceptibility.[74-77] Fetal resorptions occurred after exposure on days 8 and 11 of gestation, skeletal anomalies after exposure on day 8 or 9, and visceral anomalies (including situs inversus) only when exposure occurred on day 8 (Figure 16-4).[77]

Initially, teratogenicity associated with nitrous oxide was thought to result from its oxidation of vitamin B_{12}, which cannot then function as a coenzyme for methionine synthase.[78] Transmethylation from methyltetrahydrofolate to homocysteine to produce tetrahydrofolate (THF) and methionine is catalyzed by methionine synthase (Figure 16-5). Thus, methionine synthase inhibition could cause a decrease in THF (which could result in reduced DNA synthesis) and decreased methionine levels (which could impair methylation reactions). Nitrous oxide rapidly inactivates methionine synthase in both animals[79] and humans.[80] Prolonged human exposure to nitrous oxide leads to neurologic and hematologic symptoms, the latter probably resulting from decreased DNA synthesis.[78] The hematologic—but not the neurologic—changes are prevented by the administration of folinic acid (5-formyl THF) with the nitrous oxide, with the goal of restoring DNA synthesis.

Considerable evidence indicates that methionine synthase inhibition and a consequent lack of THF are not solely responsible for the teratogenic effects of nitrous oxide. First, maximal inhibition of methionine synthase activity occurs at concentrations of nitrous oxide that are much lower than those required to produce teratogenic effects.[81,82] Second, folinic acid, which bypasses the effect of methionine synthase inhibition on THF formation (Figure 16-5), partially prevents only one of the structural abnormalities (i.e., minor skeletal defects) produced by nitrous oxide.[83,84] Third, the administration of isoflurane or halothane with nitrous oxide prevents almost all of the teratogenic effects but does not prevent the decrease in methionine synthase activity.[84,85] Fourth, studies using an in vitro rat whole embryo culture system have shown

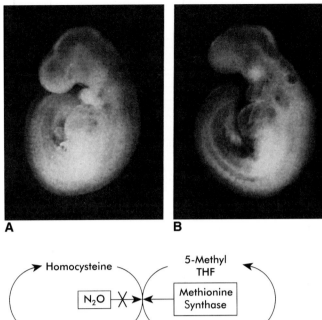

A   B   C

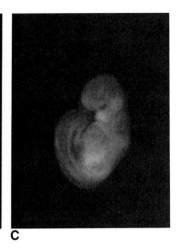

FIGURE 16-4. Effects of nitrous oxide on day 9 rat embryos grown in culture. **A,** Normal day 11 embryo. **B,** Day 11 embryo treated with 75% nitrous oxide for 24 hours from day 9. The embryo has a relatively small head as compared with other parts of the body. **C,** Day 11 embryo similarly treated with 75% nitrous oxide on day 9. The embryo is smaller than normal and is severely malformed. (From Baden JM, Fujinaga M. Effects of nitrous oxide on day 9 rat embryos grown in culture. Br J Anaesth 1991; 66:500-3.)

FIGURE 16-5. Pathway showing the inhibition of methionine synthase by nitrous oxide and its potential metabolic consequences (e.g., decreased DNA synthesis and impaired methylation reactions). *THF,* Tetrahydrofolate. (Courtesy of M. Fujinaga, Palo Alto, Calif.)

that supplementation of nitrous oxide with methionine (but not with folinic acid) almost completely prevents growth restriction and all malformations with the exception of situs inversus.[86] Additional studies have implicated alpha$_1$-adrenergic receptor stimulation in the production of situs inversus by nitrous oxide.[76,86-88] Postulated mechanisms by which sympathetic stimulation might produce adverse reproductive effects include a decrease in uterine blood flow and overstimulation of G-protein–dependent membrane signal transduction pathways.[89]

The etiology of nitrous oxide teratogenicity in rats is clearly complex and multifactorial. Determination of the relative roles of methionine deficiency and sympathetic stimulation must await the results of further studies. Although nitrous oxide is considered a weak teratogen in rats and mice, reproductive effects occur only after prolonged exposure to high concentrations that are unlikely to be encountered in clinical anesthesia.

Human Studies

Occupational Exposure to Waste Anesthetic Agents. Epidemiologic surveys dating from the 1960s and 1970s suggested that reproductive hazards (e.g., spontaneous abortion, congenital anomalies) were associated with operating room and dental surgery work.[90-94] These hazards were attributed to exposure to trace concentrations of anesthetic agents, principally nitrous oxide. Critical reviews of these studies questioned their conclusions. The reviewers noted the response bias, inappropriate control groups, lack of verification of medical data, and exposure to multiple environmental factors.[95-97] The most consistent risk associated with occupational exposure was for spontaneous abortion, which carried

a relative risk ratio of 1.3 (this is a 30% increase in risk as compared with the control population). The risk for congenital anomalies (1.2) had borderline statistical significance.[95,97] These relative risks are well within the range that might be explained by bias or uncontrolled variables.[97] For example, the relative risk of second-trimester abortion among women who drink one or two alcoholic drinks per day is 1.98; this risk increases to 3.53 with more than three drinks daily.[98] Similarly, cigarette smoking carries a relative risk of 1.8 for spontaneous abortion.[99]

More recent studies have failed to confirm an association between operating room work and increased reproductive risk.[100,101] Pregnancy outcomes were comparable in exposed and nonexposed operating room nurses when questionnaire information was matched with objective data obtained from medical records and registries of abortions, births, and congenital anomalies.[100] Similarly, in a 10-year prospective survey of all female physicians in the United Kingdom, Spence[101] found no differences in reproductive outcome when anesthesiologists were compared with other working female physicians. Although these studies may have missed an increased incidence of very early abortion, their data do not support a statistically demonstrable reproductive hazard resulting from operating room exposure to anesthetic agents.

It remains possible that the higher waste levels of nitrous oxide encountered in dentists' offices pose a reproductive risk.[93,102,103] In 1980, Cohen et al.[93] reported a doubling of the spontaneous abortion rate among exposed female chair-side assistants and the wives of exposed male dentists. The incidence of birth defects among the children of exposed dental assistants also was slightly increased as compared with that of nonexposed assistants. However, the validity of this finding is doubtful; the incidence of anomalies among the offspring of nonexposed dentists was similar to that of the exposed assistants. Moreover, the expected dose-response relationship did not exist in this study. Overall, the epidemiologic data do not support an increased risk of congenital anomalies with chronic exposure to nitrous oxide. Most recently, reduced fertility was reported among female dental assistants working with nitrous oxide in an unscavenged environment for more than 5 hours per week.[103] However, because the affected group contained only 19 individuals, it is difficult to draw firm conclusions from these data.

Studies of Operations Performed During Pregnancy. In 1963, Smith[104] reviewed the obstetric records of 18,493 pregnant women. Sixty-seven (0.36%) had had operations during pregnancy; only 10 procedures occurred during the first trimester. Fetal mortality was 11.2%, with the poorest survival occurring after operations for appendiceal abscess and cervical incompetence. In 1965, Shnider and Webster[105] examined the records of 9073 obstetric patients; 147 (1.6%) of this group had had operations during pregnancy. Preterm delivery followed operation in 8.8% of patients, and the incidences of perinatal mortality and low birth weight (LBW) infants were increased in patients who had surgery during pregnancy. More recently, Brodsky et al.[2] surveyed 12,929 pregnant dental assistants and wives of male dentists, 2% of whom had operations during gestation. Spontaneous abortions were more common in the surgical group than in the control group (8% versus 5.1% during the first trimester and 6.9% versus 1.4% during the second trimester, respectively). None of these three studies reported an increased incidence of congenital anomalies among infants of women who underwent surgery during pregnancy. Two additional studies[106,107] that focused on the risks associated with nitrous oxide exposure during early pregnancy found no increase in the incidence of congenital abnormalities or spontaneous abortions.

Duncan et al.[108] used health insurance data to study the entire Manitoba population between 1971 and 1978, matching 2565 women who had operations during pregnancy with similar controls who did not undergo surgery. Anesthesia was classified as nil (18%), general (57%), spinal/nerve block (2%), or local (24%). Although the incidence of congenital anomalies was similar in the surgical and control groups, spontaneous abortion was more common among women who had general anesthesia for surgery during the first or second trimesters. This was true for both gynecologic procedures (relative risk ratio, 2.00) and nongynecologic procedures (relative risk ratio, 1.58). Unfortunately, too few gynecologic or other major procedures were performed with other types of anesthesia to relate fetal loss to anesthetic technique. As in most studies, it is difficult to separate the effects of the anesthetic technique from that of the surgical procedure.[109]

In the largest study to date, Mazze and Källén[1] linked data from three Swedish health care registries—the Medical Birth Registry, the Registry of Congenital Malformations, and the Hospital Discharge Registry—for the years 1973 to 1981. Among the population of 720,000 pregnant women, 5405 (0.75%) had nonobstetric surgery, including 2252 who had procedures during the first trimester. (Cervical cerclage was excluded from analysis.) Of the women who had surgery, 54% received general anesthesia, which included nitrous oxide in 97% of cases. The authors examined the following adverse outcomes: (1) congenital anomalies; (2) stillborn infants; (3) infants dead at 168 hours; and (4) LBW (less than 2500 g) or very low birth weight (VLBW) (less than 1500 g) infants. There was no difference between surgical and control patients with regard to the incidence of stillbirth or the overall incidence of congenital anomalies (Figure 16-6). Although the overall rate of anomalies among infants of women who had first-trimester operations did not increase, this group had a higher-than-expected incidence of neural tube defects (6.0 observed versus 2.5 expected).[110] Five of the six mothers whose infants had these defects were among the 572 women who had surgery during gestational weeks 4 to 5, which is the period of neural tube formation; the authors cautioned that this finding could have been a chance association.[110] However, if a true causal relationship exists between neural tube defects and anesthesia at this stage of gestation, it could represent an eightfold to ninefold increase in the risk for this anomaly (i.e., an absolute risk of almost 1%). Other positive findings

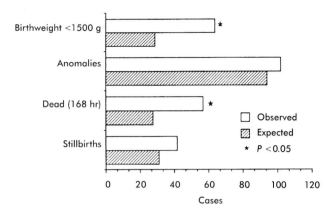

FIGURE 16-6. Total number of observed and expected adverse outcomes among women having nonobstetric operations during pregnancy. Incidences of infants with a birth weight of less than 1500 g and of infants born alive who died within 168 hours of birth were significantly increased. (From Mazze RI, Källén B. Reproductive outcome after anesthesia and operation during pregnancy: A registry study of 5405 cases. Am J Obstet Gynecol 1989; 161:1178.)

included an increased incidence of LBW and VLBW infants in the surgical group, which resulted from both preterm delivery and intrauterine growth restriction.[1] A predictable consequence of preterm delivery was an increased number of liveborn infants who died within the first 168 hours of life. Finally, no anesthetic technique or operation was associated with a significantly increased number of adverse outcomes.

A case-control study of infants born in Atlanta between 1968 and 1980 obtained information regarding first-trimester exposure to general anesthesia among the mothers of 694 infants with major CNS defects and 2984 control mothers.[111] A striking association was found between general anesthesia exposure and hydrocephalus in conjunction with another major defect (the strongest association was with hydrocephalus and eye defects). Limitations of this study include its retrospective nature and a lack of information regarding the types of surgery, the anesthetic agents used, and the presence or absence of complications. The authors cautioned that further studies are necessary to confirm their data.

In summary, although anesthesia and surgery are associated with increased incidences of abortion, intrauterine growth restriction, and perinatal mortality, these often can be attributed to the procedure, the site of surgery (e.g., proximity to the uterus), and/or the underlying maternal condition. Evidence does not suggest an overall increase in congenital abnormalities or a clear relationship between outcome and type of anesthesia.

BEHAVIORAL TERATOLOGY

It is well known that some teratogens produce enduring behavioral abnormalities without any observable morphologic changes. The CNS may be especially sensitive to such influences during the period of myelination, which in humans extends from the fourth intrauterine month to the second postnatal month. Several studies have shown that brief intrauterine exposure to halothane adversely affects postnatal learning behavior and causes CNS degeneration and decreased brain weight in rats.[112-114] In rats, the fetal nervous system is most susceptible to the effects of halothane during the second trimester.[112] Prenatal administration of systemic drugs—including barbiturates, meperidine, and promethazine—also has resulted in behavioral changes in animals,[115-117] whereas no effect has been noted with the administration of lidocaine.[55] Investigations of the effects of maternally administered analgesics at delivery have revealed transient, dose-related depression of newborn behavior.

Jevtovic-Todorovic et al.[118] have noted that currently used general anesthetic agents act by two principal mechanisms: the potentiation of gamma-aminobutyric acid (GABA)$_A$ receptors and the antagonism of N-methyl-D-aspartate (NMDA) receptors. Recent evidence suggests that drugs that act by either of these mechanisms induce widespread neuronal apoptosis in the developing rat brain when administered during the period of synaptogenesis (i.e., the brain growth-spurt period).[118-120] Jevtovic-Todorovic et al.[118] recently observed that the administration of a general anesthetic "cocktail" (midazolam, isoflurane, and nitrous oxide) to 7-day-old infant rats in doses sufficient to maintain general anesthesia for 6 hours resulted in widespread apoptotic neurodegeneration in the developing brain, deficits in hippocampal synaptic function, and persistent memory/learning impairments. They concluded that these deficits are "subtle enough to be easily overlooked" but may persist into adolescence and adulthood.[118] The implications, if any, for the human fetus during the maternal administration of general anesthesia are unknown.

Fetal Effects of Anesthesia

MAINTENANCE OF FETAL WELL-BEING

The most serious fetal risk associated with maternal surgery during pregnancy is that of intrauterine asphyxia. Because fetal oxygenation depends on maternal oxygenation, maintenance of normal maternal arterial oxygen tension, oxygen-carrying capacity, oxygen affinity, and uteroplacental perfusion are critical.

Maternal and Fetal Oxygenation

Transient mild-to-moderate decreases in maternal Pao$_2$ are well tolerated by the fetus, because fetal hemoglobin is present in high concentration and has a high affinity for oxygen. Severe maternal **hypoxemia** results in fetal hypoxia and, if persistent, may cause fetal death. Any complication that causes profound maternal hypoxemia (e.g., difficult intubation, esophageal intubation, pulmonary aspiration, high level of regional block, systemic local anesthetic toxicity) is a potential threat to the fetus.

Older studies of isolated human placental vessels suggested that **hyperoxia** might cause uteroplacental vasoconstriction, with potential impairment of fetal oxygen delivery.[121,122] This fear has proven to be unfounded, because studies in pregnant women have demonstrated improved fetal oxygenation with increasing maternal Pao$_2$.[123-125] Fetal Pao$_2$ never exceeds 60 mm Hg, even when maternal Pao$_2$ increases to 600 mm Hg, because of a large maternal-fetal oxygen tension gradient.[29] Thus, intrauterine retrolental fibroplasia and premature closure of the ductus arteriosus cannot result from high levels of maternal Pao$_2$. In a preliminary study, McClaine et al.[125] recently observed that the maternal administration of general anesthesia in gravid ewes produced an initial—but not a sustained—increase in fetal systemic oxygenation and sustained increases in fetal cerebral oxygenation.

Maternal Carbon Dioxide and Acid-Base Status

Maternal **hypercapnia** can cause fetal acidosis, because fetal Paco$_2$ correlates directly with maternal Paco$_2$. Although mild fetal respiratory acidosis is of little consequence, severe acidosis can cause fetal myocardial depression and hypotension.

Maternal **hyperventilation** with low maternal Paco$_2$ and high pH can adversely affect fetal oxygenation by means of several mechanisms.[126-128] **Respiratory** or **metabolic alkalosis** can compromise maternal-fetal oxygen transfer by causing umbilical artery constriction[126] and by shifting the maternal oxyhemoglobin dissociation curve to the left.[127] In addition, positive-pressure hyperventilation, independent of changes in Paco$_2$, may reduce uterine blood flow and cause fetal acidosis.[128] This most likely is a consequence of mechanical ventilation, whereby increased intrathoracic pressure decreases venous return and cardiac output, which in turn decreases uteroplacental perfusion. Thus hyperventilation should be avoided in the pregnant surgical patient. Rather, the Paco$_2$ should be kept in the normal range for pregnancy.

Uteroplacental Perfusion

Maternal **hypotension** from any cause can jeopardize uteroplacental perfusion and cause fetal asphyxia. The most common causes of hypotension in the pregnant patient during surgery include the following: (1) deep levels of general anesthesia; (2) sympathectomy with high levels of spinal or epidural blockade; (3) aortocaval compression; (4) hemorrhage; and (5) hypovolemia. In monkeys, prolonged hypotension (i.e., blood pressure less than 75 mm Hg) caused by deep halothane anesthesia resulted in fetal hypoxia, acidosis, and hypotension.[129] After experiencing as many as 5 hours of severe partial asphyxia in utero (pH < 7.00 for at least 1 hour), newborns were depressed and experienced seizures. Postnatal survival was poor, and pathologic brain changes included swelling, necrosis, and hemorrhage. The clinical course and neuropathologic findings in these animals resembled those of infants known to have suffered severe intrauterine asphyxia who died within a few days of birth. Despite these alarming data, several reports have attested to the safety of inducing moderate degrees of hypotension during pregnancy, usually to facilitate neurosurgical procedures.[130-132] Fetal and neonatal outcomes were unaffected in several cases in which maternal systolic blood pressure was kept in the 70 to 80 mm Hg range, even when pressures as low as 50 mm Hg were permitted briefly. In such circumstances, the risk to the fetus must be balanced against the risk of uncontrolled bleeding or maternal stroke.

The multiple factors that influence uteroplacental blood flow are discussed in detail in Chapter 3. Of particular relevance to the pregnant surgical patient are drugs that cause uterine vasoconstriction, such as sympathomimetic agents with predominantly alpha-adrenergic effects[133] or toxic doses of local anesthetics.[134] Preoperative anxiety and light anesthesia increase circulating catecholamines, which may impair uterine blood flow.[135] Drugs that cause uterine hypertonus (e.g., ketamine in early pregnancy in doses greater than 2 mg/kg,[136] alpha-adrenergic agonists,[133] toxic doses of local anesthetics[134]) may increase uterine vascular resistance, which decreases uteroplacental perfusion.

Recent evidence has challenged the historic view that the mixed-adrenergic agonist ephedrine is preferred to the alpha-adrenergic agonist phenylephrine for the treatment of hypotension during the administration of regional anesthesia in obstetric patients.[137-139] A meta-analysis of randomized controlled trials of ephedrine versus phenylephrine for the treatment of hypotension during spinal anesthesia for cesarean section resulted in the following conclusions: (1) there was no difference between phenylephrine and ephedrine for the prevention and treatment of maternal hypotension; (2) maternal bradycardia was more likely to occur with phenylephrine than with ephedrine; (3) women given phenylephrine had neonates with higher umbilical arterial blood pH measurements than those given ephedrine; and (4) there was no difference between the two vasopressors in the incidence of true fetal acidosis (i.e., umbilical arterial blood pH < 7.20).[138] Cooper et al.[139] randomized 147 patients to receive phenylephrine, ephedrine, or both phenylephrine and ephedrine for the maintenance of maternal arterial pressure during spinal anesthesia for elective cesarean section. Fetal acidosis was more frequent in the women who received ephedrine. The authors speculated that "increased fetal metabolic rate, secondary to ephedrine-induced beta-adrenergic stimulation, was the most likely mechanism for the increased incidence of fetal acidosis in the ephedrine group."[139]

FETAL EFFECTS OF INHALATION AGENTS

The volatile halogenated anesthetic agents can affect the fetus directly (by depressing the fetal cardiovascular system or CNS) or indirectly (by causing maternal hypoxia or hypotension). Studies in gravid ewes have shown minimal fetal effects with maternal administration of moderate concentrations of volatile agents.[140,141] Uterine perfusion was maintained during the inhalation of 1.0 and 1.5 MAC halothane or isoflurane, because uterine vasodilation compensated for small decreases in maternal blood pressure.[140,141] Higher concentrations (e.g., 2.0 MAC) given for prolonged periods induced marked maternal hypotension. Consequently, decreased uteroplacental blood flow resulted in fetal hypoxia, decreased fetal cardiac output, and fetal acidosis.[140]

The effects of anesthesia on the stressed fetal lamb remain uncertain. In one study, the administration of 1% halothane to the mothers of asphyxiated fetal lambs caused severe fetal hypotension, worsening of fetal acidosis, and decreases in cerebral blood flow and oxygen delivery.[142] In other studies, acidosis that was less severe or of a shorter duration was associated with the maintenance of fetal cardiac output and a preservation of the balance between oxygen supply and demand.[143-145] The protective compensatory mechanisms that exist during asphyxia may be abolished by high but not low concentrations of volatile agents.

The relevance of these data for the mother undergoing surgery during pregnancy is not clear. Clinical experience does not support avoiding volatile agents, provided that maternal hypotension is prevented. Indeed, their depressant effect on myometrial contractility may be beneficial. If intraoperative fetal heart rate (FHR) monitoring reveals signs of fetal distress, it may be advisable to discontinue the volatile agent until the fetal condition improves.

FETAL EFFECTS OF SYSTEMIC DRUGS

Opioids and induction agents decrease FHR variability, possibly to a greater extent than do the inhalation agents.[146-149] This most likely signals the presence of an anesthetized fetus and is not a cause for concern in the absence of maternal hypotension or other abnormalities. Fetal respiratory depression is relevant only if cesarean delivery is to be performed at the same time as the surgical procedure. Even then, high-dose opioid anesthesia need not be avoided when it is indicated for maternal reasons (e.g., cardiac disease). The pediatrician should be informed of maternal drug administration so that preparations can be made to ventilate the neonate mechanically.

Maternal administration of muscle relaxants and reversal agents typically has not proved to be problematic for the fetus.[148] It has been suggested that rapid intravenous injection of an anticholinesterase agent might stimulate acetylcholine release, which might cause increased uterine tone and thus precipitate preterm labor.[150] Although this concern is theoretical, slow administration of an anticholinesterase agent (after prior injection of an anticholinergic agent) has been recommended.[29] Atropine rapidly crosses the placenta and, when given in large doses, causes fetal tachycardia and loss of FHR variability.[151] Although neither atropine nor glycopyrrolate significantly affects FHR when standard clinical doses are administered alone,[152] glycopyrrolate is often recommended, because it crosses the placenta less readily and may be a more effective antisialagogue. Although limited transplacental passage of neostigmine is expected, significant transfer occasionally may occur. One case report described mild fetal bradycardia when neostigmine was administered with glycopyrrolate during emergence from general anesthesia at 31 weeks' gestation.[153] This did not occur during the administration of a second general anesthetic to the same patient 4 days later, when atropine was administered with neostigmine, presumably because atropine undergoes greater placental transfer than glycopyrrolate. Because the effects of reversal agents are unpredictable, the monitoring of FHR is necessary to guide appropriate maternal drug administration.

Sodium nitroprusside and esmolol have been used during pregnancy to induce hypotension during surgical procedures. Standard doses of nitroprusside have proved to be safe for the fetus,[130,131] and the risk of fetal cyanide toxicity appears to be low, provided tachyphylaxis does not occur and the total dose is limited.[154] The use of esmolol during pregnancy remains controversial. Ostman et al.[155] observed minimal fetal effects after the administration of esmolol in gravid ewes, whereas Eisenach and Castro[156] observed significant decreases in FHR and blood pressure as well as a modest reduction in fetal PaO_2. Fetal effects dissipated rapidly in the first study, but they persisted for 30 minutes or more in the second. Two case reports have described small decreases in FHR but no morbidity when esmolol was administered with nitroprusside during neurosurgical procedures.[157,158] By contrast, severe fetal distress followed the administration of esmolol at 38 weeks' gestation to correct maternal supraventricular tachycardia.[159] Because fetal tachycardia preceded the onset of severe bradycardia in this case, the authors speculated that fetal compromise resulted from decreased maternal cardiac output rather than from fetal beta-adrenergic receptor blockade.

Prevention of Preterm Labor

Most epidemiologic studies of nonobstetric surgery during pregnancy have reported an increased incidence of abortion and preterm delivery.[1,105,106,160] It is unclear whether the surgery, manipulation of the uterus, or the underlying condition is responsible. In a study of 778 women who underwent appendectomy during pregnancy, Mazze and Källén[160] found that 22% delivered in the week after surgery when this occurred between 24 and 36 weeks' gestation. If pregnancy continued beyond a week after surgery, there was no further increase in preterm birth. Although their database was unsuitable for determining the incidence of preterm delivery before 24 weeks' gestation, a similar increase appeared likely. Second-trimester procedures and those that do not involve uterine manipulation carry the lowest risk for preterm labor.[161]

Although the volatile halogenated agents depress myometrial irritability and theoretically are advantageous for abdominal procedures, evidence does not suggest that any anesthetic agent or technique influences the risk of preterm labor. The prophylactic use of tocolytic agents is controversial; they are not without risk, and it is unclear whether they affect outcome.[162] Selective administration to those patients at greatest risk (e.g., those undergoing cervical cerclage) has been suggested.[162] (The anesthetic implications of tocolytic therapy are discussed in Chapter 34.) Monitoring for uterine contractions should be performed with an external tocodynamometer intraoperatively (when technically feasible) and for several days postoperatively; this allows immediate tocolytic therapy to be instituted, if appropriate. Additional surveillance is necessary in patients who receive potent postoperative analgesics, because they may be unaware of mild uterine contractions.

PRACTICAL CONSIDERATIONS

Timing of Surgery

Elective surgery should not be performed during pregnancy. When possible, surgery should be avoided during the first trimester, especially during the period of organogenesis. The second trimester is the optimal time to perform surgery, because the risk of preterm labor is lowest. Urgent operation is often indicated for abdominal emergencies, some malignancies, and neurosurgical and cardiac conditions. The management of most surgical conditions should be the same in pregnant and nonpregnant patients.[161,163,164] In the most common abdominal emergency, which is appendicitis, maternal morbidity and perinatal loss increase when maternal disease is advanced.[161,163,164] Perforation may be more common in pregnant patients than in nonpregnant patients, because diagnostic difficulties may delay operation. Generalized peritonitis may also be more likely, because increased steroid levels during pregnancy may suppress the normal inflammatory response and prevent the "walling off" of the appendix by the omentum.[164]

In the event of a serious maternal illness, the remote fetal risks associated with anesthesia and operation are of secondary importance. The primary goal is to preserve the life of the mother. Hypothermia,[165,166] induced hypotension,[130,131] cardiopulmonary bypass,[167] and liver transplantation[168] all of which theoretically pose major risks to the fetus, have been associated with successful neonatal outcomes. The decision to perform simultaneous cesarean delivery depends on a number of factors, including the stage of gestation, the risk to the mother of a trial of labor at a later date, and the presence of intraabdominal sepsis. Cesarean delivery may be performed immediately before the surgical procedure to avoid fetal risks associated with special patient positioning (e.g., the sitting or prone position),[169,170] prolonged anesthesia, major intraoperative blood loss, maternal hyperventilation, deliberate hypotension, or cardiopulmonary bypass.[167]

Diagnosis and Surgical Approach

Accurate diagnosis, especially of an acute abdominal crisis, can prove extremely difficult during pregnancy.[164] Box 16-2 lists some of the conditions that must be considered in the differential diagnosis of abdominal pain during pregnancy. Nausea, vomiting, constipation, and distention are common symptoms of both normal pregnancy and abdominal pathology. Abdominal tenderness may be indistinguishable from ligamentous or uterine contraction pain. Anatomic land-

---

Box 16-2 NONOBSTETRIC ABDOMINAL CRISES IN PREGNANCY

MEDICAL CONDITIONS

Abdominal crises due to systemic disease
• Sickle cell disease
• Diabetic ketoacidosis
• Porphyria
Renal disease
• Glomerulonephritis
• Pyelonephritis
Pulmonary disease
• Basal pneumonia with pleurisy
Cholecystitis and pancreatitis (early, uncomplicated)
Myocardial infarction, pericarditis
Drug addiction (withdrawal symptoms)

SURGICAL CONDITIONS

GYNECOLOGIC PROBLEMS

Ovarian cyst/tumor
• Rupture
• Torsion
• Hemorrhage
• Infection
Torsion of a fallopian tube
Tuboovarian abscess
Uterine myoma
• Degeneration
• Infection
• Torsion

NONGYNECOLOGIC PROBLEMS

Acute appendicitis
Acute cholecystitis and its complications
Acute pancreatitis and its complications
Intestinal obstruction
Trauma with visceral injury or hemorrhage
Vascular accidents (e.g., ruptured abdominal aneurysm)
Peptic ulcer

Modified from Fainstat T, Bhat N. Surgical resolution of nonobstetric abdominal crises complicating pregnancy. In: Baden JM, Brodsky JB, editors. The Pregnant Surgical Patient. Mount Kisko, New York, Futura Publishing, 1985:154.

---

marks change as the uterus enlarges and are more variable than in the nonpregnant patient. For example, the appendix rotates counterclockwise; thus, as term approaches, the tip typically lies over the right kidney (Figure 16-7).[171,172] Because the white blood cell count in normal pregnancy can reach 15,000/mm³, it must be markedly elevated to be helpful diagnostically. Additional delay results from the reluctance to perform necessary studies involving radiation. Mazze and Källén[160] reported the misdiagnosis of appendicitis during pregnancy in 36% of all cases, with a lower rate (23%) during the first trimester than during the last two trimesters (43%).

Often, the correct diagnosis is determined only at operation. The selection of the procedure and choice of incision is influenced by the stage of gestation, the nature of the surgical problem, the certainty of the probable diagnosis, and the experience of the surgeon. Laparoscopy is performed during pregnancy for both diagnostic and therapeutic surgery with increasing frequency (vide infra). Laparotomy continues to be performed for many abdominal conditions that occur during the later stages of pregnancy. A vertical paramedian incision over the site of maximal tenderness may be selected for

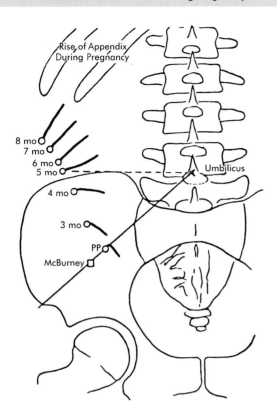

FIGURE 16-7. Changes in position and direction of the appendix during pregnancy. (From Baer JL, Reis RA, Arens RA. Appendicitis in pregnancy with changes in position and axis of normal appendix in pregnancy. JAMA 1932; 98:1359.)

appendectomy,[164] whereas a long vertical midline incision may be preferable when the diagnosis is unclear.

LAPAROSCOPY

Although pregnancy was once regarded as an absolute contraindication to laparoscopy, in recent years laparoscopy has been performed during pregnancy with increasing frequency.[173-185] In a 1994 survey of laparoendoscopic surgeons, Reedy et al.[173] obtained data about 413 laparoscopies performed during pregnancy and reviewed an additional 55 previously published cases. Among the cases surveyed, 48% were cholecystectomies, 28% were adnexal operations, 16% were appendectomies, and 8% were diagnostic procedures. Thirty-two percent of cases were performed in the first trimester, with 54% and 13% performed in the second and third trimesters, respectively. For both pregnant and nonpregnant patients, the benefits of laparoscopic surgery over conventional surgery include shorter hospitalization, less postoperative pain, and faster return to normal activities, including earlier return of normal gastrointestinal function.[174] However, concerns exist regarding fetal well-being, especially regarding the following risks: (1) uterine or fetal trauma; (2) fetal acidosis from absorbed carbon dioxide; and (3) decreased maternal cardiac output and uteroplacental perfusion resulting from increased intraabdominal pressure. In some animal studies,[186,187] maternal and fetal acidosis and tachycardia have occurred during intraabdominal insufflation, perhaps because maternal ventilation was guided by measurements of end-tidal rather than arterial carbon dioxide levels. A marked increase in $PaCO_2$ to end-tidal CO_2 gradient developed during CO_2 insufflation in gravid ewes, which suggests that $PaCO_2$ should be used to guide ventilation if maternal and fetal acidosis are to be avoided.[188] By contrast, clinical studies and clinical

experience suggest that capnography alone is an adequate monitor to guide ventilation during laparoscopic surgery in pregnant patients.[189] In one clinical study, there was no difference in the pH, the $PaCO_2$, or the arterial to end-tidal carbon dioxide pressure gradient before, during, or after termination of the pneumoperitoneum during laparoscopy.[189]

Uteroplacental perfusion decreased by 61% in one study in which gravid ewes were subjected to a CO_2 pneumoperitoneum at a pressure of 20 mm Hg (although there were no adverse fetal consequences),[190] whereas it remained unchanged in a second study in which intraabdominal pressure was only 13 mm Hg, despite a prolonged period of insufflation.[191] Steinbrook and Bhavani-Shankar[192] used thoracic electrical bioimpedance cardiography to measure changes in cardiac output in four pregnant women undergoing laparoscopic cholecystectomy. The authors observed hemodynamic changes similar to those that typically occur during laparoscopic surgery in nonpregnant patients (i.e., decrease in cardiac index with concurrent increases in mean arterial pressure and systemic vascular resistance). A gasless laparoscopic technique employing a whole abdominal-wall lift has been used successfully in seven pregnant women who underwent adnexal cyst resection with epidural anesthesia.[193]

Reported clinical experiences with laparoscopy during pregnancy generally have been favorable; complications such as intraoperative perforation of the uterus with the Verres needle have occurred rarely.[173] Moreover, most investigators have reported no difference in maternal and fetal outcome between laparoscopy and laparotomy and consider the former a safe procedure during pregnancy.[173,175-182] By contrast, Amos et al.[183] urged caution in a case series in which fetal death followed four out of seven laparoscopic surgeries.

Careful surgical and anesthetic techniques are critical to avoid problems associated with the pregnancy state and the special hazards of laparoscopy. The surgeon should be experienced with the technique, and the anesthesiologist must be aware of the accompanying cardiorespiratory changes that occur. The Society of American Gastrointestinal Endoscopic Surgeons[194] has issued its "Guidelines for Laparoscopic Surgery During Pregnancy," which recommend the following: (1) deferring surgery until the second trimester; (2) obtaining preoperative obstetric consultation; (3) using intermittent pneumatic compression devices to prevent thrombosis resulting from lower extremity stasis; (4) monitoring fetal and uterine status, as well as maternal end-tidal CO_2 and arterial blood gas measurements; (5) using an open technique to enter the abdomen; (6) avoiding aortocaval compression; (7) maintaining low pneumoperitoneum pressures (preferably 8 to 12 mm Hg but not to exceed 15 mm Hg); and (8) protecting the uterus with a lead shield if intraoperative cholangiography is planned.

General anesthesia has been used in the vast majority of cases, with only occasional mention of the use of epidural anesthesia.[173,184] Steinbrook et al.[185] described their anesthetic technique for 10 cases of laparoscopic cholecystectomy at the Brigham and Women's Hospital. They administered general anesthesia with a rapid-sequence induction followed by endotracheal intubation and positive-pressure ventilation to maintain end-tidal CO_2 between 32 and 36 mm Hg. Anesthesia was maintained with a muscle relaxant, an opioid, and a volatile halogenated agent, but nitrous oxide was avoided to prevent bowel distention and to allow a higher concentration of inspired oxygen. The pneumoperitoneum resulted in increased peak airway pressure (Figure 16-8) and decreased total lung compliance, which changed progressively with advancing gestation.

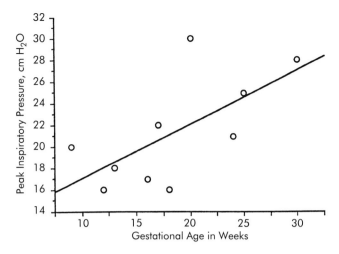

FIGURE 16-8. Peak inspiratory pressure during laparoscopic cholecystectomy during pregnancy as a function of gestational age. The best-fit line by linear regression is shown ($Y = 12.1 + 0.5X$; $R^2 = 0.43$). Peak inspiratory pressure tends to increase with advancing gestation. (From Steinbrook RA, Brooks DC, Datta S. Laparoscopic cholecystectomy during pregnancy. Surg Ensdosc 1996; 10:511-5.)

Use of the Trendelenburg position exacerbates these changes, further decreases FRC, and makes hypoxemia from airway closure more likely. Hyperventilation, which may be necessary to maintain normal maternal $PaCO_2$, may reduce uteroplacental perfusion and affect fetal oxygenation. Hypotension can result from pneumoperitoneum, aortocaval compression, or use of the reverse Trendelenburg position, and a vasopressor (e.g., ephedrine, phenylephrine) may be needed to maintain maternal blood pressure during laparoscopy.[185] As with conventional surgery, fetal well-being is best preserved by maintaining maternal oxygenation, acid-base status, and hemodynamic measurements within normal pregnancy limits. The FHR and uterine tone should be monitored both before and after surgery (vide infra), but this may not be possible during peritoneal insufflation except by means of the transvaginal route.[185]

ELECTROCONVULSIVE SHOCK THERAPY DURING PREGNANCY

The treatment of major psychiatric disorders during pregnancy is problematic, and optimal management remains controversial.[195,196] The risk of congenital malformations in the fetus exposed to psychotropic medications in utero must be balanced with the high rate of relapse that results from the discontinuation of psychotropic medications in pregnant women with mood disorders.[196] Because these medications present a low but increased risk of teratogenicity, the American Psychiatric Association has endorsed electroconvulsive shock therapy (ECT) as a treatment for major depression and bipolar disorders during all three trimesters of pregnancy,[197] and some physicians have suggested that it is "the treatment method of choice, especially when rapid control of depressive symptoms is needed."[195]

Published case reports represent the only available source of information regarding the effects of ECT during pregnancy. Moreno et al.[198] reported a case of miscarriage following the third ECT treatment in a patient at 8 weeks' gestation. The authors implicated ECT as a cause of the miscarriage; however, other possible causes of spontaneous abortion and the physical and psychologic condition of the patient could not be discarded as causative factors.

Miller[199] reviewed the details of 300 published reports of the use of ECT during pregnancy between 1924 and 1991. In 14 (4.7%) cases, ECT was begun in the first trimester; in 36 (12%), ECT was begun in the second trimester; and in 31 (10%), ECT was begun in the third trimester. In 219 (73%), cases the timing was not identified. Complications were reported in 28 (9.3%) cases. The major complications included self-limited FHR abnormalities (five cases), vaginal bleeding (five cases), uterine contractions (two cases), and abdominal pain (three cases). All babies in these cases were born healthy. Additional complications included preterm labor (four cases, although none of these immediately followed ECT), miscarriage (five cases), and stillbirth and neonatal death (three cases). The overall incidence of miscarriage was 1.6%—a rate much lower than that of the general population—which suggested that ECT is not a significant risk factor for miscarriage. Factors other than ECT were considered responsible for the stillbirths and neonatal deaths. There were five cases of congenital anomalies, but neither the pattern nor the number of anomalies suggested that ECT was a determining factor in the abnormalities.

Anesthetic agents commonly used during ECT include barbiturates, succinylcholine, and anticholinergics (e.g., glycopyrrolate); these agents have a long history of safe use during pregnancy. Ishikawa et al.[200] reported their management of a pregnant women whose third ECT was complicated by sustained uterine contractions (and fetal bradycardia) that were refractory to tocolytic agents. At the sixth ECT, general anesthesia was maintained with sevoflurane and oxygen, and uterine contractions were significantly diminished.[200]

Guidelines for ECT during pregnancy have been published.[199,201] In brief, an obstetric consultation should be obtained before the initiation of ECT. Tocodynamometry should be used to confirm the absence of uterine contractions within the hour before ECT. The procedure should be postponed if uterine contractions, cervical dilation, or vaginal bleeding are present. Adequate intravascular hydration should be assured, and 30 mL of 0.3 M sodium citrate should be administered 15 to 20 minutes before ECT. Endotracheal intubation should be considered if the patient is beyond the first trimester of pregnancy. Uterine displacement should be maintained in patients at more than 20 weeks' gestation, and the FHR should be monitored immediately before and after ECT. The patient should also be monitored for uterine contractions and vaginal bleeding after ECT.

Fetal Monitoring During Surgery

Continuous FHR monitoring (using transabdominal Doppler) is feasible beginning at approximately 18 weeks' gestation.[202,203] However, technical problems may limit the use of continuous FHR monitoring between 18 and 22 weeks' gestation. Transabdominal monitoring may not be possible during abdominal procedures or when the mother is very obese; use of transvaginal Doppler ultrasonography may be considered in selected cases. The American College of Obstetricians and Gynecologists recently opined that "the decision to use [intraoperative] fetal monitoring should be individualized, and each case warrants a team approach for optimal safety of the woman and her baby."[204]

FHR variability, which typically is a good indicator of fetal well-being, is present by 25 to 27 weeks' gestation. Changes in the baseline FHR and FHR variability caused by anesthetic agents or other drugs must be distinguished from changes that result from fetal hypoxia.[148,149] Persistent severe fetal bradycardia typically indicates true fetal distress.

Intraoperative FHR monitoring requires the presence of someone who can interpret the tracing. In addition, there should be a plan that addresses how to proceed in the event of persistent fetal distress, including whether to perform emergency cesarean delivery. The greatest value of intraoperative FHR monitoring is that it allows for the optimization of the maternal condition if the fetus show signs of compromise. In one case, decreased FHR variability was associated with maternal hypoxia, but this resolved when maternal oxygenation improved (Figure 16-9).[147] An unexplained change in FHR mandates the evaluation of maternal position, blood pressure, oxygenation, and acid-base status and the inspection of the surgical site to ensure that neither surgeons nor retractors are impairing uterine perfusion.

Anesthetic Management

PREOPERATIVE MANAGEMENT

Premedication may be necessary to allay maternal anxiety. Precautions against acid aspiration should include administration of an H_2-receptor antagonist and 30 mL of a clear antacid before the induction of anesthesia.

CHOICE OF ANESTHESIA

The choice of anesthesia should be guided by maternal indications and should take into consideration the site and the nature of the surgery. No study has correlated improved fetal outcome with any anesthetic technique. When possible, local or regional anesthesia (with the exception of paracervical block) is preferred; this permits the administration of drugs with no laboratory or clinical evidence of teratogenesis. In addition, maternal respiratory complications occur less frequently with local and regional anesthetic techniques. These techniques are suitable for cases involving cervical cerclage, urologic or lower extremity procedures, and operations on the arm or hand. Most abdominal operations require general anesthesia, because the incision typically extends to the upper abdomen, which creates an unacceptable risk of aspiration in a pregnant patient with an unprotected airway.

PREVENTION OF AORTOCAVAL COMPRESSION

Beginning at 18 to 20 weeks' gestation, the pregnant patient should be transported on her side, and the uterus should be displaced leftward when she is positioned on the operating table.

MONITORING

Maternal monitoring should include noninvasive or direct blood pressure measurement, electrocardiography, pulse oximetry, capnography, temperature monitoring, and the use of a nerve stimulator. The FHR and uterine activity should be monitored both during and after surgery when technically feasible.

ANESTHETIC TECHNIQUE

General anesthesia mandates endotracheal intubation beginning at approximately 18 to 20 weeks' gestation or earlier if gastrointestinal function is abnormal. Denitrogenation (i.e., preoxygenation) should precede the application of cricoid pressure, rapid-sequence induction, and endotracheal intubation. Drugs with a history of safe use during pregnancy include thiopental, morphine, meperidine, fentanyl, succinylcholine, and most of the nondepolarizing muscle relaxants. Many obstetric anesthesiologists would now add propofol to the list of "safe" drugs for use during pregnancy.

A commonly used technique employs a high concentration of oxygen, a muscle relaxant, and an opioid and/or a moderate concentration of a volatile halogenated agent. Scientific evidence does not support avoiding nitrous oxide during pregnancy,[22] particularly after the sixth week of gestation. Omission of nitrous oxide may increase fetal risk if inadequate anesthesia results or if a high dose of a volatile agent results in maternal hypotension. A cautious approach would restrict nitrous oxide administration to a concentration of 50% or less and would limit its use in extremely long operations. Hyperventilation should be avoided; rather, end-tidal CO_2 should be maintained in the normal range for pregnancy.

Before the administration of spinal or epidural anesthesia, rapid intravenous infusion of 1 L of crystalloid seems prudent, although the anesthesiologist should not assume that this will prevent maternal hypotension. Appropriate vasopressors should be available to treat hypotension if it occurs. The usual precautions must be taken to guard against a high block and systemic local anesthetic toxicity.

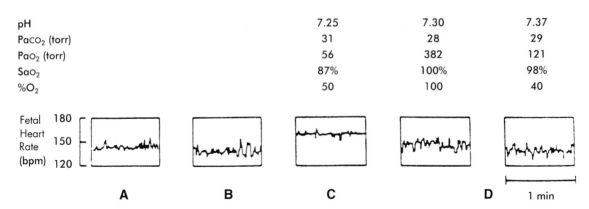

		7.25	7.30	7.37
pH		7.25	7.30	7.37
PaCO₂ (torr)		31	28	29
PaO₂ (torr)		56	382	121
SaO₂		87%	100%	98%
%O₂		50	100	40

FIGURE 16-9. Serial samples of the fetal heart rate tracing in a patient undergoing eye surgery. **A** and **B,** Baseline fetal heart rate of 140 bpm with normal beat-to-beat variability. **C,** Fetal tachycardia and decrease in beat-to-beat variability during inadvertent maternal hypoxemia (maternal PaO₂ = 56 mm Hg). **D,** After correction of maternal ventilation, baseline fetal heart rate and variability return. (From Katz JD, Hook R, Barash PG. Fetal heart rate monitoring in pregnant patients undergoing surgery. Am J Obstet Gynecol 1976; 125:267.)

Regardless of the technique used, avoidance of hypoxemia, hypotension, acidosis, and hyperventilation are the most critical elements of anesthetic management.

POSTOPERATIVE MANAGEMENT

The FHR and uterine activity should be monitored during recovery from anesthesia. Adequate analgesia should be obtained with systemic or spinal opioids. Prophylaxis against venous thrombosis should be considered.

KEY POINTS

- A significant number of women undergo anesthesia and surgery during pregnancy for procedures unrelated to delivery.
- Maternal risks are associated with the anatomic and physiologic changes of pregnancy (e.g., difficult intubation, aspiration) and with the underlying maternal disease.
- The diagnosis of abdominal conditions often is delayed during pregnancy, which increases the risk of maternal and fetal morbidity.
- Maternal catastrophes involving severe hypoxia, hypotension, and acidosis pose the greatest acute risk to the fetus.
- Other fetal risks associated with surgery include increased fetal loss, increased incidence of preterm labor, growth restriction, and low birth weight. Clinical studies suggest that anesthesia and surgery during pregnancy do not increase the risk of congenital anomalies.
- It is unclear whether adverse fetal outcomes result from the anesthetic, the operation, or the underlying maternal disease.
- No anesthetic agent is a proven teratogen in humans, although some anesthetic agents, specifically nitrous oxide, are teratogenic in animals under certain conditions.
- Many anesthetic agents have been used for anesthesia during pregnancy, with no demonstrable differences in maternal or fetal outcome.
- The anesthetic management of the pregnant surgical patient should focus on the avoidance of hypoxemia, hypotension, acidosis, and hyperventilation.

REFERENCES

1. Mazze RI, Källén B. Reproductive outcome after anesthesia and operation during pregnancy: A registry study of 5405 cases. Am J Obstet Gynecol 1989; 161:1178-85.
2. Brodsky JB, Cohen EN, Brown BW, et al. Surgery during pregnancy and fetal outcome. Am J Obstet Gynecol 1980; 138:1165-7.
3. Manley S, De Kelaita G, Joseph NJ. Preoperative pregnancy testing in ambulatory surgery. Anesthesiology 1995; 83:690-3.
4. Azzam FJ, Padda GS, DeBoard JW, et al. Preoperative pregnancy testing in adolescents. Anesth Analg 1996; 82:4-7.
5. Malviya S, D'Errico C, Reynolds P, et al. Should pregnancy testing be routine in adolescent patients prior to surgery? Anesth Analg 1996; 83:854-8.
6. American Society of Anesthesiologists. Practice Guidelines for Preanesthetic Evaluation. Park Ridge, Ill, American Society of Anesthesiologists, 1997.
7. Barron WM. The pregnant surgical patient: Medical evaluation and management. Ann Intern Med 1984; 101:683-91.
8. Cohen SE. Physiologic alterations of pregnancy: Anesthetic implications. In: Barash PG, editor. American Society of Anesthesiologists Refresher Courses in Anesthesiology. Vol. 21. Philadelphia, JB Lippincott, 1993:51-64.
9. Gin T, Chan MTV. Decreased minimum alveolar concentration of isoflurane in pregnant humans. Anesthesiology 1994; 81:829-32.
10. Chan MTV, Mainland P, Gin T. Minimum alveolar concentrations of halothane and enflurane are decreased in early pregnancy. Anesthesiology 1996; 85:782-6.
11. Capeless EL, Clapp JF. Cardiovascular changes in early phase of pregnancy. Am J Obstet Gynecol 1989; 161:1449-53.
12. Gerbasi FR, Bottoms S, Farag A, et al. Increased intravascular coagulation associated with pregnancy. Obstet Gynecol 1990; 75:385-9.
13. Gin T, Mainland P, Chan MTV, et al. Decreased thiopental requirements in early pregnancy. Anesthesiology 1997; 86:73-8.
14. Leighton BL, Cheek TG, Gross JB, et al. Succinylcholine pharmacodynamics in peripartum patients. Anesthesiology 1986; 64:202-5.
15. Sturrock JE, Nunn JF. Mitosis in mammalian cells during exposure to anesthetics. Anesthesiology 1975; 43:21-33.
16. Sturrock J, Nunn JF. Effects of halothane on DNA synthesis and the presynthetic phase (G1) in dividing fibroblasts. Anesthesiology 1976; 45:413-20.
17. Sturrock J, Nunn JF. Cytotoxic effects of procaine, lignocaine and bupivacaine. Br J Anaesth 1979; 51:273-81.
18. Sullivan FM. General discussion. Pediatrics 1974; 53:798-9.
19. Wilson JG. Environment and Birth Defects. New York, Academic Press, 1973:1-82.
20. Moore KL. The Developing Human. Philadelphia, WB Saunders, 1988:143.
21. Shepard TH. Catalog of Teratogenic Agents. 7th ed. Baltimore, Md, The Johns Hopkins University Press, 1992.
22. Fujinaga M, Baden JM. Maternal and fetal effects of anesthesia. In: Healy TEJ, Cohen PJ, editors. A Practice of Anesthesia. Sevenoaks, Kent, England, Edward Arnold, 1995:400-17.
23. Roberts CJ, Lowe CR. Where have all the conceptions gone? Lancet 1975; 1:498-9.
24. Rushton DI. The nature and causes of spontaneous abortions with normal karyotypes. In: Kalter H, editor. Issues and Reviews in Teratology. Vol. 3. New York, Plenum Press, 1985:21-63.
25. Haring OM. Effects of prenatal hypoxia on the cardiovascular system in the rat. Arch Path 1965; 80:351-6.
26. Haring OM. Cardiac malformations in rats induced by exposure of the mother to carbon dioxide during pregnancy. Circ Res 1960; 8:1218-27.
27. Geber WF. Developmental effects of chronic maternal and audiovisual stress on the rat fetus. J Embryol Exp Morphol 1966; 16:1-16.
28. Grabowski CT. Teratogenic significance of ionic and fluid imbalance. Science 1963; 142:1064-5.
29. Levinson G, Shnider SM. Anesthesia for surgery during pregnancy. In: Shnider SM, Levinson G, editors. Anesthesia for Obstetrics. Baltimore, Md, Williams & Wilkins, 1993:259-80.
30. Mole RH. Radiation effects on prenatal development and their radiological significance. Br J Radiol 1979; 52:89-101.
31. Brent RL. The effects of embryonic and fetal exposure to x-ray, microwaves, and ultrasound. Clin Obstet Gynecol 1983; 26:484-510.
32. Geber WF, Schramm LC. Congenital malformations of the central nervous system produced by narcotic analgesics in the hamster. Am J Obstet Gynecol 1975; 123:705-13.
33. Jurand A. Malformations of the central nervous system induced by neurotropic drugs in mouse embryos. Dev Growth Differentiation 1980; 22:61-78.
34. Harpel HS, Gautieri RF. Morphine induced fetal malformations. I. Exencephaly and axial skeletal fusion. J Pharm Sci 1968; 57:1590-7.
35. Jurand A, Martin LVH. Teratogenic potential of two neurotropic drugs, haloperidol and dextromoramide, tested on mouse embryos. Teratology 1990; 42:45-54.
36. Ciociola AA, Gautieri RF. Evaluation of the teratogenicity of morphine sulfate administered via a miniature implantable minipump. J Pharm Sci 1983; 72:742-5.
37. Fujinaga M, Mazze RI. Teratogenic and postnatal developmental studies of morphine in Sprague-Dawley rats. Teratology 1988; 38:401-10.
38. Fujinaga M, Stevenson JB, Mazze RI. Reproductive and teratogenic effects of fentanyl in Sprague-Dawley rats. Teratology 1986; 34:51-7.

39. Fujinaga M, RI Mazze, EC Jackson, et al. Reproductive and teratogenic effects of sufentanil and alfentanil in Sprague-Dawley rats. Anesth Analg 1988; 67:166-9.

40. Martin LVH, Jurand A. The absence of teratogenic effects of some analgesics used in anaesthesia. Anaesthesia 1992; 47:473-6.

41. McColl JD, Globus M, Robinson S. Drug induced skeletal malformations in the rat. Experientia 1963; 19:183-4.

42. Finnel RH, Shields HE, Taylor SM, et al. Strain differences in phenobarbital-induced teratogenesis in mice. Teratology 1987; 35:177-85.

43. Tonge SR. Permanent alterations in catecholamine concentrations in discrete areas of brain in the offspring of rats treated with methylamphetamine and chlorpormazine. Br J Pharmacol 1973; 47:425-7.

44. Robson JM, Sullivan FM. The production of foetal abnormalities in rabbits by imipramine. Lancet 1963; 1:638-9.

45. Heinonen OP, Slone D, Shapiro S. Birth Defects and Drugs in Pregnancy. Littleton, Mass, Publishing Sciences Group, 1977.

46. Briggs GC, Freeman RK, Yaffe SJ. Drugs in Pregnancy and Lactation. 3rd ed. Baltimore, Md, Williams & Wilkins, 1990.

47. Milkovich L, Van den Berg BJ. Effects of prenatal meprobamate and chlordiazepoxide hydrochloride on human embryonic and fetal development. N Engl J Med 1974; 291:1268-71.

48. Hartz SC, Heinonen OP, Shapiro S, et al. Antenatal exposure to meprobamate and chlordiazepoxide in relation to malformations, mental development, and childhood mortality. N Engl J Med 1975; 292: 726-8.

49. Safra MJ, Oakley GP. Association between cleft lip with or without cleft palate and prenatal exposure to diazepam. Lancet 1975; 2:478-80.

50. Saxén I, Saxén L. Association between maternal intake of diazepam and oral clefts. Lancet 1975; 2:498.

51. Rosenberg L, Mitchell AA, Parsells JL, et al. Lack of correlation of oral clefts to diazepam use during pregnancy. N Engl J Med 1983; 309:1282-5.

52. Shiono PH, Mills JL. Oral clefts and diazepam use during pregnancy. N Engl J Med 1984; 311:919-20.

53. Weber LWD. Benzodiazepines in pregnancy: Academic debate or teratogenic risk? Biol Res Pregnancy 1985; 16:151-67.

54. Fujinaga M, Mazze RI. Reproductive and teratogenic effects of lidocaine in Sprague-Dawley rats. Anesthesiology 1986; 65:626-32.

55. Teiling AKY, Mohammed AK, Minor BG, et al. Lack of effects of prenatal exposure to lidocaine on development of behavior in rats. Anesth Analg 1987; 66:533-41.

56. Fujinaga M, Baden JM, Mazze RI. Developmental toxicity of nondepolarizing muscle relaxants in cultured rat embryos. Anesthesiology 1992; 76:999-1003.

57. Jacobs RM. Failure of muscle relaxants to produce cleft palate in mice. Teratology 1971; 4:25-30.

58. Skarpa M, Dayan AD, Follenfant M, et al. Toxicity testing of atracurium. Br J Anaesth 1983; 55:27S-9S.

59. Jago RH. Arthrogryposis following treatment of maternal tetanus with muscle relaxants. Arch Dis Child 1970; 45:227-9.

60. Basford A, Fink BR. Teratogenicity of halothane in the rat. Anesthesiology 1968; 29:1167-73.

61. Pope WDB, Halsey MJ, Lansdown ABG, et al. Fetotoxicity in rats following chronic exposure to halothane, nitrous oxide, or methoxyflurane. Anesthesiology 1978; 48:11-6.

62. Wharton RS, Mazze RI, Baden JM, et al. Fertility, reproduction and postnatal survival in mice chronically exposed to halothane. Anesthesiology 1978; 48:167-74.

63. Mazze RI. Fertility, reproduction, and postnatal survival in mice chronically exposed to isoflurane. Anesthesiology 1985; 63:663-7.

64. Wharton RS, Wilson AI, Mazze RI, et al. Fetal morphology in mice exposed to halothane. Anesthesiology 1979; 51:532-7.

65. Mazze RI, Wilson AI, Rice SA, et al. Fetal development in mice exposed to isoflurane. Teratology 1985; 32:339-45.

66. Wharton RS, Mazze RI, Wilson AI. Reproduction and fetal development in mice chronically exposed to enflurane. Anesthesiology 1981; 54:505-10.

67. Mazze RI, Fujinaga M, Rice SA, et al. Reproductive and teratogenic effects of nitrous oxide, halothane, isoflurane, and enflurane in Sprague-Dawley rats. Anesthesiology 1986; 64:339-44.

68. Fink BR, Shepard TH, Blandau RJ. Teratogenic activity of nitrous oxide. Nature 1967; 214:146-8.

69. Shephard TH, Fink BR. Teratogenic activity of nitrous oxide in rats. In: Fink BR, editor. Toxicity of Anesthetics. Baltimore, Md, Williams & Wilkins, 1968:308-23.

70. Bussard DA, Stoelting RK, Peterson C, et al. Fetal changes in hamsters anesthetized with nitrous oxide and halothane. Anesthesiology 1974; 41:275-8.

71. Mazze RI, Wilson AI, Rice SA, et al. Reproduction and fetal development in rats exposed to nitrous oxide. Teratology 1984; 30:259-65.

72. Lane GA, Nahrwold ML, Tait AR, et al. Anesthetics as teratogens: Nitrous oxide is teratogenic, xenon is not. Science 1980; 210:899-901.

73. Vieira E, Cleaton-Jones P, Austin JC. Effects of low concentrations of nitrous oxide on rat fetuses. Anesth Analg 1980; 59:175-7.

74. Fujinaga M, Baden JM, Mazze RI. Susceptible period of nitrous oxide teratogenicity in Sprague-Dawley rats. Teratology 1989; 40:439-44.

75. Fujinaga M, Baden JM, Shephard TH, et al. Nitrous oxide alters body laterality in rats. Teratology 1990; 41:131-5.

76. Fujinaga M, Baden JM. Critical period of rat development when sidedness of asymmetric body structures is determined. Teratology 1991; 44:453-62.

77. Baden JM, Fujinaga M. Effects of nitrous oxide on day 9 rat embryos grown in culture. Br J Anaesth 1991; 66:500-3.

78. Chanarin I. Cobalamins and nitrous oxide: A review. J Clin Pathol 1980; 33:909-16.

79. Koblin DD, Watson JE, Deady JE, et al. Inactivation of methionine synthetase by nitrous oxide in mice. Anesthesiology 1981; 54:318-24.

80. Koblin DD, Waskell L, Watson JE, et al. II. Nitrous oxide inactivates methionine synthetase in human liver. Anesth Analg 1982; 61:75-8.

81. Baden JM, Rice SA, Serra M, et al. Thymidine and methionine syntheses in pregnant rats exposed to nitrous oxide. Anesth Analg 1983; 62:738-41.

82. Baden JM, Serra M, Mazze RI. Inhibition of rat fetal methionine synthase by nitrous oxide. Br J Anaesth 1987; 59:1040-3.

83. Keeling PA, Rocke DA, Nunn JF, et al. Folinic acid protection against nitrous oxide teratogenicity in the rat. Br J Anaesth 1986; 58:528-34.

84. Mazze RI, Fujinaga M, Baden JM. Halothane prevents nitrous oxide teratogenicity in Sprague-Dawley rats; folinic acid does not. Teratology 1988; 38:121-7.

85. Fujinaga M, Baden JM, Yhap EO, et al. Reproductive and teratogenic effects of nitrous oxide, isoflurane, and their combination in Sprague-Dawley rats. Anesthesiology 1987; 67:960-4.

86. Fujinaga M, Baden JM. Methionine prevents nitrous oxide-induced teratogenicity in rat embryos grown in culture. Anesthesiology 1994; 81:184-9.

87. Fujinaga M, Baden JM. Evidence for an adrenergic mechanism in the control of body symmetry. Dev Biol 1991; 143:203-5.

88. Fujinaga M, Maze M, Hoffman BB, et al. Activation of alpha-1 adrenergic receptors modulates the control of left/right sidedness in rat embryos. Dev Biol 1992; 150:419-21.

89. Fujinaga M, Baden JM, Suto A, et al. Preventive effects of phenoxybenzamine on nitrous oxide-induced reproductive toxicity in Sprague-Dawley rats. Teratology 1991; 43:151-7.

90. Cohen EN, Belville JW, Brown BW. Anesthesia, pregnancy, and miscarriage: A study of operating room nurses and anesthetists. Anesthesiology 1971; 35:343-7.

91. Knill-Jones RP, Moir DD, Rodrigues LV, et al. Anaesthetic practice and pregnancy: Controlled survey of women anaesthetists in the United Kingdom. Lancet 1972; 2:1326-8.

92. Cohen EN, Brown BW, Bruce DL, et al. Occupational disease among operating room personnel: A national study. Anesthesiology 1974; 41:321-40.

93. Cohen EN, Brown BW, Wu ML, et al. Occupational disease in dentistry and chronic exposure to trace anesthetic gases. J Am Dent Assoc 1980; 101:21-31.

94. Spence AA, Cohen EN, Brown BW. Occupational hazards for operating room-based physicians. JAMA 1977; 283:955-9.

95. Buring JE, Hennekens CH, Mayrent SL, et al. Health experiences of operating room personnel. Anesthesiology 1985; 62:325-30.

96. Tannenbaum TN, Goldberg RJ. Exposure to anesthetic gases and reproductive outcome. J Occup Med 1985; 27:659-68.

97. Mazze RI, Lecky JH. The health of operating room personnel (editorial). Anesthesiology 1985; 62:226-8.

98. Harlap S, Shiono PH. Alcohol, smoking, and incidence of spontaneous abortions in the first and second trimesters. Lancet 1980; 2:173-6.

99. Kline J, Stein ZA, Susser M, et al. Smoking: A risk factor for spontaneous abortion. N Engl J Med 1977; 297:793-6.

100. Ericson HA, Källén B. Hospitalization for miscarriage and delivery outcome among Swedish nurses working in operating rooms 1973-1978. Anesth Analg 1985; 64:981-8.

101. Spence AA. Environmental pollution by inhalation anaesthetics. Br J Anaesth 1987; 59:96-103.

102. Brodsky JB, Cohen EN. Health experiences of operating room personnel. Anesthesiology 1985; 63:461-3.

103. Rowland AS, Baird DD, Weinberger CR, et al. Reduced fertility among women employed as dental assistants exposed to high levels of nitrous oxide. N Engl J Med 1992; 327:993-7.

104. Smith BE. Fetal prognosis after anesthesia during gestation. Anesth Analg 1963; 42:521-6.

105. Shnider SM, Webster GM. Maternal and fetal hazards of surgery during pregnancy. Am J Obstet Gynecol 1965; 92:891-900.

106. Crawford JS, Lewis M. Nitrous oxide in early human pregnancy. Anaesthesia 1986; 41:900-5.

107. Aldridge IM, Tunstall ME. Nitrous oxide and the fetus: A review and the results of a retrospective study of 175 cases of anaesthesia for insertion of a Shirodkar suture. Br J Anaesth 1986; 58:1348-56.

108. Duncan PG, Pope WDB, Cohen MM, et al. Fetal risk of anesthesia and surgery during pregnancy. Anesthesiology 1986; 64:790-4.

109. Cohen SE. Risk of abortion following general anesthesia for surgery during pregnancy: Anesthetic or surgical procedure (letter). Anesthesiology 1986; 65:706.

110. Källén B, Mazze RI. Neural tube defects and first trimester operations. Teratology 1990; 41:717-20.

111. Sylvester GC, Khoury MJ, Lu X, et al. First trimester anesthesia exposure and the risk of central nervous system defects: A population-based case-control study. Am J Public Health 1994; 84:1757-60.

112. Smith RF, Bowman RE, Katz J. Behavioral effects of exposure to halothane during early development in the rat. Anesthesiology 1978; 49:319-23.

113. Levin ED, Bowman RE. Behavioral effects of chronic exposure to low concentrations of halothane during development in rats. Anesth Analg 1986; 65:653-9.

114. Chalon J, Hillman D, Gross S, et al. Intrauterine exposure to halothane increases murine postnatal autotolerance to halothane and reduces brain weight. Anesth Analg 1983; 62:565-7.

115. Armitage SG. The effects of barbiturates on the behavior of rat offspring as measured in learning and reasoning situations. J Comp Physiol Psychol 1952; 45:146-52.

116. Chalon J, Walpert L, Ramanathan S, et al. Meperidine-promethazine combination and learning function of mice and of their progeny. Can Anaesth Soc J 1982; 29:612-6.

117. Hoffeld DR, McNew J, Webster RL. Effect of tranquilizing drugs during pregnancy on activity of offspring. Nature 1968; 218:357-8.

118. Jevtovic-Todorovic V, Hartman RE, Izumi Y, et al. Early exposure to common anesthetic agents causes widespread neurodegeneration in the developing rat brain and persistent learning deficits. J Neurosci 2003; 23:876-82.

119. Ikonomidou C, Bosch F, Miksa M, et al. Blockade of NMDA receptors and apoptotic neurodegeneration in the developing brain. Science 1999; 283:70-4.

120. Ishimaru MJ, Ikonomidou C, Tenkova TI, et al. Distinguishing excito-toxic from apoptotic neurodegeneration in the developing rat brain. J Comp Neurol 1999; 408:461-76.

121. Nyberg R, Westin B. The influence of oxygen tension and some drugs on human placental vessels. Acta Physiol Scand 1957; 39:216-27.

122. Panigel M. Placental perfusion experiments. Am J Obstet Gynecol 1962; 84:1664-83.

123. Khazin AF, Hon EH, Hehre FW. Effects of maternal hyperoxia on the fetus. I. Oxygen tension. Am J Obstet Gynecol 1971; 109:628-37.

124. Walker A, Maddern L, Day E, et al. Fetal scalp tissue oxygen tension measurements in relation to maternal dermal oxygen tension and fetal heart rate. J Obstet Gynecol Br Commonw 1971; 78:1-12.

125. McClaine RJ, Booth JV, Schultz JR, et al. Effects of maternal general anesthesia on fetal physiology (abstract). Anesthesiology 2003; 98:A1.

126. Motoyama EK, Rivard G, Acheson F, et al. The effect of changes in maternal pH and Pco_2 on the Po_2 of fetal lambs. Anesthesiology 1967; 28:891-903.

127. Kamban JR, Handte RE, Brown WU, et al. The effect of normal and preeclamptic pregnancies on the oxyhemoglobin dissociation curve. Anesthesiology 1986; 65:426-7.

128. Levinson G, Shnider SM, de Lorimier AA, et al. Effects of maternal hyperventilation on uterine blood flow and fetal oxygenation and acid-base status. Anesthesiology 1974; 40:340-7.

129. Brann AW, Myers RE. Central nervous system findings in the newborn monkey following severe in utero partial asphyxia. Neurology 1975; 25:327-38.

130. Donchin Y, Amirav B, Sahar A, et al. Sodium nitroprusside for aneurysm surgery in pregnancy. Br J Anaesth 1978; 50: 849-51.

131. Rigg D, McDonogh A. Use of sodium nitroprusside for deliberate hypotension during pregnancy. Br J Anaesth 1981; 53:985-7.

132. Newman B, Lam AM. Induced hypotension for clipping of a cerebral aneurysm during pregnancy. Anesth Analg 1986; 65:675-8.

133. Ralston DH, Shnider SM, de Lorimier AA. Effects of equipotent ephedrine, metaraminol, mephentermine and methoxamine on uterine blood flow in the pregnant ewe. Anesthesiology 1974; 40:354-70.

134. Greiss FC, Still JG, Anderson SG. Effects of local anesthetic agents on the uterine vasculature and myometrium. Am J Obstet Gynecol 1976; 124:889-99.

135. Shnider SM, Wright RG, Levinson G, et al. Uterine blood flow and plasma norepinephrine changes during maternal stress in the pregnant ewe. Anesthesiology 1979; 50:524-7.

136. Oats JN, Vasey DP, Waldron BA. Effects of ketamine on the pregnant uterus. Br J Anaesth 1979; 51:1163-6.

137. Mercier FJ, Riley ET, Frederickson WL, et al. Phenylephrine added to prophylactic ephedrine infusion during spinal anesthesia for elective cesarean section. Anesthesiology 2001; 95:668-74.

138. Lee A, Ngan Kee WD, Gin T. A quantitative, systematic review of randomized controlled trials of ephedrine versus phenylephrine for the management of hypotension during spinal anesthesia for cesarean delivery. Anesth Analg 2002; 94:920-6.

139. Cooper DW, Carpenter M, Mowbray P, et al. Fetal and maternal effects of phenylephrine and ephedrine during spinal anesthesia for cesarean delivery. Anesthesiology 2002; 97:1582-90.

140. Palahniuk RJ, Shnider SM. Maternal and fetal cardiovascular and acid-base changes during halothane and isoflurane anesthesia in the pregnant ewe. Anesthesiology 1974; 41:462-72.

141. Bachman CR, Biehl DR, Sitar D, et al. Isoflurane potency and cardiovascular effects during short exposures in the foetal lamb. Can Anaesth Soc J 1986; 33:41-7.

142. Palahniuk RJ, Doig GA, Johnson GN, et al. Maternal halothane anesthesia reduces cerebral blood flow in the acidotic sheep fetus. Anesth Analg 1980; 59:35-9.

143. Cheek DBC, Hughes SC, Dailey PA, et al. Effect of halothane on regional cerebral blood flow and cerebral metabolic oxygen consumption in the fetal lamb in utero. Anesthesiology 1987; 67:361-6.

144. Yarnell R, Biehl DR, Tweed WA, et al. The effect of halothane anaesthesia on the asphyxiated foetal lamb in utero. Can Anaesth Soc J 1983; 30:474-9.

145. Baker BW, Hughes SC, Shnider SM, et al. Maternal anesthesia and the stressed fetus: Effects of isoflurane on the asphyxiated fetal lamb. Anesthesiology 1990; 72:65-70.

146. Johnson ES, Colley PS. Effects of nitrous oxide and fentanyl anesthesia on fetal heart-rate variability intra-and postoperatively. Anesthesiology 1980; 52:429-30.

147. Katz JD, Hook R, Barash PG. Fetal heart rate monitoring in pregnant patients undergoing surgery. Am J Obstet Gynecol 1976; 125:267-9.

148. Liu PL, Warren TM, Ostheimer GW, et al. Foetal monitoring in parturients undergoing surgery unrelated to pregnancy. Can Anaesth Soc J 1985; 32:525-32.

149. Immer-Bansi A, Immer FF, Henle S, et al. Unnecessary emergency caesarean section due to silent CTG during anaesthesia? Br J Anaesth 2001; 87:791-3.

150. McNall PG, Jafarnia MR. Management of myasthenia gravis in the obstetrical patient. Am J Obstet Gynecol 1965; 93:518-25.

151. Hellman LM, Johnson HL, Tolles WE, et al. Some factors affecting the fetal heart rate. Am J Obstet Gynecol 1961; 82:1055-64.

152. Abboud T, Raya J, Sadri S, et al. Fetal and maternal cardiovascular effects of atropine and glycopyrrolate. Anesth Analg 1983; 62:426-30.

153. Clark RB, Brown MA, Lattin DL. Neostigmine, atropine and glycopyrrolate: Does neostigmine cross the placenta? Anesthesiology 1996; 84:450-2.

154. Naulty J, Cefalo RC, Lewis PE. Fetal toxicity of nitroprusside in the pregnant ewe. Am J Obstet Gynecol 1981; 139:708-11.

155. Ostman PL, Chestnut DH, Robillard JE, et al. Transplacental passage and hemodynamic effects of esmolol in the gravid ewe. Anesthesiology 1988; 69:738-41.

156. Eisenach JC, Castro MI. Maternally administered esmolol produces beta-adrenergic blockade and hypoxemia in sheep. Anesthesiology 1989; 71:718-22.

157. Larson CP Jr, Shuer LM, Cohen SE. Maternally administered esmolol decreases fetal as well as maternal heart rate. J Clin Anesth 1990; 2: 427-9.

158. Losasso TJ, Muzzi DA, Cucchiara RF. Response of fetal heart rate to maternal administration of esmolol. Anesthesiology 1991; 74:782-4.

159. Ducey JP, Knape KG. Maternal esmolol administration resulting in fetal distress and cesarean section in a term pregnancy. Anesthesiology 1992; 77:829-32.

160. Mazze RI, Källén B. Appendectomy during pregnancy: A Swedish registry study of 778 cases. Obstet Gynecol 1991; 77:835-40.

161. McKellar DP, Anderson CT, Boynton CJ, et al. Cholecystectomy during pregnancy without fetal loss. Surg Gynecol Obstet 1992; 174:465-8.

162. Ferguson JE II, Albright GA, Ueland K. Prevention of preterm labor following surgery. In: Baden JM, Brodsky JB, editors. The Pregnant Surgical Patient. Mount Kisco, NY, Futura Publishing, 1985:223-46.

163. Fainstat T, Bhat N. Surgical resolution of nonobstetric abdominal crises complicating pregnancy. In: Baden JM, Brodsky JB, editors. The Pregnant Surgical Patient. Mount Kisco, NY, Futura Publishing, 1985: 149-76.

164. Cherry SH. The pregnant patient: Need for surgery unrelated to pregnancy. Mount Sinai J Med 1991; 58:81-4.

165. Hehre FW. Hypothermia for operations during pregnancy. Anesth Analg 1965; 44:424-8.

166. Stånge K, Halldin M. Hypothermia in pregnancy. Anesthesiology 1983; 58:460-1.

167. Strickland RA, Oliver WC, Chantigian RC, et al. Anesthesia, cardiopulmonary bypass, and the pregnant patient. Mayo Clin Proc 1991; 66: 411-29.

168. Merritt WT, Dickstein R, Beattie C, et al. Liver transplantation during pregnancy: Anesthesia for two procedures in the same patient with successful outcome of pregnancy. Transplant Proc 1991; 23:1996-7.

169. Buckley TA, Yau GHM, Poon WS, et al. Caesarean section and ablation of a cerebral arterio-venous malformation. Anaesth Intensive Care 1990; 18:248-51.

170. Whitburn RH, Laishley RS, Jewkes DA. Anaesthesia for simultaneous caesarean section and clipping of intracerebral aneurysm. Br J Anaesth 1990; 64:642-5.

171. Baer JL, Reis RA, Arens RA. Appendicitis in pregnancy with changes in position and axis of normal appendix in pregnancy. JAMA 1932; 98:1359-64.

172. Babaknia A, Hossein P, Woodruff JD. Appendicitis during pregnancy. Obstet Gynecol 1977; 1:40-4.

173. Reedy MB, Galan HL, Richards WE. Laparoscopy during pregnancy. A survey of laparoendoscopic surgeons. J Reprod Med 1997; 42:33-8.

174. Fatum M, Rojansky N. Laparoscopic surgery during pregnancy. Obstet Gynecol Surv 2001; 56:50-9.

175. Reedy MB, Källén B, Kuehl TJ. Laparoscopy during pregnancy: A study of five fetal outcome parameters with use of the Swedish Health Registry. Am J Obstet Gynecol 1997: 177;673-9.

176. Affleck DG, Handrahan D, Egger MJ, et al. The laparoscopic management of appendicitis and cholelithiasis during pregnancy. Am J Surg 1999; 178:523-529.

177. Gouldman JW, Sticca RP, Rippon MB, et al. Laparoscopic cholecystomy in pregnancy. Am Surg 1998; 64:93-7.

178. Tazuke SI, Nezhat FR, Nezhat CH, et al. Laparoscopic management of pelvic pathology during pregnancy. J Am Assoc Gynecol Laparosc 1997; 4:605-8.

179. Gurbuz AT, Peetz ME. The acute abdomen in the pregnant patient. Is there a role for laparoscopy? Surg Endosc 1997; 11:98-102.

180. Wishner JD, Zolfaghari D, Wohlgemuth SD, et al. Laparoscopic cholecystectomy in pregnancy. A report of 6 cases and review of the literature. Surg Endosc 1996; 10:314-8.

181. Lemaire BM, van Erp WF. Laparoscopic surgery during pregnancy. Surg Endosc 1997; 11:15-18.

182. Eichenberg BJ, Vanderlinden J, Miguel C, et al. Laparoscopic cholecystectomy in the third trimester of pregnancy. Am Surg 1996; 62:874-7.

183. Amos JD, Schorr SJ, Norman PF, et al. Laparoscopic surgery during pregnancy. Am J Surg 1996; 171:435-7.

184. Costantino GN, Vincent GJ, Mukalian GG, et al. Laparoscopic cholecystectomy in pregnancy. J Laparoendosc Surg 1994; 4:161-4.

185. Steinbrook RA, Brooks DC, Datta S. Laparoscopic cholecystectomy during pregnancy. Surg Endosc 1996; 10:511-6.

186. Southerland LC, Duke T, Gollagher JM, et al. Cardiopulmonary effects of abdominal CO_2 insufflation in pregnancy: Fetal and maternal parameters in the sheep model (abstract). Can J Anaesth 1994; 41:A59.

187. Galan HL, Reedy MB, Bean JD, et al. Maternal and fetal effects of laparoscopic insufflation (abstract). Anesthesiology 1994; 81:A1159.

188. Cruz AM, Southerland LC, Duke T, et al. Intraabdominal carbon dioxide insufflation in the pregnant ewe. Anesthesiology 1996; 85:1395-1402.

189. Bhavani-Shankar K, Steinbrook RA, Brooks DC, et al. Arterial to end-tidal carbon dioxide pressure difference during laparoscopic surgery in pregnancy. Anesthesiology 2000; 93:370-3.

190. Barnard JM, Chaffin D, Droste S, et al. Fetal response to carbon dioxide peritoneum in the pregnant ewe. Obstet Gynecol 1995; 85:669-74.

191. Barnard J, Chaffin D, Phernetton T. Maternal and fetal effects of a prolonged CO_2 peritoneum in the gravid ewe (abstract). Am J Obstet Gynecol 1995; 172:320.

192. Steinbrook RA, Bhavani-Shankar K. Hemodynamics during laparoscopic surgery in pregnancy. Anesth Analg 2001; 93:1570-1.

193. Tanaka H, Futamura N, Takubo S, et al. Gasless laparoscopy under epidural anesthesia for adnexal cysts during pregnancy. J Reprod Med 1999;44:929-32.

194. Society of American Gastrointestinal Endoscopic Surgeons (SAGES). SAGES Guidelines for Laparoscopic Surgery During Pregnancy (October 2000). Available at: http://www.sages.org/sg_pub23.html. Accessed: September 22, 2003.

195. Repke JT, Berger NG. Electroconvulsive therapy in pregnancy. Obstet Gynecol 1984; 63:39S-41S.

196. Altshuler LL, Cohen L, Szuba MP, et al. Pharmacological management of psychiatric illness during pregnancy: Dilemmas and guidelines. Am J Psychiatry 1996; 153:592-605.

197. American Psychiatric Association: Task Force on ECT. The practice of ECT: Recommendations for treatment, training and privileging. Convuls Ther 1990; 6:85-120.

198. Moreno ME, Muñoz JM, Valderrabanos JS, et al. Electroconvulsive therapy in the first trimester of pregnancy. J ECT 1998; 14:251-4.

199. Miller LJ. Use of electroconvulsive therapy during pregnancy. Hosp Comm Psych 1994; 45:444-50.

200. Ishikawa T, Kawahara S, Saito T, et al. Anesthesia for electroconvulsive therapy during pregnancy: A case report. Masui 2001; 50:991-7.

201. Rabheru K. The use of electroconvulsive therapy in special patient populations. Can J Psych 2001; 46:710-9.

202. Biehl DR. Foetal monitoring during surgery unrelated to pregnancy. Can Anaesth Soc J 1985; 32:455-9.

203. Pederson H, Morishima HO, Finster M. Anesthesia for the pregnant woman undergoing surgery. Semin Anaesth 1982; 1:177-83.

204. American College of Obstetricians and Gynecologists Committee on Obstetric Practice. Nonobstetric Surgery in Pregnancy. ACOG Committee Opinion No. 284, August 2003.

Part VI
Labor and Vaginal Delivery

Medical and social connotations of pain have evolved through history. Since 1847 these interpretations often influenced obstetric anesthesia. During most of the nineteenth century, patients and physicians believed that an individual's physical sensitivity to pain varied with education, social standing, and acculturation. Like the princess in Grimm's fairy tale who could feel a pea through 40 mattresses, refined women experienced more pain than "savages." As American suffragette Elizabeth Cady Stanton observed, "refined, genteel, civilized women have worse labor pain." Commenting on her own nearly painless delivery, Stanton once quipped, "Am I not almost a savage?" Upper class women often cited their sensitivity to pain as evidence of cultural superiority, and they used this fact to justify their need for obstetric anesthesia.[1]

As the nineteenth century came to a close, the social connotations of the pain also changed. Many still maintained that civilized women experienced more pain than savages. On the other hand, "sensitivity" to pain now began to signify physical deterioration rather than cultural superiority. Thus one medical book published in 1882 ascribed painful labor to "the abuses of civilization, its dissipations, and the follies of fashion." Its author, an American obstetrician named Engelmann, suggested that the idle life of upper class women led to a "relaxed condition of the uterus and abdominal walls (and) a greater tendency to malposition." He suggested that the rigorous physical life of lower class women and "savages" prepared their bodies better for childbirth.[2]

Social and cultural interpretations of childbirth pain took yet another turn in 1943, with publication of the book Revelation of Childbirth. Its author, Grantly Dick-Read, subsequently republished his book in the United States with the title, Childbirth Without Fear. It marked the beginning of the natural childbirth movement.

Dick-Read combined snippets of ideas from earlier concepts to formulate his own theory. He agreed with early nineteenth century physiologists that savages have less pain than "modern women." Unlike Engelmann, Dick-Read attributed this sensitivity to cultural rather than physical factors. According to Dick-Read, modern women had painful deliveries only because the church and culture had taught them to expect it. He said that women should be reeducated and taught that childbirth is a natural physiologic process. He opined that women would then cease to fear childbirth and thereby have less pain. Dick-Read's method, the basis for childbirth education, was a prenatal program that toughened the body with exercise and prepared the mind with facts. In yet another variation, French obstetrician Fernand Lamaze substituted Pavlovian conditioning for Dick-Read's childbirth education.[3] With Dick-Read and Lamaze, many of the social concepts of childbirth pain came full circle.

Donald Caton, M.D.

REFERENCES

1. Lawrence C. The nervous system and society in the Scottish enlightenment. In Barnes B, Shapin S, editors. Natural Order in Historical Studies of Scientific Culture. London, Sage Publications, 1979:19-40.
2. Engelmann GJ. Labor Among Primitive Peoples: Showing the Development of the Obstetric Science of Today from the Natural and Instinctive Customs of all Races, Civilized and Savage, Past and Present. St. Louis, JH Chambers, 1882:130.
3. Dick-Read G. Revelation of Childbirth. London, Heinemann, 1943.

Chapter 17

Obstetric Management of Labor and Vaginal Delivery

Dwight J. Rouse, M.D., M.S.P.H. · Frank J. Zlatnik, M.D.

THE PROCESS OF LABOR AND DELIVERY

Labor, which is also called parturition, is the physiologic process by which sufficiently frequent and strong uterine contractions cause thinning (i.e., effacement) and dilation of the cervix, thereby permitting passage of the fetus from the uterus through the birth canal.

Onset of Labor

TIMING

Fewer than 10% of pregnancies end on the expected date of delivery (EDD), but the majority of births occur within 7 days of the EDD. In the United States, approximately 10% of births occur preterm (before 37 weeks' gestation), and approximately 5% of carefully dated pregnancies remain undelivered at 42 weeks' gestation (14 days after the EDD).

MECHANISM

The cause of the onset of labor in women—either term or preterm—remains unknown. In other mammalian species, a decline in serum progesterone in association with increasing estrogen concentrations is followed by increased prostaglandin production, an increase in oxytocin receptors, and an increase in myometrial gap junction formation. In sheep, the fetus apparently triggers parturition by a surge in fetal cortisol production. In women, progesterone concentrations do not fall before the onset of labor, and no surge in fetal cortisol secretion occurs. The laboring human uterus does manifest increased prostaglandin production, an increase in oxytocin receptors, and increased myometrial gap junction formation.[1,2] As more is learned, it is likely that the apparent interspecies discrepancies will be resolved and that a unifying concept of the onset of mammalian labor will emerge. Preterm and post-term deliveries both constitute important obstetric problems, and when more is understood about the mechanism of the onset of labor, new approaches to preventing the preterm and post-term onset of parturition may evolve.

Stages of Labor

By convention, labor is divided into three stages. The first stage begins with the maternal perception of regular, painful uterine contractions and ends with the complete dilation of the cervix. Complete cervical dilation is the dilation necessary to allow movement of the fetus from the uterus into the vagina. At term gestation, 10 cm approximates complete cervical dilation. Preterm fetuses require less than 10 cm cervical dilation. The second stage of labor begins with the complete dilation of the cervix and ends with the birth of the baby. The third stage begins with the birth of the baby and ends with the delivery of the placenta. The first stage of labor can be considered the *cervical* stage, the second stage the *pelvic* stage (reflecting the descent of the fetus through the pelvis), and the third stage the *placental* stage.

Components of Labor and Delivery

When the events that occur during labor and vaginal delivery are considered, it is helpful to think about the three components of the process: (1) the **powers** (uterine contractions and, in the second stage, the addition of voluntary maternal expulsive efforts); (2) the **passageway** (the bony pelvis and the soft tissues contained therein); and (3) the **passenger** (the fetus). The interaction of these three components determines the success or failure of the process.

THE POWERS

The uterus, which is a smooth-muscle organ, contracts throughout gestation with variable frequency. The parturient verifies the onset of labor when she perceives regular, uncomfortable uterine contractions. In some women, the uterus remains relatively quiescent until the abrupt onset of labor. In others, the uterus contracts several times per hour for days without causing pain or even a clear perception of uterine contractions.

During labor, the frequency, duration, and intensity of uterine contractions increase. During early labor, the contractions may occur every 5 to 7 minutes, last 30 to 40 seconds, and develop intrauterine pressures of 20 to 30 mm Hg above basal tone (10 to 15 mm Hg). Late in the first stage of labor, contractions typically occur every 2 to 2½ minutes, last 50 to 70 seconds, and are of 40 to 60 mm Hg intensity. This increased intensity reflects a more widespread propagation of the contractions, with the recruitment of increased numbers of myometrial cells.

Retraction accompanies contraction as the myometrial cells shorten. The walls of the upper, contractile portion of the uterus thicken. Cervical dilation and effacement reflect the traction placed on the cervix by the contracting uterus. The passive lower uterine segment enlarges and becomes thinner as cervical tissue is pulled over the fetal presenting part by traction from the upper portion of the uterus. At the end of the first stage of labor, no cervix is palpable on vaginal examination. Additional uterine contractions force the fetus to descend through the birth canal, assuming there is no mechanical obstruction. At this time, the parturient perceives an urge to defecate. Her expulsive efforts add to the force of uterine contractions to hasten descent and shorten the second stage of labor.

THE PASSAGEWAY

The fetus must be of such size and conformation that there is no mechanical mismatch with the bony pelvis. (At times, an ovarian or uterine tumor [e.g., leiomyoma], cervical cancer, or a vaginal septum may impede passage of the fetus through the birth canal, but these situations are unusual.)

Four pelvic types have been described on the basis of the shape of the pelvic inlet (the plane bounded by the upper inner pubic symphysis, the linea terminalis of the iliac bones, and the sacral promontory) (Table 17-1).[3] The type and size of the pelvis constitute important predictors of the success of vaginal delivery.

The most common pelvic type and the one best suited for childbirth is the **gynecoid** pelvis. The flexed fetal head presents a circle to the bony pelvis; a pelvis with gynecoid features best accommodates this circle. The inlet is round or oval, with the transverse diameter only slightly greater than the anterior-posterior diameter. The pelvic sidewalls are straight and do not converge, the ischial spines are not prominent, the sacrum is hollow, and the subpubic arch is wide. The absence of prominent ischial spines is an important feature, because the distance between them—the transverse diameter of the midpelvis—is the narrowest pelvic dimension. The other pelvic types are less favorable for vaginal delivery.

Although radiographic pelvimetry provides much more information regarding pelvic dimensions and features than can be obtained by clinical pelvimetry alone, it has only a limited place in clinical management. In the absence of a history of pelvic fracture or musculoskeletal disease (e.g., a dwarfing condition), there are few circumstances in which the apparent pelvic anatomy precludes a trial of labor. A pelvis with smaller-than-average dimensions may be adequate for a particular fetus if the head is well-flexed, sufficient molding (i.e., overlapping of the unfused skull bones) has occurred, and the labor is strong; thus radiographic pelvimetry does not always predict the presence or absence of cephalopelvic disproportion.[4] Further, there is some risk associated with radiographic pelvimetry. In addition to the potential for point mutations in the maternal oocytes and fetal germ cells, there is a small but apparently real increase in the incidence of malignancy and leukemia in children who were exposed to diagnostic radiation in utero. Some obstetricians continue to use radiographic pelvimetry in cases of fetal breech presentation. The hope is to save a parturient from a long, futile labor and a hazardous delivery. Computed tomography is associated with less radiation exposure than traditional radiographic pelvimetry.

THE PASSENGER

Fetal size and the relationship of the fetus to the maternal pelvis affect labor progress. The **lie** of the fetus (the relationship of the long axis of the fetus to the long axis of the mother) can be either transverse or longitudinal. In the former, vaginal delivery is impossible unless the fetus is very immature.

The **presentation** denotes that portion of the fetus overlying the pelvic inlet. The presentation may be cephalic, breech, or shoulder. Cephalic presentations are further subdivided into vertex, brow, or face presentations, according to the degree of flexion of the neck. In more than 95% of labors at term, the presentation is cephalic, and the fetal head is well flexed (i.e., vertex presentation).

The **position** of the fetus denotes the relationship of a specific fetal bony point to the maternal pelvis. In vertex presentations, that bony point is the occiput. During vaginal examination, palpation of the lambdoidal sutures permits determination of the fetal position. Positions of the occiput in early labor are listed in Box 17-1.

Other markers for position include the sacrum for the breech presentation, the mentum for the face presentation, and the acromion for the shoulder presentation. (See Chapter 35 for a discussion of nonvertex presentations.)

TABLE 17-1	FEATURES DETERMINED BY CLINICAL PELVIMETRY RELATED TO PELVIC TYPE			
	Pelvic Type			
Suboptimal Features	**Gynecoid**	**Android**	**Anthropoid**	**Platypelloid**
Promontory reached (diagonal conjugate ≤ 12 cm)	−	±	−	+
Sacrum flat/forward (versus curved)	−	+	−	+
Spines prominent (found by medical student)	−	+	+	−
Sacrosciatic notch narrow (≤ 2 fingerbreadths)	−	+	−	−
Subpubic arch narrow (acute angle)	−	+	+	−

+, Present; −, absent; ±, variable.

From Zlatnik FJ. Normal labor and delivery and its conduct. In Scott JR, DiSaia PJ, Hammond CB, Spellacy WN, editors. Danforth's Obstetrics and Gynecology. 6th ed. Philadelphia, JB Lippincott, 1990;161-88.

THE MECHANISM OF LABOR

The mechanism of labor refers to the changes in fetal conformation and position that occur during descent through the birth canal during the late first stage and second stage of labor (Box 17-2).

The first cardinal movement is **engagement**. Engagement denotes passage of the biparietal diameter (BPD) (i.e., the widest transverse diameter of the fetal head) through the plane of the pelvic inlet. A direct clinical determination of engagement cannot be made, but obstetricians assume that engagement has occurred if the leading bony point of the fetal head is palpable at the level of the ischial spines. This is true because the distance between the leading bony point and the BPD is typically less than the distance between the ischial spines and the plane of the pelvic inlet. If the leading bony point is at the level of the spines, the vertex is said to be at *zero station*. If the leading bony point is 1 cm *above* the level of the spines, the station is designated as −1. Similarly, +1, +2, and +3 indicate that the leading bony point is 1, 2, or 3 cm *below* the ischial spines (Figure 17-1). At +5 station, delivery is imminent. Station refers to palpation of the leading *bony* point. Often marked edema of the scalp (e.g., caput succedaneum) occurs during labor. In such cases, the bony skull may be 2 to 3 cm higher than the scalp.

The second cardinal movement is **descent,** although it is artificial to separate descent from the other movements, because descent occurs throughout the birth process.

The third cardinal movement is **flexion**. A very small fetus can negotiate the average maternal pelvis without increased flexion. However, under the usual circumstances at term, the force from above and resistance from below enhance flexion of the occiput (Figure 17-2).

The fourth cardinal movement is **internal rotation**. At the level of the midpelvis, the fetus meets the narrowest pelvic dimension, which is the transverse diameter between the ischial spines. Because the BPD of the fetal head is slightly smaller than the suboccipitobregmatic diameter, in most labors the vertex negotiates the midpelvis with the sagittal suture in an anterior-posterior direction. If this did not occur, a larger-than-necessary diameter would be forced to pass through the narrowest portion of the pelvis. Internal rotation describes the change in the position of the vertex from occiput transverse or oblique to anterior-posterior. The occiput tends to rotate to the roomiest part of the pelvis; thus, in gynecoid pelves, the fetus is delivered as an occiput anterior.

The final cardinal movement is **extension**, which occurs as the fetal head delivers (Figure 17-3). Subsequently, the occiput rotates to the side of the back as the shoulders pass through the midpelvis in an oblique diameter. The anterior shoulder moves under the pubic symphysis. With gentle downward traction, it passes from the birth canal, and expulsion of the remainder of the fetus occurs.

This description recounts events in the typical gynecoid pelvis. Abnormalities of the pelvis affect the mechanism of labor in specific ways. In an **anthropoid** pelvis, the anterior-posterior diameter of the pelvic inlet exceeds the transverse diameter. Often internal rotation to the occiput posterior position rather than the occiput anterior position occurs.

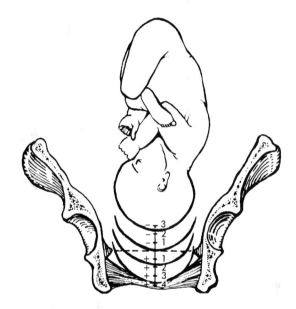

FIGURE 17-1. Stations of the fetal head. (From Zlatnik FJ. Normal labor and delivery and its conduct. In Scott JR, DiSaia PJ, Hammond CB, Spellacy WN, editors. Danforth's Obstetrics and Gynecology. 7th ed. Philadelphia, JB Lippincott, 1994:116.)

Box 17-1 POSITIONS OF THE OCCIPUT IN EARLY LABOR, LISTED BY DECREASING FREQUENCY

1. Left occiput transverse (LOT)
2. Right occiput transverse (ROT)
3. Left occiput anterior (LOA)
4. Right occiput posterior (ROP)
5. Right occiput anterior (ROA)
6. Left occiput posterior (LOP)
7. Occiput anterior (OA)
8. Occiput posterior (OP)

Box 17-2 THE CARDINAL MOVEMENTS OF LABOR

- Engagement
- Descent
- Flexion
- Internal rotation
- Extension

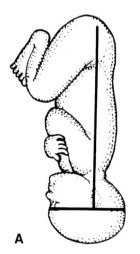
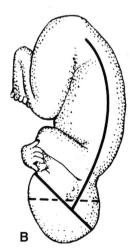

A   **B**

FIGURE 17-2. A, Relation of the head to the vertebral column before flexion. **B,** Relation of the head to the vertebral column after flexion. (From Zlatnik FJ. Normal labor and delivery and its conduct. In Scott JR, DiSaia PJ, Hammond CB, Spellacy WN, editors. Danforth's Obstetrics and Gynecology. 6th ed. Philadelphia, JB Lippincott, 1990:174.)

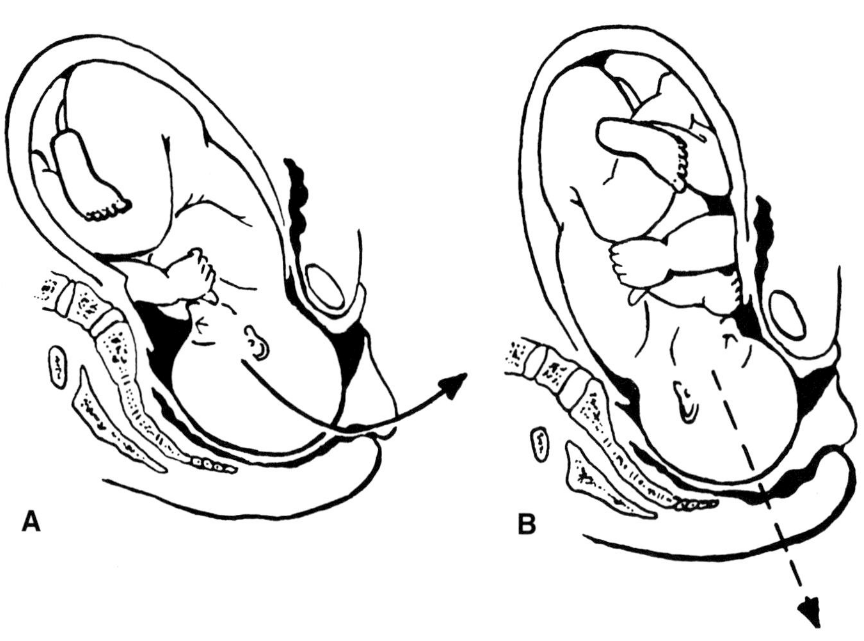

FIGURE 17-3. Vertex presentations. **A,** Occiput anterior position. **B,** Occiput posterior position. (From Zlatnik FJ. Normal labor and delivery and its conduct. In Scott JR, DiSaia PJ, Hammond CB, Spellacy WN, editors. Danforth's Obstetrics and Gynecology. 6th ed. Philadelphia, JB Lippincott, 1990:174.)

Because the pelvis is narrow transversely, further descent of the vertex occurs with the occiput in the posterior position. Delivery occurs with the occiput in the posterior position, or rotation to the occiput anterior position occurs just before delivery. In cases of persistent occiput posterior position, delivery occurs by flexion rather than extension of the fetal head (Figure 17-3).

In **platypelloid** pelves, internal rotation may not take place. The widest diameter is the transverse diameter, and descent of the vertex may occur with the occiput in the transverse position; rotation to the occiput anterior position occurs only at delivery.

Clinical Course

ADMISSION

When a patient enters the labor and delivery unit, the first question that must be asked is, "Why?" Did she come because of regular, painful uterine contractions; decreased fetal activity; vaginal bleeding; ruptured membranes; or some other reason? If the tentative diagnosis is labor, is she at term?

The time of the onset of labor and the presumed status of the membranes should be determined. Observation of the patient's demeanor coupled with the assessment of cervical effacement and dilation will signal whether the patient is in early or advanced labor. Examination of the cervix is deferred in patients with vaginal bleeding, unless placenta previa has been ruled out. Cervical examination may also be deferred in patients with premature rupture of membranes and no labor.

The obstetrician also directs attention to the second patient: the fetus. Abdominal examination is used to establish presentation and an estimate of fetal size. With most obstetric services, external electronic fetal heart rate (FHR) monitoring is used on admission to assess fetal condition. The baseline rate and variability and the presence or absence of accelerations and decelerations are of interest.

SUBSEQUENT CARE

The maternal vital signs and FHR are recorded periodically. In some obstetric services, continuous electronic FHR is used universally; with other services, it is monitored by intermit-

tent auscultation in low-risk patients. Recording the FHR every 30 minutes in the first part of the first stage of labor, every 15 minutes in the latter part of the first stage, and every 5 minutes in the second stage is perfectly acceptable. During early labor, the patient may ambulate or assume any position of comfort on the labor bed or in a chair. During advanced labor, women choose to lie down. Choices concerning analgesia or anesthesia are made according to the patient's wishes. Figure 17-4 shows a flow sheet that may be useful for physician charting during labor.

During labor, those providing obstetric care must focus on two critical questions. First, is the fetus tolerating labor in a satisfactory fashion, or is there fetal distress (see Chapter 8)? Second, is the labor progress normal?

LABOR PROGRESS: THE FRIEDMAN CURVE

One of the central tasks of those providing intrapartum care is to determine whether labor is progressing normally and, if not, to determine the significance of the delay and what the response should be. Parity is an important determinant of labor length. (Parity refers to previous pregnancies of at least 20 weeks' gestation. A pregnant woman who is gravida 2, para 1 is pregnant for the second time, and her first pregnancy resulted in delivery after 20 weeks' gestation.) Unpublished data from the University of Iowa Hospitals and Clinics indicate that approximately 50% of nulliparous women and more than 75% of parous women deliver within 12 hours of the spontaneous onset of labor; 8% of nulliparous women and only 2% of parous women remain undelivered at 24 hours.

A generation of obstetricians is indebted to Emanuel Friedman, whose landmark studies of labor provide a framework for judging labor progress. Friedman's approach was straightforward: He graphed cervical dilation on the y axis and elapsed time on the x axis for thousands of labors. He considered nulliparous and parous patients separately, and he determined the statistical limits of normal (Table 17-2).[5]

The curve of cervical dilation over time is S-shaped (Figure 17-5). Most consider Friedman's most important contribution to be his separation of the latent phase from the active phase of the first stage of labor. Many hours of regular, painful uterine contractions may take place with little appreciable

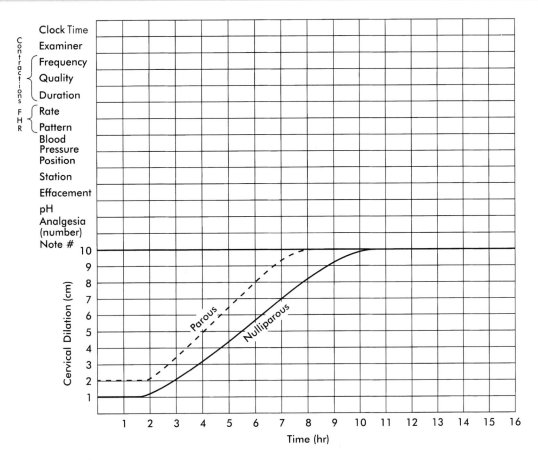

FIGURE 17-4. Flowsheet for charting labor progress. (From Zlatnik FJ. Normal labor and delivery and its conduct. In Scott JR, DiSaia PJ, Hammond CB, Spellacy WN, editors. Danforth's Obstetrics and Gynecology. 7th ed. Philadelphia, JB Lippincott, 1994:107.)

TABLE 17-2	LABOR LENGTH			
Stage of Labor	**Mean**	**Median**	**Mode**	**Limit**
Nulliparous				
First stage (hr)	14.4	12.3	9.5	—
Latent phase (hr)	8.6	7.5	6.0	20
Active phase (hr)	4.9	4.0	3.0	12
Maximum slope (cm/hr)	3.0	2.7	1.5	1.2
Second stage (hr)	1.0	0.8	0.6	2.5
Parous				
First stage (hr)	7.7	6.5	5.1	—
Latent phase (hr)	5.3	4.5	3.5	14
Active phase (hr)	2.2	1.8	1.5	5.2
Maximum slope (cm/hr)	5.7	5.2	4.5	1.5
Second stage (hr)	0.2	0.2	0.1	0.8

Important limits are enclosed in boxes; see text for discussion.
Modified from Zlatnik FJ. Normal labor and delivery and its conduct. In Scott JR, DiSaia PJ, Hammond CB, Spellacy WN, editors. Danforth's Obstetrics and Gynecology. 6th ed. Philadelphia, JB Lippincott, 1990:161-88.

change in the cervix. During this latent (or preparatory) phase, the cervix may efface and become softer. Quite abruptly, the active (or dilation) phase begins, and regular increases in cervical dilation are expected over time. The transition from the latent to the active phase of the first stage of labor does not occur at an arbitrary cervical dilation but rather is known—*in retrospect*—by the change of slope in the

cervical dilation curve. Peisner and Rosen[6] evaluated the progress of labor for 1060 nulliparous women and 639 parous women. When they excluded women with protracted or arrested labor, they noted that 60% of the women had reached the latent-active phase transition by 4 cm and 89% by 5 cm of cervical dilation.

A *nulliparous* woman may labor for 20 hours without achieving appreciable cervical dilation; 14 hours is the limit of the latent phase in the *parous* woman. Difficulty in assigning length to the latent phase lies not with its end (determined by the change in slope of the cervical dilation curve) but rather with its beginning. The onset of labor is self-reported by the parturient. The uterus contracts throughout gestation, and the degree of prelabor uterine activity and its perception are variable. Often both the patient and the physician are uncertain as to exactly when labor started.

According to Friedman, in the active phase of the first stage of labor, a nulliparous woman's cervix should dilate at a rate of at least 1.2 cm per hour, and a parous woman's cervix should dilate at least 1.5 cm per hour. (The slopes of the dilation curves in Figure 17-4 represent these lower limits of normal.) If a woman's cervix fails to dilate at the appropriate rate during the active phase of labor, she is said to have **primary dysfunctional labor.** Graphically, her cervical dilation "falls off the curve." If cervical dilation ceases during a 2-hour period in the active phase of labor, a **secondary arrest of dilation** has occurred. More contemporary studies have reported slower rates of cervical dilation and the absence of a deceleration phase.[7,8]

Abnormalities of the latent phase and active phase differ in associated factors, apparent etiologies, and significance.

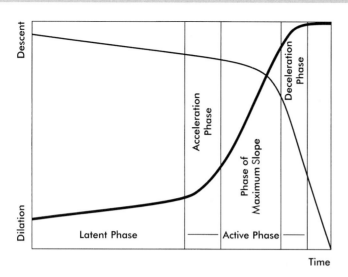

FIGURE 17-5. The Friedman curve. (From Friedman EA. Patterns of labor as indicators of risk. Clin Obstet Gynecol 1973; 16:172-83.)

A prolonged latent phase is more likely if labor begins "before the cervix is ready."[5,9] Just as there is a wide range of prelabor uterine activity, so too is there a wide range of cervical softness, effacement, and dilation at the start of labor. In some women, appreciable cervical softening, effacement, and dilation take place in late pregnancy; thus, when clinical labor begins, the cervix may already be 3 to 4 cm dilated and completely effaced. Alternatively, in other women, there is no cervical effacement or dilation at the start of labor. Given these differences, it is not surprising that varying amounts of uterine contractile work are needed to cause dilation of the cervix. The most common factor associated with a prolonged latent phase is an "unripe" cervix at the start of labor. Some women with a prolonged latent phase are not in true labor at all but are in "false labor"; this diagnosis is made in retrospect. After hours of regular, painful contractions, uterine activity may cease without appreciable cervical dilation having occurred. Several hours or days later, the patient reappears in true labor. During the latent phase of labor, it is not known with certainty whether a woman is in true or false labor.

A prolonged latent phase alone is not associated with fetal distress or cephalopelvic disproportion. However, primary dysfunctional labor and arrest of dilation during the active phase may indicate cephalopelvic disproportion.[5,10,11] Friedman's original work suggested that an arrest of dilation during the active phase was associated with the need for cesarean delivery nearly half of the time. More recent studies suggest a lower percentage, but it is clear that women who experience active-phase arrest of dilation are more likely to require abdominal delivery than women with normal labor progress during the active phase. Friedman's analysis suggested that active phase abnormalities pose a threat to the fetus, especially if they are combined with operative vaginal delivery.[12] A more recent study of women who delivered in this era of electronic FHR monitoring and decreased frequency of midforceps deliveries suggested that arrest disorders by themselves do not have adverse perinatal consequences.[11]

In summary, the prevailing view is that delays in the latent phase of the first stage of labor do not predict fetopelvic disproportion or the need for cesarean delivery, although conflicting data exist.[13] By contrast, delays in the active phase do predict fetopelvic disproportion, although not with precision. Given current obstetric practice and fetal monitoring tech-

niques, it is unlikely that first-stage labor abnormalities are intrinsically associated with neonatal depression at delivery.

AMNIOTOMY

The intact chorioamniotic membranes serve as the vessel that contains the amniotic fluid and helps protect the uterine contents from the microbial flora of the vagina. The amniotic fluid provides mechanical protection for the fetus and umbilical cord and allows growth and movement.

In the absence of intervention, the membranes generally rupture at the onset of labor or near full cervical dilation. If the membranes are intact, should they be artificially ruptured during the course of labor? If so, when? Because there is concern regarding infection once the membranes are ruptured, the performance of an amniotomy commits the mother to delivery. Because of this, it should not be done during the latent phase of labor, except in one of two circumstances: (1) there is an indication for effecting delivery; and/or (2) the patient is close to her EDD, the cervix is favorable, and the physician can confidently predict that labor will progress easily. Advantages of amniotomy during the active phase of the first stage of labor are that the ruptured membranes permit the placement of a fetal ECG electrode, which can provide more consistent information than external FHR monitoring; the amniotic fluid can be inspected for the presence or absence of meconium; and amniotomy shortens the first stage of labor.[14,15] Disadvantages of amniotomy during the active phase of the first stage of labor are that it may result in increased scalp edema (i.e., caput succedaneum, which has no clinical significance) and that there may be an increased likelihood of variable decelerations of the FHR. If there is a nonvertex presentation or the vertex is high in the pelvis and not well applied to the cervix, amniotomy is deferred to decrease the risk of prolapse of the umbilical cord.

SECOND STAGE OF LABOR

When the cervix has been completely retracted to form the lower uterine segment and is therefore not palpable on vaginal examination, full or complete dilation has been achieved, and the second stage of labor begins. Strong uterine contractions coupled with voluntary expulsive efforts by the parturient cause the fetal presenting part to descend through the pelvis, which results in delivery. At complete cervical dilation, there is frequently an increase in bloody show, the parturient may vomit, and, in the absence of anesthesia, she may complain that she needs to defecate. This sensation of needing to "bear down" encourages strong Valsalva maneuvers during uterine contractions. The effect of this sensation on the efficiency of "pushing" efforts during the second stage is reflected by the recent suggestion that acceptable durations of the second stage vary not only by parity but also by the presence or absence of epidural anesthesia.[16] A second stage longer than 2 hours in length may be considered prolonged for a nulliparous woman without epidural anesthesia, but 3 hours are granted if the patient has epidural anesthesia. For the parous patient the time limits are 1 and 2 hours, respectively.

The contemporary obstetrician is less concerned about the elapsed time during the second stage of labor than were earlier obstetricians. A generation ago, the teaching was that a long second stage meant trouble.[17] It often did, for at least two reasons. First, if cephalopelvic disproportion existed, the second stage was prolonged; this often resulted in a difficult operative vaginal delivery and serious fetal trauma. Second, cord compression may become severe with descent of the presenting part during the second stage of labor. If FHR monitoring was not performed conscientiously, considerable fetal/neonatal distress occurred in association with delayed delivery. Although the cord arterial pH varies inversely with the length of the second stage of labor,[18] the contemporary view is that the second stage of labor does not need to be terminated at any arbitrary time interval provided progress in descent continues and the FHR pattern does not indicate fetal distress. Clearly it is inappropriate to perform a difficult forceps delivery or vacuum extraction simply because an arbitrary time limit has elapsed.[19]

If the parturient is allowed to choose her own positions during labor and delivery, she does not stay in one place.[20] Without instruction from birth attendants, the parturient frequently chooses to walk or sit in a chair during early labor. Late in the first stage, however, she often returns to the labor bed. During the second stage of labor, some women assume the squatting position, whereas others, with their legs supported by the nurse and the father of the baby, assume a semi-sitting position. The goal is to achieve a position in which the parturient's bearing-down efforts are most effective. The patient should avoid the supine position, which results in aortocaval compression. Aortocaval compression seems to be less severe with the patient in the semi-sitting position, and it is avoided altogether with the patient in the left lateral position. Indeed, it is perfectly acceptable for the patient to push and deliver while remaining in the left lateral position. A vaginal examination during a contraction may provide information as to which position is best for a particular individual.

As the fetal head distends the perineum shortly before delivery, an episiotomy may be cut. This incision extends directly posteriorly from six o'clock (midline), or it extends in a 45-degree angle to either side (mediolateral). The former causes less discomfort, is more anatomic, and is easier to repair than the latter. The mediolateral episiotomy's advantage is that extension through the anal sphincter and rectal mucosa is less likely to occur, but its major disadvantage is that it may cause severe postpartum pain. (If the patient has an epidural catheter in place, the anesthesiologist may give additional local anesthetic or opioid epidurally to provide postpartum analgesia.)

The place of episiotomy in contemporary obstetrics is controversial.[21] For most of this century, episiotomy was advocated not only to shorten labor but also to protect the woman against the subsequent development of uterine prolapse, cystocele, and rectocele. An episiotomy hastens delivery, but only by a few minutes. Pelvic relaxation probably reflects the passage of the fetus through the levator sling rather than the presence or absence of an episiotomy at delivery. Tears involving the anal sphincter (third degree) and rectal mucosa (fourth degree) are more common after midline episiotomy than if episiotomy is not performed; in the absence of an episiotomy, however, anterior periurethral lacerations are almost inevitable. Although the latter rarely cause immediate problems, it is unknown whether they have any long-term effects on urethral support. No long-term scientifically valid data exist to help with obstetric decision making. Given the recognized association between midline episiotomies and third- and fourth-degree tears and the recognition that these tears may be associated with long-term morbidity, episiotomy use has become more restrictive in some obstetric services during the past 20 years.[22] Episiotomies certainly are not routinely required. However, if operative vaginal delivery of a large fetus is indicated (e.g., genuine fetal distress), an episiotomy

should not be routinely avoided. It is possible that the mediolateral operation may regain popularity given the current obstetric interest in avoiding anal sphincter/rectal injury.

THIRD STAGE OF LABOR

The third stage of labor begins with the delivery of the baby and ends with the delivery of the placenta. The placenta typically separates from the uterine wall within a few contractions after delivery of the baby, and expulsion follows a few minutes later. Signs of placental separation are listed in Box 17-3.

When the placenta has separated from the uterine wall, gentle traction on the umbilical cord, coupled with suprapubic pressure to elevate the uterus, serves to deliver the placenta and membranes. In the absence of excessive bleeding, the obstetrician waits for the signs of placental separation before attempting to deliver it. If traction is exerted on the umbilical cord before the placenta has separated, problems result. The least serious—but nonetheless embarrassing—complication involves separating the umbilical cord from the placenta. This tear in the cord results in bleeding, which is of no concern because the blood is fetal-placental blood that would be discarded; however, the obstetrician's reputation for gentleness suffers as the detached segment of umbilical cord is held with the placenta remaining in situ. A much more serious problem is uterine inversion, which can occur in a case of fundal implantation of the placenta. If the placenta has not separated and the umbilical cord does not break, excessive traction turns the uterus inside out; this results in severe hemorrhage (see Chapter 37).

If the placenta has not separated after 30 minutes or if significant bleeding occurs before 30 minutes, manual removal of the placenta is indicated. Although some obstetricians advocate performing this procedure with sedation or analgesia, we prefer regional or general anesthesia. Sublingual or intravenous administration of **nitroglycerin** may provide uterine relaxation, which facilitates manual removal of a retained placenta. The obstetrician's hand is then passed into the uterine cavity, and the edge of the placenta is identified. The hand is used as a trowel to separate the placenta from the uterine wall. If the obstetrician cannot easily develop a plane between the placenta and the uterine wall, the diagnosis of **placenta accreta** should be considered. Placenta accreta typically results in severe hemorrhage, which almost always mandates emergency hysterectomy (see Chapter 37).

After the placenta has been removed manually, uterotonic agents are administered to decrease bleeding. **Oxytocin** is given intravenously in a dilute solution (e.g., 20 units added to 1 L of intravenous fluid), or 10 units are given intramuscularly. Bolus intravenous injection of oxytocin can cause hypotension and should be avoided.[23]

If the uterus does not respond to oxytocin, other ecbolic agents can be tried. **Methylergonovine** (Methergine, 0.2 mg) has long been available for intramuscular administration. It contracts vascular smooth muscle and may cause hypertension. Methylergonovine should not be given intravenously except in cases of severe, life-threatening hemorrhage. In such

---

Box 17-3 SIGNS OF PLACENTAL SEPARATION

- The uterus rises in the maternal abdomen.
- The shape of the uterus changes from discoid to globular.
- The umbilical cord lengthens.
- A gush of blood frequently occurs.

cases, physicians should give the drug slowly and carefully monitor the maternal blood pressure.

15-Methylprostaglandin F$_{2\text{-alpha}}$ (carboprost, Hemabate) is a newer ecbolic agent. Given intramuscularly, 0.25 mg of 15-methylprostaglandin F$_{2\text{-alpha}}$ has been demonstrated to be an effective uterotonic agent when other drugs have failed.[24] It can also cause hypertension, but the hypertension is typically not as severe as that associated with administration of methylergonovine. More important, 15-methylprostaglandin F$_{2\text{-alpha}}$ may cause bronchospasm, and it probably should be avoided in patients with asthma.

Most obstetricians in the United States do not use ecbolic agents until the placenta has been delivered, whereas European obstetricians typically administer an ecbolic agent immediately after delivery of the infant or even with delivery of the anterior shoulder. The timing probably does not matter.[25] At most deliveries, the placenta is expelled soon after delivery of the baby. Immediately after the delivery of the placenta, if the obstetrician suspects an abnormality, the hand can be passed into the uterine cavity without causing undue discomfort. Within several minutes, however, the cervix and birth canal contract. Subsequent uterine exploration typically requires the administration of anesthesia.

FOURTH STAGE OF LABOR

Many obstetricians consider the 60 minutes after delivery of the placenta to be the fourth stage of labor. Labor is completed, but this designation emphasizes that the patient must be watched carefully for bleeding. More than 90% of cases of postpartum hemorrhage result from uterine atony. If uterine atony is not identified during the first hour after delivery, it is unlikely to occur subsequently. The patient should be evaluated frequently to be certain that excessive bleeding is not occurring and that the uterus remains contracted. Considerable blood loss can occur in the presence of "normal" vital signs; a modest increment in additional blood loss can then be followed by profound shock. Uterine relaxation and excessive bleeding after delivery are treated with uterine massage and further ecbolic administration (see Chapter 37).

LABOR PROGRESS: FIVE MANAGEMENT QUESTIONS

The purpose of this section is to provide a personal, step-by-step approach to the management of the laboring woman by serially posing and answering five critical questions:

1. Is the patient in labor? If the answer to this question is "no," we're in the wrong chapter. If the answer is "yes," certain factors must be considered before proceeding. Is the patient at term? If she is preterm, is she a candidate for tocolytic therapy? If the patient is at term, are there medical or obstetric conditions that affect management? Abnormal fetal size or presentation, twin gestation, preeclampsia, and vaginal bleeding are obstetric factors that may alter management from the outset. If a singleton vertex presentation is identified in an uncomplicated patient, the physician proceeds to the following question.
2. Is the labor progress abnormal? If progress is normal according to the Friedman curve, no problem exists. If progress is abnormal, the physician proceeds to the following question.
3. Is the abnormality in the active phase? An apparent prolongation of the latent phase may represent false labor. By itself, a prolonged latent phase does not predict cephalopelvic disproportion or perinatal depression.

Therefore, in the absence of some other indication for effecting delivery, the obstetrician should not administer oxytocin or perform amniotomy, which would involve committing the patient to a long labor with the risk of failure and the potential need for an unnecessary cesarean section. Long latent phases *do increase* patient anxiety and fatigue; reassurance is essential. At this point, ambulation and opioid sedation are alternatives that may be selected on an individual basis, with strong input from the woman. If false labor has occurred, contractions will cease over time, or else the patient will enter the active phase. If primary dysfunctional labor is the diagnosis or if a secondary arrest of dilation has occurred during the active phase, the physician is faced with an abnormality that may indicate cephalopelvic disproportion, which is a mechanical obstruction to delivery. The next question can then be asked.

4. Is the fetus tolerating labor? Although the FHR pattern should be monitored from admission, a delay in the active phase of labor calls for a reassessment. If fetal distress is present, the physician should effect delivery. If not, the next question is asked.
5. Does the pelvis appear to be adequate for this baby? An active-phase delay indicates either insufficient uterine contractile effort to dilate the cervix or a mechanical obstruction to delivery. Obviously this is a critical issue, because the therapeutic alternatives are very different. If the pelvis is clinically small and/or the fetus is large and the labor seems strong (e.g., intense uterine contractions occurring every 2 minutes), the choice is cesarean section. If the fetopelvic relationship is favorable for vaginal delivery and the contractions are infrequent, the choice is intravenous oxytocin, amniotomy, or both. In the vast majority of cases, however, the obstetrician is uncertain as to whether oxytocin augmentation will result in successful vaginal delivery or whether cesarean section will ultimately be required despite oxytocin augmentation. Given the uncertainty of mechanical obstruction versus insufficient uterine activity as the problem, the proper choice typically is to administer oxytocin to correct the latter, a decision that recognizes that, if the former is present, the attempt will ultimately fail. Recent data support longer periods of oxytocin augmentation for nonprogressive active phase labor (at least 4 to 6 hours) provided the FHR pattern is reassuring.[26]

The benefit of intravenous oxytocin administration in delays that occur during the active phase of the first stage of labor is that most times it will succeed and cesarean section will be avoided.[11] The risks of oxytocin stimulation are both maternal and fetal. If mechanical obstruction to delivery exists, increased uterine activity predisposes the patient to uterine rupture, which is one of the gravest obstetric complications. Multiparity and a scarred uterus are also predisposing factors.[27,28] Oxytocin has an antidiuretic effect, and in the past there were reports of water intoxication with seizures and even coma and death as iatrogenic complications of its use. In these cases, oxytocin was administered over many hours (often days) in electrolyte-free solutions, with little attention paid to maternal urinary output; infusion of electrolyte-containing solutions and close attention to the parturient's fluid balance should make this a theoretical rather than a practical concern. However, **uterine hyperstimulation** is a real concern when infusing oxytocin. The force generated during uterine contractions interrupts blood flow through the intervillous space. (Placental perfusion occurs during periods of uterine relaxation, and uterine contractions can be considered as episodes of "fetal breath-holding.") If the contractions are occurring very frequently (e.g., at intervals less than 2 minutes apart), there may be insufficient time between contractions for placental gas exchange, the fetus may become hypoxemic, and fetal distress may result. Continuous observation permits a timely diagnosis of uterine hyperstimulation. Decreasing the infusion rate or temporarily stopping the infusion promptly corrects the problem.

Currently, in the United States, oxytocin for stimulating or augmenting labor is given intravenously as a dilute solution (10 U/L of electrolyte-containing fluid), typically by infusion pump. Electronic FHR monitoring is used, and a physician or nurse remains in constant attendance. Although the foregoing procedures are quite uniform from service to service, the selected *doses* of oxytocin are not.

The variability in protocols for oxytocin stimulation of labor reflects a confusing literature.[27-32] The goal is to increase uterine activity efficiently to dilate the cervix without causing fetal distress as a result of uterine hyperstimulation. However, the best way to do this is unclear. Recommended starting doses of oxytocin vary from 1 to 6 mU/min, and then additional drug is administered until a satisfactory labor pattern is achieved. Dosage increments typically vary from 1 to 6 mU at intervals of 15 to 30 minutes. In the only randomized, double-blinded study of oxytocin dosing, increasing the dose of oxytocin by 4.5 mU/min every 30 minutes resulted in a significantly shorter duration of labor than increasing it by 1.5 mU/min every 30 minutes, with no adverse maternal or fetal-neonatal effects.[33]

The Active Management of Labor

Dystocia, which is also called abnormal labor progress, is exceeded only by repeat cesarean section as an indication for abdominal delivery in the United States. Concern for the high cesarean section rate has created interest in the remarkable results achieved with the use of active management of labor at the National Maternity Hospital in Dublin, Ireland.[27,34] Components of the active management of labor include the following: (1) a rigorous definition of labor; (2) early amniotomy; (3) constant nursing attendance; (4) the demand for continued progress in cervical dilation (1 cm or more per hour); (5) vigorous oxytocin stimulation for lack of progress; and (6) a "guarantee" that the parturient's stay in the labor unit will last no longer than 12 hours. In Dublin, these practices were associated with a cesarean birth rate of less than 5%; however, the rate has been higher in recent years.

The introduction of the active management of labor in other obstetric services has been associated with lower cesarean rates than those among historic controls. One prospective randomized trial indicated that active management shortened labor, decreased the incidence of cesarean section for dystocia, and resulted in fewer maternal infectious complications without increasing maternal or neonatal morbidity.[35] Two other randomized trials confirmed shorter labors with active management but differed regarding its effect on the rate of cesarean delivery.[36,37]

SPECIAL SITUATIONS

Premature Rupture of Membranes

Premature rupture of the membranes (PROM) is defined as a rupture of the fetal membranes (i.e., the chorioamnion) before the onset of labor. It may occur preterm (before 37 weeks' gestation) or at term.

PRETERM PROM

The most significant complication of preterm PROM is preterm birth.[38] Although the length of the latent period (that interval between membrane rupture and the onset of labor) is inversely related to the length of gestation, only one in five women with preterm PROM have latent periods that exceed one week. Indeed, PROM is the precipitating factor in one third of preterm deliveries. Other risks for preterm PROM include chorioamnionitis and prolapse of the umbilical cord. If membrane rupture occurs during the second trimester and if there is a long exposure of the fetus to oligohydramnios, there is a risk of pulmonary hypoplasia and orthopedic deformities.

Current management of preterm PROM is conservative. After the diagnosis is confirmed by inspection and nitrazine and fern testing,[39] electronic FHR monitoring is used to identify variable decelerations that signal umbilical cord compression. The mother is also evaluated for fever and uterine tenderness, which may indicate chorioamnionitis. If these are absent, the clinician awaits the onset of labor or the subsequent development of infection. The adjunctive use of maternally administered corticosteroids to enhance fetal pulmonary maturity and/or antibiotics to prevent chorioamnionitis and delay the onset of labor is common[40-42]; tocolytic therapy is ineffective in this situation.[43] On many obstetric services, delivery is effected routinely at 34 weeks (a point beyond which the rate of severe neonatal morbidity and mortality is very low) or after documentation of fetal pulmonary maturity.

TERM PROM

Approximately 10% of term pregnancies are complicated by PROM; the natural history is summarized in Table 17-3.[44]

Although chorioamnionitis is more likely to occur preterm than at term, no clear relationship exists between the length of the latent period and chorioamnionitis in the preterm patient.[45] By contrast, chorioamnionitis at term is more likely if the latent period exceeds 24 hours. The relationship between prolonged latency and chorioamnionitis accounts for the usual practice in the United States of oxytocin induction of labor if the woman with PROM at term is not in labor by six to 12 hours after membrane rupture. Hannah et al.[46] conducted a trial comparing induction with expectancy in

TABLE 17-3	THE NATURAL HISTORY OF PREMATURE RUPTURE OF THE MEMBRANES AT TERM

Elements	Percent
Prevalence	10
Spontaneous labor within 24 hours	90
If cervix unfavorable and no labor at 6 hours, percent laboring by 24 hours	60
Chorioamnionitis	
Latent period < 24 hours	1-2
Latent period > 24 hours	5-10
Significant neonatal infection if chorioamnionitis present	10

Modified from Zlatnik FJ. Management of premature rupture of membranes at term. Obstet Gynecol Clin North Am 1992; 19:353-64.

more than 5000 women with PROM at term; they found similar rates of cesarean delivery and neonatal infection in the two groups. Oxytocin induction resulted in a lower rate of maternal infection than expectant management.

CHORIOAMNIONITIS

If chorioamnionitis develops, the uterus must be emptied. Intrapartum antibiotic administration improves the outcome for both mother and baby.[47] Ampicillin and gentamycin often are chosen to combat group B streptococcus and *Escherichia coli*, which are important neonatal pathogens. Because no relationship exists between the number of hours that chorioamnionitis has been present and perinatal outcome,[48-50] chorioamnionitis alone is not an indication for abdominal delivery. Antibiotics, oxytocin, and close observation of the mother and fetus are indicated.

Induction of Labor

Induction of labor can be defined as a surgical or medical intervention that leads to uterine contractions that progressively dilate the cervix. Because elective and indicated inductions differ in terms of eligibility criteria and the methods used, they are considered separately.

ELECTIVE INDUCTION

The rationale for elective induction of labor is convenience, both for the patient and for the physician. Because it is elective, the delivery should be easily accomplished, and the risks should approach zero. Requirements for elective induction of labor include the following: (1) a parous patient; (2) a singleton vertex presentation; (3) a certain gestation of at least 39 weeks; (4) a favorable cervix; and (5) no contraindications to labor and vaginal delivery. Table 17-4 presents the Bishop score,[51] which helps quantitate favorability of the cervix; the higher the score, the shorter the labor and the less likely induction will fail. In Bishop's hands, a score of 9 or greater was not associated with failure. Friedman et al.[52] determined that the Bishop score primarily predicts the latent phase of labor. This is not surprising, because a high Bishop score indicates that the cervix is ready to dilate with uterine contractions (i.e., the cervix will soon enter the active phase). By contrast, a low score suggests that many hours of uterine contractions may be needed to soften and efface the cervix. When the components of the Bishop score are considered separately in terms of their effects on the latent phase, dilation is most

critical. Effacement, station, and consistency are each half as important, and position has little effect.[52]

With a favorable cervix, elective induction is begun by performing amniotomy with or without concomitant oxytocin administration, which some reserve for the patient who is not contracting 4 to 6 hours after amniotomy. Amniotomy typically is performed early in the morning and followed by delivery in the afternoon. Elective inductions have been criticized by some physicians because of the possibilities of induction failure and iatrogenic prematurity.[53] If candidates are selected with careful attention to the previously listed requirements, elective induction is both convenient and safe.

INDICATED INDUCTION

Indicated induction of labor is performed when delivery is indicated for maternal or fetal reasons and both can tolerate labor and vaginal delivery. Indicated inductions of labor often arise in the setting of a medical or obstetric complication such as diabetes mellitus, preeclampsia, intrauterine growth restriction, or the post-term pregnancy. By definition, the physician is dealing with a complicated pregnancy when performing an indicated induction of labor; therefore, close maternal and fetal monitoring are indicated. When considering the critical question of whether induction should be undertaken, the obstetrician must weigh the perinatal risks of continued intrauterine versus extrauterine existence and must also consider the potential adverse maternal consequences of induction, including an increased risk of infection and/or cesarean delivery.

If the Bishop score is favorable, amniotomy alone will suffice as a means of inducing labor. Often, however, the cervix is not favorable, and induction typically is accomplished with oxytocin administration combined with amniotomy. In some cases, if the cervix is unfavorable, oxytocin may be infused for one day, with the membranes intact. The infusion is stopped in the evening, and the patient is permitted to eat. The membranes are ruptured, and the oxytocin infusion is started again the following morning. Some obstetricians have advocated vaginal or cervical prostaglandins for the induction of labor; however, it is unclear that they offer an advantage over intravenous oxytocin for this purpose.[54]

When induction of labor is indicated in the setting of an unfavorable cervix, the obstetrician may attempt to increase the Bishop score before beginning the induction. Both osmotic cervical dilators and pharmacologic techniques are effective in improving the Bishop score.[55,56] Typically these adjunctive measures are instituted the evening before the planned induction. The most common pharmacologic method involves the topical application of prostaglandin E_2, either in the vagina or in the cervical canal. Prostaglandin E_2 has a local effect in the initiation of the softening, effacement, and dilation of the cervix, and it also has an oxytocin-like effect on the myometrium. Women treated with prostaglandin E_2 frequently develop contractions and labor before amniotomy or oxytocin administration. The same is true for misoprostol, which is a prostaglandin E_1 analogue that is now widely used for cervical ripening and labor induction.[57]

Although these and other studies have noted a change in cervical status after the use of these adjunctive measures, it is unclear whether these pharmacologic methods decrease the ultimate need for cesarean delivery.[57,58] Because the rationale for cervical ripening agents is to decrease the likelihood of failed induction, the ultimate place for such therapies remains to be established.

TABLE 17-4	THE BISHOP CERVIX SCORE			
	Score			
Component	**0**	**1**	**2**	**3**
Dilation (cm)	0	1-2	3-4	5+
Effacement (%)	0-30	40-50	60-70	80+
Station	−3	−2	−1/0	+1
Consistency	Firm	Medium	Soft	
Position	Posterior	Mid	Anterior	

From Bishop EH. Pelvic scoring for elective induction. Obstet Gynecol 1964; 24:266-8.

Operative Vaginal Delivery

Cesarean section has become a too-frequent solution to labor room problems. This safe operation certainly is preferable to the continuation of labor in the setting of genuine fetal distress or to the performance of a difficult and traumatic vaginal delivery. Unfortunately, however, more traditional obstetric interventions (e.g., labor, additional labor, operative vaginal delivery) are often bypassed in favor of cesarean section, perhaps more for medicolegal than for medical concerns. The appropriate use of operative vaginal delivery techniques requires an accurate assessment of the situation, technical skills, and an honest and humble physician.

VERTEX PRESENTATION

A carefully selected and performed forceps or vacuum-assisted delivery shortens the second stage of labor in cases of fetal distress, maternal illness or exhaustion, and/or undue prolongation of labor with little or no progress (Box 17-4). The station of the presenting vertex is critical to the safety of the procedure for mother and baby. The current American College of Obstetricians and Gynecologists classification permits a more rational approach to operative vaginal delivery than was available previously.[59,60]

For any operative vaginal delivery, adequate anesthesia is required. Outlet operative deliveries are perfectly safe for both mother and fetus. The low station effectively rules out cephalopelvic disproportion, and little traction is required. Outlet operative deliveries shorten the second stage by only a few minutes. Sustained fetal bradycardia is a common indication for outlet operative delivery.

An experienced physician may safely perform low-station operative deliveries in cases of fetal distress or maternal illness or exhaustion. The higher the head, the harder the pull. Rotations increase the likelihood of vaginal tears.[60]

Midpelvic deliveries reflect a more complicated problem.[61,62] If the station is overestimated, the vertex may be barely engaged. The hollow of the sacrum is incompletely filled. Midpelvic deliveries should be regarded as "trials." The obstetrician must avoid excessive traction and be willing to abandon the attempt in favor of cesarean section if delivery does not proceed easily.

Although operative vaginal delivery was traditionally accomplished with obstetric forceps, there has been recent interest in the soft plastic cup vacuum extractor.[63-66] It is unclear which is better. The vacuum extractor is easier to apply, especially if the obstetrician is uncertain of the position

of the occiput, and it most likely is associated with less maternal trauma. Forceps—but not the vacuum extractor—permits the correction of deflection or slight abnormalities of position that may impede progress. The vacuum extractor is more apt to slip off; whether this enhances safety is unknown. Neonatal results are comparable, but retinal hemorrhages, which are of uncertain significance, are more likely with vacuum extraction. The obstetrician should be trained in both techniques and should individualize their use.

Persistent occiput-posterior positions often occur in anthropoid and android pelves. In modern obstetrics, most of these infants are delivered with the occiput posterior. Extension of the episiotomy is a frequent complication in this circumstance, which argues for the consideration of a mediolateral episiotomy.

Deep transverse arrests of the occiput traditionally were managed by rotation and delivery with Kielland's forceps. Current trainees typically have little experience with this instrument, and they are more likely to select the vacuum extractor in this circumstance.

NONVERTEX PRESENTATIONS

A persistent brow presentation or a transverse lie mandates cesarean delivery. Most face presentations and selected breech presentations can be safely delivered vaginally.[67] However, in response to a large international multicenter trial in which planned vaginal delivery was associated with worse perinatal outcomes than planned cesarean delivery,[68] the American College of Obstetricians and Gynecologists now recommends cesarean delivery for the persistent singleton breech at term unless delivery is imminent.[69]

FETAL DEATH

If fetal death has occurred, the obstetrician no longer has two patients, making maternal safety the only concern. Although placenta previa or absolute cephalopelvic disproportion may indicate cesarean delivery, the obstetrician is often more willing to choose a more complicated operative vaginal delivery than if the fetus were living.

Shoulder Dystocia

With vertex presentations, most mechanical difficulties are resolved with delivery of the head; once the head is delivered, the remainder of the fetus follows easily. In as many as 3% of vaginal deliveries, this is not the case. After delivery of the (often large) head, it seems to be "sucked" back to the perineum. With maternal pushing and gentle traction, nothing happens. In this case, the anterior shoulder is trapped above the pubic symphysis. *Shoulder dystocia* is the name for this serious complication. Recognition that shoulder dystocia exists is often followed by equanimity giving way to panic. If delivery is not accomplished soon, umbilical cord compression may result in asphyxia. Excessive traction on the fetal head may result in damage to the brachial plexus (e.g., Erb's palsy), which may be permanent or temporary. During the manipulations undertaken to effect delivery, a fracture of the clavicle or humerus may result.

Risk factors for shoulder dystocia are those that predict or reflect mechanical difficulty (Box 17-5).[70-73] Women with diabetes mellitus are predisposed to shoulder dystocia, not only because fetal macrosomia is more common but also because the fetus of a mother with diabetes has a shoulder circumference that is disproportionately large relative to head

---

Box 17-4 FORCEPS CLASSIFICATION

OUTLET FORCEPS

Scalp is visible.
Skull has reached the pelvic floor, and head is on the perineum.
Sagittal suture is in the anterior-posterior diameter or within 45 degrees (e.g., occiput anterior, left occiput anterior, right occiput posterior).

LOW FORCEPS

Station is +2 or greater.
Hollow of the sacrum is filled.

MIDFORCEPS

Vertex is engaged, but the station is 0 or +1.

Box 17-5 RISK FACTORS FOR SHOULDER DYSTOCIA

- Fetal macrosomia
- Maternal diabetes mellitus
- Delayed active phase of labor
- Prolonged second stage of labor
- Operative vaginal delivery

circumference. Desultory labor may be a harbinger of mechanical mismatch, and operative vaginal delivery can exacerbate the situation.

Appropriate management of shoulder dystocia begins with the recognition that there is sufficient time to deliver the baby safely. Regional anesthesia is ideal but not essential. Extension of the episiotomy should be considered. (The anterior shoulder is stuck behind the pubic symphysis. Increased room posteriorly does not *directly* permit delivery, but it does permit vaginal manipulations that may be necessary to effect delivery.) Table 17-5 lists a personal plan of management for shoulder dystocia, but other choices are available.[70,73,74]

If suprapubic pressure (directed toward the floor) coupled with gentle traction on the head is not efficacious, the mother's thighs are removed from their supports and are hyperflexed alongside her abdomen. This maneuver (i.e., the McRoberts maneuver) elevates the symphysis in a cephalad direction and often frees the impacted shoulder and allows easy delivery. If the McRoberts maneuver is not successful, vaginal manipulations are undertaken to get the position of the shoulders into an oblique diameter of the pelvis or to deliver the posterior arm. Despite previous assumptions to the contrary, vaginal delivery of the head does not necessarily commit one to vaginal birth of the baby. In the words of Yogi Berra, "It ain't over till it's over." Although we do not have personal experience with cephalic replacement (i.e., the Zavanelli maneuver), its potential use must be kept in mind. If all measures have failed, the "tape is rewound," and the mechanism of labor is reversed. The position of the vertex is made occiput anterior, flexion is achieved, and the head is elevated, which may be facilitated by tocolysis (e.g., 100 µg of sublingual or intravenous nitroglycerin or 0.25 mg of subcutaneous terbutaline) or general anesthesia with a volatile halogenated agent. After the fetal head has been placed back into the vagina, prompt cesarean section is performed.[74]

TABLE 17-5	MANAGEMENT OF SHOULDER DYSTOCIA
Maneuver	**Desired Result**
Suprapubic pressure	Anterior shoulder dislodged from above pubic symphysis
Hyperflexion of maternal thighs alongside abdomen (McRoberts maneuver)	Cephalad rotation of pubic symphysis
Intravaginal pressure on posterior shoulder	Anterior-posterior position of shoulders transformed to oblique position
Delivery of posterior arm	Once accomplished, added room permits delivery
Cephalic replacement (Zavanelli maneuver)	Delivery by cesarean section

- The outcome of labor reflects the interaction of three components: the powers, the passageway, and the passenger.
- Assuming that the fetus is tolerating labor satisfactorily, the most important obstetric determination is whether the patient is in the latent or the active phase of the first stage of labor.
- Amniotomy shortens labor.
- Oxytocin is the most valuable obstetric drug, but there are conflicting opinions regarding the ideal dosage regimen for induction and/or augmentation of labor.
- Expectancy is the standard choice for the preterm patient with premature rupture of membranes; induction of labor generally is undertaken in patients exhibiting this condition at term.
- Elective induction of labor is an appropriate choice for a parous patient with a favorable cervix.
- The declining numbers of operative vaginal deliveries reflect medicolegal concerns rather than new scientific information.

REFERENCES

1. Casey ML, MacDonald PC. Biomedical processes in the initiation of parturition: Decidual activation. Clin Obstet Gynecol 1988; 31:533-52.
2. Garfield RE. Control of myometrial function in preterm versus term labor. Clin Obstet Gynecol 1984; 27:572-91.
3. Zlatnik FJ. Normal labor and delivery and its conduct. In: Scott JR, Di Saia PJ, Hammond CB, Spellacy WN, editors. Danforth's Obstetrics and Gynecology. 7th ed. Philadelphia, JB Lippincott, 1994:161-88.
4. Laube DW, Varner MW, Cruikshank DP. A prospective evaluation of x-ray pelvimetry. JAMA 1981; 246:2187-8.
5. Friedman EA. Labor: Clinical Evaluation and Management. 2nd ed. New York, Appleton-Century-Crofts, 1978.
6. Peisner DB, Rosen MG. Transition from latent to active labor. Obstet Gynecol 1986; 68:448-51.
7. Kelly G, Peaceman AM, Colangelo L, Rademaker A. Normal nulliparous labor: Are Friedman's definitions still relevant? (abstract) Am J Obstet Gynecol 2000; 182:S129.
8. Zhang J, Troendle J, Yancey M. Reassessing the labor curve in nulliparous women. Am J Obstet Gynecol 2002; 187:824-8.
9. Peisner DP, Rosen MG. Latent phase of labor in normal patients: A reassessment. Obstet Gynecol 1985; 66:644-8.
10. Bottoms SF, Sokol RJ, Rosen MG. Short arrest of cervical dilatation: A risk for maternal/fetal/infant morbidity. Am J Obstet Gynecol 1981; 140:108-13.
11. Bottoms SF, Hirsch VJ, Sokol RJ. Medical management of arrest disorders of labor: A current overview. Am J Obstet Gynecol 1987; 156:935-9.
12. Friedman EA. Patterns of labor as indicators of risk. Clin Obstet Gynecol 1973; 16:172-83.
13. Chelmow D, Kilpatrick SJ, Laros RK. Maternal and neonatal outcomes after prolonged latent phase. Obstet Gynecol 1993; 81:486-91.
14. Fraser WD, Marcoux S, Moutquin JM, et al. Effect of early amniotomy on the risk of dystocia in nulliparous women. N Engl J Med 1993;328:1145-9.
15. Johnson N, Lilford R, Guthrie K, et al. Randomised trial comparing a policy of early with selective amniotomy in uncomplicated labour at term. Br J Gynaecol 1997; 104:340-6.
16. American College of Obstetricians and Gynecologists. Dystocia and the Augmentation of Labor. ACOG Technical Bulletin No. 218. December, 1995.
17. Hellman LM, Prystowsky H. The duration of the second stage of labor. Am J Obstet Gynecol 1952; 63:1223-33.

18. Katz M, Lunenfeld E, Meizner I, et al. The effect of the duration of second stage of labour on the acid-base state of the fetus. Br J Obstet Gynecol 1987; 94:425-30.

19. Cohen WR. Influence of the duration of second stage labor on perinatal outcome and puerperal morbidity. Obstet Gynecol 1977; 49:266-9.

20. Carlson JM, Diehl JA, Sachtleben-Murray M, et al. Maternal position during parturition in normal labor. Obstet Gynecol 1986; 68:443-7.

21. Thorp JM, Bowes WA. Episiotomy: Can its routine use be defended? Am J Obstet Gynecol 1989; 160:1027-30.

22. Bansal RK, Tan WM, Ecker JL, et al. Is there a benefit to episiotomy at spontaneous vaginal delivery? A natural experiment. Am J Obstet Gynecol 1996;175:897-901.

23. Hendricks CH, Brenner WE. Cardiovascular effects of oxytocic drugs used postpartum. Am J Obstet Gynecol 1970; 108:751-9.

24. Hayashi RH, Castillo MS, Noah ML. Management of severe postpartum hemorrhage due to uterine atony using an analogue of prostaglandin F_2 alpha. Obstet Gynecol 1981; 58:426-9.

25. Jackson KW, Allbert JR, Schemmer GK, et al. A randomized controlled trial comparing oxytocin administration before and after placental delivery in the prevention of postpartum hemorrhage. Am J Obstet Gynecol 2001; 185:873-7.

26. Rouse DJ, Owen J, Savage KG, Hauth JC. Active phase labor arrest: Revisiting the two-hour minimum. Obstet Gynecol 2001; 98:550-4.

27. O'Driscoll K, Meagher D. Active Management of Labour: The Dublin Experience. 2nd ed. London, Bailliere Tindall, 1986.

28. Satin AJ, Leveno KJ, Sherman ML, et al. High versus low dose oxytocin for labor stimulation. Obstet Gynecol 1992; 80:111-6.

29. Seitchik J, Castillo M. Oxytocin augmentation of dysfunctional labor. I. Clinical data. Am J Obstet Gynecol 1982; 144:899-905.

30. Xenakis EM, Langer O, Piper JM, et al. Low-dose versus high-dose oxytocin augmentation of labor: A randomized trial. Am J Obstet Gynecol 1995; 173:1874-8.

31. Satin AJ, Hankins GDV, Yeomans ER. A prospective study of two dosing regimens of oxytocin for the induction of labor in patients with unfavorable cervices. Am J Obstet Gynecol 1991; 165:980-4.

32. Blakemore KJ, Qin N, Petrie RH, Paine LL. A prospective comparison of hourly and quarter-hourly oxytocin dose increase intervals for the induction of labor at term. Obstet Gynecol 1990; 75:757-61.

33. Merrill DC, Zlatnik FJ. Randomized, double-masked comparison of oxytocin dosage in induction and augmentation of labor. Obstet Gynecol 1999; 94:455-63.

34. O'Driscoll K, Foley M, MacDonald D. Active management of labor as an alternative to cesarean section for dystocia. Obstet Gynecol 1984; 63:485-90.

35. Lopez-Zeno JA, Peaceman AM, Adashek JA, Socol ML. A controlled trial of a program for the active management of labor. N Engl J Med 1992; 326:450-4.

36. Frigoletto FD, Lieberman E, Lang JM, et al. A clinical trial of active management of labor. N Engl J Med 1995; 333:745-50.

37. Rogers R, Gilson GJ, Miller AC, et al. Active management of labor: Does it make a difference? Am J Obstet Gynecol 1997; 177:599-605.

38. Malee MP. Expectant and active management of preterm premature rupture of membranes. Obstet Gynecol Clin North Am 1992; 19:309-15.

39. Gregg AR. Introduction to premature rupture of membranes. Obstet Gynecol Clin North Am 1992; 19:241-9.

40. Mercer BM, Arheart KL. Antimicrobial therapy in expectant management of preterm premature rupture of the membranes. Lancet 1995; 346:1271-9.

41. Lovett SM, Weiss JD, Diogo MJ, et al. A prospective, double-blind, randomized, controlled clinical trial of ampicillin-sulbactam for preterm premature rupture of membranes in women receiving antenatal corticosteroid therapy. Am J Obstet Gynecol 1997; 176:1030-8.

42. Crowley P. Corticosteroids after preterm premature rupture of membranes. Obstet Gynecol Clin North Am 1992; 19:317-26.

43. Ohlsson A. Treatments of preterm premature rupture of the membranes: A meta-analysis. Am J Obstet Gynecol 1989; 160:890-906.

44. Zlatnik FJ. Management of premature rupture of membranes at term. Obstet Gynecol Clin North Am 1992; 19:353-64.

45. Johnson JWC, Daikoku NH, Niebyl JR, et al. Premature rupture of the membranes and prolonged latency. Obstet Gynecol 1981; 57:547-56.

46. Hannah ME, Ohlsson A. Farine D, et al. Induction of labor compared with expectant management for prelabor rupture of the membranes at term. N Engl J Med 1996; 334:1005-10.

47. Gibbs RS, Dinsmoor MJ, Newton ER, Ramamurthy RS. A randomized trial of intrapartum versus immediate postpartum treatment of women with intra-amniotic infection. Obstet Gynecol 1988; 72:823-8.

48. Gibbs RS, Castillo MS, Rodgers PJ. Management of acute chorioamnionitis. Am J Obstet Gynecol 1980; 136:709-13.

49. Hauth JC, Gilstrap LC, Hankins GDV, Connor KD. Term maternal and neonatal complications of acute chorioamnionitis. Obstet Gynecol 1985; 66:59-62.

50. Rouse DJ, for the National Institute of Child Health Development and Maternal-Fetal Medicine Units Network. Maternal-Fetal Medicine Units Cesarean Registry: Fetal-neonatal outcome in relationship to chorioamnionitis and its duration (abstract). Am J Obstet Gynecol 2002; 187:S221.

51. Bishop EH. Pelvic scoring for elective induction. Obstet Gynecol 1964; 24:266-8.

52. Friedman EA, Niswander KR, Bayonet-Rivera NP, Sachtleben MR. Relation of prelabor evaluation to inducibility and the course of labor. Obstet Gynecol 1966; 28:495-501.

53. Rayburn WF, Zhang J. Rising rates of labor induction: Present concerns and future strategies. Obstet Gynecol 2002; 100:164-7.

54. American College of Obstetricians and Gynecologists. Induction of Labor. ACOG Practice Bulletin No. 10, November 1999.

55. Cross WG, Pitkin RM. Laminaria as an adjunct in induction of labor. Obstet Gynecol 1978; 51:606-8.

56. Bernstein P. Prostaglandin E_2 gel for cervical ripening and labour induction: A multicentre placebo-controlled trial. Can Med Assoc J 1991; 145:1249-54.

57. Sanchez-Ramos L, Kaunitz AM, Wears RL, et al. Misoprostol for cervical ripening and labor induction: A meta-analysis. Obstet Gynecol 1997; 89:633-42.

58. Owen J, Winkler CL, Harris BA, et al. A randomized double-blind trial of prostaglandin E_2 gel for cervical ripening and meta-analysis. Am J Obstet Gynecol 1991; 165:991-6.

59. American College of Obstetricians and Gynecologists. Operative Vaginal Delivery. ACOG Practice Bulletin No. 17, June 2000.

60. Hagadorn-Freathy AS, Yeomans ER, Hankins GDV. Validation of the 1988 ACOG forceps classification system. Obstet Gynecol 1991; 77: 356-60.

61. Bashore RA, Phillips WH, Brinkman CR. A comparison of the morbidity of midforceps and cesarean delivery. Am J Obstet Gynecol 1990; 162:1428-34.

62. Robertson PA, Laros RK, Zhao RL. Neonatal and maternal outcome in lowpelvic and midpelvic operative deliveries. Am J Obstet Gynecol 1990; 162:1436-42.

63. Berkus MD, Ramamurthy RS, O'Connor PS, et al. Cohort study of silastic obstetric vacuum cup deliveries. I. Safety of the instrument. Obstet Gynecol 1985; 66:503-9.

64. Dell DL, Sightler SE, Plauche WC. Soft cup vacuum extraction: A comparison of outlet delivery. Obstet Gynecol 1985; 66:624-8.

65. Broekhuizen FF, Washington JM, Johnson F, Hamilton PR. Vacuum extraction versus forceps delivery: Indications and complications, 1979-1984. Obstet Gynecol 1987; 69:338-42.

66. Williams MC, Knuppel RA, O'Brien WF, et al. A randomized comparison of assisted vaginal delivery by obstetric forceps and polyethylene vacuum cup. Obstet Gynecol 1991; 78:789-94.

67. Weiner CP. Vaginal breech delivery in the 1990s. Clin Obstet Gynecol 1992; 35:559-69.

68. Hannah ME, Hannah WJ, Hewson SA, et al., for the Term Breech Trial Collaborative Group. Planned caesarean section versus planned vaginal birth for breech presentation at term: A randomized multicentre trial. Lancet 2000; 356:1375-83.

69. American College of Obstetricians and Gynecologists. Mode of term singleton breech delivery. ACOG Committee Opinion #265. December 2001.

70. O'Leary JA, Leonetti HB. Shoulder dystocia: Prevention and treatment. Am J Obstet Gynecol 1990; 162:5-9.

71. Gross TL, Sokol RJ, Williams T, Thompson K. Shoulder dystocia: A fetal-physician risk. Am J Obstet Gynecol 1987; 156:1408-14.

72. Langer O, Berkus MD, Huff RW, Samueloff A. Shoulder dystocia: Should the fetus weighing 4000 grams be delivered by cesarean section? Am J Obstet Gynecol 1991; 165:831-7.

73. ACOG Committee on Practice Bulletins-Gynecology, The American College of Obstetrician and Gynecologists. ACOG practice bulletin clinical management guidelines for obstetrician-gynecologists. Number 40, November 2002. Obstet Gynecol 2002; 100:1045-9.

74. Sandberg EC. The Zavanelli maneuver extended: Progression of a revolutionary concept. Am J Obstet Gynecol 1988; 158:1347-52.

Chapter 18

The Pain of Childbirth and Its Effect on the Mother and the Fetus

James C. Eisenach, M.D.

The gate control theory of pain, described nearly 40 years ago by Melzack and Wall,[1] has revolutionized our understanding of the mechanisms of pain and analgesia. This theory states that the transmission of pain does not follow a dedicated, hard-wired path without control. Rather, the transmission of pain signals from the peripheral nerves through the spinal cord is regulated by the activity of other peripheral nerves, interneurons in the spinal cord, and central supraspinal centers (Figure 18-1). This theory suggests that active local processes within the spinal cord can either *open* the gate, which allows for the transmission of pain to higher centers, or *close* the gate, thereby preventing such transmission.

Subsequently, gate control theory has been expanded and refined. We now recognize that neural circuits and intraneural mechanisms regulate sensitivity at peripheral afferent terminals; along the conducting axons of peripheral nerves; in the spinal cord, pons, medulla, and thalamus; and at cortical sites of pain transmission and projection. The elegantly simplistic gate control diagram has been replaced by the concept of a *neuromatrix:* a remarkably fluid system with the capability of undergoing rapid change.[2] For example, peripheral application of capsaicin to the skin results in alterations in spinal gating mechanisms within 10 minutes so that a light touch signal is interpreted as burning pain.[3]

Gate control theory led to an explosion of research into mechanisms of chronic pain and its treatment, yet it has had little impact on our understanding of labor pain. Obstetric pain is likely the most common form of severe pain, affecting nearly 50% of the population. However, there has been virtually no development of analgesics other than local anesthetics to treat labor pain, and little fundamental research has been done to help us understand the neurophysiologic basis and gate control mechanisms for this pain. This discrepancy in interest and focus has led to vastly different approaches to the treatment of chronic and obstetric pain. A patient with chronic pain typically undergoes a sophisticated physical assessment of sensory function upon which systemic drug therapy is based.[4] The clinician may choose from nearly a dozen different classes of analgesics to treat chronic pain. Further, the pharmaceutical industry is expending enormous resources to introduce more drugs in these classes in addition to drugs that act on other receptors or enzymes. By contrast, laboring women receive no physical assessment of sensory function, and less than a handful of systemic drugs are available to them, most of which have an efficacy that does not differ from placebo in randomized controlled trials. The primary pharmacologic option for pain relief during labor is based on anatomic blockade of neural traffic with a local anesthetic. There is little pharmaceutical industry interest in developing new drugs for the treatment of intrapartum pain. Therefore, one might consider labor pain as an unmet medical need.[5]

This chapter examines the reasons for this paradox in our understanding and approach to labor pain and then reviews the basis for current therapy (anatomy), the basis for future therapy (neurophysiology), and the effects of labor pain on the mother and the baby.

EXISTENCE AND SEVERITY

The existence of chronic pain, which often lacks an obvious outward cause, is now unquestioned. By contrast, the existence of labor pain, which is accompanied by visible tissue injury, is often denied. Dick-Read[6] suggested that labor is a natural process, is not considered painful by women in primitive cultures, and should not be treated pharmacologically as a pain syndrome but rather should be handled with education and preparation. Psychoprophylaxis was further popularized by Lamaze,[7] and this method forms the basis for most of the prepared childbirth training in the developed world. Although modern prepared childbirth training clearly acknowledges the existence of pain in labor, many individuals and scientific thought leaders consider labor pain to be minor and unimportant. I was surprised by a speaker at a recent international symposium on the neurophysiologic basis of labor pain, who began her discussion by stating that the labor and delivery of her children were not that painful and that we should focus on more important matters, such as chronic pelvic pain!

Although labor is painless in a few women, the vast majority consider it painful, and a clear majority rate it as severe pain. Melzack,[8] one of the authors of the gate control theory

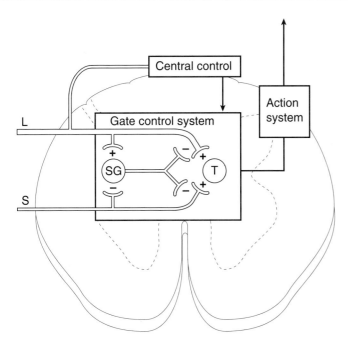

FIGURE 18-1. Gate control theory of pain. Activity in small-diameter afferents *(S)* stimulates transmission cells in the spinal cord *(T)*, which send signals supraspinally and results in the perception of pain. Small-diameter afferents also inhibit cells in the spinal cord substantia gelatinosa *(SG)*, the activity of which reduces excitatory input to T cells. Activity in large-diameter afferents *(L)* also stimulates T cells in a manner that is perceived as nonpainful and excites SG cells to "close the gate" and reduce S afferent activation of T cells. The gate mechanism is under regulation by central sites. (From Melzack R, Wall PD. Pain mechanisms: A new theory. Science 1965; 150:971-5.)

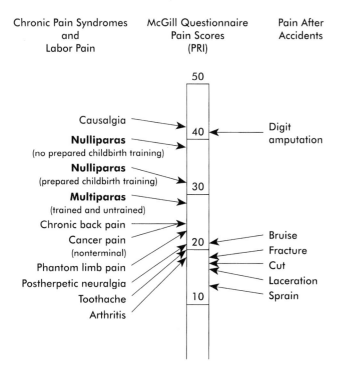

FIGURE 18-2. A comparison of pain scores using the McGill Pain Questionnaire. Scores were obtained from women in labor, patients in a general hospital clinic, and patients in the emergency department after an accident involving a traumatic injury. Note the modest difference in pain scores between nulliparous women with and without prepared childbirth training. *PRI*, The pain rating index, which represents the sum of the rank values of all the words chosen from 20 sets of pain descriptors. (Modified from Melzack R. The myth of painless childbirth [The John J. Bonica Lecture]. Pain 1984; 19:321-37.)

of pain, developed a questionnaire to assess the intensity and emotional impact of pain. Using this tool, he observed that labor pain was rated as more painful than cancer pain and that, among nulliparous women with no prepared childbirth training, it was nearly as painful as amputation of a digit without anesthesia (Figure 18-2).[8]

Melzack was not the first to make this observation. The severity of labor pain was recognized by the Romans, who termed delivery the *poena magna*—the "great pain" or "great punishment." More than 30 years before Melzack's quantification of labor pain, Hardy and Javert[9,10] quantified labor pain intensity by training subjects to match labor pain with the sensation of noxious heat applied to the skin from a radiant heat source. Several women achieved "ceiling pain" values—resulting in second-degree burns to the skin—when they attempted to match the intensity of uterine contraction pain.[9] These investigators reported a close positive correlation between cervical dilation and assessment of pain in individual women. Logistic regression of their original data[9] indicates a high likelihood of severe pain as labor progresses, with a time course closely associated with that of cervical dilation (Figure 18-3). Others have noted that uterine pressure during contractions accounts for more than 90% of variation in labor pain intensity.[11] These observations are consistent with the conclusion that cervical distention is the primary cause of pain during the first stage of labor.

There is considerable variability in the rated intensity of pain during labor. Nearly 25% of women consider it to be minimal or mild, and 23% of women consider it very severe or intolerable.[12] The reasons for this large variability are manifold. Although nulliparous women rate pain as more severe than parous women, differences are small and of questionable clinical relevance.[12] There is a correlation between intensity of pain during menses and labor pain, especially back pain,[12] although the reason for this correlation is unknown. In one study, 10% of women stated that they had never had pain before childbirth, and this subgroup experienced significantly less pain during labor and delivery,[13] which suggests that individual differences in the experience of pain during labor may reflect individual differences in perception of all types of pain. This is supported

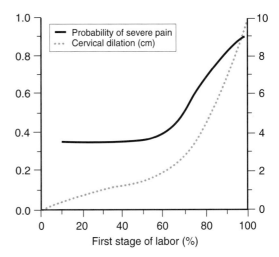

FIGURE 18-3. Likelihood of severe pain during labor. A significant minority of women (approximately one third) have severe pain (pain score >6) in early labor, and the proportion of women with severe pain increases to nearly 90% later in labor, in close relationship with cervical dilation. (Data adapted from Hardy JD, Javert CT. Studies on pain: Measurements of pain intensity in childbirth. J Clin Invest 1949; 28:153-62.)

by the recent observation that the rating of pain intensity in response to a noxious heat stimulus predicts interindividual variability in pain assessment after cesarean section.[14]

The reasons why some people perceive little pain and others more pain from the same stimulus remain unclear. A recent study involving brain imaging and a fixed acute noxious heat stimulus showed a strong correlation between verbal pain assessment and degree of activation of various cortical brain regions, especially the contralateral somatosensory cortex and anterior cingulate cortex.[15] Of interest is that the degree of activation of the thalamus was essentially identical in all subjects, which suggests that differences in perceived pain resulted from differences in modulation at *supra*thalamic levels rather than in peripheral nerves or spinal cord mechanisms. The situation in labor may be more complex. For example, there is a large polymorphism in the genes that regulate cytokine production and function, and this polymorphism affects pregnancy outcome.[16] Cytokines can also alter pain response, and it is possible that interindividual differences in labor pain may partially reflect genetic differences in cytokine production or response.

In summary, some women have painless labor, but many women experience severe pain during labor and delivery; thus it is medically appropriate to offer safe and effective means of analgesia to laboring women. The close correlation between cervical dilation and severity of pain implies that the two may be causally linked and that the likelihood of a woman requesting analgesia increases as she approaches the second stage of labor.

PERSONAL SIGNIFICANCE AND MEANING

The International Association for the Study of Pain has defined pain as "an unpleasant sensory and emotional experience associated with actual or potential tissue damage, or described in terms of such damage."[17] Clearly, this reflects an intensity-discriminatory component and an emotional-cognitive component, with powerful interactions between the two. We typically focus heavily on the former, assuming that labor pain is severe and therefore should be treated pharmacologically, while largely ignoring coping strategies and the personal meaning of labor pain, which varies considerably among women.[18]

Although many women rate the pain of labor and delivery as severe, the terms they use to more fully describe this pain reflect its emotional meaning. In a pioneering study of

the quantification of pain from experimental dilation of the cervix, Bajaj et al.[19] compared pain descriptors among women in labor, those with experimental cervical dilation, those undergoing spontaneous abortion, and those with dysmenorrhea (Table 18-1). Women with dysmenorrhea used words that indicate suffering, such as "punishing" and "wretched," whereas those in labor did not. Some authors have drawn parallels between pain from mountain climbing, which is associated with a sense of euphoria, and the pain of labor.[18] As noted by one woman, "You mature and become a stronger personality when you've had a baby and have gone through the pain. I think that is the purpose of it, what the meaning of life is ... to protect our children, to be stronger, a way of managing everyday life and become stronger...."[20] However, other women see no meaning to the pain of labor and see no reason why it should not be treated. Many other processes that involve pain (e.g., trauma, severe dental disease, cancer) are a considered a "normal" part of human life. These conditions are rarely considered to have a spiritual meaning, thereby making labor pain unique.

In summary, there are large interindividual differences in how women experience the personal significance or meaning of labor pain. These different perceptions can lead to a long-term sense of failure and guilt when pharmacologic pain relief is provided or emotional trauma when it is withheld.

ANATOMIC BASIS

First Stage of Labor

Several lines of evidence suggest that pain during the first stage of labor is transduced by afferents with peripheral terminals in the cervix and lower uterine segment rather than the uterine body, as is often depicted (Figure 18-4). Uterine body afferents fire in response to distention, but in the absence of inflammation, distention of the uterine body has no or minimal effect on behavior in laboratory animals.[21,22] These observations suggest that afferents in the uterine body may be an important site of chronic inflammatory disease and chronic pelvic pain but that they are much less relevant to acute obstetric and uterine cervical pain. In addition, afferents to the uterine body regress during normal pregnancy, whereas those to the cervix and lower uterine segment do not.[23] This denervation of the myometrium may protect against preterm labor by limiting alpha$_1$-adrenergic receptor stimulation by locally released norepinephrine. Javert and Hardy[9] reproduced the pain of uterine contractions in women during labor

TABLE 18-1	WORD DESCRIPTORS FROM THE MCGILL PAIN QUESTIONNAIRE USED TO DESCRIBE PAIN FROM THE UTERUS AND CERVIX			
Pain descriptors	**Balloon distention of the cervix**[19]	**Labor**[130]	**Abortion**[131]	**Dysmennorhea**[19]
Sensory	Shooting, boring, sharp, hot, dull, taut	Throbbing, shooting, sharp, cramping, aching, taut	Cutting, cramping, tugging, pulling, aching	Pulsing, beating, shooting, pricking, boring, drilling, sharp, cutting, pinching, pressing, cramping, tugging, pulling, hot, stinging, dull, hurting, heavy, taut
Affective		Exhausting, tiring, frightening, grueling	Tiring	Tiring, sickening, punishing, wretched
Evaluative	Annoying		Intense	Annoying, intense
Miscellaneous	Drawing, squeezing	Tearing	Numb, squeezing	Piercing, drawing, squeezing, nagging

by manual distention of the cervix. Bonica later confirmed that women undergoing cesarean section under local field block anesthesia experience pain from cervical distention (which mimics that of labor pain) but do not experience pain from uterine distention.[24]

The uterine cervix has a dual innervation; afferents innervating the endocervix and lower uterine segment have cell bodies in thoracolumbar dorsal root ganglia (DRG), whereas afferents innervating the vaginal surface of the cervix and upper vagina have cell bodies in sacral DRG.[25] These two innervations result in different sensory input and referral of pain. Pelvic afferents that innervate the vaginal surface of the cervix are almost exclusively C fibers, with the majority containing the peptides substance P (sP) and calcitonin gene-related peptide (CGRP). These afferents express alpha and beta estrogen receptors and have an innervation pattern that is not affected by pregnancy.[26-28] Stimulation of the vaginal surface of the cervix in rats results in antinociception, lordosis, ovulation, and a hormonal state of pseudopregnancy, all of which are related to mating behaviors in this species.[29] In rats, these vaginal afferent terminals are activated only during delivery and not during labor, which suggests that they are not relevant to the pain of the first stage of labor.[30] By contrast, dilation of the endocervix in rats results in the activation of afferents entering the lower thoracic spinal cord and nociception rather than antinociception. These afferents are mostly or exclusively C fibers[31] and are activated during the first stage of labor, suggesting that they are relevant to pain during this period.

More than 70 years ago, experiments in dogs allowed Cleland[32] to identify T11-12 as the segmental level of entry into the spinal cord of afferents transmitting the pain of the first stage of labor.[32] Because dysmenorrhea is abolished in women by the destruction of the superior or inferior hypogastric plexus,[33] he reasoned that these sensory afferents were likely intermingled with sympathetic efferents, and he subsequently demonstrated that analgesia during the first stage of labor could be achieved with bilateral lumbar paravertebral blocks of the sympathetic chain.[32] Pain of the first stage of labor is transmitted by afferents that pass through the paracervical region, the hypogastric nerve and plexi, and the lumbar sympathetic chain and that have cell bodies in T10-L1 DRG (Figure 18-5).

Classical teaching states that pain-transmitting C and A-delta fibers enter the spinal cord through the dorsal roots and terminate in a dense network of synapses in the ipsilateral superficial laminae (I and II) of the dorsal horn, with minimal rostrocaudal extension of fibers. Whereas this is true for somatic afferents, visceral C fiber afferents enter the cord primarily—but not exclusively—through the dorsal roots and terminate in a loose network of synapses in the superficial and deep dorsal horn and the ventral horn. These afferents even cross to the contralateral dorsal horn, with extensive rostrocaudal extension of fibers (Figure 18-5). This anatomic difference underlies the precise localization of somatic pain and the diffuse localization of visceral pain, which may cross the midline; it may also determine the potency or efficacy of drugs that must reach afferent terminals, such as opioids given intrathecally. For example, the intrathecal doses required to treat postcesarean (somatic) pain and labor (visceral) pain are similar for lipophilic agents such as fentanyl or sufentanil, perhaps because these drugs can extensively penetrate the lipid-rich environment of the spinal cord. By contrast, a much larger intrathecal dose of the hydrophilic agent morphine is required to treat the visceral pain of labor than is needed to treat the somatic pain that occurs after cesarean section.

Classical teaching states that pain-transmitting projection neurons in the spinal cord dorsal horn send axons that cross to the contralateral ventral spinothalamic tract (stimulating neurons in the thalamus) with projections to the somatosensory cortex, where pain is perceived. In addition to the thalamus, these spinal neurons also send axons through the spinoreticular and spinomesencephalic tracts, with inputs to areas of vigilance (locus coeruleus, reticular formation), cardiorespiratory regulation (nucleus tractus solitarius, caudal medulla), and reflex descending inhibition (periaqueductal gray, locus coeruleus and subcoeruleus, nucleus raphe magnus, rostral

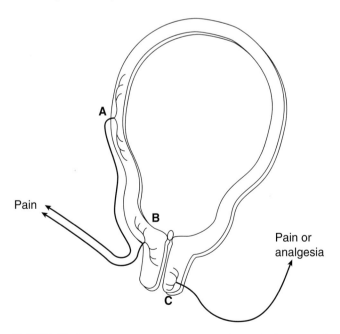

FIGURE 18-4. Uterocervical afferents activated during the first stage of labor. Uterine body afferents (A) partially regress during pregnancy and may contribute to the pain of the first stage of labor. However, the major input is from afferents in the lower uterine segment and endocervix (B). By contrast, at least in animals, the activation of afferents that innervate the vaginal surface of the cervix (C) result in analgesia, not pain, and they enter the spinal cord in sacral areas rather than at the site of referred pain in labor.

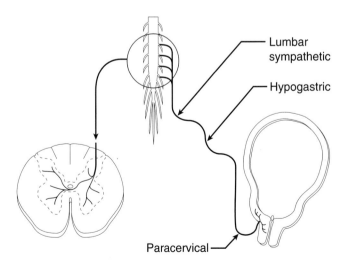

FIGURE 18-5. Pathways of the first stage of labor. Uterocervical afferents pass through the paracervical ganglion, the hypogastric nerve, and the lumbar sympathetic chain, entering the spinal cord in the T10-L1 region. Unlike somatic afferents, these visceral afferents terminate in the deep dorsal horn and the ventral horn of the spinal cord and cross the midline to the contralateral side.

medial medulla, cerebellum). Thalamic activation from painful stimuli not only results in the activation of the somatosensory cortex but also of areas of memory (prefrontal cortex), motor response (M1 motor cortex), and emotional response (insular cortex, anterior cingulate cortex) (Figure 18-6).

Brain imaging studies have not been performed in women in labor or in those undergoing experimental or therapeutic uterine cervical distention. Studies of patients undergoing esophageal distention suggest that visceral stimulation activates areas in the brain that are similar—but not identical—to those in patients undergoing somatic stimulation.[34] When stimuli are matched for levels of intensity, visceral stimulation is perceived to be more unpleasant than somatic stimulation. The region of the anterior cingulate cortex activated during visceral stimulation is more rostral than that activated during somatic stimulation and is immediately adjacent to a region activated by fear and distress.[34]

Implications of the anatomic basis for pain during the first stage of labor are that this pain is amenable to blockade of peripheral afferents (by paracervical block, paravertebral sympathetic nerve block, or epidural block of the T10-L1 dermatomes) or to blockade of spinal cord transmission of pain by intrathecal injection of local anesthetics or opioids. In addition, the widespread distribution of visceral synapses in the spinal cord imply that intrathecally administered drugs (e.g., opioids) that must reach these terminals to produce analgesia must have physicochemical properties that facilitate penetration deep into the cord.

Second Stage of Labor

Pain during the second stage of labor reflects the activation of the same afferents activated during the first stage of labor plus afferents that innervate the vaginal surface of the cervix, the vagina, and the perineum. These additional afferents course through the pudendal nerve with DRG at S2-S4, and they are somatic in nature. Thus, the pain specific to the second stage of labor is precisely localized to the vagina and perineum, and it reflects distention, ischemia, and frank injury, either by stretching to the point of disruption or by surgical incision of the perineum. Studies in animals demonstrate an antinociceptive effect of mechanical stimulation of the vaginal surface of the cervix and other behaviors related to mating and ovulation. Studies in nonpregnant women indicate a minor analgesic effect of mechanical self-stimulation of the vaginal surface of the cervix[35]; this effect may result from the stimulation of C fibers, because it is reduced in women with a high oral intake of capsaicin, which can reduce the activity of such fibers.[36] The relevance—if any—of this minor effect in reducing the pain of the second stage of labor is questionable and has not been examined. However, it does provide evidence that noxious input during labor may activate endogenous analgesia (vide infra).

Implications of the anatomic basis for the pain of the second stage of labor are that analgesia can be obtained by a combination of methods used to treat the pain of the first stage plus pudendal nerve block or extension of epidural blockade from T10 to S4.

NEUROPHYSIOLOGIC BASIS

Peripheral Afferent Terminals

Visceral nociceptors, such as those that transduce the pain of the first stage of labor, are activated by stretching and distention but, unlike somatic afferents, are not activated by cutting. With each uterine contraction, pressure is transmitted to distort and stretch the uterine cervix, thereby leading to the activation of these nerve terminals. How mechanical distention results in the depolarization of the nerve terminal and the generation of an action potential is not entirely known, but three mechanisms are likely:

1. A variety of ion channels respond to distortion of the cell membrane, and one of them—brain sodium channel-1 (BNC-1) or acid-sensing ion channel-2 (ASIC-2)—is exclusively expressed in sensory afferents and might directly depolarize the nerve terminal by opening its channel when the membrane is distorted (Figure 18-7).[37]
2. Mechanical distortion may result in the acute release of a short-acting neurotransmitter that directly and transiently stimulates ion channel receptors on nerve terminals. This

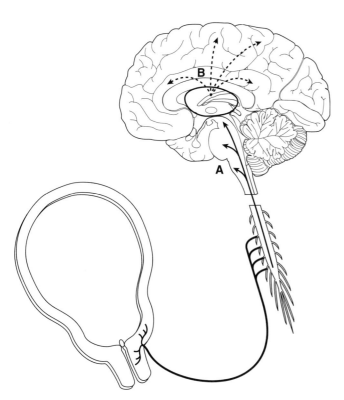

FIGURE 18-6. Supraspinal pain pathways activated by the pain of the first stage of labor. Ascending pathways project to the pons and the medulla *(A),* thereby activating centers of cardiorespiratory control and descending pathways as well as the thalamus *(B),* which in turn sends projections to anterior cingulate, motor, somatosensory, and limbic regions *(dotted lines).*

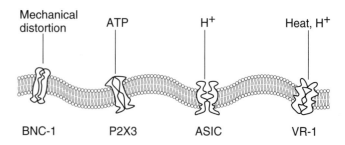

FIGURE 18-7. Afferent nerve endings contain multiple excitatory ligand-gated ion channels, including those that respond to mechanical distortion *(BNC-1,* brain sodium channel-1), ATP *(P2X3,* purinergic receptors), hydrogen ions *(ASIC,* acid-sensing ion channels), or heat *(VR-1,* vanilloid receptor type 1).

has not yet been examined in the uterine cervix. However, it is known that the bladder urothelium releases adenosine triphosphate when it is stretched, and adenosine triphosphate directly stimulates a type of ligand-gated ion channel—P2X3—on sensory afferents in the bladder wall.[38] Because P2X3 receptors are widely expressed in C fibers,[39] it is possible that this mechanism might be responsible for the pain that results from the acute distention of the uterine cervix.

3. Local ischemia during contractions may result in gated or spontaneous activity of other ion channels. Some of these ion channels—the ASIC family—respond directly to the low pH that occurs during ischemia.[40] Other classes of ion channels may be activated to open spontaneously. For example, the vanilloid receptor-1 (VR-1) can be stimulated by capsaicin, which is the active ingredient in hot chili pepper. It is likely that VR-1 receptors (which also respond to noxious heat) are expressed on visceral afferent terminals, given that the application of capsaicin or heat to the distal esophagus results in pain in humans.[41] VR-1 receptor-gated ion channels are not normally open in the absence of high temperature or capsaicin-like ligands. However, low pH shifts the temperature response of these receptors so that they open their channel at body temperature.[42]

Uterine cervical afferents (including the C fibers that innervate the vaginal surface of the cervix), contain sP, CGRP, and the enzyme nitric oxide synthase.[43] C fibers can be divided into two groups: (1) those that contain sP and CCRP and respond to nerve growth factor by actions on tyrosine kinase A receptors; and (2) those that do not contain these peptides but that contain somatostatin and respond to glial-derived growth factor by actions on a c-ret complex.[44] This is a rough classification at best, with some overlap, and further definition of C fiber subtypes will likely occur as more markers and neuropeptides are examined. Other compounds commonly contained in C fiber terminals include glutamate, vasoactive intestinal peptide, and neuropeptide Y. The variable role of C fiber subtypes in the transmission of pain is also unclear. Given that somatostatin typically inhibits sP release and pain transmission,[45,46] it is quite possible that the net transmission of nociception at the spinal cord level reflects a complex interaction between excitatory and inhibitory C fiber subtypes.

Implications of peripheral afferent neurophysiology in the pain of the first stage of labor are that the multiple ion channels that transduce the mechanical signal of cervical stretching to an electrical signal that generates the perception of pain are largely unexplored and may yield new targets for local or systemic drug delivery to treat this pain. In addition, our understanding of the classification, function, and relevance to pain of different C fiber subtypes is in its infancy. Research involving endocervical C fiber subtypes may identify new targets for the treatment of labor pain.

ROLE OF SENSITIZATION

Peripheral afferent terminals, like other parts of the sensory system, are not fixed but can change their response properties during various conditions. Especially important is inflammation (Figure 18-8), which can result in direct stimulation of afferent terminals by low pH. Also, the release of bradykinin stimulates selective ligand-gated ion channels on these terminals.[47] In addition, peripheral inflammation sensitizes afferent terminals by changing the properties of the terminals themselves; this is a process that

can result over a short time in a change in genes that are expressed by these nerve fibers, thereby leading to a large amplification of pain signaling.

Although peripheral inflammation is most commonly considered a major part of the pain that results from acute postoperative and chronic arthritic conditions, it may also play an essential role in labor pain. The cervical ripening process and labor itself both result from local synthesis and release of a variety of inflammatory products. This has been recognized clinically for many years, leading to the application of inflammatory mediators (e.g., prostaglandin [PG]E₂) to the cervix to prepare for the induction of labor and the administration of inhibitors of synthesis of inflammatory mediators (e.g., indomethacin) to stop preterm labor.

PGE_2 is an especially important sensitizing agent for uterine cervical afferents. In most species, the onset of labor is triggered by a sudden decrease in circulating estrogen concentrations. This removes a tonic block on expression of cyclooxygenase and results in an increase in local prostaglandin production, especially PGE_2.[48] PGE_2 is central to a variety of processes that are activated to allow for the ripening of the uterine cervix and its dilation during labor. Thus, during the 24 to 72 hours preceding the onset of labor, collagen becomes disorganized in the cervix as a result of activation of prostaglandin receptors and the activity of inflammatory cytokines (mostly interleukin-1-beta and tumor necrosis factor-alpha) and matrix metalloproteinases (especially types 2 and 9).[49,50] A series of studies in the rat paw have demonstrated that PGE_2 induces peripheral sensitization in a sex-independent manner by activation of protein kinase A[51] and nitric oxide synthase.[52]

Cytokines and growth factors are also released into the uterine cervix just before and during labor. The cytokine interleukin-1-beta enhances cyclooxygenase activity and sP release in DRG and the spinal cord.[53,54] Tumor necrosis factor-alpha increases the spontaneous activity of afferent

Cervical ripening factors:

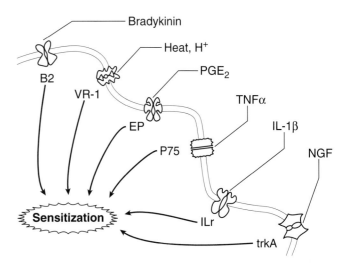

FIGURE 18-8. Effects of inflammation from cervical ripening on afferent terminals. A variety of factors—including bradykinin, heat and hydrogen ions, prostaglandins (including *PGE₂*), tumor necrosis factor-alpha (*TNFα*), interleukin-1-beta (*IL-1β*), and nerve growth factor (*NGF*)—act on their cognate receptors to sensitize nerve endings and amplify the perception and degree of pain from nerve stimulation. *B₂*, Bradykinin-2 receptor; *EP*, prostaglandin E receptor; *ILr*, interleukin-1 receptor; *p75*, p75 TNF-alpha receptor; *trkA*, tyrosine kinase A; *VR-1*, vanilloid-1 receptor.

fibers[55] and enhances CGRP release and VR-1 receptor expression in DRG cells in culture.[56] Nerve growth factor also induces mechanical hypersensitivity.[57] These sensitizing substances (prostaglandins, cytokines, and growth factors) signal peripheral nerves in a manner that results in a host of changes in DRG cell number, peptide expression and release, receptor and ion channel expression, and biophysical properties. For example, multiple sodium (Na^+) channel subtypes exist, and inflammatory mediators alter their expression,[58,59] thereby resulting in more rapid, repetitive firing capability[60] and spontaneous afferent activity.[61]

Implications of the peripheral sensitization of cervical afferents during labor are as follows: (1) Braxton-Hicks contractions, prior to the onset of this inflammatory process, are as powerful as labor contractions but are painless; (2) pain may increase as labor progresses as a result of sensitization; and (3) inflammatory mediators may provide new targets to treat labor pain.

INHIBITORY RECEPTORS

Given the multiplicity of direct excitatory and sensitizing mechanisms on peripheral terminals, a more plausible target for peripheral pain treatment is endogenous inhibitory receptors expressed on afferent terminals (Figure 18-9). Opioid receptors have achieved the widest attention. Although mu-opioid receptors are expressed in some afferents in the setting of inflammation,[62] the efficacy of the local instillation of morphine has been disappointing,[63] with the exception of intra-articular injection.[64] Similarly, we have observed that mu-opioid receptor agonists produce antinociception to uterine cervical distention by actions in the central nervous system but not in the periphery.[65]

It has been suggested that kappa-opioid receptor agonists may effectively treat visceral pain. Unlike somatic afferents, visceral afferents—at least to the gastrointestinal tract—express kappa-opioid receptors.[66] Similarly, it has been observed that kappa-opioid receptor agonists produce antinociception to uterine cervical distention by actions in the peripheral nervous system.[31,65]

Kappa-opioid receptor agonists may be especially attractive for the treatment of labor pain given that pharmaceutical firms are developing drugs of this class that are restricted to the periphery, with few central side effects[67,68] and presumably little potential for placental transfer. It has recently been observed that one of these new agents effectively treats chronic visceral pain from pancreatitis in patients receiving poor analgesia from mu-opioid receptor agonists.[69]

Estrogen and progesterone can alter the analgesic response to opioids. In most cases involving somatic stimulation, tonic estrogen treatment reduces the efficacy of mu- but not kappa-opioid receptor agonists.[70] Further, kappa-opioid receptor agonists have greater analgesic efficacy in women than in men.[71] In animals, tonic estrogen exposure reduces the inhibition of responses to uterine cervical distention by morphine but not by the kappa-opioid receptor agonist U-50488.[72] Of interest is that the inhibitory action of intrathecal morphine against responses to uterine cervical distention is unaffected by tonic estrogen exposure,[73] which is consistent with the observation that intrathecal opioids relieve the pain of the first stage of labor.

Implications of inhibitory receptors on afferent terminals are that kappa-opioid but not mu-opioid receptor agonists may produce pain relief by actions in the periphery. Such selective peripherally restricted drugs are under development for the systemic treatment of visceral pain. In addition, estrogen-dependent inhibition of the supraspinal (but not the spinal) analgesic action of mu-opioid receptor agonists may underlie the poor effect of systemic opioids[74] and the complete effect of intrathecal opioids[75] to relieve the pain of the first stage of labor.

Peripheral Nerve Axons

Much of our current approach to labor pain relies on our knowledge of the course of afferent axons and their entry level in the spinal cord, and includes the local injection of local anesthetics to block conduction of afferent traffic. Traditionally axons have been considered conduits that allow for the propagation of action potentials by the transitory opening of Na^+ channels. Recently it has become clear that not only are there a variety of subtypes of Na^+ channels but also that axons are replete with other ion channels that modulate transmission.

Of the numerous voltage-gated Na^+ channel subtypes, studies have focused on three that are expressed in sensory afferents.[76] Two of these, NaV1.8 and NaV1.9, are relatively resistant to blockade by tetrodotoxin (TTX-R), the latter often being called "persistent" due to its very slow inactivation kinetics.[77] Inflammation and injury to nerves decrease the TTX-R current density in afferent cell bodies.[78] Some investigators have suggested that NaV1.8 is selectively trafficked to the periphery after injury and inflammation[78] and that reducing NaV1.8 expression reduces hypersensitivity.[79] Others, using sucrose gap measurements of compound action potential, have demonstrated a shortened refractory period and a decrease in delayed depolarization following nerve injury[80,81] that is consistent with the increased expression of rapidly repriming TTX-S channels and the decreased expression of kinetically slow TTX-R channels, respectively. These studies have primarily focused on peripheral nerve injury models of chronic pain, but Na^+ channel subtype expression can change rapidly, and neither the subtypes nor their change during the cervical inflammation of labor have been studied.

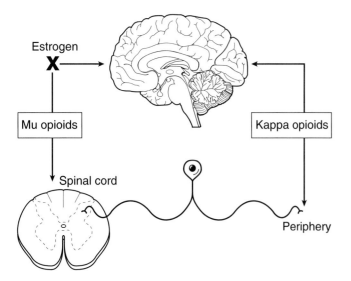

FIGURE 18-9. Kappa-opioid receptor agonists act primarily at visceral afferent terminals in the periphery and in the supraspinal central nervous system to provide analgesia during the first stage of labor, whereas mu-opioid receptor agonists act in the spinal cord and the supraspinal central nervous system. Estrogens block the effect of mu-opioid receptor agonists at supraspinal sites.

Several pharmaceutical firms have large discovery programs to produce Na$^+$ channel subtype-selective blockers that could improve both the safety and efficacy of treatment of labor pain, because they would not interact with Na$^+$ channels in the brain, heart, or motor nerve fibers. Some investigators have noted that amitriptyline and its derivatives, when injected around peripheral nerves, produce neural blockade with a duration that is two to five times longer than that provided by the longest-acting local anesthetic.[82,83] Whether this reflects interactions with Na$^+$ channel subtypes has not yet been investigated, but should toxicity studies be negative, it is conceivable that very long-lasting analgesia from such agents would allow for the use of alternative single-injection techniques (e.g., paravertebral block) for the treatment of labor pain.

A surprisingly large number of ion channels are expressed on axons and can alter neural conduction. Two examples are provided here. First, a short burst of nerve firing results in a transient refractory period, when the nerve is less susceptible to stimulation because of membrane hyperpolarization. This phenomenon, which dampens high-frequency nerve activity, results from the activation of a Na$^+$/K$^+$ exchange pump and is itself reduced in intensity by a hyperpolarization-induced current termed I$_h$. Drugs that block this opposing I$_h$ current enhance the hyperpolarization from the Na$^+$/K$^+$ exchange pump, reduce nerve traffic,[84] and produce prolonged analgesia.[85] Second, VR-1 receptors themselves are present on the axons of C fibers, and injection (around the nerve) of drugs that desensitize these receptors without first stimulating them fails to induce acute pain from receptor stimulation but produces very long periods of selective sensory analgesia without motor effects.[86] The mechanisms by which VR-1 receptor desensitization alters the transmission of action potentials is under investigation.

Implications of the neurophysiology of axonal transmission of labor pain are that Na$^+$ channel subtype-selective agents—or those that affect other ion channels expressed on axons—may provide safer and more selective tools for regional analgesic techniques.

Spinal Cord

When action potentials invade the central terminals of C and A-delta fiber afferents in the spinal cord, voltage-gated calcium channels as well as intracellular calcium channels open, and intracellular calcium concentrations increase, thereby leading to a multistep process of neurotransmitter docking and fusion with the plasma membrane and neurotransmitter release.[87] Inhibition of these calcium channels produces analgesia. Recent studies in animals suggest that at least one agent that interacts with calcium channels—gabapentin—produces antinociception to visceral stimulation.[88] Painful stimulation results in the release of multiple excitatory neurotransmitters in the spinal cord, including amino acids (glutamate, aspartate) and peptides (especially sP, CGRP, neurokinin A) that interact with specific receptors on spinal cord neurons. Although the stimulation of neurokinin receptors is necessary for the perception of moderate to severe pain,[89] a complex and poorly understood interplay exists among these released neurotransmitters in pain transmission. The same afferents may contain multiple neurotransmitters and release them differentially according to firing frequency, and the response of the postsynaptic receptor to one neurotransmitter can be modulated by another postsynaptic receptor. For this reason, factors that influence firing frequency (e.g., the I$_h$ current) can have a profound impact on net stimulation in the spinal cord.

The release of neurotransmitters at sensory afferent terminals is under powerful presynaptic control by receptors that act primarily to alter the release of intracellular calcium when an action potential arrives. Some of these are excitatory; for example, acetylcholine amplifies neurotransmitter release by actions on nicotinic acetylcholine receptors.[90] Gamma-aminobutyric acid (GABA) is the key endogenous inhibitory neurotransmitter in the nervous system, and GABA receptors powerfully reduce afferent terminal release of neurotransmitters.[91] Multiple compounds produce analgesia by enhancing the release of GABA at afferent terminals in the spinal cord; this leads to yet more complicated effects of intrathecally administered agonists. For example, acetylcholine can *enhance* the afferent terminal release of neurotransmitters by actions on nicotinic receptors or *reduce* neurotransmitter release by the enhancement of GABA release[92] via stimulation of muscarinic receptors.[93] The net effect of acetylcholine appears to be inhibitory, which is indicated by the analgesic effect of intrathecal injection of the cholinesterase inhibitor neostigmine.[94]

The inhibition of neurotransmitter release from primary afferent terminals is also the primary mechanism of action of the neurotransmitter enkephalin, which is released by spinal cord interneurons, and norepinephrine, which is released by axons descending from pontine centers. These substances act on mu-opioid and alpha$_2$-adrenergic receptors, respectively, to reduce neurotransmitter release.[95,96] This activity underlies the rationale for the intrathecal administration of opioids and alpha$_2$-adrenergic agonists to treat labor pain.

Amino acids and peptides released from sensory afferents stimulate a heterogeneous group of spinal cord neurons, including neurons that project to supraspinal structures, interneurons that modulate transmission at the afferent terminal itself (the gate of the gate control theory), and interneurons that stimulate motor and sympathetic nervous system reflexes. Of primary interest in the field of chronic pain is the activation of N-methyl-D-aspartate (NMDA) receptors by large and sustained glutamate release from intensely noxious stimulation, which leads to a sustained depolarization and enhanced excitability of projection neurons (Figure 18-10).[97] Although intrathecal injection of NMDA receptor antagonists (e.g., ketamine) has been restricted because of concerns about neurotoxicity,[98] systemic infusion of magnesium sulfate

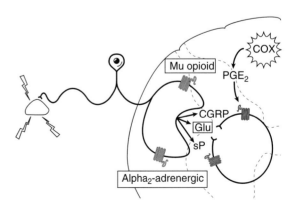

FIGURE 18-10. Pain transmission in the spinal cord. Excitatory transmission occurs directly by release of amino acids such as glutamate (*Glu*) and peptides (*sP*, substance P; *CGRP*, calcitonin gene-related peptide) and indirectly via activation of enzymes such as cyclooxygenase (*COX*) in nearby glia, which synthesize prostaglandins, including *PGE$_2$*. Inhibitory mechanisms are primarily presynaptic, with mu-opioid and alpha$_2$-adrenergic receptors being the most common (or at least the most studied).

produces postoperative analgesia.[99] Magnesium is an endogenous inhibitory modulator of NMDA receptors, and it is conceivable that magnesium sulfate, which is commonly administered systemically for obstetric indications, may have a minor effect on labor pain.

Just as sensitization processes occur with inflammation in the periphery, sensitization and amplification of pain signaling occurs at the spinal cord level during periods of prolonged, intense nociception, as occurs during labor. Some of these processes are a direct consequence of receptors (e.g., NMDA receptors) that are activated only with high intensity and prolonged stimulation or by long-term effects of simultaneous activation of glutamate and sP receptors on the same cell by co-released neurotransmitters. Others reflect the synthesis and release of classic "inflammatory" substances by glial cells in the spinal cord from prolonged afferent stimulation, such as nitric oxide and prostaglandins, especially PGE_2. Indeed, some nonsteroidal antiinflammatory drugs produce analgesia by actions in the central nervous system (probably the spinal cord), either exclusively (e.g., acetaminophen) or primarily (e.g., aspirin).[100]

Spinal sensitization processes also represent an interesting target for the novel treatment of labor pain. More than 70 years ago, Cleland[32] noted the presence of hypersensitivity to light touch on the skin of dermatomes T11 and T12 in women in labor, which likely represents the hypersensitivity of spinal cord neurons receiving both visceral input from the cervix and skin input at these levels.[101] He also noted that this hypersensitivity disappeared when visceral stimulation to these dermatomes was blocked by paravertebral injection of local anesthetic,[32] which is consistent with the reliance of hypersensitivity upon ongoing C fiber input.[102] Recently the intrathecal injection of the cyclooxygenase inhibitor ketorolac has been introduced into experimental human trials,[103] and preliminary observations that intrathecal administration of a cyclooxygenase inhibitor results in reduced response to uterine cervical distention suggest that this treatment warrants examination for the treatment of labor pain.

Implications of the neurophysiologic basis for labor pain in the spinal cord are that purely inhibitory mechanisms (e.g., opioid and alpha$_2$-adrenergic receptors) can be mimicked by the intrathecal injection of agonists to these receptors for labor analgesia, whereas the more complex intrathecal actions of other agents (e.g., acetylcholine) are less predictable. Central sensitization mechanisms in the spinal cord most certainly occur during labor, and future treatments may target those mechanisms.

Ascending Projections

Spinal cord neurons project to multiple brainstem sites as well as the thalamus. More than 25 years ago, it was noted that descending systems—activated primarily by stimulation of the nucleus raphe magnus, the periaqueductal gray, and the locus coeruleus—could reduce pain transmission, as described in the gate control theory.[104] Activation of descending pathways results in the spinal release of endogenous ligands for serotonergic, opioid, and alpha$_2$-adrenergic receptor-mediated analgesia, respectively. Spillover of neurotransmitters in cerebrospinal fluid has been used as a measure of activation of these systems, and studies measuring these substances have shown no increase in enkephalin—but an increase in norepinephrine—in laboring women.[105] These descending systems can be activated by psychoprophylactic methods,[106] and it is conceivable that agents that prolong or intensify the action of these ligands, such as enkephalinase inhibitors or blockers of monoamine reuptake, might further enhance analgesia by descending pathways.[107]

Brainstem activation by the pain of labor leads to other reflexes, such as increased sympathetic nervous system activity, increased respiratory drive, and, with prolonged activation, stimulation of descending pathways that amplify rather than reduce pain transmission at the spinal cord.[108,109] The circuitry and pharmacology of such pain-enhancing systems in the brainstem and their potential applications for treatment are under current investigation.

Our understanding of the areas of the brain activated during labor pain is limited, although studies of other types of experimental visceral nociception in healthy volunteers indicate that visceral pain is considered more unpleasant than somatic pain, which reflects the greater activation of centers of negative emotions, including fear.[34] Perception of pain is powerfully modulated in the brain. In normal volunteers, a simple noxious heat stimulus evokes a similar degree of activation of the thalamus in everyone (i.e., the pain signaling system from the periphery to the thalamus is similar), but it results in greatly differing degrees of cortical activation, which is directly correlated with the verbal assessment of pain intensity.[15] Distraction methods within the same individual do not alter thalamic activation from noxious stimulation, but they reduce cortical activation and pain report,[110] which supports a suprathalamic mechanism of psychoprophylaxis to reduce pain.

Implications of the neurophysiologic basis of labor pain and ascending projections are that multiple supraspinal sites are activated by pain. Some of these sites stimulate potentially detrimental cardiorespiratory reflexes. Other sites send descending projections that either reduce or enhance pain transmission in the spinal cord; some of these sites may be targeted for the provision of analgesia. In addition, there is emerging evidence that the suprathalamic modulation of pain signals accounts for interindividual differences in pain perception and response and for the efficacy of psychoprophylaxis.

EFFECT ON THE MOTHER

Obstetric Course

Several aspects of labor pain can affect the course of labor and delivery (Figure 18-11). The most commonly cited is the fact that pain increases sympathetic nervous system activity, which results in increased plasma concentrations of catecholamines, especially epinephrine. Provision of analgesia decreases plasma concentrations of epinephrine and its beta-adrenergic tocolytic effect on the myometrium. This may underlie the observations by some investigators who have noted, either anecdotally or under controlled conditions, a shift from a dysfunctional to a normal labor pattern in some women when analgesia is achieved with paravertebral[32,111] or epidural[112] block or with systemic meperidine analgesia.[113] In addition, the abrupt reduction in plasma concentrations of epinephrine that follows the rapid onset of intrathecal opioid analgesia may result in an acute reduction of beta-adrenergic tocolysis and a transient period of uterine hyperstimulation, which in some cases may lead to transient fetal stress and bradycardia.[114]

Ferguson's reflex involves neural input from ascending spinal tracts (especially from sacral sensory input) to the midbrain, thereby resulting in enhanced oxytocin release. Although spontaneous labor and delivery occur in women with spinal cord injury (which disrupts this tract[115]), some have argued that regional analgesia can inhibit this reflex and prolong labor, especially the second stage. However, strong evidence for this does not exist. Some studies have noted a reduction in plasma oxytocin concentrations with epidural local anesthetic[116] or intrathecal opioid[117] analgesia, whereas others have failed to note such a reduction.[118]

Papka[23] suggested that afferent terminals in the lower uterine segment and cervix may play an important secretory (efferent) function to regulate labor. Afferent terminals contain many substances that can *stimulate* (sP, glutamate, vasoactive intestinal peptide) or *inhibit* (CGRP, nitric oxide) myometrial activity, and these substances can be released locally into the cervix and lower uterine segment when terminals are depolarized by tissue distortion during contractions. In addition, depolarization of an afferent terminal can result in an action potential that, upon reaching a site of branching of the nerve, invades adjacent branches and travels distally to depolarize terminals of the same nerve in distant areas. This axon reflex has long been recognized in somatic nerves and, because visceral nerves may have more extensive arborizations, may result in the widespread release of these transmitters from local stimulation. It is tempting to speculate that these axon reflexes are more profoundly affected when local anesthetic is administered closer to the terminals (as occurs with paracervical and paravertebral blocks[111]), which are associated with the more rapid progress of cervical dilation and labor than occurs when local anesthetic is administered further from the terminals (e.g., with epidural block). This would imply that the net effect of afferent terminal-released substances inhibits rather than accelerates labor.

In summary, neural stimulation through pain pathways results in the release of substances that either drive (oxytocin)

or brake (epinephrine) uterine activity and cervical dilation; therefore, the effect of analgesia on the course of labor can vary between individuals. In addition, axon reflexes can result in the release of neurotransmitters from afferents into the lower uterine segment and cervix, which drive or brake uterine activity and cervical dilation. These reflexes can be affected differentially depending on how close to the nerve terminals that the local anesthetic is deposited.

Cardiac and Respiratory Effects

Labor results in stresses on cardiovascular and respiratory function. Pain and stress result in the activation of the sympathetic nervous system, reflected in increased plasma catecholamine concentrations, with a resultant increase in cardiac output and peripheral vascular resistance and a reduction in uteroplacental perfusion. Even transient stress may cause dramatic increases in plasma concentrations of norepinephrine and decreases in uterine blood flow (Figure 18-12). Plasma epinephrine concentrations in women with painful labor are similar to those observed after an intravenous bolus of 15 μg of epinephrine,[119] a dose that reduces uterine blood flow in animals by as much as 50%.[120] Effective analgesia (provided by either epidural local anesthetic[121] or intrathecal opioid administration[122]) results in large (50%) decreases in catecholamine concentrations in maternal blood. By contrast, regional anesthetic techniques do not alter neonatal concentrations of catecholamines, which are thought to be important to adaptation to extrauterine life.[123]

The intermittent pain of uterine contractions also stimulates respiration and results in periods of intermittent hyperventila-

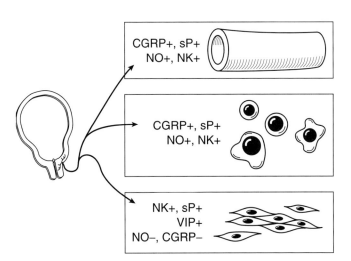

FIGURE 18-11. Aspects of pain that may affect the course of labor. In addition to indirect effects (e.g., beta-adrenergic tocolysis from increased secretion of epinephrine, increased release of oxytocin via Ferguson's reflex), depolarization of afferent terminals in the lower uterine segment and cervix can directly alter aspects of labor. Substances released by nerve terminals include those that increase local blood flow (*CGRP*, calcitonin gene-related peptide; *sP*, substance P; *NO*, nitric oxide; *NK*, neurokinin), those that stimulate immune cell function, and those that stimulate (+) or inhibit (–) myometrial smooth muscle activity, including vasoactive intestinal peptide (*VIP*).

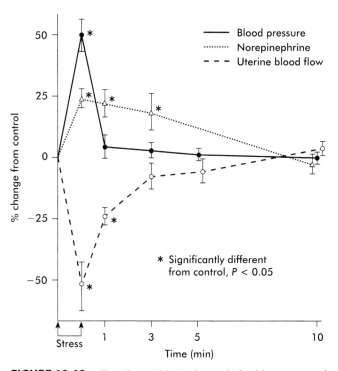

FIGURE 18-12. Effect of a painful stimulus on the hind leg on maternal blood pressure, norepinephrine concentrations, and uterine blood flow in gravid ewes. The increased blood pressure was transient, but plasma norepinephrine concentrations remained elevated for several minutes, which is reflected in the slow return of uterine blood flow to normal. (From Shnider SM, Wright RG, Levinson G, et al. Uterine blood flow and plasma norepinephrine changes during maternal stress in the pregnant ewe. Anesthesiology 1979; 50:524-7.)

tion. In the absence of supplemental oxygen administration, compensatory periods of hypoventilation between contractions result in transient periods of maternal hypoxemia and, in some cases, fetal hypoxemia (Figure 18-13). Treatment of pain with epidural analgesia abolishes the increase in net minute ventilation during labor and its accompanying increase in oxygen consumption.[124]

Clearly acute and intermittent severe pain stresses the cardiovascular and respiratory systems. These stresses are well tolerated by healthy parturients with normal uteroplacental perfusion, and some authors have indicated that they are of no concern or relevance in uncomplicated labor.[18] However, these effects may lead to maternal or fetal decompensation when disease is present, and effective analgesia is especially important in such cases.

In summary, activation of the sympathetic nervous system and intermittent periods of hyperventilation commonly occur with severe pain in labor, can have detrimental maternal and fetal effects, and are reduced or abolished with the provision of effective analgesia.

Psychologic Effects

The meaning of labor pain varies considerably among women, and it is greatly influenced by psychosocial and environmental factors *(vide supra)*. Although pain relief has a minor effect on overall maternal satisfaction with the labor and delivery process,[125] it can have profound effects in individual women. It has been argued that if a woman understands the origin of her pain and sees the labor and delivery process as positive and nonthreatening, she may undergo pain without suffering.[18] Indeed, a small proportion (< 5%) of women who request and receive epidural analgesia during labor describe a sense of deprivation from a lack of experience of labor in its entirety,[126] and some may even seek psychiatric counseling as a result.[127]

On the other hand, unrelieved severe labor pain can have several negative psychologic and physical consequences, including depression and negative thoughts about sexual relationships.[8,12] In a 5-year study in Sweden, 43 women requested elective cesarean section because of fear of labor and vaginal delivery.[128] Some countries (e.g., Brazil) have traditionally had an extremely high (> 80%) elective cesarean section rate among upper-class women because of their concern for the potential for reduced sexual function after vaginal delivery. Frank psychotic reactions resembling posttraumatic stress disorder can occur after childbirth, although the rate is < 1%.[129]

Implications of the psychologic effects of labor pain are that a small proportion of women can be psychologically harmed by either providing or withholding analgesia, which underscores the tremendous variability in the meaning of labor pain and both individual and environmental influences upon this meaning.

EFFECT ON THE FETUS

Labor pain itself has no direct effects on the fetus, because there are no direct neural connections from the mother to the fetus. However, labor pain can affect multiple systems that determine uteroplacental perfusion: (1) uterine contraction frequency and intensity, by the effect of pain on the release of oxytocin and epinephrine; (2) uterine artery vasoconstriction, by the effect of pain on the release of norepinephrine and epinephrine; and (3) maternal oxyhemoglobin desaturation, which may result from intermittent hyperventilation followed by hypoventilation *(vide supra)*. These effects are well tolerated in normal circumstances and are effectively blocked by analgesia. Analgesia may be especially important to fetal well-being when these effects of labor pain impinge on situations of limited uteroplacental reserve.

SUMMARY

Pain during the first stage of labor results from the stimulation of visceral afferents that innervate the lower uterine segment and cervix, intermingle with sympathetic efferents, and enter the spinal cord at the T10-L1 segments. Pain during the second stage of labor results from the additional stimulation of somatic afferents that innervate the vagina and perineum, travel in the pudendal nerve, and enter the spinal cord at the S2-S4 segments. These pain signals are processed in the spinal cord and are transmitted to brainstem, midbrain, and thalamic sites, the latter with projections to the cortex, which results in the sensory-emotional experience of pain. Current obstetric anesthesia practice relies nearly exclusively on the blocking of pain transmission by deposition of local anesthetic—with or without adjuncts—along the afferent nerves from sites near the peripheral afferent terminals to sites near their central terminals.

We are at the dawn of a new understanding of the neurophysiology of visceral pain in general and labor pain in particular. There is considerable academic and pharmaceutical research targeting the following: (1) the normal ionic transduction mechanisms and processes of sensitization in peripheral afferent terminals; (2) the rich pharmacology of inhibition available in the spinal cord and brainstem; and (3) the mechanisms by which conscious distraction methods function to relieve pain and how those methods can be amplified. Labor pain is an intensely variable and personal experience, and it is essential that the anesthesiologist play a flexible role within this context.

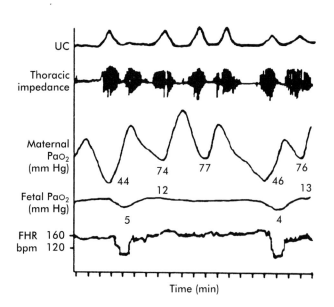

FIGURE 18-13. Maternal and fetal hypoxemia during hypoventilation between contractions that are associated with maternal hyperventilation. *UC,* Uterine contraction. (From Bonica JJ. Labour pain. In Wall PD, Melzack R, editors. Textbook of Pain. Churchill Livingstone, Edinburgh, 1984, as redrawn from Huch A, Huch R, Schneider H, Rooth GL. Continuous transcutaneous monitoring of fetal oxygen tension during labour. Br J Obstet Gynaecol 1977; 84[suppl]:1-39.)

KEY POINTS

- Labor pain exists and is severe in many women, with a close correlation between cervical dilation and pain during the first stage.
- The first stage of labor includes visceral pain from the lower uterine segment and endocervix, which results in hypersensitivity to convergent somatic dermatomes. This pain is most likely amplified over time as a result of the sensitization of peripheral and central pain-signaling pathways. The second stage of labor results in somatic pain from the vagina and perineum and is briefer than the first.
- Afferent terminals transduce a mechanical process into electrical signals, and these are likely amplified by the release of prostaglandins, cytokines, and growth factors into the cervix as part of the normal disruption of collagen that allows the cervix to soften and dilate.
- Pain transmission in the spinal cord is not hard wired; it is remarkably and rapidly plastic, and it is altered by local neuronal activity that releases mu-opioid receptor agonists and descending pathways that release alpha$_2$-adrenergic and serotonergic receptor agonists.
- There are large individual differences in pain perception that likely reflect differences at suprathalamic sites. The activation of suprathalamic sites is the primary mechanism of action for distraction methods of analgesia.
- Labor pain alters obstetric course and cardiac and respiratory function in a complex manner that normally is well tolerated, that can sometimes be detrimental to the mother or the fetus, and that is alleviated by analgesia.
- Labor pain carries meaning, which most other severe pain does not. The treatment of labor pain should be applied within this context.

REFERENCES

1. Melzack R, Wall PD. Pain mechanisms: A new theory. Science 1965; 150:971-5.
2. Melzack R. From the gate to the neuromatrix. Pain 1999; Suppl 6:S121-6.
3. Simone DA, Baumann TK, LaMotte RH. Dose-dependent pain and mechanical hyperalgesia in humans after intradermal injection of capsaicin. Pain 1989; 38:99-107.
4. Woolf CJ, Max MB. Mechanism-based pain diagnosis. Issues for analgesic drug development. Anesthesiology 2001; 95:241-9.
5. Eisenach JC. The treatment of pain: remaining challenges and future opportunities. Can J Anaesth 2002; 49:R1-3.
6. Dick-Read GP. Childbirth without fear. New York, Harper, 1953.
7. Lamaze F. Qu'est-ce que l'accouchement sans douleur par la methode psychoprophyactique? Ses principes, sa realisation, ses resultats. Paris, Savouret Connaitre, 1956.
8. Melzack R. The myth of painless childbirth (The John J. Bonica Lecture). Pain 1984; 19:321-37.
9. Javert CT, Hardy JD. Influence of analgesics on pain intensity during labor (with a note on "natural childbirth"). Anesthesiology 1951; 12:189-215.
10. Hardy JD, Javert CT. Studies on pain: Measurements of pain intensity in childbirth. J Clin Invest 1949; 28:153-62.
11. Algom D, Lubel S. Psychophysics in the field: Perception and memory for labor pain. Percept Psychophys 1994; 55:133-41.
12. Melzack R, Taenzer P, Feldman P, Kinch RA. Labour is still painful after prepared childbirth training. Can Med Assoc J 1981; 125:357-63.
13. Niven CA, Gijsbers KJ. Do low levels of labour pain reflect low sensitivity to noxious stimulation? Soc Sci Med 1989; 29:585-8.
14. Granot M, Lowenstein L, Yarnitsky D, et al. Postcesarean section pain prediction by preoperative experimental pain assessment. Anesthesiology 2003; 98:1422-6.
15. Coghill RC, McHaffie JG, Yen Y-F. Neural correlates of inter-individual differences in the subjective experience of pain. Proc Natl Acad Sci USA 2003; 100:8538-42.
16. Reid JG, Simpson NA, Walker RG, et al. The carriage of pro-inflammatory cytokine gene polymorphisms in recurrent pregnancy loss. Am J Reprod Immunol 2001; 45:35-40.
17. Merskey H. Pain terms: a list with definitions and a note on usage. Recommended by the International Association for the Study of Pain (IASP) Subcommittee on Taxonomy. Pain 1979; 6:249-52.
18. Lowe NK. The nature of labor pain. Am J Obstet Gynecol 2002; 186:S16-24.
19. Bajaj P, Drewes AM, Gregersen H, et al. Controlled dilatation of the uterine cervix. An experimental visceral pain model. Pain 2002; 99: 433-42.
20. Lundgren I, Dahlberg K. Women's experience of pain during childbirth. Midwifery 1998; 14:105-10.
21. Robbins A, Sato Y, Hotta H, Berkley KJ. Responses of hypogastric nerve afferent fibers to uterine distention in estrous or metestrous rats. Neurosci Lett 1990; 110:82-5.
22. Bradshaw HB, Temple JL, Wood E, Berkley KJ. Estrous variations in behavioral responses to vaginal and uterine distention in the rat. Pain 1999; 82:187-97.
23. Papka RE, Shew RL. Neural input to the uterus and influence on uterine contractility. In: Garfield RE, Tabb TN, editors. Control of Uterine Contractility. London, CRC Press, Inc., 1993:375-99.
24. Bonica JJ, Chadwick HS. Labour pain. In: Wall PD, Melzack R, editors. Textbook of Pain. 2nd ed. New York, Churchill Livingstone, 1989: 482-99.
25. Berkley KJ, Robbins A, Sato Y. Functional differences between afferent fibers in the hypogastric and pelvic nerves innervating female reproductive organs in the rat. J Neurophysiol 1993; 69:533-44.
26. Papka RE, Storey-Workley M, Shughrue PJ, et al. Estrogen receptor-α and -β immunoreactivity and mRNA in neurons of sensory and autonomic ganglia and spinal cord. Cell Tissue Res 2001; 304:193-214.
27. Papka RE, Storey-Workley M. Estrogen receptor-α and -β coexist in a subpopulation of sensory neurons of female rat dorsal root ganglia. Neurosci Lett 2002; 319:71-4.
28. Pokabla MJ, Dickerson IM, Papka RE. Calcitonin gene-related peptide-receptor component protein expression in the uterine cervix, lumbosacral spinal cord, and dorsal root ganglia. Peptides 2002; 23:507-14.
29. Komisaruk BR, Wallman J. Antinociceptive effects of vaginal stimulation in rats: Neurophysiological and behavioral studies. Brain Res 1977; 137:85-107.
30. Papka RE, Hafemeister J, Puder BA, et al. Estrogen receptor-α and neural circuits to the spinal cord during pregnancy. J Neurosci Res 2002; 70:808-16.
31. Sandner-Kiesling A, Pan HL, Chen SR, et al. Effect of kappa opioid agonists on visceral nociception induced by uterine cervical distention in rats. Pain 2002; 96:13-22.
32. Cleland JGP. Paravertebral anaesthesia in obstetrics. Surg Gynecol Obstet 1933; 57:51-62.
33. Cotte G. Sur le traitement des dysmenorrhees rebelles par la sympathectomie hypogastrique periarterielle ou la section du nerf presacre. Lyon Med 1925; LVI:153.
34. Strigo IA, Duncan GH, Boivin M, Bushnell MC. Differentiation of visceral and cutaneous pain in the human brain. J Neurophysiol 2003; 89:3294-303.
35. Whipple B, Komisaruk BR. Elevation of pain threshold by vaginal stimulation in women. Pain 1985; 21:357-67.
36. Whipple B, Martinez-Gomez M, Oliva-Zarate L, et al. Inverse relationship between intensity of vaginal self-stimulation-produced analgesia and level of chronic intake of a dietary source of capsaicin. Physiol Behav 1989; 46:247-52.
37. Lingueglia E, de Weille JR, Bassilana F, et al. A modulatory subunit of acid sensing ion channels in brain and dorsal root ganglion cells. J Biol Chem 1997; 272:29778-83.
38. Cockayne DA, Hamilton SG, Zhu QM, et al. Urinary bladder hyporeflexia and reduced pain-related behaviour in P2X$_3$-deficient mice. Nature 2000; 407:1011-5.

39. Burnstock G. P2X receptors in sensory neurones. Br J Anaesth 2000; 84:476-88.

40. Waldmann R, Champigny G, Lingueglia E, et al. H(+)-gated cation channels. Ann N Y Acad Sci 1999; 868:67-76.

41. Drewes AM, Schipper KP, Dimcevski G, et al. Multimodal assessment of pain in the esophagus: A new experimental model. Am J Physiol Gastrointest Liver Physiol 2002; 283:G95-103.

42. Julius D, Basbaum AI. Molecular mechanisms of nociception. Nature 2001; 413:203-10.

43. Papka RE, McNeill DL, Thompson D, Schmidt HHHW. Nitric oxide nerves in the uterus are parasympathetic, sensory, and contain neuropeptides. Cell Tissue Res 1995; 279:339-49.

44. Bennett DL, Michael GJ, Ramachandran N, et al. A distinct subgroup of small DRG cells express GDNF receptor components and GDNF is protective for these neurons after nerve injury. J Neurosci 1998; 18:3059-72.

45. Kim SJ, Chung WH, Rhim H, et al. Postsynaptic action mechanism of somatostatin on the membrane excitability in spinal substantia gelatinosa neurons of juvenile rats. Neuroscience 2002; 114:1139-48.

46. Carlton SM, Du JH, Zhou ST, Coggeshall RE. Tonic control of peripheral cutaneous nociceptors by somatostatin receptors. J Neurosci 2001; 21:4042-9.

47. Linhart O, Obreja O, Kress M. The inflammatory mediators serotonin, prostaglandin E_2 and bradykinin evoke calcium influx in rat sensory neurons. Neuroscience 2003; 118:69-74.

48. Sato T, Michizu H, Hashizume K, Ito A. Hormonal regulation of PGE_2 and COX-2 production in rabbit uterine cervical fibroblasts. J Applied Physiol 2001; 90:1227-31.

49. Lyons CA, Beharry KD, Nishihara KC, et al. Regulation of matrix metalloproteinases (type IV collagenases) and their inhibitors in the virgin, timed pregnant, and postpartum rat uterus and cervix by prostaglandin E_2-cyclic adenosine monophosphate. Am J Obstet Gynecol 2002; 187:202-8.

50. Stygar D, Wang H, Vladic VS, et al. Increased level of matrix metalloproteinases 2 and 9 in the ripening process of the human cervix. Biol Reprod 2002; 67:889-94.

51. Aley KO, Levine JD. Role of protein kinase A in the maintenance of inflammatory pain. J Neurosci 1999; 19:2181-6.

52. Aley KO, McCarter G, Levine JD. Nitric oxide signaling in pain and nociceptor sensitization in the rat. J Neurosci 1998; 18:7008-14.

53. Samad TA, Moore KA, Sapirstein A, et al. Interleukin-1beta-mediated induction of COX-2 in the CNS contributes to inflammatory pain hypersensitivity. Nature 2001; 410:471-5.

54. Inoue A, Ikoma K, Morioka N, et al. Interleukin-1beta induces substance P release from primary afferent neurons through the cyclooxygenase-2 system. J Neurochem 1999; 73:2206-13.

55. Leem J-G, Bove GM. Mid-axonal tumor necrosis factor-alpha induces ectopic activity in a subset of slowly conducting cutaneous and deep afferent neurons. J Pain 2002; 3:45-9.

56. Winston J, Toma H, Shenoy M, Pasricha PJ. Nerve growth factor regulates VR-1 mRNA levels in cultures of adult dorsal root ganglion neurons. Pain 2001; 89:181-6.

57. Rueff A, Dawson AJLR, Mendell LM. Characteristics of nerve growth factor induced hyperalgesia in adult rats: Dependence on enhanced bradykinin-1 receptor activity but not neurokinin-1 receptor activation. Pain 1996; 66:359-72.

58. Waxman SG, Kocsis JD, Black JA. Type III sodium channel mRNA is expressed in embryonic but not adult spinal sensory neurons, and is reexpressed following axotomy. J Neurophysiol 1994; 72:466-70.

59. Kim CH, Oh Y, Chung JM, Chung K. The changes in expression of three subtypes of TTX sensitive sodium channels in sensory neurons after spinal nerve ligation. Mol Brain Res 2001; 95:153-61.

60. Black JA, Cummins TR, Plumpton C, et al. Upregulation of a silent sodium channel after peripheral, but not central, nerve injury in DRG neurons. J Neurophysiol 1999; 82:2776-85.

61. Liu CN, Wall PD, Ben Dor E, et al. Tactile allodynia in the absence of C-fiber activation: Altered firing properties of DRG neurons following spinal nerve injury. Pain 2000; 85:503-21.

62. Mousa SA, Zhang Q, Sitte N, et al. β-endorphin-containing memory-cells and μ-opioid receptors undergo transport to peripheral inflamed tissue. J Neuroimmunol 2001; 115:71-8.

63. Picard PR, Tramèr MR, McQuay HJ, Moore RA. Analgesic efficacy of peripheral opioids (all except intra-articular): A qualitative systematic review of randomised controlled trials. Pain 1997; 72:309-18.

64. Kalso E, Tramèr MR, Carroll D, et al. Pain relief from intra-articular morphine after knee surgery: A qualitative systematic review. Pain 1997; 71:127-34.

65. Sandner-Kiesling A, Eisenach JC. Pharmacology of opioid inhibition to noxious uterine cervical distention. Anesthesiology 2002; 97:966-71.

66. Sengupta JN, Su X, Gebhart GF. Kappa, but not μ or δ, opioids attenuate responses to distention of afferent fibers innervating the rat colon. Gastroenterology 1996; 111:968-80.

67. Gebhart GF, Su X, Joshi S, et al. Peripheral opioid modulation of visceral pain. Ann N Y Acad Sci 2000; 909:41-50.

68. Binder W, Walker JS. Effect of the peripherally selective kappa-opioid agonist, asimadoline, on adjuvant arthritis. Br J Pharmacol 1998; 124:647-54.

69. Eisenach JC, Carpenter R, Curry R. Analgesia from a peripherally active kappa-opioid receptor agonist in patients with chronic pancreatitis. Pain 2003; 101:89-95.

70. Cicero TJ, Nock B, O'Connor L, Meyer ER. Role of steroids in sex differences in morphine-induced analgesia: Activational and organizational effects. J Pharmacol Exp Ther 2002; 300:695-701.

71. Gear RW, Miaskowski C, Gordon NC, et al. Kappa-opioids produce significantly greater analgesia in women than in men. Nature Med 1996; 2:1248-50.

72. Sandner-Kiesling A, Eisenach JC. Estrogen reduces efficacy of μ- but not κ-opioid agonist inhibition in response to uterine cervical distention. Anesthesiology 2002; 96:375-9.

73. Shin SW, Eisenach JC. Intrathecal morphine reduces the visceromotor response to acute uterine cervical distention in an estrogen-independent manner. Anesthesiology 2003; 98:1467-71.

74. Olofsson C, Ekblom A, Ekman-Ordeberg G, et al. Lack of analgesic effect of systemically administered morphine or pethidine on labour pain. Br J Obstet Gynaecol 1996; 103:968-72.

75. Leighton BL, DeSimone CA, Norris MC, Ben-David B. Intrathecal narcotics for labor revisited: The combination of fentanyl and morphine intrathecally provides rapid onset of profound, prolonged analgesia. Anesth Analg 1989; 69:122-5.

76. Goldin AL, Barchi RL, Caldwell JH, et al. Nomenclature of voltage-gated sodium channels. Neuron 2000; 28:365-8.

77. Renganathan M, Cummins TR, Waxman SG. Nitric oxide blocks fast, slow, and persistent Na^+ channels in C-type DRG neurons by S-nitrosylation. J Neurophysiol 2002; 87:761-75

78. Gold MS, Weinreich D, Kim CS, et al. NaV1.8 mediates neuropathic pain via redistribution in the axons of uninjured afferents (abstract). Soc Neurosci 2001; 55:6.

79. Lai J, Gold MS, Kim CS, et al. Inhibition of neuropathic pain by decreased expression of the tetrodotoxin-resistant sodium channel, NaV1.8. Pain 2002; 95:143-52.

80. Nonaka T, Honmou O, Sakai J, et al. Excitability changes of dorsal root axons following nerve injury: implications for injury-induced changes in axonal Na(+) channels. Brain Res 2000; 859:280-5.

81. Sakai J, Honmou O, Kocsis JD, Hashi K. The delayed depolarization in rat cutaneous afferent axons is reduced following nerve transection and ligation, but not crush: Implications for injury-induced axonal Na+ channel reorganization. Muscle Nerve 1998; 21:1040-7.

82. Gerner P, Mujtaba M, Sinnott CJ, Wang GK. Amitriptyline *versus* bupivacaine in rat sciatic nerve blockade. Anesthesiology 2001; 94:661-7.

83. Gerner P, Mujtaba M, Khan M, et al. *N*-phenylethyl amitriptyline in rat sciatic nerve blockade. Anesthesiology 2002; 96:1435-42.

84. Dalle C, Schneider M, Clergue F, et al. Inhibition of the I_h current in isolated peripheral nerve: A novel mode of peripheral antinociception? Muscle Nerve 2001; 24:254-61.

85. Chaplan SR, Guo HQ, Lee DH, et al. Neuronal hyperpolarization-activated pacemaker channels drive neuropathic pain. J Neurosci 2003; 23:1169-78.

86. Kissin I, Bright CA, Bradley EL. Selective and long-lasting neural blockade with resiniferatoxin prevents inflammatory pain hypersensitivity. Anesth Analg 2002; 94:1253-8.

87. Ludwig M, Sabatier N, Bull PM, et al. Intracellular calcium stores regulate activity-dependent neuropeptide release from dendrites. Nature 2002; 418:85-9.

88. Feng Y, Cui ML, Willis WD. Gabapentin markedly reduces acetic acid-induced visceral nociception. Anesthesiology 2003; 98:729-33.

89. Cao YQ, Mantyh PW, Carlson EJ, et al. Primary afferent tachykinins are required to experience moderate to intense pain. Nature 1998; 392:390-4.

90. Khan IM, Marsala M, Printz MP, et al. Intrathecal nicotinic agonist-elicited release of excitatory amino acids as measured by in vivo spinal microdialysis in rats. J Pharmacol Exp Ther 1996; 278:97-106.

91. Riley RC, Trafton JA, Chi SI, Basbaum AI. Presynaptic regulation of spinal cord tachykinin signaling via $GABA_B$ but not $GABA_A$ receptor activation. Neuroscience 2001; 103:725-37.

92. Li DP, Chen SR, Pan YZ, et al. Role of presynaptic muscarinic and $GABA_B$ receptors in spinal glutamate release and cholinergic analgesia in rats. J Physiol 2002; 543:807-18.

93. Baba H, Kohno T, Okamoto M, et al. Muscarinic facilitation of GABA release in substantia gelatinosa of the rat spinal dorsal horn. J Physiol 1998; 508:83-93.

94. Lauretti GR, Hood DD, Eisenach JC, Pfeifer BL. A multi-center study of intrathecal neostigmine for analgesia following vaginal hysterectomy. Anesthesiology 1998; 89:913-8.

95. Lombard M-C, Besson J-M. Attempts to gauge the relative importance of pre- and postsynaptic effects of morphine on the transmission of noxious messages in the dorsal horn of the rat spinal cord. Pain 1989; 37:335-45.

96. Kuraishi Y, Hirota N, Sato Y, et al. Noradrenergic inhibition of the release of substance P from the primary afferents in the rabbit spinal dorsal horn. Brain Res 1985; 359:177-82.

97. Headley PM, Grillner S. Excitatory amino acids and synaptic transmission: The evidence for a physiological function. Trends Pharmacol Sci 1990; 11:205-11.

98. Karpinski N, Dunn J, Hansen L, Masliah E. Subpial vacuolar myelopathy after intrathecal ketamine: Report of a case. Pain 1997; 73:103-5.

99. Wilder-Smith CH, Knöpfli R, Wilder-Smith OHG. Perioperative magnesium infusion and postoperative pain. Acta Anaesth Scand 1997; 41:1023-7.

100. Svensson CI, Yaksh TL. The spinal phospholipase-cyclooxygenase-prostanoid cascade in nociceptive processing. Annu Rev Pharmacol Toxicol 2002; 42:553-83.

101. Roza C, Laird JM, Cervero F. Spinal mechanisms underlying persistent pain and referred hyperalgesia in rats with an experimental ureteric stone. J Neurophysiol 1998; 79:1603-12.

102. Ossipov MH, Lopez Y, Nichols ML, et al. The loss of antinociceptive efficacy of spinal morphine in rats with nerve ligation injury is prevented by reducing spinal afferent drive. Neurosci Lett 1995; 199:87-90.

103. Eisenach JC, Curry R, Hood DD, Yaksh TL. Phase I safety assessment of intrathecal ketorolac. Pain 2002; 99:599-604.

104. Basbaum AI, Fields HL. Endogenous pain control mechanisms: Review and hypothesis. Ann Neurol 1978; 4:451-62.

105. Eisenach JC, Dobson CE, Inturrisi CE, et al. Effect of pregnancy and pain on cerebrospinal fluid immunoreactive enkephalins and norepinephrine in healthy humans. Pain 1990; 43:149-54.

106. Benedetti F, Arduino C, Amanzio M. Somatotopic activation of opioid systems by target-directed expectations of analgesia. J Neurosci 1999; 19:3639-48.

107. Millan MJ. The role of descending noradrenergic and serotoninergic pathways in the modulation of nociception: Focus on receptor multiplicity. In: Dickenson A, Besson JM, editors. Handbook of Experimental Pharmacology: The Pharmacology of Pain. Berlin Heidelberg, Springer-Verlag, 1997:385-446.

108. Zhuo M, Sengupta JN, Gebhart GF. Biphasic modulation of spinal visceral nociceptive transmission from the rostroventral medial medulla in the rat. J Neurophysiol 2002; 87:2225-36.

109. Al Chaer ED, Traub RJ. Biological basis of visceral pain: Recent developments. Pain 2002; 96:221-5.

110. Jones AK, Kulkarni B, Derbyshire SW. Pain mechanisms and their disorders. Br Med Bull 2003; 65:83-93.

111. Leighton BL, Halpern SH, Wilson DB. Lumbar sympathetic blocks speed early and second stage induced labor in nulliparous women. Anesthesiology 1999; 90:1039-46.

112. Moir DD, Willocks J. Management of incoordinate uterine action under continuous epidural analgesia. BMJ 1967; 3:396-400.

113. Riffel HD, Nochimson DJ, Paul RH, Hon EH. Effects of meperidine and promethazine during labor. Obstet Gynecol 1973; 42:738-45.

114. Clarke VT, Smiley RM, Finster M. Uterine hyperactivity after intrathecal injection of fentanyl for analgesia during labor: A cause of fetal bradycardia. Anesthesiology 1994; 81:1083.

115. Hingson RA, Hellman LM. Anatomic and physiologic considerations. In: Hingson RA, Hellman LM, editors. Anesthesia for Obstetrics. Philadelphia, JB Lippincott, 1956:74.

116. Rahm VA, Hallgren A, Hogberg H, et al. Plasma oxytocin levels in women during labor with or without epidural analgesia: A prospective study. Acta Obstet Gynecol Scand 2002; 81:1033-9.

117. Stocche RM, Klamt JG, Antunes-Rodrigues J, et al. Effects of intrathecal sufentanil on plasma oxytocin and cortisol concentrations in women during the first stage of labor. Reg Anesth Pain Med 2001; 26:545-50.

118. Scull TJ, Hemmings GT, Carli F, et al. Epidural analgesia in early labour blocks the stress response but uterine contractions remain unchanged. Can J Anaesth 1998; 45:626-30.

119. Leighton BL, Norris MC, Sosis M, et al. Limitations of epinephrine as a marker of intravascular injection in laboring women. Anesthesiology 1987; 66:688-91.

120. Hood DD, Dewan DM, James FM. Maternal and fetal effects of epinephrine in gravid ewes. Anesthesiology 1986; 64:610-3.

121. Shnider SM, Abboud TK, Artal R, et al. Maternal catecholamines decrease during labor after lumbar epidural anesthesia. Am J Obstet Gynecol 1983; 147:13-5.

122. Cascio M, Pygon B, Bernett C, Ramanathan S. Labour analgesia with intrathecal fentanyl decreases maternal stress. Can J Anaesth 1997; 44:605-9.

123. Jouppila R, Puolakka J, Kauppila A, Vuori J. Maternal and umbilical cord plasma noradrenaline concentrations during labour with and without segmental extradural analgesia, and during caesarean section. Br J Anaesth 1984; 56:251-4.

124. Hagerdal M, Morgan CW, Sumner AE, Gutsche BB. Minute ventilation during and oxygen consumption during labor with epidural analgesia. Anesthesiology 1983; 59:425-57.

125. Hodnett ED. Pain and women's satisfaction with the experience of childbirth: A systematic review. Am J Obstet Gynecol 2002; 186:S160-72.

126. Billewicz-Driemel AM, Milne MD. Long-term assessment of extradural analgesia for pain relief in labour. II. Sense of deprivation after extradural analgesia in labour: Relevant or not? Br J Anaesth 1976; 48:139-44.

127. Stewart DE. Psychiatric symptoms following attempted natural childbirth. Can Med Assoc J 1982; 127:713-6.

128. Ryding E. Psychosocial indications for cesarean section. Acta Obstet Gynecol Scand 1991; 70:47-9.

129. Ballard CG, Stanley AK. Post traumatic stress disorder after childbirth. Br J Psych 1995; 166:525-8.

130. Niven C, Gijsbers K. A study of labour pain using the McGill Pain Questionnaire. Soc Sci Med 1984; 19:1347-51.

131. Wells N. Pain and distress during abortion. Health Care Women Int 1991; 12:293-302.

Chapter 19
Childbirth Preparation and Nonpharmacologic Analgesia

Marie E. Minnich, M.D., M.M.M.

Pregnant women and their support person(s) obtain information regarding childbirth and analgesia from many sources, including obstetricians, childbirth preparation classes, lay periodicals, books and pamphlets, family, friends and—increasingly—the Internet. Anesthesiologists should be familiar with this information. Patients' preparation and understanding or misunderstanding will influence their birth experiences. Knowledge of the information and biases held by patients will help anesthesiologists in their interactions with pregnant women. Prepared childbirth training provides undeniable benefits to the pregnant woman and her support person. However, prepared childbirth training should not be equated with nonpharmacologic analgesia.[1] Some childbirth preparation instructors discourage the use of medications during labor and delivery, whereas others make a nonbiased presentation of the advantages and disadvantages of various analgesic techniques. The information contained in this chapter should provide a basis for informed discussion among patients, nurses, obstetricians, and anesthesiologists.

PAIN TRANSMISSION AND PERCEPTION

Anesthesiologists are indebted to John Bonica[2] for his thorough discussion of the pain of childbirth. Investigators have used sophisticated questionnaires[3,4] and visual analog scales[5] to evaluate the maternal perception of pain during parturition. Melzack et al.[6,7] used the McGill Pain Questionnaire to measure the intensity of labor pain in nulliparous and parous women. They noted that labor pain is one of the most intense pains studied with this questionnaire (see Figure 18-2). Parous women had lower scores than nulliparous women, but responses varied widely (Figures 19-1 and 19-2). Prepared childbirth training resulted in a modest decrease in the average pain score among nulliparous women, but it clearly did not eliminate pain in these women.[6,7]

CHILDBIRTH PREPARATION

History
The history of modern childbirth preparation began in the first half of the twentieth century; however, it is important to review earlier changes in obstetric practice to understand the perceived need for a new approach. Before the mid-nineteenth century, childbirth occurred at home in the company of family and friends. The specialty of obstetrics developed in an effort to decrease maternal mortality. Interventions initially developed for the management of complications became accepted and practiced as routine obstetrics. Physicians first gave anesthesia for childbirth during this period. The 1848 meeting of the American Medical Association included reports of the use of ether and chloroform in approximately 2000 obstetric cases.[8] The combination of morphine and scopolamine (i.e., twilight sleep) was introduced in the early twentieth century. These techniques were widely used, and influential women demanded that they be made available to all parturients.[9] Together, these developments moved childbirth from the home and family unit to the hospital environment.[10] Despite their desire for analgesia/anesthesia for labor and delivery, women began to resent the fact that they were not active participants in childbirth.

Beck et al.[11] have written a detailed history of childbirth preparation. Dick-Read[12,13] reported the earliest method in his books *Natural Childbirth* and *Childbirth Without Fear*. In his original publication, he asserted his belief that childbirth was not inherently painful. He opined that the pain of childbirth results from a "fear-tension-pain-syndrome." He believed—and taught—that antepartum instruction regarding muscle relaxation and elimination of fear would prevent labor pain. He later established antenatal classes that included groups of mothers and fathers. Some readers incorrectly concluded that he advocated a return to primitive obstetrics, but this was not the case. Review of his practice reveals that he used the available obstetric techniques—analgesia, anesthesia, episiotomy, forceps, and abdominal delivery—as appropriate for the individual patient. However, he cautioned against the routine use of these procedures, and he encouraged active participation of mothers in the delivery of their infants. Unfortunately, he did not use the scientific method to validate his beliefs.

Although Dick-Read was the earliest proponent of natural childbirth, it was Fernand Lamaze[14] who introduced the Western world to psychoprophylaxis. His publications were based on techniques he observed while traveling in Russia. Although his theories ostensibly were translations of teachings later published in the West by Velvovsky et al.,[15] they contained substantial differences and modifications. The "Lamaze method" became popular in the United States after Marjorie Karmel[16] described her childbirth experience under the care of Dr. Lamaze. Within a year of the publication of her popular book, the American Society for Psychoprophylaxis

McGill Pain Scores of 87 Nulliparas

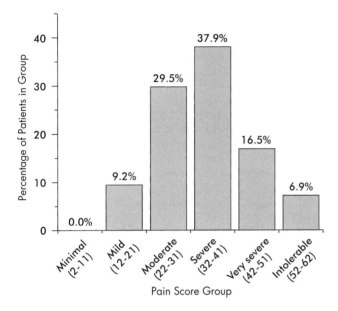

FIGURE 19-1. The severity of pain during labor as assessed by the McGill Pain Questionnaire for 87 nulliparous women. (Modified from Melzack R, Taezner P, Feldman P, Kinch RA. Labour is still painful after prepared childbirth training. Can Med Assoc J 1981; 125:357-63.)

McGill Pain Scores of 54 Multiparas

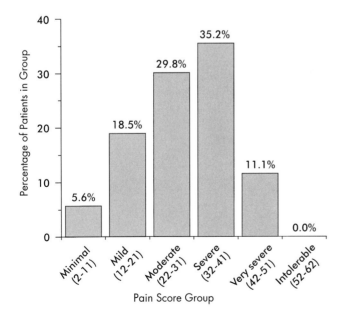

FIGURE 19-2. The severity of pain during labor as assessed by the McGill Pain Questionnaire for 54 parous women. (Modified from Melzack R, Taezner P, Feldman P, Kinch RA. Labour is still painful after prepared childbirth training. Can Med Assoc J 1981; 125:357-63.)

in Obstetrics was born. Lamaze and Karmel published their experience at a time when organizations such as the International Childbirth Education Association and the La Leche League were formed.[17] These organizations actively and aggressively encouraged a renewed emphasis on family-centered maternity care, and society was ripe for the ideas and theories promoted by these organizations. Women were ready to actively participate in childbirth and to have an input in the decisions regarding obstetric and anesthetic interventions. Childbirth preparation methods were taught and used extensively, despite a lack of scientific validation of their efficacy.

In 1975, Leboyer[18] described a modification of natural childbirth in his book, *Birth Without Violence*. He advocated childbirth in a dark, quiet room; gentle massage of the newborn without routine suctioning; and a warm bath soon after birth. He opined that these maneuvers result in a less shocking first-separation experience and a healthier, happier infancy and childhood. Although there are few controlled studies of this method, published observations do not support his claim of superiority.[19,20]

Physicians were the initial advocates of the various natural childbirth methods. Obstetricians had become increasingly aware that analgesic and anesthetic techniques were not harmless, and they supported the use of natural childbirth methods.[11] Subsequently, natural childbirth, like the methods of obstetric analgesia introduced earlier in the century, was actively promoted by lay groups rather than physicians.[21] Lay publications, national advocacy groups, and formal instruction of patients accounted for the increased interest in psychoprophylaxis and other techniques associated with natural childbirth.

Goals and Advantages

The major goals of childbirth education that were initially promoted by Dick-Read are taught with little modification in formal childbirth preparation classes today. Most current classes credit Lamaze with the major components of childbirth preparation, even though Dick-Read was the first to promote patient education, relaxation training, breathing exercises, and paternal participation.[11] Box 19-1 describes the stated goals of current childbirth preparation classes. In addition, some instructors and training manuals claim other benefits of childbirth preparation (Box 19-2). The reviews of Beck and Hall[22] and Lindell[23] conclude that much of the research on the efficacy of childbirth education does not meet the fundamental requirements of the scientific method. Despite these shortcomings, childbirth preparation classes are and likely will continue to be widely available and attended.

The effect of childbirth education on attitude and childbirth experience depends in part on the social class to which the mother belongs. Most investigators have found that childbirth classes have a positive effect on the attitudes of both parents in all social classes, but this effect is more pronounced among "working class"[24] and indigent women[25]; this probably

---

Box 19-1 GOALS OF CHILDBIRTH PREPARATION

• Patient education regarding pregnancy, labor, and delivery
• Relaxation training
• Instruction in breathing techniques
• Father/support person participation
• Early parental bonding

reflects the greater availability and use of other educational materials by middle- and upper-class women. Childbirth classes often are the only—or at least the primary—source of information for working class and indigent women.

Limitations

Limitations of the widespread application of psychoprophylaxis and other childbirth preparation methods remain. Proponents assume that these techniques are easily used during labor and delivery, but Copstick et al.[26] concluded that this assumption is not valid. Patients were able to use the coping techniques in the early first stage of labor, but the use of these coping skills became less and less common as labor progressed. By the onset of the second stage, less than one third of mothers were able to use any of the breathing or postural techniques taught during their childbirth classes.[26] The method of preparation influences the ability of the pregnant woman to use the breathing and relaxation techniques. Bernardini et al.[27] observed that self-taught pregnant women are less likely to practice the techniques during the prenatal period or to use the techniques during labor.

Childbirth preparation classes may create false expectations. If a woman does not enjoy the "normal" delivery discussed during classes, she may experience a sense of failure or inferiority. Both Stewart[28] and Guzman Sanchez et al.[29] have discussed the psychologic reactions of women who were unable to use psychoprophylaxis successfully during labor and delivery. In addition, several women have written about their disappointment with the dogmatic approach of their childbirth instructors; these women described instructors who rigidly defined the "correct" way to have a "proper birth experience."[30-32]

Box 19-2 PURPORTED BENEFITS OF CHILDBIRTH PREPARATION

- Increased maternal control and cooperation
- Decreased maternal anxiety
- Decreased maternal pain
- Decreased maternal need for analgesia/anesthesia
- Shorter labor
- Decreased maternal morbidity
- Decreased fetal stress/distress
- Strengthened family relationships as a result of the shared birth experience

---

Effects

Little scientific evidence supports the efficacy of childbirth preparation. Psychology, nursing, obstetric, anesthesia, and lay journals provide extensive discussions of childbirth preparation, but most articles represent uncontrolled clinical experience. Outcome studies often do not include a group of patients who were randomized to an untreated or a placebo-control group, and statistical analysis often is incomplete. Despite these shortcomings, supporters of childbirth preparation assume that it offers benefits for mother and child. Table 19-1 summarizes a few of the studies of the efficacy of Lamaze and other childbirth preparation techniques. The findings are not consistent. Some authors have reported a *decreased* use of analgesics[33-36] or regional anesthesia,[33-36,37] shorter labor,[38] decreased performance of instrumental[33,35,37] and cesarean[37] delivery, and less frequent fetal distress,[37] whereas others have reported *no change* in the use of analgesics[37-41] or regional anesthesia,[39,41] length of labor,[34,35,37,39-41] performance of instrumental[39-41] and cesarean[35,39-41] delivery, and incidence of fetal distress.[35,36,38,39] These diverse findings may reflect different patient populations, poor study design, or researcher bias.

To elucidate the effect of the coping techniques taught in childbirth classes, several investigators have attempted to quantify changes in pain threshold, pain perception, anxiety levels, and physiologic responses to standardized stimuli. Several studies have evaluated nonpregnant, nulliparous women in laboratory settings,[42-45] and another study evaluated pregnant women in the antepartum, intrapartum, and postpartum periods.[46] Conclusions varied depending on the stimuli applied, the coping techniques studied, and the parameters analyzed. Together, these studies suggest that *practicing* the techniques is important to outcome and that newer cognitive techniques (e.g., systematic desensitization, sensory transformation) may be more effective than traditional Lamaze techniques of varied breathing patterns and relaxation. Further studies may help refine childbirth preparation to maximize the positive psychophysiologic effects.

NONPHARMACOLOGIC ANALGESIC TECHNIQUES

Nonpharmacologic analgesic techniques range from those that require minimal specialized equipment and training and that are available to all patients to those that are offered only by institutions that have the necessary equipment and personnel

---

TABLE 19-1   EFFECTS OF CHILDBIRTH PREPARATION

Reference	Analgesic Use	Regional Anesthesia	Length of Labor	Cesarean Delivery Rate	Instrumental Delivery Rate	Fetal Distress	Oxytocin Use
Patton et al.[39]	NC	NC	NC	NC	NC	NC	↑
Hetherington[33]	↓	↓	—	—	↓	—	—
Zax et al.[34]	↓	↓	NC	—	—	—	—
Scott et al.[35]	↓	↓	NC	NC	↓	NC	NC
Hughey et al.[37]	NC	↓	NC	↓	↓	↓	NC
Sturrock et al.[40]	NC	—	NC	NC	NC	—	—
Brewin et al.[41]	NC	NC	NC	NC	NC	—	—
Delke et al.[38]	NC	—	↓	—	—	NC	NC
Rogers[36]	↓	—	—	—	—	NC	—

NC, No change; ↑, increased; ↓, decreased; —, not studied/reported.

trained in their use (Box 19-3). Although the literature is not replete with studies that fulfill the requirements of the scientific method, numerous articles elucidate the various techniques that are thought to reduce pain and enhance the progress of labor.[47] Gentz[48] recently reviewed published information about alternative therapies for pain management during labor. This comprehensive review provides anesthesiologists with a foundation for discussion with patients and providers. However, insufficient clinical evidence exists to form the basis for an in-depth discussion of some of the recent therapeutic suggestions, including music therapy, aromatherapy, and chiropractic, among others. These analgesic techniques may provide intangible benefits that are not easily documented by a rigid scientific method. Parturients may consider these benefits an integral and important part of their labor experience.

Emotional Support

Some techniques that require minimum equipment and specialized training are taught as integral components of childbirth preparation classes. Emotional support is essential to the process of a satisfying childbirth experience; typically the parturient's husband or friend provides this support.[49-51] This support appears most helpful for the parturient who lives in a stable family unit. At least one study noted that husband participation was associated with decreased maternal anxiety and medication requirements.[49] Others have found that emotional support provided by unfamiliar individuals (e.g., doulas) also has a positive effect.[52-56] Several studies have evaluated the benefits of emotional support provided by doulas or other unrelated individuals on the length of labor,[52,54-56] oxytocin use,[54] requirements for analgesia and/or anesthesia,[54-56] incidence of operative delivery,[52,54,55] and maternal morbidity.[52-54] In some studies, individual companions (doulas) were assigned to a parturient,[52-54,56] whereas another study allowed the parturient to converse with other patients, including those who had recently delivered.[55] These studies all suggested that a patient's sense of isolation adversely affects her perception of labor. Further, the companionship of another woman who is not part of the medical establishment may decrease a parturient's anxiety more effectively than the companionship provided by her husband. These studies are fascinating and have important implications for obstetric care. The patient populations studied represent special situations, and the results may not be reproduced in all patient populations. Further studies should be performed to determine whether the same effects are seen in other hospital settings (e.g., hospitals that encourage husband participation during childbirth). If the decreased incidence of instrumental delivery and cesarean section and decreased maternal and perinatal morbidity are confirmed in subsequent studies, these findings may prompt a change in the approach to the laboring patient.

Meanwhile, all parturients should have access to emotional support, whether it is provided by the husband, a family member, a labor companion (e.g., doula), or professional hospital staff.

Touch and Massage

Various touch and massage techniques are discussed with women and their support persons during childbirth preparation classes. These may include effleurage, counterpressure to alleviate back discomfort, light stroking, or merely a reassuring pat.[47] There has been minimal scientific study of the effects of touch and massage[57-59] on labor progress and outcome; nonetheless, they provide a comfort appreciated by women during labor. These measures may be used by the parturient, her support person, or the professional staff members providing intrapartum care.[59] These techniques are easily discontinued if the parturient desires. In some cases, touch and massage may reduce discomfort. More often, touch and massage transmit a sense of caring, which fosters a sense of security and well-being.

Therapeutic Use of Heat and Cold

Another simple technique for alleviating labor pain is the therapeutic use of temperature (hot or cold) applied to various regions of the body. Warm compresses may be placed on localized areas, or a warm blanket may cover the entire body. Alternatively, icepacks may be placed on the low back or perineum to decrease pain perception. The therapeutic use of heat and cold during labor has not been studied in a rigorous scientific manner. The use of superficial heat and cold for comfort is widespread (if not completely understood), and it has no discernible risk for the mother or the fetus.[47]

Hydrotherapy

Hydrotherapy may involve a simple shower or tub bath, or it may include the use of a whirlpool or large tub specially equipped for pregnant patients. Box 19-4 lists the purported benefits of hydrotherapy. Several authors[47,60,61] have discussed the intrapartum benefits of hydrotherapy (e.g., decreased anxiety and pain, increased contraction efficiency). Two randomized, controlled studies[62,63] and a matched-control study[64] demonstrated a decreased incidence of operative delivery, perineal trauma, and analgesia use. However, in a more recent randomized, controlled trial, Eckert et al.[65] observed no significant differences in maternal outcome measures. In addition, although neonatal outcomes were equivalent, infants in the water bath group required significantly more resuscitative measures than women in the control group. Robertson et al.[66] noted no significant association between water baths during labor and the occurrence of chorioamnionitis or endometritis. Some authors contend that bathing, showering, and other

---

Box 19-3 NONPHARMACOLOGIC ANALGESIC TECHNIQUES

MINIMAL TRAINING/ EQUIPMENT	SPECIALIZED TRAINING/EQUIPMENT
• Emotional support	• Biofeedback
• Touch and massage	• Transcutaneous electrical nerve stimulation (TENS)
• Therapeutic use of heat and cold	• Acupuncture
• Hydrotherapy	• Hypnosis
• Vertical position	

Box 19-4 PURPORTED BENEFITS OF HYDROTHERAPY

• Reduced anxiety
• Relaxation
• Decreased pain
• Decreased blood pressure
• Increased efficiency of uterine contractions
• Rotation of occiput posterior position to occiput anterior

hydrotherapy maneuvers are comfort measures with little risk to the mother or the infant, if appropriate monitoring continues during the water immersion.

Vertical Position

Several authors have studied the effects of various positions on pain perception and labor outcome. These positions are broadly categorized as vertical (e.g., sitting, standing, walking, squatting) or horizontal (e.g., supine, lateral). Box 19-5 lists the rationale for the use of the upright posture during labor. The vertical position is associated with decreased pain,[67-69] especially in early labor, or no change in pain perception.[70,71] Length of labor is either unaffected[69-72] or decreased,[68,73] and most studies have observed no demonstrable difference in the incidence of instrumental delivery.[69-72] In a prospective, randomized study, Bloom et al.[71] noted that walking did *not* shorten the duration of the first stage of labor, reduce the requirement for oxytocin augmentation, reduce the use of analgesia, or decrease the requirement for operative delivery. They concluded that "walking neither enhanced nor impaired active labor and was not harmful to the mothers or their infants."[71]

Nonetheless, many obstetricians and nurses believe that ambulation is associated with shorter labors that require less analgesia. Ambulation may not produce shorter, less painful labor; rather, it is possible that shorter, less painful labor allows continued ambulation. Collis et al.[74] found that maternal ambulation had no significant effect on length of labor, analgesic requirements, or method of delivery in patients receiving combined spinal-epidural analgesia.

There is renewed interest in the squatting or modified squatting position and its increased comfort for women during childbirth. Most authors[75-79] have noted that Western women have insufficient muscular strength and stamina to maintain an unsupported squatting position for any length of time. Gardosi et al.[76] designed and studied a birth cushion that allows for a modified, supported squat, which resulted in an increased incidence of spontaneous delivery and a decreased incidence of perineal tears. Others have yet to substantiate the results of this initial trial.

Some studies have evaluated the use of a birth chair to facilitate delivery in the sitting position.[69,72,80] These studies noted no difference in the length of the second stage, the mode of delivery, perineal trauma, or neonatal Apgar scores. However, two studies[69,72] reported greater intrapartum blood loss and an increased incidence of postpartum hemorrhage.

Ambulation and change of position (especially with use of the vertical position) appear to aid maternal comfort without causing risk to the fetus. It is unclear whether birthing cushions or stools confer any benefit to the mother or the baby.

Biofeedback

Biofeedback is a convenient and effective relaxation method that is used as an adjunct to the relaxation training taught in Lamaze and other childbirth education programs. Two biofeedback procedures may be applicable to the laboring woman: skin-conductance (autonomic) and electromyographic (voluntary muscle) relaxation. St. James-Roberts et al.[81] demonstrated that electromyographic but not skin-conductance biofeedback techniques could be taught effectively in Lamaze classes. They noted no difference in length of the first stage of labor, use of epidural anesthesia, incidence of instrumental delivery, or neonatal Apgar scores among electromyographic, skin-conductance, and control groups. Duchene[82] reported decreased pain perception during labor and delivery, use of fewer medications, and shorter labor (not statistically significant) with electromyographic biofeedback; there was no difference in neonatal Apgar scores. Approximately 40% of study patients requested and received epidural analgesia. Biofeedback training does not appear to confer substantial benefit beyond that of traditional relaxation training taught in childbirth education classes.

Transcutaneous Electrical Nerve Stimulation

There are four types of publications concerning the efficacy and suitability of transcutaneous electrical nerve stimulation (TENS) as an analgesic technique for labor: (1) case studies,[83,84] (2) TENS-only studies,[85-88] (3) TENS versus control studies,[89-94] and (4) TENS versus TENS-placebo studies, with or without a control group.[95-100] The following summary does not include observations from case reports and TENS-only trials. Harrison et al.[99] noted a shorter labor in those patients who received TENS and who required no additional analgesics. All other authors observed no effect on the length of labor, the use of other analgesics, and the incidence of instrumental delivery. Pain perception was unchanged in most studies, except that Erkkola et al.[94] noted increased pain perception in early labor (cervical dilation < 7 cm) in patients receiving TENS, and Vincenti et al.[91] observed decreased pain perception.

Advantages of TENS are that it is easy to use and discontinue, it is noninvasive, and it has no demonstrable harmful effects on the fetus. The only stated disadvantage is the occasional interference with electronic fetal heart rate monitoring. Patients tend to rate the device as helpful, despite the fact that it does not decrease the use of additional analgesics. Widespread use of TENS does not seem warranted.

Acupuncture/Acupressure

Traditional Chinese medicine includes extensive use of acupuncture. Given the fact that acupuncture can provide analgesia, there is interest in its use for intrapartum analgesia. Some studies have examined traditional (i.e., manual) acupuncture,[101] whereas others have studied electroacupuncture or both methods.[102-104] Given the lack of widespread use in obstetric patients, there is a lack of standardization of the proper acupuncture points to be stimulated. Each of these studies[101-104] examined specific—but diverse—acupuncture points to relieve abdominal, back, and perineal pain, and the results are conflicting. At one extreme, Wallis et al.[103] found acupuncture ineffective, whereas Umeh[101] and Pei and Huang[104] concluded that it is a valuable analgesic technique. Some authors felt that the placement and maintenance of acupuncture needles was cumbersome and poorly accepted by patients, whereas others considered the time required to place and secure the needles to be well spent. Cultural differences among the patient populations may help explain some

---

Box 19-5 PURPORTED BENEFITS OF UPRIGHT POSITION

• Maternal comfort and relaxation
• Facilitation of fetal head engagement and rotation
• Increased pelvic diameter
• Decreased incidence of perineal tears

of this disparity. In addition, the varied levels of experience of these acupuncturists may have influenced the results. Acupressure has been touted as an effective noninvasive technique that uses pressure at traditional acupuncture points.[105] However, it is unlikely that either acupuncture or acupressure will gain widespread acceptance by Western society for intrapartum analgesia.

Hypnosis

The use of hypnosis for obstetric analgesia is not new.[106] Early proponents touted its safety for the mother and the fetus, decreased analgesic requirements, and shorter labor as the major advantages of intrapartum hypnosis. Whether hypnosis differs substantially from other childbirth preparation techniques is an unresolved controversy. Fee and Reilley[107] concluded that the breathing and relaxation exercises used in childbirth preparation do not represent a hypnotic trance; support for their conclusion is provided by the successful teaching of childbirth preparation exercises to women who are not susceptible to hypnosis. However, women susceptible to hypnosis may achieve a state much like a hypnotic trance when using these same exercises.

Instruction in the techniques of self-hypnosis before the onset of labor or, alternatively, availability of the hypnotist during labor is time consuming for the hypnotist. Proponents previously suggested that successful hypnosis training should begin early in the third trimester. More recently, Oster[108] suggested that training may begin as late as 3 to 6 weeks before the expected date of delivery. Neither individual nor group sessions have proved to be superior. In addition, Rock et al.[109] found that hypnosis could be introduced to untrained, nonvolunteer patients during labor. On average, this added approximately 45 minutes of additional care, and all but 3 of 22 patients in the experimental group required additional analgesia. Some studies[110] found that hypnosis did not decrease analgesic requirements, but others[111] noted that hypnosis resulted in decreased analgesic requirements and a tendency toward less perineal trauma.

Childbirth preparation and hypnosis seem to result in similar effects on obstetric outcome. Harmon et al.[112] combined hypnosis and skill mastery with childbirth education. Experimental patients with a high susceptibility to hypnosis had decreased use of opioid, tranquilizer, and oxytocic medications, shorter first and second stages of labor, and a higher incidence of spontaneous delivery. Patients with a low susceptibility to hypnosis did not gain substantial advantage from the addition of hypnosis to the routine childbirth education provided for the control group.

In summary, hypnosis has at least three limitations: (1) antepartum training sessions are required; (2) trained hypnotherapists must be available during labor; and (3) it offers no clear benefit. Therefore hypnosis is unlikely to attain widespread use.

IMPLICATIONS FOR THE ANESTHESIOLOGIST

Childbirth preparation classes and nonpharmacologic analgesic techniques are not comparable with regional analgesia/anesthesia for the relief of labor pain. Thus some might wonder whether it is important or useful for anesthesiologists to have knowledge of these techniques. If our only obligation to the obstetric patient is a technical one (i.e., to eliminate pain safely with the use of regional anesthesia), perhaps knowledge of these techniques is superfluous. However, the practice of obstetric anesthesia should not be limited to the performance of pain-relieving procedures; our contributions to the care of the obstetric patient and her family should extend beyond the administration of regional anesthesia.

Much has been written in professional and lay journals concerning the "proper childbirth experience." Each patient's expectations concerning labor influence her childbirth experience. Yarrow[113] described the results of a nonscientific poll of 72,000 readers of *Parents Magazine*, which revealed that there is an undeniable movement toward more family-centered maternity care. Women currently view childbirth from the perspective of educated consumers: they expect to have choices and a degree of control during childbirth. We may not always be comfortable with this situation, but it is a reality for modern obstetric practice. Our challenge is to provide safe, effective analgesia in a nonthreatening, "home-like" environment. We are not solely responsible for a patient's childbirth experience, but our interactions with the patient, her family, and her obstetrician will influence her perception of childbirth.

Anesthesiologists must become effective educators as well as health care providers. Patients should have realistic expectations regarding the pain of labor and the variability of individual labor patterns. They should be encouraged to define success as a positive childbirth experience regardless of the mode of delivery, use of analgesia and anesthesia, or other arbitrary definitions. An obstetrician gave the following advice to prospective mothers[114]:

> If you do end up choosing some form of pain relief during labor, do not feel inadequate if a friend had her baby without assistance. Some labors are more intense than others. Ultimately, holding your baby in your arms is more important than the method you used to bring her into the world.

Anesthesiologists may effectively provide similar advice. Unfortunately, anesthesiologists have had little involvement in prenatal education classes. Their active participation in childbirth education classes may help patients receive more accurate information concerning the risks and benefits of analgesia/anesthesia for labor, vaginal delivery, and cesarean section. Anesthesiologists can encourage childbirth instructors to prepare patients for the unexpected and to acknowledge that the commonly described "typical" labor may, in fact, be atypical. Well-informed patients are more likely to accept the interventions that may become necessary during labor. Women with medical or obstetric diseases that may increase anesthetic risk should be encouraged to discuss these problems with an anesthesiologist before the onset of labor; thus we must develop procedures to facilitate antepartum consultation. In summary, the active participation of the anesthesiologist in childbirth education will cause women to perceive the anesthesiologist as an integral part of the obstetric care team.

Some nonpharmacologic analgesic techniques may have benefits other than decreased pain perception. For example, some obstetricians and nurses believe that ambulation and subsequent squatting (or use of a birth cushion) shortens labor and increases the rate of spontaneous vaginal delivery. If this is true, we should attempt to develop and use analgesic techniques that take advantage of these relatively simple maneuvers. For example, the use of intrathecal opioids for early labor allows for continued ambulation and the use of showers and/or tubs. Some techniques of epidural analgesia allow sitting with support. Finally, epidural analgesia/anesthesia does not eliminate the beneficial effects of other comfort measures (e.g., massage, continued emotional support from family and friends).

Whenever possible, anesthesiologists should provide safe anesthetic care that is compatible with reasonable patient expectations. Future studies concerning the efficacy of childbirth education, nonpharmacologic analgesic techniques, and regional anesthetic techniques should evaluate the patient's overall experience and satisfaction rather than limit evaluation to the usual measures of obstetric outcome.[115] In an editorial that accompanied the study by Bloom et al.[71], Cefalo and Bowes[116] commented, "In the end, the nurses, midwives, and physicians who attend a woman with compassion, understanding, and professionalism are the most important factors in the management of any labor."

KEY POINTS

- Childbirth preparation does not eliminate the pain of labor or substantially reduce the use of analgesia/anesthesia, but it does decrease the anxiety associated with labor.
- Emotional support provided by doulas decreases the use of analgesics, the length of labor, and the incidence of forceps and abdominal deliveries in selected patient populations.
- Biofeedback, transcutaneous electrical nerve stimulation, acupuncture, and hypnosis do not provide significant benefits beyond other childbirth preparation techniques, although transcutaneous electrical nerve stimulation is well received by patients.
- Some maneuvers (e.g., ambulation, squatting) taught as techniques to decrease pain may help shorten labor and hasten spontaneous delivery.
- Anesthesiologists should become active participants in childbirth education. Anesthesiologists should encourage and facilitate the honest discussion of the risks and benefits of the analgesic/anesthetic techniques available at their hospitals.
- No nonpharmacologic technique consistently provides the quality of intrapartum pain relief that is provided by regional analgesia/anesthesia.

REFERENCES

1. Ziemer MM. Does prepared childbirth mean pain relief? Top Clin Nurs 1980; 2:19-26.
2. Bonica JJ, McDonald JS. The Pain of Childbirth. In: Bonica JJ, editor. The Management of Pain. 2nd ed. Philadelphia, Lea & Febiger, 1990:1313-43.
3. Melzack R. The McGill Pain Questionnaire: Major properties and scoring methods. Pain 1975; 1:277-99.
4. Reading AE. A comparison of the McGill Pain Questionnaire in chronic and acute pain. Pain 1982; 13:185-92.
5. Scott J, Huskisson EC. Graphic representation of pain. Pain 1976; 2:175-84.
6. Melzack R. Taenzer P, Feldman P, Kinch RA. Labour is still painful after prepared childbirth training. Can Med Assoc J 1981; 125:357-63.
7. Melzack R. The myth of painless childbirth (the John J. Bonica lecture). Pain 1984; 19:321-37.
8. Speert H. Obstetrics and Gynecology in America: A History. Baltimore, Md, Waverly Press, 1980.
9. Wertz RW, Wertz DC. Lying-In: A History of Childbirth in America. New York, The Free Press, 1977.
10. Devitt N. The transition from home to hospital birth in the United States, 1930-1960. Birth Fam J 1977; 4:47-58.
11. Beck NC, Geden EA, Brouder GT. Preparation for labor: A historical perspective. Psychosom Med 1979; 41:243-58.
12. Dick-Read G. Natural Childbirth. London, Heinemann, 1933.
13. Dick-Read G. Childbirth Without Fear. New York, Harper & Brothers, 1944.
14. Lamaze F. Painless Childbirth (Celestin LR, translator). London, Burke, 1958.
15. Velvovsky I, Platonov K, Ploticher V, Shugom E, editors. Painless Childbirth Through Psychoprophylaxis (Myshne DA, translator). Moscow, Foreign Languages Publishing House, 1960.
16. Karmel M. Thank You, Dr. Lamaze. New York, Lippincott, 1959.
17. Karmel M. Thank You, Dr. Lamaze. 2nd ed. New York, Harper & Row, 1981:7-8.
18. Leboyer F. Birth Without Violence. New York, Alfred A. Knopf, 1975.
19. Nelson NM, Enkin MW, Saigal S, et al. A randomized clinical trial of the Leboyer approach to childbirth. N Engl J Med 1980; 302:655-60.
20. Saigal S, Nelson NM, Bennett KJ, Enkin MW. Observations on the behavioral state of newborn infants during the first hour of life. Am J Obstet Gynecol 1981; 139:715-9.
21. Pitcock CD, Clark RB. From Fanny to Fernand: The development of consumerism in pain control during the birth process. Am J Obstet Gynecol 1992; 167:581-7.
22. Beck NC, Hall D. Natural childbirth: A review and analysis. Obstet Gynecol 1978; 52:371-9.
23. Lindell SG. Education for childbirth: A time for change. J Obstet Gynecol Neonatal Nurs 1988; 17:108-12.
24. Nelson MK. The effect of childbirth preparation on women of different social classes. J Health Soc Behav 1982; 23:339-52.
25. Zacharias JF. Childbirth education classes: Effects on attitudes toward childbirth in high-risk indigent women. JOGN Nurs 1981; 10:265-7.
26. Copstick S, Hayes RW, Taylor KE, Morris NF. A test of a common assumption regarding the use of antenatal training during labour. J Psychosom Res 1985; 29:215-8.
27. Bernardini JY, Maloni JA, Stegman CE. Neuromuscular control of childbirth-prepared women during the first stage of labor. JOGN Nurs 1983; 12:105-11.
28. Stewart DE. Psychiatric symptoms following attempted natural childbirth. Can Med Assoc J 1982; 127:713-6.
29. Guzman Sanchez A, Segura Ortega L, Panduro Baron JG. Psychological reaction due to failure using the Lamaze method. Int J Gynaecol Obstet 1985; 23:343-6.
30. Ephron N. Having a baby after 35. New York, New York Times Sunday Magazine, November 26, 1978.
31. Behan M. Childbirth machisma. Parenting, April 1988, 53-7.
32. Crittendon D. Knock me out with a truck. Wall Street Journal, November 6, 1992, A14.
33. Hetherington SE. A controlled study of the effect of prepared childbirth classes on obstetric outcomes. Birth 1990; 17:86-90.
34. Zax M, Sameroff AJ, Farnum JE. Childbirth education, maternal attitudes, and delivery. Am J Obstet Gynecol 1975; 123:185-90.
35. Scott JR, Rose NB. Effect of psychoprophylaxis (Lamaze preparation) on labor and delivery in primiparas. N Engl J Med 1976; 294:1205-7.
36. Rogers CH. Type of medications used in labor by Lamaze and non-Lamaze prepared subjects and the effect on newborn Apgar scores using analysis of variance. Thesis, University of Alabama (Huntsville), 1981.
37. Hughey MJ, McElin TW, Young T. Maternal and fetal outcome of Lamaze-prepared patients. Obstet Gynecol 1978; 51:643-7.
38. Delke I, Minkoff H, Grunebaum A. Effect of Lamaze childbirth preparation on maternal plasma beta-endorphin immunoreactivity in active labor. Am J Perinatol 1985; 2:317-9.
39. Patton LL, English EC, Hambleton JD. Childbirth preparation and outcomes of labor and delivery in primiparous women. J Fam Pract 1985; 20:375-8.
40. Sturrock WA, Johnson JA. The relationship between childbirth education classes and obstetric outcome. Birth 1990; 17:82-5.
41. Brewin C, Bradley C. Perceived control and the experience of childbirth. Br J Clin Psychol 1982; 21:263-9.
42. Worthington EL, Martin GA. A laboratory analysis of response to pain after training in three Lamaze techniques. J Psychosom Res 1980; 24:109-16.

43. Manderino MA, Bzdek VM. Effects of modeling and information on reactions to pain: A childbirth-preparation analogue. Nurs Res 1984; 33:9-14.

44. Geden E, Beck NC, Brouder G, et al. Self-report and psychophysiological effects of Lamaze preparation: An analogue of labor pain. Res Nurs Health 1985; 8:155-65.

45. Geden EA, Beck NC, Anderson JS, et al. Effects of cognitive and pharmacologic strategies on analogued labor pain. Nurs Res 1986; 35:301-6.

46. Whipple B, Josimovich JB, Komisaruk BR. Sensory thresholds during the antepartum, intrapartum and postpartum periods. Int J Nurs Stud 1990; 27:213-21.

47. Simkin P. Reducing pain and enhancing progress in labor: A guide to non-pharmacologic methods for maternity care givers. Birth 1995; 22:161-71.

48. Gentz BA. Alternative therapies for the management of pain in labor and delivery. Clin Obstet Gynecol 2001; 44:704-32.

49. Henneborn WJ, Cogan R. The effect of husband participation on reported pain and probability of medication during labor and birth. J Psychosom Res 1975; 19:215-22.

50. Keirse MJNC, Enkin M, Lumley J. Social and professional support during labor. In: Chalmers I, Enkin M, Keirse MJNC, editors. Effective Care in Pregnancy and Childbirth. New York, Oxford University Press, 1989:805-14.

51. Bertsch TD, Nagishima-Whalen L, Dykeman S, et al. Labor support by first-time fathers: Direct observations. J Psychosom Obstet Gynecol 1990; 11:251-60.

52. Sosa R, Kennell J, Klaus M, et al. The effect of a supportive companion on perinatal problems, length of labor, and mother-infant interaction. N Engl J Med 1980; 303:597-600.

53. Klaus MH, Kennell JH, Robertson SS, Sosa R. Effects of social support during parturition on maternal and infant mortality. BMJ 1986; 293:585-7.

54. Kennell J, Klaus M, McGrath S, et al. Continuous emotional support during labor in a US hospital: A randomized controlled trial. JAMA 1991; 265:2197-201.

55. Skibsted L, Lange AP. The need for pain relief in uncomplicated deliveries in an alternative birth center compared to an obstetric delivery ward. Pain 1992; 48:183-6.

56. Hofmeyer GJ, Nikodem VC, Wolman W, et al. Companionship to modify the clinical birth environment: Effects on progress and perceptions of labour and breast-feeding. Br J Obstet Gynecol 1991; 98:756-64.

57. Birch ER. The experience of touch received during labor: Postpartum perceptions of therapeutic value. J Nurse Midwifery 1986; 31:270-6.

58. Penny KS. Postpartum perceptions of touch received during labor. Res Nurs Health 1979; 2:9-16.

59. Chang M-Y, Wang S-Y, Chen C-H. Effects of massage on pain and anxiety during labour: A randomized controlled trial in Taiwan. J Adv Nurs 2002; 38:68-73.

60. Odent M. Birth under water. Lancet 1983; 2:1476-7.

61. Milner I. Water baths for pain relief in labour. Nurs Times 1988; 84: 38-40.

62. Rush J, Burlock S, Lambert K, et al. The effects of whirlpool baths in labor: A randomized, controlled trial. Birth 1996; 23:136-43.

63. Schorn M, McAllister J, Blanco J. Water immersion and the effect on labor. Nurse-Midwifery 1993; 38:336-42.

64. Aird I, Luckas M, Buckett W, et al. Effects of intrapartum hydrotherapy on labor related parameters. Aust NZ J Obstet Gynaecol 1997; 37: 137-42.

65. Eckert K, Turnbull D, MacLennan A. Immersion in water in the first stage of labor: A randomized controlled trial. Birth 2001; 28:84-93.

66. Robertson PA, Huang LJ, Croughan-Minihane MS, Kilpatrick SJ. Is there an association between water baths during labor and the development of chorioamnionitis or endometritis? Am J Obstet Gynecol 1998; 178:1215-21.

67. Melzack R, Belanger E, Lacroix R. Labor pain: Effect of maternal position on front and back pain. J Pain Symptom Manage 1991; 6:476-80.

68. Andrews CM, Chrzanowski M. Maternal position, labor, and comfort. Appl Nurs Res 1990; 3:7-13.

69. Waldenstroem RNM, Gottvall K. A randomized trial of birthing stool or conventional semirecumbent position for second-stage labor. Birth 1991; 18:5-10.

70. Gardosi J, Sylvester S, Lynch C. Alternative positions in second stage of labour: A randomized controlled trial. Br J Obstet Gynaecol 1989; 96:1290-6.

71. Bloom SL, McIntire DD, Kelley MA, et al. Lack of effect of walking on labor and delivery. N Engl J Med 1998; 339:76-9.

72. Stewart P, Spiby H. A randomized study of the sitting position for delivery using a newly designed obstetric chair. Br J Obstet Gynaecol 1989; 96:327-33.

73. Liu YC. The effects of the upright position during childbirth. Image J Nurs Sch 1989; 21:14-8.

74. Collis RE, Harding SA, Morgan BM. Effect of maternal ambulation on labour with low-dose combined spinal-epidural analgesia. Anaesthesia 1999; 54:535-9.

75. Johnson N, Johnson VA, Gupta JK. Maternal positions during labor. Obstet Gynecol Surv 1991; 46:428-34.

76. Gardosi J, Hutson N, Lynch C. Randomized, controlled trial of squatting in the second stage of labour. Lancet 1989; 2:74-7.

77. Gupta JK, Leal CB, Johnson N, Lilford RJ. Squatting in the second stage of labour (letter). Lancet 1989; 2:561-2.

78. Kakol K. Position in labor: Does mother know best? Prof Nurs 1989; 4:481-4.

79. Samra JS, Tang LC, Obhrai MS. Birth in the squatting position (letter). Lancet 1989; 2:1150-1.

80. Shannahan MK, Cottrell BH. The effects of birth chair delivery on maternal perceptions. J Obstet Gynecol Neonatal Nurs 1989; 18:323-6.

81. St. James-Roberts I, Chamberlain G, Haran FJ, Hutchinson CM. Use of electromyographic and skin-conductance biofeedback relaxation training to facilitate childbirth in primiparae. J Psychosom Res 1982; 26:455-62.

82. Duchene P. Effects of biofeedback on childbirth pain. J Pain Symptom Manag 1989; 4:117-23.

83. Keenan DL, Simonsen L, McCrann DJ. Transcutaneous electrical nerve stimulation for pain control during labor and delivery. A case report. Phys Ther 1985; 65:1363-4.

84. Lea P. Delivering women from labor pain. Can Nurse 1992; 88:17-9.

85. Augustinsson LE, Bohlin P, Bundsen P, et al. Pain relief during delivery by transcutaneous electrical nerve stimulation. Pain 1977; 4:59-65.

86. Stewart P. Transcutaneous nerve stimulation as a method of analgesia in labour. Anaesthesia 1979; 34:357-60.

87. Grim LC, Morey SH. Transcutaneous electrical nerve stimulation for relief of parturition pain: A clinical report. Phys Ther 1985; 65:337-40.

88. Robson JE. Transcutaneous nerve stimulation for pain relief in labour. Anaesthesia 1979; 34:357-60.

89. Bundsen P, Peterson LE, Selstam U. Pain relief in labor by transcutaneous electrical nerve stimulation: A prospective matched study. Acta Obstet Gynecol Scand 1981; 60:459-68.

90. Bundsen P, Ericson K, Peterson LE, Thiringer K. Pain relief in labor by transcutaneous electrical nerve stimulation: Testing of a modified stimulation technique and evaluation of the neurological and biochemical condition of the newborn infant. Acta Obstet Gynecol Scand 1982; 61:129-36.

91. Vincenti E, Cervellin A, Mega M, et al. Comparative study between patients treated with transcutaneous electric stimulation and controls during labour. Clin Exp Obstet Gynecol 1982; 9:95-7.

92. Harrison RF, Shore M, Woods T, et al. A comparative study of transcutaneous electrical nerve stimulation (TENS), entonox, pethidine + promazine and lumbar epidural for pain relief in labor. Acta Obstet Gynecol Scand 1987; 66:9-14.

93. Chia YT, Arulkumaran S, Chua S, Ratnam SS. Effectiveness of transcutaneous electric nerve stimulator for pain relief in labour. Asia-Oceania J Obstet Gynaecol 1990; 16:145-51.

94. Erkkola R, Pikkola P, Kanto J. Transcutaneous nerve stimulation for pain relief during labour: A controlled study. Ann Chir Gynaecol 1980; 69:273-7.

95. Nesheim BI. The use of transcutaneous nerve stimulation for pain relief during labor: A controlled clinical study. Acta Obstet Gynecol Scand 1981; 60:13-6.

96. Thomas IL, Tyle V, Webster J, Neilson A. An evaluation of transcutaneous electrical nerve stimulation for pain relief in labour. Aust NZ J Obstet Gynaecol 1988; 28:182-9.

97. Lee EWC, Chung IWY, Lee JYL, et al. The role of transcutaneous electrical nerve stimulation in management of labour in obstetric patients. Asia-Oceania J Obstet Gynaecol 1990; 16:247-54.

98. Van der Ploeg J, Vervest H, Liem A, et al. Transcutaneous nerve stimulation (TENS) during the first stage of labour: A randomized clinical trial. Pain 1996; 68:75-8.

99. Harrison RF, Woods T, Shore M, et al. Pain relief in labour using transcutaneous electrical nerve stimulation (TENS): A TENS/TENS placebo controlled study in two parity groups. Br J Obstet Gynaecol 1986; 93:739-46.

100. Carroll D, Tramer M, McQuay H, et al. Transcutaneous electrical nerve stimulation in labour pain: A systemic review. Br J Obstet Gynaecol 1997; 104:169-75.

101. Umeh BUO. Sacral acupuncture for pain relief in labour: Initial clinical experience in Nigerian women. Acupunct Electrother Res 1986; 11:147-51.

102. Abouleish E, Depp R. Acupuncture in obstetrics. Anesth Analg 1975; 54:83-8.
103. Wallis L, Shnider SM, Palahniuk RJ, Spivey HL. An evaluation of acupuncture analgesia in obstetrics. Anesthesiology 1974; 41:596-601.
104. Pei DE, Huang YL. Use of acupuncture analgesia during childbirth. J Tradit Chin Med 1985; 5:253-5.
105. Jimenez S. Acupressure: Pain relief at your fingertips. Int J Childbirth Educ 1996; 10:7-10.
106. August RV. Hypnosis in Childbirth. New York, McGraw-Hill, 1961.
107. Fee FA, Reilley RR. Hypnosis in obstetrics: A review of techniques. J Am Soc Psychosom Dent Med 1982; 29:17-29.
108. Oster MI. Contemporary methods in hypnotic preparation for childbirth. CRNA 2000; 11:160-6.
109. Rock NL, Shipley TE, Campbell C. Hypnosis with untrained, nonvolunteer patients in labor. Int J Clin Exp Hypn 1969; 17:25-36.
110. Freeman RM, Macaulay AJ, Eve L, Chamberlain GVP. Randomized trial of self hypnosis for analgesia in labour. BMJ 1986; 292:657-8.
111. Letts P, Baker P, Ruderman J, et al. The use of hypnosis in labor and delivery: A preliminary study. J Womens Health Gend Based Med 1993; 2:335-41.
112. Harmon TM, Hynan MT, Tyre TE. Improved obstetric outcomes using hypnotic analgesia and skill mastery combined with childbirth education. J Consult Clin Psychol 1990; 58:525-30.
113. Yarrow L. Giving birth: 72,000 moms tell all. Parents 1992; 67:148-59.
114. Stevenson-Smith F, Salmon DK. Pain relief during labor. Parents 1993; 68:127.
115. MacArthur C, Lewis M, Knox EG. Evaluation of obstetric analgesia and anaesthesia: Long-term maternal recollections. Int J Obstet Anesth 1993; 2:3-11.
116. Cefalo RC, Bowes WA. Managing labor: Never walk alone (editorial). N Engl J Med 1998; 339:117-8.

Chapter 20

Systemic Analgesia: Parenteral and Inhalational Agents

Marsha L. Wakefield, M.D.

Systemic drugs have been used to decrease the pain of childbirth since 1847, when James Young Simpson used diethyl ether to anesthetize a parturient with a deformed pelvis. A heightened awareness of neonatal effects and an increased desire by women to actively participate in childbirth have prompted physicians to abandon heavy sedation during labor and to abandon the administration of general anesthesia during uncomplicated vaginal delivery. Epidural and spinal anesthesia provide effective maternal pain relief with few adverse effects on the infant. Epidural and spinal analgesic techniques have replaced systemic analgesics as the preferred techniques for many patients.

In 1997, Hawkins et al.[1] published the results of a survey of obstetric anesthetic practice in the United States for the year 1992 and compared the results with those of a 1981 survey. Fewer patients received no analgesia in 1992 than in 1981. However, in 1992, systemic medications (e.g., opioids, barbiturates, tranquilizers) remained the most frequently used form of analgesia despite a substantial increase in the use of regional anesthesia. There was a 100% increase in the use of epidural analgesia during the decade between 1981 and 1992. A smaller proportion of women received regional anesthesia for labor and delivery in the smaller facilities (i.e., those with less than 500 births per year) than in the larger facilities. Regional anesthesia was unavailable in 20% of the smallest hospitals in the 1992 survey. Oyston[2] made similar observations in a 1995 survey of obstetric units in Ontario. In 66 of 142 hospitals, intramuscular and intravenous opioids were the only types of analgesia available.

The use of systemic analgesic drugs remains common practice for several reasons. First, some conditions (e.g., hemorrhage, coagulopathy) contraindicate the administration of epidural or spinal anesthesia. Second, regional anesthesia is not available in all hospitals, especially smaller facilities. Third, epidural or spinal anesthesia is not without risk, and some women decline these techniques. Alternatively, some women choose to receive a systemic analgesic drug during early labor and opt for regional anesthesia as pain becomes more intense.

PARENTERAL OPIOIDS

Opioids are the most widely used systemic medications for labor analgesia. Use of these drugs does not require the use of specialized equipment or personnel. These drugs allow the parturient to better tolerate the pain of labor, but typically they do not provide complete analgesia. Systemic opioids have become less popular because of the frequency of maternal side effects (e.g., nausea, vomiting, delayed gastric emptying, dysphoria, drowsiness, hypoventilation) and the potential for adverse neonatal effects.

Although systemic opioids have long been used for labor analgesia, there is little scientific evidence to suggest that one drug is intrinsically better than another for this use; most often the selection of an opioid is based on institutional tradition and/or personal preference (Table 20-1). The efficacy of systemic opioid analgesia and the incidence of side effects are largely dose dependent rather than drug dependent.

Because of their lipid solubility and low molecular weight (less than 500 daltons), all opioids easily cross the placenta by diffusion and are associated with the risks of neonatal respiratory depression and neurobehavioral changes. Neonatal metabolism and elimination of drugs are prolonged as compared with adults; opioids may also cause fetal effects in utero. The blood-brain barrier is less well developed as compared with that of the adult. Opioids may result in decreased beat-to-beat variability

TABLE 20-1	OPIOIDS USED FOR LABOR ANALGESIA			
Drug	**Usual dose (IV/IM)**	**Onset (IV/IM)**	**Duration**	**Comments**
Meperidine	25 mg IV/50 mg IM	5-10 min IV/40-45 min IM	2-3 hr	Active metabolite is normeperidine; neonatal effects most likely if delivery occurs between 1 and 4 hr after administration
Morphine	2-5 mg IV/10 mg IM	5 min IV/20-40 min IM	3-4 hr	Infrequent use during labor; greater respiratory depression in neonate than with meperidine
Fentanyl	25-50 μg IV/100 μg IM	2-3 min IV/10 min IM	30-60 min	Short-acting, potent respiratory depressant; used as continuous infusion and/or PCA; cumulative effect with large doses over time
Nalbuphine	10-20 mg IV/IM	2-3 min IV/15 min IM/SQ	3-6 hr	Agonist/antagonist; less nausea and vomiting than with meperidine
Butorphanol	1-2 mg IV/IM	5-10 min IV/10-30 min IM	3-4 hr	Agonist/antagonist; maternal sedation similar to meperidine plus phenothiazine
Pentazocine	20-40 mg IV/IM	2-3 min IV/15-20 min IM/SQ	2-3 hr	Agonist/antagonist; psychomimetic effects possible with usual doses but more frequent after large doses; infrequent use during labor

IM, Intramuscular; *IV*, intravenous; *PCA*, patient-controlled analgesia; *SQ*, subcutaneous.

of the fetal heart rate (FHR); however, this change usually does not reflect a worsening of fetal oxygenation or acid-base status. The likelihood of neonatal respiratory depression depends on the dose and timing of administration. Even in the absence of obvious neonatal depression at birth, there may be subtle changes in neonatal neurobehavior for several days.[3] The long-term clinical significance of these neurobehavioral changes is unclear. Reynolds et al.[4] recently performed a meta-analysis of studies that have compared epidural analgesia with systemic opioid analgesia using meperidine, butorphanol, or fentanyl. The authors concluded that lumbar epidural analgesia was associated with "improved neonatal acid-base status, suggesting that placental exchange is well preserved in association with maternal sympathetic blockade and good analgesia."

Modes of Administration

INTERMITTENT BOLUS DOSES

Opioids may be given subcutaneously or intramuscularly, but they are more often administered intravenously, either intermittently or by continuous intravenous infusion. The route and timing of administration influence maternal uptake and placental transfer. **Subcutaneous** and **intramuscular** injections have the advantage of simplicity. Of course, intramuscular injection is painful. Absorption varies with the site of injection, and injection is followed by a delay in the onset of analgesia. Subcutaneous or intramuscular injection results in analgesia of variable onset, quality, and duration.

Advantages of **intravenous** administration include the following: (1) less variability in the peak plasma concentration of drug; (2) faster onset of analgesia; and (3) the ability to titrate dose to effect. The intravenous route is generally preferred, because absorption is less certain after intramuscular injection.

PATIENT-CONTROLLED ANALGESIA

Patient-controlled analgesia (PCA) is widely used in the management of postoperative pain. Although continuous intravenous infusion of opioids has been used for at least four decades, the growing popularity of PCA for postoperative analgesia has prompted the use of this technique for labor analgesia. Purported advantages of PCA include the following: (1) superior pain relief with lower doses of drug; (2) less risk of maternal respiratory depression (as compared with bolus intravenous administration); (3) less placental transfer of drug; (4) less need for antiemetic agents; and (5) higher patient satisfaction.[5] Smaller, more frequent dosing should result in a more stable plasma drug concentration and a more consistent analgesic effect.[6]

PCA for labor is not without limitations. Despite frequent administration, small doses of opioid may not always be effective for the fluctuating intensity of labor pain, especially in the late first or second stage of labor.[7] Moreover, the risk to the fetus and neonate remains unclear; studies have used variable methods of neonatal assessment. Variable doses and dosing intervals have been used, including the continuous infusion-PCA combination and PCA bolus alone. Meperidine, nalbuphine, fentanyl, and, more recently, remifentanil have been the opioids most frequently used for PCA administration. However, the most appropriate drug, drug dose, and dosing schedules have not been defined (Table 20-2).

PCA offers an attractive alternative for labor analgesia in hospitals in which epidural anesthesia is unavailable or when epidural anesthesia is contraindicated or unsuccessful. The mother can tailor the administration of analgesia according to her individual needs. Although PCA may result in higher patient satisfaction than other methods of opioid administration, most studies have not demonstrated either a reduced use of drug or improved analgesia with PCA as compared with intravenous administration of an opioid by the obstetric nurse.

TABLE 20-2	OPIOIDS USED FOR INTRAVENOUS PATIENT-CONTROLLED ANALGESIA DURING LABOR	
Drug	**Patient-Controlled Dose**	**Lockout Period (min)**
Meperidine	10-15 mg	8-20
Nalbuphine	1-3 mg	6-10
Fentanyl	10-25 μg	8-12
Remifentanil (boluses only)	0.4-0.5 μg/kg	2-3
Remifentanil (infusion with patient-controlled boluses)	0.05 μg/kg/min basal infusion with bolus doses of 0.25 μg/kg	5

Meperidine

Meperidine (pethidine, Demerol) is the opioid most widely used for labor analgesia worldwide. Although there are significant doubts about meperidine's analgesic efficacy and ongoing concerns about its maternal, fetal, and neonatal side effects, administration of the drug has "the virtue of familiarity and low cost."[8] There is no convincing evidence that alternative opioids are better than meperidine.[8] Meperidine is a synthetic opioid that readily crosses the placenta by passive diffusion, and it achieves equilibrium between maternal and fetal compartments within 6 minutes.[9] The usual dose is 25 to 50 mg intravenously or 50 to 100 mg intramuscularly every 2 to 4 hours. The onset of analgesia is within 5 minutes of intravenous administration and within 45 minutes of intramuscular administration. A phenothiazine is often administered with meperidine to diminish nausea and vomiting.

The half-life of meperidine is 2½ to 3 hours in the mother and 18 to 23 hours in the neonate.[10,11] Meperidine is metabolized in the liver to normeperidine, meperidic acid, and normeperidic acid. Normeperidine is a pharmacologically active metabolite that is a potent respiratory depressant; it also crosses the placenta. In addition, maternally administered meperidine is metabolized by the neonate, who produces a significant amount of normeperidine. The half-life of normeperidine in the neonate is approximately 60 hours.[12]

The timing of the administration of meperidine affects the risk of neonatal depression at birth. Maximal fetal tissue uptake of meperidine occurs approximately 2 to 3 hours after maternal administration. Thus, from the pharmacologic standpoint, the best timing for birth after maternal administration of meperidine would be within the first hour *or* more than 4 hours after a single intravenous dose. Studies have shown that infants born 2 to 3 hours after maternal administration of meperidine have an increased risk of respiratory depression.[13,14]

After administration of a single dose of meperidine (or in patients with a short administration-to-delivery interval), neonatal depression is proportional to the total amount of meperidine transferred to the fetus before delivery. However, normeperidine concentrations *increase* as meperidine concentrations decrease over time. Normeperidine is more slowly excreted than meperidine, and it tends to accumulate in maternal plasma after multiple doses of meperidine.[15] The concentrations of normeperidine may become clinically significant after the administration of multiple doses of meperidine or in patients with a prolonged administration-to-delivery interval. Normeperidine may account in part for the subtle changes in neonatal neurobehavior that may be present for as long as 3 to 5 days after meperidine administration[15-19]; these changes include decreased duration of wakefulness, decreased duration of non-rapid eye movement sleep, and decreased attentiveness. An alteration in infant breast-feeding behavior has been noted after the administration of 100 mg of meperidine during labor.[20] These changes have occurred despite high Apgar scores at birth, and the long-term significance of these subtle changes in behavior is unclear.

Like other opioids, meperidine may cause decreased FHR variability. The maximum effect on FHR variability occurs 25 minutes after intravenous administration and 40 minutes after intramuscular administration. Variability of the FHR typically recovers within 60 minutes.[21,22] It is widely believed that meperidine (as well as other opioids) may slow labor when given during the latent phase; it does not slow the active phase of the first stage of labor. By decreasing the maternal concentrations of circulating catecholamines, administration of meperidine may accelerate labor in some patients.

PATIENT-CONTROLLED ADMINISTRATION

Erskine et al.[23] compared PCA meperidine (0.3 mg/kg bolus with a 10-minute lockout) with pentazocine (0.15 mg/kg bolus with a 10-minute lockout). A third group of patients received intramuscular meperidine. Analgesia was satisfactory with both methods of PCA. There were fewer maternal side effects with pentazocine. There were no differences in neonatal assessment among the three groups of infants, which included the measurement of Apgar scores and neurobehavioral testing on days 1 and 5 of life.

Rayburn et al.[7] compared PCA meperidine (10 mg bolus with a 20-minute lockout) with nurse-administered meperidine (25 to 50 mg intravenously) given every 3 hours as requested. After 2 hours, the total dose of meperidine used was greater in the PCA group. No significant differences were found in maternal side effects, analgesia, or sedation. A total of 5 of 31 infants in the PCA group and 3 of 33 infants in the nurse-administered group received naloxone; this was most common when the total dose exceeded 100 mg in either group. There was no difference between the two groups in neonatal neurobehavioral assessment at 2 to 4 hours and 24 hours after delivery.[7]

Morphine

Earlier in this century, morphine was often administered in combination with scopolamine to provide "twilight sleep" during labor and delivery. Significant maternal and neonatal complications occurred with the use of large doses. Maternal analgesia was obtained, but the price included excessive maternal sedation and neonatal respiratory depression.

Today, the usual dose for maternal analgesia is 2 to 5 mg intravenously or 5 to 10 mg intramuscularly. The onset of analgesia is within 3 to 5 minutes after intravenous administration and within 20 to 40 minutes after intramuscular administration. The peak effect is reached approximately 20 minutes after intravenous administration and 1 to 2 hours after intramuscular administration.[24]

Morphine is metabolized primarily by conjugation in the liver to morphine-3-glucuronide (M3G), which is the major metabolite and lacks analgesic effect. M3G is highly water soluble and is excreted by the kidneys.[25] If renal function is normal, 66% of the injected dose of morphine is cleared in the urine within 6 hours, and 90% is cleared within 24 hours.[26]

Morphine rapidly crosses the placenta. Gerdin et al.[27] demonstrated that the fetomaternal blood concentration ratio is 0.96 at 5 minutes, and it approaches 1.0 over time. Fetal effects depend on dose and gestational age. The more immature the fetal liver, the less effectively morphine is metabolized. In addition, morphine may more readily cross the blood-brain barrier of the immature fetus. As is the case with other opioids, maternal administration of morphine may result in decreased FHR variability; however, a consistent change in FHR unique to morphine has not been noted.

Olofsson et al.[28] assessed the analgesic efficacy of intravenous morphine during labor. They administered repeated doses of 0.05 mg/kg of intravenous morphine after every third contraction up to a limit of 0.2 mg/kg. The decrease in overall pain intensity—as assessed by a visual analogue scale—was clinically insignificant. However, the number of women who experienced back pain decreased significantly after morphine administration. The investigators suggested that systemically administered opioids do not effectively relieve the intermittent visceral pain that occurs during labor.

Gerdin et al.[25] found that morphine kinetics differed between pregnant and nonpregnant women. They noted a larger plasma clearance, a shorter elimination half-life, an earlier peak M3G plasma level, and a higher M3G/morphine ratio in parturients. The rapid maternal elimination of morphine decreased the period of fetal intrauterine exposure to the drug. They observed no cases of neonatal depression as judged by Apgar scores. Gerdin et al.[25,27] also suggested that the short maternal elimination half-life of morphine should prompt the reevaluation of morphine as an analgesic agent in obstetric patients on the basis of pharmacokinetic parameters.

Way et al.[29] gave intramuscular morphine (0.05 mg/kg) or meperidine (0.5 mg/kg) to a group of newborns. The infants who received morphine showed greater respiratory depression when response to CO_2 was measured. The researchers attributed the greater respiratory depression to a greater permeability of the neonatal brain to morphine. Currently morphine is administered infrequently during labor and vaginal delivery.

Fentanyl

Fentanyl (Sublimaze) is a highly lipid-soluble, highly protein-bound synthetic opioid with an analgesic potency 75 to 100 times that of morphine and 800 times that of meperidine. Interest in its use for obstetric analgesia/anesthesia developed because of its rapid onset, short duration of action, and lack of active metabolites. Large doses of fentanyl may result in accumulation of drug. With large doses, fentanyl does not behave as a short-acting drug.

Because of its lipid solubility, fentanyl crosses biologic membranes (e.g., the placenta) rapidly. Craft et al.[30] noted that the intravenous administration of fentanyl (50, 75, or 100 μg) did not affect maternal or fetal cardiovascular function, uterine tone, uterine blood flow, or maternal or fetal acid-base status in gravid ewes. Fentanyl was detected in fetal blood within 1 minute, and concentrations peaked at 5 minutes. Maternal concentrations remained 2.5 times those of the fetal concentrations from 5 to 60 minutes after drug injection.

Eisele et al.[31] gave fentanyl 1 μg/kg to pregnant women who received either regional or general anesthesia for cesarean section. Fentanyl resulted in improved maternal analgesia without appreciable hemodynamic changes. The average umbilical/maternal fentanyl concentration ratio was 0.31.

Administration of fentanyl did not affect Apgar scores, umbilical cord blood gas and pH measurements, or neurobehavioral scores at 4 and 24 hours.

Smith et al.[32] observed that intravenous fentanyl 50 μg had temporary depressant effects on fetal biophysical parameters. Breathing movements were abolished in all fentanyl-exposed fetuses ($n = 12$) at 10 minutes after fentanyl administration, but the fetal breathing movements returned to baseline by 20 minutes. A gradual decrease in the FHR baseline was also observed in the fentanyl group during the first 40 minutes after fentanyl administration. A reduction in beat-to-beat FHR variability was observed for 30 minutes in 8 of 12 fetuses exposed to fentanyl, and a sinusoidal FHR pattern was observed for 30 minutes in two fetuses. None of the FHR alterations persisted beyond 40 minutes. None of the changes in the fetal biophysical parameters resulted in any apparent effect on neonatal condition at delivery.[32]

Rayburn et al.[33] administered fentanyl in doses of 50 to 100 μg intravenously as often as every hour at maternal request during active labor. The cumulative doses ranged from 50 to 600 μg. All patients experienced transient analgesia (onset within 5 minutes and a duration of 45 minutes) and sedation. Administration of fentanyl resulted in a decrease in FHR variability that lasted 30 minutes. The authors performed neonatal assessment on both the infants exposed to fentanyl and a control group of infants not exposed to any analgesic drugs. They observed no difference between groups in Apgar scores, incidence of respiratory depression, neonatal vital signs, or Neurologic and Adaptive Capacity Scores at 2 to 4 hours and 24 hours after delivery. Of the total, 1 of 137 infants in the fentanyl group and 1 of 112 infants in the control group received naloxone.[33]

Rayburn et al.[34] also randomized 105 healthy pregnant women at term to receive either intravenous fentanyl (50 to 100 μg every hour) or meperidine (25 to 50 mg every 2 to 3 hours). This was a nonblinded study. The authors stated that "the analgesics were rated equivalent in efficacy." However the two drugs may have been similarly *ineffective*, given the fact that both groups had a mean pain score of 6/10 at 4 to 7 cm cervical dilation and 9/10 at 8 to 10 cm dilation. Maternal nausea, vomiting, and prolonged sedation occurred less frequently in the fentanyl group. Naloxone was administered to 1 of 49 infants in the fentanyl group versus seven of 56 infants in the meperidine group ($P < 0.05$). The two groups of infants had similar Neurologic and Adaptive Capacity Scores at 2 to 4 hours and 24 hours after delivery.

PATIENT-CONTROLLED ADMINISTRATION

Rayburn et al.[35] compared PCA fentanyl (10 μg/hour continuous infusion plus a 10 μg bolus with a 12-minute lockout) with nurse-administered fentanyl (50 μg loading dose plus 50 to 100 μg every hour as needed) for labor analgesia. Analgesia and sedation were equivalent in the two groups; however, both groups had incomplete pain relief during late labor. Neonatal outcomes were similar for the two groups as judged by Apgar scores, the need for naloxone, and neonatal neuroadaptive testing.

Morley-Forster and Weberpals[36] retrospectively reviewed the outcomes of 32 neonates whose mothers received PCA fentanyl during labor. Fourteen (44%) of the infants had a 1-minute Apgar score of less than 6. At 5 minutes, all had an Apgar score greater than 7 (except for three infants who had received naloxone). Gestational age, birth weight, method of delivery, PCA duration, time from last dose to delivery, and dose and rate of fentanyl infusion were not predictive of low 1-minute Apgar scores. However, the total dose of fentanyl received by the mothers of infants requiring naloxone was significantly higher than that of the mothers whose infants did not require naloxone (770 ± 233 μg versus 298 ± 287 μg). In summary, these authors noted a 44% incidence of "moderately depressed" neonates (i.e., Apgar scores of less than 6 at 1 minute) after exposure to PCA fentanyl. Prospective studies are needed to define the optimal use of PCA fentanyl during labor.

Nalbuphine

Nalbuphine (Nubain) is a mixed agonist/antagonist opioid analgesic. Nalbuphine and morphine result in similar respiratory depression at equianalgesic doses. However, nalbuphine demonstrates a ceiling effect for respiratory depression with increasing doses. Maximal respiratory depression occurs with a 30-mg dose in the average adult. Nalbuphine results in no further increase in respiratory depression with doses greater than 30 mg.

Nalbuphine is approximately 0.7 to 0.8 times as potent as morphine for the relief of acute pain.[37] The usual dose is 10 to 20 mg every 4 to 6 hours. The onset of analgesia occurs within 2 to 3 minutes of intravenous administration and within 15 minutes of intramuscular or subcutaneous administration. The duration of analgesia ranges from 3 to 6 hours.

Wilson et al.[38] evaluated the pharmacokinetics of nalbuphine during parturition. Intravenous administration of nalbuphine resulted in a fetal-maternal plasma concentration ratio that varied from 0.37 to 6.03, and the mean elimination half-life was approximately 2½ hours. Nonetheless, they observed no adverse neonatal effects. Wilson et al.[39] also performed a randomized, double-blind comparison of intramuscular nalbuphine 20 mg and meperidine 100 mg for labor analgesia. There was no difference between the two groups in the efficacy of analgesia. Nalbuphine was associated with less maternal nausea and vomiting than meperidine, but it tended to produce more maternal sedation and dizziness. The mean umbilical vein/maternal vein ratio of drug was higher for nalbuphine (0.78 ± 0.03) than for meperidine (0.61 ± 0.02). Neonatal neurobehavioral scores were lower in the nalbuphine group at 2 to 4 hours, but there was no significant difference between groups at 24 hours. The authors concluded that "nalbuphine does not offer a substantial improvement over pethidine for pain relief in labour."[39]

Nicolle et al.[40] evaluated the transplacental transfer and pharmacokinetics of nalbuphine in the neonate. They found that the fetal-maternal ratio was high (0.74) and that it did not correlate with the administered dose of nalbuphine. The estimated plasma half-life in the neonate was calculated at 4.1 hours. This half-life is longer than in adults and, more importantly, longer than that of naloxone administered intravenously. The investigators also noted a flattening of FHR variability in 54% of fetuses; this was seen 5 minutes after intravenous injection and 15 minutes after intramuscular injection of nalbuphine and lasted for 10 to 35 minutes after the administration of the drug. The changes did not correlate with maternal dose or cord blood nalbuphine concentrations. Analgesia in the same group of parturients was rated as effective in only 54% of patients (44% acceptable and 10% excellent). Relaxation but not pain relief was described by 43%. However, 78% of the same group of parturients were willing to have the same treatment in a subsequent labor.[40]

Giannina et al.[41] compared the effects of meperidine and nalbuphine on intrapartum FHR tracings. They found that nalbuphine significantly decreased the number of accelerations of 10 and 15 beats per minute and also the time spent in episodes of high variation, long-term variation, and short-term variation. Meperidine had no significant effect on any FHR characteristic.

Decreases in FHR variability, sinusoidal FHR patterns, fetal tachycardia, and fetal bradycardia have all been reported following the maternal administration of nalbuphine during labor. One case of severe fetal bradycardia after maternal nalbuphine administration did not resolve until naloxone was given intravenously to the mother.[42] Fetal acoustic stimulation response does not appear to be affected by low-dose nalbuphine (5 mg subcutaneously). This test may be useful as a means of evaluating fetal well-being in the presence of an altered FHR tracing after systemic opioid administration.[43]

PATIENT-CONTROLLED ADMINISTRATION

Frank et al.[44] compared PCA nalbuphine (3 mg intravenous bolus with a 10-minute lockout) with meperidine (15 mg intravenous bolus with a 10-minute lockout). Analgesia was better in the nalbuphine group. There was no difference in maternal sedation, maternal cardiorespiratory changes, or the progress of labor. There was no difference between the two groups of infants in Apgar scores, time to sustained respiration, or modified neurobehavioral assessment at 6 to 10 hours after delivery.[44]

Podlas and Breland[5] compared PCA nalbuphine (1 mg intravenous bolus with a 6- to 10-minute lockout) with nurse-administered nalbuphine (10 to 20 mg intravenously every 4 to 6 hours by request). Analgesia was judged satisfactory in both groups, but patients clearly preferred the PCA mode. Approximately 93% of women in the PCA group (but only 64% of women in the intermittent bolus group) reported that they would ask for this method of analgesia again. Apgar scores were similar between groups, and the interval between the last dose and delivery did not affect Apgar scores. No infant required the administration of naloxone.

Butorphanol

Butorphanol is an opioid with agonist-antagonist properties that resemble those of pentazocine. It is five times as potent as morphine and 40 times as potent as meperidine.[45,46] The typical dose during labor is 1 to 2 mg intravenously or intramuscularly. Butorphanol is 95% metabolized in the liver to inactive metabolites. Excretion is primarily renal, with a small contribution from the biliary system. Butorphanol and morphine result in similar respiratory depression at equianalgesic doses, but, as is the case with nalbuphine, a ceiling effect is noted with butorphanol. Butorphanol 2 mg produces respiratory depression similar to that which occurs with morphine 10 mg or meperidine 70 mg. However, butorphanol 4 mg results in less respiratory depression than morphine 20 mg or meperidine 140 mg.[45,46]

Atkinson et al.[47] compared butorphanol 1 to 2 mg with fentanyl 50 to 100 μg given intravenously as frequently as every 1 to 2 hours for labor analgesia. Both patients and nurses rated analgesia better with butorphanol than with fentanyl. The reduction in pain with butorphanol was more significant in the parous patients. Patients receiving fentanyl required more doses than patients in the butorphanol group. Likewise, more patients in the fentanyl group later received epidural anesthesia. There was no difference between groups in uterine activity, adverse maternal effects, or adverse fetal effects.[47]

Maduska and Hajghassemali[48] compared butorphanol (1 to 2 mg) with meperidine (40 to 80 mg) for labor analgesia. Butorphanol and meperidine resulted in analgesia of similar efficacy. They noted rapid placental transfer of butorphanol, with a mean umbilical vein/maternal vein concentration ratio of 0.84 at 1½ to 3½ hours after intramuscular injection. The authors observed no differences between groups in FHR during labor, Apgar scores, time to sustained respiration, and umbilical cord blood gas and acid-base measurements. Likewise, Hodgkinson et al.[49] performed a double-blind assessment of intravenous butorphanol (1 or 2 mg) and meperidine (40 or 80 mg) for labor analgesia. Both drugs provided adequate maternal pain relief, but there were fewer maternal side effects (e.g., nausea, vomiting, dizziness) in the butorphanol groups. There was no difference between groups in Apgar scores or neonatal neurobehavioral scores. Finally, Quilligan et al.[50] performed a double-blind comparison of intravenous butorphanol (1 or 2 mg) and meperidine (40 or 80 mg) during labor; they noted better analgesia at 30 minutes and 1 hour after the administration of butorphanol. There was no difference in Apgar scores between the two groups of infants.

Butorphanol offers excellent analgesia with some sedation, an effect that is similar to that of the combination of meperidine and a phenothiazine. It has a short half-life and inactive metabolites. These properties, combined with a ceiling effect on maternal respiratory depression and favorable neurobehavioral outcomes in the neonate, make butorphanol a useful agent for labor analgesia.

Pentazocine

Pentazocine (Talwin) has both agonist and weak antagonist properties. Pentazocine 30 to 60 mg is equipotent to morphine 10 mg. Peak analgesia occurs within 10 minutes after intravenous administration, and plasma levels peak at 15 to 60 minutes after intramuscular administration.[51] A ceiling effect for respiratory depression occurs at doses of 40 to 60 mg. Clinical studies have demonstrated that a single injection of meperidine 100 mg or pentazocine 40 to 45 mg produces similar degrees of neonatal respiratory depression. However, repeated maternal doses of pentazocine do not increase neonatal respiratory depression proportionally, whereas the respiratory depression with repeated doses of meperidine is cumulative.[52,53] Psychomimetic effects may occur with standard doses, but they occur more frequently after larger doses. The potential for psychomimetic side effects has limited the popularity of pentazocine in obstetrics.

Congeners of Fentanyl

SUFENTANIL

Sufentanil is a derivative of fentanyl with increased potency and lipophilicity. Although it has been widely used for both epidural and intrathecal analgesia during labor, its potency has limited its systemic use during labor. A 10 µg dose of sufentanil did not provide satisfactory analgesia when given intravenously or epidurally, but it was effective when administered intrathecally.[54]

ALFENTANIL

Alfentanil is another fentanyl derivative with a potency that is greater than morphine but less than fentanyl. Alfentanil is less lipophilic and more highly protein-bound than other opioids. Its limited volume of distribution results in a rapid onset and a short duration of action. Despite these benefits, alfentanil has been associated with a greater depression of neonatal neurobehavioral scores than meperidine.[55] Morley-Foster et al.[56] compared PCA fentanyl (20 µg bolus with a 5-minute lockout and a 20 µg/hr basal infusion) and PCA alfentanil (200 µg bolus with a 5-minute lockout and a 200 µg/hr basal infusion) in a group of laboring women in whom epidural analgesia was contraindicated. PCA fentanyl provided better pain relief during late labor than did PCA alfentanil. There was no difference between the two groups in the quality of analgesia during early labor, maternal side effects, or neonatal outcome. Despite its more rapid onset, "alfentanil did not prove as effective for PCA analgesia in labor as fentanyl."[56]

REMIFENTANIL

Remifentanil is an ultrashort-acting synthetic mu-opioid receptor agonist with a rapid onset of action (approximately 1 minute) after intravenous administration. It is rapidly metabolized by plasma and tissue esterases to an inactive metabolite, and this process is not dependent on renal or hepatic function. Unlike other opioids, the context-sensitive half-life is constant (3½ minutes), so the drug does not accumulate, even after prolonged administration. Kan et al.[57] evaluated the intravenous infusion of remifentanil during the administration of epidural anesthesia for cesarean section. They concluded that the transplacental transfer of remifentanil occurs rapidly, but the drug is redistributed and metabolized quickly in the fetus. In theory, remifentanil's rapid onset of action and lack of accumulation suggest that it might be an ideal choice for intravenous PCA during labor.

Most of the support for the administration of remifentanil during labor comes from reports of its use in parturients in whom lumbar epidural analgesia was contraindicated. Remifentanil has been administered by a pure PCA bolus mode and also via continuous basal infusion with supplemental PCA boluses. Some reports have described effective analgesia, whereas others have described ineffective analgesia. The efficacy of intravenous PCA is primarily dependent on the amount of the bolus dose. If the bolus is too small, the patient loses confidence in the technique; if it is too large, side effects are more likely to occur. A variety of doses and delivery regimens have been used in an attempt to find the best combination.

Volikas and Male[58] used a pure PCA technique, allowing remifentanil bolus doses of 0.5 µg/kg with a 5-minute lockout. They compared this regimen to PCA meperidine, using bolus doses of 10 mg with a 10-minute lockout. The authors observed significantly lower mean hourly and postpartum pain scores in the remifentanil group. However, the study was terminated after the enrollment of 17 subjects because of an unacceptably high number of low Apgar scores in the meperidine group. Low Apgar scores were not observed in the remifentanil group.

Volamanen et al.[59] determined the median effective PCA bolus dose of remifentanil to be 0.4 µg/kg, with a wide individual variation (0.2 to 0.8 µg/kg). These investigators described effective analgesia but noted mild maternal sedation in all 17 subjects, maternal oxygen desaturation (< 94%) in 10 of 17 women, and reduced beat-to-beat variability of the

FHR in 4 of 17 patients. The changes in FHR variability resolved within 15 minutes of discontinuing the remifentanil.

Olufolabi et al.[60] used PCA bolus doses from 0.25 µg/kg to a maximum of 0.5 µg/kg (with a 2-minute lockout) in four parturients. As labor progressed, the authors observed inadequate analgesia with significant opioid-related side effects. They concluded that remifentanil is an "unsuitable analgesic for labor." By contrast, Thurlow and Waterhouse[61] reported adequate analgesia with 20-µg PCA bolus doses of intravenous remifentanil (with a 2-minute lockout) in two parturients.

Roelants et al.[62] utilized a continuous basal infusion of 0.05 µg/kg/min with supplemental bolus doses of 25 µg with a 5-minute lockout. All patients remained alert or easily arousable and were satisfied with their analgesia. Others have used a basal infusion with bolus doses between 0.2 µg/kg and 1.0 µg/kg. However, at the higher doses, both supplemental oxygen and treatment for nausea have been needed. One case report described a 34-hour intravenous remifentanil infusion for labor that was initiated at a dose of 0.05 µg/kg/min; as labor progressed, the infusion dose was increased to 0.15 to 0.2 µg/kg/min.[63] The infusion was continued through spontaneous delivery and episiotomy repair. The infant (delivered at 33 weeks' gestation) had Apgar scores of 5 and 7 at 1 and 5 minutes, respectively. Deep variable FHR decelerations were noted before delivery, and a nuchal cord was present at delivery. Naloxone was not required by the infant after brief nasopharyngeal suctioning and positive-pressure ventilation. The neonatal depression at delivery may or may not have been related to the remifentanil, because there were other confounding factors at delivery.[63]

In summary, remifentanil has been used for intravenous labor analgesia most effectively in the bolus PCA or continuous infusion with bolus PCA mode. Potential advantages include better titration of analgesia and better neonatal outcome as compared with other opioids. There is huge interindividual variation in the dose required, and dose requirements increase as labor progresses. The best dose and/or dosing regimen remains undetermined. Potential disadvantages include maternal sedation and oxygen desaturation. These patients need to be constantly monitored. Supplemental oxygen easily corrects the oxygen desaturation but will not correct the underlying decrease in respiratory rate with the corresponding increase in Pa_{CO_2}. Although remifentanil is rapidly metabolized and/or redistributed by the fetus, it may be preferable to discontinue remifentanil 15 minutes before delivery to minimize the incidence of newborn respiratory depression. Remifentanil has been used effectively as a method of managing labor pain in patients in whom epidural analgesia has been considered to be contraindicated. Additional controlled studies of large numbers of patients are needed to determine if it is a suitable method of pain management for healthy patients undergoing uncomplicated labor and delivery.

OPIOID ANTAGONISTS

Naloxone (Narcan) is the opioid antagonist of choice to reverse the neonatal effects of maternal opioid administration. There is no neonatal benefit to the maternal administration of naloxone during labor or just before delivery. This practice antagonizes maternal analgesia during labor or at delivery without causing a decrease in opioid-related maternal side effects[64]; at best, it provides uncertain and/or incomplete reversal of the depressive effects on the neonate. When maternal administration of an opioid is anticipated to result in neonatal respiratory depression, it is best to administer naloxone directly to the newborn. Naloxone reverses opioid depression of newborn minute ventilation and increases the slope of the CO_2-response curve in infants affected by the maternal administration of an opioid.[65] Naloxone may precipitate a withdrawal reaction in the newborn of the opioid-dependent mother. The recommended dose is 0.1 mg/kg of a 1 mg/mL or 0.4 mg/mL solution. Naloxone should be given intravenously or intratracheally, if possible. It may also be given intramuscularly or subcutaneously; however, absorption of the agent may be delayed and unpredictable in the infant who is stressed and vasoconstricted.[66]

NONSTEROIDAL ANTIINFLAMMATORY DRUGS

Ketorolac is a prostaglandin synthetase inhibitor that is most often administered for postoperative analgesia. In theory, it may suppress uterine contractions, and it may cross the placenta and cause closure of the fetal ductus arteriosus. There are few data about the administration of ketorolac during labor. Walker et al.[67] gave ketorolac 10 mg intramuscularly to 31 women during labor, and they subsequently measured maternal and cord blood concentrations of the drug. They observed that the cord blood concentration was typically between 10% and 20% of the concentration in maternal blood. Subsequently, Walker et al.[68] randomized 128 women to receive either ketorolac 10 mg, meperidine 50 mg, or meperidine 100 mg intramuscularly during labor. Patients who received ketorolac had the highest pain scores, although the authors noted that all three treatments were "relatively ineffective in relieving labour pain." Women who received ketorolac had less sedation than women who received meperidine. In addition, infants exposed to ketorolac had higher 1-minute Apgar scores than infants exposed to meperidine. There was no significant difference between groups in the duration of labor. The authors suggested that prostaglandin synthetase inhibitors "may have a subsidiary role in the management of labour pain." More published data regarding the efficacy and safety of ketorolac in pregnant women are needed.

BARBITURATES

During very early labor, anxiety may be managed with either intramuscular or oral barbiturates. The most commonly used barbiturates for this indication are pentobarbital (Nembutal) 100 to 200 mg orally or intramuscularly and secobarbital (Seconal) 100 mg orally or intramuscularly (Table 20-3). Because the primary effect of barbiturates is sedation, their use is limited to the treatment of anxiety. A dose of barbiturate may provide a welcomed night's sleep in a patient with prodromal labor. The maximum sedative effect typically occurs approximately 1 hour after oral administration and 30 minutes after intramuscular administration. Barbiturates have no analgesic effect when given alone, and they may have an antianalgesic effect when given without an opioid in the presence of pain. These doses of pentobarbital and secobarbital have minimal effects on maternal ventilation and uterine tone.[69]

All barbiturates are lipid soluble and readily cross the placenta, and they are measurable in the fetal blood soon after administration to the mother. When administration is limited to early labor, a single dose of barbiturate rarely results in

TABLE 20-3   SEDATIVES AND NONOPIOID ADJUNCTS USED FOR LABOR

Class	Drug	Usual dose	Onset	Duration	Comments
Barbiturates	Pentobarbital (Nembutal)	100-200 mg PO/IM	30-60 min		Possible antianalgesic effect if used alone
	Secobarbital (Seconal)	100 mg PO/IM			Useful only in very early or latent phase labor
Phenothiazines	Promethazine (Phenergan)	25 mg IV/50 mg IM	20 min	4-5 hr	Possible contribution to maternal hypotension; antiemetic effect; wide use in combination with opioids
	Propiomazine (Largon)	20-40 mg IV/IM	15-30 min IV, 40-60 min IM	1-2 hr IV, 3-4 hr IM	Shorter onset and duration than promethazine; maternal hypotension; respiratory depression greater than with promethazine
Antihistamines	Hydroxyzine (Vistaril)	50 mg IM	30 min	4 hr	Used to prevent nausea and vomiting with opioids; painful on injection; no IV formulation
Benzodiazepines	Diazepam (Valium)	2-5 mg IV/10 mg IM	5 min	1-2 hr/3-4 hr	Used as treatment for eclamptic seizures; has an active metabolite; prolonged half-life in neonate; neonatal depression possibly prolonged; neonatal hypotonia and impaired thermogenesis; use in labor is rare
	Lorazepam (Ativan)	1-2 mg IV/2-4 mg IM	20-40 min	6-8 hr	Shorter elimination half-life but longer clinical effect; not used in obstetrics
	Midazolam (Versed)	1-2 mg IV in increments	3-5 min	1-2 hr	Water soluble; good amnesia; short half-life; not used for labor; primarily used as an adjunct after cesarean delivery
Dissociative	Ketamine (Ketalar)	10-20 mg IV in increments; up to 1 mg/kg over 30 min	30-60 sec	5 min	Psychomimetic effects with higher doses; not useful for first-stage labor; used just before delivery or as an adjunct to regional anesthesia; higher doses possibly lead to loss of consciousness and increased uterine tone

IM, Intramuscular; *IV,* intravenous; *PO,* oral.

neonatal depression. There is a greater likelihood of neonatal depression if the mother delivers shortly after the administration of a barbiturate or if the mother receives both a barbiturate and a systemic analgesic drug.[69]

PHENOTHIAZINES

Phenothiazines are often used in combination with opioids in obstetric patients. These drugs produce sedation and reduce nausea and vomiting. Some physicians contend that the phenothiazines potentiate the analgesic effects of opioids, but others argue that there is little objective evidence of potentiation.[70] Phenothiazines rapidly cross the placenta and may result in decreased beat-to-beat variability of the FHR. However, clinical doses of these drugs do not seem to cause

neonatal respiratory depression. Large studies that include neurobehavioral assessment are lacking.

Some phenothiazines (e.g., chlorpromazine, promazine, prochlorperazine) are rarely used in obstetrics, because they cause substantial alpha-adrenergic receptor blockade, which may cause maternal hypotension.[71]

Promethazine

Promethazine (Phenergan) is one of the most commonly used phenothiazines. When given intravenously in a dose of 25 to 50 mg, it has a rapid onset and produces effective sedation, with few side effects (Table 20-3). Promethazine is a mild respiratory stimulant; it results in a modest increase in the minute volume of ventilation and the ventilatory response to

CO_2. This may counteract the respiratory depressant action of meperidine but by a mechanism that does not involve opioid receptors. Promethazine appears in the fetal blood within 1 to 2 minutes of maternal intravenous administration, and it reaches equilibrium in 15 minutes.[71]

Propiomazine

Unlike promethazine, propiomazine (Largon) is a mild respiratory depressant in adults. The ventilatory response to a CO_2 challenge is depressed after propiomazine alone; this effect is additive to the respiratory depression caused by the administration of an opioid. However, propiomazine results in little if any neonatal respiratory depression.[72] Powe et al.[73] showed that propiomazine and promethazine provided similar maternal sedation and similar potentiation of meperidine analgesia. Another study noted that the administration of propiomazine 20 mg with meperidine 50 mg resulted in more effective analgesia and sedation than did meperidine alone and that 97% of the infants had an Apgar score of 7 or higher at 1 minute.[73] Propiomazine has a shorter onset and duration than promethazine (Table 20-3).[73,74]

HYDROXYZINE

Hydroxyzine (Vistaril) is an antihistamine agent; it is not a phenothiazine. Hydroxyzine is used to provide sedation and to prevent maternal nausea and vomiting, and it often is administered in combination with an opioid. The standard dose is 25 to 50 mg intramuscularly (Table 20-3). It is not administered intravenously, because intravenous administration is irritating to the veins and is associated with a high degree of thrombophlebitis. Intramuscular administration is also somewhat painful.

Some studies have suggested that the administration of both hydroxyzine and meperidine results in better analgesia and greater sedation than does the administration of meperidine alone. The administration of hydroxyzine does not seem to result in neonatal respiratory depression.[75]

SCOPOLAMINE

Scopolamine is an anticholinergic agent. In the distant past, it was widely used to provide sedation and amnesia in obstetric patients, and it was often given in combination with an opioid to produce "twilight sleep." Agitation and excitement were common side effects; these, in addition to amnesia, are undesirable effects during labor and vaginal delivery. Scopolamine rapidly crosses both the maternal blood-brain barrier and the placenta. It does not cause maternal or neonatal respiratory depression. Scopolamine increases the FHR and may decrease beat-to-beat FHR variability.[76] Maternal administration of physostigmine reverses the maternal sedation and the decreased FHR variability associated with scopolamine.[77,78]

METOCLOPRAMIDE

Metoclopramide often is administered to treat maternal nausea and vomiting and to accelerate gastric emptying before cesarean section. At least two studies have noted that metoclopramide may provide some analgesia during labor.[79,80] Vella et al.[79] observed that the administration of metoclopramide reduced requirements for nitrous oxide during labor. Similarly, women who received both meperidine and metoclopramide had slightly better pain scores than women who received meperidine alone. Administration of metoclopramide did not cause maternal sedation.[79] Rosenblatt et al.[80] observed that the administration of metoclopramide resulted in a decreased duration of labor, a decreased use of morphine, and lower pain scores as compared with the administration of saline-placebo in women undergoing prostaglandin-induced termination of pregnancy during the second trimester.

BENZODIAZEPINES

Benzodiazepines have been used for sedation in obstetric patients but have never achieved widespread use during labor because of significant side effects (Table 20-3). **Diazepam** (Valium) readily crosses the placenta and may accumulate in the fetus. The fetal concentration typically equals or exceeds the maternal concentration. Diazepam has a long elimination half-life of 24 to 48 hours, and its main metabolite (n-methyl-diazepam) is an active compound that is slightly less potent than diazepam, with an elimination half-life of 51 to 120 hours.[81]

Although diazepam may decrease systemic opioid requirements during labor, it is a costly gain. The administration of diazepam (with or without opioids) during labor has been associated with neonatal hypotonicity, hypoactivity, and respiratory depression.[82] Diazepam impairs neonatal temperature regulation and the neonatal response to metabolic stress.[83,84] Many of the neonatal effects may be dose related. When smaller doses (2.5 to 10 mg intravenously) were used in patients who received regional anesthesia for cesarean section, Rolbin et al.[85] found that small doses did not alter Apgar scores or umbilical cord blood gas and acid-base measurements. They observed decreased muscle tone at 4 hours but not 24 hours after delivery.

Lorazepam (Ativan) is another benzodiazepine that is an anticonvulsant, anxiolytic, and amnesic drug. Its half-life is 12 hours, but, in contrast with diazepam, its primary metabolite is a pharmacologically inactive glucuronide. McAuley et al.[86] gave lorazepam 2 mg or placebo during early labor in nulliparous women. Subsequently, they gave meperidine 100 mg as needed for analgesia. Analgesia was better in the lorazepam group. There was an increased incidence of respiratory depression in the lorazepam group, although this difference was not statistically significant. There was no significant difference between groups in neonatal neurobehavioral testing. Diminished recall of labor was more common in the lorazepam group.[86]

Midazolam (Versed) is a benzodiazepine with several advantages. It is water soluble, causes less pain with intravenous or intramuscular injection than diazepam, and has a rapid onset and a short duration of action, and its metabolites are inactive. There is little information about the use of midazolam as an adjunct to labor analgesia. Studies have evaluated the administration of midazolam before cesarean section and have noted that it rapidly crosses the placenta. The umbilical vein/maternal vein ratio is approximately 0.65, and the neonatal elimination half-life is 6.3 hours.[87] Neonates exposed to the higher doses required for the induction of general anesthesia showed a higher incidence of respiratory depression as well as decreased body tone and temperature as compared with infants exposed to thiopental.[88,89] Because midazolam is a potent amnesic, physicians must be aware of its potential to reduce maternal recall of labor and delivery[90]; most women want to remember the childbirth experience.

KETAMINE

Ketamine is a phencyclidine derivative. Small doses administered intravenously or intramuscularly provide a dissociative state of analgesia with or without amnesia; larger doses (e.g., 1 mg/kg) are used to induce general anesthesia. Ketamine is best avoided in the preeclamptic patient, because it causes sympathetic nervous system stimulation and may exacerbate hypertension; however, it is the induction agent of choice for patients with hypovolemia or asthma.

Ketamine produces a dose-related effect on uterine tone. With clinical doses, this effect is of little or no clinical significance. With larger doses (e.g., 1.5 to 2.0 mg/kg), uterine tone may increase by as much as 40%. Small doses of ketamine do not result in neonatal depression; high doses have been associated with low Apgar scores and abnormal neonatal muscle tone.[91]

Intravenous ketamine has a rapid onset of action (i.e., approximately 30 seconds) and a short duration of action (i.e., 3 to 5 minutes). Therefore, ketamine is not very useful for analgesia during the first stage of labor. However, ketamine may provide effective analgesia just before vaginal delivery. The anesthesiologist may administer a small (10 to 20 mg) dose of ketamine to a patient with no regional anesthesia or as an adjunctive agent to a patient with unsatisfactory regional anesthesia (Table 20-3). The dose may be repeated at intervals of 2 to 5 minutes. The total dose should not exceed 1 mg/kg during a 30-minute period. When it is used in this manner, ketamine results in a low incidence of maternal hallucinations; however, amnesia is common. The anesthesiologist must maintain continual verbal contact with the patient. It is critical that the patient remain awake and that she be able to protect her airway. (Editor's note: I am familiar with a case of maternal aspiration in a patient who received intravenous ketamine analgesia for vaginal delivery.)

INHALATION ANALGESIA

In the United States, the use of inhalation analgesia for labor and/or vaginal delivery is uncommon. Although many of the inhalation anesthetic agents used in surgery have been tried for pain relief during childbirth, only nitrous oxide remains in regular use. A recent survey from Ontario, Canada, noted that nitrous oxide analgesia was available in 75% of hospitals. Hospitals without the availability of epidural analgesia were more likely to have nitrous oxide analgesia than those with epidural analgesia (89% versus 70%).[2] In Great Britain, nitrous oxide (mixed 1:1 with oxygen) may be administered by unsupervised midwives in settings in which regional anesthesia is not available.

Nitrous Oxide

Intermittent inhalation of nitrous oxide can provide analgesia for labor, but it does not completely eliminate the pain of contractions. In recent years, the efficacy of Entonox (50% nitrous oxide with 50% oxygen) for labor analgesia has been questioned. Several studies of intrapartum analgesia have noted that 30% to 40% of mothers reported little or no benefit from Entonox.[92] Others argue that, when properly timed, inhalation of 50% nitrous oxide provides significant pain relief in as many as half of parturients.[93] To achieve substantial pain relief with nitrous oxide, maternal cooperation is required. There must be an analgesic concentration of nitrous oxide in the blood (and thus the brain) at the peak of the contraction. The patient is encouraged to breathe the mixture of 50% nitrous oxide in oxygen from the very beginning of the contraction and to continue until the end of the contraction. Nitrous oxide does not interfere with uterine activity.[94]

Suitable equipment must be available to provide safe and satisfactory inhalation analgesia with nitrous oxide. An apparatus that limits the concentration of nitrous oxide (e.g., a nitrous oxide/oxygen blender or a premixed 1:1 cylinder) is required, and it must be checked periodically to prevent the unintentional administration of a high concentration of nitrous oxide and a hypoxic concentration of gas. Inhalation may occur through a mask or a mouthpiece with a one-way valve to limit pollution of the labor suite with unscavenged gases.

Environmental pollution from the unscavenged nitrous oxide may be significant.[95] It is unclear whether occupational exposure to subanesthetic concentrations of nitrous oxide results in significant health risks for health care workers.[96,97]

Some physicians have expressed concern about the possibility of diffusion hypoxia after the administration of a nitrous oxide/oxygen mixture, which may lead to hypoxemia during labor. Carstoniu et al.[98] compared parturients breathing 50% nitrous oxide in oxygen (Nitronox) with a similar group of women breathing compressed air. The maternal SaO_2 measurements between contractions were slightly higher in the nitrous oxide/oxygen group than in the group breathing compressed air. Unfortunately, there was no difference between the two groups in mean pain scores. By contrast, other physicians have observed episodes of maternal hypoxemia with the use of nitrous oxide analgesia during labor.[99,100] Some studies have also suggested that the combined use of nitrous oxide and opioids increases the risk of maternal hypoxemia during labor.[101,102] Physicians, midwives, and nurses must be aware of the additive effects of inhalation agents and systemic opioids and/or sedatives leading to the increased potential for hypoxemia.

With the intermittent inhalation of nitrous oxide, accumulation over time is negligible, and the neonate eliminates most of the gas within minutes of birth, principally by means of the lungs.[103] Used in this way, nitrous oxide does not depress neonatal respiration or affect neonatal neurobehavior.[104] If neonatal respiratory depression occurs, the infant should be ventilated with 100% oxygen, which results in the rapid elimination of nitrous oxide.

Volatile Halogenated Agents

All volatile halogenated anesthetic agents cause a dose-related relaxation of uterine smooth muscle.[106] The extent of depression of uterine activity is directly proportional to the dose for each agent. Administration of 0.5 MAC of halothane, enflurane, or isoflurane significantly diminishes spontaneous uterine activity, but it does not affect the uterine smooth muscle response to oxytocin. Administration of a greater concentration of a volatile halogenated agent may decrease the uterine smooth muscle response to the administration of oxytocin.[106,107]

Abboud et al.[108] compared the administration of 0.25% to 1.25% **enflurane** in oxygen with the administration of 30% to 60% nitrous oxide in oxygen during the second stage of labor. Approximately 89% of the women in the enflurane group and 76% of the women in the nitrous oxide group rated their analgesia as satisfactory. Obstetricians rated the enflurane as more effective than the nitrous oxide. Four (7%) of the women in the enflurane group and five (10%) of the women in the nitrous oxide group experienced amnesia. Estimated blood loss was similar in the two groups. There was no difference between the two groups in the 1- and 5-minute Apgar scores. In addition, there was no significant difference between groups in umbilical cord blood gas and acid-base measurements.[108]

Subsequently, Abboud et al.[109] performed a similar study of **isoflurane**. Women in the isoflurane group received 0.2% to 0.7% of isoflurane in oxygen, and women in the nitrous oxide group received 30% to 60% nitrous oxide in oxygen. The authors noted that "isoflurane and nitrous oxide were given similarly high scores by mothers, anesthesiologists and obstetricians." Again, estimated blood loss was similar in the two groups. There was no significant difference between the two groups of infants in Apgar scores, umbilical cord blood gas and acid-base measurements, and neurobehavioral scores.[109]

Arora et al.[110] compared the administration of Entonox (50% nitrous oxide in oxygen) with the administration of a mixture of Entonox and 0.25% isoflurane for analgesia during the first stage of labor. As expected, the nitrous oxide/isoflurane mixture provided better pain relief than nitrous oxide alone. The women used these methods for variable intervals during labor, and some also received intramuscular diamorphine; these variables confounded the limited evaluation of the newborns. Wee et al.[111] also reported significantly improved pain relief with 0.2% isoflurane plus Entonox as compared with Entonox alone. No statistically significant difference in drowsiness was noted. Neonatal evaluation was limited to an assessment of Apgar scores, which did not differ between groups. Two other studies noted that the intermittent inhalation of isoflurane (0.75% in oxygen) and enflurane (1.0% in oxygen) provided better first-stage analgesia than 50% nitrous oxide in oxygen. In both studies, use of the volatile halogenated agent was associated with increased drowsiness.[112,113] Ross et al.[114] studied 221 women who used 0.25% isoflurane with Entonox. These patients self-administered the mixture while in labor after Entonox alone had become inadequate for pain relief. No mother became unduly sedated or lost consciousness while breathing the mixture, and there was no increase in the need for neonatal resuscitation except in babies whose mothers had also received an opioid.[114]

Desflurane is an inhalation agent that is notable for a rapid onset of and recovery from anesthesia. In addition, desflurane undergoes minimal metabolism. Swart et al.[115] randomized 60 healthy parturients to receive either 1.0% to 4.5% desflurane in oxygen or 30% to 60% nitrous oxide in oxygen during the second stage of labor. The authors stated that "desflurane and nitrous oxide received similar analgesia scores from mothers, anesthesiologists, and obstetricians," but they did not provide data regarding the efficacy of these two techniques. All newborns were vigorous at 5 minutes and had normal acid-base measurements; the two groups of infants also had similar neurobehavioral scores. Eight women in the desflurane group and one woman in the nitrous oxide group had amnesia for the delivery ($P < 0.05$).

Several problems limit the routine use of inhalational analgesia during labor: (1) the need for specialized vaporizers; (2) concern regarding pollution of the labor and delivery environment with waste anesthetic gases; (3) incomplete analgesia; (4) the potential for maternal amnesia; and (5) the potential for the loss of protective airway reflexes and pulmonary aspiration of gastric contents. This last problem is the greatest concern to some anesthesiologists, prompting them to ban inhalation analgesia during both the first and second stages of labor in their hospitals.

KEY POINTS

- All systemic analgesic drugs rapidly cross the placenta. These drugs may result in a transient decrease in the variability of the fetal heart rate.
- Both meperidine and its active metabolite normeperidine may cause neonatal respiratory and neurobehavioral depression.
- Physicians should not give naloxone to the mother to prevent neonatal respiratory depression. Rather, if the infant shows evidence of opioid-induced respiratory depression, naloxone should be given directly to the infant.
- Barbiturates are useful only for sedation during early, prodromal labor.
- Benzodiazepines have limited application for labor and vaginal delivery.
- Ketamine is not used for analgesia during the first stage of labor. Small doses of ketamine may provide analgesia for delivery in patients with no regional anesthesia or in patients with unsatisfactory regional anesthesia.
- Inhalation analgesia is infrequently used during the first stage of labor in the United States. Inhalation analgesia (e.g., 40% to 50% nitrous oxide in oxygen) may provide modest analgesia for delivery in patients with no regional anesthesia or as a supplement in patients with unsatisfactory regional anesthesia.
- The administration of inhalational analgesia places the anesthesiologist and the patient on a "slippery slope." A well-intentioned desire to provide effective analgesia places the patient at risk for loss of consciousness; however, during the administration of systemic analgesic drugs, it is imperative that the patient remain awake and retain her protective airway reflexes.

REFERENCES

1. Hawkins JL, Gibbs CP, Orleans M, et al. Obstetric anesthesia workforce survey, 1981 versus 1992. Anesthesiology 1997; 87:135-43.
2. Oyston J. Obstetrical anesthesia in Ontario. Can J Anaesth 1995; 45:1117-25.
3. Spielman FJ. Systemic analgesics during labor. Clin Obstet Gynecol 1987; 30:495-503.
4. Reynolds F, Sharma SK, Seed PT. Analgesia in labour and fetal acid-base balance: A meta-analysis comparing epidural with systemic opioid analgesia. BJOG 2002; 109:1344-53.
5. Podlas J, Breland BD. Patient-controlled analgesia with nalbuphine during labor. Obstet Gynecol 1987; 70:202-4.
6. McIntosh DG, Rayburn WF. Patient-controlled analgesia in obstetrics and gynecology. Obstet Gynecol 1991; 78:1129-35.
7. Rayburn W, Leuschen MP, Earl R, et al. Intravenous meperidine during labor: A randomized comparison between nursing and patient-controlled administration. Obstet Gynecol 1989; 74:702-4.

8. Bricker L, Lavender T. Parenteral opioids for labor pain relief: A systematic review. Am J Obstet Gynecol 2002; 186:S94-109.

9. Shnider SM, Way EL, Lord MJ. Rate of appearance and disappearance of meperidine in fetal blood after administration of narcotic to the mother (abstract). Anesthesiology 1966; 27:227-8.

10. Kuhnert BR, Kuhnert PM, Tu AL, et al. Meperidine and normeperidine levels following meperidine administration during labor. I. Mother. Am J Obstet Gynecol 1979; 133:904-13.

11. Caldwell J, Notarianni LJ. Disposition of pethidine in childbirth (letter). Br J Anaesth 1978; 50:307-8.

12. Caldwell J, Wakile LA, Notarianni LJ, et al. Maternal and neonatal disposition of pethidine in childbirth: A study using quantitative gas chromatography-mass spectrometry. Life Sci 1978; 22:589-96.

13. Shnider SM, Moya F. Effect of meperidine on the newborn infant. Am J Obstet Gynecol 1964; 89:1008-15.

14. Kuhnert BJ, Kuhnert PM, Philipson EH, Syracuse CD. Disposition of meperidine and normeperidine following multiple doses during labor. II. Fetus and neonate. Am J Obstet Gynecol 1985; 151:410-5.

15. Belfrage P, Boréus LO, Hartvig P, et al. Neonatal depression after obstetrical analgesia with pethidine: The role of the injection-delivery time interval and of the plasma concentrations of pethidine and norpethidine. Acta Obstet Gynecol Scand 1981; 60:43-9.

16. Stechler G. Newborn attention as affected by medication during labor. Science 1964; 144:315-7.

17. Hodgkinson R, Bhatt M, Wang CN. Double-blinded comparison of neurobehavior of neonates following the administration of different doses of meperidine to the mother. Can Anaesth Soc J 1978; 25:405-11.

18. Belsey EM, Rosenblatt DB, Lieberman BA, et al. The influence of maternal analgesia in neonatal behaviour. I. Pethidine. Br J Obstet Gynaecol 1981; 88:398-406.

19. Kuhnert BR, Linn PL, Kennard MJ, et al. Effects of low doses of meperidine on neonatal behavior. Anesth Analg 1985; 63:301-8.

20. Nissen E, Widstrom AM, Matthiesen AS, et al. Effects of routinely given pethidine during labour on infants' developing breastfeeding behaviors. Effects of dose-delivery time interval and various concentrations of pethidine/norpethidine in cord plasma. Acta Paediatr 1997; 86:210-8.

21. Kariniemi V, Pirkko A. Effects of intramuscular pethidine on fetal heart rate variability. Br J Obstet Gynaecol 1981; 88:718-20.

22. Petrie RH, Yeh SY, Murata Y, et al. The effects of drugs on fetal heart rate variability. Am J Obstet Gynecol 1978; 130:294-9.

23. Erskine WA, Dick A, Morrell DF, et al. Self-administered intravenous analgesia during labour: A comparison between pentazocine and pethidine. S Afr Med J 1985; 87:764-7.

24. Stoelting RK. Opioid agonists and antagonists. In: Stoelting RK. Pharmacology and Physiology in Anesthetic Practice. 2nd ed. Philadelphia, JB Lippincott, 1991:74-82.

25. Gerdin A, Salmonson T, Lindberg B, Rane A. Maternal kinetics of morphine during labor. J Perinat Med 1990; 18:479-87.

26. Brunk FS, Delle M. Morphine metabolism in man. Clin Pharmacol Ther 1974; 16:51.

27. Gerdin E, Rane A, Lindberg B. Transplacental transfer of morphine in man. J Perinat Med 1990; 18:305

28. Olofsson C, Ekblom A, Ekman-Ordeberg G, et al. Analgesic efficacy of intravenous morphine in labour pain: A reappraisal. Int J Obstet Anesth 1996; 5:176-80.

29. Way WL, Costley EC, Way EL. Respiratory sensitivity of the newborn infant to meperidine and morphine. Clin Pharm Ther 1965; 6:454-61.

30. Craft JB, Coaldrake LA, Bolan JC, et al. Placental passage and uterine effects of fentanyl. Anesth Analg 1983; 62:894-8.

31. Eisele JH, Wright R, Rogge P. Newborn and maternal fentanyl levels at cesarean section. Anesth Analg 1982; 61:179-80.

32. Smith CV, Rayburn WF, Allen KV, et al. Influence of intravenous fentanyl on fetal biophysical parameters during labor. J Matern Fetal Med 1996; 5:89-92.

33. Rayburn W, Rathke A, Leuschen P, et al. Fentanyl citrate analgesia during labor. Am J Obstet Gynecol 1989; 161:202-6.

34. Rayburn WF, Smith CV, Parriott JE, Woods RE. Randomized comparison of meperidine and fentanyl during labor. Obstet Gynecol 1989; 74:604-6.

35. Rayburn WF, Smith CV, Leuschen MP, et al. Comparison of patient-controlled and nurse-administered analgesia using intravenous fentanyl during labor. Anesth Rev 1991; 18:31-6.

36. Morley-Forster PK, Weberpals J. Neonatal effects of patient-controlled analgesia using fentanyl in labor. Int J Obstet Anesth 1998; 7:103-7.

37. Fahmy NR. Agonist/antagonist opioid analgesics: Nalbuphine hydrochloride. In: Estafanous FG, editor. Opioids in Anesthesia. London, Butterworth, 1984:20-7.

38. Wilson SJ, Errick JK, Balkon J. Pharmacokinetics of nalbuphine during parturition. Am J Obstet Gynecol 1986; 155:340-4.

39. Wilson CM, McClean E, Moore J, Dundee JW. A double-blind comparison of intramuscular pethidine and nalbuphine in labour. Anaesthesia 1986; 41:1207-13.

40. Nicolle E, Devillier P, Delanoy B, et al. Therapeutic monitoring of nalbuphine: Transplacental transfer and estimated pharmacokinetics in the neonate. Eur J Clin Pharmacol 1996; 49:485-9.

41. Giannina G, Guzman ER, Yu-Ling L, et al. Comparison of the effects of meperidine and nalbuphine on intrapartum fetal heart rate tracings. Obstet Gynecol 1995; 86:441-5.

42. Roumen FJME, Aardenburg R, da Costa AJ, Maertzdorf WJ. Fetal bradycardia following administration of nalbuphine during labor. J Matern Fetal Med 1994; 3:27-30.

43. Poehlmann S, Stubblefield P, Pinette M. Effect of labor analgesia with nalbuphine hydrochloride on fetal response to vibroacoustic stimulation. J Reprod Med 1995; 40:707-10.

44. Frank M, McAteer EJ, Cattermole R, et al. Nalbuphine for obstetric analgesia: A comparison of nalbuphine with pethidine for pain relief in labour when administered by patient-controlled analgesia. Anaesthesia 1987; 42:697-703.

45. Nagashima H, Karamanian A, Malovany R, et al. Respiratory and circulatory effects of intravenous butorphanol and morphine. Clin Pharm Ther 1976; 19:738-45.

46. Kallos T, Caruso FS. Respiratory effects of butorphanol and pethidine. Anaesthesia 1979; 34:633-7.

47. Atkinson BD, Truitt LJ, Rayburn WF, et al. Double-blind comparison of intravenous butorphanol (Stadol) and fentanyl (Sublimaze) for analgesia during labor. Am J Obstet Gynecol 1994; 171:993-8.

48. Maduska AL, Hajghassemali M. A double-blind comparison of butorphanol and meperidine in labour: Maternal pain relief and effects on the newborn. Can Anaesth Soc J 1978; 25:398-404.

49. Hodgkinson R, Huff RW, Hayashi RH, Hussain FJ. Double-blind comparison of maternal analgesia and neonatal neurobehavior following intravenous butorphanol and meperidine. J Int Med Res 1979; 7:224-30.

50. Quilligan EJ, Keegan KA, Donahue MJ. Double-blind comparison of intravenously injected butorphanol and meperidine in parturients. Int J Gynaecol Obstet 1980; 18:363-7.

51. Jaffe JH, Martin WR. Opioids with mixed actions: Partial agonists. In: Gilman AG, Rall TW, Nies AS, Taylor P, editors. The Pharmacological Basis of Therapeutics. 8th ed. New York, Pergamon Press, 1990:512-4.

52. Moore J, Ball HG. A sequential study of intravenous analgesic treatment during labour. Br J Anaesth 1974; 46:365-72.

53. Refstad SO, Lindbaek E. Ventilatory depression of the newborn of women receiving pethidine or pentazocine. Br J Anaesth 1980; 52:265-71.

54. Camann WR, Denney RA, Holby ED, Datta S. A comparison of intrathecal, epidural, and intravenous sufentanil for labor analgesia. Anesthesiology 1992; 77:884-7.

55. Shannon KT, Ramanathan S. Systemic medication for labor analgesia. Obstet Pain Manage 1995; 2:1-6.

56. Morley-Foster PK, Reid DW, Vandeberghe H. A comparison of patient-controlled analgesia fentanyl and alfentanil for labor analgesia. Can J Anaesth 2000; 47:113-9.

57. Kan RE, Hughes SC, Rosen MA, et al. Intravenous remifentanil: Placental transfer, maternal and neonatal effects. Anesthesiology 1998; 88:1467-74.

58. Volikas I, Male D. A comparison of pethidine and remifentanil patient-controlled analgesia for labour. Int J Obstet Anesth 2001; 10:86-90.

59. Volamanen P, Akural EI, Raudaskoski T, et al. Remifentanil in obstetric analgesia: A dose finding study. Anesth Analg 2002; 94:913-7.

60. Olufolabi AJ, Booth JV, Wakeling HG, et al. A preliminary investigation of remifentanil as a labor analgesic. Anesth Analg 2000; 91:606-8.

61. Thurlow JA, Waterhouse P. Patient-controlled analgesia in labour using remifentanil in two parturients with platelet abnormalities. Br J Anaesth 2000; 84:411-3.

62. Roelants F, De Franceschi E, Veyckemans F, et al. Patient-controlled intravenous analgesia using remifentanil in the parturient. Can J Anaesth 2001; 48:175-8.

63. Owen MD, Poss MJ, Dean LS, et al. Prolonged intravenous remifentanil infusion for labor analgesia. Anesth Analg 2002; 94:918-9.

64. Girvan CB, Moore J, Dundee JW. Pethidine compared with pethidine-naloxone administered during labor. Br J Anaesth 1976; 48:563-9.

65. Gerhardt T, Bancalari E, Cohen H, Rocha LF. Use of naloxone to reverse narcotic respiratory depression in the newborn infant. J Pediatr 1977; 90:1009-12.

66. American Heart Association and American Academy of Pediatrics. Textbook of Neonatal Resuscitation. Kattwinkel J, Niermeyer S, Denson S, Zaichkin J, and AHA/AAP Neonatal Resuscitation Program Steering Committee, editors. 2000:7-3.

67. Walker JJ, Johnstone J, Lloyd J, et al. The transfer of ketorolac tromethamine from maternal to foetal blood. Eur J Clin Pharmacol 1988; 34:509-11.

68. Walker JJ, Johnston J, Fairlie FM, et al. A comparative study of intramuscular ketorolac and pethidine in labour pain. Eur J Obstet Gynecol Reprod Biol 1992; 46:87-94.

69. McDonald JS. Preanesthetic and intrapartal medications. Clin Obstet Gynecol 1977; 20:447-59.

70. McQuitty FM. Relief of pain in labour: A controlled double-blind trial comparing pethidine and various phenothiazine derivatives. J Obstet Gynaecol Br Commonw 1967; 74:925-8.

71. Clark RB, Seifen AB. Systemic medication during labor and delivery. Obstet Gynecol Annu 1983; 12:165-97.

72. Eisenstein JI, Rubin EJ, Arnold M, et al. Propiomazine hydrochloride in obstetrics. Am J Obstet Gynecol 1964; 88:606-11.

73. Powe CE, Kien IM, Fromhagen C, et al. Propiomazine hydrochloride in obstetrical analgesia. JAMA 1962; 181:290-4.

74. Ullery JC, Bair JR. Maternal-fetal effects of propiomazine-meperidine analgesia. Am J Obstet Gynecol 1962; 84:1051-6.

75. Zsigmond EK, Patterson RI. Double-blind evaluation of hydroxyzine hydrochloride in obstetric anesthesia. Anesth Analg 1967; 46:275-80.

76. Boehm FH, Growdon JH. The effect of scopolamine on fetal heart rate baseline variability. Am J Obstet Gynecol 1974; 120:1099-104.

77. Boehm FH, Ehilmez A, Smith BE. Physostigmine's effect on diminished fetal heart rate variability caused by scopolamine, meperidine and propiomazine. J Perinat Med 1977; 5:214-22.

78. Smith DB, Clark RB, Stephens SR, et al. Physostigmine reversal of sedation in parturients. Anesth Analg 1976; 55:478-80.

79. Vella L, Francis D, Houlton P, Reynolds F. Comparison of the antiemetics metoclopramide and promethazine in labour. BMJ 1985; 290:1173-5.

80. Rosenblatt WH, Cioffi AM, Sinatra R, Silverman DG. Metoclopramide-enhanced analgesia for prostaglandin-induced termination of pregnancy. Anesth Analg 1992; 75:760-3.

81. Mandelli M, Tognoni G, Garatini S. Clinical pharmacokinetics of diazepam. Clin Pharmacokinet 1978; 3:72-91.

82. McAllister CB. Placental transfer and neonatal effects of diazepam when administered to women just before delivery. Br J Anaesth 1980; 52:423-7.

83. Cree JE, Meyer J, Hailey DM. Diazepam in labour: Its metabolism and effect on the clinical condition and thermogenesis of the newborn. BMJ 1973; 4:251-5.

84. Owen JR, Irani SF, Blair AW. Effect of diazepam administered to mothers during labour on temperature regulation of the neonate. Arch Dis Child 1972; 47:107-10.

85. Rolbin SH, Wright RG, Shnider SM, et al. Diazepam during cesarean section: Effects on neonatal Apgar scores, acid-base status, neurobehavioral assessment, and maternal and fetal plasma norepinephrine levels. Abstracts of Scientific Papers, Annual Meeting, American Society of Anesthesiologists, New Orleans, 1977:449.

86. McAuley DM, O'Neill MP, Moore J, Dundee JW. Lorazepam premedication for labour. Br J Obstet Gynecol 1982; 89:149-54.

87. Bach V, Carl P, Ravlo O, et al. A randomized comparison between midazolam and thiopental for elective cesarean section anesthesia. III. Placental transfer and elimination in neonates. Anesth Analg 1989; 68:238-42.

88. Bland BAR, Lawes EG, Duncan PW, et al. Comparison of midazolam and thiopental for rapid sequence anesthetic induction for elective cesarean section. Anesth Analg 1987; 66:1165-8.

89. Ravlo O, Carl P, Crawford ME, et al. A randomized comparison between midazolam and thiopental for elective cesarean section anesthesia. II. Neonates. Anesth Analg 1989; 68:234-7.

90. Seidman SF, Marx GF. Midazolam in obstetric anesthesia. Anesthesiology 1987; 67:443-4.

91. Akamatsu TJ, Bonica JJ, Rehmet R, et al. Experiences with the use of ketamine for parturition. I. Primary anesthesia for vaginal delivery. Anesth Analg 1974; 53:284-7.

92. Yentis SM. The use of Entonox® for labour pain should be abandoned. Int J Obstet Anesth 2001: 10:25-28.

93. Rosen M. Recent advances in pain relief in childbirth: Inhalation and systemic analgesia. Br J Anaesth 1971; 43:837-48.

94. Marx GF, Katsnelson T. The introduction of nitrous oxide into obstetrics. Obstet Gynecol 1992; 80:715-8.

95. Mills GH, Singh D, Longan M, et al. Nitrous oxide exposure on the labour ward. Int J Obstet Anesth 1996; 5:160-4.

96. Bernow J, Bjordal J, Wiklund KE. Pollution of delivery ward air by nitrous oxide: Effects of various modes of room ventilation, excess and close scavenging. Acta Anaesthesiol Scand 1984; 28:119-23.

97. Munley AJ, Railton R, Gray WM, Carter KB. Exposure of midwives to nitrous oxide in four hospitals. BMJ 1986; 293:1063-4.

98. Carstoniu J, Levytam S, Norman P, et al. Nitrous oxide in labour: Safety and efficacy assessed by a double-blind placebo controlled study. Anesthesiology 1994; 80:30-5.

99. Lin DM, Reisner LS, Benumof J. Hypoxemia occurs intermittently and significantly with nitrous oxide labor analgesia (abstract). Anesth Analg 1989; 68:S167.

100. Lucas DN, Siemaszko O, Yentis SM. Maternal hypoxemia associated with the use of Entonox in labour. Int J Obstet Anesth 2000; 9:270-2.

101. Deckart R, Fembacher PM, Schneider KTM, Graeff H. Maternal arterial oxygen saturation during labor and delivery: Pain dependent alteration and effects on the newborn. Obstet Gynecol 1987; 70:21-5.

102. Irestadt L. Current status for nitrous oxide for obstetric pain relief. Acta Anesthesiol Scand 1994; 38:711-2.

103. Brownridge P. Treatment options for the relief of pain during childbirth. Drugs 1991; 41:69-80.

104. Stefani SJ, Hughes SC, Shnider SM, et al. Neonatal neurobehavioral effects of inhalation analgesia for vaginal delivery. Anesthesiology 1982; 56:351-5.

105. Munson ES, Embro WJ. Enflurane, isoflurane, and halothane and isolated human uterine muscle. Anesthesiology 1977; 46:11-4.

106. Marx GF, Kim YO, Lin CC, et al. Postpartum uterine pressures under halothane or enflurane anesthesia. Obstet Gynecol 1978; 51:695-8.

107. Abadir AR, Humayen SG, Calvello D, Gintautas J. Effects of isoflurane and oxytocin on gravid human uterus in vitro (abstract). Anesth Analg 1987; 66:S1.

108. Abboud TK, Shnider SM, Wright RG, et al. Enflurane analgesia in obstetrics. Anesth Analg 1981; 60:133-7.

109. Abboud TK, Gangolly J, Mosaad P, Crowell D. Isoflurane in obstetrics. Anesth Analg 1989; 68:388-91.

110. Arora S, Turnstall M, Ross J. Self-administered mixture of Entonox and isoflurane in labour. Int J Obstet Anesth 1992; 1:199-202.

111. Wee MYK, Hasan MA, Thomas TA. Isoflurane in labor. Anaesthesia 1993; 48:369-72.

112. McLeod DD, Ramayya GP, Turnstall ME. Self-administered isoflurane in labour. Anaesthesia 1985; 40:424-6.

113. McGuiness C, Rosen M. Enflurane as an analgesic in labour. Anaesthesia 1984; 39:24-6.

114. Ross JA, Tunstall ME, Campbell DM, et al. The use of 0.25% isoflurane premixed in 50% nitrous oxide and oxygen for pain relief in labour. Anaesthesia 1999; 54:1166-72.

115. Swart F, Abboud TK, Zhu J, et al. Desflurane analgesia in obstetrics: Maternal and neonatal effects (abstract). Anesthesiology 1991; 75:A844.

Chapter 21
Epidural and Spinal Analgesia/Anesthesia

I. LOCAL ANESTHETIC TECHNIQUES

Linda S. Polley, M.D. · Beth Glosten, M.D.

Epidural and spinal analgesia are the most effective methods of intrapartum pain relief in current clinical practice.[1-4] During the first stage of labor, pain results primarily from uterine contractions and cervical dilation. Painful impulses are transmitted by means of visceral afferent nerve fibers, which travel with sympathetic nerve fibers and enter the spinal cord at the tenth, eleventh, and twelfth thoracic and first lumbar spinal segments. During the first stage of labor, segmental lumbar epidural analgesia can be tailored to block the pain that results from uterine contractions and cervical dilation. Extension of epidural analgesia to include the distribution of the pudendal nerve (i.e., the second, third, and fourth sacral segments) alleviates the pain caused by the distention of the vagina and perineum during the second stage of labor.

Epidural analgesia provides complete analgesia in the majority of laboring women.[3,5] In a survey of 1000 consecutive patients who chose a variety of analgesic techniques for labor and vaginal delivery (including nonpharmacologic methods, transcutaneous electrical nerve stimulation, intramuscular meperidine, inhalation of nitrous oxide, epidural analgesia, and a combination of these techniques), pain relief and overall satisfaction with the birth experience were greater in patients who received epidural analgesia.[4] Similarly, randomized studies that have compared epidural analgesia with systemic opioids and/or inhalation analgesia (i.e., nitrous oxide) have shown that pain scores are lower and patients are more satisfied with epidural analgesia.[3,6-9]

The provision of analgesia for labor may result in other benefits. Effective epidural analgesia reduces maternal plasma concentrations of catecholamines (Figure 21-1).[10] Decreased alpha- and beta-adrenergic receptor stimulation may result in improved uteroplacental perfusion and more effective uterine activity.[11,12]

Painful uterine contractions result in maternal hyperventilation,[13] which causes maternal respiratory alkalosis, a leftward shift of the oxyhemoglobin dissociation curve, increased maternal hemoglobin oxygen affinity, and reduced oxygen

delivery to the fetus (Figure 21-2).[14] Hypocarbia also leads to hypoventilation between contractions, which can cause a decrease in maternal Pa_{O_2}. Effective epidural analgesia blunts this "hyperventilation-hypoventilation cycle."[15]

Epidural analgesia is not used by all laboring women. Surveys of obstetric anesthesia practice in the United States reveal that the use of epidural analgesia has increased over the past two decades. In 1981, 16% of laboring women in the United States received epidural analgesia;[16] use was somewhat greater among hospitals delivering more than 1500 babies per year. In 1997, a majority of parturients in the United States chose to receive neuraxial (epidural, spinal, or combined spinal-epidural) analgesia.[17] In the United Kingdom, the epidural analgesia rate among laboring women is approximately 24%.[18] The availability of skilled anesthesia care providers influences the epidural analgesia rate.[19] Other factors include the information and advice provided to pregnant women by obstetricians, nurses, and childbirth education instructors. Obstetric complications,[4] as well as the personal and cultural expectations of a laboring woman, also have an impact on the patient's childbirth experience and the use of epidural analgesia (see Chapters 18 and 19). The optimum epidural analgesia rate is unknown.

In contemporary clinical practice, healthcare costs have assumed significant importance. A recent study estimated the expected cost to society of epidural analgesia for labor to be $259 to $338 greater than the expected cost of intravenous analgesia.[20] Another study concluded that the anesthesiologist's labor cost per patient receiving epidural analgesia was $325 with intermittent anesthesiologist staffing and $728 with 24-hour-a-day dedicated anesthesiologist staffing of Labor and Delivery.[21] A major problem of such analyses is the difficulty of determining the total value of epidural analgesia. The presence of an epidural catheter not only provides superior pain relief during labor, but it also can be used to facilitate the administration of epidural anesthesia for emergency cesarean section. Hawkins et al.[22] observed that the maternal case-fatality rate for general anesthesia was 16.7 times that for regional anesthesia among obstetric patients undergoing cesarean section in the United States for the years 1985 to 1990.

Ideally, the anesthesiologist should tailor the analgesic technique to meet the patient's individual needs. The risks and benefits of the various epidural and spinal analgesic techniques should be assessed for each patient. Good technique requires thoughtful preparation and meticulous attention to detail to ensure maternal and fetal safety.

EPIDURAL ANALGESIA/ANESTHESIA

Indications
Epidural analgesia is indicated to treat the pain experienced by a woman in labor. Controversy exists regarding when it is appropriate to begin epidural analgesia during labor in an individual patient. Some obstetricians contend that "early" epidural analgesia (e.g., before 5 cm cervical dilation) may interfere with uterine contractions and slow the progress of labor (see Section III of this chapter). The American College of Obstetricians and Gynecologists (ACOG) recently reaffirmed the earlier opinion published jointly with the American Society of Anesthesiologists (ASA). Namely, the ACOG and the ASA have stated that "in the absence of a medical contraindication, maternal request is a sufficient medical indication for pain relief during labor" and that "decisions regarding analgesia should be closely coordinated among the obstetrician, the anesthesiologist, the patient, and skilled support personnel."[23] We believe that epidural analgesia is an appropriate treatment for the pain of even early labor (defined as regular uterine contractions that cause progressive effacement and dilation of the uterine cervix); we do not require a minimum cervical dilation before the administration of epidural analgesia.[10,11,24,25] However, if a patient in early labor requests epidural analgesia, we may first administer either a spinal or epidural opioid alone or an epidural opioid combined with a very dilute solution of local anesthetic to avoid large cumulative doses of local anesthetic (see Section II of this chapter).

Epidural analgesia may facilitate an atraumatic vaginal breech delivery, the vaginal delivery of twin infants, and vaginal delivery of a preterm infant (see Chapters 34 and 35). By providing effective pain relief, epidural analgesia facilitates the control of blood pressure in preeclamptic women (see Chapter 44). Epidural analgesia also blunts the hemodynamic effects of uterine contractions (e.g., sudden increase in preload) and the associated pain response (tachycardia, increased systemic vascular resistance, hypertension, hyperventilation) in patients with other medical complications (e.g., mitral stenosis, spinal cord injury, intracranial neurovascular disease, asthma) (see Chapters 40, 48, and 51).

Contraindications
Box 21-1 lists the contraindications to epidural and spinal analgesia. Some anesthesiologists have suggested that the presence of systemic maternal infection or preexisting neurologic disease is a relative contraindication. However, most cases of systemic infection (especially if properly treated) or neurologic disease do not contraindicate the administration of epidural analgesia (see Chapters 36 and 48). It is also controversial whether mild or isolated abnormalities in tests of blood coagulation preclude the use of epidural analgesia (see Chapter 42). The anesthesiologist should consider the risks and benefits of epidural analgesia for each patient individually.

Preparation
The anesthesiologist should first perform a thorough preanesthetic evaluation and obtain informed consent (Boxes 21-2 and 21-3). The preanesthetic evaluation should include a review of maternal obstetric and medical conditions that may influence anesthetic management. A directed physical examination should include a baseline blood pressure measurement and an

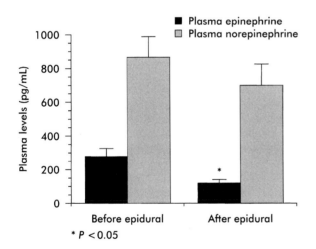

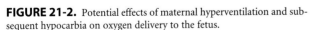

FIGURE 21-1. Influence of epidural analgesia on maternal plasma concentrations of catecholamines during labor. (Modified from Shnider SM, Abboud TK, Artal R, et al. Maternal catecholamines decrease during labor after lumbar epidural anesthesia. Am J Obstet Gynecol 1983; 147:13-5.)

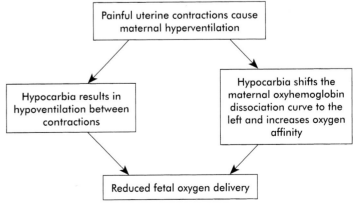

FIGURE 21-2. Potential effects of maternal hyperventilation and subsequent hypocarbia on oxygen delivery to the fetus.

assessment of the maternal airway and back. The preanesthetic evaluation also should include an assessment of the fetus (e.g., gestational age, fetal growth, fetal presentation, fetal well-being). Ideally, the anesthesiologist should consult with the obstetrician before the administration of epidural analgesia.

Informed consent should include a frank discussion about anesthetic procedures and risks. Although it may be best for this information to be transmitted before the onset of labor (e.g., during antenatal classes),[26] this is not always feasible. Some anesthesiologists fear that distressed, desperate, or sedated parturients may not understand the discussion of anesthetic procedures. However, adequacy of consent can be demonstrated not only by documentation of information provided to the patient but also by the lack of patient objection to a procedure and the cooperation provided by the patient during the procedure.[27] We do not find it difficult to explain the procedure and the risks of epidural analgesia to a laboring woman. The preanesthetic evaluation allows the physician to communicate a sense of concern and to demonstrate a commitment to the patient's care. Most laboring women understand the need for informed consent, and they appreciate the opportunity to participate in decisions regarding their care. Surveys of postpartum women have revealed that most parturients want to know the possible complications of epidural analgesia, even those that are rare but serious.[28,29]

Resuscitation equipment, drugs, and supplies must be immediately available for the management of a serious complication of epidural analgesia (e.g., hypotension, total spinal anesthesia, systemic local anesthetic toxicity) (Box 21-4).[30] Emergency airway equipment should be checked before the administration of epidural analgesia. We often administer supplemental oxygen during placement of the epidural catheter and during establishment of the epidural block. Our goals are to increase fetal oxygen content and increase fetal

---

Box 21-1 CONTRAINDICATIONS TO EPIDURAL AND SPINAL ANALGESIA

- Patient refusal or inability to cooperate
- Increased intracranial pressure secondary to a mass lesion
- Skin or soft tissue infection at the site of needle placement
- Frank coagulopathy
- Uncorrected maternal hypovolemia (e.g., hemorrhage)
- Inadequate training in or experience with the technique

Box 21-2 CHECKLIST BEFORE THE PLACEMENT OF AN EPIDURAL CATHETER AND THE ADMINISTRATION OF EPIDURAL ANALGESIA

1. The patient requests epidural analgesia for pain relief (or for relief of anticipated pain, as in cases of the planned induction of labor).
2. A preanesthetic evaluation is performed, which includes an assessment of the patient's medical and anesthetic history.
3. The risks of epidural analgesia are discussed with the patient, and informed consent is obtained.
4. The obstetrician is consulted to confirm the following:
   - That the patient is in labor and the obstetrician is committed to delivering the infant; and
   - That all relevant obstetric issues are understood (e.g., gestational age, intrauterine growth restriction, fetal presentation, risk of obstetric hemorrhage, previous cesarean delivery).
5. An assessment of fetal well-being is performed in consultation with the obstetrician.

---

tolerance of a reduction in uteroplacental perfusion if severe hypotension or local anesthetic toxicity occurs.[31]

MONITORS

During the initiation of epidural analgesia, we monitor all patients with an automatic blood pressure cuff and either an

---

Box 21-3 ADMINISTRATION OF EPIDURAL ANALGESIA FOR LABOR: A TECHNIQUE

1. Informed consent is obtained, and the obstetrician is consulted.
2. Monitoring includes the following:
   - Blood pressure every 1 to 2 minutes for 15 minutes after giving a bolus of local anesthetic;
   - Continuous maternal heart rate monitoring during induction of anesthesia;
   - Continuous fetal heart rate monitoring; and
   - Continual verbal communication.
3. The patient is hydrated with 500 mL of Ringer's lactate solution.
4. The patient assumes a lateral decubitus or sitting position.
5. The epidural space is identified with a loss-of-resistance technique.
6. The epidural catheter is threaded 3 to 5 cm into the epidural space.
7. A test dose of 3 mL of 1.5% lidocaine with 1:200,000 epinephrine or 3 mL of 0.25% bupivacaine with 1:200,000 epinephrine is injected after careful aspiration and after a uterine contraction (to minimize the chance of confusing tachycardia that results from pain with tachycardia as a result of intravenous injection of the test dose).
8. If the test dose is negative, one or two 5-mL doses of 0.25% bupivacaine are injected to achieve a cephalad sensory level of approximately T10.*
9. After 15 to 20 minutes, the block is assessed by means of loss of sensation to cold or pinprick. If no block is evident, the catheter is replaced. If the block is asymmetric, the epidural catheter is withdrawn 0.5 to 1.0 cm, and an additional 5 to 10 mL of the same bupivacaine solution is injected. If the block remains inadequate, the catheter is replaced.
10. The patient is cared for in the lateral or semilateral position to avoid aortocaval compression.
11. Subsequently, maternal blood pressure is measured every 5 to 15 minutes. The fetal heart rate is monitored continuously.
12. The level of analgesia and the intensity of motor block are assessed every 1 to 2 hours.

*At the University of Michigan, a high-volume, low-concentration technique is used to establish epidural analgesia. Specifically, four 5-mL doses of bupivacaine 0.05% with fentanyl 3 µg/mL (i.e., a total dose of 20 mL) are injected to achieve a cephalad sensory level of T10.

Box 21-4 RESUSCITATION EQUIPMENT AND DRUGS THAT SHOULD BE AVAILABLE DURING ADMINISTRATION OF EPIDURAL ANALGESIA

DRUGS	EQUIPMENT
Thiopental	Oxygen supply
Succinylcholine	Self-inflating bag and mask for
Ephedrine	positive-pressure ventilation
Atropine	Masks
Epinephrine	Oral and nasal airways
Phenylephrine	Laryngoscopes
Calcium chloride	Endotracheal tubes
Sodium bicarbonate	Suction (including the
Naloxone	necessary supplies)
	Intravenous catheters and fluids
	Syringes and needles

electrocardiogram or a pulse oximeter to facilitate continuous assessment of the maternal heart rate (Box 21-3). Maternal blood pressure is measured every 1 to 2 minutes after the administration of the test and therapeutic doses of local anesthetic. Subsequently (15 minutes after administration of a bolus dose of local anesthetic), maternal blood pressure is measured every 5 to 15 minutes. Continuous pulse oximetry is used in selected patients (e.g., patients with asthma or cardiovascular disease). Rarely, invasive hemodynamic monitoring is necessary. The sensory level of analgesia and the intensity of motor block are assessed after the administration of the test and therapeutic doses of local anesthetic. Subsequently, sensory level and motor block are assessed every 1 to 2 hours (Box 21-5).[32]

When possible, we monitor the fetal heart rate (FHR) continuously during placement of the catheter and administration of epidural analgesia. The ASA Task Force on Obstetrical Anesthesia[30] has stated the following:

> The fetal heart rate should be monitored by a qualified individual before and after administration of regional analgesia for labor. The Task Force recognizes that *continuous* electronic recording of the fetal heart rate may not be necessary in every clinical setting and may not be possible during placement of a regional anesthetic.

The ACOG has provided no specific guidelines regarding the use of FHR monitoring during epidural analgesia.[33] Of course, the anesthesiologist cannot predict when hypotension will occur during the administration of regional anesthesia. Because of this, we believe that continuous electronic FHR monitoring should be performed both *during* (if possible) and *after* the administration of epidural analgesia in all laboring women.

In some cases, the mother's position or maternal obesity precludes the use of an external monitor (e.g., Doppler ultrasonography) to monitor the FHR during placement of the catheter. In such cases (especially when there is concern regarding fetal well-being), it is helpful for the obstetrician to place a fetal scalp electrode to monitor the FHR. It is especially important to monitor the FHR continuously during and after the epidural injection of local anesthetic solution. Some anesthesiologists have suggested the use of the FHR monitor to assess maternal heart rate during the administration of an epinephrine-containing test dose.[34] We prefer to use a separate monitor of maternal heart rate so that FHR monitoring is not interrupted.

INTRAVENOUS HYDRATION

Placement of an intravenous catheter (preferably 18-gauge or larger) and correction of hypovolemia with intravenous hydration are necessary before the administration of epidural analgesia to prevent hypotension that can result from sympathetic blockade. Most anesthesiologists administer approximately 500 mL of Ringer's lactate (without dextrose) to prevent a significant decrease in blood pressure and uteroplacental perfusion.[35-37] Severe hypotension is less likely with the contemporary administration of a dilute solution of local anesthetic for epidural

---

Box 21-5 ASSESSMENT OF MOTOR BLOCK

1. Complete—unable to move feet or knees
2. Almost complete—able to move feet only
3. Partial—just able to move knees
4. None—full flexion of knees and feet

From Bromage PR. Epidural Analgesia. Philadelphia, WB Saunders, 1978:144.

---

analgesia. However, deterioration in FHR patterns has been observed when the fluid preload was omitted.[38] We continue to give a 500-mL fluid bolus before the administration of epidural analgesia in laboring women at the University of Michigan. Rarely, hydration should be guided by the measurement of central venous or pulmonary artery pressure.

Ringer's lactate (without dextrose) is the most commonly used intravenous fluid in laboring women, both for bolus administration and maintenance infusion. However, in a prospective randomized trial of 106 laboring women that underwent spontaneous vaginal delivery, the administration of Ringer's lactate with 5% glucose for *maintenance* hydration reduced umbilical cord acidemia and hypercarbia without changes in cord blood levels of glucose or base excess.[39] Additional studies are needed. However, anesthesiologists and obstetricians should continue to avoid the *bolus* administration of dextrose-containing solutions in laboring women.

MATERNAL POSITION

Either the lateral decubitus or the sitting position can be used during identification of the epidural space (see Chapter 11). The lateral position has some advantages over the sitting position: (1) it seems intuitive that uteroplacental perfusion is better in the lateral position[40]; (2) orthostatic hypotension is less likely; (3) the lateral position often facilitates continuous FHR monitoring during placement of the catheter; and (4) some patients find this position more comfortable.[41] However, one study demonstrated a greater reduction in maternal cardiac output with maximal lumbar flexion in the lateral decubitus position than in the sitting position during identification of the epidural space in laboring women.[42] The authors speculated that maximal lumbar flexion in the lateral decubitus position results in concealed aortocaval compression. In contrast, they suggested that the uterus falls forward (and thus does not cause aortocaval compression) when the patient assumes the sitting flexed position. They recommended that "the tight fetal curl position be avoided," especially when the patient assumes the lateral decubitus position for identification of the epidural space.[42]

In obese women, the sitting position is often advantageous. It may provide better respiratory mechanics, help the anesthesiologist identify midline and bony landmarks, and improve maternal comfort during placement of the epidural catheter.[41] Maternal position during placement of the epidural catheter does not seem to affect the incidence of unintentional dural puncture. However, adoption of the lateral recumbent head-down position for epidural catheter placement may reduce the incidence of epidural venous puncture.[43] The skill of the anesthesiologist is also important.

Aortocaval compression must be avoided at all times. The gravid uterus can occlude the inferior vena cava and aorta when the parturient assumes the supine position.[44-47] This position may cause maternal hypotension[48,49] and decreased uteroplacental perfusion,[40,50] even in the absence of anesthesia. Increased venous tone in the lower extremities helps overcome partial occlusion of the inferior vena cava in unanesthetized pregnant women. If maternal hydration is inadequate and if aortocaval compression is not avoided, the onset of anesthesia-induced sympathetic blockade will result in decreased venous return, decreased cardiac output, and decreased uteroplacental perfusion.[47] The avoidance of aortocaval compression is essential to maintain normal cardiac output and uteroplacental perfusion.[47,48,51]

Some anesthesiologists contend that maternal position after epidural catheter placement affects the efficacy of epidural analgesia, although this is a matter of some dispute *(vide infra)*. Beilen et al.[52] recently observed that the placement of the parturient in the supine position with a 30-degree leftward tilt was associated with better epidural analgesia than maintenance of the left lateral decubitus position in laboring women.

Test Dose

Epidural catheter placement may be complicated by blood vessel or dural puncture. The anesthesiologist must recognize the unintentional intravenous or subarachnoid placement of the needle or catheter to prevent possible local anesthetic toxicity and high or total spinal anesthesia. Simple aspiration of the catheter is not adequate to identify all cases of intravascular or intrathecal placement of the catheter.[53-55] The purpose of the test dose is to give a dose of drug that allows the recognition of intravenous or subarachnoid placement of the catheter but does not result in systemic toxicity or total spinal anesthesia. The ideal test dose must be readily available, safe, and effective. It should have a high sensitivity (i.e., a low rate of false negatives) and a high specificity (i.e., a low rate of false positives) (Box 21-6).

The test dose should allow easy identification of **subarachnoid (intrathecal)** placement of the catheter without causing total spinal anesthesia and hemodynamic compromise. Bupivacaine (7.5 to 12.5 mg) and lidocaine (45 to 60 mg) have been used.[56-58] (Ropivacaine 15 mg is *not* a useful intrathecal test dose because of a slow onset of motor block after intrathecal injection.[59]) Subarachnoid injection of a hyperbaric solution of local anesthetic typically produces a rapid onset of sacral analgesia with some evidence of motor block (Figure 21-3).[56] Unfortunately, the hyperbaric lidocaine test dose as described by Abraham et al.[56] is not available commercially. In a study of older, nonpregnant patients receiving continuous spinal anesthesia for surgery, Colonna-Romano and Lingaraju[58] used the commercially available test dose of lidocaine 45 mg plus epinephrine 15 μg (without dextrose). The authors concluded that the best method of detecting intrathecal injection is an assessment of motor function (straight-leg raising) 4 minutes after the test-dose injection. The application of these data to pregnant patients is unclear. Richardson et al.[60] described the

rapid onset (1 to 3 minutes) of high levels of spinal anesthesia with motor block and hypotension in five parturients who had received a test dose that included lidocaine 45 mg plus epinephrine 15 μg (without dextrose). This solution is slightly hypobaric relative to cerebrospinal fluid (CSF) at body temperature; thus the upright posture of these parturients during the injection may have contributed to the high levels of spinal anesthesia. The anesthesiologist must recognize the possible range of responses to the dose of local anesthetic used to assess the position of an epidural catheter and should perform a careful assessment of sensory, motor, and sympathetic function 3 to 5 minutes after administration of the test dose before concluding that the test dose is negative.

If there is uncertainty regarding the response to the test dose, the anesthesiologist can repeat the test dose, replace the catheter, or inject only small doses of local anesthetic. Rarely the catheter may migrate from the epidural to the subarachnoid space during labor.[61,62] Thus, a test dose should be repeated before each supplemental bolus injection of local anesthetic.

The ideal method for excluding **intravenous** placement of the catheter is controversial. Blood vessel puncture (indicated by aspiration of blood or blood-tinged fluid through the epidural catheter) occurs in 9% to 20% of obstetric patients,[63,64] and intravenous placement of an epidural catheter occurs in approximately 7% to 8.5% of obstetric patients.[65] Failure to recognize intravenous placement of the epidural catheter and subsequent intravenous injection of a large dose of local anesthetic may lead to systemic local anesthetic toxicity, with central nervous system (CNS) symptoms, seizures, cardiovascular collapse, and death.[62,66] In normal volunteers and sedated surgical patients, intravenous injection of 15 μg of epinephrine (3 mL of a 1:200,000 solution) reliably causes tachycardia (i.e., an increase in heart rate of approximately 30 bpm within 20 to 40 seconds).[67,68]

However, some anesthesiologists have expressed several concerns regarding the use of an epinephrine-containing test dose in laboring women. First, intravenous epinephrine may cause a transient decline in uterine blood flow from alpha-receptor mediated constriction of the uterine artery (Figure 21-4).[69-71] However, this decrease in uterine blood flow is comparable to

---

Box 21-6 SUGGESTED EPIDURAL TEST DOSE REGIMENS

SUBARACHNOID

Lidocaine 45 to 60 mg
Bupivacaine 7.5 to 12.5 mg

INTRAVENOUS

Changes in heart rate and/or blood pressure
• Epinephrine 15 μg
• Isoproterenol 5 μg

Subjective symptoms
• Local anesthetic alone
  1. 2-Chloroprocaine 1.5 mg/kg
  2. Lidocaine 100 mg
• Fentanyl 100 μg

Doppler changes (1 to 2 mL of air), used only with single-orifice epidural catheters

References 56, 57, 67, 68, 78-80, 83-89.

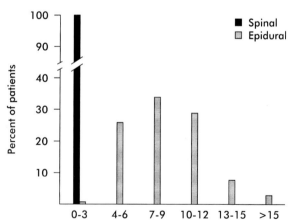

FIGURE 21-3. Percent of pregnant patients who demonstrated objective evidence of anesthesia (defined as the loss of sensation to pinprick) after epidural injection of 2 to 3 mL of hyperbaric 1.5% lidocaine with 1:200,000 epinephrine *(hatched bars)* (*n* = 250) or after intrathecal injection of 2 mL of hyperbaric 1.5% lidocaine with 1:200,000 epinephrine *(solid bar)* (*n* = 15). (From Abraham RA, Harris AP, Maxwell LG, et al. The efficacy of 1.5% lidocaine with 7.5% dextrose and epinephrine as an epidural test dose for obstetrics. Anesthesiology 1986: 64:116-9.)

that which occurs during a uterine contraction. Youngstrom et al.[72] noted that this intravenous dose of epinephrine did not worsen fetal condition in acidotic fetal lambs. Any transient effect of epinephrine on uterine blood flow likely represents a less-severe insult than systemic local anesthetic toxicity.

Second, some anesthesiologists argue that the epinephrine-containing test dose lacks specificity. The maternal tachycardic response to intravenous injection of epinephrine cannot always be distinguished from other causes of tachycardia during labor (e.g., pain during a uterine contraction) (Figure 21-5).[34,73,74] Cartwright et al.[74] noted that 12% of laboring women had an increase in heart rate of at least 30 bpm after epidural injection of 3 mL of 0.5% bupivacaine *without* epinephrine. One study suggested that the positive-predictive value of a tachycardic response to an epinephrine-containing test dose is 55% to 73%.[75] This study suggested that if a positive heart rate response to an epinephrine-containing test dose occurs in 20% of patients, 5% to 9% of epidural catheters would be identified incorrectly as intravascular and removed unnecessarily. Colonna-Romano and Nagaraj[55] concluded that the intravenous injection of an epinephrine-containing test dose results in "a sudden and fast acceleration in maternal heart rate within one minute." Thus, careful assessment of the rate of increase in maternal heart rate may help distinguish a contraction-induced increase in heart rate from the effect of intravenously injected epinephrine, thereby improving the specificity of the epinephrine test.[55] It is unclear whether such an assessment is practical clinically.[76]

Third, some anesthesiologists argue that the epinephrine-containing test dose also lacks sensitivity (the ability to elicit a predictable increase in heart rate). An increase in maternal heart rate of 25 bpm occurring within 2 minutes of drug injection and lasting at least 15 seconds was observed in only 5 of 10 laboring women who received 15 µg of epinephrine intravenously (Figure 21-6).[77] Detection of intravenous epinephrine was improved when the authors retrospectively defined a positive maternal tachycardic response as a 10-bpm increase over the maximum maternal heart rate measured during the 2 minutes preceding the epinephrine injection. Others have confirmed that these revised criteria improve the sensitivity of the epinephrine-containing test dose in laboring women.[75] The usefulness of an epinephrine-containing test dose also improves if additional information is obtained. One group gave intravenous injections of *either* bupivacaine 12.5 mg with epinephrine 12.5 µg *or* normal saline to laboring women. They correctly identified the test solution in 39 of 40 women when they assessed maternal heart rate, blood pressure, uterine contractions, the timing of injection, the presence of analgesia, and subjective signs and symptoms of intravascular injection (e.g., palpitations, lightheadedness, dizziness).[78] The tachycardic response to intravenous epinephrine is absent in patients who have received a beta-adrenergic receptor antagonist.[67]

Other means of identifying intravascular placement of an epidural catheter have been proposed (Box 21-6). Intravenous administration of isoproterenol 5 µg consistently results in tachycardia in pregnant women.[79,80] Data from animals[71,81] and noninvasive measurements in parturients[80] suggest that isoproterenol is devoid of the adverse effects of epinephrine on uterine blood flow, and limited neurotoxicity evaluations

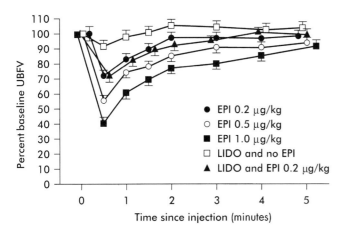

FIGURE 21-4. The effect of intravenous epinephrine, lidocaine, and lidocaine with epinephrine on uterine artery blood flow velocity *(UBFV)* in the pregnant guinea pig. The dose of lidocaine was 0.4 mg/kg. *EPI,* Epinephrine; *LIDO,* lidocaine. Values are presented as mean ± SEM percentage of baseline. (From Chestnut DH, Weiner CP, Martin JG, et al. Effect of intravenous epinephrine on uterine artery blood flow velocity in the pregnant guinea pig. Anesthesiology 1986; 65:633-6.)

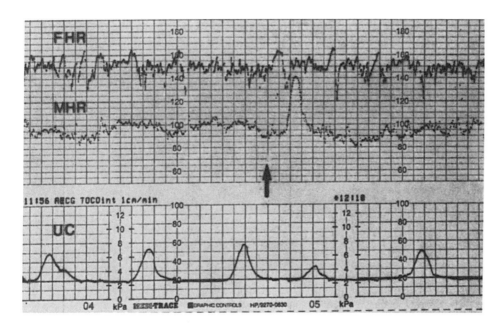

FIGURE 21-5. Heart rate of a laboring patient *(MHR)*, fetal heart rate *(FHR)*, and uterine contractions *(UC)* are shown. This tracing was obtained with the use of an FHR monitor with dual heart rate capacity. Note the variability of the MHR with uterine contractions. An intravenous injection of bupivacaine 12.5 mg and epinephrine 12.5 µg was given *(arrow)*. Note the marked increase in MHR in response to intravenous injection of the test dose. The maternal tachycardia had a duration of approximately 40 seconds. (From Van Zundert AA. Vaes LE, De Wolf AM. ECG monitoring of mother and fetus during epidural anesthesia. Anesthesiology 1987; 66:584-5.)

have not revealed adverse effects.[81] Marcus et al.[82] randomized 80 laboring women to receive three doses of bupivacaine 0.125% with sufentanil 7.5 µg and either epinephrine 12.5 µg or isoproterenol 5 µg; the authors observed no clinical evidence of neurotoxicity. However, isoproterenol has not been approved for epidural or intrathecal administration. Given the lack of adequate information regarding potential neurotoxicity, we do not recommend the use of isoproterenol as an epidural test dose.

Leighton et al.[83] have advocated the use of air as an objective marker of intravascular injection. Intravenous injection of 1 or 2 mL of air through a single-orifice catheter consistently produces changes in heart sounds as detected by the use of precordial Doppler ultrasound.[83] (The external FHR monitor can be used for this purpose.) False-negative results may occur when small volumes of air are injected through multiorifice epidural catheters; thus the air test is not a reliable intravenous test when multi-orifice epidural catheters are used.[84,85]

Subjective CNS symptoms have also been evaluated as a means for recognizing the unintentional intravenous injection of epidural medications. Colonna-Romano et al.[86] administered either intravenous saline, lidocaine 100 mg, or 2-chloroprocaine 100 mg to laboring women. Blinded observers recorded the occurrence of CNS symptoms (i.e., dizziness, tinnitus, funny taste) after intravenous injection of local anesthetic. Lidocaine 100 mg was determined to have the

potential to be a reliable marker of intravenous injection when the symptoms of tinnitus and funny taste were considered (sensitivity 100%, specificity 81%). 2-Chloroprocaine was found to be less reliable (sensitivity, 81% to 94%; specificity, 69% to 81%). In volunteers, a dose of 1.5 mg/kg of 2-chloroprocaine was necessary to produce a probability of 90% that the subject would report symptoms of intravenous injection.[87]

Some anesthesiologists advocate the administration of fentanyl 100 µg to test for intravenous injection.[88] Morris et al.[89] evaluated the accuracy and reliability of the fentanyl test dose in a double-blind study in which either intravenous or epidural fentanyl 100 µg was administered to parturients. The investigators observed for the presence of sedation, dizziness, euphoria, and analgesia. They found dizziness to be the most reliable symptom of intravenous fentanyl injection, with a sensitivity of 92% and a specificity of 92%.

Some situations reduce the reliability of subjective symptoms as a signal of intravenous injection of a drug. Tests that rely on the self-reporting of subjective symptoms require clear communication with the patient and thus are less useful when the anesthesiologist and patient speak different languages. Exhaustion and/or prior opioid administration also may affect the reliability of the test.

Lastly, the choice of epidural catheter may affect the reliability of the epidural test dose. Multi-orifice epidural catheters have three potential sites of exit for injected fluid

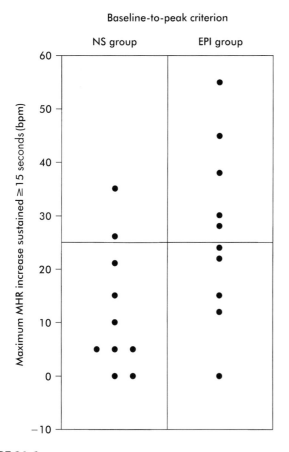

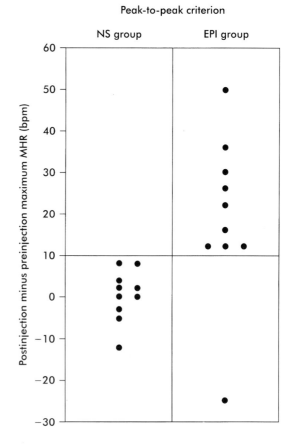

FIGURE 21-6.   Maximum maternal heart rate *(MHR)* changes after intravenous injection of 15 µg of epinephrine *(EPI group)* or saline *(NS group)*. Baseline-to-peak criterion for a positive heart rate response to epinephrine was prospectively defined as an increase in heart rate of more than 25 bpm above that at the time of epinephrine injection, which occurred within 120 seconds of drug injection. Peak-to-peak criterion for a positive heart rate response was retrospectively defined as an increase in heart rate of more than 10 bpm during the 2 minutes after the injection as compared with the maximum MHR recorded during the 2 minutes preceding the injection. (From Leighton BL, Norris MC, Sosis M, et al. Limitations of epinephrine as a marker of intravascular injection in laboring women. Anesthesiology 1987: 66:688-91.)

or air, and the orifices may lie within two different body compartments. If injected too slowly, air or fluid will preferentially exit the proximal orifice. The speed of injection used in clinical practice typically exceeds that required to ensure that fluid will exit all three orifices. On the other hand, air must be injected at a much greater speed to ensure that it exits all three orifices; this speed is not practical for clinical use. The distal orifice is both the most difficult to test and the one most likely to be positioned outside of the epidural space.[85] Clearly, every dose injected through a multi-orifice catheter must be fractionated and considered a "test dose."

In summary, no perfect test dose exists. Because most anesthesiologists currently give laboring patients small doses of a dilute solution of local anesthetic, some argue that a test dose is unnecessary. Norris et al.[90] recently concluded that, when using a multi-orifice epidural catheter, a regimen that includes observation, aspiration, and incremental drug injection obviates the need for a specific test dose to exclude intravenous placement of the catheter. However, this conclusion depends heavily on the use of small doses of local anesthetic. Laboring women may need large doses of local anesthetic for operative delivery. In some cases, large doses are administered for emergency cesarean section. We want to determine as soon as possible that the epidural catheter is correctly positioned within the epidural space. In addition, the epinephrine-containing test dose provides an objective marker of intravascular injection, which has stood the test of time. Thus we typically give a test dose that includes either 7.5 mg of bupivacaine or 45 to 60 mg of lidocaine with 15 μg of epinephrine.

Prevention of local anesthetic toxicity and high spinal anesthesia should also include several other steps:
1. Observe for the passive return of blood or CSF through the catheter.
2. Aspirate before each injection.
3. Give the test dose *after* a uterine contraction.
4. Maintain verbal contact with the patient, and look for subjective symptoms and objective signs of intravenous or subarachnoid injection of the local anesthetic.
5. Do not inject more than 5 mL of local anesthetic as a single bolus, and never inject a bolus dose of local anesthetic that could cause systemic toxicity or total spinal anesthesia.
6. Have a low threshold for repeating the test dose or replacing the epidural catheter if uncertainty exists regarding the catheter location. If little or no block is produced after the injection of an appropriate dose of local anesthetic, assume

that the local anesthetic was injected intravenously and remove the catheter.

Even with these precautions, local anesthetic toxicity may occur.[61,62,91,92] The anesthesiologist must have the skill and equipment to treat convulsions, total spinal anesthesia, and cardiovascular collapse.

Choice of Local Anesthetic

During labor, the ideal epidural local anesthetic would provide a rapid onset of effective analgesia with minimal motor blockade, minimal risk of maternal toxicity, and negligible effect on uterine activity and uteroplacental perfusion. It would undergo limited transplacental transfer and thus have minimal effect on the fetus and newborn. Finally, this ideal agent would have a long duration of action. Although this perfect local anesthetic does not exist, each local anesthetic used in obstetrics has useful features.

BUPIVACAINE

Bupivacaine, an amide local anesthetic, is the local anesthetic that is used most often during the administration of epidural analgesia for labor. After epidural administration of bupivacaine during labor, the patient first perceives some pain relief within approximately 8 to 10 minutes,[93] but approximately 20 minutes are required to achieve the peak effect. Epidural administration of 8 to 10 mL of 0.25% to 0.5% bupivacaine provides approximately 2 hours of analgesia (Table 21-1).[5] When dilute solutions are used, bupivacaine produces excellent sensory analgesia with minimal motor blockade, and tachyphylaxis occurs rarely.[5] A 0.125% solution is often adequate during early labor, and a 0.25% solution is effective during active labor in most patients. These concentrations can be reduced with the addition of an opioid. At the University of Michigan, we establish epidural analgesia by giving a large volume (20 mL) of a very dilute solution of bupivacaine (0.05%) with fentanyl 3 μg/mL.

Bupivacaine is highly protein bound, which limits transplacental transfer. The umbilical vein:maternal vein concentration ratio is approximately 0.3.[94]

An association between the use of epidural bupivacaine during labor and FHR decelerations has been reported.[95,96] In one study, 8 of 42 fetuses whose mothers received 0.5% bupivacaine epidurally had late FHR decelerations as compared with 3 of 47 fetuses whose mothers received 1.5% lidocaine and none of 34 fetuses whose mothers received 2% 2-chloroprocaine during labor.[95] These FHR decelerations were not

TABLE 21-1 EPIDURAL ANALGESIA FROM 10 ML OF 0.25% BUPIVACAINE WITH AND WITHOUT EPINEPHRINE 1:300,000		
Parameter	Bupivacaine alone (n = 50)	Bupivacaine with epinephrine (n = 50)
Highest sensory dermatome	T10 ± 0.3	T10 ± 0.3
Onset of considerable or complete analgesia (minutes)	8.7 ± 0.8	5.8 ± 0.6*
Duration of analgesia (minutes)†	92 ± 5	123 ± 7*
Number of patients who required 5 mL of additional bupivacaine for effective analgesia	18	9*

Values are expressed as mean ± SEM.
*P < 0.05 compared with plain bupivacaine group.
†Includes some patients who delivered before regression of analgesia.
Modified from Eisenach JC, Grice SC, Dewan DM. Epinephrine enhances analgesia produced by epidural bupivacaine during labor. Anesth Analg 1987; 66:447-51.

associated with maternal hypotension. Others have described an association between "bupivacaine bradycardia" and increased uterine tone.[97] These FHR decelerations do not seem to result from the systemic absorption of bupivacaine, and they appear to occur only in laboring women. Loftus et al.[98] did not observe FHR decelerations in women who received epidural bupivacaine for elective cesarean section, despite the use of larger doses of bupivacaine and more extensive sympathetic blockade. Of interest, one study noted that the administration of either epidural bupivacaine or intrathecal sufentanil was followed by a similar incidence of FHR decelerations (23% and 22%, respectively) in laboring women.[99] Other studies have not observed an increased incidence of FHR decelerations after the epidural administration of bupivacaine during labor.[100,101] Further, the reports of FHR decelerations after bupivacaine did not demonstrate adverse neonatal outcome; thus the significance of these decelerations is unclear. There are no published data about the relationship between the concentration of bupivacaine used for intrapartum epidural analgesia and the incidence of FHR decelerations. At the University of Michigan, such events have been rare since we decreased the concentration of local anesthetic used for epidural analgesia in laboring women.

ROPIVACAINE

Ropivacaine is an amide local anesthetic that is similar to bupivacaine in structure and pharmacodynamics.[102] Ropivacaine is a homolog of bupivacaine and mepivacaine, but, unlike these other local anesthetics, it is formulated as the single-levorotary enantiomer rather than as a racemic mixture (see Chapter 12). Studies in vitro and in vivo suggest that ropivacaine is less cardiodepressant and arrhythmogenic than bupivacaine when equal doses are compared.[103-105] Studies of pregnant sheep suggest that clinically relevant plasma concentrations of ropivacaine do not adversely affect uterine blood flow.[106] Ropivacaine is cleared more rapidly than bupivacaine after intravenous administration in both pregnant and nonpregnant sheep. Consequently, a larger dose of drug—but *not* a higher plasma concentration—is required to produce systemic toxicity.[107] These findings would suggest that ropivacaine has a greater margin of safety than bupivacaine for situations in which unintentional intravenous injection occurs in pregnant women. However, many previous investigations assumed that ropivacaine and bupivacaine are equipotent; subsequent studies have demonstrated that ropivacaine is 40% less potent than bupivacaine.[108,109] When ropivacaine concentrations are adjusted for this potency difference, there is no clear advantage for ropivacaine in terms of the risk of systemic toxicity.[108]

In reality, systemic toxicity is not a major concern with the contemporary use of a dilute solution of local anesthetic for epidural analgesia during labor. It is of note that several studies comparing equal concentrations of ropivacaine and bupivacaine given by patient-controlled epidural analgesia (PCEA) have not found any significant difference in clinical efficacy between the two local anesthetics.[110-113] Other studies that adjusted for the potency difference and compared equipotent concentrations (e.g., 0.0625% bupivacaine versus 0.1% ropivacaine) also found no difference in clinical efficacy.[114,115] It is important to recognize that potency is an unchanging property of a drug, whereas clinical efficacy is influenced by multiple variables. For example, ropivacaine has a longer duration of analgesia than bupivacaine,[108] which

may offset its lesser potency when administered by continuous epidural infusion.

Studies conducted in vitro[116] and early clinical studies[117,118] suggested that ropivacaine may be associated with less motor block than bupivacaine; this would be a desirable characteristic of a local anesthetic used for epidural analgesia during labor. However, these studies also compared equal concentrations of ropivacaine and bupivacaine, and the decreased motor block may reflect the decreased potency of ropivacaine. A study of the relative motor-blocking potencies of epidural ropivacaine and bupivacaine showed that ropivacaine was 40% less potent than bupivacaine in terms of motor block,[119] which corresponds to the relative analgesic potencies of the two drugs.[108,109] Several clinical studies[120,121] and a well-conducted meta-analysis of studies comparing epidural ropivacaine and bupivacaine[122] did not demonstrate an advantage for ropivacaine in terms of decreased motor block.

It is difficult to justify the increased cost of ropivacaine without clear patient benefit. There is no definitive evidence of increased patient safety or decreased motor block when ropivacaine is used to provide epidural analgesia in laboring women, and there is no significant difference between ropivacaine and bupivacaine in obstetric or neonatal outcome.[122] By contrast, ropivacaine offers increased patient safety in nonobstetric settings in which high concentrations and greater volumes of drugs are administered (e.g., brachial plexus blockade).

LEVOBUPIVACAINE

Levobupivacaine is the purified levorotary enantiomer of racemic bupivacaine and has been available for clinical use since 1999. Like ropivacaine, both preclinical and clinical studies have suggested that levobupivacaine has less potential for cardiotoxicity than bupivacaine when equal concentrations of the two drugs are compared.[123-125] Again, toxicity can be properly evaluated only when equi*potent* concentrations of drug are compared. Levobupivacaine has been compared to bupivacaine in laboring women and has been found to be only slightly less potent than bupivacaine, with a potency ratio of 0.98 (95% confidence internal, 0.67 to 1.41).[126] Other studies have suggested that levobupivacaine and ropivacaine have similar potency.[127,128] When considered together, these observations are confusing, given the clear evidence that ropivacaine is less potent than bupivacaine. Unfortunately, no single study has evaluated all three drugs in laboring women. Additional studies are needed to assess the relative potency of levobupivacaine as compared with bupivacaine and ropivacaine.

LIDOCAINE

Lidocaine is an amide local anesthetic with a duration between that of bupivacaine and 2-chloroprocaine. During labor, the administration of a 0.75% to 1.5% solution of lidocaine typically provides satisfactory analgesia, but it may not provide analgesia comparable to that provided by bupivacaine.[129]

At delivery, the umbilical vein:maternal vein lidocaine concentration ratio is approximately twice that of bupivacaine.[130,131] Early studies discouraged the epidural administration of lidocaine in pregnant women.[132,133] In 1974, Scanlon et al.[132] reported that the epidural administration of lidocaine or mepivacaine during labor was associated with abnormal neonatal neurobehavioral examinations as compared with infants of mothers who received no analgesia.

Subsequently, several larger, carefully controlled studies have demonstrated that the epidural administration of lidocaine, bupivacaine, or 2-chloroprocaine results in similar neonatal outcome.[134,135] Although some investigators have observed subtle differences in neurobehavior between infants exposed to lidocaine and those exposed to other local anesthetics, these differences are within the inherent variability of the examinations and are not clinically significant. Other factors (e.g., mode of delivery) appear to be much more important determinants of neonatal condition.

2-CHLOROPROCAINE

2-Chloroprocaine is an ester local anesthetic with a rapid onset of action. Epidural administration of 5 to 10 mL of 2% 2-chloroprocaine provides effective analgesia for approximately 40 minutes. Unfortunately, the short duration of action limits its usefulness during labor. In addition, the epidural administration of 2-chloroprocaine adversely affects the efficacy of subsequently administered epidural bupivacaine and opioids.[136,137] This adverse effect may occur even when small doses of 2-chloroprocaine are administered as a test dose (e.g., 40 mg as an intrathecal test followed by 100 mg as an intravenous test).

Administration of either 2% or 3% 2-chloroprocaine is most useful when the anesthesiologist needs to extend epidural anesthesia rapidly for operative vaginal or cesarean delivery. 2-Chloroprocaine has a very short half-life in maternal and fetal blood[138]; this feature makes it an attractive agent for cases of fetal distress, because the placental transfer of 2-chloroprocaine is not increased by the presence of fetal acidosis.[139]

Epidural injection of large volumes of 2-chloroprocaine (Nesacaine-MPF) has been associated with back pain (perhaps from the binding of calcium by added *ethylenediamine tetraacetic acid* [EDTA], resulting in muscle spasm).[140] All published cases occurred in nonpregnant patients. McLoughlin and DiFazio[141] reported back pain in one patient who received 35 mL of 2% 2-chloroprocaine epidurally for postpartum tubal ligation. The formulation of 2-chloroprocaine (also named Nesacaine-MPF) currently marketed for epidural injection does not contain EDTA or other preservatives. It is packaged in colored vials to reduce the oxidation of the 2-chloroprocaine.

EPINEPHRINE

Some anesthesiologists add a low dose of epinephrine (1:200,000 to 1:800,000) to the solution of local anesthetic. The addition of epinephrine hastens the onset of epidural bupivacaine analgesia,[93,142] and it has a modest bupivacaine-sparing effect,[143] perhaps as a result of the stimulation of alpha-adrenergic receptors in the spinal cord (Table 21-1).[93,142] The addition of epinephrine to the local anesthetic has a variable effect on the systemic uptake of the local anesthetic in obstetric patients.[144-148] The systemic absorption of epinephrine may increase maternal heart rate and may also result in a transient decrease in uterine activity as a result of beta-adrenergic receptor stimulation.[93,149,150] However, some studies have shown that the addition of epinephrine to either bupivacaine or lidocaine does not prolong labor as compared with the epidural administration of bupivacaine or lidocaine alone.[149,151] Epidural administration of an epinephrine-containing local anesthetic solution does not adversely affect intervillous blood flow[152] or neonatal outcome.[142,144] One disadvantage of the use of epinephrine is that it increases the intensity of motor block.[151] For this reason, we do not routinely administer epinephrine-containing local anesthetic solutions during labor.

Maintenance of Epidural Analgesia

INTERMITTENT BOLUS INJECTION

Painful labor lasts several hours in most parturients; therefore, a single epidural injection of local anesthetic typically does not provide adequate analgesia for the duration of labor. Supplemental doses of local anesthetic are necessary to maintain epidural analgesia in most women (Table 21-2). Before giving an additional therapeutic dose, the anesthesiologist should first exclude migration of the epidural catheter into a blood vessel or the subarachnoid space. The spread and quality of analgesia may change with repeat epidural injections of local anesthetic. After several injections, blockade of the sacral segments, intense motor block, or both may develop.[151] The sensory level and the intensity of motor block should be assessed and recorded before and after each bolus injection of local anesthetic.

CONTINUOUS EPIDURAL INFUSION

A continuous epidural infusion of a dilute solution of local anesthetic is a popular technique for the maintenance of epidural analgesia during labor. The potential benefits of continuous epidural infusion include the following: (1) the maintenance of a stable level of analgesia; (2) a more stable maternal heart rate and blood pressure, with a decreased risk of hypotension; and (3) a less frequent need to give bolus doses of local anesthetic, which may reduce the risk of systemic local anesthetic toxicity.

Published studies have suggested that the continuous epidural infusion and intermittent bolus injection techniques have comparable safety. In theory, maintenance of a constant

TABLE 21-2	MAINTAINING AN EPIDURAL BLOCK: INTERMITTENT INJECTION AND CONTINUOUS INFUSION TECHNIQUES		
Drug	**Intermittent injection**	**Continuous infusion**
Bupivacaine	5-10 mL of a 0.125%-0.375% solution every 60-120 min	0.0625%-0.25% solution given at a rate of 8-15 mL/hr
Ropivacaine	5-10 mL of a 0.125%-0.25% solution every 60-120 min	0.125%-0.25% solution given at a rate of 6-12 mL/hr
Lidocaine	5-10 mL of a 0.75%-1.5% solution every 60-90 min	0.5%-1.0% solution given at a rate of 8-15 mL/hr
2-Chloroprocaine	5-10 mL of a 1%-2% solution every 45-60 min	0.75% solution given at a rate of 27 mL/hr

References 96, 120, 121, 129, 153-156, 158.

level of anesthesia should promote maternal hemodynamic stability and improve fetal and neonatal outcome. Only one published study has suggested a trend toward less frequent hypotension and a decreased incidence of abnormal FHR patterns during the continuous epidural infusion of bupivacaine as compared with intermittent bolus injections of bupivacaine.[153] However, neonatal outcome was the same in both groups. Other studies have not demonstrated a decreased incidence of maternal hypotension, fewer FHR abnormalities, or improved neonatal outcome with the continuous epidural infusion technique.[96,154]

Controlled trials of intrapartum epidural analgesia maintained by either intermittent bolus injection or continuous infusion of bupivacaine have consistently demonstrated that women require fewer bolus injections with the continuous infusion technique.[153-155] The continuous infusion technique increases the time between bolus injections and results in increased patient satisfaction.[155,156] This is advantageous in a busy obstetric anesthesia practice, where an anesthesiologist is not always available to give an additional bolus dose of local anesthetic immediately after the onset of recurrent pain.

Most studies suggest that the continuous epidural infusion technique results in the administration of a greater total dose of bupivacaine,[154-157] but this does not seem to result in greater maternal venous or umbilical venous bupivacaine concentrations at delivery.[155,157] The continuous epidural infusion of bupivacaine often results in satisfactory perineal analgesia, which obviates the need for a bolus dose of local anesthetic at delivery. Unfortunately, a prolonged epidural infusion of 10 to 14 mL/hr of 0.125% bupivacaine also may cause significant motor block.[153,154,156-158] The administration of a larger volume (e.g., 12 to 18 mL/hr) of a more dilute (0.075%) bupivacaine solution may provide good analgesia with less motor block.[156] Titration of the dose of bupivacaine to meet the individual needs of each patient (rather than administration of the same dose to all patients) may also help minimize motor block while providing effective analgesia.

Abboud et al.[158] observed that the continuous epidural infusion of bupivacaine (0.125% at 14 mL/hr), lidocaine (0.75% at 14 mL/hr), and 2-chloroprocaine (0.75% at 27 mL/hr) all provided similar maternal analgesia and neonatal outcome. Others have found that the analgesia provided by the epidural infusion of bupivacaine (0.125%) is superior to that provided by lidocaine (0.75%).[129] In practice, it is difficult to obtain satisfactory results with the continuous epidural infusion of 2-chloroprocaine. Analgesia may regress rapidly, and the epidural administration of 2-chloroprocaine adversely affects the response to other epidural agents. We do not administer a continuous epidural infusion of 2-chloroprocaine at the University of Michigan.

Migration of the epidural catheter into the subarachnoid, subdural, or intravenous space can occur with either the intermittent bolus injection or continuous infusion technique. If the epidural catheter should migrate into a vein during the continuous epidural infusion of a dilute solution of local anesthetic, it is unlikely that the patient will have symptoms of local anesthetic toxicity; rather, the level of anesthesia will regress. Because of this, the anesthesiologist should suspect the intravenous migration of an epidural catheter when a patient unexpectedly complains of pain during the continuous infusion of a local anesthetic during labor.

Migration of the epidural catheter into the subdural or subarachnoid space should result in a slow ascent of the level of anesthesia and an increased density of motor block. These observations apply to the epidural infusion of a 0.125% solution of bupivacaine at a modest rate (e.g., 10 to 15 mL/hr). The continuous infusion of a more concentrated solution or the use of a more rapid rate of infusion most likely reduces the margin of safety.

The use of a continuous epidural infusion technique does not obviate the need for frequent assessment of the patient. The anesthesiologist should assess the patient every 1 to 2 hours, and this procedure should include assessing the quality of analgesia and progress of labor, determining and recording the sensory level and intensity of motor block, and reviewing the maternal blood pressure measurements and FHR tracing for the previous hour. An inappropriately high level of anesthesia signals the administration of an excessive dose of local anesthetic or subdural or subarachnoid migration of the catheter. A low level of anesthesia may signal intravenous migration of the catheter, movement of the catheter outside of the epidural space, or administration of an inadequate dose of local anesthetic.

EQUIPMENT

Anesthesiologists should consider other precautions to enhance the safety of a continuous epidural infusion technique. The use of an infusion pump identical to that used for the intravenous administration of other drugs increases the chance that a nurse or physician will inject oxytocin, magnesium sulfate, or another drug into the epidural space unintentionally. Thus we recommend the use of an infusion pump that differs from the pumps used by the nursing staff and that is used exclusively for continuous epidural infusion. The pump should be easy to use, reliable, adjustable, and sturdy.

The anesthesiologist should also use infusion tubing (which connects the pump to the epidural catheter) that is unique for the epidural administration of a drug. The presence of an injection side-port increases the likelihood of unintentional epidural administration of the wrong drug; thus we recommend the use of tubing that does not have an injection side-port. A less desirable alternative is to wrap tape over the injection side-port on the tubing. In any case, the epidural catheter and tubing should be clearly labeled with the word "epidural."

Each labor unit must have a clear policy as to who may adjust the rate of infusion. At the University of Michigan, only anesthesia personnel make changes in the content and rate of the infusion unless maternal or fetal distress exists, in which case the pump is turned off by the nurse or obstetrician and the anesthesiologist is notified.

Use of the continuous infusion technique also requires careful preparation of the solution of local anesthetic. Either the anesthesiologist or a hospital pharmacist may prepare the solution. Sterile technique and preservative-free saline should be used to dilute the solution of local anesthetic. The anesthesiologist who prepares the solution should always double-check the syringe contents before beginning the infusion.

PATIENT-CONTROLLED EPIDURAL ANALGESIA

Studies have evaluated the use of PCEA in laboring women.[120,159-162] With this technique, each patient can adjust her level of analgesia (Table 21-3). Gambling et al.[160] observed that PCEA with 0.125% bupivacaine (with or without epinephrine) resulted in analgesia similar to that provided by the intermittent bolus injection or continuous epidural infusion of the same solution (Figure 21-7). PCEA has been associated with greater maternal satisfaction as compared with both intermittent bolus injection[160] (Figure 21-8) and continuous epidural infusion.[162]

In the majority of studies, the use of PCEA results in a lower average hourly dose of bupivacaine than does a continuous epidural infusion of bupivacaine.[159,161-164] One study found no difference in volume requirements between the two modes of administration.[165] However, studies have demonstrated a wide range of bupivacaine dose requirements among individual patients. This underscores the principle that intrapartum analgesic requirements vary among patients, and it also illustrates an advantage of the PCEA technique, which is that the dose of local anesthetic is titrated to effect.[163,166,167]

A wide variety of infusion regimens have been described for use with PCEA (Table 21-3). Gambling et al.[169] used a solution of 0.125% bupivacaine plus epinephrine 1:400,000 and fentanyl 2.5 µg/mL, and they compared several bolus doses with varying lockout intervals. They found no difference in block characteristics between a small bolus dose with a short lockout interval (2-mL dose, 10-minute lockout) and a larger bolus dose with a longer lockout interval (6-mL dose, 30-minute lockout). Ferrante et al.[163] found that when a 3-mL bolus dose is offered (with a 10-minute lockout), the use of a 6 mL/hr background infusion (as compared with no

background infusion or an infusion of 3 mL/hr) decreased the need for supplemental doses administered by an anesthesiologist without increasing motor block or altering other block characteristics. In the absence of a basal infusion, larger doses (12-mL bolus dose and a 25-minute lockout) provide better analgesia and maternal satisfaction than smaller doses (4-mL bolus and an 8-minute lockout).[170]

Many women appreciate the sense of autonomy associated with the use of PCEA. However, this technique is best reserved for patients who are willing and able to understand that they are in control of their analgesia. The anesthesiologist and nurse must not forget to monitor the patient. The intravascular or subarachnoid migration of an epidural catheter can occur. Likewise, the patient may experience inadequate analgesia. Moreover, an error in programming the PCEA pump may occur. Finally, the anesthesiologist should give attention to the previously discussed precautions regarding the choice of equipment and supplies.

Anesthesia for Vaginal Delivery

During the second stage of labor, pain results from distention of the pelvic floor, vagina, and perineum. Pain impulses are transmitted to the spinal cord by means of somatic nerve

TABLE 21-3	MAINTAINING AN EPIDURAL BLOCK: RECIPES FOR PATIENT-CONTROLLED EPIDURAL ANALGESIA			
Anesthetic solution	**Basal infusion rate (mL/hour)**	**Bolus dose (mL)**	**Lockout interval (minutes)**	**Maximum hourly dose (mL)**
Bupivacaine, 0.125%	4	4	20	16
Bupivacaine, 0.125%, plus fentanyl, 2 µg/mL	6	3	10	24
Bupivacaine, 0.25%	0	3	5-20	12
Bupivacaine, 0.11%, plus fentanyl, 2 µg/mL	10	5	10	30
Bupivacaine, 0.0625%, plus fentanyl, 2 µg/mL, plus clonidine, 4.5 µg/mL	0	4	15	16
Ropivacaine, 0.125%	6	4	10	30

References 120, 159, 161, 163, 168.

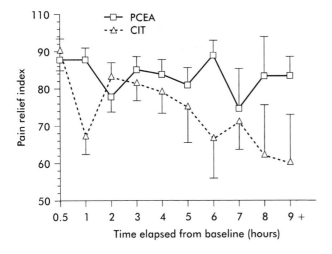

FIGURE 21-7. Analgesia over time in laboring women who received either patient-controlled epidural analgesia (PCEA) (n = 30) or conventional intermittent top-up injections (CIT) (n = 28). Pain relief index = 100 − ([actual pain score/baseline pain score] × 100). No differences in analgesia existed between the groups. (From Gambling DR, McMorland GH, Yu P, Laszlo C. Comparison of patient-controlled epidural analgesia and conventional intermittent "top-up" injections during labor. Anesth Analg 1990: 70:256-61.)

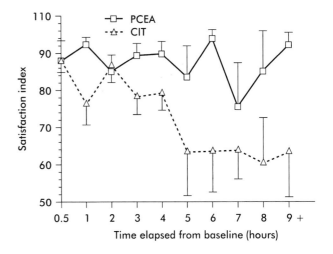

FIGURE 21-8. Patient satisfaction over time in laboring women who received either patient-controlled epidural analgesia (PCEA) (n = 30) or conventional intermittent top-up injections (CIT) (n = 28). Satisfaction index = 100 − ([actual satisfaction score/baseline satisfaction score] × 100). PCEA use was associated with significantly better patient satisfaction. (From Gambling DR, McMorland GH, Yu P, Laszlo C. Comparison of patient-controlled epidural analgesia and conventional intermittent "top-up" injections during labor. Anesth Analg 1990: 70:256-61.)

fibers that enter the cord at S2 to S4. These somatic nerve fibers are larger than the visceral afferent nerve fibers that transmit the pain of the first stage of labor. Blockade of these nerve fibers may require a more concentrated solution and/or a greater volume of local anesthetic than is required during the first stage of labor[171]; this often creates a dilemma for the anesthesiologist. Administration of a more concentrated solution of local anesthetic results in more intense motor block at a time when maternal expulsive efforts are helpful.

The continuous epidural infusion of bupivacaine often results in the gradual development of sacral analgesia. Likewise, several epidural injections of 0.25% bupivacaine (given every 60 to 90 minutes) may result in sacral analgesia.[151] If analgesia is not adequate for the second stage of labor, the anesthesiologist can give additional doses of local anesthetic to augment perineal analgesia (Box 21-7). Some anesthesiologists contend that the use of the sitting position helps facilitate the onset of perineal analgesia. Published studies suggest that maternal position does not consistently affect the spread of local anesthetic in the epidural space[172-174]; rather, the administration of a larger volume of local anesthetic solution facilitates the onset of sacral analgesia.[175] Unfortunately, this also results in a higher (i.e., more cephalad) sensory level of analgesia, and the patient should be observed for evidence of hemodynamic or respiratory compromise.

Dense anesthesia is often required for delivery, especially if the obstetrician performs an episiotomy or a forceps or vacuum-extraction delivery. After administration of a test dose, we give 5 to 15 mL of 1% to 2% lidocaine or 2% to 3% 2-chloroprocaine. We inject this "delivery dose" when the fetal head is visible on the perineum during pushing or when the obstetrician has decided to proceed with instrumental delivery. The anesthesiologist should monitor the maternal blood pressure carefully, especially if excessive blood loss occurs in a patient with extensive anesthesia.

Occasionally a parturient will tolerate the pain of labor until late in the first stage (i.e., more than 8 cm cervical dilation) and then request analgesia. Advanced labor does not preclude the placement of a lumbar epidural catheter, especially in a nulliparous woman. A nulliparous parturient may have a second stage of labor that lasts 2 to 3 hours. Another option is to administer **combined spinal-epidural (CSE)** analgesia. A long spinal needle is placed through a properly sited epidural needle, a small dose of local anesthetic (e.g., bupivacaine 2.5 mg, with or without an opioid) is injected, the spinal needle is removed, and an epidural catheter is placed.[176] The advantages of this technique are that it provides a rapid onset of spinal analgesia with sacral coverage for advanced labor, and it includes the placement of an epidural catheter

for use if the extent or duration of the spinal analgesia is inadequate. One disadvantage is that testing for possible subarachnoid placement cannot be done until the intrathecal analgesia subsides. For this reason, we do not advocate the CSE technique in parturients with morbid obesity, a potentially difficult airway, or a nonreassuring FHR pattern. In these women, it is essential to verify catheter position at the time of placement to avoid the risks of general anesthesia for urgent cesarean section.

A **caudal epidural** catheter, which facilitates the onset of sacral analgesia, is an option for analgesia late in labor. Caudal analgesia was the first form of regional analgesia used during labor.[177] However, caudal analgesia is used infrequently in modern obstetric anesthesia practice. Disadvantages of this technique include the following: (1) increased technical difficulty; (2) increased local anesthetic dose requirement during the first stage; and (3) the risk of injecting the local anesthetic into the fetus.[178] Anatomic variations of the caudal canal decrease the rate of success for caudal analgesia during labor (an 8% failure rate).[179] Because of the risk of fetal toxicity from direct injection of local anesthetic into the fetal scalp, some physicians recommend the performance of a rectal examination to ensure that the needle has been sited correctly within the caudal epidural space. A test dose must be administered to exclude intravenous or subarachnoid placement of the caudal needle or catheter. Sacral analgesia adequate for labor and delivery can be achieved with an injection of 12 to 15 mL of 0.25% bupivacaine, 1.0% to 1.5% lidocaine, or 2% 2-chloroprocaine.

Some anesthesiologists favor the **double-catheter** technique for selected patients. A lumbar epidural catheter can be used to provide analgesia during the first stage of labor, followed by the use of a caudal epidural catheter to provide analgesia during the second stage. Ideally the lumbar epidural catheter should be placed at the first or second lumbar interspace; this increases the likelihood of providing a true **segmental block** during the first stage of labor. This technique is most useful in cases in which an extensive sympathectomy (e.g., aortic stenosis, primary pulmonary hypertension) must be avoided. Moreover, some anesthesiologists favor this technique in cases in which a rapid onset of sacral analgesia may be required (e.g., breech presentation, multiple gestation).

SPINAL ANALGESIA/ANESTHESIA

In most cases, a single-shot subarachnoid injection of local anesthetic is not suitable for the first stage of labor. A single-shot injection has a finite duration, and multiple injections result in an increased risk of postdural puncture headache (PDPH). Alternatively, a single subarachnoid injection of an opioid may be appropriate (see Section II of this chapter).

Placement of a catheter in the subarachnoid space allows the anesthesiologist to administer continuous spinal analgesia/anesthesia by intermittent bolus injection or continuous infusion of a local anesthetic. This technique has been described for use in patients in whom placement of an epidural catheter is problematic (e.g., in patients with morbid obesity or abnormal vertebral anatomy, such as kyphoscoliosis).[180,181] Early reports of this technique described the use of a standard epidural catheter placed through an 18- or 19-gauge needle.[182] Very small (e.g., 28- to 32-gauge) catheters were developed for insertion through small (e.g., 22- to 26-gauge) spinal needles. Unfortunately, several cases of **cauda equina syndrome** (associated with the use of spinal microcatheters during

---

Box 21-7 ANESTHESIA FOR VAGINAL DELIVERY

- Lumbar epidural catheter in place: Supplemental anesthesia with 5 to 15 mL of 1%-2% lidocaine or 2%-3% 2-chloroprocaine
- Caudal epidural catheter in place: Supplemental anesthesia with 12 to 15 mL of 1%-2% lidocaine or 2%-3% 2-chloroprocaine
- Spinal anesthesia: Intrathecal injection of 25 to 50 mg of hyperbaric lidocaine, 4 to 6 mg hyperbaric tetracaine, or 6 to 8 mg hyperbaric bupivacaine (a larger dose is given if the obstetrician plans a "trial of forceps," in which case cesarean delivery may be necessary)
- Combined spinal-epidural anesthesia: Intrathecal injection of 2.5 to 5 mg bupivacaine followed by placement of an epidural catheter for use if the spinal anesthesia is insufficient

surgery in nonpregnant patients) prompted the Food and Drug Administration to remove these microcatheters from the market.[183] The etiology of these neurologic deficits is unclear. Some anesthesiologists have suggested that neurologic injury results from the maldistribution of local anesthetic within the subarachnoid space.[183] The very slow rate of injection through a caudally directed microcatheter may lead to the pooling of local anesthetic solution in the terminal part of the dural sac. If the local anesthetic solution is hyperbaric, the neighboring elements of the cauda equina experience prolonged exposure to a high concentration of local anesthetic and a hyperglycemic, hyperosmotic marinade (e.g., 550 to 800 mOsm). Permanent neural damage may occur from the combination of tissue dehydration and a toxic concentration of local anesthetic. It is unclear whether this complication is unique to the use of microcatheters.

Early clinical studies have suggested that the subarachnoid injection of 1.0 mL of 1.0% lidocaine[184] or 0.5 to 1.5 mL of 0.25% bupivacaine[185,186] provides satisfactory analgesia for labor. Analgesia can be maintained with **intermittent injections** of 1.0% lidocaine[184] or 0.25% bupivacaine or with a **continuous infusion** of 0.125% bupivacaine at a rate of 1.5 mL/hr.[185] At the University of Michigan, we administer our standard epidural solution (0.05% bupivacaine plus fentanyl 3 µg/mL) at an initial rate of 3 mL/hour and titrate the rate of infusion to the individual patient's needs. Low doses (e.g., 0.2 to 0.5 mL) of hyperbaric solution (e.g., 0.75% bupivacaine or 5% lidocaine) have also been used to provide continuous spinal analgesia during labor.[182,186] Patient-controlled spinal analgesia for labor has been described.[187] If intrathecal local anesthetics are used for intrapartum analgesia, the sensory level and the intensity of motor block should be monitored. Moreover, the anesthesiologist must be prepared to treat hypotension and other complications associated with high spinal anesthesia.

The anesthesiologist may give single-shot spinal anesthesia for vaginal delivery in a patient who does not have epidural anesthesia and who requires perineal anesthesia. A "saddle block" can be administered to achieve blockade of the sacral spinal segments; a small dose of a hyperbaric local anesthetic solution is adequate for this purpose (Box 21-7). A saddle block may be advantageous in the patient with a preterm fetus or a vaginal breech presentation. In these cases, dense perineal relaxation may facilitate an atraumatic vaginal delivery. A saddle block also provides excellent anesthesia for an outlet/low forceps delivery. A higher level (T10) of anesthesia often is required for a midforceps delivery. Unlike what occurs with epidural anesthesia, patient position for this type of delivery significantly affects the intrathecal spread of a hyperbaric solution of local anesthetic. We administer the block with the patient in the sitting position to promote caudad spread of the hyperbaric local anesthetic, and we administer the local anesthetic immediately after a uterine contraction to decrease the likelihood of an unexpected high block. The anesthesiologist should determine and record the sensory level and should be prepared to manage the unexpected case of high spinal anesthesia.

Clear communication between the obstetrician and anesthesiologist is essential. If the obstetrician is certain that the application of forceps (or vacuum extraction) will result in a successful delivery, a saddle block will likely provide satisfactory anesthesia. However, in some cases, the obstetrician will perform a trial of forceps. We alter our technique when giving spinal anesthesia for a trial of forceps. If the trial fails, cesarean delivery follows. In some cases, we give a dose of local anesthetic appropriate for cesarean delivery (e.g., 1.6 mL of hyperbaric 0.75% bupivacaine). Alternatively, a saddle block can be administered using the CSE technique. If spinal anesthesia is inadequate for the planned procedure, additional local anesthetic can be given through the epidural catheter.

COMPLICATIONS

Hypotension

With the onset of sympathetic blockade, peripheral venodilation and increased venous capacitance result in decreased venous return to the heart, which may result in decreased maternal blood pressure and cardiac output. *Hypotension* is often defined as a 20% to 30% decrease in systolic blood pressure (as compared with baseline) or a systolic blood pressure of less than 100 mm Hg. Without prophylactic hydration, the epidural administration of 4 to 6 mL of 0.5% bupivacaine results in hypotension in approximately 17% of laboring women.[188] Modest hypotension rarely results in adverse consequences in young, nonpregnant patients. However, during pregnancy, uteroplacental perfusion depends on the maintenance of normal maternal blood pressure. Uncorrected hypotension results in decreased uteroplacental perfusion. If hypotension is severe and prolonged, hypoxia and acidosis will develop in the fetus.[188]

The prevention of hypotension includes volume expansion before the induction of epidural analgesia and avoidance of aortocaval compression. Treatment includes the administration of additional intravenous crystalloid, the placement of the mother in the full lateral (and Trendelenburg) position, and the administration of supplemental oxygen. If these measures do not result in the prompt restoration of blood pressure or if hypotension is severe, the anesthesiologist should give 5 to 10 mg of ephedrine intravenously.[189-192] The FHR is monitored continuously. Ephedrine crosses the placenta and may cause an increase in FHR and an increase in FHR variability (e.g., saltatory FHR pattern).[193,194]

Inadequate Analgesia

The failure rate for epidural analgesia ranges from 1.5% to 5.0%, depending on the skill of the anesthesiologist.[179,188,195] Successful location of the epidural space is not always possible, and satisfactory analgesia does not always occur, even when the epidural space has been identified correctly. Patient factors (e.g., obesity, abnormal lumbar spine anatomy, depth of the epidural space[196]) increase the likelihood of an unsatisfactory result. Unfortunately, failure to provide adequate analgesia not only results in a dissatisfying experience for the patient but also may result in litigation.[197] The risk of failed anesthesia and the potential need to place a second epidural catheter should be discussed with the patient during the preanesthetic evaluation, before placement of the first epidural catheter.

Typically, small doses of local anesthetic are used for epidural analgesia during labor; thus the resulting block may be asymmetric or have missed segments (Box 21-8). Crawford[195] observed this complication in 15.4% of patients who received 8 mL of 0.25% bupivacaine. An advantage of using a dilute solution of local anesthetic is the ability to increase the volume administered to ensure adequate analgesic spread. Maternal position has only a small effect on the development of an asymmetric block.[198,199] Husemeyer and White[199] gave 10 mL of 1.5% lidocaine epidurally to pregnant women who were in the lateral position; they observed only a slightly greater spread (two to three spinal segments) of anesthesia on the dependent side. Others have observed that posture has little influence on the spread of local anesthetic within the epidural space.[173,200] It is likely that the position of the epidural catheter in relation to other epidural space structures (e.g., connective tissue, fatty tissue, blood vessels) affects the spread and quality of analgesia. Anatomic barriers (e.g., a longitudinal connective tissue band between the dura and ligamentum flavum) or placement of the catheter tip in the anterior epidural space or paravertebral space may explain some cases of single nerve root, unilateral, or asymmetric block.[201-204]

The type of epidural catheter used, choice of air versus saline for loss of resistance, and the depth of placement in the epidural space may affect the rate of success. The rate of satisfactory, symmetric epidural block is higher with multi-orifice catheters than with single-orifice catheters.[205] (In theory, a disadvantage of the multi-orifice catheter is that the orifices may be in different locations. For example, one orifice may be within the epidural space when another is within an epidural vein.[206]) Use of air for loss of resistance may result in air bubbles in the epidural space, which may adversely affect the quality of analgesia.[207,208] Shallow placement (i.e., 2 cm for single-orifice catheters[209] and 3 cm for multi-orifice catheters[210]) increases the likelihood of block failure as a result of movement of the catheter outside of the epidural space. Relatively deep placement (i.e., 7 to 8 cm for either type of catheter) increases the chance of intravenous placement.[209,210]

If epidural analgesia during labor is unilateral or asymmetric, the administration of a large volume of a dilute solution (e.g., 10 mL of 0.0625% to 0.125% bupivacaine) may result in a symmetric block. Moreover, withdrawal of the catheter 0.5 to 1 cm, followed by the administration of additional local anesthetic, may result in a more satisfactory spread of local anesthetic. However, the anesthesiologist should always consider the replacement of the epidural catheter in patients with unsatisfactory epidural analgesia.

Pain often becomes more intense as labor progresses. An epidural block that was adequate at 4 cm cervical dilation may not be adequate at 8 cm cervical dilation. The anesthesiologist should be aware of the progress of the patient's labor when assessing an inadequate block. The patient may need a larger dose of local anesthetic; a 5- to 10-mL bolus of 0.125% or 0.25%

Box 21-8 MANAGING AN INADEQUATE EPIDURAL BLOCK

1. Perform an honest evaluation of the anesthetic:
   - Is the catheter really in the epidural space?
   - If in doubt, replace the catheter.
2. If the catheter is in the epidural space but the block is asymmetric:
   - Withdraw the catheter 0.5-1.0 cm, place the less-blocked side in the dependent position, and increase the volume (and decrease the concentration) of local anesthetic.
   - If these maneuvers are unsuccessful, replace the catheter.
3. If the catheter is in the epidural space but the patient feels pain because of a change in the nature of her labor:
   - Ask the obstetrician to evaluate the progress of labor.
   - Check for bladder distention.
   - Increase the volume and/or concentration of local anesthetic, or add an opioid to the solution of local anesthetic.
   - Do not use an opioid to cover up a misplaced catheter.

---

bupivacaine is often adequate. Alternatively, an opioid may be added to the solution of local anesthetic (see Section II of this chapter). This is especially helpful if the patient is experiencing back pain because the fetus is in the occiput posterior position. Inadequate analgesia may result from migration of the epidural catheter into a vein or movement of the catheter outside of the epidural space.[211] Before giving a bolus dose of local anesthetic, the anesthesiologist should give a test dose to exclude intravenous migration of the catheter. The response to the bolus dose should be assessed, and the catheter should be replaced (with the patient's consent) if no block is obtained.

Intravascular Injection of Local Anesthetic

The incidence of fatal systemic toxic reactions to local anesthetics apparently has declined since 1984.[22] Nonetheless, systemic toxicity remains a serious potential complication during the administration of epidural anesthesia in obstetric patients. Chadwick[197] noted that maternal convulsions (as a result of the unintentional intravascular injection of local anesthetic) were the single most common untoward event in obstetric-anesthesia–related malpractice claims (see Chapter 29). Convulsions resulted in serious damage to the mother or newborn in 74% of cases.

Intravenous injection of a large dose of local anesthetic causes CNS symptoms (e.g., restlessness, dizziness, tinnitus, perioral paresthesia, difficulty speaking, seizures, loss of consciousness). Cardiovascular effects may progress from increased blood pressure (as a result of sympathetic stimulation) to bradycardia, depressed ventricular function, and ventricular tachycardia and fibrillation. Bupivacaine cardiotoxicity may be fatal in pregnant women[66] (see Chapter 12). Factors that increase the risk of local anesthetic toxicity in pregnant women include the following: (1) the frequent use of bupivacaine in this population; (2) a decreased maternal concentration of plasma proteins (e.g., alpha-1-acid glycoprotein), which results in a higher free concentration of local anesthetic[212]; (3) more frequent cannulation of an epidural vein in obstetric patients[63,64,213]; (4) the rapid onset of hypoxemia during hypoventilation or apnea; and (5) the technical difficulty associated with the administration of effective cardiopulmonary resuscitation in pregnant women.[214,215]

Box 21-9 lists guidelines for the management of the unintentional intravascular injection of local anesthetic. In the past, bretylium was recommended for the treatment of bupivacaine-induced ventricular arrhythmias.[216] However, the world's natural supply of bretylium is nearly exhausted,[217] and the drug is no longer available; it has been deleted from the Advanced Cardiovascular Life Support (ACLS) algorithm for ventricular fibrillation/pulseless ventricular tachycardia. Currently there are no specific guidelines for the pharmacologic treatment of bupivacaine cardiotoxicity in parturients. Amiodarone is listed as the preferred antiarrhythmic agent in the most current ACLS algorithm, and it now seems to be the drug of choice for the treatment of bupivacaine-induced ventricular arrhythmias.

Unintentional Dural Puncture

The incidence of unintentional dural puncture during attempted identification of the epidural space ranges from less than 1.0% to 7.6% in obstetric patients.[5,195,218] The incidence depends in part on the skill of the anesthesiologist.[5,195] Crawford[5,195] observed an incidence of 13% if the anesthesiologist had performed fewer than 10 epidural blocks, 6% if

Box 21-9 MANAGEMENT OF UNINTENTIONAL INTRAVENOUS INJECTION OF LOCAL ANESTHETIC

- Be aware that hypoxemia and acidosis develop rapidly during convulsions. Stop convulsions with a barbiturate or benzodiazepine and/or succinylcholine.
- Administer 100% oxygen to maintain maternal oxygenation. Use positive-pressure ventilation if necessary. Tracheal intubation will facilitate ventilation and help protect the airway, but the administration of oxygen before intubation should not be delayed.
- Monitor maternal blood pressure, electrocardiogram, and fetal heart rate.
- Support blood pressure with intravenous fluids and vasopressors.
- Provide cardiopulmonary resuscitation if necessary. Delivery of the fetus may facilitate successful resuscitation of the mother.
- Treat bradycardia with atropine. Treat ventricular tachycardia and ventricular fibrillation per Advanced Cardiovascular Life Support (ACLS) guidelines.
- Prevent maternal respiratory and metabolic acidosis.

the anesthesiologist had performed 10 to 49 blocks, 2% if the anesthesiologist had performed 60 blocks, and 1.2% if the anesthesiologist had performed more than 100 blocks. Dural puncture may be detected at the time of insertion of the epidural needle or after placement of the catheter. If dural puncture is detected with the epidural needle, the anesthesiologist can remove the needle and place an epidural catheter at another interspace. Local anesthetic (injected epidurally) may pass through the dural puncture site and into the subarachnoid space, which will result in an unexpected high block.[62] One advantage to the placement of an epidural catheter after unintentional dural puncture is that saline or blood can be injected through the epidural catheter to prevent a PDPH (see Chapter 32). However, some anesthesiologists question the wisdom of performing a prophylactic epidural blood patch through an epidural catheter placed earlier during labor.

Another option for the management of unintentional dural puncture is the placement of a catheter in the subarachnoid space and the administration of continuous spinal analgesia for labor and delivery. We reserve this technique for patients at high risk for repeat dural puncture or in cases in which it may be difficult to enter either the epidural or subarachnoid space successfully at an alternative interspace (e.g., in obese women or in patients with abnormal anatomy of the lumbar spine). It is important to include a label that clearly identifies this catheter as a spinal catheter to decrease the likelihood of injecting an epidural dose of local anesthetic into the subarachnoid space. Most evidence suggests that the introduction of a subarachnoid catheter and the administration of continuous spinal analgesia do *not* decrease the likelihood of PDPH in obstetric patients.[186,219,220]

If dural puncture is not recognized until CSF is aspirated from the catheter or if administration of the test dose results in spinal anesthesia, the anesthesiologist has two options: (1) the placement of an epidural catheter at an alternative interspace, or (2) the administration of continuous spinal anesthesia through the existing catheter.

Unexpected High Block

An unexpected high level of anesthesia may result from one of two situations. First, a high (or total) spinal block results after the unintentional placement of the catheter in either the subarachnoid or subdural space, followed by the injection of an epidural dose of local anesthetic through that catheter. Second, the epidural catheter may migrate into the subarachnoid or subdural space during the course of labor and delivery. Crawford[62] reported six cases of high or total spinal block in a series of nearly 27,000 cases of lumbar epidural anesthesia administered during labor (an incidence of approximately 1 in 4500). Paech et al.[221] reported eight cases of unexpectedly high block in a series of 10,995 epidural blocks in obstetric patients (an incidence of approximately 1 in 1400). Two patients required intubation and mechanical ventilation.

Aspiration alone is an inadequate method of excluding subarachnoid placement of the catheter.[53] Administration of an appropriate test dose and careful assessment of the patient's response to the test dose should minimize the chance of unintentional injection of a large dose of local anesthetic into the subarachnoid space.

High or total spinal anesthesia results in hypotension, dyspnea, the inability to speak, and loss of consciousness. Evidence of spinal anesthesia may be apparent shortly after intrathecal injection of a local anesthetic, but the maximal spread may not be evident for several minutes. This underscores the need for the anesthesiologist to carefully assess the effects of both the test and therapeutic doses on the mother and fetus.[222] If total spinal anesthesia should occur, the anesthesiologist must be prepared to maintain oxygenation, ventilation, and circulation (Box 21-10). Immediate management includes avoidance of aortocaval compression, ventilation with 100% oxygen, endotracheal intubation, and administration of intravenous fluids and ephedrine to support the blood pressure as needed. The FHR should be monitored continuously.

A high block may also result from **subdural injection** of a local anesthetic.[222-225] The subdural space is the potential space between the dura mater and the arachnoid mater. A retrospective review of 2182 epidural catheters placed in nonobstetric patients demonstrated that the clinical signs of subdural catheter placement occurred in approximately 0.82% of patients.[223] Subdural injection of local anesthetic typically results in an unexpectedly high (but patchy) block with an onset time that is intermediate between spinal and epidural anesthesia (i.e., 10 to 20 minutes). Cranial spread is more extensive than caudal spread of the local anesthetic; thus sacral analgesia typically is absent. The block may involve the cranial nerves. (The subdural space, unlike the epidural space, extends intracranially.) Thus apnea and unconsciousness can occur during a subdural block. A subdural block results in less-intense motor block than that which occurs with high or

Box 21-10 MANAGEMENT OF TOTAL SPINAL ANESTHESIA

- High spinal anesthesia may occur several minutes after an epidural injection of local anesthetic. Communicate with the patient. Agitation, dyspnea, and difficulty speaking may herald the onset of total spinal anesthesia.
- Avoid aortocaval compression.
- Administer 100% oxygen to the mother.
- Provide positive-pressure ventilation, preferably through an endotracheal tube.
- Monitor maternal blood pressure, electrocardiogram, and fetal heart rate.
- Support maternal circulation with intravenous fluids and ephedrine as needed. Do not hesitate to give epinephrine, if needed.

total spinal anesthesia.[224] This may reflect the limited spread of the local anesthetic within the subdural space, which helps spare the anterior motor fibers.[226] Subdural block results in less severe hypotension than that which occurs with high or total spinal anesthesia, most likely because subdural injection results in a slower onset of anesthesia (Table 21-4). The unpredictable spread of local anesthetic, the delayed onset of maximal spread (as compared with spinal anesthesia), the patchy nature of the block, and the sacral sparing make it difficult to use a subdural catheter safely during labor and delivery. If we suspect that a catheter is positioned within the subdural space, we replace it with an epidural catheter.

An unexpected high block may result from the migration of an epidural catheter into the subdural or subarachnoid space.[226] It is unclear how a soft epidural catheter can penetrate the dura. Disposable epidural needles are sharp, and insertion of the needle into the epidural space may result in an unrecognized nick in the dura, which may represent a site for delayed migration of the catheter into the subdural or subarachnoid space. Subdural or subarachnoid injection of local anesthetic also may occur if a multi-orifice catheter is used and one orifice is located within the epidural space while another is located within the subdural or subarachnoid space. In this situation, the force of injection determines the ultimate destination of the local anesthetic.

During the continuous infusion of a local anesthetic, a gradual increase in the level of anesthesia and intensity of motor block may herald the subarachnoid infusion of the local anesthetic solution. When the anesthesiologist gives a bolus dose of local anesthetic, the response should be compared with the patient's response to earlier bolus doses.

Extensive Motor Block

Clinically significant motor block may occur after repeated bolus doses[151] or after many hours of a continuous infusion[227] of epidural bupivacaine. The administration of bupivacaine with epinephrine results in a greater likelihood of dense motor block than the administration of bupivacaine alone.[151] Extensive motor block is often bothersome for the patient,[228] and it may impair maternal expulsive efforts during the second stage of labor and increase the likelihood of instrumental vaginal delivery (see Section III of this chapter). Some obstet-ricians argue that pelvic floor relaxation prevents internal rotation of the fetal head and increases the likelihood of an abnormal position of the vertex at delivery. In addition, some anesthesiologists contend that motor block increases the likelihood that the mother will assume an unnatural position, which may increase the risk of postpartum back pain.[229,230]

If intense motor blockade develops during the continuous epidural infusion of a local anesthetic, the infusion can be discontinued for a short period (e.g., 30 minutes). Subsequently, the infusion can be restarted at a reduced rate or with a more dilute solution of local anesthetic. Extensive motor blockade does not occur when a very dilute solution of local anesthetic in combination with an opioid is administered.

Urinary Retention

Urinary retention may occur during labor, and it may be difficult for a laboring woman to feel the urge to void or to coordinate urination during the administration of epidural analgesia. Nurses and physicians should observe for evidence of a distended bladder, especially if the patient complains of suprapubic pain during a contraction. The patient's inability to void and bladder distention should prompt catheterization to empty the bladder.

Urinary retention may also occur after vaginal delivery, with or without epidural analgesia. Grove[231] observed some degree of bladder dysfunction in 14.2% of women who had a normal delivery and in 37.5% of women who underwent instrumental vaginal delivery, all without epidural analgesia. Crawford[5] evaluated the incidence of urinary retention in a population of women who had received epidural analgesia with bupivacaine 0.25% to 0.5% with epinephrine for labor and delivery; this complication was observed in 6.8% of women who had undergone spontaneous vaginal delivery and in 17.3% of women who had undergone instrumental vaginal delivery. A more recent study of postpartum urinary retention in a large series of patients (n = 3364) who received either bupivacaine 0.25% with epinephrine 1:200,000 or bupivacaine 0.125% with 10 μg sufentanil noted a lower incidence of this complication (0.9%).[232] Although the use of epidural analgesia was not randomized, a higher incidence of urinary retention was found among those women who received epidural analgesia (2.7%) as compared with those who did not (0.1%).

TABLE 21-4	CLINICAL FEATURES OF EPIDURAL, SUBDURAL, AND SPINAL BLOCKS		
	Epidural block	**Subdural block**	**Spinal block**
Onset time	Slow	Intermediate	Rapid
Spread	As expected	Higher than expected; may extend intracranially, but sacral sparing is common	Higher than expected; may extend intracranially, and a sacral block is typically present
Nature of block	Segmental	Patchy	Dense
Motor block	Minimal	Minimal	Dense
Hypotension	Less than spinal, and dependent on the extent of the block	Intermediate between spinal and epidural, and dependent on the extent of the block	Likely

The role of epidural analgesia in the etiology of postpartum urinary retention is unclear. Obstetric factors (e.g., long labor, edema, instrumental delivery, perineal trauma, hematoma, pain) may predispose women to difficulty with voiding.[233] Some of these factors are also indications for the use of epidural analgesia, which may result in selection bias. Dense or prolonged epidural anesthesia suppresses the urge to void. Postpartum patients should be observed for urinary retention. A prolonged inability to void mandates catheterization of the bladder to prevent overdistention.

Unexpected Prolonged Block

Rarely the duration of epidural anesthesia exceeds the time expected. Most cases of unexpected prolonged block follow the epidural administration of a high concentration of local anesthetic with epinephrine.[234] Abnormal neurologic findings after the administration of epidural anesthesia should prompt the anesthesiologist to look for evidence of peripheral nerve injury or an epidural hematoma or abscess (see Chapter 33). Factors that argue against the presence of an epidural hematoma or abscess include the following: (1) the absence of back pain; (2) a unilateral block; and (3) regression (rather than progression) of the symptoms. Peripheral nerve injuries typically result in a neurologic deficit in the distribution of a specific peripheral nerve. Neurologic or neurosurgical consultation should be obtained if there is any question about the etiology of a prolonged block. Avoiding the use of a high concentration of local anesthetic should help minimize the incidence of this side effect during and after labor and vaginal delivery.

Back Pain

Back pain is a common complaint during pregnancy and the puerperium, and it often results from the exaggerated lumbar lordosis of pregnancy. However, other factors may predispose a woman to backache after delivery. Grove[231] observed back pain in 40% of women who had had a spontaneous vaginal delivery and 25% of women who had undergone instrumental vaginal delivery, all without epidural analgesia. Other studies have reported the occurrence of postpartum backache in 3% to 45% of women who received epidural analgesia for labor and delivery.[195,218] Factors proposed to increase the risk of postpartum backache after the administration of epidural analgesia include the following: (1) the use of a large needle; (2) supraspinous ligament hematoma; (3) difficult identification of the epidural space; (4) prolonged assumption of an unnatural position during labor and delivery; and (5) sacroiliac strain as a result of moving the lower extremities before resolution of anesthesia.[62,179,230]

MacArthur et al.[229,230] have suggested that the administration of epidural analgesia increases the risk of postpartum back pain. Data collected from a retrospective review of 11,701 case records and patient questionnaires (mailed 1 to 9 years after delivery) demonstrated a significant association between the use of intrapartum epidural analgesia and persistent, postpartum back pain (epidural analgesia, 19%; no epidural analgesia, 11%). The excess back pain associated with epidural analgesia was unaffected by the mode of delivery, but an increased incidence of back pain occurred only among those women who had experienced labor. The authors suggested the following[229]:

The backache is not solely a consequence of epidural anaesthesia but is probably due to a combination of muscular relaxation and postural stress in labour. The problem now is to determine in precise detail the mechanisms that result in backache and to refine the management of epidural anaesthesia in labour.

This retrospective study suffers not only from patient **recall bias** (i.e., patients with a problem are much more likely to complete and return the questionnaire) but also from **selection bias** in the epidural and nonepidural groups. Patients who select epidural analgesia for labor may have obstetric, orthopedic, social, or other unidentified factors that predispose them to postpartum back pain. In addition, details of anesthetic management were not described in either article. If large doses of a concentrated solution of local anesthetic were used, motor block and analgesia may have allowed women to adopt positions that predisposed them to back strain.

In an attempt to assess anesthetic factors that might contribute to postpartum backache, Russell et al.[235] randomly assigned laboring women requesting epidural analgesia to receive either bupivacaine alone or bupivacaine plus an opioid. Despite the expected differences in motor block, the incidence of backache did not differ between the two anesthetic groups (bupivacaine alone, 39%; bupivacaine plus opioid, 30%). In addition, the incidence of backache in both epidural groups was similar to that found in a nonrandomized control group of women who labored without epidural analgesia (31%). Antepartum backache predicted the occurrence of postpartum backache.[235]

All prospective reports have failed to show a significant relationship between the use of epidural analgesia and long-term backache. Breen et al.[236] observed no difference in the incidence of postpartum backache among women who delivered vaginally with or without epidural analgesia. Factors that predicted postpartum backache included a history of back pain and greater body weight. A Canadian study evaluated patients after delivery and assessed the presence of postpartum backache as a function of patient-selected intrapartum analgesia.[237] The rate of low back pain was greater in the epidural group (53%) than in the nonepidural group (43%) on only the first postpartum day. The rates were similar on postpartum day 7 and at 6 weeks. These authors suggested that the increased incidence of backache immediately after delivery may have resulted from tissue trauma during needle placement. A follow-up study of the same patients 1 year after delivery revealed a similar rate of backache among the epidural and nonepidural patients.[238] Similarly, more recent studies have observed no difference in the incidence of long-term backache between women who received epidural analgesia and those who received alternative forms of pain relief.[239,240]

In summary, these prospective studies have consistently shown that no causal relationship exists between the use of epidural analgesia and the development of long-term postpartum backache.

Pelvic Floor Injury

Few studies have evaluated the possible effects of epidural analgesia on postpartum pelvic floor function. Sartore et al.[241] observed no significant difference in the incidence of stress urinary incontinence, anal incontinence, or vaginal prolapse 3 months after vaginal delivery in 140 primiparous women who either did or did not receive epidural analgesia. The authors matched these women according to several factors, including duration of labor and method of delivery. Any factor that might increase the likelihood of instrumental vaginal delivery might be expected to increase the risk of pelvic floor injury and subsequent pelvic floor dysfunction (see Section III of this chapter). However, to our knowledge, there is no evidence that epidural analgesia per se predisposes to pelvic floor injury. Further studies—with longer periods of follow-up—would be of interest to both physicians and patients.

OTHER EFFECTS OF EPIDURAL ANALGESIA FOR LABOR

Neonatal Outcome

Thalme et al.[242] observed that newborns whose mothers received epidural analgesia had higher pH measurements and less metabolic acidosis in the first hour of life as compared with newborns whose mothers received systemic opioid analgesia. Pello et al.[101] observed similar umbilical arterial blood pH and base deficit measurements in the newborns of mothers who did and did not receive epidural analgesia (Figure 21-9). Contemporary studies have demonstrated no difference in neonatal outcome (as assessed by Apgar scores and umbilical cord blood pH measurements) among infants of mothers who were randomized to receive either epidural bupivacaine or systemic meperidine[3,7]; however, maternal analgesia in these two groups was not equivalent. Sharma et al.[243] randomized patients to receive either epidural analgesia or patient-controlled analgesia (PCA) with intravenous meperidine. These authors used PCA in an effort to achieve analgesia similar to that provided by epidural analgesia. Some infants in the PCA meperidine group required the reversal of neonatal respiratory depression with naloxone, but other indices of newborn outcome (Apgar scores and umbilical cord blood pH measurements) were similar.[243]

Reynolds et al.[244] recently performed a meta-analysis of studies comparing epidural analgesia versus systemic opioid analgesia, in which umbilical cord blood gas analysis was performed at delivery. Fetal base excess, the most specific index of the metabolic component of fetal acid-base balance, was higher in the epidural group than in the control group. The authors concluded the following:

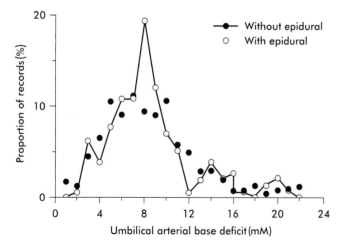

FIGURE 21-9. Distribution of umbilical arterial base deficit values in the newborns of mothers who did ($n = 240$) and did not ($n = 154$) receive epidural analgesia for labor. No differences existed between the two groups. (From Pello LC, Rosevear SK, Dawes GS, et al. Computerized fetal heart rate analysis in labor. Obstet Gynecol 1991; 78:602-10.)

Expectant mothers can be reassured that, although epidural analgesia may be associated with some short term maternal side effects, it does not exacerbate fetal acidosis, and if anything, may partially protect the fetus from fetal hypoxia. It is important to dispel the notion that epidural analgesia is in some way harmful to babies.

Tests of neonatal neurobehavior after exposure to various methods of maternal analgesia have produced conflicting results. Using the Early Neonatal Neurobehavior Scale, Scanlon et al.[132] reported lower scores among newborns whose mothers received either epidural mepivacaine or lidocaine as compared with newborns whose mothers received no analgesia. Abboud et al.[95] observed no significant difference in the Early Neonatal Neurobehavior Scale scores among newborns whose mothers received epidural bupivacaine, lidocaine, 2-chloroprocaine, or no analgesia. Thorp et al.[7] assessed labor outcome after the maternal administration of either intravenous meperidine or epidural bupivacaine. They did not observe any difference between groups in neonatal Neurologic and Adaptive Capacity Scores at 2 and 24 hours after delivery.[7] The Neurologic and Adaptive Capacity Scores assessment was intended to discriminate between neonatal asphyxia and drug effects but has been found to be unreliable.[245] Other studies have demonstrated better neurobehavioral performance among the newborns of mothers who received regional analgesia as compared with infants whose mothers received systemic opioids or general anesthesia.[246,247]

Body Temperature Changes

Epidural analgesia can affect maternal body temperature. When epidural analgesia is established, a decrease in maternal core temperature results from heat redistribution from the core to the relatively cool periphery and may cause thermoregulatory shivering.[248] Some clinical studies have not found an association between core temperature and shivering during epidural analgesia,[249] most likely because many other factors may affect the shivering response. Skin temperature increases during epidural anesthesia,[248] which may suppress shivering during hypothermia.[250] The addition of an opioid to the local anesthetic solution also affects the shivering response.[251-253] At least one study has suggested that the epidural administration of epinephrine increases shivering[251]; the etiology of this response is unknown. Some[251,254]—but not all[255]—studies have suggested that the temperature of the epidural injectate affects the incidence of shivering, perhaps through the stimulation of spinal cord thermoreceptors. However, the epidural injection of large volumes of cold saline does not trigger shivering in volunteers.[256]

Clinical studies have noted a gradual increase in core temperature over several hours in laboring women receiving epidural anesthesia, which was not observed in women receiving no analgesia, inhaled nitrous oxide, or parenteral opioids.[257-259] The increase in core temperature typically is small (less than 1.0° C, with a maximum temperature of approximately 38° C) and is greatest in women who labor in rooms with relatively warm ambient temperatures (i.e., 23 to 29° C).[258] In a retrospective study, Herbst et al.[260] identified the use of epidural analgesia as a risk factor for intrapartum fever, along with prolonged labor and a prolonged interval from rupture of membranes to delivery. There are several reasons why temperatures may be higher in women who receive epidural analgesia. These women already may have had a longer labor and may therefore be at higher risk for infection, such as chorioamnionitis; thus the lack of randomization to analgesic technique in some of these reports introduces the potential for selection bias. Alternatively, epidural analgesia may alter maternal temperature regulation; thus a greater core temperature is "tolerated" in the presence of an epidural block. In volunteer subjects, epidural analgesia increases the threshold for thermoregulatory sweating and, presumably by means of sympathectomy, it can prevent sweating and evaporative heat loss in the part of the body affected by the block.[261] Consequently, laboring patients with epidural analgesia who are in a warm environment would likely have a small increase in core temperature.

The significance of these small temperature changes is unclear, but an increase in fetal temperature and FHR can occur, and it may be difficult to distinguish this temperature change from one indicating infection. (However, systemic infection typically results in a larger increase in maternal temperature, which is often accompanied by shivering or shaking chills.) One retrospective, nonrandomized study found a higher rate of neonatal sepsis evaluations among infants of women who had received epidural analgesia during labor.[262] Subsequent retrospective reviews have found that epidural analgesia during labor is associated with more neonatal sepsis evaluations but *not* more neonatal sepsis.[263,264] Nulliparity and dysfunctional labor, two situations in which epidural analgesia is often employed, are also associated with maternal fever.[265] One recent study implicated chorioamnionitis but *not* epidural analgesia as a cause of maternal fever in laboring women.[266] In summary, the overall high rate of neonatal sepsis evaluations among these otherwise healthy populations suggests that the criteria used for sepsis evaluations are inappropriate and need to be reevaluated.

KEY POINTS

- Neuraxial analgesia is the most effective form of intrapartum analgesia currently available. In most cases, maternal request for pain relief represents a sufficient indication for the administration of epidural analgesia.
- The safe administration of neuraxial analgesia requires a thorough (albeit directed) preanesthetic evaluation and the immediate availability of appropriate resuscitation equipment.
- The administration of the test dose should allow the anesthesiologist to recognize most cases of unintentional subarachnoid or intravascular placement of the epidural catheter. All therapeutic doses of local anesthetic should be administered incrementally.
- Bupivacaine is the local anesthetic most often used for epidural analgesia during labor. Ropivacaine and levobupivacaine are satisfactory (albeit more expensive) alternatives. Most anesthesiologists reserve 2-chloroprocaine and lidocaine for cases that require the rapid extension of anesthesia for vaginal or cesarean delivery.
- The most common complication of neuraxial analgesia is hypotension. Prophylaxis and treatment include the avoidance of aortocaval compression, intravenous hydration, and the administration of ephedrine as needed.

REFERENCES

1. Howell CJ, Chalmers I. A review of prospectively controlled comparisons of epidural with non-epidural forms of pain relief during labour. Int J Obstet Anes 1992; 1:93-110.
2. Morgan B, Bulpitt CJ, Clifton P, Lewis PJ. Effectiveness of pain relief in labour: Survey of 1000 mothers. Br Med J 1982; 285:689-90.
3. Philipsen T, Jensen NH. Epidural block or parenteral pethidine as analgesic in labour: A randomized study concerning progress in labour and instrumental deliveries. Eur J Obstet Gynecol Reprod Biol 1989; 30:27-33.
4. Paech MJ. The King Edward Memorial Hospital 1,000 mother survey of methods of pain relief in labour. Anaesth Intensive Care 1991; 19:393-9.
5. Crawford JS. Lumbar epidural block in labour: A clinical analysis. Br J Anaesth 1972; 44:66-74.
6. Ramin SM, Gambling DR, Lucas MJ, et al. Randomized trial of epidural versus intravenous analgesia during labor. Obstet Gynecol 1995; 86: 783-9.
7. Thorp JA, Hu DH, Albin RM, et al. The effect of intrapartum epidural analgesia on nulliparous labor: A randomized, controlled, prospective trial. Am J Obstet Gynecol 1993; 169:851-8.
8. Chestnut DH, McGrath JM, Vincent RD, et al. Does early administration of epidural analgesia affect obstetric outcome in nulliparous women who are in spontaneous labor? Anesthesiology 1994; 80:1201-8.
9. Chestnut DH, Vincent RD, McGrath JM, et al. Does early administration of epidural analgesia affect obstetric outcome in nulliparous women who are receiving intravenous oxytocin? Anesthesiology 1994; 80:1193-200.
10. Shnider SM, Abboud TK, Artal R, et al. Maternal catecholamines decrease during labor after lumbar epidural anesthesia. Am J Obstet Gynecol 1983; 147:13-5.
11. Lederman RP, Lederman E, Work BA, McCann DS. The relationship of maternal anxiety, plasma catecholamines, and plasma cortisol to progress in labor. Am J Obstet Gynecol 1978; 132:495-500.
12. Lederman RP, Lederman E, Work B, McCann DS. Anxiety and epinephrine in multiparous women in labor: Relationship to duration of labor and fetal heart rate pattern. Am J Obstet Gynecol 1985; 153:870-7.
13. Jouppila R, Hollmen A. The effect of segmental epidural analgesia on maternal and foetal acid-base balance, lactate, serum potassium and creatine phosphokinase during labour. Acta Anaesth Scand 1976; 20:259-68.
14. Levinson G, Shnider SM, deLorimier AA, Steffenson JL. Effects of maternal hyperventilation on uterine blood flow and fetal oxygenation and acid-base status. Anesthesiology 1974; 40:340-7.
15. Peabody JL. Transcutaneous oxygen measurement to evaluate drug effects. Clin Perinatol 1979; 6:109-21.
16. Gibbs CP, Krischer J, Peckham BM, et al. Obstetric anesthesia: A national survey. Anesthesiology 1986; 65:298-306.
17. Hawkins JL, Beaty BR, Gibbs CP. Update on obstetric anesthesia practices in the United States (abstract). Anesthesiology 1999; 90:A53.
18. Burnstein R, Buckland R, Pickett JA. A survey of epidural analgesia for labour in the United Kingdom. Anaesthesia 1999; 54:634-40.
19. Davies MW, Harrison JC, Ryan TDR. Current practice of epidural analgesia during normal labour. A survey of maternity units in the United Kingdom. Anaesthesia 1993; 48:63-5.
20. Macario A, Scibetta WC, Navarro J, et al. Analgesia for labor pain: A cost model. Anesthesiology 2000; 92:841-50.
21. Bell ED, Penning DH, Cousineau EF, et al. How much labor is in a labor epidural? Manpower cost and reimbursement for an obstetric analgesia service in a teaching institution. Anesthesiology 2000; 92:851-8.
22. Hawkins JL, Koonin LM, Palmer SK, et al. Anesthesia-related deaths during obstetric delivery in the United States, 1979-1990. Anesthesiology 1997; 86:277-84.
23. American College of Obstetricians and Gynecologists Committee on Obstetric Practice. Analgesia and cesarean delivery rates. ACOG Committee Opinion No. 269. Obstet Gynecol 2002; 99:369-70.
24. Rogers R, Gilson G, Kammerer-Doak D. Epidural analgesia and active management of labor: Effects on length of labor and mode of delivery. Obstet Gynecol 1999; 93:995-8.
25. Holt RO, Diehl SJ, Wright JW. Station and cervical dilation at epidural placement in predicting cesarean risk. Obstet Gynecol 1999; 93:281-4.
26. Swan HD, Borshoff DC. Informed consent: Recall of risk information following epidural analgesia in labour. Anaesth Intensive Care 1994; 22:139-41.
27. Knapp RM. Legal view of informed consent for anesthesia during labor (letter). Anesthesiology 1990; 72:211.
28. Pattee C, Ballantyne M, Milne B. Epidural analgesia for labour and delivery: Informed consent issues. Can J Anaesth 1997; 44:918-23.

29. Jackson A, Henry R, Avery N, et al. Informed consent for labour epidurals: What labouring women want to know. Can J Anaesth 2000; 47:1068-73.

30. Practice Guidelines for Obstetrical Anesthesia: A report by the American Society of Anesthesiologists Task Force on Obstetrical Anesthesia. Anesthesiology 1999; 90:600-11.

31. Paulick RP, Meyers RL, Rudolph AM. Effect of maternal oxygen administration on fetal oxygenation during graded reduction of umbilical or uterine blood flow in fetal sheep. Am J Obstet Gynecol 1992; 167:233-9.

32. Bromage PR. Epidural analgesia. Philadelphia, PA, WB Saunders, 1978:144.

33. ACOG technical bulletin. Fetal heart rate patterns: Monitoring, interpretation, and management. Int J Gynaecol Obstet 1995; 51:65-74.

34. Chestnut DH, Weiner CP. Monitoring maternal heart rate during epidural injection of a test dose containing epinephrine (letter). Anesthesiology 1986; 64:839-40.

35. Collins KM, Bevan DR, Beard RW. Fluid loading to reduce abnormalities of fetal heart rate and maternal hypotension during epidural analgesia in labour. Br Med J 1978; 2:1460-1.

36. Ramanathan S, Masih A, Rock I, et al. Maternal and fetal effects of prophylactic hydration with crystalloids or colloids before epidural anesthesia. Anesth Analg 1983; 62:673-8.

37. Zamora JE, Rosaeg OP, Lindsay MP, et al. Haemodynamic consequences and uterine contractions following 0.5 or 1.0 litre crystalloid infusion before obstetric epidural analgesia. Can J Anaesth 1996; 43:347-52.

38. Kinsella SM, Pirlet M, Mills MS, et al. Randomized study of intravenous fluid preload before epidural analgesia during labour. Br J Anaesth 2000; 85:311-3.

39. Fisher AJ, Huddleston JF. Intrapartum maternal glucose infusion reduces umbilical cord acidemia. Am J Obstet Gynecol 1997; 177:765-9.

40. Suonio S, Simpanen A-L, Olkkonen H, et al. Effect of the left lateral recumbent position compared with the supine and upright positions on placental blood flow in normal late pregnancy. Ann Clin Res 1976; 8:22-6.

41. Vincent RD, Chestnut DH. Which position is more comfortable for the parturient during identification of the epidural space? Int J Obstet Anesth 1991; 1:9-11.

42. Andrews PJD, Ackerman WE, Juneja MM. Aortocaval compression in the sitting and lateral decubitus positions during extradural catheter placement in the parturient. Can J Anaesth 1993; 40:320-4.

43. Bahar M, Chanimov M, Cohen ML, et al. Lateral recumbent head-down posture for epidural catheter insertion reduces intravascular injection. Can J Anesth 2001; 48:48-53.

44. Bieniarz J, Crottogini JJ, Curuchet E, et al. Aortocaval compression by the uterus in late human pregnancy. II. An arteriographic study. Am J Obstet Gynecol 1968; 100:203-17.

45. Calvin S, Jones OW III, Knieriem K, et al. Oxygen saturation in the supine hypotensive syndrome. Obstet Gynecol 1988; 71:872-7.

46. Kerr MG, Scott DB, Samuel E. Studies of the inferior vena cava in late pregnancy. Br Med J 1964; 1:532-3.

47. Scott DB. Inferior vena caval occlusion in late pregnancy and its importance in anaesthesia. Br J Anaesth 1968; 40:120-8.

48. Eckstein K-L, Marx GF. Aortocaval compression and uterine displacement. Anesthesiology 1974; 40:92-6.

49. Marx GF, Husain FJ, Shiau HF. Brachial and femoral blood pressures during the prenatal period. Am J Obstet Gynecol 1980; 136:11-3.

50. Ellington C, Katz VL, Watson WJ, et al. The effect of lateral tilt on maternal and fetal hemodynamic variables. Obstet Gynecol 1991; 77:201-3.

51. Ueland K, Hansen J. Maternal cardiovascular dynamics. II. Posture and uterine contractions. Am J Obstet Gynecol 1969; 103:1-7.

52. Beilin Y, Abramovitz SE, Zahn J, et al. Improved epidural analgesia in the parturient in the 30° tilt position. Can J Anaesth 2000; 47:1176-81.

53. Troop M. Negative aspiration for cerebral spinal fluid does not assure proper placement of epidural catheter. J Am Assoc Nurse Anesth 1992; 60:301-3.

54. Palkar NV, Boudreaux RC, Mankad AV. Accidental total spinal block: A complication of an epidural test dose. Can J Anaesth 1992; 39:1058-60.

55. Colonna-Romano P, Nagaraj L. Tests to evaluate intravenous placement of epidural catheters in laboring women: A prospective clinical study. Anesth Analg 1998; 86:985-8.

56. Abraham RA, Harris AP, Maxwell LG, et al. The efficacy of 1.5% lidocaine with 7.5% dextrose and epinephrine as an epidural test dose for obstetrics. Anesthesiology 1986; 64:116-9.

57. Prince GD, Shetty GR, Miles M. Safety and efficacy of a low volume extradural test dose of bupivacaine in labour. Br J Anaesth 1989; 62:503-8.

58. Colonna-Romano P, Lingaraju N. Diagnostic accuracy of an intrathecal test dose in epidural analgesia. Can J Anaesth 1994; 41:572-4.

59. Ngan Kee WD, Khaw KS, Lee BB, et al. The limitations of ropivacaine with epinephrine as an epidural test dose in parturients. Anesth Analg 2001; 92:1529-31.

60. Richardson MG, Lee AC, Wissler RN. High spinal anesthesia after epidural test dose administration in five obstetric patients. Reg Anesth 1996; 21:119-23.

61. Philip JH, Brown WU. Total spinal anesthesia late in the course of obstetric bupivacaine epidural block. Anesthesiology 1976; 44:340-1.

62. Crawford JS. Some maternal complications of epidural analgesia for labour. Anaesthesia 1985; 40:1219-25.

63. Mannion D, Walker R, Clayton K. Extradural vein puncture: An avoidable complication. Anaesthesia 1991; 46:585-7.

64. Verniquet AJW. Vessel puncture with epidural catheters. Anaesthesia 1980; 35:660-2.

65. Mulroy MF, Norris MC, Liu SS. Safety steps for epidural injection of local anesthetics: Review of the literature and recommendations. Anesth Analg 1997; 85:1346-56.

66. Albright GA. Cardiac arrest following regional anesthesia with etidocaine or bupivacaine. Anesthesiology 1979; 51:285-7.

67. Guinard JP, Mulroy MF, Carpenter RL, et al. Test doses: Optimal epinephrine content with and without acute beta-adrenergic blockade. Anesthesiology 1990; 73:386-92.

68. Moore DC, Batra MS. The components of an effective test dose prior to epidural block. Anesthesiology 1981; 55:693-6.

69. Hood DD, Dewan DM, James FM III. Maternal and fetal effects of epinephrine in gravid ewes. Anesthesiology 1986; 64:610-3.

70. Chestnut DH, Weiner CP, Martin JG, et al. Effect of intravenous epinephrine on uterine artery blood flow velocity in the pregnant guinea pig. Anesthesiology 1986; 65:633-6.

71. Marcus MAE, Vertommen JD, Van Aken H, et al. Hemodynamic effects of intravenous isoproterenol versus epinephrine in the chronic maternal-fetal sheep preparation. Anesth Analg 1996; 82:1023-6.

72. Youngstrom P, Hoyt M, Veille JC, et al. Effects of intravenous test dose epinephrine on fetal sheep during acute fetal stress and acidosis. Reg Anesth 1990; 15:237-41.

73. Chestnut DH, Owen CL, Brown CK, et al. Does labor affect the variability of maternal heart rate during induction of epidural anesthesia? Anesthesiology 1988; 68:622-5.

74. Cartwright PD, McCarroll SM, Antzaka C. Maternal heart rate changes with a plain epidural test dose. Anesthesiology 1986; 65:226-8.

75. Colonna-Romano P, Lingaraju N, Godfrey SD, et al. Epidural test dose and intravascular injection in obstetrics: Sensitivity, specificity, and lowest effective dose. Anesth Analg 1992; 75:372-6.

76. Mulroy M, Glosten B. The epinephrine test dose in obstetrics: Note the limitations (editorial). Anesth Analg 1998; 86:923-5.

77. Leighton BL, Norris MC, Sosis M, et al. Limitations of epinephrine as a marker of intravascular injection in laboring women. Anesthesiology 1987; 66:688-91.

78. Gieraerts R, Van Zundert A, De Wolf A, et al. Ten mL bupivacaine 0.125% with 12.5 µg epinephrine is a reliable epidural test dose to detect inadvertent intravascular injection in obstetric patients. A double-blind study. Acta Anaesthesiol Scand 1992; 36:656-9.

79. Leighton BL, DeSimone CA, Norris MC, et al. Isoproterenol is an effective marker of intravenous injection in laboring women. Anesthesiology 1989; 71:206-9.

80. Marcus MAE, Vertommen JD, Van Aken H, et al. Hemodynamic effects of intravenous isoproterenol versus saline in the parturient. Anesth Analg 1997; 84:1113-6.

81. Norris MC, Arkoosh VA, Knobler R. Maternal and fetal effects of isoproterenol in the gravid ewe. Anesth Analg 1997; 85:389-94.

82. Marcus MAE, Vertommen JD, Van Aken H, et al. The effects of adding isoproterenol to 0.125% bupivacaine on the quality and duration of epidural analgesia in laboring parturients. Anesth Analg 1998; 86:749-52.

83. Leighton BL, Norris MC, DeSimone CA, et al. The air test as a clinically useful indicator of intravenously placed epidural catheters. Anesthesiology 1990; 73:610-3.

84. Leighton BL, Topkis WG, Gross JB, et al. Multiport epidural catheters: Does the air test work? Anesthesiology 2000; 92:1617-20.

85. Power I, Thorburn J. Differential flow from multihole epidural catheters. Anaesthesia 1988; 43:876-8.

86. Colonna-Romano P, Lingaraju N, Braitman LE. Epidural test dose: Lidocaine 100 mg, not chloroprocaine, is a symptomatic marker of IV injection in labouring parturients. Can Anaesth Soc J 1993; 40:714-7.

87. Rathmell JP, Viscomi CM, Ashikaga T. Detection of intravascular epidural catheters using 2-chloroprocaine. Influence of local anesthetic dose and nalbuphine premedication. Reg Anesth 1997; 22:113-8.

88. Yoshii WY, Miller M, Rottman RL, et al. Fentanyl for epidural intravascular test dose in obstetrics. Reg Anesth 1993; 18:296-9.

89. Morris GF, Lang SA. Can parturients distinguish between intravenous and epidural fentanyl? Can J Anaesth 1994; 41:667-72.

90. Norris MC, Fogel ST, Dalman H, et al. Labor epidural analgesia without an intravascular "test dose." Anesthesiology 1998; 88:1495-501.

91. McLean BY, Rottman RL, Kotelko DM. Failure of multiple test doses and techniques to detect intravascular migration of an epidural catheter. Anesth Analg 1992; 74:454-6.

92. Paech MJ. Inadvertent spinal anaesthesia with 0.125% bupivacaine and fentanyl during labour. Anaesth Intensive Care 1990; 18:400-12.

93. Eisenach JC, Grice SC, Dewan DM. Epinephrine enhances analgesia produced by epidural bupivacaine during labor. Anesth Analg 1987; 66:447-51.

94. Belfrage P, Berlin A, Raabe N, et al. Lumbar epidural analgesia with bupivacaine in labor. Am J Obstet Gynecol 1975; 123:839-44.

95. Abboud TK, Khoo SS, Miller F, et al. Maternal, fetal, and neonatal responses after epidural anesthesia with bupivacaine, 2-chloroprocaine, or lidocaine. Anesth Analg 1982; 61:638-44.

96. Eddleston JM, Maresh M, Horsman EL, et al. Comparison of the maternal and fetal effects associated with intermittent or continuous infusion of extradural analgesia. Br J Anaesth 1992; 69:154-8.

97. Steiger RM, Nageotte MP. Effect of uterine contractility and maternal hypotension on prolonged decelerations after bupivacaine epidural anesthesia. Am J Obstet Gynecol 1990; 163:808-12.

98. Loftus JR, Holbrook RH, Cohen SE. Fetal heart rate after epidural lidocaine and bupivacaine for elective cesarean section. Anesthesiology 1991; 75:406-12.

99. Nielsen PE, Erickson JR, Abouleish EI, et al. Fetal heart rate changes after intrathecal sufentanil or epidural bupivacaine for labor analgesia: Incidence and clinical significance. Anesth Analg 1996; 83:742-6.

100. McGrath J, Chestnut D, Debruyn C. The effect of epidural bupivacaine versus intravenous nalbuphine on fetal heart rate tracings (abstract). Anesthesiology 1992; 77:A984.

101. Pello LC, Rosevear SK, Dawes GS, et al. Computerized fetal heart rate analysis in labor. Obstet Gynecol 1991; 78:602-10.

102. Katz JA, Bridenbaugh PO, Knarr DC, et al. Pharmacodynamics and pharmacokinetics of epidural ropivacaine in humans. Anesth Analg 1990; 70:16-21.

103. Santos AC, Arthur GR, Pedersen H, et al. Systemic toxicity of ropivacaine during ovine pregnancy. Anesthesiology 1991; 75:137-41.

104. Pitkanen M, Feldman HS, Arthur GR, et al. Chronotropic and inotropic effects of ropivacaine, bupivacaine, and lidocaine in the spontaneously beating and electrically paced isolated, perfused rabbit heart. Reg Anesth 1992; 17:183-92.

105. Moller R, Covino BG. Cardiac electrophysiologic properties of bupivacaine and lidocaine compared with those of ropivacaine, a new amide local anesthetic. Anesthesiology 1990; 72:322-9.

106. Santos AC, Arthur GR, Roberts DJ, et al. Effect of ropivacaine and bupivacaine on uterine blood flow in pregnant ewes. Anesth Analg 1992; 74:62-7.

107. Santos AC, Arthur GR, Wlody D, et al. Comparative systemic toxicity of ropivacaine and bupivacaine in nonpregnant and pregnant ewes. Anesthesiology 1995; 82:734-40.

108. Polley LS, Columb MO, Naughton NN, et al. Relative analgesic potencies of ropivacaine and bupivacaine for epidural analgesia in labor: Implications for therapeutic indexes. Anesthesiology 1999; 90:944-50.

109. Capogna G, Celleno D, Fusco P, et al. Relative potencies of bupivacaine and ropivacaine for analgesia in labour. Br J Anaesth 1999; 82:371-3.

110. Owen MD, D'Angelo R, Gerancher JC, et al. 0.125% ropivacaine is similar to 0.125% bupivacaine for labor analgesia using patient-controlled epidural infusion. Anesth Analg 1998; 86:527-31.

111. Meister GC, D'Angelo R, Owen M, et al. A comparison of epidural analgesia with 0.125% ropivacaine with fentanyl versus 0.125% bupivacaine with fentanyl during labor. Anesth Analg 2000; 90:632-7.

112. Owen MD, Thomas JA, Smith T, et al. Ropivacaine 0.075% and bupivacaine 0.075% with fentanyl 2 μg/ml are equivalent for labor epidural analgesia. Anesth Analg 2002; 94:179-83.

113. Chua NP, Sia AT, Ocampo CE. Parturient-controlled epidural analgesia during labour: bupivacaine vs. ropivacaine. Anaesthesia 2001; 56:1169-73.

114. Fernández-Guisasola J, Serrano ML, Cobo B, et al. A comparison of 0.0625% bupivacaine with fentanyl and 0.1% ropivacaine with fentanyl for continuous epidural labor analgesia. Anesth Analg 2001; 92:1261-5.

115. Parpaglioni R, Capogna G, Celleno D. A comparison between low-dose ropivacaine and bupivacaine at equianalgesic concentrations for epidural analgesia during the first stage of labor. Int J Obstet Anesth 2000; 9:83-6.

116. Bader AM, Datta S, Flanagan H, et al. Comparison of bupivacaine-and ropivacaine-induced conduction blockade in the isolated rabbit vagus nerve. Anesth Analg 1989; 68:724-7.

117. Brockway MS, Bannister J, McClure JH, et al. Comparison of extradural ropivacaine and bupivacaine. Br J Anaesth 1991; 66:31-7.

118. Griffin RP, Reynolds F. Extradural anaesthesia for caesarean section: A double-blind comparison of 0.5% ropivacaine with 0.5% bupivacaine. Br J Anaesth 1995; 74:512-6.

119. Lacassie HJ, Columb MO, Lacassie HP, et al. The relative motor blocking potencies of epidural bupivacaine and ropivacaine in labor. Anesth Analg 2002; 95:204-8.

120. Owen MD, D'Angelo R, Gerancher JC, et al. 0.125% ropivacaine is similar to 0.125% bupivacaine for labor analgesia using patient-controlled epidural infusion. Anesth Analg 1998; 86:527-31.

121. Stienstra R, Jonker TA, Bourdrez P, et al. Ropivacaine 0.25% versus bupivacaine 0.25% for continuous epidural analgesia in labor: A double-blind comparison. Anesth Analg 1995; 80:285-9.

122. Halpern SH, Walsh V. Epidural ropivacaine versus bupivacaine for labor: A meta-analysis. Anesth Analg 2003; 96:1473-9.

123. Vanhoutte F, Vereecke J, Verbeke N, et al. Stereoselective effects of the enantiomers of bupivacaine on the electrophysiological properties of the guinea-pig papillary muscle. Br J Pharmacol 1991; 103:1275-81.

124. Gristwood R, Bardsley H, Baker H, et al. Reduced cardiotoxicity of levobupivacaine compared with racemic bupivacaine (Marcaine): New clinical evidence. Exp Opin Invest Drugs 1994; 3:1209-12.

125. Bardsley H, Gristwood R, Baker H, et al. A comparison of the cardiovascular effects of levobupivacaine and rac-bupivacaine following intravenous administration to healthy volunteers. Br J Clin Pharmacol 1998; 46:245-9.

126. Lyons G, Columb M, Wilson RC, et al. Epidural pain relief in labour: Potencies of levobupivacaine and racemic bupivacaine. Br J Anaesth 1998; 81:899-901.

127. Polley LS, Columb MO, Naughton NN, et al. Relative analgesic potencies of levobupivacaine and ropivacaine for epidural analgesia in labor. Anesthesiology 2003; 99:1354-8.

128. Benhamou D, Ghosh C, Mercier FJ. A randomized sequential allocation study to determine the minimum effective analgesic concentration of levobupivacaine and ropivacaine in patients receiving epidural analgesia for labor. Anesthesiology 2003; 99:1383-6.

129. Milaszkiewicz R, Payne N, Loughnan B, et al. Continuous extradural infusion of lignocaine 0.75% vs bupivacaine 0.125% in primiparae: Quality of analgesia and influence on labour. Anaesthesia 1992; 47:1042-6.

130. Kennedy RL, Bell JU, Miller RP, et al. Uptake and distribution of lidocaine in fetal lambs. Anesthesiology 1990; 72:483-9.

131. Biehl D, Shnider SM, Levinson G, et al. Placental transfer of lidocaine: Effects of fetal acidosis. Anesthesiology 1978; 48:409-12.

132. Scanlon JW, Brown WJ Jr, Weiss JB, et al. Neurobehavioral responses of newborn infants after maternal epidural anesthesia. Anesthesiology 1974; 40:121-8.

133. Scanlon JW, Ostheimer GW, Lurie AO, et al. Neurobehavioral responses and drug concentrations in newborns after maternal epidural anesthesia with bupivacaine. Anesthesiology 1976; 45:400-5.

134. Abboud TK, Kim KC, Noueihed R, et al. Epidural bupivacaine, chloroprocaine, or lidocaine for cesarean section: Maternal and neonatal effects. Anesth Analg 1983; 62:914-9.

135. Kuhnert BR, Harrison MJ, Linn PL, et al. Effects of maternal epidural anesthesia on neonatal behavior. Anesth Analg 1984; 63:301-8.

136. Grice SC, Eisenach JC, Dewan DM. Labor analgesia with epidural bupivacaine plus fentanyl: Enhancement with epinephrine and inhibition with 2-chloroprocaine. Anesthesiology 1990; 72:623-8.

137. Corke BC, Carlson CG, Dettbarn WD. The influence of 2-chloroprocaine on the subsequent analgesic potency of bupivacaine. Anesthesiology 1984; 60:25-7.

138. Kuhnert BR, Kuhnert PM, Philipson EH, et al. The half-life of 2-chloroprocaine. Anesth Analg 1986; 65:273-8.

139. Philipson EH, Kuhnert BR, Syracuse CD. Fetal acidosis, 2-chloroprocaine, and epidural anesthesia for cesarean section. Am J Obstet Gynecol 1985; 151:322-4.

140. Fibuch EE, Opper SE. Back pain following epidurally administered Nesacaine-MPF. Anesth Analg 1989; 69:113-5.

141. McLoughlin TM, DiFazio CA. More on back pain after Nesacaine-MPF (letter). Anesth Analg 1990; 71:562-3.

142. Abboud TK, Sheik-ol-Eslam A, Yanagi T, et al. Safety and efficacy of epinephrine added to bupivacaine for lumbar epidural analgesia in obstetrics. Anesth Analg 1985; 64:585-91.

143. Polley LS, Columb MO, Naughton NN, et al. Effect of epidural epinephrine on the minimum local analgesic concentration of epidural bupivacaine in labor. Anesthesiology 2002; 96:1123-8.

144. Abboud TK, David S, Nagappala S, et al. Maternal, fetal, and neonatal effects of lidocaine with and without epinephrine for epidural anesthesia in obstetrics. Anesth Analg 1984; 63:973-9.

145. Brose WG, Cohen SE. Epidural lidocaine for cesarean section: Effect of varying epinephrine concentration. Anesthesiology 1988; 69:936-40.

146. Ohno H, Watanabe M, Saitoh J, et al. Effect of epinephrine concentration on lidocaine disposition during epidural anesthesia. Anesthesiology 1988; 68:625-8.

147. Reynolds F, Taylor G. Plasma concentrations of bupivacaine during continuous epidural analgesia in labour: The effect of adrenaline. Br J Anaesth 1971; 43:436-40.

148. Reynolds F, Laishley R, Morgan B, et al. Effect of time and adrenaline on the feto-maternal distribution of bupivacaine. Br J Anaesth 1989; 62:509-14.

149. Craft JB Jr, Epstein BS, Coakley CS. Effect of lidocaine with epinephrine versus lidocaine (plain) on induced labor. Anesth Analg 1972; 51:243-6.

150. Matadial L, Cibils LA. The effect of epidural anesthesia on uterine activity and blood pressure. Am J Obstet Gynecol 1976; 125:846-54.

151. Yarnell RW, Ewing DA, Tierney E, et al. Sacralization of epidural block with repeated doses of 0.25% bupivacaine during labor. Reg Anesth 1990; 15:275-9.

152. Albright GA, Jouppila R, Hollmen AI, et al. Epinephrine does not alter human intervillous blood flow during epidural anesthesia. Anesthesiology 1981; 54:131-5.

153. Lamont RF, Pinney D, Rodgers P, et al. Continuous versus intermittent epidural analgesia. Anaesthesia 1989; 44:893-6.

154. Bogod DG, Rosen M, Rees GA. Extradural infusion of 0.125% bupivacaine at 10 mL/hr to women during labour. Br J Anaesth 1987; 59:325-30.

155. Li DF, Rees GAD, Rosen M. Continuous extradural infusion of 0.0625% or 0.125% bupivacaine for pain relief in primigravid labour. Br J Anaesth 1985; 57:264-70.

156. Hicks JA, Jenkins JG, Newton MC, et al. Continuous epidural infusion of 0.075% bupivacaine for pain relief in labour. Anaesthesia 1988; 43:289-92.

157. Smedstad KG, Morison DH. A comparative study of continuous and intermittent epidural analgesia for labour and delivery. Can J Anaesth 1988; 35:234-41.

158. Abboud TK, Afrasiabi A, Sarkis F, et al. Continuous infusion epidural analgesia in parturients receiving bupivacaine, chloroprocaine, or lidocaine: Maternal, fetal, and neonatal effects. Anesth Analg 1984; 63:421-8.

159. Gambling DR, Yu P, McMorland GH, et al. A comparative study of patient controlled epidural analgesia (PCEA) and continuous infusion epidural analgesia (CIEA) during labor. Can J Anaesth 1988; 35:249-54.

160. Gambling DR, McMorland GJ, Yu P, et al. Comparison of patient-controlled epidural analgesia and conventional intermittent "top-up" injections during labor. Anesth Analg 1990; 70:256-61.

161. Purdie J, Reid J, Thorburn J, et al. Continuous extradural analgesia: Comparison of midwife top-ups, continuous infusions and patient controlled administration. Br J Anaesth 1992; 68:580-4.

162. Sia AT, Chong JL. Epidural 0.2% ropivacaine for labour analgesia: Parturient-controlled or continuous infusion? Anaesth Intensive Care 1999; 27:154-8.

163. Ferrante FM, Rosinia FA, Gordon C, et al. The role of continuous background infusions in patient-controlled epidural analgesia for labor and delivery. Anesth Analg 1994; 79:80-4.

164. Curry PD, Pacsoo C, Heap DG. Patient-controlled epidural analgesia in obstetric anaesthetic practice. Pain 1994; 57:125-8.

165. Smedvig JP, Soreide E, Gjessing L. Ropivacaine 1 mg/ml, plus fentanyl 2 µg/ml for epidural analgesia during labour: Is mode of administration important? Acta Anaesthiol Scand 2001; 45:595-9.

166. Tan S, Reid J, Thorburn J. Extradural analgesia in labour: Complications of three techniques of administration. Br J Anaesth 1994; 73:619-23.

167. Gambling DR, Bogod D. Controversies in obstetric anaesthesia: Epidural infusions in labour should be abandoned in favour of patient-controlled epidural analgesia. Int J Obstet Anesth 1996; 5:59-63.

168. D'Angelo R. Epidural PCA during labor. American Society of Anesthesiologists Newsletter 2001; 65:16-8.

169. Gambling DR, Huber CJ, Berkowitz J, et al. Patient-controlled epidural analgesia in labour: Varying bolus dose and lockout interval. Can J Anaesth 1993; 40:211-7.

170. Bernard JM, Le Roux D, Vizquel L, et al. Patient-controlled epidural analgesia during labor: The effects of the increase in bolus and lockout interval. Anesth Analg 2000; 90:328-32.

171. Capogna G, Celleno D, Lyons G, et al. Minimum local analgesic concentration of extradural bupivacaine increases with progression of labour. Br J Anaesth 1998; 80:11-3.

172. Merry A, Cross JA, Mayadeo SV, et al. Posture and the spread of extradural analgesia in labour. Br J Anaesth 1983; 55:303-7.

173. Park WY, Hagins FM, Macnamara TE. Lateral position and epidural anesthetic spread. Anesth Analg 1983; 62:278-9.

174. Park WY. Factors influencing distribution of local anesthetics in the epidural space. Reg Anesth 1988; 13:49-57.

175. Erdemir HA, Sopper LE, Sweet RB. Studies of factors affecting peridural anesthesia. Anesth Analg 1965; 44:400-4.

176. Stacey RGW, Watt S, Kadim MY, et al. Single space combined spinal-extradural technique for analgesia in labour. Br J Anaesth 1993; 71:499-502.

177. Galley AH. Continuous caudal analgesia in obstetrics. Anaesthesia 1949; 4:154-68.

178. Sinclair JC, Fox HA, Lentz JF, et al. Intoxication of the fetus by a local anesthetic. A newly recognized complication of maternal caudal anesthesia. N Engl J Med 1965; 273:1173-7.

179. Dawkins CJM. An analysis of the complications of extradural and caudal block. Anaesthesia 1969; 24:554-63.

180. Moran DH, Johnson MD. Continuous spinal anesthesia with combined hyperbaric and isobaric bupivacaine in a patient with scoliosis. Anesth Analg 1990; 70:445-7.

181. Milligan KR, Carp H. Continuous spinal anaesthesia for caesarean section in the morbidly obese. Int J Obstet Anesth 1992; 1:111-3.

182. Elam JO. Catheter subarachnoid block for labor and delivery: A differential segmental technic employing hyperbaric lidocaine. Anesth Analg 1970; 49:1007-15.

183. Rigler ML, Drasner K, Krejcie TC, et al. Cauda equina syndrome after continuous spinal anesthesia. Anesth Analg 1991; 72:275-81.

184. Huckaby T, Skerman JH, Hurley RJ, et al. Sensory analgesia for vaginal deliveries: A preliminary report of continuous spinal anesthesia with a 32-gauge catheter. Reg Anesth 1991; 16:150-3.

185. McHale S, Mitchell V, Howsam S, et al. Continuous subarachnoid infusion of 0.125% bupivacaine for analgesia during labor. Br J Anaesth 1992; 69:634-6.

186. Norris MC, Leighton BL. Continuous spinal analgesia after unintentional dural puncture in parturients. Reg Anesth 1990; 15:285-7.

187. Pavy TJG. Patient-controlled spinal analgesia for labour and caesarean delivery. Anaesth Intensive Care 2001; 29:58-61.

188. Hollmen A, Jouppila R, Pihlajaniemi R, et al. Selective lumbar epidural block in labour: A clinical analysis. Acta Anaesth Scand 1977; 21:174-81.

189. Shnider SM, deLorimier AA, Holl JW, et al. Vasopressors in obstetrics. I. Correction of fetal acidosis with ephedrine during spinal hypotension. Am J Obstet Gynecol 1968; 1102:911-9.

190. Tong C, Eisenach JC. The vascular mechanism of ephedrine's beneficial effect on uterine perfusion during pregnancy. 1992; 76:792-8.

191. Ralston DH, Shnider SM, deLorimier AA. Effects of equipotent ephedrine, metaraminol, mephentermine, and methoxamine on uterine blood flow in the pregnant ewe. Anesthesiology 1974; 40:354-70.

192. James FM, Greiss FC Jr, Kemp RA. An evaluation of vasopressor therapy for maternal hypotension during spinal anesthesia. Anesthesiology 1970; 33:25-34.

193. Hughes SC, Ward MG, Levinson G, et al. Placental transfer of ephedrine does not affect neonatal outcome. Anesthesiology 1985; 63:217-9.

194. Wright RG, Shnider SM, Levinson G, et al. The effect of maternal administration of ephedrine on fetal heart rate and variability. Obstet Gynecol 1981; 57:734-8.

195. Crawford JS. The second thousand epidural blocks in an obstetric hospital practice. Br J Anaesth 1972; 44:1277-87.

196. Narang VPS, Linter SPK. Failure of extradural blockade in obstetrics: A new hypothesis. Br J Anaesth 1988; 60:402-4.

197. Chadwick HS. An analysis of obstetric anesthesia cases from the American Society of Anesthesiologists closed claims project database. Int J Obstet Anesth 1996; 5:258-63.

198. Apostolou GA, Zarmakoupis PK, Mastrokostopoulos GT. Spread of epidural anesthesia and the lateral position. Anesth Analg 1981; 60:584-6.

199. Husemeyer RP, White DC. Lumbar extradural injection pressures in pregnant women: An investigation of relationships between rate of injection, injection pressures and extent of analgesia. Br J Anaesth 1980; 52:55-60.

200. Norris MC, Leighton BL, DeSimone CA, et al. Lateral position and epidural anesthesia for cesarean section. Anesth Analg 1988; 67:788-90.

201. Savolaine ER, Pandya JB, Greenblatt SH, Conover SR. Anatomy of the human lumbar epidural space: New insights using CT-epidurography. Anesthesiology 1988; 68:217-20.

202. McCrae AF, Whitfield A, McClure JH. Repeated unilateral epidural blockade. Anaesthesia 1992; 47:859-61.

203. Blomberg RG, Olsson SS. The lumbar epidural space in patients examined with epiduroscopy. Anesth Analg 1989; 68:157-60.
204. Asato F, Goto F. Radiographic findings of unilateral epidural block. Anesth Analg 1996; 83:519-22.
205. D'Angelo R, Foss ML, Livesay CH. A comparison of multiport and uniport epidural catheters in laboring patients. Anesth Analg 1997; 84:1276-9.
206. Beck H, Brassow F, Doehn M, et al. Epidural catheters of the multi-orifice type: Dangers and complications. Acta Anaesthesiol Scand 1986; 30:549-55.
207. Dalens B, Bazin JE, Haberer JP. Epidural bubbles as a cause of incomplete analgesia during epidural anesthesia. Anesth Analg 1987; 66:679-83.
208. Beilin Y, Arnold I, Telfeyan C, et al. Quality of analgesia when air versus saline is used for identification of the epidural space in the parturient. Reg Anesth Pain Med 2000; 25:596-9.
209. D'Angelo R, Berkebile BL, Gerancher JC. Prospective examination of epidural catheter insertion. Anesthesiology 1996; 84:88-93.
210. Beilin Y, Bernstein HH, Zucker-Pinchoff B. The optimal distance that a multi-orifice epidural catheter should be threaded into the epidural space. Anesth Analg 1995; 81:301-4.
211. Crosby ET. Epidural catheter migration during labour: An hypothesis for inadequate analgesia. Can J Anaesth 1990; 37:789-93.
212. Wulf H, Munstedt P, Maier C. Plasma protein binding of bupivacaine in pregnant women at term. Acta Anaesthesiol Scand 1991; 35:129-33.
213. Kenepp NB, Gutsche BB. Inadvertent intravascular injections during lumbar epidural anesthesia (letter). Anesthesiology 1981; 54:172-3.
214. Lee RV, Rodgers BD, White LM, et al. Cardiopulmonary resuscitation of pregnant women. Am J Med 1986; 81:311-8.
215. Marx GF. Cardiopulmonary resuscitation of late-pregnant women (letter). Anesthesiology 1982; 56:156.
216. Kasten GW, Martin ST. Bupivacaine cardiovascular toxicity: Comparison of treatment with bretylium and lidocaine. Anesth Analg 1985; 64:911-6.
217. American Heart Association. Part 6: Advanced cardiovascular life support. Section 1: Introduction to ACLS 2000: Overview of recommended changes in ACLS from the Guidelines 2000 Conference. Circulation 2000; 102:I-86-9.
218. Ong B, Cohen MM, Cumming M, et al. Obstetrical anaesthesia at Winnipeg women's hospital 1975-83: Anaesthetic techniques and complications. Can J Anaesth 1987; 34:294-9.
219. Jeskins GD, Moore PAS, Cooper GM, et al. Long term morbidity following dural puncture in an obstetric population. Int J Obstet Anesth 2001; 10:17-24.
220. Spiegel JE, Tsen LC, Segal S. Requirement for and success of epidural blood patch after intrathecal catheter placement for unintentional dural puncture (abstract). Anesthesiology 2001; 94:A76.
221. Paech MJ, Godkin R, Webster S. Complications of obstetric epidural analgesia and anaesthesia: A prospective analysis of 10,995 cases. Int J Obstet Anesth 1998; 7:5-11.
222. Morgan B. Unexpectedly extensive conduction blocks in obstetric epidural analgesia. Anaesthesia 1990; 45:148-52.
223. Lubenow T, Keh-Wong E, Kristof K, et al. Inadvertent subdural injection: A complication of an epidural block. Anesth Analg 1988; 67:175-9.
224. Lee A, Dodd KW. Accidental subdural catheterisation. Anaesthesia 1986; 41:847-9.
225. Boys JE, Norman PF. Accidental subdural analgesia: A case report, possible clinical implications and relevance to "massive extradurals." Br J Anaesth 1975; 47:1111-3.
226. Abouleish E, Goldstein M. Migration of an extradural catheter into the subdural space. Br J Anaesth 1986; 58:1194-7.
227. Chestnut DH, Vandewalker GE, Owen CL, et al. The influence of continuous epidural bupivacaine analgesia on the second stage of labor and method of delivery in nulliparous women. Anesthesiology 1987; 66:774-80.
228. Russell R. Assessment of motor blockade during epidural analgesia in labour. Int J Obstet Anesth 1992; 1:230-4.
229. MacArthur C, Lewis M, Knox EG, et al. Epidural anaesthesia and long term backache after childbirth. Br Med J 1990; 301:9-12.
230. MacArthur C, Lewis M, Knox EG. Investigation of long term problems after obstetric epidural anaesthesia. Br Med J 1992; 304:1279-82.
231. Grove LH. Backache, headache and bladder dysfunction after delivery. Br J Anaesth 1973; 45:1147-9.
232. Olofsson CIJ, Ekblom AOA, Edman-Ordeberg GE, et al. Post-partum urinary retention: A comparison between two methods of epidural analgesia. Eur J Obstet Gynecol Reprod Biol 1996; 71:31-4.
233. Liang CC, Wong SY, Tsay PT, et al. The effect of epidural analgesia on postpartum urinary retention in women who deliver vaginally. Int J Obstet Anesth 2002; 11:164-9.
234. Cuerden C, Buley R, Downing JW. Delayed recovery after epidural block in labour: A report of four cases. Anaesthesia 1977; 32:773-6.
235. Russell R, Dundas R, Reynolds F. Long term backache after childbirth: Prospective search for causative factors. BMJ 1996; 312:1384-8.
236. Breen TW, Ransil BJ, Groves PA, et al. Factors associated with back pain after childbirth. Anesthesiology 1994; 81:29-34.
237. MacArthur A, MacArthur C, Weeks S. Epidural anaesthesia and low back pain after delivery: A prospective cohort study. BMJ 1995; 311:1336-9.
238. MacArthur AJ, MacArthur C, Weeks SK. Is epidural anesthesia in labor associated with chronic low back pain? A prospective cohort study. Anesth Analg 1997; 85:1066-70.
239. Howell CJ, Kidd C, Roberts W, et al. A randomised controlled trial of epidural compared with non-epidural analgesia in labour. Br J Obstet Gynaecol 2001; 108:27-33.
240. Howell CJ, Dean T, Lucking L, et al. Randomised study of long term outcome after epidural versus non-epidural analgesia during labour. BMJ 2002; 325:357-61.
241. Sartore A, Pregazzi R, Bortoli P, et al. Effects of epidural analgesia during labor on pelvic floor function after vaginal delivery. Acta Obstet Gynecol Scand 2003; 82:143-6.
242. Thalme B, Belfrage P, Raabe N. Lumbar epidural analgesia in labour. Acta Obstet Gynecol Scand 1974; 53:27-35.
243. Sharma SK, Sidawi JE, Ramin SM, et al. Cesarean delivery: A randomized trial of epidural versus patient-controlled meperidine analgesia during labor. Anesthesiology 1997; 87:487-94.
244. Reynolds F, Sharma SK, Seed PT. Analgesia in labour and fetal acid-base balance: A meta-analysis comparing epidural with systemic opioid analgesia. BJOG 2002; 109:1344-53.
245. Halpern SH, Littleford JA, Brockhurst NJ, et al. The neurologic and adaptive capacity score is not a reliable method of newborn evaluation. Anesthesiology 2001; 94:958-62.
246. Dailey PA, Baysinger CL, Levinson G, et al. Neurobehavioral testing of the newborn infant. Clin Perinatol 1982; 9:191-213.
247. Hodgkinson R, Marx GF, Kim SS, et al. Neonatal neurobehavioral tests following vaginal delivery under ketamine, thiopental, and extradural anesthesia. Anesth Analg 1977; 56:548-53.
248. Hynson JM, Sessler DI, Glosten B, et al. Thermal balance and tremor patterns during epidural anesthesia. Anesthesiology 1991; 74:680-90.
249. Kapusta L, Confino E, Ismajovich B, et al. The effect of epidural analgesia on maternal thermoregulation in labor. Int J Gynaecol Obstet 1985; 23:185-9.
250. Benzinger TH, Pratt AW, Kitzinger C. The thermostatic control of human metabolic heat production. Proc Natl Acad Sci USA 1961; 47:730-9.
251. Shehabi Y, Gatt S, Buckman T, et al. Effect of adrenaline, fentanyl and warming of injectate on shivering following extradural analgesia in labour. Anaesth Intensive Care 1990; 18:31-7.
252. Juneja M, Ackerman WE, Heine MF, et al. Butorphanol for the relief of shivering associated with extradural anesthesia in parturients. J Clin Anesth 1992; 4:390-3.
253. Brownridge P. Shivering related to epidural blockade with bupivacaine in labour, and the influence of epidural pethidine. Anaesth Intensive Care 1986; 14:412-7.
254. Ponte J, Collett BJ, Walmsley A. Anaesthetic temperature and shivering in epidural anaesthesia. Acta Anaesthesiol Scand 1986; 30:584-7.
255. Webb PJ, James FM III, Wheeler AS. Shivering during epidural analgesia in women in labor. Anesthesiology 1981; 55:706-7.
256. Ponte J, Sessler DI. Extradurals and shivering: Effects of cold and warm extradural saline injections in volunteers. Br J Anaesth 1990; 64:731-3.
257. Camann WR, Hortvet LA, Hughes N, et al. Maternal temperature regulation during extradural analgesia for labour. Br J Anaesth 1991; 67:565-8.
258. Macaulay JH, Bond K, Steer PJ. Epidural analgesia in labor and fetal hyperthermia. Obstet Gynecol 1992; 80:665-9.
259. Fusi L, Steer PJ, Maresh MJA, et al. Maternal pyrexia associated with the use of epidural analgesia in labour. Lancet 1989; 1:1250-2.
260. Herbst A, Wolner-Hanssen P, Ingemarsson I. Risk factors for fever in labor. Obstet Gynecol 1995; 86:790-4.
261. Glosten B, Savage M, Rooke GA, et al. Epidural anesthesia and the thermoregulatory responses to hyperthermia: Preliminary observations in volunteer subjects. Acta Anaesthesiol Scand 1998; 42:442-6.
262. Lieberman E, Lang JM, Frigoletto F, et al. Epidural analgesia, intrapartum fever, and neonatal sepsis evaluation. Pediatrics 1997; 99:415-9.
263. Goetzl L, Cohen A, Frigoletto F, et al. Maternal epidural use and neonatal sepsis evaluation in afebrile mothers. Pediatrics 2001; 108:1099-102.

264. Yancey MK, Zhang J, Schwarz J, et al. Labor epidural analgesia and intrapartum maternal hyperthermia. Obstet Gynecol 2001; 98:763-70.

265. Philip J, Alexander JM, Sharma SK, et al. Epidural analgesia during labor and maternal fever. Anesthesiology 1999; 90:1271-5.

266. Vallejo MC, Kaul B, Adler LJ, et al. Chorioamnionitis, not epidural analgesia, is associated with maternal fever during labour. Can J Anaesth 2001; 48:1122-6.

Chapter 21
Epidural and Spinal Analgesia/Anesthesia

II. OPIOID TECHNIQUES
Edward T. Riley, M.D. · Brian K. Ross, Ph.D., M.D.

During labor, the ideal analgesic technique would be safe for the mother and fetus, would not interfere with the progress of labor and delivery, and would provide flexibility in response to changing conditions. In addition, the ideal agent would provide consistent pain relief, have a long duration of action, minimize undesirable side effects, and minimize physician involvement. No single local anesthetic is an ideal analgesic agent during labor. Disadvantages of epidural and spinal local anesthetic techniques include hypotension, motor block, nonspecific sensory block, shivering, and the risk of cardiovascular collapse (e.g., from high spinal anesthesia or systemic local anesthetic toxicity).

The afferent nerve fibers that transmit pain impulses during labor include the visceral and somatic sensory fibers. During the **first stage of labor,** pain primarily results from dilation of the cervix and distention of the lower uterine segment, which occurs with uterine contractions. These pain impulses are transmitted by means of afferent A-delta and C fibers, which are **visceral afferent nerves** that accompany the sympathetic nerves and enter the spinal cord at T10 to L1. The visceral pain of uterine contractions is described as dull and aching; although severe, it is poorly localized by the patient. Visceral pain is transmitted by slow-conducting fibers that are easier to block than somatic nerve fibers. During the **second stage of labor,** pain results from distention of the pelvic floor, vagina, and perineum. Pain impulses are transmitted to the spinal cord by means of **somatic nerve fibers** that enter the spinal cord at S2 to S4. Somatic pain is transmitted by rapidly conducting fibers that are more difficult to block. The pain is sharp and well localized by the patient.

The visceral and somatic nerve fibers that transmit the pain of labor enter the dorsal horn of the spinal cord, where the initial level of pain modulation naturally occurs. Two decades ago, investigators identified dense concentrations of opiate receptors in the dorsal horn of the spinal cord. The application of small doses of an opioid to these receptor sites results in a specific and profound opioid response.[1,2] By contrast, systemic opioid administration activates multiple peripheral receptors, which results in analgesia that is tainted by the occurrence of unwanted side effects.

The introduction of intraspinal opioids appeared to fulfill the prediction made by Benjamin Rush in 1818: "A medicine would be discovered which should suspend sensibility altogether and leave irritability or powers of motion unimpaired."[3] In this section we explore how spinal opioids by themselves and in combination with local anesthetics bring us closer to achieving this goal.

MECHANISM OF ACTION

In 1979, investigators first reported dramatic pain relief after the epidural and intrathecal administration of opioids in humans.[4,5] Intraspinal morphine administration results in long-lasting pain relief with little if any effect on voluntary motor function or sympathetic tone. Intraspinal opioid administration provides excellent analgesia under certain circumstances, but this technique does not provide anesthesia (i.e., the complete absence of sensation). Likewise, intraspinal opioids provide effective pain relief in some but not all circumstances in obstetric patients.

Intraspinal opioid administration exploits the pharmacology of pain-modulating and pain-relieving systems that exist within the spinal cord (Figure 21-10). Opioids block the transmission of pain-related information by binding at presynaptic and postsynaptic receptor sites in the dorsal horn of the spinal cord (i.e., Rexed laminae I, II, and V) (Figure 21-11) and in the brainstem nuclei, periventricular gray matter, medial thalamus, and perhaps components of the vagal system. The modulation of pain in the spinal cord is the result of opioid binding at several different subtypes of opioid receptors (Table 21-5).

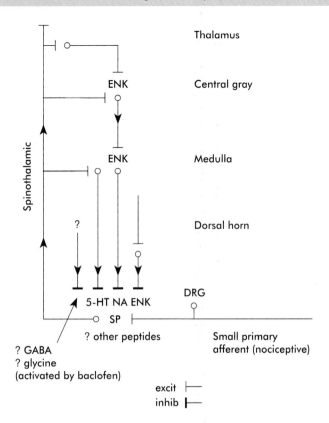

FIGURE 21-10. Model of pain transmission. Proposed excitatory *(excit)* and inhibitory *(inhib)* pathways and transmitters. Primary afferent nociceptive impulses are conducted by way of the dorsal root ganglion to spinothalamic and spinoreticular neurons in the dorsal horn, with substance P as the transmitter. *DRG,* Dorsal root ganglion; *SP,* substance P; *5-HT,* serotonin; *NA,* noradrenaline (norepinephrine); *ENK,* enkephalin; *GABA,* gamma-amino butyric acid. (From Cousins MJ, Cherry DA, Gourlay GK. Acute and chronic pain: Use of spinal opioids. In Cousins MJ, Bridenbaugh PO, editors. Neural Blockade in Clinical Anesthesia and Management of Pain. 2nd ed. Philadelphia, PA JB Lippincott, 1988:961.)

The effects of opioids are defined not only by their relative affinity for various receptors and the location of those receptors in the central nervous system (CNS) but also by the opioids' ability to reach those receptors. If given epidurally, opioids reach the receptor sites by penetrating the dura, passing through the cerebrospinal fluid (CSF), and entering the superficial laminae of the dorsal horn, where the receptors are located (Figure 21-12). The movement of opioids into the CSF also accounts for the occurrence of side effects.

The transmembrane movement of opioids, like that of local anesthetics, is modulated by the physicochemical properties of these drugs. **Lipid solubility** is a major determinant of opioid action. An increased lipid solubility allows a drug to diffuse rapidly to its site of action, which results in a more rapid onset of analgesia. For example, fentanyl is highly lipid soluble (600 times more lipid soluble than morphine), and it has a more rapid onset of action than morphine.[6] However, this increased lipid solubility of fentanyl is a double-edged sword: fentanyl also diffuses away from the site of action more quickly and thus has a shorter duration of action than morphine.

The relationships between lipid solubility and onset, potency, and duration of action are complex. For example, sufentanil, which is even more lipid soluble than fentanyl, also has a rapid onset of action (possibly faster than fentanyl), but it has a longer duration of action than fentanyl when given intrathecally.[7]

Onset, potency, and duration are also affected by other physiochemical properties, including **molecular weight, pKa, and protein binding** (Table 21-6). For instance, the lower the pKa, the greater the percentage of opioid that exists in the uncharged form (i.e., the anionic base) at a pH of 7.4. In the uncharged form, opioids penetrate the dura mater and dorsal horn more easily, which results in a more rapid onset of analgesia.

The physicochemical properties of opioids determine not only their rate of absorption but also their movement within the CSF. The speed and extent of rostral spread of the opioid in the CSF determines the incidence and severity of its side effects. Hydrophilic agents (i.e., those that are not very lipid soluble) are retained in the CSF; these agents may move a great distance within the subarachnoid space before they diffuse into the lipid tissues of the spinal cord. Hydrophilic agents (e.g., metrizamide) move from the lumbar subarachnoid space to the medulla within 30 minutes of injection.[8] This suggests that relatively large quantities of hydrophilic opioids (e.g., morphine) travel freely in the CSF and gain access to the respiratory centers on the ventral surface of the medulla. The rostral spread of opioid within the subarachnoid space may then result in respiratory depression. By contrast, the more lipid-soluble agents (e.g., fentanyl, sufentanil) penetrate tissues rapidly, which both limits the amount of opioid that moves cephalad and hastens the clearance of drug from the CSF (Figure 21-13).[9]

In summary, the beneficial and worrisome effects of intraspinal opioids depend on the following: (1) the opioid receptor that is activated (i.e., mu, kappa, delta); (2) the amount of opioid administered; (3) the opioid lipid solubility; and (4) the rate of movement and clearance of the opioid in the CSF.

EPIDURAL OPIOIDS

Epidural opioids frequently are used in conjunction with local anesthetics to provide analgesia during labor. Animal studies suggest that, when both an opioid and a local anesthetic are given epidurally, they interact synergistically to provide effective pain relief.[10] This allows for the administration of a smaller dose of each drug, which should decrease the incidence and/or severity of side effects. For example, epidural administration of a local anesthetic alone can provide adequate analgesia throughout labor, but the concentration of local anesthetic needed to maintain analgesia often results in significant motor block. Epidural administration of an opioid alone provides moderate analgesia during early labor, but the dose needed to maintain analgesia is accompanied by significant side effects (e.g., pruritus, nausea, perhaps neonatal depression). In addition, epidural administration of an opioid alone provides inadequate analgesia during the advanced phase of the first stage of labor as well as during the second stage.[11] By combining an opioid with a less-concentrated solution of local anesthetic, adequate analgesia can be provided throughout labor with less motor block, nausea, and pruritus and with no neonatal depression.[12]

To understand the interaction of local anesthetics and opioids when they are delivered together into the epidural space, it is important to understand how opioids act alone in the epidural space. **Morphine** was one of the first opioids used for labor analgesia. Hughes et al.[11] compared the epidural administration of morphine (2.0, 5.0, and 7.5 mg) with epidural bupivacaine 0.5% (Figure 21-14). Morphine was effective

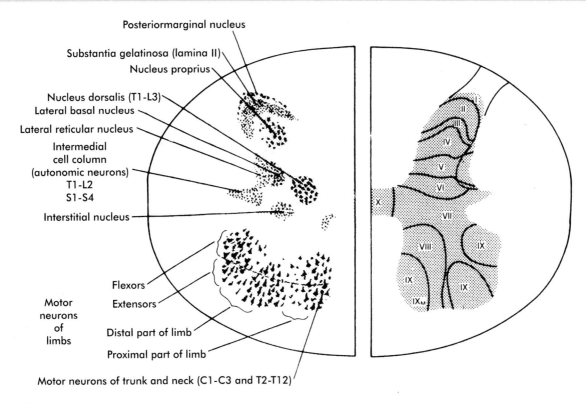

FIGURE 21-11. Architecture of the spinal cord, showing the Rexed laminae and gray matter nuclei. (From Ross BK, Hughes SC. Epidural and spinal narcotic analgesia. Clin Obstet Gynecol 1987; 30:552-65.)

TABLE 21-5	SUBTYPES OF OPIOID RECEPTORS	
Receptor type	**Physiologic response**	**Receptor agonist**
Mu	Analgesia, miosis, bradycardia, respiratory depression	Morphine, meperidine, fentanyl, sufentanil
Kappa	Sedation	Nalbuphine, butorphanol
Sigma	Tachycardia, tachypnea, hypertonia	Phencyclidine
Delta	Analgesia (?)	Enkephalins, DADL*
Epsilon	?	

*Alpha-ala₂, alpha-leu₅-enkephalin.

*Alpha-ala$_2$, alpha-leu$_5$-enkephalin.

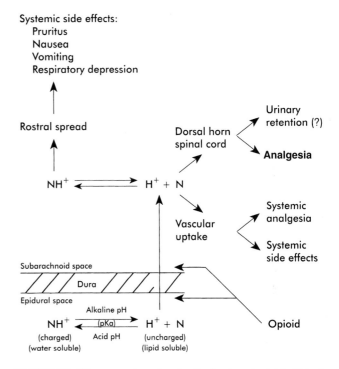

FIGURE 21-12. Factors that affect the distribution of opioid within the neuraxis and their important effects. (From Ross BK, SC. Epidural and spinal narcotic analgesia. Clin Obstet 1987;30:552-65.)

only at the highest dose (7.5 mg), but this dose resulted in significant side effects.

During the second stage of labor, epidural morphine, even in large doses, does not provide adequate analgesia. In addition to inconsistent analgesia, morphine suffers from a delayed onset of action (30 to 60 minutes), a property that few laboring women find attractive. Administration of a larger dose does not hasten the onset significantly, but it increases the risk of side effects. The delayed onset likely reflects morphine's lipid insolubility.

Epidural morphine administration results in significant levels of drug in both maternal and umbilical cord blood (Figure 21-15). Nydell-Lindahl et al.[13] concluded that the administration of a modest dose (4 to 6 mg) of morphine, a relatively short interval between injection and delivery, or

both could increase the risk of neonatal depression, especially in preterm infants.

Because of the slow onset of action, inconsistent analgesia, and frequent side effects associated with epidural morphine, investigators soon evaluated the epidural administration of the more lipophilic agents (e.g., **fentanyl**,[6] **sufentanil**,[14]

alfentanil,[15] **meperidine**[16]). The extremely lipid-soluble agents (e.g., fentanyl, sufentanil) have a rapid onset of action. Permeability is not a rate-limiting factor, and increasing the concentration gradient (through administration of a larger dose) facilitates faster entry into the spinal cord. The same properties that facilitate a rapid onset also result in a shorter duration of action. The increased lipid solubility results in

TABLE 21-6	OPIOIDS USED TO PROVIDE EPIDURAL ANALGESIA DURING LABOR			
Opioid	**Lipid solubility***	**Dose**	**Onset (minutes)**	**Duration (hours)**
Morphine	1.4	3-5 mg	30-60	4-12
Meperidine	39	25-50 mg	5-10	2-4
Methadone	116	5 mg	15-20	6-8
Butorphanol	140	2-4 mg	10-15	6-12
Diamorphine	280	5 mg	9-15	6-12
Fentanyl	816	50-100 μg	5-10	1-2
Sufentanil	1727	5-10 μg	5-10	1-3

*Octanol-water partition coefficient.

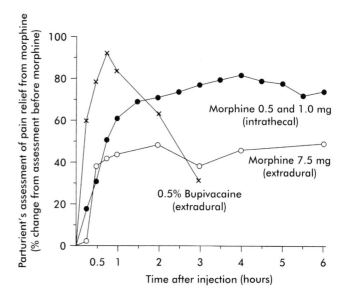

FIGURE 21-14. Maternal pain relief (before delivery) after epidural administration of 10 mL of 0.5% bupivacaine, epidural administration of 7.5 mg of morphine, or intrathecal injection of 0.5 or 1 mg of morphine. (From Abboud TK, Shnider SM, Dailey PA, et al. Intrathecal administration of hyperbaric morphine for the relief of pain in labour. Br J Anaesth 1984; 56:1351-60.)

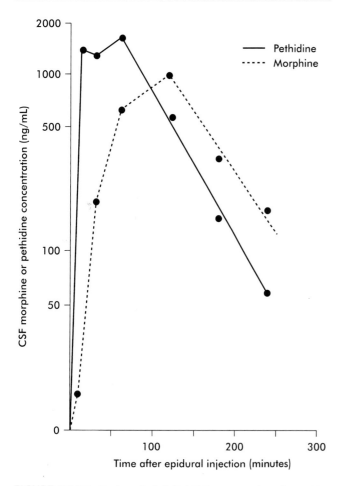

FIGURE 21-13. Cerebrospinal fluid (CSF) concentration of morphine and pethidine (meperidine) as a function of time after lumbar epidural administration. A 10-mL solution containing both morphine (10 mg) and pethidine (50 mg) was administered by means of a lumbar catheter. CSF was sampled from the C7 to T1 interspace at the times indicated. (From Gourlay GK, Cherry DA, Plummer JL, et al. The influence of drug polarity on the absorption of opioid drugs into CSF and subsequent cephalad migration following lumbar epidural administration: Application to morphine and pethidine. Pain 1987;31:297-305.)

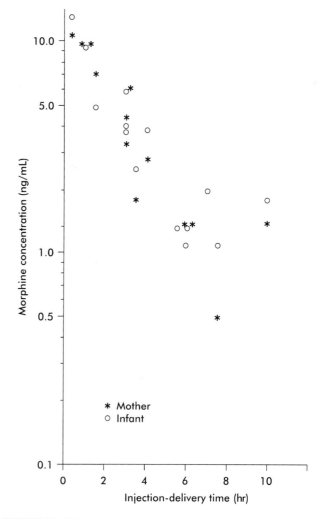

FIGURE 21-15. Maternal and newborn blood concentrations of morphine after epidural morphine administration. (From Nybell-Lindahl G, Carlsson C, Ingemarsson I, et al. Maternal and fetal concentrations of morphine after epidural administration during labor. Am J Obstet Gynecol 1981; 139:20-1.)

increased systemic absorption, which limits the duration of analgesia. Epidural administration of 150 to 200 μg of fentanyl[6] provides satisfactory labor analgesia for only 60 to 90 minutes. In addition, the lipid-soluble agents—when given alone—resemble morphine in their inability to provide adequate analgesia during advanced labor.

The primary limitation of epidural opioids is that they may relieve visceral pain during the first stage of labor, but they are less effective in the treatment of somatic pain during advanced labor (including the second stage), and they clearly do not provide adequate analgesia for operative delivery. By contrast, local anesthetic techniques provide dense somatic analgesia but often do not provide selective visceral analgesia. For these reasons, the combination of a dilute solution of local anesthetic with a lipid-soluble opioid may be a superior alternative. The administration of both a local anesthetic and an opioid hastens the onset and prolongs the duration of analgesia and results in fewer side effects than the administration of an equipotent dose of local anesthetic or opioid alone.

Justins et al.[6] observed that the addition of 80 μg of fentanyl to a solution of 0.5% bupivacaine resulted in more rapid and complete analgesia than the epidural administration of 0.5% bupivacaine alone. The epidural administration of fentanyl results in significant systemic absorption of the drug. Some investigators have suggested that the improved analgesia results from a supraspinal action rather than from a primary spinal action. However, Reynolds and O'Sullivan[17] helped refute this argument. They observed that patients who received 80 μg of fentanyl with the initial epidural dose of 0.25% bupivacaine had more rapid, complete, and prolonged analgesia than did patients who received 80 μg of fentanyl intravenously. Likewise, D'Angelo et al.[18] recently demonstrated that epidural but not intravenous fentanyl reduced epidural bupivacaine requirements in laboring women. Polley et al.[19] determined that the median effective local analgesic concentration (EC_{50}) of epidural bupivacaine in laboring women was reduced from 0.064% to 0.034% when fentanyl was co-administered epidurally rather than intravenously. These studies strongly suggest that epidural fentanyl provides analgesia primarily through a spinal site of action.

The addition of an opioid allows the anesthesiologist to give a more dilute solution of local anesthetic to provide excellent analgesia during labor. Published studies have demonstrated that epidural fentanyl[19,20] and sufentanil[21] decrease epidural bupivacaine requirements during labor in a dose-dependent fashion (Figure 21-16). Advantages of a decreased total dose of local anesthetic include the following: (1) a decreased risk of systemic local anesthetic toxicity; (2) a decreased risk of high or total spinal anesthesia; (3) decreased plasma concentrations of local anesthetic in the fetus and neonate; and (4) a decreased intensity of motor block. (Intense motor block likely prolongs the second stage of labor and increases the incidence of instrumental vaginal delivery.)

Administration of a dilute solution of local anesthetic requires the use of a continuous epidural infusion technique to maintain adequate analgesia. The continuous epidural infusion technique has supplanted the intermittent bolus injection technique in many hospitals. Studies have demonstrated that even a prolonged epidural infusion of fentanyl or sufentanil is safe for both the mother and fetus.[22-24] Elliot[23] observed that the continuous epidural infusion of 0.125% bupivacaine with fentanyl 4 μg/mL provided more effective analgesia than the continuous epidural infusion of either 0.125% or 0.25% bupivacaine alone. The addition of fentanyl did not affect the

method of delivery or neonatal outcome. Chestnut et al.[25] reported that the continuous epidural infusion of 0.0625% bupivacaine and 0.0002% fentanyl (2 μg/mL) at a rate of 12.5 mL/hr produced analgesia similar to that provided by the epidural infusion of 0.125% bupivacaine alone. Women in the bupivacaine-fentanyl group had less-intense motor block than women who received bupivacaine alone. There was no difference between the two groups in the duration of the second stage of labor or the method of delivery; however, the continuous epidural infusion was discontinued at the onset of the second stage of labor in both groups. Subsequently, Chestnut et al.[26] observed that the continuous epidural infusion of 0.0625% bupivacaine and 0.0002% fentanyl until delivery did not prolong the second stage of labor or increase the incidence of instrumental vaginal delivery as compared with the discontinuation of the epidural infusion at the onset of full cervical dilation in a similar group of patients. However, patients who received epidural bupivacaine-fentanyl until delivery only had partial analgesia during the second stage of labor. It remains unclear whether dilute local anesthetic-opioid solutions can be used to provide *total* analgesia throughout labor without affecting the progress of labor or the method of delivery. Nonetheless, it seems intuitive that a decreased motor block is advantageous. At Stanford University Hospital, most laboring women prefer to have little or no motor block during the administration of epidural analgesia. Surprisingly, not all studies have confirmed that decreased motor block results in improved maternal satisfaction scores.[27]

Published studies suggest that lipid-soluble opioids are superior to morphine when used in combination with a local anesthetic for epidural analgesia in laboring women. In theory, three lipid-soluble opioids—fentanyl, sufentanil, and alfentanil—may be combined with a local anesthetic to provide effective epidural analgesia. Loftus et al.[28] evaluated the addition of either fentanyl (75-μg bolus followed by a continuous epidural infusion of 1.5 μg/mL) or sufentanil (15-μg bolus followed by a continuous epidural infusion of 0.25 μg/mL) to 0.25% bupivacaine (12-mL bolus followed by an epidural infusion of a 0.125% solution at 10 mL/hr). The authors made the following observations:

1. Although they administered fentanyl and sufentanil in a ratio of 5.7:1, the ratio of fentanyl to sufentanil in maternal

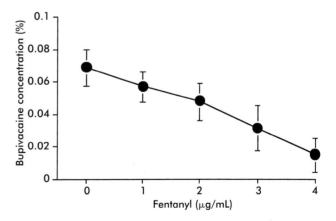

FIGURE 21-16. The effect of epidural fentanyl on the minimum local anesthetic concentration (defined as the effective concentration in 50% of subjects [EC_{50}]) for epidural bupivacaine analgesia during labor. Data are expressed as median concentrations with 95% confidence intervals. (Data from Lyons G, Columb M, Hawthorne L, Dresner M. Extradural pain relief in labour: Bupivacaine sparing by extradural fentanyl is dose dependent. Br J Anaesth 1997; 78:493-6.)

venous plasma was 27:1. This suggests that higher plasma concentrations of drug result from a given dose of fentanyl than from an equivalent dose of sufentanil.

2. The umbilical vein:maternal vein concentration ratios were 0.37 for fentanyl and 0.81 for sufentanil. When viewed in isolation, these data would suggest that placental transfer of sufentanil is greater than that of fentanyl.

3. Fentanyl was detected in most umbilical artery blood samples, whereas sufentanil was detected in only one of nine samples.

4. Neonatal outcome was uniformly good, as determined by Apgar scores and umbilical cord blood gas and pH measurements. However, the 24-hour Neurologic and Adaptive Capacity Scores were somewhat lower in the fentanyl group. It is unclear whether these differences were *clinically* significant.

5. Pain scores were similar in the two groups, except for better pain scores in the sufentanil group at 20 and 120 minutes.

Together, these data suggest that both drugs are safe and effective but that sufentanil may provide slightly better analgesia with slightly less neonatal neurobehavioral depression.

Epidural sufentanil administration results in small concentrations in the fetal circulation because of its high lipid solubility and its large volume of distribution. When epidural sufentanil is absorbed systemically, it has a larger volume of distribution than fentanyl. Therefore, epidural sufentanil administration results in a relatively lower plasma concentration of drug. When transferred across the placenta, sufentanil again has a larger volume of distribution and a correspondingly lower fetal blood concentration of drug as compared with fentanyl. (This remains true even though the umbilical vein/maternal vein ratio for sufentanil is higher than that for fentanyl.) The somewhat better analgesia provided by sufentanil probably results from its greater potency (i.e., greater affinity for opioid receptors) and its greater lipid solubility (which results in better penetration into the spinal cord).

To our knowledge, no study has compared alfentanil with sufentanil for epidural analgesia during labor. However, it is likely that epidural alfentanil would not be as effective or safe as epidural sufentanil. Alfentanil has less lipid solubility and potency than sufentanil. It is logical to assume that sufentanil would be superior to alfentanil in providing epidural analgesia in laboring women.

Meperidine may be used effectively alone (without a local anesthetic), in part because it possesses local anesthetic properties.[29] When given during labor, epidural meperidine 100 mg provides analgesia similar to that provided by 0.25% bupivacaine, with less motor blockade. However, this dose of epidural meperidine produces more sedation, nausea, and pruritus than epidural bupivacaine. Handley and Perkins[30] observed that the addition of 25 mg of meperidine to 10 mL of 0.125%, 0.187%, or 0.25% bupivacaine provided adequate analgesia for the first stage of labor. The use of the more concentrated solutions (i.e., 0.187% and 0.25% bupivacaine) did not enhance the quality or duration of analgesia, but it did hasten the onset of analgesia (10 to 20 minutes versus 20 to 30 minutes). Brownridge et al.[31] noted that the addition of 25 mg of meperidine to 0.125% bupivacaine produced adequate analgesia without adverse effect on neonatal Neurologic and Adaptive Capacity Scores. They also observed that the epidural administration of meperidine effectively prevents or treats the shivering that often occurs during labor.[31,32] No study has compared epidural meperidine with other bupiva-

caine/opioid combinations. At the University of Washington, patients who request epidural analgesia during latent-phase or early active-phase labor typically receive 25 mg of epidural meperidine, which is diluted in 5 mL of saline. These patients often receive a second—and in some cases a third—25-mg dose of epidural meperidine 2 hours after the previous dose. This regimen results in few side effects, and patient satisfaction is high. However, more research is needed to help determine the role of epidural meperidine in obstetric anesthesia practice.

Butorphanol is a lipid-soluble opioid agonist-antagonist, with weak mu-receptor and strong kappa-receptor activity. Kappa receptors appear to be involved in the modulation of visceral pain; therefore kappa-receptor agonists should be useful agents for the relief of labor pain, which has a significant visceral component.[33-35] Somnolence is the most prominent side effect of epidural butorphanol. Hunt et al.[33] evaluated the epidural administration of either 1, 2, or 3 mg of butorphanol with 0.25% bupivacaine in laboring women. The addition of butorphanol to bupivacaine hastened the onset and prolonged the duration of analgesia as compared with epidural bupivacaine alone. The authors concluded that the optimal dose of butorphanol was 2 mg. Of concern was the observation of a transient sinusoidal fetal heart rate (FHR) pattern in the 3-mg group that was not unlike that seen after the intravenous administration of butorphanol.[34] However, there was no difference among groups in Apgar scores, umbilical cord blood gas and pH measurements, or neurobehavioral scores. Abboud et al.[35] observed that the addition of 1 or 2 mg of butorphanol to 0.25% bupivacaine improved the quality and duration of analgesia as compared with the epidural administration of bupivacaine alone. All infants were vigorous and had normal umbilical blood gas and pH measurements as well as normal neurobehavioral scores. The authors observed few maternal side effects. However, some anesthesiologists have noted that the epidural administration of butorphanol results in somnolence and occasional dysphoria, which are side effects of kappa-receptor stimulation. Additional studies that include both maternal psychometric assessment and an assessment of neonatal outcome are needed.

Although the addition of an opioid to either lidocaine or bupivacaine results in at least an additive—if not a synergistic—effect, this may not be true with 2-chloroprocaine. 2-Chloroprocaine or one of its metabolites (e.g., 4-amino-2-chlorobenzoic acid) impairs the subsequent analgesic action of epidural bupivacaine, fentanyl, and morphine.[36-39] When given after 2-chloroprocaine, epidural fentanyl provides less-effective (of shorter duration) postcesarean analgesia than when given after lidocaine.[39] However, 2-chloroprocaine has less inhibitory effect on the efficacy of epidural fentanyl in laboring women. Epidural fentanyl (60 μg) decreases the EC_{50} of 2-chloroprocaine during labor from 0.43% to 0.26% (a 40% reduction).[40] This same dose of fentanyl decreases the EC_{50} of epidural bupivacaine during labor by 55%.[20] Therefore, fentanyl augments epidural bupivacaine analgesia slightly more than it augments analgesia provided by epidural 2-chloroprocaine.

The addition of **epinephrine** may increase the efficacy of epidural opioids,[41] but the enhanced effect is insufficient to make epidural opioids (without local anesthetic) an attractive regimen for the duration of labor. Epinephrine appears to potentiate the analgesia provided by the epidural administration of local anesthetics and opioids. Epinephrine likely causes vasoconstriction and decreased epidural blood flow, which delays the elimination of the drugs from the neuraxis. The addition of epinephrine to a local anesthetic typically results in an increased density of motor block. Epinephrine is also absorbed systemically; subsequent stimulation of beta$_2$ uterine receptors may result in a slowing of labor.[42]

Epinephrine may also enhance analgesia by means of the direct stimulation of alpha$_2$-adrenoreceptors and the inhibition of the release of substance P in the dorsal horn.[43] Studies have evaluated the epidural administration of **clonidine,** another alpha$_2$-adrenoreceptor agonist.[44-49] Epidural administration of clonidine alone provides modest analgesia, and clonidine may enhance the analgesia provided by the epidural administration of other drugs (e.g., local anesthetics, opioids). Unlike epinephrine, clonidine does not increase the motor block that results from the epidural administration of a local anesthetic, but it does potentiate both the quality and duration of analgesia.[47-49]

In summary, the apparent advantages of the addition of an opioid to an epidural solution of local anesthetic include the following: (1) decreased total dose of anesthetic; (2) decreased motor block; (3) decreased shivering; and (4) increased patient satisfaction. Some anesthesiologists contend that local anesthetic-opioid techniques result in a decreased risk of hypotension, but this is unproved. Likewise, it is unclear whether local anesthetic/opioid techniques can provide total analgesia during the second stage of labor without affecting the progress of labor and the method of delivery (see Section III of this chapter). Other adjuncts (e.g., clonidine) may prove useful in the future. Because epinephrine increases epidural local-anesthetic–induced motor block, we do not recommend its use when providing epidural anesthesia for labor. However, other anesthesiologists have a different view, and some consider epinephrine a useful adjunct, especially when added to a very dilute solution of local anesthetic with an opioid.

INTRATHECAL OPIOIDS

The ideal analgesic agent for labor would provide a rapid onset of pain relief, have a long duration of action, minimize undesirable side effects (e.g., motor block, hypotension), preserve proprioception, and have no effect on the fetus. Of the analgesic options used clinically, intrathecal opioids perhaps come closest to achieving these goals (Table 21-7).

However, some disadvantages are associated with the intrathecal administration of opioids alone. Single doses of the lipid-soluble opioids have a limited duration of action (1 to 2 hours). Additional doses require repeat dural punctures or the presence of an intrathecal catheter (both of which increase the risk of postdural puncture headache [PDPH] to unacceptable levels). In addition, intrathecal opioids alone do not provide adequate analgesia during the second stage of labor.

TABLE 21-7	OPIOIDS USED TO PROVIDE INTRATHECAL ANALGESIA DURING LABOR	
Drug	**Dose**	
Morphine	0.25-0.3 mg	
Fentanyl	15-30 µg	
Sufentanil	5-10 µg	
Meperidine	10 mg	

Early studies demonstrated that the intrathecal administration of 0.5 to 2 mg of **morphine** reliably produced analgesia during the first stage of labor, but the analgesia was less reliable during the second stage of labor and during instrumental vaginal delivery.[50,51] Intrathecal administration of these relatively large doses of morphine resulted in a high incidence of side effects, including somnolence, nausea and vomiting, pruritus, and respiratory depression (Table 21-8). Abouleish[52] reported a case of life-threatening respiratory depression 1 hour after delivery and 7 hours after the administration of 1 mg of hyperbaric intrathecal morphine.

In 1984, Nordberg et al.[53] demonstrated that the intrathecal administration of as little as 0.25 mg of morphine resulted in high CSF concentrations of the drug (Figure 21-17). The intrathecal administration of small doses of morphine has considerable appeal with regard to avoiding side effects, especially respiratory depression. However, morphine alone has a prolonged onset and is unacceptable for many laboring women. (Editor's Note: In the first edition of this text, Dr. Ross endorsed the use of intrathecal morphine in laboring women. He noted that the intrathecal administration of 0.25 to 0.30 mg of morphine provides analgesia for much of the first stage of labor [i.e., 4 to 8 hours or until the patient has a cervical dilation of 6 to 8 cm]. He also noted that the concurrent epidural injection of a small dose of local anesthetic [e.g., 3 mL of 0.25% bupivacaine with 1:200,000 epinephrine] results in a significant potentiation of analgesia. In the second edition, Dr. Riley clearly favored the intrathecal administration of a lipid-soluble opioid rather than morphine during labor. Subsequently, some anesthesiologists have advocated the co-administration of small doses of intrathecal bupivacaine, fentanyl, and morphine in laboring women,[54] but this is not yet common practice. Clearly we have not yet determined the ideal drug, dose, and/or combination of drugs for intrapartum intrathecal analgesia.)

Intrathecal injection of a more lipid-soluble opioid results in a more rapid onset of analgesia, with fewer side effects. Several studies have demonstrated the efficacy of intrathecal **sufentanil** and **fentanyl** in laboring women.[55-64] When used alone, intrathecal sufentanil or fentanyl provides analgesia with a rapid onset (usually within 2 or 3 minutes) and a duration of 70 to 100 minutes. Intrathecal administration of a lipid-soluble opioid provides analgesia with a significantly faster onset than that provided by epidural bupivacaine analgesia, and it results in no motor block.[57] Intrathecal administration of 10 µg of sufentanil provides satisfactory analgesia in 90% to

TABLE 21-8	PERCENTAGE OF PATIENTS EXPERIENCING ADVERSE SIDE EFFECTS AFTER INTRATHECAL INJECTION OF 0.5 OR 1.0 MG OF MORPHINE		
Side effects	**0.5 mg** **(n = 12)**	**1 mg** **(n = 18)**	**Overall incidence** **(n = 30)**
Pruritus	58%	94%	80%
Nausea/vomiting	50%	56%	53%
Urinary retention	42%	44%	43%
Drowsiness	33%	50%	43%
Respiratory depression	0%	6%	3%

Modified from Abboud TK, Shnider SM, Dailey PA, et al. Intrathecal administration of hyperbaric morphine for the relief of pain in labour. Br J Anaesth 1984; 56: 1351-60.

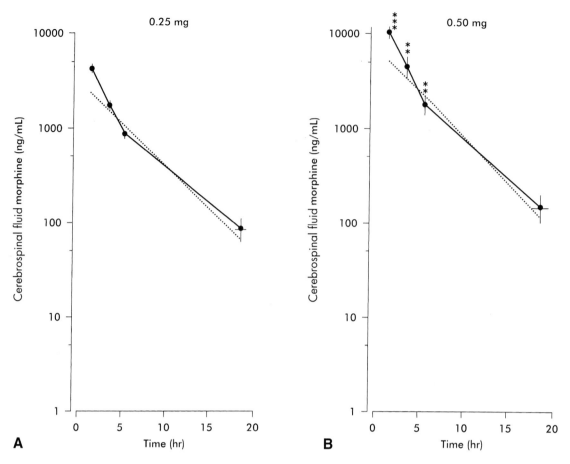

FIGURE 21-17. Cerebrospinal fluid morphine concentrations versus time after a single intrathecal dose of either 0.25 mg (**A**) or 0.50 mg (**B**) of morphine. (From Nordberg G, Hedner T, Mellstrand T, Dahlstrom B, Pharmacokinetic aspects of intrathecal morphine analgesia. Anesthesiology 1984; 60:448-54.)

95% of nulliparous women when administered before 5 cm cervical dilation. (Published studies have suggested that the effective dose of intrathecal sufentanil for 50% of patients [ED_{50}] is approximately 2 to 4 µg, and the effective dose for 95% of patients [ED_{95}] is 9 to 15 µg.[59-61] The ED_{50} of intrathecal fentanyl is approximately 14 to 18 µg;[62,63] the ED_{95} is most likely 20 to 30 µg.)

Unfortunately, the duration of analgesia is brief (i.e., 70 to 100 minutes). In one study, the addition of morphine 0.25 mg to sufentanil 10 µg prolonged the duration of intrathecal sufentanil analgesia by only 20 minutes.[64]

This problem (i.e., brief duration) may be overcome by the placement of a spinal catheter, which allows repeated intrathecal injection of a lipid-soluble opioid. However, the Food and Drug Administration (FDA) has removed the small-gauge spinal microcatheters from the market. (Studies of the safety of small-gauge spinal microcatheters in obstetric patients are in progress.) An epidural catheter can be placed in the subarachnoid space, but this technique results in a high incidence of PDPH. Thus the unavailability of the small-gauge spinal microcatheters and the unacceptable PDPH rate with the larger epidural catheters limit the intrathecal administration of a lipid-soluble opioid to a single injection. Typically this injection is given during the administration of combined spinal-epidural (CSE) analgesia *(vide infra)*. With this technique, the patient receives the benefit of the initial intrathecal injection of a lipid-soluble opioid, and an epidural catheter is placed to allow for the administration of additional drug(s) as needed.

An alternative drug is **meperidine.** Meperidine is unique among the opioids in that it possesses weak local anesthetic properties[29] and has been used in large doses (e.g., 1 mg/kg) as the sole agent to provide spinal anesthesia for surgical procedures.[65] Intrathecal administration of meperidine (10 to 20 mg) results in effective labor analgesia within 2 to 12 minutes, with a duration of 1 to 3 hours. Honet et al.[55] compared the efficacy of intrathecal meperidine 10 mg, fentanyl 10 µg, or sufentanil 5 µg in 65 laboring women. These three regimens resulted in a similar onset (less than 5 minutes) and duration (80 to 100 minutes) of effective analgesia. However, the meperidine group had significantly lower pain scores after cervical dilation had progressed beyond 6 cm. As labor advances, the nature of pain becomes increasingly somatic; only meperidine also functions as a spinal anesthetic. This helps explain why meperidine may provide more effective analgesia during advanced labor, including the second stage. However, we observed that the intrathecal administration of both sufentanil and a local anesthetic was superior to intrathecal meperidine alone for the relief of pain during labor.[66]

In Great Britain, some anesthetists have advocated the intrathecal administration of **diamorphine** (heroin). This drug is unavailable for clinical use in the United States. Kestin et al.[67] observed that the intrathecal administration of diamorphine (0.2 to 0.5 mg) provided good to excellent analgesia in 90% of laboring women. The mean duration of analgesia was approximately 100 minutes. However, 75% of patients had pruritus, nausea, and vomiting. By contrast, Sneyd et al.[68] observed prolonged analgesia after the intrathecal administration of diamorphine 2.5 mg, with a lesser incidence of side effects.

Intrathecal opioids alone provide effective analgesia during early labor,[69] but they do not provide effective analgesia during advanced labor. This may result from the fact that advanced labor causes more severe pain and/or the fact that the pain of advanced labor is somatic rather than visceral. To treat the more intense pain of advanced labor, it has become common practice to add a small dose of bupivacaine to fentanyl or sufentanil. In two nonrandomized studies, patients with a cervical dilation of more than 6 cm received intrathecal sufentanil 10 µg and bupivacaine 2.5 mg as part of a CSE technique. All of the patients received effective analgesia, and a majority did not require additional local anesthetic administered through the epidural catheter before delivery.[70,71] When given to patients in early labor, the addition of bupivacaine 2.5 mg to sufentanil 10 µg results in a higher sensory level and a greater incidence of hypotension than does the administration of intrathecal sufentanil alone.[72] Some anesthesiologists have suggested decreasing the dose of bupivacaine. Sia et al.[72] recommended "that the dose of local anaesthetic be reduced or omitted to improve the haemodynamic profile as well as the success of maternal ambulation in labour." Joos and Van Steenberge[73] claimed that the intrathecal administration of sufentanil 5 µg with bupivacaine 1 mg resulted in excellent analgesia in 94% of laboring women, with minimal motor block and a 4% incidence of hypotension. However, these authors did not stratify their results for patients in early versus advanced labor. It is our experience that women in advanced labor need the full 2.5-mg dose of bupivacaine. The dose of intrathecal bupivacaine remains a matter of a clinical judgment. We recommend co-administration of 0 to 1.25 mg of intrathecal bupivacaine during early labor and 2.0 to 2.5 mg of bupivacaine during late labor.

Recent data suggest that, when giving intrathecal bupivacaine, a smaller dose of opioid may be as effective as the larger doses that have been used in the past.[74,75] Stocks et al.[74] found that the ED_{50} of intrathecal bupivacaine alone for labor analgesia was 2.0 mg. The co-administration of 5, 15, or 25 µg of fentanyl lowered the ED_{50} to 0.7 mg to 0.9 mg. However, there was no significant difference in the ED_{50} of intrathecal bupivacaine with any of the doses of fentanyl that were studied (i.e., the smallest dose was as effective as the largest dose for reducing the ED_{50} of intrathecal bupivacaine). These investigators also observed less pruritus with the smallest dose (5 µg) of fentanyl. As a result, we have reduced the amount of opioid that we give with intrathecal bupivacaine.

Intrathecal administration of both sufentanil and a small dose of bupivacaine results in prolonged analgesia as compared with intrathecal sufentanil alone. Campbell et al.[76] demonstrated that the intrathecal administration of both sufentanil 10 µg and bupivacaine 2.5 mg provided analgesia with an average duration of 148 minutes, but sufentanil or bupivacaine alone provided analgesia for only 114 and 70 minutes, respectively. None of these patients experienced clinically significant hypotension or motor block. Subsequently, Campbell et al.[77] observed that **epinephrine** prolonged the average duration of intrathecal sufentanil-bupivacaine analgesia from 145 to 188 minutes. However, four (20%) of the 20 patients in the epinephrine group developed clinically significant motor block. Epinephrine is not required to provide effective intrathecal analgesia; thus we do not recommend the addition of epinephrine when providing intrathecal opioid analgesia. Alternatively, the addition of **clonidine** 30 µg

to intrathecal sufentanil prolongs analgesia by 30 to 40 minutes without causing motor block in laboring women.[78,79] However, Mercier et al.[79] demonstrated that the addition of intrathecal clonidine 30 µg to sufentanil 5 µg resulted in an increased incidence of hypotension. By contrast, Gautier et al.[78] noted that clonidine 30 µg did not affect the incidence of hypotension in laboring women who received intrathecal sufentanil.

The co-administration of a small dose of intrathecal morphine may prolong the analgesia provided by intrathecal bupivacaine and a lipophilic opioid. Yeh et al.[54] recently observed that the addition of morphine 0.15 mg to intrathecal bupivacaine 2.5 mg and fentanyl 25 µg prolonged the mean ± SD duration of analgesia from 148 ± 44 minutes to 252 ± 63 minutes. We are aware of several groups of anesthesiologists—who rely solely on intrathecal injections for labor analgesia—who now use this combination of agents in their clinical practice.

With epidural catheter-based techniques that are commonly used today, the duration of analgesia from the initial intrathecal injection is not an important issue. Further analgesia can be provided with a continuous epidural infusion, a patient-controlled epidural infusion pump, or a combination of the two. These techniques have proved safe and effective.[80-82]

When intrathecal opioid analgesia is provided, it seems best to inject an isobaric solution of the opioid. Two studies have demonstrated inadequate analgesia when sufentanil was given in a hyperbaric solution.[83,84] It is probably necessary for the opioid to penetrate the spinal cord rather than the nerve roots. Injection of a hyperbaric solution of opioid below the level of the spinal cord is less likely to provide adequate analgesia.

COMPLICATIONS AND SIDE EFFECTS

Neurotoxicity

Clinicians should exercise caution before injecting any agent into the epidural or subarachnoid space; the potential for irritation or outright damage to neural structures always must be considered. The anesthesiologist should be especially careful before injecting a new agent into the subarachnoid space, because it is far less forgiving than the epidural space.

Preservative-free morphine (which is commercially available for epidural and intrathecal administration) has no deleterious effect on neural tissue.[85] There are few laboratory studies of the effects of fentanyl on neural tissue. However, this drug has been administered to a large number of patients, with no published reports of neurotoxicity. Thus it is reasonable to conclude that either epidural or intrathecal administration of modest doses of fentanyl does not cause neurotoxicity.

Few studies have evaluated the safety of other agents that have been administered into the epidural and subarachnoid spaces. Rawal et al.[86] demonstrated histologic changes in sheep that are consistent with neurotoxicity after the intrathecal administration of 7.5 µg/kg of sufentanil every 6 hours for 72 hours. Smaller doses (i.e., 0.75 µg/kg) resulted in only mild changes. These doses are much larger than those used in clinical practice, and the clinical relevance of these observations is unclear. To our knowledge, there are no published reports of neurologic deficits after the epidural or intrathecal administration of sufentanil in humans.

Unfortunately, clinicians continue to administer agents that have not undergone adequate evaluation in animal models. Yaksh and Collins[87] correctly noted that "studies in animals should precede human use of spinally administered drugs."

Effect on Progress of Labor

Some controversy remains regarding whether epidural or spinal analgesia prolongs labor and increases the incidence of operative delivery (see Section III of this chapter). The cause-and-effect relationship between the use of these analgesic techniques and prolonged labor is unclear. Severe discomfort during early labor may signal abnormal labor and may predict an increased risk of FHR abnormalities and operative delivery.[88]

Intense motor block prolongs the second stage of labor and increases the incidence of instrumental vaginal delivery.[89] A growing body of evidence suggests that the use of a dilute solution of local anesthetic with an opioid—which results in less motor block than the epidural administration of a more concentrated solution of local anesthetic—results in a decreased likelihood of operative delivery. A large prospective, randomized trial from the United Kingdom demonstrated a significant reduction in the incidence of instrumental vaginal delivery with the use of a low-dose epidural technique.[90] Decreased motor block is also advantageous, in part because most patients prefer little motor block during labor.

Sensory Changes

In one of the early studies of intrathecal opioid administration during labor, Cohen et al.[56] observed sensory changes in women who received intrathecal sufentanil. Subsequent studies have demonstrated that these sensory changes do not result from a local anesthetic effect of sufentanil. Sensory changes do not predict the quality or duration of analgesia or the degree of hemodynamic change.[58] Further, intrathecal sufentanil does not cause a sympathectomy.[91] Wang et al.[92] have provided the best explanation for these sensory changes. They showed that intrathecal opioids block the afferent information from A-delta and C fibers to the spinal cord but that efferent nerve impulses are unaffected. These sensory changes can be clinically significant, especially when they extend to the cervical dermatomes. In such cases, patients may feel that they cannot breathe or swallow; this can be quite distressing. Fortunately, neither intrathecal sufentanil nor fentanyl affects the efferent limb of the nervous system, and motor function is *not* impaired. These patients should be reassured that respiratory efforts are not impaired and that these symptoms will subside in 30 to 60 minutes.[93]

In addition to sensory changes, two recent case reports have described mental status changes, aphasia, and automatisms after the intrathecal injection of sufentanil.[94,95] These symptoms seem to be related to an opioid effect. In one case, the symptoms were partially reversed by naloxone.[95]

Hypotension

Several studies have described a decrease in blood pressure after intrathecal opioid administration in laboring women.[56,58] Initially some investigators concluded that intrathecal opioids exerted a local anesthetic effect, which resulted in a sympathectomy. However, subsequent studies have demonstrated that the decreased blood pressure results from pain relief rather than from a sympathectomy.[91] However, sympathetic blockade can be expected if either a local anesthetic or clonidine is administered intrathecally with the opioid.

Nausea and Vomiting

It is difficult to determine the incidence of nausea and vomiting as a direct side effect of epidural and intrathecal opioid administration. Other causes of nausea and vomiting in the parturient include pregnancy itself, the pain of labor, and systemic opioids, which are often administered before intrathecal or epidural opioids. The cause of nausea mediated by neuraxial opioid administration is unclear, but it may be caused by the modulation of afferent input at the area postrema (i.e., the chemoreceptor trigger zone) or at the nucleus of the tractus solitarius, which is a key relay station in the visceral sensory network.[96] Of interest is that nausea is less common after epidural or intrathecal opioid administration during labor than after the administration of the same drugs for postcesarean analgesia. Norris et al.[97] noted that women who received epidural or intrathecal opioid analgesia during labor had an incidence of nausea of only 1.0% and 2.4%, respectively. Although the incidence of nausea is low, treatment should be available. **Metoclopramide** 10 mg intravenously is very effective and has few significant side effects. A partial explanation for metoclopramide's efficacy may be that it promotes gastric emptying. In our experience, **ondansetron** (Zofran) is effective for the treatment of opioid-induced nausea in laboring women, and it also has few side effects. **Droperidol** is effective for the treatment of nausea, but it has the most significant side effects of the three drugs (e.g., dysphoria, akathisia, oculogyric crisis). Pregnant women may be especially vulnerable to these side effects.[98] In addition, the FDA has issued a "black box" warning because of concern that the administration of droperidol may result in an increased risk of cardiac arrhythmias.

Pruritus

Pruritus is the most common side effect of epidural or intrathecal opioid administration.[14,56] Intrathecal opioid administration seems to be associated with a higher incidence of pruritus than epidural opioid administration (41.4% versus 1.3% in one study[97]).

Two options to decrease the incidence of pruritus are administration of a lower dose of opioid[54] and/or co-administration of a local anesthetic.[99] With epidural opioid administration, both the incidence and severity of pruritus seem to be dose-dependent.[19] However, even small doses of intrathecal opioids may result in significant pruritus.[100] It is our unproved observation that the intrathecal administration of a lipid-soluble opioid (e.g., sufentanil) results in segmental pruritus. For example, our patients often complain of perineal and truncal pruritus after intrathecal sufentanil administration.[56] By contrast, patients more often complain of facial pruritus after intrathecal morphine administration.

The cause of the pruritus is unclear, but it appears to be unrelated to histamine release. Pruritus may result from a perturbation of sensory input, which results from rostral spread of the opioid within the CSF to the level of the trigeminal nucleus or subnucleus caudalis.[96,101] A disruption of sensory modulation is consistent with the observation that a similar pattern of pruritus is seen in medical conditions in which sensory modulation is disturbed (e.g., diabetic neuropathy, multiple sclerosis).[102]

The treatment of pruritus varies. Some anesthesiologists give **diphenhydramine** (25 mg intravenously) to treat pruritus, despite the probability that this side effect is unrelated to histamine release. Any benefit may result from the modest sedation that follows the administration of this drug. Intravenous administration of **naloxone** (0.1 to 0.4 mg) or **nalbuphine** (2.5 to 5 mg) typically results in a prompt, dramatic relief of symptoms. At Stanford University Hospital, we rarely need to treat pruritus that occurs after intrathecal sufentanil administration. For those patients who require treatment, we give small doses (i.e., 2.5 mg) of nalbuphine, which may be repeated as necessary. The advantage of nalbuphine is that it is less likely to reverse the intrathecal or epidural opioid analgesia.[103]

Respiratory Depression

The administration of opioids by *any* route entails some risk of respiratory depression. When giving an opioid epidurally or intrathecally, factors that affect the risk of respiratory depression include the choice of drug (including its pharmacokinetics), the dose, and its interaction with opioids and other CNS depressants administered intravenously. With intraspinal opioids, the most important factor affecting the onset of respiratory depression is the lipid solubility of the drug.[104] In general, if respiratory depression is going to occur, it will occur within 2 hours of the injection of a lipid-soluble opioid such as fentanyl and sufentanil. When a lipid-soluble opioid gains access to the CSF, it is quickly absorbed by lipophilic body tissues. Subsequent clearance and elimination resemble those associated with intravenous injection of the same drug. Thus, with intraspinal injection of a lipid-soluble opioid, the "time window" for respiratory depression is short. Conversely, with a hydrophilic drug such as morphine, the onset of respiratory depression is delayed. Once a hydrophilic drug such as morphine enters the CSF, it tends to stay in the CSF. Rostral migration and absorption into the respiratory centers occur over several hours; thus respiratory depression may not occur until 6 to 12 hours after injection of the drug (Figure 21-18).

The dose of opioid is a major determinant of the risk of respiratory depression. Rarely, respiratory arrest follows the intrathecal administration of 10 μg of sufentanil.[105,106] However, most cases of clinically significant respiratory depression occur with larger doses of drug (e.g., intrathecal sufentanil 15 μg). Such large doses are unnecessary. Further, the administration of larger doses may *not* result in better (or more prolonged) analgesia. In a study of female volunteers, Lu et al.[107] observed that doses of intrathecal sufentanil greater than 12.5 μg did not result in a proportionate increase in either the intensity or the duration of analgesia. However, the administration of larger doses of sufentanil resulted in dose-related increases in serum sufentanil concentrations, which may worsen respiratory depression. Herman et al.[108] concluded that the ED_{95} of intrathecal sufentanil for laboring women is approximately 9 μg. Arkoosh et al.[59] reported that the calculated ED_{95} for intrathecal sufentanil is approximately 15 μg. However, they concluded that a dose of 10 μg should produce satisfactory analgesia in 90% to 95% of laboring women. Together, published studies suggest that doses of intrathecal sufentanil greater than 10 μg are unnecessary. (Editor's Note: In my practice, when I balance the quality of analgesia versus the risk of respiratory depression, the preferred dose of intrathecal sufentanil is approximately 7.5 μg, and the preferred dose of intrathecal fentanyl is 20 to 25 μg.)

Another risk factor is previous parenteral opioid administration. Three case reports implicated prior intravenous opioid administration as a contributing factor to the respiratory arrest that occurred after intrathecal sufentanil administration in laboring women.[109,110] Atkinson et al.[111] found an increased need for supplemental oxygen among patients who received intravenous meperidine before receiving intrathecal sufentanil during labor.

The increased respiratory drive that occurs during pregnancy—which continues well into the postpartum period—probably adds a degree of protection for the parturient.[112] Epidural and intraspinal opioids can be used safely in the parturient as long as adequate monitoring is available. Monitoring (e.g., assessment of somnolence and respiratory

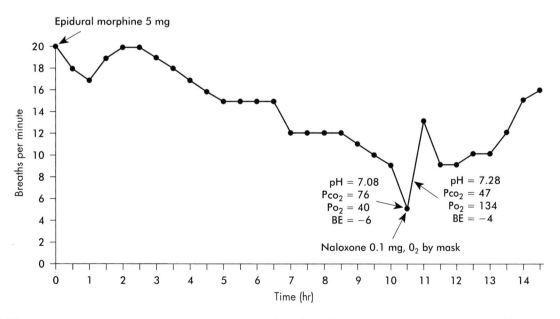

FIGURE 21-18. Respiratory rate of an obstetric patient who received 5 mg of morphine after cesarean section and who experienced delayed respiratory depression. (From Leicht CH, Hughes SC, Dailey PA, et al Epidural morphine sulfate for analgesia after cesarean section: A prospective report of 1000 patients [abstract]. Anesthesiology 1986; 65:A366.)

rate) should continue for at least 2 hours after intrathecal sufentanil or fentanyl administration and for at least 16 hours after intrathecal morphine administration. The use of pulse oximetry is not necessary for most patients provided that small doses are administered, nursing assessment occurs at frequent intervals, and the patient has not received other opioids or CNS depressants. (However, some anesthesiologists advocate the use of pulse oximetry in patients who have received intrathecal morphine for postcesarean analgesia.)

Urinary Retention

Urinary retention is a troublesome side effect of neuraxial opioids. The etiology may be the rapid onset of detrusor muscle relaxation that results from the sacral spinal action of opioids.[113] The onset of urinary retention appears to parallel the onset of analgesia. It is difficult to determine the magnitude of this problem during labor, because parturients often require catheterization for other reasons.

Delayed Gastric Emptying

Labor may result in delayed gastric emptying, which may be exacerbated by opioid administration.[114] Intravenous or intramuscular opioid administration results in delayed gastric emptying in laboring women. By contrast, clinically useful doses of epidural fentanyl have little effect on gastric emptying during labor.[115-117] However, intrathecal fentanyl administration seems to delay gastric emptying more than epidural fentanyl.[116] Delayed gastric emptying may predispose a patient to nausea and vomiting. In addition, it may result in a greater volume of gastric contents, which—in theory—might be problematic in patients who require the induction of general anesthesia for emergency cesarean section.

Recrudescence of Herpes Simplex Viral Infection

Genital herpes infection (herpes simplex virus-2 [HSV-2]) is the most common form of herpes viral infection during pregnancy.[118] The common cold sore or fever blister (HSV labialis or HSV-1) is the manifestation of the reactivation of latent HSV-1 infection. Reactivation of HSV-1 can occur after exposure to ultraviolet light, fever, immunosuppression, or trauma. In a retrospective study, Crone et al.[119] first noted an increased incidence of recurrent HSV-1 infection in pregnant women who received epidural morphine for postcesarean analgesia. The incidence of the reactivation of HSV-1 infection was approximately 10% in patients who received epidural morphine for postcesarean analgesia as compared with an incidence of less than 1% in similar patients who did not receive epidural morphine. Two prospective studies have confirmed this observation.[120,121] Case reports also have associated intraspinal meperidine and fentanyl with the subsequent recurrence of HSV-1 infection.[122,123]

The mechanism of HSV-1 reactivation after intraspinal opioid administration remains unclear. Proposed theories include the following: (1) the skin trigger mechanism, whereby the pruritus and ensuing scratching triggers reactivation[124]; (2) the ganglion trigger theory, whereby the exogenous opioid spreads rostrally and binds to trigeminal nerve opioid receptors, which alters the sensory modulation and results in reactivation[125]; and (3) an altered immunologic response.[126] Recent observations by Boyle[121] cast doubt on the first theory. Also, the third theory seems unlikely, because patients who undergo cesarean section without epidural morphine rarely experience reactivation of HSV-1 infection.

To our knowledge, postcesarean reactivation of HSV-1 infection following intraspinal opioid administration has not resulted in clinically significant maternal or neonatal complications. In addition, we are unaware of any study that has determined whether epidural or intrathecal opioid administration during labor increases the incidence of recurrent HSV-1 infection after vaginal delivery.

Postdural Puncture Headache

In the past, the risk of PDPH limited the use of spinal anesthetic techniques in obstetric patients. The use of noncutting, pencil-point spinal needles (e.g., Whitacre, Sprotte) has substantially reduced the incidence of PDPH after intrathecal opioid administration. In a prospective but nonrandomized study, Norris et al.[97] evaluated outcomes for 924 women who chose either epidural or CSE analgesia during labor. There was no difference in the incidence of PDPH between the two groups, although there was a higher incidence of unintentional dural puncture in the epidural analgesia group. When providing CSE analgesia, the anesthesiologist can use the spinal needle to confirm the position of the epidural needle, which may help prevent unintentional dural puncture with the epidural needle.

Fetal Side Effects

Epidural and intrathecal opioids may affect the fetus in either (or both) of two ways. First, systemic absorption of the opioid is followed by transplacental transfer of the drug, which may result in a *direct* effect on the fetus. Second, the effects on the mother produced by an opioid may affect the fetus *indirectly*.

Direct fetal effects may include intrapartum effects on the FHR as well as possible respiratory depression after delivery. Epidural opioid administration has little effect on the FHR.[28,127,128] Systemic absorption of an opioid may result in neonatal respiratory depression; this occurs more often after intravenous administration of opioids during labor.[129,130] When given by continuous epidural infusion, epidural opioid administration rarely results in accumulation of the drug and subsequent neonatal respiratory depression.[22-24] Bader et al.[22] noted that a continuous epidural infusion of 0.125% bupivacaine with fentanyl 2 μg/mL over a period of 1 to 15 hours did not appear to result in significant fetal drug accumulation or adverse neonatal effects. (In this study, the maximal cumulative dose of fentanyl was 300 μg.) Porter et al.[24] assessed whether the addition of fentanyl 2.5 μg/mL to an epidural infusion of 0.0625% bupivacaine affected neonatal condition. The mean ± SD maternal dose of fentanyl was 183 ± 75 μg, with a range of 53 to 400 μg. The addition of fentanyl did not depress neonatal respiration or adversely affect neurobehavioral scores or other indices of neonatal welfare. Loftus et al.[28] observed only a modest reduction in Neurologic and Adaptive Capacity Scores at 24 hours in babies whose mothers had received epidural fentanyl during labor. Babies exposed to sufentanil during labor had somewhat higher Neurologic and Adaptive Capacity Scores at 24 hours, and sufentanil was detected in the umbilical artery in only one of nine samples (*vide supra*).

Intrathecal administration of an opioid during labor has even less direct effects on the fetus than epidural administration. Smaller doses of opioid are administered, and less drug is absorbed systemically.

The **indirect fetal effects** of epidural and intrathecal opioids may be more significant. Obviously, if the mother has severe respiratory depression and hypoxemia, fetal hypoxemia and hypoxia will follow.[110] More common is the occurrence of fetal bradycardia after intrathecal administration of a lipid-soluble opioid. Several case reports have described abrupt fetal bradycardia after intrathecal administration of either sufentanil or fentanyl.[131-133] The presumed etiology is that the rapid onset of analgesia results in decreased plasma concentrations of catecholamines.[134] Epinephrine causes uterine relaxation by stimulating beta$_2$-adrenergic uterine receptors. Decreased circulating concentrations of epinephrine may result in increased uterine tone. Because uteroplacental perfusion occurs during periods of uterine diastole (i.e., uterine relaxation), uterine hypertonus may result in decreased uteroplacental perfusion and fetal hypoxia.

Published observations suggest that uterine hypertonus and fetal bradycardia may follow the administration of either intrathecal or epidural analgesia during labor. Nielsen et al.[135] assessed FHR tracings after the administration of either intrathecal sufentanil or epidural bupivacaine during labor. They observed no difference in the incidence of FHR abnormalities (i.e., recurrent late decelerations and/or bradycardia; 22% in the intrathecal sufentanil group versus 23% in the epidural bupivacaine group).

Fortunately, fetal bradycardia after labor analgesia does not appear to have a detrimental effect on the outcome of labor. Albright and Forster[136] retrospectively reviewed outcomes for 2560 women who delivered at their hospital between March 1995 and April 1996. Approximately half of the patients received CSE analgesia (including 10 to 15 µg of intrathecal sufentanil), and the other half received either systemic opioids or no medication. There was no difference between the two groups in the incidence of emergency cesarean section (1.3% versus 1.4%, respectively). Mardirosoff et al.[137] recently performed a systematic review of reports of randomized comparisons of intrathecal opioid analgesia versus *any* non-intrathecal opioid regimen in laboring women. The authors noted that intrathecal opioid analgesia appeared to result in a significant increase in the risk of fetal bradycardia (odds ratio, 1.8; 95% confidence interval, 1.0 to 3.1). However, the risk of cesarean section for FHR abnormalities was similar in the two groups (6.0% versus 7.8%).[137]

Given the risk of fetal bradycardia with neuraxial analgesia in laboring women, the FHR should be monitored during and after the administration of either epidural or intrathecal analgesia. The occurrence of fetal bradycardia should result in prompt efforts to achieve fetal resuscitation in utero. Such measures should include the following: (1) relief of aortocaval compression; (2) discontinuation of intravenous oxytocin; (3) administration of supplemental oxygen; (4) treatment of maternal hypotension, if present; and (5) fetal scalp stimulation.

Persistent uterine hypertonus should also prompt the administration of a tocolytic drug to achieve uterine relaxation. In the past, most physicians administered **terbutaline** intravenously for this purpose. Mercier et al.[138] described the use of intravenous **nitroglycerin** to treat FHR abnormalities that resulted from uterine hypertonus. The authors described consistent success after the administration of one or two doses (60 to 90 µg) of nitroglycerin. In theory, nitroglycerin is an ideal drug for use in this setting. Significant hypotension

occurs infrequently and is easily treated. In addition, nitroglycerin has a short duration of action; thus labor resumes shortly after cessation of the hypertonus. (By contrast, the administration of terbutaline may result in a prolonged tocolytic effect.) Unfortunately, we have not had similar success with nitroglycerin in our practice; perhaps this results from our unwillingness to wait more than 2 to 3 minutes before using another drug to achieve uterine relaxation. Buhimschi et al.[139] recently observed that three doses of sublingual nitroglycerin (800 µg per dose) did not reduce uterine activity or tone in laboring women, despite reducing maternal blood pressure approximately 20%. Nonetheless, sublingual nitroglycerin (400 µg per dose) is our first choice for the treatment of uterine hypertonus.[140] We administer terbutaline if there is no evidence of uterine relaxation within 2 to 3 minutes. Of course, it is prudent to make preparations for emergency cesarean delivery should the fetal bradycardia not resolve quickly.

NEW TECHNIQUES FOR LABOR ANALGESIA

Combined Spinal-Epidural Analgesia

CSE analgesia has gained increasing popularity during the last several years. With this technique, the anesthesiologist first places an epidural needle in the epidural space. A spinal needle is then introduced through the epidural needle into the subarachnoid space. An opioid is injected into the subarachnoid space, the spinal needle is withdrawn, and an epidural catheter is placed. The epidural catheter can be used later, or an infusion can be started immediately.

The CSE technique has become especially popular in obstetric anesthesia practice.[141] We administer CSE analgesia in patients who are in either early or advanced labor. In early labor, a small dose of intrathecal sufentanil alone (5 to 10 µg) provides complete (or nearly complete) analgesia—without any motor block—for almost 2 hours. As labor progresses and becomes more painful, both a local anesthetic and an opioid can be administered through the epidural catheter to provide and maintain analgesia until delivery. During advanced labor, the administration of intrathecal sufentanil (5 to 7.5 µg) plus a small dose of isobaric bupivacaine (2.5 mg) provides a rapid onset of excellent analgesia in most patients.[70,142] This small dose of bupivacaine results in little motor block.[66,76] Co-administration of both sufentanil and bupivacaine typically provides more than 2 hours of satisfactory analgesia, and many patients do not require additional drug(s) to be administered through the epidural catheter. For many patients, this represents the only regimen that provides a rapid onset of complete analgesia without significant motor block.

In theory, the incidence of PDPH should be higher with CSE analgesia than with epidural analgesia alone. The administration of CSE analgesia includes deliberate dural puncture in all patients plus the risk of unintentional dural puncture with the epidural needle. Norris et al.[97] found no difference in the overall incidence of headache between patients who received either CSE analgesia or epidural analgesia alone. However, women who requested epidural analgesia alone were significantly more likely to have an unintentional dural puncture than those who requested CSE analgesia. When providing CSE analgesia, the anesthesiologist can use the spinal needle to confirm the position of the epidural needle, which may help prevent unintentional dural puncture with the epidural needle.

Another concern is the potential for unintentional placement of the epidural catheter in the subarachnoid space. In laboratory studies performed on isolated portions of human dura, it was impossible to force an 18-gauge epidural catheter through a dural hole made by a spinal needle of 26-gauge size or smaller.[143] One Swedish physician observed "only one catheter penetration of the dura . . . during a 6-year period in which about 4000 CSE blocks were performed."[144] This incidence of intrathecal catheters is probably not different than what would be expected using a traditional epidural technique.

Finally, some anesthesiologists have expressed concern that an epidurally administered drug may pass through the dural hole and lead to an unintentional high block. This most likely is not a significant problem clinically. Suzuki et al.[145] assessed the effect of dural puncture with a 26-gauge needle on the spread of analgesia after the epidural injection of a local anesthetic. Twenty patients underwent dural puncture with a 26-gauge Whitacre needle, and 20 patients received epidural analgesia without dural puncture. No drug was injected at the time of dural puncture. The caudal spread of analgesia was significantly greater in the dural puncture group, but there was no difference between the two groups in the cranial spread of analgesia. The authors concluded that only a small amount of local anesthetic moved into the subarachnoid space through the dural hole made by a 26-gauge Whitacre needle; this resulted in a greater caudal but not a greater cephalad spread of local anesthetic.[145]

Patient-Controlled Epidural Analgesia

In most cases, either an anesthesiologist or a certified registered nurse anesthetist manages the continuous epidural infusion of local anesthetic, with or without an opioid. Ideally, the anesthesia care provider will titrate the epidural infusion to the needs of each individual patient. Pain varies greatly among individuals and during the course of labor and delivery in an individual patient. Some women want to participate more actively in all aspects of their intrapartum care, including the provision of pain relief during labor. Patient-controlled epidural analgesia (PCEA) allows the parturient to titrate the delivery of analgesic drugs to minimize periods of either inadequate or excessive analgesia. Published studies have suggested that PCEA provides effective analgesia and results in high patient satisfaction.[146-150] Some—but not all—studies suggest that PCEA reduces drug use and manpower requirements. Gambling et al.[146] demonstrated that PCEA resulted in a 26% decrease in the total dose of 0.125% bupivacaine used as compared with a fixed-rate continuous epidural infusion.

Investigators have suggested that the safety of PCEA is enhanced by the epidural administration of a dilute solution of local anesthetic and opioid; this should result in less risk than the administration of larger doses of either agent alone. The most common PCEA solution is 0.125% bupivacaine with 1 to 3 μg/mL of fentanyl. During the administration of PCEA, Ferrante et al.[150] observed that the addition of fentanyl to a 0.125% solution of bupivacaine decreased the hourly bupivacaine requirement during the first (8.8 mg versus 15.8 mg) and second (6.8 mg versus 17.2 mg) stages of labor.

Published studies have not reported significant maternal or fetal and neonatal complications of PCEA. Although contemporary infusion pumps are very reliable, mishaps can occur.[151] One disadvantage of either fixed-rate or patient-controlled epidural infusion techniques is that they encourage less-frequent contact between the anesthesia care provider and the patient. The use of these techniques does not obviate the need for a skilled anesthesia care provider who is readily available to manage complications.

Continuous Spinal Analgesia

Continuous spinal analgesia is an old technique that has several advantages over single-shot spinal analgesia. The continuous spinal technique allows greater control over the dose of drug and the onset and duration of analgesia. Historically, its major disadvantage in obstetric patients was the high incidence of PDPH, which resulted from the use of an epidural needle to place a large-gauge catheter. The renewed interest in intrathecal opioid administration during labor has resulted in a resurgence of interest in the use of continuous spinal analgesia in obstetric patients. In 1989, the introduction of small-gauge spinal microcatheters (i.e., 28- and 32-gauge) appeared to be a boon for continuous spinal analgesia. These microcatheters allowed the anesthesiologist to provide continuous spinal analgesia with a very low risk of PDPH. Several investigators gained substantial experience with the continuous intrathecal administration of local anesthetic alone, local anesthetic-opioid combinations, and opioid alone.[67,152,153]

Unfortunately, several reports soon appeared that noted permanent neurologic sequelae after the use of these microcatheters.[154-157] Laboratory studies have suggested that injury results from a nonuniform distribution of local anesthetic within the subarachnoid space.[155,157] In 1992, the FDA issued a safety alert announcing its decision "to remove from the market all small-bore catheters distributed for continuous spinal anesthesia" (i.e., 27-gauge or smaller).[158] Until studies have documented the safety of microcatheters for intrathecal drug delivery, this technique should not be used. Studies of safety and efficacy are in progress.

A PRACTICAL GUIDE TO INTRATHECAL AND EPIDURAL OPIOID ADMINISTRATION DURING LABOR

Intrathecal Opioids

Pregnant women, especially those who are nulliparous, often experience significant discomfort during the latent phase of labor. Many anesthesiologists and obstetricians prefer to avoid the epidural administration of a local anesthetic during early labor. In the past, the analgesic options during early labor were limited to psychoprophylactic techniques (e.g., Lamaze) and the systemic administration of opioids, with their attendant complications. With the introduction of intrathecal opioid analgesia, anesthesiologists currently can offer an alternative technique that provides superior analgesia to parturients who are not yet in active labor. In addition, women with significant medical disease are ideal candidates for intrathecal opioid administration.

During the initiation of neuraxial analgesia at Stanford University Hospital, we prefer intrathecal opioids over epidural opioids for two reasons. First, the intrathecal route allows for the administration of a smaller dose of drug. Second, intrathecal opioid analgesia has a more rapid onset and is more reliable than epidural opioid analgesia. Intrathecal administration of sufentanil 5 to 10 μg or fentanyl 20 to 30 μg (using the needle-through-needle CSE technique) provides excellent analgesia for almost 2 hours or until the second stage of labor approaches.

Box 21-11 describes our technique for the use of intrathecal sufentanil during early labor. An 18-gauge, 89-mm Tuohy-Schliff epidural needle is placed using a standard loss-of-resistance technique, and a 26-gauge, 127-mm pencil-point needle is passed through the epidural needle into the subarachnoid space. Sufentanil 5 to 10 μg is administered intrathecally. The spinal needle is removed, and an epidural catheter is threaded into the epidural space so that continuous epidural analgesia can be administered when more dense analgesia is required. At that time, we initiate epidural analgesia with 10 to 15 mL of 0.125% bupivacaine, with or without an epidural bolus of sufentanil.

If the patient is in the active phase of labor or approaching the second stage, we add 2.5 mg of bupivacaine to the intrathecal dose of sufentanil. This reliably provides a rapid onset of excellent analgesia with little motor block. (We use isobaric bupivacaine; hyperbaric bupivacaine settles too low in the sacrum and does not reliably provide analgesia of similar quality.[83,84]) Ropivacaine (2 to 4 mg) may be substituted for bupivacaine, but this more expensive local anesthetic offers no clinical advantage over bupivacaine when given intrathecally.[159]

If we perform the CSE technique during the active phase of labor, we typically begin an epidural infusion of 0.0625% bupivacaine and sufentanil 0.33 μg/mL at 10 to 15 mL/hr shortly after giving the intrathecal sufentanil; the only exceptions would be for those women who are expected to deliver within 1 hour. However, we almost always place an epidural catheter immediately after intrathecal opioid injection. Too often a woman will require more analgesia before delivery, even if she is completely dilated at the time of the block. In addition, the epidural catheter allows for the augmentation or extension of anesthesia in patients who require instrumental vaginal (e.g., forceps, vacuum extraction) or cesarean delivery.

Some anesthesiologists allow patients to ambulate after the administration of an intrathecal opioid.[160-165] (Some anesthesiologists have specifically suggested that intrathecal sufentanil 5 μg with bupivacaine 1.25 mg may be a good choice for parturients who desire to ambulate during early labor.[166]) Supervised ambulation seems safe for both the mother and fetus, provided the mother retains adequate motor function, proprioception, and balance. Unfortunately, no test reliably predicts who may ambulate safely. In addition, some patients may experience postural hypotension. Therefore, patients should wait approximately 20 minutes after receiving either an intrathecal or epidural bolus injection of drug, and they should sit on the side of the bed for 1 or 2 minutes before standing up. In addition, patients should ambulate only with assistance. At Stanford University Hospital, patients are encouraged to ambulate (with assistance) to the bathroom or to a chair, but they are not allowed to walk unsupervised or in the hallway. It remains unclear whether ambulation affects the outcome of labor and method of delivery in patients who receive CSE analgesia.[164,165,167,168]

Epidural Opioids

The following is a reliable regimen for the administration of epidural analgesia alone. After placement of the epidural catheter, a total dose of 12 to 15 mL of 0.125% bupivacaine with 10 μg of sufentanil is given in two or three fractionated doses over several minutes. This produces satisfactory analgesia in most patients. In our judgment, this regimen does not require the administration of a separate test dose, although this is a matter of some dispute (see Section I in this chapter). Intravenous administration of 12 to 15 mL of 0.125% bupivacaine over several minutes is unlikely to result in systemic toxicity. (A test dose that includes 3 mL of 1.5% lidocaine with epinephrine will increase the severity of motor block.) If there is no evidence of spinal anesthesia after administration of the first 4 or 5 mL of 0.125% bupivacaine, it can be assumed that the catheter is not placed in the subarachnoid space. If the patient develops the expected sensory level after the administration of 12 to 15 mL of 0.125% bupivacaine, it can be assumed that the catheter is not intravenous in its location.

If this initial dose of 12 to 15 mL of 0.125% bupivacaine does not provide satisfactory analgesia, we give additional 5-mL boluses of either 0.125% or 0.25% bupivacaine. When the patient is comfortable and the sensory level appears to be stable, we begin a continuous epidural infusion of 0.0625% bupivacaine with fentanyl 2 μg/mL or sufentanil 0.33 μg/mL at a rate of 10 to 15 mL/hr (Table 21-9). This regimen provides excellent analgesia with few side effects and little motor block, even with a prolonged infusion. In most patients, maintenance of the epidural infusion until delivery will maintain satisfactory analgesia while preserving adequate strength for maternal pushing during the second stage of labor.[169]

Monitoring

Adequate monitoring is essential after epidural or intrathecal opioid administration. During labor, the best monitors are medical personnel who remain at the bedside. Respiratory rate, heart rate, blood pressure, sedation, and FHR should be evaluated at regular intervals during labor and for approximately 2 hours after epidural or intrathecal administration of a lipophilic spinal opioid. Pulse oximetry should be used in high-risk cases.

Administration of epidural or intrathecal morphine mandates monitoring for a longer interval (i.e., at least 16 hours) because of the risk of delayed respiratory depression. The use of standard postpartum orders helps promote safety during and after the administration of either epidural or intrathecal morphine. Standard orders help ensure that none of the important areas of care are overlooked unintentionally; these orders should be tailored to the specific institution (Box 21-12).[170]

When epidural or intrathecal opioids are administered, resuscitation drugs and equipment must be immediately available. Thorough, ongoing training of nursing personnel also is essential.

Box 21-11   SUGGESTED APPROACH TO USE OF INTRATHECAL SUFENTANIL DURING EARLY LABOR

- Combined spinal-epidural technique
  - 18-gauge Tuohy-Schliff epidural needle—89 mm long
  - 26-gauge pencil-point needle—127 mm long
- Intrathecal sufentanil (5 to 10 μg)
- Epidural catheter placed immediately after intrathecal sufentanil injection
- Injection of local anesthetic through the epidural catheter at time of recurrent pain
  - 10 to 15 mL of 0.125% bupivacaine
    - No epidural bolus of sufentanil if less than 1 hour after intrathecal sufentanil
    - Epidural bolus of sufentanil 10 μg if more than 1 hour after intrathecal sufentanil
  - Epidural infusion of 0.0625% bupivacaine with sufentanil 0.33 μg/mL at 10 to 15 mL/hr

TABLE 21-9	INFUSION REGIMENS FOR CONTINUOUS EPIDURAL ANALGESIA DURING LABOR

	Drug			
	Bupivacaine	**Bupivacaine-fentanyl**	**Bupivacaine-butorphanol**	**Bupivacaine-sufentanil**
Loading dose				
Bupivacaine	0.125%-0.25%	0.125%-0.25%	0.125%-0.25%	0.0625%-0.125%
Opioid	None	2.5-5 µg/mL	0.2 mg/mL	1.0 µg/mL
Volume	10-15 mL	10-15 mL	10-15 mL	10-15 mL
Infusion				
Bupivacaine	0.125%-0.25%	0.0625%-0.125%	0.0625%-0.125%	0.031%-0.125%
Opioid	None	1-2 µg/mL	0.1 mg/mL	0.2-0.33 µg/mL
Rate	10-15 mL/hr	10-15 mL/hr	8-12 mL/hr	10-15 mL/hr

Modified from Naulty JS. Continuous infusions of local anesthetics and narcotics for epidural analgesia in the management of labor. Anesthesiol Clin 1990; 28:17-24.

Box 21-12 SUGGESTED ELEMENTS OF INTRASPINAL OPIOID ORDERS*

DRUG

A section describing the agent administered, the dose given, the route of administration (intrathecal/epidural), and the time administered. It should be clear that intravenous access is required and that no systemic opioids should be administered during the prescribed interval without the order of the anesthesiologist.

(Epidural/spinal) _____ (drug) _____ mg was administered at _____ (time) on _____ (date).

Maintain intravenous access (drip, peripheral heparin lock) for at least 16 hours after epidural/spinal opioid administration.

No other systemic opioids may be given except as ordered by the anesthesiologist.

MONITORING

A section describing the monitoring appropriate for the patient population and the drugs administered.

Respiratory rate and sedation scale every hour for 16 hours

Respiratory monitor for first 16 hours _____ Yes _____ No

If apnea monitor ordered, discontinue monitor after 16 hours if:
• patient conscious and alert; and
• no respiratory depression during the past 16 hours.

SIDE EFFECTS

A section describing the treatment of side effects (e.g., respiratory depression, nausea and vomiting, itching, urinary retention).

Naloxone 0.4 mg at bedside.

If patient is found apneic, give naloxone 0.4 mg intravenously and call anesthesiologist stat.

If patient has a respiratory rate < 10/min and/or a sedation score of 3:
• give naloxone 0.1 mg intravenously and call anesthesiologist stat; and
• may repeat every 5 minutes × 2.

For severe itching, nalbuphine 2.5 mg intravenously every 30 minutes, up to a total dose of 10 mg.

If not effective, give naloxone 0.1 mg intravenously.

May repeat every 10 minutes × 5.

Metoclopramide 5 mg intravenously slowly for nausea and vomiting.

May repeat every 6 hours × 3.

If first dose not effective within 30 minutes, ondansetron 4 mg intravenously.

For urinary retention, "in and out" bladder catheter as needed.

ANALGESIA

Additional analgesia may be necessary for breakthrough pain, so drugs and doses of acceptable analgesics must be specified.

Call anesthesiologist for inadequate analgesia.

Another option is as follows:

Morphine sulfate, 1 to 2 mg intravenously every 1 to 2 hours as needed for pain (hold for respiratory rate ≤ 10) or nalbuphine 5 to 10 mg intravenously every 2 to 3 hours

16 hours after epidural/intrathecal opioid administration, pain medications should be given as ordered by the obstetrician.

*Editor's Note: In the first edition of this text, Dr. Ross advocated standardized orders for parturients who have received intraspinal opioids. However, some of these orders (e.g., hourly monitoring of respiratory rate and sedation score for 16 to 24 hours) apply primarily to patients who have received intraspinal morphine. Most obstetric anesthesiologists advocate less restrictive orders for patients who have received a lipid-soluble opioid intraspinally (i.e., either epidurally or intrathecally) during labor. The specifics of the orders should be institution-specific and cannot be generalized to fit all environments.

KEY POINTS

- During early labor, intrathecal or epidural opioid administration allows the anesthesiologist to provide excellent analgesia while avoiding the side effects associated with the administration of local anesthetics. Some anesthesiologists allow patients to ambulate after intrathecal opioid administration.

- Intrathecal opioids alone may provide excellent analgesia during the first stage of labor. The lipid-soluble opioids have largely supplanted morphine for intrathecal administration during labor. Intrathecal administration of a lipid-soluble opioid is especially useful when administered as part of a combined spinal-epidural technique. During advanced labor, it is helpful to add a small dose of bupivacaine (i.e., 1.0 to 2.5 mg) to the lipid-soluble opioid.

- Epidural administration of a local anesthetic-opioid solution allows the anesthesiologist to provide excellent analgesia while decreasing the total dose of local anesthetic and minimizing the side effects of each agent. Perhaps the major advantage of this technique is that the severity of motor block can be minimized during labor.

- The most common side effects of epidural or intrathecal opioid administration are pruritus and nausea and vomiting. Fetal bradycardia and respiratory depression are the most serious complications of these techniques. Patients who have received epidural or intrathecal morphine are at highest risk for delayed respiratory depression, and these patients should be observed for at least 16 hours after the epidural or intrathecal administration of morphine.

REFERENCES

1. Atweh S, Kuhar M. Autoradiographic localization of opiate receptors in rat brain. I. Spinal cord and lower medulla. Brain Res 1977; 53:53-67.
2. Pert C, Kuhar M, Snyder S. Opiate receptor: Autoradiographic localization in rat brain. Proc Natl Acad Sci USA 1976; 73:3729-33.
3. Heaton C. The history of anesthesia and analgesia in obstetrics. J Hist Med Allied Sci 1946; 1:567-72.
4. Wang J, Nauss L, Thomas J. Pain relief by intrathecally applied morphine in man. Anesthesiology 1979; 50:149-51.
5. Behar M, Magora F, Olshwang D, Davidson J. Epidural morphine in treatment of pain. Lancet 1979; 1:527-8.
6. Justins DM, Francis D, Houlton PG, Reynolds F. A controlled trial of extradural fentanyl in labour. Br J Anaesth 1982; 54:409-14.
7. Gaiser RR, Cheek TG, Gutsche BB. Comparison of three different doses of intrathecal fentanyl and sufentanil for labor analgesia. J Clin Anesth 1998; 10:488-93.
8. Drayer B, Rosenbaum A. Studies of the third circulation: Amipaque CT cisternography and ventriculography. J Neurosurg 1978; 48:946-56.
9. Gourlay GK, Cherry DA, Plummer JL, et al. The influence of drug polarity on the absorption of opioid drugs into CSF and subsequent cephalad migration following lumbar epidural administration: Application to morphine and pethidine. Pain 1987; 31:297-305.
10. Vercauteren M, Meert TF. Isobolographic analysis of the interaction between epidural sufentanil and bupivacaine in rats. Pharmacol Biochem Behav 1997; 58:237-42.
11. Hughes SC, Rosen MA, Shnider SM, et al. Maternal and neonatal effects of epidural morphine for labor and delivery. Anesth Analg 1984; 63:319-24.
12. Vertommen JD, Vandermeulen E, Van Aken H, et al. The effects of the addition of sufentanil to 0.125% bupivacaine on the quality of analgesia during labor and on the incidence of instrumental deliveries. Anesthesiology 1991; 74:809-14.
13. Nydell-Lindahl G, Carlsson C, Ingemarsson I, et al. Maternal and fetal concentrations of morphine after epidural administration during labor. Am J Obstet Gynecol 1981; 139:20-1.
14. Steinberg RB, Powell G, Hu XH, Dunn SM. Epidural sufentanil for analgesia for labor and delivery. Reg Anesth 1989; 14:225-8.
15. Heytens L, Cammu H, Camu F. Extradural analgesia during labour using alfentanil. Br J Anaesth 1987; 59:331-7.
16. Baraka A, Maktabi M, Noueihid R. Epidural meperidine-bupivacaine for obstetric analgesia. Anesth Analg 1982; 61:652-6.
17. Reynolds F, O'Sullivan G. Epidural fentanyl and perineal pain in labour. Anaesthesia 1989; 44:341-4.
18. D'Angelo R, Gerancher JC, Eisenach JC, Raphael BL. Epidural fentanyl produces labor analgesia by a spinal mechanism. Anesthesiology 1998; 88:1519-23.
19. Polley LS, Columb MO, Naughton NN, et al. Effect of intravenous versus epidural fentanyl on the minimum local analgesic concentration of epidural bupivacaine in labor. Anesthesiology 2000; 93:122-8.
20. Lyons G, Columb M, Hawthorne L, Dresner M. Extradural pain relief in labour: Bupivacaine sparing by extradural fentanyl is dose dependent. Br J Anaesth 1997; 78:493-6.
21. Polley LS, Columb MO, Wagner DS, Naughton NN. Dose-dependent reduction of the minimum local analgesic concentration of bupivacaine by sufentanil for epidural analgesia in labor. Anesthesiology 1998; 89:626-32.
22. Bader AM, Fragneto R, Terui K, et al. Maternal and neonatal fentanyl and bupivacaine concentrations after epidural infusion during labor. Anesth Analg 1995; 81:829-32.
23. Elliott RD. Continuous infusion epidural analgesia for obstetrics: Bupivacaine versus bupivacaine-fentanyl mixture. Can J Anaesth 1991; 38:303-10.
24. Porter J, Bonello E, Reynolds F. Effect of epidural fentanyl on neonatal respiration. Anesthesiology 1998; 89:79-85.
25. Chestnut DH, Owen CL, Bates JN, et al. Continuous infusion epidural analgesia during labor: A randomized, double-blind comparison of 0.0625% bupivacaine/0.0002% fentanyl versus 0.125% bupivacaine. Anesthesiology 1988; 68:754-9.
26. Chestnut DH, Laszewski LJ, Pollack KL, et al. Continuous epidural infusion of 0.0625% bupivacaine-0.0002% fentanyl during the second stage of labor. Anesthesiology 1990; 72:613-8.
27. Calow C, Dresner M, Bamber J, Freeman J. Does motor block influence satisfaction with epidural analgesia? (abstract). Int J Obstet Anesth 1998; 7:195-6.
28. Loftus JR, Hill H, Cohen SE. Placental transfer and neonatal effects of epidural sufentanil and fentanyl administered with bupivacaine during labor. Anesthesiology 1995; 83:300-8.
29. Jaffe RA, Rowe MA. A comparison of the local anesthetic effects of meperidine, fentanyl, and sufentanil on dorsal root axons. Anesth Analg 1996; 83:776-81.
30. Handley G, Perkins G. The addition of pethidine to epidural bupivacaine in labour: Effect of changing bupivacaine strength. Anaesth Intensive Care 1992; 20:151-5.
31. Brownridge P, Plummer J, Mitchell J, Marshall P. An evaluation of epidural bupivacaine with and without meperidine in labor. Reg Anesth 1992; 17:15-21.
32. Brownridge P. Shivering related to epidural blockade with bupivacaine in labour, and the influence of epidural pethidine. Anaesth Intensive Care 1986; 14:412-7.
33. Hunt CO, Naulty JS, Malinow AM, et al. Epidural butorphanol-bupivacaine for analgesia during labor and delivery. Anesth Analg 1989; 68:323-7.
34. Hatjis CG, Meis PJ. Sinusoidal fetal heart rate pattern associated with butorphanol administration. Obstet Gynecol 1986; 67:377-80.
35. Abboud TK, Afrasiabi A, Zhu J, et al. Epidural morphine or butorphanol augments bupivacaine analgesia during labor. Reg Anesth 1989; 14:115-20.
36. Corke B, Carlson C, Dettbarn W. The influence of 2-chloroprocaine on the subsequent analgesic potency of bupivacaine. Anesthesiology 1984; 60:25-7.
37. Grice SC, Eisenach JC, Dewan DM. Labor analgesia with epidural bupivacaine plus fentanyl: Enhancement with epinephrine and inhibition with 2-chloroprocaine. Anesthesiology 1990; 72:623-8.
38. Chestnut DH, Geiger M, Bates JN, Choi WW. The influence of pH-adjusted 2-chloroprocaine on the quality and duration of subsequent epidural bupivacaine analgesia during labor: A randomized, double-blind study. Anesthesiology 1989; 70:437-41.

39. Camann WR, Hartigan PM, Gilbertson LI, et al. Chloroprocaine antagonism of epidural opioid analgesia: A receptor-specific phenomenon? Anesthesiology 1990; 73:860-3.

40. Polley LS, Columb MO, Lyons G, Nair SA. The effect of epidural fentanyl on the minimum local analgesic concentration of epidural chloroprocaine in labor. Anesth Analg 1996; 83:987-90.

41. Skjoldebrand A, Garle M, Gustafsson LL, et al. Extradural pethidine with and without adrenaline during labour: Wide variation in effect. Br J Anaesth 1982; 54:415-20.

42. Dounas M, O'Kelly BO, Jamali S, et al. Maternal and fetal effects of adrenaline with bupivacaine (0.25%) for epidural analgesia during labour. Eur J Anaesthesiol 1996; 13:594-8.

43. Fleetwood-Walker S, Mitchell R, Hope P, et al. A µ-receptor mediates the selective inhibition by noradrenaline of nociceptive responses of identified dorsal horn neurones. Brain Res 1985; 334:243-54.

44. Yaksh TL, Reddy SV. Studies in the primate on the analgesic effects associated with intrathecal actions of opiates, alpha-adrenergic agonists and baclofen. Anesthesiology 1981; 54:451-67.

45. Eisenach JC, De Kock M, Klimscha W. Alpha(2)-adrenergic agonists for regional anesthesia. A clinical review of clonidine (1984-1995). Anesthesiology 1996; 85:655-74.

46. Huntoon M, Eisenach JC, Boese P. Epidural clonidine after cesarean section. Appropriate dose and effect of prior local anesthetic. Anesthesiology 1992; 76:187-93.

47. Buggy DJ, MacDowell C. Extradural analgesia with clonidine and fentanyl compared with 0.25% bupivacaine in the first stage of labour (comments). Br J Anaesth 1996; 76:319-21.

48. Cigarini I, Kaba A, Bonnet F, et al. Epidural clonidine combined with bupivacaine for analgesia in labor. Effects on mother and neonate. Reg Anesth 1995; 20:113-20.

49. O'Meara ME, Gin T. Comparison of 0.125% bupivacaine with 0.125% bupivacaine and clonidine as extradural analgesia in the first stage of labour. Br J Anaesth 1993; 71:651-6.

50. Baraka A, Noueihid R, Hajj S. Intrathecal injection of morphine for obstetric analgesia. Anesthesiology 1981; 54:136-40.

51. Abboud TK, Shnider SM, Dailey PA, et al. Intrathecal administration of hyperbaric morphine for the relief of pain in labour. Br J Anaesth 1984; 56:1351-60.

52. Abouleish E. Apnoea associated with the intrathecal administration of morphine in obstetrics. A case report. Br J Anaesth 1988; 60:592-4.

53. Nordberg G, Hedner T, Mellstrand T, Dahlstrom B. Pharmacokinetic aspects of intrathecal morphine analgesia. Anesthesiology 1984; 60:448-54.

54. Yeh HM, Chen LK, Shyu MK, et al. The addition of morphine prolongs fentanyl-bupivacaine spinal analgesia for the relief of labor pain. Anesth Analg 2001; 92:665-8.

55. Honet JE, Arkoosh VA, Norris MC, et al. Comparison among intrathecal fentanyl, meperidine, and sufentanil for labor analgesia. Anesth Analg 1992; 75:734-9.

56. Cohen SE, Cherry CM, Holbrook RH Jr, et al. Intrathecal sufentanil for labor analgesia: Sensory changes, side effects, and fetal heart rate changes. Anesth Analg 1993; 77:1155-60.

57. D'Angelo R, Anderson MT, Philip J, Eisenach JC. Intrathecal sufentanil compared to epidural bupivacaine for labor analgesia. Anesthesiology 1994; 80:1209-15.

58. Riley ET, Ratner EF, Cohen S. Intrathecal sufentanil for labor analgesia: Do sensory changes predict better analgesia and greater hypotension? Anesth Analg 1997; 84:346-51.

59. Arkoosh VA, Cooper M, Norris MC, et al. Intrathecal sufentanil dose response in nulliparous patients. Anesthesiology 1998; 89:364-70.

60. Foss ML, Nelson KE, D'Angelo R, et al. Dose response study of intrathecal sufentanil in laboring patients (abstract.) Anesthesiology 1997; 87:A898.

61. Camann W, Abouleish A, Eisenach J, et al. Intrathecal sufentanil and epidural bupivacaine for labor analgesia: Dose-response of individual agents and in combination. Reg Anesth Pain Med 1998; 23:457-62.

62. Palmer CM, Cork RC, Hays R, et al. The dose-response relation of intrathecal fentanyl for labor analgesia. Anesthesiology 1998; 88:355-61.

63. D'Angelo R, Nelson K, Meister G, et al. Dose response study of spinal fentanyl in early labor (abstract). Anesthesiology 1998; 89:A1069.

64. Grieco WM, Norris MC, Leighton BL, et al. Intrathecal sufentanil labor analgesia: The effects of adding morphine or epinephrine. Anesth Analg 1993; 77:1149-54.

65. Kafle SK. Intrathecal meperidine for elective caesarean section: A comparison with lidocaine. Can J Anaesth 1993; 40:718-21.

66. Yeh J, Cohen S, Riley E. Evaluation of sensory, motor and hemodynamic changes with intrathecal bupivacaine, sufentanil and meperidine (abstract). Proceedings of the Annual Meeting of the Society for Obstetric Anesthesia and Perinatology, Bermuda, 1997.

67. Kestin IG, Madden AP, Mulvein JT, Goodman NW. Analgesia for labour and delivery using incremental diamorphine and bupivacaine by means of a 32-gauge intrathecal catheter. Br J Anaesth 1992; 68:244-7.

68. Sneyd J, Meyer-Witting M. Intrathecal diamorphine (heroin) for obstetric analgesia. Int J Obstet Anesth 1992; 1:153-5.

69. Lim EH, Sia AT, Wong K, Tan HM: Addition of bupivacaine 1.25 mg to fentanyl confers no advantage over fentanyl alone for intrathecal analgesia in early labour. Can J Anaesth 2002; 49:57-61.

70. Abouleish A, Abouleish E, Camann W. Combined spinal-epidural analgesia in advanced labour. Can J Anaesth 1994; 41:575-8.

71. Viscomi CM, Rathmell JP, Mason SB, et al. Analgesic efficacy and side effects of subarachnoid sufentanil-bupivacaine administered to women in advanced labor. Reg Anesth 1996; 21:424-9.

72. Sia ATH, Chong JL, Tay DHB, et al. Intrathecal sufentanil as the sole agent in combined spinal-epidural analgesia for the ambulatory parturient. Can J Anaesth 1998; 45:620-5.

73. Joos S, Van Steenberge A. Does anesthesiology, like history, repeat itself? (letter). Anesthesiology 1998; 89:542.

74. Stocks GM, Hallworth SP, Fernando R, et al. Minimum local analgesic dose of intrathecal bupivacaine in labor and the effect of intrathecal fentanyl. Anesthesiology 2001; 94:593-8.

75. Wong CA, Scavone BM, Loffredi M, et al. The dose-response of intrathecal sufentanil added to bupivacaine for labor analgesia. Anesthesiology 2000; 92:1553-8.

76. Campbell DC, Camann WR, Datta S. The addition of bupivacaine to intrathecal sufentanil for labor analgesia. Anesth Analg 1995; 81:305-9.

77. Campbell DC, Banner R, Crone LA, et al. Addition of epinephrine to intrathecal bupivacaine and sufentanil for ambulatory labor analgesia. Anesthesiology 1997; 86:525-31.

78. Gautier PE, De Kock M, Fanard L, et al. Intrathecal clonidine combined with sufentanil for labor analgesia. Anesthesiology 1998; 88:651-6.

79. Mercier FJ, Dounas M, Bouaziz H, et al. The effect of adding a minidose of clonidine to intrathecal sufentanil for labor analgesia. Anesthesiology 1998; 89:594-601.

80. Norris MC. Are combined spinal-epidural catheters reliable? Int J Obstet Anesth 2000; 9:3-6.

81. Gaiser RR, Lewin SB, Cheek TG, Gutsche BB. Effects of immediately initiating an epidural infusion in the combined spinal and epidural technique in nulliparous parturients. Reg Anesth Pain Med 2000; 25:223-7.

82. al-Mufti R, Morey R, Shennan A, Morgan B. Blood pressure and fetal heart rate changes with patient-controlled combined spinal epidural analgesia while ambulating in labour. Br J Obstet Gynaecol 1997; 104:554-8.

83. Ferouz F, Norris MC, Arkoosh VA, et al. Baricity, needle direction, and intrathecal sufentanil labor analgesia. Anesthesiology 1997; 86:592-8.

84. Gage JC, D'Angelo R, Miller R, Eisenach JC. Does dextrose affect analgesia or the side effects of intrathecal sufentanil? Anesth Analg 1997; 85:826-30.

85. Abouleish E, Barmada M, Nemoto E, et al. Acute and chronic effects of intrathecal morphine in monkeys. Br J Anaesth 1981; 53:1027-32.

86. Rawal N, Nuutinen L, Raj PP, et al. Behavioral and histopathologic effects following intrathecal administration of butorphanol, sufentanil, and nalbuphine in sheep. Anesthesiology 1991; 75:1025-34.

87. Yaksh TL, Collins JG. Studies in animals should precede human use of spinally administered drugs. Anesthesiology 1989; 70:4-6.

88. Wuitchik M, Bakal D, Lipshitz J. Relationships between pain, cognitive activity and epidural analgesia during labor. Pain 1990; 41:125-32.

89. Chestnut DH, Vandewalker GE, Owen CL, et al. The influence of continuous epidural bupivacaine analgesia on the second stage of labor and method of delivery in nulliparous women. Anesthesiology 1987; 66:774-80.

90. Comparative Obstetric Mobile Epidural Trial (COMET) Study Group UK. Effect of low-dose mobile versus traditional epidural techniques on mode of delivery: A randomised controlled trial. Lancet 2001; 358:19-23.

91. Riley ET, Walker D, Hamilton CL, Cohen SE. Intrathecal sufentanil for labor analgesia does not cause a sympathectomy. Anesthesiology 1997; 87:874-8.

92. Wang C, Chakrabarti MK, Whitwam JG. Specific enhancement by fentanyl of the effects of intrathecal bupivacaine on nociceptive afferent but not on sympathetic efferent pathways in dogs. Anesthesiology 1993; 79:766-73.

93. Hamilton CL, Cohen SE. High sensory block after intrathecal sufentanil for labor analgesia. Anesthesiology 1995; 83:1118-21.

94. Scavone BM. Altered level of consciousness after combined spinal-epidural labor analgesia with intrathecal fentanyl and bupivacaine. Anesthesiology 2002; 96:1021-2.

95. Fragneto RY, Fisher A. Mental status change and aphasia after labor analgesia with intrathecal sufentanil/bupivacaine. Anesth Analg 2000; 90:1175-6.

96. Bromage P, Camporesi E, Durant P, Neilsen C. Nonrespiratory side effects of epidural morphine. Anesth Analg 1982; 61:490-5.

97. Norris MC, Grieco WM, Borkowski M, et al. Complications of labor analgesia: Epidural versus combined spinal epidural techniques. Anesth Analg 1994; 79:529-37. (Published erratum appears in Anesth Analg 1994; 79:1217.)

98. Thorpe S, Smith A. A case of postoperative anxiety due to low dose droperidol used with patient-controlled analgesia. Int J Obstet Anesth 1996; 5:283-4.

99. Asokumar B, Newman LM, McCarthy RJ, et al. Intrathecal bupivacaine reduces pruritus and prolongs duration of fentanyl analgesia during labor: A prospective, randomized controlled trial. Anesth Analg 1998; 87:1309-15.

100. Norris MC, Fogel ST, Holtmann B. Intrathecal sufentanil (5 vs. 10 µg) for labor analgesia: Efficacy and side effects. Reg Anesth Pain Med 1998; 23:252-7.

101. Hu J, Dostrovsky J, Sessle B. Functional properties of neurons in cat trigeminal subnucleus caudalis (medullary dorsal horn). J Neurophysiol 1981; 45:173-92.

102. Ballantyne J, Loach A, Carr D. Itching after epidural and spinal opiates. Pain 1988; 33:149-60.

103. Cohen SE, Ratner EF, Kreitzman TR, et al. Nalbuphine is better than naloxone for treatment of side effects after epidural morphine. Anesth Analg 1992; 75:747-52.

104. Chaney MA. Side effects of intrathecal and epidural opioids. Can J Anaesth 1995; 42:891-903.

105. Greenhalgh CA. Respiratory arrest in a parturient following intrathecal injection of sufentanil and bupivacaine. Anaesthesia 1996; 51:173-5.

106. Katsiris S, Williams S, Leighton BL, Halpern S. Respiratory arrest following intrathecal injection of sufentanil and bupivacaine in a parturient. Can J Anaesth 1998; 45:880-3.

107. Lu JK, Schafer PG, Gardner TL, et al. The dose-response pharmacology of intrathecal sufentanil in female volunteers. Anesth Analg 1997; 85:372-9.

108. Herman NL, Calicott R, Van Decar TK, et al. Determination of the dose-response relationship for intrathecal sufentanil in laboring patients. Anesth Analg 1997; 84:1256-61.

109. Lu J, Manullang T, Staples M, et al. Maternal respiratory arrests, severe hypotension, and fetal distress after administration of intrathecal, sufentanil, and bupivacaine after intravenous fentanyl. Anesthesiology 1997; 87:170-2.

110. Ferouz F, Norris MC, Leighton BL. Risk of respiratory arrest after intrathecal sufentanil. Anesth Analg 1997; 85:1088-90.

111. Atkinson P, Huffnagle H, Arkoosh V, et al. How common is respiratory depression in laboring patients who receive intrathecal sufentanil alone or following IV opioids? Anesthesiology 1997; 87:A828.

112. Bromage P, Camporesi E, Durant P, Neilsen C. Rostral spread and epidural morphine. Anesthesiology 1982; 36:165-85.

113. Rawal N, Mollefors K, Axelsson K, et al. An experimental study of urodynamic effects of epidural morphine and of naloxone reversal. Anesth Analg 1983; 62:641-7.

114. Holdsworth JD. Relationship between stomach contents and analgesia in labour. Br J Anaesth 1978; 50:1145-8.

115. Zimmermann DL, Breen TW, Fick G. Adding fentanyl 0.0002% to epidural bupivacaine 0.125% does not delay gastric emptying in laboring parturients. Anesth Analg 1996; 82:612-6.

116. Kelly MC, Carabine UA, Hill DA, Mirakhur RK. A comparison of the effect of intrathecal and extradural fentanyl on gastric emptying in laboring women. Anesth Analg 1997; 85:834-8.

117. Porter JS, Bonello E, Reynolds F. The influence of epidural administration of fentanyl infusion on gastric emptying in labour. Anaesthesia 1997; 52:1151-6.

118. Stagno S, Whitley R. Herpes virus infections of pregnancy. II. Herpes simplex virus and varicella-zoster virus infections. N Engl J Med 1985; 313:1327-30.

119. Crone LA, Conly JM, Clark KM, et al. Recurrent herpes simplex virus labialis and the use of epidural morphine in obstetric patients. Anesth Analg 1988; 67:318-23.

120. Crone LA, Conly JM, Storgard C, et al. Herpes labialis in parturients receiving epidural morphine following cesarean section. Anesthesiology 1990; 73:208-13.

121. Boyle RK. Herpes simplex labialis after epidural or parenteral morphine: A randomized prospective trial in an Australian obstetric population. Anaesth Intensive Care 1995; 23:433-7.

122. Valley MA, Bourke DL, McKenzie AM. Recurrence of thoracic and labial herpes simplex virus infection in a patient receiving epidural fentanyl. Anesthesiology 1992; 76:1056-7.

123. Acalovschi I. Herpes simplex after spinal pethidine (letter). Anaesthesia 1986; 41:1271-2.

124. Glaser T, Gotlieg-Stematsky T. Clinical Aspects, Human Herpes Virus Infections. New York, NY, Marcel Dekker, 1982:1-40.

125. Scott P, Fischer H. Spinal opiate analgesia and facial pruritus: A neural theory. Postgrad Med J 1982; 58:531-5.

126. Gieraerts R, Navalgund A, Vaes L, et al. Increased incidence of itching and herpes simplex in patients given epidural morphine after cesarean section. Anesth Analg 1987; 66:1321-4.

127. Viscomi CM, Hood DD, Melone PJ, Eisenach JC. Fetal heart rate variability after epidural fentanyl during labor. Anesth Analg 1990; 71:679-83.

128. Wilhite AO, Moore CH, Blass NH, Christmas JT. Plasma concentration profile of epidural alfentanil. Bolus followed by continuous infusion technique in the parturient: Effect of epidural alfentanil and fentanyl on fetal heart rate. Reg Anesth 1994; 19:164-8.

129. Smith CV, Rayburn WF, Allen KV, et al. Influence of intravenous fentanyl on fetal biophysical parameters during labor. J Matern Fetal Med 1996; 5:89-92.

130. Rayburn WF, Smith CV, Parriott JE, Woods RE. Randomized comparison of meperidine and fentanyl during labor. Obstet Gynecol 1989; 74:604-6.

131. Clarke VT, Smiley RM, Finster M. Uterine hyperactivity after intrathecal injection of fentanyl for analgesia during labor: A cause of fetal bradycardia? (letter). Anesthesiology 1994; 81:1083.

132. Friedlander JD, Fox HE, Cain CF, et al. Fetal bradycardia and uterine hyperactivity following subarachnoid administration of fentanyl during labor. Reg Anesth 1997; 22:378-81.

133. Kahn L, Hubert E. Combined spinal epidural (CSE) analgesia, fetal bradycardia, and uterine hypertonus (letter). Reg Anesth Pain Med 1998; 23:111-2.

134. Cascio M, Pygon B, Bernett C, Ramanathan S. Labour analgesia with intrathecal fentanyl decreases maternal stress. Can J Anaesth 1997; 44:605-9.

135. Nielsen PE, Erickson JR, Abouleish EI, et al. Fetal heart rate changes after intrathecal sufentanil or epidural bupivacaine for labor analgesia: Incidence and clinical significance. Anesth Analg 1996; 83:742-6.

136. Albright GA, Forster RM. Does combined spinal-epidural analgesia with subarachnoid sufentanil increase the incidence of emergency cesarean delivery? Reg Anesth 1997; 22:400-5.

137. Mardirosoff C, Dumont L, Boulvain M, Tramer MR. Fetal bradycardia due to intrathecal opioids for labor analgesia: A systematic review. BJOG 2002; 109:274-81.

138. Mercier FJ, Dounas M, Bouaziz H, et al. Intravenous nitroglycerin to relieve intrapartum fetal distress related to uterine hyperactivity: A prospective observational study. Anesth Analg 1997; 84:1117-20.

139. Buhimschi CS, Buhimschi IA, Malinow AM, Weiner CP. Effects of sublingual nitroglycerin on human uterine contractility during the active phase of labor. Am J Obstet Gynecol 2002; 187:235-8.

140. Bell E. Nitroglycerin and uterine relaxation (letter). Anesthesiology 1996; 85:683.

141. Rawal N, Van Zundert A, Holmstrom B, Crowhurst JA. Combined spinal-epidural technique. Reg Anesth 1997; 22:406-23.

142. Viscomi CM, Rathmell JP, Pace NL. Duration of intrathecal labor analgesia: Early versus advanced labor. Anesth Analg 1997; 84:1108-12.

143. Rawal N, Schollin J, Wesstrom G. Epidural versus combined spinal epidural block for cesarean section. Acta Anaesth Scand 1988; 32:61-6.

144. Svante Linden. Personal communication cited by Abouleish E, Rawal N, Shaw J, et al. Intrathecal morphine 0.2 mg versus epidural bupivacaine 0.125% or their combination: Effects on parturients. Anesthesiology 1991; 74:711-6.

145. Suzuki N, Koganemaru M, Onizuka S, Takasaki M. Dural puncture with a 26-gauge spinal needle affects spread of epidural anesthesia. Anesth Analg 1996; 82:1040-2.

146. Gambling DR, Yu P, Cole C, et al. A comparative study of patient controlled epidural analgesia (PCEA) and continuous infusion epidural analgesia (CIEA) during labour. Can J Anaesth 1988; 35:249-54.

147. Gambling DR, McMorland GH, Yu P, Laszlo C. Comparison of patient-controlled epidural analgesia and conventional intermittent "top-up" injections during labor. Anesth Analg 1990; 70:256-61.

148. Paech MJ, Pavy TJ, Sims C, et al. Clinical experience with patient-controlled and staff-administered intermittent bolus epidural analgesia in labour. Anaesth Intensive Care 1995; 23:459-63.

149. Lysak SZ, Eisenach JC, Dobson CE. Patient-controlled epidural analgesia during labor: A comparison of three solutions with a continuous infusion control (comments). Anesthesiology 1990; 72:44-9.

150. Ferrante FM, Lu L, Jamison SB, Datta S. Patient-controlled epidural analgesia: Demand dosing. Anesth Analg 1991; 73:547-52.

151. White P. Mishaps with patient-controlled analgesia. Anesthesiology 1987; 66:81-3.

152. Johnson MD, Hurley RJ, Gilbertson LI, Datta S. Continuous micro-catheter spinal anesthesia with subarachnoid meperidine for labor and delivery. Anesth Analg 1990; 70:658-61.

153. Huckaby T, Skerman JH, Hurley RJ, Lambert DH. Sensory analgesia for vaginal deliveries: A preliminary report of continuous spinal anesthesia with a 32-gauge catheter. Reg Anesth 1991; 16:150-3.

154. Drasner K, Rigler ML, Sessler DI, Stoller ML. Cauda equina syndrome following intended epidural anesthesia. Anesthesiology 1992; 77:582-5.

155. Rigler ML, Drasner K. Distribution of catheter-injected local anesthetic in a model of the subarachnoid space. Anesthesiology 1991; 75:684-92.

156. Drasner K, Rigler ML. Repeat injection after a "failed spinal": At times, a potentially unsafe practice (letter). Anesthesiology 1991; 75:713-4.

157. Ross BK, Coda B, Heath CH. Local anesthetic distribution in a spinal model: A possible mechanism of neurologic injury after continuous spinal anesthesia. Reg Anesth 1992; 17:69-77.

158. FDA Safety Alert. Cauda equina syndrome associated with use of small-bore catheters in continuous spinal anesthesia. May 29, 1992.

159. Levin A, Datta S, Camann WR. Intrathecal ropivacaine for labor analgesia: A comparison with bupivacaine. Anesth Analg 1998; 87:624-7.

160. Collis RE, Baxandall ML, Srikantharajah ID, et al. Combined spinal epidural analgesia with ability to walk throughout labour (letter). Lancet 1993; 341:767-8. (Published erratum appears in Lancet 1993; 341:1038.)

161. Shennan A, Cooke V, Lloyd-Jones F, et al. Blood pressure changes during labour and whilst ambulating with combined spinal epidural analgesia. Br J Obstet Gynaecol 1995; 102:192-7.

162. Al-Mufti R, Morey R, Shennan A, Morgan B. Blood pressure and fetal heart rate changes with patient-controlled combined spinal epidural analgesia while ambulating in labour. Br J Obstet Gynaecol 1997; 104:554-8.

163. Parry MG, Fernando R, Bawa GPS, Poulton BB. Dorsal column function after epidural and spinal blockade: Implications for the safety of walking following low-dose regional analgesia for labour. Anaesthesia 1998; 53:382-403.

164. Nageotte M, Larson D, Rumney P, et al. A prospective randomized study of intrapartum epidural versus combination intrathecal/epidural anesthesia with or without ambulation (abstract). Am J Obstet Gynecol 1997; 176:S22.

165. May AE, Elton DC. Ambulatory extradural analgesia in labour reduces risk of caesarean section (abstract). Br J Anaesth 1996; 77:692P.

166. Sia ATH, Chong JL, Chiu JW. Combination of intrathecal sufentanil 10 μg plus bupivacaine 2.5 mg for labor analgesia: Is half the dose enough? Anesth Analg 1999; 88:362-6.

167. Bloom SL, McIntire DD, Kelly MA, et al. Lack of effect of walking on labor and delivery. N Engl J Med 1998; 339:76-9.

168. Cefalo RC, Bowes WA. Managing labor: Never walk alone (editorial). N Engl J Med 1998; 339:117-8.

169. Stoddart AP, Nicholson KE, Popham PA. Low dose bupivacaine/fentanyl epidural infusions in labour and mode of delivery. Anaesthesia 1994; 49:1087-90.

170. Ready L, Oden R, Chadwick H, et al. Development of an anesthesiology-based postoperative pain management service. Anesthesiology 1988; 68:100-6.

Chapter 21
Epidural and Spinal Analgesia/Anesthesia

III. EFFECT ON THE PROGRESS OF LABOR AND METHOD OF DELIVERY

David H. Chestnut, M.D.

Epidural analgesia/anesthesia during labor is associated with an increased risk of prolonged labor and operative delivery.* Controversy exists as to whether there is a cause-and-effect relationship between the use of these analgesic techniques and prolonged labor or operative delivery. Our understanding of this subject has been limited by the difficulty of performing controlled trials in which patients are randomized to receive epidural analgesia or an alternative form of pain relief. Further, epidural analgesia is not a generic procedure. Conclusions regarding the effect of one technique on the progress of labor may not be applicable to other techniques.

Retrospective studies suffer from selection bias. In some cases, distinguishing between anesthesia administered for pain relief during labor and anesthesia administered in preparation for operative delivery is difficult. Moreover, women at increased risk for prolonged labor and operative delivery are more likely to request and receive epidural analgesia during labor than women who have a rapid, uncomplicated labor.[1,2] Wuitchik et al.[1] observed a relationship between pain and cognitive activity during early labor and the subsequent progress of labor in 115 healthy nulliparous women. During the latent phase, higher levels of pain were predictive of longer latent and active phases of labor. "Distress-related thoughts" during latent-phase labor also predicted a longer latent phase, active phase, and second stage of labor. Those women who reported "horrible" or "excruciating" pain during the latent phase were more than twice as likely to require instrumental delivery than women who only had "discomfort." In addition, those patients who reported "distress" rather than "coping" had a 2.6-fold increase in the incidence of instrumental delivery, a fivefold increase in the incidence of abnormal fetal heart rate (FHR) patterns, and a fourfold increase in the require-

*The term *operative delivery* refers to both cesarean section and instrumental vaginal delivery (e.g., forceps delivery, vacuum extraction).

ment for pediatric assistance during neonatal resuscitation.[1] Other studies have noted that laboring women who subsequently undergo cesarean delivery require higher doses of intravenous opioids and/or epidural local anesthetics for pain relief during labor.[3-5] Therefore, the early onset of severe pain may predict an increased risk of abnormal labor, FHR abnormalities, and operative delivery. Likewise, the requirement for high doses of analgesic agents may predict an increased risk of cesarean section.

Published studies suffer from other limitations. For example, many studies include both nulliparous and parous women. The duration of labor is longer and the incidence of operative delivery is higher in nulliparous women than in parous women. Most studies also do not consider the effect of obstetric management. For example, some obstetricians are more reluctant to augment labor with oxytocin than others. The early, aggressive use of oxytocin may decrease the likelihood of prolonged labor and operative delivery in patients who receive epidural analgesia. When labor progresses slowly, "the psychology of prolonged and nonprogressive labor dominates management strategies, as physicians, patients, and families become exhausted and frustrated with the lack of progress."[6]

Neuhoff et al.[6] retrospectively reviewed the records of 607 nulliparous women at term gestation who delivered at their hospital. The authors divided the patients into two groups: (1) clinic patients (n = 192), whose obstetric care was provided primarily by obstetric residents; and (2) private patients (n = 415), whose obstetric care was provided by physicians or nurse-midwives in private practice. Approximately 42% of patients in both groups received epidural analgesia during labor. However, 5.2% of patients in the clinic group versus 17.1% of patients in the private group underwent cesarean section (P < 0.001) (Table 21-10). More striking was the difference between the groups in the incidence of cesarean section for dystocia (0.5% in the clinic group versus 13.7% in the private group, P < 0.001). Among women who received

| TABLE 21-10 | MODE OF DELIVERY AND EPIDURAL USE |

	Clinic (n = 192)	Private (n = 415)	P value
Cesarean rate			
Total	5.2%	17.1%	< 0.001
Failure to progress	0.5%	13.7%	< 0.001
Vaginal delivery			
Vacuum/forceps	14.6%	13.7%	—
Spontaneous	80.2%	69.2%	< 0.005
Epidural use			
Total	41.6%	41.7%	—
Placed before 4 cm	20.0%	18.5%	—

From Neuhoff D, Burke MS, Porreco RP. Cesarean birth for failed progress in labor. Obstet Gynecol 1989; 73:915-20. Reprinted with permission from the American College of Obstetricians and Gynecologists.

epidural analgesia, approximately 70% of patients in both the clinic and private groups received intravenous oxytocin. The authors acknowledged, "It was difficult in this retrospective review to tell which came first; that is, oxytocin augmentation requiring epidural anesthesia or epidural anesthesia followed by oxytocin augmentation."[6]

Likewise, Guillemette and Fraser[7] observed marked obstetrician variation in cesarean section rates, despite similarities in the use of oxytocin and epidural analgesia. Segal et al.[8] concluded that obstetric practice style is a major determinant of the cesarean section rate. For example, Fraser et al.[9] observed a temporal variation in the incidence of cesarean section. The incidence peaked in the evening, which was consistent with the hypothesis of obstetrician convenience. Further, De Regt et al.[10] suggested that private physicians may be more concerned about adverse outcomes and potential litigation than resident physicians.[9]

FIRST STAGE OF LABOR

Kilpatrick and Laros[11] retrospectively evaluated the length of the first and second stages of labor in 6991 parturients with a singleton gestation and a vertex presentation at 37 to 42 weeks' gestation. All women delivered spontaneously, without the use of oxytocin. The authors concluded that the use of regional anesthesia significantly prolonged the first and second stages of labor in both nulliparous and parous women (Table 21-11).

In 1992, Howell and Chalmers[12] reviewed prospectively controlled comparisons of epidural with nonepidural forms of pain relief during labour.[13-27] The authors concluded that these data "do not permit any firm conclusions about the effects of epidural block on the duration of the first stage of labour." However, they noted that oxytocin was used more frequently in patients who received epidural analgesia in the two trials for which that information was available (Table 21-12). (A 1999 meta-analysis concluded that epidural bupivacaine analgesia may increase the likelihood of oxytocin augmentation of spontaneous labor.[28])

Thorp et al.[29] randomized 93 nulliparous women to receive either epidural bupivacaine or intravenous meperidine analgesia. The mean ± standard deviation (SD) duration of the first stage of labor was 676 ± 394 minutes in the epidural group versus 519 ± 279 minutes in the meperidine group (P < 0.05). The authors did not report the mean interval between randomization and the onset of full cervical dilation in the two groups, and some women were receiving intravenous oxytocin at the time of randomization (i.e., nine in the epidural group versus three in the meperidine group).

Ramin et al.[30] randomized 1330 women of mixed parity to receive either epidural bupivacaine-fentanyl or intravenous meperidine analgesia during labor. Among the 664 women randomized to an offer of epidural analgesia, 232 (35%) did not receive the allocated treatment. Approximately half refused the offer of epidural analgesia, and the remaining half delivered before epidural analgesia could be administered. Among the 666 women randomized to an offer of meperidine analgesia, 229 (34%) were not treated according to the allocated protocol. Approximately half of those women requested and received epidural analgesia because the meperidine provided inadequate pain relief. The authors did not report data on the duration of labor among all 1330 patients. Among protocol-compliant patients, the interval from admission to delivery was approximately 1½ hours longer in women who received epidural analgesia than in those who received meperidine. Moreover, women in the epidural group were more likely to receive oxytocin augmentation (i.e., 32% in the epidural group versus 23% in the meperidine group).

Sharma et al.[31] subsequently randomized 459 nulliparous women in spontaneous labor at term to receive either epidural bupivacaine-fentanyl or intravenous meperidine analgesia. Women in the epidural group had a longer mean ± SD interval from initiation of analgesia to complete cervical

| TABLE 21-11 | LENGTHS OF THE FIRST AND SECOND STAGES OF LABOR |

	No regional anesthesia		Regional anesthesia	
Group	First stage (hr)	Second stage (min)	First stage (hr)	Second stage (min)
Nulliparous				
Mean ± SD	8.1 ± 4.3	54 ± 39	10.2 ± 4.4	79 ± 53
Limit	16.6	132	19.0	185
Parous				
Mean ± SD	5.7 ± 3.4	19 ± 21	7.4 ± 3.8	45 ± 43
Limit	12.5	61	14.9	131

All means are significantly different (P < 0.0001).
Modified from Kilpatrick SJ, Laros RK. Characteristics of normal labor. Obstet Gynecol 1989; 74:85-7. Reprinted with permission from the American College of Obstetricians and Gynecologists.

TABLE 21-12   EFFECT OF EPIDURAL ANALGESIA ON THE DURATION OF THE FIRST STAGE OF LABOR

	Epidural	Control	P value
Thalme et al.[15]			
Proportion > 8 hours	8 of 12	9 of 12	NS
Oxytocin augmentation	4 of 12	1 of 12	NS
Jouppila and Hollmén[17]			
Mean (range) minutes	402 (120-1040)	245 (90-480)	NS
Bratteby et al.[18]			
Mean (range) hours			
Continuous	8.6 (3-15)		NS
Intermittent	8.3 (3-15)		
Paracervical		7.4 (3-14)	
Nitrous oxide		6.4 (2-11)	
Oxytocin augmentation	19 of 34	6 of 39	< 0.01
Jouppila et al.[19]			
Mean (range) minutes	189 (123-355)	330 (120-630)	NS
Robinson et al.[20]			
Mean ± SD hours			
Nulliparous	8.2 ± 3.5	8.3 ± 3.1	NS
Parous	6.0 ± 3.0	6.4 ± 4.2	NS
Ryhänen et al.[25]			
Mean ± SD minutes	341 ± 190	320 ± 210	NS
Philipsen and Jensen[26]			
Median (range) minutes	197 (10-580)	180 (25-925)	NS
Thorp et al.[29]			
Mean ± SD minutes	676 ± 394	519 ± 279	< 0.05

Modified from Howell CJ, Chalmers I. A review of prospectively controlled comparisons of epidural with non-epidural forms of pain relief during labour. Int J Obstet Anesth 1992; 1:93-110.

dilation (302 ± 189 minutes in the epidural group versus 261 ± 188 minutes in the intravenous meperidine group, $P = 0.03$). Subsequently these investigators performed a secondary analysis of this randomized trial, and they noted that the active phase of the first stage of labor was 1 hour longer in the epidural group than in the intravenous meperidine group (6.0 ± 3.2 hours versus 5.0 ± 3.2 hours, $P < 0.001$).[32]

By contrast, Bofill et al.[33] observed no difference in the duration of the first stage of labor—or in the requirement for oxytocin augmentation of labor—among 100 term nulliparous women in spontaneous labor who were randomized to receive either epidural bupivacaine or intravenous butorphanol analgesia. These investigators followed a protocol that included early amniotomy, early diagnosis of desultory labor, and aggressive use of intravenous oxytocin. Leighton and Halpern[34] performed a meta-analysis of both randomized controlled trials and prospective cohort studies in which patients received either epidural analgesia or parenteral opioids during labor. They noted that the duration of the first stage of labor was slightly but not significantly longer in women who received epidural analgesia.

Analgesia During the Latent Phase

Some obstetricians contend that epidural analgesia is more likely to prolong the first stage of labor if it is administered during the latent phase. Friedman and Sachtleben[35] retrospectively evaluated the progress of labor in 330 parturients who received early caudal anesthesia (i.e., before 7 cm cervical dilation) at their hospital between January 1955 and December 1957. The authors evaluated nulliparous and parous women separately. They observed no difference in the duration of either the first or the second stage of labor between the

two groups of women who received early caudal epidural anesthesia and the two control groups. The authors stated the following[35]:

Other factors, reputed to effect slowing of labor, such as administration of the caudal too early...were examined. The anticipated actions could not be verified. Slowing of cervical dilation by the premature application of caudal anesthesia was certainly observed in this series. That the overall data should not reflect this seemed rather odd.

The authors concluded that "caudal anesthesia does not necessarily affect the course of labor."[35] Nonetheless, they stated that "proper administration entails withholding it until the active phase of labor is entered."[35]

Read et al.[36] assessed the progress of labor in 1355 consecutive Caucasian women who had a vaginal delivery at their hospital. Some 405 of these women received lumbar epidural analgesia with either 0.25% or 0.375% bupivacaine. The other women received either meperidine or no analgesia. The authors did not note the method of group assignment, and no evidence suggests that they randomly assigned either the method or the timing of analgesia. The authors concluded, "There can be no reasonable doubt that epidural analgesia delays the progress of labor, particularly if it is given early, in the latent phase."[36]

At the University of Iowa, we performed two studies to determine whether early administration of epidural analgesia prolongs labor in healthy nulliparous women with a singleton fetus in a vertex presentation. The first study included women who were receiving oxytocin for induction or augmentation of labor at the time of the request for epidural analgesia.[37] The second study included women in spontaneous labor.[38] In both studies, randomization occurred only after the following conditions were met: (1) the patient had requested pain relief;

(2) an epidural catheter had been placed; and (3) the cervix was at least 3 but less than 5 cm dilated. Patients were randomized to receive either early or late epidural analgesia. Patients in the early epidural group received 3 mL of 1.5% lidocaine with epinephrine followed by 0.25% bupivacaine as needed 5 minutes after randomization. Patients in the late group received nalbuphine 10 mg intravenously. Late-group patients could receive a second dose of nalbuphine, on request, at least 1 hour after the first dose. Late-group patients did not receive epidural analgesia until the cervix was at least 5 cm dilated or until at least 1 hour had elapsed after the second dose of nalbuphine. Patients in both groups received a continuous epidural infusion of 0.125% bupivacaine after the cervix was at least 5 cm dilated.

In the first study, 150 patients were randomized to receive either early or late epidural analgesia.[37] There was no difference between groups in the duration of the first or second stage of labor. (These results are consistent with earlier observations suggesting that regional anesthesia does not affect the uterine contractile response to oxytocin,[39] although this is a matter of some dispute.[40]) Likewise, in the second study, early administration of epidural analgesia did not prolong the first stage of labor or increase the number of patients who required oxytocin augmentation of labor. The mean ± SD interval between randomization and the onset of complete cervical dilation was 329 ± 197 minutes in the early group and 359 ± 214 minutes in the late group. Fifty-three (31%) of 172 women in the early group and 62 (38%) of 162 women in the late group required intravenous oxytocin after randomization.

Similarly, Brody et al.[41] observed that the early administration of epidural analgesia (i.e., before 5 cm cervical dilation) did not prolong the first stage of labor or increase the requirement for intravenous oxytocin as compared with the delayed administration of epidural analgesia (i.e., after 5 cm cervical dilation) in 103 nulliparous women during spontaneous labor at term. Other studies have observed that the administration of epidural analgesia before 4 cm cervical dilation does not prolong labor as compared with administration of epidural analgesia after 4 cm cervical dilation.[42,43] (One study noted that women who received epidural analgesia before 4 cm cervical dilation had a *shorter* labor than women who received epidural analgesia after 4 cm cervical dilation.[43]) There are few published data regarding the effects of epidural analgesia administered during *very early* labor (i.e., before 2 to 3 cm cervical dilation) on the subsequent progress of labor.

The aforementioned studies do not necessarily confirm that early epidural analgesia has no effect on the duration of the first stage of labor. However, they suggest that the effect, if any, of early epidural analgesia does not differ from that of intravenous opioids. Some investigators have suggested that opioids may decrease uterine activity and prolong the first stage of labor.[44-46]

Crawford[47] discussed the controversy regarding the administration of analgesia during the latent phase of labor:

There is a reluctance among obstetricians and midwives— but not, I suggest, among anaesthetists—to acknowledge that the contractions of the latent phase can be painful. The reluctance doubtless stems partly from the ... fallacy that the administration of the powerful central nervous system depressants or of regional blockade will retard, or possibly even temporarily halt, progress through the latent phase. However, if this view were valid, the search for ways to counter the threat of onset of premature labor would surely have ended successfully decades ago. Of themselves neither systemic analgesics, tranquilizers, or sedatives, nor block of the sensory nerve supply of the uterus has more than an evanescent depressant effect on uterine activity.[48] It seems likely that the misapprehension arose from the fact that in the past mothers given such therapy were coincidentally rendered mildly hypotensive, possibly owing to aortocaval compression and a degree of peripheral vasodilation. A fall in blood pressure from a normotensive level is the factor that can most reliably be expected to cause uterine hypotonia and a reduction in the rate of contractions. The conclusion to be drawn is that if the mother requests relief from pain, it should be provided, by any mutually agreed technique. There is no justification for debate about whether she is in the latent or the active phase of labour.

Choice of Local Anesthetic

Some physicians have suggested that the choice of local anesthetic may affect the uterine response to epidural analgesia.[49] For example, some studies have noted a transient decrease in uterine activity after the epidural administration of lidocaine[50,51] but not bupivacaine.[52-54] Willdeck-Lund et al.[55] observed a transient decrease in uterine activity after the epidural administration of lidocaine with epinephrine, bupivacaine with epinephrine, or bupivacaine alone. Abboud et al.[56,57] observed no difference in uterine activity or the duration of the first stage of labor in women who received intermittent bolus injections or a continuous epidural infusion of bupivacaine, 2-chloroprocaine, or lidocaine during labor. It is unlikely that the choice of local anesthetic affects the progress of the first stage of labor.

Epinephrine-Containing Local Anesthetic Solutions

The epidural administration of a local anesthetic with epinephrine is followed by systemic absorption of both drugs. Some physicians have expressed concern that the epinephrine may exert a beta-adrenergic tocolytic effect. Early studies, which used large doses of epinephrine, suggested that the caudal epidural administration of local anesthetic with epinephrine prolonged the first stage of labor and increased the number of patients who required oxytocin augmentation of labor.[58,59] Subsequently, most studies have suggested that the addition of 1:200,000 to 1:800,000 epinephrine to the local anesthetic solution does not affect the progress of labor or method of delivery.[60-66] One exception is the study by Dounas et al.[67] They observed that nulliparous women who received epidural bupivacaine with 1:200,000 epinephrine (i.e., 5 µg/mL) had a longer first stage of labor than women who received epidural bupivacaine without epinephrine (i.e., 414 ± 49 minutes versus 296 ± 24 minutes). However, epidural bupivacaine with 1:600,000 epinephrine did not prolong the first stage of labor.

Maternal Circulation

Schellenberg[53] suggested that aortocaval compression is responsible for the transient decrease in uterine activity that occurs after the administration of epidural anesthesia in some patients. He concluded that this effect does not occur if aortocaval compression is avoided.

Cheek et al.[68] observed that women who received a 1000-mL bolus of normal saline experienced a transient decrease in uterine activity *before* the administration of epidural analgesia. By contrast, women who received maintenance fluid only (i.e., 125 mL/hr) or a 500-mL bolus did not demonstrate any change in uterine activity. Subsequently, there was no decrease in uterine activity after the administration of epidural anesthesia in any of the three groups. In fact, the women who received maintenance fluid had an *increase* in uterine activity during the 20 minutes after the initiation of epidural blockade. Zamora et al.[69] made similar observations. Miller et al.[70] concluded the following:

> One hypothesis offered to explain this phenomenon is that the fluid bolus inhibits antidiuretic hormone release from the posterior pituitary gland. Since this organ also releases oxytocin, the production of that hormone might also be transiently suppressed. This may partially explain the transient changes in uterine contractility observed in association with epidural analgesia. Nevertheless, the benefits of hydration before the administration of an epidural block are well established and should not be avoided because of concern that uterine activity might be transiently depressed.

Epidural and Intrathecal Opioids

Most[71-78]—but not all[79,80]—studies have noted normal progress of labor after epidural or intrathecal opioid administration. Interpretation of these studies is clouded by the fact that most patients also received an epidural local anesthetic. Abouleish et al.[79] observed that intrathecal morphine administration appeared to prolong the first stage of labor. One group of patients received intrathecal morphine 0.2 mg, a second group received epidural bupivacaine 0.125%, and a third group received both intrathecal morphine and epidural bupivacaine. The mean ± SEM duration of the first stage of labor was longer in both groups that received intrathecal morphine than in the group that received epidural bupivacaine alone (i.e., 10.5 ± 1.3 hours and 11.1 ± 0.2 hours versus 6.5 ± 0.8 hours, respectively). Potential mechanisms by which opioids might interfere with labor include an effect on spinal cord centers that may control uterine contractility (as has been observed for other visceral organs[81]) and opioid-induced central depression of endogenous oxytocin secretion.[82] It is unlikely that the uterine depressant effect of morphine is mediated by activation of uterine opioid receptors.[83,84]

Most contemporary studies suggest that combined spinal-epidural (CSE) analgesia (i.e., intrathecal fentanyl or sufentanil followed by epidural bupivacaine) does *not* prolong the first stage of labor as compared with epidural analgesia alone.[75-78] Some anesthesiologists have suggested that the intrathecal administration of a lipid-soluble opioid may result in increased uterine tone. The presumed etiology is that the rapid onset of analgesia results in a decreased maternal plasma concentration of epinephrine. Epinephrine causes uterine relaxation by stimulating beta$_2$-adrenergic uterine receptors; thus a decreased plasma concentration of epinephrine may result in increased uterine tone. It is unclear whether this accelerates the first stage of labor. Tsen et al.[77] observed that CSE analgesia was associated with *more rapid* cervical dilation than epidural analgesia alone. However, others have been unable to confirm this observation.[78]

Other Factors

In a prospective but nonrandomized study, Rahm et al.[85] observed that epidural analgesia (bupivacaine with sufentanil) during the first stage of labor was associated with a decline in plasma oxytocin levels at 60 minutes as compared with healthy controls who did not receive epidural analgesia. Behrens et al.[86] observed that epidural analgesia during the first stage of labor significantly reduced the release of prostaglandin F$_2$ and "impede[d] the normal progressive increase in uterine activity." By contrast, Nielsen et al.[87] measured upper and lower uterine segment intrauterine pressures for 50 minutes before and after the administration of epidural bupivacaine analgesia in 11 nulliparous women during spontaneous labor. The authors observed no significant difference in the number of contractions before and after epidural analgesia. They also observed significantly greater intrauterine pressure measurements in the upper uterine segment than in the lower segment (consistent with fundal dominance) both before and after epidural analgesia. Further, fundal dominance increased after epidural analgesia as compared with the preanalgesia period.

Summary

Epidural analgesia seems to reduce uterine activity in some patients, but it results in enhanced uterine activity in others.[88] It is unclear whether a prolonged first stage is harmful for the mother or fetus. Wittels[89] stated, "Prolonged duration of labor is often quoted as an adverse maternal event; however, duration alone is of little significance if labor pain is adequately controlled and fetal/neonatal well-being is preserved." It is more important to determine whether epidural analgesia increases the likelihood of operative delivery or adverse neonatal outcome.

SECOND STAGE OF LABOR AND METHOD OF VAGINAL DELIVERY

Howell and Chalmers[12] reviewed data for the duration of the second stage of labor and the incidence of instrumental vaginal delivery in studies in which an attempt had been made to randomize patients to receive epidural or nonepidural analgesia during the first stage of labor (Tables 21-13 and 21-14). They separated the studies in which epidural analgesia was maintained throughout the second stage from those in which epidural analgesia was maintained during the first stage only. One study deserves a separate comment: Robinson et al.[20] allocated 386 women during pregnancy to one of three groups, but only 134 (36%) of these women were included in subsequent published studies. The authors included only 93 women in their comparison of epidural versus nonepidural analgesia. Thus this study has at least two major flaws. First, the allocation occurred before the final consent was obtained. Second, the two groups of patients were not similar. Approximately 56% of the women in the epidural group but only 19% of the women in the control group underwent induction of labor, which is a risk factor for prolonged labor and operative delivery. This suggests a "biased dropout from the original randomized cohorts."[12]

Interpretation of these studies is clouded by the fact that most studies did not assess the quality of analgesia during the second stage of labor. Further, most authors did not define the criteria for the performance of instrumental vaginal delivery. Often it is difficult to distinguish indicated instrumental deliveries from elective instrumental deliveries. An obstetrician is more likely to perform an elective instrumental delivery in a patient with satisfactory anesthesia than in a patient without anesthesia. Nonetheless, the weight of evidence suggests that women who receive effective epidural anesthesia during the second stage of labor are more likely to undergo instrumental vaginal delivery than women who do not receive epidural anesthesia.

Other studies have specifically assessed the effect of maintaining epidural analgesia until delivery with regard to the duration of the second stage and the incidence of operative

TABLE 21-13 EFFECT OF EPIDURAL ANALGESIA ON THE DURATION OF THE SECOND STAGE OF LABOR

	Epidural	Control	P value
Epidural block continued through the second stage			
Noble et al.[13]			
Proportion > 30 minutes	64 of 100	32 of 102	< 0.01
Thalme et al.[15]			
Proportion > 60 minutes	6 of 12	4 of 12	NS
Mean (variance) minutes	50 (N/A)	60 (N/A)	
Bratteby et al.[18]			
Mean (range) minutes			
Continuous	59 (5-150)		NS
Intermittent	52 (10-135)		
Paracervical		51 (8-120)	
Nitrous oxide		20 (1-51)	
Robinson et al.[20]			
Mean ± SD hours			
Nulliparous	0.9 ± 0.4	0.7 ± 0.3	< 0.01
Parous	0.5 ± 0.3	0.3 ± 0.2	< 0.01
Thorp et al.[29]			
Mean ± SD minutes	115 ± 71	54 ± 45	< 0.05
Epidural block during the first stage only			
Jouppila and Hollmén[17]			
Mean (range) minutes	12.1 (1-31)	14.8 (4-58)	NS
Jouppila et al.[19]			
Mean (range) minutes	9.5 (4-17)	15.0 (8-32)	NS
Ryhänen et al.[25]			
Mean ± SD minutes	18.6 ± 14.2	5.8 ± 3.4	NS
Philipsen and Jensen[26]			
Median (range) minutes	47 (5-274)	37 (5-150)	NS

Modified from Howell CJ, Chalmers I. A review of prospectively controlled comparisons of epidural with non-epidural forms of pain relief during labour. Int J Obstet Anesth 1992; 1:93-110.

TABLE 21-14 EFFECT OF EPIDURAL ANALGESIA ON THE INCIDENCE OF ASSISTED VAGINAL DELIVERY

	Experimental		Control		Odds ratio (95% confidence interval)
	n	**%**	**n**	**%**	
Block maintained during the second stage of labor					
Bratteby[24]	16 of 36	44.4	7 of 41	17.1	3.6 (1.3-9.6)
Noble et al.[13]	30 of 100	30	6 of 102	5.9	5.2 (2.5-10.6)
Buchan et al.[14]	5 of 10	50	0 of 10	0	12.6 (1.8-90.6)
Thalme et al.[15]	6 of 14	42.9	4 of 14	28.6	1.8 (0.4-8.3)
Robinson et al.[20]	22 of 45	48.9	9 of 48	18.8	3.8 (1.6-9.0)
Thorp et al.[29]	9 of 48	18.8	5 of 45	11.1	—
Typical odds ratio (95% confidence interval)					4.2 (2.7-6.6)
Block discontinued for the second stage of labor					
Philipsen and Jensen[26]	14 of 57	24.6	14 of 54	25.9	0.9 (0.4-2.2)
Jouppila[16]	1 of 12	8.3	1 of 12	8.3	1.0 (0.1-17.0)
Jouppila et al.[19]	0 of 8	0	0 of 10	0	1.0 (1.0-1.0)
Typical odds ratio (95% confidence interval)					0.9 (0.4-2.1)

Modified from Howell CJ, Chalmers I. A review of prospectively controlled comparisons of epidural with non-epidural forms of pain relief during labour. Int J Obstet Anesth 1992; 1:93-110.

delivery.[90-95] In these studies, all patients received epidural analgesia during the first stage of labor, but they were randomized to receive either additional local anesthetic or no additional local anesthetic during the second stage.

In a randomized trial, Johnsrud et al.[91] observed no difference in the duration of the second stage of labor or the incidence of instrumental vaginal delivery between women who continued to receive an epidural infusion of 0.25% bupivacaine during the second stage and similar women whose infusion was discontinued at the onset of the second stage. However, there was no significant difference between the two groups in the quality of analgesia during the second stage.

At the University of Iowa, we performed three randomized, double-blind studies in which healthy, nulliparous women receiving a continuous epidural infusion of local anesthetic were randomized to receive either additional local anesthetic or saline-placebo during the second stage of labor.[92-94] In all three studies, instrumental vaginal deliveries were performed for obstetric indications only. In the first study, we compared obstetric outcome in nulliparous women who continued to receive an epidural infusion of 0.75% lidocaine beyond a cervical dilation of 8 cm with the obstetric outcome of similar women who received saline-placebo.[92] Maintenance of the epidural lidocaine infusion until delivery did not prolong the second stage of labor (73 ± 63 minutes in the lidocaine group versus 76 ± 48 minutes in the saline-placebo group). Unfortunately, the continuous epidural infusion of lidocaine did not reliably provide second-stage analgesia. Women who continued to receive lidocaine until delivery did not consistently perceive that they had better analgesia than women who received saline-placebo.

In the second study, we compared outcome in nulliparous women who continued to receive an epidural infusion of 0.125% bupivacaine beyond a cervical dilation of 8 cm with the outcome of similar women who received saline-placebo.[93] Maintenance of the epidural bupivacaine infusion until delivery resulted in profound analgesia that was clearly superior to that provided by the saline-placebo. Epidural bupivacaine infusion prolonged the second stage of labor (124 ± 70 minutes versus 94 ± 54 minutes, $P < 0.05$) and nearly doubled the incidence of instrumental vaginal delivery (52% versus 27%, $P < 0.05$). In retrospect, it seems likely that some women in the bupivacaine group had an excessive density of neural blockade. However, prolongation of the second stage did not increase the incidence of cesarean section, and it did not affect Apgar scores or umbilical cord blood gas and pH measurements at delivery.

In the third study, maintenance of an epidural infusion of 0.0625% bupivacaine and 0.0002% fentanyl beyond full cervical dilation neither prolonged the second stage nor increased the incidence of instrumental vaginal delivery.[94] However, it provided second-stage analgesia that was only marginally better than that experienced by women who received saline-placebo.

Collectively, these three studies illustrate two fundamental principles of obstetric anesthesia. First, epidural analgesia during labor is not a generic procedure. Second, epidural administration of a local anesthetic (with or without an opioid) during the second stage is not synonymous with the provision of effective analgesia.[96]

Continuous Epidural Infusion

The continuous epidural infusion of local anesthetic results in a more stable level of analgesia and is also more convenient

for the anesthesiologist. Unfortunately, the use of this technique may tempt the anesthesiologist to place the patient on automatic pilot. As a result, the anesthesiologist may be less likely to individualize patient management. If the anesthesiologist tries to eliminate the need for supplemental bolus injections, some patients will receive more local anesthetic than they need. Studies have confirmed that the continuous epidural infusion of local anesthetic results in the administration of a higher total dose of local anesthetic than occurs with intermittent epidural bolus injections (Table 21-15).[97-104] Patients who receive a prolonged epidural infusion of 0.125% or 0.25% bupivacaine are at risk for the development of significant motor block. Bogod et al.[98] observed that patients who received a continuous epidural infusion of 0.125% bupivacaine had a higher incidence of leg weakness than patients who received intermittent bolus injections of 0.5% bupivacaine. Smedstad and Morison[101] noted an increased incidence of instrumental vaginal delivery in nulliparous women who received a continuous epidural infusion of 0.25% bupivacaine as compared with similar patients who received intermittent bolus injections of 0.25% bupivacaine. Other studies have not confirmed that the continuous epidural infusion of local anesthetic results in an increased incidence of instrumental vaginal delivery. Aquilina and Carli[104] observed no difference in the incidence of instrumental vaginal delivery among nulliparous women who received either a continuous epidural infusion of 0.125% bupivacaine or intermittent epidural boluses of 0.25% bupivacaine. However, there was a twofold increase in the incidence of rotational forceps delivery in the continuous infusion group.

Van der Vyver et al.[105] performed a meta-analysis of randomized controlled trials that compared patient-controlled epidural analgesia (PCEA) with the continuous epidural infusion of local anesthetic. They noted that patients who received PCEA required lower total doses of local anesthetic and had less motor block than those patients who received a continuous epidural infusion. Recently, a preliminary study suggested that PCEA with 0.0625% bupivacaine and fentanyl 2 μg/mL was associated with a lower incidence of instrumental vaginal delivery than continuous epidural infusion of 0.125% bupivacaine with fentanyl 2 μg/mL.[106] It is unclear whether the difference in outcome resulted from the use of a patient-controlled infusion or the administration of a more dilute solution of bupivacaine.

Concentration of Local Anesthetic

Epidural administration of a concentrated solution of local anesthetic may result in relaxation of the pelvic floor, which may interfere with the internal rotation of the fetal head during labor. Skeletal muscle relaxation may not only increase the risk of fetal head malposition (e.g., occiput posterior, occiput transverse) but also may result in decreased maternal expulsive efforts. Epidural administration of a dilute solution of local anesthetic results in less motor block, fewer cases of malposition of the vertex, and fewer instrumental vaginal deliveries than does the administration of a more concentrated solution.[107-112]

The addition of an opioid to the solution of local anesthetic allows the administration of a decreased total dose of local anesthetic, which results in less motor block.[74,112,113] Decreased motor block does not consistently shorten the second stage of labor or reduce the incidence of instrumental vaginal delivery.[74,113] In a randomized, double-blind study, we

| TABLE 21-15 | STUDIES THAT HAVE COMPARED CONTINUOUS EPIDURAL INFUSION VERSUS INTERMITTENT EPIDURAL BOLUS INJECTION OF BUPIVACAINE DURING LABOR |

	Continuous infusion	Intermittent bolus	P value
Total dose of bupivacaine*			
Nadeau and Elliot[97]	88 ± ?	26 ± ?	?
Bogod et al.[98]	178 ± 83	130 ± 69	< 0.005
Gaylard et al.[99]	198 ± 63	111 ± 54	< 0.001
Hicks et al.[100]	135 ± 59	118 ± 47	NS
Smedstad and Morison[101]	161 ± 71	87 ± 54	< 0.001
Eddleston et al.[102]	1.53 ± 0.13	0.22 ± 0.12	NS
Method of delivery			
Bogod et al.[98]			
Spontaneous	15 (30%)	17 (34%)	NS
Instrumental vaginal	26 (52%)	23 (46%)	
Cesarean	9 (18%)	10 (20%)	
Gaylard et al.[99]			
Spontaneous	13 (43%)	13 (43%)	NS
Instrumental vaginal	10 (33%)	12 (40%)	
Cesarean	7 (23%)	5 (17%)	
Hicks et al.[100]			
Spontaneous	14 (37%)	18 (51%)	NS
Instrumental vaginal	17 (45%)	14 (40%)	
Cesarean	7 (19%)	3 (9%)	
Smedstad and Morison[101]			
Spontaneous	5 (18%)	15 (52%)	< 0.05
Instrumental vaginal	15 (54%)	7 (24%)	
Cesarean	8 (29%)	7 (24%)	
Eddleston et al.[102]			
Spontaneous	19 (48%)	24 (60%)	NS
Instrumental vaginal	15 (38%)	10 (25%)	
Cesarean	6 (15%)	6 (15%)	
Lamont et al.[103]			
Spontaneous	105 (56%)	106 (55%)	NS
Instrumental vaginal	60 (32%)	56 (29%)	
Cesarean	23 (12%)	31 (16%)	
Aquilina and Carli[104]			
Spontaneous	536 (47%)	409 (51%)	NS
Instrumental vaginal	387 (34%)	238 (30%)	
Cesarean	202 (18%)	145 (18%)	
Rotational forceps	87 (8%)	35 (4%)	< 0.005

*Results are expressed as mean ± SD mg of bupivacaine except in the study by Eddleston et al.,[102] who expressed results as mean ± SEM mg/kg.

assessed the analgesic efficacy of the continuous epidural infusion of 0.0625% bupivacaine and 0.0002% fentanyl versus 0.125% bupivacaine alone in 80 nulliparous women.[74] A similar proportion of women in each group had excellent or good analgesia during the first and second stages of labor. Women in the bupivacaine-only group were more likely to have motor block at full cervical dilation. However, the less intense motor block experienced by women in the bupivacaine-fentanyl group did not significantly shorten the second stage (112 ± 64 minutes in the bupivacaine-fentanyl group versus 124 ± 69 minutes in the bupivacaine-only group) or result in a decreased incidence of instrumental vaginal delivery. One criticism of this study is that the epidural infusion was discontinued at full cervical dilation in both groups. Thus, it is possible that we lost the opportunity to detect a difference between groups in the duration of the second stage and in the method of delivery.

Vertommen et al.[114] performed a multicenter randomized study of epidural bolus administration of 0.125% bupivacaine with 1:800,000 epinephrine, with and without sufentanil, in 695 parturients of mixed parity. There was no difference between the two groups in the duration of the second stage of labor (33 ± 24 minutes in the sufentanil group versus 27 ± 21 minutes in the control group). Women in the sufentanil group had a decreased incidence of instrumental vaginal delivery (24% versus 36%, $P < 0.01$). The authors attribute this reduction to the decreased total dose of bupivacaine (34 ± 17 versus 42 ± 19 mg) and the decreased intensity of motor block in the sufentanil group. The large size of this study commands attention; however, there were several limitations. First, the study's design was least stringent with regard to the indications for instrumental delivery. The authors did not prohibit the performance of elective instrumental vaginal deliveries, and they did not distinguish between elective and indicated instrumental deliveries. Second, both groups of patients received very small total doses of bupivacaine. Anesthesiologists should ask whether such small doses of bupivacaine would provide effective analgesia in their patients.

Third and perhaps most important, the authors did not specifically assess and report the quality of analgesia during the second stage of labor. In an accompanying editorial, I noted that "no published study has shown that one can consistently provide effective analgesia *throughout the second stage of labor* without increasing the risk of instrumental delivery."[96]

The Comparative Obstetric Mobile Epidural Trial (COMET) Study Group[170] randomly assigned 1054 nulliparous women requesting epidural analgesia to receive a traditional ($n = 353$), a low-dose CSE ($n = 351$), or a low-dose epidural infusion technique ($n = 350$). The spontaneous vaginal delivery rate was 35% in the traditional epidural group, 43% in the low-dose CSE group (odds ratio, 1.38; 95% confidence interval, 1.01 to 1.89), and 43% in the low-dose infusion group (odds ratio, 1.39; 95% confidence interval, 1.01 to 1.90). The increased likelihood of spontaneous vaginal delivery in the two low-dose groups resulted from a reduction in the incidence of instrumental vaginal delivery in those two groups. There was no difference among the three groups in the incidence of cesarean section.[170]

Angle et al.[172] performed a meta-analysis to examine the impact of low- versus high-dose epidural analgesia on the method of delivery. They observed that the odds of instrumental vaginal delivery were significantly reduced in patients who received low-dose epidural analgesia.

Why should anesthesiologists give attention to the effects of analgesia on the method of vaginal delivery? A properly performed outlet- or low-forceps delivery does not increase the risk of adverse neonatal outcome.[117-120] However, a difficult midforceps delivery likely results in increased neonatal risk.[118-121] Instrumental delivery also results in an increased risk of maternal trauma (e.g., third- and fourth-degree vaginal lacerations, which are associated with a small but not negligible risk of rectovaginal fistula). Robinson et al.[122] observed that epidural analgesia was associated with an increased rate of severe perineal trauma because of the more frequent use of instrumental vaginal delivery and episiotomy in nulliparous patients who received epidural analgesia. Regardless of the magnitude of these risks, many women want to minimize the likelihood of operative delivery, and they perceive that an increased risk of instrumental vaginal delivery is undesirable.[97]

Robinson et al.[123] observed an increased incidence of malposition of the occiput at delivery in those patients who received epidural analgesia before engagement of the fetal head. By contrast, Yancey et al.[124] observed that the administration of on-demand epidural analgesia did not result in an increased frequency of malposition of the fetal head at delivery in nulliparous women.

Maternal Expulsive Efforts

Some—but not all—studies suggest that delayed pushing may result in an increased likelihood of spontaneous vaginal delivery.[125-130] Early pushing (i.e., before the mother feels the urge to push or before the fetal head is visible at the perineum) often results in maternal exhaustion, and it may result in more frequent FHR decelerations as compared with delayed pushing.[130] Fraser et al.[128] performed a multicenter, randomized controlled trial of delayed pushing in 1862 laboring nulliparous women with epidural analgesia. Delayed pushing resulted in a reduced risk of difficult delivery; the greatest effect was on the risk of midpelvic procedures. Further, spontaneous vaginal delivery occurred more frequently in the women who had delayed pushing. In addition, abnormal

umbilical cord blood pH (< 7.10 arterial or < 7.15 venous) occurred more frequently in the delayed pushing group.

It seems reasonable to allow uterine contractile forces to do most of the work in promoting the descent of the fetal head. Almost two decades ago, Crawford[47] made the following recommendation:

> The tenets of good practice should surely be that the mother should not be encouraged to bear down unless she feels the urge to do so or, at the earliest, until the fetal presenting part is powerfully distending the perineum, and, if there is no evidence of fetal distress or undue maternal fatigue, that there is no justification for undertaking an assisted delivery. Fetal distress and maternal fatigue will occur much less frequently if mothers are well hydrated, are not encouraged prematurely to bear down, and are by appropriate positioning not exposed to aortocaval compression.

Use of Oxytocin

Delayed pushing is of no benefit unless there is adequate uterine activity to promote the descent of the fetal head. Scull et al.[131] demonstrated that epidural bupivacaine analgesia does not affect the maternal plasma concentration of oxytocin during the first stage of labor. However, other studies have suggested that epidural analgesia results in decreased maternal release of oxytocin and decreased uterine activity during either the first[85] or second[132,133] stage of labor. Goodfellow and Studd[126] observed that an increased intravenous dose of oxytocin plus delayed pushing resulted in a decreased incidence of instrumental vaginal delivery in nulliparous women who were receiving epidural analgesia.

Saunders et al.[134] evaluated obstetric outcome in 226 women with adequate epidural bupivacaine (0.375%) analgesia in whom full cervical dilation had been achieved without prior oxytocin augmentation. The authors randomized these patients to receive either intravenous oxytocin or placebo after the diagnosis of full cervical dilation. The mothers were encouraged to begin expulsive efforts once the fetal head was visible at the perineum or after 1 hour had elapsed since the diagnosis of full cervical dilation. Forceps delivery was performed after 1 hour of maternal pushing unless delivery was imminent. Intravenous infusion of oxytocin resulted in a shorter second stage of labor, a decreased number of nonrotational forceps deliveries, and less perineal trauma, but it did not result in a decreased number of *rotational* forceps deliveries performed for malposition of the occiput.

Duration of the Second Stage

Some studies have suggested that a prolonged second stage of labor results in progressive fetal acidosis.[135] In the past, few obstetricians allowed the second stage to progress beyond 2 hours. Most contemporary studies have suggested that a delay in the second stage is not harmful to the infant or mother provided that the following are true: (1) electronic FHR monitoring confirms the absence of fetal distress; (2) the mother is well hydrated and has adequate analgesia; and (3) there is ongoing progress in the descent of the fetal head.[136-138] The American College of Obstetricians and Gynecologists (ACOG) has defined a prolonged second stage as lasting more than 3 hours in nulliparous women with regional anesthesia and more than 2 hours in nulliparous women without regional anesthesia. For parous women, the ACOG has defined a prolonged second stage as more than 2 hours in those with regional anesthesia and more than 1 hour in those without regional anesthesia.[139]

Kadar et al.[140] concluded that, for most patients, little benefit is gained by allowing the second stage of labor to exceed 3 hours. Paterson et al.[141] evaluated the second stage of labor in 25,069 women who delivered an infant of at least 37 weeks' gestation, with a vertex presentation, after the spontaneous onset of labor. The authors concluded the following:

> In multiparae not using epidural analgesia the likelihood of spontaneous vaginal delivery after one hour in the second stage was low, but in those multiparae using epidural analgesia and in all nulliparae there was no clear cut-off point for expectation of spontaneous delivery in the near future; they continued to give birth at a steady rate over several hours. While maternal and fetal conditions are satisfactory, intervention should be based on the rate of progress rather than the elapsed time since full cervical dilation.

Summary

Epidural administration of a dilute solution of local anesthetic results in fewer cases of malposition of the vertex and fewer instrumental vaginal deliveries than administration of a more concentrated solution. Maintenance of total anesthesia likely prolongs the second stage of labor. A prolonged second stage itself does not seem to result in harm to the mother or infant provided that the mother has effective analgesia, is well hydrated, and is not exhausted and that the fetus shows no evidence of distress. Derham et al.[137] concluded the following:

> Associations with poor outcome are more likely related to the injudicious use of forceps just because a defined period of time has passed. Prolonged duration should be seen as a marker of potential obstetric problems and greater attention paid to progress in the second stage as judged by the rate of descent and rotation.

Obstetricians should be encouraged to avoid an arbitrary termination of the second stage of labor.

THIRD STAGE OF LABOR

Rosaag et al.[142] retrospectively reviewed the outcomes of all of the 7468 women who underwent vaginal delivery at their hospital between 1996 and 1999. The authors observed that epidural analgesia was not associated with a prolonged third stage of labor. However, the duration of the third stage of labor was shorter in women who received epidural analgesia and subsequently required manual removal of the placenta. The authors suggested that epidural analgesia "provided a 'permissive' role." In other words, epidural analgesia likely facilitated and/or encouraged earlier intervention by the obstetrician.[142]

CESAREAN SECTION

Noble et al.[13] assessed obstetric outcome in 245 patients randomized to receive either epidural bupivacaine (0.5%) analgesia or "conventional" analgesia (e.g., pethidine, nitrous oxide, or no analgesia). The authors included the following comments[13]:

> Of 245 selected patients, 43 had to be removed from the trial after labor ensued.... Most of the patients removed from the non-epidural group were apparently experiencing severe pain; they were usually primigravidae whose baby presented in the occipito-posterior position.... The majority of patients

removed from the epidural group were apparently normal and usually multigravidae; their labors were so rapid it was not possible to arrange for an epidural block.

In other words, low-risk patients were excluded from the epidural group, but high-risk patients were excluded from the nonepidural group. Nonetheless, there was only one cesarean section in the epidural group as compared with three in the control group. The authors' candid comments illustrate that, even when a prospective, randomized study is performed, it is difficult to maintain conditions that allow for the comparison of patients at equal risk for abnormal labor and operative delivery.

Philipsen and Jensen[26] randomized 111 women to receive either epidural bupivacaine (0.375%) or intramuscular meperidine analgesia during labor. Undergoing cesarean section were 10 (17%) of 57 women in the epidural group versus 6 (11%) of 54 women in the meperidine group; 9 women (16%) in the epidural group versus 3 women (6%) in the meperidine group underwent cesarean section for dystocia. These differences were not statistically significant, but the authors did not enroll a sufficient number of patients to exclude the possibility that epidural analgesia causes an increased incidence of cesarean section.

Thorp et al.[143] retrospectively reviewed records for 711 consecutive nulliparous women at term gestation, all of whom had a cephalic fetal presentation and a spontaneous onset of labor. All patients were managed according to the principles of active management of labor. Women in the epidural group had a less favorable cervical dilation at admission (3.0 ± 1.4 versus 4.8 ± 2.6 cm), were more likely to undergo oxytocin augmentation of labor (73% versus 27%), had a longer total duration of labor (8.6 ± 3.1 hours versus 4.7 ± 2.8 hours), and delivered larger babies (3400 ± 466 g versus 3255 ± 456 g). The incidence of cesarean section for dystocia was 10.3% in the epidural group versus 3.8% in the nonepidural group. The authors listed three mechanisms by which epidural analgesia might increase the incidence of cesarean section for dystocia. First, they suggested that "a decrease in uterine activity without appropriate intervention with oxytocin could result in more cesarean sections for dystocia."[143] Second, they suggested that "relaxation of the pelvic diaphragm could predispose fetuses in a cephalic presentation to minor malpresentations such as occipitoposterior, deflexion, and asynclitism."[143] Third, the authors stated that "epidural analgesia could decrease the maternal stimulus and ability to push during the second stage."[143] They did not acknowledge the possibility that the reasons some—but not all—women request and receive epidural analgesia may reflect or predict a greater likelihood of abnormal labor and an increased risk for operative delivery.

Subsequently, Thorp et al.[144] performed a similar retrospective review of 500 consecutive nulliparous women. In this study, the incidence of cesarean section for dystocia was 11.4% in the epidural group as compared with 2.4% in the nonepidural group. In both studies, there was no difference between the epidural and nonepidural groups in the incidence of cesarean section for fetal distress. The authors stated, "The greatest effect of epidural analgesia on the incidence of cesarean section for dystocia was observed in nulliparas who dilated at slower rates (< 1 cm/hr) in early labor and who had epidural analgesia placed at 5 cm or less of cervical dilation."[144] They concluded that "epidural analgesia in first labors may have contributed significantly to the cesarean epidemic."[144] (*Consumer Reports* cited this study in an article titled "Too Many Cesareans."[145])

Lieberman et al.[146] performed a retrospective study of 1733 nulliparous women in spontaneous labor at term. Using a multivariate logistic regression analysis, the authors observed that women who received epidural analgesia were 3.7 times more likely to undergo a cesarean section. Further, the authors stated that "the greatest increase in cesarean risk was noted when epidural analgesia was administered earlier in labor."[146]

By contrast, in a retrospective study of 7317 women of mixed parity, Ploeckinger et al.[147] observed no significant increase in the incidence of cesarean section in women who received epidural analgesia. Likewise, Loncar et al.[148] retrospectively reviewed obstetric outcome for all 7315 women who delivered at the University of Alabama at Birmingham Hospital between January 1994 and December 1996. After controlling for confounding variables (e.g., parity, gestational age, size of infant), the authors concluded that the use of intrapartum epidural analgesia was not associated with an increased risk of cesarean delivery (adjusted odds ratio, 1.02; 95% confidence interval, 0.87 to 1.21).

Thorp et al.[29] randomized 93 indigent nulliparous women to receive either epidural bupivacaine (0.125% to 0.25%) or intravenous meperidine analgesia during labor. Epidural bupivacaine provided analgesia that was clearly superior to that provided by intravenous meperidine. Twelve (25%) of 48 women in the epidural group—versus 1 (2%) of 45 women in the meperidine group—underwent cesarean delivery. Among the 12 women in the epidural group who underwent cesarean delivery, 11 received epidural analgesia before 5 cm cervical dilation. The authors concluded that "this adverse effect of epidural analgesia on labor and delivery may be limited by delaying the epidural placement to a cervical dilatation of 5 cm."[29] Unfortunately, the authors also assumed responsibility for decisions regarding the method of delivery. The decision to perform a cesarean delivery is a subjective one, and it was impossible to blind the obstetricians to the group assignment.

Four prospective, randomized trials were performed at the University of Texas Southwestern Medical Center at Dallas.[30,31,149,150] Ramin et al.[30] randomized 1330 women of mixed parity to receive either epidural bupivacaine-fentanyl or intravenous meperidine analgesia during labor (vide supra). Approximately one third of the women in each group did not receive the allocated treatment. When the authors evaluated outcome according to intention-to-treat, they observed that 60 (9%) of the 664 women in the epidural group versus 35 (5%) of the 666 women in the meperidine group underwent operative delivery for dystocia. However, these results are misleading; the authors defined operative delivery as either cesarean section or low forceps delivery. Within the intention-to-treat analysis, the authors did not report the number of cesarean deliveries in the two groups; thus it is unclear whether there was an increased incidence of cesarean delivery in the women randomized to an offer of epidural analgesia.

Subsequently, Sharma et al.[149] randomized 715 women of mixed parity in spontaneous labor at term to receive either epidural analgesia or patient-controlled intravenous analgesia (PCIA) with meperidine. (The authors chose PCIA so that fewer patients in the meperidine group would "cross over" to the epidural group.) Enrollment and randomization occurred when the patients were admitted from the triage area to the nurse-midwifery service at Parkland Hospital. Subsequently, an anesthesiologist offered epidural analgesia to those women randomized to the epidural group but not to those randomized to the PCIA group. Epidural analgesia was initiated with small boluses of 0.25% bupivacaine and was maintained with a continuous epidural infusion of 0.125% bupivacaine with 2 µg/mL fentanyl. The PCIA was initiated with 50 mg meperidine and 25 mg promethazine and was maintained by patient-controlled boluses of 10 to 15 mg of meperidine every 10 minutes. Among the 358 women who were randomized to an offer of epidural analgesia, 243 actually received epidural analgesia. Of the remaining 115 women, 78 labored rapidly and never requested or received epidural analgesia, and the remaining 37 refused epidural analgesia. Among the 357 women who were randomized to an offer of PCIA, 259 women completed the study as allocated. Of the remaining 98 women, 73 labored rapidly and did not receive any analgesia, 20 refused PCIA, and five who had received meperidine PCIA "crossed over" to epidural analgesia because of inadequate pain relief.

Using an intention-to-treat analysis, the authors observed no difference between the two groups in the incidence of cesarean section (i.e., 4% in the epidural group and 5% in the PCIA group). When the authors evaluated outcome among the nulliparous women, they again noted no difference between the two groups in the incidence of cesarean section (i.e., 5% in the epidural group and 6% in the PCIA group). Women in the epidural group had lower pain scores during both the first and second stages of labor, and women in the PCIA group had higher sedation scores. (Women in the PCIA group were "visibly sedated but . . . invariably arousable."[149]) There was no difference between the two groups in neonatal outcome except that more babies in the PCIA group received naloxone to reverse respiratory depression at birth. The authors also noted no difference between the two groups in the incidence of cesarean section when they evaluated outcomes for protocol-compliant patients (i.e., 5% in the epidural analgesia group and 6% in the PCIA group).[149]

In this group's third randomized trial,[150] patients were randomized to receive either CSE or intravenous meperidine analgesia during labor. Profound fetal bradycardia, which prompted emergency cesarean section within 1 hour of intrathecal administration of sufentanil, occurred in 8 of 400 parturients who received CSE analgesia versus none of 352 women who received intravenous meperidine ($P < 0.01$). However, CSE analgesia did not increase the overall incidence of cesarean section or the incidence of cesarean section for dystocia in either nulliparous or parous women.

Sharma et al.[31] recently reported this group's fourth randomized trial (vide supra), which was limited to nulliparous women in spontaneous labor at term. Some 459 women were randomly assigned to receive either epidural bupivacaine-fentanyl or PCIA with meperidine. There was no difference between the two groups in the incidence of cesarean section (i.e., 7% in the epidural group versus 9% in the PCIA group). More women randomized to receive epidural analgesia underwent instrumental vaginal delivery than those randomized to receive PCIA (12% in the epidural group versus 3% in the PCIA group, $P < 0.001$).

Three other recent studies observed no increase in the overall incidence of cesarean section in nulliparous women randomized to receive epidural bupivacaine analgesia as compared with similar women randomized to receive intravenous or intramuscular opioid analgesia.[33,151,152] A 1994 meta-analysis suggested a strong association between epidural analgesia and an increased risk of cesarean section.[153] However, a 1998 meta-analysis of randomized controlled trials did not support the hypothesis that epidural analgesia causes an increase in the cesarean section rate.[154] Likewise, a 2002 meta-analysis of both randomized controlled trials and prospective cohort studies concluded that epidural analgesia does not affect the incidence of cesarean section.[34]

At the University of Iowa, we performed two studies to assess the effect of the *timing* of epidural analgesia on the incidence of cesarean section (*vide supra*). Early administration of epidural analgesia (i.e., between 3 and 5 cm cervical dilation) did *not* increase the incidence of cesarean section in nulliparous women who were in spontaneous labor or in those who were receiving oxytocin for induction or augmentation of labor as compared with women who received epidural analgesia after 5 cm cervical dilation.[37,38]

Some physicians have questioned whether prospective, randomized studies provide an accurate representation of the effect of epidural analgesia on the method of delivery in clinical practice. Is it possible that these studies introduce a Hawthorne effect that affects the results of the study? (The Hawthorne effect may be defined as the appearance or disappearance of a phenomenon on initiation of a study to confirm or exclude its existence.) An alternative study design is to assess obstetric outcome immediately before and after a sentinel event, such as the introduction of an epidural analgesia service in a given hospital.[155-161] For example, Gribble and Meier[155] compared obstetric outcomes for two 15-month periods: September 1, 1986, through December 1, 1987 (a period in which epidural analgesia was not available), and May 1, 1989, through August 1, 1990 (a period in which epidural analgesia was available 24 hours per day). During the 17-month interim, anesthesiologists introduced an epidural analgesia service at the authors' hospital (St. Joseph's Hospital in Marshfield, Wisconsin). The authors assessed obstetric outcomes for those patients with a singleton gestation in a vertex presentation who underwent a trial of labor and who

had not had a previous cesarean delivery. The authors evaluated obstetric outcomes only for those patients whose obstetrician practiced at St. Joseph's Hospital during both 15-month periods. The before group included 1298 patients, and the after group included 1084 patients. Approximately 48% of the patients in the after group received intrapartum epidural analgesia. Approximately 9% of the women in the before group and 8% of the women in the after group underwent cesarean section. There was no significant difference between the two groups when the patients were stratified into subgroups according to parity and indication for cesarean section. The authors concluded that "the availability of on-demand epidural analgesia for patients in labor did not increase the primary cesarean rate."[155]

One limitation of this study design is that it assumes that there were no other changes in obstetric management during the after period. DeMott and Sandmire[162] observed that the incidence of cesarean section in nulliparous women in Green Bay, Wisconsin, decreased from 9% between 1986 and 1987 to 7% between 1989 and 1990. The authors stated that their patients did not receive epidural analgesia, and they wondered, "if epidural analgesia had not been instituted at the Marshfield Clinic . . . in 1988, would they have experienced a similar decrease in the cesarean rate for nulliparous patients over the contemporary period of time?"[162] In other words, they suggested that the introduction of epidural analgesia may have prevented a decrease in the cesarean section rate at the Marshfield Clinic.

Other studies noted no increase in the overall incidence of cesarean section (or the incidence of cesarean section for dystocia) during the period immediately after the abrupt introduction of an epidural analgesia service in those hospitals (Figures 21-19 and 21-20).[156-160] In one study, the decreased incidence of cesarean section primarily reflected an increased number of patients who underwent vaginal birth after cesarean section (VBAC) after the introduction of an epidural

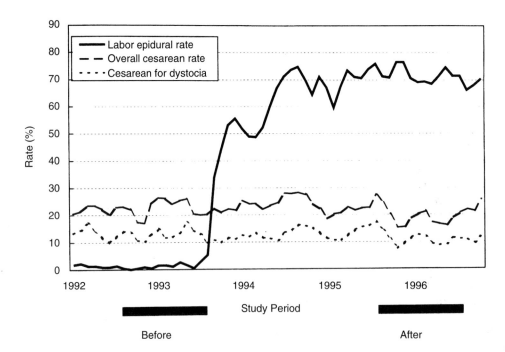

FIGURE 21-19. Epidural analgesia and cesarean delivery rates for nulliparous women who delivered at Tripler Army Medical Center for the years 1992-1996. (From Zhang J, Yancey MK, Klebanoff MA, et al. Does epidural analgesia prolong labor and increase risk of cesarean delivery? A natural experiment. Am J Obstet Gynecol 2001; 185:128-34.)

analgesia service.[156] This observation prompts two comments. First, the availability of epidural analgesia encourages more women to attempt VBAC (see Chapter 23). Second, it is important to consider the impact of epidural analgesia on the total population. For example, the provision of adequate analgesia often allows the obstetrician to manage labor aggressively. An exhausted patient in severe pain may beg the obstetrician to perform cesarean section, despite the fact that she remains in the latent phase and has not undergone an adequate trial of labor. The provision of effective analgesia allows the obstetrician to administer oxytocin, which facilitates an adequate trial of labor. Likewise, some obstetricians allow a trial of labor in patients with a breech presentation only if the patient agrees to receive epidural analgesia.

Iglesias et al.[163] assessed the success of a program designed to reduce the incidence of cesarean section in a rural Canadian community hospital. In 1985, the investigators revised their criteria for the diagnosis of dystocia, and they began to encourage VBAC. Overall, the cesarean section rate decreased from 23% in 1985 to 13% in 1989 (*P* = 0.001). Meanwhile, the overall rate of epidural analgesia increased from 35% in 1985 to 57% in 1989 (*P* < 0.001). The authors concluded that "the availability of epidural analgesia was an important factor in encouraging the acceptance of VBAC and oxytocin use."[163]

Socol et al.[164] evaluated the impact of three initiatives to decrease the cesarean section rate at Northwestern Memorial Hospital, a university hospital that provides care primarily for private patients. First, they strongly encouraged VBAC. Second, after the 1988 calendar year, they circulated records showing the cesarean section rate of every obstetrician to each attending physician. Third, they recommended the active management of labor as the preferred method of labor management for term nulliparous women. The rates of total, primary, and repeat cesarean deliveries decreased from 27%, 18%, and 9% in 1986 to 17%, 11%, and 6%, respectively, in 1991 (*P* < 0.0001 for all three comparisons). Meanwhile, the use of epidural analgesia increased from 28% in 1986 to 48% in 1991 (*P* < 0.0001). There was no change in the incidence of instrumental vaginal delivery (13% in 1986 versus 13% in 1991).

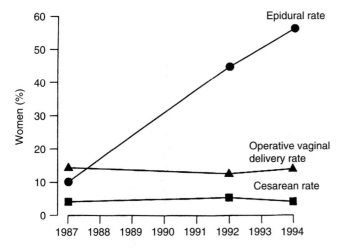

FIGURE 21-20. Epidural analgesia and cesarean and instrumental vaginal delivery rates for 1000 consecutive nulliparous women in spontaneous labor at term in three different years at the National Maternity Hospital in Dublin, Ireland. (From Impey L, MacQuillan K, Robson M. Epidural analgesia need not increase operative delivery rates. Am J Obstet Gynecol 2000; 182:358-63.)

Lagrew and Morgan[165] evaluated the impact of a similar program to decrease the cesarean delivery rate at Saddleback Hospital, a private hospital in California. The total, primary, and repeat cesarean delivery rates declined from 31%, 18%, and 13% in 1988 to 15%, 10%, and 5%, respectively, in 1994 (*P* < 0.0001 for all three comparisons). Meanwhile, the epidural analgesia rate increased from 62% in 1988 to 76% in 1994 (*P* < 0.0001). In these three studies,[163-165] the physicians successfully reduced the incidence of cesarean section while increasing the use of epidural analgesia during labor. Further, a second study[166] from Saddleback Hospital evaluated obstetric outcome for 16,230 deliveries between May 1988 and July 1995. The authors divided obstetricians into two groups, depending on whether their individual cesarean section rates were greater than 15% (the control group) or less than 15% (the target group). Obstetricians in the target group used epidural analgesia *more often* than obstetricians in the control group. In other words, the target group of obstetricians was able to achieve a *lower* cesarean section rate despite their *greater* use of epidural analgesia.[166]

Conversely, Johnson and Rosenfeld[167] observed that an abrupt decrease in the use of epidural analgesia at their hospital in 1994 did not result in a decreased incidence of cesarean delivery in their patients.

Obstetricians in the United States have long admired the low rate of cesarean section at the National Maternity Hospital in Dublin, Ireland. Obstetricians at this hospital were the first physicians to advocate the active management of labor (see Chapter 17). Some obstetricians in the United States have suggested that the low cesarean section rate in Dublin has resulted in part from the infrequent use of epidural analgesia during labor. Impey et al.[159] compared obstetric outcome for the first 1000 nulliparous women (term gestation, singleton fetus, cephalic presentation, spontaneous labor) who delivered at the National Maternity Hospital in 1987 with the outcome for a similar group of women who delivered in 1992 and 1994. The epidural analgesia rate increased from 10% in 1987 to 45% in 1992 and 57% in 1994. In each of these three years, 82% of women underwent spontaneous vaginal delivery. The cesarean section rate was 4% in 1987, 5% in 1992, and 4% in 1994 (*P* = NS) (Figure 21-20). The authors concluded the following[159]:

> The consistency of the operative delivery rates in three years with very different epidural rates suggests that epidural analgesia does not increase the cesarean delivery rate and that, with appropriate management of the second stage, it may not have to increase instrumental vaginal delivery rates. Further, it can be administered early and allowed to continue until after delivery.

Segal et al.[161] performed a meta-analysis of studies reporting the cesarean delivery rate immediately before and after a rapid change in the availability of epidural analgesia. The authors observed no significant change in the overall cesarean delivery rate following an abrupt increase in the availability of epidural analgesia.

Many practitioners believe—as I do—that the epidural administration of a dilute solution of local anesthetic (e.g., 0.0625% to 0.125% bupivacaine) is less likely to increase the cesarean section rate than is the administration of a more concentrated solution (e.g., 0.25% to 0.5% bupivacaine). Naulty et al.[108] evaluated the effect of changes in epidural analgesia practice (over time) on obstetric outcome at George Washington University Hospital. In the first group of patients, epidural analgesia was administered with intermittent bolus doses of either 1.5% lidocaine or 0.25% to 0.5% bupivacaine. Patients in this group typically did not receive additional local anesthetic during the second stage of labor. In the second group, the authors began epidural analgesia with a bolus dose of 0.25% bupivacaine with fentanyl 5 µg/mL, and they maintained analgesia until delivery with a continuous epidural infusion of 0.125% to 0.25% bupivacaine with fentanyl 2 µg/mL. In the third group, the authors began epidural analgesia by injecting 10 mL of 0.125% bupivacaine with sufentanil 0.5 µg/mL, and they maintained analgesia with a continuous epidural infusion of 0.03% to 0.06% bupivacaine with sufentanil 0.3 µg/mL. After the first change in technique, there was a significant *increase* in the proportion of women who received epidural analgesia for labor, but there was a significant *decrease* in the proportion of laboring women who underwent either outlet-forceps delivery or cesarean section. After the second change in technique, there was a further decrease in the incidence of cesarean section and midforceps delivery, but the rate of outlet-forceps delivery did not change further.

Similarly, Parker[109] evaluated the effect of changes in epidural analgesia practice (over time) on obstetric outcome at Barnes Hospital. The first group of patients received intermittent epidural bolus doses of 0.375% bupivacaine with 1:200,000 epinephrine, the second group received intermittent bolus doses of 0.25% bupivacaine, and the third group received intermittent bolus doses of 0.125% bupivacaine with fentanyl. Women who received 0.125% bupivacaine with fentanyl had a decreased incidence of fetal head malposition and cesarean section as compared with similar women whose analgesia was maintained with either 0.25% or 0.375% bupivacaine.

Olofsson et al.[168] randomized 1000 women of mixed parity—who requested epidural analgesia during labor—to receive either 0.25% bupivacaine with 1:200,000 epinephrine or 0.125% bupivacaine with sufentanil. The incidence of cesarean section was 15% in the high-dose bupivacaine group and 10% in the low-dose bupivacaine group ($P < 0.05$).

In these last three studies, the role of the epidural opioid in promoting a decreased incidence of cesarean section is unclear. In one prospective randomized study, 12 (32%) of 38 women who received epidural bupivacaine with fentanyl underwent cesarean section as compared with only two (6%) of 34 women who received bupivacaine alone.[169] Nageotte et al.[170] randomly assigned 761 nulliparous women in spontaneous labor at term who requested epidural analgesia to receive either CSE analgesia or epidural analgesia alone. Women who received epidural analgesia alone received an epidural bolus of 0.25% bupivacaine with 50 µg of fentanyl followed by a continuous epidural infusion of 0.125% bupivacaine with 2 µg/mL of fentanyl. Women who received CSE analgesia received 10 µg of intrathecal sufentanil followed by a continuous epidural infusion of 0.0625% bupivacaine with 2 µg/mL of fentanyl. Among the women who received CSE analgesia, approximately half were discouraged from walking, and the remaining half were encouraged to walk. There was no significant difference between the two groups in the incidence of cesarean section. However, there was a modest decrease in the incidence of instrumental vaginal delivery among the women who received CSE analgesia. Among all women, dystocia requiring cesarean section was significantly more likely when analgesia was administered with the fetal vertex at a negative (i.e., high) station. (One other study suggested that administration of epidural analgesia with the fetal vertex at a high station predicts an increased risk of cesarean section.[171]) Nageotte et al.[170] were unable to assess whether ambulation affected outcomes in the CSE group. (Likewise, it

remains unclear whether walking or standing shortens the duration of either the first[172-175] or second[176] stages of labor in patients receiving epidural analgesia.)

May and Elton[177] reported a preliminary study suggesting that CSE analgesia may result in a decreased incidence of cesarean section as compared with epidural analgesia alone. By contrast, the COMET study[116] *(vide supra)* demonstrated no difference in the incidence of cesarean section among 1054 nulliparous women who received either a traditional, a low-dose CSE, or a low-dose epidural infusion technique during labor.

CONCLUSIONS AND RECOMMENDATIONS

An unacceptably high number of American women involuntarily experience severe pain during labor. As noted by the American Society of Anesthesiologists and the ACOG, "There is no other circumstance where it is considered acceptable for a person to experience severe pain, amenable to safe intervention, while under a physician's care."[178] Unfortunately, labor represents one of the few circumstances in which the provision of effective analgesia is alleged to interfere with the parturient's and obstetrician's goal (i.e., spontaneous vaginal delivery). Dense regional anesthesia may adversely affect the progress of labor in some patients. Anesthesiologists should identify those methods of analgesia that provide the most effective pain relief without increasing the risk of cesarean section. Cesarean section results in an increased risk of maternal morbidity and mortality, and it is more expensive than vaginal delivery. However, recent randomized trials suggest that the contemporary use of epidural analgesia does *not* increase the cesarean section rate.[31,33,147-150] Further, even if it were shown that the contemporary use of epidural analgesia results in a small increase in the cesarean section rate, it is unclear how many women—who currently choose epidural analgesia— would voluntarily opt for nothing or intravenous opioid analgesia, which is less effective and provides marked sedation.

It is appropriate for anesthesiologists to provide substantial (albeit not always total) pain relief during both the first and second stages of labor. Among women in spontaneous labor, it seems reasonable to delay the administration of epidural analgesia until labor is well established. However, it is unnecessary to withhold analgesia until the patient has achieved an arbitrary cervical dilation during the first stage of labor, and it is inhumane to discontinue analgesia altogether during the second stage. Most women strongly dislike a dense motor block, and many prefer to maintain some sensation of uterine contractions and perineal pressure, especially during the second stage of labor. Some women benefit from a less intense block, and almost all women benefit from coaching and encouragement during the second stage.

Physicians do not need to withhold pain relief to achieve an acceptable cesarean delivery rate. I disagree with the recent ACOG recommendation that, "when feasible, obstetric practitioners should delay the administration of epidural analgesia in nulliparous women until the cervical dilation reaches 4-5 cm. . . ."[179,180] Fortunately, the ACOG added that they have "no desire to limit the use of epidural analgesia by women in labor."[179] Further, the ACOG stated that "the decision of when to [administer] epidural analgesia should be made individually with each patient, [and that] . . . women in labor should not be required to reach 4-5 cm of cervical dilation before receiving epidural analgesia."[180] Maternal-fetal factors and obstetric management—not the use of epidural analgesia—are the most important determinants of the cesarean delivery rate.[8,181,182]

KEY POINTS

- Epidural analgesia/anesthesia during labor is associated with an increased risk of prolonged labor and operative delivery. Controversy exists regarding whether there is a cause-and-effect relationship between the use of these analgesic techniques and prolonged labor or operative delivery. The presence of severe pain during early labor—and/or increased local anesthetic/opioid dose requirements—may signal an increased risk for prolonged labor and operative delivery.

- Epidural analgesia during labor is not a generic procedure. Conclusions regarding the effect of one technique on the progress of labor may not be applicable to other techniques.

- Maintenance of total anesthesia likely prolongs the second stage of labor, and it may increase the incidence of instrumental vaginal delivery.

- Epidural administration of a dilute solution of local anesthetic (with or without an opioid) is less likely to result in prolonged labor and malposition of the fetal vertex than epidural administration of a more concentrated solution of local anesthetic.

- Among women in spontaneous labor, it seems reasonable to delay the administration of epidural analgesia until labor is well established. However, it is unnecessary to await an arbitrary cervical dilation of 5 cm. Further, it is inhumane to discontinue analgesia altogether during the second stage of labor.

- Several retrospective, population-based studies suggest that the introduction of an epidural analgesia service or the increased use of epidural analgesia does *not* increase the cesarean section rate. Further, recent randomized controlled trials suggest that the contemporary use of epidural analgesia does *not* increase the cesarean section rate.

- In some patients, the use of epidural analgesia may increase the likelihood of vaginal delivery. For example, the availability of epidural analgesia may encourage women with a history of previous cesarean section to attempt vaginal birth after cesarean section.

- Even if it were shown that the contemporary use of epidural analgesia results in a small increase in the cesarean section rate, it is unclear how many women—who currently choose epidural analgesia—would voluntarily opt for nothing or intravenous opioid analgesia, which is less effective and provides marked sedation.

- Maternal-fetal factors and obstetric management—not the use of epidural analgesia—are the most important determinants of the cesarean section rate.

REFERENCES

1. Wuitchik M, Bakal D, Lipshitz J. The clinical significance of pain and cognitive activity in latent labor. Obstet Gynecol 1989; 73:35-42.
2. Palmer S, Lobo A, Tinnell C. Pain and duration of latent phase labor predicts the duration of active phase labor (abstract). Anesthesiology 1996; 85:A858.
3. Alexander JM, Sharma SK, McIntire DD, et al. Intensity of labor pain and cesarean delivery. Anesth Analg 2001; 92:1524-8.
4. Hess PE, Pratt SD, Soni AK, et al. An association between severe labor pain and cesarean delivery. Anesth Analg 2000; 90:881-6.
5. Panni MK, Segal S. Local anesthetic requirements are greater in dystocia than in normal labor. Anesthesiology 2003; 98:957-63.
6. Neuhoff D, Burke MS, Porreco RP. Cesarean birth for failed progress in labor. Obstet Gynecol 1989; 73:915-20.
7. Guillemette J, Fraser WD. Differences between obstetricians in caesarean section rates and the management of labour. Br J Obstet Gynaecol 1992; 99:105-8.
8. Segal S, Blatman R, Doble M, Datta S. The influence of the obstetrician in the relationship between epidural analgesia and cesarean section for dystocia. Anesthesiology 1999; 91:90-6.
9. Fraser W, Usher RH, McClean FH, et al. Temporal variation in rates of cesarean section for dystocia: Does "convenience" play a role? Am J Obstet Gynecol 1987; 156:300-4.
10. De Regt RH, Minkoff HL, Feldman J, Schwarz RH. Relation of private or clinic care to the cesarean birth rate. N Engl J Med 1986; 315:619-24.
11. Kilpatrick SJ, Laros RK. Characteristics of normal labor. Obstet Gynecol 1989; 74:85-7.
12. Howell CJ, Chalmers I. A review of prospectively controlled comparisons of epidural with non-epidural forms of pain relief during labour. Int J Obstet Anaesth 1992; 1:93-110.
13. Noble AD, Craft IL, Bootes JAH, et al. Continuous lumbar epidural analgesia using bupivacaine: A study of the fetus and newborn child. J Obstet Gynaecol Br Commonw 1971; 78:559-63.
14. Buchan PC, Milne MK, Browning MCK. The effect of continuous epidural blockade on plasma 11-hydroxycorticosteroid concentrations in labour. J Obstet Gynaecol Br Commonw 1973; 80:974-7.
15. Thalme B, Belfrage P, Raabe N. Lumbar epidural analgesia in labour. I. Acid-base balance and clinical condition of mother, fetus and newborn child. Acta Obstet Gynecol Scand 1974; 53:27-35.
16. Jouppila R. The effect of segmental epidural analgesia on maternal growth hormone, insulin, glucose and free fatty acids during labour. Ann Chir Gynaecol 1976; 65:398-404.
17. Jouppila R, Hollmén A. The effect of segmental epidural analgesia on maternal and foetal acid-base balance, lactate, serum potassium and creatine phosphokinase during labour. Acta Anaesth Scand 1976; 20:259-68.
18. Bratteby LE, Andersson L, Swanström S. Effect of obstetric regional analgesia on the change in respiratory frequency in the newborn. Br J Anaesth 1979; 51:41S-5S.
19. Jouppila R, Jouppila P, Moilanen K, Pakarinen A. The effect of segmental epidural analgesia on maternal prolactin during labour. Br J Obstet Gynaecol 1980; 87:234-8.
20. Robinson JO, Rosen M, Evans JM, et al. Maternal opinion about analgesia for labour: A controlled trial between epidural block and intramuscular pethidine combined with inhalation. Anaesthesia 1980; 35:1173-81.
21. Swanström S, Bratteby LE. Metabolic effects of obstetric regional analgesia and of asphyxia in the newborn infant during the first two hours after birth. I. Arterial blood glucose concentrations. Acta Paediatr Scand 1981; 70:791-800.
22. Swanström S, Bratteby LE. Metabolic effects of obstetric regional analgesia and of asphyxia in the newborn infant during the first two hours after birth. II. Arterial plasma concentrations of glycerol, free fatty acids and beta-hydroxybutyrate. Acta Paediatr Scand 1981; 70:801-9.
23. Swanström S, Bratteby LE. Metabolic effects of obstetric regional analgesia and of asphyxia in the newborn infant during the first two hours after birth. III. Adjustment of arterial blood gases and acid-base balance. Acta Paediatr Scand 1981; 70:811-8.
24. Bratteby LE. Short-and long-term effects on the infant of obstetric regional anesthesia. Acta Anaesthesiol Scand 1983; 27(suppl 78):36.
25. Ryhänen P, Jouppila R, Lanning M, et al. Effect of segmental epidural analgesia on changes in peripheral blood leucocyte counts, lymphocyte subpopulations, and *in vitro* transformation in healthy parturients and their newborns. Gynecol Obstet Invest 1984; 17:202-7.
26. Philipsen T, Jensen NH. Epidural block or parenteral pethidine as analgesic in labour: A randomized study concerning progress in labour

and instrumental deliveries. Eur J Obstet Gynecol Reprod Biol 1989; 30:27-33.

27. Philipsen T, Jensen NH. Maternal opinion about analgesia in labour and delivery: A comparison of epidural blockade and intramuscular pethidine. Eur J Obstet Gynecol Reprod Biol 1990; 34:205-10.

28. Zhang J, Klebanoff MA, DerSimonian R. Epidural analgesia in association with duration of labor and mode of delivery: A quantitative review. Am J Obstet Gynecol 1999; 180:970-7.

29. Thorp JA, Hu DH, Albin RM, et al. The effect of intrapartum epidural analgesia on nulliparous labor: A randomized, controlled, prospective trial. Am J Obstet Gynecol 1993; 169:851-8.

30. Ramin SM, Gambling DR, Lucas MJ, et al. Randomized trial of epidural versus intravenous analgesia during labor. Obstet Gynecol 1995; 86:783-9.

31. Sharma SK, Alexander JM, Messick G, et al. A randomized trial of epidural analgesia versus intravenous meperidine analgesia during labor in nulliparous women. Anesthesiology 2002; 96:546-51.

32. Alexander JM, Sharma SK, McIntire DD, Leveno KJ. Epidural analgesia lengthens the Friedman active phase of labor. Obstet Gynecol 2002; 100:46-50.

33. Bofill JA, Vincent RD, Ross EL, et al. Nulliparous active labor, epidural analgesia, and cesarean delivery for dystocia. Am J Obstet Gynecol 1997; 177:1465-70.

34. Leighton BL, Halpern SH. The effects of epidural analgesia on labor, maternal, and neonatal outcomes: A systematic review. Am J Obstet Gynecol 2002; 186:S69-77.

35. Friedman EA, Sachtleben MR. Caudal anesthesia: The factors that influence its effect on labor. Obstet Gynecol 1959; 13:442-50.

36. Read MD, Hunt LP, Anderton JM, Lieberman BA. Epidural block and the progress and outcome of labour. J Obstet Gynecol 1983; 4:35-9.

37. Chestnut DH, Vincent RD, McGrath JM, et al. Does early administration of epidural analgesia affect obstetric outcome in nulliparous women who are receiving intravenous oxytocin? Anesthesiology 1994; 80:1193-1200.

38. Chestnut DH, McGrath JM, Vincent RD, et al. Does early administration of epidural analgesia affect obstetric outcome in nulliparous women who are in spontaneous labor? Anesthesiology 1994; 80:1201-8.

39. Henry JS, Kingston MB, Maughan GB. The effect of epidural anesthesia on oxytocin-induced labor. Am J Obstet Gynecol 1967; 97:350-9.

40. Alexander JM, Lucas MJ, Ramin SM, et al. The course of labor with and without epidural analgesia. Am J Obstet Gynecol 1998; 178:516-20.

41. Brody SC, Grobman WA, Peaceman AM. The impact on labor of delaying epidural analgesia in nulliparous patients: A randomized trial (abstract). Am J Obstet Gynecol 1997; 176:S22.

42. Luxman D, Wolman I, Groutz A, et al. The effect of early epidural block administration on the progression and outcome of labor. Int J Obstet Anesth 1998; 7:161-4.

43. Rogers R, Gilson G, Kammerer-Doak D. Epidural analgesia and active management of labor: Effects on length of labor and mode of delivery. Obstet Gynecol 1999; 93:995-8.

44. Friedman EA. Effects of drugs on uterine contractility. Anesthesiology 1965; 26:409-22.

45. Petrie RH, Yeh S, Barron BA, et al. Dose-response effects of intravenous meperidine on uterine activity. J Matern Fetal Med 1993; 2:159-64.

46. Yoo KY, Lee J, Kim HS, Jeong SW. The effects of opioids on isolated human pregnant uterine muscles. Anesth Analg 2001; 92:1006-9.

47. Crawford JS. The stages and phases of labour: An outworn nomenclature that invites hazard. Lancet 1983; 2:271-2.

48. Studd JWW, Crawford JS, Duignan NM, et al. Effect of lumbar epidural analgesia on the fate of cervical dilatation and the outcome of labour of spontaneous onset. Br J Obstet Gynaecol 1980; 87:1015-21.

49. Lowensohn RI, Paul RH, Fales S, et al. Intrapartum epidural anesthesia: An evaluation of effects on uterine activity. Obstet Gynecol 1974; 44:388-93.

50. Zador G, Nilsson BA. Low dose intermittent epidural anaesthesia with lidocaine for vaginal delivery. II. Influence on labour and foetal acid-base status. Acta Obstet Gynaecol Scand 1974; 34(suppl):17-30.

51. Zador G, Nilsson BA. Continuous drip lumbar epidural anaesthesia with lidocaine for vaginal delivery. II. Influence on labour and foetal acid-base status. Acta Obstet Gynecol Scand 1974; 34(suppl):41-9.

52. Crawford JS. Patient management during extradural anaesthesia for obstetrics. Br J Anaesth 1975; 74:273-7.

53. Schellenberg JC. Uterine activity during lumbar epidural analgesia with bupivacaine. Am J Obstet Gynecol 1977; 127:26-31.

54. Gal D, Choudhry R, Ung KA, et al. Segmental epidural analgesia for labor and delivery. Acta Obstet Gynecol Scand 1979; 58:429-31.

55. Willdeck-Lund G, Lindmark G, Nilsson BA. Effect of segmental epidural analgesia upon the uterine activity with special reference to the use of different local anaesthetic agents. Acta Anaesth Scand 1979; 23:519-28.

56. Abboud TK, Khoo SS, Miller F, et al. Maternal, fetal, and neonatal responses after epidural anesthesia with bupivacaine, 2-chloroprocaine, or lidocaine. Anesth Analg 1982; 61:638-44.

57. Abboud TK, Afrasiabi A, Sarkis F, et al. Continuous infusion epidural analgesia in parturients receiving bupivacaine, chloroprocaine, or lidocaine: Maternal, fetal, and neonatal effects. Anesth Analg 1984; 63:421-8.

58. Gunther RE, Bauman J. Obstetrical caudal anesthesia. I. A randomized study comparing 1% mepivacaine with 1% lidocaine plus epinephrine. Anesthesiology 1969; 31:5-19.

59. Gunther RE, Bellville JW. Obstetrical caudal anesthesia. II. A randomized study comparing 1% mepivacaine with 1% mepivacaine plus epinephrine. Anesthesiology 1972; 37:288-98.

60. Craft JB, Epstein BS, Coakley CS. Effect of lidocaine with epinephrine versus lidocaine (plain) on induced labor. Anesth Analg 1972; 51:243-6.

61. Abboud TK, David S, Nagappala S, et al. Maternal, fetal, and neonatal effects of lidocaine with and without epinephrine for epidural anesthesia in obstetrics. Anesth Analg 1984; 63:973-9.

62. Abboud TK, Shiek-ol-Eslam A, Yanagi T, et al. Safety and efficacy of epinephrine added to bupivacaine for lumbar epidural analgesia in obstetrics. Anesth Analg 1985; 64:585-91.

63. Abboud TK, DerSakissian L, Terrasi J, et al. Comparative maternal, fetal, and neonatal effects of chloroprocaine with and without epinephrine for epidural anesthesia in obstetrics. Anesth Analg 1987; 66:71-5.

64. Eisenach JC, Grice SC, Dewan DM. Epinephrine enhances analgesia produced by epidural bupivacaine during labor. Anesth Analg 1987; 66:447-51.

65. Grice SC, Eisenach JC, Dewan DM. Labor analgesia with epidural bupivacaine plus fentanyl: Enhancement with epinephrine and inhibition with 2-chloroprocaine. Anesthesiology 1990; 72:623-8.

66. Yau G, Gregory MA, Gin T, Oh TE. Obstetric epidural analgesia with mixtures of bupivacaine, adrenaline and fentanyl. Anaesthesia 1990; 45:1020-3.

67. Dounas M, O'Kelly B, Jamali S, et al. Maternal and fetal effects of adrenaline with bupivacaine (0.25%) for epidural analgesia during labour. Eur J Anaesth 1996; 13:594-8.

68. Cheek TG, Samuels P, Tobin M, Gutsche BB. Rapid intravenous saline infusion decreases uterine activity in labor, epidural analgesia does not (abstract). Anesthesiology 1989; 71:A884.

69. Zamora JE, Rosaeg OP, Lindsay MP, Crossan ML. Acute intravenous hydration prior to epidural analgesia for labour: Effects of two volumes of lactated Ringer's solution on uterine contractions and maternal hemodynamics (abstract). Anesth Analg 1995; 80:S578.

70. Miller AC, DeVore JS, Eisler EA. Effects of anesthesia on uterine activity and labor. In: Shnider SM, Levinson G, editors. Anesthesia for Obstetrics. 3rd ed. Baltimore, MD, Williams & Wilkins, 1993:53-69.

71. Baraka A, Noueihid R, Hajj S. Intrathecal injection of morphine for obstetric analgesia. Anesthesiology 1981; 54:136-40.

72. Abboud TK, Shnider SM, Dailey PA, et al. Intrathecal administration of hyperbaric morphine for the relief of pain in labour. Br J Anaesth 1984; 56:1351-60.

73. Dailey PA, Brookshire GL, Shnider SM, et al. The effects of naloxone associated with the intrathecal use of morphine in labor. Anesth Analg 1984; 64:658-66.

74. Chestnut DH, Owen CL, Bates BN, et al. Continuous infusion epidural analgesia during labor: A randomized, double-blind comparison of 0.0625% bupivacaine/0.0002% fentanyl versus 0.125% bupivacaine. Anesthesiology 1988; 68:754-9.

75. Groves PA, Sarna MC, Foley L, Oriol NE. The effect of intrathecal sufentanil and ultra-low-dose epidural bupivacaine on labor progress (abstract). Anesth Analg 1995; 80:S163.

76. Pan PH, Fragneto R, Moore C, Ross V. Do obstetric outcomes differ between early combined spinal-epidural and epidural anesthesia in nulliparous patients receiving intravenous oxytocin? (abstract). Anesthesiology 1996; 85:A854.

77. Tsen LC, Thue B, Datta S, Segal S. Is combined spinal-epidural analgesia associated with more rapid cervical dilation in nulliparous patients when compared with conventional epidural analgesia? Anesthesiology 1999; 91:920-5.

78. Norris MC, Fogel ST, Conway-Long C. Combined spinal-epidural versus epidural labor analgesia. Anesthesiology 2001; 95:913-20.

79. Abouleish E, Rawal N, Shaw J, et al. Intrathecal morphine 0.2 mg versus epidural bupivacaine 0.125% or their combination: Effects on parturients. Anesthesiology 1991; 74:711-6.

80. Roux M, Wattrisse G, Subtil D, et al. A comparison of early combined spinal epidural analgesia vs epidural analgesia on labor stage duration and obstetric outcome (abstract). Anesthesiology 1996; 85:A851.

81. Rawal N, Möllefors K, Axelsson K, et al. An experimental study of urodynamic effects of epidural morphine and of naloxone reversal. Anesth Analg 1983; 62:641-7.

82. Bicknell RJ, Leng G. Russell JA, et al. Hypothalamic opioid mechanisms controlling oxytocin neurons during parturition. Brain Res Bull 1988; 20:743-9.

83. Sivalingam T, Pleuvry BJ. Actions of morphine, pethidine, and pentazocine on the oestrus and pregnant rat uterus in vitro. Br J Anaesth 1985; 57:430-3.

84. Faletti A, Chaud MA, Gimeno MAF, Gimeno AL. Morphine diminishes the constancy of spontaneous uterine contractions, antagonizes the positive inotropic effects of prostaglandin E_2, but not of prostaglandin $F_{2\alpha}$ and inhibits prostaglandin E and F outputs from the uterus of ovariectomized rats. Prostaglandins Leukot Essent Fatty Acids 1988; 34:147-51.

85. Rahm VA, Hallgren A, Hogberg H, et al. Plasma oxytocin levels in women during labor with or without epidural analgesia: A prospective study. Acta Obstet Gynecol Scand 2002; 81:1033-9.

86. Behrens O, Goeschen K, Luck HJ, Fuchs AR. Effects of lumbar epidural analgesia on prostaglandin F_2 release and oxytocin secretion during labor. Prostaglandins 1993; 45:285-96.

87. Nielsen PE, Abouleish E, Meyer BA, Parisi VM. Effect of epidural analgesia on fundal dominance during spontaneous active-phase nulliparous labor. Anesthesiology 1996; 84:540-4.

88. Moir DD, Willocks J. Management of incoordinate uterine action under continuous epidural analgesia. Br Med J 1967; 3:396-400.

89. Wittels B. Does epidural anesthesia affect the course of labor and delivery? Semin Perinatol 1991; 15:358-67.

90. Phillips KC, Thomas TA. Second stage of labour with or without extradural analgesia. Anaesthesia 1983; 38:872-6.

91. Johnsrud ML, Dale PO, Lövland B. Benefits of continuous infusion epidural analgesia throughout vaginal delivery. Acta Obstet Gynecol Scand 1988; 67:355-8.

92. Chestnut DH, Bates JN, Choi WW. Continuous infusion epidural analgesia with lidocaine: Efficacy and influence during the second stage of labor. Obstet Gynecol 1987; 69:323-7.

93. Chestnut DH, Vandewalker GE, Owen CL, et al. The influence of continuous epidural bupivacaine analgesia on the second stage of labor and method of delivery in nulliparous women. Anesthesiology 1987; 66:774-80.

94. Chestnut DH, Laszewski LJ, Pollack KL, et al. Continuous epidural infusion of 0.0625% bupivacaine-0.0002% fentanyl during the second stage of labor. Anesthesiology 1990; 72:613-8.

95. Luxman D, Wolman I, Niv D, et al. Effect of second-stage 0.25% epidural bupivacaine on the outcome of labor. Gynecol Obstet Invest 1996; 42:167-70.

96. Chestnut DH. Epidural anesthesia and instrumental vaginal delivery (editorial). Anesthesiology 1991; 74:805-8.

97. Nadeau S, Elliott RD. Continuous bupivacaine infusion during labour: Effects on analgesia and delivery (abstract). Can Anaesth Soc J 1985; 32:S70.

98. Bogod DG, Rosen M, Rees GAD. Extradural infusion of 0.125% bupivacaine at 10 mL h^{-1} to women during labour. Br J Anaesth 1987; 59:325-30.

99. Gaylard DG, Wilson IH, Balmer HGR. An epidural infusion technique for labour. Anaesthesia 1987; 42:1098-101.

100. Hicks JA, Jenkins JG, Newton MC, Findley IL. Continuous epidural infusion of 0.075% bupivacaine for pain relief in labour. Anaesthesia 1988; 43:289-92.

101. Smedstad KG, Morison DH. A comparative study of continuous and intermittent epidural analgesia for labour and delivery. Can J Anaesth 1988; 35:234-41.

102. Eddleston JM, Maresh M, Horsman EL, et al. Comparison of the maternal and fetal effects associated with intermittent or continuous infusion of extradural analgesia. Br J Anaesth 1992; 69:154-8.

103. Lamont RF, Pinney D, Rodgers P, Bryant TN. Continuous versus intermittent epidural analgesia: A randomised trial to observe obstetric outcome. Anaesthesia 1989; 44:893-6.

104. Aquilina RJ, Carli F. Epidural bupivacaine infusions versus intermittent top-ups: Effects on analgesia and mode of delivery in 1947 primiparae (abstract). Int J Obstet Anesthesia 1994; 3:111-2.

105. van der Vyver M, Halpern S, Joseph G. Patient-controlled epidural analgesia versus continuous infusion for labour analgesia: A meta-analysis. Br J Anaesth 2002; 89:459-65.

106. Sharma SK, Alexander JM, Wiley J, Leveno KJ. The effects of patient-controlled epidural analgesia versus continuous infusion epidural analgesia on the course of labor and delivery (abstract). Anesthesiology 2001; 94:A24.

107. Turner MJ, Silk JM, Alagesan K, et al. Epidural bupivacaine concentration and forceps delivery in primiparae. J Obstet Gynaecol 1988; 9:122-5.

108. Naulty JS, March MG, Leavitt KL, et al. Effect of changes in labor analgesic practice on labor outcome (abstract). Anesthesiology 1992; 77:A979.

109. Parker RK. Influence of labor epidural management on outcome in obstetrics (abstract). Reg Anesth 1992; 17(suppl):31.

110. Murphy JD, Henderson K, Bowden MI, et al. Bupivacaine versus bupivacaine plus fentanyl for epidural analgesia: Effect on maternal satisfaction. BMJ 1991; 302:564-7.

111. Stoddart AP, Nicholson KEA, Popham PA. Low dose bupivacaine/fentanyl epidural infusions in labour and mode of delivery. Anaesthesia 1994; 49:1087-90.

112. James KS, McGrady E, Quasim I, Patrick A. Comparison of epidural bolus administration of 0.25% bupivacaine and 0.1% bupivacaine with 0.0002% fentanyl for analgesia during labour. Br J Anaesth 1998; 81:507-10.

113. Russell R, Reynolds F. Epidural infusion of low-dose bupivacaine and opioid in labour: Does reducing motor block increase the spontaneous delivery rate? Anaesthesia 1996; 51:266-73.

114. Vertommen JD, Vandermeulen E, Van Aken H, et al. The effects of addition of sufentanil to 0.125% bupivacaine on the quality of analgesia during labor and on the incidence of instrumental deliveries. Anesthesiology 1991; 74:809-14.

115. Comparative Obstetric Mobile Epidural Trial (COMET) Study Group UK. Effect of low-dose mobile versus traditional epidural techniques on mode of delivery: A randomized controlled trial. Lancet 2001; 358:19-23.

116. Angle P, Halpern S, Morgan A. Effect of low-dose mobile versus high-dose epidural techniques on the progress of labor: A meta-analysis (abstract). Anesthesiology (Supplement) 2002; 96:P-52.

117. Livnat EJ, Fejgin M, Scommegna A, et al. Neonatal acid-base balance in spontaneous and instrumental vaginal deliveries. Obstet Gynecol 1978; 52:549-51.

118. McBride WG, Black BP, Brown CJ, et al. Method of delivery and developmental outcome at five years of age. Med J Aust 1979; 1:301-4.

119. Friedman EA, Sachtleben-Murray MR, Dahrouge D, Neff RK. Long-term effects of labor and delivery on offspring: A matched-pair analysis. Am J Obstet Gynecol 1984; 150:941-5.

120. Gilstrap LC, Hauth JC, Schiano S, Connor KD. Neonatal acidosis and method of delivery. Obstet Gynecol 1984; 63:681-5.

121. Dierker LJ, Rosen MG, Thompson K, Lynn P. Midforceps deliveries: Long-term outcome of infants. Am J Obstet Gynecol 1986; 154:764-8.

122. Robinson JN, Norwitz ER, Cohen AP, et al. Epidural analgesia and third-or fourth-degree lacerations in nulliparas. Obstet Gynecol 1999; 94:259-62.

123. Robinson CA, Macones GA, Roth NW, Morgan MA. Does station of the fetal head at epidural placement affect the position of the fetal vertex at delivery? Am J Obstet Gynecol 1996; 175:991-4.

124. Yancey MK, Zhang J, Schweitzer DL, et al. Epidural analgesia and fetal head malposition at vaginal delivery. Obstet Gynecol 2001; 97:608-12.

125. Maresh M, Choong KH, Beard RW. Delayed pushing with lumbar epidural analgesia in labour. Br J Obstet Gynaecol 1983; 90:623-7.

126. Goodfellow CF, Studd C. The reduction of forceps in primagravidae with epidural analgesia: A controlled trial. Br J Clin Pract 1979; 33:287-8.

127. Vause S, Congdon HM, Thornton JG. Immediate and delayed pushing in the second stage of labour for nulliparous women with epidural analgesia: A randomized controlled trial. Br J Obstet Gynaecol 1998; 105:186-8.

128. Fraser WD, Marcoux S, Krauss I, et al. Multicenter, randomized, controlled trial of delayed pushing for nulliparous women in the second stage of labor with continuous epidural analgesia. Am J Obstet Gynecol 2000; 182:1165-72.

129. Fitzpatrick M, Harkin R, McQuillan K, et al. A randomized clinical trial comparing the effects of delayed versus immediate pushing with epidural analgesia on mode of delivery and faecal continence. BJOG 2002; 109:1359-65.

130. Hansen SL, Clark SL, Foster JC. Active pushing versus passive fetal descent in the second stage of labor: A randomized controlled trial. Obstet Gynecol 2002; 99:29-34.

131. Scull TJ, Hemmings GT, Carli F, et al. Epidural analgesia in early labour blocks the stress response but uterine contractions remain unchanged. Can J Anaesth 1998; 45:626-30.

132. Goodfellow CF, Hull MGR, Swaab DF, et al. Oxytocin deficiency at delivery with epidural analgesia. Br J Obstet Gynaecol 1983; 90:214-9.

133. Bates RG, Helm CW, Duncan A, Edmonds DK. Uterine activity in the second stage of labour and the effect of epidural analgesia. Br J Obstet Gynaecol 1985; 92:1246-50.

134. Saunders NJSG, Spiby H, Gilbert L, et al. Oxytocin infusion during second stage of labour in primiparous women using epidural analgesia: A randomised double blind placebo controlled trial. BMJ 1989; 299:1423-6.

135. Katz M, Lunenfeld E, Meizner I, et al. The effect of the duration of the second stage of labour on the acid-base state of the fetus. Br J Obstet Gynaecol 1987; 94:425-30.

136. Saunders NSG, Paterson CM, Wadsworth J. Neonatal and maternal morbidity in relation to the length of the second stage of labour. Br J Obstet Gynaecol 1992; 99:381-5.

137. Derham RJ, Crowhurst J, Crowther C. The second stage of labour: Durational dilemmas. Aust NZ J Obstet Gynaecol 1991; 31:31-6.

138. Menticoglou SM, Manning F, Harman C, Morrison I. Perinatal outcome in relation to second-stage duration. Am J Obstet Gynecol 1995; 173:906-12.

139. American College of Obstetricians and Gynecologists Committee on Obstetrics: Maternal and Fetal Medicine. Obstetric Forceps. ACOG Committee Opinion No. 71, 1989.

140. Kadar N, Cruddas M, Campbell S. Estimating the probability of spontaneous delivery conditional on time spent in the second stage. Br J Obstet Gynaecol 1986; 93:568-76.

141. Paterson CM, Saunders NSG, Wadsworth J. The characteristics of the second stage of labour in 25,069 singleton deliveries in the North West Thames Health Region, 1988. Br J Obstet Gynaecol 1992; 99:377-80.

142. Rosaeg OP, Campbell N, Crossan ML. Epidural analgesia does not prolong the third stage of labour. Can J Anaesth 2002; 49:490-2.

143. Thorp JA, Parisi VM, Boylan PC, Johnston DA. The effect of continuous epidural analgesia on cesarean section for dystocia in nulliparous women. Am J Obstet Gynecol 1989; 161:670-5.

144. Thorp JA, Eckert LO, Ang MS, et al. Epidural analgesia and cesarean section for dystocia: Risk factors in nulliparas. Am J Perinatol 1991; 8:402-10.

145. Too many cesareans. Consumer Reports Feb 1991, 120-6.

146. Lieberman E, Lang JM, Cohen A, et al. Association of epidural analgesia with cesarean delivery in nulliparas. Obstet Gynecol 1996; 88:993-1000.

147. Ploeckinger B, Ulm MR, Chalubinski K, Gruger W. Epidural anaesthesia in labour: Influence on surgical delivery rates, intrapartum fever and blood loss. Gynecol Obstet Invest 1995; 39:24-7.

148. Loncar JM, Rouse DJ, Owen J, et al. Does intrapartum epidural analgesia increase the cesarean delivery rate? (abstract). Am J Obstet Gynecol 1998; 178:S175.

149. Sharma SK, Sidawi JE, Ramin SM, et al. Cesarean delivery: A randomized trial of epidural versus patient-controlled meperidine analgesia during labor. Anesthesiology 1997; 87:487-94.

150. Gambling DR, Sharma SK, Ramin SM, et al. A randomized study of combined spinal-epidural analgesia versus intravenous meperidine during labor: Impact on cesarean delivery rate. Anesthesiology 1998; 89:1336-44.

151. Clark A, Carr D, Loyd G, et al. The influence of epidural analgesia on cesarean delivery rates: A randomized, prospective trial. Am J Obstet Gynecol 1998; 179:1527-33.

152. Loughnan BA, Carli F, Romney M, et al. Randomized controlled comparison of epidural bupivacaine versus pethidine for analgesia in labour. Br J Anaesth 2000; 84:715-9.

153. Morton SC, Williams MS, Keeler EB, et al. Effect of epidural analgesia for labor on the cesarean delivery rate. Obstet Gynecol 1994; 83:1045-52.

154. Halpern SH, Leighton BL, Ohlsson A, et al. Effect of epidural vs parenteral opioid analgesia on the progress of labor: A meta-analysis. JAMA 1998; 280:2105-10.

155. Gribble RK, Meier PR. Effect of epidural analgesia on the primary cesarean rate. Obstet Gynecol 1991; 78:231-4.

156. Larson DD. The effect of initiating an obstetric anesthesiology service on rate of cesarean section and rate of forceps delivery (abstract). Society for Obstetric Anesthesia and Perinatology 1992:13.

157. Lyon DS, Knuckles G, Whitaker E, Salgado S. The effect of instituting an elective labor epidural program on the operative delivery rate. Obstet Gynecol 1997; 90:135-41.

158. Fogel ST, Shyken JM, Leighton BL, et al. Epidural labor analgesia and the incidence of cesarean delivery for dystocia. Anesth Analg 1998; 87:119-23.

159. Impey L, MacQuillan K, Robson M. Epidural analgesia need not increase operative delivery rates. Am J Obstet Gynecol 2000; 182:358-63.

160. Zhang J, Yancey MK, Klebanoff MA, et al. Does epidural analgesia prolong labor and increase risk of cesarean delivery? A natural experiment. Am J Obstet Gynecol 2001; 185:128-34.

161. Segal S, Su M, Gilbert P. The effect of a rapid change in availability of epidural analgesia on the cesarean delivery rate: A meta-analysis. Am J Obstet Gynecol 2000; 183:974-8.

162. DeMott RK, Sandmire HK. Effect of epidural analgesia on the primary cesarean rate (letter). Obstet Gynecol 1992; 79:155-6.

163. Iglesias S, Burn R, Saunders LD. Reducing the cesarean section rate in a rural community hospital. Can Med Assoc J 1991; 145:1459-64.

164. Socol ML, Garcia PM, Peaceman AM, Dooley SL. Reducing cesarean births at a primarily private university hospital. Am J Obstet Gynecol 1993; 168:1748-58.

165. Lagrew DC, Morgan MA. Decreasing the cesarean section rate in a private hospital: Success without mandated clinical changes. Am J Obstet Gynecol 1996; 174:184-91.

166. Lagrew DC, Adashek JA. Lowering the cesarean section rate in a private hospital: Comparison of individual physicians' rates, risk factors, and outcomes. Am J Obstet Gynecol 1998; 178:1207-14.

167. Johnson S, Rosenfeld JA. The effect of epidural anesthesia on the length of labor. J Fam Pract 1995; 40:244-7.

168. Olofsson C, Ekblom A, Ekman-Ordeberg G, Irestedt L. Obstetric outcome following epidural analgesia with bupivacaine-adrenaline 0.25% or bupivacaine 0.125% with sufentanil: A prospective randomized controlled study in 1000 parturients. Acta Anesthesiol Scand 1998; 42:284-92.

169. Lysak SZ, Eisenach JC, Dobson CE. Patient-controlled epidural analgesia during labor: A comparison of three solutions with a continuous infusion control. Anesthesiology 1990; 72:44-9.

170. Nageotte MP, Larson D, Rumney PJ, et al. Epidural analgesia compared with combined spinal-epidural analgesia during labor in nulliparous women. N Engl J Med 1997; 337:1715-9.

171. Holt RO, Diehl SJ, Wright JW. Station and cervical dilation at epidural placement in predicting cesarean risk. Obstet Gynecol 1999; 93:281-4.

172. Collis RE, Harding SA, Morgan BM. Effect of maternal ambulation on labour with low-dose combined spinal-epidural analgesia. Anaesthesia 1999; 54:535-9.

173. Asselineau D. Does ambulation under epidural analgesia during labor modify the conditions of fetal extraction? Contracept Fertil Sex 1996; 24:505-8.

174. Vallejo MC, Firestone LL, Mandell GL, et al. Effect of epidural analgesia with ambulation on labor duration. Anesthesiology 2001; 95:857-61.

175. Sandefo I, Lebrun T, Polin B, Olle D. Epidural analgesia and labor: Lack of efficacy of walking on labor duration due to short duration of walking time (letter). Anesthesiology 2002; 97:525.

176. Golara M, Plaat F, Shennan AH. Upright versus recumbent position in the second stage of labour in women with combined spinal-epidural analgesia. Int J Obstet Anesth 2002; 11:19-22.

177. May AE, Elton CD. Ambulatory extradural analgesia in labour reduces risk of caesarean section. Br J Anaesth 1996; 77:692P-3P.

178. American Society of Anesthesiologists and American College of Obstetricians and Gynecologists. Pain Relief During Labor. 1992 (revised in 2000).

179. American College of Obstetricians and Gynecologists Committee on Obstetric Practice. Analgesia and Cesarean Delivery Rates. ACOG Committee Opinion No. 269. 2002.

180. American College of Obstetricians and Gynecologists. Obstetric Analgesia and Anesthesia. ACOG Practice Bulletin No. 36. 2002.

181. Chestnut DH. Does epidural analgesia during labor affect the incidence of cesarean delivery? Reg Anesth 1997; 22:495-9.

182. Chestnut DH. Epidural analgesia and the incidence of cesarean section: Time for another close look (editorial). Anesthesiology 1997; 87:472-6.

Chapter 22

Alternative Regional Anesthetic Techniques: Paracervical Block, Lumbar Sympathetic Block, Pudendal Nerve Block, and Perineal Infiltration

David H. Chestnut, M.D.

Epidural and spinal analgesia/anesthesia are the most flexible analgesic techniques available for obstetric patients. The anesthesiologist may use an epidural or a spinal technique to provide effective analgesia during the first and/or second stage of labor. Subsequently, the epidural or spinal technique may be used to provide profound anesthesia for either vaginal or cesarean delivery. Unfortunately, some maternal conditions (e.g., coagulopathy, hemorrhage) contraindicate the administration of epidural and spinal anesthesia. Many parturients do not have access to epidural and spinal anesthesia, and others do not want epidural or spinal anesthesia. The purpose of this chapter is to discuss alternative regional anesthetic techniques for labor and vaginal delivery.

PARACERVICAL BLOCK

During the first stage of labor, pain results primarily from dilation of the cervix and distention of the lower uterine segment and upper vagina. Pain impulses are transmitted from the upper vagina, cervix, and lower uterine segment by visceral afferent nerve fibers that join the sympathetic chain at L2 to L3 and enter the spinal cord at T10 to L1. Some obstetricians perform paracervical block to provide analgesia during the first stage of labor. The goal is to block transmission through the paracervical ganglion—also known as *Frankenhäuser's ganglion*—which lies immediately lateral and posterior to the cervicouterine junction.

Paracervical block does not adversely affect the progress of labor. Further, it provides excellent analgesia without the annoying sensory and motor blockade that may occur during epidural and spinal anesthesia. This technique does not block somatic sensory fibers from the lower vagina, vulva, and perineum. Thus it does not relieve the pain caused by distention of these structures during the second stage of labor.

In 1945, Rosenfeld[1] introduced obstetric paracervical block in the United States. Subsequently, paracervical block became a popular technique for analgesia during labor. In 1981, approximately 5% of obstetric patients in the United States received paracervical block.[2] Approximately 12% of parturients received paracervical block during labor in Sweden between 1983 and 1986,[3] and in some parts of Scandinavia it remains the most frequently used form of regional analgesia during labor. In the United States, the decline in the popularity of paracervical block has resulted from both fear of fetal complications and the increased popularity of epidural and spinal anesthetic techniques. American and European medical journals have reported more than 50 perinatal deaths associated with paracervical block.[4-7] As early as 1963, Nyirjesy et al.[4] stated, "We feel that the high incidence of infant complications found in this study warrants the discontinuation of the obstetric use of paracervical block in our own practice." In 1986, Shnider[8] opined that paracervical block during labor "should be largely abandoned." Subsequently, he recommended that this technique be avoided in cases of uteroplacental insufficiency or preexisting fetal distress. He acknowledged that "there may be exceptions if other anesthetic techniques are contraindicated or pose a greater hazard to the mother or fetus."[7] As recently as 1997, 2% to 6% of parturients in the United States received paracervical block during labor. The highest incidence (6%) occurred in hospitals with less than 500 deliveries per year.[9]

Some obstetricians argue that in the absence of fetal bradycardia, paracervical block has few adverse effects on the infant. Jensen et al.[10] randomly assigned 117 nulliparous women to receive either paracervical block with 12 mL of 0.25% bupivacaine or 75 mg of meperidine intramuscularly. Women in the paracervical block group had significantly better analgesia than women in the meperidine group at 20, 40, and 60 minutes. During the first 60 minutes, pain relief was complete or acceptable in 78% of the women in the paracervical block group as compared with 31% of the women in the meperidine group. Two fetuses in the paracervical block group and one in the meperidine group had transient brady-cardia. A total of 6 infants in the paracervical block group versus 16 in the meperidine group ($P < 0.05$) had fetal/neonatal distress, which the authors defined as an umbilical arterial blood pH of 7.15 or less and/or a 1-minute Apgar score of 7 or less.[10] (Few physicians agree that a 1-minute Apgar score of 7 is a sign of neonatal distress.)

Kangas-Saarela et al.[11] compared neonatal neurobehavioral responses in 10 infants whose mothers received bupivacaine paracervical block with 12 infants whose mothers received no analgesia. The authors performed paracervical block while each patient lay in a left lateral position, and they limited the depth of the injection to 3 mm or less. They observed no significant differences between groups in the neurobehavioral responses at 3 hours, 1 day, 2 days, or 4 to 5 days after delivery. The authors concluded that properly performed paracervical block does not adversely affect newborn behavior or neurologic function.[11]

Technique

Paracervical block is performed with the patient in a modified lithotomy position. The uterus should be displaced leftward during performance of the block. This may be accomplished by placing a folded pillow beneath the patient's right buttock. The physician uses a needle guide to define and limit the depth of the injection and to decrease the risk of vaginal or fetal injury. The obstetrician introduces the needle and needle guide into the vagina with the left hand for the left side of the pelvis and with the right hand for the right side (Figure 22-1). The needle and needle guide are introduced into the left or right lateral vaginal fornix, near the cervix, at the 4 o'clock or

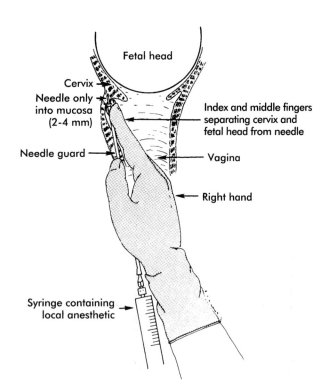

FIGURE 22-1. Technique of paracervical block. Notice the position of the hand and fingers in relation to the cervix and fetal head. There is no undue pressure applied at the vaginal fornix by the fingers or the needle guide, and the needle is inserted at a shallow depth. (From Abouleish E. Pain Control in Obstetrics. New York, JB Lippincott, 1977:344.)

8 o'clock position. The needle is advanced through the vaginal mucosa to a depth of 2 to 3 mm.[12] The obstetrician should aspirate before each injection of local anesthetic. A total of 5 to 10 mL of local anesthetic, without epinephrine, is injected on each side.[13] Some obstetricians recommend giving incremental doses of local anesthetic on each side (e.g., 2.5 to 5 mL of local anesthetic between the 3 and 4 o'clock positions, followed by 2.5 to 5 mL between the 4 and 5 o'clock positions).[12,14,15]

After injecting the local anesthetic in either the left or right lateral vaginal fornix, the physician should wait 5 to 10 minutes and observe the fetal heart rate (FHR) before injecting the local anesthetic on the opposite side.[15] Some obstetricians do not endorse this recommendation. Van Dorsten et al.[16] randomized 42 healthy parturients at term to two methods of paracervical block. The study group experienced a 10-minute interval between injections of local anesthetic on the left and right sides of the vagina. The control group had almost simultaneous injection on the left and right sides. No cases of fetal bradycardia occurred in either group. The authors concluded that patient selection and lateral positioning after the block have a more important role in the prevention of postparacervical block fetal bradycardia than does spacing the injections of local anesthetic. However, because the authors studied only 42 patients and had no cases of fetal bradycardia in either group, they could not exclude the possibility that incremental injection might reduce the incidence of fetal bradycardia in a larger series of patients.

Choice of Local Anesthetic

The physician should administer small volumes of dilute solutions of local anesthetic. There is no reason to inject more than 10 mL of local anesthetic on each side. Further, there is no indication for the use of concentrated solutions such as 2% lidocaine, 0.5% bupivacaine, or 3% 2-chloroprocaine. Nieminen and Puolakka[17] observed that paracervical block with 10 mL of 0.125% bupivacaine (5 mL on each side) provided analgesia similar to that provided by 10 mL of 0.25% bupivacaine.

The choice of local anesthetic is controversial. The North American manufacturers of bupivacaine have stated that bupivacaine is contraindicated for the performance of paracervical block. In contrast, many European obstetricians—especially those in Finland—prefer bupivacaine for this procedure. Bupivacaine is more cardiotoxic in pregnant women than are other local anesthetics, and some investigators have suggested that bupivacaine results in a higher incidence of fetal bradycardia or adverse outcome than other local anesthetics used for paracervical block. Teramo[6] reviewed 50 cases of perinatal death associated with paracervical block; the local anesthetic was bupivacaine in at least 29 of the 50 cases.

Some physicians have suggested that 2-chloroprocaine is the local anesthetic of choice for paracervical block. Published studies suggest but do not prove that postparacervical block fetal bradycardia occurs less frequently with 2-chloroprocaine than with amide local anesthetics.[14,18-20] Weiss et al.[18] performed a double-blind study in which they randomized 60 patients to receive 20 mL of either 2% 2-chloroprocaine or 1% lidocaine for paracervical block. Bradycardia occurred in 1 of the 29 fetuses in the 2-chloroprocaine group compared with 5 of 31 fetuses in the lidocaine group ($P = 0.14$). LeFevre[20] retrospectively observed that fetal bradycardia occurred after 2 of 33 (6%) paracervical blocks performed with 2-chloroprocaine versus 44 of 361 (12%) paracervical blocks performed with mepivacaine ($P = 0.29$).

2-Chloroprocaine undergoes rapid enzymatic hydrolysis. Thus it has the shortest intravascular half-life among the local anesthetics used clinically. This rapid metabolism seems advantageous in the event of unintentional intravascular or fetal injection. Philipson et al.[19] performed paracervical block with 10 mL of 1% 2-chloroprocaine in 16 healthy parturients. At delivery, only trace concentrations of 2-chloroprocaine were detected in 1 (6%) of the maternal samples and 4 (25%) of the umbilical cord venous blood samples. The authors concluded the following[19]:

> In all of the studies of paracervical block with 2-chloroprocaine, there were no cases in which the abnormal fetal heart rate patterns were associated with depressed neonates. This is in contrast to the studies with amide local anesthetics and may be explained by the rapid enzymatic inactivation of 2-chloroprocaine.

Some obstetricians dislike 2-chloroprocaine because of its relatively short duration of action. However, in one study the mean duration of analgesia was 40 minutes after paracervical administration of either 2-chloroprocaine or lidocaine.[18] Philipson and Kuhnert[21] suggested that if paracervical block with 2-chloroprocaine has a shorter duration than the amide local anesthetics, "frequent contact with the anesthetist or obstetrician provides opportunities for additional support and reassurance of the patient."

Maternal Complications

Maternal complications are uncommon but may be serious (Box 22-1).[22-25] Systemic local anesthetic toxicity may result from direct intravascular injection or rapid systemic absorption of the local anesthetic. Postpartum neuropathy may be a complication of direct sacral plexus trauma, or it may result from hematoma formation. Retropsoal and subgluteal abscesses are rare but may result in major maternal morbidity or mortality.[24,25]

Fetal Complications

In some cases, severe fetal injury results from direct injection of local anesthetic into the fetal scalp.[7,26,27] Fetal scalp injection of 10 or 20 mL of local anesthetic undoubtedly results in systemic local anesthetic toxicity. This complication may result in fetal death. Fetal scalp injection seems more likely to occur when the obstetrician performs paracervical block in the presence of advanced (i.e., more than 8 cm) cervical dilation.

Bradycardia is the most common fetal complication. Fetal bradycardia typically develops within 2 to 10 minutes after the injection of local anesthetic. Most cases resolve within 5 to 10 minutes, but some cases of bradycardia persist for as long

---

Box 22-1 MATERNAL COMPLICATIONS OF PARACERVICAL BLOCK

Vasovagal syncope
Laceration of the vaginal mucosa
Systemic local anesthetic toxicity
Parametrial hematoma
Postpartum neuropathy
Paracervical, retropsoal, and subgluteal abscess

---

as 30 minutes. Published studies have noted an incidence of bradycardia that varies between 0% and 70%.[15,20,28-34] These figures represent extremes on either side of the true incidence of this complication. Some studies have overstated the problem by defining bradycardia as a baseline FHR of less than 120 bpm. (A baseline FHR of 110 bpm does *not* necessarily indicate fetal distress.) Experienced obstetricians clearly do not encounter clinically significant fetal bradycardia after 70% of their paracervical blocks. It is equally clear that the incidence of clinically significant fetal bradycardia is not zero. Rosen[34] recently reviewed four randomized controlled trials published between 1975 and 2000, and he estimated that the incidence of postparacervical block fetal bradycardia is approximately 15%. Further, it is difficult to teach this technique without placing some fetuses at risk.

Shnider et al.[30] reported that fetal bradycardia occurred after 24% of 845 paracervical blocks administered to 705 patients with either 1% mepivacaine, 1% lidocaine, or 1% propitocaine. Neonatal depression occurred significantly more often among infants who had FHR changes after paracervical block when compared with both a control group and a group of infants with no FHR changes after paracervical block. In contrast, Carlsson et al.[31] performed 523 paracervical blocks with 0.125% or 0.25% bupivacaine in 469 women. Of the total, 9 (1.9%) fetuses had bradycardia, but all 9 neonates had a 5-minute Apgar score of 9 or 10.

Goins[32] noted that fetal bradycardia occurred in 24 (13%) of 182 patients who received paracervical block with 20 mL of 1% mepivacaine between 1988 and 1990. He compared neonatal outcome for these patients with neonatal outcome for 343 patients who received other analgesic/anesthetic techniques. There was a slightly higher incidence of low Apgar scores at 1 and 5 minutes in the paracervical block group, but the difference was not statistically significant.

LeFevre[20] observed fetal bradycardia after 46 (11%) of 408 paracervical blocks. Fetal bradycardia was more common in those patients with nonreassuring FHR tracings before the performance of paracervical block. Ranta et al.[33] observed fetal bradycardia after only 5 (2%) of 248 paracervical blocks with 10 mL of 0.25% bupivacaine (5 mL on each side).

ETIOLOGY

The etiology of fetal bradycardia after paracervical block is unclear. Investigators have offered at least four theories that might explain the etiology of fetal bradycardia.

Reflex Bradycardia

Manipulation of the fetal head, the uterus, or the uterine blood vessels during performance of the block may cause reflex fetal bradycardia.[29]

Direct Fetal Central Nervous System and Myocardial Depression

The performance of paracervical block results in the injection of large volumes of local anesthetic close to the uteroplacental circulation. Local anesthetic rapidly crosses the placenta[35] and may cause fetal central nervous system (CNS) depression, myocardial depression, and/or umbilical vasoconstriction. Puolakka et al.[36] observed that the most common abnormality after paracervical block was the disappearance of FHR accelerations. They speculated that FHR changes result from rapid transplacental passage of local anesthetic into the fetal circulation, followed by a direct toxic effect of the local anesthetic on the FHR regulatory centers.

Some investigators have suggested that fetal bradycardia results from a direct toxic effect of the local anesthetic on the fetal heart.[37,38] Shnider et al.[37] reported that in four cases of fetal bradycardia, fetal scalp blood mepivacaine concentrations were higher than peak concentrations in maternal arterial blood. Asling et al.[38] made similar observations in six of seven cases of fetal bradycardia. They suggested that local anesthetic reaches the fetus by a more direct route than maternal systemic absorption, and they speculated that high fetal concentrations of local anesthetic result from local anesthetic diffusion across the uterine arteries. This would result in local anesthetic concentrations in intervillous blood that are higher than concentrations in brachial arterial blood. High fetal concentrations would then result from the passive diffusion of local anesthetic across the placenta.

High fetal concentrations of local anesthetic also may result from fetal acidosis and ion trapping.[39,40] Local anesthetics are weak bases, and if a fetus develops acidosis, increasing amounts of local anesthetic will cross the placenta, regardless of the site of maternal injection. It also is possible that the obstetrician may directly inject local anesthetic into uterine blood vessels.

Most studies have noted that local anesthetic concentrations in the fetus are consistently *lower* than those in the mother after paracervical block.[13] Further, fetal bradycardia has not consistently occurred in documented cases of fetal local anesthetic toxicity. Freeman et al.[41] injected 300 mg of mepivacaine directly into the fetal scalp of two anencephalic fetuses. The QRS complex widened, the P-R interval lengthened, and both fetuses died, but fetal bradycardia did not occur before fetal death. In contrast, the authors observed no widening of the QRS complex or lengthening of the P-R interval in normal fetuses that had bradycardia after paracervical block. Rather, the fetal electrocardiogram (ECG) changes were consistent with sinoatrial node suppression with a wandering atrial pacemaker. The authors concluded that a mechanism other than direct fetal myocardial depression is responsible for fetal bradycardia after paracervical block.

Increased Uterine Activity

Increased uterine activity results in decreased uteroplacental perfusion. Fishburne et al.[42] noted that direct uterine arterial injection of bupivacaine consistently caused a significant increase in uterine tone in gravid ewes. Uterine arterial injection of 2-chloroprocaine did not affect myometrial tone, whereas lidocaine resulted in an intermediate effect.

Myometrial injection of a local anesthetic also may cause increased uterine activity. Morishima et al.[43] performed paracervical block with either lidocaine or 2-chloroprocaine in pregnant baboons with normal and acidotic fetuses. A transient increase in uterine activity and a significant reduction in uterine blood flow occurred after paracervical block in 73% of the mothers. Approximately 33% of the normal fetuses and all of the acidotic fetuses had bradycardia after paracervical block. The acidotic fetuses had more severe bradycardia, greater hypoxemia, and slower recovery of oxygenation when compared with fetuses that were well oxygenated before paracervical block. The authors concluded that postparacervical block fetal bradycardia is in part a result of increased uterine activity, decreased uteroplacental perfusion, and decreased oxygen delivery to the fetus. They also concluded that paracervical block should be avoided in the presence of fetal distress.

Uterine and/or Umbilical Artery Vasoconstriction

The deposition of local anesthetic in close proximity to the uterine arteries may cause uterine artery vasoconstriction, with a subsequent decrease in uteroplacental perfusion. At least two studies noted that lidocaine and mepivacaine caused vasoconstriction of human uterine arteries in vitro.[44,45] (These studies were performed before recognition of the importance of intact endothelium during investigation of vascular smooth muscle response.) Similarly, Norén et al.[46,47] noted that bupivacaine caused concentration-dependent contraction of uterine arterial smooth muscle from rats and pregnant women. The calcium entry-blocking drugs verapamil and nifedipine decreased the vascular smooth muscle contraction caused by bupivacaine. The authors concluded that the use of bupivacaine for paracervical block may cause uterine artery vasoconstriction, especially when the bupivacaine is injected close to the uterine arteries. Further, they suggested that the administration of a calcium entry-blocking drug may successfully eliminate this vasoconstrictive effect of bupivacaine. (Although these studies were performed in 1991, the authors did not mention whether they preserved, removed, or even observed the presence of the vascular endothelium. The presence of vascular endothelium may alter the response of vascular smooth muscle to local anesthetics.[48])

Greiss et al.[49] observed that intraaortic injection of lidocaine or mepivacaine resulted in decreased uterine blood flow in gravid ewes. Similarly, Fishburne et al.[42] noted that direct uterine arterial injection of lidocaine, bupivacaine, or 2-chloroprocaine decreased uterine blood flow in gravid ewes. They concluded that only paracervical block "would be expected to produce the high, sustained uterine arterial concentrations of anesthetic drugs that cause the significant reductions in uterine blood flow which we now feel are the etiology of fetal bradycardia."[42] More recently, Manninen et al.[50] observed that paracervical injection of 10 mL of 0.25% bupivacaine resulted in an increase in the uterine artery pulsatility index (PI)—an estimate of uterine vascular resistance—in healthy nulliparous women, suggesting that paracervical block may result in uterine artery vasoconstriction.

In contrast, Puolakka et al.[36] used ^{133}Xe to measure intervillous blood flow before and after the performance of paracervical block with 10 mL of 0.25% bupivacaine in 10 parturients. They observed no decrease in mean intervillous blood flow in these patients. Further, they observed minimal change in intervillous blood flow in the three patients who had fetal bradycardia after paracervical block. Using Doppler ultrasonography, Räsänen and Jouppila[51] observed no significant change in either uterine or umbilical artery PI after the performance of paracervical block with 10 mL of 0.25% bupivacaine in 12 healthy parturients. However, fetal bradycardia occurred in two patients, and in those two cases a marked increase in the umbilical artery PI occurred.

Baxi et al.[52] performed paracervical block with 20 mL of 1% lidocaine in 10 pregnant patients. They observed a decrease in fetal transcutaneous Po_2 5 minutes after injecting lidocaine in each of the 10 patients. There was a maximum decline in transcutaneous Po_2 at 11.5 minutes, and transcutaneous Po_2 returned to baseline by approximately 31 minutes. Some but not all of the patients had increased uterine activity after paracervical block. In contrast, Jacobs et al.[53] observed a consistent, sustained decrease in fetal transcutaneous Po_2 after only 1 of 10 paracervical blocks performed with 10 mL of

0.25% bupivacaine. The authors attributed their good results to the following precautions: (1) performance of paracervical block only in healthy mothers with normal pregnancies, (2) administration of a small dose of bupivacaine, (3) a limited depth of injection, (4) administration of bupivacaine in four incremental injections (i.e., two injections on each side), and (5) use of the left lateral position immediately after performance of the block. More recently, Kaita et al.[54] observed that paracervical injection of 10 mL of 0.25% bupivacaine in 10 healthy parturients resulted in a slight (clinically insignificant) increase in fetal SaO_2, as measured by fetal pulse oximetry.

In summary, most observers currently believe that postparacervical block bradycardia results from decreased uteroplacental and/or fetoplacental perfusion. Decreased uteroplacental perfusion may result from increased uterine activity and/or a direct vasoconstrictive effect of the local anesthetic. Likewise, decreased umbilical cord blood flow may result from increased uterine activity and/or umbilical cord vasoconstriction. Regardless of the etiology, the severity and duration of fetal bradycardia correlate with the incidence of fetal acidosis and subsequent neonatal depression. Freeman et al.[41] reported a significant decrease in pH and an increase in base deficit only in fetuses with bradycardia of longer than 10 minutes' duration.

Physician Complications
The performance of paracervical block requires the physician to make several blind needle punctures within the vagina. The needle guide does not consistently protect the physician from a needle-stick injury. Thus the performance of paracervical block may entail a risk of physician exposure to human immunodeficiency virus (HIV) or another virus.

Recommendations
It is difficult for me to offer enthusiasm for the performance of paracervical block in contemporary obstetric practice. Nonetheless, there most likely remain some circumstances in which paracervical block is an appropriate technique. I offer the following recommendations for safe practice:

1. Perform paracervical block only in healthy parturients at term who have no evidence of uteroplacental insufficiency or fetal distress.
2. Continuously monitor the FHR and uterine activity before, during, and after performance of paracervical block. Perform paracervical block only in patients with a reassuring FHR tracing. An obvious exception would be a patient whose fetus has an anomaly incompatible with life (e.g., anencephaly).
3. Do not perform paracervical block when the cervix is dilated 8 cm or more.
4. Establish intravenous access before performing paracervical block.
5. Maintain left uterine displacement while performing the block.
6. Limit the depth of injection to approximately 3 mm.
7. Aspirate before each injection of local anesthetic.
8. After injecting the local anesthetic on one side, wait 5 to 10 minutes and observe the FHR before injecting the local anesthetic on the opposite side.
9. Administer small volumes of a dilute solution of local anesthetic. 2-Chloroprocaine is the agent of choice.

10. Avoid the administration of epinephrine-containing local anesthetic solutions.
11. Monitor the mother's blood pressure after performance of the block. Maintain normal maternal blood pressure.
12. If fetal bradycardia should occur, try to achieve fetal resuscitation in utero. Discontinue oxytocin, administer supplemental oxygen, and ensure that the patient is on her left side. Determine the fetal scalp blood pH or perform operative delivery if the fetal bradycardia persists beyond 10 minutes.

LUMBAR SYMPATHETIC BLOCK
In 1927, Dellepiane and Badino[55] first described the use of paravertebral lumbar sympathetic block in obstetric patients. In 1933, Cleland[56] introduced the procedure in the United States when he demonstrated that lower uterine and cervical visceral afferent sensory fibers join the sympathetic chain at L2 to L3. Subsequently, this procedure was used as an effective—if not popular—method of first-stage analgesia in some hospitals.[57-60] Like paracervical block, paravertebral lumbar sympathetic block interrupts the transmission of pain impulses from the cervix and lower uterine segment to the spinal cord. Lumbar sympathetic block provides analgesia during the first stage of labor but does not relieve pain during the second stage.[61] It provides analgesia comparable to that provided by paracervical block but with less risk of fetal bradycardia.

Lumbar sympathetic block may have a favorable effect on the progress of labor. Hunter[62] reported that lumbar sympathetic block *accelerated* labor in 20 of 39 patients with a normal uterine contractile pattern before performance of the block. (Indeed, some of those patients had a 5- to 15-minute period of uterine hypertonus after the block.) Further, he observed that lumbar sympathetic block converted an abnormal uterine contractile pattern to a normal pattern in 14 of 19 patients. He concluded that lumbar sympathetic block represents "one of the most reliable methods reported to actively convert an abnormal labor pattern to a normal pattern." More recently, Leighton et al.[63] randomized 39 healthy nulliparous women at term to receive either epidural analgesia or lumbar sympathetic block. The women who received lumbar sympathetic block had a more rapid rate of cervical dilation during the first 2 hours of analgesia, a shorter second stage of labor, and a nonsignificant trend toward a decreased incidence of cesarean section for dystocia. However, there was no difference between groups in the rate of cervical dilation during the active phase of the first stage of labor.

Anesthesiologists may successfully perform lumbar sympathetic block when a history of previous back surgery precludes the successful administration of epidural anesthesia.[64] Some anesthesiologists offer lumbar sympathetic block to prepared childbirth enthusiasts who desire first-stage analgesia without any motor block or loss of perineal sensation. Meguiar and Wheeler[65] stated that the primary usefulness of lumbar sympathetic block is "in cases where continuous lumbar epidural analgesia is refused or contraindicated." They administered 20 mL of 0.5% bupivacaine with 1:200,000 epinephrine to 40 nulliparous women. Among these 40 women, 38 experienced good analgesia, and 28 patients delivered before resolution of the block. Pain recurred before delivery in the remaining 12 women; the mean duration of analgesia was 283 ± 103 minutes in those patients.[65] Leighton et al.[63] administered the same dose of bupivacaine, but they observed a shorter duration of analgesia than that observed by Meguiar and Wheeler.[65]

During the last two decades, lumbar sympathetic block all but disappeared from obstetric anesthesia practice in the United States, for several reasons. Anesthesiologists may minimize motor block during epidural anesthesia by giving dilute solutions of local anesthetic, with or without an opioid. For those few patients who want to retain full perineal sensation, anesthesiologists may give an opioid alone, either intrathecally or epidurally. Thus there are few patients for whom lumbar sympathetic block holds unique advantages. Further, the procedure often is painful, and few anesthesiologists have acquired and maintained proficiency in performing lumbar sympathetic block in obstetric patients.

Lumbar sympathetic block remains an attractive technique in a small number of patients.[64] Alternatively, Nair and Henry[66] recently described the performance of bilateral paravertebral block for women in whom epidural analgesia is contraindicated.

Technique

With the patient in the sitting position, a 10-cm, 22-gauge needle is used to identify the transverse process on one side of the second lumbar vertebra. The needle is then withdrawn, redirected, and advanced another 5 cm so that the tip of the needle is at the anterolateral surface of the vertebral column, just anterior to the medial attachment of the psoas muscle. It is possible to place the needle within a blood vessel or the subarachnoid space; thus the anesthesiologist must aspirate before injecting the local anesthetic. Two 5-mL increments of local anesthetic solution are then injected, and the procedure is repeated on the opposite side of the vertebral column.

Complications

Modest hypotension occurs in 5% to 15% of patients.[62,63,65] The incidence of hypotension can be reduced by giving 500 mL of Ringer's lactate intravenously before performing the block. Less common maternal complications include systemic local anesthetic toxicity, total spinal anesthesia, retroperitoneal hematoma, Horner's syndrome,[67] and postdural puncture headache (PDPH).[68]

Fetal complications are unlikely unless hypotension or increased uterine activity results in decreased uteroplacental perfusion.

PUDENDAL NERVE BLOCK

During the second stage of labor, pain results from distention of the lower vagina, vulva, and perineum. The pudendal nerve includes somatic nerve fibers from the anterior primary divisions of the second, third, and fourth sacral nerves, and it represents the primary source of sensory innervation for the lower vagina, vulva, and perineum. The pudendal nerve also provides motor innervation to the perineal muscles and to the external anal sphincter.

In 1916, King[69] reported the use of pudendal nerve block for vaginal delivery. This procedure did not become popular until 1953 and 1954, when Klink[70] and Kohl[71] described the anatomy and reported modified techniques. Obstetricians often perform pudendal nerve block in patients without epidural or spinal anesthesia. The goal is to block the pudendal nerve distal to its formation by the anterior divisions of S2

to S4 but proximal to its division into its terminal branches (i.e., dorsal nerve of the clitoris, perineal nerve, and inferior hemorrhoidal nerve). Pudendal nerve block may provide satisfactory anesthesia for spontaneous vaginal delivery and perhaps for outlet-forceps delivery, but it provides inadequate anesthesia for mid-forceps delivery, postpartum examination and repair of the upper vagina and cervix, and manual exploration of the uterine cavity.[72]

Efficacy and Timing

The efficacy of pudendal nerve block varies depending on the experience of the obstetrician. Unilateral or bilateral failure is common. Thus obstetricians typically perform simultaneous infiltration of the perineum, especially if the obstetrician delays the performance of pudendal nerve block until delivery. Scudamore and Yates[73] reported a bilateral success rate of approximately 50% after use of the transvaginal route and approximately 25% after use of the transperineal route. They concluded the following[73]:

> The term "pudendal block" is often a misnomer .... If this limitation were more widely appreciated, then many mothers would be spared the unnecessary pain which is caused when relatively complicated procedures are attempted under inadequate anesthesia.

In the United States, most obstetricians perform pudendal nerve block immediately before delivery. This practice reflects their concern that perineal anesthesia prolongs the second stage of labor. An advantage to early pudendal nerve block is that the obstetrician may repeat the block on one or both sides if it should fail, provided the maximum safe dose of local anesthetic is not exceeded. European obstetricians seem more willing to perform pudendal nerve block at the onset of the second stage of labor. Langhoff-Roos and Lindmark[74] administered pudendal block before or just after complete cervical dilation in 551 (64%) of 865 women. In a nonrandomized study, Zador et al.[75] evaluated obstetric outcome in 24 patients who received pudendal block when the cervix was completely dilated and in 24 patients who did not receive pudendal block. Pudendal block slightly prolonged the second stage of labor, but it did not increase the incidence of instrumental vaginal delivery.

It is barbaric to withhold analgesia during the second stage of labor. Obstetricians need not delay the administration of pudendal nerve block until delivery. Rather, for those patients without epidural or spinal analgesia, it seems appropriate to perform pudendal nerve block when the patient complains of vaginal and perineal pain.

Technique

The transvaginal approach is more popular than the transperineal approach in the United States. The obstetrician uses a needle guide (either the Iowa trumpet or the Kobak needle guide) to prevent injury to the vagina and fetus. In contrast to the technique for paracervical block, the needle must protrude 1.0 to 1.5 cm beyond the needle guide to allow adequate penetration for injection of the local anesthetic. The obstetrician introduces the needle and needle guide into the vagina with the left hand for the left side of the pelvis and with the right hand for the right side (Figure 22-2). The needle is introduced through the vaginal mucosa and sacrospinous ligament, just medial and posterior to the ischial spine. The pudendal artery lies in close proximity to the pudendal nerve;

thus the obstetrician must aspirate before and during the injection of local anesthetic. The obstetrician typically injects 7 to 10 mL of local anesthetic solution on each side. (Some obstetricians inject 3 mL of local anesthetic just above the ischial spine on each side.[76]) The obstetrician should pay attention to the total dose of local anesthetic given, especially when repetitive pudendal nerve block or both pudendal nerve block and perineal infiltration are performed.

Choice of Local Anesthetic

Rapid maternal absorption of the local anesthetic occurs after the performance of pudendal nerve block.[75,77,78] Zador et al.[75] detected measurable concentrations of lidocaine in maternal venous and fetal scalp capillary blood within 5 minutes of the injection of 20 mL of 1% lidocaine. They detected peak concentrations between 10 and 20 minutes after injection. Kuhnert et al.[78] reported that after pudendal nerve block, neonatal urine concentrations of lidocaine and its metabolites were similar to those measured in neonatal urine after epidural administration of lidocaine.

Some physicians favor the administration of 2-chloroprocaine. Its rapid onset of action provides an advantage when pudendal nerve block is performed immediately before delivery. Its rapid metabolism and short intravascular half-life decrease the likelihood of maternal or fetal systemic toxicity. 2-Chloroprocaine has the disadvantage of a short duration of action. However, if the obstetrician performs pudendal nerve block with 2-chloroprocaine at the onset of the second stage of labor, the block can be repeated as needed. When the block is performed immediately before delivery, the brief duration of action of 2-chloroprocaine is not a disadvantage for the experienced obstetrician.

Merkow et al.[79] evaluated neonatal neurobehavior in infants whose mothers received 30 mL of 0.5% bupivacaine, 1% mepivacaine, or 3% 2-chloroprocaine for pudendal nerve block and perineal infiltration before delivery. There was an improved neonatal response to pinprick at 4 hours in the mepivacaine group; otherwise there were no significant differences among groups in neurobehavioral scores at 4 and 24 hours after delivery.

Regardless of the choice of local anesthetic, there is no indication for the administration of a concentrated solution. For example, it is unnecessary—and perhaps dangerous—to give 0.5% bupivacaine, 2% lidocaine, or 3% 2-chloroprocaine. Rather, the obstetrician should use 2% 2-chloroprocaine or 1% lidocaine.

Some obstetricians contend that the addition of epinephrine to the local anesthetic solution improves the quality of pudendal nerve block. Langhoff-Roos and Lindmark[74] reported a randomized, double-blind study of 865 patients who received pudendal nerve block with 16 mL of 1% mepivacaine, 1% mepivacaine with epinephrine, or 0.25% bupivacaine. Mepivacaine with epinephrine provided effective anesthesia more often and also caused a greater "loss of the urge to bear down" than did the other two local anesthetic solutions. However, there was no significant difference among groups in the duration of the second stage or the incidence of instrumental vaginal delivery. Schierup et al.[80] randomized 151 patients to receive pudendal block with 20 mL of 1% mepivacaine, with or without epinephrine. The addition of epinephrine did not improve the quality of anesthesia. The results showed that 64 of 75 patients (85%) in the epinephrine group and 69 of 76 patients (91%) in the no-epinephrine group had excellent or good pain relief. The addition of epinephrine slightly prolonged the interval between pudendal block administration and delivery. Maternal venous blood mepivacaine concentrations were slightly higher in the no-epinephrine group, but there was no difference between groups in umbilical cord blood concentrations of mepivacaine.

Complications

Maternal complications are uncommon but may be serious (Box 22-2). Systemic local anesthetic toxicity may result from either direct intravascular injection or systemic absorption of an excessive dose of local anesthetic. Toxicity may occur if the obstetrician exceeds the safe dose of local anesthetic during repetitive injections performed to obtain a successful block. Vaginal, ischiorectal, and retroperitoneal hematomas may result from trauma to the pudendal artery.[81] These hematomas typically are small and rarely require operative intervention. Subgluteal and retropsoal abscesses are rare but can result in significant morbidity or mortality.[24,25,82]

Fetal complications are rare. The primary fetal complications result from fetal trauma and/or direct fetal injection of local anesthetic.[7,27]

As with paracervical block, the performance of pudendal block requires the obstetrician to make several blind needle punctures within the vagina. The needle guide does not uniformly protect the physician from a needle-stick injury. Thus performance of pudendal block may entail a risk of physician exposure to HIV or another virus.

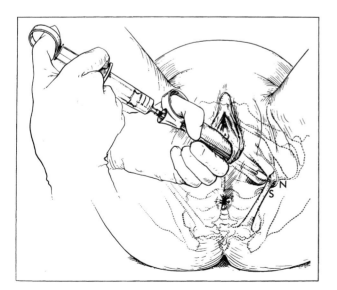

FIGURE 22-2. Local infiltration of the pudendal nerve. Transvaginal technique showing the needle extended beyond the needle guard and passing through the sacrospinous ligament (S) to reach the pudendal nerve (N). (From Cunningham FG, MacDonald PC, Gant NF, et al. Williams Obstetrics, 20th ed. Stamford, Conn, Appleton and Lange, 1997:389.)

Box 22-2 MATERNAL COMPLICATIONS OF PUDENDAL NERVE BLOCK
Laceration of the vaginal mucosa
Systemic local anesthetic toxicity
Vaginal and ischiorectal hematoma
Retropsoal and subgluteal abscess

PERINEAL INFILTRATION

Perineal infiltration is perhaps the most common local anesthetic technique used for vaginal delivery. Given the frequent failure of pudendal nerve block, obstetricians often perform pudendal nerve block and perineal infiltration simultaneously. Perineal infiltration also may be required in patients with unsatisfactory epidural anesthesia. The obstetrician injects several milliliters of local anesthetic solution into the posterior fourchette. There are no large nerve fibers to be blocked; thus a rapid onset of anesthesia occurs. However, perineal infiltration provides anesthesia only for episiotomy and repair. Often there is inadequate anesthesia, even for these limited procedures. Moreover, perineal infiltration provides no muscle relaxation.

Choice of Local Anesthetic

Philipson et al.[83] evaluated the pharmacokinetics of lidocaine after perineal infiltration. They gave 1% or 2% lidocaine without epinephrine during the crowning phase of the second stage of labor in 15 healthy parturients. The mean ± SD dose of lidocaine was 79 ± 3 mg, and the mean drug-to-delivery interval was 7.8 ± 7.0 minutes. The authors detected lidocaine in maternal plasma as early as 1 minute after injection. Peak maternal plasma concentrations of lidocaine occurred between 3 and 15 minutes after injection. Despite the administration of small doses of lidocaine and the short drug-to-delivery intervals, there was rapid placental transfer of significant amounts of lidocaine. The mean fetal:maternal lidocaine concentration ratio of 1.32 was significantly higher than the ratio reported after administration of lidocaine for paracervical block, pudendal nerve block, or epidural anesthesia for vaginal delivery or cesarean section. There was a significant correlation between the fetal:maternal lidocaine concentration ratio and the length of the second stage of labor. The authors speculated that fetal tissue acidosis increased the fetal:maternal lidocaine ratio after perineal infiltration in this study. Finally, they noted the persistence of lidocaine and its pharmacologically active metabolites for at least 48 hours after delivery.[83]

Subsequently, Philipson et al.[84] evaluated the placental transfer of 2-chloroprocaine after perineal administration of 1% or 2% 2-chloroprocaine shortly before delivery. The mean ± SD dose of 2-chloroprocaine was 81.8 ± 27.0 mg, and the mean drug-to-delivery interval was 6.7 ± 4.3 minutes. Perineal infiltration of 2-chloroprocaine provided adequate anesthesia for episiotomy repair except in two patients who required additional local anesthetic for repair of a fourth-degree laceration. The authors did not detect 2-chloroprocaine in maternal plasma after infiltration or at delivery. Further, they detected 2-chloroprocaine at delivery in only one umbilical cord venous blood sample, and they detected no 2-chloroprocaine in neonatal plasma. In contrast, the authors consistently detected the drug's metabolite, chloroaminobenzoic acid, in maternal plasma, umbilical cord venous plasma, and neonatal urine. The fetal:maternal ratio of chloroaminobenzoic acid (0.80) was similar to that reported after the administration of 2-chloroprocaine for paracervical block and epidural anesthesia for cesarean section. The authors suggested that very little—if any—unchanged 2-chloroprocaine reaches the fetus after perineal infiltration. They concluded that 2-chloroprocaine may be preferable to lidocaine for antepartum perineal infiltration.[84]

Complications

The obstetrician must take care to avoid injection of the local anesthetic into the fetal scalp. Kim et al.[85] reported one case of newborn lidocaine toxicity after maternal perineal infiltration of 6 mL of 1% lidocaine before vaginal delivery. Similarly, DePraeter et al.[86] reported a case of neonatal lidocaine toxicity in a newborn whose mother received perineal infiltration with 10 mL of 2% lidocaine 4 minutes before delivery. In both cases, the infants were initially vigorous but required endotracheal intubation 15 minutes after delivery. No lidocaine was detected in umbilical cord blood, but neonatal blood samples revealed concentrations of 14 μg/mL and 13.8 μg/mL at 2 hours and 6.5 hours, respectively. Small scalp puncture wounds suggested that the lidocaine toxicity resulted from direct fetal scalp injection. Kim et al.[85] suggested that the presence of a molded head in the occiput posterior position may predispose to unintentional direct injection of the fetal scalp. These two cases support the recommendation of 2-chloroprocaine for perineal infiltration.

KEY POINTS

- **Paracervical block and lumbar sympathetic block provide effective analgesia for the first stage of labor. Neither technique relieves pain during the second stage.**
- **Fetal bradycardia is the most common complication of paracervical block.**
- **Paracervical block is contraindicated in patients with uteroplacental insufficiency or preexisting fetal distress.**
- **For patients without epidural or spinal anesthesia, it is appropriate to perform pudendal nerve block when the patient complains of pelvic floor pain.**
- **Pudendal nerve block may provide satisfactory anesthesia for spontaneous vaginal delivery and outlet-forceps delivery, but it provides inadequate anesthesia for mid-forceps delivery, postpartum repair of the cervix, and manual exploration of the uterine cavity.**
- **Perineal infiltration provides anesthesia only for episiotomy and repair.**
- **It is unnecessary—and perhaps dangerous—to give concentrated solutions of local anesthetic for paracervical block, pudendal nerve block, or perineal infiltration.**
- **Some cases of fetal injury result from direct fetal scalp injection of local anesthetic during attempted paracervical block, pudendal nerve block, or perineal infiltration.**
- **2-Chloroprocaine most likely is the safest choice of local anesthetic for paracervical block, pudendal nerve block, and perineal infiltration.**
- **The performance of either paracervical block or pudendal nerve block requires the obstetrician to make several blind needle punctures within the vagina. Thus there is a risk of physician needle-stick injury during the performance of either procedure.**

REFERENCES

1. Rosenfeld SS. Paracervical anesthesia for the relief of labor pains. Am J Obstet Gynecol 1945; 50:529-35.
2. Gibbs CP, Krischer J, Peckham BM, et al. Obstetric anesthesia: A national survey. Anesthesiology 1986; 65:298-306.
3. Gerdin E, Cnattingius S. The use of obstetric analgesia in Sweden 1983-1986. Br J Obstet Gynaecol 1990; 97:789-96.
4. Nyirjesy I, Hawks BL, Hebert JE, et al. Hazards of the use of paracervical block anesthesia in obstetrics. Am J Obstet Gynecol 1963; 87:231-5.
5. Rosefsky JB, Petersiel ME. Perinatal deaths associated with mepivacaine paracervical-block anesthesia in labor. N Engl J Med 1968; 278:530-3
6. Teramo K. Effects of obstetrical paracervical blockade on the fetus. Acta Obstet Gynecol Scand 1971; 16 (suppl):1-55.
7. Shnider SM, Levinson G, Ralston DH. Regional anesthesia for labor and delivery. In Shnider SM, Levinson G, editors. Anesthesia for Obstetrics, 3rd ed. Baltimore, Williams & Wilkins, 1993:135-53.
8. Shnider SM. Criticizes paracervical block for analgesia during labor. Ob Gyn News, Apr 1986.
9. Hawkins JL, Beaty BR, Gibbs CP. Update on U.S. OB anesthesia practices (abstract). Anesthesiology 1997; 91:A1060.
10. Jensen F, Qvist I, Brocks V, et al. Submucous paracervical blockade compared with intramuscular meperidine as analgesia during labor: A double-blind study. Obstet Gynecol 1984; 64:724-7.
11. Kangas-Saarela T, Jouppila R, Puolakka J, et al. The effect of bupivacaine paracervical block on the neurobehavioural responses of newborn infants. Acta Anaesthesiol Scand 1988; 32:566-70.
12. Jägerhorn M. Paracervical block in obstetrics: An improved injection method. Acta Obstet Gynecol Scand 1975; 54:9-27.
13. Cibils LA, Santonja-Lucas JJ. Clinical significance of fetal heart rate patterns during labor. III. Effect of paracervical block anesthesia. Am J Obstet Gynecol 1978; 130:73-100.
14. Freeman DW, Arnold NI. Paracervical block with low doses of chloroprocaine: Fetal and maternal effects. JAMA 1975; 231:56-7.
15. King JC, Sherline DM. Paracervical and pudendal block. Clin Obstet Gynecol 1981; 24:587-95.
16. Van Dorsten JP, Miller FC, Yeh SY. Spacing the injection interval with paracervical block: A randomized study. Obstet Gynecol 1981; 58:696-702.
17. Nieminen K, Puolakka J. Effective obstetric paracervical block with reduced dose of bupivacaine. Acta Obstet Gynecol Scand 1997; 76:50-4.
18. Weiss RR, Halevy S, Almonte RO, et al. Comparison of lidocaine and 2-chloroprocaine in paracervical block: Clinical effects and drug concentrations in mother and child. Anesth Analg 1983; 62:168-73.
19. Philipson EH, Kuhnert BR, Syracuse CB, et al. Intrapartum paracervical block anesthesia with 2-chloroprocaine. Am J Obstet Gynecol 1983; 146:16-22.
20. LeFevre ML. Fetal heart rate pattern and postparacervical fetal bradycardia. Obstet Gynecol 1984; 64:343-6.
21. Philipson EH, Kuhnert BR. Letter to the editor. Acta Obstet Gynecol Scand 1984; 63:187.
22. Gaylord TG, Pearson JW. Neuropathy following paracervical block in the obstetric patient. Obstet Gynecol 1982; 60:521-5.
23. Mercado AO, Naz JF, Ataya KM. Postabortal paracervical abscess as a complication of paracervical block anesthesia. J Reprod Med 1989; 34:247-9.
24. Hibbard LT, Snyder EN, McVann RM. Subgluteal and retropsoal infection in obstetric practice. Obstet Gynecol 1972; 39:137-50.
25. Svancarek W, Chirino O, Schaefer G, Blythe JG. Retropsoas and subgluteal abscesses following paracervical and pudendal anesthesia. JAMA 1977; 237:892-4.
26. O'Meara OP, Brazie JV. Neonatal intoxication after paracervical block (letter). N Engl J Med 1968; 278:1127-8.
27. Chase D, Brady JP. Ventricular tachycardia in a neonate with mepivacaine toxicity. J Pediatr 1977; 90:127-9.
28. Teramo K, Widholm O. Studies of effect of anaesthetics on foetus. I. Effect of paracervical block with mepivacaine upon foetal acid-base values. Acta Obstet Gynecol Scand 1967; 46 (suppl 2):1-39.
29. Rogers RE. Fetal bradycardia associated with paracervical block anesthesia in labor. Am J Obstet Gynecol 1970; 106:913-6.
30. Shnider SM, Asling JH, Holl JW, Margolis AJ. Paracervical block anesthesia in obstetrics. I. Fetal complications and neonatal morbidity. Am J Obstet Gynecol 1970; 107:619-25.
31. Carlsson BM, Johansson M, Westin B. Fetal heart rate pattern before and after paracervical anesthesia: A prospective study. Acta Obstet Gynecol Scand 1987; 66:391-5.
32. Goins JR. Experience with mepivacaine paracervical block in an obstetric private practice. Am J Obstet Gynecol 1992; 167:342-5.
33. Ranta P, Jouppila P, Spalding M, et al. Paracervical block: A viable alternative for labor pain relief? Acta Obstet Gynecol Scand 1995; 74:122-6.
34. Rosen MA. Paracervical block for labor analgesia: A brief historic review. Am J Obstet Gynecol 2002; 186:S127-30.
35. Gordon HR. Fetal bradycardia after paracervical block: Correlation with fetal and maternal blood levels of local anesthetic (mepivacaine). N Engl J Med 1968; 279:910-4.
36. Puolakka J, Jouppila R, Jouppila P, Puukka M. Maternal and fetal effects of low-dosage bupivacaine paracervical block. J Perinat Med 1984; 12:75-84.
37. Shnider SM, Asling JH, Margolis AJ, et al. High fetal blood levels of mepivacaine and fetal bradycardia (letter). N Engl J Med 1968; 279:947-8.
38. Asling JH, Shnider SM, Morgolis AJ, et al. Paracervical block anesthesia in obstetrics. II. Etiology of fetal bradycardia following paracervical block anesthesia. Am J Obstet Gynecol 1970; 107:626-34.
39. Brown WU, Bell GC, Alper MH. Acidosis, local anesthetics, and the newborn. Obstet Gynecol 1976; 48:27-30.
40. Biehl D, Shnider SM, Levinson G, Callender K. Placental transfer of lidocaine: Effects of fetal acidosis. Anesthesiology 1978; 48:409-12.
41. Freeman RK, Gutierrez NA, Ray ML, et al. Fetal cardiac response to paracervical block anesthesia. Part I. Am J Obstet Gynecol 1972; 113:583-91.
42. Fishburne JI, Greiss FC, Hopkinson R, Rhyne AL. Responses of the gravid uterine vasculature to arterial levels of local anesthetic agents. Am J Obstet Gynecol 1979; 133:753-61.
43. Morishima HO, Covino BG, Yeh MN, et al. Bradycardia in the fetal baboon following paracervical block anesthesia. Am J Obstet Gynecol 1981; 140:775-80.
44. Cibils LA. Response of human uterine arteries to local anesthetics. Am J Obstet Gynecol 1976; 126:202-10.
45. Gibbs CP, Noel SC. Response of arterial segments from gravid human uterus to multiple concentrations of lignocaine. Br J Anaesth 1977; 49:409-12.
46. Norén H, Lindblom B, Källfelt B. Effects of bupivacaine and calcium antagonists on the rat uterine artery. Acta Anaesthesiol Scand 1991; 35:77-80.
47. Norén H, Lindblom B, Källfelt B. Effects of bupivacaine and calcium antagonists on human uterine arteries in pregnant and non-pregnant women. Acta Anaesthesiol Scand 1991; 35:488-91.
48. Halevy S, Freese KJ, Liu-Barnett M, Altura BM. Endothelium-dependent local anesthetics action on umbilical vessels. FASEB 1991; J5:A1421.
49. Greiss FC, Still JG, Anderson SG. Effects of local anesthetic agents on the uterine vasculature and myometrium. Am J Obstet Gynecol 1976; 124:889-99.
50. Manninen T, Aantaa R, Salonen M, Pirhonen J, Palo P. A comparison of the hemodynamic effects of paracervical block and epidural anesthesia for labor analgesia. Acta Anaesthesiol Scand 2000; 44:441-5.
51. Räsänen J, Jouppila P. Does a paracervical block with bupivacaine change vascular resistance in uterine and umbilical arteries? J Perinat Med 1994; 22:301-8.
52. Baxi LV, Petrie RH, James LS. Human fetal oxygenation following paracervical block. Am J Obstet Gynecol 1979; 135:1109-12.
53. Jacobs R, Stalnacke B, Lindberg B, Rooth G. Human fetal transcutaneous Po_2 during paracervical block. J Perinat Med 1982; 10:209-14.
54. Kaita TM, Nikkola EM, Rantala MI, Ekblad UU, Salonen MAO. Fetal oxygen saturation during epidural and paracervical analgesia. Acta Obstet Gynecol Scand 2000; 79:336-40.
55. Dellepiane G, Badino P. L'anestesia paravertebrale in ostetricia e ginecologia. Clin Ostet 1927; 29:537-58.
56. Cleland JGP. Paravertebral anaesthesia in obstetrics: Experimental and clinical basis. Surg Gynecol Obstet 1933; 57:51-62.
57. Shumacker HB, Manahan CP, Hellman LM. Sympathetic anesthesia in labor. Am J Obstet Gynecol 1943; 45:129.
58. Jarvis SM. Paravertebral sympathetic nerve block: A method for the safe and painless conduct of labor. Am J Obstet Gynecol 1944; 47:335-42.
59. Reich AM. Paravertebral lumbar sympathetic block in labor: A report on 500 deliveries by a fractional procedure producing continuous conduction anesthesia. Am J Obstet Gynecol 1951; 61:1263-76.
60. Cleland JGP. Continuous peridural and caudal analgesia in obstetrics. Analg Anesth 1949; 28:61-76.
61. Bonica JJ. Principles and Practice of Obstetric Analgesia and Anesthesia. Philadelphia, FA Davis, 1967:520-6.
62. Hunter CA. Uterine motility studies during labor: Observations on bilateral sympathetic nerve block in the normal and abnormal first stage of labor. Am J Obstet Gynecol 1963; 85:681-6.
63. Leighton BL, Halpern SH, Wilson DB. Lumbar sympathetic blocks speed early and second stage induced labor in nulliparous women. Anesthesiology 1999; 90:1039-46.

64. Suelto MD, Shaw DB. Labor analgesia with paravertebral lumbar sympathetic block. Reg Anesth Pain Med 1999; 24:179-81.

65. Meguiar RV, Wheeler AS. Lumbar sympathetic block with bupivacaine: Analgesia for labor. Anesth Analg 1978; 57:486-90.

66. Nair V, Henry R. Bilateral paravertebral block: A satisfactory alternative for labour analgesia. Can J Anesth 2001; 48:179-84.

67. Wills MH, Korbon GA, Arasi R. Horner's syndrome resulting from a lumbar sympathetic block. Anesthesiology 1988; 68:613-4.

68. Artuso JD, Stevens RA, Lineberry PJ. Postdural puncture headache after lumbar sympathetic block: A report of two cases. Regional Anesth 1991; 16:288-91.

69. King R. Perineal anesthesia in labor. Surg Gynecol Obstet 1916; 23: 615-8.

70. Klink EW. Perineal nerve block: An anatomic and clinical study in the female. Obstet Gynecol 1953; 1:137-46.

71. Kohl GC. New method of pudendal nerve block. Northwest Med 1954; 53:1012-3.

72. Hutchins CJ. Spinal analgesia for instrumental delivery: A comparison with pudendal nerve block. Anaesthesia 1980; 35:376-7.

73. Scudamore JH, Yates MJ. Pudendal block—a misnomer? Lancet 1966; 1:23-4.

74. Langhoff-Roos J, Lindmark G. Analgesia and maternal side effects of pudendal block at delivery: A comparison of three local anesthetics. Acta Obstet Gynecol Scand 1985; 64:269-73.

75. Zador G, Lindmark G, Nilsson BA. Pudendal block in normal vaginal deliveries. Acta Obstet Gynecol Suppl 1974; 34:51-64.

76. Cunningham FG, MacDonald PC, Gant NF, et al. Williams Obstetrics, 20th ed. Stamford, Appleton & Lange, 1997: 387-8.

77. Shnider SM, Way EL. Plasma levels of lidocaine (Xylocaine) in mother and newborn following obstetrical conduction anesthesia: Clinical applications. Anesthesiology 1968; 29:951-8.

78. Kuhnert BR, Knapp DR, Kuhnert PM, Prochaska AL. Maternal, fetal, and neonatal metabolism of lidocaine. Clin Pharmacol Ther 1979; 26: 213-20.

79. Merkow AJ, McGuinness GA, Erenberg A, Kennedy RL. The neonatal neurobehavioral effects of bupivacaine, mepivacaine, and 2-chloroprocaine used for pudendal block. Anesthesiology 1980; 52:309-12.

80. Schierup L, Schmidt JF, Jensen AT, Rye BAO. Pudendal block in vaginal deliveries: Mepivacaine with and without epinephrine. Acta Obstet Gynecol Scand 1988; 67:195-7.

81. Kurzel RB, Au AH, Rooholamini SA. Retroperitoneal hematoma as a complication of pudendal block: Diagnosis made by computed tomography. West J Med 1996; 164:523-5.

82. Wenger DR, Gitchell RG. Severe infections following pudendal block anesthesia: Need for orthopaedic awareness. J Bone Joint Surg 1973; 55:202-7.

83. Philipson EH, Kuhnert BR, Syracuse CD. Maternal, fetal, and neonatal lidocaine levels following local perineal infiltration. Am J Obstet Gynecol 1984; 149:403-7.

84. Philipson EH, Kuhnert BR, Syracuse CD. 2-Chloroprocaine for local perineal infiltration. Am J Obstet Gynecol 1987; 157:1275-8.

85. Kim WY, Pomerance JJ, Miller AA. Lidocaine intoxication in a newborn following local anesthesia for episiotomy. Pediatrics 1979; 64:643-5.

86. DePraeter C, Vanhaesebrouch P, De Praeter N, Govaert P. Episiotomy and neonatal lidocaine intoxication (letter). Eur J Pediatr 1991; 150: 685-6.

Chapter 23
Vaginal Birth After Cesarean Section

David H. Chestnut, M.D.

In 1916, Edward Cragin[1] stated, "Once a cesarean, always a cesarean." This edict has had a profound impact on obstetric practice in the United States. The cesarean section rate increased from 5.5% of all deliveries in 1970 to 10.4% in 1975, 16.5% in 1980, and 22.7% in 1985 (Figure 23-1).[2,3] In 1988, 967,000 cesarean sections—24.7% of all deliveries—were performed in the United States.[3,4] Much of this increase in the cesarean section rate resulted from repeat cesarean sections.[5] In contemporary practice, elective repeat cesarean deliveries account for approximately one third of all cesarean sections.[3] Cesarean section currently is the most frequently performed operation in the United States, and *previous* cesarean section is the most common indication.

Most United States physicians ignored Cragin's subsequent statement: "Many exceptions occur."[1] Vaginal birth after cesarean section (VBAC) has been common practice in Western European countries for many years. In 1981 the National Institute of Child Health and Human Development Conference on Childbirth concluded that VBAC is an appropriate option for many women.[6] In 1994 the American College of Obstetricians and Gynecologists (ACOG) concluded the following[7]:

> The concept of routine repeat cesarean birth should be replaced by a specific decision process between the patient and the physician for a subsequent mode of delivery....In the absence of a contraindication, a woman with one previous cesarean delivery with a lower uterine segment incision should be counseled and encouraged to undergo a trial of labor in her current pregnancy.

Rosen et al.[8] modified Cragin's original dictum as follows: "Once a cesarean, a trial of labor should precede a second cesarean except in the most unusual circumstances." The VBAC rate sharply increased from 2.2% in 1970 to 28.3% in 1995.[3] This change in practice helped reduce the overall cesarean section rate to 20.7% in 1996 (Figure 23-1).[3] However, in recent years the safety of VBAC has undergone further scrutiny. Consequently, the VBAC rate decreased from 28.3% in 1995 to 20.6% in 2000 and 16.5% in 2001.[10] Meanwhile, in 2001 the overall cesarean section rate increased to 24.4%, which approximates the peak rate of 24.7% in 1988.

PRIMARY CESAREAN SECTION: CHOICE OF UTERINE INCISION

Obstetric practice in 1916 hardly resembled obstetric practice today. In 1916, only 1% to 2% of all infants were delivered by cesarean section. Most cesarean sections were performed in patients with a contracted bony pelvis, and obstetricians uniformly performed a classic uterine incision (i.e., a long vertical incision in the upper portion of the uterus) (Figure 23-2). A patient with a classic uterine incision is at high risk for catastrophic uterine rupture during a subsequent pregnancy. Such uterine rupture may occur before or during labor, and it often results in maternal and perinatal morbidity or mortality.

In 1922, De Lee and Cornell[11] advocated the performance of a vertical incision in the lower uterine segment. Unfortunately, low-vertical incisions rarely are confined to the lower uterine segment. Such incisions often extend to the body of the uterus, which does not heal as well as the lower uterine segment. Kerr[12] later advocated the performance of a low-*transverse* uterine incision (Figure 23-2). A low-transverse uterine incision results in less blood loss and is easier to repair than a classic uterine incision.[13] Further, a low-transverse uterine incision is more likely to heal satisfactorily and maintain its integrity during a subsequent pregnancy. Thus obstetricians prefer to make a low-transverse uterine incision during most cesarean sections.

Obstetricians reserve the low-vertical incision for patients whose lower uterine segment does not have enough width to allow safe delivery. Preterm parturients may have a narrow lower uterine segment. In these patients, delivery through a transverse uterine incision may cause an extension of the incision into the vessels of the broad ligament. For example, a patient with preterm labor at 26 weeks' gestation may undergo cesarean section because of a breech presentation, and the obstetrician may perform a low-vertical incision to facilitate an atraumatic delivery of the fetal head.

Obstetricians rarely perform a classic uterine incision in modern obstetric practice. An obstetrician may perform a classic uterine incision when the need for extensive intrauter-ine manipulation of the fetus (e.g., delivery of a fetus with a transverse lie) is anticipated. Some obstetricians prefer a classic uterine incision in patients with an anterior placenta previa. In such cases, the performance of a classic incision allows the obstetrician to avoid cutting through the placenta, which may result in significant hemorrhage.

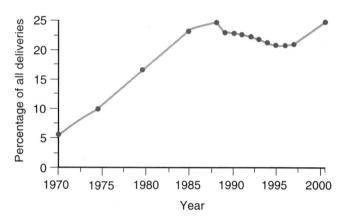

FIGURE 23-1. Incidence of cesarean section in the United States.[2-4,9,10]

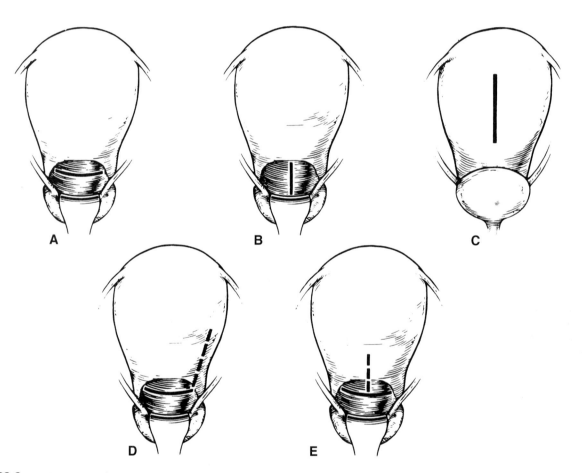

FIGURE 23-2. Uterine incisions for cesarean delivery. **A,** Low transverse incision. The bladder is retracted downward, and the incision is made in the lower uterine segment, curving gently upward. If the lower segment is poorly developed, the incision also can curve sharply upward at each end to avoid extending into the ascending branches of the uterine arteries. **B,** Low vertical incision. The incision is made vertically in the lower uterine segment after reflecting the bladder, avoiding extension into the bladder below. If more room is needed, the incision can be extended upward into the upper uterine segment. **C,** Classic incision. The incision is entirely within the upper uterine segment and can be at the level shown or in the fundus. **D,** J incision. If more room is needed when an initial trans-verse incision has been made, either end of the incision can be extended upward into the upper uterine segment and parallel to the ascending branch of the uter-ine artery. **E,** T incision. More room can be obtained in a transverse incision by an upward midline extension into the upper uterine segment. (From Depp R. Cesarean delivery. In Gabbe SG, Niebyl JR, Simpson JL, editors. Obstetrics: Normal and Problem Pregnancies, 4th ed. New York, Churchill Livingstone, 2002:552.)

RATIONALE FOR VBAC

A trial of labor is successful in 60% to 80% of women who had a low-transverse uterine incision performed during a previous cesarean section.[14-20] Flamm et al.[16] performed a large multicenter study of VBAC. Among 5733 women who attempted VBAC, 4291 (75%) delivered vaginally. Some 10 of 5733 patients experienced uterine rupture, an incidence of 0.2%. There were no maternal deaths among the patients who underwent a trial of labor, but there were two maternal deaths among the 9365 patients who underwent *elective* repeat cesarean section.[16] Flamm et al.[19] subsequently performed another prospective multicenter study of VBAC. Of 7229 patients, 5022 (70%) had a trial of labor and 2207 underwent elective repeat cesarean section. Some 3746 (75%) of the women who opted for a trial of labor delivered vaginally. The rate of uterine rupture was 0.8%. The incidence of postpartum transfusion, the incidence of postpartum fever, and the duration of hospitalization were significantly *lower* in the trial-of-labor group than in the elective repeat cesarean group.

Why might a patient choose VBAC rather than elective repeat cesarean section? The direct costs of vaginal delivery are less than those for elective repeat cesarean section.[4] Further, successful VBAC allows the mother to avoid the risks of cesarean section. There is no published study in which patients were randomized to undergo repeat cesarean section or a trial of labor that proves that maternal and neonatal outcome is better with the latter. But some studies have suggested that maternal morbidity occurs less frequently with VBAC than with repeat cesarean section.[7,8,19] In 1991, Rosen et al.[8] performed a meta-analysis of 31 studies to evaluate the association between route of delivery after cesarean section and maternal and perinatal morbidity and mortality. There was no significant difference in the rates of uterine scar dehiscence or rupture between women who attempted VBAC and those who underwent elective repeat cesarean section. Maternal febrile morbidity was significantly lower among women who attempted VBAC than among those who underwent elective repeat cesarean section.

Successful VBAC also avoids the neonatal risks of elective cesarean section. Inappropriate assessment of fetal maturity occasionally results in the delivery of a preterm infant. Thus elective cesarean section results in some cases of iatrogenic neonatal respiratory distress. When Rosen et al.[8] excluded patients whose fetuses died antepartum, weighed less than 750 g at delivery, and/or had congenital anomalies incompatible with life, they found no difference in perinatal mortality between those who attempted VBAC and those who underwent elective repeat cesarean section.

In contrast, McMahon et al.[21] performed a population-based longitudinal study of 6138 women in Nova Scotia who had previously undergone cesarean section and who delivered a single live infant between 1986 and 1992. Some 3249 women attempted VBAC, and 2889 women chose a repeat cesarean section. There were no maternal deaths. There was no difference between the two groups in the incidence of "minor complications" (i.e., puerperal fever, transfusion, wound infection). However, "major complications" (i.e., hysterectomy, uterine rupture, operative injury) were nearly twice as likely among women who attempted VBAC than among women who underwent elective repeat cesarean section. There was no difference between the two groups in perinatal mortality or morbidity.

However, two perinatal deaths occurred after uterine rupture in the trial-of-labor group.

More recently, Lydon-Rochelle et al.[22] conducted a population-based, retrospective cohort analysis of obstetric outcome for all (i.e., 20,095) nulliparous women who gave birth to a live singleton infant by cesarean section in civilian hospitals in the State of Washington between 1987 and 1996 and who subsequently delivered a second singleton child during the same period. They observed that spontaneous labor was associated with a tripling of the risk of uterine rupture (i.e., a uterine rupture rate of 5.2 per 1000 women who had a spontaneous onset of labor *versus* 1.6 per 1000 women who underwent elective repeat cesarean delivery without labor). Further, the incidence of infant death was over 10 times as high among the 91 women who had uterine rupture when compared with the 20,004 who did not (i.e., a 5.5% incidence of infant death versus a 0.5% incidence).[22]

ELIGIBILITY CRITERIA

Indication for Previous Cesarean Section

A high likelihood of success is expected with VBAC, even in women in whom the indication for previous cesarean section was dystocia or failure to progress in labor. Rosen and Dickinson[23] performed a meta-analysis of 29 studies of VBAC. Among patients whose previous cesarean section was performed for dystocia or cephalopelvic disproportion, the average rate of successful vaginal delivery was 67%. Seitchik and Rao[24] reported 58 patients who had received oxytocin augmentation of labor before undergoing cesarean section for dystocia in a previous pregnancy; 40 (69%) of those patients delivered vaginally during a subsequent pregnancy.

History of More Than One Cesarean Section

Some obstetricians accept the safety of a trial of labor after one low-transverse cesarean section, but they follow a modified version of Cragin's original dictum: "*Twice* a section, always a section."[25] Some studies have suggested that patients with more than one previous cesarean section may safely attempt VBAC.[16,26-29] However, Caughey et al.[30] observed that women with a history of two prior cesarean deliveries have an almost five-fold greater risk of uterine rupture during a trial of labor than women with only one previous cesarean section. The ACOG[31] concluded that "women with two previous low-transverse cesarean deliveries and no contraindications who wish to attempt VBAC may be allowed a trial of labor." However, the ACOG noted that these women "should be advised that the risk of uterine rupture increases as the number of cesarean deliveries increases." There are few published data regarding VBAC in patients with a history of *more than two* cesarean sections.

Previous Low Vertical Incision

Some obstetricians allow a trial of labor after a previous low-vertical uterine incision, provided that there is documentation that the uterine incision was confined to the lower uterine segment. (Low-vertical uterine incisions often extend above the lower uterine segment, especially when performed in preterm patients.) Naef et al.[32] retrospectively reviewed outcome for 174 women who attempted VBAC after a previous low-vertical cesarean section. Approximately 144 (83%) women delivered vaginally. Uterine rupture occurred in two (1.1%) of the patients. The authors concluded that "the likelihood of successful outcome and the incidence of complications are comparable to those of published experience with a trial of labor after a previous low-segment transverse incision."[32] Adair et al.[33] made similar observations. The ACOG has stated: "Whether [a] trial of labor should be encouraged for patients with...a low-vertical uterine incision is controversial." [31] Nonetheless, the ACOG has concluded that "women with a vertical incision within the lower uterine segment that does not extend into the fundus are candidates for VBAC."[31]

Twin Gestation

Some obstetricians believe that uterine overdistention, which occurs with twin gestation, increases the risk of uterine rupture in patients with a history of previous cesarean section. Strong et al.[34] reported 25 patients with twin gestation who attempted VBAC; 18 (72%) delivered both infants vaginally. There were no significant differences in maternal morbidity or neonatal morbidity/mortality among these 25 patients when compared with 31 similar patients who underwent elective repeat cesarean section. Miller[35] compared outcome for 92 women with twin gestation who attempted VBAC *versus* outcome for 118 women who underwent repeat cesarean section without a trial of labor. A trial of labor resulted in vaginal delivery of both infants in 64 (70%) of the patients. There were no differences between the two groups in maternal or neonatal morbidity or mortality, except that women in the trial-of-labor group had a decreased incidence of postpartum endometritis and a decreased length of hospitalization. Some obstetricians have suggested that a patient with twin gestation should attempt VBAC only if there is a vertex presentation for twin A.[34]

Breech Presentation

Ophir et al.[36] reviewed their experience with 47 patients with breech presentation who attempted VBAC; 37 (79%) patients delivered vaginally. Sarno et al.[37] reported successful vaginal delivery in 13 (48%) of 27 patients with breech presentation who attempted VBAC. Breech presentation itself does not result in an increased risk of uterine rupture. Most obstetricians choose the route of delivery according to their philosophy regarding the management of breech presentation. Many obstetricians do not allow a trial of labor in *any* patient with a breech presentation. Thus many patients with breech presentation undergo elective cesarean section, with or without a history of previous cesarean section.

Unknown Uterine Scar

For some patients, there is no documentation of the type of incision performed during a previous cesarean section. Some obstetricians require documentation of the type of previous uterine incision before they allow a patient to attempt VBAC. At least two studies have concluded that a trial of labor does not significantly increase maternal or perinatal morbidity/mortality in patients with an unknown uterine scar.[38,39] Perhaps this is true because most patients with an unknown uterine scar had a low-transverse uterine incision at previous cesarean section. Ultrasound examination may help the obstetrician con-

firm the presence of a low-transverse uterine scar in pregnant patients with an unknown uterine scar.[40]

Suspected Macrosomia

It is difficult to make a reliable antepartum diagnosis of fetal macrosomia. Flamm and Goings[41] evaluated obstetric outcome in 301 patients who attempted VBAC and whose infants weighed more than 4000 g at delivery. Among the 240 patients whose infants weighed between 4000 and 4500 g, 139 (58%) delivered vaginally. Among the 61 patients whose infants weighed more than 4500 g, 26 (43%) delivered vaginally. These authors pooled their data with four other studies of VBAC in women with macrosomic infants. Among 807 women who attempted VBAC and delivered macrosomic infants, 556 (69%) delivered vaginally. They concluded that suspected fetal macrosomia does not contraindicate VBAC in nondiabetic pregnant women. (Diabetic patients with fetal macrosomia have an increased risk for shoulder dystocia.) They emphasized that "care should be taken to ensure that crude estimates of 'macrosomia' are not used to discourage women with normal-size infants from pursuing vaginal birth after cesarean."[41] In 1994 the ACOG concluded that an estimated fetal weight of more than 4000 g does not contraindicate VBAC.[7] However, in 1999, the ACOG included suspected macrosomia on the list of VBAC eligibility criteria that are controversial.[31]

Size of Hospital

VBAC can be performed safely in community hospitals that have the personnel and other resources needed for the timely management of obstetric emergencies such as uterine rupture. Holland et al.[18] observed a vaginal delivery rate of 71% among those women who attempted VBAC in three non-university level-II hospitals in Mississippi. However, most studies of VBAC have been conducted in university or tertiary-level hospitals with in-house obstetricians, anesthesia providers, and operating room staff. The ACOG has noted that "the safety of [a] trial of labor is less well documented in smaller community hospitals or facilities where resources may be more limited."[31] Accordingly, in 1999 the ACOG revised its guidelines as follows[31]:

> Because uterine rupture maybe catastrophic, VBAC should be attempted in institutions equipped to respond to emergencies with physicians immediately available to provide emergency care.

The ACOG has defended this guideline by noting that "VBAC is a completely elective procedure that allows for reasonable precautions in assuming this small but significant risk [of uterine rupture]."[42] The ACOG has also noted that "the operational definition of 'immediately available' personnel and facilities remains the purview of each local institution...."[42] However, this requirement for the immediate availability of physicians and other personnel clearly represents a more stringent standard than the "readily available" requirement included in other published guidelines for obstetric care.

Zlatnik[43] earlier made the following comments regarding performance of VBAC in a community hospital:

> If a timely cesarean section cannot be performed in a community hospital, VBAC is out of the question, but the larger question is: Should obstetrics continue to be practiced there? Timely cesarean section is an essential option for all laboring women.

Summary of Eligibility Criteria

Eligibility criteria can be summarized as follows:

1. Previous cesarean section for dystocia or cephalopelvic disproportion does not contraindicate a trial of labor.
2. A history of one or two previous low-transverse cesarean deliveries does not contraindicate a trial of labor.
3. A previous low-vertical incision or an estimated fetal weight of more than 4000 g does not contraindicate a trial of labor, but the ACOG has acknowledged that this is controversial. There is insufficient evidence to determine the safety of VBAC in patients with multiple gestation or breech presentation.[31]
4. A previous classic or T-shaped uterine incision contraindicates a trial of labor.
5. VBAC need not be confined to university hospitals and other large medical centers. However, ACOG guidelines require that physicians and other personnel be "immediately available" to provide emergency care.[31]

IMPLEMENTATION OF VBAC

Flamm et al.[16] concluded that if all eligible women underwent a trial of labor after previous cesarean section, obstetricians could avoid performing over 200,000 cesarean sections in the United States each year. Pickhardt et al.[44] reviewed the clinical course and outcome of all parturients who attempted VBAC at the University of Mississippi Medical Center. They identified no single criterion or optimal clusters of factors that would allow the obstetrician to predict a successful or failed VBAC in an individual patient. They concluded the following[44]:

> It seems appropriate to encourage a trial of labor *in almost all* patients with prior low-segment incisions (transverse or vertical) regardless of their obstetric history or their recent clinical parameters. Exceptions to this policy would be the infrequent, carefully selected patient deemed to be at too great a risk for trial of labor on the basis of medical and/or obstetric consideration(s).

Why have most eligible patients continued to undergo elective repeat cesarean section? The low frequency of VBAC has resulted from both physician and patient preference. VBAC requires more physician effort than does elective repeat cesarean section. Flamm et al.[16] stated, "Clearly, in any practice setting, it is easier for a physician to perform a scheduled 40-minute operation than to stay up all night with a laboring patient." In some cases, physician reimbursement is greater for elective repeat cesarean section than for VBAC, despite the fact that VBAC requires greater physician effort.

Stafford[4] reviewed the impact of nonclinical factors on the performance of repeat cesarean section in the State of California. In 1986, there were 45,425 deliveries among women with a history of previous cesarean section. VBAC occurred in only 10.9% of those women, and no group of California hospitals had a VBAC rate higher than 29.2%. He observed that "proprietary hospitals, with the greatest incentive to maximize reimbursement, had the highest repeat cesarean section rates." Nonteaching hospitals and hospitals with low-volume obstetric services had lower VBAC rates than teaching hospitals and hospitals with high-volume obstetric services. Likewise, Hueston and Rudy[45] observed that women who undergo elective repeat cesarean section are more likely to have private insurance than women who attempt VBAC. Stafford[4] concluded the following:

Because a cesarean section is nearly twice as costly as a vaginal birth… the higher repeat cesarean section rates associated with proprietary hospitals, non-teaching hospitals, and low-volume hospitals contribute to increased health care expenditures.

In contrast, Clark et al.[46] assessed both the direct and indirect costs of VBAC. They concluded that "any economic savings for the healthcare system of a policy of trial of labor are at best marginal, even in a tertiary care center with a success rate for vaginal birth after cesarean of 70%." Further, they stated that "a policy of trial of labor does not result in any cost saving under most birthing circumstances encountered in the United States today."[46] The ACOG has acknowledged that "the difficulty in accessing the cost-benefit of VBAC is that the costs are not all incurred by one entity."[31]

Some women reject VBAC because they have experienced prolonged, painful labor during previous pregnancies. They fear that they will again experience a prolonged, painful labor and ultimately require a repeat cesarean section. This fear is more common in women who have delivered in smaller hospitals without the availability of epidural analgesia during labor. Other women reject VBAC because they prefer to schedule the date of elective repeat cesarean delivery. (A scheduled, elective cesarean section allows the patient to arrange for a relative or friend to come and provide childcare.) Kirk et al.[47] questioned 160 women regarding factors affecting their choice between VBAC and elective repeat cesarean section. They concluded that "social exigencies appeared to play a more important role than an assessment of the medical risks in making these decisions." Similarly, Joseph et al.[48] concluded that fear and inconvenience are the most common deterrents to VBAC. Finally, some women reject a trial of labor because of their concern regarding the adverse effects of labor and vaginal delivery on the maternal pelvic floor, with the risk of subsequent problems such as urinary and fetal incontinence.

Some insurance carriers have required that eligible women with a history of previous cesarean section attempt VBAC in subsequent pregnancies. These carriers deny partial or full reimbursement to women who choose elective repeat cesarean section unless there is a medical reason to perform repeat cesarean section. The ACOG has encouraged VBAC in eligible patients, but it is "opposed to any interference by insurers with the patient's right to consider the options and choose based upon the informed consent process."[49] Others have agreed that hospitals and insurers should *not* mandate a trial of labor for pregnant women with a history of previous cesarean delivery.[50] Chervenak and McCullough[51] concluded that obstetricians should recommend VBAC but perform elective repeat cesarean section if the patient prefers the latter. The ACOG has concluded the following[31]:

> After thorough counseling that weighs the individual benefits and risks of VBAC, the ultimate decision to attempt this procedure or undergo a repeat cesarean delivery should be made by the patient and her physician.

RISKS OF VBAC

What is the risk of uterine rupture during VBAC? A lower uterine segment scar is relatively avascular, and massive hemorrhage rarely follows separation of a lower segment scar. In contrast, rupture of a classic uterine scar may result in massive intraperitoneal bleeding. Unfortunately, there is some inconsistency and confusion in reports of the incidence of asymptomatic uterine scar dehiscence as opposed to frank uterine rupture. Uterine scar dehiscence may be defined as a uterine wall defect that does not result in fetal distress or excessive hemorrhage and that does not require emergency cesarean section or postpartum laparotomy. In contrast, uterine rupture is a uterine wall defect that results in fetal distress and/or maternal hemorrhage sufficient to require cesarean section or postpartum laparotomy.[17] Using these definitions, Farmer et al.[17] noted that among 7598 patients who attempted VBAC at their hospital between 1983 and 1989, the incidence of uterine scar dehiscence was 0.7% and the incidence of uterine rupture was 0.8%.

Some obstetricians have suggested that published studies underestimate the risks of VBAC. Scott[52] reported 12 women from Salt Lake City who experienced clinically significant uterine rupture during attempted VBAC. Similarly, Jones et al.[53] reported eight Denver women who experienced uterine rupture during attempted VBAC. There were no maternal deaths, but three women required obstetric hysterectomy. Four perinatal deaths and at least two cases of severe neurologic impairment occurred. Some of the women did not experience optimal obstetric management. (Scott's series included two women who labored at home.) Nonetheless, Scott[52] noted that "vaginal birth after cesarean, although usually successful, is not always uncomplicated."

Most obstetricians want to avoid unnecessary repeat cesarean section, but they fear that they will be found liable if an adverse event occurs during attempted VBAC. In one case, a jury awarded a verdict of 98.5 million dollars because of a delayed diagnosis of uterine rupture.[54] Phelan[55] cited another court decision that—in his opinion—will have a "chilling effect on the future of VBAC." In this case, the fetal heart rate (FHR) was normal until it abruptly decreased to 80 beats per minute at a cervical dilation of 9 cm. The interval between the onset of the deceleration and emergency cesarean delivery was 27 minutes. At delivery, the fetal head was found in the left adnexa. The mother required transfusion, and the child now suffers from developmental delay and cerebral palsy. The court found that the defendants were negligent in their failure to deliver the infant in a timely manner and to provide adequate informed consent. The court also concluded that "the ACOG 30-minute rule represented the maximum period of elapse" and did not represent the minimum standard of care. As a result of this verdict, Phelan[55] proposed the use of a VBAC consent form that includes the following statement: "I understand that if my uterus ruptures during my VBAC, there may not be sufficient time to operate and to prevent the death of or permanent brain injury to my baby." Flamm[56] noted that "widespread implementation of this or similar consent forms essentially would mean the end of VBAC [and that] in some parts of the country, the pendulum seems to be swinging back toward routine repeat cesarean." Flamm[56] also noted the following:

> On a national level, giving up VBAC would mean performing an additional 100,000 cesareans every year. It is unlikely this huge number of operations could be performed without any serious complications and perhaps even some maternal deaths.

In contrast, Greene[57] wrote a sobering editorial on the risks of VBAC. He acknowledged that the study by Lydon-Rochelle et al.[22] was an observational study of the results of clinical practice and not a randomized trial. However, Greene[57] noted that the study's troubling results "reflect broad experience in a wide range of clinical-practice settings," and he stated that "there is no reason to believe that improvements in clinical care can substantially reduce the risks of uterine rupture and perinatal mortality." Greene[57] concluded his editorial with the following opinion:

> After a through discussion of the risks and benefits of attempting a vaginal delivery after cesarean section, a patient might ask, "But doctor, what is the safest thing for my baby?" Given the findings of Lydon-Rochelle et al., my unequivocal answer: elective repeated cesarean section.

OBSTETRIC MANAGEMENT

In an editorial, Pitkin[58] made the following statement regarding VBAC:

> The message seems clear: Many women with previous cesarean can be delivered vaginally, and thereby gain substantial advantage, but neither the decision for trial labor nor management during that labor should be arrived at in a cavalier or superficial manner.

Intravenous Access and Availability of Blood

It seems prudent to recommend the early establishment of intravenous access in women who attempt VBAC. Moreover, cross-matched blood should be readily available for these patients.

Fetal Heart Rate Monitoring

Continuous electronic FHR monitoring represents the best means of detecting uterine rupture.[59-61] Rodriguez et al.[60] reviewed 76 cases of uterine rupture at their hospital. Fetal distress occurred in 59 of the 76 patients and was the most reliable sign of uterine rupture. At the University of Alabama at Birmingham Hospital, we continuously monitor the FHR in all patients who attempt VBAC.

Intrauterine Pressure Monitoring

The intrauterine pressure catheter provides a quantitative measurement of uterine tone both during and between contractions. Some obstetricians contend that an intrauterine pressure catheter should be used in all patients who attempt VBAC. They argue that a loss of intrauterine pressure and cessation of labor will signal the occurrence of uterine rupture. In one study,[60] 39 patients had an intrauterine pressure catheter at the time of uterine rupture. None of these patients had an apparent decrease in resting uterine tone or cessation of labor, but four patients experienced an increase in baseline uterine tone. In these four cases, the increase in baseline uterine tone was associated with severe variable FHR decelerations that prompted immediate cesarean section. The authors concluded that the information obtained by the use of the intrauterine pressure catheter did not assist obstetricians in making the diagnosis of uterine rupture.[60]

Of course, the obstetrician may use an intrauterine pressure catheter for other reasons in these patients. For example, it may be prudent to place an intrauterine pressure catheter in patients who receive oxytocin.

Use of Prostaglandin Gel

Lydon-Rochelle et al.[22] observed a uterine rupture rate of 24.5 per 1000 women who attempted VBAC with prostaglandin-induced labor. Subsequently, the ACOG Committee on Obstetric Practice concluded that "the risk of uterine rupture during VBAC . . . is substantially increased with the use of various prostaglandin cervical ripening agents for the induction of labor, and their use for this purpose is discouraged."[62] The ACOG also reaffirmed its position that "misoprostol should not be used in patients with a previous cesarean delivery or major uterine surgery."[62]

Oxytocin Augmentation of Labor

Some obstetricians have long argued that the administration of oxytocin increases the likelihood of uterine rupture during VBAC. However, several studies[14,26,63,64] have suggested that obstetricians may safely use oxytocin to augment labor in patients who attempt VBAC. Horenstein and Phelan[63] prospectively studied 732 patients who attempted VBAC at their hospital between July 1, 1982, and June 30, 1983. Among the 289 patients who received oxytocin, 200 (69%) delivered vaginally, compared with 395 (89%) of the 443 patients who did not receive oxytocin. Uterine scar dehiscence occurred in 3% and 2% of patients in the oxytocin and no-oxytocin groups, respectively. There was no difference between the two groups in other indices of maternal morbidity or perinatal morbidity or mortality. Phelan et al.[26] evaluated the use of oxytocin in their patients who underwent a trial of labor after *two* cesarean sections. Approximately 284 (57%) of these 501 patients received oxytocin, which did not significantly increase the incidence of uterine scar dehiscence. Rosen et al.[8] performed a meta-analysis of 31 studies of VBAC. They noted that the use of oxytocin did not increase the risk of uterine scar dehiscence or rupture during VBAC.

In contrast, Lydon-Rochelle et al.[22] observed an increased risk of uterine rupture among women who underwent induction of labor without prostaglandins but presumably *with* oxytocin. Zelop et al.[65] observed an increased rate of uterine rupture in women receiving oxytocin induction of labor for attempted VBAC when compared with similar women attempting VBAC with spontaneous labor. Further, the rate of uterine rupture was also increased in women receiving oxytocin for *augmentation* of labor, but the difference was not statistically significant. The ACOG has concluded that the "use of oxytocin . . . for VBAC requires close patient monitoring."[31]

ANESTHETIC MANAGEMENT

Historically there has been concern that epidural anesthesia during labor might delay the diagnosis of uterine scar dehiscence or rupture.[66-68] Some obstetricians have contended that epidural anesthesia masks the pain of uterine scar separation or rupture. Plauché et al.[66] stated, "Regional anesthesia, such as epidural anesthesia, blunts the patient's perception of symptoms and the physician's ability to elicit signs of early uterine rupture." Others have argued that the sympathectomy associated with epidural anesthesia attenuates the maternal compensatory response to the hemorrhage associated with uterine rupture. For example, sympathectomy might prevent the compensatory tachycardia and vasoconstriction that occur during hemorrhage. However, there is an emerging consensus that these concerns do not preclude administration of epidural analgesia, for several reasons.

First, pain, uterine tenderness, and tachycardia have low *sensitivity* as diagnostic symptoms and signs of lower uterine

segment scar dehiscence or rupture. Some uterine scars separate painlessly. Many obstetricians have discovered an asymptomatic lower uterine segment scar dehiscence at the time of elective repeat cesarean section. Molloy et al.[69] reported eight cases of uterine rupture among 1781 patients who attempted VBAC. None of these eight patients had abdominal pain, but all eight had FHR abnormalities. Uppington[59] reported six cases of uterine scar dehiscence or rupture among 222 women who attempted VBAC. There were four cases of lower uterine segment scar dehiscence or rupture in women without epidural anesthesia. Only one of these four women had pain, only two had uterine tenderness, and none had tachycardia. Fetal distress was the most common sign of uterine rupture. Johnson and Oriol[61] reviewed 14 studies of VBAC published between 1980 and 1989. Among 10,967 patients who attempted VBAC, 1623 patients received epidural anesthesia. Among those who experienced uterine rupture, 5 of 14 patients (35%) with epidural anesthesia experienced abdominal pain as compared with 4 of 23 patients (17%) without epidural anesthesia. Fetal distress was the most common sign of uterine rupture among patients who did and did not receive epidural anesthesia. None of these authors observed that epidural anesthesia delayed the diagnosis of uterine rupture.

Second, pain, uterine tenderness, and tachycardia have low *specificity* as diagnostic symptoms and signs of lower uterine segment scar dehiscence. Case et al.[70] reported 20 patients with a history of previous cesarean section in whom the indication for urgent repeat cesarean section was severe hypogastric pain and/or tenderness. At surgery, they confirmed the presence of scar dehiscence in only one of the 20 patients. Eckstein et al.[71] suggested that the unexpected development of pain during previously successful epidural anesthesia might be indicative of uterine rupture. Crawford[72] referred to this phenomenon as the "epidural sieve." Others have described patients who received epidural anesthesia and who subsequently complained of pain and tenderness secondary to uterine scar rupture.[73-76] I have provided anesthesia care for several patients in whom the first suggestion of scar separation was the sudden and unexpected development of "breakthrough pain" despite the continuous epidural infusion of bupivacaine. Thus epidural anesthesia may improve the specificity of abdominal pain as a symptom of uterine scar separation or rupture.

Third, most cases of lower uterine segment scar dehiscence do *not* result in severe hemorrhage. For example, only one of Uppington's six patients had intrapartum vaginal bleeding.[59] However, if significant bleeding should occur, epidural anesthesia may attenuate the maternal compensatory response to hemorrhage. We observed that epidural anesthesia (median sensory level of T9) significantly worsened maternal hypotension, uterine blood flow, and fetal oxygenation during untreated hemorrhage (20 mL/kg) in gravid ewes.[77] Intravascular volume replacement promptly eliminated the differences between groups in maternal mean arterial pressure, cardiac output, and fetal Pao_2. Maternal heart rate did not change significantly during hemorrhage in the control animals. However, there was a significant decrease in maternal heart rate during hemorrhage in the animals who received epidural anesthesia.[77] Perhaps maternal bradycardia should prompt suspicion of maternal hemorrhage in patients with epidural anesthesia.

Fourth, several published series have reported the successful use of epidural anesthesia in women undergoing

VBAC.* There is little evidence that epidural anesthesia decreases the likelihood of vaginal delivery or that epidural anesthesia adversely affects maternal or neonatal outcome in women who have uterine scar separation or rupture. Flamm et al.[15] reported a multicenter study of 1776 patients who attempted VBAC. Approximately 134 of 181 women (74%) who received epidural anesthesia delivered vaginally as compared with 1180 of 1595 women (74%) who did not receive epidural anesthesia. Phelan et al.[78] reported that among patients who received both oxytocin augmentation and epidural anesthesia, 69% delivered vaginally. This did not differ from the incidence of vaginal delivery among patients who received oxytocin *without* epidural anesthesia. Other investigators have reported smaller studies suggesting a decreased rate of vaginal delivery among patients who received epidural anesthesia.[79,80] However, this effect was limited to patients who received oxytocin for the induction or augmentation of labor. These authors concluded that epidural anesthesia does *not* decrease the likelihood of successful VBAC.

Fifth, some obstetricians favor the use of epidural anesthesia because it facilitates postpartum uterine exploration to assess the integrity of the uterine scar.[13] Meehan et al.[81] earlier supported routine palpation of the uterine scar. However, Meehan et al.[82] subsequently acknowledged that it is not necessary to repair all such defects. Many obstetricians manage asymptomatic uterine scar dehiscence with "expectant observation."[13] Thus they argue that routine palpation of the uterine scar is unnecessary after successful VBAC.

Sixth, epidural anesthesia provides rapid access to safe, surgical anesthesia if cesarean section and/or postpartum laparotomy should be required.[83]

Finally, it is inhumane to deny effective analgesia to women who attempt VBAC. Further, many women are more likely to attempt VBAC if they know that they will receive effective pain relief during labor.[7,31] Thus the availability—and frequent use—of epidural analgesia may decrease the incidence of unnecessary repeat cesarean section.

The ACOG[31] has concluded that VBAC does *not* contraindicate the use of epidural anesthesia. In my judgment, the availability of epidural analgesia is an essential component to a successful VBAC program.

It seems reasonable to provide analgesia—but not total anesthesia—during labor in these patients. In my practice, we give a dilute solution of local anesthetic during the first stage of labor so that the patient retains some sensation in the event of uterine rupture. We establish analgesia with 5-mL bolus doses of 0.25% bupivacaine, and we maintain analgesia with a continuous epidural infusion of 0.125% bupivacaine. Some anesthesiologists prefer to give these patients even more dilute solutions of local anesthetic (e.g., 0.0625% bupivacaine with fentanyl).

---

*References 14-17, 26-28, 39, 59, 72, 78-80

KEY POINTS

- Cesarean section is the most frequently performed operation in the United States, and previous cesarean section is the most common indication.
- A trial of labor is successful in 60% to 80% of women who had a low-transverse uterine incision performed during previous cesarean section.

- Previous cesarean section for cephalopelvic disproportion or dystocia does not contraindicate a trial of labor.
- The ACOG has stated that physicians, anesthesia providers, and other personnel must be immediately available to provide emergency care for patients attempting VBAC.
- Hospitals and insurers should not mandate a trial of labor for pregnant women with a history of previous cesarean delivery.
- Continuous electronic FHR monitoring represents the best means of detecting uterine rupture.
- Obstetricians may use oxytocin to augment labor in patients who attempt VBAC; however, uterine hyperstimulation should be avoided.
- Women are more likely to attempt VBAC if they know that they will receive effective analgesia during labor.
- Epidural analgesia does not delay the diagnosis of uterine rupture, and it does not decrease the likelihood of successful VBAC.

REFERENCES

1. Cragin EB. Conservatism in obstetrics. New York Med J 1916; 104:1-3.
2. American College of Obstetrics and Gynecologists. Issues in Women's Health Media Kit: 1998. Washington, DC, 1998.
3. American College of Obstetrics and Gynecologists. Issues in Women's Health Media Kit: 1999. Washington, DC, 1999.
4. Stafford RS. The impact of nonclinical factors on repeat cesarean section. JAMA 1991; 265:59-63.
5. Taffel SM, Placek PJ, Liss T. Trends in the United States cesarean section rate and reasons for the 1980-85 rise. Am J Pub Health 1987; 77:955-9.
6. United States Department of Health and Human Services; Public Health Service; National Institutes of Health. Repeat cesarean birth. In Cesarean Childbirth. NIH Publication No. 82-2067. Washington DC, United States Government Printing Office, 1981; 351-74.
7. American College of Obstetricians and Gynecologists Committee on Obstetric Practice. Vaginal Delivery After a Previous Cesarean Birth. ACOG Committee Opinion No. 143. Washington, DC, October 1994.
8. Rosen MG, Dickinson JC, Westhoff CL. Vaginal birth after cesarean: A meta-analysis of morbidity and mortality. Obstet Gynecol 1991; 77:465-70.
9. Porreco RP, Thorp JA. The cesarean birth epidemic: Trends, causes, and solutions. Am J Obstet Gynecol 1996; 175:369-74.
10. Brink S. Too posh to push: Cesarean sections have spiked dramatically: Progress or convenience? U.S. News and World Report, August 5, 2002.
11. De Lee JB, Cornell EL. Low cervical cesarean section (laparotrachelotomy). JAMA 1922; 79:109-12.
12. Kerr JMM. The technique of cesarean section, with special reference to the lower uterine segment incision. Am J Obstet Gynecol 1926; 12:729-34.
13. Depp R. Cesarean delivery. In Gabbe SG, Niebyl JR, Simpson JL, editors. Obstetrics: Normal and Problem Pregnancies, 4th ed. New York, Churchill Livingstone, 2002: 539-606.
14. Flamm BL, Dunnett C, Fischermann E, Quilligan EJ. Vaginal delivery following cesarean section: Use of oxytocin augmentation and epidural anesthesia with internal tocodynamic and internal fetal monitoring. Am J Obstet Gynecol 1984; 148:759-63.
15. Flamm BL, Lim OW, Jones C, et al. Vaginal birth after cesarean section: Results of a multicenter study. Am J Obstet Gynecol 1988; 158:1079-84.
16. Flamm BL, Newman LA, Thomas SJ, et al. Vaginal birth after cesarean delivery: Results of a 5-year multicenter collaborative study. Obstet Gynecol 1990; 76:750-4.
17. Farmer RM, Kirschbaum T, Potter D, et al. Uterine rupture during trial of labor after previous cesarean section. Am J Obstet Gynecol 1991; 165:996-1001.
18. Holland JG, Dupre AR, Blake PG, et al. Trial of labor after cesarean delivery: Experience in the non-university level II regional hospital setting. Obstet Gynecol 1992; 79:936-9.

19. Flamm BL, Goings JR, Liu Y, Wolde-Tsadik G. Elective repeat cesarean delivery versus trial of labor: A prospective multicenter study. Obstet Gynecol 1994; 83:927-32.

20. Miller DA, Diaz FG, Paul RH. Vaginal birth after cesarean: A 10-year experience. Obstet Gynecol 1994; 84:255-8.

21. McMahon MJ, Luther ER, Bowes WA, Olshan AF. Comparison of a trial of labor with an elective second cesarean section. N Engl J Med 1996; 335:689-95.

22. Lydon-Rochelle M, Holt VL, Easterling TR, Martin DP. Risk of uterine rupture during labor among women with a prior cesarean delivery. N Engl J Med 2001; 345:3-8.

23. Rosen MG, Dickinson JC. Vaginal birth after cesarean: A meta-analysis of indicators for success. Obstet Gynecol 1990; 76:865-9.

24. Seitchik J, Rao VRR. Cesarean delivery in nulliparous women for failed oxytocin-augmented labor: Route of delivery in subsequent pregnancy. Am J Obstet Gynecol 1982; 143:393-7.

25. Roberts LJ. Elective section after two sections: Where's the evidence? Br J Obstet Gynaecol 1991; 98:1199-1202.

26. Phelan JP, Ahn MO, Diaz F, et al. Twice a cesarean, always a cesarean? Obstet Gynecol 1989; 73:161-5.

27. Pruett KM, Kirshon B, Cotton DB, Poindexter AN. Is vaginal birth after two or more cesarean sections safe? Obstet Gynecol 1988; 72:163-5.

28. Novas J, Myers SA, Gleicher N. Obstetric outcome of patients with more than one previous cesarean section. Am J Obstet Gynecol 1989; 160:364-7.

29. Asakura H, Myers SA. More than one previous cesarean delivery: A 5-year experience with 435 patients. Obstet Gynecol 1995; 85:924-9.

30. Caughey AB, Shipp TD, Repke JT, et al. Rate of uterine rupture during a trial of labor in women with one or two prior cesarean deliveries. Am J Obstet Gynecol 1999; 181:872-6.

31. American College of Obstetricians and Gynecologists Practice Bulletin. Vaginal birth after previous cesarean delivery. American College of Obstetricians and Gynecologists Clinical Management Guidelines for Obstetricians-Gynecologists. Washington, DC, Number 5, July 1999.

32. Naef RW, Ray MA, Chauhan SP, et al. Trial of labor after cesarean delivery with a lower-segment, vertical uterine incision: Is it safe? Am J Obstet Gynecol 1995; 172:1666-74.

33. Adair CD, Sanchez-Ramos L, Whitaker D, et al. Trial of labor in patients with a previous lower uterine vertical cesarean section. Am J Obstet Gynecol 1996; 174:966-70.

34. Strong TH, Phelan JP, Ahn MO, Sarno AP. Vaginal birth after cesarean delivery in the twin gestation. Am J Obstet Gynecol 1989; 161:29-32.

35. Miller DA, Mullin P, Hou D, Paul RH. Vaginal birth after cesarean section in twin gestation. Am J Obstet Gynecol 1996; 175:194-8.

36. Ophir E, Oettinger M, Yagoda A, et al. Breech presentation after cesarean section: Always a section? Am J Obstet Gynecol 1989; 161:25-8.

37. Sarno AP, Phelan JP, Ahn MO, Strong TH. Vaginal birth after cesarean delivery: Trial of labor in women with breech presentation. J Reprod Med 1989; 34:831-3.

38. Beall M, Eglinton GS, Clark SL, Phelan JP. Vaginal delivery after cesarean section in women with unknown types of uterine scar. J Reprod Med 1984; 29:31-5.

39. Pruett KM, Kirshon B, Cotton DB. Unknown uterine scar and trial of labor. Am J Obstet Gynecol 1988; 159:807-10.

40. Lonky NM, Worthen N, Ross MG. Prediction of cesarean section scars with ultrasound imaging during pregnancy. J Ultrasound Med 1989; 8:15-9.

41. Flamm BL, Goings JR. Vaginal birth after cesarean section: Is suspected fetal macrosomia a contraindication? Obstet Gynecol 1989; 74:694-7.

42. Anonymous. ACOG calls for 'immediately available' VBAC services. ASA Newsl 1999; 63:21.

43. Zlatnik FJ. VBAC and the community hospital revisited. Iowa Perinat Lett 1989; 10:20.

44. Pickhardt MG, Martin JN, Meydrech EF, et al. Vaginal birth after cesarean delivery: Are there useful and valid predictors of success or failure? Am J Obstet Gynecol 1992; 166:1811-9.

45. Hueston WJ, Rudy M. Factors predicting elective repeat cesarean delivery. Obstet Gynecol 1994; 83:741-4.

46. Clark SL, Scott JR, Porter TF, et al. Is vaginal birth after cesarean less expensive than repeat cesarean delivery? Am J Obstet Gynecol 2000; 182:599-602.

47. Kirk EP, Doyle KA, Leigh J, Garrard ML. Vaginal birth after cesarean or repeat cesarean section: Medical risks or social realities? Am J Obstet Gynecol 1990; 162:1398-405.

48. Joseph GF, Stedman CF, Robichaux AG. Vaginal birth after cesarean section: The impact of patient resistance to a trial of labor. Am J Obstet Gynecol 1991; 164:1441-7.

49. Kaminetzky HA. The patient's right to choose. ACOG Newsletter, September 1989.

50. Sachs BP, Kobelin C, Castro MA, Frigoletto F. The risks of lowering the cesarean-delivery rate. N Engl J Med 1999; 340:54-7.

51. Chervenak FA, McCullough LB. An ethically justified algorithm for offering, recommending, and performing cesarean delivery and its application in managed care practice. Obstet Gynecol 1996; 87:302-5.

52. Scott JR. Mandatory trial of labor after cesarean delivery: An alternative viewpoint. Obstet Gynecol 1991; 77:811-4.

53. Jones RO, Nagashima AW, Hartnett-Goodman MM, Goodlin RC. Rupture of low transverse cesarean scars during trial of labor. Obstet Gynecol 1991; 77:815-7.

54. Freeman G, editor. $98.5 million verdict in missed uterine rupture. OB-GYN Malpractice Prev 1996; 3:41-8.

55. Phelan JP. VBAC. Time to reconsider? OBG Management 1996; November:62-8.

56. Flamm BL. Once a cesarean, always a controversy. Obstet Gynecol 1997; 90:312-5.

57. Greene MF. Vaginal delivery after cesarean section: Is the risk acceptable? (editorial) N Engl J Med 2001; 345:54-5.

58. Pitkin RM. Once a cesarean? (editorial). Obstet Gynecol 1991; 77:939.

59. Uppington J. Epidural analgesia and previous caesarean section. Anaesthesia 1983; 38:336-41.

60. Rodriguez MH, Masaki DI, Phelan JP, Diaz FG. Uterine rupture: Are intrauterine pressure catheters useful in the diagnosis? Am J Obstet Gynecol 1989; 161:666-9.

61. Johnson C, Oriol N. The role of epidural anesthesia in trial of labor. Regional Anesth 1990; 15:304-8.

62. American College of Obstetricians and Gynecologists Committee on Obstetric Practice. Induction of labor for vaginal birth after cesarean delivery. Washington, DC. ACOG Committee Opinion Number 271, April 2002.

63. Horenstein JM, Phelan JP. Previous cesarean section: The risks and benefits of oxytocin usage in a trial of labor. Am J Obstet Gynecol 1985; 151:564-9.

64. Flamm BL, Goings JR, Fuelberth NJ, et al. Oxytocin during labor after previous cesarean section: Results of a multicenter study. Obstet Gynecol 1987; 70:709-12.

65. Zelop CM, Shipp TD, Repke JT, et al. Uterine rupture during induced or augmented labor in gravid women with one prior cesarean delivery. Am J Obstet Gynecol 1999; 181:882-6.

66. Plauché WC, Von Almen W, Muller R. Catastrophic uterine rupture. Obstet Gynecol 1984; 64:792-7.

67. Abraham R, Sadovsky E. Delay in the diagnosis of rupture of the uterus due to epidural anesthesia in labor. Gynecol Obstet Invest 1992; 33:239-40.

68. Tehan B. Abolition of the extradural sieve by addition of fentanyl to extradural bupivacaine. Br J Anaesth 1992; 69:520-1.

69. Molloy BG, Sheil O, Duignan NM. Delivery after caesarean section: Review of 2176 consecutive cases. Br Med J 1987; 294:1645-7.

70. Case BD, Corcoran R, Jeffcoate N, Randle GH. Caesarean section and its place in modern obstetric practice. J Obstet Gynaecol Br Commonw 1971; 78:203-14.

71. Eckstein KL, Oberlander SG, Marx GF. Uterine rupture during extradural blockade. Can Anaesth Soc J 1973; 20:566-8.

72. Crawford JS. The epidural sieve and MBC (minimal blocking concentration): A hypothesis. Anaesthesia 1976; 31:1277-80.

73. Carlsson C, Nybell-Lindahl G, Ingemarsson I. Extradural block in patients who have previously undergone caesarean section. Br J Anaesth 1980; 52:827-30.

74. Rowbottom SJ, Tabrizian I. Epidural analgesia and uterine rupture during labour. Anaesth Intens Care 1994; 22:79-80.

75. Kelly MC, Hill DA, Wilson DB. Low dose epidural bupivacaine/fentanyl infusion does not mask uterine rupture. Internat J Obstet Anesth 1997; 6:52-4.

76. Rowbottom SJ, Critchley LAH, Gin T. Uterine rupture and epidural analgesia during trial of labour. Anaesthesia 1997, 52:483-8.

77. Vincent RD, Chestnut DH, Sipes SL, et al. Epidural anesthesia worsens uterine blood flow and fetal oxygenation during hemorrhage in gravid ewes. Anesthesiology 1992; 76:799-806.

78. Phelan JP, Clark SL, Diaz F, Paul RH. Vaginal birth after cesarean. Am J Obstet Gynecol 1987; 157:1510-5.

79. Stovall TG, Shaver DC, Solomon SK, Anderson GD. Trial of labor in previous cesarean section patients, excluding classical cesarean sections. Obstet Gynecol 1987; 70:713-7.

80. Sakala EP, Kaye S, Murray RD, Munson LJ. Epidural analgesia: Effect on the likelihood of a successful trial of labor after cesarean section. J Reprod Med 1990; 35:886-90.

81. Meehan FP, Moolgaoker AS, Stallworthy J. Vaginal delivery under caudal analgesia after caesarean section and other major uterine surgery. Br Med J 1972; 2:740-2.

82. Meehan FP, Burke G, Kehoe JT, Magani IM. True rupture/scar dehiscence in delivery following prior section. Int J Gynecol Obstet 1990; 31:249-55.

83. Bucklin BA. Vaginal birth after cesarean delivery. Anesthesiology 2003; 99:1444-8.

Chapter 24
Postpartum Tubal Sterilization

Joy L. Hawkins, M.D.

Many parous women choose tubal ligation for permanent contraception. Half are performed postpartum (approximately 350,000 annually in the United States) and half as ambulatory interval procedures.[1] The purpose of this chapter is to discuss the considerations and controversies regarding the administration of anesthesia during the postpartum period.

ASA GUIDELINES

The American Society of Anesthesiologists (ASA) has published "Practice Guidelines for Obstetrical Anesthesia,"[2] which includes a discussion of postpartum tubal ligation. (See Appendix B at the end of the text.) The Task Force recommendations can be summarized as follows:

1. "Evaluation of the patient for postpartum tubal ligation should include assessment of hemodynamic status (e.g., blood loss) and consideration of anesthetic risks."
2. "The patient planning to have an elective postpartum tubal ligation within 8 hours of delivery should have no oral intake of solid food during labor, and postpartum until the time of surgery."
3. "Both the timing of the procedure and the decision to use a specific anesthetic technique (i.e., regional versus general) should be individualized, based on anesthetic and/or obstetric risk factors and patient preferences."
4. "The procedure should not be attempted at a time when it might compromise other aspects of patient care."

SURGICAL CONSIDERATIONS

Tubal sterilization can be performed satisfactorily at any time, but the early postpartum period has several advantages for women who have had an uncomplicated vaginal delivery.[3] The patient avoids the cost and inconvenience of a second hospital visit. The uterine fundus remains near the umbilicus for several days postpartum, which allows easy access to the fallopian tubes. Rates of serious complications (e.g., bowel laceration, vascular injury) are lower during minilaparotomy than during laparoscopy.[4]

Postpartum tubal ligation is not wise if the patient is ambivalent regarding permanent sterilization. Women who undergo postpartum sterilization may have an increased probability of regret when compared with women who undergo interval sterilization.[5]

There are at least two potential disadvantages to *immediate* postpartum sterilization. First, multiparous women are at increased risk for uterine atony and postpartum hemorrhage. (This risk decreases substantially 12 hours after delivery.) Second, immediate surgery results in sterilization before assessment of the newborn is complete.

Several techniques are used for postpartum tubal sterilization (Figure 24-1).[6] The failure rate is lowest (approximately 0.75%) if some form of tubal resection occurs.[7] With the **Irving** procedure, the obstetrician buries the cut ends of the tubes in the myometrium and mesosalpinx. This technique is least likely to fail, but it requires more extensive exposure and increases the risk of hemorrhage. The **Pomeroy** procedure is simplest. The surgeon ligates a loop of oviduct and excises the loop above the suture. With the **Parkland** procedure, the obstetrician ligates the tube proximally and distally and then excises the midsegment. The last two methods are most commonly performed during postpartum tubal ligations. Regardless of the technique, the obstetrician should document that fimbriae are present to preclude ligation of another structure such as the round ligament. The excised portions typically are sent to a pathologist for verification.

NONMEDICAL ISSUES

Nonmedical issues affect decisions regarding the timing of tubal sterilization. The obstetrician must obtain and document informed consent for surgery.[8] Tubal ligation should be considered an irreversible procedure. Therefore most obstetricians require a discussion with the patient before labor and delivery. Physicians should be aware of state laws or insurance regulations that may require a specific interval between obtaining consent and performance of sterilization procedures. Regulations often do not allow the woman to give consent while in labor or immediately after delivery. For example, the Medicaid reimbursement program includes the following requirements for sterilization[9]:
- The patient must be at least 21 years of age and mentally competent when consent is obtained.
- Informed consent may not be obtained while the patient is in labor or during childbirth.

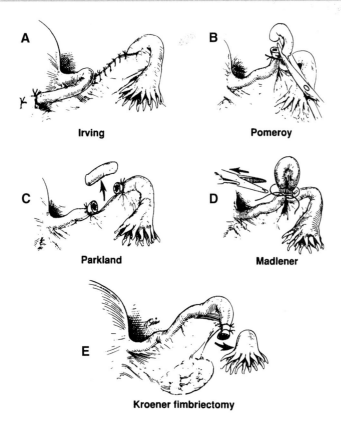

FIGURE 24-1. Techniques for tubal sterilization. **A,** Irving procedure. The medial cut end of the oviduct is buried in the myometrium posteriorly, and the distal cut end is buried in the mesosalpinx. **B,** Pomeroy procedure. A loop of oviduct is ligated, and the knuckle of tube above the ligature is excised. **C,** Parkland procedure. A midsegment of tube is separated from the mesosalpinx at an avascular site, and the separated tubal segment is ligated proximally and distally and then excised. **D,** Madlener procedure. A knuckle of oviduct is crushed and then ligated without resection; this technique has an unacceptably high failure rate of approximately 7%. **E,** Kroener procedure. The tube is ligated across the ampulla, and the distal portion of the ampulla, including all of the fimbria, is resected; some studies have reported an unacceptably high failure rate with this technique. (From Cunningham FG, MacDonald PC, Gant NF, et al. Williams Obstetrics, 20th ed. Stamford, Conn, Appleton & Lange, 1997:1376.)

- Consent may not be obtained while the patient is undergoing an abortion or under the influence of alcohol or other substances.
- A total of 30 days must pass between the date the consent is signed and the date the procedure is performed. (Exceptions to the 30-day waiting period can be made for preterm delivery or emergency abdominal surgery.)
- Consent is valid for only 180 days.

In some cases the obstetrician may schedule a patient for a postpartum tubal ligation because of a fear that the patient will not return for interval tubal sterilization 6 weeks postpartum. Concerns regarding patient compliance should not prompt the performance of postpartum tubal ligation in patients with significant medical or obstetric complications.

PREOPERATIVE EVALUATION

The patient scheduled for postpartum tubal ligation requires a thorough preoperative evaluation, and a reevaluation should be performed even if the patient is known to the anesthesia providers as a result of the provision of labor analgesia. A cursory evaluation should not be performed simply because the patient is young and healthy. Patients with pregnancy-

induced hypertension may safely receive regional or general anesthesia for postpartum tubal ligation provided that there is no evidence of pulmonary edema, oliguria, or thrombocytopenia.[10]

Physicians and nurses often underestimate blood loss during delivery. Excessive blood loss from uterine atony is not uncommon in multiparous patients. The presence of orthostatic changes in blood pressure and heart rate should be excluded, especially if an *immediate* postpartum procedure is to be performed. At the University of Colorado, if surgery is performed the next day, we determine the hematocrit several hours after delivery (to allow for equilibration) and compare it with the antepartum measurement. We do not obtain a hematocrit before an *immediate* postpartum tubal sterilization (performed less than 8 hours after delivery), provided that the antepartum hematocrit was acceptable, there are no orthostatic changes, and there was no evidence of excessive blood loss during delivery.

No absolute value of hematocrit requires a delay of surgery, but physical signs of hemodynamic instability or laboratory evidence of excessive blood loss should prompt postponement of the procedure until 6 to 8 weeks postpartum. Fever may signal the presence of endometritis or urinary tract infection and also may require postponement of surgery until a later date. Finally, the condition of the neonate should be confirmed just before surgery to exclude any unexpected problems.

Often mothers are concerned that medications administered during surgery might affect their ability to breast-feed or that these medications might harm the neonate. Any drug present in the mother's blood will be present in breast milk, with the concentration dependent on factors such as protein binding, lipid solubility, and degree of ionization.[11] Typically the amount of drug present in breast milk is small. Opioids, barbiturates, and propofol administered during anesthesia are excreted in insignificant amounts. (See Chapter 13 for a detailed discussion of interactions between drugs and breast-feeding.)

RISK OF ASPIRATION

Historically, anesthesiologists have considered maternal aspiration the major risk associated with anesthesia for postpartum tubal ligation, although the evidence for this is scant and conflicting.[12] Several factors may place the pregnant woman at increased risk for aspiration. Some but not all of these factors are resolved at delivery. The placenta is the primary site of progesterone production, and progesterone concentrations fall rapidly after the delivery of the placenta (Figure 24-2).[13,14] Typically progesterone concentrations decline within 2 hours of delivery, and by 24 hours postpartum, progesterone concentrations are similar to those found during the luteal phase of the menstrual cycle.

Two important questions to address during the preanesthetic evaluation are: (1) What is the duration of the fast for solids? (2) Were parenteral opioids administered during labor?

Gastric Emptying

Several studies have assessed gastric emptying in pregnant and postpartum women. O'Sullivan et al.[15] used an epigastric impedance technique to compare gastric emptying times for solids and liquids in women during the third trimester of

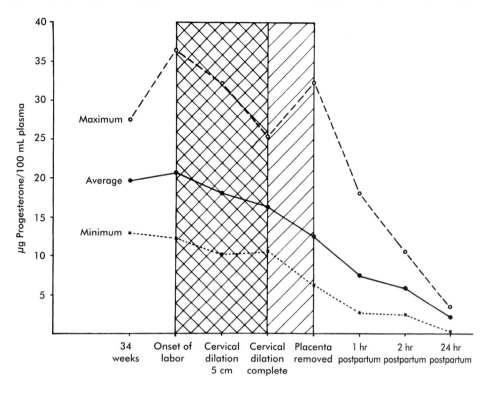

FIGURE 24-2. Average progesterone concentrations with the highest and lowest measurements of 13 pregnant women at given time intervals. (From Llauro JL, Runnebaum B, Zander J. Progesterone in human peripheral blood before, during and after labor. Am J Obstet Gynecol 1968; 101:871.)

pregnancy, in women during the first hour postpartum, and in nonpregnant controls. They observed that the overall rate of emptying was slower in the postpartum patients than in pregnant or nonpregnant patients. When they separated those patients who had received opioids in labor from those who had not, they found that the women who had *not* received opioids had rates of gastric emptying that were similar to those of nonpregnant controls. They concluded that the rate of gastric emptying in postpartum women is delayed *only* if opioids have been administered during labor.

Other studies have used the paracetamol absorption technique to assess gastric emptying. Macfie et al.[16] compared women in all three trimesters of pregnancy with nonpregnant controls and found no significant delay in gastric emptying at any time during pregnancy. Gin et al.[17] studied women on the first and third days after delivery and at 6 weeks postpartum. They found comparable times to peak concentration of paracetamol in all three groups. They concluded that gastric emptying was no different in the immediate postpartum period than 6 weeks later, and they recommended that "the approach to prophylaxis against acid aspiration should be more consistent between nonpregnant and postpartum patients." Whitehead et al.[18] observed no significant delay in gastric emptying during the first, second, or third trimesters of pregnancy or between 18 and 48 hours postpartum when compared with gastric emptying in nonpregnant controls. However, they observed that gastric emptying was significantly delayed during the first 2 hours after vaginal delivery. (At least 4 of the 17 women studied received intramuscular meperidine during labor.) The authors did not measure gastric emptying between 2 and 18 hours postpartum. They concluded, "The presence of delayed gastric emptying in the immediate (within 2 hours) postpartum period confirms that strict precautions against acid aspiration... should be provided to mothers who are newly delivered and requiring anaesthesia."[18]

Sandhar et al.[19] used applied potential tomography to measure gastric emptying in 10 patients at term gestation, 2 to 3 days

postpartum, and 6 weeks postpartum. (The 6-week measurement served as each woman's control value.) All measurements were made after administration of an H_2-receptor antagonist. The times to 50% emptying after ingestion of 400 mL of water were not different among the three periods of testing (Figure 24-3).

Wong et al.[20] assessed gastric emptying in nonlaboring pregnant women at term gestation, after ingestion of either 50 or 300 mL of water, by using two techniques: (1) serial assessment of acetaminophen absorption, and (2) use of ultrasonography to determine gastric antrum cross-sectional areas. Gastric emptying was significantly faster after ingestion of 300 mL of water, consistent with the observation that a liquid meal may actually accelerate gastric emptying. Kubli et al.[21] compared the effects of isotonic "sport drinks" versus water on residual gastric volume in women in early labor. Women who received isotonic "sports drinks" had similar gastric volumes

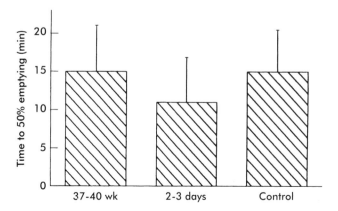

FIGURE 24-3. Mean (SEM) times to 50% gastric emptying (min). No significant differences were noted between term pregnant, postpartum, and nonpregnant control women. (From Sandhar BK, Elliott RH, Windram I, Rowbotham DJ. Peripartum changes in gastric emptying. Anaesthesia 1992; 47:197.)

and a similar incidence of vomiting as compared with those who received water, but the ingestion of "sport drinks" prevented the increase in ketone production that occurred in the control (water) group.

Altogether, these studies suggest that gastric emptying of liquids is not delayed during the postpartum period unless an opioid has been administered. In contrast, Jayaram et al.[22] found that 39% of postpartum patients, but no nonpregnant patients presenting for gynecologic surgery, had solid food particles in the stomach, as demonstrated by ultrasonography. Body mass index was significantly greater in the postpartum patients, which suggests that weight may have been a factor. However, 4 hours after a standardized meal, 95% of postpartum women—compared with only 19% of nonpregnant subjects—still had solid food particles in the stomach. Prior administration of an opioid did not seem to be a risk factor in this study. Scrutton et al.[23] randomized 94 women presenting in early labor to receive either a light diet or water only during labor. The mothers who ate a light diet had significantly larger gastric antrum cross-sectional areas (determined by ultrasonography) and were twice as likely to vomit at or around delivery as those who had water only. Also, the volumes vomited were significantly larger in the women who ate a light diet.

In summary, the preponderance of evidence suggests that (1) administration of an opioid increases the likelihood of delayed gastric emptying during the early postpartum period, (2) gastric emptying of *solids* is delayed during labor in all parturients, and (3) gastric emptying of clear liquids is probably *not* delayed unless parenteral opioids were administered. However, there are few data on gastric emptying during the first 8 hours postpartum.

During the preoperative assessment, the anesthesiologist should determine when solids were last consumed and whether opioids have been administered *by any route*. Systemic absorption of an opioid occurs after epidural administration. However, published studies have provided conflicting results regarding the effect of epidural opioid administration on gastric emptying. Wright et al[24] observed that epidural administration of 10 mL of 0.375% bupivacaine with fentanyl 100 µg caused a modest prolongation of gastric emptying during labor when compared with epidural administration of bupivacaine alone. However, Kelly et al.[25] found that intrathecal, but *not* epidural, fentanyl delayed gastric emptying. Metoclopramide may not accelerate gastric emptying in patients who have received an opioid.

Gastric Volume and pH

The conventional wisdom is that a gastric volume of more than 25 mL and a gastric pH of less than 2.5 are risk factors for aspiration pneumonitis. Coté[26] noted that this dogma was derived from unpublished animal studies and that it assumes that every milliliter of gastric fluid is directed into the trachea. A marked disparity exists between the incidence of patients labeled "at risk" and the incidence of patients with clinically significant aspiration pneumonitis.

Blouw et al.[27] measured gastric volume and pH in nonpregnant women undergoing gynecologic surgery and postpartum women 9 to 42 hours after delivery. They found no significant difference between the two groups. Approximately 75% of women in both groups had a gastric pH of less than 2.5. When the combination of volume and pH was used to determine the risk of aspiration, 64% of the control patients but only 33% of postpartum patients were at risk. They concluded that postpartum patients are not at greater risk than nonpregnant patients undergoing elective surgery, once 8 hours have elapsed after delivery. (They did not examine patients earlier than 8 hours after delivery.) However, they acknowledged that a large number of patients in both groups are at risk.

James et al.[28] attempted to determine the "safe" interval after delivery. They compared postpartum women 1 to 8 hours, 9 to 23 hours, and 24 to 45 hours after delivery with a control group of nonpregnant women undergoing elective surgery. There were no significant differences between the group of patients undergoing elective surgery and any of the postpartum groups (Table 24-1). Approximately 60% of *all* patients were considered "at risk" for aspiration pneumonitis. The investigators concluded that there was no difference in the risk for sequelae if aspiration should occur, but they speculated that hormonal changes or mechanical factors might make aspiration more likely during the postpartum period.

Finally, Lam et al.[29] administered 150 mL of water to 50 women 2 to 3 hours before tubal ligation that was performed 1 to 5 days postpartum. Another 50 postpartum and 50 nonpregnant women fasted after midnight. The authors found no differences in gastric pH or volume among the postpartum-water group, the postpartum-fasted group, and the group of nonpregnant controls undergoing elective surgery.

In conclusion, there is little evidence that postpartum women are at greater risk for sequelae of aspiration than patients undergoing elective surgery based *solely* on pregnancy-induced changes in gastric pH and volume.

Gastroesophageal Reflux

Women in the third trimester of pregnancy have decreased lower esophageal barrier pressures as compared with nonpregnant controls.[30] Those with symptoms of heartburn have even lower pressures and a higher incidence of gastric reflux. Vanner and Goodman[31] asked parturients to swallow a pH electrode to measure lower esophageal pH at term and on the second postpartum day. Patients were placed in four positions: supine with tilt, left lateral, right lateral, and lithotomy, and were then asked to perform a Valsalva and other maneuvers to promote reflux. A total of 17 of 25 patients had reflux at term, whereas only 5 of 25 had reflux after delivery. The investigators concluded that the incidence of reflux returns toward normal by the second day after delivery. (This is an arguable conclusion, given the fact that they did not determine the incidence of reflux before or 6 to 8 weeks after pregnancy.)

TABLE 24-1	GASTRIC VOLUME AND pH AT INTERVALS AFTER DELIVERY		
	Vol > 25 mL (%)	pH < 2.5 (%)	At risk* (%)
Group 1 (1-8 hr)	73	100	73
Group 2 (9-23 hr)	40	100	40
Group 3 (24-45 hr)	73	80	67
Group 4 (control)	67	80	60

*Gastric contents with pH less than 2.5 and volume greater than 25 mL.
(From James CF, Gibbs CP, Banner T. Postpartum perioperative risk of aspiration pneumonia. Anesthesiology 1984; 61:757-8.)

Summary

No data indicate that the postpartum patient's safety is enhanced by delaying surgery or is compromised by proceeding immediately after delivery. This has led to confusion and inconsistency in the development of policies for the performance of postpartum tubal ligation.[32] No time interval guarantees that the postpartum patient is free of risk for aspiration. It is probably prudent to use some form of aspiration prophylaxis in all patients undergoing postpartum tubal ligation. However, significant aspiration pneumonitis is so rare that it will be difficult to document cost-effectiveness and decreased rates of morbidity and mortality from the use of these measures. H_2-receptor antagonists and antacids do not decrease the *possibility* of regurgitation and aspiration, but they may make the *consequences* less severe. Metoclopramide may decrease the incidence of reflux by increasing lower esophageal sphincter tone.[30] None of these medications can guarantee that gastric contents will not enter the lungs. Aspiration is best prevented by an experienced anesthesiologist using careful airway management and/or by use of regional anesthetic techniques.

Performance of an *immediate* postpartum tubal ligation (within 8 hours of delivery) may decrease both the length of the hospital stay and hospital costs.[33] In this era of health care cost-containment, any decision to postpone surgery that requires an extra day of hospitalization must be evaluated carefully. If gastric emptying time and gastric volume and pH are no different in the postpartum patient than in nonpregnant women, should we wait 8 hours or more after delivery before performing a postpartum tubal ligation? Reasons for an 8-hour delay might include the following. First, women may remain at increased risk for gastroesophageal reflux immediately after delivery. Second, delays in gastric emptying caused by the antepartum administration of opioids will subside. Third, an 8-hour delay allows the administration of aspiration prophylaxis drugs, although these also might be given during labor. Fourth, maximal hemodynamic stress and potential instability occur immediately postpartum when central blood volume suddenly increases because of contraction of the evacuated uterus, relief of aortocaval compression, and loss of the low-resistance placental circuit. (The patient with cardiovascular disease is at greatest risk for hemodynamic decompensation immediately postpartum.) Fifth, if there are concerns about excessive blood loss at delivery, an 8-hour delay allows the physician to assess serial hemodynamic measurements (including the presence or absence of orthostatic changes), obtain an equilibrated postpartum hematocrit, and if necessary, restore intravascular volume. Sixth, delay allows a more thorough evaluation of the infant. Finally, delay allows the woman to assess her decision fully.

In summary, we perform immediate postpartum tubal ligation in patients who have a functioning epidural catheter in place. We give these patients an H_2-receptor antagonist and metoclopramide intravenously during labor, and we administer a clear (nonparticulate) antacid after delivery, just before going to the operating room. In other patients who do not want (or are unable to receive) epidural analgesia for labor, we give an H_2-receptor antagonist and metoclopramide intravenously after delivery and wait at least 2 hours for maximal effect. Patients should be NPO for solids for 8 hours, similar to that for nonpregnant patients undergoing elective surgery. Before surgery we monitor blood loss and assess orthostatic vital signs. We then give a clear antacid just before going to the operating room. Most of these patients (without preexisting epidural analgesia) receive spinal anesthesia for postpartum tubal ligation. However, we are willing to provide general anesthesia using rapid-sequence induction with cricoid pressure.

ANESTHETIC MANAGEMENT

Local, general, or regional anesthesia may be used successfully for postpartum tubal sterilization. Physiology remains altered in the postpartum patient and requires some modification in anesthetic technique. It seems reasonable to give all postpartum patients some form of aspiration prophylaxis. This may include a clear (nonparticulate) antacid, an H_2-receptor antagonist, and/or metoclopramide to increase lower esophageal sphincter tone and hasten gastric emptying. Metoclopramide also may prevent emesis during and after surgery. Patients with additional risk factors for aspiration (e.g., morbid obesity, diabetes mellitus) warrant prophylaxis with all three classes of drugs.

Local Anesthesia

Local anesthesia is used for more than 75% of tubal sterilizations worldwide, although regional anesthesia is most often administered for postpartum tubal sterilization in the United States.[3] Several reports have documented the efficacy and safety of local anesthesia for postpartum or laparoscopic tubal ligation in the hospital operating room, a free-standing outpatient facility, or the obstetrician's office. An anesthesiologist may or may not be involved. Cruikshank et al.[34] described the use of intraperitoneal lidocaine for postpartum tubal ligation. After intravenous administration of diazepam, lidocaine 100 mg was used to infiltrate the skin and subcutaneous tissue. The peritoneum was entered, and 400 mg of lidocaine (80 mL of 0.5% solution) was instilled into the peritoneal cavity. A Pomeroy tubal ligation was performed 5 minutes later. All patients had complete peritoneal anesthesia, and all patients stated they would have the same procedure again. None recalled any pain or discomfort 24 hours later. Signs of lidocaine toxicity were absent, and the maximum blood level obtained was 5.3 µg/mL. Surgeons rated the conditions excellent.

Poindexter et al.[35] described almost 3000 laparoscopic tubal sterilization procedures performed with local anesthesia in an ambulatory surgical facility. After intravenous sedation with midazolam (5 to 10 mg) and fentanyl (50 to 100 µg), the skin was infiltrated with 10 mL of 0.5% bupivacaine. After insertion of the trocar, the abdomen was insufflated with nitrous oxide. Each tube was sprayed with 5 mL of 0.5% bupivacaine, and a Silastic ring was applied. Patients were discharged home after approximately 1 hour in the post-anesthesia care unit (PACU). The authors reported a technical failure rate of 0.14% and no unintended laparotomies or intraoperative complications. They reported that this technique reduced surgical time by 33% and cost by 68% to 85% when compared with general anesthesia. They presented no data regarding patient satisfaction. The authors also made no comment on the use of pulse oximetry or blood pressure monitors, but 4% of patients required oxygen therapy for "adequate tissue perfusion." This study was done in the 1980s, before many ambulatory surgery facilities had sedation guidelines in place.

General Anesthesia

Much of the impetus for performing sterilization procedures under local anesthesia came from two reports[36,37] in 1983 indicating that morbidity and mortality were much higher when general anesthesia was used. The first report[36] involved 3500 interval laparoscopic tubal sterilizations at nine university medical centers. Among all patients, the risk of intraoperative or postoperative complications was 1.75%, but the risk was five times higher with general anesthesia than with local anesthesia. (In this report, local anesthesia included local, epidural, and spinal anesthesia.) The reason for the difference was unclear. In the second report,[37] the Centers for Disease Control examined deaths attributed to tubal sterilization procedures from 1977 to 1981. They included both immediate postpartum laparotomies and interval laparoscopic procedures. Of the 29 deaths, 11 followed complications of general anesthesia and were caused by hypoventilation or cardiorespiratory arrest. (Aspiration was not reported.) Among the 6 patients whose deaths were definitely attributed to hypoventilation, none had been intubated, and 5 of the 11 deaths attributed to general anesthesia occurred during postpartum laparotomy. Of these, only one woman had been intubated; all others underwent mask ventilation. The authors concluded, "It appears that for tubal sterilization, like abortion, the greatest risk of death is that associated with the anesthesia used during the procedure."

In the 20 years since those reports, appropriate airway management with endotracheal intubation has become standard practice. Adequate monitoring of ventilation—by using ASA standards—should help prevent morbidity and mortality associated with general anesthesia. At the University of Colorado, we perform a rapid-sequence induction (with cricoid pressure) and intubate all patients who receive general anesthesia for postpartum tubal ligation.

Should the anesthesiologist use an inhalation or an intravenous technique to maintain general anesthesia for postpartum tubal ligation? Marx et al.[38] measured postpartum uterine activity and the response to oxytocin with different concentrations of halothane or enflurane (Figure 24-4). Impaired spontaneous uterine activity occurred at 0.5 minimum alveolar concentration (MAC) of both agents, and loss of the response to oxytocin occurred near 1.0 MAC. Spontaneous contractions reappeared when anesthetic concentrations were reduced below these levels. Parous women are at risk for post-

partum uterine atony, and administration of a high concentration of a volatile halogenated agent may precipitate postpartum hemorrhage. The anesthesiologist should not give a high concentration of a volatile halogenated agent during the postpartum period.

Two studies have determined the MAC of isoflurane during the postpartum period.[39,40] Chan et al.[39] found a positive correlation between MAC and the length of time after delivery, with nonpregnant values achieved by 72 hours postpartum. Zhou et al.[40] determined that MAC was approximately 0.75% in the first 12 hours postpartum and 1.04% in patients who were 12 to 24 hours postpartum. No significant difference in MAC existed between the latter group and a control group of nonpregnant gynecologic patients. Together these results demonstrate that the reduced MAC observed during pregnancy persists for a variable period between 12 and 36 hours postpartum.

Propofol has some advantages (e.g., rapid awakening, decreased incidence of emesis) that make it attractive for short sterilization procedures. When propofol was used for induction and maintenance of anesthesia for cesarean section, breast milk samples obtained at 4 and 8 hours postpartum had a low concentration of the drug, which suggested a negligible neonatal exposure to propofol.[41] Use of sodium thiopental for induction of anesthesia also results in negligible neonatal exposure during subsequent breast-feeding.

Alterations occur in the activity of both depolarizing and nondepolarizing muscle relaxants during the postpartum period. Evans and Wroe[42] described the changes in plasma cholinesterase activity during pregnancy. A rapid fall in activity occurred during the first trimester. This low level of activity was maintained until delivery and was followed by an even lower level of activity during the first week postpartum. Ganga et al.[43] found that a lower dose of succinylcholine was required to achieve 80% twitch suppression in postpartum patients than in nonpregnant women. Time to recovery also was prolonged and correlated with lower cholinesterase activity in the postpartum patients. Leighton et al.[44] studied four groups of patients: nonpregnant, nonpregnant using oral contraceptives, term pregnant, and postpartum women. Cholinesterase activity was significantly

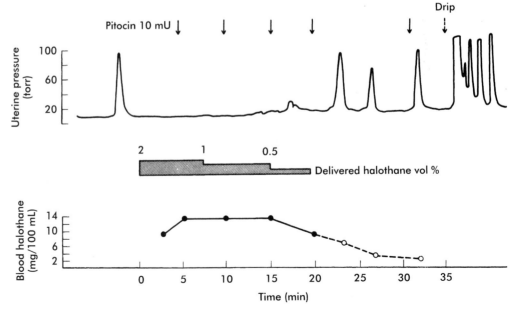

FIGURE 24-4. Halothane anesthesia blocked the normal response to oxytocin when arterial blood levels exceeded 10.5 mg/100 mL or approximately 0.8 MAC. (From Marx GF, Kim YI, Lin CC, et al. Postpartum uterine pressures under halothane or enflurane anesthesia. Obstet Gynecol 1978; 51:697.)

lower in both term pregnant and postpartum women. Recovery time was 25% longer in the postpartum patients than in other groups (685 sec versus approximately 500 sec). Although a 3-minute prolongation of paralysis may not seem clinically significant, it could be important if airway difficulties occur.[44]

Metoclopramide prolongs neuromuscular block with succinylcholine by 135% to 228% because of its inhibition of plasma cholinesterase.[45] Cimetidine and ranitidine do not affect the plasma cholinesterase activity or the duration of action of succinylcholine.[46]

Several studies have evaluated the use of the nondepolarizing muscle relaxants rocuronium, mivacurium, vecuronium, atracurium, and cisatracurium in postpartum patients. Rocuronium's duration of action is prolonged by approximately 25% in postpartum patients,[47] and mivacurium's duration of action is prolonged approximately 20%.[48] Vecuronium's duration of action is prolonged by more than 50% in postpartum patients.[49] In contrast, the duration of action for atracurium is unchanged[50] (Figure 24-5) and that of cisatracurium is significantly shorter in the postpartum period.[51] These changes could be clinically significant during a short procedure. Khuenl-Brady et al.[50] suggested that a relative decrease in hepatic blood flow and/or competition between vecuronium and steroid hormones for hepatic uptake may interfere with the hepatic clearance of vecuronium in postpartum women. Gin et al.[52] recently concluded that the duration of action for rocuronium is not prolonged in postpartum women if lean body mass—rather than total body weight—is used to calculate dose. They speculated that the prolonged duration noted earlier[47] might be explained by relative drug overdose if the dose of rocuronium is based on the patient's temporarily increased body weight.[52]

Regional Anesthesia

Spinal and epidural anesthesia both provide excellent operating conditions for postpartum tubal ligation. Airway obstruction, hypoventilation, and aspiration are much less likely during and after regional anesthesia. A sensory level of T4 is needed to block visceral pain during exposure and manipulation of the fallopian tubes. The choice between spinal and epidural anesthesia is a matter of personal preference for the patient and the anesthesiologist.

When the performance of postpartum tubal ligation is anticipated in a parous patient, I encourage administration of **epidural analgesia** for labor and delivery. The epidural anesthetic can be extended for immediate postpartum tubal ligation if appropriate. I avoid administration of parenteral opioids during labor if immediate postpartum tubal ligation is planned. Immediate postpartum tubal ligation may save the patient the cost and inconvenience of an extra day in the hospital, allow her to eat shortly after delivery (and surgery), and allow her to avoid the apprehension of undergoing a surgical procedure the following day. The avoidance of opioids helps maintain normal gastric emptying, which should decrease the risk of aspiration during postpartum surgery. If the patient is stable and personnel are available, the procedure may be performed immediately after delivery, after moving the patient to the operating room. The obstetrician must exclude excessive intrapartum blood loss and document that the patient has given informed consent. Additional intravenous crystalloid is administered, and the sensory level is extended with a concentration of local anesthetic suitable for surgical anesthesia. Appropriate sedative drugs also may be given, if desired. The anesthesiologist should be cautious about giving sedative drugs that may cause prolonged postpartum amnesia. Most women want to remember their first several hours of contact with their newborn. In some cases, peripartum administration of a benzodiazepine may cause retrograde amnesia, and the patient may not recall childbirth.[53]

If surgery is not performed immediately, the catheter may be left in place for delayed postpartum tubal ligation. Several studies have evaluated the efficacy of using a previously placed epidural catheter for a tubal ligation performed several hours after delivery. Vincent and Reid[54] found that the mean delivery-to-surgery interval was shorter in those patients who had adequate epidural anesthesia than in those without adequate anesthesia (10.6 versus 14.8 hours). The chance of successful epidural anesthesia was greatest if the catheter was reinjected within 4 hours of delivery. In contrast, Lawlor et al.[55] reported an 87% success rate, with no difference in the catheter placement-to-surgery interval between the successful-epidural and failed-epidural groups (21.4 versus 20.5 hours). In this study each epidural catheter was threaded 4 to 7.5 cm into the epidural space. Similarly, Goodman et al.[56] had an overall success rate of 92% in the reactivation of epidural catheters. The success rate was 93% among patients who underwent surgery

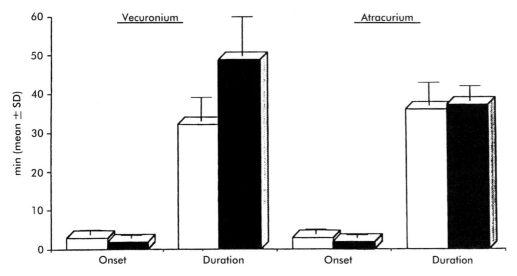

FIGURE 24-5. Onset and duration of action of vecuronium (0.1 mg/kg) and atracurium (0.5 mg/kg) in postpartum *(solid bar)* and nonpregnant control *(open bar)* patients. $P < 0.001$. (From Khuenl-Brady KS, Koller J, Mair P, et al. Comparison of vecuronium- and atracurium-induced neuromuscular blockade in postpartum and nonpregnant patients. Anesth Analg 1991; 72:112.)

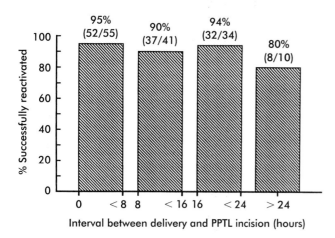

FIGURE 24-6. Rate of successful reactivation of epidural catheters for various intervals between delivery and the incision for postpartum tubal ligation. (From Goodman EJ, Dumas SD. The rate of successful reactivation of labor epidural catheters for postpartum tubal ligation surgery. Regional Anesth Pain Med 1998; 23:258–61.)

less than 24 hours after delivery but was only 80% among the 10 patients who underwent surgery more than 24 hours after delivery—a nonsignificant difference (Figure. 24-6). Clinical experience suggests that if the anesthesiologist uses an epidural catheter placed for labor, the risk of failure may be greater if surgery is delayed more than 10 hours after delivery. To assure maximal success when using a multi-orifice catheter, the anesthesiologist should thread the catheter 4 to 6 cm into the epidural space and have the patient assume a deflexed position before taping the catheter to the skin.[57,58]

Epidural anesthesia requires the use of large volumes of local anesthetic and thereby introduces the risk of intravascular injection and cardiotoxicity.[59] Epidural anesthesia also is time consuming; the induction of epidural anesthesia may require *more* time than the tubal ligation itself. **Spinal anesthesia** is simple to perform and rapid in onset and provides dense sensory and motor block. In one study,[60] spinal anesthesia for postpartum tubal ligation was associated with lower professional fees and operating room charges than attempted reactivation of an epidural catheter placed during labor. The ability to reinject a catheter intraoperatively is not necessary for a short procedure such as postpartum tubal ligation, and there is no need for prolonged postoperative analgesia. With the availability of small-gauge (25- or 27-gauge) pencil-point or noncutting spinal needles, the risk of postdural puncture headache (PDPH) is small. Some anesthesiologists have suggested that the incidence of PDPH in obstetric patients is no different after spinal anesthesia with a 25-gauge Whitacre needle than after planned epidural anesthesia (Table 24-2).

Local anesthetic requirements for spinal and epidural anesthesia are decreased during pregnancy, but studies have demonstrated a return to nonpregnant requirements by 36 hours postpartum. Assali and Prystowsky[61] demonstrated a return to nonpregnant requirements by 36 to 48 hours postpartum. Abouleish[62] prospectively compared the dose of spinal bupivacaine required for cesarean section with that required for postpartum tubal ligation. He noted that 30% more bupivacaine was required to achieve a T4 dermatomal level in women who were 8 to 24 hours postpartum. The reason for the rapid decrease in sensitivity to local anesthetics is unclear but may be related to the rapid fall in progesterone levels after delivery of the placenta.

Group*	Number of Anesthetics	Incidence of Postdural Puncture Headache
26 g Quincke	2256	5.2%
27 g Quincke	852	2.5%
25 g Whitacre	1000	1.1%
17 g Epidural	21,578	1.3%

TABLE 24-2 RISK OF POSTDURAL PUNCTURE HEADACHE AFTER SPINAL AND EPIDURAL ANESTHESIA IN OBSTETRIC PATIENTS

*A versus D, and B versus D: $P < 0.05$; C versus D: not significant.
(From Hurley RJ, Lambert D, Hertwig L, Datta S. Postdural puncture headache in the obstetric patient: Spinal vs epidural anesthesia [abstract]. Anesthesiology 1992; 77:A1018.)

Datta et al.[63] examined plasma and cerebrospinal fluid (CSF) progesterone concentrations and spinal lidocaine requirements in nonpregnant, term pregnant, and postpartum women 12 to 18 hours after delivery. Compared with nonpregnant women, plasma progesterone levels were 60 times higher in the pregnant women but only seven times higher in the postpartum women. CSF progesterone concentrations were eight times higher in term pregnant women and three times higher in postpartum women than in nonpregnant women. Intrathecal lidocaine requirements were similar in pregnant and postpartum patients, even though plasma and CSF progesterone concentrations were lower in the postpartum women. The authors suggested "that a minimum level of progesterone in the CSF and/or plasma is necessary for this heightened local anesthetic activity" associated with progesterone. Together these studies suggest that local anesthetic requirements return to nonpregnant requirements 12 to 36 hours after delivery.[61-63]

Huffnagle et al.[64] gave subarachnoid lidocaine 75 mg to postpartum women to determine whether age, weight, height, body-mass index, vertebral column length, or time from delivery to placement of the block correlated with the spread of sensory block. Only patient height had a weak positive correlation, and it accounted for less than 15% of the variance in height of block. Because of the large variation in the spread of sensory block within patients of the same height, the investigators concluded that there was little use in adjusting the dose of local anesthetic on that basis.

Many anesthesiologists have discontinued the use of hyperbaric lidocaine for spinal anesthesia because of concern about transient neurologic symptoms (TNS). Philip et al.[65] compared spinal administration of hyperbaric 5% lidocaine with hyperbaric 0.75% bupivacaine for postpartum tubal ligation; they observed a 3% incidence of TNS with lidocaine as compared with a 7% incidence with bupivacaine—a nonsignificant difference. In an accompanying editorial, Schneider and Birnbach[66] acknowledged that "there are no very short-acting hyperbaric spinal local anesthetics that have taken the place of lidocaine for these short procedures and many believe that spinal bupivacaine lasts too long to be a reasonable choice of anesthetic for a procedure that will last < 20 min." However, they concluded, "Because pregnant patients represent a population that lies to the extreme in terms of the criteria for safety and lack of morbidity, we believe that for the present, there is still insufficient safety evidence to suggest that spinal hyperbaric 5% lidocaine be routinely used in obstetrics."[66]

TABLE 24-3	CHARACTERISTICS OF MEPERIDINE VERSUS LIDOCAINE FOR SPINAL ANESTHESIA FOR POSTPARTUM TUBAL LIGATION	
	Meperidine	**5% lidocaine**
Surgical duration (min)	30	28
Maximal height sensory block	T3 (C8-T6)	T3 (C6-T5)
Mean duration motor block (min)	83	134*
PACU time to discharge (min)	39	91*
Time to first analgesic (min)	398	86*

*$P < 0.0001$.
(From Curran C, Dickerson SE, Bailey SL. Efficacy of intrathecal meperidine as the sole anesthetic for postpartum tubal ligation [abstract]. Anesthesiology 1992; 77:A1004.)

In a dose-response study, Huffnagle et al.[67] found that 7.5 mg hyperbaric bupivacaine—injected intrathecally in the lateral position—provided adequate surgical anesthesia for postpartum tubal ligation with "a minimum duration of motor block and recovery time."

Postpartum women seem to be at decreased risk for hypotension during spinal anesthesia as compared with pregnant women. Abouleish[62] gave ephedrine to correct maternal hypotension in 83% of pregnant women who received spinal bupivacaine anesthesia for cesarean section. In contrast, only 7% of postpartum women who received spinal anesthesia for tubal ligation required ephedrine. Pregnant women undergo an autotransfusion immediately after delivery. The increased intravascular volume and the lack of aortocaval compression may help protect postpartum patients from hypotension during spinal anesthesia. Sharma et al.[68] compared the use of crystalloid with the use of 6% hetastarch for the prevention of hypotension during spinal anesthesia for postpartum tubal ligation. They observed a 52% incidence of hypotension in the crystalloid group and a 16% incidence in the hetastarch group. However, they acknowledged that the increased expense of colloid might not be justifiable. Suelto et al.[69] compared normotensive and hypertensive patients receiving hyperbaric lidocaine for postpartum tubal ligation and found no difference in the use or dose of ephedrine for treatment of hypotension.

Preservative-free intrathecal meperidine can be used as an alternative to local anesthetic for postpartum tubal ligation.[70,71] The typical dose is 1 mg per kg prepregnant weight (50 to 80 mg) for cesarean section or tubal ligation. With an onset time of 3 to 5 minutes and a duration of 30 to 60 minutes, meperidine compares favorably with 5% lidocaine (Table 24-3). In one study,[71] patients who received meperidine (50 to 80 mg) had a shorter recovery room stay, longer postoperative pain relief, and less motor block than patients who received 5% lidocaine (60 to 90 mg). In another study[72] that compared lidocaine 70 mg with meperidine 60 mg for postpartum tubal ligation, patients who received meperidine had more pruritus but longer postoperative analgesia (448 versus 83 minutes). There was no difference in nausea, oxyhemoglobin desaturation, or patient satisfaction between groups. Intrathecal meperidine may be an excellent alternative to lidocaine for postpartum tubal ligation.

Box 24-1 summarizes a personal approach to anesthetic management for postpartum tubal ligation.

Box 24-1 ANESTHETIC MANAGEMENT FOR POSTPARTUM TUBAL LIGATION

INTRAPARTUM MANAGEMENT

Encourage use of epidural analgesia.
Avoid administration of parenteral opioids.
Keep NPO except for clear liquids.
Give aspiration prophylaxis if the procedure is to be performed immediately after delivery.

TIMING OF SURGERY

Consider performing surgery immediately postpartum if the patient is hemodynamically stable and has received aspiration prophylaxis.
An epidural catheter placed for labor may provide more reliable anesthesia if used within 10 hours of delivery.

EPIDURAL ANESTHESIA

Use 3% 2-chloroprocaine unless a longer procedure is planned.
If a catheter placed during labor is used, beware of an increased risk of failure if the delivery-to-surgery interval is prolonged.
Give fentanyl 50 to 100 μg via the catheter at the end of the procedure.

SPINAL ANESTHESIA

It is the preferred technique for *delayed* postpartum tubal ligation or for *immediate* surgery in patients who did not have an epidural catheter placed before delivery.
Use a small-gauge, noncutting, pencil-point spinal needle.
Give lidocaine 75 mg with fentanyl 10 to 25 μg, or give bupivacaine 7.5 mg with fentanyl 10 to 25 μg

GENERAL ANESTHESIA

Perform a rapid-sequence induction with cricoid pressure.
Intubate the patient, and control ventilation.
Avoid high concentrations of a volatile halogenated agent.
Monitor neuromuscular blockade if nondepolarizing agents are used.

Postoperative Analgesia

Postpartum tubal ligation produces modest postoperative pain of short duration. Patients typically receive one dose of parenteral opioid postoperatively, followed by oral analgesics. Optimal analgesia encourages early ambulation, interaction with the neonate, and early discharge from the hospital. An oral nonsteroidal antiinflammatory drug (NSAID) such as ibuprofen may be given to supplement other analgesics. Two studies demonstrated that intrathecal meperidine provided 6 to 8 hours of profound postoperative analgesia.[71,72] In one study, the addition of 25 μg of fentanyl to intrathecal lidocaine at the time of surgery provided better analgesia than lidocaine alone for 4 hours postoperatively.[73] When epinephrine 0.2 mg was added to lidocaine with fentanyl 10 μg for spinal anesthesia, the duration of complete and effective analgesia was prolonged and the incidence of pruritus was decreased, but the time to complete motor recovery was prolonged.[74] Campbell et al.[75] used 0.1 mg intrathecal morphine and found complete relief of postoperative pain without any increase in side effects as compared with a saline control. Although it is effective, spinal morphine analgesia should be used with caution because these patients may be discharged soon after postpartum tubal ligation, before the risk of delayed respiratory depression has lapsed.

Local anesthetic infiltration of the mesosalpinx with bupivacaine or topical application of a local anesthetic to the fallopian tubes significantly decreases opioid requirements postoperatively.[76] These are simple, rapid techniques that can be used by the obstetrician. Wittels et al.[77] reported that use of multi-modal therapy with spinal or epidural anesthesia, intravenous ketorolac 60 mg, intravenous metoclopramide 10 mg, and infiltration of the incised skin, fallopian tabes, and mesosalpinx with 0.5% bupivacaine prevented pain, nausea, and painful uterine cramping in both the immediate postoperative period and for 7 days after postpartum tubal ligation in 9 of 10 patients. The manufacturer (Roche) of ketorolac has stated that ketorolac is contraindicated in nursing mothers because of the *possible* adverse effects of prostaglandin synthetase inhibitors on neonates. In contrast, the American Academy of Pediatrics considers ketorolac to be compatible with breast-feeding.[78]

KEY POINTS

- **Postpartum tubal sterilization is an elective procedure. No data indicate that the postpartum patient's safety is enhanced by delaying surgery or compromised by proceeding with tubal ligation immediately after delivery.**
- **Postpartum sterilization offers the advantages of convenience for the patient and technical simplicity for the surgeon.**
- **Postpartum patients do not have lower gastric pH or higher gastric volumes than nonpregnant patients undergoing elective surgery. Some studies suggest that gastric emptying is delayed postpartum only if the patient has received an opioid analgesic.**
- **The incidence of gastroesophageal reflux returns toward normal by the second postpartum day.**
- **Anesthetic drugs do not appear in breast milk in amounts that affect the neonate.**
- **The duration of succinylcholine-, rocuronium-, mivacurium-, and vecuronium-induced neuromuscular blockade is prolonged during the postpartum period. In contrast, the duration of action for atracurium is unchanged and that of cisatracurium is shorter.**
- **An epidural catheter placed for labor may be used for postpartum tubal ligation, but the risk of failure may be greater if surgery is delayed more than 10 hours after delivery.**
- **Spinal anesthesia is preferred for delayed postpartum tubal ligation, regardless of whether the patient had an epidural catheter placed for labor.**
- **The local anesthetic dose for spinal anesthesia returns to nonpregnant requirements by 12 to 36 hours postpartum.**

REFERENCES

1. Westhoff C, Davis A. Tubal sterilization: Focus on the U.S. experience. Fertil Steril 2000;73:913-22.
2. Practice Guidelines for Obstetrical Anesthesia: A report by the American Society of Anesthesiologists' Task Force on Obstetrical Anesthesia. Anesthesiology 1999; 90:600-11.
3. Pati S, Cullins V. Female sterilization, evidence. Obstet Gynecol Clin North Am 2000; 27:859-99.
4. World Health Organization, Task Force on Female Sterilization, Special Programme of Research, Development and Research Training in Human Reproduction. Minilaparotomy or laparoscopy for sterilization: A multicenter, multinational randomized study. Am J Obstet Gynecol 1982; 143:645-54.
5. Hillis SC, Marchbanks PA, Tylor LR, et al. Poststerilization regret: Findings from the United States collaborative review of sterilization. Obstet Gynecol 1999; 93:889-94.
6. Cunningham FG, MacDonald PC, Gant NF, et al. Williams Obstetrics, 20th ed. Stamford, Conn, Appleton & Lange, 1997:1375-81.
7. Peterson HB, Zhisen X, Hughes JM, et al. The risk of pregnancy after tubal sterilization: Findings from the U.S. Collaborative Review of Sterilization. Am J Obstet Gynecol 1996; 174:1161-70.
8. American College of Obstetricians and Gynecologists Committee on Technical Bulletins. Sterilization. ACOG Technical Bulletin #222. Washington, DC, 1996.
9. Medicaid. Sterilizations, hysterectomies and abortions. Consent form, Form no. 91860 MED-178 (rev Feb 6, 1979).
10. Vincent RD, Martin RQ. Postpartum tubal ligation after pregnancy complicated by preeclampsia or gestational hypertension. Obstet Gynecol 1996; 88:119-22.
11. Ito S. Drug therapy: drug therapy for breast-feeding women. NEJM 2000; 343:118-25.
12. Bucklin BA, Smith CV. Postpartum tubal ligation: Safety, timing, and other implications for anesthesia. Anesth Analg 1999; 89:1269-74.
13. Deshpande GN, Turner AK, Sommerville IF. Plasma progesterone and pregnanediol in human pregnancy, during labour and post-partum. J Obstet Gynaecol Br Emp 1960; 67:954-61.
14. Llauro JL, Runnebaum B, Zander J. Progesterone in human peripheral blood before, during and after labor. Am J Obstet Gynecol 1968; 101:867-73.
15. O'Sullivan GM, Sutton AJ, Thompson SA, et al. Noninvasive measurement of gastric emptying in obstetric patients. Anesth Analg 1987; 66:505-11.
16. Macfie AG, Magides AD, Richmond MN, Reilly CS. Gastric emptying in pregnancy. Br J Anaesth 1991; 67:54-7.
17. Gin T, Cho AMW, Lew JKL, et al. Gastric emptying in the postpartum period. Anaesth Intens Care 1991; 19:521-4.
18. Whitehead EM, Smith M, Dean Y, O'Sullivan G. An evaluation of gastric emptying times in pregnancy and the puerperium. Anaesthesia 1993; 48:53-7.
19. Sandhar BK, Elliott RH, Windram I, Rowbotham DJ. Peripartum changes in gastric emptying. Anaesthesia 1992; 47:196-8.
20. Wong CA, Loffredi M, Ganchiff JN, et al. Gastric emptying of water in term pregnancy. Anesthesiology 2002; 96:1395-1400.
21. Kubli M, Scrutton MJ, Seed PT, et al. An evaluation of isotonic "sport drinks" during labor. Anesth Analg 2002; 94:404-8.
22. Jayaram A, Bowen MP, Deshpande S, Carp HM. Ultrasound examination of the stomach contents of women in the postpartum period. Anesth Analg 1997; 84:522-6.
23. Scrutton MJ, Metcalfe GA, Lowy C, et al. Eating in labour: A randomized controlled trial assessing the risks and benefits. Anaesthesia 1999;54: 329-34.
24. Wright PMC, Allen RW, Moore J, Donnelly JP. Gastric emptying during lumbar extradural analgesia in labor: Effect of fentanyl supplementation. Br J Anaesth 1992; 68:248-51.
25. Kelly MC, Carabine UA, Hill DA, Mirakhur RK. A comparison of the effect of intrathecal and extradural fentanyl on gastric emptying in laboring women. Anesth Analg 1997; 85:834-6.
26. Coté CJ. Aspiration: An overrated risk in elective patients. In Stoelting RK, Barash PG, Gallagher TJ, editors. Advances in Anesthesia. St Louis, Mosby, 1992:5-6.
27. Blouw R, Scatliff J, Craig DB, Palahniuk RJ. Gastric volume and pH in postpartum patients. Anesthesiology 1976; 45:456-7.
28. James CF, Gibbs CP, Banner T. Postpartum perioperative risk of aspiration pneumonia. Anesthesiology 1984; 61:756-9.

29. Lam KK, So HY, Gin T. Gastric pH and volume after oral fluids in the postpartum patient. Can J Anaesth 1993; 40:218-21.

30. Brock-Utne JG, Dow TGB, Welman S, et al. The effect of metoclopramide on the lower oesophageal sphincter in late pregnancy. Anaesth Intens Care 1978; 6:26-9.

31. Vanner RG, Goodman NW. Gastro-oesophageal reflux in pregnancy at term and after delivery. Anaesthesia 1989; 44:808-11.

32. Bogod DG. The postpartum stomach: When is it safe? (editorial). Anaesthesia 1994; 49:1-2.

33. Barton ACH, Spielman FJ, Onder R, Mayer DC. Timing of postpartum sterilization: Complications and cost-savings of early tubal ligations. Anesthesiology 1996; 85:A896.

34. Cruikshank DP, Laube DW, DeBacker LJ. Intraperitoneal lidocaine anesthesia for postpartum tubal ligation. Obstet Gynecol 1973; 42:127-30.

35. Poindexter AN, Abdul-Malak M, Fast JE. Laparoscopic tubal sterilization under local anesthesia. Obstet Gynecol 1990; 75:5-8.

36. DeStefano F, Greenspan JR, Dicker RC, et al. Complications of interval laparoscopic tubal sterilization. Obstet Gynecol 1983; 61:153-8.

37. Peterson HB, DeStefano F, Rubin GL, et al. Deaths attributable to tubal sterilization in the United States, 1977 to 1981. Am J Obstet Gynecol 1983; 146:131-6.

38. Marx GF, Kim YI, Lin CC, et al. Postpartum uterine pressures under halothane or enflurane anesthesia. Obstet Gynecol 1978; 51:695-8.

39. Chan MTV, Gin T. Postpartum changes in the minimum alveolar concentration of isoflurane. Anesthesiology 1995; 82:1360-3.

40. Zhou HH, Norman P, DeLima LGR, Mehta M, Bass D. The minimum alveolar concentration of isoflurane in patients undergoing bilateral tubal ligation in the postpartum period. Anesthesiology 1995; 82:1364-8.

41. Dailland P, Cockshott ID, Lirzin JD, et al. Intravenous propofol during cesarean section: Placental transfer, concentrations in breast milk, and neonatal effects: A preliminary study. Anesthesiology 1989; 71:827-34.

42. Evans RT, Wroe JM. Plasma cholinesterase changes during pregnancy. Anaesthesia 1980; 35:651-4.

43. Ganga CC, Heyduk JV, Marx GF, Sklar GS. A comparison of the response to suxamethonium in postpartum and gynaecological patients. Anaesthesia 1982; 37:903-6.

44. Leighton BL, Cheek TG, Gross JB, et al. Succinylcholine pharmacodynamics in peripartum patients. Anesthesiology 1986; 64:202-5.

45. Kao YJ, Turner DR. Prolongation of succinylcholine block by metoclopramide. Anesthesiology 1989; 70:905-8.

46. Woodworth GE, Sears DH, Grove TM, et al. The effect of cimetidine and ranitidine on the duration of action of succinylcholine. Anesth Analg 1989; 68:295-7.

47. Puhringer FK, Sparr HJ, Mitterschiffthaler G, et al. Extended duration of action of rocuronium in postpartum patients. Anesth Analg 1997; 84:352-4.

48. Gin T, Derrick JL, Chan MTV, et al. Postpartum patients have slightly prolonged neuromuscular block after mivacurium. Anesth Analg 1998; 86:82-5.

49. Hawkins JL, Adenwala J, Camp C, Joyce TH. The effect of H_2-receptor antagonist premedication on the duration of vecuronium-induced neuromuscular blockade in postpartum patients. Anesthesiology 1989; 71:175-7.

50. Khuenl-Brady KS, Koller J, Mair P, et al. Comparison of vecuronium and atracurium-induced neuromuscular blockade in postpartum and nonpregnant patients. Anesth Analg 1991; 72:110-3.

51. Pan PH, Moore C. Comparison of cisatracurium-induced neuromuscular blockade between immediate postpartum and nonpregnant patients. J Clin Anesth 2001; 13:112-7.

52. Gin T, Chan MTV, Chan KL, et al. Prolonged neuromuscular block after rocuronium in postpartum patients. Anesth Analg 2002; 94:686-9.

53. Camann W, Cohen MB, Ostheimer GW. Is midazolam desirable for sedation in parturients (letter)? Anesthesiology 1986; 65:441.

54. Vincent RD, Reid RW. Epidural anesthesia for postpartum tubal ligation using epidural catheters placed during labor. J Clin Anesth 1993; 5:289-91.

55. Lawlor M, Weiner M, Fantauzzi M, Johnson C. Efficacy of epidural anesthesia for post-partum tubal ligation utilizing indwelling labor epidural catheters. Reg Anesth 1994; 19:54.

56. Goodman EJ, Dumas SD. The rate of successful reactivation of labor epidural catheters for postpartum tubal ligation surgery. Reg Anesth Pain Med 1998; 23:258-61.

57. Beilin Y, Bernstein HH, Zucker-Pinchoff B. The optimal distance that a multiorifice epidural catheter should be threaded into the epidural space. Anesth Analg 1995; 81:301-4.

58. Hamilton CL, Riley ET, Cohen SE. Changes in the position of epidural catheters associated with patient movement. Anesthesiology 1997; 86:778-84.

59. Abouleish EI, Elias M, Nelson C. Ropivacaine-induced seizure after extradural anaesthesia. Br J Anaesth 1998; 80:843-4.

60. Viscomi CM, Rathmell JP. Labor epidural catheter reactivation or spinal anesthesia for delayed postpartum tubal ligation: A cost comparison. J Clin Anesth 1995; 7:380-3.

61. Assali NS, Prystowsky H. Studies on autonomic blockade. I. Comparison between the effects of tetraethylammonium chloride (TEAC) and high selective spinal anesthesia on blood pressure of normal and toxemic pregnancy. J Clin Invest 1950; 29:1354-66.

62. Abouleish EI. Postpartum tubal ligation requires more bupivacaine for spinal anesthesia than does cesarean section. Anesth Analg 1986; 65: 897-900.

63. Datta S, Hurley RJ, Naulty JS, et al. Plasma and cerebrospinal fluid progesterone concentrations in pregnant and nonpregnant women. Anesth Analg 1986; 65:950-4.

64. Huffnagle S, Norris MC, Leighton BL, et al. Do patient variables influence the subarachnoid spread of hyperbaric lidocaine in the postpartum patient? Reg Anesth 1994; 19:330-4.

65. Philip J, Sharma SK, Gottumukkala VNR, et al. Transient neurologic symptoms after spinal anesthesia with lidocaine in obstetric patients. Anesth Analg 2001; 92:405-9.

66. Schneider MC, Birnbach DJ. Lidocaine neurotoxicity in the obstetric patient: Is the water safe? Anesth Analg 2001; 92:287-90.

67. Huffnagle SL, Norris MC, Huffnagle HJ, et al. Intrathecal hyperbaric bupivacaine dose response in postpartum tubal ligation patients. Reg Anesth Pain Med 2002; 27:284-8.

68. Sharma SK, Gajraj NM, Sidawi JE. Prevention of hypotension during spinal anesthesia: A comparison of intravascular administration of hetastarch versus lactated Ringer's solution. Anesth Analg 1997; 84:111-4.

69. Suelto MD, Vincent RD, Larmon JE, et al. Spinal anesthesia for postpartum tubal ligation after pregnancy complicated by preeclampsia or gestational hypertension. Reg Anesth Pain Med 2000; 25:170-3.

70. Chen BJ, Liao KT, Kwan WF, et al. Fixed dose of spinal meperidine and lidocaine for postpartum tubal ligation (abstract). Anesthesiology 1995; 83:A842.

71. Curran C, Dickerson SE, Bailey SL. Efficacy of intrathecal meperidine as the sole anesthetic for postpartum tubal ligation (abstract). Anesthesiology 1992; 77:A1004.

72. Norris MC, Honet JE, Leighton BL, et al. A comparison of meperidine and lidocaine for spinal anesthesia for postpartum tubal ligation. Reg Anesth 1996; 21:84-8.

73. Durkan WJ, Leicht CH, Evans DH. Postoperative analgesia after intrathecal fentanyl-lidocaine for postpartum tubal ligation surgery (abstract). Anesthesiology 1990; 73:A932.

74. Malinow AM, Mokriski BLK, Nomura MK, et al. Effect of epinephrine on intrathecal fentanyl analgesia in patients undergoing postpartum tubal ligation. Anesthesiology 1990; 73:381-5.

75. Campbell DC, Riben CM, Rooney ME, et al. Intrathecal morphine for postpartum tubal ligation postoperative analgesia. Anesth Analg 2001; 93:1006-11.

76. Alexander CD, Wetchler BV, Thompson RE. Bupivacaine infiltration of the mesosalpinx in ambulatory surgical laparoscopic tubal sterilization. Can J Anaesth 1987; 34:362-5.

77. Wittels B, Faure EAM, Chavez R, et al. Effective analgesia after bilateral tubal ligation. Anesth Analg 1998; 87:619-23.

78. American Academy of Pediatrics Committee on Drugs. The transfer of drugs and other chemicals into human milk. Pediatrics 1994; 93: 137-50.

Part VII
Cesarean Section

During most of the nineteenth century, physicians performed very few cesarean sections because the mortality rate was so high. For example, in his case books, John Snow mentions more than 90 patients anesthetized for vaginal delivery, but not one cesarean section.[1] The procedure was reserved for desperate situations. One physician quipped that a woman had a better chance of surviving an abdominal delivery if she performed the surgery herself, or if her abdomen were accidentally ripped open by the horn of a bull.[2]

Hemorrhage and infection caused most deaths. The use of anesthesia allowed surgeons to develop techniques to deal with these problems. Italian surgeon, Eduardo Porro, made the first important innovation in 1876. To limit hemorrhage he excised the uterus after delivering the child. Others had left the uterine incision open in the belief that it would heal better. In 1882, German surgeon, Max Sänger, advised closing the uterus with sutures, thereby obviating the need for hysterectomy. Sänger, benefiting from the advances in bacteriology, also devised techniques to limit the risk of infection.[3]

In 1910 J. Whitridge Williams of John Hopkins, still called cesarean section a "dangerous procedure" despite the fact that the maternal mortality rate had fallen to 10%. He performed it only for the most severe cases of contracted pelvis.[2,4] In fact, Williams warned that a cesarean section "should never be performed when the child is dead or in serious danger." Even in 1970, cesarean section rates remained below 7% in the United States, and less than 2% in many European countries.[5]

With few agents to choose from, anesthetic techniques for cesarean section also evolved slowly. Regional anesthesia was not available before 1900. Ether and chloroform were the only two potent agents available for general anesthesia until the addition of cyclopropane. Until curare was introduced to clinical practice, use of these agents necessitated achieving an anesthetic depth sufficient to obtain abdominal relaxation.

Only in the past four decades have there been incentives to develop better anesthetic techniques for cesarean section. First, obstetricians began to perform cesarean section more often to deal with fetal and maternal problems. Second, physicians developed a better understanding of the physiology of pregnancy, especially the nature of risks associated with anesthesia. Third, anesthesiologists and obstetricians began to place greater emphasis on the well-being of the neonate, which required the development of anesthetic techniques that would protect the mother but have the least possible effect on the child.

Donald Caton, M.D.

REFERENCES

1. Ellis RH. The Case Books of Dr. John Snow. London, Wellcome Institute for the History of Medicine, 1994, supplement # 14.
2. Williams JW. Obstetrics: A Text-Book for the Use of Students and Practitioners. New York, D. Appleton and Co, 1904:400-11.
3. O'Dowd M, Philipp EE. The History of Obstetrics and Gynaecology. New York, The Parthenon Publishing Group, 1994:157-65.
4. Loudon I. Death in Childbirth: An International Study of Maternal Care and Maternal Mortality, 1800-1950. New York, Oxford University Press, 1992:132-9.
5. Hellman LM, Pritchard JA, Wynn RM. Williams Obstetrics. New York, Appleton-Century-Crofts, 1971:1007-167.

Chapter 25
Anesthesia for Cesarean Section

Krzysztof M. Kuczkowski, M.D. ·
Laurence S. Reisner, M.D. · Dennis Lin, M.D.

The cesarean section rate in the United States now exceeds 24% (see Figure 23-1).[1,2] The anesthetic care given during cesarean delivery is the culmination of almost all of the principles of obstetric anesthesia. The anesthesiologist must safely provide anesthesia for the mother without compromising the condition of the fetus and newborn. During the last several decades, the incidence of anesthesia-related maternal mortality in the United States has declined.[3] The incidence of maternal deaths from other causes also has declined.[4] Anesthesia remains responsible for approximately 3% to 12% of all maternal deaths.[3,5-8] The majority of these deaths occur during general anesthesia and result from failed intubation, failed ventilation and oxygenation, and/or pulmonary aspiration of gastric contents.[3,6] Associated factors include obesity, hypertensive disorders of pregnancy, and emergently performed procedures.[6] Many anesthesiologists have recommended the administration of regional anesthesia when possible and that general anesthesia be used only when it is absolutely necessary (see Chapter 26).[9,10]

These principles have been incorporated into clinical practice. In 1997, Hawkins et al.[11] compared the results of their survey of obstetric anesthesia practice in the United States for the year 1992 with those for the year 1981. Only 17% of women undergoing cesarean section received general anesthesia, 40% received spinal anesthesia, and 44% received epidural anesthesia. This reflects a significant decrease in the use of general anesthesia and a significant increase in the use of epidural anesthesia since 1981. In comparison, at the University of California, San Diego, 1364 cesarean sections were performed during 1991 and 1992, and only 7.6% of these patients received general anesthesia (Figure 25-1).

Tsen et al.[12] reviewed the anesthetic technique used for all cesarean sections performed at the Brigham and Women's Hospital between 1990 and 1995. The use of general anesthesia for cesarean section decreased from 7.2% in 1990 to 3.6% in 1995. The authors noted that contemporary graduates of anesthesiology residency programs have limited experience with the administration of general anesthesia for cesarean section in parturients with or without a difficult airway. They also noted that the few patients who require general anesthesia for cesarean section are more likely to have diseases that may complicate anesthetic management.

PREPARATION FOR ANESTHESIA

Preanesthetic Medication

Nonobstetric patients often receive other medications before the administration of anesthesia. The goals of preanesthetic medication typically are as follows: (1) to dry secretions; (2) to prevent vagal activity; (3) to provide anxiolysis; (4) to ensure analgesia for uncomfortable anesthetic procedures; and (5) to provide a basal level of analgesia for surgery. Most women do not require sedative drugs before the administration of anesthesia for cesarean section, and they are usually avoided until after delivery of the infant. They offer little to the patient receiving general anesthesia, and verbal reassurance often will suffice for the patient receiving regional anesthesia. If necessary, the anesthesiologist may give a small dose of a benzodiazepine (e.g., midazolam 0.5 to 2 mg or diazepam 2 to 5 mg) and/or an opioid (e.g., fentanyl 25 to 50 μg) intravenously. Alternatively, a small oral dose of diazepam (e.g., 5 mg) may be given 1 to 2 hours before elective cesarean section. Small doses of these drugs should result in minimal fetal and neonatal depression.[13,14] A major disadvantage of the benzodiazepines is their potential for amnesia; most patients want to remember their childbirth experience.

In selected cases, it is not unreasonable to administer an anticholinergic agent, which decreases secretions and lessens the likelihood of bradycardia during either regional or general anesthesia. Atropine readily crosses the placenta and results in an increased fetal heart rate (FHR), with decreased beat-to-beat variability.[15] By contrast, glycopyrrolate does not readily cross the placenta, and it is the anticholinergic agent of choice.[16] Unfortunately, the anticholinergic agents result in decreased lower esophageal sphincter tone.[17] Moreover, most patients dislike the mouth dryness that follows the administration of an anticholinergic agent. We do not routinely give an anticholinergic agent before the administration of either regional or general anesthesia for cesarean section. When it is indicated, glycopyrrolate may be given intramuscularly 30 to 60 minutes before the induction of anesthesia or intravenously just before the administration of anesthesia. Some anesthesiologists give scopolamine transdermally to minimize the nausea that often accompanies intrathecal or epidural administration of an opioid.[18] All patients should also receive pharmacologic aspiration prophylaxis *(vide infra)*. One commonly used agent—metoclopramide—also has an antiemetic effect, and it increases lower esophageal sphincter tone and reduces gastric volume by increasing gastric peristalsis.

Intravenous Fluids

Most patients should receive an intravenous bolus of crystalloid, although those who receive general anesthesia may require less volume. Before giving regional anesthesia, we give 15 to 20 mL/kg of a balanced salt solution (e.g., Ringer's lactate or 0.9% saline) to maintain adequate intravascular volume after the onset of sympathetic blockade. The bolus of intravenous fluid is most effective if it is given within 30 minutes of induction of anesthesia; otherwise the crystalloid redistributes to other body compartments. Recently some anesthesiologists have questioned the efficacy of hydration for the prevention of hypotension during the administration of regional anesthesia. Rout et al.[19] noted that the incidence of hypotension was reduced only from 71% in patients without prehydration to 55% in patients who received intravenous fluid administration as the primary method of prophylaxis during the administration of spinal anesthesia for elective cesarean section. This study does not suggest that intravenous hydration should be omitted but rather that additional means of preventing hypotension are necessary. It also suggests that,

in an urgent situation, it is not necessary to wait for the fluid bolus to be completed before proceeding with regional anesthesia.

Prophylactic hydration may not only decrease the incidence of hypotension but may also result in improved uteroplacental perfusion. Crino et al.[20] observed that rapid intravenous infusion of crystalloid resulted in a selective increase in blood flow to the placental implantation site in gravid ewes near term. They also demonstrated "both an increase in oxygen delivery and a decrease in vascular resistance at the placental implantation site when concurrent maternal hemodilution, and therefore volume expansion, occurred after crystalloid infusion." They concluded that "this study provides additional evidence that the placental vasculature may not be maximally dilated under all conditions and confirms that certain interventions can indeed improve placental blood flow and oxygen delivery."

Although glucose is a useful component of maintenance fluid administration during labor, its use in bolus or resuscitative fluid therapy may be detrimental to the fetus. Rapid infusion of a large glucose load results in both maternal and fetal hyperglycemia and hyperinsulinemia. When the infant is delivered and its activity level is increased, the use of glucose is escalated. However, the insulin has a longer half-life, and the neonate is at risk for hypoglycemia during the second hour of life.[21] Jaundice is also more prevalent among infants whose mothers received a large glucose infusion before cesarean delivery.

Administration of a large bolus of crystalloid may exacerbate the decrease in colloid osmotic pressure that occurs during the first 6 to 12 hours postpartum.[22] This change has little clinical significance for healthy patients, but it may predispose patients with preeclampsia or cardiovascular disease to the development of pulmonary edema. Balanced salt solutions remain the preferred volume expander in the United States. Some anesthesiologists in other countries prefer to give a synthetic colloid (e.g., dextran, hydroxyethyl starch) for this pur-

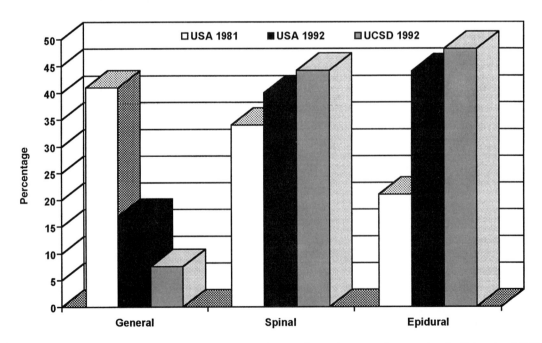

FIGURE 25-1. Anesthetic techniques administered for cesarean section in the United States in 1981 and 1992 and at the University of California San Diego *(UCSD)* in 1992. (The 1981 United States data were obtained from Gibbs CP, Krischer J, Peckman BM, et al. Obstetric anesthesia: A national survey. Anesthesiology 1986; 65:298-306; the 1992 United States data were obtained from Hawkins JL, Gibbs CP, Orleans M, et al. Obstetric anesthesia work force survey, 1981 versus 1992. Anesthesiology 1997; 87:135-43.)

pose.[23-27] These solutions remain in the intravascular space for a longer time than crystalloids, and a decreased volume is required to achieve equivalent volume expansion. However, these solutions are expensive, and some surgeons argue that they alter blood rheology and platelet function, which may result in increased blood loss.[28] Moreover, dextran is associated with a small but definite risk of anaphylaxis. Ueyama et al.[26] evaluated the efficacy of crystalloid and colloid preload in patients receiving spinal anesthesia for elective cesarean section. Although the incidence of hypotension was lower in patients who received 1.0 L of hydroxyethyl starch solution, the authors concluded that the "augmentation of blood volume with preloading, regardless of the fluid used, must be large enough to result in a significant increase in cardiac output for effective prevention of hypotension."[26]

The typical amount of blood loss during cesarean section is 500 to 1000 mL.[29,30] Administration of a volatile halogenated agent may result in increased blood loss,[31,32] although this is a matter of some dispute.[33] Given the fact that pregnancy typically results in a 30% to 50% increase in maternal blood volume, most patients do not require transfusion. Unfortunately, blood loss in some cases may be substantial, and blood and blood products should be readily available. It is satisfactory to perform a type and screen (rather than a full cross-match) for most patients,[34] and the alternative use of a "hold clot" may be safe in some practices (see Chapter 37).[35]

Maternal Position

Aortocaval compression must be avoided before and during the performance of cesarean section (Box 25-1).[36] When the pregnant woman lies supine, the gravid uterus compresses the aorta and the inferior vena cava against the bodies of the lumbar vertebrae. Aortocaval compression results in decreased uteroplacental perfusion by one or more of three mechanisms. First, it results in decreased venous return, which may cause decreased maternal cardiac output and blood pressure. Second, the obstruction of uterine venous drainage increases uterine venous pressure and decreases uterine artery perfusion pressure. Third, the compression of the aorta or common iliac arteries results in decreased uterine artery perfusion pressure. Therefore, it is necessary to maintain left uterine displacement before and during the performance of cesarean section, regardless of the anesthetic technique.[37] This may be easily accomplished by placing a wedge (e.g., folded blanket) beneath the right buttock. Alternatively, a gas-powered inflatable device constructed from materials available in most hospitals can be used.[38] The qualitative effectiveness of the technique can be assessed by palpating the right femoral pulse while manually lifting the uterus and displacing it to the left. If the pulse quality increases significantly, the method for left uterine displacement is probably not as efficient as imagined. Some anesthesiologists assess the adequacy of left uterine displacement by monitoring blood pressure or SaO_2 on a lower extremity.

Monitoring

Automated blood pressure cuffs are invaluable for the rapid and frequent determination of blood pressure during cesarean section (Box 25-2). We often place an intra-arterial catheter in patients with severe preeclampsia or cardiovascular disease.

The American Society of Anesthesiologists (ASA) "Standards for Basic Anesthetic Monitoring" require that "a quantitative method of assessing oxygenation such as pulse oximetry" be used during the administration of either regional or general anesthesia for surgery.[39] It is especially important to monitor SaO_2 during the induction of general anesthesia. Likewise, it is important to monitor SaO_2 after the administration of sedative drugs in patients who have received regional anesthesia for cesarean section. Sedation may increase the risk of respiratory arrest during regional anesthesia.[40,41] Gauthier et al.[41] concluded that "the combination of spinal anesthesia and midazolam has a modest synergistic effect on the decrease in tidal volume, minute ventilation, and mean inspiratory flow rate."

The ASA also requires "continual monitoring for the presence of expired carbon dioxide" during the administration of general anesthesia.[39] End-tidal carbon dioxide analysis allows rapid verification of correct placement of the endotracheal tube within the trachea. Failure to detect carbon dioxide should immediately signal the occurrence of esophageal intubation. Anesthesiologists should use a quantitative method of end-tidal carbon dioxide analysis during the administration of general anesthesia for cesarean section. It is best to avoid hyperventilation in pregnant patients (see Chapter 3). Anesthesiologists may also use capnography to monitor respiration during the administration of regional anesthesia.

The ASA requires the continuous display of the electrocardiogram (ECG) during the administration of anesthesia for surgery. Some anesthesiologists have noted the occurrence of ECG changes (e.g., ST-segment depression in the lateral leads) during cesarean section. These changes occur in as many as 25% to 65% of patients, and they are most common after the delivery of the infant.[42-44] In some patients, the ST-segment changes are consistent with changes that occur as a result of myocardial ischemia. The cause or causes of these changes are unclear. Investigators have speculated that acute hypervolemia, tachycardia, venous air embolism, coronary vasospasm, vasopressor administration, and/or amniotic fluid embolism might be responsible. Mathew et al.[43] combined Holter monitoring with transthoracic echocardiography in women who underwent either cesarean or vaginal delivery. The authors observed that ST-segment depression was common during cesarean section and that it did not vary according to the anesthetic technique. However, transthoracic echocardiography did not provide any evidence of regional wall motion abnormalities. Further, the authors did not observe ST-segment depression during vaginal delivery. One study revealed that creatine phosphokinase MB-fraction was negative in women experiencing ST-segment depression at cesarean section.[45] Likewise,

---

Box 25-1   LEFT UTERINE DISPLACEMENT

- Allows adequate venous return
  - Helps maintain maternal cardiac output and blood pressure
  - Avoids increased uterine venous pressure
- Minimizes compression of the aorta
- Prevents a decrease in uterine artery perfusion pressure

Box 25-2   INTRAOPERATIVE MONITORING

- Blood pressure
- Oxygen saturation (pulse oximeter)
- Precordial stethoscope
- End-tidal carbon dioxide
- Electrocardiogram
- Nerve stimulator (during general anesthesia)
- Temperature (during general anesthesia)
- Fetal heart rate

other studies have suggested that these ECG changes do not signal the occurrence of clinically significant myocardial dysfunction.[44] The etiology of these changes remains unclear, and the possibility of transient rate-related subendocardial ischemia has not been completely excluded. Of interest is that baseline maternal heart rate may be predictive of maternal hypotension in patients receiving spinal anesthesia for elective cesarean section.[46]

Some anesthesiologists have called attention to the frequent occurrence of Doppler ultrasonographic evidence of venous air embolism during cesarean section (see Chapter 38).[47-49] Doppler ultrasonography is a sensitive method for the diagnosis of venous air embolism. Unfortunately, it is probably too sensitive, because it detects clinically insignificant emboli as small as 0.1 mL. We do not routinely use Doppler ultrasound to monitor for evidence of venous air embolism during cesarean section; rather, we rely on the triad of chest pain, oxyhemoglobin desaturation, and arrhythmia to diagnose hemodynamically significant venous air embolism.[50] It seems prudent to maintain adequate intravascular volume and to place the patient in 5 to 10 degrees of reverse Trendelenburg position after the start of surgery.[49] It may be prudent to use Doppler ultrasound to look for evidence of venous air embolism in patients with a known intracardiac shunt.

It is unnecessary to measure cardiac output during the administration of anesthesia for most patients undergoing cesarean section. In some patients with severe preeclampsia or cardiovascular disease, the anesthesiologist may place a pulmonary artery catheter to allow for the measurement of filling pressures and cardiac output. In selected cases, noninvasive Doppler ultrasonographic measurement of cardiac output provides helpful information.

When possible, the anesthesiologist should monitor the FHR before, during, and after the administration of anesthesia for cesarean section. If the membranes are intact (e.g., elective cesarean section), Doppler ultrasonography can be used to monitor the FHR until it is time to prepare and drape the abdomen for surgery. If the membranes are ruptured, a fetal scalp ECG electrode can be used to monitor the FHR until delivery. Continuous FHR monitoring allows both the anesthesiologist and the obstetrician to evaluate the effects of maternal position, anesthesia, hypotension, and other drugs on the fetus. Changes in the FHR may prompt pharmacologic therapy; in some cases, such changes may dictate immediate delivery. By contrast, a reassuring FHR tracing allows the obstetrician to perform delivery without haste.[51]

PREVENTION OF MATERNAL COMPLICATIONS

Aspiration

All patients should receive acid aspiration prophylaxis, regardless of the planned anesthetic for cesarean section (see Chapter 30). In one large survey from Sweden, the incidence of aspiration was approximately 15 per 10,000 cases of general anesthesia for cesarean section, which was three times greater than that for patients who received general anesthesia for nonobstetric surgery.[52] Aspiration was the cause of death in one third of the 67 women who died as the result of general anesthesia for obstetric cases in the United States between 1979 and 1990.[3] Although the risk of aspiration is greater during general anesthesia than during regional anesthesia, a patient may still vomit and aspirate gastric contents while receiving regional anesthesia.

Means of preventing aspiration include the following: (1) avoidance of general anesthesia; (2) performance of awake intubation in the patient with a difficult airway; and (3) application of cricoid pressure, rapid-sequence induction of general anesthesia, and intubation with a cuffed endotracheal tube. A few anesthesiologists recommend the use of an orogastric or nasogastric tube to empty the stomach. This is uncomfortable for the awake patient, and it is unlikely that this technique removes all gastric contents. Of course, the anesthesiologist should attempt to empty the stomach after the induction of general anesthesia. At the end of surgery, the anesthesiologist should confirm the full return of neuromuscular function, and the patient should be extubated only when she is awake and responds to verbal commands.

Additional means of prophylaxis include pharmacologic therapy to decrease gastric volume and increase gastric pH. The simplest method is the administration of an oral antacid before the administration of anesthesia. Suspension (e.g., particulate-containing) antacids may cause pulmonary injury similar to that caused by the aspiration of gastric acid and are not recommended.[53] A clear antacid (e.g., 0.3 M sodium citrate) is preferred.[54] Alka-Seltzer Gold and Bicitra both contain sodium citrate as the active ingredient.

The administration of an H_2-receptor antagonist increases gastric pH.[55] Unfortunately, an H_2-receptor antagonist does not alter the pH of existing gastric contents. Rout et al.[56] observed that the intravenous administration of ranitidine 50 mg and the oral administration of sodium citrate 30 mL resulted in a greater increase in gastric pH than the administration of sodium citrate alone, provided at least 30 minutes had elapsed from the time of ranitidine administration until intubation. The combination of ranitidine and sodium citrate reduced the number of patients at risk for acid aspiration at the time of intubation and during extubation.[57]

The proton pump inhibitor omeprazole also reduces gastric acidity. However, one study suggested that it may be less effective than either ranitidine or famotidine.[57] Twice as many patients in the omeprazole group had a gastric pH of 2.5 or less (21% versus 8% and 10%, respectively), and the omeprazole-treated patients also had a greater residual gastric volume. In another study, Stuart et al.[58] concluded the following:

> Ranitidine and omeprazole administered intravenously were equally effective adjuncts to sodium citrate in reducing gastric acidity for emergency Caesarean section. Compared with sodium citrate alone, the addition of either ranitidine, omeprazole or metoclopramide alone did not reduce gastric volume, while small reductions in gastric volume were seen with the addition of metoclopramide and either ranitidine or omeprazole.

Metoclopramide accelerates gastric emptying in nonpregnant patients.[59] At least one study has documented its efficacy during early pregnancy,[60] but it is unclear whether it reliably empties the stomach before the performance of cesarean section at term.[61] Metoclopramide also increases lower esophageal sphincter tone, which may provide some additional protection against the aspiration of gastric contents. Finally, metoclopramide has an antiemetic effect, and many anesthesiologists give it to prevent or treat nausea and vomiting during the administration of regional anesthesia for cesarean section.[62,63] We routinely give metoclopramide to our patients before cesarean section.

Difficult Intubation

The anesthesiologist must perform a careful and thorough evaluation of the airway in every patient who presents for cesarean section (see Chapter 31). The examination should include an assessment of the following: (1) the visibility of the oropharyngeal structures; (2) the hyomental or thyromental distance; and (3) neck (atlantooccipital) mobility.[64] The anesthesiologist should have a definite plan for the management of both the recognized and the unrecognized difficult airway, and this plan should be reviewed frequently. The equipment required for alternative methods of securing the airway should be readily available in all anesthetizing locations.

Hypotension

Hypotension is perhaps the most common complication of regional anesthesia in obstetric patients. Hypotension results from the following: (1) increased venous capacitance and pooling of a major portion of the blood volume in the lower extremities and the splanchnic bed; and (2) decreased systemic vascular resistance. Uteroplacental perfusion depends on maintenance of normal maternal blood pressure. One definition of hypotension in obstetric patients is a decrease in systolic blood pressure of at least 25% or any systolic blood pressure less than 100 mm Hg.[65,66] Hypertensive women may require higher perfusion pressures to maintain adequate uteroplacental blood flow. Maintenance of normal maternal blood pressure during spinal or epidural anesthesia results in better umbilical cord blood gas and acid-base measurements at cesarean delivery.[67] Of course, it is difficult to determine the mother's baseline blood pressure if she has not received prenatal care or if she arrives in active labor. Assessment of the FHR often helps the anesthesiologist assess the effect of a change in blood pressure on uteroplacental perfusion.

Measures to prevent hypotension include the following: (1) administration of fluids before the administration of regional anesthesia; (2) left uterine displacement; and (3) administration of a prophylactic vasopressor. In our practice, ephedrine is the preferred vasopressor for the prophylaxis or treatment of most cases of hypotension in obstetric patients. Laboratory and clinical studies have confirmed that ephedrine maintains or restores uterine blood flow when it is given to maintain or restore maternal blood pressure.[68,69] Tong and Eisenach[70] documented that the presence of functional endothelium alters the vascular response to the vasopressors ephedrine and metaraminol. The authors concluded that "ephedrine may spare uterine perfusion during pregnancy due to more selective constriction of systemic vessels than that caused by metaraminol."

In the past, most obstetric anesthesiologists have avoided the administration of an alpha-adrenergic agonist, because laboratory studies suggest that these agents increase uterine vascular resistance and reduce uteroplacental perfusion. However, clinical studies have suggested that small doses of an alpha-adrenergic agonist (e.g., 20 to 40 μg of intravenous phenylephrine) may be given safely for the prevention or treatment of hypotension during the administration of regional anesthesia for cesarean section.[71,72] Lee et al.[73] recently performed a quantitative, systematic review of randomized controlled trials of ephedrine versus phenylephrine for the treatment of hypotension during spinal anesthesia for cesarean section. The authors made the following observations: (1) there was no difference between phenylephrine and ephedrine for the prevention and treatment of maternal hypotension; (2) maternal bradycardia was more likely to occur with phenylephrine than with ephedrine; (3) neonates whose mothers received phenylephrine had higher umbilical arterial blood pH measurements than those whose mothers received ephedrine; and (4) there was no difference between the two vasopressors in the incidence of true fetal acidosis (i.e., umbilical arterial blood pH measurements < 7.2). The authors concluded that their systematic review "does not support the traditional idea that ephedrine is the preferred choice for the management of maternal hypotension during spinal anesthesia for elective cesarean section in healthy, nonlaboring women."[73] Subsequently, Cooper et al.[74] performed a randomized, double-blind study of ephedrine versus phenylephrine for the treatment of maternal hypotension during spinal anesthesia for cesarean section. The authors observed more cases of fetal acidosis in women who received ephedrine than in those who received phenylephrine. These observations are somewhat puzzling given the laboratory evidence that ephedrine protects uteroplacental perfusion better than phenylephrine. Ephedrine crosses the placenta and increases the FHR.[75] Cooper et al.[74] speculated that "increased fetal metabolic rate, secondary to ephedrine-induced beta-adrenergic stimulation, [is] the most likely mechanism for the increased incidence of acidosis in the ephedrine group." However, the preponderance of evidence suggests that ephedrine does not adversely affect neonatal outcome.[75]

Nonetheless, in our practice, ephedrine remains the preferred vasopressor agent for the treatment of most episodes of maternal hypotension, in part because of its ease of use and its long history of safety for both mother and baby. An alpha-adrenergic agonist is preferred in those patients who may not tolerate tachycardia caused by ephedrine (e.g., patients with mitral stenosis or asymmetric septal hypertrophy).

Many anesthesiologists believe that the prophylactic administration of ephedrine helps prevent the hemodynamic consequences that accompany the rapid onset of sympathectomy during spinal anesthesia (Figure 25-2).[76-85] Studies have demonstrated that prophylactic intramuscular ephedrine decreases the incidence of hypotension associated with spinal anesthesia[76] but not that associated with epidural anesthesia.[77] Loughrey et al.[78] evaluated the efficacy and dose-response

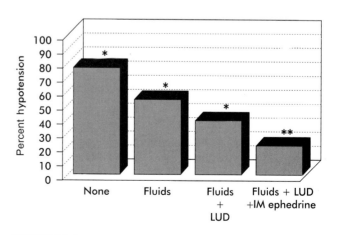

FIGURE 25-2. Efficacy of hypotension prophylaxis during administration of spinal anesthesia for cesarean section. *LUD,* Left uterine displacement. (*Modified from Clark RB, Thompson CH. Prevention of spinal hypotension associated with cesarean section. Anesthesiology 1976; 45:670-4; **Modified from Gutsche B. Prophylactic ephedrine preceding spinal analgesia for cesarean section. Anesthesiology 1976; 45:462-5.)

of prophylactic intravenous ephedrine for the prevention of maternal hypotension during the administration of spinal anesthesia for cesarean section, and they concluded that a prophylactic intravenous bolus of 12 mg of ephedrine (followed by rescue boluses as needed) results in a lower incidence of hypotension than the administration of rescue doses of ephedrine alone. Simon et al.[79] observed that a single 15- or 20-mg bolus dose of intravenous ephedrine decreased the incidence of maternal hypotension more effectively than a single 10-mg dose. However, Ngan Kee et al.[80] observed that the smallest effective prophylactic dose of ephedrine was 30 mg. Even this dose did not completely eliminate hypotension, nausea, vomiting, and fetal acidosis, and it caused reactive hypertension in some patients.

Other studies have suggested that the prophylactic intravenous administration of modest doses of ephedrine is *not* effective for the prevention of spinal hypotension.[81] Lee et al.[85] performed a quantitative systematic review of the efficacy and safety of prophylactic ephedrine to prevent hypotension during spinal anesthesia for cesarean delivery. The authors concluded that prophylactic ephedrine is more effective than control for preventing hypotension during spinal anesthesia for elective cesarean delivery, but they did not confirm a clinically relevant positive effect on neonatal outcome. The authors concluded that published studies do not support the routine use of prophylactic ephedrine to prevent adverse effects of maternal hypotension during the administration of spinal anesthesia for cesarean delivery. Nonetheless, some anesthesiologists continue to advocate the administration of 25 to 50 mg of ephedrine intramuscularly before the administration of spinal anesthesia or 5 to 10 mg of ephedrine intravenously immediately after the intrathecal injection of a local anesthetic. We do not administer prophylactic ephedrine unless the patient has a low baseline blood pressure (i.e., systolic blood pressure less than 105 mm Hg) before the administration of spinal anesthesia.

During the administration of regional anesthesia for cesarean section, hypotension is more likely to occur in women who are not in labor than in women who are in labor.[77] The treatment of hypotension includes the following: (1) exaggerated left uterine displacement; (2) administration of additional intravenous fluids; (3) intravenous administration of ephedrine in bolus doses of 5 to 10 mg; and (4) administration of supplemental oxygen.[72]

High Spinal Anesthesia

High or total spinal anesthesia may occur as the result of an unintentional intrathecal injection of an epidural dose of local anesthetic or extensive rostral spread of a subarachnoid block. The likelihood of an intended epidural dose leading to high spinal anesthesia is approximately 1 in 50,000.[86] The manifestations include complete sensory and motor blockade and hypotension, bradycardia, unconsciousness, loss of protective airway reflexes, and respiratory arrest. As devastating as this situation may appear, prompt intervention by the anesthesiologist should prevent any significant or lasting sequelae. Treatment includes endotracheal intubation, positive-pressure ventilation with 100% oxygen, and maintenance of maternal circulation (e.g., left uterine displacement, elevation of the legs, intravenous administration of ephedrine and fluids). The anesthesiologist should not hesitate to give epinephrine if a compromised patient does not respond to initial doses of ephedrine.

During the administration of epidural anesthesia, the anesthesiologist should administer a test dose to exclude unintentional subarachnoid injection of local anesthetic. The test dose should contain a dose of local anesthetic that is capable of producing a detectable but not excessive level of spinal anesthesia (e.g., 30 to 60 mg of lidocaine, 7.5 to 10 mg of bupivacaine). The anesthesiologist should wait an adequate time (e.g., 3 to 5 minutes) before concluding that the test dose is negative.

During the administration of epidural anesthesia, an unexpected high block may result from subdural (i.e., epiarachnoid) placement of the catheter (see Chapter 21). The management of this complication is similar to that for high or total spinal anesthesia.[87] Further use of the catheter should be abandoned, because appropriate doses of either local anesthetics or opioids have not been established for this route of administration.

Local Anesthetic Toxicity

Central nervous system and cardiovascular toxicity may occur if an epidural dose of local anesthetic is injected unintentionally into an epidural vein; convulsions, unconsciousness, arrhythmias, and cardiovascular collapse may ensue. The treatment of local anesthetic toxicity is similar to that for total spinal anesthesia, but more potent cardiac stimulation with epinephrine, as well as closed-chest cardiac massage and defibrillation, may be required. Resuscitation may prove to be quite difficult if bupivacaine is the local anesthetic, because some evidence suggests that pregnancy enhances the cardiovascular toxicity of bupivacaine.[88] Polymorphic undulating ventricular tachycardia may occur.[89]

The prevention of local anesthetic toxicity includes the administration of a test dose to help exclude the unintentional intravenous injection of local anesthetic. Many anesthesiologists include a small dose (e.g., 15 µg) of **epinephrine** as a marker of intravenous injection.[90] Unfortunately, cyclic changes in maternal heart rate during labor complicate the interpretation of the epinephrine test dose.[91,92] In addition, some anesthesiologists fear that the intravenous injection of epinephrine may decrease uteroplacental perfusion and precipitate fetal distress. Fortunately, the decreased uteroplacental perfusion is transient, and no evidence suggests that the intravenous injection of 15 µg of epinephrine adversely affects fetal and neonatal outcome.[93]

Some anesthesiologists have suggested the use of **isoproterenol** as an alternative marker of intravascular injection. Small doses of isoproterenol reliably produce maternal tachycardia, with little or no decrease in uterine blood flow.[94,95] Isoproterenol is not packaged in a convenient format for use as a test dose; it must be diluted and added to the local anesthetic solution. Further, there are few data regarding the toxicology of the epidural or spinal injection of isoproterenol.[96]

Leighton and Gross[97] have suggested the use of **air** as a test dose. They inject 1 or 2 mL of air epidurally, and they use a precordial Doppler ultrasound probe to detect unintentional intravenous injection. In our judgment, this method is inconvenient and not suitable for routine clinical use.

We inject an epinephrine-containing test dose through the epidural catheter, and then we use the ECG and/or pulse oximeter to look for a change in maternal heart rate. If unequivocal maternal tachycardia occurs, we remove the catheter and replace it at an alternative interspace. If maternal tachycardia does *not* occur, we evaluate the patient for the presence of spinal anesthesia 3 to 5 minutes after the injection of the test dose. (We also test for a narrow, three- to four-segment band of epidural analgesia.) After we have determined that spinal anesthesia has not occurred, we administer the therapeutic dose of local anesthetic in incremental bolus doses. Of course, we aspirate before giving each dose of local anesthetic.

If the patient has an equivocal episode of tachycardia within 60 seconds of receiving the test dose, we aspirate again. If aspiration is negative, we administer a second test dose 3 to 5 minutes later. If that second test dose is negative, we proceed with the incremental injection of the therapeutic dose. In reality, every dose should be considered a test dose; the anesthesiologist should continuously observe for evidence of systemic toxicity. It is important to maintain continual verbal contact with the patient during and after the administration of a local anesthetic.

Failed Regional Anesthesia

Common causes of **failed spinal anesthesia** include the following: (1) omission of the local anesthetic from the drug mixture; (2) administration of an inadequate dose of local anesthetic; (3) placement of the drug in a space other than the subarachnoid space; (4) pooling of a hyperbaric drug with lack of cephalad spread (usually associated with use of the sitting position or injection in a dural root sleeve); and (5) on rare occasions, a low-potency drug lot.

Management depends on the clinical circumstances and patient preference. If delivery is urgent or if the patient does not wish to undergo a second attempt at spinal anesthesia, general anesthesia may be administered. Failed spinal anesthesia, followed by the administration of general anesthesia, occurs in approximately 1% of the cases of planned spinal anesthesia for cesarean section at our institution. If delivery is not urgent, the anesthesiologist may perform a second spinal anesthetic. A patient should be encouraged to accept another attempt at spinal anesthesia if she has a difficult airway or a medical condition that would make general anesthesia a poor choice. If there is evidence of little or no anesthesia, we give the same dose of local anesthetic as that used for the first attempt. Case reports and laboratory studies have suggested that the maldistribution of local anesthetic may be responsible for cases of persistent neurologic injury (e.g., cauda equina syndrome) after the administration of continuous spinal anesthesia with hyperbaric lidocaine.[98,99] It is unclear whether these concerns apply to the administration of single-shot spinal anesthesia.[84] Nonetheless, it seems prudent to look for evidence of sacral block before performing a second spinal anesthetic. Evidence of sacral blockade suggests that the maldistribution of local anesthetic may be the cause of the failed spinal anesthesia; thus the anesthesiologist should alter the patient's position during and after the administration of a second spinal anesthetic.

Failed epidural anesthesia occurs in approximately 2% to 6% of cases.[101] A failed epidural anesthetic may fall into one of two categories. The attempt may produce no anesthesia at all, in which case the catheter most likely is not in the epidural space. Alternatively, the patient may have patchy, incomplete epidural anesthesia that is inadequate for cesarean delivery. Causes of failure include the following: (1) displacement of the catheter from the epidural space; (2) malposition of the catheter within the epidural space; (3) anatomic barriers to the diffusion of local anesthetic[102,103]; and (4) administration of an inadequate concentration and/or volume of local anesthetic.

In cases of failed epidural anesthesia, the epidural anesthetic can be repeated or spinal or general anesthesia can be given as dictated by clinical circumstances and patient preference. Often it is helpful for the obstetrician to inject several milliliters of local anesthetic into the affected area in patients with evidence of a partial block. Performance of a second epidural procedure also is reasonable. However, a large dose of local anesthetic often has already been administered, and the anesthesiologist must be alert for signs of local anesthetic toxicity. In addition, much time has elapsed, and the obstetrician, anesthesiologist, and patient often become impatient. In these cases, the administration of spinal anesthesia is an attractive alternative. There are two potential problems with this approach. First, the spinal needle may encounter a collection of local anesthetic solution within the epidural space. The anesthesiologist may presume that the local anesthetic solution represents cerebrospinal fluid (CSF) and may inject the spinal drug epidurally. To our knowledge, no one has documented the incidence of this problem. However, there are several reports of a second and more serious problem: high spinal anesthesia.[104,105] Presumably, the large volume of local anesthetic within the epidural space results in a decreased volume in the lumbar subarachnoid space, which predisposes the patient to high spinal anesthesia. In our hospital, approximately 5% of planned epidural anesthetics require conversion to spinal anesthesia for cesarean section. We have observed that high spinal anesthesia occurred in three of 27 (11%) of these patients.[105] Physicians should thus exercise caution when giving spinal anesthesia after failed epidural anesthesia.

Persistent Neurologic Deficit

Persistent neurologic deficit is rare after the proper administration of spinal or epidural anesthesia. The unintentional subarachnoid injection of a large dose of 2-chloroprocaine (Nesacaine-CE) has resulted in several cases of persistent neurologic deficit.[106,107] Subsequent investigations suggested that the antioxidant sodium (meta)bisulfite and the low pH of the solution were responsible.[108] However, a recent study suggested that bisulfite was the "scapegoat" for 2-chloroprocaine neurotoxicity.[109] Current preparations of 2-chloroprocaine (Nesacaine-MPF) have a higher pH and contain no antioxidant or preservatives.

GENERAL CONSIDERATIONS

Supplemental oxygen should be administered to improve maternal and fetal oxygenation during administration of either general or regional anesthesia.[110] Supplemental oxygen may also reduce the frequency and severity of maternal nausea during regional anesthesia.[111] One of the arguments for providing supplemental oxygen to the mother during cesarean section is to optimize neonatal outcome. However, the need for routine administration of supplemental oxygen during elective cesarean section has become a matter of some dispute.[112-114] Khaw et al.[112] assessed the effects of a high-inspired oxygen fraction during elective caesarean section with spinal anaesthesia on maternal and fetal oxygenation and lipid peroxidation. The authors observed that breathing a high-inspired concentration of oxygen caused a modest increase in fetal oxygenation but also caused a concomitant increase in oxygen free-radical activity in both the mother and fetus.[112] The clinical relevance of the increase in oxygen free-radical activity is unclear, and further investigation seems warranted. Maternal comfort during oxygen administration is also an issue. Cogliano et al.[114] assessed the acceptability of oxygen administered by face mask versus nasal cannulae. The authors found that the use of the face mask impeded communication, and they concluded that nasal cannulae may be a "more patient-acceptable" method of providing supplemental oxygen.

The presence of a support person (e.g., the father of the baby) currently is standard practice in most hospitals in the United States. This individual often makes a significant contribution to the comfort of the awake patient who has received regional anesthesia, and he or she may provide effective emotional support and may serve as a translator in cases of language difficulty. This person is not present to watch surgery, videotape neonatal resuscitation, or assist during the administration of general anesthesia. Some anesthesiologists prefer to first administer regional anesthesia and then invite the support individual into the operating room just before the start of surgery. It should be emphasized that the guest must leave the operating room immediately on the request of medical personnel; this may be necessary if the patient has inadequate regional anesthesia and requires the administration of general anesthesia.

Once the infant is delivered and the umbilical cord is clamped, oxytocin should be administered to hasten uterine involution and reduce blood loss.[115] Bolus intravenous administration of oxytocin may cause maternal hypotension and tachycardia and should be avoided.[116] Rather, the anesthesiologist should place 10 to 20 U of oxytocin in 1000 mL of crystalloid and administer 40 to 80 mU/min.

If uterine atony does not respond to oxytocin infusion, an ergot preparation (e.g., methylergonovine 0.2 mg intramuscularly) or a prostaglandin (e.g., 15-methyl prostaglandin $F_{2-alpha}$ 250 μg intramuscularly or intramyometrially) may be required. Ergot derivatives exert a tetanic uterotonic effect. These drugs may produce severe hypertension, especially when given after a vasopressor.[117] Rarely, these drugs may precipitate myocardial ischemia or a cerebrovascular accident.[118] Methylergonovine should be given intravenously only in cases of life-threatening hemorrhage, and it should be given slowly, over a period of 60 seconds or longer.

The most commonly used prostaglandin is carboprost tromethamine (15-methyl prostaglandin $F_{2-alpha}$). Side effects of this drug include nausea, vomiting, diarrhea, fever, tachypnea, tachycardia, hypertension, and bronchoconstriction.[119] This agent is best avoided in patients with asthma.

After delivery, many obstetricians prefer to exteriorize the uterus, because this maneuver allows for excellent exposure of the uterine incision during closure. Unfortunately, it also results in traction on the peritoneum, which often results in pain and/or nausea during regional anesthesia or hemodynamic changes during general anesthesia. It is unclear why manipulation of the viscera results in discomfort in patients with a high level of sensory blockade.[100] Uterine exteriorization also may increase the incidence of venous air embolism.[48]

Sedation may be required during cesarean delivery with regional anesthesia, for a variety of reasons (e.g., anxiety, nausea, discomfort from the procedure, sensation of pressure or tugging, "restless legs" or attempted movement in the presence of motor blockade, discomfort from lying on the operating table). We try to avoid the administration of sedative drugs before delivery of the infant. Reassurance and encouragement are often adequate, but there are times when phar-

macologic intervention is appropriate. The inhalation of analgesic concentrations (e.g., 40% to 50%) of nitrous oxide in oxygen is often sufficient and does not result in neonatal depression. Low-dose ketamine (0.25 mg/kg) provides some analgesia (and perhaps amnesia) without compromising maternal reflexes or the neonate. Small doses of fentanyl (50 to 100 μg) may be administered intravenously, if required. Likewise, alfentanil or remifentanil may prove useful in this situation, although these drugs have undergone little evaluation in obstetric patients.[121] Metoclopramide, ondansetron, or a small dose of droperidol may be given to treat nausea,[62,63,122] and a small dose of a benzodiazepine can be given to treat maternal anxiety and restlessness. We prefer to delay administration of a benzodiazepine until after delivery. (Some anesthesiologists have suggested the use of music to decrease intraoperative requirements for sedative drugs in awake patients.[123] To our knowledge, no study has evaluated the use of intraoperative music for patients undergoing cesarean section. It is possible that the reassurance provided by the baby's father or another support person may be more helpful than music.)

Often it is difficult for an anesthesiologist to acknowledge that regional anesthesia is inadequate for surgery. It is essential that the patient remain responsive to verbal commands and retain all protective airway reflexes. Aggressive attempts to provide sedation and supplemental analgesia can easily lead to a state equivalent to general anesthesia. This places the patient at risk for hypoventilation, airway obstruction, and pulmonary aspiration of gastric contents. If modest sedation and small doses of an analgesic prove inadequate, it is more prudent and much safer to acknowledge the inadequacy of regional anesthesia and administer general anesthesia. If regional anesthesia is inadequate but delivery is imminent, it is reasonable to allow the obstetrician to accomplish the delivery. After the infant is delivered, the anesthesiologist should proceed with general anesthesia. Of course, this should include the application of cricoid pressure, rapid-sequence induction, and intubation with a cuffed endotracheal tube.

Standards and methods of postanesthesia recovery should be identical to those used for patients who undergo surgery in the main operating suite of the hospital. The monitoring capabilities, level of training of personnel, and emergency equipment should be equivalent. Patient recovery may take place in a specified postanesthesia care unit or in a patient room, as long as the care provided is equivalent to that provided elsewhere in the hospital. If a patient requires ventilatory support, some anesthesiologists prefer to transfer that patient to the postanesthesia care unit in the main operating suite.

CHOICE OF ANESTHETIC TECHNIQUE

The anesthesiologist should consider the indication for cesarean section (Box 25-3), the urgency of the procedure, the health of the mother and fetus, and the desires of the mother. Spinal anesthesia is an appropriate choice for most elective and urgent cesarean sections in patients without preexisting epidural anesthesia. Often it is possible to extend preexisting epidural anesthesia for emergency cesarean section. In addition, epidural anesthesia is preferred when physicians want to minimize the likelihood of maternal hypotension[124] or when intense motor blockade of the thoracoabdominal segments is not desired (e.g., in patients with respiratory compromise).

Box 25-3 INDICATIONS FOR CESAREAN SECTION

- Repeat cesarean section
  - Scheduled
  - Failed attempt at vaginal delivery
- Dystocia
- Abnormal presentation
  - Transverse lie
  - Breech presentation
  - Multiple gestation
- Fetal stress/distress
- Deteriorating maternal medical illness
  - Preeclampsia
  - Heart disease
  - Pulmonary disease
- Hemorrhage
  - Placenta previa
  - Placental abruption

Box 25-4 SPINAL ANESTHESIA FOR CESAREAN SECTION

- Metoclopramide 10 mg intravenously
- Clear antacid orally
- Intravascular volume expansion with Ringer's lactate or normal saline (15-20 mL/kg)
- Application of monitors
- Supplemental oxygen by face mask or nasal prongs
- Prophylactic intramuscular ephedrine (25-50 mg) in patients with a baseline systolic blood pressure of less than 105 mm Hg
- Lumbar puncture at L3-L4
  - Right lateral or sitting position
- 25- or 24-gauge Sprotte needle or 27- or 25-gauge Whitacre needle
- Bupivacaine 12 mg in 8.25% dextrose
  - Morphine 0.1-0.25 mg for postoperative analgesia
- Left uterine displacement
- Aggressive treatment of hypotension
  - Exaggerated left uterine displacement
  - Intravenous fluids
  - Ephedrine and/or low-dose phenylephrine

The choice of anesthesia is more difficult in cases of fetal stress and distress (see Chapter 26). Obstetricians worry that the anesthesiologist may not be able to provide regional anesthesia with sufficient speed to allow for a timely delivery or that regional anesthesia may result in hypotension and impaired uteroplacental perfusion. Clinical studies suggest that the administration of regional anesthesia does not result in increased risk to the fetus, even in cases of modest fetal distress.[125,126] However, general anesthesia is indicated for a stat cesarean section when time is of the essence. In all cases, the anesthesiologist and obstetrician must weigh the severity of fetal compromise against the maternal risks of general anesthesia.

The choice of anesthetic technique for patients with a medical illness depends on the nature of the disorder and the maternal condition. Severe maternal hemorrhage typically dictates the administration of general anesthesia (see Chapter 37). It is acceptable to administer regional anesthesia in patients with a diagnosis of placenta previa who show no evidence of hypovolemia. The anesthesiologist must be ready to replace significant blood loss, because these patients are at risk for bleeding from the lower uterine segment implantation site and placenta accreta.[127,128]

Local anesthesia (e.g., abdominal field block) rarely may be advantageous when anesthesia personnel are unavailable to administer anesthesia for emergency cesarean section. Likewise, local anesthesia may be advantageous for the patient with debilitating disease or for the patient who is in extremis. Local anesthesia also may be a valuable adjunct in some patients with incomplete epidural or spinal anesthesia.

Spinal Anesthesia

Spinal anesthesia offers the advantages of simplicity, rapid onset, and dense neural blockade. It is associated with negligible maternal risk of systemic local anesthetic toxicity, minimal transfer of drug to the infant, and negligible risk of local anesthetic depression of the infant.[129] Many anesthesiologists contend that spinal anesthesia results in a better quality of anesthesia than does epidural anesthesia. It is especially well suited for the patient undergoing elective cesarean section and for many cases of emergency cesarean section (e.g., in patients with dystocia or a footling breech presentation). The introduction of noncutting, pencil-point spinal needles has significantly reduced the incidence of postdural puncture headache in obstetric patients.

Most spinal anesthetics are administered as a single injection procedure. Although the rapid onset of anesthesia is often advantageous, the rapid onset of sympathetic blockade may result in abrupt, severe hypotension. If surgery is longer than anticipated, supplemental analgesia or general anesthesia may be required. However, if the procedure is shorter than anticipated, the recovery time may be prolonged. There is limited published experience with continuous spinal anesthesia, which allows for the administration of spinal anesthesia for prolonged surgery.[130]

TECHNIQUE

We give 30 mL of 0.3 M sodium citrate to increase gastric fluid pH (Box 25-4). In most patients, we give metoclopramide 10 mg intravenously to prevent nausea. Whenever it is possible, a bolus (15 to 20 mL/kg) of Ringer's lactate or other balanced salt solution is given intravenously shortly before the block is administered. On occasion, we administer 25 to 50 mg of ephedrine into the deltoid muscle to help prevent hypotension in patients with a low baseline blood pressure (i.e., systolic blood pressure less than 105 mm Hg). We also give supplemental oxygen by face mask to all patients receiving spinal (or epidural) anesthesia for cesarean section.

We often perform spinal anesthesia with the patient in the right lateral decubitus position. This helps ensure the presence of a similar level of anesthesia bilaterally, given the fact that the patient will be positioned with a wedge beneath her right hip.[131] The parturient's enlarged hips tend to tilt the spinal column in a head-down direction, which favors the more cephalad spread of a hyperbaric drug. This results in a more rapid onset of sensory block to the sixth thoracic dermatome and may lead to an earlier decline in blood pressure.[132] We use the sitting position if landmarks cannot be palpated easily in the lateral position or when speed is important. (Of interest, Yun et al.[133] observed that the severity and duration of hypotension were greater when combined spinal-epidural [CSE] anesthesia for cesarean section was administered in the sitting position as compared with the administration of CSE anesthesia in the lateral position. The reason for this difference was unclear.)

Lumbar puncture is performed at the L3 to L4 or the L2 to L3 interspace. The choice of needle is a matter of individual preference. We use a small-gauge pencil-point needle (usually 24- to 27-gauge Sprotte or Pencan needle) to minimize the likelihood of a postdural puncture headache (PDPH).[133-136]

Pregnant women require less local anesthetic to achieve a given level of anesthesia than do nonpregnant women. Both mechanical and hormonal factors are likely responsible for the decreased local anesthetic dose requirements during pregnancy.[137] The selection of a local anesthetic, with or without adjuvant drugs, depends on the anticipated duration of surgery, the plan for postoperative analgesia, and the preference of the anesthesiologist (Table 25-1).

Among the ester-linked local anesthetic agents are procaine (Novocain) and tetracaine (Pontocaine). Procaine has rapid onset, but the duration of surgical anesthesia is only 30 to 60 minutes. Tetracaine is a more potent agent, with an onset of 5 to 10 minutes and a duration of approximately 120 minutes. Some anesthesiologists combine procaine and tetracaine to gain both a rapid onset and a long duration.[138]

The amide local anesthetic lidocaine (Xylocaine) has been used for spinal anesthesia for cesarean section because of its rapid onset and short duration of action (45 to 75 minutes). However, some anesthesiologists now avoid the use of hyperbaric lidocaine for spinal anesthesia because of concern about the association between hyperbaric lidocaine and transient neurologic symptoms (see Chapter 12).

Spinal bupivacaine (Marcaine, Sensorcaine) has a rapid onset of action similar to lidocaine but a duration intermediate between lidocaine and tetracaine. Patients have a faster recovery with bupivacaine than with tetracaine, because the motor blockade resolves simultaneously with the sensory blockade.[139]

Ropivacaine (Naropin) is an amide local anesthetic agent with a duration intermediate between lidocaine and tetrocaine.[140] Ropivacaine is less potent than bupivacaine when given for spinal anesthesia.[141] Khaw et al.[142] randomized 72 patients undergoing elective cesarean section to receive CSE anesthesia with 10, 15, 20, or 25 mg of spinal ropivacaine diluted to 3 mL with normal saline. The authors concluded that ropivacaine was a "suitable agent" for spinal anesthesia for cesarean delivery, and they determined that the effective dose to produce 50% response and the effective dose to produce 95% response for spinal ropivacaine were 16.7 and 26.8 mg, respectively.[142] Subsequently, these investigators observed that hyperbaric spinal ropivacaine (25 mg) produced a more rapid block with faster recovery and fewer requirements for supplemental epidural anesthesia than did the same dose of plain ropivacaine in women receiving spinal anesthesia for elective cesarean section.

The newest local anesthetic agent in obstetric anesthesia practice is levobupivacaine (Chirocaine), which is the pure S(−)-enantiomer of racemic bupivacaine. Clinical studies have established that the dose-response for spinal levobupivacaine is similar to that for racemic bupivacaine.[144-146] In a randomized, double-blind, crossover study, Alley et al.[146] concluded that levobupivacaine has equivalent clinical effi-

cacy to racemic bupivacaine when given intrathecally in volunteers in doses from 4 to 12 mg.

In most cases, anesthesiologists administer these local anesthetics as hyperbaric solutions. The quality of the block may be enhanced by the addition of epinephrine.[147] Epinephrine also prolongs the duration of tetracaine spinal anesthesia by 30% to 50%. Some controversy exists as to whether epinephrine prolongs the duration of spinal anesthesia with lidocaine or bupivacaine.[148,149]

Some anesthesiologists alter the dose of a drug according to the height or weight of the patient. Others give a single, fixed dose for the majority of obstetric patients. We favor the latter approach and give 12 mg of hyperbaric bupivacaine, 60 mg of hyperbaric lidocaine, or 9 mg of hyperbaric tetracaine. The dose is decreased slightly for very short patients, and it is increased slightly if the block is performed in the sitting position. **Bupivacaine** remains our preferred local anesthetic for most patients undergoing cesarean section. We frequently include 10 to 20 μg of fentanyl to enhance the quality of the block[150] and a small dose (0.1 to 0.25 mg) of preservative-free morphine to provide postoperative analgesia. Alternatively, some anesthesiologists administer intrathecal meperidine 80 to 100 mg as a single agent for spinal anesthesia for cesarean section. With this regimen, the patient may have effective analgesia for as long as 6 hours after surgery.[151]

After the drug(s) is(are) injected and the needle is removed, the patient is placed supine with left uterine displacement. We typically give supplemental oxygen by face mask, but we use nasal cannulae when the patient will not accept the face mask. The blood pressure and heart rate are determined every minute for the next 10 minutes, because hypotension, tachycardia, or bradycardia may occur suddenly. If a fetal scalp ECG electrode is not in place, the FHR should be monitored by Doppler ultrasonography before the abdomen is prepared for surgery. Spinal anesthesia may result in a decrease in maternal cardiac output before delivery; cardiac output typically increases after the uterus is emptied. However, modest hypotension and tachycardia may occur during the administration of oxytocin after delivery.[152,153] These changes do not represent a threat to the healthy patient, but they may cause adverse sequelae in the patient with cardiovascular disease.

Initially, the operating table should be level, or it should be adjusted to achieve a slight degree of Trendelenburg position. This should result in a sensory level of approximately T4 in most patients. (A mid- or high-thoracic level is required even though the obstetrician will perform a lower abdominal skin incision. Traction on the peritoneum and uterine exteriorization frequently cause discomfort during surgery.) The patient may complain of dyspnea with the onset of a high-thoracic sensory level of anesthesia. Dense motor blockade of the abdominal muscles and some of the intercostal muscles typically occurs. The patient also loses her sense of thoracic proprioception, and she does not feel her chest rise and fall. In addition, the enlarged uterus pushes the abdominal contents against the diaphragm, which increases the work of breathing in the supine position. If the patient can speak clearly in a normal voice, it is unlikely that there is ventilatory compromise. Sedative or opioid drugs should not be administered to allay the feeling of dyspnea unless the intent is to intubate the patient. Rarely a patient with a macrosomic infant or multiple gestation may experience clinically significant respiratory distress even though the level of anesthesia is within the desired range. We have found that gentle bag-and-mask ventilation

TABLE 25-1	DRUGS USED FOR SPINAL ANESTHESIA FOR CESAREAN SECTION	
Drug	Dosage range (mg)	Duration (min)
Lidocaine	60-75	45-75
Bupivacaine	7.5-15.0	60-120
Tetracaine	7.0-10.0	120-180
Procaine	100-150	30-60
Adjuvant drugs		
Epinephrine	0.1-0.2	—
Morphine	0.1-0.25	360-1080
Fentanyl	0.010-0.025	180-240

with oxygen provides welcomed relief until delivery; the respiratory distress typically disappears after the uterus is emptied. If there is any doubt about the status of the patient's protective airway reflexes or her ability to maintain ventilation, an endotracheal tube should be inserted after performing a rapid-sequence induction of general anesthesia.

Epidural Anesthesia

The popularity of epidural anesthesia for cesarean section has increased during the last two decades, in part because of the more frequent use of epidural analgesia during labor. With epidural anesthesia, the local anesthetic agent gains access to the nerve roots in the region of the dural cuffs by absorption through the arachnoid villi that penetrate the dura in this location.[154] Therefore, the spread of anesthesia is volume dependent and not related to specific gravity differences between the local anesthetic solution and the CSF. With epidural anesthesia, a solution of local anesthetic with a much larger volume than that used for spinal anesthesia is necessary. In addition, the absolute dose is 5 to 10 times greater than that used for spinal anesthesia.

One of the major advantages of epidural anesthesia is that the local anesthetic agent can be administered in incremental doses and that the total dose can be titrated to the desired sensory level. This, coupled with the slower onset of anesthesia, allows the maternal cardiovascular system to compensate for the occurrence of sympathetic blockade. The result is a decreased risk of severe hypotension and a decreased risk of reduced uteroplacental perfusion. This makes epidural anesthesia the anesthetic technique of choice for many women with severe preeclampsia or cardiovascular disease.

The use of a continuous technique allows the anesthesiologist to give additional local anesthetic to maintain anesthesia, regardless of the duration of surgery. Epidural anesthesia results in less-intense motor blockade than does spinal anesthesia. This is advantageous for patients with multiple gestation or pulmonary disease. (In these patients, a high level of motor blockade may impair ventilation.) In addition, the lower extremity "muscle pump" may remain intact, which may reduce the incidence of thromboembolic disease. The anesthesiologist may give an opioid through the epidural catheter to provide postoperative analgesia. PDPH should not occur unless unintentional dural puncture occurs. The frequency of unintentional dural puncture is 1 in 200 to 1 in 500 cases in experienced hands.[155] Admittedly, a higher incidence of unintentional dural puncture occurs in training institutions. Unfortunately, if unintentional dural puncture occurs with a 16- or 18-gauge epidural needle, the incidence of PDPH is 50% to 85%.[156,157]

The slower onset of epidural anesthesia is disadvantageous in some situations (e.g., a patient with a footling breech presentation and active labor). After giving the test dose, the anesthesiologist must wait 3 to 5 minutes before giving the therapeutic dose in incremental bolus doses. Depending on the local anesthetic that has been chosen, another 10 to 20 minutes are required before the onset of surgical anesthesia. Epidural anesthesia requires the administration of large doses of local anesthetic, which results in some risk of systemic local anesthetic toxicity. The epidural needle or catheter may enter an epidural vein in as many as 9% of pregnant women.[158] In addition, an epidural catheter subsequently may migrate into a blood vessel during labor or surgery. Thus, the anesthesiologist must aspirate before giving each dose of local

anesthetic, and each dose should be considered a test dose. Finally, the systemic absorption of the local anesthetic results in a greater placental transfer of drug than occurs with spinal anesthesia. However, this does not affect neonatal neurobehavior and is of little clinical significance when appropriate doses are administered.[159]

Unintentional subarachnoid injection of a large dose of local anesthetic results in high or total spinal anesthesia. Prompt maternal resuscitation should prevent maternal mortality. Resuscitation should include the following: (1) intubation with a cuffed endotracheal tube; (2) positive-pressure ventilation with 100% oxygen; (3) left uterine displacement; (4) administration of fluids and vasopressors as needed to support maternal circulation; and (5) aspiration and lavage of the subarachnoid space.[160] In some cases, it may be necessary for the obstetrician to empty the uterus (i.e., immediate cesarean section) to facilitate maternal resuscitation.

TECHNIQUE

Patient preparation and monitoring are similar to that used for spinal anesthesia (Box 25-5). We give a similar bolus (15 to 20 mL/kg) of crystalloid intravenously. When extending epidural anesthesia established during labor, we give a smaller bolus of crystalloid. Because epidural anesthesia results in a slower onset of sympathetic blockade, we do not administer prophylactic ephedrine.

Chapter 11 includes a detailed discussion of the technique that is used to identify the epidural space. Although it is possible to give both the test and therapeutic doses of local anesthetic through the needle, most anesthesiologists prefer to place a catheter and use a continuous technique. The catheter is gently aspirated to look for the presence of blood or CSF; a test dose of local anesthetic is then administered. Because we include 15 µg of epinephrine in the test dose, we look for immediate evidence of tachycardia or hypertension, which signals intravenous injection of the test dose. We also question the patient for symptoms of intravenous injection of local anesthetic. We then wait 3 to 5 minutes before looking for evidence of spinal anesthesia.

We believe that the test dose should be administered through the epidural catheter rather than through the needle

---

Box 25-5 EPIDURAL ANESTHESIA FOR CESAREAN SECTION

- Metoclopramide 10 mg intravenously
- Clear antacid orally
- Intravascular volume expansion with Ringer's lactate or normal saline (15-20 mL/kg)
- Application of monitors
- Supplemental oxygen by face mask or nasal prongs
- Epidural catheter at L2-L3 or L3-L4
- Left uterine displacement
- Test dose

- Therapeutic dose
  - 5-mL boluses of 2% lidocaine + 1:400,000 epinephrine
  - Alternatively, 5-mL boluses of 0.5% bupivacaine, 0.5% ropivacaine, or 3% 2-chloroprocaine (Boluses of lidocaine or 2-chloroprocaine every 1-2 minutes, boluses of bupivacaine or ropivacaine every 2-5 minutes)
- Aggressive treatment of hypotension
  - Exaggerated left uterine displacement
  - Intravenous fluids
  - Ephedrine and/or low-dose phenylephrine

before insertion of the catheter. Administration of a test dose through the needle results in some evidence of epidural anesthesia, which confuses the interpretation of the subsequent test dose administered through the catheter.

Approximately 3 to 5 minutes after the administration of the test dose, there should be no significant change in heart rate or blood pressure and no evidence of motor blockade or dense sensory blockade. (A small band of anesthesia should be evident in the lower thoracic and upper lumbar dermatomes.) The therapeutic dose is then administered. The pregnant woman requires approximately 1 mL of local anesthetic solution for each segment of desired blockade.[161] A T4 level is desired for cesarean section; 18 segments require blockade, and most patients require 20 to 25 mL of local anesthetic. We give 5 mL of local anesthetic as the first therapeutic bolus dose. We wait at least 2 minutes and observe for evidence of intravascular or spinal injection before giving the next aliquot of local anesthetic.

The local anesthetic agents used by most anesthesiologists include lidocaine (1.5% to 2%), 2-chloroprocaine (3%), bupivacaine (0.5%), and ropivacaine (0.5%) (Table 25-2). Epidural administration of 0.75% bupivacaine is *not* recommended because of its association with maternal cardiotoxicity.[162] Ropivacaine is a relatively new local anesthetic that shares many similarities with bupivacaine but has less cardiac toxicity. Clinical studies comparing 0.5% ropivacaine with 0.5% bupivacaine have demonstrated similar patterns of anesthesia with less motor blockade in the women who received epidural ropivacaine for cesarean section. Umbilical cord blood gas and pH measurements, Apgar scores, and neonatal neurobehavioral scores also were similar.[163,164] Mepivacaine, which has a potency similar to lidocaine, has been used infrequently, because one study suggested that it might have adverse neonatal affects.[165] Subsequent studies have suggested that the epidural administration of mepivacaine does not adversely affect the infant.[166] Etidocaine rarely is used in obstetric patients; it results in a profound motor blockade that persists even after the sensory blockade has receded.[167] Levobupivacaine, the pure S(−)-enantiomer of racemic bupivacaine, has a potency similar to bupivacaine, although it produces a sensory block that tends to be of slightly longer duration when given epidurally.[144]

The choice of drug depends on the desired onset of action, the expected duration of surgery, and the condition of the

mother and fetus. 2-Chloroprocaine produces anesthesia most rapidly, whereas bupivacaine, levobupivacaine, and ropivacaine have the slowest onsets of action. Lidocaine has an intermediate onset of action. The durations of surgical anesthesia are approximately 40 to 50 minutes for 2-chloroprocaine, 75 to 100 minutes for lidocaine, and 120 to 180 minutes for bupivacaine, levobupivacaine, and ropivacaine.

Some anesthesiologists administer a combination of drugs either simultaneously or in sequence. The combination of bupivacaine and 2-chloroprocaine does not seem to enhance the quality of anesthesia.[168] If epidural opioid administration is planned for postoperative analgesia, 2-chloroprocaine should not be given. Administration of 2-chloroprocaine adversely affects the subsequent efficacy of epidural opioid analgesia.[169]

Many anesthesiologists include epinephrine with the solution of local anesthetic. Typically, the concentration of epinephrine is 1:200,000 or 1:400,000 (i.e., 5.0 or 2.5 µg/mL). Purported advantages of epinephrine include the following: (1) decreased vascular absorption of the local anesthetic; (2) improved quality of anesthesia; and (3) prolonged duration of the block. It is especially helpful to include epinephrine with a solution of lidocaine. Epidural administration of lidocaine without epinephrine does not consistently result in satisfactory anesthesia for cesarean section. Some anesthesiologists worry that systemic absorption of the epinephrine may result in adverse hemodynamic effects.[170,171] Alahuhta et al.[172] used Doppler ultrasonography and M-mode echocardiography to evaluate the hemodynamic effects of epidural bupivacaine with epinephrine before cesarean section. The addition of epinephrine resulted in a decrease in maternal diastolic pressure, but it did not affect systolic pressure or uterine blood flow.

We prefer to give lidocaine with epinephrine (1:400,000) to most patients. We add the epinephrine to a solution of plain lidocaine just before giving the lidocaine epidurally; this allows us to inject a lidocaine-epinephrine solution with a higher pH and less sodium (meta)bisulfite than the commercially prepared solutions of lidocaine with epinephrine. In some cases, we first give 6 to 10 mL of 0.5% bupivacaine to obtain a T10 sensory level. After 15 minutes, we administer 15 to 20 mL of 2% lidocaine with epinephrine in incremental doses. This technique results in a dense neural block of the lower abdomen. When time does not permit this approach, we inject 2% lidocaine with epinephrine from the beginning.

The addition of 1 mEq of sodium bicarbonate to each 10 mL of lidocaine hastens the onset of epidural lidocaine anesthesia; alkalinized lidocaine has an onset of action similar to that for 2-chloroprocaine.[173-175] The addition of bicarbonate results in the generation of carbon dioxide; the alkalinized lidocaine has activity similar to the lidocaine hydrocarbonate solutions available in countries other than the United States.[175] Unfortunately, the rapid onset of action also increases the likelihood of hypotension.[176] However, use of alkalinized lidocaine does not adversely affect neonatal outcome.[177] Either 2-chloroprocaine or alkalinized lidocaine with epinephrine is a good choice when it is necessary to extend preexisting epidural anesthesia for an urgent cesarean section.

It may be necessary to give additional doses of local anesthetic during surgery, depending on the drug selected and the duration of the procedure. De Leon-Casasola et al.[178] compared a continuous epidural infusion of 2-chloroprocaine with intermittent bolus injections of either bupivacaine or 2-chloroprocaine for the maintenance of epidural anesthesia during cesarean section. Both methods provided adequate

TABLE 25-2	DRUGS USED FOR EPIDURAL ANESTHESIA FOR CESAREAN SECTION	
Drug	Dosage range (mg)	Duration (min)*
Lidocaine 2% with epinephrine	300-500	75-100
2-Chloroprocaine 3%	450-750	40-50
Bupivacaine 0.5%	75-125	120-180
Ropivacaine 0.5%	75-125	120-180
Adjuvant drugs		
Morphine	3-4	720-1440
Fentanyl	0.05-0.10	120-240
Meperidine	50-75	240-720

*For the local anesthetics, the duration is defined as the time to two-segment regression. For the adjuvant drugs, the duration is defined as the duration of analgesia (or time to first request for a supplemental analgesic drug).

surgical anesthesia, but the continuous infusion group had less need for ephedrine to maintain blood pressure, and they had a shorter recovery room stay. This technique may be advantageous in situations in which 2-chloroprocaine is administered as the primary local anesthetic for cesarean section.

Opioids are administered epidurally to enhance intraoperative analgesia and to provide postoperative analgesia. Some anesthesiologists administer 50 to 100 μg of fentanyl with the initial therapeutic dose of local anesthetic.[179,180] Others delay the administration of fentanyl or morphine until after the umbilical cord is clamped.[181,182] The administration of 50 to 100 μg of fentanyl before delivery does not seem to adversely affect the neonate.[179,180] One study suggested that the lowest effective dose is 75 μg[179]; this technique seems most advantageous when 0.5% bupivacaine is given as the primary local anesthetic. We typically administer 2% lidocaine with epinephrine, and it is rarely necessary for us to give fentanyl epidurally before delivery of the infant. After delivery, we give 50 to 100 μg of fentanyl epidurally as needed. We also give a single dose of morphine (3 to 4 mg) to provide postoperative analgesia.[181,183]

Combined Spinal-Epidural Anesthesia

In 1981, Brownridge[184] first described the administration of combined spinal-epidural (CSE) anesthesia for elective cesarean section. He inserted an epidural catheter at the L1 to L2 interspace, and he gave a test dose of local anesthetic. He then performed spinal anesthesia at the L3 to L4 interspace. He used the epidural catheter to extend the level of the block, if necessary, and to provide postoperative analgesia. Subsequently, others have modified this technique by locating the epidural space with the Tuohy needle, inserting a long spinal needle through the Tuohy needle, injecting the local anesthetic intrathecally, and then inserting the epidural catheter.[185,186]

The distance from the tip of the epidural needle to the posterior wall of the dural sac in the midline varies from 0.30 to 1.05 cm. Further, the anteroposterior diameter of the dural sac varies considerably during flexion and extension of the spinal column.[187] The necessary length of protrusion of the spinal needle beyond the tip of the epidural needle has been the subject of debate and typically varies from 10 to 16 mm.[187] Joshi et al.[188] reported that the length of spinal needle protrusion should be greater than 13 mm. On the other hand, Vandermeersch[189] considers a protrusion of at least 17 mm to be optimal.

The type of spinal needle may also influence the success rate of the CSE technique. A variety of special CSE needle sets are available commercially. Of interest is that, in a European survey, it was reported that special CSE needle sets were used by only 31% of anesthesiologists; the remainder used their own combination of epidural needles and extra-long spinal needles.[187] Eldor et al.[190] have described a modification that includes the addition of a small, separate conduit for the spinal needle. With this modification, the epidural catheter can be inserted before the anesthesiologist performs a dural puncture with the spinal needle. The Espocan CSEA needle set (B. Braun, Inc., Bethlehem, PA) allows a different exit point for the passage of the epidural catheter and the spinal needle. A "back eye" at the epidural needle curve near its bevel permits the passage of the spinal needle, whereas the epidural catheter enters the epidural space through the "regular" needle eye.

Thus the point of dural contact by the epidural catheter is at some distance from the dural hole, which might reduce the risk of epidural catheter penetration through the hole in the dura.[187] However, the latter is highly unlikely when a 20-gauge epidural catheter and a small-gauge (i.e., 25-gauge or smaller) noncutting spinal needle are used. To our knowledge there is only one published report of presumed, unintentional insertion of an epidural catheter through the dural puncture site.[191]

With the needle-through-needle CSE technique, the tip of the spinal needle may scrape against the inner wall of the Tuohy-Schliff needle, and concern has been raised that metal particles might be introduced into the subarachnoid space. However, Herman et al.[192] did not find any evidence of metal particles produced by use of the needle-through-needle CSE technique. Curiously, it is not always possible to place a needle within the subarachnoid space when using the single interspace technique; thus some anesthesiologists have suggested that the epidural and spinal techniques should be performed at separate interspaces.

The advantage of the CSE technique is that the rapid onset and density of spinal anesthesia can be combined with the versatility of epidural anesthesia.[194] The epidural catheter allows the anesthesiologist to maintain anesthesia for prolonged surgery and to provide postoperative analgesia. Davies et al.[195] compared the use of CSE anesthesia with epidural anesthesia alone for elective cesarean section. Patients who received the CSE technique had a more rapid onset of anesthesia and more intense motor blockade than those who received epidural anesthesia alone. Pain scores were lower during performance of the block and at the time of delivery in the CSE group than in the epidural-only group. There was no difference between groups in the incidence of maternal hypotension, nausea, backache, or headache; in the use of supplemental analgesics for postoperative pain; or in overall patient satisfaction. These authors and others have observed that the CSE technique results in a low incidence of PDPH.[195,196]

The CSE technique has become increasingly popular in contemporary obstetric anesthesia practice, and it may be preferred when both a rapid onset of dense neural blockade and the ability to prolong the duration of anesthesia are desired.[194] Several authors have reported a very low incidence of PDPH associated with CSE anesthesia, which may reflect the fact that the epidural needle, which must be correctly placed first, serves as the introducer for the spinal needle. This typically insures a one-time, small dural puncture by the spinal needle.[187,195,196] The low incidence of PDPH seems advantageous in patients with a history of PDPH, given the association between previous PDPH and recurrent PDPH.[187,197] Further, the appearance of the CSF in the hub of the spinal needle indirectly confirms the correct placement of the epidural needle, which is of increased importance in patients with difficult anatomic landmarks and/or increased skin-epidural space distance.[198] Some anesthesiologists have suggested that the CSE technique is cumbersome and time-consuming. However, new CSE trays have eliminated many equipment limitations and thus have reduced preparation and procedure times. With experience, the entire procedure should not take longer than approximately 4 to 5 minutes.[199]

General Anesthesia

General anesthesia continues to fulfill an important role in the care of patients undergoing cesarean section (Box 25-6).

Box 25-6 INDICATIONS FOR GENERAL ANESTHESIA FOR CESAREAN SECTION

- Dire fetal distress in the absence of preexisting epidural anesthesia
- Acute maternal hypovolemia
- Significant coagulopathy
- Inadequate regional anesthesia
- Maternal refusal of regional anesthesia

Box 25-7 GENERAL ANESTHESIA FOR CESAREAN SECTION

H_2-receptor antagonist or proton pump inhibitor and/or metoclopramide intravenously
Clear antacid orally
Left uterine displacement
Application of monitors
Denitrogenation (administration of 100% oxygen)
- Traditional 3-5 minutes versus four vital-capacity breaths
Cricoid pressure
Intravenous induction
- Thiobarbiturate, propofol, ketamine, or etomidate
- Succinylcholine (rocuronium or vecuronium if succinylcholine is contraindicated)
Intubation with a 6.0- to 7.0-mm cuffed endotracheal tube
Administration of 30% to 50% nitrous oxide in oxygen and a low concentration (e.g., 0.5 minimum alveolar concentration [MAC]) of a volatile halogenated agent
After delivery
- Increased concentration of nitrous oxide, with or without a low concentration of a volatile halogenated agent
- Opioid
- Intravenous hypnotic agent (e.g., benzodiazepine, barbiturate, propofol), if needed
- Muscle relaxant (e.g., succinylcholine boluses or infusion, rocuronium, mivacurium, cisatracurium, vecuronium)
Extubation awake with intact airway reflexes

There are few if any absolute contraindications to the administration of general anesthesia for cesarean section; however, we prefer to avoid general anesthesia in patients with a difficult airway or a history of malignant hyperthermia or severe asthma.

When giving general anesthesia for cesarean section, the anesthesiologist should attempt to minimize the maternal risk of aspiration and the risk of neonatal depression (Box 25-7). When possible, measures to reduce and/or alkalinize gastric contents should be instituted before the patient is transferred to the operating table. After the patient is placed on the operating table, a wedge or a folded blanket is placed beneath the right hip to ensure left uterine displacement. Appropriate monitors, including a nerve stimulator, are applied. The patient should then breathe 100% oxygen through a well-fitting face mask. Approximately 3 to 5 minutes is the ideal interval to achieve denitrogenation (termed the traditional or T method). When time is of the essence, the patient may take four vital-capacity breaths of 100% oxygen (termed the 4DB/30 sec method) just before the induction of anesthesia (see Chapter 31).[165] Of interest is that Baraka et al.[201] demonstrated that an eight-deep-breaths-in-60-seconds method of preoxygenation (termed the 8DB/60 sec method) results in a slower rate of hemoglobin desaturation (to $SaO_2 = 95\%$) during apnea than the traditional method. Benumof[202] noted that the authors hypothesized that "the 8DB/60 sec method might

result in a greater store of oxygen in the alveolar compartment compared to the [traditional] method by either causing an increase in flow rate into or the volume of the compartment." Benumof[202] agreed that the 8DB/60 sec method of preoxygenation described by Baraka et al.[201] might be best with regard to both efficacy and efficiency. However, he postulated that the answer as to why the 8DB/60 sec method resulted in slower hemoglobin desaturation than the T method might be the result of an increase in oxygen in the blood compartment rather than in the alveolar compartment.

Adequate denitrogenation is essential, because the parturient's decreased functional residual capacity and increased oxygen consumption result in a rapid onset of hypoxemia during apnea. Baraka et al.[203] speculated that the head-up position, which tends to increase functional residual capacity, might improve the margin of safety. They compared the use of the head-up and supine positions for denitrogenation before the induction of anesthesia in pregnant and non-pregnant women. Although the use of the head-up position prolonged the interval between the onset of apnea and oxyhemoglobin desaturation (i.e., SaO_2 less than 95%) in nonpregnant women, the head-up position resulted in no benefit for pregnant women.

A small dose of a nondepolarizing muscle relaxant may be given 3 to 5 minutes before induction to prevent fasciculations after the administration of succinylcholine. Alternatively, this small dose may serve as a priming dose if a nondepolarizing agent will be used to achieve muscle relaxation. Although this may be accomplished with any of the available agents, d-tubocurarine 3 mg is the recommended drug for this purpose. Anecdotal reports suggest that small doses of the other intermediate acting agents (e.g., vecuronium) may result in partial paralysis in some patients.[204] We rarely give a defasciculating dose or a priming dose of a nondepolarizing muscle relaxant, for several reasons. First, we prefer to avoid the risk of partial paralysis in an awake patient. Second, some evidence suggests that succinylcholine provides more rapid and profound relaxation in the absence of a small dose of a nondepolarizing relaxant, although this is a matter of some dispute.[205] Third, if the patient has received magnesium sulfate for tocolysis or seizure prophylaxis, defasciculation is unnecessary because of the effect of magnesium at the neuromuscular junction.[206] Indeed, administration of a small dose of a nondepolarizing muscle relaxant is hazardous in a hypermagnesemic patient.

Induction of anesthesia is performed after the abdomen has been prepared and draped and the obstetrician is ready to begin surgery, and a rapid-sequence induction is used. This requires that a qualified assistant apply pressure to the cricoid cartilage to occlude the esophagus until an endotracheal tube has been inserted correctly, the cuff has been inflated, and ventilation of the lungs has been verified.

INDUCTION AGENTS

When choosing an induction agent, the primary goals are as follows: (1) to preserve maternal blood pressure, cardiac output, and uterine blood flow; (2) to minimize fetal and neonatal depression; and (3) to ensure maternal hypnosis and amnesia.

Thiopental

The barbiturates (e.g., thiopental, methohexital, thiamylal) are the most popular induction agents for cesarean section. Extensive published data have confirmed the safety of thiopental for the induction of anesthesia in obstetric patients. Thiopental provides prompt, reliable induction of anesthesia; it has few adverse effects on airway irritability; its pharmacokinetics are well understood; and it results in a smooth emergence from anesthesia. The preferred dose is 4 mg/kg. Thiopental is both a negative inotrope and a vasodilator, but this dose is unlikely to have an adverse hemodynamic effect on the normal pregnant woman. However, this dose may result in a significant decline in cardiac output and blood pressure in hypovolemic patients.

Thiopental rapidly crosses the placenta, and it can be detected in umbilical venous blood within 30 seconds of administration. The umbilical venous blood concentration peaks in 1 minute. The umbilical venous:maternal venous blood concentration ratio approaches 1.0 by the time of delivery.[207] Equilibration of umbilical venous and arterial blood concentrations begins to occur quickly. The umbilical artery:umbilical vein concentration ratio ranges from 0.46 with induction-to-delivery (I-D) intervals of 4 to 7 minutes[208] to 0.87 with I-D intervals of 8 to 22 minutes.[209] These data suggest that the equilibrium of the thiopental in the fetus is a relatively rapid process and can be expected by the time of delivery. However, with doses of less than 4 mg/kg, peak barbiturate concentrations in the fetal brain rarely exceed the threshold for depression. Umbilical venous blood thiopental concentrations are well below the arterial plasma concentrations of thiopental necessary to produce anesthesia in adults (i.e., 39 to 42 µg/mL).[207] Larger doses of thiopental (e.g., 8 mg/kg) do produce significant neonatal depression.[210]

Several theories have been proposed to explain the scenario of an unconscious mother with an awake neonate. These include the following: (1) preferential uptake of thiopental by the fetal liver, which is the first organ perfused by blood from the umbilical vein[210,211]; (2) the higher relative water content of the fetal brain[212]; (3) rapid redistribution of the drug into maternal tissues, which causes a rapid reduction in the maternal-to-fetal concentration gradient; (4) nonhomogeneity of blood flow in the intervillous space; and (5) progressive dilution by admixture with the various components of the fetal circulation.[213] Because of this rapid equilibration of thiopental and a lack of a significant concentration of thiopental in the fetal brain, there is no advantage in delaying delivery until thiopental concentrations decline. However, there is no evidence of an adverse effect of thiopental on the fetus when the I-D time is prolonged.

Propofol

Propofol is an intravenous agent that allows a rapid, smooth induction of anesthesia. It attenuates the cardiovascular response to laryngoscopy and intubation more effectively than does thiopental.[214-216] Propofol may be administered by continuous intravenous infusion for the maintenance of anesthesia. Perhaps its major advantage is the rapid awakening that follows the discontinuation of an infusion of propofol. Moreover, intravenous infusion of propofol allows the anesthesiologist to give 100% oxygen. Some studies have noted that the administration of propofol results in a greater decrease in blood pressure than does thiopental.[217] (Decreased blood pressure results in decreased uteroplacental perfusion.) Other studies have not observed significant hypotension after the administration of propofol (2.0 to 2.8 mg/kg) before cesarean section.[218-221] Likewise, these studies noted that the administration of propofol does not adversely affect umbilical cord blood gas and pH measurements at delivery.[218-222] Alon

et al.[223] observed that the administration of thiopental but not propofol resulted in decreased uterine blood flow in gravid ewes. Unfortunately, administration of propofol and succinylcholine resulted in marked maternal bradycardia, and one animal experienced a sinus arrest.

Propofol is a lipophilic agent with a low molecular weight, and it rapidly crosses the placenta. Dailland et al.[222] observed that the umbilical venous:maternal venous blood concentration ratio at delivery was 0.70. The authors also observed that propofol was rapidly cleared from the neonatal circulation, and they detected low concentrations of propofol in breast milk.

Most studies have noted that the administration of propofol and thiopental result in similar Apgar and neurobehavioral scores. However, Celleno et al.[224] observed that the administration of propofol 2.8 mg/kg resulted in lower Apgar scores and lower neurobehavioral scores at 1 hour after delivery as compared with the administration of thiopental. The two groups of infants had similar neurobehavioral scores by 4 hours after delivery.

Propofol is more expensive than other induction agents. In addition, propofol provides an excellent vehicle for the growth of bacteria, and, for this reason, it should be used promptly after its withdrawal from the ampule. Propofol does not offer significant advantages over thiopental during rapid-sequence induction of general anesthesia in most obstetric patients. However, propofol blunts the hypertensive response to laryngoscopy and intubation more effectively than the other induction agents; thus it may be a good choice for the induction of general anesthesia in hypertensive patients.[225]

Ketamine

Ketamine is also an excellent choice for the induction of general anesthesia for cesarean section. The usual dose is 1.0 mg/kg. It has a rapid onset of action, it provides both analgesia and hypnosis, and it reliably provides amnesia. In addition, its sympathomimetic properties are advantageous in patients with asthma or modest hypovolemia. Ketamine also is an excellent choice in cases of severe fetal distress; 100% oxygen can be administered until delivery, with a low risk of maternal awareness and recall. Clinical studies have suggested that the use of ketamine is associated with a decreased incidence of maternal awareness as compared with the administration of thiopental alone or of a combination of smaller doses of thiopental and ketamine.[226,227]

When a dose of 1 mg/kg is used for induction, systolic blood pressure increases by approximately 14% immediately after the induction of anesthesia and by approximately 30% after laryngoscopy and intubation.[228] These hemodynamic changes result from ketamine's indirect sympathomimetic activity; thus ketamine should be avoided in hypertensive patients. However, ketamine also results in direct myocardial depression and in decreased cardiac output and hypotension if the patient has severe hypovolemia.[229]

Large doses of ketamine increase uterine tone. However, an induction dose of 1 mg/kg does not increase uterine tone.[230-232] Ketamine rapidly crosses the placenta, and it reaches a maximum concentration in the fetus approximately 1½ to 2 minutes after administration.[233] Bernstein et al.[234] observed similar umbilical cord blood gas and pH measurements and Apgar scores after the administration of ketamine and thiopental for the induction of general anesthesia for elective cesarean section. Further, Hodgkinson et al.[235] observed slightly better neurobehavioral scores in infants whose mothers received ketamine 1 mg/kg as compared with infants exposed to thiopental. Ketamine is a very useful induction agent in obstetric patients.

Some anesthesiologists hesitate to use ketamine because of its psychotropic properties. After the administration of ketamine, dreaming is common. Large doses of ketamine can cause dysphoria and hallucinations during emergence from anesthesia. The concomitant administration of a benzodiazepine reduces or eliminates these side effects.[236]

Etomidate

Etomidate is an intravenous induction agent that has been used in obstetric anesthesia practice since 1979. The usual dose is 0.2 to 0.3 mg/kg. Etomidate produces a rapid onset of anesthesia in one arm-to-brain circulation time. It undergoes rapid hydrolysis, which results in a rapid recovery period. Etomidate causes little cardiovascular depression; thus it is an excellent choice in patients with hemodynamic instability. Gregory and Davidson[237] observed that the administration of etomidate before elective cesarean section did not adversely affect umbilical cord blood gas and pH measurements or Apgar scores. Downing et al.[238] observed that infants exposed to etomidate 0.3 mg/kg had better acid-base measurements and better overall condition than infants exposed to thiopental 3.5 mg/kg. Unfortunately, intravenous injection of etomidate may result in pain and myoclonus, which can be severe.[239] Etomidate may also result in the suppression of neonatal serum cortisol concentrations, although it is unclear whether this level of suppression is clinically significant.[240]

Midazolam

Midazolam is a short-acting, water-soluble benzodiazepine that has few adverse hemodynamic effects and provides hypnosis and amnesia. Midazolam rapidly crosses the placenta, although it may not cross as rapidly as thiopental and diazepam.[241] Crawford et al.[242] observed that midazolam and thiopental resulted in similar maternal hemodynamic responses when they were used for the induction of general anesthesia for elective cesarean section. Ravlo et al.[243] observed that infants exposed to midazolam or thiopental had similar Apgar scores. By contrast, Bland et al.[244] observed a higher incidence of low Apgar scores and increased time-to-spontaneous respiration in infants exposed to midazolam as compared with similar infants exposed to thiopental. Umbilical cord blood gas measurements did not differ between the two groups. At 2 hours of life, infants exposed to midazolam had lower neurobehavioral scores for body temperature, general body tone, and arm recoil; these differences did not persist at 4 hours after delivery.[244] There are few indications for the use of midazolam for the induction of general anesthesia for cesarean section. It should be used only when there are relative or absolute contraindications to the use of other agents.

MUSCLE RELAXANTS

The depolarizing agent **succinylcholine** 1.0 to 1.5 mg/kg remains the muscle relaxant of choice for most patients. This dose provides complete muscle relaxation and optimal conditions for laryngoscopy and intubation within approximately 45 seconds of intravenous administration. Succinylcholine is highly ionized and water soluble, and only small amounts cross the placenta. Maternal administration of succinylcholine rarely affects neonatal neuromuscular function. One study noted that only doses that exceed 300 mg result in significant placental transfer, and the exposed infants did not exhibit signs of muscle weakness.[245] Administration of suc-

cinylcholine may result in neonatal apnea in infants of women with homozygotic atypical pseudocholinesterase deficiency.[246]

Succinylcholine is rapidly metabolized by plasma pseudocholinesterase. Pseudocholinesterase activity decreases 30% during pregnancy, but recovery from succinylcholine is not prolonged. The parturient's increased volume of distribution offsets the effect of the decreased pseudocholinesterase activity.[247] The administration of metoclopramide may also result in a prolongation of succinylcholine-induced neuromuscular blockade.[248] The anesthesiologist should confirm the return of neuromuscular function before giving additional doses of muscle relaxant.

Rocuronium is a suitable alternative to succinylcholine when a nondepolarizing agent is preferred for rapid-sequence induction of general anesthesia for cesarean section.[249] Abouleish et al.[250] found that the maximal effect was achieved 98 seconds after the administration of a dose of 0.6 mg/kg and that they were able to reverse neuromuscular blockade satisfactorily at the conclusion of cesarean section in all patients. Further, conditions for laryngoscopy and intubation were suitable at 79 seconds when they used 4 to 6 mg/kg of thiopental for the induction of anesthesia. Magorian et al.[251] demonstrated that a larger dose of rocuronium (0.9 or 1.2 mg/kg) results in an onset of paralysis similar to that provided by succinylcholine but that the duration of action is prolonged.

Vecuronium may be administered when the use of succinylcholine is contraindicated; however, it has a significantly slower onset of action. Hawkins et al.[252] studied the use of two vecuronium regimens for rapid-sequence induction of anesthesia before elective cesarean section. One group of women received 10 μg/kg of vecuronium as a priming dose followed by 100 μg/kg 4 to 6 minutes later; the other group received 200 μg/kg as a single bolus. The onset time for both groups (177 seconds and 175 seconds, respectively) was much longer than that for succinylcholine. Moreover, the duration of blockade was prolonged (73 minutes in the priming-dose group and 115 minutes in the other group).

Atracurium is a less desirable agent for rapid-sequence induction of anesthesia. The high dose required for a rapid onset of action may result in significant histamine release and hypotension. The isomer **cisatracurium** does not have these undesirable side effects, but its relatively slow onset makes it undesirable for use during rapid-sequence induction of general anesthesia.

Regardless of the choice of muscle relaxant, laryngoscopy and intubation should not be attempted until adequate muscle relaxation has occurred. The use of a nerve stimulator allows an objective assessment of the onset of paralysis and also guides the administration of additional doses of muscle relaxant.

Only very small amounts of the nondepolarizing muscle relaxants cross the placenta; thus the infant is rarely affected. Clinical studies have confirmed that the maternal administration of a muscle relaxant does not affect Apgar or neurobehavioral scores.[253,254]

INTUBATION

In most cases, the anesthesiologist should not attempt ventilation before insertion of the endotracheal tube. There are two exceptions to this dictum. First, positive-pressure ventilation may be needed when oxyhemoglobin desaturation occurs before the onset of adequate muscle relaxation. Second, in unexpected cases of difficult intubation, positive-pressure ventilation is needed between the first and second attempts at laryngoscopy.

A short-handled laryngoscope is advantageous, because it prevents contact with the enlarged maternal breasts. A 6.0- to 7.0-mm endotracheal tube is the preferred size for most pregnant patients. After intubation, the presence of end-tidal carbon dioxide and bilateral breath sounds should be verified. At that time, surgery may begin.

AWARENESS DURING ANESTHESIA

The anesthesiologist must recognize the risk of maternal awareness between induction of general anesthesia and delivery of the infant. The desire to minimize neonatal depression must be balanced against the risk of maternal awareness. If another agent is not given after the induction of anesthesia, the incidence of awareness increases in direct proportion to the I-D interval. Administration of 50% nitrous oxide in oxygen *without* another agent results in maternal awareness in 12% to 26% of cases.[255-257] Awareness is inhumane for the mother and results in high maternal concentrations of catecholamines, which result in uterine artery vasoconstriction and reduced oxygen delivery to the fetus.[258] Some anesthesiologists have questioned whether it is appropriate for the obstetrician to begin surgery immediately after endotracheal intubation.[259] EEG spectrum analysis[260] and brainstem auditory evoked potentials[261] can alert the anesthesiologist to a patient who has inadequate anesthesia, but this technology is not yet suitable for the conditions under which most general anesthetics are given for obstetric cases. Some physicians have advocated use of the Bispectral Index (BIS), a multivariate processed electroencephalographic assessment, to help the anesthesiologist titrate the doses of anesthetic agents administered during cesarean section to ensure adequate maternal hypnosis without increasing the risk of neonatal depression.[262] Lubke et al.[263] reported that the Bispectral Index reflects direct and indirect memory function during cesarean section. However, there is insufficient evidence to support the routine use of the Bispectral Index or other similar electroencephalographic variables to monitor the depth of general anesthesia for cesarean section.

Anesthesiologists may choose one of several options to prevent maternal awareness. A common approach is to administer 50% nitrous oxide in oxygen in combination with a low concentration of a volatile halogenated agent (e.g., halothane 0.5%, isoflurane 0.6%, enflurane 1.0%, desflurane 3.0%, sevoflurane 1.0%).[264-268] This method is simple and reduces the incidence of maternal awareness to less than 1%. A low concentration of a volatile halogenated agent is adequate for most patients, because pregnancy decreases anesthetic requirements by as much as 30% to 40%. Predelivery administration of a low concentration of a volatile halogenated agent does not adversely affect neonatal condition, and it does not significantly increase maternal blood loss.[269]

Earlier studies suggested that a maternal inspired oxygen concentration of 60% resulted in improved fetal oxygenation as compared with the administration of lesser concentrations of oxygen.[270,271] This prompted the recommendation that all women receive at least 50% oxygen during the administration of general anesthesia for cesarean section. Piggott et al.[272] noted that the administration of 100% oxygen resulted in higher umbilical venous blood P_{O_2} and higher 1-minute Apgar scores as compared with the administration of 50% oxygen. Women who received 100% oxygen also received a higher concentration of isoflurane (1.8% for 5 minutes and

1.2% thereafter) without maternal awareness or excessive bleeding. This study supports the administration of 100% oxygen and a higher concentration of a volatile halogenated agent in cases of fetal distress. Lawes et al.[273] questioned the need to administer 50% oxygen for *elective* cesarean section. They observed no difference in neonatal oxygenation or outcome between infants whose mothers received 33% oxygen and infants whose mothers received 50% oxygen.

Intravenous techniques used to prevent maternal awareness include the administration of repeat boluses of thiopental[274] or the use of ketamine, midazolam, or propofol for the induction and maintenance of anesthesia. In one study, when ketamine 1.5 mg/kg was used as the only anesthetic agent, there were no cases of maternal awareness when the I-D interval was less than 10 minutes.[275] Another successful approach to avoiding maternal awareness has been to combine ketamine and thiopental.[276]

In most cases, we give 30% to 50% nitrous oxide in oxygen and a low concentration (0.5 minimum alveolar concentration [MAC]) of a volatile halogenated agent (e.g., halothane, enflurane, isoflurane, sevoflurane, desflurane).

MAINTENANCE OF ANESTHESIA

After delivery, we increase the concentration of nitrous oxide. Some anesthesiologists decrease or discontinue the administration of the volatile halogenated agent to allow for optimal uterine involution. However, the uterus should contract adequately in response to oxytocin despite the administration of a low concentration of a volatile halogenated agent. Studies have noted that sevoflurane[267] and desflurane[268] are equally as effective as the other volatile agents but without demonstrable advantage during the administration of anesthesia for cesarean section. We discontinue the volatile halogenated agent only if there is evidence of uterine atony that is unresponsive to oxytocin. We then administer modest doses of opioid as needed to maintain adequate maternal anesthesia.

Some physicians have expressed concern that opioids may accumulate in the breast milk or colostrum. Steer et al.[277] measured fentanyl concentrations in colostrum after maternal administration of fentanyl 2 μg/kg. The peak concentration (0.4 ng/mL) occurred at 45 minutes, and fentanyl was undetectable 10 hours later. Thus a modest dose of opioid administered during cesarean section does not place the infant at risk for sedation.

Muscle relaxation may be maintained with any of the nondepolarizing agents or with an infusion of succinylcholine. Two studies have noted that the duration of action of vecuronium is prolonged in postpartum patients.[278,279] We prefer to give cisatracurium for the maintenance of muscle relaxation. Both cisatracurium and atracurium are metabolized by the Hofmann elimination reaction and by nonspecific plasma esterase hydrolysis. **Mivacurium** is a short- to intermediate-acting nondepolarizing muscle relaxant that is hydrolyzed by plasma cholinesterase. It has an onset time of approximately 2.5 minutes, and its duration of action is approximately twice that of succinylcholine. Its duration is only 30% to 40% of the duration of atracurium and vecuronium. Mivacurium's duration of action does not correlate with plasma cholinesterase activity, which may reflect other routes of metabolism and/or excretion.[280] Its properties suggest that it would be a suitable choice for the maintenance of muscle relaxation during cesarean section.

At the end of surgery, residual nondepolarizing neuromuscular blockade is reversed with neostigmine, edrophonium, or pyridostigmine; an anticholinergic agent also is administered to blunt the muscarinic side effects. The upper airway is suctioned, and extubation is performed when the patient has regained her protective reflexes, can maintain her own airway, and responds appropriately to verbal commands.

Local Anesthesia

The use of local infiltration anesthesia as the primary anesthetic technique for cesarean section is an all but forgotten art.[281-283] Local infiltration often is used to provide supplemental anesthesia in patients with inadequate epidural anesthesia, but it is rarely used as the primary anesthetic technique. Admittedly, there are few indications for this technique in modern obstetric practice. The obstetrician may use this technique when a skilled anesthesia care provider is not immediately available to provide general or regional anesthesia for a patient with severe fetal distress. In addition, it may be the most appropriate technique for the rare parturient who is in extremis. We recently used local anesthesia for a patient with a severe coagulopathy and a known difficult airway who required an emergency cesarean section at our hospital.

It is possible to perform the entire procedure with local infiltration, provided the obstetrician makes a midline abdominal incision, makes minimal use of retractors, and does not exteriorize the uterus. Alternatively, the obstetrician might begin surgery and deliver the infant with the aid of local infiltration. Temporary hemostasis may be achieved until an anesthesia care provider arrives, and surgery may be completed after the induction of general anesthesia.

Local infiltration is performed in sequential steps as the operation progresses (Box 25-8). Time must be allowed for the local anesthetic to penetrate and exert its effect before proceeding to the next step. We recommend the administration of 0.5% lidocaine; the use of a more concentrated solution is likely to result in systemic toxicity.

Bonica[284] described six steps for local infiltration: (1) intracutaneous; (2) subcutaneous; (3) intrarectus; (4) parietal peritoneal; (5) visceral peritoneal; and (6) paracervical. A 25-gauge spinal needle is used to make the intracutaneous injection; the needle is inserted just below the umbilicus and is directed in the midline toward the symphysis pubis. Approximately 10 mL of local anesthetic is required to create a skin wheal that extends from the symphysis pubis to the umbilicus. The subcutaneous injection is also performed for the full length of the planned incision. Approximately 10 to 20 mL of local anesthetic is injected subcutaneously.

Box 25-8 LOCAL INFILTRATION ANESTHESIA FOR CESAREAN SECTION

1. Professional support person with patient
2. Infiltration with lidocaine 0.5% (total dose should not exceed 500 mg)
3. Intracutaneous injection in the midline from the umbilicus to the symphysis pubis
4. Subcutaneous injection
5. Incision down to the rectus fascia
6. Rectus fascia blockade
7. Parietal peritoneum infiltration and incision
8. Visceral peritoneum infiltration and incision
9. Paracervical injection
10. Uterine incision and delivery
11. Administration of general endotracheal anesthesia for uterine repair and closure, if needed

---

Ideally, the obstetrician should then wait approximately 3 to 4 minutes before making the skin incision.

A vertical skin incision is made between the umbilicus and the symphysis pubis and is extended down to the rectus fascia. The obstetrician then infiltrates local anesthetic into the rectus fascia and rectus muscles by making three to five laterally directed injections on each side. The needle should have an angle of 10 to 15 degrees to the skin and should pass between the layers of the rectus sheath. The needle is inserted a distance of 3 to 5 cm, aspiration is performed, and 2 to 3 mL of local anesthetic are injected at each site. An additional 1 mL is then injected as the needle is withdrawn. The obstetrician should also make oblique injections at the upper and lower poles of the incision. The local anesthetic will spread freely in the rectus sheath, but it takes 4 to 5 minutes for anesthesia to become complete. It is also necessary to infiltrate generously in the suprapubic area to ensure blockade of the branches of the iliohypogastric nerve. The disadvantage of this method of rectus block is that it requires a large volume (40 to 50 mL) of local anesthetic solution. An alternative method that provides less-effective analgesia but requires less volume and time is to raise a longitudinal paramedian wheal in the rectus fascia on each side of the midline and to then infiltrate the suprapubic region.

Next the obstetrician extends the incision through the rectus sheath. At this time, the peritoneum may be grasped with a forceps clamp. If pain occurs, the parietal peritoneum may be infiltrated with 5 to 10 mL of local anesthetic and then incised. The surgeon must use gentle surgical technique. The visceral peritoneum overlying the area of the uterine incision is injected with 10 mL of local anesthetic, and it is incised and reflected appropriately. Although incision through the lower uterine segment is not very painful, some surgeons prefer to inject 5 to 10 mL of local anesthetic in each paracervical region to block pain impulses from the uterus and cervix. A uterine incision is then made, and the infant is delivered. The surgeon must avoid forceful retraction and blunt dissection of tissue planes. Uterine manipulation should be kept to a minimum. A person at the head of the table who can provide coaching and reassurance to the mother is invaluable.

The major disadvantages of local anesthesia are patient discomfort and the potential for systemic toxicity, given that approximately 100 mL of local anesthetic solution is required. This is problematic, because a skilled anesthesia care provider may not be present to assist with resuscitation of the mother. Another disadvantage is that time is required for maximal anesthesia to develop. This time may be sacrificed when fetal distress is the indication for cesarean section, but the mother likely will suffer greater discomfort. Finally, local infiltration does not provide satisfactory operating conditions if the obstetrician encounters a complication of surgery (e.g., uterine atony, uterine laceration, broad ligament hematoma).

EFFECTS OF ANESTHESIA ON THE FETUS AND NEONATE

The placental transfer of drugs administered to the mother may directly affect the fetus. These drugs may cause clinically apparent depression of the infant at delivery or subtle neurobehavioral changes during the first several hours after birth. Maternal hypotension or the administration of uterine artery vasoconstrictive drugs results in decreased uteroplacental blood flow, which may cause fetal hypoxia and acidosis. Maternal hypoxemia also adversely affects the fetus.

Clinical studies have demonstrated no significant difference in umbilical cord blood gas and pH measurements between infants exposed to general or regional anesthesia for elective[285-292] or emergency[126] cesarean section. The anesthesiologist should attempt to prevent conditions that may cause fetal hypoxemia and acidosis by doing the following: (1) providing left uterine displacement to prevent aortocaval compression; (2) ensuring adequate maternal oxygenation; (3) avoiding maternal hyperventilation; (4) avoiding excessive doses of anesthetic agents; and (5) treating hypotension promptly.

One factor that may affect oxygenation and acid-base status at delivery is the uterine-incision-to-delivery (U-D) interval. Crawford et al.[293,294] emphasized that the U-D interval is more important than the I-D interval in determining the biochemical and clinical condition of the neonate. The performance of the uterine incision may precipitate myometrial contraction, which results in decreased uteroplacental perfusion. A U-D interval of longer than 3 minutes is associated with an increased incidence of low umbilical cord blood pH measurements and low Apgar scores, regardless of the anesthetic technique.[295] Bader et al.[296] observed that a prolonged U-D interval is associated with a corresponding increase in umbilical artery catecholamine concentrations. They observed that umbilical arterial pH measurements were significantly lower in infants with higher umbilical arterial blood catecholamine concentrations. The obstetrician should minimize the U-D interval, regardless of the type of anesthesia that is used.

During the administration of regional anesthesia, a prolonged I-D interval does not adversely affect neonatal acid-base measurements or Apgar scores, provided that hypotension is prevented or treated promptly.[295] The combination of uncorrected hypotension and a prolonged I-D interval results in neonatal acidosis.[297]

During the administration of general anesthesia, the I-D interval may also affect neonatal condition. Datta et al.[295] observed a higher incidence of neonatal acidosis and low 1-minute Apgar scores when the I-D interval exceeded 8 minutes in patients who received general anesthesia. Earlier studies included similar observations, although patients received inspired oxygen concentrations of only 25% to 33%,

and some of the patients did not have left uterine displacement.[298,299] Crawford et al.[293] concluded that, if the maternal inspired concentration of oxygen is 65% to 70% and both aortocaval compression and hypotension are prevented, an I-D interval during general anesthesia of as long as 30 minutes does not significantly affect umbilical cord blood gas and acid-base measurements at delivery. However, other studies have suggested that a high inspired concentration of oxygen does not offset the disadvantage of a prolonged I-D interval.[300,301]

A prolonged I-D interval results in greater fetal exposure to nitrous oxide and the volatile halogenated agent. Thus a prolonged I-D interval may result in a greater risk of neonatal depression at delivery, despite the presence of normal umbilical cord blood gas and acid-base measurements.[302]

Some clinical studies have shown no differences in Apgar scores between infants of mothers who received either general or epidural anesthesia for elective cesarean section.[285-287,303,304] Other studies have shown lower 1-minute Apgar scores for infants exposed to general anesthesia.[126,288,305,306] Abboud et al.[304] observed no differences in Apgar scores at 1 and 5 minutes among infants delivered by cesarean section with either general or regional anesthesia, but they noted that infants exposed to general anesthesia had lower neurobehavioral scores at 15 minutes and 2 hours after delivery. At 24 hours, there was no significant difference between groups in neurobehavioral scores. Marx et al.[126] observed lower 1-minute Apgar scores in infants of mothers who received general anesthesia for emergency cesarean section as compared with similar infants whose mothers received regional anesthesia. However, there was no difference between groups in 5-minute Apgar scores (Figure 25-3).

Ong et al.[306] retrospectively evaluated the outcomes of infants delivered by cesarean section over a 9-year period. There was an increased incidence of low 1-minute Apgar scores among infants exposed to general anesthesia for elective cesarean section. Further, there was an increased incidence of low 1- and 5-minute Apgar scores among infants exposed to general anesthesia for emergency cesarean section; many of these infants required intubation and positive-pressure ventilation. However, the authors observed no difference in

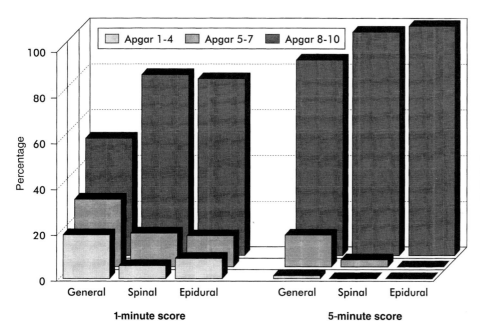

FIGURE 25-3. Neonatal condition after cesarean section for fetal distress. (Modified from Marx GF, Luykx WM, Cohen S. Fetal-neonatal status following cesarean section for fetal distress. Br J Anaesth 1984; 56:1009-13.)

the ultimate neonatal outcome. They concluded that infants exposed to general anesthesia are more likely to be depressed and require active resuscitation than those exposed to regional anesthesia for cesarean section. However, the increased incidence of neonatal depression does not reflect an increased risk of asphyxia.

Nitrous oxide has been implicated as a cause of neonatal depression. Nitrous oxide rapidly crosses the placenta.[302] Fetal uptake, as demonstrated by an increasing umbilical artery: umbilical vein ratio of nitrous oxide, continues during the first 20 minutes after the induction of anesthesia. One study that evaluated the administration of 70% nitrous oxide suggested that a long I-D interval is associated with neonatal depression at delivery[307]; this may result from the anesthetic effect of nitrous oxide and diffusion hypoxia. However, effective ventilation with 100% oxygen results in the rapid elimination of nitrous oxide from the infant, and effective resuscitation typically results in a high 5-minute Apgar score.

Uncorrected hypotension during regional anesthesia results in fetal and neonatal acidosis.[308] Single-shot spinal anesthesia results in a greater likelihood of severe hypotension than does epidural anesthesia. Volume expansion, left uterine displacement, and prophylactic ephedrine are used to prevent hypotension during spinal anesthesia.[73,309,310] In the absence of hypotension, the administration of spinal anesthesia does not adversely affect umbilical cord blood pH measurements or Apgar scores.[73,292,309,311] However, severe or uncorrected hypotension may result in lower umbilical cord blood pH measurements.[292] Corke et al.[297] observed that hypotension that lasted for 2 minutes was associated with a slightly lower umbilical artery pH during spinal anesthesia. However, these brief episodes of hypotension did not affect Apgar or neurobehavioral scores. Roberts et al.[312] observed that a greater incidence of fetal acidemia occurs with spinal and CSE anesthesia for elective cesarean section than with epidural or general anesthesia. However, Apgar scores were 8 or greater at 1 minute in all groups. Spinal anesthesia does not adversely affect the newborn infant, provided that hypotension is treated promptly and adequately and adequate maternal oxygenation is maintained.

The slower onset of epidural anesthesia results in a lower incidence of hypotension. Although hypotension occurs in some patients who receive epidural anesthesia, it typically is less severe and easier to treat than that associated with spinal anesthesia. Epidural anesthesia does not adversely affect neonatal outcome, provided that hypotension is treated promptly and adequately.[81]

Some physicians have expressed concern that the placental transfer of local anesthetic agents may adversely affect the fetus and the neonate. Administration of spinal anesthesia requires a small dose of local anesthetic agent, and the infant is exposed to low concentrations of drug.[129] However, in 1974, Scanlon et al.[313] reported lower neurobehavioral scores in infants whose mothers received epidural lidocaine or mepivacaine during labor. They noted that the infants had lower scores for habituation and muscle tone than did the control infants during the first few hours of life. In other words, the infants were alert but floppy. Subsequent studies have observed that the epidural administration of lidocaine for cesarean section does not adversely affect neurobehavioral scores.[314,315] Only Kuhnert et al.[316] observed subtle differences in the neurobehavioral scores of neonates whose mothers received epidural lidocaine. Several studies have concluded that the epidural administration of bupivacaine or 2-chloroprocaine

does not affect neonatal neurobehavioral scores.[304,314,317,318] In summary, the administration of epidural anesthesia does not significantly affect neonatal neurobehavior. Other considerations should dictate the anesthesiologist's choice of anesthetic technique and anesthetic agents.

KEY POINTS

- More than 24% of all infants born in the United States are delivered by cesarean section.
- The majority of cesarean sections are performed with spinal or epidural anesthesia.
- The major maternal risks of general anesthesia are failed intubation, failed ventilation, and pulmonary aspiration of gastric contents.
- Hypotension is more common during spinal anesthesia than during epidural anesthesia, and it is more common during epidural anesthesia than during general anesthesia.
- The prevention or prompt treatment of maternal hypotension is necessary to ensure optimal neonatal outcome.
- The administration of continuous epidural anesthesia allows the anesthesiologist to titrate the dose of local anesthetic agent to the desired level of anesthesia, and it allows the anesthesiologist to minimize the incidence of severe hypotension.
- A uterine incision-to-delivery interval of more than 3 minutes is associated with an increased likelihood of neonatal acidosis at delivery, regardless of the anesthetic technique.
- Infants exposed to general anesthesia have lower 1-minute Apgar scores than infants exposed to regional anesthesia. However, after effective resuscitation and ventilation with 100% oxygen, these infants have 5-minute Apgar scores that do not differ from those of infants exposed to regional anesthesia.
- The administration of spinal or epidural anesthesia does not result in clinically significant changes in neonatal neurobehavior.
- Rarely, local infiltration anesthesia may be used as the primary anesthetic technique for cesarean section.

REFERENCES

1. American College of Obstetrics and Gynecologists. Issues in Women's Health Media Kit. Washington, DC, 1998.
2. Depp R. Cesarean delivery. In: Gabbe S, Niebyl JR, Simpson JL, editors. Obstetrics: Normal and Problem Pregnancies. 3rd ed. New York, Churchill Livingstone, 2002:538-606.
3. Hawkins JL, Koonin LM, Palmer SK, Gibbs CP. Anesthesia-related deaths during obstetric delivery in the United States, 1979-1990. Anesthesiology 1997; 86:277-84.
4. Koonin LM, MacKay AP, Berg CJ, et al. Pregnancy-related mortality surveillance—United States. 1987-1990. MMWR CDC Surveill Summ 1997; 46:17-36.

5. Sachs BP, Oriol NE, Ostheimer GW, et al. Anesthetic-related maternal mortality, 1954 to 1985. J Clin Anesth 1989; 1:333-8.

6. Hibbard BM, Anderson MM, O'Drife JO, et al, editors. Report on Confidential Enquiries into Maternal Deaths in the United Kingdom 1991-1993. London, England, HMSO, 1996.

7. Hawkins JL, Birnbach DJ. Maternal mortality in the United States: Where are we going and how will we get there? Anesth Analg 2001; 93:1-3.

8. Panchal S, Arria AM, Labhsetwar SA. Maternal mortality during hospital admission for delivery: A retrospective analysis using a state-maintained database. Anesth Analg 2001; 93:134-41.

9. Conklin KA. Can anesthetic-related maternal mortality be reduced? Am J Obstet Gynecol 1990; 163:253-4.

10. Morgan BM, Magni V, Goroszenuik T. Anaesthesia for emergency caesarean section. Br J Obstet Gynaecol 1990; 97:420-4.

11. Hawkins JL, Gibbs CP, Orleans M, et al. Obstetric anesthesia work force survey, 1981 versus 1992. Anesthesiology 1997; 87:135-43.

12. Tsen LC, Pitner R, Camann WR. General anesthesia for cesarean section at a tertiary care hospital 1990-1995: Indications and implications. Int J Obstet Anesth 1998; 7:147-52.

13. Kanto J, Sjowall S, Erkkola R, et al. Placental transfer and maternal midazolam kinetics. Clin Pharmacol Ther 1983; 33:786-91.

14. Eisele JH, Wright R, Rogge P. Newborn and maternal fentanyl levels at cesarean section. Anesth Analg 1982; 61:179-80.

15. Parer JT. Fetal heart rate. In: Creasy RK, Resnik R, editors. Maternal-Fetal Medicine: Principles and Practice. 2nd ed. Philadelphia, PA, WB Saunders, 1989:314-43.

16. Murad SHN, Conklin KA, Tabsh KMH, et al. Atropine and glycopyrrolate: Hemodynamic effects and placental transfer in the pregnant ewe. Anesth Analg 1981; 60:710-4.

17. Brock-Utne JG, Rubin J, Welman S, et al. The effect of glycopyrrolate (Robinul) on the lower oesophageal sphincter. Can Anaesth Soc J 1978; 25:144-6.

18. Kotelko DM, Rottman RL, Wright WC, et al. Transdermal scopolamine decreases nausea and vomiting following cesarean section in patients receiving epidural morphine. Anesthesiology 1989; 71:675-8.

19. Rout CC, Rocke DA, Levin J, et al. A re-evaluation of the role of crystalloid preload in the prevention of hypotension associated with spinal anesthesia for elective cesarean section. Anesthesiology 1993; 79:262-9.

20. Crino JP, Harris AP, Parisi VM, Johnson TRB. Effect of rapid intravenous crystalloid infusion on uteroplacental blood flow and placental implantation-site oxygen delivery in the pregnant ewe. Am J Obstet Gynecol 1993; 168:1603-9.

21. Kenepp NB, Kumar S, Shelley WC, et al. Fetal and neonatal hazards of maternal hydration with 5% dextrose before caesarean section. Lancet 1982; 1:1150-2.

22. Gonik B, Cotton D, Spillman, et al. Peripartum colloid osmotic pressure changes: Effects of controlled fluid management. Am J Obstet Gynecol 1985; 151:812-5.

23. Wennberg E, Frid I, Haljamae H, et al. Comparison of Ringer's acetate with 3% dextran 70 for volume loading before extradural caesarean section. Br J Anaesth 1990; 65:654-60.

24. Siddik SM, Aouad MT, Kai GE, et al. Hydroxyethylstarch 10% is superior to Ringer's solution for preloading before spinal anesthesia for cesarean section. Can J Anaesth 2000; 47:616-21.

25. Weeks S. Reflections on hypotension during cesarean section under spinal anesthesia: Do we need to use colloid? Can J Anaesth 2000; 47:607-10.

26. Ueyama H, He Y, Tanigami H, et al. Effects of crystalloid and colloid preload on blood volume in the parturient undergoing spinal anesthesia for elective cesarean section. Anesthesiology 1999; 91:1571-6.

27. Loughrey YR, Datta S, Tsen LC. Hypotension prophylaxis for caesarean section. Anaesthesia 2002; 57:284-313.

28. Strauss RG, Stansfield C, Henriksen RA, Villhauer PJ. Pentastarch may cause fewer effects on coagulation than hetastarch. Transfusion 1988; 28:257-60.

29. Ueland K. Maternal cardiovascular dynamics. VII. Intra-partum blood volume changes. Am J Obstet Gynecol 1976; 126:671-7.

30. Duthie SJ, Ghosh A, Ng A, Ho PC. Intra-operative blood loss during elective lower segment caesarean section. Br J Obstet Gynaecol 1992; 99:364-7.

31. Gilstrap LC, Hauth JC, Hankins GDV, Patterson AR. Effect of type of anesthesia on blood loss at cesarean section. Obstet Gynecol 1987; 69:328-32.

32. Andrews WW, Ramin SM, Maberry MC, et al. Effect of type of anesthesia on blood loss at elective repeat cesarean section. Am J Perinatol 1992; 9:197-200.

33. Hood DD, Holubec DM. Elective repeat cesarean section: Effect of anesthesia type on blood loss. J Reprod Med 1990; 35:368-72.

34. Reisner LS. Type and screen for cesarean section: A prudent alternative. Anesthesiology 1983; 58:476-8.

35. Cousins LM, Teplick FB, Poeltler DM. Pre-cesarean blood bank orders: A safe and less expensive approach. Obstet Gynecol 1996; 87:912-6.

36. Bienarz J, Crottogini JJ, Curuchet E, et al. Aortocaval compression by the uterus in late human pregnancy. Am J Obstet Gynecol 1968; 100:203-17.

37. Milsom I, Forssman L, Biber B, et al. Maternal haemodynamic changes during caesarean section: A comparison of epidural and general anaesthesia. Acta Anaesthesiol Scand 1985; 29:161-7.

38. Endler GC, Donath RW. Inflation device to prevent aortocaval compression during pregnancy. Anesth Analg 1985; 64:1015-6.

39. American Society of Anesthesiologists. Standards for Basic Intra-Operative Monitoring. Park Ridge, IL. (Last amended October 21, 1998)

40. Caplan RA, Ward JR, Posner K, Cheney FW. Unexpected cardiac arrest during spinal anesthesia: A closed claims analysis of predisposing factors. Anesthesiology 1988; 68:5-11.

41. Gauthier RA, Dyck B, Chung F, et al. Respiratory interaction after spinal anesthesia and sedation with midazolam. Anesthesiology 1992; 77:909-14.

42. Palmer CM, Norris MC, Giudici MC, et al. Incidence of electrocardiographic changes during cesarean delivery under regional anesthesia. Anesth Analg 1990; 70:36-40.

43. Mathew JP, Fleischer LA, Rinehouse JA, et al. ST segment depression during labor and delivery. Anesthesiology 1992; 77:635-41.

44. Burton A, Camann W. Electrocardiographic changes during cesarean section: A review. Int J Obstet Anesth 1996; 5:47-53.

45. Ross RM, Baker T. Cardiac enzymes in patients undergoing caesarean section. Can J Anaesth 1995; 42:46-50.

46. Frolich MA, Caton D. Baseline heart rate may predict hypotension after spinal anesthesia in prehydrated obstetrical patients. Can J Anaesth 2002; 49:185-9.

47. Malinow AM, Naulty JS, Hunt CO, et al. Precordial ultrasonic monitoring during cesarean delivery. Anesthesiology 1987; 66:816-9.

48. Handler JS, Bromage PR. Venous air embolism during cesarean delivery. Reg Anesth 1990; 15:170-3.

49. Fong J, Gadalla F, Druzin M. Venous emboli occurring during caesarean section: The effect of patient position. Can J Anaesth 1991; 38:191-5.

50. Fong J, Gadalla F, Pierri MK, Druzin M. Are Doppler-detected venous emboli during cesarean section air emboli? Anesth Analg 1990; 71:254-7.

51. Robson SC, Boys RJ, Rodeck C, Morgan B. Maternal and fetal hemodynamic effects of spinal and extradural anesthesia for elective caesarean section. Br J Anaesth 1992; 68:54-9.

52. Olsson GL, Hallen B, Hambraeus-Jonzon K. Aspiration during anaesthesia: A computer-aided study of 185,358 anaesthetics. Acta Anaesthesiol Scand 1986; 30:84-92.

53. Gibbs CP, Schwartz DJ, Wynne JW, et al. Antacid pulmonary aspiration in the dog. Anesthesiology 1979; 51:380-5.

54. Dewan DM, Floyd HM, Thistlewood JM, et al. Sodium citrate pretreatment in elective cesarean section patients. Anesth Analg 1985; 64:34-7.

55. Hodgkinson R, Glassenberg R, Joyce TH, et al. Comparison of cimetidine (Tagamet) with antacid for safety and effectiveness in reducing gastric acidity before elective cesarean section. Anesthesiology 1983; 59:86-90.

56. Rout CC, Rocke DA, Gouws E. Intravenous ranitidine reduces the risk of acid aspiration of gastric contents at emergency cesarean section. Anesth Analg 1993; 76:156-61.

57. Lin CJ, Huang CL, Hsu HW, Chen TL. Prophylaxis against acid aspiration in regional anesthesia for elective cesarean section: A comparison between oral single-dose ranitidine, famotidine and omeprazole assessed with fiberoptic gastric aspiration. Acta Anaesthesiol Sin 1996; 34:179-84.

58. Stuart JC, Kan AF, Rowbottom SJ, et al. Acid aspiration prophylaxis for emergency caesarean section. Anaesthesia 1996; 51:415-21.

59. Manchikanti L, Marrero TC, Roush JR. Preanesthetic cimetidine and metoclopramide for acid aspiration prophylaxis in elective surgery. Anesthesiology 1984; 61:48-54.

60. Wyner J, Cohen SE. Gastric volume in early pregnancy: Effects of metoclopramide. Anesthesiology 1982; 57:202-12.

61. Cohen SE, Jasson J, Talafre, ML, et al. Does metoclopramide decrease the volume of gastric contents in patients undergoing cesarean section? Anesthesiology 1984; 61:604-7.

62. Chestnut DH, Vandewalker GE, Owen CL, et al. Administration of metoclopramide for the prevention of nausea and vomiting during epidural anesthesia for elective cesarean section. Anesthesiology 1987; 66:563-6.

63. Lussos SA, Bader A, Thornhill ML, Datta S. The antiemetic efficacy and safety of prophylactic metoclopramide for elective cesarean delivery during spinal anesthesia. Reg Anesth 1992; 17:126-30.

64. Frerk CM. Predicting difficult intubation. Anaesthesia 1991; 46:1005-8.

65. Hon EH, Reid BL, Hehre FW. The electronic evaluation of the fetal heart rate. II. Changes with maternal hypotension. Am J Obstet Gynecol 1960; 79:209-15.

66. Huovinen K, Lehtovirta P, Forss M, et al. Changes in placental intervillous blood flow measured by the 133Xenon method during lumbar epidural block for elective caesarean section. Acta Anaesthesiol Scand 1979; 23:529-33.

67. Datta S, Alper M, Ostheimer GW, Weiss JB. Methods of ephedrine administration and nausea and hypotension during spinal anesthesia for cesarean section. Anesthesiology 1982; 56:68-70.

68. Ralston DH, Shnider SM, deLorimer AA. Effects of equipotent ephedrine, metaraminol, mephentermine, and methoxamine on uterine blood flow in the pregnant ewe. Anesthesiology 1974; 40:354-70.

69. Hollmen AI, Jouppila R, Albright GA, et al. Intervillous blood flow during caesarean section with prophylactic ephedrine and epidural anaesthesia. Acta Anaesthesiol Scand 1984; 28:396-400.

70. Tong C, Eisenach JC. The vascular mechanism of ephedrine's beneficial effect on uterine perfusion during pregnancy. Anesthesiology 1992; 76:792-8.

71. LaPorta RF, Arthur GR, Datta S. Phenylephrine in treating maternal hypotension due to spinal anesthesia for caesarean delivery: Effects on neonatal catecholamine concentrations, acid base status and Apgar scores. Acta Anaesthesiol Scand 1995; 39:901-5.

72. McKinlay J, Lyons G. Obstetric neuraxial anaesthesia: Which pressor agents should we be using? Int J Obstet Anesth 2002; 11:117-21.

73. Lee A, Ngan Kee WD, Gin T. A quantitative, systematic review of randomized controlled trials of ephedrine versus phenylephrine for the management of hypotension during spinal anesthesia for cesarean delivery. Anesth Analg 2002; 94:920-6.

74. Cooper DW, Carpenter M, Mowbray P, et al. Fetal and maternal effects of phenylephrine and ephedrine during spinal anesthesia for cesarean delivery. Anesthesiology 2002; 97:1582-90.

75. Hughes SC, Ward MG, Levinson G, et al. Placental transfer of ephedrine does not affect neonatal outcome. Anesthesiology 1985; 63:217-9.

76. Gutsche B. Prophylactic ephedrine preceding spinal analgesia for cesarean section. Anesthesiology 1976; 45:462-5.

77. Brizgys RV, Dailey PA, Shnider SM, et al. The incidence and neonatal effects of maternal hypotension during epidural anesthesia for cesarean section. Anesthesiology 1987; 67:782-6.

78. Loughrey JP, Walsh F, Gardiner J. Prophylactic intravenous bolus ephedrine for elective caesarean section under spinal anaesthesia. Eur J Anaesthesiol 2002; 19:63-8.

79. Simon L, Provenchere S, de Saint Blanquat L, et al. Dose of prophylactic intravenous ephedrine during spinal anesthesia for cesarean section. J Clin Anesth 2001; 13:366-9.

80. Ngan Kee WD, Khaw KS, Lee BB, et al. A dose-response study of prophylactic intravenous ephedrine for the prevention of hypotension during spinal anesthesia for cesarean delivery. Anesth Analg 2000; 90:1390-5.

81. King SW, Rosen MA. Prophylactic ephedrine and hypotension associated with spinal anesthesia for cesarean delivery. Int J Obstet Anesth 1998; 7:18-21.

82. Vercauteren MP, Coppejans HC, Hoffmann VH, et al. Prevention of hypotension by a single 5-mg dose of ephedrine during small-dose spinal anesthesia in prehydrated cesarean delivery patients. Anesth Analg 2000; 90:324-7.

83. Tsen LC, Boosalis P, Segal S, et al. Hemodynamic effects of simultaneous administration of intravenous ephedrine and spinal anesthesia for cesarean delivery. J Clin Anesth 2000; 12:378-82.

84. Turkoz A, Togal T, Gokdeniz R, et al. Effectiveness of intravenous ephedrine infusion during spinal anaesthesia for caesarean section based on maternal hypotension, neonatal acid-base status and lactate levels. Anaesth Intensive Care 2002; 30:316-20.

85. Lee A, Ngan Kee WD, Gin T. Prophylactic ephedrine prevents hypotension during spinal anesthesia for cesarean delivery but does not improve neonatal outcome: A quantitative systematic review. Can J Anaesth 2002; 49:588-99.

86. Scott DB, Hibbard BM. Serious non-fatal complications associated with extradural block in obstetric practice. Br J Anaesth 1990; 64:537-41.

87. Chadwick HS, Bernards CM, Kovarik DW, Tomlin JJ. Subdural injection of morphine for analgesia following cesarean section: A report of three cases. Anesthesiology 1992; 77:590-4.

88. Morishima HO, Pedersen H, Finster M, et al. Bupivacaine toxicity in pregnant and nonpregnant ewes. Anesthesiology 1985; 63:134-9.

89. Kasten GW, Martin ST. Bupivacaine cardiovascular toxicity: Comparison of treatment with bretylium and lidocaine. Anesth Analg 1985; 64:911-6.

90. Moore DC, Batra MS. The components of an effective test dose prior to an epidural block. Anesthesiology 1981; 55:693-6.

91. Cartwright PD, McCarroll SM, Antzaka C. Maternal heart rate changes with plain epidural test dose. Anesthesiology 1986; 65:226-8.

92. Chestnut DH, Owen CL, Brown CK, et al. Does labor affect the variability of maternal heart rate during induction of epidural anesthesia? Anesthesiology 1988; 68:622-5.

93. Youngstrom P, Hoyt M, Veille JC, et al. Effects of intravenous test dose epinephrine on fetal sheep during acute fetal stress and acidosis. Reg Anesth 1991; 15:237-41.

94. Marcus MAE, Vertommen JD, Van Aken H, Wouters PF. Hemodynamic effects of intravenous isoproterenol versus epinephrine in the chronic maternal-fetal sheep preparation. Anesth Analg 1996; 82:1023-6.

95. Marcus MAE, Vertommen JD, Van Aken H, et al. Hemodynamic effects of intravenous isoproterenol versus saline in the parturient. Anesth Analg 1997; 84:1113-6.

96. Marcus MAE, Vertommen JD, Van Aken H, Van Lommel F. Light microscopic neuropathological observations after intrathecal bolus injections of isoproterenol (abstract). Anesthesiology 1994; 81:A1175.

97. Leighton BL, Gross JB. Air: An effective indicator of intravenously located epidural catheters. Anesthesiology 1989; 71:848-51.

98. Drasner K, Rigler M. Repeat injection after a "failed spinal": At times a potentially unsafe practice. Anesthesiology 1991; 75:713-4.

99. Ross BK, Coda B, Heath CH. Local anesthetic distribution in a spinal model: A possible mechanism of neurologic injury after continuous spinal anesthesia. Reg Anesth 1992; 17:69-77.

100. Abouleish E. Cauda equina syndrome, continuous spinal anesthesia and repeated spinal block: Is there a relationship? Reg Anesth 1992; 17:356-7.

101. Collins VJ. Epidural anesthesia. In: Collins VJ, editor. Principles of Anesthesiology: General and Regional Anesthesia. 3rd ed. Philadelphia, PA, Lea & Febiger, 1993:571-610.

102. Blomberg R. The dorsomedian connective tissue band in the lumbar epidural space of humans: An anatomical study using epiduroscopy in autopsy cases. Anesth Analg 1986; 65:747-52.

103. Luyendijk W. The plica mediana dorsalis of the dura mater and its relation to lumbar peridurography (canalography). Neuroradiology 1976; 11:147-9.

104. Stone PA, Thorburn J, Lamb KSR. Complications of spinal anaesthesia following extradural block for caesarean section. Br J Anaesth 1989; 62:335-7.

105. Furst SR, Reisner LS. Risk of high spinal anesthesia following failed epidural block for cesarean delivery. J Clin Anesth 1995; 7:71-4.

106. Reisner LS, Hochman BN, Plumer MH. Persistent neurologic deficit and adhesive arachnoiditis following intrathecal 2-chloroprocaine injection. Anesth Analg 1980; 59:452-4.

107. Ravindran R, Bond VK, Tasch MD, et al. Prolonged neural blockade following regional anesthesia with 2-chloroprocaine. Anesth Analg 1980; 59:447-51.

108. Gissen AJ, Datta S, Lambert D. The chloroprocaine controversy II. Is chloroprocaine neurotoxic? Reg Anesth 1984; 9:135-45.

109. Taniguchi M, Bollen AW, Drasner K. Sodium bisulfite: Scapegoat for chloroprocaine neurotoxicity? Anesthesiology 2004; 100:85-91.

110. Ramanathan S, Gandhi S, Arismendy J, et al. Oxygen transfer from mother to fetus during cesarean section under epidural anesthesia. Anesth Analg 1982; 61:576-81.

111. Ratra CK, Badola RP, Bhargava KP. A study of factors concerned in emesis during spinal anaesthesia. Br J Anaesth 1972; 44:1208-11.

112. Khaw KS, Wang CC, Ngan Kee WD, et al. Effects of high inspired oxygen fraction during elective caesarean section under spinal anaesthesia on maternal and fetal oxygenation and lipid peroxidation. Br J Anaesth 2002; 88:18-23.

113. Backe SK. Oxygen and elective caesarean section. Br J Anaesth 2002; 88:4-5.

114. Cogliano MS, Graham AC, Clark VA. Supplementary oxygen administration for elective caesarean section under spinal anaesthesia. Br J Anaesth 2002; 57:66-9.

115. Munn MB, Owen J, Vincent R, et al. Comparison of two oxytocin regimens to prevent uterine atony at cesarean delivery: A randomized controlled trial. Obstet Gynecol 2001; 98:386-90.

116. Secher NJ, Arnsbo P, Wallin L. Haemodynamic effects of oxytocin (syntocinon) and methyl ergometrine (methergin) on the systemic and pulmonary circulations of pregnant anaesthetized women. Acta Obstet Gynecol Scand 1978; 57:97-103.

117. Casady GN, Moore DC, Bridenbaugh LD. Postpartum hypertension after the use of vasoconstrictor and oxytocic drugs. JAMA 1960; 172:1011-5.

118. Ko WJ, Ho HN, Chu SH. Postpartum myocardial infarction rescued with an intraaortic balloon pump and extracorporeal membrane. Int J Cardiol 1998; 63:81-4.

119. Eklund B, Carlson LA. Central and peripheral circulatory effects and metabolic effects of different prostaglandins given IV to man. Prostaglandins 1980; 20:333-47.

120. Kehlet H. Modification of responses to surgery by neural blockade: Clinical implications. In: Cousins MJ, Bridenbaugh PO, editors. Neural Blockade in Clinical Anesthesia and Management of Pain. 2nd ed. Philadelphia, PA, JB Lippincott, 1988:145-88.

121. Kan RE, Hughes SC, Rosen MA, et al. Intravenous remifentanil: Placental transfer, maternal and neonatal effects. Anesthesiology 1998; 88:1467-74.

122. Pan PH, Moore CH. Intraoperative antiemetic efficacy of prophylactic ondansetron versus droperidol for cesarean section patients under epidural anesthesia. Anesth Analg 1996; 83:982-6.

123. Koch ME, Kain ZN, Ayoub C, Rosenbaum SH. The sedative and analgesic sparing effect of music. Anesthesiology 1998; 89:300-6.

124. Robson SC, Boys RJ, Rodeck C, Morgan B. Maternal and fetal haemodynamic effects of spinal and extradural anaesthesia for elective caesarean section. Br J Anaesth 1992; 68:54-9.

125. Gale R, Zalkinder-Luboshitz I, Slater PE. Increased neonatal risk from the use of general anesthesia in emergency cesarean section: A retrospective analysis of 374 cases. J Reprod Med 1982; 27:715-9.

126. Marx GF, Luykx WM, Cohen S. Fetal-neonatal status following caesarean section for fetal distress. Br J Anaesth 1984; 56:1009-13.

127. Clark SL, Koonings PP, Phelan JP. Placenta previa/accreta and prior cesarean section. Obstet Gynecol 1985; 66:89-92.

128. Chestnut DH, Dewan DM, Redick LF, et al. Anesthetic management for obstetric hysterectomy: A multi-institutional study. Anesthesiology 1989; 70:607-10.

129. Kuhnert BR, Philipson EH, Pimental R, et al. Lidocaine disposition in mother, fetus, and neonate after spinal anesthesia. Anesth Analg 1986; 65:139-44.

130. Robson SC, Samsoon G, Boys RJ, et al. Incremental spinal anaesthesia for elective caesarean section: Maternal and fetal haemodynamic effects. Br J Anaesth 1993; 70:634-8.

131. Sprague DH. Effects of position and uterine displacement on spinal anesthesia for cesarean section. Anesthesiology 1976; 44:164-6.

132. Inglis A, Daniel M, McGrady E. Maternal position during the induction of spinal anaesthesia for caesarean section. A comparison of right lateral and sitting positions. Anaesthesia 1995; 50:363-5.

133. Yun EM, Marx GF, Santos AC. The effects of maternal position during induction of combined spinal-epidural anesthesia for cesarean delivery. Anesth Analg 1998; 87:614-8.

134. Lynch J, Krings-Ernst I, Strick K, et al. Use of a 25-gauge Whitacre needle to reduce the incidence of postdural puncture headache. Br J Anaesth 1991; 67:690-3.

135. Ross BK, Chadwick HS, Mancuso JJ, Benedetti C. Sprotte needle for obstetric anesthesia: Decreased incidence of post-dural puncture headache. Reg Anesth 1992; 17:29-33.

136. Mayer DC, Quance D, Weeks SK. Headache after spinal anesthesia for cesarean section: A comparison of the 27-gauge Quincke and 24-gauge Sprotte needles. Anesth Analg 1992; 75:377-80.

137. Datta S, Lambert DH, Gregus J, et al. Differential sensitivities of mammalian nerve fibers during pregnancy. Anesth Analg 1983; 62:1070-2.

138. Chantigian RC, Datta S, Burger GA, et al. Anesthesia for cesarean delivery utilizing spinal anesthesia: Tetracaine versus tetracaine and procaine. Reg Anesth 1984; 9:195-9.

139. Lussos SA, Datta S. Anesthesia for cesarean delivery. I. General considerations and spinal anesthesia. Int J Obstet Anesth 1992; 1:79-91.

140. Casati A, Santorsola R, Cerchierini E, Moizo E. Ropivacaine. Minerva Anestesiol 2001; 67:15-9.

141. Malinovsky JM, Charles F, Kick O, et al. Intrathecal anesthesia: Ropivacaine versus bupivacaine. Anesth Analg 2000; 91:1457-60.

142. Khaw KS, Ngan Kee WD, Wong EL, et al. Spinal ropivacaine for cesarean section: A dose-finding study. Anesthesiology 2001; 95:1346-50.

143. Khaw KS, Ngan Kee WD, Wong M, et al. Spinal ropivacaine for cesarean delivery: A comparison of hyperbaric and plain solutions. Anesth Analg 2002; 94:680-5.

144. Foster RH, Markham A. Levobupivacaine: A review of its pharmacology and use as a local anaesthetic. Drugs 2000; 59:551-79.

145. Glaser C, Marhofer P, Zimpfer G, et al. Levobupivacaine versus racemic bupivacaine for spinal anesthesia. Anesth Analg 2002; 94:194-8.

146. Alley EA, Kopacz DJ, McDonald SB, Liu SS. Hyperbaric spinal levobupivacaine: A comparison to racemic bupivacaine in volunteers. Anesth Analg 2002; 94:188-93.

147. Abouleish EI. Epinephrine improves the quality of spinal hyperbaric bupivacaine for cesarean section. Anesth Analg 1987; 66:395-400.

148. Leicht CH, Carlson SA. Prolongation of lidocaine spinal anesthesia with epinephrine and phenylephrine. Anesth Analg 1986; 65:365-9.

149. Spivey DL. Epinephrine does not prolong lidocaine spinal anesthesia in term parturients. Anesth Analg 1985; 64:468-70.

150. Shende D, Cooper GM, Bowden MI. The influence of intrathecal fentanyl on the characteristics of subarachnoid block for caesarean section. Anaesthesia 1998; 53:702-10.

151. Camann WR, Bader AM. Spinal anesthesia for cesarean delivery with meperidine as the sole agent. Int J Obstet Anesth 1992; 1:156-8.

152. Ueland K, Gills RE, Hansen JM. Maternal cardiovascular dynamics I. Cesarean section under subarachnoid block anesthesia. Am J Obstet Gynecol 1968; 100:42-54.

153. Johnstone M. The cardiovascular effect of oxytocic drugs. Br J Anaesth 1972; 44:826-33.

154. Shantha TR, Evans JA. The relationship of epidural anesthesia to neural membranes and arachnoid villi. Anesthesiology 1972; 37:543-57.

155. Dawkins CJM. An analysis of the complications of extradural and caudal block. Anaesthesia 1969; 24:554-63.

156. Craft JB, Epstein BS, Coakley CS. Prophylaxis of dural puncture headache with epidural saline. Anesth Analg 1973; 52:228-31.

157. Brownridge P. The management of headache following accidental dural puncture in obstetric patients. Anaesth Intensive Care 1983; 11:4-15.

158. Verniquet AJW. Vessel puncture with epidural catheters. Anaesthesia 1980; 35:660-2.

159. Abboud TK, Nagappala S, Murakawa K, et al. Comparison of the effects of general and regional anesthesia for cesarean section on neonatal neurologic and adaptive capacity scores. Anesth Analg 1985; 64: 996-1000.

160. Covino BG, Marx GF, Finster M, Zsigmond EK. Prolonged sensory/motor deficits following inadvertent spinal anesthesia (editorial). Anesth Analg 1980; 59:399-400.

161. Bromage PR. Epidural Analgesia. Philadelphia, PA, WB Saunders, 1978:513-600.

162. Albright G. Cardiac arrest following regional anesthesia with etidocaine or bupivacaine (editorial). Anesthesiology 1979; 51:285-6.

163. Griffin RP, Reynolds F. Extradural anaesthesia for caesarean section: A double-blind comparison of 0.5% ropivacaine with 0.5% bupivacaine. Br J Anaesth 1995; 74:512-6.

164. Datta S, Camann W, Bader A, et al. Clinical effects and maternal and fetal plasma concentrations of epidural ropivacaine versus bupivacaine for cesarean section. Anesthesiology 1995; 82:1346-52.

165. Brown WU, Bell GC, Lurie AO, et al. Newborn blood levels of lidocaine and mepivacaine in the first postnatal day following maternal epidural anesthesia. Anesthesiology 1975; 42:698-707.

166. Abboud TK, Moore MJ, Jacobs J, et al. Epidural mepivacaine for cesarean section: Maternal and neonatal effects. Reg Anesth 1987; 12:76-9.

167. Winnie AP, Masters RW, Durrani Z, Patel KP. Motor block outlasts sensory block: A unique characteristic of etidocaine. Reg Anesth 1984; 9:146-53.

168. Cohen SE, Thurlow A. Comparison of a chloroprocaine-bupivacaine mixture with chloroprocaine and bupivacaine used individually for obstetric epidural analgesia. Anesthesiology 1979; 51:288-92.

169. Camann WR, Hartigan PM, Gilbertson LI, et al. Chloroprocaine antagonism of epidural opioid analgesia: A receptor-specific phenomenon? Anesthesiology 1990; 73:860-3.

170. Skjoldebrand A, Eklund J, Lunell NO, et al. The effect on uteroplacental blood flow of epidural anaesthesia containing adrenaline for caesarean section. Acta Anaesthesiol Scand 1990; 34:85-9.

171. Marx GF, Elstein ID, Schuss M, et al. Effects of epidural block with lignocaine and lignocaine-adrenaline on umbilical artery velocity wave ratios. Br J Obstet Gynaecol 1990; 97:517-20.

172. Alahuhta S, Rasanen J, Jouppila R, et al. Effects of extradural bupivacaine with adrenaline for caesarean section on uteroplacental and fetal circulation. Br J Anaesth 1991; 67:678-82.

173. DiFazio CA, Carron H, Grosslight KR, et al. Comparison of pH-adjusted lidocaine solutions for epidural anesthesia. Anesth Analg 1986; 65:760-4.

174. Fernando R, Jones HM. Comparison of plain and alkalinized local anesthetic mixtures of lignocaine and bupivacaine for elective extradural caesarean section. Br J Anaesth 1991; 67:699-703.

175. Wong K, Strichartz GR, Raymond SA. On the mechanisms of potentiation of local anesthetics by bicarbonate buffer: Drug structure-activity studies on isolated peripheral nerve. Anesth Analg 1993; 76:131-43.

176. Parnass SM, Curran MJA, Becker GL. Incidence of hypotension associated with epidural anesthesia using alkalinized and nonalkalinized lidocaine for cesarean section. Anesth Analg 1987; 66:1148-50.

177. Guay J, Gaudreault P, Boulanger A, et al. Lidocaine hydrocarbonate and lidocaine hydrochloride for cesarean section: Transplacental passage and neonatal effects. Acta Anaesthesiol Scand 1992; 36:722-7.

178. De Leon-Casasola OA, Lema MJ, Emrich L, Syed N. Continuous 2-chloroprocaine infusion versus intermittent bolus injections of bupivacaine or 2-chloroprocaine for epidural anesthesia in cesarean delivery. Reg Anesth 1991; 16:154-60.

179. Helbo-Hansen HS, Bang U, Lindholm P, Klitgaard NA. Maternal effects of adding fentanyl to 0.5% bupivacaine for caesarean section. Int J Obstet Anesth 1993; 2:21-6.

180. Helbo-Hansen HS, Bang U, Lindholm P, Klitgaard NA. Neonatal effects of adding fentanyl to 0.5% bupivacaine for caesarean section. Int J Obstet Anesth 1993; 2:27-33.

181. Chadwick HS, Ready LB. Intrathecal and epidural morphine sulfate for postcesarean analgesia: A clinical comparison. Anesthesiology 1988; 68:925-9.

182. Naulty JS, Datta S, Ostheimer GW, et al. Epidural fentanyl for postcesarean delivery pain management. Anesthesiology 1985; 63:694-8.

183. Rosen MA, Hughes SC, Shnider SM, et al. Epidural morphine for relief of postoperative pain of cesarean delivery. Anesth Analg 1983; 62:666-72.

184. Brownridge P. Epidural and subarachnoid analgesia for elective caesarean section. Anaesthesia 1981; 36:70.

185. Rawal N. Single segment combined subarachnoid and epidural block for caesarean section. Can Anaesth Soc J 1986; 33:254-5.

186. Carrie LES. Combined spinal-epidural anesthesia for cesarean section. Tech Reg Anesth Pain Manage 1997; 1:118-22.

187. Rawal N, Holmstrom B, van Zundert A, et al. The combined spinal-epidural technique. In: Birnbach DJ, Gatt SP, Datta S, editors. Textbook of Obstetric Anesthesia. New York, NY, Churchill Livingstone, 2000:157-82.

188. Joshi G, McCaroll S. Evaluation of combined spinal-epidural anaesthesia using two different techniques. Reg Anesth 1994; 19:169-74.

189. Vandermeersch E. Combined spinal-epidural anaesthesia. Baillieres Clin Anaesth 1993; 7:691-708.

190. Eldor J, Guedj P, Goyal Y. Combined spinal and epidural needle (letter). Anesth Analg 1992; 74:169-70.

191. Robbins PM, Fernando R, Lim GH. Accidental intrathecal insertion of an extradural catheter during combined spinal-extradural anaesthesia for caesarean section. Br J Anaesth 1995; 75:355-7.

192. Herman N, Molin J, Knape KG. No additional metal particle formation using the needle-through-needle combined epidural/spinal technique. Acta Anaesthesiol Scand 1996; 40:227-31.

193. Lyons G, MacDonald R, Mikl B. Combined epidural/spinal anaesthesia for caesarean section: Through the needle or in separate spaces? Anaesthesia 1992; 47:199-201.

194. Choi DH, Kim JA, Chung IS. Comparison of combined spinal epidural anesthesia and epidural anesthesia for cesarean section. Acta Anaesthesiol Scand 2000; 44:214-9.

195. Davies SJ, Paech MJ, Welch H, et al. Maternal experience during epidural or combined spinal-epidural anesthesia for cesarean section: A prospective, randomized trial. Anesth Analg 1997; 85:607-13.

196. Kumar CM. Combined subarachnoid and epidural block for caesarean section. Can J Anaesth 1986; 33:329-30.

197. Kuczkowski KM, Benumof JL. Post-dural puncture syndrome in an elderly patient with remote history of previous post-dural puncture syndrome. Acta Anaesthesiol Scand 2002; 46:1049-50.

198. Kuczkowski KM, Benumof J.L. Repeat cesarean section in a morbidly obese parturient: A new anesthetic option. Acta Anaesthesiol Scand 2002; 46:753-4.

199. Rawal N, Schollin J, Wesstrom G. Epidural versus combined spinal epidural block for caesarean section. Acta Anaesthesiol Scand 1988; 32:61-6.

200. Norris MC, Dewan DM. Preoxygenation for cesarean section: A comparison of two techniques. Anesthesiology 1985; 62:287-9.

201. Baraka AS, Taha SK, Aouad MT, et al. Preoxygenation: Comparison of maximal breathing and tidal volume breathing techniques. Anesthesiology 1999; 91:612-6.

202. Benumof JL. Preoxygenation. Anesthesiology 1999; 91:603-5.

203. Baraka AS, Hanna MT, Jabbour SI, et al. Preoxygenation of pregnant and nonpregnant women and the head-up versus supine position. Anesth Analg 1992; 75:757-9.

204. Cherala S, Eddie D, Halpern M, Shevde K. Priming with vecuronium in obstetrics (letter). Anaesthesia 1987; 42:1021.

205. Cook WP, Schultetus RR, Caton D. A comparison of d-tubocurarine pretreatment and no pretreatment in obstetric patients. Anesth Analg 1987; 66:756-60.

206. DeVore JS, Asrani R. Magnesium sulfate prevents succinylcholine induced fasciculations in toxemic parturients. Anesthesiology 1980; 52:76-7.

207. Kosaka Y, Takahashi T, Mark LC. Intravenous thiobarbiturate anesthesia for caesarean section. Anesthesiology 1969; 31:489-506.

208. Schepens P, Heyndrickx A. Placental transfer of thiopental. Eur J Toxicol 1975; 58:87-93.

209. Morgan DJ, Blackman GL, Paull JD, Wolf LJ. Pharmacokinetics and plasma binding of thiopental. II. Studies at cesarean section. Anesthesiology 1981; 54:474-80.

210. Finster M, Mark LC, Morishima HO, et al. Plasma thiopental concentrations in the newborn following delivery under thiopental-nitrous oxide anesthesia. Am J Obstet Gynecol 1966; 95:621-9.

211. Finster M, Morishima HO, Mark LC, et al. Tissue thiopental concentrations in the fetus and newborn. Anesthesiology 1972; 36:155-8.

212. Flowers CE Jr. The placental transmission of barbiturates and thiobarbiturates and their pharmacological action on the mother and the infant. Am J Obstet Gynecol 1959; 78:730-40.

213. Born GVR, Dawes GS, Mott JC, Widdicombe JG. Changes in the heart and lungs at birth. Cold Spring Harb Symp Quant Biol 1954; 19:102-8.

214. Peltz B, Sinclair DM. Induction agents for caesarean section: A comparison of thiopentone and ketamine. Anaesthesia 1973; 28:37-42.

215. Harris CE, Murray AM, Anderson JM, et al. Effects of thiopentone, etomidate, and propofol on the hemodynamic response to tracheal intubation. Anaesthesia 1988; 43(Suppl):32-6.

216. Gin T, Gregory MA, Oh TE. The hemodynamic effects of propofol and thiopentone for induction of caesarean section. Anaesth Intensive Care 1990; 18:175-9.

217. Grounds RM, Twigley AJ, Carli F, et al. The haemodynamic effects of intravenous induction: Comparison of the effects of thiopentone and propofol. Anaesthesia 1985; 40:735-40.

218. Abboud TK, Zhu J, Richardson M, et al. Intravenous propofol vs thiamylal-isoflurane for caesarean section: Comparative maternal and neonatal effects. Acta Anaesthesiol Scand 1995; 39:205-9.

219. Moore J, Bill KM, Flynn RJ, et al. A comparison between propofol and thiopentone as induction agents in obstetric anaesthesia. Anaesthesia 1989; 44:753-7.

220. Gregory MA, Gin T, Yau G, et al. Propofol infusion anaesthesia for caesarean section. Can J Anaesth 1990; 37:514-20.

221. Yau G, Gin T, Ewart MC, et al. Propofol for induction and maintenance of anaesthesia at caesarean section: A comparison with thiopentone/enflurane. Anaesthesia 1991; 46:20-3.

222. Dailland P, Cockshott ID, Lirzin JD, et al. Intravenous propofol during cesarean section: Placental transfer, concentrations in breast milk, and neonatal effects—A preliminary study. Anesthesiology 1989; 71:827-34.

223. Alon E, Ball RH, Gille MH, et al. Effects of propofol and thiopental on maternal and fetal cardiovascular and acid-base variables in the pregnant ewe. Anesthesiology 1993; 78:562-76.

224. Celleno D, Capogna G, Tomassetti M, et al. Neurobehavioural effects of propofol on the neonate following elective caesarean section. Br J Anaesth 1989; 62:649-54.

225. Gin T. Propofol during pregnancy. Acta Anaesthesiol Sin 1994; 32:127-32.

226. Schultetus RR, Hill CR, Dharamraj CM, et al. Wakefulness during cesarean section after anesthetic induction with ketamine, thiopental, or ketamine and thiopental combined. Anesth Analg 1986; 65:723-8.

227. McDonald JS, Mateo CV, Reed EC. Modified nitrous oxide or ketamine hydrochloride for cesarean section. Anesth Analg 1972; 51:975-83.

228. Horwitz LD. Effects of intravenous anesthetic agents on left ventricular function in dogs. Am J Physiol 1977; 232:H44-8.

229. Galloon S. Ketamine for obstetric delivery. Anesthesiology 1976; 44:522-4.

230. Marx GF, Hwang HS, Chandra PC. Postpartum uterine pressures with different doses of ketamine. Anesthesiology 1979; 50:163-6.

231. Oates JN, Vasey DP, Waldron BA. Effects of ketamine on the pregnant uterus. Br J Anaesth 1979; 51:1163-6.

232. Ellington A, Haram K, Sagen N, Solheim E. Transplacental passage of ketamine after intravenous administration. Acta Anaesthiol Scand 1977; 21:41-4.

233. Bernstein K, Gisselsson L, Jacobsson T, Ohrlander S. Influence of two different anaesthetic agents on the newborn and the correlation between foetal oxygenation and induction-delivery time in elective caesarean section. Acta Anaesthesiol Scand 1985; 29:157-60.

234. Hodgkinson R, Marx GF, Kim SS, Miclat NM. Neonatal neurobehavioral tests following vaginal delivery under ketamine, thiopental, and extradural anesthesia. Anesth Analg 1977; 56:548-53.

235. Ellington A, Haram K, Sagen N. Ketamine and diazepam as anesthesia for forceps delivery: A comparative study. Acta Anaesthesiol Scand 1977; 21:37-40.

236. Gregory MA, Davidson DG. Plasma etomidate levels in mother and fetus. Anaesthesia 1991; 46:716-8.

237. Downing JW, Buley RJR, Brock-Utne JG, Houlton PC. Etomidate for induction of anaesthesia at caesarean section: Comparison with thiopentone. Br J Anaesth 1979; 51:135-9.

238. Laughlin TP, Newberg LA. Prolonged myoclonus after etomidate anesthesia. Anesth Analg 1985; 64:80-2.

239. Reddy BK, Pizer B, Bull PT. Neonatal serum cortisol suppression by etomidate compared with thiopentone, for elective cesarean section. Eur J Anaesthesiol 1988; 5:171-6.

240. Bach V, Carl P, Ravlo O, Crawford ME, et al. A randomized comparison between midazolam and thiopental for elective cesarean section anesthesia. III. Placental transfer and elimination in neonates. Anesth Analg 1989; 68:238-42.

241. Crawford ME, Carl P, Bach V, et al. A randomized comparison between midazolam and thiopental for elective cesarean section anesthesia. I. Mothers. Anesth Analg 1989; 68:229-33.

242. Ravlo O, Carl P, Crawford ME, et al. A randomized comparison between midazolam and thiopental for elective cesarean section anesthesia. II. Neonates. Anesth Analg 1989; 68:234-7.

243. Bland BAR, Lawes EG, Duncan PW, et al. Comparison of midazolam and thiopental for rapid sequence anesthetic induction for elective cesarean section. Anesth Analg 1987; 66:1165-8.

244. Doze VA, Shafer A, White PF. Propofol-nitrous oxide versus thiopental-isoflurane-nitrous oxide for general anesthesia. Anesthesiology 1988; 69:63-71.

245. Kvisselgard N, Moya F. Investigation of placental thresholds to succinylcholine. Anesthesiology 1961; 22:7-10.

246. Baraka A, Haroun S, Bassili M, Abu-Hailder G. Response of the newborn to succinylcholine injection in homozygotic atypical mothers. Anesthesiology 1985; 43:115-6.

247. Leighton BL, Cheek TG, Gross JB, et al. Succinylcholine pharmacodynamics in peripartum patients. Anesthesiology 1986; 64:202-5.

248. Kao YJ, Turner DR. Prolongation of succinylcholine block by metoclopramide. Anesthesiology 1988; 63:983-6.

249. Levy DM, Cooper G. Non-depolarising neuromuscular blockers can be used routinely instead of suxamethonium at induction of general anaesthesia for caesarean section. Int J Obstet Anesth 1999; 8:266-72.

250. Abouleish E, Abboud T, Lechevalier J, et al. Rocuronium (Org 9426) for cesarean section. Br J Anaesth 1994; 73:336-41.

251. Magorian T, Flannery KB, Miller RD. Comparison of rocuronium, succinylcholine, and vecuronium for rapid-sequence induction of anesthesia in adult patients. Anesthesiology 1993; 79:913-8.

252. Hawkins JL, Johnson TD, Kabicek MA, et al. Vecuronium for rapid sequence intubation for cesarean section. Anesth Analg 1990; 71:185-90.

253. Dailey PA, Fisher DM, Shnider SM, et al. Pharmacokinetics, placental transfer and neonatal effects of vecuronium and pancuronium administered during cesarean section. Anesthesiology 1984; 60:569-74.

254. Flynn PJ, Frank M, Hughes R. Use of atracurium in caesarean section. Br J Anaesth 1984; 56:599-604.

255. Warren TM, Datta S, Ostheimer GW, et al. Comparison of the maternal and neonatal effects of halothane, enflurane, and isoflurane for cesarean delivery. Anesth Analg 1983; 62:516-20.

256. Crawford JS. Awareness during operative obstetrics under general anesthesia. Br J Anaesth 1971; 43:179-82.

257. Abboud TK, Kim SH, Henriksen EH, et al. Comparative maternal and neonatal effects of halothane and enflurane for cesarean section. Acta Anaesthesiol Scand 1985; 29:663-8.

258. Morishima HO, Pederson H, Finster M. Influence of maternal physiologic stress on the fetus. Am J Obstet Gynecol 1978; 131:286-90.

259. King HK, Ashley S, Brathwaite D, et al. Adequacy of general anesthesia for cesarean section. Anesth Analg 1993; 77:84-8.

260. Gaitini L, Vaida S, Collins G, et al. Awareness detection during cesarean section under general anaesthesia using EEG spectrum analysis. Can J Anaesth 1995; 42:377-81.

261. Schwender D, Madler C, Klassing S, et al. Mid-latency auditory evoked potentials and wakefulness during caesarean section. Eur J Anaesth 1995; 12:171-9.

262. Yeo SN, Lo WK. Bispectral Index in assessment of adequacy of general anaesthesia for lower segment caesarean section. Anaesth Intensive Care 2002; 30:36-40.

263. Lubke GH, Kerssens C, Gershon RY, et al. Memory formation during general anesthesia for emergency cesarean section. Anesthesiology 2000; 92:1029-34.

264. Moir DD. Anaesthesia for caesarean section: An evaluation of a method using low concentrations of halothane and 50 percent of oxygen. Br J Anaesth 1970; 42:136-42.

265. Tunstall ME. The reduction of amnesic wakefulness during caesarean section. Anaesthesia 1979; 34:316-9.

266. Abboud TK, D'Onofrio L, Reyes A, et al. Isoflurane or halothane for cesarean section: Comparative maternal and neonatal effects. Acta Anaesthiol Scand 1989; 33:578-81.

267. Gambling DR, Sharma SK, White PF, et al. Use of sevoflurane during elective caesarean birth: A comparison with isoflurane and spinal anesthesia. Anesth Analg 1995; 81:90-5.

268. Abboud TK, Zhu M, Peres E, et al. Desflurane: A new volatile anesthetic for cesarean section. Maternal and neonatal effects. Acta Anaesthesiol Scand 1995; 39:723-6.

269. Bogod DG, Rosen M, Rees GAD. Maximum FIO2 during caesarean section. Br J Anaesth 1988; 61:255-62.

270. Marx GF, Mateo CV. Effects of different oxygen concentrations during general anaesthesia for elective caesarean section. Can Anaesth Soc J 1971; 18:587-93.

271. Rorke MJ, Davey DA, DuToit HJ. Foetal oxygenation during caesarean section. Anaesthesia 1968; 23:585-96.

272. Piggott SE, Bogod DG, Rosen M, et al. Isoflurane with either 100% oxygen or 50% nitrous oxide in oxygen for caesarean section. Br J Anaesth 1990; 65:325-9.

273. Lawes EG, Newman B, Campbell MJ, et al. Maternal inspired oxygen concentration and neonatal status for caesarean section under general anaesthesia: Comparison of effects of 33% or 50% oxygen in nitrous oxide. Br J Anaesth 1988; 61:250-4.

274. Mark LC. The dilemma of general anesthesia for cesarean section: Adequate fetal oxygenation vs. maternal awareness during operation. Anesthesiology 1982; 56:405-6.

275. Baraka A, Louis F, Dalleh R. Maternal awareness and neonatal outcome after ketamine induction for caesarean section. Can J Anaesth 1990; 37:641-4.

276. Krissel J, Dick WF, Leyser KH, et al. Thiopentone, thiopentone/ketamine, and ketamine for induction of anaesthesia in caesarean section. Eur J Anaesth 1994; 11:115-22.

277. Steer PL, Biddle CJ, Marley WS, et al. Concentration of fentanyl in colostrum after an analgesic dose. Can J Anaesth 1992; 39:231-5.

278. Khuenl-Brady KS, Kollin J, Mair P, et al. Comparison of vecuronium and atracurium induced neuromuscular blockade in postpartum and nonpregnant patients. Anesth Analg 1991; 72:110-3.

279. Camp CE, Tessem J, Adenwala J, Joyce TH III. Vecuronium and prolonged neuromuscular blockade in postpartum patients. Anesthesiology 1987; 67:1006-8.

280. Stoelting R. Pharmacology and Physiology in Anesthetic Practice. Philadelphia, PA, JB Lippincott, 1992:217-8.

281. Ranney B, Stanage WF. Advantages of local anesthesia for cesarean section. Obstet Gynecol 1975; 45:163-7.

282. Friedman AJ, Haseltine FP, Berkowitz RL. Pregnancy in a patient with cystic fibrosis and idiopathic thrombocytopenic purpura. Obstet Gynecol 1980; 55:511-4.

283. Cooper MG, Feeney EM, Joseph M, McGuinness JJ. Local anaesthetic infiltration for caesarean section. Anaesth Intensive Care 1989; 17:198-201.

284. Bonica JJ. Local-regional analgesia for abdominal delivery. In: Bonica JJ, editor. Obstetric Analgesia and Anesthesia. Philadelphia, PA, FA Davis, 1967:527-38.

285. Fox GS, Smith JB, Namba Y, Johnson RC. Anesthesia for cesarean section: Further studies. Am J Obstet Gynecol 1979; 133:15-9.

286. James FM, Crawford JS, Hopkinson R, et al. A comparison of general anesthesia and lumbar epidural analgesia for elective cesarean section. Anesth Analg 1977; 56:228-35.

287. Downing JW, Houlton PC, Barclay A. Extradural analgesia for caesarean section: A comparison with general anaesthesia. Br J Anaesth 1979; 51:367-73.

288. Crawford JS, Davies P. Status of neonates delivered by elective cesarean section. Br J Anaesth 1982; 54:1015-22.

289. Milsom I, Forssman L, Biber B, et al. Maternal haemodynamic changes during caesarean sections: A comparison of epidural and general anesthesia. Acta Anaesthesiol Scand 1985; 29:161-7.

290. Shyken JM, Smeltzer JS, Baxi LV, et al. A comparison of the effect of epidural, general, and no anesthesia on funic acid-base values by stage of labor and type of delivery. Am J Obstet Gynecol 1990; 163:802-7.

291. Evans CM, Murphy JF, Gray OP, Rosen M. Epidural versus general anaesthesia for elective caesarean section: Effect on Apgar score and acid-base status of the newborn. Anaesthesia 1989; 44:778-82.

292. Datta S, Brown WU Jr. Acid-base status in diabetic mothers and their infants following general or spinal anesthesia for cesarean section. Anesthesiology 1977; 47:272-6.

293. Crawford JS, Burton M, Davies P. Anaesthesia for caesarean section: Further refinements of a technique. Br J Anaesth 1973; 45:726-32.

294. Crawford JS, Davies P. A return to trichloroethylene for obstetric anaesthesia. Br J Anaesth 1975; 47:482-90.

295. Datta S, Ostheimer GW, Weiss JB, et al. Neonatal effect of prolonged anesthetic induction for cesarean section. Obstet Gynecol 1981; 58: 331-5.

296. Bader AM, Datta S, Arthur GR, et al. Maternal and fetal catecholamines and uterine incision-to-delivery interval during elective cesarean section. Obstet Gynecol 1990; 75:600-3.

297. Corke BC, Datta S, Ostheimer GW, et al. Spinal anesthesia for caesarean section: The influence of hypotension on neonatal outcome. Anaesthesia 1982; 37:658-62.

298. Fothergill RJ, Robertson A, Bord RA. Neonatal acidaemia related to procrastination at caesarean section. J Obstet Gynaecol Br Commonw 1971; 78:1010-23.

299. Magno R, Selstein U, Karlsson K. Anesthesia for cesarean section. II. Effects of induction-delivery interval on the respiratory adaptation of the newborn in elective cesarean section. Acta Anaesthesiol Scand 1975; 19:250-9.

300. Kivalo I, Timonem S, Castren O. The influence of anesthesia and the induction-delivery interval on the newborn delivered by cesarean section. Ann Chir Gynaecol Fenn 1971; 60:71-5.

301. Robertson A, Fothergill RJ, Hall RA, et al. Effects of anesthesia with a high oxygen concentration on the acid-base state of babies delivered at elective cesarean section. S Afr Med J 1974; 48:2309-13.

302. Marx GF, Joshi CW, Orkin LR. Placental transmission of nitrous oxide. Anesthesiology 1970; 32:429-32.

303. Zagorzycki MT, Brinkman CR. The effect of general and epidural anesthesia upon neonatal Apgar scores in repeat cesarean section. Surg Gynecol Obstet 1982; 155:641-5.

304. Abboud TK, Najappala S, Murakawa K, et al. Comparison of the effects of general and regional anesthesia for cesarean section on neonatal neurologic and adaptive capacity scores. Anesth Analg 1985; 64:996-1000.

305. Apgar V, Holaday DA, James LS, et al. Comparison of regional and general anesthesia in obstetrics. JAMA 1957; 165:2155-61.

306. Ong BY, Cohen MM, Palahniuk RJ. Anesthesia for cesarean section: Effects on neonates. Anesth Analg 1989; 68:270-5.

307. Finster M, Poppers PJ. Safety of thiopental used for induction of general anesthesia in elective cesarean section. Anesthesiology 1968; 29:190-1.

308. Ralston DH, Shnider SM. The fetal and neonatal effects of regional anesthesia in obstetrics. Anesthesiology 1978; 48:34-64.

309. Caritis SN, Abouleish E, Edelstone DI, Mueller-Heubach E. Fetal acid-base state following spinal or epidural anesthesia for cesarean section. Obstet Gynecol 1980; 56:610-5.

310. Kang YG, Abouleish E, Caritis S. Prophylactic intravenous ephedrine infusion during spinal anesthesia for cesarean section. Anesth Analg 1982; 61:839-42.

311. Datta S, Kitzmiller JL, Naulty JS, et al. Acid-base status of diabetic mothers and their infants following spinal anesthesia for cesarean section. Anesth Analg 1982; 61:662-5.

312. Roberts SW, Leveno KJ, Sidawi JE, et al. Fetal acidemia associated with regional anesthesia for elective cesarean delivery. Obstet Gynecol 1995; 85:79-83.

313. Scanlon JW, Brown WU, Weiss JB, Alper MH. Neurobehavioral responses of newborn infants after maternal epidural anesthesia. Anesthesiology 1974; 40:121-8.

314. Abboud TK, Kim KC, Noueihed R, et al. Epidural bupivacaine, chloroprocaine, or lidocaine for cesarean section: Maternal and neonatal effects. Anesth Analg 1983; 62:914-9.

315. Kileff ME, James FM, Dewan DM, Floyd HM. Neonatal neurobehavioral responses after epidural anesthesia for cesarean section using lidocaine and bupivacaine. Anesth Analg 1984; 63:413-7.

316. Kuhnert BR, Harrison MJ, Linn PL, Kuhnert PM. Effects of maternal epidural anesthesia on neonatal behavior. Anesth Analg 1984; 63:301-8.

317. Kuhnert BR, Kennard MJ, Linn PL. Neonatal neurobehavior after epidural anesthesia for cesarean section: A comparison of bupivacaine and chloroprocaine. Anesth Analg 1988; 67:64-8.

318. Kangas-Saarela T, Jouppila R, Alabuhta S, et al. The effect of lumbar epidural analgesia on neurobehavioral responses of newborn infants. Acta Anaesthesiol 1989; 33:320-5.

Chapter 26
Anesthesia for Fetal Distress

David H. Chestnut, M.D.

Occasionally I hear a statement similar to the following: "This patient is 42 years old, and she is having her first child; this is a premium pregnancy." I respond, "True, true, but those statements are unrelated. Every pregnancy is a premium pregnancy."

Fetal heart rate (FHR) abnormalities often prompt the performance of an emergency cesarean section. The anesthesiologist must be prepared to provide anesthesia expeditiously but safely.

DEFINITION

Parer and Livingston[1] acknowledged that "fetal distress is a widely used but poorly defined term." They defined *fetal distress* as follows: "Progressive fetal asphyxia that, if not corrected or circumvented, will result in decompensation of the physiologic responses (primarily redistribution of blood flow to preserve oxygenation of vital organs) and cause permanent central nervous system and other damage or death."

Unfortunately, as used clinically, the term *fetal distress* is imprecise and nonspecific, has a low positive predictive value, and often is associated with the delivery of an infant who is in good condition at birth.[2] The American College of Obstetricians and Gynecologists (ACOG) has suggested that the term *fetal distress* be replaced with the term *nonreassuring fetal status* and that obstetricians further describe the reason for concern (e.g., repetitive variable decelerations, fetal bradycardia, biophysical profile score of 2). The ACOG has noted the following: "Whereas *fetal distress* implies an ill fetus, *nonreassuring fetal status* describes the clinician's interpretation of data regarding fetal status (i.e., the clinician is not reassured by the findings)."[2]

Nonetheless, in clinical practice, many obstetricians continue to use the term *fetal distress* to describe a wide range of FHR abnormalities. In some cases, the global use of the term *fetal distress* has resulted in unnecessarily urgent delivery under general anesthesia, when consideration of the severity of the FHR abnormality may have permitted administration of a safer anesthetic for the mother (e.g., regional anesthesia).[2] Most maternal deaths that result from anesthesia occur during emergency cesarean section.

LABORATORY STUDIES

Several studies have examined the effects of anesthetic agents on acidotic fetal lambs. Palahniuk et al.[3] used an inflated occlusion loop to cause partial umbilical cord compression in gravid ewes. This resulted in fetal metabolic and respiratory acidosis, with a decrease in mean ± SEM fetal arterial pH from 7.34 ± 0.14 to 7.05 ± 0.04. Each ewe was then anesthetized with 4% halothane in oxygen. After paralysis with succinylcholine and endotracheal intubation, anesthesia was maintained with 1% halothane in oxygen for 15 minutes. Maternal administration of halothane caused marked fetal hypotension, further reduced mean fetal arterial pH to 6.85 ± 0.05, and reduced fetal cerebral blood flow and oxygen delivery.

Yarnell et al.[4] also used an umbilical cord occlusion loop to cause hypoxia and acidosis in fetal lambs. After umbilical cord occlusion had caused fetal arterial pH to decline to between 7.10 and 7.15, each ewe was anesthetized with 1.5% halothane, and ventilation was controlled mechanically. Umbilical cord occlusion alone significantly increased fetal mean arterial pressure (MAP) and cerebral blood flow and decreased FHR and cardiac output. Maternal administration of 1.5% halothane for 15 minutes resulted in a decrease of fetal MAP to control, but there was no significant change in fetal cardiac output, cerebral blood flow, or arterial pH (mean ± SEM pH was 7.14 ± 0.03 before and 7.09 ± 0.03 after 15 minutes of halothane). The authors concluded that "low levels of halothane anaesthesia in a stable maternal preparation do not cause further deterioration in the asphyxiated foetus if the duration of anaesthesia is less than 15 minutes."[4] They acknowledged that their results differed from those in the earlier study.[3] They also noted that the inhalation induction used by Palahniuk et al.[3] necessitated a longer exposure to halothane and may have resulted in higher halothane concentrations.

Swartz et al.[5] performed a similar study with three groups of pregnant sheep. Again, an umbilical cord occlusion loop was slowly inflated until fetal arterial pH had decreased to between 7.08 and 7.13. Group A animals—the control group—received no anesthesia. Group B animals received intravenous sodium thiopental 3 mg/kg followed by 50% nitrous oxide and 0.5% halothane in oxygen for 15 minutes. Group C animals received intravenous sodium thiopental

3 mg/kg followed by 1% halothane in oxygen for 15 minutes. Umbilical cord occlusion alone increased fetal MAP and decreased FHR. The administration of general anesthesia in groups B and C abolished the fetal hypertension and bradycardia produced by umbilical cord occlusion, but it did not significantly alter fetal cerebral or myocardial blood flow. During the administration of anesthesia (or oxygen alone in group A), fetal pH progressively decreased in each group. The authors concluded that, in cases of fetal asphyxia, "general anesthesia will not improve the fetal condition and rapid delivery is essential."[5]

Cheek et al.[6] used adjustable uterine artery occlusion to effect hypoxia and acidosis in fetal lambs. They gradually tightened the uterine artery occluder until either transient fetal bradycardia occurred or uterine blood flow was reduced to 50% of control. Next they adjusted the occluder to achieve a stable fetal acidosis (i.e., fetal pH between 7.10 and 7.20). They subsequently administered 5% halothane by face mask for the induction of general anesthesia, and they gave succinylcholine to facilitate endotracheal intubation. After intubation, they controlled ventilation mechanically and administered 1% halothane for 15 minutes. Uterine artery occlusion significantly decreased FHR and hemoglobin oxygen saturation and increased fetal $Paco_2$, MAP, and cerebral, myocardial, and adrenal blood flow. Mean ± SEM fetal arterial pH before and after halothane was 7.14 ± 0.02 and 7.02 ± 0.03, respectively. Halothane abolished the fetal hypertension and bradycardia produced by uterine artery occlusion, but it did not significantly reduce fetal cerebral, myocardial, or adrenal blood flow or cerebral oxygen delivery (Table 26-1). Uterine artery occlu-

sion decreased cerebral oxidative metabolism, but no further significant change occurred after the administration of halothane. The authors concluded that maternal administration of low concentrations of halothane for 15 to 20 minutes "does not abolish normal fetal responses to asphyxia and maintains regional cerebral blood flow, cerebral oxygen supply, and lower cerebral metabolic oxygen consumption . . . ."[6]

Subsequently, Baker et al.[7] used a similar protocol to study the effects of isoflurane. Uterine artery occlusion was performed to achieve a stable fetal acidosis, and each ewe was then anesthetized with 4% isoflurane in oxygen by mask. Succinylcholine was administered to facilitate endotracheal intubation. Ventilation was controlled mechanically, and each ewe received 1% isoflurane for 15 minutes. Uterine artery occlusion significantly decreased FHR, hemoglobin oxygen saturation, and pH and increased fetal $Paco_2$ and cerebral, myocardial, and adrenal blood flow. Administration of isoflurane further increased fetal $Paco_2$ and decreased mean ± SEM fetal arterial pH from 7.16 ± 0.01 to 6.99 ± 0.03, but it did not alter fetal Pao_2 or hemoglobin oxygen saturation. Brainstem and total cerebral blood flow returned toward control during the administration of isoflurane (Table 26-2). Uterine artery occlusion decreased cerebral oxygen delivery, but no further change occurred during the administration of isoflurane. An insignificant decrease in cerebral oxygen consumption occurred during uterine artery occlusion, and there was a further significant decrease during the administration of isoflurane. The authors concluded that "although the increase in blood flow to the brainstem and total brain was blunted, the balance between cerebral oxygen supply and demand remained favorable."[7]

TABLE 26-1	CEREBRAL METABOLIC MEASUREMENTS*		
Variable	**Control**	**Asphyxia**	**Asphyxia + halothane**
Arterial O_2 (mL/100 mL)	6.0 ± 0.5	2.8 ± 0.2[‡]	3.4 ± 0.4[‡]
Cerebral A-V O_2 difference (mL/100 mL)	2.2 ± 0.2	1 ± 0.2[‡]	0.8 ± 0.2[‡]
Cerebral blood flow[†] (mL × g^{-1} × min^{-1})	193 ± 22	304 ± 33[‡]	285 ± 23[‡]
Cerebral O_2 delivery[†] (mL × 100 g^{-1} × min^{-1})	11.2 ± 1.1	8.3 ± 0.8	9.7 ± 1.5
Cerebral O_2 consumption[§] (mL × 100 g^{-1} × min^{-1})	4.1 ± 0.6	2.8 ± 0.4[‡]	2.0 ± 0.3[‡]

*Mean ± SE (n = 9; except[†], where n = 7).
[†]$P < 0.05$, significantly different from control.
[§]Hemisphere.
From Cheek DBC, Hughes SC, Dailey PA, et al. Effect of halothane on regional cerebral blood flow and cerebral metabolic oxygen consumption in the fetal lamb in utero. Anesthesiology 1987; 67:361-6.

TABLE 26-2	CEREBRAL METABOLIC MEASUREMENTS		
Variable	**Control**	**Asphyxia**	**Asphyxia + isoflurane**
Total brain blood flow (mL × 100 g^{-1} × min^{-1}) (8)	196 ± 24	346 ± 46*	267 ± 43
O_2 content (mL/dL)			
Axillary artery (8)	6.21 ± 0.63	2.81 ± 0.28*	2.65 ± 0.51*
Sagittal sinus (6)	4.38 ± 0.71	1.88 ± 0.25*	2.19 ± 0.63*
C(a-v) O_2 (mL/dL) (6)	2.13 ± 0.14	0.94 ± 0.09*	0.83 ± 0.16*
$CMRo_2$ (mL O_2 × 100 g^{-1} × min^{-1})(6)	3.54 ± 0.65	2.54 ± 0.35	1.73 ± 0.22*
O_2 delivery (mL O_2 × 100 g^{-1} × min^{-1})(6)	10.00 ± 2.93	6.66 ± 1.34	6.43 ± 1.99

*$P < 0.05$, versus control.
Values in parentheses are the number of observations.
From Baker BW, Hughes SC, Shnider SM, et al. Maternal analgesia and the stressed fetus: Effects of isoflurane on the asphyxiated fetal lamb. Anesthesiology 1990; 72:65-70.

Pickering et al.[8] used umbilical cord occlusion to evaluate the effects of sodium thiopental and ketamine on acidotic fetal lambs. Each ewe received either high-dose sodium thiopental (10 mg/kg), low-dose sodium thiopental (6 mg/kg), high-dose ketamine (4 mg/kg), or low-dose ketamine (2 mg/kg). Fetal blood pressure tended to increase with acidosis and returned toward or below control values after the administration of either sodium thiopental or ketamine. High-dose sodium thiopental produced the greatest fetal hypotension and the greatest reduction in fetal pH. Both high-dose sodium thiopental and high-dose ketamine significantly reduced fetal cerebral blood flow and cerebral oxygen delivery. Low-dose ketamine seemed to better preserve cerebral blood flow than low-dose thiopental, although the difference between the two groups was not statistically significant. Both doses of sodium thiopental but neither dose of ketamine caused marked fetal tachycardia. The authors concluded that "in the presence of foetal asphyxia, low-dose ketamine may be preferable to thiopentone as an induction drug."[8]

Leicht et al.[9] used the model of uterine artery occlusion to compare the effects of sodium thiopental and ketamine on acidotic fetal lambs. They induced anesthesia with either sodium thiopental (4 mg/kg) or ketamine (3 mg/kg). Subsequently, they administered either drug intravenously "in doses sufficient to keep the animals anesthetized" for 15 minutes. Induction of anesthesia with either agent caused no significant change in fetal blood pressure, cerebral blood flow, or cerebral metabolic oxygen consumption. However, fetal PaO_2 increased significantly with the administration of oxygen before and after the induction of anesthesia. They concluded that there is "no clear difference between ketamine and sodium thiopental in rapid sequence induction of general anesthesia in the presence of fetal asphyxia."[9]

Swartz et al.[10] also studied the effects of ketamine on acidotic fetal lambs. They inflated an umbilical cord occlusion loop until fetal pH had decreased to between 7.12 and 7.15. Subsequently, one group of animals received no anesthesia while continuing to breathe humidified oxygen. A second group received ketamine (3 mg/kg) intravenously, and ventilation was controlled with 100% oxygen. These animals received a second dose of ketamine (1 mg/kg) 10 minutes after induction to maintain anesthesia for the duration of the 15-minute study period. Ketamine abolished the fetal hypertension and bradycardia produced by partial umbilical cord occlusion. By contrast, ketamine did not worsen fetal arterial blood gas or pH measurements and did not alter cerebral or myocardial blood flow. The authors concluded that ketamine-oxygen anesthesia "does not cause further deterioration in the acidotic fetal lamb" and that "ketamine is a safe anesthetic agent in acute fetal distress."[10]

Friesen et al.[11] evaluated the effect of lidocaine on cardiac output and regional blood flow in normal and acidotic fetal lambs. Normal fetuses with arterial lidocaine concentrations of 1.5 to 3.4 µg/mL had no change in cardiac output or regional blood flow. By contrast, acidotic fetuses with arterial lidocaine concentrations of 1.3 to 1.5 µg/mL experienced tachycardia and increased cerebral blood flow as compared with control acidotic fetuses that did not receive lidocaine. Lidocaine did not alter fetal blood pressure or acid-base status. The authors speculated that a direct vasodilating effect of lidocaine on cerebral vessels may have resulted in increased cerebral blood flow. They concluded that a fetal blood lidocaine concentration of 1.5 µg/mL "does not produce significant deterioration in acidotic foetuses." The failure of

lidocaine to reduce fetal blood pressure—as occurred with the administration of halothane in earlier studies of acidotic fetal lambs[3,6]—prompted the authors to suggest that regional anesthesia might promote better neonatal outcomes in situations of fetal distress.[11]

Morishima et al.[12] also studied the effects of lidocaine in mature acidotic fetal lambs. They partially occluded the umbilical cord to reduce the fetal PaO_2 to approximately 15 mm Hg, and they adjusted the occlusion to maintain this level of PaO_2 for at least 90 minutes before maternal infusion of either lidocaine (0.1 mg/kg/min) or saline-control for 180 minutes. A third group of animals received lidocaine without umbilical cord occlusion. Maternal infusion of lidocaine resulted in a steady-state maternal arterial lidocaine concentration of approximately 2.15 µg/mL. Fetal plasma lidocaine concentrations were between 1.0 and 1.5 µg/mL. Most arterial and tissue lidocaine concentrations were higher in acidotic fetuses than in normal fetuses. Partial umbilical cord occlusion significantly decreased FHR and increased fetal cerebral, myocardial, and adrenal blood flow. Neither lidocaine nor saline-control significantly altered the fetal response to umbilical cord occlusion. The authors concluded that lidocaine, in modest concentrations, does not alter the fetal response to asphyxia. However, placental transfer of lidocaine is enhanced by fetal acidosis.

By contrast, Morishima et al.[13] subsequently observed that similar fetal concentrations of lidocaine significantly increased fetal $PaCO_2$ and decreased fetal pH, blood pressure, and cerebral, myocardial, and adrenal blood flow in acidotic preterm fetal lambs. The authors concluded that "the immature fetus loses its cardiovascular adaptation to asphyxia when exposed to clinically acceptable plasma concentrations of lidocaine obtained transplacentally from the mother."[13]

Santos et al.[14] observed that maternal intravenous infusion of bupivacaine did not alter the changes in fetal blood pressure and acid-base status that occur during partial umbilical cord occlusion in preterm fetal lambs. However, bupivacaine abolished the compensatory increase in myocardial and cerebral blood flow. The authors were unable to determine whether these effects resulted from bupivacaine-induced inhibition of nitric oxide synthesis.

These studies of acidotic fetal lambs do not perfectly mimic clinical practice. First, physicians should use caution when extrapolating animal studies to clinical practice. Second, if fetal distress results from increased uterine activity, volatile halogenated anesthetic agents will decrease uterine activity, which may improve uteroplacental blood flow. Uterine relaxation also may relieve compression of the umbilical cord. In these animal studies, umbilical cord or uterine artery occlusion remained constant during the administration of anesthesia. Third, in cases of severe fetal compromise, the duration of fetal anesthetic exposure is clearly less than 15 to 180 minutes. A skilled obstetrician can deliver the infant within 1 or 2 minutes after making the skin incision. Such brief exposure to a volatile halogenated anesthetic agent should not influence the neonatal outcome significantly. Fourth, maternal-fetal intravenous infusion of lidocaine should not be equated with the administration of spinal or epidural anesthesia, which may produce maternal hemodynamic changes unrelated to the maternal and fetal blood concentrations of lidocaine. Fifth, although one study[14] suggests that the effects of bupivacaine may be less severe than those of lidocaine in acidotic preterm fetal lambs, readers should exercise caution when comparing the results of two laboratory studies performed a decade apart. Neither study directly compared the effect of bupivacaine versus the effect of lidocaine, and lidocaine has enjoyed a long history of safe use in pregnant patients. Finally, these studies did not address the hypothesis that anesthetic agents (e.g., barbiturates, ketamine) may protect the fetal brain from neurologic damage during hypoxia.[15,16]

CLINICAL STUDIES

Few clinical studies have evaluated the anesthetic management of patients with fetal distress. Gale et al.[17] retrospectively reviewed the records of 374 women who underwent cesarean section at their hospital between 1977 and 1980. Some 205 women underwent elective cesarean section, and the remaining 169 women underwent nonelective cesarean section. There was no difference in neonatal outcome between women who received general anesthesia and those who received epidural anesthesia for elective cesarean section. By contrast, among the women who underwent nonelective cesarean section, 23 of 91 mothers who received general anesthesia had infants who required "respiratory assistance" after delivery as compared with only 10 of 78 infants whose mothers received epidural anesthesia ($P < 0.05$).

Marx et al.[18] evaluated the anesthetic management of 126 women who underwent cesarean section for fetal distress. The obstetrician preoperatively determined the fetal scalp blood pH in each case, and the mother selected the anesthetic technique. Seventy-one women received general anesthesia, and 55 received regional anesthesia. (Among those 55 women, 33 received spinal anesthesia, and 22 received an extension of epidural anesthesia with 3% 2-chloroprocaine.) Each cesarean section began within 20 minutes of the last fetal scalp pH determination. No patient experienced clinically significant hypotension or required vasopressor treatment. At delivery, umbilical arterial and venous blood gas and pH measurements and 5-minute Apgar scores were similar in the general and regional anesthesia groups (Table 26-3), and 1-minute Apgar scores were significantly higher in the regional anesthesia group. Umbilical arterial blood pH measurements were higher than the last scalp blood pH measurement in 80% and 63% of the regional and general anesthesia cases, respectively. In five cases, the umbilical arterial blood pH was substantially less than the last scalp blood pH, but the authors did not identify the anesthetic technique for those five cases. The authors concluded that "regional analgesia provides maternal and fetal advantages, even in the presence of fetal distress."[18]

Similarly, Ramanathan et al.[19] evaluated their experience with the administration of anesthesia for 101 patients with fetal distress. Of these, 67 women received general anesthesia, and 34 women received an extension of epidural anesthesia with 3% 2-chloroprocaine. Some 97% of babies in the epidural anesthesia group and 79% of babies in the general anesthesia group had an umbilical venous blood pH measurement that was higher than the preoperative scalp blood pH measurement. The authors concluded that the rapid extension of epidural anesthesia "does not adversely affect the neonatal outcome regardless of the type of abnormal fetal heart rate pattern."[19]

Eisenach[20] combined the data from the aforementioned two studies (Table 26-4).[18,19] Review of those data suggests that infants of mothers who received regional anesthesia fared at least as well as those infants whose mothers received general anesthesia. However, there are limitations to the application of these studies. First, both were retrospective studies. The

patients were not randomized to receive either regional or general anesthesia. When any retrospective study is interpreted, the potential for selection bias must be considered. Is it possible that either the general or regional anesthesia group included a higher percentage of patients whose fetuses deteriorated between the last scalp pH determination and the induction of anesthesia? Second, severe fetal distress clearly was not present in each case. In the study by Marx et al.,[18] the mean ± SD fetal scalp pH measurements for the two groups were 7.20 ± 0.05 and 7.20 ± 0.04, respectively. Thus, some of the fetuses in both groups most likely did not require urgent cesarean delivery. Third, Marx et al.[18] reported no cases of clinically significant hypotension. In clinical practice, the emergency administration of spinal anesthesia results in hypotension in some patients. Spinal anesthesia is associated with a rapid onset of sympathectomy, and, in emergency cases, there is limited time to expand the maternal intravascular volume before the induction of anesthesia. Finally, some anesthesiologists may not be able to provide safe, effective regional anesthesia as quickly as that provided by the authors of these studies.

Mokriski and Malinow[21] randomized 66 patients who required general anesthesia for emergency cesarean section to receive either halothane or isoflurane (i.e., 0.7 minimum alveolar concentration [MAC]) with 50% nitrous oxide and oxygen until delivery. The mean ± SD induction-to-delivery interval was 5.3 ± 3 minutes in both the halothane and isoflurane groups. There was no difference between the two groups in Apgar scores, umbilical arterial or venous blood gas and pH

TABLE 26-3	FETAL BIOCHEMICAL DATA*	
Parameter	General anesthesia ($n = 71$)	Regional anesthesia ($n = 55$)
SC pH	7.204 ± 0.053	7.198 ± 0.043
UV pH	7.286 ± 0.050	7.282 ± 0.054
UA pH	7.221 ± 0.057	7.220 ± 0.053
UV P_{CO_2} (kPa)	5.75 ± 0.97	5.64 ± 0.80
UA P_{CO_2} (kPa)	6.61 ± 1.37	6.73 ± 1.10
UV P_{O_2} (kPa)	3.86 ± 1.14	3.52 ± 0.93
UA P_{O_2} (kPa)	2.39 ± 0.94	2.18 ± 0.69

*All data are reported as mean ± SD.
SC, Scalp capillary blood; UA, umbilical artery blood; UV, umbilical vein blood.
From Marx GF, Luykx WM, Cohen S. Fetal-neonatal status following caesarean section for fetal distress. Br J Anaesth 1984; 56:1009-13.

TABLE 26-4	FETAL DISTRESS: REGIONAL VERSUS GENERAL ANESTHESIA	
Parameter	General anesthesia ($n = 134$)	Regional anesthesia ($n = 93$)
Scalp pH	7.18	7.20
Umbilical venous pH at delivery	7.26	7.28
Percentage of newborns with improved pH at delivery	71%	87%

From Eisenach JC. Fetal stress/distress. Probl Anesth 1989; 3:19-31. Data combined from studies by Marx et al.[18] and Ramanathan et al.[19]

measurements, or incidence of newborn acidosis. The authors did not determine fetal scalp blood pH before the induction of anesthesia, and they did not include a third group of patients who did not receive a volatile halogenated agent. Thus, the authors could not eliminate "the possibility that both drugs exaggerate fetal acidosis to a similar degree."[21] Neither this study nor laboratory studies favor one volatile halogenated agent over another in cases of fetal distress.

OBSTETRIC MANAGEMENT

The diagnosis of fetal distress should prompt the obstetrician and the anesthesiologist to attempt fetal resuscitation in utero (Box 26-1).

Maternal Position

Unfortunately, some obstetricians and nurses allow parturients to remain supine during labor. Uteroplacental perfusion and fetal condition often improve after the patient has assumed the lateral decubitus position.

The obstetrician should perform a vaginal examination to determine whether umbilical cord prolapse has occurred. Fetal distress may also result from intrauterine compression of the umbilical cord, perhaps against the bony pelvis. Umbilical cord compression can be alleviated by having the patient move into one of a variety of positions (e.g., left lateral decubitus, right lateral decubitus, Trendelenburg, knee-chest). In some cases of cord compression, the fetus will tolerate the left but not the right lateral decubitus position or vice versa.

Supplemental Oxygen

Most obstetricians advocate the maternal administration of supplemental oxygen at the first sign of fetal distress. Contrary to earlier reports, it seems unlikely that supplemental oxygen causes uterine vasoconstriction. Administration of supplemental oxygen *increases* fetal oxygenation and helps maintain fetal oxidative metabolism during periods of decreased umbilical and uteroplacental perfusion in pregnant sheep.[22,23] Similarly, the administration of supplemental oxygen increases fetal transcutaneous P_{O_2} during labor in both healthy and high-risk parturients.[24] However, there is little objective evidence that maternal administration of supplemental oxygen improves neonatal outcome in cases of fetal distress during labor.[25] In a randomized, controlled trial of healthy parturients undergoing normal labor, Thorp et al.[26]

observed lower umbilical arterial blood pH measurements in newborn infants exposed to supplemental maternal oxygen for more than 10 minutes during the second stage of labor as compared with control infants and infants exposed to supplemental maternal oxygen for less than 10 minutes. Khaw et al.[27] observed that the administration of supplemental oxygen ($F_iO_2 = 0.6$) to healthy women undergoing elective cesarean section resulted in a modest increase in fetal oxygenation but caused an increase in both maternal and fetal oxygen free radical activity. It is unclear whether these observations apply to situations of fetal distress or if the evidence of increased free radical activity is a marker of adverse neonatal outcome.[28]

Maternal Circulation

If an intravenous bolus of crystalloid is needed, a non-dextrose-containing balanced salt solution (e.g., Ringer's lactate) should be used.[29,30] Bolus administration of a dextrose-containing solution may cause maternal hyperglycemia; fetal hyperglycemia, hyperinsulinemia, and metabolic acidosis; and neonatal hypoglycemia.[31-34] In addition, in a model of asphyxia in sheep, fetal hyperglycemia was associated with the rapid development of acidosis, decreased cerebral oxygen consumption, and evidence of worsened cerebral function.[35]

If maternal hypotension occurs, **ephedrine** is the preferred vasopressor for most patients. However, **phenylephrine** seems preferable in parturients with preexisting maternal tachycardia or in patients in whom maternal tachycardia would be detrimental.[36]

Discontinuation of Oxytocin

Intravenous administration of oxytocin is a common cause of uterine hyperactivity and decreased uteroplacental perfusion. Oxytocin should be discontinued at the first sign of fetal distress, regardless of the presence of uterine hypertonus.

Tocolysis

Some obstetricians give an intravenous bolus injection of a tocolytic agent (e.g., a beta-adrenergic agent, magnesium sulfate) to aid fetal resuscitation.[37-40] The beta-adrenergic tocolytic agents do not directly increase uteroplacental perfusion; rather, these agents may improve uteroplacental perfusion indirectly by relaxing the uterus. It is helpful to consider uteroplacental perfusion in the same way as myocardial perfusion. Myocardial perfusion occurs during diastole, between contractions. Likewise, uteroplacental perfusion occurs during uterine diastole, between uterine contractions.

Ingemarsson et al.[38] gave an intravenous bolus of 0.25 mg of **terbutaline** to 33 women with prolonged fetal bradycardia. The FHR increased after injection of terbutaline in 30 cases, and 23 women subsequently delivered vigorous infants vaginally. Patriarco et al.[39] randomized 20 patients with fetal distress to receive either no medication or 0.25 mg of terbutaline subcutaneously. At delivery, there was significant improvement in the acid-base status of the fetuses in the terbutaline group but not in the control group (Figure 26-1). Hanley et al.[40] performed a meta-analysis of the published studies of pharmacologic tocolysis for intrauterine fetal resuscitation. They noted that the mean umbilical arterial blood pH at cesarean delivery was significantly higher in patients who received terbutaline before delivery than in patients who did not.

Box 26-1 OBSTETRIC MANAGEMENT OF FETAL DISTRESS

- Optimize maternal position.
  - Avoid or relieve aortocaval compression.
  - Change position to relieve umbilical cord compression.
- Administer supplemental oxygen.
- Maintain maternal circulation.
  - Give non-dextrose-containing balanced salt solution.
  - Treat hypotension with ephedrine.
- Discontinue oxytocin.
- Consider administration of a tocolytic agent for treatment of uterine hyperactivity.
- Consider saline amnioinfusion to relieve umbilical cord compression.

Administration of a tocolytic agent undoubtedly improves fetal condition in cases of uterine hyperactivity, and this treatment may allow the obstetrician to avoid cesarean section altogether. Unfortunately, in some cases the anesthesiologist must administer an emergency anesthetic to a patient who has just received a bolus injection of a beta-adrenergic agent.

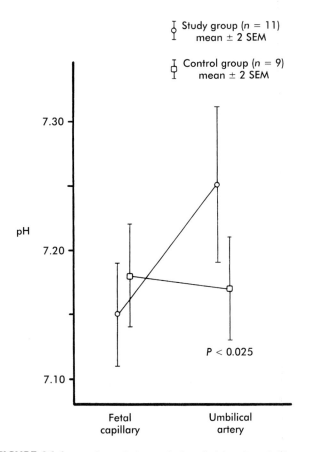

FIGURE 26-1. pH change before and after administration of either no medication or terbutaline 0.2 mg subcutaneously. (From Patriarco MS, Viechnicki BM, Hutchinson TA, et al. A study on intrauterine fetal resuscitation with terbutaline. Am J Obstet Gynecol 1987; 157:384-7.)

Bell[41] reported the successful use of sublingual **nitroglycerin** spray to relax the uterus in a patient who had experienced uterine hyperstimulation and late FHR decelerations during intravenous administration of oxytocin (Figure 26-2). One advantage of nitroglycerin is that its systemic effects are brief. The sublingual route of administration is convenient and obviates the need to prepare an intravenous infusion.

Saline Amnioinfusion

The obstetrician may infuse a bolus of normal saline into the uterine cavity to relieve umbilical cord compression (Figure 26-3).[42,43] Likewise, the obstetrician may perform saline amnioinfusion in patients with thick, meconium-stained amniotic fluid.[44]

ANESTHETIC MANAGEMENT

Preanesthetic Evaluation

Every woman admitted to the labor and delivery unit is a potential candidate for the emergency administration of anesthesia. Ideally, an anesthesia care provider will evaluate every patient shortly after admission; unfortunately, that is not possible in most hospitals. In some hospitals, the obstetrician or nurse completes a short questionnaire that targets specific components of the patient's history and physical examination that are relevant to anesthesia practice.[45] The obstetrician should obtain antepartum consultation from an anesthesiologist when factors that place the patient at increased risk for complications from anesthesia are detected.[46]

In some cases, the anesthesiologist is asked to give an emergency anesthetic to a parturient who has not undergone preanesthetic evaluation. In cases of dire fetal distress, the anesthesiologist may need to perform that evaluation even as other preparations are made for anesthesia (e.g., the establishment of intravenous access and the placement of the blood pressure cuff, pulse oximeter probe, and electrocardiogram [ECG] electrodes). In some cases, the degree of urgency may affect the duration and extent of the preanesthetic evaluation. However, the anesthesia care provider should not compromise

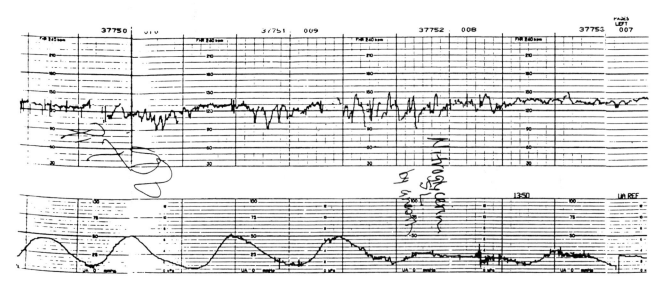

FIGURE 26-2. Use of sublingual nitroglycerin spray to relax the uterus in a patient who had experienced uterine hyperstimulation and late fetal heart rate decelerations during intravenous administration of oxytocin. (From Bell E. Nitroglycerin and uterine relaxation [letter]. Anesthesiology 1996; 85:683.)

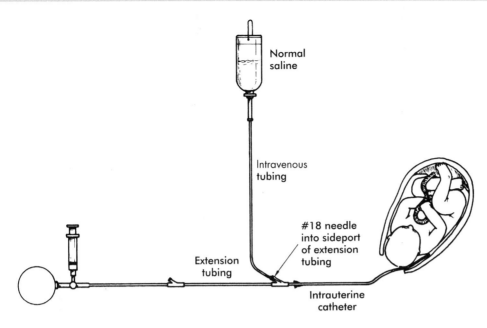

FIGURE 26-3. Materials for saline amnioinfusion. (From Miyazaki FS, Nevarez F. Saline amnioinfusion for relief of repetitive variable decelerations: A prospective randomized study. Am J Obstet Gynecol 1985; 153:301-6.)

maternal safety and should obtain critical information from every patient. For example, the anesthesiologist should obtain information regarding previous medical and anesthetic history from every patient; similarly, he or she should evaluate the airway and the potential difficulty of intubation in every patient.

Preparation for Anesthesia

When possible, the following precautions should be taken before the administration of every emergency obstetric anesthetic, regardless of the planned anesthetic technique (Box 26-2):

1. **Antacid.** Administer a clear antacid (e.g., 30 mL of 0.3 M sodium citrate). I also give metoclopramide 10 mg intravenously to all patients except those who require stat cesarean section.
2. **Position.** Avoid aortocaval compression. Optimize the position of the patient's head and neck to facilitate successful laryngoscopy and endotracheal intubation, if needed.
3. **Supplemental oxygen.** Administer supplemental oxygen before, during, and after the induction of either general or regional anesthesia.
4. **Maternal circulation.** Establish good intravenous access. If an intravenous bolus of crystalloid is needed, administer a non-dextrose-containing balanced salt solution. If maternal hypotension occurs, **ephedrine** is the preferred vasopressor for most patients. If the patient's blood pressure does not improve with ephedrine, 50-μg bolus doses of **phenylephrine** may be given. (However, phenylephrine seems preferable in parturients with preexisting maternal tachycardia or in patients in whom maternal tachycardia would be detrimental.[36]) **Epinephrine** should be given in the rare case of catastrophic hypotension.

5. **Maternal monitors.** Apply maternal monitors, including a blood pressure cuff, ECG leads, and a pulse oximeter probe. In cases of general anesthesia, plan to monitor end-tidal CO_2 and neuromuscular function.
6. **FHR monitoring.** Monitor the FHR in the operating room. Amniotomy has occurred in most cases of acute fetal distress; thus a fetal scalp (or buttock) ECG lead can be used to monitor the FHR before, during, and after the induction of anesthesia for emergency cesarean section. The circulating nurse can reach under the drapes to disconnect the ECG lead immediately before delivery of the infant. If the nurse has difficulty disconnecting the ECG lead from the fetal scalp, the lead can be disconnected from the maternal leg plate, and the obstetrician may deliver the ECG lead through the uterine incision. Delivery of the infant is not a sterile procedure, and delivery of the ECG lead along with the infant should not increase the risk of maternal infection.

During my 10 years of practice at the University of Iowa Hospitals and Clinics, we left the fetal scalp ECG lead in place and monitored the FHR until delivery, without evidence of an increased incidence of maternal infection. At the University of Alabama at Birmingham Hospital, our obstetric population primarily consists of indigent patients who have a high risk of postcesarean endometritis and wound infection. Our obstetricians believe that delivery of the scalp ECG lead with the infant results in an increased incidence of postcesarean infection in this population; thus they prefer to remove the scalp ECG lead immediately before they make the skin incision in patients who receive regional anesthesia and just before induction in patients who receive general anesthesia.

Continuous FHR monitoring is useful for at least three reasons. First, the FHR abnormality often resolves. In some

---

Box 26-2 PREPARATION FOR ANESTHESIA

1. Administer a clear antacid (e.g., 30 mL of 0.3 M sodium citrate).
2. Optimize maternal position.
   - Avoid aortocaval compression.
   - Optimize position of the patient's head and neck (i.e., the sniffing position).
3. Administer supplemental oxygen.
4. Maintain maternal circulation.
   - Establish good intravenous access.
   - Give a non-dextrose-containing balanced salt solution.
   - Treat hypotension with ephedrine.
   - If the patient's blood pressure does not improve with ephedrine, give phenylephrine or epinephrine.
5. Apply maternal monitors.
6. Monitor the fetal heart rate.
7. Reassure the infant's mother and father.

cases, the obstetrician will forego the performance of a cesarean section. In other cases, the obstetrician may continue with plans to perform a cesarean section, but continuous FHR monitoring may facilitate the use of regional anesthesia. For example, an improved FHR tracing allows the anesthesiologist to wait for an extension of adequate epidural anesthesia. Alternatively, an improved FHR tracing allows the anesthesiologist to administer spinal or epidural anesthesia de novo.

Second, continuous FHR monitoring may guide management in cases of failed intubation. If failed intubation occurs and there is no evidence of ongoing severe fetal distress, both the anesthesiologist and the obstetrician will have greater confidence in a decision to awaken the patient and proceed with an alternative anesthetic technique. By contrast, if there is evidence of ongoing dire fetal distress, the anesthesiologist may decide to provide general anesthesia by means of face mask or laryngeal mask airway ventilation, and the obstetrician may proceed with cesarean section (see Chapter 31).

Third, intraoperative FHR monitoring allows the obstetrician to modify the surgical technique according to the urgency of delivery. Petrikovsky et al.[47] reported their experience with intraoperative FHR monitoring during cesarean section for fetal distress. In one case, an abnormal FHR tracing markedly improved after the induction of general anesthesia, and this knowledge allowed the obstetrician to perform a difficult dissection without haste.

7. **Reassurance of the parents.** The emotional needs of the infant's mother and father are important. Parental distress often accompanies fetal distress. The anesthesiologist is often the best person to reassure distressed parents. All members of the obstetric care team should remember that unnecessary chaos need not accompany urgency.

Choice of Anesthetic Technique

Moore et al.[48] prospectively studied the effects of the timing of cesarean section on the neonatal outcomes of 261 consecutive patients who underwent cesarean section for fetal distress. They divided these patients into those for whom the decision-to-delivery interval was less than 30 minutes and those for whom the decision-to-delivery interval was more than 30 minutes. At delivery, the mean umbilical arterial blood pH measurements for the two groups were 7.23 ± 0.09 and 7.25 ± 0.08, respectively ($P < 0.02$). The umbilical venous blood pH measurements were 7.28 ± 0.08 and 7.31 ± 0.07, respectively ($P < 0.004$). Umbilical blood acidemia (i.e., umbilical arterial blood pH < 7.15, umbilical venous blood pH < 7.20) was more common among those patients whose decision-to-delivery time was less than 30 minutes (16% versus 7%, $P < 0.001$), but the incidence of low 5-minute Apgar scores (3% versus 1%) and the rate of admission to the neonatal intensive care unit (20% versus 21%) were similar. In another study of patients undergoing emergency cesarean section for a variety of indications, MacKenzie and Cooke[49] observed a trend toward improved umbilical arterial blood pH measurements with a more prolonged decision-to-delivery interval in patients with and without evidence of fetal distress. In a retrospective study, Schauberger et al.[50] observed an increased incidence of low Apgar scores in patients with a decision-to-incision interval of less than 30 minutes. In all three studies, the rapid delivery group most likely included those patients with the most severe FHR abnormalities. Nonetheless,

Moore et al.[48] concluded the following: ". . . utilizing traditionally accepted indicators of fetal distress, immediate neonatal outcome is not influenced by the decision-to-delivery time."

In contrast, Dunphy et al.[51] retrospectively reviewed data for 104 consecutive patients who underwent cesarean section for fetal distress during labor. The median decision-to-delivery time was 34 minutes. The authors observed no significant correlation between the decision-to-delivery interval and the 1- and 5-minute Apgar scores or the umbilical cord arterial and venous blood acid-base measurements. However, there was a significant association between the decision-to-delivery interval and admission to the special care unit. The relative risk of admission to the special care unit doubled when the decision-to-delivery interval was extended from 10 to 35 minutes. Likewise, Korhonen and Kariniemi[52] observed better neonatal outcomes with a shorter decision-to-delivery interval. Among 60 cases with the operating team in the hospital, the decision-to-delivery interval was 13.5 ± 0.7 minutes. Among 41 cases with the operating team on call from home, the decision-to-delivery interval was 23.6 ± 0.9 minutes. Three fetuses in the latter group died in utero, and a fourth infant suffered hypoxic ischemic encephalopathy. Chauhan et al.[53] retrospectively assessed the impact of the decision-to-incision interval in 117 patients who underwent emergency cesarean section for suspected fetal distress. The authors observed a more frequent occurrence of three markers of adverse outcome in patients with a decision-to-incision time of more than 30 minutes: (1) lower mean umbilical arterial blood pH; (2) increased incidence of umbilical arterial blood pH < 7.00; and (3) greater likelihood of admission to the neonatal intensive care unit.

Harris[45] defined emergency cesarean sections as "all cesarean sections that are not performed on a scheduled elective basis." Further, he divided emergency cesarean sections into three categories: stable, urgent, and stat (Table 26-5). (Lucas et al.[54] described a similar classification system but used terminology different from that used by Harris.) **Stable** emergency cesarean sections are performed in patients with stable maternal and fetal physiology but who require cesarean section before destabilization occurs. One example is the patient with chronic uteroplacental insufficiency. Such patients may present to the labor and delivery unit after a nonreactive nonstress test or a positive contraction stress test. Another example is the patient who presents with a footling breech presentation, ruptured membranes, and no labor; the obstetrician may want to perform cesarean section to avoid the risks of umbilical cord prolapse and fetal head entrapment. Anesthetic decisions for these patients do not differ from those for patients scheduled for elective cesarean section, with two exceptions. First, the anesthesiologist may delay surgery (e.g., for 6 to 8 hours after the ingestion of solid food) to allow gastric emptying. Second, I prefer epidural anesthesia in patients with chronic uteroplacental insufficiency. The relatively slow onset decreases the likelihood of severe hypotension. The slow onset also allows the anesthesiologist to titrate the sensory level.

Urgent cesarean sections are performed in those patients in whom maternal and/or fetal physiology is unstable but not immediately life-threatening to the mother or fetus. Examples of circumstances that call for urgent cesarean section include the following: (1) cord prolapse *without* fetal distress; and (2) variable FHR decelerations with prompt recovery and normal FHR variability.

TABLE 26-5	CATEGORIES OF EMERGENCY CESAREAN SECTION

Examples	Preferred anesthetic technique
Stable	
Chronic uteroplacental insufficiency	Epidural, spinal
Abnormal fetal presentation with ruptured membranes (not in labor)	
Urgent	
Dystocia	Extension of preexisting epidural anesthesia or spinal
Failed trial of forceps	
Active genital herpes infection with rupture of membranes	
Previous classic cesarean section and active labor	
Cord prolapse without fetal distress	
Variable decelerations with prompt recovery and normal fetal heart rate variability	
Stat	
Massive maternal hemorrhage	General unless preexisting epidural anesthesia can be extended satisfactorily
Ruptured uterus	
Cord prolapse with fetal bradycardia	
Agonal fetal distress (e.g., prolonged bradycardia or late decelerations with no fetal heart rate variability)	

Modified from Harris AP. Emergency cesarean section. In Rogers MC, editor. Current Practice in Anesthesiology. Toronto, Canada, BC Decker, 1990:361-6.

Stat cesarean sections are performed in those patients with conditions that are immediately life-threatening for the mother and/or fetus. Examples of circumstances that should prompt stat cesarean section include the following: (1) prolonged fetal bradycardia; and (2) late FHR decelerations with no FHR variability.

The assignment of an individual patient to either the urgent or stat category may affect the decision regarding the choice of anesthetic technique. In some cases, it may be unclear—and arguable—if the patient requires urgent or stat cesarean section. Most FHR abnormalities do not reflect agonal fetal distress; thus few patients require stat cesarean section.

The fifth edition of *Guidelines for Perinatal Care*[55] includes the following statement regarding the timing of cesarean section:

Any hospital providing an obstetric service should have the capability of responding to an obstetric emergency. No data correlate the timing of intervention with outcome, and there is little likelihood that any will be obtained. However, in general, the consensus has been that hospitals should have the capability of beginning a cesarean delivery within 30 minutes of the decision to operate. Some indications for cesarean delivery can be appropriately accommodated in greater than 30 minutes. Conversely, examples of indications that may mandate more expeditious delivery include

hemorrhage from placenta previa, abruptio placentae, prolapse of the umbilical cord, and uterine rupture.

In 1992 and 1998, the ACOG issued a committee opinion entitled, "Anesthesia for Emergency Deliveries."[46] (See appendix at the end of this chapter.) That document can be summarized as follows:

1. "Failed intubation and pulmonary aspiration of gastric contents continue to be leading causes of maternal morbidity and mortality from anesthesia."
2. "The obstetric care team should be alert to the presence of risk factors that place the parturient at increased risk for complications from emergency general or regional anesthesia."
3. When risk factors are identified, the obstetrician should obtain antepartum consultation from an anesthesia care provider. (For this recommendation to be effective, anesthesiologists should establish procedures to facilitate antepartum consultation.)
4. The obstetrician and the anesthesiologist should develop "strategies . . . to minimize the need for emergency induction of general anesthesia in women for whom this would be especially hazardous." Such strategies may include the early establishment of intravenous access and the early placement of an epidural or spinal catheter.
5. If a patient is at high risk for complications from anesthesia (e.g., prior failed intubation), the obstetrician should strongly consider the wisdom of referring that patient to a hospital with personnel who can provide appropriate anesthesia care on a 24-hour basis.
6. In emergency obstetric cases, "the maternal as well as the fetal status must be considered . . . . Although there are some situations in which general anesthesia is preferable to regional anesthesia, the risk of general anesthesia must be weighed against the benefit for those patients who have a greater potential for complications."
7. Some fetuses with nonreassuring FHR patterns are diagnosed as experiencing fetal distress. However, "the term 'fetal distress' is imprecise, nonspecific, and has little positive predictive value. The character of the fetal heart rate abnormality should be considered when the urgency of the delivery and the type of anesthesia to be administered are determined."
8. "Cesarean deliveries that are performed for a nonreassuring fetal heart rate pattern do not necessarily preclude the use of regional anesthesia."

Hawkins et al.[56] noted that the estimated rate of maternal death from complications of general anesthesia during cesarean section increased from 20.0 deaths per million general anesthetics between 1979 and 1984 to 32.3 deaths per million between 1985 and 1990. In contrast, the estimated rate of death from complications of regional anesthesia during cesarean section decreased from 8.6 per million regional anesthetics between 1979 and 1984 to 1.9 per million between 1985 and 1990. Further, the case fatality rate for general anesthesia was 2.3 times that for regional anesthesia between 1979 and 1984, and it increased to 16.7 times that for regional anesthesia between 1985 and 1990. Similarly, between 1991 and 1993, all of the direct anesthetic deaths associated with cesarean section in the United Kingdom occurred in women who received general anesthesia.[57] Demographic and personal characteristics associated with an increased risk of maternal death include the following: (1) non-white ethnicity; (2) poor socioeconomic status; (3) obesity; and (4) age of more than 35 years.[58-60]

In cases of emergency cesarean section, it is important that the anesthesiologist ask the obstetrician two questions: (1) What is the diagnosis?; and 2) How quickly should the baby be delivered?[61] (Stated another way, what is the degree of urgency?) It is critical that the obstetrician clearly communicate the severity of the FHR abnormality.[62] Most anesthesiologists are not experts in FHR monitoring; thus the obstetrician must identify those cases that require urgent cesarean section as opposed to those cases that require stat cesarean section. Likewise, the anesthesiologist must clearly communicate concerns. The anesthesiologist and the obstetrician will be more likely to agree on a decision to give regional anesthesia if the anesthesiologist suspects that intubation may be difficult.

EXTENSION OF EPIDURAL ANESTHESIA

I encourage the early administration of epidural anesthesia in patients at high risk for operative delivery. Such cases include but are not limited to patients with breech presentation, multiple gestation, preeclampsia, diabetes mellitus, selected forms of cardiac disease, and evidence of intrauterine fetal stress (e.g., intrauterine growth restriction, oligohydramnios). Early use and maintenance of epidural anesthesia facilitate the extension of epidural anesthesia for emergency cesarean section. Morgan et al.[63] successfully anticipated 87% of 360 consecutive emergency cesarean sections, and the early establishment of epidural anesthesia allowed for the successful extension of epidural anesthesia in 70% of those 360 cases. Riley and Papasin[64] performed a retrospective study in which they identified two factors associated with the failed extension of epidural anesthesia for emergency cesarean section: (1) an increased requirement for supplemental boluses of local anesthetic during labor; and (2) anesthetic care provided by an attending anesthesiologist who was not a specialist in obstetric anesthesia.

If an epidural catheter has been placed earlier, a partial level of anesthesia already exists, and there is hemodynamic stability, the extension of epidural anesthesia is appropriate for either instrumental vaginal delivery or cesarean section. I give an intravenous bolus of Ringer's lactate and inject 15 to 20 mL of 3% **2-chloroprocaine** epidurally in 5-mL increments over 2 to 3 minutes while the urethral catheter is inserted and the abdomen is prepared and draped. 2-Chloroprocaine has a rapid onset of action, and it is rapidly metabolized by both the mother and fetus. In addition, fetal acidosis does not enhance the placental transfer of 2-chloroprocaine.[65] (Fetal acidosis enhances the placental transfer of amide local anesthetics,[66,67] but the clinical significance is arguable.) Although 2-chloroprocaine provides surgical anesthesia most rapidly, **lidocaine with epinephrine** also can be administered successfully. Price et al.[68] administered 20 mL of 2% lidocaine with 1:200,000 epinephrine for the extension of epidural anesthesia in 36 patients who required emergency cesarean section. "Despite a wide range of initial analgesic sensory levels, the technique produced blocks that were dense with adequate anesthesia for surgery in all patients within 12.5 min[utes]."[68] Gaiser et al.[69,70] advocate the administration of 1.5% lidocaine with freshly added epinephrine (1:200,000) and sodium bicarbonate (2 mL of bicarbonate per 23 mL of local anesthetic). The onset of anesthesia is approximately 2 minutes *slower* with this regimen than with 2-chloroprocaine.[69,70] Alkalinization of lidocaine with epinephrine hastens the onset of anesthesia,[71] but the faster onset may be offset by the additional time required for preparation of the solution.[72] Thus, when time is of the essence, 3% 2-chloroprocaine remains the local anesthetic agent of choice for the extension of epidural anesthesia

for emergency cesarean section. In my judgment, 0.5% bupivacaine is an unsatisfactory choice in this setting,[73] although others have a different view.[74]

After the administration of either 2-chloroprocaine or lidocaine, satisfactory anesthesia is often present when the surgeon is ready to make the skin incision. If not, the ongoing FHR tracing dictates whether a delay is acceptable. If there is partial but incomplete epidural anesthesia, the obstetrician may provide supplemental anesthesia by performing local infiltration with a dilute solution of local anesthetic (e.g., either 1% 2-chloroprocaine or 0.5% lidocaine); this may serve as a temporizing measure. Some anesthesiologists provide supplemental analgesia with 10-mg intravenous doses of ketamine.[45] If supplemental local infiltration is ineffective, the anesthesiologist should be prepared to administer general anesthesia. Surgery should not be delayed in the presence of ongoing severe fetal distress.

ADMINISTRATION OF SPINAL ANESTHESIA

The use of spinal anesthesia for urgent cesarean section remains controversial in some hospitals. Obstetricians have two concerns. First, they worry that the anesthesiologist will be unable to provide spinal anesthesia quickly and thus will delay surgery. Second, they worry that the emergency administration of spinal anesthesia, with its rapid onset of sympathectomy, will result in maternal hypotension and worsened fetal condition. However, laboring women who receive spinal anesthesia for cesarean section have a lower incidence of hypotension as compared with women who are not in labor.[75]

Before giving spinal anesthesia to a patient who requires urgent cesarean section, consideration should be given to the following questions: (1) Could the fetal distress be a result of a concealed placental abruption, with unrecognized hypovolemia?; (2) Can anesthesia be achieved quickly, without delaying surgery?; (3) Can severe hypotension be avoided?; and (4) If severe maternal hypotension should occur, does the surgeon have sufficient skill to accomplish rapid delivery? Nonetheless, I have developed an increased enthusiasm for the administration of spinal anesthesia in patients who require urgent cesarean section. I ensure the presence of good intravenous access and give a bolus of a non-dextrose-containing crystalloid as rapidly as possible. However, I do *not* delay the administration of spinal anesthesia until the infusion of 1500 mL of crystalloid as I would for a non-urgent cesarean section. Rout et al.[76] concluded, "Though fluid preloading will reduce the incidence of postspinal hypotension, the reduction is not sufficient to justify delay in commencing spinal anesthesia when this is the most appropriate method of anesthesia for the patient."

I assure the obstetrician that, if I encounter unexpected technical difficulty, I will proceed with an alternative technique. (In a teaching hospital, the most experienced person available should administer the spinal anesthetic; this is not a good case for the inexperienced first-year resident.) Typically I use a 25-gauge Whitacre needle, but if the patient is obese and time is of the essence, I may use a larger (e.g., 22-gauge) needle. On one occasion, I deliberately used an 18-gauge epidural needle to ensure rapid performance of spinal anesthesia in a morbidly obese patient with a prolapsed umbilical cord.

Typically I give hyperbaric **bupivacaine** 12 mg. Unlike epidural bupivacaine, spinal bupivacaine has a rapid onset of action. Finally, I give ephedrine prophylactically, and I treat hypotension aggressively. With these safeguards, severe hypotension is rare.

Some anesthesiologists advocate the administration of continuous spinal anesthesia for urgent cesarean section in patients with a difficult airway.[77,78]

GENERAL ANESTHESIA

Rapid-sequence induction of general anesthesia is preferred for many cases of stat cesarean section. The technique typically does not differ from that used for nonemergent cases, with the following exceptions.

First, in situations of dire fetal distress, it is acceptable to forego 3 to 5 minutes of denitrogenation and ask the mother to take four maximally deep breaths of 100% oxygen before the induction of general anesthesia.[79]

Second, **ketamine** is the preferred induction agent for many of these cases. Laboratory and clinical data do not clearly favor one induction agent over another; however, laboratory studies[8-10] hint that ketamine is a better choice than sodium thiopental. Further, patients with fetal distress often are hypovolemic, and ketamine is preferred to sodium thiopental in such patients.

Third, the presence of dire fetal distress prompts me to give a higher inspired concentration of oxygen (60% to 100%) than that given in nonemergency cases. Early studies suggested that an increase in the maternal PaO_2 above 300 mm Hg failed to produce a corresponding increase in umbilical arterial and venous blood PO_2.[80-82] (Harris[45] correctly noted that "there is no currently available method to measure the maternal PaO_2 instantaneously and ensure that it is indeed greater that 300 mm Hg in a given patient.") Other authors criticized these studies for not ensuring relief from aortocaval compression and for not ensuring that all patients were adequately anesthetized.[83-85] Subsequent studies have suggested that the maternal administration of 100% oxygen increases umbilical cord venous and arterial blood PO_2 as compared with lesser inspired concentrations of oxygen.[83,85]

Rapid-sequence induction of general anesthesia should not be performed indiscriminately. A history and/or suspicion of difficult intubation should prompt the anesthesiologist to perform either awake intubation or regional anesthesia, despite the presence of fetal distress. The mother should not be endangered to deliver a distressed fetus. Rarely, if there is a contraindication to rapid-sequence induction of general anesthesia, local infiltration may be needed as the primary anesthetic technique.[86-88] This technique is not ideal, and it is never easy. Unfortunately, many obstetricians currently have no experience with this technique, and the anesthesiologist must serve as a consultant. In such cases, the following advice should be provided to the obstetrician. First, the obstetrician should plan to perform a vertical skin incision, which will provide the best exposure in a patient with no skeletal muscle relaxation. Second, the obstetrician will need to give a large volume (e.g., 60 to 80 mL) of local anesthetic to provide some semblance of satisfactory anesthesia. To give this large volume of local anesthetic without causing systemic local anesthetic toxicity, the obstetrician should use a dilute solution of local anesthetic (e.g., 1% 2-chloroprocaine or 0.5% lidocaine).

In some cases, the anesthesiologist is asked to provide emergency induction of anesthesia in a patient with no intravenous access. Two reports have described the use of **sevoflurane** for the inhalation induction of general anesthesia for emergency cesarean section in three patients with no intravenous access.[89,90] The advantages of sevoflurane include its nonpungent odor, a low incidence of airway irritability, and its low blood-gas solubility coefficient, which facilitates the rapid induction of general anesthesia. Schaut et al.[89] called attention to the historical use of cyclopropane for the induction and maintenance of general anesthesia for emergency cesarean section. I question whether it is ever acceptable to administer general anesthesia for cesarean section in a patient with no intravenous access,[91-93] although this is a matter of some dispute.[94]

Postpartum Evaluation

All members of the obstetric care team should be aware of the mother's special needs postpartum. In one study,[95] women who underwent emergency cesarean section were more than six times more likely to develop postpartum depression than women who underwent spontaneous or instrumental vaginal delivery.

KEY POINTS

- The term *fetal distress* is imprecise and nonspecific, has a low positive predictive value, and is often associated with the delivery of an infant who is in good condition.
- The diagnosis of fetal distress should prompt the obstetrician and the anesthesiologist to attempt fetal resuscitation in utero.
- Attempts at fetal resuscitation should include relief from aortocaval compression, the administration of supplemental oxygen, the restoration and maintenance of maternal circulation, and the discontinuation of intravenous oxytocin.
- Most maternal deaths resulting from anesthesia occur during emergency cesarean section.
- The obstetrician and anesthesiologist should develop "strategies . . . to minimize the need for emergency induction of general anesthesia."[46]
- When possible, the fetal heart rate should be monitored before, during, and after the administration of anesthesia for emergency cesarean section.
- Emergency cesarean sections fall into three categories: stable, urgent, and stat.
- The anesthesiologist may safely give regional anesthesia for most emergency cesarean sections.

REFERENCES

1. Parer JT, Livingston EG. What is fetal distress? Am J Obstet Gynecol 1990; 162:1421-7.
2. American College of Obstetricians and Gynecologists Committee on Obstetric Practice. Inappropriate use of the terms fetal distress and birth asphyxia. ACOG Committee Opinion No. 197. Washington, DC, 1998.
3. Palahniuk RJ, Doig GA, Johnson GN, Pash MP. Maternal halothane anesthesia reduces cerebral blood flow in the acidotic sheep fetus. Anesth Analg 1980; 59:35-9.
4. Yarnell R, Biehl DR, Tweed WA, et al. The effect of halothane anaesthesia on the asphyxiated foetal lamb in utero. Can Anaesth Soc J 1983; 30:474-9.
5. Swartz J, Cummings M, Pucci W, Biehl D. The effects of general anaesthesia on the asphyxiated foetal lamb in utero. Can Anaesth Soc J 1985; 32:577-82.

6. Cheek DBC, Hughes SC, Dailey PA, et al. Effect of halothane on regional cerebral blood flow and cerebral metabolic oxygen consumption in the fetal lamb in utero. Anesthesiology 1987; 67:361-6.

7. Baker BW, Hughes SC, Shnider SM, et al. Maternal anesthesia and the stressed fetus: Effects of isoflurane on the asphyxiated fetal lamb. Anesthesiology 1990; 72:65-70.

8. Pickering BG, Palahniuk RJ, Coté J, et al. Cerebral vascular responses to ketamine and thiopentone during foetal acidosis. Can Anaesth Soc J 1982; 29:463-7.

9. Leicht CH, Baker BW, Rosen MA, et al. The effect of ketamine or sodium thiopental rapid sequence induction on the asphyxiated fetal lamb (abstract). Anesthesiology 1986; 65:A387.

10. Swartz J, Cumming M, Biehl D. The effect of ketamine anaesthesia on the acidotic fetal lamb. Can J Anaesth 1987; 34:233-7.

11. Friesen C, Yarnell R, Bachman C, et al. The effect of lidocaine on regional blood flows and cardiac output in the non-stressed and the stressed foetal lamb. Can Anaesth Soc J 1986; 33:130-7.

12. Morishima HO, Santos AC, Pedersen H, et al. Effect of lidocaine on the asphyxial responses in the mature fetal lamb. Anesthesiology 1987; 66:502-7.

13. Morishima HO, Pedersen H, Santos AC, et al. Adverse effects of maternally administered lidocaine on the asphyxiated preterm fetal lamb. Anesthesiology 1989; 71:110-5.

14. Santos AC, Yun EM, Bobby PD, et al. The effects of bupivacaine, L-nitro-L-arginine-methyl ester, and phenylephrine on cardiovascular adaptations to asphyxia in the preterm fetal lamb. Anesth Analg 1997; 85:1299-306.

15. Rurak DW, Taylor SM. Oxygen consumption in fetal lambs after maternal administration of sodium pentobarbital. Am J Obstet Gynecol 1986; 154:674-8.

16. Hoffman WE, Pelligrino D, Werner C, et al. Ketamine decreases plasma catecholamines and improves outcome from incomplete cerebral ischemia in rats. Anesthesiology 1992; 76:755-62.

17. Gale R, Zalkinder-Luboshitz I, Slater PE. Increased neonatal risk from the use of general anesthesia in emergency cesarean section: A retrospective analysis of 374 cases. J Reprod Med 1982; 27:715-9.

18. Marx GF, Luykx WM, Cohen S. Fetal-neonatal status following caesarean section for fetal distress. Br J Anaesth 1984; 56:1009-13.

19. Ramanathan J, Ricca DM, Sibai BM, Angel JJ. Epidural vs. general anesthesia in fetal distress with various abnormal fetal heart rate patterns (abstract). Anesth Analg 1988; 67:S180.

20. Eisenach JC. Fetal stress/distress. Probl Anesth 1989; 3:19-31.

21. Mokriski BK, Malinow AM. Neonatal acid-base status following general anesthesia for emergency abdominal delivery with halothane or isoflurane. J Clin Anesth 1992; 4:97-100.

22. Edelstone DI, Peticca BB, Goldblum LJ. Effects of maternal oxygen administration on fetal oxygenation during reductions in umbilical blood flow in fetal lambs. Am J Obstet Gynecol 1985; 152: 351-8.

23. Paulick RP, Meyers RL, Rudolph AM. Effect of maternal oxygen administration on fetal oxygenation during graded reduction of umbilical or uterine blood flow in fetal sheep. Am J Obstet Gynecol 1992; 167:233-9.

24. Willcourt RJ, King JC, Queenan JT. Maternal oxygenation administration and the fetal transcutaneous PO_2. Am J Obstet Gynecol 1983; 146:714-5.

25. Thurlow JA, Kinsella SM. Intrauterine resuscitation: Active management of fetal distress. Int J Obstet Anesth 2002; 11:105-16.

26. Thorp JA, Trobough T, Evans R, Hedrick J, Yeast JD. The effect of maternal oxygen administration during the second stage of labor on umbilical cord blood gas values: A randomized controlled prospective trial. Am J Obstet Gynecol 1995; 172:465-74.

27. Khaw KS, Wang CC, Ngan Kee WD, Pang CP, Rogers MS. Effects of high inspired oxygen fraction during elective caesarean section under spinal anaesthesia on maternal and fetal oxygenation and lipid peroxidation. Br J Anaesth 2002; 88:18-23.

28. Backe SK, Lyons G. Oxygen and elective caesarean section (editorial). Br J Anaesth 2002; 88:4-5.

29. Thomas P, Buckley P, Fox M. Maternal and neonatal blood glucose after crystalloid loading for epidural caesarean section. Anaesthesia 1984; 39:1240-2.

30. Chestnut DH, Bates JN, Choi WW. Effect of intravenous administration of Ringer's lactate on maternal capillary blood glucose before elective cesarean section. J Reprod Med 1987; 32:191-3.

31. Kenepp NB, Shelley WC, Gabbe SG, et al. Fetal and neonatal hazards of maternal hydration with 5% dextrose before caesarean section. Lancet 1982; 1:1150-2.

32. Mendiola J, Grylack LJ, Scanlon JW. Effects of intrapartum maternal glucose infusion on the normal fetus and newborn. Anesth Analg 1982; 61:32-5.

33. Grylack LJ, Chu SS, Scanlon JW. Use of intravenous fluids before cesarean section: Effects on perinatal glucose, insulin, and sodium homeostasis. Obstet Gynecol 1984; 63:654-8.

34. Philipson EH, Kalhan SC, Riha MM, Pimentel R. Effects of maternal glucose infusion on fetal acid-base status in human pregnancy. Am J Obstet Gynecol 1987; 157:866-73.

35. Blomstrand S, Hrbek A, Karlsson K, et al. Does glucose administration affect the cerebral response to fetal asphyxia? Acta Obstet Gynecol Scand 1984; 63:345-53.

36. McKinlay J, Lyons G. Obstetric neuraxial anaesthesia: Which pressor agents should we be using? Int J Obstet Anesth 2002; 11:117-21.

37. Reece EA, Chervenak FA, Romero R, Hobbins JC. Magnesium sulfate in the management of acute intrapartum fetal distress. Am J Obstet Gynecol 1984; 148:104-6.

38. Ingemarsson I, Arulkumaran S, Ratnam SS. Single injection of terbutaline in term labor. I. Effect on fetal pH in cases with prolonged bradycardia. Am J Obstet Gynecol 1985; 153:859-65.

39. Patriarco MS, Viechnicki BM, Hutchinson TA, et al. A study on intrauterine fetal resuscitation with terbutaline. Am J Obstet Gynecol 1987; 157:384-7.

40. Hanley ML, Ananth CV, Vintziceos AM. The intrapartum use of tocolysis for fetal distress: A meta-analysis (abstract). Am J Obstet Gynecol 1997; 176:S149.

41. Bell E. Nitroglycerin and uterine relaxation (letter). Anesthesiology 1996; 85:683.

42. Miyazaki FS, Taylor NA. Saline amnioinfusion for relief of variable or prolonged decelerations: A preliminary report. Am J Obstet Gynecol 1983; 146:670-8.

43. Miyazaki FS, Nevarez F. Saline amnioinfusion for relief of repetitive variable decelerations: A prospective randomized study. Am J Obstet Gynecol 1985; 153:301-6.

44. Wenstrom KD, Parsons MT. The prevention of meconium aspiration in labor using amnioinfusion. Obstet Gynecol 1989; 73:647-51.

45. Harris AP. Emergency cesarean section. In: Rogers MC, editor. Current Practice in Anesthesiology. Toronto, Canada, BC Decker, 1990:361-6.

46. American College of Obstetricians and Gynecologists Committee on Obstetrics: Maternal and Fetal Medicine. Anesthesia for Emergency Deliveries. ACOG Committee Opinion No. 104. Washington, DC, 1992. (This opinion was reaffirmed in 1998.)

47. Petrikovsky BM, Cohen M, Tancer ML. Usefulness of continuous fetal heart rate monitoring during cesarean section. Am J Obstet Gynecol 1989; 161:36-7.

48. Moore TR, Gilbert WM, Resnik R, Stevenson RC. A prospective study of the 30 minute rule in the timing of cesarean delivery for fetal distress (abstract). Am J Obstet Gynecol 1992; 166(suppl):400.

49. MacKenzie IZ, Cooke I. Prospective 12 month study of 30 minute decision to delivery intervals for "emergency" cesarean section. BMJ 2001; 322:1334-5.

50. Schauberger CW, Rooney BL, Beguin EA, et al. Evaluating the thirty minute interval in emergency cesarean sections. J Am Coll Surg 1994; 179:151-5.

51. Dunphy BC, Robinson JN, Sheil OM, et al. Caesarean section for fetal distress, the interval from decision to delivery, and the relative risk of poor neonatal condition. J Obstet Gynaecol 1991; 11:241-4.

52. Korhonen J, Kariniemi V. Emergency cesarean section: The effect of delay on umbilical arterial gas balance and Apgar scores. Acta Obstet Gynecol Scand 1994; 73:782-6.

53. Chauhan SP, Roach H, Naef RW, et al. Cesarean section for suspected fetal distress: Does the decision-incision time make a difference? J Reprod Med 1997; 42:347-52.

54. Lucas DN, Yentis SM, Kinsella SM, et al. Urgency of caesarean section: A new classification. J R Soc Med 2000; 93:346-50.

55. Hauth JC, Merenstein GB, editors. Guidelines for Perinatal Care. 4th ed. American Academy of Pediatrics and American College of Obstetricians and Gynecologists, Elk Grove Village, IL, 2002:147.

56. Hawkins JL, Koonin LM, Palmer SK, Gibbs CP. Anesthesia-related deaths during obstetric delivery in the United States, 1979-1990. Anesthesiology 1997; 86:277-84.

57. Hibbard BM, Anderson MM, Drife JO, et al. Report on Confidential Enquiries into Maternal Deaths in the United Kingdom 1991-1993. London, England, Her Majesty's Stationery Office, 1996.

58. Kaunitz AM, Hughes JM, Grimes DA, et al. Causes of maternal mortality in the United States. Obstet Gynecol 1985; 65:605-12.

59. Endler GC, Mariona FG, Sokol RJ, Stevenson LB. Anesthesia-related maternal mortality in Michigan, 1972 to 1984. Am J Obstet Gynecol 1988; 159:187-93.

60. Oriol NE. Maternal mortality: USA view. In: Van Zundert A, Ostheimer GW, editors. Pain Relief and Anesthesia in Obstetrics. New York, NY, Churchill Livingstone, 1996:745-56.

61. Spielman FJ, Mayer DC. Clear head, steady hands: Anesthesia for emergency cesarean delivery (editorial). Am J Anesthesiol 2001; 28:328-30.

62. Tuffnell DJ, Wilkinson K, Beresford N. Interval between decision and delivery by caesarean section: Are current standards achievable? BMJ 2001; 322:1330-3.

63. Morgan BM, Magni V, Goroszenuik T. Anaesthesia for emergency cesarean section. Br J Obstet Gynaecol 1990; 97:420-4.

64. Riley ET, Papasin J. Epidural catheter function during labor predicts anesthetic efficacy for subsequent cesarean delivery. Int J Obstet Anesth 2002; 11:81-4.

65. Philipson EH, Kuhnert BR, Syracuse CD. Fetal acidosis, 2-chloroprocaine, and epidural anesthesia for cesarean section. Am J Obstet Gynecol 1985; 151:322-4.

66. Brown WU, Bell GC, Alper MH. Acidosis, local anesthetics, and the newborn. Obstet Gynecol 1976; 48:27-30.

67. Biehl D, Shnider SM, Levinson G, Callender K. Placental transfer of lidocaine: Effects of fetal acidosis. Anesthesiology 1978; 48:409-12.

68. Price ML, Reynolds F, Morgan BM. Extending epidural blockade for emergency caesarean section: Evaluation of 2% lignocaine with adrenaline. Int J Obstet Anesth 1991; 1:13-8.

69. Gaiser RR, Cheek TG, Gutsche BB. Epidural lidocaine versus 2-chloroprocaine for fetal distress requiring urgent cesarean section. Int J Obstet Anesth 1994; 3:208-10.

70. Gaiser RR, Cheek TG, Adams HK, Gutsche BB. Epidural lidocaine for cesarean delivery of the distressed fetus. Int J Obstet Anesth 1998; 7:27-31.

71. Lam DTC, Ngan Kee WD, Shaw KS. Extension of epidural blockade in labour for emergency caesarean section using 2% lidocaine with epinephrine and fentanyl, with or without alkalinisation. Anaesthesia 2001; 56:777-98.

72. Lucas DN, Borra PJ, Yentis SM. Epidural top-up solutions for emergency caesarean section: A comparison of preparation times. Br J Anaesth 2000; 84:494-6.

73. Dickson MAS, Jenkins J. Extension of epidural blockade for emergency caesarean section: Assessment of a bolus dose of bupivacaine 0.5% 10 mL following an infusion of 0.1% for analgesia in labour. Anaesthesia 1994; 94:636-8.

74. Lucas DN, Ciccone GK, Yentis SM. Extending low-dose epidural analgesia for emergency caesarean section: A comparison of three solutions. Anaesthesia 1999; 54:1173-7.

75. Clark RB, Thompson DS, Thompson CH. Prevention of spinal hypotension associated with cesarean section. Anesthesiology 1976; 45:670-4.

76. Rout CC, Rocke DA, Levin J, et al. A reevaluation of the role of crystalloid preload in the prevention of hypotension associated with spinal anesthesia for elective cesarean section. Anesthesiology 1993; 79:262-9.

77. Malan TP, Johnson MD. The difficult airway in obstetric anesthesia: Techniques for airway management and the role of regional anesthesia. J Clin Anesth 1988; 1:104-11.

78. Ranasinghe JS, Ranasinghe N, Bailur N, Gallardo C. Use of continuous spinal anesthesia for an urgent cesarean delivery. Am J Anesthesiol 2001; 28:341-3.

79. Norris MC, Dewan DM. Preoxygenation for cesarean section: A comparison of two techniques. Anesthesiology 1985; 62:827-9.

80. Rorke MJ, Davey DA, Du Toit HJ. Fetal oxygenation during caesarean section. Anaesthesia 1968; 23:585-96.

81. Baraka A. Correlation between maternal and fetal Po_2 and Pco_2 during caesarean section. Br J Anaesth 1970; 42:434-8.

82. Marx GF, Mateo CV. Effects of different oxygen concentrations during general anaesthesia for elective caesarean section. Can Anaesth Soc J 1971; 18:587-93.

83. Ramanathan S, Gandhi S, Arismendy J, et al. Oxygen transfer from mother to fetus during cesarean section under epidural anesthesia. Anesth Analg 1982; 61:576-81.

84. Crawford JS. Fetal well-being and maternal awareness (editorial). Br J Anaesth 1988; 61:247-9.

85. Bogod DG, Rosen M, Rees GAD. Maximum F_IO_2 during caesarean section. Br J Anaesth 1988; 61:255-62.

86. Ranney B, Stanage W. Advantages of local anesthesia for cesarean section. Obstet Gynecol 1975; 45:163-7.

87. Cooper MG, Feeney EM, Joseph M, McGuinness JJ. Local anaesthetic infiltration for caesarean section. Anaesth Intensive Care 1989; 17:198-212.

88. Leiberman JR, Cohen A, Wiznitzer A, et al. Cesarean section by local anesthesia in patients with familial dysautonomia. Am J Obstet Gynecol 1991; 165:110-1.

89. Schaut DJ, Khona R, Gross JB. Sevoflurane inhalation induction for emergency cesarean section in a parturient with no intravenous access. Anesthesiology 1997; 86:1392-4.

90. Simon GR, Wilkins CJ, Smith I. Sevoflurane induction for emergency caesarean section: Two case reports in women with needle phobia. Int J Obstet Anesth 2002; 11:296-300.

91. Bhavani-Shankar K, Camann WR. Letter to the editor: The practice of using sevoflurane inhalation induction for emergency cesarean section and a parturient with no intravenous access. Anesthesiology 1998; 88:275-6.

92. Sitzman BT. Letter to the editor: The practice of using sevoflurane inhalation induction for emergency cesarean section and a parturient with no intravenous access. Anesthesiology 1998; 88:276.

93. Gambling DR, Reisner LS. Letter to the editor: The practice of using sevoflurane inhalation induction for emergency cesarean section and a parturient with no intravenous access. Anesthesiology 1998; 88:276-7.

94. Levy DM. Inhalational induction of anaesthesia for caesarean section: Not to be sniffed at? Int J Obstet Anesth 2002; 11:235-7.

95. Boyce PM, Todd AL. Increased risk of postnatal depression after emergency caesarean section. Med J Aust 1992; 157:172-4.

Appendix

American College of Obstetricians and Gynecologists Committee Opinion: Anesthesia for Emergency Deliveries*

Failed intubation and pulmonary aspiration of gastric contents continue to be leading causes of maternal morbidity and mortality from anesthesia. The risk of these complications can be reduced by the following: (1) careful antepartum assessment to identify patients at risk; (2) greater use of regional anesthesia when possible; and (3) appropriate selection and preparation of patients who require general anesthesia for delivery.

ANTEPARTUM RISK ASSESSMENT

The obstetric care team should be alert to the presence of risk factors that place the parturient at increased risk for complications from emergency general or regional anesthesia. These factors include—but are not limited to—marked obesity, severe facial and neck edema, extremely short stature, a short neck, difficulty opening the mouth, a small mandible, protuberant teeth, arthritis of the neck, anatomic abnormalities of the face or mouth, a large thyroid, asthma, serious medical or obstetric complications, and a history of problems with anesthetics.

When such risk factors are identified, a provider who is credentialed to provide general and regional anesthesia should be consulted in the antepartum period to allow for joint development of a plan of management that includes optimal location for delivery. Strategies can thereby be developed to minimize the need for the emergency induction of general anesthesia in women for whom this would be especially hazardous. For those patients at risk, consideration should be given to the planned placement during early labor of an intravenous line and an epidural or spinal catheter (with confirmation that the catheter is functional). If a patient at unusual risk of complications from anesthesia is identified (e.g., prior failed intubation), strong consideration should be given to antepartum referral of the patient to allow for delivery at a hospital that can manage such anesthesia on a 24-hour basis.

EMERGENCY ANESTHESIA

The need for expeditious abdominal delivery cannot always be anticipated. When preparing for the rapid initiation of anesthesia, both the maternal and the fetal status must be considered. Oral nonparticulate antacids should be administered immediately before the induction of general or major regional anesthesia to decrease the mother's risk of developing aspiration pneumonitis.

Although there are some situations in which general anesthesia is preferable to regional anesthesia, the risk of general anesthesia must be weighed against the benefit for those patients who have a greater potential for complications. Examples of circumstances in which a rapid induction of general anesthesia may be indicated include the following: (1) prolapsed umbilical cord with severe fetal bradycardia; and (2) active hemorrhage in a hemodynamically unstable mother.

In some cases, a nonreassuring fetal heart rate pattern is diagnosed as fetal distress, and delivery is performed immediately. The term *fetal distress* is imprecise, nonspecific, and has little positive predictive value. The character of the fetal heart rate abnormality should be considered when the urgency of the delivery and the type of anesthesia to be administered are determined. Cesarean deliveries that are performed for a nonreassuring fetal heart rate pattern do not necessarily preclude the use of regional anesthesia.

---

*From American College of Obstetricians and Gynecologists Committee on Obstetrics: Maternal and Fetal Medicine. Anesthesia for Emergency Deliveries. ACOG Committee Opinion No. 104. Washington, DC, 1992. (This opinion was reaffirmed in 1998.)

Chapter 27
Postoperative Analgesia: Systemic Techniques

Robert K. Parker, D.O.

Pain can be defined as "an unpleasant sensory and emotional experience associated with actual or potential tissue damage, or described in terms of such damage."[1] All cultures have attempted to control pain. The ability to sense pain after an injury has some benefit. For example, withdrawal from a noxious stimulus (e.g., heat, fire) prevents serious injury. Pain also promotes immobility, which encourages rest, healing, and recuperation.[2] However, there are several disadvantages of postoperative pain. Complete immobility predisposes patients to atelectasis, pneumonia, and thromboembolic complications.[3] In obstetric patients, persistent pain interferes with the early postpartum interaction between mother and baby.

During the management of postoperative pain, the physician must balance pain relief with undesirable side effects. For obstetric patients, side effects may be direct (e.g., nausea, vomiting, sedation) or indirect (e.g., interference with maternal-infant bonding, excretion of medication in breast milk). Effective pain relief does not necessarily make the patient completely insensible to the fact that surgery was performed; rather, it allows a degree of comfort that promotes physical recovery and a sense of well-being.

HISTORICAL PERSPECTIVE

Historically, the surgeon has prescribed postoperative pain medications when writing the general postoperative orders. In 1973, Marks and Sachar[4] noted that 73% of postoperative patients experienced distressing pain despite the use of intramuscular opioids. They concluded that most physicians prescribed inadequate doses of analgesics at infrequent intervals. Austin et al.[5] observed that the duration of the minimum effective analgesic concentration of meperidine was only 35% of the prescribed 4-hour dosing interval. In a review of nursing practice, Short et al.[6] found that only 29% of the maximum prescribed dose of morphine and only 17% of the maximum prescribed dose of meperidine were actually administered to a group of elderly men who had undergone elective surgery. Only 1 of 56 patients received 100% of the prescribed dose of analgesic; no other patient received more than 63% of the prescribed analgesic, and 29% of the patients received no analgesic.

Anxiety and stress may worsen pain. Anxiolytic agents may potentiate the pain relief provided by analgesics, but these drugs should be used properly. Health care providers often misunderstand which drugs provide analgesia and which drugs provide anxiolysis. Loper et al.[7] questioned 370 physician house staff and intensive care unit nurses regarding the administration of analgesic and anxiolytic agents. A total of 50% of the physicians and 75% of the nurses incorrectly indicated that pancuronium was an effective anxiolytic, and 5% and 8%, respectively, incorrectly indicated that pancuronium was also an effective analgesic agent. Likewise, 78% of the physicians and 44% of the nurses incorrectly responded that diazepam was an effective analgesic agent. The authors aptly entitled their article "Paralyzed with pain: The need for education."

Patients' fears and misconceptions also predispose them to inadequate pain relief. Egbert et al.[8] first demonstrated the beneficial effects of patient education in the reduction of postoperative opioid requirements and the shortening of hospital stays. Before surgery, Owen et al.[9] questioned 259 patients regarding their expectations about postoperative pain. Subsequently, they questioned the same patients regarding their experiences after surgery. A majority (56%) anticipated moderate, severe, or unbearable pain, and 71% expected "a lot of relief" or "complete relief" from prescribed analgesics. A total of 65% indicated that they would wait until the pain was severe before requesting an analgesic, but 76% expected the nurse to administer the medication immediately; 77% of patients were prescribed analgesics "on demand." Intermittent intramuscular injections of morphine (maximum, 10 mg) or meperidine (maximum, 100 mg) were prescribed, with a stipulated interval of 3 to 4 hours. During the first 24 hours after surgery, patients received an average of only 2.7 injections. Approximately one fourth of the patients subsequently indicated that they had received effective pain control, but more than half indicated that they had experienced pain for most or all of the time. Other studies[10-12] have identified similar problems. Wallace[11] demonstrated reduced postoperative pain and emotional distress in patients who had received specific and accurate preoperative instruction regarding postoperative pain and pain relief as compared with patients who did not receive similar instruction. Several investigators have described strategies to improve preoperative patient education, which should facilitate the control of pain after surgery.[12,13] Unfortunately, many cesarean sections are performed as unscheduled, emergency procedures, and these strategies must be modified for the obstetric population.

OPIOID ADMINISTRATION

Intramuscular and Subcutaneous Administration

Postoperative opioid requirements vary widely among patients for a variety of reasons. The intramuscular and subcutaneous routes of administration typically do not provide the flexibility needed to respond to those varied requirements. In many hospitals, these routes of administration are used for the majority of patients with postoperative pain. Advantages of the intramuscular and subcutaneous routes include ease of administration and low cost. Unfortunately, analgesia may be inadequate because of the failure to achieve and maintain an adequate concentration of drug at the opioid receptor sites. One study evaluated blood concentrations of meperidine after scheduled intramuscular injections in women recovering from abdominal hysterectomy or cholecystectomy. Peak blood concentrations varied as much as fivefold, and the times to peak plasma concentrations varied as much as sevenfold.[5] Although one may intend to give the drug intramuscularly, computerized tomographic analysis has demonstrated that as much as 85% of the drug may be deposited subcutaneously rather than intramuscularly.[14]

Austin et al.[5] plotted blood meperidine concentrations versus the quality of analgesia. They noted a steep curve between no analgesia and complete analgesia. In a second study, these investigators gave intramuscular injections of meperidine on demand.[15] Patients varied widely in the blood meperidine concentrations needed to provide effective analgesia. However, for each individual patient, the meperidine concentration that provided pain relief remained relatively consistent for the first 2 days after surgery. Of interest, the authors were unable to demonstrate a significant correlation between body weight and blood concentrations of meperidine. This observation argues against the common practice of dosing on the basis of body weight.

Varied pharmacodynamics also contribute to the varied opioid requirements among patients. Some patients undoubtedly have a higher pain tolerance than others. High scores on anxiety and neuroticism scales are associated with low pain tolerance (as evidenced by high analgesic requirements).[15,16] Anxiety may make pain more intolerable, and pain may increase anxiety. Spielberger et al.[17] delineated two types of anxiety: (1) state anxiety, an emotional state that varies in intensity and fluctuates with time; and (2) trait anxiety, a personality characteristic that remains stable over time. Scott et al.[18] assessed various preoperative predictors of postoperative pain; they observed a linear relationship between the level of state anxiety and the severity of postoperative pain. The patient's ability to cope also affects the use of opioids. Anxious patients tend to request and consume more opioids after surgery than passive patients. Unfortunately, there remains no clinically useful method for predicting the analgesic requirements of an individual patient.

Multiple schemes for prescribing intramuscular opioids have been devised. Clinical practice is based more on tradition than on science. The literature is replete with reports of a variety of regimens, but the recurring theme is that of unpredictable efficacy.

Intravenous Administration

In 1963, Roe[19] demonstrated that small intravenous bolus doses of opioid provided more effective postoperative pain relief than did the intramuscular administration of larger doses of drug. Unfortunately, this results in a brief duration of analgesia. The intravenous administration of larger bolus doses (in an effort to increase the duration of analgesia) results in an increased incidence of side effects.

CONTINUOUS INTRAVENOUS INFUSION

Church[20] described a method of circumventing the problems of intermittent intravenous injections. A drip regulator controlled the infusion of meperidine at a rate of 0.3 mg/kg/hr. As a safety measure, only the hourly dose was added to a drip chamber, and the infusion was continued only if the respiratory rate was higher than 10 breaths per minute.

Stapleton et al.[21] assessed another regimen for the intravenous infusion of meperidine. They gave a loading dose of 1 mg/min for 45 minutes followed by 0.53 mg/min for 28 minutes. A maintenance infusion of 0.4 mg/min was used for the remainder of the 32-hour study period. Their goal was to maintain a steady-state blood concentration of meperidine, and they plotted the meperidine concentrations versus the pain scores. The minimum blood meperidine concentration needed to relieve severe pain was approximately 0.46 µg/mL, but there was considerable variation in the blood concentrations of meperidine associated with moderate pain.

Rutter et al.[22] assessed morphine requirements immediately after surgery and used each patient's individual requirements as a guideline for comparing intravenous infusion, scheduled intramuscular injection, and intramuscular injection on patient request. Intravenous infusion provided better pain relief at a lower total dose than either of the intramuscular methods but at the expense of a slightly more blunted mental state.

Catley et al.[23] compared the use of intravenous morphine infusion with the use of either epidural or intercostal bupivacaine for postoperative analgesia. Using pulse oximetry, they observed 456 episodes of pronounced oxyhemoglobin desaturation (SaO_2 less than 80%) in 10 of 16 patients who received a continuous intravenous infusion of morphine. Conversely, SaO_2 did not decline to less than 87% in any of the patients treated with regional analgesia. Marshall et al.[24] compared the continuous intravenous infusion of morphine with saline-placebo in patients recovering from cholecystectomy. The dose of morphine was determined according to the patient's weight. Both groups had equal access to a fixed dose of supplemental intramuscular morphine as desired. There was no difference between groups in the amount of supplemental morphine required during the first 24 hours. Further, patients in the continuous morphine group required more supplemental morphine during the 24 hours after discontinuation of the infusion. The authors suggested that this may have reflected the development of tolerance in those patients. Patients in the morphine infusion group also had more side effects than those in the saline-placebo group.

Nimmo and Todd[25] evaluated the continuous intravenous infusion of fentanyl. An intravenous infusion of either fentanyl 1.5 µg/kg/hr, fentanyl 0.5 µg/kg/hr, or dextrose-placebo was begun 1 to 2 hours before elective abdominal hysterectomy in 24 patients. All patients were allowed intramuscular injection of Cyclimorph (morphine 10 mg and cyclizine 50 mg) on demand. Patients who received the larger dose of fentanyl demanded fewer supplemental intramuscular boluses than did the placebo group, but they received a greater total dose of opioid.

These studies demonstrate a common theme. Despite the use of a continuous opioid infusion (either as a fixed dose or a dose based on weight), these investigators could not identify an ideal dose that would provide adequate analgesia without supplemental bolus doses or side effects. Stanski[26] demonstrated that changes in surgical stimulation cause fluctuations in dose requirements during the intravenous infusion of opioid during surgery. Likewise, fluctuations in painful stimulation can be expected after surgery. Opioid requirements may be minimal during periods of inactivity, but dose requirements increase during periods of heightened activity. It may be futile to attempt to maintain a steady-state opioid concentration to relieve postoperative pain during periods of changing painful stimuli.

Patient-Controlled Analgesia

Sechzer[27] described the analgesic response to small intravenous doses of opioids given by a nurse in response to a patient's demands. This technique of intravenous "on-demand analgesia" resulted in consistent pain relief with low total doses of opioid. Sechzer[27] confirmed the cyclical nature of pain and the varied dose requirements among patients, but he also confirmed the consistency of opioid requirements in an individual patient.

This intermittent intravenous bolus-dose technique resulted in additional work for nursing personnel, which made this technique impractical. Investigators began to develop instruments that would allow patients to self-administer small intravenous boluses on demand. These early instruments (the Demand Dropmaster, the Analgesic-Demand System, and the Demanalg) were quite cumbersome.[28-30] The first commercially available device was the Cardiff Palliator.[31] Subsequently, Keeri-Szanto[32] recognized that patient-controlled analgesia (PCA) provides both pharmacologic and nonpharmacologic benefits. The author noted that the majority of patients "adapted successfully to up to four-fold variations in drug delivery," but that 21% of patients "triggered the apparatus in response to some clue other than the amount of drug received." Keeri-Szanto[32] referred to these patients as *placebo reactors*. The author also recognized that a patient's sense of autonomy significantly increases the efficacy of a given dose of drug.

Because of concerns regarding abuse potential, inappropriate use, dangerous side effects, and lack of patient understanding, Hull and Sibbald[33] developed a sophisticated, cumbersome, and expensive PCA device that included a series of electronic fail-safe circuits. This device communicated with patients by means of messages that could be recorded in the patient's own language and limited the dose according to the patient's respiratory rate. Subsequently, investigators began using PCA as a research tool. These studies did not use a physician-chosen endpoint for analgesia; rather, the patient defined the endpoints of analgesia. Tamsen et al.[34-37] observed that there was no correlation between analgesic concentrations of drug and age, gender, body weight, or the rate of elimination of drug. Dose requirements and therapeutic concentrations varied widely among patients, although individual patient plasma concentrations remained relatively constant with the self-administration of morphine or meperidine during the early postoperative period.

Studies have demonstrated that intravenous PCA provides better pain relief than intramuscular opioid administration in nonobstetric patients.[38-40] In contrast, studies in obstetric patients have demonstrated that intravenous PCA and intramuscular opioid administration provide comparable pain relief after cesarean section.[41-43] However, intravenous PCA provides more immediate pain relief, fewer side effects, and greater satisfaction than intramuscular opioid administration in both obstetric and nonobstetric patients.[38-43] When given a choice, most patients prefer intravenous PCA over intramuscular opioid administration.

Ferrante et al.[44] developed a statistical model to compare the efficacy of intravenous PCA with that of traditional intramuscular opioids. They found that intravenous PCA was no more effective than intramuscular opioids. Patients self-administered opioids to "moderate" levels of pain relief with PCA. The authors suggested that some patients may not envision the possibility of complete postoperative analgesia, and these patients dose themselves according to their expectations. Experience suggests that the effective use of PCA requires effective nurse education and patient instruction (Box 27-1).

It is unclear whether PCA has a dose-sparing effect. Some[43,48-50] but not all[38,40-42,51] studies have noted that intravenous PCA results in the administration of a decreased total dose of opioid. This discrepancy may result in part from the use of different drugs and varied endpoints in these studies. Some studies have also not included appropriate controls.

Some physicians have expressed concern regarding the potential for opioid abuse and addiction during the use of PCA. Graves et al.[52] concluded that their patients used PCA "for pain relief, not for euphoria, and did not exhibit sedation or respiratory depression." To my knowledge, there are no published cases of the development of addiction after the short-term use of PCA for postoperative analgesia in obstetric patients. In general, if opioids are discontinued or tapered within 3 weeks of surgery, physical dependence does not

---

Box 27-1 REQUIREMENTS FOR SAFE, EFFECTIVE USE OF PATIENT-CONTROLLED ANALGESIA (PCA)

NURSE EDUCATION

- Patients may best control their pain once they have achieved a reasonable level of wakefulness and comfort after surgery.
- Patients must be mentally and physically capable of managing their own pain.

PATIENT EDUCATION

CONCEPTS OF PAIN MANAGEMENT

- Treat discomfort. Delayed treatment may result in severe pain, which may interfere with recovery and result in greater overall opioid use.
- Anticipate painful stimuli. Greater activity leads to greater discomfort. Pretreatment with an opioid may diminish fluctuations in pain.
- Postoperative opioids used to treat pain have very little addiction potential.[45,46]

HOW DOES PCA WORK?

- Small doses of opioid given on demand may minimize peaks and troughs in pain relief.
- Overdose is rare. The dose is prescribed by the physician. The lockout interval permits the onset of action before administration of another dose.
- Safety of PCA is a function of patient participation. Only the patient should activate the PCA device.[47]

develop.[53] Lee et al.[54] demonstrated that the coadministration of nalbuphine or naloxone blocked the development of tolerance and dependence to morphine in laboratory animals. Unlike naloxone, the coadministration of nalbuphine did not attenuate the antinociceptive effect of morphine and produced less-intense signs of morphine withdrawal.

There is a lack of consensus regarding the most appropriate drug for intravenous PCA. Morphine and meperidine are the most commonly prescribed opioids. In addition, the use of the very lipid-soluble opioids (fentanyl, sufentanil, alfentanil), agonist-antagonist agents (butorphanol, buprenorphine, nalbuphine), and other opioids (hydromorphone, oxymorphone, methadone) has been described (Table 27-1).[55]

There remains controversy regarding the use of a continuous basal (background) infusion in conjunction with intravenous PCA. In theory, the use of PCA alone should accommodate the wide variability of dose requirements among individual patients. However, patients who are sedated (as a result of residual anesthetic drugs) or fatigued after surgery may underdose themselves when using a PCA delivery system. In addition, distressing pain may occur with increased physical activity, even in patients who are comfortable at rest.[4,5,56] Sinatra et al.[57] demonstrated decreased pain during movement when a basal infusion of morphine or oxymorphone was added to intravenous PCA therapy in patients recovering from cesarean section. The improved pain relief was accompanied by an increase in the incidence of nausea and vomiting. Owen et al.[58] did not observe any advantage to the use of a fixed-rate basal opioid infusion during intravenous PCA therapy in patients recovering from gynecologic surgery.

We evaluated the use of three different infusion rates of morphine during PCA therapy in patients recovering from gynecologic surgery. The use of a basal (background) infusion did not improve pain relief but resulted in an increased total dose of opioid and an increased severity of side effects.[59] Subsequently, we observed that the addition of a basal infusion during the nighttime hours did not improve sleep,

decrease nocturnal awakening as a result of pain, or decrease opioid requirements in patients who received PCA therapy during recovery from abdominal hysterectomy. Most patients found it convenient to self-administer opioid when they were awakened because of activity in the room. Only 8% of patients found that it was inconvenient to use PCA during the nighttime hours.[60] In the two studies, 85% of all patients achieved adequate analgesia without any change in their PCA regimen and without major side effects.

The inherent safety of a PCA delivery system results from the fact that the patient determines when she needs an additional dose of analgesic drug. If a patient becomes excessively sedated, the number of self-administered bolus doses will decrease; this reduces the potential for opioid-induced respiratory depression. The inherent safety of the technique is diminished when a patient is obligated to receive a continuous infusion of opioid as part of a combined PCA-basal infusion regimen.[61] Moreover, the potential for programming errors is increased when multiple changes are required in the PCA prescription.[62,63] When prescribing PCA therapy for patients recovering from cesarean section, it is best to use PCA alone, *without* a basal infusion of opioid. A continuous basal infusion should be added only if pain relief is inadequate despite appropriate PCA use. This scheme may need to be modified and a basal infusion included for patients who are opioid dependent.

When beginning intravenous PCA after cesarean section, I prescribe patient-controlled bolus doses of morphine, 1 to 1.5 mg, with an 8-minute lockout interval. This regimen provides satisfactory analgesia with few side effects in most obstetric patients. The dose and lockout interval may be adjusted to accommodate those few patients who experience unsatisfactory analgesia.

There is no need to change the PCA prescription to wean a patient from intravenous PCA. Painful stimuli diminish with time after surgery. Patients using PCA appropriately will administer bolus doses less frequently as the pain decreases. Alternatively, an oral analgesic may be prescribed at regular intervals while the patient continues to use PCA. The patient will administer fewer bolus doses of opioid, and PCA may then be discontinued.

Finally, the operative procedure and the needs and capabilities of the individual patient should be considered before choosing the route and technique of drug administration. For example, most patients do not require PCA after postpartum tubal ligation. Moreover, PCA is useless if the patient is incapable of using the device. I have observed two patients in wrist restraints who were wearing a "wristwatch" PCA device.

Intravenous PCA is not readily available at all institutions. The success of intravenous PCA underscores the efficacy of "on-demand" analgesia. The concept of "on-demand" analgesia should not be limited to intravenous administration but should also apply to intramuscular, subcutaneous, and oral administration.

TABLE 27-1	GUIDELINES REGARDING THE BOLUS DOSE, LOCK-OUT INTERVAL, AND CONTINUOUS INFUSION RATE FOR VARIOUS OPIOID ANALGESICS WHEN USING A PCA SYSTEM		
Drug	Bolus dose (mg)	Lockout interval (minutes)	Continuous infusion (mg/hr)
Agonists			
Fentanyl	0.015-0.05	3-10	0.02-0.1
Hydromorphone	0.1-0.5	5-15	0.2-0.5
Meperidine	5-15	5-15	5-40
Methadone	0.5-3.0	10-20	—
Morphine	0.5-3.0	5-20	1-10
Oxymorphone	0.2-0.8	5-15	0.1-1
Sufentanil	0.003-0.015	3-10	—
Agonist-antagonists			
Buprenorphine	0.03-0.2	10-20	—
Nalbuphine	1-5	5-15	1-8
Pentazocine	5-30	5-15	6-40

Modified from Lubenow TR, Ivankovich AD, McCarthy RJ. Management of acute postoperative pain. In Barash PG, Cullen BF, Stoelting RK, editors. Clinical Anesthesia. 3rd ed. Philadelphia, PA, JB Lippincott-Raven, 1997:1320.

Oral Administration

Oral administration of analgesics is the mainstay of pain management for patients undergoing outpatient surgery. In the past, oral opioid administration after intraabdominal surgery was deferred until the patient tolerated oral intake of liquids. Patients who have undergone cesarean section experience a faster return of bowel function than patients who have undergone other abdominal procedures. Many obstetricians have relaxed restrictions regarding oral intake during the early postoperative period. For example, most obstetricians do not require the patient to pass flatus before they begin a clear liquid diet after cesarean section. In our hospital, oral opioid analgesics are used (albeit somewhat sparingly) to supplement intrathecal or epidural opioid analgesia after cesarean section. Some patients receive an oral opioid analgesic before discharge from the postanesthesia care unit. We have observed few side effects associated with the early administration of oral analgesics, and we have not observed an increased incidence of nausea, vomiting, or delayed bowel function in these patients.

Oral analgesics have limitations during the early postoperative period. The absorption of oral analgesic drugs is somewhat unpredictable during this time. Changes in gastric emptying may occur after any abdominal operation. Operations on abdominal viscera (other than the stomach or duodenum) result in gastric retention for 6 to 24 hours postoperatively.[64] Delayed gastric emptying results in delayed absorption of drug. The stress of surgery may result in increased gastric acid content, which may also limit the absorption of oral opioids. The first-pass hepatic effect and liver inactivation of drug limit the efficacy of oral analgesics, although this disadvantage is not limited to the early postoperative period. Further, oral analgesics are of no value in patients with persistent nausea and vomiting. Of interest, in a prospective, randomized trial, Asao et al.[65] recently observed that gum chewing three times per day (beginning on the first postoperative morning) enhanced recovery from postoperative ileus in patients recovering from laparoscopic colectomy.

The effective use of oral analgesics may be accomplished with on-demand, combination therapy. Multimodal therapy begun in the operating room should continue throughout the postoperative period. For example, transition from intravenous PCA to oral agents may be accomplished by starting a nonsteroidal antiinflammatory drug (NSAID) or acetaminophen, with or without an opioid. We commonly begin by giving one oral acetaminophen tablet with oxycodone every 4 hours (on schedule) plus one tablet every 4 hours on patient demand. The flexible dosing allows the patient to participate in her pain management. A patient may find that she needs only the scheduled oral medication or possibly two tablets every 4 hours or one tablet every 2 hours. The patient subsequently weans herself from intravenous PCA. When intravenous PCA demands diminish and are replaced with oral agents, the intravenous PCA is discontinued. We encourage the maintenance of preemptive analgesia. Specifically, I explain to patients that oral analgesics (i.e., "pain pills") should have been called "discomfort pills": you take them for discomfort so that you do not experience pain.

Side Effects

Opioid receptor-mediated side effects (e.g., nausea, pruritus) may occur independent of dose. Severe side effects may reflect a relative overdose. Side effects rarely signal an allergic reaction.

Most side effects are self-limiting. An opioid-receptor antagonist may be administered to relieve annoying side effects. The mixed agonist-antagonist nalbuphine is especially useful (vide infra). Alternatively, there may be some benefit to the administration of a different opioid. One study[66] demonstrated a higher incidence of adynamic ileus after cesarean section in patients using intravenous PCA as compared with patients receiving intramuscular opioid analgesia, despite similar total doses of drug.

NONOPIOID ANALGESICS

NSAIDs are also used to provide postoperative analgesia.[67] They are rarely satisfactory as sole agents for the relief of pain in patients recovering from abdominal surgery.[68] When they are used as a part of a multimodal approach to the treatment of postoperative pain, NSAIDs may improve overall analgesia[69] and provide some opioid dose-sparing effect.[70-72] For example, some investigators have suggested that NSAIDs may enhance intraspinal opioid analgesia without increasing the risk of sedation, pruritus, or respiratory depression (see Chapter 28). (It is unclear whether the opioid dose-sparing effect consistently decreases the incidence and/or severity of opioid-mediated side effects.) The NSAIDs exert an antiinflammatory effect at the incision site, and they also may relieve the discomfort of uterine cramping after vaginal delivery.[73,74] In one study, continuous intravenous infusion of ketorolac (105 mg over 24 hours) resulted in a 30% reduction in the dose of PCEA meperidine, but it did not significantly improve pain relief, reduce opioid-related side effects, or change patient outcome in women recovering from cesarean section.[75] Huang et al.[76] observed that tenoxicam, an injectable NSAID (available outside the United States) reduced uterine cramping and meperidine consumption without increasing side effects in patients recovering from cesarean delivery.

Nonselective NSAIDs inhibit cyclooxygenase (COX-1 and COX-2) enzymes involved in prostaglandin synthesis. The COX-1 (expressed isoform) enzyme is active throughout the body, and its inhibition may result in adverse gastrointestinal, renal, and antiplatelet effects. Conversely, the COX-2 (inducible isoform) enzyme is expressed in association with pain and inflammation; its inhibition results in the observed antiinflammatory and analgesic effects.[77-79] Oral COX-1 inhibitors (e.g., ibuprofen) have been widely used for providing analgesia after both cesarean and vaginal delivery. Ketorolac, an injectable COX-1 inhibitor, is used postoperatively when patients are unable to tolerate oral agents. Some physicians are reluctant to administer COX-1 NSAIDs for routine postpartum analgesia because of concern that these agents might inhibit platelet function and cause increased postpartum bleeding. The oral COX-2 selective NSAIDs (e.g., rofecoxib, celecoxib, valdecoxib) are finding their way into obstetric clinical practice but have not been studied extensively in humans. Currently, they are not recommended for intrapartum use. Transfer of these drugs into breast milk is likely, and their effects on the newborn are unclear. We are beginning to use the COX-2 selective agents *after* cesarean section, but we avoid their use in patients who plan to breastfeed. Parecoxib, an injectable pro-drug (or precursor) of valdecoxib, is currently undergoing human trials in the United States, but it has not yet received approval by the United States Food and Drug Administration (FDA). Parecoxib 20 mg compares favorably with ketorolac 30 mg and morphine 4 mg in patients recovering from lower abdominal gynecologic surgery.[78]

Propacetamol (a pro-drug of acetaminophen) has been administered in parts of Europe since 1985 for the treatment of postoperative pain. Acetaminophen is a potent analgesic, but it loses much of its effect when given orally because of its first-pass hepatic metabolism. Intravenous administration of propacetamol is currently undergoing phase III trials in the United States.

ADJUNCTIVE AGENTS, MUTIMODAL THERAPY, AND PREEMPTIVE ANALGESIA

For many years, some surgeons have injected local anesthetic at the incision site at the end of surgery. Ejlersen et al.[80] observed that preincisional lidocaine infiltration provided more effective postoperative analgesia than postincisional lidocaine infiltration in patients who had undergone elective inguinal herniorrhaphy. These findings support the hypothesis that "prevention of hyperalgesia and/or central nervous system hyperexcitability owing to the afferent barrage from the surgical area is of major importance in reducing acute pain."[80] Amide local anesthetics possess potent, long-lasting antiinflammatory properties.[81] Preincisional administration of an amide local anesthetic may not only provide neural blockade but may also result in the inhibition of inflammatory changes in the surrounding tissues. However, Pavy et al.[82] observed that preoperative skin infiltration with 0.5% bupivacaine did *not* enhance postoperative analgesia in patients who received spinal anesthesia for elective cesarean section. The authors speculated that the lack of difference in pain scores between the two groups resulted from the high quality of analgesia provided by intrathecal morphine (0.25 to 0.3 mg).

Kee et al.[83] observed that patients who received ketamine for the induction of general anesthesia for cesarean section required less morphine during the first 24 hours after surgery as compared with patients who received thiopental. The authors suggested that ketamine may have exerted both a direct and a preemptive analgesic effect. Woolf and Chong[84] and Ochroch et al.[85] have reviewed the subject of preemptive analgesia.

A growing number of anesthesiologists use a balanced, multimodal approach when providing postoperative analgesia.[86] Addressing specific pain pathways and targets using a variety of modalities and drugs takes advantage of additive and synergistic effects while potentially reducing the incidence and/or severity of side effects observed with larger doses of any individual drug. Recent studies have demonstrated the advantages of the preoperative administration of NSAIDs,[87-90] acetaminophen,[91] and sustained-release opioids such as oxycodone,[92] but these regimens have not been specifically studied in patients undergoing cesarean delivery. Local anesthetic infiltration of the incisional area by either continuous[93] or patient-controlled[94] instillation improves pain relief both at rest and with activity. Iliohypogastric and ilioinguinal nerve blocks also reduce morphine requirements after cesarean section.[95]

Stress and anxiety potentiate pain and hinder pain-coping mechanisms. In theory, methods that reduce stress and alleviate anxiety should also reduce pain. As anesthesiologists, we often provide care for patients with preoperative fear and anxiety, which cause physiologic alterations such as hypertension, tachycardia, hyperventilation, sweating, and peripheral vasoconstriction. The patient with unresolved fear and anxiety is at risk for similar physiologic changes during the postoperative period. Such patients may experience more severe pain than patients who are not fearful or anxious. Patient education, as well as reassurance and support from family and medical personnel, may reduce this enhancement of postoperative pain.

Benzodiazepines may also be used to reduce anxiety. Unfortunately, these drugs are potent amnestic agents, and they provide retrograde amnesia in some patients. Camann et al.[96] reported several cases of retrograde amnesia in women who received 2 to 7 mg of midazolam after the umbilical cord was clamped at cesarean delivery; these women had no recall of the birth of their babies. Most women want to remember their first interactions with their newborn infant, so physicians should use caution in the administration of benzodiazepines during the puerperium.

Metoclopramide is a central and peripheral dopamine antagonist with peripheral cholinergic properties. Anesthesiologists often give metoclopramide to accelerate gastric emptying before the induction of general anesthesia. Metoclopramide is also an effective antiemetic agent. Studies have demonstrated that metoclopramide reduces the pain of renal colic,[97] and it is an effective analgesic adjunct during labor[98] and prostaglandin $F_{2-alpha}$-induced abortion.[99] Metoclopramide may enhance analgesia by reducing uterine smooth muscle spasm[99]; thus some investigators have speculated that it may decrease the pain of uterine cramping after cesarean delivery. At some institutions, anesthesiologists routinely prescribe scheduled doses of metoclopramide to potentiate analgesia and reduce nausea during and after the administration of neuraxial opioids or intravenous PCA for postcesarean analgesia. In some cases, droperidol—a neuroleptic butyrophenone used clinically for antiemesis and sedation—is given to reduce nausea and vomiting and to potentiate analgesia with intravenous PCA morphine.[100] Safety concerns regarding droperidol, including its potential to prolong the QT interval (Torsades de Pointes) and cause sudden death, have prompted the FDA to issue a "black box" warning, which is the most serious warning for an FDA-approved drug. It is now recommended that an electrocardiogram be obtained before the administration of droperidol and that continuous electrocardiographic monitoring be utilized for 2 hours thereafter.

A recent study demonstrated that prophylactic ondansetron reduced the incidence of postoperative nausea and vomiting but did not improve overall patient satisfaction in women receiving PCA morphine after cesarean delivery.[101]

Nalbuphine, an opioid agonist-antagonist, effectively reverses the respiratory depression that results from the administration of high doses of fentanyl during general anesthesia.[102] Nalbuphine either maintains or enhances analgesia when it is used to treat the nausea and pruritus that accompany epidural or intrathecal opioid analgesia in patients recovering from cesarean section.[103] I have successfully administered nalbuphine intravenously to alleviate the nausea, vomiting, and pruritus experienced by patients using intravenous morphine or meperidine PCA, and I have not noted any increase in PCA demands or complaints of inadequate analgesia. At least two studies have described the patient-controlled intravenous administration of nalbuphine for postoperative analgesia.[104,105] In both studies, nalbuphine provided satisfactory pain relief (comparable to that provided by morphine and meperidine) with few side effects. I have prescribed patient-controlled intravenous nalbuphine for those patients with a prior history of side effects during the use of opioid agonists.

OPIOIDS IN BREAST MILK

In the year 150 AD, Soranus of Ephesus[106] encouraged wet nurses to abstain from drugs and alcohol to avoid adverse effects on the infant. There is little objective information regarding the effects of maternally administered analgesics on breast-fed infants.

Breast milk is a suspension of protein and fat in a mineral-carbohydrate solution synthesized from the maternal circulation. Breast milk begins as colostrum, which is manufactured as early as the twelfth week of gestation. Colostrum, which is a thick, yellowish fluid, is high in protein and low in fat content as compared with mature milk. Colostrum comprises approximately 85% of breast milk during the first 2 to 3 days after delivery; approximately 7 to 123 mL (an average of 37 mL) of colostrum are made during the first 24 hours. Parity affects the production of breast milk; parous women produce greater amounts of all forms of breast milk. Most women produce approximately 500 mL of milk per day by day 5.[107]

Transitional milk comprises approximately 85% of breast milk by day 3. Breast milk subsequently fluctuates in its composition until approximately day 14, when 80% is mature breast milk, which is high in fat and low in protein content.[108]

Drug excretion into milk may occur when a drug is bound to the milk proteins or adheres to the milk fat globules.[107] Several factors may influence drug excretion into breast milk. The breast stores a minimal quantity of milk. The act of breast-feeding results in milk production, letdown, and secretion, as well as increased breast blood flow. The timing of breast-feeding (relative to drug administration) influences the amount of drug that appears in breast milk. If the infant feeds when the mother's blood level of drug is high, more drug is transferred to the breast milk as it is manufactured.[108] Breast milk content also influences the amount of drug that crosses from maternal plasma. Lipid-soluble drugs are less likely to accumulate in colostrum (which has a relatively low fat content) than in mature milk. Likewise, opioids (most of which are weak bases) are less likely to accumulate in colostrum (pH of 7.4) than in mature breast milk (pH of 7.0).[109]

The critical issue may not be the drug content of breast milk but rather the effect of the drug on the newborn. The extent of systemic absorption after oral administration to the infant, the infant's ability to metabolize the drug, and the infant's ability to excrete the drug or its metabolites should be considered. If metabolism or excretion is delayed, a drug that is found in low concentrations in breast milk may accumulate in the infant. In general, preterm infants do not tolerate drugs as well as term infants, for several reasons: (1) preterm infants have immature organ systems; (2) preterm infants have less total body protein available for drug binding; and (3) preterm infants have less body fat content, which increases the likelihood that lipid-soluble drugs will gain access to the brain.[110]

The American Academy of Pediatrics Committee on Drugs[111] has compiled a list of drugs that are transferred to human breast milk. These drugs are divided into those that contraindicate breast-feeding (category 1), those that require the temporary interruption of breast-feeding (category 2), and those that are compatible with breast-feeding (category 3) (Table 27-2).

There is little information regarding the effects of PCA on breast-feeding infants. Steer et al.[114] observed that fentanyl concentrations were higher in colostrum than in maternal serum after the intravenous administration of fentanyl 2 μg/kg during cesarean section or postpartum tubal ligation. Colostrum fentanyl concentrations were greatest at 45 minutes after intravenous administration, but fentanyl was "virtually undetectable" (0.08 ng/mL or less) 10 hours later. The authors provided a calculation of the "worst-case example" of fentanyl delivery to a 3-kg infant; they concluded that "it would be surprising if such a low dose would produce any deleterious effects." Koehntop et al.[116] determined that neonates who were less than 14 days old were more suscepti-

ble to respiratory depression at low plasma fentanyl concentrations than older infants, children, and adults.

Wittels et al.[117] evaluated neonatal neurobehavior in breast-fed infants whose mothers received intravenous PCA with either morphine or meperidine (followed by the oral administration of the same opioid) for postcesarean analgesia. On the third day of life, neonates in the morphine group scored significantly higher than neonates in the meperidine group. The authors suggested that breast-milk meperidine and normeperidine have a greater potential for producing neonatal central nervous system depression because of increased enteral bioavailability and accumulation. Among patients receiving PCA morphine after cesarean section, colostrum concentrations of morphine and morphine-6-glucuronide are negligible as compared with maternal plasma concentrations.[118]

The effects of maternal medication can be minimized by giving attention to the following principles: (1) avoiding the administration of drugs with a long plasma half-life; (2) when possible, delaying drug administration until just after an episode of breast-feeding; (3) observing the neonate for abnormal signs or symptoms (e.g., change in feeding or sleep patterns, somnolence, decreased muscle tone, increased irritability); and (4) when possible, choosing drugs that have the least potential for excretion into breast milk and accumulation in the neonate or that are known to be tolerated by the newborn. The American Academy of Pediatrics Committee on Drugs[111] lists butorphanol, codeine, fentanyl, methadone, and morphine as maternally administered opioids that typically are compatible with breast-feeding. The manufacturer of ketorolac (Roche) has stated that ketorolac is contraindicated in nursing mothers because of the *possible* adverse effects of prostaglandin synthetase inhibitors in neonates. By contrast, the American Academy of Pediatrics considers the use of ketorolac to be compatible with breast-feeding.[111]

NEW MODALITIES OF SYSTEMIC DRUG ADMINISTRATION

After a period of decline,[119,120] the introduction of new drugs has increased during the last decade. Approximately 10 years (and $802 million) are required to take a new drug from discovery through clinical testing, development, and regulatory approval.[121] The drug industry is currently giving attention to the development of new drug delivery systems. The goals of new methods of administration include the following: (1) the precise, controlled delivery of the prescribed dose; (2) a rapid onset of action; (3) the avoidance of first-pass hepatic metabolism; (4) the maintenance of a steady-state concentration of drug; (5) an improved side-effect profile; and (6) improved patient compliance. The ultimate goal is to deliver a drug to a specific receptor target without affecting the rest of the body.

The transdermal route of administration has several advantages: (1) decreased gastrointestinal degradation; (2) decreased first-pass hepatic metabolism; (3) stable plasma concentrations; and (4) improved patient compliance. Some transdermal systems allow the delivery of a bolus of drug at the time of initial application followed by a constant release to maintain a stable plasma concentration. Transdermal delivery systems currently are used to administer a variety of drugs, including scopolamine, nitroglycerin, clonidine, estradiol, nicotine, and fentanyl. Investigators are evaluating the transdermal administration of other opioids and NSAIDs. I apply transdermal scopolamine before cesarean section in patients who have a strong history of hyperemesis gravidarum or motion

TABLE 27-2   SYSTEMIC ANALGESICS AND LACTATION[111-115]

Analgesic	Category	Milk: plasma ratio	Newborn tolerance
Nonopioid			
Acetaminophen	3	1.9	Well tolerated
Aspirin	3	0.08	Caution in early infancy
Ibuprofen	3	0.01	Well tolerated
Ketorolac	3	0.025-0.037	The manufacturer has stated that the use of ketorolac is contraindicated in nursing mothers; this contradicts the American Academy of Pediatrics assessment that the administration of ketorolac is usually compatible with breast-feeding.
Opioid			
Butorphanol	3	1.9 (oral) 0.7 (intramuscular)	No reports of adverse effects
Codeine	3	2.5	Possible accumulation
Fentanyl	3	>1	Well tolerated
Heroin	3	>1	Possible addiction
Hydromorphone	—	No data	No data
Meperidine	3	1.4	Prolonged half-life
Methadone	3	0.83	CAUTION: Withdrawal symptoms possible with abrupt cessation
Morphine	3	0.23-5.07	Possible accumulation
Nalbuphine	—	No data	No data
Oxycodone	—	3.4	Periodic sleeplessness; failure to feed
Oxymorphone	—	No data	No data
Pentazocine	—	Minimal excretion	No data
Propoxyphene	3	0.50	Poor muscle tone reported

sickness. The currently available formulation provides 1.5 mg of scopolamine over 72 hours. I inform patients of the potential for dry mouth and impaired acuity of near vision; I also inform patients that these effects may persist for several hours, even after removal of the transdermal delivery device.

Most patients tolerate the transdermal administration of fentanyl.[122-125] Steinberg et al.[126] reported a case of acute toxic delirium in a patient using transdermal fentanyl. Rose et al.[127] reported a case of fentanyl overdose as a result of cutaneous hyperthermia. One limitation of the transdermal method is the potential for ongoing transdermal absorption of drug after removal of the transdermal patch; this results in a slow decline in plasma concentrations of fentanyl and norfentanyl, which is an inactive fentanyl metabolite.

The skin provides a fairly substantial barrier to the passive transdermal absorption of a drug. Chemical enhancers may be used to facilitate absorption of the drug. Constant electrical current applied to the skin (iontophoresis) is also used to diminish the skin barrier. These techniques have been used to facilitate the transdermal administration of morphine, hydromorphone, insulin, and a luteinizing-hormone–releasing hormone agonist.[128-130]

The oral and nasal transmucosal methods of the delivery of drugs have been used for both medicinal and recreational purposes for many years. Transmucosal delivery includes the following advantages: (1) simplicity; (2) speed; (3) decreased gastrointestinal degradation; and (4) decreased first-pass hepatic metabolism. Oral or nasal transmucosal administration of a lipophilic agent may result in plasma concentrations that approach those resulting from intravenous administration of the drug. Penetration enhancers (e.g., sodium glycocholate) may be added to facilitate the absorption of large proteins and peptides.[131] Studies have evaluated the use of intranasal fentanyl and intranasal butorphanol for postoperative analgesia.[132,133]

Future research is likely to involve attempts to deliver a drug to a specific target. Drug carriers (e.g., liposomes) may facilitate the administration and release of a drug in specific locations. Further, it may be possible to deliver a drug to its target in an inactive form (pro-drug); at the desired site of action, the drug may then be converted chemically or enzymatically to its active form. These new techniques may minimize side effects and systemic toxicity.

KEY POINTS

- Patient education increases the efficacy of systemic opioid analgesic techniques after surgery. Patients should understand the importance of effective pain relief, and they should receive instruction in the use of patient-controlled delivery systems.
- Patients have wide variations in analgesic requirements after surgery.
- Preemptive analgesia and multimodal therapies may enhance postoperative pain relief.
- The use of patient-controlled bolus doses, with an appropriate lockout interval, is satisfactory for the majority of patients using intravenous patient-controlled analgesia. A continuous basal infusion should be added only when pain relief is inadequate despite appropriate patient-controlled analgesia use.
- A patient may breast-feed while receiving systemic opioids after cesarean section. However, the newborn should be observed for signs and symptoms of drug transfer and accumulation.

REFERENCES

1. Merskey II, Albe-Fessard DG, Bonica JJ, et al. (IASP Subcommittee on Taxonomy). Pain terms: A list with definitions and notes on usage. Pain 1979; 6:249-52.
2. Wall PD. On the relation of injury to pain. Pain 1979; 6:253-64.
3. Bromage PR, Camporesi EM, Chestnut D. Epidural narcotics for postoperative analgesia. Anesth Analg 1980; 59:473-80.
4. Marks RM, Sachar EJ. Undertreatment of medical inpatients with narcotic analgesics. Ann Intern Med 1973; 78:173-81.
5. Austin KL, Stapleton JV, Mather LE. Multiple intramuscular injections: A major source of variability in analgesic response to meperidine. Pain 1980; 8:47-62.
6. Short LM, Burnett ML, Egbert AM, Parks LH. Medicating the postoperative elderly: How do nurses make their decisions? J Gerontol Nurs 1990; 16:12-7.
7. Loper K, Butler S, Nessly M, Wild L. Paralyzed with pain: The need for education. Pain 1989; 37:315-7.
8. Egbert LD, Battit GE, Welch CE, Bartlett MK. Reduction of postoperative pain by encouragement and instruction of patients. N Engl J Med 1964; 270:825-7.
9. Owen H, McMillan V, Rogowski D. Postoperative pain therapy: A survey of patients' expectations and their experience. Pain 1990; 41:303-7.
10. Donovan BD. Patient attitudes to postoperative pain relief. Anaesth Intensive Care 1983; 11:125-9.
11. Wallace LM. Surgical patients' expectations of pain and discomfort: Does accuracy of expectations minimize post-surgical pain and distress? Pain 1985; 22:363-73.
12. Lavies N, Hart L, Rounsefell B, Runciman W. Identification of patient, medical and nursing staff attitudes to postoperative opioid analgesia: Stage 1 of a longitudinal study of postoperative analgesia. Pain 1992; 48:313-9.
13. Ready LB, Oden R, Chadwick HS, et al. Development of an anesthesiology-based postoperative pain management service. Anesthesiology 1988; 68:100-6.
14. Cockshott WP, Thompson GT, Howlett LJ, Seeley ET. Intramuscular or intralipomatous injections? N Engl J Med 1982; 307:356-8.
15. Austin KL, Stapleton JV, Mather LE. Relationship between blood meperidine concentrations and analgesic response. Anesthesiology 1980; 53:460-6.
16. Lim AT, Edis G, Kranz H, et al. Postoperative pain control: Contributions of psychological factors and transcutaneous electrical stimulation. Pain 1983; 17:179-88.
17. Spielberger CD, Auerbach S, Wadsworth M, et al. Emotional reactions to surgery. J Consult Clin Psychol 1973; 40:33-8.
18. Scott LE, Clum GA, Peoples JB. Preoperative predictors of postoperative pain. Pain 1983; 15:283-93.
19. Roe BB. Are postoperative narcotics necessary? Arch Surg 1963; 87: 912-5.
20. Church JJ. Continuous narcotic infusions for relief of postoperative pain. Br Med J 1979; 1:977-9.
21. Stapleton JV, Austin KL, Mather LE. A pharmacokinetic approach to postoperative pain: Continuous infusion of pethidine. Anaesth Intensive Care 1979; 7:25-32.
22. Rutter PC, Murphy F, Dudley HA. Morphine: Controlled trial of different methods of administration for postoperative pain relief. Anaesthesia 1985; 40:1086-92.
23. Catley DM, Thornton C, Jordan C, et al. Pronounced, episodic oxygen desaturation in the postoperative period: Its association with ventilatory pattern and analgesic regimen. Anesthesiology 1985; 63:20-8.
24. Marshall HUW, Porteous C, McMillan I, et al. Relief of pain by infusion of morphine after operation: Does tolerance develop? Br Med J 1985; 291:19-21.
25. Nimmo WS, Todd JG. Fentanyl by constant rate IV infusion for postoperative analgesia. Br J Anaesth 1985; 57:250-4.
26. Stanski DR. Narcotic pharmacokinetics and dynamics: The basis of infusion applications. Anaesth Intensive Care 1987; 15:23-6.
27. Sechzer PH. Objective measurement of pain. Anesthesiology 1968; 29:209-10.
28. Forrest WH, Smethurst PWR, Kienitz ME. Self-administration of intravenous analgesics. Anesthesiology 1970; 33:363-5.
29. Sechzer PH. Studies in pain with the analgesic-demand system. Anesth Analg 1971; 50:1-10.
30. Keeri-Szanto. Apparatus for demand analgesia. Can Anaesth Soc J 1971; 18:581-2.
31. Evans JM, Rosen M, MacCarthy J, Hogg MIJ. Apparatus for patient-controlled administration of intravenous narcotics during labor. Lancet 1976; 1:17-8.
32. Keeri-Szanto. Drugs or drums: What relieves postoperative pain? Pain 1979; 6:217-30.
33. Hull CJ, Sibbald A. Control of postoperative pain by interactive demand analgesia. Br J Anaesth 1981; 53:385-91.
34. Tamsen A, Hartvig P, Fagerlund C, et al. Patient-controlled analgesic therapy: Clinical experience. Acta Anaesth Scand 1982; 74:157-60.
35. Tamsen A, Hartvig P, Fagerlund C, Dahlstrom B. Patient-controlled analgesic therapy. Part I. Pharmacokinetics of pethidine in the pre- and postoperative periods. Clin Pharmacokinet 1982; 7:149-63.
36. Tamsen A, Hartvig P, Fagerlund C, Dahlstrom B. Patient-controlled analgesic therapy. Part II. Individual analgesic demand and analgesic plasma concentrations of pethidine in postoperative pain. Clin Pharmacokinet 1982; 7:164-75.
37. Dahlstrom B, Tamsen A, Paalzow L, Hartvig P. Patient-controlled analgesic therapy. Part IV: Pharmacokinetics and analgesic plasma concentrations of morphine. Clin Pharmacokinet 1982; 7:266-79.
38. Bollish SJ, Collins CL, Kirking DM, Bartlett RH. Efficacy of patient-controlled vs. conventional analgesia for postoperative pain. Clin Pharmacol 1985; 4:48-52.
39. Egbert AM, Parks LH, Short LM. Randomized trial of postoperative patient-controlled analgesia vs. intramuscular narcotics in frail elderly men. Arch Intern Med 1990; 150:1897-903.
40. Berde CB, Lehn BM, Yee JD, et al. Patient-controlled analgesia in children and adolescents: A randomized, prospective comparison with intramuscular administration of morphine for postoperative analgesia. J Pediatr 1991; 118:460-6.
41. Eisenach JC, Grice SC, Dewan DM. Patient-controlled analgesia following cesarean section: A comparison with epidural and intramuscular narcotics. Anesthesiology 1988; 68:444-8.
42. Harrison DM, Sinatra R, Morgese L, Chung JH. Epidural narcotic and patient-controlled analgesia for post-cesarean section pain relief. Anesthesiology 1988; 68:454-7.
43. Rayburn WF, Geranis BJ, Ramadei CA, et al. Patient-controlled analgesia for post-cesarean pain. Obstet Gynecol 1988; 72:136-9.
44. Ferrante FM, Orav EJ, Rocco AG, Gallo J. A statistical model for pain in patient-controlled analgesia and conventional intramuscular opioid regimens. Anesth Analg 1988; 67:457-61.
45. Jick H, Miettinen OS, Shapiro S, et al. Comprehensive drug surveillance (letter). JAMA 1980; 213:1455.
46. Porter J, Jick H. Addiction rare in patients treated with narcotics (letter). N Engl J Med 1980; 302:123.
47. Workerlin G, Larson CP. Spouse-controlled analgesia (letter). Anesth Analg 1990; 70:119.
48. Brewington KC. Patient-controlled analgesia in gynecology oncology surgery. Ala Med 1989; 59:5-17.
49. Bennett R, Batenhorst R, Vivens BA, et al. Patient-controlled analgesia: A new concept of postoperative pain relief. Ann Surg 1982; 195:700-5.
50. Graves DA, Foster TS, Batenhorst R, et al. Patient-controlled analgesia. Ann Intern Med 1983; 99:360-6.
51. Dahl JB, Daugaard JJ, Larsen HV, et al. Patient-controlled analgesia: A controlled trial. Acta Anaesth Scand 1987; 31:744-7.
52. Graves DA, Arrigo JM, Foster TS, et al. Relationship between plasma morphine concentrations and pharmacologic effects in postoperative patients using patient-controlled analgesia. Clin Pharmacol 1985; 4:41-7.
53. Benedetti C. Opioid analgesia: Recent advances in systemic administration. Satellite Symposium of the 5th World Congress on Pain, Venice, July 1987.
54. Lee S, Wang J, Ho S, Tao P. Nalbuphine coadministered with morphine prevents tolerance and dependence. Anesth Analg 1997; 84:810-5.
55. Lubenow TR, McCarthy RJ, Ivankovich AD. Management of acute postoperative pain. In: Barash PG, Cullen BF, Stoelting RK, editors. Clinical Anesthesia. 2nd ed. Philadelphia, PA, JB Lippincott, 1992:1559.
56. Donovan M, Dillon P, McGuire L. Incidence and characteristics of pain in a sample of medical-surgical inpatients. Pain 1987; 30:69-78.
57. Sinatra R, Chung KS, Silverman DG, et al. An evaluation of morphine and oxymorphone administered via patient-controlled analgesia (PCA) or PCA plus basal infusion in postcesarean-delivery patients. Anesthesiology 1989; 71:502-7.
58. Owen H, Szekely SM, Plummer JL, et al. Variables of patient controlled analgesia. II. Concurrent infusion. Anaesthesia 1989; 44:11-3.
59. Parker RK, Holtmann B, White PF. Patient-controlled analgesia: Does a concurrent opioid infusion improve pain management after surgery? JAMA 1991; 266:1947-52.
60. Parker RK, Holtmann B, White PF. Effects of a nighttime opioid infusion with PCA therapy on patient comfort and analgesic requirements after abdominal hysterectomy. Anesthesiology 1992; 76:362-7.

61. McKenzie R. Patient-controlled analgesia (PCA) (letter). Anesthesiology 1988; 69:1027.

62. White PF. Mishaps with patient-controlled analgesia. Anesthesiology 1987; 66:81-3.

63. White PF, Parker RK. Is the risk of using a "basal" infusion with patient-controlled analgesia therapy justified? (letter) Anesthesiology 1992; 76:489.

64. Kelly KA. Gastric motility after gastric operations. In: Nyhus LM, editor. Surgery Annual. New York, NY, Appleton-Century Crofts, 1974:103-23.

65. Asao T, Kuwano H, Nakamura J, et al. Gum chewing enhances early recovery from postoperative ileus after laparoscopic colectomy. J Am Coll Surg 2002; 195:30-2.

66. LaRosa JA, Saywell Jr RM, Zollinger TW, et al. The incidence of adynamic ileus in postcesarean patients. Patient-controlled analgesia versus intramuscular analgesia. J Reprod Med 1993; 38:293-300.

67. Carlborg I, Lindoff C, Hellman A. Diclofenac versus pethidine in the treatment of pain after hysterectomy. Eur J Anesthesiol 1987; 4:241-7.

68. Waters J, Hullander M, Kraft A, et al. Post-cesarean pain relief with ketorolac tromethamine and epidural morphine (abstract). Anesthesiology 1992; 77:A813.

69. Sun HL, Wu CC, Lin MS, Chang CF. Effects of epidural morphine and intramuscular diclofenac combination in postcesarean analgesia: A dose-range study. Anesth Analg 1993; 76:284-8.

70. Hodsman NBA, Burns J, Blyth A, et al. The morphine sparing effects of diclofenac sodium following abdominal surgery. Anaesthesia 1987; 42:1005-8.

71. Gillies GWA, Kenny GNC, Bullingham RES, McArdle CS. The morphine sparing effect of ketorolac tromethamine: A study of a new, parenteral nonsteroidal antiinflammatory agent after abdominal surgery. Anaesthesia 1987; 42:727-31.

72. O'Hara DA, Franciullo G, Hubbard L, et al. Evaluation of the safety and efficacy of ketorolac versus morphine by patient-controlled analgesia for postoperative pain. Pharmacotherapy 1997; 17:891-9.

73. Bloomfield SS, Barden TP, Mitchell J. Naproxen, aspirin and codeine in postpartum uterine pain. Clin Pharmacol Ther 1977; 21:414-21.

74. Sunshine A, Zighelboim I, Olson NZ, et al. A comparative oral analgesic study of ibuprofen, aspirin, and placebo in postpartum pain. J Clin Pharmacol 1985; 25:374-80.

75. Pavy TJG, Paech MJ, Evans SF. The effect of intravenous ketorolac on opioid requirement and pain after cesarean delivery. Anesth Analg 2001; 92:1010-4.

76. Huang YC, Tsai SK, Huang CH, et al. Intravenous tenoxicam reduces uterine cramps after cesarean delivery. Can J Anaesth 2002; 49:384-7.

77. Cheer SM, Goa KL. Parecoxib (parecoxib sodium). Drugs 2001; 61:1133-41.

78. Tang JU, Li S, White PF, et al. Effect of parecoxib, a novel intravenous cyclooxygenase type-2 inhibitor, on the postoperative opioid requirement and quality of pain control. Anesthesiology 2002; 96:1305-9

79. Hawkey CJ. COX-2 inhibitors. Lancet 1999; 353:307-14.

80. Ejlersen E, Andersen HB, Eliasen K, Mogensen T. A comparison between preincisional and postincisional lidocaine infiltration and postoperative pain. Anesth Analg 1992; 74:495-8.

81. McGregor RR, Thorner RE, Wright DM. Lidocaine inhibits granulocyte adherences and prevents delivery in inflammatory sites. Blood 1980; 56:203-9.

82. Pavy TJG, Gambling DR, Kliffer AP, et al. Effect of preoperative skin infiltration with 0.5% bupivacaine on postoperative pain following cesarean section under spinal anesthesia. Int J Obstet Anesth 1994; 3:199-202.

83. Kee WD, Khaw KS, Ma ML, et al. Postoperative analgesic requirement after cesarean section: A comparison of anesthetic induction with ketamine or thiopental. Anesth Analg 1997; 85:1294-8.

84. Woolf CJ, Chong M-S. Preemptive analgesia: Treating postoperative pain by preventing the establishment of central sensitization. Anesth Analg 1993; 77:362-79.

85. Ochroch EA, Mardini IA, Gottschalk A. The role of NSAIDs in preemptive analgesia. Anesth Analg 2003. In press.

86. Halpern SH, Walsh VL. Multimodal therapy for post-cesarean delivery pain. Reg Anesth Pain Med 2001; 26:298-300.

87. Desjardins PJ, Grossman EH, Kuss ME, et al. The injectable cyclooxygenase-2-specific inhibitor parecoxib sodium has analgesic efficacy when administered preoperatively. Anesth Analg 2001; 93:721-7.

88. Reuben SS, Fingeroth R, Krushell R, Maciolek H. Evaluation of the safety and efficacy of the perioperative administration of rofecoxib for total knee arthroplasty. J Arthroplasty 2002; 17:26-31.

89. Reuben SS, Bhopatkar S, Maciolek H, et al. The preemptive analgesic effect of rofecoxib after ambulatory arthroscopic knee surgery. Anesth Analg 2002; 94:55-9.

90. Desjardins PJ, Shu VS, Recker DP, et al. A single preoperative oral dose of valdecoxib, a new cyclooxygenase-2 specific inhibitor, relieves postoral surgery or bunionectomy pain. Anesthesiology 2002; 97:565-73.

91. Issioui T, Klein KW, White PF, et al. The efficacy of premedication with celecoxib and acetaminophen in preventing pain after otolaryngologic surgery. Anesth Analg 2002; 94:1188-93.

92. Reuben SS, Steinberg RB, Maciolek H, Joshi W. Preoperative administration of controlled-release oxycodone for the management of pain after ambulatory laparoscopic tubal ligation surgery. J Clin Anesth 2002; 14:223-7.

93. Givens VA, Lipscomb GH, Meyer NL. A randomized trial of postoperative wound irrigation with local anesthetic for pain after cesarean delivery. Am J Obstet Gynecol 2002; 186:1188-91.

94. Fredman B, Shapiro A, Zohar E. The analgesic efficacy of patient-controlled ropivacaine instillation after cesarean delivery. Anesth Analg 2000; 91:1436-40.

95. Bell EA, Jones BP, Olufolabi AJ, et al. Iliohypogastric-ilioinguinal peripheral nerve block for post-cesarean delivery analgesia decreases morphine use but not opioid-related side effects. Can J Anaesth 2002; 49:694-700.

96. Camann W, Cohen MB, Ostheimer GW. Is midazolam desirable for sedation in parturients? (letter) Anesthesiology 1986; 65:441.

97. Hedenbro JL, Olsson AM. Metoclopramide and ureteric colic. Acta Chir Scand 1988; 154:439-40.

98. Vella L, Francis D, Houlton P, Reynolds F. Comparison of the antiemetics metoclopramide and promethazine in labor. Br Med J 1985; 290:1173-5.

99. Rosenblatt WH, Cioffi AM, Sinatra R, et al. Metoclopramide: An analgesic adjunct to patient-controlled analgesia. Anesth Analg 1991; 73:553-5.

100. Freedman GM, Kreitzer JM, Reuben SS, Eisenkraft JB. Improving patient-controlled analgesia: Adding droperidol to morphine sulfate to reduce nausea and vomiting and potentiate analgesia. Mount Sinai J Med 1995; 62:222-5.

101. Cherian VT, Smith I. Prophylactic ondansetron does not improve patient satisfaction in women using PCA after caesarean section. Br J Anaesth 2001; 87:502-4.

102. Moldenhauer CC, Roach GW, Finlayson DC, et al. Nalbuphine antagonism of ventilatory depression following high-dose fentanyl anesthesia. Anesthesiology 1986; 62:216-8.

103. Cohen SE, Ratner EF, Kreitzman TR, et al. Nalbuphine is better than naloxone for treatment of side effects after epidural morphine. Anesth Analg 1992; 75:747-52.

104. Sprigge JS, Otton PE. Nalbuphine versus meperidine for post-operative analgesia: A double-blind comparison using the patient-controlled analgesic technique. Can Anaesth Soc J 1983; 30:517-21.

105. Bahar M, Rosen M, Vickers MD. Self-administered nalbuphine, morphine and pethidine: Comparison, by route, following cholecystectomy. Anaesthesia 1985; 40:529-32.

106. Soranus. Gynecology (translation). Baltimore, MD, Johns Hopkins University Press, 1956.

107. Yaffe SJ. Introduction. In: Briggs GG, Freeman RK, Yaffe SJ, editors. Drugs in Pregnancy and Lactation. 3rd ed. Baltimore, MD, Williams & Wilkins, 1990:XV.

108. Riordan J. Drugs and breast-feeding. In: Riordan J, Auerbach K, editors. Breast-feeding and Human Lactation. Boston, MA, Jones & Bartlett, 1993:138.

109. Feldman S, Pickering LK. Pharmacokinetics of drugs in human milk. In: Howell RR, Morris FH, Pickering LK, editors. Human Milk in Infant Nutrition and Health. Springfield, IL, Charles C. Thomas, 1986:256-78.

110. Lawrence RA. Breast-feeding: A Guide for the Medical Profession. 3rd ed. St. Louis, MO, Mosby, 1989:263-7.

111. American Academy of Pediatrics Committee on Drugs. The transfer of drugs and other chemicals into human milk. Pediatrics 2001; 108:776-89.

112. Pittman KA, Smyth RD, Losada M, et al. Human perinatal distribution of butorphanol. Am J Obstet Gynecol 1980; 138:797-800.

113. Lawrence RA. Breast-feeding: A Guide for the Medical Profession. 3rd ed. St. Louis, MO, Mosby, 1989:520-5; 573-5.

114. Steer PL, Biddle CJ, Marley WS, et al. Concentration of fentanyl in colostrum after analgesic dose. Can J Anaesth 1992; 39:231-5.

115. Rathmell JP, Viscomi CM, Ashburn MA. Management of nonobstetric pain during pregnancy and lactation. Anesth Analg 1997; 85:1074-87.

116. Koehntop DE, Rodman JH, Brundage DM, et al. Pharmacokinetics of fentanyl in neonates. Anesth Analg 1986; 65:227-32.

117. Wittels B, Scott DT, Sinatra RS. Exogenous opioids in human breast milk and acute neonatal neurobehavior: A preliminary study. Anesthesiology 1990; 73:864-9.

118. Baka NE, Bayoumeu F, Boutroy MJ, Laxenaire MC. Colostrum morphine concentrations during postcesarean intravenous patient-controlled analgesia. Anesth Analg 2002; 94:184-7.
119. Grabowski HG. Public policy and pharmaceutical innovation. Health Care Financing Rev 1982; 4:75-87.
120. May MS, Wardell WM, Lasagna L. New drug development during and after a period of regulatory change: Clinical research activity of major United States pharmaceutical firms, 1958 to 1979. Clin Pharmocol Ther 1983; 33:691-700.
121. Di Masi JA, Hansen RW, Grabowski HG. The price of innovation: new estimates of drug development costs. J Health Econ 2003; 22:151-85.
122. Duthie DJR, Rowbotham DJ, Wyld R, et al. Plasma fentanyl concentrations during transdermal delivery of fentanyl to surgical patients. Br J Anaesth 1988; 60:614-8.
123. Caplan RA, Ready LB, Oden RV, et al. Transdermal fentanyl for postoperative pain management. JAMA 1989; 261:1036-9.
124. Gourlay GK, Kowalski SR, Plummer JL, et al. The transdermal administration of fentanyl in the treatment of postoperative pain: Pharmacokinetics and pharmacodynamics. Pain 1989; 37:193-202.
125. Sevarino FB, Naulty JS, Sinatra R, et al. Transdermal fentanyl for postoperative pain management in patients recovering from abdominal gynecologic surgery. Anesthesiology 1992; 77:463-6.
126. Steinberg RB, Gilman DE, Johnson F. Acute toxic delirium in a patient using transdermal fentanyl. Anesth Analg 1992; 75:1014-6.
127. Rose PG, Macfee MS, Boswell MV. Fentanyl transdermal system overdose secondary to cutaneous hyperthermia. Anesth Analg 1993; 77:390-1.
128. Meyer BR, Kreis W, Eschbach J, et al. Transdermal versus subcutaneous leuprolide: A comparison of acute pharmacodynamic effect. Clin Pharmacol Ther 1990; 48:340-5.
129. Meyer BR, Katzeff HL, Eschbach JC, et al. Transdermal delivery of human insulin to albino rabbits using electrical current. Am J Med Sci 1989; 297:321-5.
130. Ashburn MA, Stephen RL, Ackerman E, et al. Iontophoretic delivery of morphine for postoperative analgesia. J Pain Symptom Manage 1992; 7:27-33.
131. Lee WA, Longnecker JP. Intranasal delivery of proteins and peptides. Biopharm 1988; 4:30-7.
132. Striebel HW, Koenigs D, Kramer J. Postoperative pain management by intranasal demand-adapted fentanyl titration. Anesthesiology 1992; 77:281-5.
133. Abboud TK, Zhu J, Gangolly J, et al. Transnasal butorphanol: A new method for pain relief in post-cesarean section pain. Acta Anaesthesiol Scand 1991; 35:14-8.

Chapter 28

Postoperative Analgesia: Epidural and Spinal Techniques

Chakib M. Ayoub, M.D. · Raymond S. Sinatra, M.D., Ph.D.

Poorly controlled pain interferes with ambulation, breast-feeding, and early maternal-infant bonding after cesarean delivery. These activities are also hampered by the excess sedation and other side effects associated with the intramuscular administration of analgesic agents. Nursing mothers are especially concerned about neonatal exposure to analgesic drugs, and some women tend to avoid medications—especially opioid analgesics—that may accumulate in breast milk.[1]

In the United States, most cesarean sections are performed with regional anesthesia,[2] and the administration of epidural and intrathecal opioids has become a popular means of augmenting intraoperative anesthesia and optimizing postoperative analgesia.[3] More than 90% of obstetric anesthesiologists administer intraspinal opioids in this setting.[3] (In this chapter, the terms *intraspinal* and *neuraxial* both refer to either the epidural or intrathecal administration of opioids.)

Among patients who receive epidural anesthesia, the indwelling epidural catheter facilitates the intermittent bolus injection or continuous epidural infusion of opioid during the intraoperative and postoperative periods. The introduction of noncutting spinal needles (e.g., Sprotte, Whitacre), which result in a low incidence of postdural puncture headache (PDPH), has led to an increase in the percentage of cesarean sections performed with spinal anesthesia.[4,5] At Yale-New Haven Hospital, more than 90% of elective cesarean sections are currently performed with spinal anesthesia.[5] More than 95% of the women undergoing these procedures receive intrathecal opioids for postoperative analgesia.

PHARMACOLOGY

The complex pharmacokinetics and receptor interactions that follow intrathecal and epidural opioid administration have been reviewed in detail elsewhere.[6-9] The identification of endogenous opioid peptides, specific opioid binding sites,[10] and receptor subtypes[11,12] has helped clarify how and where opioids act within the central nervous system (CNS). Before 1974, investigators favored the view that parenterally administered opioids either modulated pain at supraspinal centers or activated descending inhibitory pathways, without a direct effect at the spinal cord. Kitahata et al.[13] subsequently provided evidence that intrathecal morphine directly suppressed the transmission of noxious input at the first synapse between sensory afferents and nociceptive cells in Rexed laminae I, II, and V of the dorsal horn (Figure 28-1). This activity was determined to be quite selective, because laminae IV and VI neurons (which respond to non-noxious

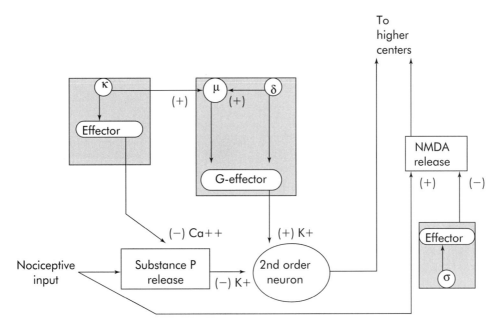

FIGURE 28-1. Overview of opioid receptor subtypes mediating spinal analgesia. Ligand-specific binding at mu (μ) and delta (δ) subtypes result in receptor conformational changes and activation (coupling) of guanosine nucleotide effector proteins. G-effector activation inhibits adenylate cyclase, resulting in decreased cAMP synthesis, increased K^+ conductance, and neuronal hyperpolarization. Kappa (κ)-receptor binding activates an uncharacteristic effector protein, which decreases the Ca^{++}-ion flux required for substance P release. Sigma (σ)-receptor subtypes modulate pain at supraspinal sites by inhibiting N-methyl-D-aspartate (NMDA) release. The μ and δ receptors may exist as a complex within the same cell. Activation of δ and κ subtypes may enhance μ receptor-mediated analgesia. (From Sinatra RS, Hord AH, Ginsberg B, Preble LM, editors. Acute Pain: Mechanisms and Management. St Louis, Mosby, 1992:3.)

cutaneous and proprioceptive stimuli) were unaffected. These observations supported autoradiographic findings in which the following were true: (1) significant opioid binding was localized within the dorsal horn[10]; and (2) reductions in neuronal responses to noxious stimuli occurred as radiolabeled morphine molecules penetrated lamina II.[14] Using animal models, researchers[12,15] reported that intrathecal morphine produced naloxone-reversible analgesia of prolonged duration and that two or more distinct opioid receptor systems were likely to be involved in the modulation of pain at the spinal level.

In 1979, Wang et al.[16] published the first report of intraspinal opioid administration in humans. In six of eight patients suffering from intractable cancer pain, intrathecal morphine (0.5 to 1.0 mg) produced complete pain relief for 12 to 24 hours, without evidence of significant sedation, respiratory depression, or impairment of neuromuscular function. Subsequently, thousands of published documents have confirmed the analgesic efficacy of intraspinal opioids.

The **epidural** route of administration is complicated by several anatomic and physiologic factors, including the following: (1) drug penetration of the dura and pia mater; (2) absorption by epidural fat; and (3) the consequences of vascular uptake and redistribution of drug to supraspinal sites.[7,8] A small portion of an epidural dose crosses the dura to enter the cerebrospinal fluid (CSF) and penetrates spinal tissue in amounts proportional to the agent's lipid solubility. Activation of spinal opioid receptors effectively blunts nociceptive input at the first synapse in the CNS. The remainder of the dose is absorbed by the vasculature, thereby producing plasma levels comparable with those achieved with intramuscular injection and providing some degree of supraspinal analgesia.[6] A bolus dose of epidural morphine 6 mg results in a clinically significant plasma concentration of 34 ng/mL 15 minutes after administration and a peak CSF concentration of approximately 1000 ng/mL at 1 hour after administration.[8]

Intrathecal administration allows injection of the drug directly into the CSF. This is a more efficient method of delivering opioid to spinal cord receptors. A bolus dose of intrathecal morphine 0.5 mg results in a CSF concentration that is greater than 10,000 ng/mL, with barely detectable plasma concentrations.[9]

Intrathecal and epidural opioids often produce **analgesia of greater intensity** than similar doses administered parenterally. The gain in potency is inversely proportional to the lipid solubility of the agent used. As the blood-brain barrier is bypassed, the hydrophilic opioids exhibit the greatest **gain in potency**.[6,17] A second advantage of intraspinal opioids is the **selectivity of analgesia**, which occurs in the absence of motor or sympathetic blockade.[6,18] Unlike local anesthetic blockade, intraspinal opioid analgesia facilitates patient ambulation while minimizing the risk of hypotension.[18]

Although opioid dose, volume of injectate, and degree of ionization are important variables, lipid solubility plays the key role in determining the onset of analgesia, the dermatomal spread, and the duration of activity.[6,7] Highly lipid-soluble opioids have a more rapid onset than more ionized water-soluble agents such as morphine.[6,7] The duration of activity is affected by the rate of clearance of the drug from the sites of activity. Lipid-soluble opioids are rapidly cleared by the vasculature, whereas water-soluble agents remain in the CSF and spinal tissues for longer periods (Figure 28-2).[6]

EPIDURAL OPIOIDS

Morphine

Morphine was the first opioid to receive Food and Drug Administration (FDA) approval for intraspinal (i.e., either epidural or intrathecal) administration. It has been widely investigated and extensively used clinically. After epidural

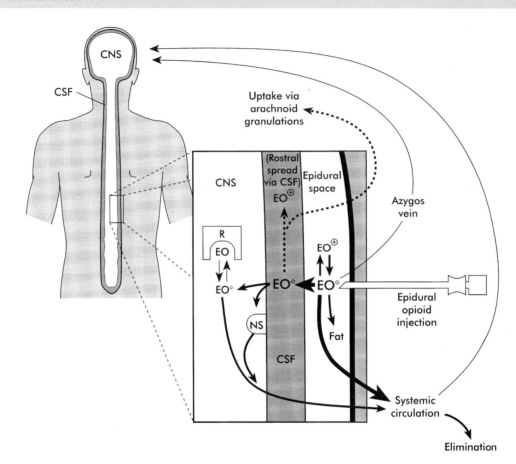

FIGURE 28-2. Factors that influence dural penetration, cerebrospinal fluid (CSF) sequestration, and vascular clearance of epidurally administered opioids. The major portion of epidurally-administered opioids *(EO)* is absorbed by epidural and spinal blood vessels or dissolved into epidural fat. Molecules taken up by the epidural plexus and azygos system may recirculate to supraspinal centers and mediate central opioid effects. A smaller percentage of uncharged molecules *(EO°)* traverse the dura and enter the CSF. Lipophilic opioids rapidly exit the CSF and penetrate into spinal tissue. As with intrathecal dosing, the majority of these molecules are either trapped within lipid membranes (nonspecific binding sites, *NS*) or are rapidly removed by the spinal vasculature. A small fraction of molecules bind to and activate opioid receptors *(R)*. Hydrophilic opioids penetrate pia-arachnoid membranes and spinal tissue slowly. A larger proportion of these molecules remain sequestered in CSF and are slowly transported rostrally. This CSF depot permits gradual spinal uptake, greater dermatomal spread, and a prolonged duration of activity. (From Sinatra RS. Pharmacokinetics and pharmacodynamics of spinal opioids. In Sinatra RS, Hord AH, Ginsberg B, Preble LM, editors. Acute Pain: Mechanisms and Management. St Louis, Mosby, 1992:106.)

administration, plasma morphine concentrations are similar to those observed after intramuscular injection; however, the onset of analgesia is delayed. The peak effect often does not occur until 60 to 90 minutes after epidural injection. This latency results from morphine's low lipid solubility, which retards penetration into spinal tissue.[6-8] Epidural morphine provides a prolonged duration of analgesia, which typically persists long after plasma concentrations have declined to subtherapeutic levels. This finding reflects the fact that significant amounts of morphine become sequestered in CSF, which functions as an aqueous drug depot.[6,8]

Fuller et al.[19] reviewed the records of 4880 women who received 2 to 5 mg of epidural morphine at the conclusion of cesarean section. The mean duration of analgesia was 23 hours, but the duration varied widely among patients. Of interest, the authors were unable to demonstrate a correlation between the dose of morphine and the duration of analgesia. Palmer et al.[20] performed a prospective, dose-response study of epidural morphine for postcesarean analgesia. They observed that the quality of analgesia improved as the dose of epidural morphine increased from 1.25 to 3.75 mg. A further increase in dose (to 5 mg) did not improve analgesia or reduce the amount of supplemental intravenous morphine that was required (Figure 28-3). Further, the authors did not observe a

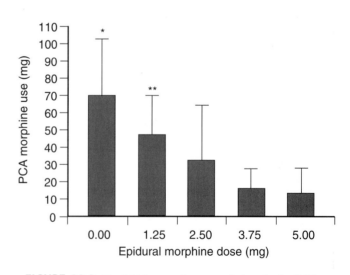

FIGURE 28-3. Total 24-hour patient-controlled analgesia *(PCA)* morphine use. Data are mean ± 95% confidence interval. Groups were significantly different ($P < 0.001$). *Group 0.0 mg was significantly different from Groups 2.5, 3.75, and 5.0 mg. **Group 1.25 was significantly different from Groups 3.75 and 5.0 mg. (From Palmer CM, Nogami WM, Van Maren G, Alves DM. Postcesarean epidural morphine: A dose-response study. Anesth Analg 2000; 90:887-91.)

clear relationship between the dose of epidural morphine and the severity of either pruritus or nausea and vomiting. This finding is somewhat inconsistent with results from earlier studies, which demonstrated dose-dependent increases in side effects; perhaps this observation may be attributed to the relatively narrow dose range of epidural morphine that was used in this study.[20]

The volume of the diluent does not appear to affect the pharmacokinetics or clinical activity of epidural morphine. The quality and duration of analgesia, need for supplemental analgesics, and incidence of side effects were similar when 4 mg of epidural morphine was administered with 2, 10, or 20 mL of sterile saline.[21]

The choice of local anesthetic used for epidural anesthesia seems to affect the subsequent efficacy of epidural morphine.[22] Parturients who receive 2-chloroprocaine as the primary local anesthetic experience unexpectedly poor postoperative analgesia that typically lasts less than 3 hours. Some anesthesiologists have speculated that this is a result of the low pH of the 2-chloroprocaine solution, although this is unproved. The occurrence of inadequate analgesia in this setting may also be related to the relatively rapid regression of 2-chloroprocaine anesthesia and the delay to peak effect of epidural morphine. It is unclear whether the addition of epinephrine to the local anesthetic affects the efficacy of epidural morphine analgesia, which occurs when epinephrine is added to *intrathecal* bupivacaine and morphine.[23]

In studies performed at Yale-New Haven[24] and Wake Forest University Hospitals,[25] patients treated with a single 5-mg dose of epidural morphine experienced more effective postcesarean analgesia than similar women who self-administered intravenous morphine or received intramuscular morphine (Figure 28-4). Cade et al.[26] reported that intermittently administered boluses of epidural morphine provided better analgesia with less drowsiness but more pruritus than a nurse-adjusted continuous intravenous infusion of meperidine or morphine. Despite a greater incidence of troublesome side effects, more patients (83% versus 74%) preferred epidural morphine to continuous intravenous opioid analgesia.

Most patients would tolerate an unintentional intravenous injection of 3 to 5 mg of morphine. However, the uninten-

tional subdural or intrathecal injection of the same dose would likely produce excessive sedation and respiratory depression.[27]

Administration of epidural morphine would be universally popular if not for troublesome side effects, including pruritus, nausea, vomiting, and delayed respiratory depression.[6,28,29] In theory, a low-dose, continuous infusion of morphine should avoid initial peak and subsequent trough CSF concentrations, thereby providing more consistent analgesia and a reduced incidence of unpleasant side effects. Leicht et al.[30] compared the epidural administration of a 5-mg bolus dose of morphine with the injection of a reduced bolus dose (2.5 mg) followed by a continuous epidural infusion of 0.5 mg/hr. Among patients who received the bolus dose, less than 50% experienced excellent analgesia, and 17% complained of severe nausea and vomiting. By contrast, patients who received a continuous epidural infusion reported superior pain relief, with no complaints of severe nausea and vomiting.

Lipophilic Opioids

The recognition that delayed respiratory depression and other side effects resulted from the rostral spread of hydrophilic morphine molecules[6-8,28] prompted the evaluation of the more lipid-soluble agents, which rapidly leave the aqueous CSF and rapidly penetrate the spinal cord (Table 28-1).[31-37]

FENTANYL

Although it is not FDA-approved for intraspinal administration, fentanyl's high analgesic efficacy and excellent safety profile have withstood the test of time. Fentanyl has become the intraspinal opioid most often administered for analgesia during labor, and, in many centers, it has supplanted morphine for the relief of postcesarean pain. Commercial preparations of fentanyl contain no preservative and are suitable for intravenous, epidural, or subarachnoid administration. Fentanyl is much more lipid soluble than morphine, and it rapidly penetrates the dura and spinal tissues.[6,18] Nevertheless, a significant portion of an epidural dose undergoes vascular absorption rather than meningeal penetration.[38]

Naulty et al.[32] reported that epidural fentanyl (50 to 100 µg) provided 4 to 5 hours of complete pain relief and significantly reduced 24-hour analgesic requirements after cesarean delivery. Subsequently, other investigators were unable to duplicate these results. Sevarino et al.[34] observed an analgesic duration of only 90 minutes and no reduction in 24-hour opioid requirements in patients who received 100 µg of epidural fentanyl during epidural lidocaine anesthesia. This discrepancy in the duration of analgesia was attributed to the potentiating effect of 0.75% bupivacaine (used in Naulty's study), which is no longer used in obstetric patients. After the resolution of motor blockade, residual quantities of bupivacaine can potentiate spinal opioid analgesia.[39,40] In addition to providing local anesthetic effects, bupivacaine may alter opioid receptor conformation and facilitate opioid binding.[39]

In contrast with bupivacaine, prior epidural injection of 2-chloroprocaine decreases the duration of epidural fentanyl analgesia, even if the 2-chloroprocaine is used only as a test dose or to supplement a block after the injection of 0.5% bupivacaine. This effect does not appear to be a pH-dependent phenomenon; rather, it may reflect antagonism caused by a metabolite of 2-chloroprocaine.[41]

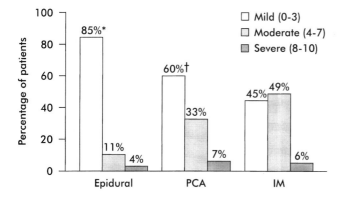

FIGURE 28-4. Percentage of patients recovering from cesarean section and treated with either epidural, patient-controlled analgesia (PCA), or intramuscular (IM) morphine and reporting mild, moderate, or severe discomfort during the 24-hour study period. *$P < 0.05$ denotes epidural versus PCA and IM. †P = NS denotes PCA versus IM. (From Harrison DM, Sinatra RS, Morgese L, et al. Epidural narcotic and PCA for postcesarean section pain relief. Anesthesiology 1988; 68:454-7.)

TABLE 28-1	SPINAL OPIOID PHYSIOCHEMISTRY AND PHARMACODYNAMICS								
Opioid	Molecular weight	Lipid solubility*	Parenteral potency	pKa	Mu-receptor affinity	Dissociation kinetics	Potency gain (epidural vs. IV or SC)	Onset of analgesia	Duration of analgesia
Morphine	285	1.4	1	7.9	Moderate	Slow	10	Delayed	Prolonged
Meperidine	247	39	0.1	8.5	Moderate	Moderate	2-3	Rapid	Intermediate
Methadone	309	116	2	9.3	High	Slow	2-3	Rapid	Intermediate
Hydromorphone	285	25	10	—	High	Slow	5	Rapid	Prolonged
Alfentanil	417	129	25	6.5	High	Very rapid	1-2	Very rapid	Short
Fentanyl	336	816	80	8.4	High	Rapid	1-2	Very rapid	Short
Sufentanil	386	1727	800	8.0	Very high	Moderate	1-1.5	Very rapid	Short

IV, Intravenous; *SC*, subcutaneous.
*Octanol-water partition coefficient at pH of 7.4.

Unlike local anesthetics, which block nerve fibers immediately adjacent to the lumbar sites of administration, opioids modulate nociception by stimulating opioid receptors within the thoracolumbar region of the spinal cord (Figure 28-5).[6] Lipophilic opioids do not spread rostrally in CSF to any great extent, and they tend to have fairly segmental analgesic profiles.[6,7] Birnbach et al.[42] observed that a larger volume of the diluent solution hastened the onset and prolonged the duration of analgesia provided by epidural fentanyl. Patients who received 50 µg of fentanyl with injectate volumes of only 1 or 2 mL often failed to develop complete analgesia. By contrast, diluent volumes of 10 mL or more were associated with a more rapid onset and a prolonged duration of analgesia (Figure 28-6). Some investigators have suggested that the administration of epidural fentanyl *before* incision may provide preemptive analgesia that improves intraoperative and postoperative analgesia.[43,44]

Fentanyl's rapid onset and short duration make it ideally suited for continuous epidural infusion. With this technique, the level of analgesia can be titrated to the pain stimulus, and the opioid effects can be terminated rapidly if problems occur. Youngstrom et al.[45] evaluated the continuous epidural infusion of fentanyl 4 µg/mL and epinephrine 1.6 µg/mL for postcesarean analgesia. Patients who received a continuous epidural infusion at a rate of 15 mL/hr obtained excellent pain relief and required few self-administered doses of intravenous opioid for the supplementation of analgesia.

Epidural fentanyl administration results in significant systemic absorption of drug, and some investigators have questioned the neuraxial specificity of epidural fentanyl analgesia.[33,46] Earlier studies suggested that subcutaneous, intravenous, and patient-controlled intravenous fentanyl provide equivalent analgesia and similar plasma concentrations as compared with the epidural administration of the drug.[46-48] The high dose requirements (40 to 80 µg/hr or 1000 to 2000 µg/day) underscore the relative inefficiency and potential toxicity of the epidural administration of fentanyl and other lipophilic opioids.[46,48] Recent evidence suggests that epidural fentanyl provides postcesarean analgesia via a spinal

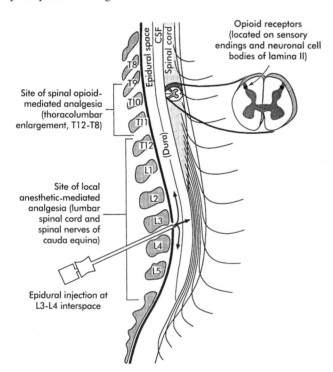

FIGURE 28-5. Relationships between epidural deposition of opioid analgesics and local anesthetics with regard to sites of activity. (From Sinatra RS. Pharmacokinetics and pharmacodynamics of spinal opioids. In Sinatra RS, Hord AH, Ginsberg B, Preble LM, editors. Acute Pain: Mechanisms and Management. St Louis, Mosby, 1992:7.)

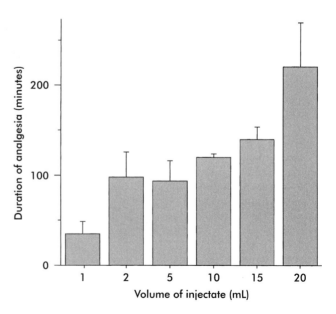

FIGURE 28-6. Duration of postcesarean analgesia provided by epidural fentanyl 50 µg administered in different volumes of normal saline. (From Birnbach DJ, Johnson MD, Arcario T, et al. Effect of diluent volume on analgesia produced by epidural fentanyl. Anesth Analg 1988; 68:808-10.)

mechanism. Cohen et al.[49] prospectively evaluated the interaction between fentanyl (administered either epidurally or intravenously) and epidural bupivacaine 0.015% with epinephrine 1 µg/mL. The authors concluded that epidural fentanyl analgesia occurs primarily by a spinal mechanism and that "the enhancement of fentanyl's efficacy by very small dose epidural bupivacaine and epinephrine requires an interaction of these drugs at the spinal level."[49]

Continuous epidural infusion and patient-controlled epidural infusion (PCEA) of fentanyl are widely used because these techniques provide a uniform level of effective analgesia, with fewer annoying side effects than are observed with epidural morphine.[32-35,50] In a prospective evaluation of 3823 patients who received epidural opioids after cesarean section, those treated with an epidural infusion of fentanyl plus epinephrine reported fewer side effects than patients who had received 4 to 5 mg of epidural morphine.[50] A single epidural dose of fentanyl may result in early-onset respiratory depression, but it does not cause delayed respiratory depression.[51,52]

SUFENTANIL

Sufentanil is a lipid-soluble opioid that has a parenteral potency five to ten times greater than fentanyl. Epidural sufentanil provides effective pain relief that is rapid in onset; however, dose requirements are high, and the duration of analgesia is relatively brief. In patients recovering from cesarean delivery, the ratio of analgesic potency of epidural sufentanil to fentanyl is approximately 5:1. After the epidural administration of equianalgesic doses of sufentanil or fentanyl, no differences in onset, quality, or duration of analgesia can be detected.[53] An epidural bolus of 25 µg of sufentanil produces less than 2 hours of complete analgesia, whereas 50 µg provides only 3 to 4 hours of pain relief.[35,54] Duration of analgesia may be extended by adding epinephrine (300 µg) to the diluent solution[55] or by increasing the injectate volume from 10 to 20 mL. However, the unintentional intravenous injection of epinephrine is not without risk. Rosen et al.[35] compared the effects of 5 mg of epidural morphine with 30, 45, or 60 µg of sufentanil in patients recovering from cesarean section (Table 28-2). Most patients who received sufentanil reported at least 50% pain relief within 15 minutes. However, the duration of analgesia among patients given 30 to 60 µg of sufentanil was only 3.9 to 5.6 hours. By contrast, patients who received morphine experienced analgesia with a median duration of 26.4 hours. The authors concluded that sufentanil "may be superior to morphine for epidural analgesia in clinical settings in which a rapid onset is desired."[35]

Sufentanil and other lipophilic opioids are rapidly absorbed from the epidural space and transported by means of the circulation to the CNS.[6,56,57] Ionescu et al.[56] reported that, apart from the first 2 minutes after epidural or intravenous injection, plasma levels of sufentanil were comparable throughout a 3-hour sampling interval. After the administration of an epidural bolus of sufentanil 50 µg in anesthetized dogs, CSF concentrations of sufentanil were 140 times greater than those found in plasma; however, the amount detected in cisternal CSF was only 5% of that measured in lumbar CSF. Peak concentrations of sufentanil were detected in plasma (0.35 ng/mL) after 6 minutes, in lumbar CSF (57 ng/mL) after 6.5 minutes, and in cisternal CSF (1.2 ng/mL) after 21 minutes.[58]

Sufentanil's rapid onset and short duration of action are desirable characteristics for continuous epidural infusion. Continuous infusion allows the anesthesiologist to titrate the level of analgesia, thereby minimizing annoying side effects and the risk of respiratory depression while avoiding peaks and troughs in analgesic effect.[59] Vascular uptake of epidurally administered sufentanil is significant, and plasma concentrations rise progressively.[59,60] For this reason, the epidural infusion most likely should be discontinued at 32 to 36 hours to prevent cumulative toxicity.

In summary, epidural sufentanil provides a rapid onset of analgesia in patients experiencing severe pain.[61] Unfortunately, epidural boluses of sufentanil offer few advantages over fentanyl and may be associated with a greater risk of acute respiratory depression.[62]

Other Epidural Opioids

Less-commonly administered epidural opioids include meperidine, hydromorphone, diamorphine, butorphanol, and nalbuphine.[36,63-86]

MEPERIDINE

Meperidine is commonly used as a parenteral analgesic in patients recovering from cesarean section. Unlike other opioids, meperidine has local anesthetic qualities. Two clinical trials compared the safety and efficacy of epidural meperidine 50 mg and intramuscular meperidine 100 mg.[68,69] Both studies noted that either route of administration provided 2.5 to 3 hours of analgesia, although the onset was faster in the epidural group. Patients preferred the epidural route of administration. Paech[36] evaluated the quality of analgesia and side effects produced by a single epidural bolus of meperidine

TABLE 28-2	ONSET AND DURATION OF EPIDURAL ANALGESIA PROVIDED BY MORPHINE AND SUFENTANIL IN PATIENTS RECOVERING FROM CESAREAN DELIVERY			
		Sufentanil		
	Morphine (5 mg)	30 µg	45 µg	60 µg
Onset of 50% pain relief (min)	52* (24-80)	15 (15-19)	15 (15-15)	15 (15-15)
Onset of 90% pain relief (min)	90* (60-202)	30 (15-38)	30 (15-45)	15 (15-19)
Duration of analgesia after first dose (hr)	26.4* (17.3-31.5)	3.9 (2.8-5.2)	4.5 (2.7-6.2)	5.6 (4.4-7.2)
Duration of analgesia after second dose (hr)	—	3.5 (2.5-5.9)	5.5 (3.9-7.0)	5.2 (4.1-6.6)

Values are median, with semiquartile range in parentheses.
*$P = 0.05$ as compared with each sufentanil group.
From Rosen MA, Dailey PA, Hughes SC, et al. Epidural sufentanil for postoperative analgesia after cesarean section. Anesthesiology 1988; 68:448-52.

50 mg or fentanyl 100 µg in 50 women recovering from cesarean section. All patients experienced highly effective pain relief, with few side effects. The onset of pain relief was slightly faster with fentanyl; however, the duration of analgesia was longer with meperidine. Ngan Kee et al.[70,71] compared different doses of epidural meperidine (12.5, 25, 50, 75, and 100 mg) as well as varying volumes of diluent in two separate studies. They concluded that meperidine 25 mg diluted in 5 mL of saline is superior to 12.5 mg and that doses of 50 mg or more offer no improvement in the quality or duration of analgesia (Figure 28-7). In contrast with the marked hemodynamic changes observed with intrathecal meperidine, epidural administration of meperidine causes minimal hemodynamic effects in pregnant women at term (Figure 28-8).[72]

The addition of epinephrine 5 µg/mL to PCEA meperidine 5 mg/mL did not improve analgesia or reduce meperidine consumption after cesarean section, but it increased the severity of nausea and pruritus. The authors attributed this observation to increased central effects as a result of enhanced transfer of drug into the CSF.[73]

HYDROMORPHONE

Hydromorphone is an hydroxylated derivative of morphine with a lipid solubility intermediate between that of morphine and meperidine.[38] Available in preservative-free solution, it provides effective epidural analgesia in patients recovering from cesarean section.[63,74,75] The quality of analgesia noted with epidural hydromorphone appears to be similar to that observed with morphine; however, its onset is faster, and its duration is somewhat shorter. On the basis of unpublished clinical observations, a ratio of 5:1 between morphine and hydromorphone has been used when administering the drug as an epidural bolus, and a ratio of 3:1 has been recommended for continuous epidural infusion.[38]

Chestnut et al.[74] evaluated the epidural administration of hydromorphone 1 mg during wound closure in patients who had received epidural lidocaine or bupivacaine anesthesia. The mean time to first request for supplemental analgesia was 13 hours, and 92% of patients reported good or excellent pain

relief. Henderson et al.[75] observed that the median duration of postcesarean analgesia provided by epidural hydromorphone 1 mg was 19.3 hours. In both studies, approximately 50% of patients reported mild-to-moderate itching, but not all required treatment. Halpern et al.[76] compared the efficacy of pain relief and the incidence and severity of side effects with epidural hydromorphone 0.6 mg versus epidural morphine 3 mg in 46 patients undergoing cesarean section. They found no overall difference between groups in quality of analgesia or severity of side effects. Pruritus was somewhat more pronounced in the hydromorphone group within the first 6 hours; at 18 hours, the incidence was higher in the morphine group. The high incidence of pruritus underscores the sensitivity of parturients to this side effect. In a study of nonpregnant patients, epidural hydromorphone administration was associated with a 75% decrease in the incidence of pruritus as compared with the epidural administration of equipotent doses of morphine.[77]

DIAMORPHINE

Diamorphine is a lipid-soluble derivative of morphine that is available for intravenous or epidural administration in the United Kingdom. It provides rapid and effective epidural analgesia, but systemic absorption is high, and the duration of activity is only 6 to 8 hours.[64] Haynes et al.[78] reported that the median duration of analgesia after epidural administration of diamorphine 5 mg was 12 hours and that parenteral morphine requirements for the treatment of breakthrough pain were negligible during the first 24 hours after surgery. Semple et al.[79] evaluated the effects of epinephrine on the vascular uptake and analgesia duration of epidural diamorphine 5 mg in patients recovering from cesarean section. Plasma levels of the principal metabolite (morphine) were lower and the duration of analgesia was longer in patients who received diamorphine plus epinephrine than in those who received diamorphine alone (12.5 hours versus 9.9 hours, respectively). Unfortunately, the addition of epinephrine resulted in a higher incidence of annoying side effects.

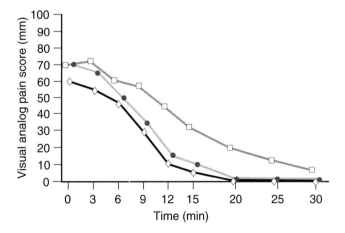

FIGURE 28-7. Visual analog pain scores (median and interquartile range) after epidural injection of meperidine 25 mg diluted to 2 mL (□), 5 mL (◇), or 10 mL (○). The area under the curve was different among groups and was greater in the 2-mL group as compared with both the 5-mL group and the 10-mL group, but there was no difference between the 5-mL group and the 10-mL group. (From Ngan Kee WD, Lam KK, Chen PP, Gin T. Epidural meperidine after cesarean section: The effect of diluent volume. Anesth Analg 1997; 85:380-4.)

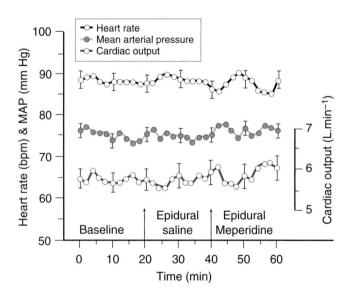

FIGURE 28-8. Heart rate, mean arterial pressure, and cardiac output recorded after the epidural administration of meperidine 50 mg. (From Khaw KS, Ngan Kee WD, Critchley LAH. Epidural meperidine does not cause hemodynamic changes in the term parturient. Can J Anaesth 2000; 47:155-9.)

BUTORPHANOL

The mixed agonist-antagonist opioids offer two theoretical advantages when administered epidurally: (1) the ability to selectively activate kappa-opioid receptors, which modulate visceral nociception[12]; and (2) a ceiling effect for respiratory depression, which should limit the reduction in respiratory drive even if opioid molecules spread rostrally to the brainstem. Unfortunately, significant sedation often occurs as a result of vascular uptake and activation of supraspinal kappa receptors.[11]

Two studies demonstrated that epidural butorphanol (2 to 4 mg) provided as many as 8 hours of postcesarean analgesia without significant pruritus.[67,80] Epidural butorphanol resulted in a dose-dependent increase in sedation. Camann et al.[81] questioned the efficacy of epidural butorphanol, noting that, in patients recovering from cesarean section, epidural butorphanol 2 mg offered few if any advantages over a similar dose given intravenously. At Yale-New Haven Hospital, we have been dissatisfied with the level of sedation associated with epidural butorphanol 4 mg. Excessive maternal somnolence detracts from the overall mission of providing selective spinal analgesia and ultimately leads to patient and nursing staff dissatisfaction.[5]

The neurologic safety of epidural butorphanol administration has not been established. In sheep, a single epidural bolus caused no problems; however, repeated intrathecal injection of 2 to 4 mg of butorphanol over a period of 3 days resulted in hind-limb paralysis and histopathologic evidence of neurotoxicity.[82] Eisenach[83] cautioned against administering butorphanol epidurally given that a catheter could migrate into the intrathecal space at any time.

NALBUPHINE

Nalbuphine is a semisynthetic opioid structurally related to oxymorphone. It has a higher lipid solubility than morphine and an activity profile in vitro that suggests moderate agonist activity at kappa-opioid receptors and antagonist activity at mu-opioid receptors. Nalbuphine provides effective analgesia in certain animal models of visceral nociception; its rapid onset and intermediate duration of action are consistent with its lipid solubility and rapid clearance.[84]

Camann et al.[85] evaluated the efficacy of epidural nalbuphine for postcesarean analgesia. Doses ranging from 10 to 30 mg provided minimal to no analgesia in patients who had received epidural 2-chloroprocaine anesthesia and a poor quality of analgesia (with a mean duration of only 77 minutes) in patients recovering from epidural lidocaine anesthesia. The major side effect was somnolence.

Parker et al.[86] studied the effect of adding 0.02, 0.04, and 0.08 mg/mL of nalbuphine to an epidural infusion of hydromorphone 0.075 mg/mL. The overall incidences of nausea (19% to 35%) and pruritus (32% to 62%) were similar in the four groups. The highest dose of nalbuphine appeared to antagonize epidural analgesia; however, the 0.04 mg/mL concentration resulted in lower nausea scores and a decreased incidence of urinary retention without affecting the efficacy of analgesia.

Epidural Opioid Combinations

One method used to hasten the onset of epidural analgesia and to provide a prolonged duration of effect is to combine fentanyl with a small dose of morphine. Cohen et al.[87] retrospectively observed that the intraoperative administration of

epidural fentanyl decreased the subsequent efficacy of epidural morphine analgesia after cesarean section. They speculated that epidural fentanyl might initiate acute tolerance or affect the pharmacokinetics and receptor-binding characteristics of morphine. In a randomized, double-blind study, Vincent et al.[88] noted that epidural fentanyl (administered immediately after delivery of the infant) improved the quality of intraoperative analgesia without worsening epidural morphine analgesia after cesarean section. Patients who received epidural fentanyl experienced less intraoperative nausea and vomiting than did patients in the control group.

The addition of sufentanil to morphine may also hasten the onset and prolong the duration of epidural analgesia.[61,89] Dottrens et al.[89] randomized patients to receive a single epidural dose of either morphine 4 mg, sufentanil 50 µg, or morphine 2 mg with sufentanil 25 µg. The morphine-sufentanil combination provided a more rapid onset of pain relief than did morphine alone. Epidural morphine and epidural morphine-sufentanil provided analgesia of similar duration (Figure 28-9). Patients who received sufentanil alone required larger doses of supplemental opioids than did patients in the other two groups.

Studies of the combination of butorphanol and morphine have provided conflicting results.[90-93] Lawhorn et al.[92] noted that the combination of epidural morphine 4 mg and butorphanol 3 mg provided a duration of analgesia similar to that provided by epidural morphine alone but with a decreased incidence of pruritus and nausea. Of interest is that these authors did not observe increased maternal somnolence in the women who received epidural butorphanol. Similarly, Wittels et al.[90] noted that patients who received epidural butorphanol 3 mg and morphine 4 mg reported superior pain control, a lower incidence of pruritus, and greater satisfaction during the first 12 hours after cesarean section than patients who received morphine alone. By contrast, Gambling et al.[93] observed that similar doses of epidural butorphanol and

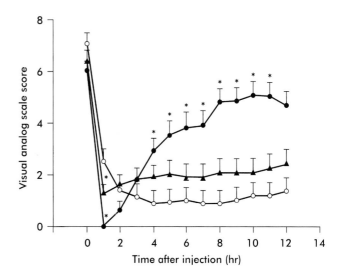

FIGURE 28-9. Pain as measured by visual analog scale before and after epidural administration of morphine 4 mg (O), sufentanil 50 µg (●), or the combination of morphine 2 mg and sufentanil 25 µg (▲) *$P < 0.05$ as compared with time-matched data points for epidural morphine administration. (From Dottrens M, Rifat K, Morel DR. Comparison of extradural administration of sufentanil, morphine and sufentanil-morphine combination after caesarean section. Br J Anaesth 1992; 69:9-12.)

morphine provided less effective analgesia than epidural morphine alone, with no reduction in the incidence of pruritus.

Patient-Controlled Epidural Analgesia

Multiple studies have compared epidural morphine versus intravenous patient-controlled analgesia (PCA) for postcesarean analgesia.[24,25] Single doses of epidural morphine provided better pain relief than that achieved with either intravenous PCA or intramuscular morphine. However, patients who self-administered intravenous morphine experienced fewer troublesome side effects, achieved more uniform and sustained analgesia, and enjoyed greater autonomy. Self-administration techniques permit the patient to titrate analgesic agents in proportion to the intensity of postsurgical discomfort; this reduces patient anxiety while increasing patient control. Thus it seems reasonable to expect that epidural opioid analgesia might be combined with a self-administration dosing regimen to provide the psychologic benefits of PCA and the superior analgesia associated with intraspinal opioids. Box 28-1 lists the potential advantages of PCEA.[94]

Chrubasik et al.[94] noted that the dose of self-administered **morphine** required to provide effective PCEA was significantly less than that used with either continuous epidural opioid or intravenous PCA techniques. Walmsley[95] reported that PCEA morphine provided high clinical efficacy and safety in more than 4000 patients recovering from a variety of surgical procedures.

Disadvantages of using morphine for PCEA include its prolonged latency and the risk of delayed respiratory depression. For this reason, more lipophilic opioids (e.g., meperidine, fentanyl, hydromorphone, sufentanil) have been evaluated for use in this setting.[96-110]

Yarnell et al.[96] noted that PCEA **meperidine** provided better postcesarean analgesia than intramuscular injections of the drug. In addition, patients who received PCEA meperidine ambulated sooner and cared for their infants earlier. The incidence of side effects was similar in the two groups. However, one patient in the PCEA group developed respiratory depression 25 minutes after receiving 75 mg of epidural meperidine in the operating room. As might be expected, PCEA meperidine was preferred over intramuscular administration by both patients and nursing staff. The authors suggested that the technique can be safely used on the ward, because respiratory depression, if it occurs, should happen soon after the epidural bolus is given.

In a recent study, Fanshawe[110] noted that PCEA meperidine (15-mg boluses with a 10-minute lockout) provided analgesia comparable to that provided by epidural morphine 4 mg. There was no difference between the two groups in the incidence of nausea and vomiting, but PCEA meperidine was associated with significantly less pruritus than epidural morphine.[110] Rosaeg et al.[97] observed that PCEA meperidine was associated with less pruritus and nausea than epidural boluses of morphine, although such therapy was more expensive and provided less effective pain control. Ngan Kee et al.[98] compared the efficacy of meperidine and fentanyl administered through either PCEA or intravenous PCA. They noted that the epidural route offered advantages for both drugs but that patient satisfaction was greatest with PCEA meperidine.

Patients using PCEA **fentanyl** typically require less drug and experience similar analgesia as compared with patients treated with a continuous epidural infusion of fentanyl.[99]

Box 28-1 POTENTIAL ADVANTAGES OF PATIENT-CONTROLLED EPIDURAL INFUSION VERSUS TRADITIONAL EPIDURAL OPIOID TECHNIQUES

VERSUS EPIDURAL OPIOID BOLUSES OR INFUSION

- Patient control and autonomy
- Increased patient satisfaction
- Decreased anxiety
- Reduced opioid requirement

VERSUS INTRAVENOUS PATIENT-CONTROLLED ANALGESIA

- Increased efficacy of analgesia
- Increased patient satisfaction
- Reduced opioid requirement
- Decreased sedation
- Shorter hospitalization (?)

Nevertheless, patients recovering from cesarean delivery may require significant amounts of PCEA fentanyl (e.g., 100-μg loading dose followed by maintenance doses approaching 50 to 75 μg/hr) to provide analgesia equal to a single 3-mg dose of epidural morphine. The advantage of PCEA fentanyl is that it involves a lower incidence of pruritus than that which occurs with epidural morphine.[100] Cooper et al.[101] found that the addition of fentanyl 2 μg/mL to 0.05% bupivacaine reduced epidural bupivacaine dose requirements by 68% while decreasing PCEA demands and improving analgesia at rest in patients recovering from cesarean delivery. Other benefits included less motor and sensory block and higher patient satisfaction. However, there was no significant difference between groups in pain scores during coughing (Figure 28-10). This study demonstrated an additive analgesic effect between 0.05% bupivacaine and fentanyl, but the authors concluded that the study failed to demonstrate any significant clinical benefit from using these two drugs in combination when compared with epidural fentanyl alone.

Parker and White[103] noted that patients who self-administered epidural **hydromorphone** required four to five times less drug than patients who received intravenous PCA hydromorphone after cesarean section (Figure 28-11). The authors speculated that the dose sparing in the PCEA group was responsible in part for a significant reduction in adverse effects, a more rapid return of bowel function, and a shortened hospital stay among patients in that group. In a second study,[104] these investigators attempted to further improve the efficacy of PCEA hydromorphone by adding 0.08% bupivacaine or by using a basal infusion of hydromorphone in patients recovering from cesarean section. These adjuvant therapies did not improve pain scores, decrease PCEA demands, or reduce 24-hour dose requirements, but were associated with either significant lower extremity sensory deficits (e.g., numbness) or a fivefold increase in nausea and vomiting. In a third study,[105] PCEA hydromorphone alone or with varying concentrations of nalbuphine was evaluated in 64 patients recovering from cesarean delivery. The addition of nalbuphine to the epidural infusate resulted in lower nausea scores and decreased urinary retention. Nalbuphine did not decrease the incidence of pruritus but was associated with a partial reversal of analgesia (Figure 28-12).

Sufentanil has also been advocated for PCEA.[106-109] In an evaluation of 441 patients recovering from cesarean section, Grass et al.[106] noted that patients using PCEA sufentanil

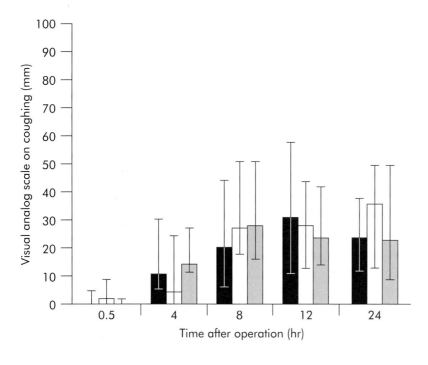

FIGURE 28-10. Pain scores on a visual analog scale for coughing. Median score and interquartile range for groups who received epidural bupivacaine *(black bar)*, fentanyl *(white bar)*, and bupivacaine plus fentanyl *(hatched bar)*. (From Cooper DW, Ryall DM, McHardy FE, et al. Patient-controlled extradural analgesia with bupivacaine, fentanyl, or a mixture of both, after caesarean section. Br J Anaesth 1996; 76:611-5.)

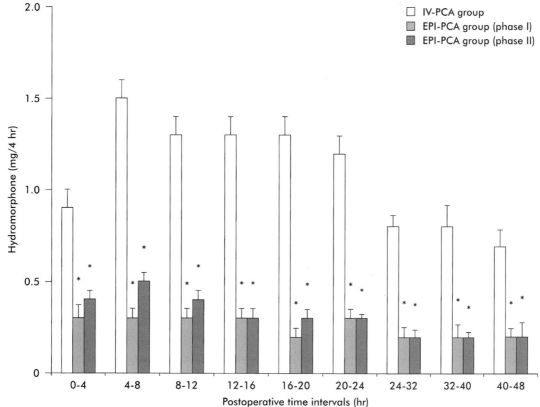

FIGURE 28-11. Postoperative hydromorphone use (mg/4-hour interval) via patient controlled analgesia (PCA) after either an intravenous (IV) or epidural (EPI) loading dose. Results are expressed as mean ± SEM. *$P < 0.05$, significantly different from IV-PCA group. (From Parker R, White P. Epidural patient-controlled analgesia: An alternative to intravenous patient-controlled analgesia for pain relief after cesarean delivery. Anesth Analg 1992; 75:245-51.)

experienced superior analgesia and had a shorter duration of hospitalization (4.3 days versus 5.0 days) as compared with similar women who received intramuscular opioids. In a follow-up study, these authors noted that PCEA sufentanil resulted in a more rapid onset of peak analgesia and better analgesia with movement than did intravenous PCA morphine.[107] The authors suggested that both the superior analgesia during movement and the decreased level of sedation provided by PCEA sufentanil resulted in improved maternal-infant bonding. They also noted that earlier ambulation and hospital discharge should reduce overall hospital costs. It was unclear whether the improved outcome resulted from the opioid, the method of administration, or both.

At Yale-New Haven Hospital, we observed that patients who used either PCEA or intravenous PCA sufentanil self-administered similar doses of drug and obtained a similar

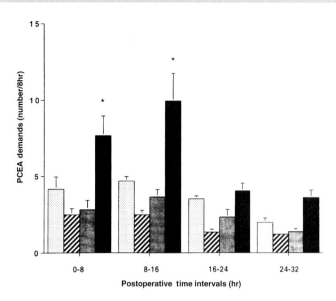

FIGURE 28-12. Number of patient controlled epidural analgesia (PCEA) demands per 8-hour interval for 32 hours after surgery. Light stippled bar, no nalbuphine; hatched bar, nalbuphine 0.02 mg/mL; dark stippled bar, nalbuphine 0.04 mg/mL; solid bar, nalbuphine 0.08 mg/mL. Values are expressed as mean ± SEM. *$P < 0.05$ as compared with control (group 1). The highest nalbuphine concentration resulted in increased PCEA demand during the study period. (From Parker R, Holtman B, White PF. Patient-controlled epidural analgesia: Interactions between nalbuphine and hydromorphone. Anesth Analg 1997; 84:757-63.)

quality of analgesia after gynecologic surgery.[108] Likewise, Cohen et al.[109] noted that PCEA sufentanil and PCEA fentanyl provided similar analgesia after cesarean section. Patients who self-administered sufentanil made fewer PCEA demands, but they had a higher incidence of dizziness and vomiting.

INTRATHECAL OPIOIDS

Morphine

Given the increased popularity of spinal anesthesia for cesarean section, intrathecal morphine is an attractive option for postcesarean analgesia. The duration of action and the side-effect profile are similar to those of epidural morphine. Of course, dose requirements are much smaller (i.e., 0.1 to 0.25 mg). This low dose requirement reflects the potency gain associated with subarachnoid deposition of drug and is advantageous in parturients who are concerned about the accumulation of opioids in breast milk. Zakowski et al.[111] examined the plasma pharmacokinetics and urinary excretion of intrathecal morphine alone (0.6 mg) and morphine plus epinephrine in patients recovering from cesarean section. Unconjugated morphine concentrations peaked at 3 hours in both groups; however, plasma concentrations were 66% lower in the epinephrine group. The peak concentration of 2.34 ng/mL was significantly lower than the peak concentration of 10 to 14 ng/mL observed 15 minutes after the epidural administration of 5 mg of morphine[112] and much lower than the minimum effective plasma concentration required with intravenous PCA morphine. Intrathecal morphine administration results in a faster onset of analgesia than does epidural morphine, but this technique still requires 45 to 60 minutes to achieve a peak effect. The duration of analgesia averages 18 to 24 hours,[6,113-115] with an estimated ED_{50} of 0.022 ± 0.053 mg.[116] Chadwick and Ready[114] observed that 150 (78%)

of 193 women who had received intrathecal morphine (0.3 to 0.5 mg) had at least 20 hours of postcesarean analgesia as compared with 113 (64%) of 176 women who had received epidural morphine (3 to 5 mg). The side effects of pruritus and nausea were similar in the two groups. Only two patients in each group had respiratory depression (i.e., a respiratory rate of less than 11 breaths per minute), and these cases did not require intervention.

Several studies have attempted to define the optimal dose of intrathecal morphine for postcesarean analgesia. Abboud et al.[113] observed prolonged postcesarean analgesia in patients who received either 0.1 or 0.25 mg of intrathecal morphine with hyperbaric bupivacaine for cesarean section. The mean durations of analgesia were 18.6 and 27.7 hours, respectively. Abouleish et al.[115] performed a prospective evaluation of intrathecal morphine 0.2 mg administered with hyperbaric bupivacaine in 856 women undergoing cesarean section. The mean duration of analgesia was 14 hours, and 58% of patients did not require additional analgesics for 24 hours. Among those who had breakthrough pain, the average dose of supplemental morphine was only 9.1 ± 0.5 mg. Huffnagle et al.[117] found that the analgesic effect of intrathecal morphine plateaus at a dose between 0.125 and 0.2 mg. Milner et al.[118] noted that 0.1 mg of intrathecal morphine produces analgesia comparable to that provided by 0.2 mg of morphine but that the lower dose (0.1 mg) results in significantly less nausea and vomiting. Likewise, Uchiyama et al.[119] observed that 0.1 mg of intrathecal morphine provides postcesarean analgesia of a duration that is comparable with that provided by 0.2 mg. Because the incidence of side effects is greater with the 0.2-mg dose, the authors concluded that 0.1 mg is the optimal dose of intrathecal morphine for postcesarean analgesia.

Dahl et al.[120] recently performed a systematic review of randomized controlled trials of intrathecal opioids in patients undergoing cesarean section (Figure 28-13). The authors recommended morphine 0.1 mg as the drug and dose of choice. The authors acknowledged that, for every 100 women receiving intrathecal morphine 0.1 mg, "43 patients will experience pruritus, 10 will experience nausea, and 12 will experience vomiting postoperatively, all of whom would not have experienced these adverse effects without treatment."[120]

The fact that small doses (0.1 to 0.2 mg) of intrathecal morphine provide effective, prolonged analgesia similar to that provided by 3 to 4 mg of epidural morphine illustrates the 20:1 potency ratio of intrathecal versus epidural morphine. A recent study compared intrathecal morphine 0.15 mg to PCEA bupivacaine 0.06% with sufentanil 1 µg/mL for postcesarean analgesia. The PCEA regimen provided better pain relief and caused less nausea and vomiting, but it was more expensive than intrathecal morphine.[121]

Paech et al.[122] recently performed a randomized comparison of intrathecal morphine 0.2 mg and PCEA meperidine for postcesarean analgesia. All participants experienced good pain relief; however, those treated with intrathecal morphine reported significantly lower pain scores at 8 and 12 hours as well as a higher incidence of severe pruritus, nausea, and drowsiness.

In summary, the intrathecal administration of a small dose of morphine provides effective analgesia for most patients, with a reasonable risk-to-benefit ratio. Some patients require small doses of parenteral opioids for supplemental analgesia during the first 24 hours.[123]

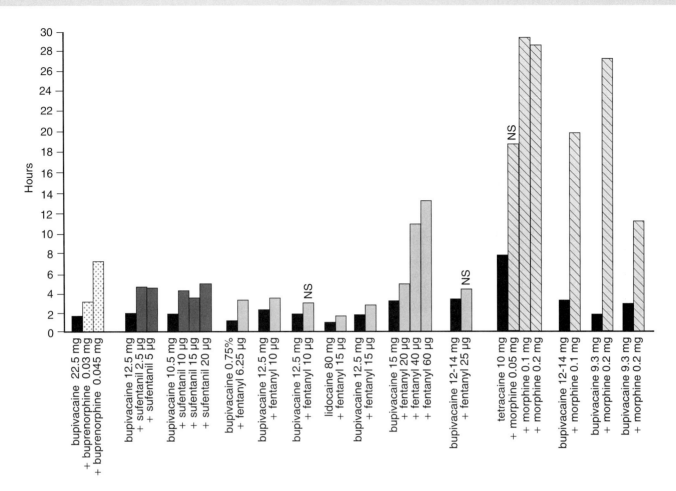

FIGURE 28-13. Time to first administration (in hours) of postoperative supplemental analgesics in patients receiving spinal anesthesia with local anesthetic alone *(solid bars)* or local anesthetic combined with buprenorphine, sufentanil, fentanyl, or morphine in varying doses *(various bars)*. *NS*, No significant difference from control. (From Dahl JB, Jeppesen IS, Jorgensen H, et al. Intraoperative and postoperative analgesic efficacy and adverse effects of intrathecal opioids in patients undergoing cesarean section with spinal anesthesia. Anesthesiology 1999; 91:1919-27.)

Lipophilic Opioids

FENTANYL

Belzarena[124] randomized 100 women presenting for elective cesarean section with spinal bupivacaine to receive either 0.25, 0.5, or 0.75 μg/kg of intrathecal fentanyl. The mean ± SD durations of analgesia ranged from 305 ± 89 minutes with 0.25 μg/kg to 787 ± 161 minutes with 0.75 μg/kg of fentanyl. However, patients who received the two higher doses experienced decreased respiratory rates and a high incidence of annoying side effects (e.g., pruritus, nausea).

These and other investigators defined the duration of analgesia as the time from the administration of fentanyl until the time that the patient first requested additional analgesia. Patients could not self-administer pain medication and may have delayed their request for a painful intramuscular injection. By contrast, we have observed that 12.5 to 25 μg of intrathecal fentanyl provides *negligible* postcesarean pain relief and that analgesia often wanes before or soon after the patient is discharged from the postanesthesia care unit (PACU). We typically initiate intravenous PCA in the PACU as the spinal anesthetic regresses. Patients commonly self-administer 50 to 75 mg of meperidine within the first 3 to 4 hours after the regression of bupivacaine-fentanyl spinal anesthesia. The primary advantage of intrathecal fentanyl is that it improves analgesia *during* cesarean section.

SUFENTANIL

Since the FDA approved its use in obstetric practice, the intrathecal administration of sufentanil has gained limited popularity. Courtney et al.[125] examined intrathecal sufentanil dose responses during and after cesarean section. Doses of 0, 10, 15, or 20 μg of intrathecal sufentanil were administered with hyperbaric bupivacaine. All three doses of sufentanil resulted in a mean duration of analgesia of approximately 3 hours. More than 90% of patients reported pruritus, but only one patient required treatment. Intrathecal sufentanil did not affect neonatal condition as assessed by umbilical cord blood gas and pH measurements and Apgar and neurobehavioral scores. Dahlgren et al.[126] compared the safety and efficacy of smaller doses of sufentanil (2.5 and 5 μg), fentanyl 10 μg, and placebo when coadministered with hyperbaric bupivacaine 12.5 mg for cesarean section. The duration of complete analgesia in patients receiving intrathecal opioids increased from approximately 1.5 hours in the placebo group to 2.5 to 3.5 hours in the three treatment groups. Sufentanil 5 μg provided the longest duration of analgesia but was associated with the highest incidence of pruritus, with 9 (45%) of 20 patients requiring treatment. Intrathecal sufentanil—but not fentanyl or placebo—reduced requirements for intraoperative antiemetics and postoperative intravenous morphine.[126]

Other Intrathecal Opioids

MEPERIDINE

Intrathecal meperidine reduces the intensity of pain associated with the regression of spinal anesthesia, provides effective postoperative analgesia of intermediate duration (4 to 5 hours),[127-129] and facilitates the transition to intravenous PCA. Feldman et al.[128] evaluated dose responses for intrathecal meperidine. They added either 10 or 20 mg of meperidine or saline-placebo to 12 mg of hyperbaric bupivacaine during the administration of spinal anesthesia for cesarean section. Both doses of meperidine effectively attenuated the discomfort associated with uterine exteriorization; however, the 20-mg dose was associated with a higher incidence of intraoperative nausea. The bupivacaine-meperidine combination did not increase the incidence of hypotension or high segmental block, and it did not delay recovery of motor function. Patients treated with either dose of meperidine reported lower pain scores and higher satisfaction with analgesia during the first 4 hours of recovery than patients who had received intrathecal saline-placebo. Similarly, Yu et al.[130] found that the addition of meperidine 10 mg to hyperbaric bupivacaine 10 mg prolonged the duration of effective analgesia in patients recovering from elective cesarean section (234 minutes in the meperidine group versus 125 minutes in the saline-placebo group). However, the incidence of intraoperative nausea and vomiting was greater in the meperidine group.

Unlike other opioids, meperidine has local anesthetic qualities. Some anesthesiologists have administered intrathecal meperidine 5% (1 mg/kg) as the sole anesthetic agent for cesarean section, noting that the mean duration of surgical anesthesia was 41.0 ± 15.5 minutes.[127,129] This technique did not depress neonatal Apgar scores.[129]

DIAMORPHINE

Diamorphine has several desirable properties that suggest that it might be a useful intrathecal analgesic agent. These include the following: (1) its high lipophilicity (octanol-water coefficient = 280), which results in a rapid onset of analgesia; and (2) a prolonged duration of analgesia as a result of the activity of the drug's major metabolites. Diamorphine is deacetylated in CSF to its active metabolites 6-mono-acetylmorphine and morphine. Intrathecal diamorphine administration is believed to incur less risk of centrally mediated side effects (e.g., respiratory depression, pruritus, urinary retention) than intrathecal morphine.[131]

Kelly et al.[131] randomized 80 women to receive intrathecal diamorphine (0.125, 0.25, or 0.375 mg) with hyperbaric bupivacaine 0.5% for cesarean section. The two higher doses of intrathecal diamorphine provided effective analgesia. The occurrence of both vomiting and pruritus was dose-related, and clinically significant respiratory depression was not observed. Husaini et al.[132] observed that intrathecal diamorphine 0.2 mg and intrathecal morphine 0.2 mg provided similar postcesarean analgesia as measured by postoperative PCA morphine requirements. However, the patients that received intrathecal morphine had a higher incidence of pruritus and drowsiness.

BUTORPHANOL

Gould et al.[73] observed that intrathecal butorphanol 0.4 mg combined with hyperbaric bupivacaine provided effective augmentation of intraoperative anesthesia and more than 8 hours of postcesarean analgesia. However, the potential neurotoxicity of this agent may preclude its use in this setting (*vide infra*).

NALBUPHINE

Culebras et al.[134] randomized 100 patients undergoing cesarean section to receive either intrathecal morphine 0.2 mg or intrathecal nalbuphine (0.2, 0.8 or 1.6 mg) with hyperbaric bupivacaine 10 mg. Intrathecal morphine provided significantly longer analgesia than did intrathecal nalbuphine. Intrathecal nalbuphine 0.8 mg provided good intraoperative and early postoperative analgesia without side effects, and administration of a larger dose (1.6 mg) did not increase efficacy. In an accompanying editorial, Yaksh and Birnbach[84] criticized this study because of their concern that "co-administration of local anesthetic, as was used by Culebras et al.,[134] may result in possible toxic interactions and alterations in pH and drug clearance, which have not been previously investigated." Further, Yaksh and Birnbach[84] concluded that, for intrathecal nalbuphine, "the evidence to support its safe use is currently insufficient."

METHADONE

Intrathecal methadone provides effective postcesarean analgesia of intermediate duration; analgesia is more prolonged than that provided by intrathecal fentanyl but shorter than that provided by intrathecal morphine. Chung et al.[135] observed that patients treated with intrathecal methadone 1 mg experienced less effective *intra*operative analgesia than individuals given intrathecal methadone 2 mg or fentanyl 12.5 μg. Methadone provided superior *post*operative analgesia. Patients who received 2 mg of methadone experienced as many as 8 hours of effective postcesarean analgesia and a significant reduction in intravenous PCA meperidine requirements throughout the 24-hour study period. Side effects included a high incidence of pruritus and a mild degree of intraoperative sedation. Somnolence was exacerbated by small doses of droperidol but not by metoclopramide.[135]

Intrathecal Opioid Combinations

Intrathecal administration of morphine in combination with a lipophilic opioid may offer some advantages. Because of morphine's delayed onset to peak analgesic effect, patients recovering from spinal lidocaine anesthesia often report breakthrough pain in the PACU. Sabilla et al.[136] found that the intrathecal combination of fentanyl 25 μg with morphine 0.1 mg provided superior postoperative analgesia as compared with fentanyl but offered no advantage over morphine alone. By contrast, Lee et al.[137] recently observed that patients who received both intrathecal fentanyl 20 μg and morphine 0.2 mg had more pain than those who received intrathecal morphine only. They concluded that the intrathecal morphine was not effective because it was not binding to the spinal opioid receptors that were occupied by the concurrently administered intrathecal fentanyl.

The rapid onset and intermediate duration of intrathecal meperidine may compensate for the latency of intrathecal morphine and provide a smooth transition during the regression of spinal anesthesia. Chung et al.[138] found that the combination of meperidine 10 mg and morphine 0.15 mg provided more uniform analgesia, higher satisfaction, and a lower requirement for intravenous opioid supplementation than either morphine or meperidine alone in patients recovering from cesarean delivery.

Tables 28-3 and 28-4 include the doses of epidural and intrathecal opioids that are administered for postcesarean

TABLE 28-3	OPIOIDS EMPLOYED FOR EPIDURAL ANALGESIA AFTER CESAREAN SECTION

Drug(s)	Dose	Onset (min)	Peak effect (min)	Duration (hr)	Advantages	Disadvantages
Epidural analgesia						
Morphine	2-4 mg	45-60	60-120	12-24	Long duration	Delayed onset, significant side effects, delayed respiratory depression
Fentanyl	50-100 µg	5	20	2-3	Very rapid onset, few side effects, may be combined with PCA	High dose requirement, short duration
Sufentanil	25-50 µg	5	15-20	2-4	Very rapid onset, may be combined with PCA	High dose requirement, short duration
Hydromorphone	0.4-0.75 mg	15	45-60	10-20	Long duration, more rapid onset than morphine	Side effect profile similar to morphine
Butorphanol	2-4 mg	15	40	2-4	Fairly rapid onset	Questionable spinal activity, excessive sedation
Meperidine	50 mg	15	30	4-6	Rapid onset, intermediate duration, few side effects, reduction in "shaking"	Nausea and vomiting
Morphine/ fentanyl	3 mg/50 µg	10	15	12-24	Rapid onset, long duration, fewer side effects than standard 5-mg dose of morphine	
Morphine/ sufentanil	3 mg/25 µg	5	15	12-24	Very rapid onset, long duration, fewer side effects than standard 5-mg dose of morphine	
Continuous fentanyl	100-µg bolus, 40-75 µg/hr	10	20	Indefinite	Rapid onset, long duration, reduced side effects	Labor intensive, infusion device necessary, maintenance of epidural catheter necessary, high dose requirement, cumulative toxicity possible
Continuous sufentanil	25-µg bolus, 20-25 µg/hr	5	15	Indefinite	Very rapid onset, long duration, reduced side effects	Labor intensive, infusion device necessary, maintenance of epidural catheter necessary, high dose requirement, cumulative toxicity possible
Continuous hydromorphone	0.4-mg bolus, 0.05-0.1 mg/hr	20	30	Indefinite	Rapid onset, reduced dose requirement as compared with intravenous PCA administration	Labor intensive, infusion device necessary, maintenance of epidural catheter necessary, high dose requirement, cumulative toxicity possible

PCA, Patient-controlled analgesia.

analgesia. Box 28-2 summarizes current practice at Yale-New Haven Hospital.

Caution must be exercised when administering a drug in the subarachnoid space, because the drug and diluent solution are placed in direct contact with the spinal cord and nerves. Drugs and diluents that are designed and proved safe for parenteral use may not be safe when administered intrathecally.[139] A number of opioid analgesics have been administered intrathecally to healthy obstetric patients without knowledge of their safety.[140] Rawal et al.[141] evaluated the behavioral and histopathologic effects of butorphanol, sufentanil, and nalbuphine after intrathecal administration in sheep. Nalbuphine caused the least evidence of irritation to neural tissue. Intrathecal administration of commercial preparations of dezocine produced neuropathologic changes in dog spinal cord.[142] Preservatives added to parenteral opioid preparations, including sodium (meta)bisulfite and disodium ethylenediaminetetraacetic acid (EDTA), are known to incite inflammatory and fibrotic changes in pia-arachnoid and spinal tissue when administered intrathecally.

INTRAOPERATIVE BENEFITS OF EPIDURAL AND INTRATHECAL OPIOIDS

Epidural and intrathecal opioids are commonly employed to enhance intraoperative analgesia. During cesarean section, many obstetricians exteriorize the uterus during closure of the hysterotomy incision. Uterine exteriorization is a potent stimulus of intraoperative nausea, vomiting, and visceral discomfort, despite high thoracic levels of anesthesia. Several studies have demonstrated an improved quality of intraoperative analgesia when a dose of 50 to 100 μg of fentanyl was added to epidural lidocaine[34,104,143,144] or bupivacaine.[145] Several studies[32,143] have demonstrated that the epidural injection of

---

TABLE 28-4   OPIOIDS EMPLOYED FOR INTRATHECAL ANALGESIA AFTER CESAREAN SECTION

Drug	Dose	Onset (min)	Peak effect (min)	Duration (hr)	Advantages	Disadvantages
Morphine	0.1-0.25 mg	30	60	12-24	Long duration	Significant side effects, delayed respiratory depression
Fentanyl	10-20 μg	5	10	2-3	Rapid onset, few side effects	Short duration
Sufentanil	5-10 μg	5	10	2-4	Rapid onset, few side effects	Short duration
Meperidine	10 mg	10	15	4-5	Rapid onset, potentiation of spinal anesthesia	Nausea and vomiting

---

Box 28-2 EPIDURAL AND SPINAL OPIOID ANALGESIA AFTER CESAREAN SECTION: CURRENT CLINICAL PRACTICE AT YALE-NEW HAVEN HOSPITAL

SPINAL ANESTHESIA FOR CESAREAN SECTION

Some patients receive a single dose of preservative-free **morphine** (0.25 mg), which is mixed with either hyperbaric bupivacaine (12.5 mg) or lidocaine (60 to 75 mg). Alternatively, we add two opioids to the local anesthetic solution: preservative-free **meperidine** (10 mg) and **morphine** (0.1 to 0.15 mg). This combination provides better analgesia than morphine alone during the first several hours after cesarean section.

All patients receive **metoclopramide** (10 mg) intravenously before the administration of spinal anesthesia. This dose of antiemetic is readministered every 6 hours for 24 hours after surgery. Patients who complain of moderate-to-severe pruritus receive intravenous **diphenhydramine** (12.5 to 25 mg), **naloxone** (0.04 to 0.08 mg), or **nalbuphine** (5 mg).

All patients are provided low-dose intravenous (IV) patient-controlled analgesia (PCA) **meperidine** (5 to 8 mg every 6 to 10 minutes as needed) for supplemental analgesia. Patients who receive the smaller (0.1 to 0.15 mg) dose of morphine are provided PCA immediately after arrival to the postpartum floor, whereas patients who receive the larger (0.25 mg) dose do not begin PCA until 8 to 12 hours after the administration of spinal anesthesia. IV PCA is continued for 24 to 36 hours, and all patients are followed by the Acute Pain Service. Standard orders include an hourly assessment of respiratory rate and level of sedation and intermittent use of pulse oximetry.

EPIDURAL ANESTHESIA FOR CESAREAN SECTION

We give most patients a small dose of epidural **fentanyl** (50 to 75 μg) to augment intraoperative anesthesia. We delay epidural fentanyl administration until after the umbilical cord is clamped in the following cases: (1) severe fetal distress; (2) thick meconium-stained amniotic fluid; (3) preterm delivery; and (4) other conditions associated with an increased risk of neonatal respiratory depression. After delivery, we give either hydromorphone (0.4 mg) or a combination of preservative-free **morphine** (2 to 3 mg) and **meperidine** (40 mg) epidurally. We add saline so that the total volume is 10 mL. This dose of hydromorphone may be readministered every 6 hours, or the morphine-meperidine may be readministered every 12 hours for 36 hours. Alternatively, the catheter may be removed, and IV PCA may be begun 6 to 12 hours after the epidural administration of opioid. Some patients receive a continuous epidural infusion of **hydromorphone** (10 μg/mL) at a dose of 0.05 to 0.1 mg/hr or a continuous epidural infusion of **fentanyl** (5 μg/mL) at a dose of 40 to 60 μg/hr. Patient-controlled bolus doses (5 to 15 μg of fentanyl or 5 to 10 μg of hydromorphone every 15 minutes) may be combined with a lower background epidural infusion rate.

We administer **metoclopramide** for the treatment of nausea and vomiting and give small doses of **diphenhydramine, naloxone,** or **nalbuphine** for the treatment of pruritus. We give a small dose of **ketorolac** (15 mg slow IV bolus every 6 hours) for breakthrough pain.

50 to 100 μg of fentanyl immediately after delivery rapidly relieved the nausea and discomfort associated with intraabdominal manipulation (e.g., uterine exteriorization, abdominal exploration, manipulation of fallopian tubes, peritoneal closure). This dose produces no change in the sensory level or the density of motor blockade, and it results in only a slight increase in maternal sedation. By contrast, Yee et al.[146] observed no difference in intraoperative analgesia or in the incidence of side effects after the administration of 25 or 50 μg of epidural fentanyl during elective cesarean section.

Anxious patients may benefit from the epidural administration of fentanyl before the skin incision. Several studies have evaluated the safety of epidural fentanyl administration before delivery. Epidural fentanyl did not affect the neonatal pattern of breathing, oxygen saturation, Apgar scores, umbilical cord blood pH, or Neurologic and Adaptive Capacity Scores. Although epidural fentanyl (1 μg/kg) had no apparent effect on neonatal outcome or neurobehavior and resulted in umbilical artery plasma concentrations that were below the limit of their assay, Preston et al.[44] suggested that epidural fentanyl administration be delayed until the umbilical cord is clamped. In a review of this study, James[147] commented: "Which is worse, a perhaps unrecognized newborn effect of epidural fentanyl, or reduced uterine blood flow from maternal stress associated with pain during a surgical procedure?"

Intrathecal fentanyl also improves the quality of intraoperative spinal anesthesia. The exact mechanisms by which intraspinal opioids decrease visceral pain and the central effects of visceral stimulation have not been defined; however, opioids are known to enhance spinal anesthetic blockade produced by intrathecal lidocaine and bupivacaine.[41] Intraspinal opioids provide selective enhancement of sensory blockade and (with the possible exception of meperidine) no enhancement of motor or sympathetic blockade. The combination of intrathecal fentanyl and hyperbaric bupivacaine provides more effective intraoperative analgesia than that provided by bupivacaine alone.[124] Doses of 12.5 to 25 μg of fentanyl decrease the level of discomfort often associated with peritoneal traction and uterine exteriorization. Patients remain alert and without evidence of hypoxemia or respiratory depression. Facial-truncal pruritus is commonly observed; however, symptoms typically are mild and do not require treatment.

Epidural meperidine, butorphanol, and sufentanil effectively reduce the incidence and severity of shivering during cesarean section.[148-152] Shivering not only causes maternal anxiety but also results in physiologic stress, including increased cardiac output, oxygen consumption, and carbon dioxide production. Sutherland et al.[151] reported an incidence of shivering of 36% in patients treated with epidural bupivacaine alone but an incidence of only 11% in those treated with epidural bupivacaine plus meperidine 25 mg. Umbilical cord blood meperidine concentrations were either undetectable or clinically insignificant, and all Apgar scores were satisfactory. Chen et al.[150] compared the addition of fentanyl 100 μg or butorphanol 2 mg to 2% lidocaine during the administration of epidural anesthesia for cesarean section. Approximately 60% of patients who received lidocaine alone experienced shivering; 50% of women who received lidocaine with fentanyl experienced shivering as compared with 7% of those who received lidocaine with butorphanol. Sevarino et al.[152] reported that epidural sufentanil 25 μg reduced the incidence of intraoperative shivering by 75% and that doses of 50 μg or more completely abolished such activity.

Some evidence suggests that intrathecal opioids may reduce the incidence of PDPH after spinal anesthesia. Eldor and Guedj[153] evaluated the administration of bupivacaine spinal anesthesia with a 26-gauge needle followed by the administration of epidural morphine for postcesarean analgesia. No headaches occurred during the administration of epidural morphine. Subsequently, five patients who complained of headache experienced a resolution of symptoms after another dose of epidural morphine. By contrast, Abboud et al.[154] observed no difference in the incidence of PDPH between patients who received both intrathecal bupivacaine and morphine 0.2 mg and those who received bupivacaine alone. The authors used a 25-gauge Quincke needle during the administration of spinal anesthesia, and both groups had a high incidence of PDPH (19% and 22%, respectively). Carney et al.[155] likewise observed that the administration of intrathecal morphine 0.15 mg did not reduce either the incidence or severity of PDPH in patients who received spinal bupivacaine anesthesia.

OTHER POSTPARTUM APPLICATIONS OF EPIDURAL AND INTRATHECAL OPIOIDS

Vaginal Delivery

Intraspinal opioid analgesia is also advantageous in patients at high risk for severe pain after a traumatic vaginal delivery. At Yale-New Haven Hospital, we offer epidural or intrathecal opioid analgesia (e.g., fentanyl, meperidine, a small dose of morphine) to patients with a third- or fourth-degree episiotomy, extensive vaginal and cervical lacerations, or a mediolateral episiotomy. Patients report effective pain relief and few side effects during the immediate postpartum period. Colburn et al.[156] evaluated the efficacy of epidural fentanyl 50 μg or saline-placebo in patients recovering from traumatic vaginal delivery. Patients treated with fentanyl had lower pain scores during the first 2 hours, a longer time to the first request for an oral opioid analgesic, and decreased analgesic requirements as compared with patients who received saline-placebo. No patient experienced urinary retention or respiratory depression, and the administration of fentanyl did not increase the incidence of nausea, pruritus, or sedation.

Tubal Ligation

Patients recovering from tubal ligation are rarely troubled by severe or prolonged discomfort and typically require minimal amounts of postoperative analgesics. Nonetheless, some investigators have advocated intrathecal opioid administration as a simple, effective method of postoperative analgesia.

Malinow et al.[157] evaluated the efficacy of fentanyl 10 μg added to spinal lidocaine with and without epinephrine 0.2 mg in 52 patients who underwent postpartum tubal ligation. The addition of fentanyl alone did not provide postoperative analgesia. However, when both epinephrine and fentanyl were added to the spinal anesthetic, the mean time to first supplemental opioid was increased to 11 hours. The authors speculated that epinephrine may delay the systemic absorption of fentanyl and thereby extend the duration of opioid-specific analgesia. They also suggested that epinephrine may contribute to analgesia at the spinal cord level by suppressing the activity of wide-dynamic-range neurons in the spinal cord.

Meperidine has local anesthetic properties and may be administered intrathecally as a sole anesthetic agent for postpartum tubal ligation. Honet et al.[158] noted that intrathecal meperidine 60 mg provided spinal anesthesia with a quality similar to that provided by intrathecal hyperbaric lidocaine 70 mg. Patients who received meperidine had significantly less postoperative pain and required less supplemental analgesia than patients who received intrathecal lidocaine. Pruritus was the only significant side effect associated with meperidine.

SIDE EFFECTS OF EPIDURAL AND INTRATHECAL OPIOIDS

Intraspinal opioid administration may result in annoying (and occasionally serious) side effects and complications, including pruritus, nausea and vomiting, urinary retention, somnolence, and respiratory depression.[159]

Pruritus

Pruritus follows intraspinal opioid administration more often in obstetric patients than in any other patient group. The incidence ranges from 40% to 80% of parturients treated with epidural and intrathecal morphine, hydromorphone, or methadone.[6,24,26,114,120] Mild pruritus, typically involving the face or chest, may occur even more frequently; however, patients may not mention it unless directly questioned. Occasionally, the intensity of itching is so annoying that it interferes with sleep and breast-feeding.[5] Severe pruritus is the most frequent cause of patient dissatisfaction after the administration of epidural and intrathecal morphine. Pruritus occurs somewhat less often after epidural or intrathecal administration of a lipid-soluble opioid.[74,75,135] Epidural fentanyl administration results in pruritus of the face and/or chest in approximately one third of patients; however, symptoms are mild and rarely require treatment.

The etiology of pruritus is unclear, but its occurrence does not reflect an acute or excessive release of histamine. Indeed, pruritus is most severe 3 to 6 hours after intraspinal morphine administration.[6,28] At this time, plasma concentrations of opioid and histamine are clinically insignificant.[160] Further, pruritus often occurs after the intraspinal administration of other opioids (e.g., fentanyl, sufentanil) that do not cause histamine release. Changes in spinal efferent outflow may indirectly release small amounts of histamine in tissues adjacent to peripheral nerve endings[161]; this finding may explain why antihistamines may provide some relief of pruritus after intraspinal opioid administration. Moreover, pruritus may reflect a unique nonsegmental reflex whereby alterations in spinal and trigeminal nerve processing of afferent information result in nociceptive input that is reinterpreted as itching.[160]

Mild facial pruritus may be relieved with cold compresses, whereas pruritus of moderate severity may respond to one or more doses of **diphenhydramine** 25 mg. Moderate-to-severe pruritus may be treated successfully with small intravenous doses of **naloxone** (0.04 to 0.08 mg), which typically relieve symptoms without reversing the analgesia.[6] Of interest, Sun[162] reported a case of acute opioid withdrawal syndrome shortly after the intravenous administration of naloxone 0.14 mg for the treatment of pruritus in a patient who had received epidural morphine 2 mg for postcesarean analgesia.

Some investigators have suggested that prostaglandins are involved in the etiology of pruritus following intraspinal opioid administration. Prostaglandins enhance C-fiber transmission to the CNS, release histamine, and potentiate the pruritus induced by histamine[163]; thus nonsteroidal antiinflammatory drugs (NSAIDs) may have a role in the treatment of pruritus. Colbert et al.[163] demonstrated that administration of rectal **diclofenac** resulted in a significant reduction in both the incidence and severity of pruritus in patients who had received intrathecal morphine. Diclofenac also reduced pain and subsequent PCA morphine consumption.[163]

Side effects of intraspinal opioids often outlast the effect of a single bolus dose of naloxone; thus a continuous intravenous infusion of naloxone may be preferable.[164] One or two ampules of naloxone (0.4 to 0.8 mg) may be added to each liter of the patient's maintenance intravenous fluid. An infusion rate of 125 mL/hr delivers 50 to 100 µg/hr of naloxone. Luthman et al.[165] evaluated the effect of a continuous naloxone infusion in patients given spinal bupivacaine plus intrathecal morphine 0.2 mg for cesarean section. Patients treated with naloxone experienced significant reductions in the frequency and severity of pruritus with no impairment in the quality or duration of pain relief.

Alternatively, some anesthesiologists prefer intravenous **nalbuphine** (3 to 10 mg) for the treatment of pruritus. One study noted excellent results with a continuous infusion of nalbuphine 5 mg/hr.[166] However, the systemic consequences of kappa-receptor agonists (e.g., oversedation) should be considered before giving such a large dose of this drug. Continuous intravenous infusion of nalbuphine 5 mg/hr represents an excessive dose that most likely would cause significant sedation. It rarely is necessary to give more than two 5-mg doses of nalbuphine to treat pruritus after a single dose of epidural morphine (3 to 4 mg) or intrathecal morphine (0.1 to 0.25 mg).

In a randomized, double-blind study, Cohen et al.[167] evaluated the efficacy of one to three doses of either naloxone 0.2 mg or nalbuphine 5 mg for the treatment of pruritus and nausea after the administration of epidural morphine 5 mg for postcesarean analgesia. The authors observed a significant decrease in the incidence of vomiting and in the severity of nausea and pruritus only in patients who received nalbuphine. A greater number of patients in the naloxone group required a second and third dose of the study drug or alternative therapy. Patients who received nalbuphine had increased sedation, whereas naloxone resulted in an increase in pain scores.

Morgan et al.[168] evaluated the efficacy of prophylactic nalbuphine in patients who received epidural morphine for postcesarean analgesia. They gave nalbuphine 20 mg at skin closure and every 6 hours thereafter. Prophylactic administration of nalbuphine did not result in decreased pruritus scores as compared with administration of saline-placebo. The nalbuphine did not antagonize epidural morphine analgesia, but it resulted in increased somnolence.

Kendrick et al.[169] evaluated the use of patient-controlled nalbuphine or naloxone to treat annoying side effects associated with epidural morphine analgesia after cesarean section. There was no difference between the two groups in pain or sedation scores; however, patients in the nalbuphine group had less pruritus and a decreased need for hospital staff intervention.

Abboud et al.[170] evaluated the efficacy of prophylactic oral **naltrexone** (a long-acting opioid antagonist) in patients who had received intrathecal morphine. They observed a significant reduction in the level of somnolence among those patients who received either 3 or 6 mg of naltrexone. Patients who received 6 mg also experienced less pruritus and nausea; however, this dose was associated with a shortened duration of postcesarean analgesia.

Borgeat et al.[171] reported that **propofol** relieved the pruritus caused by epidural and intrathecal morphine. Subhypnotic doses of intravenous propofol 10 mg provided rapid relief of mild-to-moderate pruritus; the relief lasted more than 60 minutes. The authors proposed that the antipruritus activity of propofol does not depend on the specific antagonism of opioid receptors; rather, it may result from nonselective depression of neural transmission in the spinal cord. The same group compared the efficacy of propofol 10 mg with that of naloxone 2 μg/kg for the treatment of epidural morphine-induced pruritus.[172] The overall success rate (approximately 80%) was similar in the two groups. Of interest, patients in the propofol group had significantly less postoperative pain. The authors speculated that this effect may result from propofol's inhibition of the release of excitatory amino acids that are known to be involved in the modulation of pain.[172] By contrast, Beilin et al.[173] observed that a subhypnotic dose of propofol 20 mg (administered in two divided doses 5 minutes apart) did *not* relieve pruritus caused by intrathecal morphine 0.25 mg. A recent study found that intravenous nalbuphine 3 mg was superior to intravenous propofol 20 mg for the treatment of pruritus in patients who had received intrathecal morphine for postcesarean analgesia.[174]

Ondansetron, a selective serotonin (5-hydroxytryptamine [5-HT]) receptor antagonist, has been advocated as a treatment of morphine-induced pruritus. The rationale is that the dense concentration of 5-HT$_3$ receptors has been identified in the dorsal part of the rat spinal cord—particularly in the superficial layers of the dorsal horn—and in the nucleus of the spinal tract of the trigeminal nerve in the mouse medulla. Borgeat et al.[175] observed that the administration of ondansetron 8 mg intravenously is an effective treatment for pruritus associated with intrathecal or epidural morphine. Ondansetron did not affect postoperative pain or sedation and did not cause hemodynamic changes.[175] Yeh et al.[176] observed that the prophylactic administration of ondansetron 0.1 mg/kg immediately after delivery significantly reduced the incidence of pruritus in patients who had received intrathecal morphine. However, the routine prophylactic use of this drug may be associated with unnecessary drug administration in some patients who might not have developed pruritus or who would not have requested treatment.

Ondansetron is not currently recommended for routine use in breast-feeding mothers. Ondansetron is a lipophilic drug that may be excreted in breast milk, and no studies have measured the concentration of this drug in breast milk.[176]

Horta et al.[177] studied the effect of three doses of epidural droperidol (1.25, 2.5, and 5 mg) on the incidence of pruritus in patients who also received epidural morphine. Epidural droperidol resulted in a dose-related reduction in the incidence of pruritus, which was independent of the dose-related somnolence.

Nausea and Vomiting

Although nausea and vomiting are common complaints among patients recovering from cesarean delivery, the incidence of symptoms is increased among patients treated with epidural and intrathecal opioids.[178] Depending on the agent used and the dose administered, the percentage of patients who develop nausea and vomiting ranges from 20% to 60%.[19,120,178] Some but not all of these patients require treatment. In general, patients treated with morphine and buprenorphine experience the highest incidence of nausea and vomiting,[66] whereas patients who receive a continuous fentanyl-epinephrine infusion are affected less often.[50] Nausea may result from either rostral spread of the drug in the CSF to the brainstem or vascular uptake and delivery to the vomiting center and chemoreceptor trigger zone.[6,28]

A variety of agents have been evaluated for the prevention or treatment of intraspinal opioid-induced emesis, including **metoclopramide** (10 mg) and low doses of **droperidol** (0.625 to 1.25 mg). In our experience, small doses of droperidol often result in excessive sedation in patients who have received epidural or intrathecal morphine, meperidine, or methadone.[5] Further, droperidol has been removed from the formulary in many hospitals because of FDA concerns that it may result in cardiac arrhythmias. Thus metoclopramide appears to be a better choice. It provides effective antiemesis, does not increase maternal sedation, and has no untoward effects on the neonate.[179] The use of a **transdermal scopolamine** patch may also reduce the incidence of nausea and vomiting, especially during the first 10 hours after cesarean delivery.[180] This preparation has a latency of 3 to 4 hours, and it typically is ineffective for the treatment of an acute exacerbation of nausea and vomiting.

In the presence of intractable nausea, intravenous boluses of **naloxone** (40 to 80 μg) followed by a continuous infusion of 50 to 100 μg/hr may be useful. **Ondansetron** may also be helpful in cases of intractable nausea. Doses of 2 to 4 mg intravenously every 4 to 6 hours have been advocated to reduce the incidence and severity of intraspinal opioid-induced nausea.[5] A major disadvantage of ondansetron is that it is expensive.

Glucocorticoids have various effects on the CNS; they help regulate transmitter levels, receptor densities, and neuronal configuration.[181] Numerous glucocorticoid receptors have been identified in the nucleus of the solitary tract, the nucleus of raphe, and the area postrema. These nuclei have significant activity in the regulation of nausea and vomiting, and glucocorticoids may exert an antiemetic action through these nuclei.[181] Tzeng et al.[181] evaluated the efficacy of intravenous **dexamethasone** for the prevention of nausea and vomiting in patients who received epidural morphine 3 mg for postcesarean analgesia. Both dexamethasone 8 mg and droperidol 1.25 mg significantly decreased the incidence of nausea and vomiting as compared with saline-placebo. Patients who received droperidol reported a more frequent incidence of restlessness (16%) than those who received dexamethasone.

Ho et al.[182] have advocated the prophylactic use of **acupuncture** bands bilaterally on the P-6 (HG-6) acupoint to reduce the incidence of nausea and vomiting after the administration of epidural morphine for postcesarean analgesia. According to traditional Chinese acupuncture textbooks, the P-6 acupoint is located 4 to 5 cm proximal to the transverse crease of the wrist and 1 to 1.3 cm deep from the skin, between the tendons of the flexor carpi radialis and palmaris longus.

Acupressure, a noninvasive variation of acupuncture, has been suggested as a potential nonpharmacologic, noninvasive method of preventing nausea and vomiting during and after spinal anesthesia for cesarean section. Acupressure is performed by placing a flexible strap with a spherical plastic bead on the anterior surface of the right forearm between the tendons of the flexor carpi radialis and palmaris longus.[183]

Urinary Retention

Urinary retention is a common complication of intraspinal opioid administration in nonpregnant patients. However, this is an infrequent complication in patients who are recovering from cesarean delivery; this probably reflects the common practice of maintaining an indwelling urinary catheter for the first 24 hours after surgery. Evron et al.[184] reported that patients who received epidural morphine 4 mg had greater difficulty in micturition and a greater incidence of urinary retention than patients who received an equivalent dose of epidural methadone for postcesarean analgesia. Other studies have not reported urinary retention as a complication of intraspinal opioid analgesia in patients recovering from cesarean section.

Intraspinal opioid-induced urinary retention may result from the inhibition of sacral parasympathetic outflow, which results in the relaxation of the bladder detrusor muscle and an inability to relax the sphincter.[185] This effect may be relieved with a large intravenous dose (0.8 mg) of naloxone; unfortunately, a reversal of analgesia may also occur.[6,186] Bethanechol (Urecholine) and apomorphine may also provide relief.[185] Ambulation and intermittent bladder catheterization are more practical forms of treatment in this patient population.

Respiratory Depression

Respiratory depression is the most feared complication of epidural and intrathecal opioid administration.[6,19,28]

MORPHINE

Mild respiratory depression occurs 30 to 90 minutes after the epidural administration of morphine; this results from the systemic absorption of morphine from the epidural space.[6] Delayed respiratory depression, which results from the rostral spread of morphine in the CSF, may occur 6 to 10 hours later.[28,29] After reaching the fourth ventricle, the drug rapidly equilibrates with intracranial CSF and interacts with the medullary respiratory centers to reduce the ventilatory response to carbon dioxide.

Risk factors for respiratory depression include advanced age and morbid obesity.[6] Patients recovering from cesarean section typically are young and healthy, and they rarely present with significant pulmonary disease or other risk factors that might increase the likelihood of respiratory depression. Pregnant women also have an increased concentration of progesterone, which is a respiratory stimulant[187]; this may decrease the risk of respiratory depression. Nonetheless, clinically significant respiratory depression may occur in this low-risk population. Fuller et al.[19] reported that 12 of 4880 patients who received epidural morphine for postcesarean analgesia developed clinically significant respiratory depression (i.e., a respiratory rate of less than 10 breaths per minute). Hourly nursing observation detected these 12 cases, and no sequelae occurred. Most patients responded to verbal stimulation, and only three patients required administration of naloxone.

Ostman et al.[188] continuously monitored SaO_2 during the night before surgery and the night after epidural administration of morphine 4 mg for postcesarean analgesia in six patients; they observed episodes of desaturation on both evenings. Epidural morphine administration did not cause a further (or more prolonged) reduction in SaO_2, and it did not result in a respiratory rate of less than 12 breaths per minute

in any patient. Albright[189] used an apnea monitor to assess respiratory rate for 16 hours after epidural administration of morphine, hydromorphone, or meperidine in patients who had undergone cesarean section. No patient treated with hydromorphone had a respiratory rate of less than 10 breaths per minute as compared with one patient each in the morphine and meperidine groups.

Early reports suggested that intrathecal morphine was associated with a higher incidence of delayed respiratory depression than epidural morphine.[6] This observation reflected the relatively high doses of morphine (1 to 5 mg) administered intrathecally in early clinical trials. Subsequently, investigators have demonstrated that smaller doses of intrathecal morphine provide effective analgesia with a low risk of clinically significant respiratory depression. Abboud et al.[113] evaluated CO_2 response after the intrathecal administration of morphine (either 0.1 or 0.25 mg) or the subcutaneous administration of 8 mg of morphine. Neither dose of intrathecal morphine affected CO_2 response or minute ventilation during the 24-hour observation period. By contrast, both measurements were depressed for 3 hours after subcutaneous morphine administration.

Bailey et al.[190] evaluated the dose responses of intrathecal morphine in human volunteers. Twenty healthy, young, adult male volunteers received either 0.0, 0.2, 0.4, or 0.6 mg of preservative-free intrathecal morphine. The two larger doses of morphine resulted in only a modest increase in the intensity of analgesia as compared with the 0.2-mg dose. The primary benefit of the two larger doses was a prolonged duration of effective analgesia. Intrathecal morphine produced significant, dose-related decreases in SaO_2 as detected by pulse oximetry. Maximal respiratory depression occurred 3.5 to 7.5 hours after intrathecal morphine administration. However, subjects who received 0.6 mg of intrathecal morphine "demonstrated significant depression (< 50% of baseline) of the ventilatory response to carbon dioxide up to 19.5 hours after [administration of intrathecal morphine]."[190] Administration of supplemental oxygen (2 L/min through nasal cannulae) consistently alleviated hypoxemia. The authors concluded that clinical signs and symptoms were unreliable predictors of respiratory depression. Specifically, respiratory rate, level of sedation, pupil size, and other adverse effects "did not reliably indicate when mild, moderate, or severe hypoxemia and ventilatory depression occurred."[190] These volunteers were not pregnant, and they were not subjected to an ongoing noxious stimulus (e.g., skin incision, uterine cramping). All of the volunteers were young and healthy, and they did not have altered pulmonary mechanics, which occur in patients who have undergone abdominal surgery.

Epidural administration of 3 to 4 mg of morphine or intrathecal administration of 0.1 to 0.25 mg of morphine results in a very low risk of clinically significant respiratory depression in obstetric patients. Thus, most anesthesiologists do not administer prophylactic naloxone to patients with uncomplicated recovery from cesarean section.[191] It seems prudent to administer prophylactic naloxone to morbidly obese parturients and to individuals with severe pulmonary disease. Continuous intravenous infusion of naloxone (1 μg/kg/hr) prevents delayed respiratory depression in high-risk general surgical patients without affecting the quality of analgesia.[192]

The rare patient who displays signs of somnolence, hypoventilation, and arterial desaturation should receive supplemental oxygen and an intravenous bolus dose of naloxone. An intravenous infusion of naloxone may also be justified in patients who continue to show evidence of moderate-to-severe respiratory depression. Such therapy should be maintained for as long as the patient remains symptomatic; this may be as long as 8 to 12 hours in patients who have received intrathecal or epidural morphine.

Administration of sedative drugs (e.g., droperidol, diphenhydramine) may exacerbate somnolence in patients who are pain free[5]; thus caution should be exercised when giving a sedative drug to treat the nausea or pruritus associated with epidural and intrathecal morphine.

LIPOPHILIC OPIOIDS

Single epidural or intrathecal doses of a lipophilic opioid are not associated with delayed respiratory depression.[51] By contrast, early-onset respiratory depression, which typically occurs within 30 minutes of administration, has been observed.[52,62] Epidural meperidine 75 mg resulted in clinically significant hypoventilation and hypoxemia 20 to 25 minutes after cesarean section in a previously healthy 34-year-old parturient.[193] Negre et al.[52] observed that the epidural administration of a large dose (200 µg) of fentanyl significantly depressed the ventilatory response to CO_2 at 30, 60, and 120 minutes after administration of the drug. The ventilatory response returned to baseline by 180 minutes and remained normal thereafter.

Early-onset respiratory depression results from vascular uptake of the lipophilic opioid by the epidural or subarachnoid venous plexus and rapid transport by means of the systemic circulation to brainstem respiratory centers.[6] Cohen et al.[62] evaluated the ventilatory response to CO_2 after the epidural administration of 30 or 50 µg of sufentanil after cesarean section. Patients in both groups experienced significant sedation and depression of respiratory drive. Although plasma levels of sufentanil peaked at 10 to 15 minutes, the highest sedation scores and the maximal depression of CO_2 response occurred 45 to 60 minutes after administration. The authors suggested that vascular uptake of sufentanil (and perhaps rostral CSF flow) may have been responsible for respiratory depression at the level of the brainstem. They cautioned against the administration of a bolus dose of more than 30 µg, and they advised close monitoring of patients for several hours.

In general, early-onset respiratory depression is of lesser significance than delayed-onset respiratory compromise; it is more likely to occur in a high-visibility, controlled setting (e.g., operating room, PACU, intensive care unit), where an anesthesia care provider is present or immediately available. No study has addressed the potential for delayed or progressive respiratory depression in obstetric patients treated with a continuous epidural infusion of a lipophilic opioid. Evidence from nonpregnant patients suggests that plasma levels of fentanyl (and, to a lesser extent, sufentanil) rise progressively during the course of continuous epidural infusion.[194] Of importance was the finding that fentanyl levels exceeded minimum effective plasma analgesic concentrations at 24 to 30 hours.

Monitoring

What is the most appropriate method of respiratory monitoring for patients treated with epidural or intrathecal morphine or a continuous epidural opioid infusion? No single solution is appropriate for every institution. Various noninvasive monitors have been advocated, including pulse oximetry and end-tidal P_{CO_2} monitors; none of these methods has become universally accepted. Use of an apnea monitor is associated with frequent, annoying false alarms. Apnea monitors do not detect hypoventilation, and the patient or nurse must turn off the monitor when the patient ambulates or cares for her newborn. Pulse oximeters share the disadvantages of inconvenience for the patient, frequent motion-artifact alarms, and an inability to detect hypercarbia. In their study of intrathecal morphine administration in male volunteers, Bailey et al.[190] concluded the following:

> Only pulse oximetry reliably detected inadequate oxygenation in our subjects. While monitoring postoperative patients who have received intrathecal morphine with pulse oximetry may be effective, it requires frequent nursing observation, is fraught with false positive signals, and is often impractical. Nevertheless, even if only intermittently applied and/or observed, it may represent the best method available to detect hypoxemia after intrathecal morphine, as is the case after general anesthesia. Interestingly, at times the pulse oximeter alarm alone was enough to restore adequate breathing and oxygen saturation in some subjects.

Hourly assessment of respiratory rate is the most common form of monitoring.[19] Vigilant nursing observation and documentation of an inadequate respiratory effort, a slow respiratory rate, or unusual somnolence is probably the best form of monitoring in obstetric patients.[162,178,191] In our experience, respiratory depression does not develop suddenly; rather, it is slowly progressive, and it is typically preceded by increasing maternal somnolence. With appropriate nursing staff education, hospitals can provide safe care for the majority of women who receive a modest dose of epidural (3 to 4 mg) or intrathecal (0.1 to 0.25 mg) morphine or a continuous epidural infusion of fentanyl. An anesthesia care provider should be readily available to manage complications that may arise.

Clinicians should use an increased level of surveillance after the epidural or intrathecal administration of morphine in patients who are morbidly obese or in preeclamptic women who are receiving magnesium sulfate for seizure prophylaxis. Abouleish et al.[115] detected mild respiratory depression in 8 of 856 patients who received intrathecal morphine; all 8 of these patients were markedly obese. Hypermagnesemia also increases the risk of respiratory depression. Finally, extra surveillance is recommended for healthy patients who have received intrathecal or epidural morphine in doses larger than 0.25 and 5.0 mg, respectively.

SUPPLEMENTAL ANALGESIA

Parenteral Opioids

A significant number of patients who are treated with a single dose of intrathecal or epidural morphine request additional analgesia within 8 to 12 hours of morphine administration. We do not recommend administration of a second dose of epidural morphine in patients who are receiving nursing care on the postpartum ward. One option is to give an intramuscular injection of a small dose of opioid. (The dose should be small to prevent additive respiratory depression.) Alternative therapy includes intravenous administration of a mixed agonist-antagonist such as butorphanol, nalbuphine, or dezocine.

Restricted-dose PCA may be safer than intramuscular administration of a larger dose of opioid when it is used to augment intraspinal morphine analgesia. A small dose of epidural (2 to 3 mg) or intrathecal (0.1 to 0.15 mg) morphine, combined with low-dose intravenous PCA, represents a safe, effective method of postcesarean analgesia.[195] In our judgment, this regimen is safer than the epidural or intrathecal administration of larger doses of morphine. This combination therapy provides effective and prolonged analgesia, uniformity of pain relief, a significant reduction in overall dose requirements, and a reduced incidence of pruritus and other troublesome side effects. Intraspinal morphine administration, followed by low-dose PCA, may reduce drug accumulation in breast milk, which may decrease the likelihood of altered neonatal neurobehavior. Low-dose intravenous PCA (meperidine 5 mg or morphine 0.5 mg, with a 10- to 15-minute lockout) helps establish and maintain an excellent level of analgesia without causing a significant increase in maternal sedation. However, even with these small doses, PCA meperidine is associated with more evidence of neonatal neurobehavioral depression than PCA morphine.[196] Moreover, the amount of morphine and morphine-6-glucuronide transferred into the colostrum during PCA morphine administration is negligible and clinically insignificant.[197] Therefore, morphine is the parenteral opioid of choice for postcesarean analgesia among nursing parturients.[196,197]

Nonsteroidal Antiinflammatory Drugs

NSAIDs may enhance intraspinal opioid analgesia without increasing the risk of sedation, pruritus, or respiratory depression. NSAIDs may be administered as part of a multimodal approach to the treatment of postoperative pain. After cesarean section, NSAIDs exert an antiinflammatory effect at the incision site, and they also reduce cramping pain by decreasing the intensity of uterine contractions.[198] In theory, nonselective NSAIDs may have an adverse effect on hemostasis, and they may increase the risk of postoperative bleeding.

The manufacturer (Roche) has stated that **ketorolac** is contraindicated in nursing mothers because of the possible adverse effects of prostaglandin synthetase inhibitors on neonates. In contrast, the American Academy of Pediatrics considers ketorolac to be compatible with breast-feeding.[199]

Cartwright[200] observed that the intramuscular administration of ketorolac 30 mg resulted in a faster onset and longer duration of postcesarean analgesia than the opioid agonist papaverine. However, 45% of patients withdrew from the study because of inadequate pain relief. Ketorolac should not be considered a primary analgesic; instead, small doses might be used to potentiate intraspinal opioid analgesia. Waters et al.[201] noted that ketorolac alone (60-mg load, followed by 30 mg every 6 hours) did not provide postcesarean analgesia as effectively as ketorolac plus epidural morphine (2 mg) or epidural morphine (5 mg) alone. Mok and Tzeng[202] observed that a single intramuscular dose of ketorolac 30 mg plus epidural morphine 2 mg provided more effective analgesia than epidural morphine 2 mg alone. This regimen is attractive because a single dose of ketorolac would be less likely to affect coagulation. In contrast, Cohen et al.[198] found that postcesarean analgesia provided by the combination of intravenous ketorolac and spinal morphine was not superior to that achieved when either drug was administered alone. Patients receiving spinal morphine (0.1 or 0.2 mg) required the same amount of supplemental intravenous meperidine and had similar satisfaction scores, but they had a higher incidence of pruritus. This study may be criticized for the relatively high doses of ketorolac used (60-mg bolus followed by 30 mg every 6 hours for three doses.) It is conceivable that multimodal

benefits may have been demonstrated if smaller and perhaps safer doses (e.g., 15-mg load and then 15 mg every 6 hours) had been coadministered with an even smaller, subtherapeutic dose (0.05 mg) of intrathecal morphine.

In another multimodal trial, Sun et al.[203] reported that patients treated with epidural morphine 2 mg plus intramuscular **diclofenac** 75 mg experienced superior postcesarean analgesia and required less supplemental meperidine than individuals who received either epidural morphine or intramuscular diclofenac alone. The pain associated with uterine cramping was better controlled in the diclofenac-morphine group (Figure 28-14). The decreased intensity of uterine cramping pain was not associated with uterine hypotonia or increased postpartum bleeding.

Dennis et al.[204] evaluated the use of rectal diclofenac 100 mg as an adjunct to intrathecal morphine 0.2 mg. Rectal diclofenac did not enhance analgesia, but it prolonged the time to first request for supplemental analgesia by more than 5 hours. Lim et al.[205] studied the effect of a single postcesarean dose of rectal diclofenac 100 mg in conjunction with PCEA ropivacaine 0.2% with fentanyl 2 μg/mL in 48 parturients undergoing cesarean section. Diclofenac provided effective postcesarean analgesia and reduced epidural local anesthetic/opioid requirements by 33% during the first 24 hours postoperatively. Cardoso et al.[206] evaluated the use of intramuscular diclofenac 75 mg (administered every 8 hours) as an adjunct to intrathecal morphine (0.025 to 0.1 mg) for postcesarean analgesia. Intrathecal morphine 0.025 mg combined with intramuscular diclofenac provided excellent postcesarean analgesia, with a modest incidence of pruritus. The authors concluded that there was no advantage in giving a dose of intrathecal morphine larger than 0.025 mg when combined with intramuscular diclofenac.

In another study, the use of rectal **indomethacin** 100 mg with intrathecal morphine (0.25 to 0.3 mg) plus fentanyl (10 to 15 μg) increased the mean time to first request for supplemental analgesia from 9 hours in the placebo-suppository group to 39.5 hours in the indomethacin group. Patients in the indomethacin group made fewer requests for supplemental analgesia for the duration of the study.[207] Similarly, in a retrospective study, Ambrose[208] observed that rectal

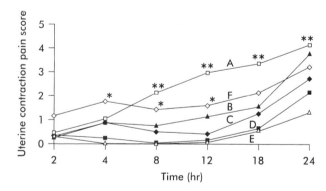

FIGURE 28-14. Uterine contraction pain scores in patients recovering from cesarean section: Groups A, B, C, D, and E received 0.5, 1, 2, 3, and 4 mg of epidural morphine, respectively, plus 75 mg of intramuscular diclofenac. Group F received 4 mg epidural morphine and intramuscular saline-placebo. *$P < 0.05$ group F versus groups D and E (4-12 hours). †$P < 0.05$ group A versus group E (8-24 hours) and group A versus group F (at 12 hours). No differences were found among groups B, C, D, and E. (From Sun HL, Wu CC, Lin MS, Chang CF. Effects of epidural morphine and intramuscular diclofenac combination in postcesarean analgesia: A dose-range study. Anesth Analg 1993; 76:284-8.)

indomethacin 50 mg reduced postcesarean opioid requirements. Yang et al.[209] have recommended the use of intrathecal morphine 0.1 mg in combination with rectal indomethacin 100 mg at the end of surgery followed by 500 mg naproxen orally twice daily. They observed that this regimen provides postcesarean analgesia of similar quality to intrathecal morphine 0.25 mg but with fewer undesirable side effects.

COX-2 Inhibitors

The cyclooxygenase-2 (COX-2) inhibitors selectively block COX-2, thereby inhibiting prostaglandin synthesis and reducing pain and inflammation following tissue injury. These drugs do not block COX-1, which maintains platelet function and gastric mucosal integrity. The COX-2 inhibitors have no effect on the bleeding time, and their efficacy in reducing pain and opioid dose requirements has been demonstrated in patients recovering from orthopedic surgery.[210] No formal studies have evaluated these agents as adjuncts to neuraxial opioid analgesia; however, one would expect efficacy similar to that reported for diclofenac and ketorolac (vide supra), with reduced risk of postoperative bleeding. At our institution, we have administered the oral suspension of **rofecoxib** 50 mg for postcesarean analgesia in patients highly sensitive to opioids. However, we avoid the COX-2 inhibitors in patients who are breast-feeding, given the lack of information regarding effects on the neonate.

Metoclopramide

Metoclopramide is an effective antiemetic for patients complaining of intraspinal opioid-induced nausea and vomiting; it also helps relieve the pain associated with uterine cramping. We have evaluated the analgesic efficacy of intravenous metoclopramide during prostaglandin-induced termination of pregnancy.[211] In this setting, the administration of metoclopramide resulted in lower pain scores, a shortened duration of labor, and a reduced requirement for PCA morphine (Figure 28-15). In contrast, metoclopramide 20 mg administered intravenously failed to improve pain scores or reduce PCA morphine requirements in patients recovering from cesarean delivery with spinal bupivacaine anesthesia.[212]

Although the mechanism of action has not been determined, metoclopramide may produce analgesia by inhibiting acetylcholinesterase, thereby increasing concentrations of acetylcholine and augmenting acetylcholine-mediated analgesia in the spinal cord. Metoclopramide-induced analgesia can be reversed by atropine but not by naloxone.[212]

Metoclopramide is a safe drug in the patient who is nursing; in fact, it is often prescribed to improve milk production in mothers of preterm infants.[213] We often give metoclopramide as an adjunct for epidural and intrathecal opioids, especially when patients complain of cramping pain or other visceral discomfort. This form of discomfort is common in patients who receive intravenous oxytocin after delivery.

Alpha-Adrenergic Agonists

Intraspinal alpha-adrenergic agonists offer the potential of effective analgesia without the nausea, pruritus, and respiratory depression associated with intraspinal opioids. Neurons in the brainstem and midbrain nuclei project to the spinal cord and modulate pain processing in the dorsal horn. A significant proportion of these descending tracts are noradrenergic; they release norepinephrine in response to noxious stimulation. Norepinephrine inhibits the release of substance P from primary afferent neurons in the dorsal horn of the spinal cord; this results in an increased pain threshold.[214] In animal models, the efficacy of intraspinal opioid analgesia is inhibited by intrathecally administered alpha-adrenergic antagonists and is augmented by both alpha-adrenergic agonists and agents that inhibit norepinephrine reuptake.[215,216]

Epidural and intrathecal alpha$_2$-adrenergic agonists provide analgesia by mimicking the activity of the descending noradrenergic system. Both laboratory studies and clinical trials have evaluated the epidural administration of the alpha$_2$-adrenergic agonist **clonidine**. Eisenach et al.[217] observed that epidural clonidine (in doses greater than 600 μg) provided rapid and reliable analgesia after cesarean section; however, the duration of complete pain relief was brief. Doses of this magnitude are associated with a number of side effects, including cardiovascular depression, altered uteroplacental perfusion, sedation, and altered release of insulin.

Narchi et al.[218] assessed the administration of smaller doses of epidural clonidine in patients recovering from cesarean section. After the regression of epidural lidocaine anesthesia, epidural doses of either 150 or 300 μg of clonidine provided more effective analgesia during the 3-hour study interval than did 10 mg of intramuscular morphine. However, the higher dose of clonidine was associated with marked sedation, obstructive apnea, and episodes of arterial oxygen desaturation.

A continuous epidural infusion of clonidine may provide a more sustained level of analgesia. This technique avoids the peak plasma concentrations associated with larger bolus doses, and it may reduce the incidence and severity of side effects. Mendez et al.[219] evaluated the safety and efficacy of epidural clonidine infusion in 60 patients who received epidural bupivacaine anesthesia for cesarean section. After delivery, patients received either a 400-μg bolus dose of epidural clonidine followed by an infusion at the rate of 10 μg/hr or an 800-μg bolus dose of clonidine followed by an infusion at 20 μg/hr. A third group received both a

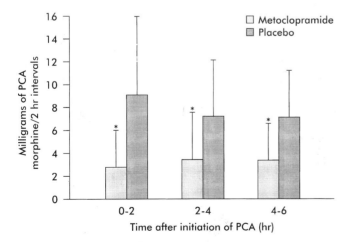

FIGURE 28-15. Patient controlled analgesia (PCA) morphine requirements in patients undergoing prostaglandin-induced abortion. The dark bar represents patients treated with intravenous metoclopramide 10 mg every 6 hours; the hatched bar represents patients receiving saline-placebo. *$P < 0.05$. (From Rosenblatt WH, Cioffi AM, Sinatra RS, Silverman DG. Metoclopramide-enhanced analgesia for prostaglandin-induced termination of pregnancy. Anesth Analg 1992; 75:760-3.)

bolus and an infusion of saline-placebo. The lower dose of clonidine provided negligible analgesia; however, patients who received the larger dose of clonidine required 50% less PCA morphine during the first 24 hours than patients treated with epidural saline. Epidural clonidine was associated with transient sedation, but other side effects were minimal.

Huntoon et al.[220] suggested that 400 μg of epidural clonidine administered when the patient first perceives pain in the PACU represents the optimal loading dose. They suggested that an infusion rate of 40 μg/hr provides more reliable analgesia and a greater reduction in PCA morphine use during the first 24 hours. These authors also noted that the prior epidural administration of 2-chloroprocaine (but not bupivacaine) attenuated the subsequent efficacy of epidural clonidine analgesia. The etiology of 2-chloroprocaine's antagonism of alpha$_2$-adrenergic analgesia is unclear, but it may have been related to the presence of the calcium chelator disodium EDTA, which may have interfered with calcium-mediated analgesic effects. The current formulation of 2-chloroprocaine (for epidural administration) does not contain EDTA.

Capogna et al.[221] observed that the addition of clonidine (75 to 150 μg) to epidural morphine 2 mg significantly increased the duration of postcesarean analgesia without increasing the risk of side effects. Mogensen et al.[222] evaluated the quality of postoperative analgesia provided by a continuous epidural infusion of morphine and 0.125% bupivacaine, with or without clonidine. The addition of clonidine resulted in improved analgesia during cough and movement. However, this three-drug combination was associated with enhanced sympathetic blockade and an increased incidence of hypotension. An isobolographic evaluation of epidural clonidine (in doses ranging from 50 to 400 μg) plus fentanyl (15 to 135 μg) did not demonstrate synergy between clonidine and fentanyl in patients recovering from cesarean delivery[223]; this study suggested that these two drugs interact in an additive rather than a synergistic manner in humans. Nonetheless, the study also suggested that clonidine and fentanyl may be combined to provide excellent analgesia, with few side effects.[223]

Aside from its use in cancer patients, there have been few clinical evaluations of intrathecal clonidine.[224-226] Filos et al.[224] reported that intrathecal clonidine 150 μg provided more than 6 hours of pain relief in patients recovering from cesarean section. Intrathecal clonidine resulted in greater sedation and a greater number of complaints of dry mouth as compared with intrathecal administration of saline-placebo. Subsequently, the same group of investigators compared 150, 300, and 450 μg of intrathecal clonidine in patients recovering from general anesthesia for elective cesarean section. They observed dose-dependent analgesia lasting 402 ± 75 minutes, 570 ± 76 minutes, and 864 ± 80 minutes, respectively. Intrathecal clonidine reduced mean arterial pressure ($21 \pm 13\%$) only in the group of patients who received 150 μg of clonidine. Relative hemodynamic stability was observed after the intrathecal administration of the two larger doses (300 and 450 μg) of clonidine; the nearly immediate onset of analgesia suggested a spinal rather than systemic site of action.[225] Benhamou et al.[226] evaluated the addition of clonidine 75 μg (with or without fentanyl 12.5 μg) to hyperbaric bupivacaine during the administration of spinal anesthesia for cesarean section. The addition of clonidine improved intraoperative analgesia without an increase in side effects. The addition of both clonidine and fentanyl further improved analgesia but resulted in an increase in sedation and pruritus.

The FDA has approved a solution of clonidine (Duraclon, Roxane Laboratories) for epidural administration in patients with severe cancer pain that is not adequately relieved by opioid analgesics alone. The package insert states that epidural clonidine "is not recommended for obstetrical, postpartum, or perioperative pain management. The risk of hemodynamic instability, especially hypotension and bradycardia, from epidural clonidine may be unacceptable in these patients. However, in a rare obstetrical, postpartum or perioperative patient, potential benefits may outweigh the possible risks."

Dexmedetomidine is an alpha$_2$-adrenergic receptor agonist. Intravenous administration of dexmedetomidine 0.4 μg/kg provided modest analgesia and reduced 24-hour morphine requirements in patients recovering from laparoscopic tubal ligation.[227] Patients treated with dexmedetomidine had higher respiratory rates and SaO$_2$ than individuals who received opioids alone; however, they also experienced side effects, including sedation and bradycardia.

The side effects (e.g., sedation, hypotension, bradycardia) that follow the intraspinal administration of clonidine or dexmedetomidine have tempered the enthusiasm for the intraspinal administration of alpha$_2$-adrenergic agonists. Future studies undoubtedly will assess the potential synergy between alpha$_2$-adrenergic agonists and opioid analgesics.[228] Intraspinal administration of more selective alpha$_2$-adrenergic agonists may be advantageous in patients recovering from cesarean section and other operative procedures.

Droperidol

Droperidol has weak alpha-adrenergic properties that may provide useful augmentation of intraspinal analgesia. Naji et al.[229] observed that patients who received a combination of epidural droperidol 2.5 mg plus morphine 4 mg experienced equivalent postoperative analgesia, with a 50% reduction in annoying side effects (e.g., pruritus, emesis, urinary retention) as compared with patients who received epidural morphine alone. Droperidol-morphine therapy was associated with an initial increase in the level of sedation; however, during the next 8 to 12 hours, sedation scores were higher in patients treated with morphine alone. This finding may reflect the greater need for supplemental antiemetics in the morphine-only group and the sedative effects associated with those agents. Sanansilp et al.[230] assessed the concurrent administration of either epidural or intravenous droperidol 2.5 mg with epidural morphine 5 mg after cesarean section. Intravenous—but not epidural—droperidol reduced the incidence of nausea and vomiting without causing an increase in sedation. Neither intravenous nor epidural droperidol reduced the incidence or severity of pruritus.

Ketamine

Ketamine interacts with both sigma-opioid and N-methyl-D-aspartate receptors and has been used as an epidural analgesic.[231,232] In laboratory animals, intrathecal ketamine was not associated with neurologic dysfunction or neuropathologic changes.[233] Naguib et al.[231] observed that epidural ketamine 30 mg provided effective analgesia of intermediate duration in general surgical patients. Despite the relatively large dose administered, no patient experienced respiratory depression or dysphoria. Four patients complained of transient burning in the back during injection; however, no neurologic complications were observed. In a double-blind study, Kawana et al.[232] noted that low-dose epidural keta-mine (4, 6, and 8 mg) provided inferior analgesia as com-pared with epidural morphine 3 mg in patients recovering from gynecologic surgery. Epidural administration of both an opioid and ketamine may activate spinal opioid and N-methyl-D-aspartate receptors, which might result in additive analgesia. This combination has not been evaluated in patients recovering from cesarean section. In a study of nonobstetric patients, Chia et al.[234] demonstrated an addi-tive analgesic effect when ketamine was added to a multi-modal PCEA regimen that also included morphine, bupivacaine, and epinephrine.

Neostigmine

Intrathecal administration of neostigmine (an anti-cholinesterase agent) inhibits the metabolism of spinally released acetylcholine and produces analgesia in animals[235-237] and humans,[238-242] without the side effect of pruritus or the risk of delayed respiratory depression. Krukowski et al.[241] noted that intrathecal neostigmine (10 to 100 µg) resulted in a dose-dependent reduction in the use of intravenous PCA morphine after cesarean section. However, their results sug-gested that intrathecal neostigmine may result in an increased incidence of nausea. Chung et al.[242] observed that intrathecal neostigmine 25 µg resulted in postcesarean anal-gesia similar to that provided by intrathecal morphine 0.1 mg but with a high incidence of nausea and vomiting. The combination of intrathecal neostigmine 12.5 µg and intrathecal morphine 0.05 mg appeared to produce better analgesia with fewer side effects than either intrathecal neostigmine 25 µg or intrathecal morphine 0.1 mg alone. Neostigmine is not approved for intrathecal administration. The high incidence of nausea that follows intrathecal neostigmine administration will likely limit its use as a sole analgesic agent. Perhaps intrathecal neostigmine may prove useful as an adjunct to other agents.

Ilioinguinal Nerve Block

Ilioinguinal nerve blocks have been used to supplement intrathecal opioid analgesia in patients recovering from cesarean section performed with a Pfannenstiel incision. Witkowski et al.[243] noted that patients who received ilioin-guinal nerve blocks had a similar quality of analgesia but less itching than patients who received either intrathecal mor-phine 0.15 mg or ilioinguinal nerve blocks plus the same dose of intrathecal morphine. There appears to be no postoperative analgesic benefit to performing either ilioinguinal nerve blocks[244] or preoperative skin infiltration with 0.5% bupiva-caine[245] in patients receiving spinal anesthesia for elective cesarean section.

CONTROVERSIES AND RELATIVE CONTRAINDICATIONS

Most patients who qualify for either spinal or epidural anes-thesia can safely receive intraspinal opioid therapy, provided that the nursing staff has received adequate education and that close patient surveillance is maintained. Intraspinal opi-oid analgesia is contraindicated in settings in which there are no standardized orders, no nursing policies and proce-dures, and no qualified clinician who is available to manage complications.

Several maternal conditions represent relative contraindi-cations to intraspinal opioid therapy. In these cases, the anes-thesiologist should assess the risks and benefits for the individual patient before deciding whether to proceed with intraspinal opioid therapy.

Herpes Simplex Virus Labialis

As much as 40% to 50% of the United States population may experience recurrent herpes simplex virus (HSV) infec-tions,[246] and exposure to epidural/intrathecal morphine may increase the risk of recrudescence. The administration of epidural morphine increases the incidence of reactivation of HSV labialis (HSVL or HSV-1) in patients recovering from cesarean section.[19,247,248] In a prospective study of 729 patients recovering from cesarean section, Crone et al.[247] observed recurrent HSV-1 infection in 13 (9.3%) of 140 patients who received epidural morphine versus only 6 (1.0%) of 583 patients who did not receive epidural morphine. Subsequently, in a randomized evaluation of seropositive parturients, these investigators noted that 19 (19.8%) of 96 patients who received epidural morphine developed oral lesions within the first 5 days after cesarean section.[248] In contrast, none of the 91 patients who received intramuscular opioids developed evidence of recurrent infection. These investigators did not determine the frequency of asymptomatic oral viral shedding. Primary HSV infection was not observed in the infants of symptomatic mothers. The authors suggested that facial pru-ritus might be linked to the reactivation of latent HSV-1 infec-tion, perhaps because of opioid activity within the trigeminal nerve ganglion. However, two subsequent prospective studies provided conflicting results. In one study, the effects of neu-raxial morphine and parenteral opioids did not differ signifi-cantly.[249] In the other study, the incidence of recurrent HSV-1 infection was 11.5 times higher with epidural morphine than with parenteral morphine.[250]

Boyle[251] suggested that intraspinal morphine may remove host repression of viral regulatory polypeptide synthesis in the central trigeminal nuclei or ganglion, thus causing the reacti-vation of HSV-1 infection. He offered the following specula-tion: "Virus replication, axonal migration and intraepithelial shedding then proceeds from nerve endings. At the same time, morphine causes a selective quantitative deficiency in cell-mediated immunity to HSV-1. The virus may then prolif-erate within the epidermis and cause a local lesion before host immune defenses can clear it."[251]

It is unclear whether all opioids are capable of reactivating HSV-1 in susceptible patients. No published study has docu-mented an increased risk of recurrent HSV-1 infection in obstetric patients who received epidural fentanyl during or after cesarean section. Valley et al.[252] reported a nonobstetric patient who had recurrent HSV-1 infection approximately 36 hours after an epidural infusion of fentanyl was initiated for postoperative analgesia.

Other factors may affect the risk of recurrent HSV-1 infec-tion, including the following: (1) intrathecal delivery of a large dose of drug (secondary to unintentional dural puncture); (2) hormonal responses to surgical trauma; (3) emotional stress; and (4) socioeconomic status. Weiss et al.[253] observed that intrathecal or epidural morphine administration did not increase the incidence of recurrent HSV-1 infection in a patient population that was heterogeneous for race and socioeconomic status. Approximately 6% of patients who received both regional anesthesia and intraspinal morphine developed recurrent lesions versus 4% of the patients who received regional anesthesia without intraspinal morphine. Of interest, 11% of patients who received general anesthesia had recurrent HSV-1 infection.

Notwithstanding these observations, the anesthesiologist should exercise caution in the administration of epidural or intrathecal morphine in parturients with a history of HSV-1 infection. Neonatal HSV infection is a serious illness, and it would be devastating for the mother to transmit this infection to her newborn. It seems prudent to notify the patient of the potential for reactivation of the virus and to discuss alternative methods of analgesia.

Human Immunodeficiency Virus

There are few data on the risks and benefits of intraspinal opioid administration in patients with human immunodeficiency virus (HIV) infection. Tom et al.[254] noted that HIV-positive patients who underwent diagnostic dural puncture followed by epidural blood patch did not experience deterioration in CNS function or evidence of CNS infection. Hughes et al.[255] observed no neurologic or infectious complications after the administration of epidural or intrathecal local anesthetics and opioids in HIV-positive parturients. Unfortunately, both of these studies assessed outcome in a small number of patients. At Yale-New Haven Hospital, HIV-positive patients are evaluated and treated on an individual basis. Patients who are HIV-positive deserve the same quality of intrapartum and postoperative analgesia as uninfected patients. We typically administer either epidural or intrathecal opioids to individuals for whom regional anesthesia is not contraindicated. In general, we avoid epidural and intrathecal opioids in HIV-positive patients with sepsis, significant depression of platelet and white blood cell count, and clinical evidence of CNS or spinal cord involvement.

Epilepsy

In general, intraspinal opioid administration does not result in an increased risk for recurrent seizures. A possible exception is the epidural administration of meperidine. Meperidine's major metabolite is normeperidine, which causes increased CNS excitability. For this reason, it seems prudent to avoid multiple doses (or a continuous infusion) of meperidine in patients with a history of a seizure disorder. Likewise, we avoid multiple doses of meperidine in preeclamptic patients.

Patients with a seizure disorder may be sensitive to hypoventilation and/or mild hypoxemia. Borgeat et al.[256] reported a case of a 30-year-old epileptic patient recovering from cesarean section who developed a tonic-clonic seizure 6 hours after the administration of epidural morphine. The authors suggested that increased CNS excitability may have resulted from an opioid-induced alteration in ventilation and that patients with a seizure disorder should be given supplemental oxygen and monitored closely.

Multiple Sclerosis

Berger and Ontell[257] reported the intrathecal administration of tetracaine and morphine 0.5 mg in a patient with slowly progressive multiple sclerosis. The patient experienced 24 hours of effective postoperative analgesia and did not experience a recurrence of multiple sclerosis during a 6-month interval after surgery. Intraspinal opioid therapy should be limited to the use of widely prescribed agents (e.g., preservative-free solutions of morphine or fentanyl). It seems prudent to avoid intraspinal opioid therapy in patients who are experiencing an exacerbation of their disease.

Substance Abuse

Patients who abuse opioids and individuals who use opioids for the treatment of chronic pain often have significant opioid tolerance as well as physical and psychologic dependency. They typically have a low pain threshold and unrealistic expectations regarding pain relief. Intrathecal or epidural opioid therapy is ideal for this patient population, because these patients benefit from prolonged, effective analgesia and are rarely troubled by annoying side effects or respiratory depression. We recommend a continuous epidural infusion of opioid in these patients; the epidural infusion should be maintained until the patient tolerates oral analgesics.

The anesthesiologist should keep the following two caveats in mind. First, although an intraspinal opioid provides effective postoperative analgesia, plasma concentrations of opioid typically are lower than those required to maintain physical and psychologic well-being. Intramuscular methadone or oral methadone elixir must also be administered to prevent symptoms of acute withdrawal. Second, epidural or intrathecal administration of a mixed agonist-antagonist should be avoided in these patients. These agents may bind to mu-opioid receptors and precipitate an acute abstinence syndrome.[258]

Asthma

Parenteral administration of opioids (especially morphine and meperidine) causes mast cells to release histamine, which may precipitate bronchospasm in asthmatic patients. Plasma histamine concentrations are not increased in patients who complain of pruritus after the epidural administration of morphine[161]; this suggests that epidural and intrathecal morphine therapy is unlikely to precipitate bronchospasm. There appears to be little risk associated with the intrathecal administration of 0.1 to 0.25 mg of morphine in patients with well-controlled asthma. However, it seems prudent to avoid epidural administration of morphine or meperidine in symptomatic parturients. These individuals—as well as those patients with mastocytosis, carcinoid syndrome, and a history of morphine-induced anaphylaxis—may be safely managed with a continuous epidural infusion of fentanyl or sufentanil.

Morbid Obesity

Morbidly obese patients and individuals with sleep apnea and Pickwickian syndrome are more likely to develop opioid-induced sedation, airway obstruction, and hypoventilation. Van Dercar et al.[259] reported a near-fatal episode of respiratory depression during the use of PCA morphine in an obese patient with sleep apnea. These patients benefit from reductions in movement-associated pain and total opioid dose, but they appear to be quite sensitive to the sedative and respiratory depressant effects of epidural and intrathecal morphine.[117] The anesthesiologist should carefully consider the risks and benefits of intraspinal opioid therapy in morbidly obese patients. We offer the following recommendations for the use of intraspinal opioids in these patients. First, they should be monitored with continuous pulse oximetry in a high-visibility setting for the first 24 hours after delivery. Second, low-flow nasal oxygen should be administered. Third, prophylactic intravenous infusion of naloxone should be considered. Fourth, sedative-hypnotic agents (e.g., diphenhydramine, droperidol) should be avoided.

EFFECTS ON OUTCOME AFTER CESAREAN SECTION

Although intraspinal opioids currently represent the "gold standard" for providing effective postcesarean analgesia, it has been difficult to demonstrate that intraspinal opioid techniques improve perioperative outcome. This difficulty may be attributed in part to the fact that most of these patients are young, healthy, and at low risk for serious perioperative morbidity and mortality. Nonetheless, intraspinal opioids provide several therapeutic advantages in these patients. Few individuals would question that a technique that safely and effectively minimizes pain and suffering should be provided for humanitarian reasons alone. Intraspinal opioid therapy facilitates earlier sitting, standing, and ambulation after cesarean section.[260] In theory, early ambulation and improved pulmonary toilet reduce the incidence of deep vein thrombosis and pneumonia after cesarean section. Pregnancy results in hypercoagulability, especially during the puerperium. Surgical trauma and postoperative immobility increase the risk for deep vein thrombosis and pulmonary embolism; thus early ambulation is especially desirable in the patient who is recovering from cesarean delivery. Improved analgesia should also facilitate the interaction between the mother and her newborn.

Cohen et al.[87] retrospectively reviewed the records of 684 healthy parturients who received one of five analgesic regimens after cesarean section: (1) epidural morphine; (2) epidural morphine plus fentanyl; (3) intrathecal morphine; (4) intramuscular opioids; or (5) PCA opioids. No evidence suggested that the intraspinal opioid techniques improved maternal outcome. Likewise, Stenkamp et al.[261] found no difference in the length of hospital stay between patients who received a single epidural dose of morphine and those who received intramuscular opioids for postcesarean analgesia.

Intraspinal opioid analgesia may be more likely to improve outcome in high-risk obstetric patients. Women with severe preeclampsia, cardiovascular disease, and morbid obesity may benefit from the reduction in cardiovascular stress and improved pulmonary function associated with effective analgesia.[262,263] Rawal et al.[263] compared the efficacy of intramuscular and epidural morphine in 30 nonpregnant, morbidly obese patients recovering from abdominal surgery. Patients in the epidural morphine group were more alert and able to walk sooner, recovered bowel function earlier, and "benefited more from vigorous physiotherapy . . ., which resulted in fewer pulmonary complications."[263]

O'Flaherty et al.[264] observed that a single epidural or intrathecal dose of fentanyl does not blunt the adrenocorticotrophic hormone and cortisol responses during cesarean section. However, other investigators have noted that a continuous epidural infusion of opioid and dilute local anesthetic attenuates coagulation abnormalities and hemodynamic and stress hormone responses in nonpregnant patients.[265-267]

Some studies have suggested that opioid-based PCEA may improve postoperative outcome.[96,98,101] These studies have noted that the use of PCEA results in decreased movement-associated pain, which should facilitate deep breathing, coughing, and early ambulation. Two studies noted that patients treated with PCEA meperidine[96] and hydromorphone[103] required less drug and had shortened times to return of bowel sounds, resumption of flatus, and resumption of a solid diet as compared with similar patients who self-administered the same drug intravenously. In a prospective study, 176 patients who received sufentanil PCEA after cesarean section had a shorter length of hospital stay than patients who received intramuscular opioids.[101]

The potential advantages that intraspinal opioid analgesia offers the neonate should also be considered. Reduced maternal doses of opioid should result in decreased opioid concentrations in breast milk. In one study, a single dose of epidural morphine 4 mg significantly reduced intravenous PCA morphine requirements in nursing mothers recovering from cesarean section, and this may have been responsible for the superior neurobehavioral scores observed in the breast-fed neonates in that group.[196]

FUTURE APPLICATIONS

The future of spinal/epidural techniques for postoperative analgesia remains unclear. Some centers have begun to limit such therapy because of reductions in reimbursement. Nevertheless, a number of modifications have been proposed to improve the safety and overall efficacy of such techniques, including the following:

1. **Minidose epidural (1 to 2 mg) or intrathecal (0.05 to 0.1 mg) morphine, combined with an alpha$_2$-adrenergic agonist and perhaps small doses of intravenous ketorolac.** This combination of agents would provide multimodal analgesia[268] while minimizing dose-dependent side effects.
2. **Continuous intrathecal administration of a lipophilic opioid.** The use of this technique depends on the reapproval of small-gauge microcatheters by the FDA. This form of therapy allows the smallest possible dose of opioid to be given, and it takes maximal advantage of the selectivity of spinal analgesia.
3. **Intrathecal administration of a lipophilic opioid sequestered in albumin, lipid solvents,[269] or liposomes.** These substances function as drug depots that permit slow, sustained release of the drug, thereby extending the duration of activity.

KEY POINTS

- Epidural or intrathecal opioid administration offers several advantages to patients recovering from cesarean section: excellent analgesia, a decrease in the total dose of opioid, a low level of sedation, and minimal accumulation of the drug in breast milk. Epidural and intrathecal opioid analgesia facilitates early ambulation and perhaps an early return of bowel function.
- Epidural and intrathecal opioids bind and activate opioid receptors in the dorsal horn of the spinal cord. Hydrophilic opioids (e.g., morphine) penetrate spinal tissues slowly, and the drug remains in solution in the cerebrospinal fluid; this results in a delayed onset and a prolonged duration of action.

- Lipophilic opioids penetrate spinal tissues rapidly. These agents are also rapidly absorbed by the systemic vasculature. Consequently, the onset of action is rapid, but the duration is relatively short.
- Single-dose intrathecal or epidural administration of a lipophilic opioid improves intraoperative analgesia, but it provides only a short duration of postcesarean analgesia. Careful monitoring is essential for the safe use of epidural and intrathecal opioid techniques.
- Pruritus is the most common side effect of epidural or intrathecal morphine administration, and it is the most frequent cause of patient dissatisfaction with this technique.
- Delayed respiratory depression is a rare but serious complication that results from rostral migration of opioid to the brainstem through the cerebrospinal fluid. Most cases of delayed respiratory depression have resulted from the epidural or intrathecal administration of morphine.
- Intravenous naloxone or nalbuphine may eliminate or reduce the severity of side effects associated with intraspinal opioids without affecting the quality or duration of analgesia.
- Patient-controlled epidural infusion offers the increased control associated with self-administration techniques, and it provides a more selective form of analgesia than intravenous patient-controlled analgesia.
- The anesthesiologist may augment intraspinal opioid analgesia with restricted-dose intravenous patient-controlled analgesia or concurrent administration of a nonsteroidal antiinflammatory drug or metoclopramide.

REFERENCES

1. Wittels B, Scott DT, Sinatra R. Exogenous opioids in human breast milk and acute neonatal neurobehavior: A preliminary study. Anesthesiology 1990; 73:684-9.
2. Hawkins JL, Gibbs CP, Orleans M, et al. Obstetric anesthesia work force survey, 1981 versus 1992. Anesthesiology 1997; 87:135-43.
3. Chen B, Kwan W, Lee C, Cantley E. A national survey of obstetric post-anesthesia care in teaching hospitals (abstract). Anesth Analg 1993; 76:S43.
4. Mayer DC, Quance D, Weeks SK. Headache after spinal anesthesia for cesarean section: A comparison of the 27-gauge Quinke and 24-gauge Sprotte needles. Anesth Analg 1992; 75:377-80.
5. Sinatra RS. Unpublished observations. Yale University School of Medicine, Department of Anesthesiology, 1993-2002.
6. Cousins MJ, Mather LE. Intrathecal and epidural administration of opioids. Anesthesiology 1984; 61:276-310.
7. Gourlay GK, Cherry DA, Plummer JL, et al. The influence of drug polarity on the absorption of opioid drugs into CSF and subsequent cephalad migration following lumbar epidural administration. Pain 1987; 31:297-305.
8. Nordberg G, Hedner T, Mellstrand T, et al. Pharmacokinetic aspects of epidural morphine analgesia. Anesthesiology 1983; 58:545-51.
9. Nordberg G, Hedner T, Mellstrand T, et al. Pharmacokinetic aspects of intrathecal morphine analgesia. Anesthesiology 1984; 60:448-54.
10. Atweh SA, Kuhar MJ. Autoradiographic localization of opiate receptors in rat brain. I. Spinal cord and lower medulla. Brain Res 1977; 124:53-67.
11. Martin WF, Eades CG, Fraser HF. Use of hindlimb reflexes of the chronic spinal dog for comparing analgesics. J Pharmacol Exp Ther 1964; 144:8-11.
12. Schmauss C, Yaksh TL. In vivo studies on spinal opiate receptor systems mediating antinociception. II. Pharmacological profiles suggesting a differential association of mu, delta, and kappa receptors. J Pharmacol Exp Ther 1984; 228:1-12.
13. Kitahata LM, Kosaka Y, Taub A. Lamina-specific suppression of dorsal horn activity by morphine sulfate. Anesthesiology 1974; 41:39-48.
14. Nishio Y, Sinatra RS, Kitahata LM, et al. Spinal cord distribution of 3H-morphine after intrathecal administration: Relationship to analgesia. Anesth Analg 1989; 68:323-7.
15. Yaksh TL, Reddy SVR. Studies in the primate on the analgesic effects associated with intrathecal actions of opiates, adrenergic agonists and baclofen. Anesthesiology 1981; 54:451-67.
16. Wang J, Nauss LA, Thomas JE. Pain relief by intrathecally applied morphine in man. Anesthesiology 1979; 50:149-50.
17. Van den Hoogen RHWM, Colpaert FC. Epidural and subcutaneous morphine, meperidine (pethidine), fentanyl and sufentanil in the rat: Analgesia and other in vivo pharmacologic effects. Anesthesiology 1987; 66:186-94.
18. Cousins MJ, Mather LE, Glynn CJ. Selective spinal analgesia. Lancet 1979; 1:1141-2.
19. Fuller JG, McMorland GH, Douglas MJ, Palmer L. Epidural morphine for analgesia after caesarean section: A report of 4,880 patients. Can J Anaesth 1990; 37:636-40.
20. Palmer CM, Nogami WM, Van Maren G, Alves DM. Postcesarean epidural morphine: A dose-response study. Anesth Analg 2000; 90:887-91.
21. Asantila R, Eklund P, Rosenberg PH. Epidural analgesia with 4 mg of morphine following caesarean section: Effect of injected volume. Acta Anaesthesiol Scand 1993; 37:764-7.
22. Eisenach JC, Schlairet TJ, Dobson CE, et al. Effect of prior anesthetic solution on epidural morphine analgesia. Anesth Analg 1991; 73:119-23.
23. Abouleish E, Rawal N, Tobon-Randall B, et al. A clinical and laboratory study to compare the addition of 0.2 mg of morphine, 0.2 mg of epinephrine, or their combination to hyperbaric bupivacaine for spinal anesthesia in cesarean section. Anesth Analg 1993; 77:457-62.
24. Harrison DM, Sinatra RS, Morgese L, et al. Epidural narcotic and PCA for postcesarean section pain relief. Anesthesiology 1988; 68:454-7.
25. Eisenach JC, Grice SC, Dewan DM. Patient controlled analgesia following cesarean section: A comparison with epidural and intramuscular narcotics. Anesthesiology 1988; 68:444-8.
26. Cade L, Ashley J, Ross W. Comparison of epidural and intravenous opioid analgesia after elective caesarean section. Anaesth Intensive Care 1992; 20:41-5.
27. Chadwick HS, Bernards CM, Kovarik DW, Tomlin JJ. Subdural injection of morphine for analgesia following cesarean section: A report of three cases. Anesthesiology 1992; 77:590-4.
28. Bromage PR, Camporesi EM, Durant PAC, et al. Rostral spread of epidural morphine. Anesthesiology 1982; 56:431-5.
29. Kafer ER, Brown JT, Scott D, et al. Biphasic depression of ventilatory responses to CO_2 following epidural morphine. Anesthesiology 1987; 58:418-27.
30. Leicht CH, Durkan WJ, Fians DH, et al. Postoperative analgesia with epidural morphine: Single bolus vs. Daymate elastomeric continuous infusion technique (abstract). Anesthesiology 1990; 73:A931.
31. Wolfe MJ, Nicholas ADG. Selective epidural analgesia. Lancet 1979; 2:150.
32. Naulty JS, Datta S, Ostheimer GW, et al. Epidural fentanyl for postcesarean delivery pain management. Anesthesiology 1985; 63:694-8.
33. Robertson K, Douglas MJ, McMorland GH. Epidural fentanyl, with and without epinephrine for postcesarean section analgesia. Can Anaesth Soc J 1985; 32:502-5.
34. Sevarino FB, McFarlane C, Sinatra RS, et al. Epidural fentanyl does not influence intravenous PCA requirements in the post-caesarean patient. Can J Anaesth 1991; 38:450-3.
35. Rosen MA, Dailey PA, Hughes SC, et al. Epidural sufentanil for postoperative analgesia after cesarean section. Anesthesiology 1988; 68:448-52.
36. Paech MJ. Post caesarean section pain relief with epidural pethidine or fentanyl. Anaesth Intensive Care 1989; 17:157-65.
37. Semple AJ, Macrae DJ, Munishankarappa S, et al. Effect of the addition of adrenaline to extradural diamorphine analgesia after caesarean section. Br J Anaesth 1988; 60:632-8.
38. De Leon-Casasola OA, Lema MJ. Postoperative epidural opioid analgesia: What are the choices? Anesth Analg 1996; 83:867-75.
39. Tejwani GA, Rattan AK, McDonald JS. Role of spinal opioid receptors in the antinociceptive interactions between intrathecal morphine and bupivacaine. Anesth Analg 1992; 74:726-34.
40. Penning JP, Yaksh TL. Interaction of intrathecal morphine with bupivacaine and lidocaine in the rat. Anesthesiology 1992; 77:1186-200.
41. Camann WR, Hartigan PM, Gilbertson LI, et al. Chloroprocaine antagonism of epidural opioid analgesia: A receptor-specific phenomenon? Anesthesiology 1990; 73:860-3.

42. Birnbach DJ, Johnson MD, Arcario T, et al. Effect of diluent volume on analgesia produced by epidural fentanyl. Anesth Analg 1988; 68:808-10.

43. Katz J, Kavanagh BP, Sandler AN, et al. Preemptive analgesia: Clinical evidence of neuroplasticity contributing to postoperative pain. Anesthesiology 1992; 77:439-46.

44. Preston P, Rosen M, Hughes SC, et al. Epidural anesthesia with fentanyl and lidocaine for cesarean section: Maternal effects and neonatal outcome. Anesthesiology 1988; 68:938-43.

45. Youngstrom P, Hoyt M, Herman M, et al. Dose-response study of continuous infusion epidural fentanyl-epinephrine for postcesarean analgesia. Anesthesiology 1990; 73:A984.

46. Glass PSA, Estok P, Ginsberg B, et al. Use of patient-controlled analgesia to compare the efficacy of epidural to intravenous fentanyl administration. Anesth Analg 1992; 74:345-51.

47. Loper KA, Ready LB, Sandler A. Epidural and intravenous fentanyl infusions are clinically equivalent following knee surgery. Anesth Analg 1990; 70:72-5.

48. Ellis JD, Millar WL, Reisner LS. A randomized double-blind comparison of epidural versus intravenous fentanyl infusion for analgesia after cesarean section. Anesthesiology 1990; 72:981-6.

49. Cohen S, Pantuck CB, Amar D, et al. The primary action of epidural fentanyl after cesarean delivery is via a spinal mechanism. Anesth Analg 2002; 94:674-9.

50. Youngstrom P, Boyd B, Rhoton F. Complaints of side effects from postcesarean epidural opioid analgesia: Fewer with fentanyl-epinephrine infusion than with morphine bolus (abstract). Anesthesiology 1992; 77:A859.

51. Lam AM, Knill RL, Thompson WR, et al. Epidural fentanyl does not cause delayed respiratory depression. Can Anaesth Soc J 1983; 30:578-9.

52. Negre I, Gueneron JP, Ecoffey C, et al. Ventilatory response to carbon dioxide after intramuscular and epidural fentanyl. Anesth Analg 1987; 66:707-10.

53. Grass JA, Sakima NT, Schmidt R, et al. A randomized, double-blind, dose-response comparison of epidural fentanyl versus sufentanil analgesia after cesarean section. Anesth Analg 1997; 85:365-71.

54. Tan S, White PF, Cohen SE. Sufentanil for postcesarean analgesia: Epidural vs. intravenous administration (abstract). Anesthesiology 1986; 65:A398.

55. Leight CH, Kelleher AJ, Robinson DE, et al. Prolongation of postoperative epidural sufentanil analgesia with epinephrine. Anesth Analg 1990; 70:323-8.

56. Ionescu IT, Taverne RHT, Houweling PL, et al. Pharmacokinetic study of extradural and intrathecal sufentanil anesthesia for major surgery. Br J Anaesth 1991; 66: 458-64.

57. DeSousa H, Stiller R. Cisternal CSF and arterial plasma levels of fentanyl, alfentanil and sufentanil after lumbar epidural injection (abstract). Anesthesiology 1989; 71:A839.

58. Stevens RA, Petty RH, Hill HF, et al. Redistribution of sufentanil to cerebrospinal fluid and systemic circulation after epidural administration in dogs. Anesth Analg 1993; 76:323-7.

59. Rosen MA, Hughes SC, Shnider SM, et al. Continuous epidural sufentanil for postoperative analgesia (abstract). Anesth Analg 1990; 70:S331.

60. Coda BA, Kawata J, Ross BK. Plasma sufentanil concentration during prolonged epidural infusion for postoperative analgesia (abstract). Anesth Analg 1993; 76:S49.

61. Seitman DT. Comparison between epidural sufentanil and epidural bupivacaine used for immediate post cesarean section relief in the patient already receiving epidural morphine (abstract). Anesthesiology 1990; 73:A989.

62. Cohen SE, Labaille T, Benhamou D, et al. Respiratory effects of epidural sufentanil after cesarean section. Anesth Analg 1992; 74:677-82.

63. Dougherty TB, Baysinger CL, Henenberger JC, et al. Epidural hydromorphone with and without epinephrine for post-operative analgesia after cesarean delivery. Anesth Analg 1989; 68:318-22.

64. Macrae DJ, Munishankarappa S, Burrow LM, et al. Double blind comparison of the efficacy of extradural diamorphine, extradural phenoperidine and intramuscular diamorphine following caesarean section. Br J Anaesth 1987; 59:354-9.

65. Beeby D, MacIntosh KC, Bailey M. Postoperative analgesia after caesarean section using epidural methadone. Anaesthesia 1984; 39:61-3.

66. Simpson KH, Madej TH, Mcdowell JM. Comparison of extradural buprenorphine and extradural morphine after caesarean section. Br J Anaesth 1988; 60:627-31.

67. Abboud TK, Moore M, Zhu J, et al. Epidural butorphanol or morphine for the relief of postcesarean section pain. Anesth Analg 1987; 66:887-93.

68. Brownridge P, Frewin DB. A comparative study of techniques of postoperative analgesia following caesarean section and lower abdominal surgery. Anaesth Intensive Care 1985; 13:123-30.

69. Perriss BW, Latham BV, Wilson IH. Analgesia following extradural and intramuscular pethidine in post-caesarean section patients. Br J Anaesth 1990; 64:355-7.

70. Ngan Kee WD, Lam KK, Chen PP, Gin T. Epidural meperidine after cesarean section: The effect of diluent volume. Anesth Analg 1997; 85:380-4.

71. Ngan Kee WD, Lam KK, Chen PP, Gin T. Epidural meperidine after cesarean section: A dose-response study. Anesthesiology 1996; 85:289-94.

72. Khaw KS, Ngan Kee WD, Critchley LAH. Epidural meperidine does not cause hemodynamic changes in the term parturient. Can J Anaesth 2000; 47:155-9.

73. Ngan Kee WD, Khaw KS, Ma ML. The effect of the addition of adrenaline to pethidine for patient-controlled epidural analgesia after caesarean section. Anaesthesia 1998; 53:1012-27.

74. Chestnut DH, Choi WW, Isbell TJ. Epidural hydromorphone for postcesarean analgesia. Obstet Gynecol 1986; 68:65-9.

75. Henderson SK, Matthew EB, Cohen H, et al. Epidural hydromorphone: A double-blind comparison with intramuscular hydromorphone for postcesarean section analgesia. Anesthesiology 1987; 66:825-30.

76. Halpern SH, Arellano R, Preston R, et al. Epidural morphine vs. hydromorphone in post-caesarean section patients. Can J Anaesth 1996; 43:595-8.

77. Chaplan SR, Duncan SR, Brodsky JB. Morphine and hydromorphone epidural analgesia. Anesthesiology 1992; 77:1090-4.

78. Haynes SR, Davidson I, Allsop JR, Dutton DA. Comparison of epidural methadone with epidural diamorphine for analgesia following caesarean section. Acta Anaesthesiol Scand 1993; 37:375-80.

79. Semple AJ, Macrae DJ, Munishankarappa S, et al. Effect of the addition of adrenaline to extradural diamorphine analgesia after caesarean section. Br J Anaesth 1988; 60:632-8.

80. Palacios QT, Jones MM, Hawkins JL, et al. Postcesarean section analgesia: A comparison of epidural butorphanol and morphine. Can J Anaesth 1991; 38:24-30.

81. Camann WR, Loferski BL, Fanciullo GJ, et al. Does epidural butorphanol offer any clinical advantage over the intravenous route? Anesthesiology 1992; 76:216-20.

82. Rawal N, Nuutinen L, Raj PP, et al. Behavioral and histopathologic effects following intrathecal administration of butorphanol, sufentanil and nalbuphine in sheep. Anesthesiology 1991; 75:1025-34.

83. Eisenach J. Opioid antagonist adjuncts to epidural morphine for postcesarean analgesia: Maternal outcomes (letter). Anesth Analg 1994; 79:611.

84. Yaksh T, Birnbach D. Intrathecal nalbuphine after cesarean delivery: Are we ready? Anesth Analg 2000; 91:505-8.

85. Camann WR, Hurley RH, Gilbertson LI, et al. Epidural nalbuphine for analgesia following caesarean delivery: Dose-response and effect of local anaesthetic choice. Can J Anaesth 1991; 38:728-32.

86. Parker RK, Holtmann B, White PF. Patient-controlled epidural analgesia: Interactions between nalbuphine and hydromorphone. Anesth Analg 1997; 84:757-63.

87. Cohen SE, Subak LL, Brose WG, et al. Epidural analgesia for cesarean section: Patient evaluations and costs of five opioid techniques. Reg Anesth 1991; 16:141-9.

88. Vincent RD, Chestnut DH, Choi WW, et al. Does epidural fentanyl decrease the efficacy of epidural morphine after cesarean delivery? Anesth Analg 1992; 74:658-63.

89. Dottrens M, Rifat K, Morel DR. Comparison of extradural administration of sufentanil, morphine and sufentanil-morphine combination after caesarean section. Br J Anaesth 1992; 69:9-12.

90. Wittels B, Glosten B, Faure EAM, et al. Opioid antagonist adjuncts to epidural morphine for postcesarean analgesia: Maternal outcomes. Anesth Analg 1993; 77:925-32.

91. Wittels B, Toledano A. The effects of epidural morphine and epidural butorphanol on maternal outcomes after cesarean delivery (letter). Anesth Analg 1998; 81:1317.

92. Lawhorn CD, McNitt JD, Fibuch EE, et al. Epidural morphine with butorphanol for postoperative analgesia after cesarean delivery. Anesth Analg 1991; 72:53-7.

93. Gambling DR, Huber C, Howell P, Kozak S. Epidural butorphanol does not reduce side-effects from epidural morphine post-caesarean section (abstract). Proc Soc Obstet Anesth Perinatol 1991; 22:17.

94. Chrubasik J, Wust H, Schulte-Monting J, et al. Relative analgesic potency of epidural fentanyl, alfentanil, and morphine in treatment of postoperative pain. Anesthesiology 1988; 68:929-33.

95. Walmsley PNH. Patient controlled epidural analgesia. In: Sinatra RS, Hord A, Ginsberg B, Preble L, editors. Acute Pain: Mechanisms and Management. St. Louis, MO, Mosby, 1992:312-20.

96. Yarnell RW, Murphy IL, Polis T, et al. Patient-controlled analgesia with epidural meperidine after cesarean section. Reg Anesth 1992; 17:329-33.

97. Rosaeg OP, Lindsay MP. Epidural opioid analgesia after caesarean section: A comparison of patient-controlled analgesia with meperidine and single bolus injection of morphine. Can J Anaesth 1994; 41: 1063-8.

98. Ngan Kee WD, Lam KK, Chen PP, Gin T. Comparison of patient-controlled epidural analgesia with patient-controlled intravenous analgesia using pethidine or fentanyl. Anaesth Intensive Care 1997; 25:126-32.

99. Boudreault D, Brasseur L, Samii K, Lemoing JP. Comparison of continuous epidural bupivacaine infusion plus either continuous epidural infusion or patient-controlled epidural injection of fentanyl for postoperative analgesia. Anesth Analg 1991; 73:132-7.

100. Yu PYH, Gambling DR. A comparative study of patient-controlled epidural fentanyl and single dose epidural morphine for post-caesarean analgesia. Can J Anaesth 1993; 40:416-20.

101. Cooper DW, Ryall DM, McHardy FE, et al. Patient-controlled extradural analgesia with bupivacaine, fentanyl, or a mixture of both, after caesarean section. Br J Anaesth 1996; 76:611-5.

102. Cohen S, Amar D, Pantuck CB, et al. Adverse effects of epidural 0.03% bupivacaine during analgesia after cesarean section. Anesth Analg 1992; 75:753-6.

103. Parker R, White P. Epidural patient-controlled analgesia: An alternative to intravenous patient controlled analgesia for pain relief after cesarean delivery. Anesth Analg 1992; 75:245-51.

104. Parker R, Sawaki Y, White PF. Epidural patient-controlled analgesia: Influence of bupivacaine and hydromorphone basal infusion on pain control after cesarean delivery. Anesth Analg 1992; 75:740-6.

105. Parker R, Holtman B, White PF. Patient-controlled epidural analgesia: Interactions between nalbuphine and hydromorphone. Anesth Analg 1997; 84:757-63.

106. Grass JA, Zuckerman RL, Tsao H, et al. Patient controlled epidural analgesia results in shorter hospital stay after cesarean section (abstract). Reg Anesth 1991; 15(suppl):26.

107. Grass JA, Harris AP, Sakima NT, et al. Pain management after cesarean section: Sufentanil PCEA versus morphine IV-PCA (abstract). Anesth Analg 1992; 74:S120.

108. Sinatra RS, Sevarino FB, Paige D, et al. Patient controlled analgesia with sufentanil: A comparison of intravenous versus epidural administration. J Clin Anesth 1996; 8:123.

109. Cohen S, Amar D, Pantuck CB, et al. Postcesarean delivery epidural patient-controlled analgesia, fentanyl or sufentanil. Anesthesiology 1993; 78:486-91.

110. Fanshawe MP. A comparison of patient controlled epidural pethidine versus single dose epidural morphine for analgesia after caesarean section. Anaesth Intensive Care 1999; 27:610-14.

111. Zakowski MI, Ramanathan S, Sharnick S. Uptake and distribution of bupivacaine and morphine after intrathecal administration in parturients: Effects of epinephrine. Anesth Analg 1992; 74:664-9.

112. Zakowski MI, Ramanathan S, Khoo P, et al. Pharmacokinetics of two-dose epidural morphine regimen for cesarean section analgesia (abstract). Anesth Analg 1991; 72:S332.

113. Abboud TK, Dror A, Mosaad P, et al. Minidose intrathecal morphine for the relief of postcesarean section pain: Safety, efficacy, and ventilatory responses to carbon dioxide. Anesth Analg 1988; 67:137-41.

114. Chadwick HS, Ready LB. Intrathecal and epidural morphine sulfate for postcesarean analgesia: A clinical comparison. Anesthesiology 1988; 68:925-9.

115. Abouleish E, Rawal N, Rashad MN. The addition of 0.2 mg subarachnoid morphine to hyperbaric bupivacaine for cesarean delivery: A prospective study of 856 cases. Reg Anesth 1991; 16:137-40.

116. Gerancher FC, Floyd H, Eisenach J. Determination of an effective dose of intrathecal morphine for pain relief after cesarean delivery. Anesth Analg 1999; 88:346-51.

117. Huffnagle HJ, Norris MC, Leighton BL, et al. A dose-response study of intrathecal morphine for post cesarean section analgesia (abstract). Anesth Analg 1997; 84:S388.

118. Milner AR, Bogod DG, Harwood RJ. Intrathecal administration of morphine for elective caesarean section. A comparison between 0.1 mg and 0.2 mg. Anaesthesia 1996; 51:871-3.

119. Uchiyama A, Ueyama H, Nakano S, et al. Low dose intrathecal morphine and pain relief following caesarean section. Int J Obstet Anesth 1994; 3:87-91.

120. Dahl JB, Jeppesen IS, Jorgensen H, et al. Intraoperative and postoperative analgesic efficacy and adverse effects of intrathecal opioids in patients undergoing cesarean section with spinal anesthesia. Anesthesiology 1999; 91:1919-27.

121. Vercauteren M, Vereecken K, La Malfa M, et al. Cost-effectiveness of analgesia after caesarean section. A comparison of intrathecal morphine and epidural PCA. Acta Anaesthesiol Scand 2002; 46:85-89.

122. Paech MJ, Pavy TJG, Orlikowski CEP, et al. Postoperative intraspinal opioids analgesia after caesarean section: A randomized comparison of subarachnoid morphine and epidural pethidine. Int J Obstet Anesth 2000; 9:238-45.

123. Palmer CM, Emerson S, Volgoropolous D, Alves D. Dose-response relationship of intrathecal morphine for postcesarean analgesia. Anesthesiology 1999; 90:437-44.

124. Belzarena SD. Clinical effects of intrathecally administered fentanyl in patients undergoing cesarean section. Anesth Analg 1992; 74:653-7.

125. Courtney MA, Hauch M, Bader AM, et al. Perioperative analgesia with subarachnoid sufentanil administration. Reg Anesth 1992; 17:274-8.

126. Dahlgren G, Hultstrand C, Jakobsson J, et al. Intrathecal sufentanil, fentanyl, or placebo added to bupivacaine for cesarean section. Anesth Analg 1997; 85:1288-93.

127. Thi TVN, Orliaguet G, Ngu TH, Bonnet F. Spinal anesthesia with meperidine as the sole agent for cesarean delivery. Reg Anesth 1994; 19:386-9.

128. Feldman JM, Griffin F, Fermo L, Raessler K. Intrathecal meperidine for pain after cesarean delivery: Efficacy and dose-response (abstract). Anesthesiology 1992; 77:A1011.

129. Kafle SK. Intrathecal meperidine for elective caesarean section: A comparison with lidocaine. Can J Anaesth 1993; 40:718-21.

130. Yu SC, Ngan Kee WD, Kwan ASK. Addition of meperidine to bupivacaine for spinal anaesthesia for caesarean section. Br J Anaesth 2002; 88:379-83.

131. Kelly MC, Carabine UA, Mirakhur RK. Intrathecal diamorphine for analgesia after caesarean section. Anaesthesia 1998; 53:231-7.

132. Husaini SW, Russell IF. Intrathecal diamorphine compared with morphine for postoperative analgesia after caesarean section under spinal anaesthesia. Br J Anaesth 1998; 81:135-9.

133. Gould DB, Singer SB, Smeltzer JS. Dose-response of subarachnoid butorphanol analgesia concurrent with bupivacaine for cesarean section. Reg Anesth 1991; 15:46.

134. Culebras X, Gaggero G, Zatloukal J, et al. Advantages of intrathecal nalbuphine, compared with intrathecal morphine, after cesarean delivery: An evaluation of postoperative analgesia and adverse effects. Anesth Analg 2000; 91:601-5.

135. Chung KS, Fermo L, Sinatra RS, et al. Perioperative efficacy of intrathecal methadone-bupivacaine for cesarean section: Comparison with fentanyl (abstract). Anesthesiology 1993; 79:A1026.

136. Sibilla C, Albertazzi P, Zatelli R, Mertinello R. Perioperative analgesia for cesarean section: Comparison of intrathecal morphine and fentanyl alone or in combination. Int J Obstet Anesth 1997; 6:43-8.

137. Lee SHR, Herman NL, Leighton BL, et al. Does IT fentanyl affect IT morphine analgesia after cesarean delivery? (abstract). Anesthesiology 2000; 92:A77.

138. Chung JH, Sinatra RS, Sevarino FB, Fermo L. Subarachnoid meperidine-morphine combination. An effective perioperative analgesic adjunct for cesarean delivery. Reg Anesth 1997; 22:119-24.

139. Eisenach JC. Of course it's safe! (editorial). Obstet Anesth Digest 1992; 12:97-9.

140. Yaksh TL, Collins JG. Studies in animals should precede human use of spinally administered drugs. Anesthesiology 1989; 70:4-6.

141. Rawal N, Nuutinen L, Raj PP, et al. Behavioral and histopathological effects following intrathecal administration of butorphanol, sufentanil, and nalbuphine in sheep. Anesthesiology 1991; 75:1025-34.

142. Coombs DW, Deroo DB, Colburn RW, et al. Toxicity of chronic analgesia in a canine model: Neuropathologic observations with dezocine lactate. Reg Anesth 1990; 15:94-102.

143. Ackerman WE, Juneja MM, Colclough GW, et al. Epidural fentanyl significantly decreases nausea and vomiting during uterine manipulation in awake patients undergoing cesarean section (abstract). Anesthesiology 1988; 69:A679.

144. Ackerman WE, Juneja MM, Kaczorowski DM, Colclough GW. A comparison of the incidence of pruritus following epidural opioid administration in the parturient. Can J Anaesth 1989; 36:388-91.

145. Gaffud MP, Bansal P, Lawton C, et al. Surgical analgesia during cesarean delivery with epidural bupivacaine and fentanyl. Anesthesiology 1986; 65:331-4.

146. Yee I, Carstoniu J, Halpern S, Pittini R. A comparison of two doses of epidural fentanyl during caesarean section. Can J Anaesth 1993; 40:722-5.

147. James FM. Comment. Obstet Anesth Digest 1989; 8:183.

148. Macintyre PE, Pavlin EC, Dwersteg JF. Effect of meperidine on oxygen consumption, carbon dioxide production, and respiratory gas exchange in postanesthesia shivering. Anesth Analg 1987; 66:751-5.

149. Juneja M, Ackerman WF, Heine MF, et al. Butorphanol for the relief of shivering associated with extradural anesthesia in parturients. J Clin Anesth 1992; 4:390-3.

150. Chen AK, Kwan WF, Harrity WV. The effect of epidural butorphanol and fentanyl on shivering during cesarean section. Reg Anesth 1991; 15:30.

151. Sutherland J, Seaton H, Lowry C. The influence of epidural pethidine on shivering during lower segment caesarean section under epidural anaesthesia. Anaesth Intensive Care 1991; 19:228-32.

152. Sevarino FB, Johnson MD, Lema MJ, et al. The effect of epidural sufentanil on shivering and body temperature in the parturient. Anesth Analg 1989; 68:530-3.

153. Eldor J, Guedj P. Epidural morphine for prophylaxis of post dural puncture headache in parturients. Reg Anesth 1992; 17:112.

154. Abboud TK, Zhu J, Reyes A, et al. Effect of subarachnoid morphine on the incidence of spinal headache. Reg Anesth 1992; 17:34-6.

155. Carney MD, Weiss JH, Norris MC, Leighton BL. Intrathecal morphine and post dural puncture headache. Anesthesiology 1990; 73:A949.

156. Colburn N, Mandell G, Rudy T. Epidural fentanyl for post-vaginal delivery pain (abstract). Anesthesiology 1990; 73:A986.

157. Malinow AM, Mokriski BLK, Nomura MK, et al. Effect of epinephrine on intrathecal fentanyl analgesia (abstract). Proc Soc Obstet Anesth Perinatol 1989; 21:8.

158. Honet JE, Costello DT, Norris MC, et al. Spinal anesthesia for postpartum tubal ligation: Meperidine vs lidocaine (abstract). Anesthesiology 1991; 75:A859.

159. Bromage PR. The price of intraspinal narcotic analgesia: Basic constraints. Anesth Analg 1981; 60:461-3.

160. Scott PV, Fischer HBJ. Intraspinal opiates and itching: A new reflex. Br Med J 1982; 284:1015-6.

161. Zakowski MI, Ramanathan S, Khoo P, et al. Plasma histamine with intraspinal morphine in cesarean section (abstract). Anesth Analg 1990; 70:S448.

162. Sun HL. Naloxone-precipitated acute opioid withdrawal syndrome after epidural morphine. Anesth Analg 1998; 86:544-5.

163. Colbert S, O'Hanlon DM, Galvin S, et al. The effect of rectal diclofenac on pruritus in patients receiving intrathecal morphine. Anaesthesia 1999; 54:948-52.

164. Dailey PA, Brookshire GL, Shnider SM, et al. Naloxone decreases side effects after intrathecal morphine for labor. Anesth Analg 1985; 64:658-66.

165. Luthman JA, Kay NH, White JB. Intrathecal morphine for post caesarean section analgesia: Does naloxone reduce the incidence of pruritus? Int J Obstet Anesth 1992; 1:191-4.

166. Chalmers PC, Lang CM, Greenhouse BB. The use of nalbuphine in association with epidural narcotics. Anesthesiol Rev 1988; 15:21-7.

167. Cohen SE, Ratner EF, Kreitzman TR, et al. Nalbuphine is better than naloxone for treatment of side effects after epidural morphine. Anesth Analg 1992; 75:747-52.

168. Morgan PJ, Mehta S, Kapala DM. Nalbuphine pretreatment in cesarean section patients receiving epidural morphine. Reg Anesth 1991; 16:84-8.

169. Kendrick WD, Birch RFH, Woods AM. Pruritus control following epidural opiates through continuous infusion plus self administration of mu antagonists versus mixed agonist-antagonists in the post cesarean section population. Anesthesiology 1990; 73:A941.

170. Abboud TK, Lee K, Zhu J, et al. Prophylactic oral naltrexone with intrathecal morphine for cesarean section: Effects on adverse reactions and analgesia. Anesth Analg 1990; 71:367-70.

171. Borgeat A, Wilder-Smith OHG, Saiah M, et al. Subhypnotic doses of propofol relieve pruritus induced by epidural and intrathecal morphine. Anesthesiology 1992; 76:510-2.

172. Saiah M, Borgeat A, Wilder-Smith OHG, et al. Epidural-morphine-induced pruritus: Propofol versus naloxone. Anesth Analg 1994; 78:1110-3.

173. Beilin Y, Bernstein HH, Zucker-Pinchoff B, et al. Subhypnotic doses of propofol do not relieve pruritus induced by intrathecal morphine after cesarean section. Anesth Analg 1998; 86:310-3.

174. Charuluxananan S, Kyokong O, Somboonviboon W, et al. Nalbuphine versus propofol for treatment of intrathecal morphine-induced pruritus after cesarean delivery. Anesth Analg 2001; 93:162-5.

175. Borgeat A, Stirnemann HR. Ondansetron is effective to treat spinal or epidural morphine-induced pruritus. Anesthesiology 1999; 90:432-6.

176. Yeh HM, Chen LK, Lin CJ, et al. Prophylactic intravenous ondansetron reduces the incidence of intrathecal morphine-induced pruritus in patients undergoing cesarean delivery. Anesth Analg 2000; 91:172-5.

177. Horta ML, Ramos L, Gonçalves ZR. The inhibition of epidural morphine-induced pruritus by epidural droperidol. Anesth Analg 2000; 90:638-41.

178. Celleno D, Costantino P, Emanuelli M, et al. Epidural analgesia during and after cesarean delivery: Comparison of five opioids. Reg Anesth 1991; 16:79-83.

179. Lussos SA, Bader AM, Thornhill ML, Datta S. The antiemetic efficacy and safety of prophylactic metoclopramide for elective cesarean delivery during spinal anesthesia. Reg Anesth 1992; 17:126-30.

180. Kotelko DM, Rottman RL, Wright WC, et al. Transderm scop decreases nausea and vomiting following cesarean in patients receiving epidural morphine. Anesthesiology 1989; 71:675-9.

181. Tzeng JI, Wang JJ, Ho ST, et al. Dexamethasone for prophylaxis of nausea and vomiting after epidural morphine for post-caesarean section analgesia: Comparison of droperidol and saline. Br J Anaesth 2000; 85:865-8.

182. Ho C-M, Hseu S-S, Tsai S-K, Lee T-Y. Effect of P6 acupressure on prevention of nausea and vomiting after epidural morphine for postcesarean section pain relief. Acta Anaesthesiol Scand 1996; 40:372-5.

183. Harmon D, Ryan M, Kelly A, Bowen M. Acupressure and prevention of nausea and vomiting during and after spinal anaesthesia for caesarean section. Br J Anaesth 2000; 84:463-7.

184. Evron S, Samueloff A, Simon A. Urinary function during epidural analgesia with methadone and morphine in postcesarean section patients. Pain 1985; 23:135-40.

185. Durant PAC, Yaksh TL. Drug effects on urinary bladder tone during spinal morphine-induced inhibition of the micturition reflex in unanesthetized rats. Anesthesiology 1988; 68:325-34.

186. Rawal N, Schott U, Dahlstrom B, et al. Influence of naloxone infusion on analgesia and respiratory depression following epidural morphine. Anesthesiology 1986; 64:194-201.

187. Lyons HA, Antonio R. The sensitivity of the respiratory center in pregnancy and after the administration of progesterone. Trans Assoc Am Physicians 1959; 72:173-80.

188. Ostman LP, Owen CL, Bates JN, et al. Oxygen saturation in patients the night prior to and the night after cesarean section during epidural morphine analgesia. Anesthesiology 1988; 69:A691.

189. Albright G. Epidural morphine, hydromorphone, and meperidine for postcesarean section pain relief utilizing a respiratory apnea monitor (abstract). Anesthesiology 1983; 59:A416.

190. Bailey PL, Rhondeau S, Schafer PG, et al. Dose-response pharmacology of intrathecal morphine in human volunteers. Anesthesiology 1993; 79:49-59.

191. Ready LB, Loper KA, Nessly M, Wild L. Postoperative epidural morphine is safe on surgical wards. Anesthesiology 1991; 75:452-6.

192. Johnson A, Bengtsson M, Soderlind K, Lofstrom JB. Influence of intrathecal morphine and naloxone intervention on postoperative ventilatory regulation in elderly patients. Acta Anaesthesiol Scand 1992; 36:435-44.

193. Rosaeg OP, Suderman V, Yarnell RW. Early respiratory depression during caesarean section following epidural meperidine. Can J Anaesth 1992; 39:71-4.

194. Geller E, Chrubasik J, Graf R, et al. A randomized double-blind comparison of epidural sufentanil versus intravenous sufentanil or epidural fentanyl analgesia after major abdominal surgery. Anesth Analg 1993; 76:1243-50.

195. Kemper PM, Treiber N. Neuraxial morphine plus PCA: A new method of postcesarean analgesia (abstract). Anesth Analg 1990; 70:S198.

196. Wittels B, Glosten B, Faure E, et al. Postcesarean analgesia using both epidural morphine and intravenous patient-controlled analgesia: Neurobehavioral outcomes among nursing neonates. Anesth Analg 1997; 85:600-6.

197. Baka NE, Bayoumeu F, Boutroy MJ, Laxenaire MC. Colostrum morphine concentrations during postcesarean intravenous patient-controlled analgesia. Anesth Analg 2002; 94:184-7.

198. Cohen SE, Desai JB, Ratner EF, et al. Ketorolac and spinal morphine for postcesarean analgesia. Int J Obstet Anesth 1996; 5:14-8.

199. American Academy of Pediatrics Committee on Drugs. The transfer of drugs and other chemicals into human milk. Pediatrics 1994; 93:137-50.

200. Cartwright DP. Analgesia after caesarean section: Ketorolac and papaveretum compared (abstract). Proc Soc Obstet Anesth Perinatol 1991; 23:107.

201. Waters J, Hullander M, Kraft A, et al. Postcesarean pain relief with ketorolac tromethamine and epidural morphine (abstract). Anesthesiology 1992; 77:A813.

202. Mok MS, Tzeng JI. Intramuscular ketorolac enhances the analgesic effect of low dose epidural morphine (abstract). Anesth Analg 1993; 76:269.

203. Sun HL, Wu CC, Lin MS, Chang CF. Effects of epidural morphine and intramuscular diclofenac combination in postcesarean analgesia: A dose-range study. Anesth Analg 1993; 76:284-8.

204. Dennis AR, Leeson-Payne CG, Hobbs GJ. Analgesia after caesarean section. The use of rectal diclofenac as an adjunct to spinal morphine. Anaesthesia 1995; 50:297-9.

205. Lim NLSH, Lo WK, Chon JL, Pan AX. Single dose diclofenac suppository reduces post-cesarean PCEA requirements. Can J Anaesth 2001; 48:383-6.

206. Cardoso MMSC, Carvalho JCA, Amaro AR, et al. Small doses of intrathecal morphine combined with systemic diclofenac for postoperative pain control after cesarean delivery. Anesth Analg 1998; 86:538-41.

207. Pavy TJG, Gambling DR, Merrick PM, Douglas MJ. Rectal indomethacin potentiates spinal morphine analgesia after caesarean delivery. Anaesth Intensive Care 1995; 23:555-9.

208. Ambrose FP. A retrospective study of the effect of postoperative indomethacin rectal suppositories on the need for narcotic analgesia in patients who had a cesarean delivery while they were under regional anesthesia. Am J Obstet Gynecol 2001; 184:1544-8.

209. Yang T, Breen TW, Archer D, Fick G. Comparison of 0.25 mg and 0.1 mg intrathecal morphine for analgesia after cesarean section. Can J Anaesth 1999; 46:856-60.

210. Gimbel JS, Brugger A, Zhao W, et al. Efficacy and tolerability of celecoxib versus hydrocodone/acetaminophen in the treatment of pain after ambulatory orthopedic surgery in adults. Clin Ther 2001; 23:228-41.

211. Rosenblatt WHO, Cioffi AM, Sinatra RS, Silverman DG. Metoclopramide-enhanced analgesia for prostaglandin-induced termination of pregnancy. Anesth Analg 1992; 75:760-3.

212. Driver RP Jr, D'Angelo R, Eisenach JC. Bolus metoclopramide does not enhance morphine analgesia after cesarean section. Anesth Analg 1996; 82:1033-5.

213. Ehrenkranz RA, Ackerman BA. Metoclopramide effect on faltering milk production by mothers of premature infants. Pediatrics 1986; 78: 614-20.

214. Kuraishi Y, Hirota N, Sato Y, et al. Noradrenergic inhibition of the release of substance P from the primary afferents in the rabbit spinal dorsal horn. Brain Res 1985; 359:177-82.

215. Taiwo YO, Fabian A, Pazoles CJ, et al. Potentiation of morphine antinociception by monoamine reuptake inhibitors in the rat spinal cord. Pain 1985; 21:329-37.

216. Kitahata LM. Spinal analgesia with morphine and clonidine. Anesth Analg 1989; 68:191-3.

217. Eisenach JC, Lysak SZ, Viscomi CM. Epidural clonidine analgesia following surgery: Phase I. Anesthesiology 1989; 71:640-6.

218. Narchi P, Benhamou D, Hamza J, Bouaziz H. Ventilatory effects of epidural clonidine during the first 3 hours after caesarean section. Acta Anaesth Scand 1992; 36:791-5.

219. Mendez RM, Eisenach JC, Kashtan K. Epidural clonidine infusion following cesarean section. Anesthesiology 1990; 73:A918.

220. Huntoon M, Eisenach JC, Boese P. Epidural clonidine after cesarean section. Anesthesiology 1992; 76:187-93.

221. Capogna G, Celleno D, Zangrillo A, et al. Addition of clonidine to epidural morphine enhances postoperative analgesia after cesarean delivery. Reg Anesth 1995; 20:57-61.

222. Mogensen T, Eliasen K, Ejlersen E, et al. Epidural clonidine enhances postoperative analgesia from a combined low-dose epidural bupivacaine and morphine regimen. Anesth Analg 1992; 75:607-10.

223. Eisenach JC, D'Angelo R, Taylor C, Hood DD. An isobolographic study of epidural clonidine and fentanyl after cesarean section. Anesth Analg 1994; 79:285-90.

224. Filos KS, Goudas LC, Patroni O, Polyzou V. Intrathecal clonidine as a sole analgesic for pain relief after cesarean section. Anesthesiology 1992; 77:267-74.

225. Filos KS, Goudas LC, Patroni O, Polyzou V. Hemodynamic and analgesic profile after intrathecal clonidine in humans. Anesthesiology 1994; 81:591-601.

226. Benhamou D, Thorin D, Brichant JF, et al. Intrathecal clonidine and fentanyl with hyperbaric bupivacaine improves analgesia during cesarean section. Anesth Analg 1998; 87:609-13.

227. Aho MS, Erkola OA, Scheinin H, et al. Effect of intravenously administered dexmedetomidine on pain after laparoscopic tubal ligation. Anesth Analg 1991; 73:112-8.

228. Motsch J, Graber E, Ludwig K. Addition of clonidine enhances postoperative analgesia from epidural morphine: A double blind study. Anesthesiology 1990; 73:1067-73.

229. Naji P, Farschtschian M, Wilder-Smith O, Wilder-Smith C. Epidural droperidol and morphine for postoperative pain. Anesth Analg 1990; 70:583-8.

230. Sananisilp V, Areewatana S, Tonsukchai N. Droperidol and the side effects of epidural morphine after cesarean section. Anesth Analg 1998; 86:532-7.

231. Naguib M, Adu-Gyamfi Y, Absood GH, et al. Epidural ketamine for postoperative analgesia. Can Anaesth Soc J 1986; 33:16-21.

232. Kawana Y, Sato H, Shimada H, et al. Epidural ketamine for postoperative pain relief after gynecologic operations: A double blind study and comparison with epidural morphine. Anesth Analg 1987; 66:735-8.

233. Brock-Utne JG, Kallichurum S, Mankowitz E, et al. Intrathecal ketamine with preservative-histological effect on spinal nerve root of baboons. S Afr Med J 1981; 61:441-2.

234. Chia YY, Liu K, Liu YC, et al. Adding ketamine in a multimodal patient-controlled epidural regimen reduces postoperative pain and analgesic consumption. Anesth Analg 1998; 86:1245-9.

235. Bouaziz H, Tong C, Eisenach JC. Postoperative analgesia from intrathecal neostigmine in sheep. Anesth Analg 1995; 80:1140-4.

236. Yaksh TL, Grafe MR, Malkmus S, et al. Studies on the safety of chronically administered intrathecal neostigmine methylsulfate in rats and dogs. Anesthesiology 1995; 82:412-27.

237. Hood DD, Eisenach JC, Tong C, et al. Cardiorespiratory and spinal cord blood flow effects of intrathecal neostigmine methylsulfate, clonidine, and their combination in sheep. Anesthesiology 1995; 82:428-35.

238. Collins JG. Spinally administered neostigmine: Something to celebrate (editorial). Anesthesiology 1995; 82:327-8.

239. Hood DD, Eisenach JC, Tuttle R. Phase I safety assessment of intrathecal neostigmine methylsulfate in humans. Anesthesiology 1995; 82:331-43.

240. Pan PM, Mok MS. Efficacy of intrathecal neostigmine for the relief of post cesarean pain (abstract). Anesthesiology 1995; 83:A786.

241. Krukowski JA, Hood DD, Eisenach JC, et al. Intrathecal neostigmine for post-cesarean section analgesia: Dose response. Anesth Analg 1997; 84:1269-75.

242. Chung C-J, Kim J-S, Park H-S, Chin Y-J. The efficacy of intrathecal neostigmine, intrathecal morphine, and their combination for post-cesarean section analgesia. Anesth Analg 1998; 87:341-6.

243. Witkowski TA, Leighton BL, Norris MC. Ilioinguinal nerve blocks: An alternative or supplement to intrathecal morphine (abstract). Anesthesiology 1990; 73:A962.

244. Huffnagle JH, Norris MC, Leighton BL, Arkoosh VA. Ilioinguinal iliohypogastric nerve blocks before or after cesarean delivery under spinal anesthesia? Anesth Analg 1996; 82:8-12.

245. Pavy TJG, Gambling DR, Kliffer AP, et al. Effect of preoperative skin infiltration with 0.5% bupivacaine on postoperative pain following cesarean section under spinal anesthesia. Int J Obstet Anesth 1994; 3:199-202.

246. James CF. Recurrence of herpes simplex virus blepharitis after cesarean section and epidural morphine. Anesth Analg 1996; 82:1094-6.

247. Crone LAL, Conly JM, Clark KM, et al. Recurrent herpes simplex virus labialis and the use of epidural morphine on obstetric patients. Anesth Analg 1988; 67:318-23.

248. Crone LAL, Conly JM, Storgard C, et al. Herpes labialis in parturients receiving epidural morphine following cesarean section. Anesthesiology 1990; 73:208-13.

249. Norris MC, Weiss J, Carney M, Leighton BL. The incidence of herpes simplex virus labialis after cesarean delivery. Int J Obstet Anesth 1994; 3:127-31.

250. Boyle RK. Herpes simplex labialis after epidural or parenteral morphine: A randomized prospective trial in an Australian obstetric population. Anaesth Intensive Care 1995; 23:433-7.

251. Boyle RK. A review of anatomical and immunological links between epidural morphine and herpes simplex labialis in obstetric patients. Anaesth Intensive Care 1995; 23:425-32.

252. Valley MA, Bourke D, McKenzie AM. Recurrence of thoracic and labial herpes simplex virus infection in a patient receiving epidural fentanyl. Anesthesiology 1992; 76:1056-7.

253. Weiss JH, Carney MD, Norris MC, et al. Incidence of recurrent herpes simplex virus labialis after cesarean section (abstract). Anesthesiology 1990; 73:A951.

254. Tom DJ, Gulevich SJ, Shapiro HM, et al. Epidural blood patch in the HIV-positive patient. Anesthesiology 1992; 76:943-7.

255. Hughes SC, Dailey PA, Landers D, et al. The HIV? parturient and regional anesthesia: Clinical and immunologic response (abstract). Anesthesiology 1992; 77:A1036.

256. Borgeat A, Biollaz J, Depierraz B, Neff R. Grand mal seizure after extradural morphine analgesia. Br J Anaesth 1988; 60:733-5.

257. Berger JM, Ontell R. Intrathecal morphine in conjunction with a combined spinal and general anesthetic in a patient with multiple sclerosis. Anesthesiology 1987; 66:400-2.

258. Weintraub SJ, Naulty SJ. Acute abstinence syndrome after epidural injection of butorphanol. Anesth Analg 1985; 64:452-3.

259. Van Dercar DH, Martinez AP, DeLisser EA. Sleep apnea syndromes: A potential contraindication for patient-controlled analgesia. Anesthesiology 1991; 74:623-4.

260. Cohen SE, Woods WA. The role of epidural morphine in the postcesarean patient: Efficacy and effects on bonding. Anesthesiology 1983; 58:500-4.

261. Stenkamp SJ, Easterling TR, Chadwick HS. Effect of epidural and intrathecal morphine on the length of stay following cesarean section. Anesth Analg 1989; 68:66-9.

262. Ramanathan J, Coleman P, Sibai B. Anesthetic modification of hemodynamic and neuroendocrine stress responses to cesarean delivery in women with severe preeclampsia. Anesth Analg 1991; 73:772-9.

263. Rawal N, Sjostrand U, Christoffersson E, et al. Comparison of intramuscular and epidural morphine for postoperative analgesia in the grossly obese: Influence on postoperative ambulation and pulmonary function. Anesth Analg 1984; 63:583-8.

264. O'Flaherty D, Popat M, Delwood L. Addition of epidural or intrathecal fentanyl for cesarean delivery does not alter the stress response (abstract). Anesth Analg 1993; 76:S306.

265. Tuman KJ, McCarthy RJ, March RJ, et al. Effects of epidural anesthesia and analgesia on coagulation and outcome after vascular surgery. Anesth Analg 1991; 73:696-704.

266. Yeager MP, Glass DD, Neff RK, et al. Epidural anesthesia and analgesia in high risk surgical patients. Anesthesiology 1987; 66:729-33.

267. Armitage EN. Postoperative pain—prevention or relief? Br J Anaesth 1989; 63:136-7.

268. Kavanagh, B, Katz J, Sandler A, et al. Preoperative multi-modal analgesia: A randomized double blind, placebo controlled study (abstract). Anesth Analg 1993; 76:S182.

269. Langerman L, Golomb E, Benita S, Tverskoy M. Intrathecal opiates: A new way for prolongation of pharmacological effect. Anesthesiology 1989; 71:A697.

Part VIII
Anesthetic Complications

James Young Simpson introduced anesthesia to obstetrics when the practice of medicine was in a period of great flux. As late as 1820, most Western medical schools were still practicing a form of medicine derived from the teachings of Galen, a second century Greek physician. According to Galenic principles, all disease originated from an imbalance among the four elements (earth, air, fire, and water), hydraulic pressures, or electrical forces. Treatment consisted of the time-honored measures of purging, bleeding, cupping, or the administration of stimulants or depressants. Simpson, Meigs, Channing and all the others involved in the early debate about obstetric anesthesia learned this style of practice as students.

Within a few years of their graduation, Galenic forms of medicine had been discredited and had disappeared. In its place Laennec, Louis and other French physicians developed principles of medical theory and practice that we use today—physical diagnosis, statistical analysis, physiology, pathology, and chemistry.[1]

Thus the introduction of anesthesia represented a significant challenge. Physicians who had once been taught to treat the pain of childbirth with bloodletting could now use ether or chloroform. They recognized the therapeutic potential of the drugs, but they also recognized their dangers and questioned their safety and effects on labor and the newborn.[2]

Evaluating the risks of anesthesia was quite different from recognizing the problems. In 1850 pharmacology was in its infancy, and medical physiology, pathology, and biochemistry were not very well developed. There was no tradition for drug testing that Simpson and Meigs could model. Their inexperience with medical science was reflected in their response to obstetric anesthesia. For example, seeking a better agent to replace ether, Simpson simply tried a series of compounds on himself and his friends until he stumbled upon one that worked—chloroform. Within a month he had administered chloroform to a patient and had published a paper. He conducted no animal studies or clinical trials, collected no data, and performed no statistical analyses of his results. His claims were reviewed by no clinical board or governmental agency, and he had no reason to fear a malpractice suit. Such an approach led to a rapid dissemination of new ideas, but it took years before anyone identified the problems associated with the new remedy, much less sorted them out. Accordingly, after the introduction of obstetric anesthesia, more than half a century passed before physicians began to develop the tools that they needed to understand the problems associated with the use of ether and chloroform.[3]

Donald Caton, M.D.

REFERENCES

1. Temkin O. Galenism, Rise and Decline of a Medical Philosophy. Ithaca, Cornell University Press, 1973.
2. Rosenberg CE. The therapeutic revolution: medicine, meaning, and social change in nineteenth-century America. In Vogel MJ, Rosenberg CE, editors: The Therapeutic Revolution: Essays in the Social History of American Medicine. Philadelphia, University of Pennsylvania Press, 1979:3-26.
3. Newman C. The Evolution of Medical Education in the Nineteenth Century. New York, Oxford University Press, 1957.

Chapter 29
Medicolegal Issues in Obstetric Anesthesia

Mark S. Williams, M.D., M.B.A., J.D. · Brian K. Ross, M.D., Ph.D. ·
Lisa Vincler Brock, J.D. · H.S. Chadwick, M.D.

For most women, childbirth is a normal physiologic process that brings great joy to themselves and their families. Expectations typically are high, and there is great disappointment when the outcome is less than perfect for the mother and infant. Anesthesiologists who provide care for obstetric patients have a unique and challenging role. Some women view anesthesia for labor as nonessential or undesirable, yet many of those women ultimately request and/or need anesthesia services. In contrast, most women have high expectations regarding both the availability and the quality of anesthesia services for labor and vaginal or cesarean delivery. Pregnant women and their families may have misconceptions regarding anesthesia options, procedures, and risks. They may be influenced by the biases and anxieties of their family and friends. Further, the process of obtaining informed consent may be problematic in patients who are experiencing severe pain during active labor. These and other factors may affect a patient's decision to seek legal remedies for real or perceived injuries or other adverse events.

The financial and emotional costs of litigation are substantial for both patients and health care providers. Patients and their families must adjust to the reality of the adverse outcome as well as to the overwhelming (and in some cases ongoing) financial costs. All medicolegal claims (both with and without merit) increase the costs of liability premiums, encourage the practice of defensive medicine, and increase the cost of health care services. Further, fear of litigation may have an adverse effect on the availability of health care services. Ultimately, society bears the cost of litigation.

Anesthesiologists should be aware of basic medicolegal issues so that they may practice risk-management strategies designed to minimize both patient dissatisfaction and legal consequences in the event of an unanticipated adverse outcome.

LAWSUITS INVOLVING CLAIMS AGAINST HEALTH CARE PROVIDERS

Theories of Liability

Every physician has a duty to provide professional services that are consistent with a minimum level of competence. This is an objective standard based on the physician's qualifications, level of expertise, and the circumstances of the particular case.[1] The failure to meet this objective standard of care may give rise to a cause of action for medical negligence. The standard of care for medical practice is dynamic and changes as the profession adopts new treatments and approaches for patient care. Therefore changes in accepted medical practice may create additional professional obligations and, in turn, additional legal duties for physicians.

Although the specific medical malpractice laws vary from state to state, several different causes of action may be brought against a physician. By way of example, we will use the laws of the state of Washington to illustrate principles of malpractice laws. Patients may sue for injuries resulting from the provision of health care by using one or more of three different theories (or causes of action): (1) medical malpractice, (2) breach of contractual promise that injury would not occur, and (3) lack of informed consent.[2] Plaintiffs (patients) commonly file lawsuits that allege improper care based on more than one of these theories (e.g., alleging both a violation of the standard of care and a lack of informed consent for the medical treatment rendered). For a plaintiff to prevail with regard to medical malpractice claims, he or she must prove that the injury resulted from the failure of the health care provider to follow the accepted standard of care. The standard of care may be defined as "that degree of care, skill, and learning expected of a reasonably prudent health care provider at that time in the profession or class to which he belongs . . . acting in the same or similar circumstances."[3] This objective standard is applied to the particular facts of the plaintiff's situation in a malpractice action.

A mistake or a bad result does not necessarily denote negligence. Similarly, unless a physician contracts otherwise with the patient (i.e., makes a promise of a specific outcome) the provision of medical care alone does not warrant or guarantee that an illness or disease will be cured. A physician is liable for a misjudgment or mistake only when it is proved to have occurred through a failure to act in accordance with the care and skill of a reasonably prudent practitioner.

Establishing Medical Malpractice

In most malpractice cases, four elements are required for proving medical negligence:

1. **Duty.** It must be shown that a duty to provide care existed (i.e., a health care provider-patient relationship existed).
2. **Breach.** It must be shown that the health care provider failed to meet his or her duty to provide reasonable care (i.e., the health care provider was negligent).
3. **Injury.** It must be shown that the patient experienced an injury that resulted in damages.
4. **Proximate cause.** It must be shown that the negligence of the health care provider proximately caused the patient's injury (there must be a sufficiently direct connection between the negligence of the health care provider and the injury experienced by the patient).[3]

If any one of these elements is missing, the plaintiff cannot establish medical malpractice. The plaintiff has the burden of proof to establish each of these elements by a "preponderance of the evidence." This quantum of proof means that a proposition is more probably true than not true (i.e., greater than 50% certainty).

If the malpractice claim involves the issue of whether a physician used a proper method of treatment, the plaintiff must use expert testimony to establish that the defendant physician violated the standard of care and that such violation probably caused plaintiff's injury.[4] Expert testimony to establish how a reasonably prudent health care practitioner would act under similar circumstances typically must be provided by an expert with the same educational background and training as the defendant physician.

In certain cases, the plaintiff may not be required to present expert testimony to prove negligence, and the burden of proof may shift to the defendant. This represents the doctrine of *res ipsa loquitor* (i.e., the thing speaks for itself). This doctrine includes three conditions: (1) the injury ordinarily does not occur in the absence of negligence; (2) the injury must be caused by an agency or instrumentality within the exclusive control of the defendant; and (3) the injury must not have been a result of any voluntary action or contribution on the part of the plaintiff.[5] Claims involving injuries sustained during administration of anesthesia (e.g., misplaced surgical instruments) have been made under this doctrine.[4,6] Nerve injury cases have been described as "custom made" for *res ipsa loquitor*.[7]

Establishing Lack of Informed Consent

A distinct cause of action based on lack of informed consent exists and underscores the high value placed on the patient's right to be fully informed of his or her choices in medical care. Historically, a physician's failure to obtain informed consent for surgery was treated as a battery (i.e., unlawful touching) claim. Both medical ethics and law recognize the concepts of patient self-determination and autonomy, which may be described as respecting the individual patient's ability to determine his or her own destiny.[8] Informed consent case law began to develop as early as 1914, but many of the existing informed consent statutes were not adopted by state legislatures until the mid-1960s or later.

These are the elements that generally are required for proving lack of informed consent:

1. The physician failed to inform the patient of a material fact or facts relating to the treatment.
2. The patient consented to the treatment without being aware or fully informed of such material fact(s).
3. A reasonably prudent patient under similar circumstances would not have consented to the treatment if informed of such material fact(s).
4. The treatment provided was the proximately caused injury to the patient.

Each of these four elements must be proved for the plaintiff to prevail on a claim of lack of informed consent. Expert testimony is necessary to prove the existence of risk of injury, its likelihood of occurrence, and the type of harm in question. For the trier of fact (judge or jury), the relevant inquiry is not whether the patient (plaintiff) would or would not have consented but what a "reasonably prudent" patient under similar circumstances would have done *if fully informed.*[9]

The doctrine of informed consent does not require a full disclosure of all possible risks; rather, it requires disclosure of only those risks that are reasonably foreseeable.[10] Courts have determined that if a risk is very small, then as a matter of law, the risk is not reasonably foreseeable for purposes of informed consent. For example, one court has held that a 0.75% risk of esophageal perforation during an esophagoscopy is not, as a matter of law, a reasonably foreseeable risk.[11] In another case, a court held that a risk of 1 in 20,000 to 1 in 50,000 is not a reasonably foreseeable risk.[12] To conclude the same "as a matter of law" means that the court conclusively decides that aspect of the claim. However, there is no clearly defined standard that can guide health care providers in defining those reasonably foreseeable risks that require disclosure in all situations. Each court decision is based on the facts of the particular case, including the evidence presented. Unless a risk is serious and unless expert testimony establishes its existence, nature, and likelihood of occurrence, the mere presence of the risk may not be "material" and so there would be no duty for the physician to disclose it. In determining whether all material facts were disclosed, testimony about the customary disclosure practices of physicians may be considered as evidence but will not necessarily resolve the issue. The determination of materiality is a two-step process: (1) the scientific nature of the risk is ascertained via expert testimony, and (2) the trier of fact then decides whether that probability is a risk that a reasonable patient would consider in deciding on treatment.[13]

Even in circumstances in which the health care providers acknowledge their failure to provide important information to the patient or the patient's legally authorized surrogate decision-maker, the jury is still asked to decide whether the patient or the patient's decision-maker would have consented to such a course of treatment despite the risk. For example, in *Barth v. Rock,* a 5-year-old patient suffered a cardiac arrest (and eventual death) after receiving general anesthesia by mask with sodium thiopental, nitrous oxide, and a succinylcholine infusion for open reduction of an arm fracture. Both the surgeon and the nurse anesthetist admitted that they failed to inform the minor patient's parents about the risks of general anesthesia. The appellate court held that the jury should have been instructed that as a matter of law there was no informed consent; however, the jury would still need to decide whether the parents would have consented to the anesthetic had they been adequately informed of the risks.[14]

If a plaintiff establishes the four elements for a cause of action based on lack of informed consent, the burden shifts to the physician to establish a defense that justifies why the material information was not provided (e.g., the insignificant nature of the risk) or why disclosure would not have altered the chosen course of treatment. In addition, the health care providers may claim that the case was a medical emergency. State laws generally supply a defense of "implied consent" for provision of necessary emergency treatment when the patient is unable to provide his or her own consent and no legally authorized surrogate decision-maker is immediately available.[15] If the health care providers' treatment was authorized under a medical emergency, they should carefully document their determination of same. The documentation in the patient's medical record should contain a description of the patient's presenting condition, its immediacy, its magnitude, and the nature of the immediate threat of harm to the patient. It is advisable for at least two health care providers to chart this information, which will support their actions in the event that a lack-of-informed-consent lawsuit is filed. The "emergency treatment" rule is limited in two respects. First, it requires that the patient needs immediate care to preserve life or health. Second, the physician may provide only that care that is reasonable in light of the patient's condition. Washington law does not define "emergency." The University of Washington's institutional definition for "emergency" is broader than only life-threatening conditions and includes potential impairment of bodily functions.

THE LITIGATION PROCESS

It is helpful for health care providers to have a basic understanding of sources of law, how lawsuits are initiated, and typical steps in the litigation process.

Sources of Law

Legal authority has multiple sources, including federal and state constitutions, federal and state statutes, federal and state regulations, and federal and state case law. **Constitutions** are the fundamental laws of a nation or state, which establish the role of government in relation to the governed. Constitutions act as philosophical touchstones for the society from which other ideas may be drawn. One example is the "right to privacy" established in case law, which flows from the constitutional recognition of individual liberty.[16] **Statutes** are the laws written and enacted by elected officials in legislative bodies. **Regulations** are written by government agencies as permitted by statutory delegation. Although regulations have the force and effect of law, they must be consistent with their enabling legislation. **Case law** refers to written opinions or decisions of judges that arise from individual lawsuits. Case law that may

be cited as legal authority (precedent) is limited to cases at the appellate level (i.e., cases appealed from trial court decisions). The vast majority of lawsuits settle before trial and only a small percentage of trial court decisions result in appeal; thus case law reflects a very small portion of actual litigation. Like medicine, the practice of law is dynamic and changes as new legislation and regulations are adopted or new case law is created. In addition, any one or several of these sources of law may be relevant to a particular case.

When creating new laws or applying the law in deciding the proper result for a particular case, a legislative body or a court also may consider other information about standards for health care providers' conduct. For example, the court may give strong weight to the Joint Commission on Accreditation of Healthcare Organizations (JCAHO) standards and find that a provider acting in accordance with JCAHO requirements was adhering to his or her professional obligations.[17] In writing legislation or court decisions, lawmakers also may defer to standards and practice guidelines adopted by professional organizations, such as the American Society of Anesthesiologists (ASA). The adoption of professional standards and practice guidelines strengthens the influence of professional organizations in the law-making process because lawmakers often are willing to defer to professional organizations' statements on standard of care and professional ethics.

The use of medical practice guidelines in malpractice litigation has been viewed not only as an important reform in clarifying the tort standard of care but also as an affirmative defense for health care providers who practice within that standard.[18] Some states—including Florida, Kentucky, Maine, and Maryland—have adopted statutes to use medical practice guidelines in such a manner.[19]

Initiation of a Lawsuit

Medical malpractice lawsuits are initiated when a plaintiff files a **Complaint** with the court. The physician receives notice of the legal action when he or she is served with a copy of the **Summons** and the Complaint. In the Complaint, the plaintiff alleges the facts giving rise to the cause(s) of action against the physician. The Complaint requires a written **Answer** to be filed (by the attorney representing the physician) with the court within a specified period of time. If a timely Answer is not filed, a default judgment may be entered against the physician (i.e., a judgment is allowed because *no response* may be treated as *no defense* to the allegations).

In civil actions against health care providers, plaintiffs frequently are motivated to sue for an award of monetary damages. Medical malpractice lawsuits may include multiple defendants, such as the treating physician, the hospital, the manufacturer of health care equipment, pharmaceutical companies, or others. Defense counsel will evaluate their clients' potential liability exposure (i.e., any aspect of care arguably not meeting the standard of care). Both plaintiff and defense counsel will weigh the perceived risks if the case proceeds to trial and will determine how much they think the case is worth. The valuation of a case may include more than assigning a dollar value; it also may include considerations such as setting a potential precedent or maintaining a business relationship.

Discovery

Discovery refers to the early phase of litigation after a lawsuit is initiated. During this phase, the litigants on both sides research the strengths and weakness of their cases by obtaining and examining medical records, by reviewing medical literature, and by interviewing and deposing witnesses including the plaintiff(s), the treating health care providers, and potential expert witnesses.

During discovery, certain methods for gathering information generally are used. These methods include interrogatories and depositions. **Interrogatories** are written questions that are served on one party from an opposing party. Interrogatories must be answered in writing, under oath, within a prescribed period of time. Failure to respond as required may result in the court issuing sanctions against the non-responding party. **Depositions** involve testimony under oath, which is recorded by a court reporter. In a deposition taken for the purpose of discovery, the attorneys representing all opposing litigants participate and ask questions of the witness. The purposes of discovery depositions include the following: (1) to obtain facts and other evidence; (2) to encourage the other side to commit to a position "on the record" (i.e., in preserved testimony); (3) to discover the names of other potential witnesses; (4) to assess how strong a witness the deposed individual may make; (5) to limit facts and issues for the lawsuit; (6) to encourage the other side to make admissions against their own interests in the lawsuit; and (7) to evaluate the case for its dollar (or other) value and potential settlement.

Trial

A trial typically consists of (1) jury selection, (2) opening statements, (3) plaintiff's trial testimony, (4) defendant's trial testimony, (5) closing arguments, (6) jury instructions given by the judge, and (7) delivery of the jury's verdict. There also may be post-verdict proceedings and motions. The lawyers for all parties file briefs with the court in advance of the trial to outline the case for the trial judge. The lawyers also prepare and argue over the content of jury instructions, seeking the best language to support their theory of the case. The judge decides which jury instructions will be given and reads them to the jurors just before jury deliberation. Attorneys frequently file motions about significant trial proceedings, such as the scope of admissible evidence. The trial judge rules on these motions outside the presence of the jury.

A jury verdict does not necessarily end the case. If a verdict in favor of the plaintiffs is reached, defense counsel may file one of the following motions: (1) to ask the court to set aside the verdict and grant a new trial; (2) to ask the court to change the verdict and enter a judgment in the defendant's favor; or (3) to ask for a reduction in the amount of damages awarded to the plaintiff(s). Defense counsel also may seek to reopen settlement negotiations or may choose to appeal the case. The plaintiff(s) may take similar post-verdict steps if the jury renders a verdict in favor of the defendant(s).

The vast majority of medical malpractice cases never go to trial. A 1991 study showed that only 2% of persons injured by physicians' negligence ever file a lawsuit.[20] Subsequently, only 10% of all medical malpractice claims go to trial.[21] Settlement negotiations result in the disposal of many cases. Other cases are dismissed by plaintiffs or are dismissed by the court on legal grounds such as **summary judgment,** when a judge may rule that a plaintiff's case is legally insufficient. Defendants win approximately 71% of medical malpractice claims.[21]

In seeking to minimize the often lengthy and costly litigation process, some states have turned to various types of alter-native dispute resolution to resolve claims against health care providers. The state of Washington has passed legislation that requires that all causes of action for damages arising from injury resulting from health care be subject to mandatory mediation prior to trial.[22]

INFORMED CONSENT

Documentation

Before providing medical care, a physician is obligated to obtain informed consent from the patient or the patient's legally authorized surrogate decision-maker. Informed consent is a process, not a form. Consent is the dialog between the patient and the health care provider in which both parties ask questions and exchange information; the end result is the patient's agreement to a specific surgical or medical intervention. The "consent form" cannot replace the exchange of information; rather, it may serve only to document the process.

Nonetheless, documentation of informed consent is critical for health care providers. Adequate documentation helps health care providers to defend their actions should patients subsequently challenge their consent for health care. Hospitals, clinics, and individual health care providers frequently choose to use standardized forms for documenting the informed consent process. Using a standardized form has several benefits: (1) it provides some uniform documentation for medical services within the institution or practice, (2) it serves as a guide for what types of information the health care provider(s) should give to their patients, and (3) it provides tangible evidence of the discussion/exchange of information between the health care provider(s) and the patient. This evidence may be especially compelling when the patient signs a statement affirming that the information was received. In some jurisdictions, a valid consent form signed by the patient may provide a direct means of defense and actually shift the burden of proof to the plaintiff who wishes to make a claim of lack of informed consent. For example, Washington law shifts the burden of proof to a patient claiming lack of informed consent if a consent form (for the treatment at issue) containing the statutory required elements is signed by the patient. In such jurisdictions, a rebuttable presumption that informed consent was obtained is created by the use of a properly executed consent form.[23]

The fact that consent is a communication *process* does not obviate the need for some type of documentation to record the conclusion of the process. This authorization for treatment is important for several reasons. As previously noted, a properly signed consent form affords a defense to an informed consent action against the provider. There may be other compelling legal reasons to document consent—including the ability to substantiate the provision of services and regulatory compliance in the patient's medical record.[24] A 1986 study noted that many anesthesia departments were not documenting their discussions with patients about either general or specific risks of anesthesia.[25] Recently there has emerged a growing awareness of the value of documenting consent for anesthesia. Some publications recommend the use of a separate standardized anesthesia consent form.[26] This may be driven by concerns stemming from cases such as *Funke v. Fieldman,* in which an anesthesiologist was held liable for failing to inform a patient of the material risks associated with spinal anesthesia. The patient brought suit after she suffered paralysis and bladder control problems attributed to injury as a result of the spinal anesthesia. She claimed that the anesthesiologist told her that the only potential complication of spinal anesthesia was headache.[27]

Specific recommendations for adequate anesthesia record keeping are included in the ASA statement, "Documentation of Anesthesia Care."[28] Adequate charting is critical to defending a malpractice claim. Without good documentation, health care providers may be unable to defend their actions successfully, even if the treatment met the medical standard of care. However, there is a lack of consensus as to whether anesthesiologists should have patients sign a separate anesthesia consent form.

Capacity to Consent/Mental Competence

To provide medical consent, a patient must be able to make an informed choice about recommended treatment. This includes understanding the risks and benefits of the treatment options, including nontreatment. Health care providers and the courts often use the terms *capacity/incapacity* and *competence/incompetence* interchangeably to describe whether a patient has the ability to make a reasoned choice regarding health care. The determination as to whether a patient has the ability to provide informed consent generally is a professional judgment made by the treating health care provider. However, if a court has made a judgment regarding a patient's capacity to make such decisions, the health care provider(s) should obtain a copy of the court order, because it may delineate whether the patient is considered able to make his or her own health care decisions. For example, a guardianship is a type of court proceeding that may have an impact on the informed consent process. If a patient has a legal guardian with the authority to make health care decisions on behalf of the patient, that guardian should be consulted about the patient's care and is the person legally authorized to provide consent.

Most states have laws that delineate who is legally authorized to provide consent for health care decisions on behalf of an incapacitated individual. State laws vary, but they typically provide a list of persons (in order of priority) who may give consent. These laws assume that legal relatives are the most appropriate surrogate decision-makers. However, the competent patient is free to select any competent adult to act as his or her health care decision-maker by executing a **Durable Power of Attorney for Health Care,** which appoints that person as his or her agent. For example, Washington law authorizes the following persons to make decisions for an incapacitated patient, in order of priority: guardian, holder of Durable Power of Attorney, spouse, adult children, parents, and adult brothers and sisters.[14] Health care providers are required to make reasonable efforts to locate a person in the highest possible category to provide consent. If there are two or more persons in the same category (e.g., adult children), then the medical treatment decision must be unanimous among those persons. These surrogate decision-makers generally are required to make "substituted judgment" decisions on behalf of the patient (i.e., they are obligated to decide as they believe the patient would, not as they may prefer). If what the patient would want under the circumstances is unknown, then the surrogate must make a decision consistent with the patient's "best interests."[29] The surrogate decision-maker has the authority to provide consent for medical treatment, including nontreatment.

Minor Patients

Existing laws regarding the ability of minors to provide their own consent for medical care may be best understood as a patchwork quilt. Both state statutes and case law may differ from state to state. There are three ways in which a minor may be deemed able to give his or her own consent for medical care: (1) by state law that permits the minor to consent for the specific type of care; (2) by a clinical determination made by the health care providers that the minor is mature and emancipated for consent purposes; and (3) by a judicial determination of emancipation.

In the past, minors were unable to provide consent for any medical treatment. Even today, for most health care decisions, a parent is still required to provide consent for medical treatment of a minor patient.[24] Thus health care providers should typically obtain consent from the minor's parents before providing nonemergency treatment unless the minor is emancipated (by either a clinical or judicial determination) or the minor is permitted by statute to consent to the type of health care sought.

In most states, minors are permitted to consent for certain types of treatment at ages lower than the age of majority or adulthood.[30] For example, in Washington a minor may consent to treatment of sexually transmitted diseases at 14 years of age and to mental health treatment at 13 years of age, even though the age of majority is 18 years.[31-34] For some medical treatment including contraception and obstetric care, case law has generally held that minors have rights of privacy and autonomy that are fundamental and equivalent to rights of adults.[35] The issue of abortion presents a more complex issue, with the courts often taking a compromise position between (1) affording minors the right to make their own decision regarding the continuation of a pregnancy and (2) according parents or guardians unchallenged authority to determine that the pregnancy will be continued to term.[36]

In addition to statutes and case law regarding a minor's ability to provide consent, there also exists a broader legal concept—the emancipated or mature minor doctrine.[30,37] This doctrine allows health care providers to determine whether a minor is emancipated for providing medical consent. Case law may not give a precise definition of an "emancipated minor," but it may list criteria that health care providers should consider. Such criteria may include the minor's age, maturity, intelligence, training, experience, economic independence, and freedom from parental control. When a minor is deemed emancipated for medical consent, the health care provider should chart the objective facts that support the emancipation decision, consistent with institutional policies and/or other legal guidance.

Some states have adopted emancipation statutes that permit minors to file for emancipation status in court.[38] Typically a minor is required to be a minimum age to file for emancipation. (In Washington the minor must be at least 16 years of age.) Once the court grants emancipation status, a minor generally has the right to give informed consent for health care. A signed copy of the court's emancipation order should be placed in the patient's medical record.

Emancipation per se does not alter the requirement that a patient provide informed consent for medical treatment, including nontreatment. Emancipation status only gives the minor patient rights (for providing consent) that are equal to those of an adult patient. The emancipated minor (like any adult patient) must have the ability to weigh the risks and the benefits of the proposed treatment or nontreatment.

Consent for Labor Analgesia

It is common practice for surgical patients to sign a preoperative consent form, which includes a statement giving consent for anesthesia. The situation in obstetrics is somewhat different in that not all laboring women require operative delivery. Several years ago, an unpublished survey of obstetric centers in the greater Seattle area revealed that approximately one half of the institutions do not require a signed consent form for obstetric procedures other than cesarean section. At many of these institutions, a separate written consent signed by the patient is not obtained before administration of anesthesia. A survey of United States and United Kingdom obstetric anesthesiologists indicated that 52% of United States anesthesiologists (but only 15% of the United Kingdom anesthetists) obtain a separate written consent for epidural analgesia during labor.[39]

In the past at the University of Washington, we did not use a consent form for obstetric or anesthetic procedures associated with labor and vaginal delivery. Since 1997 we have used such a form for obstetric and anesthetic procedures that may be desired or necessary during labor and delivery. A consent form provides a specific opportunity for the patient to ask questions. It also provides additional documentation that consent was obtained. The combined form has the additional advantage of not requiring the patient to sign multiple medicolegal documents. Although a signed consent form is not necessary, it should be standard practice for anesthesiologists to document that verbal informed consent was obtained before administration of anesthesia.

Ideally, the anesthesiologist will discuss anesthesia options before the patient is in severe pain and distress. Unfortunately, the anesthesiologist often first encounters the patient when she is in severe pain. Although the anesthesiologist may tailor the consent process according to the circumstances, the presence of maternal pain and distress does not obviate the need for the anesthesiologist to present a frank discussion of the risks of anesthesia as well as the alternatives. A recent survey of Canadian women revealed their strong preference to be informed of all possible complications of epidural anesthesia, especially serious ones, even when the risk was quite low.[40] This study and others have emphasized that parturients desire to have these discussions as early in labor as possible.

Grice et al.[41] performed a study to evaluate the ability of laboring women to recall the details of preanesthesia discussion and to determine whether verbal consent alone or a combination of verbal and written consent provided superior recall. They randomized 113 laboring women to one of two groups—verbal consent alone or verbal consent plus written consent. The verbal-plus-written consent group had significantly higher recall scores (90 ± 2) than the verbal-only group (80 ± 2). The authors noted that only two women (both in the verbal group) felt that they were unable (because of either inadequate information or situational stress) to give valid consent. The authors concluded that "the high recall scores achieved by the women in both groups suggest that the majority of laboring women are at least as mentally and physically competent to give consent as preoperative cardiac patients."

Clark et al.[42] randomized hospital inpatients to receive either an oral discussion alone or both an oral discussion and a preprinted anesthesia consent form. In contrast to the results of Grice et al.,[41] these authors found that "patients remembered less of the information concerning anesthetic risks discussed during the preoperative interview if they received a preprinted, risk-specific anesthesia consent form at the beginning of the interview." The authors speculated that "patients who see an anesthesia consent form for the first time during the preoperative interview may try to read and listen simultaneously and with their attention divided, may remember less of the preoperative discussion."[42]

Anesthesiologists have expressed concern regarding the adequacy of the informed consent process when women are experiencing the severe pain of active labor. Of interest, the absence of adequate informed consent has rarely been the primary basis for a verdict in a medical malpractice suit in cases involving analgesia during labor. In 1990, Knapp[43] searched the Lexis database and found only three cases that addressed the adequacy of informed consent for anesthesia during labor. In each case, the court ruled in favor of the defendant anesthesiologist. Knapp noted the following:

> Not one even speculated that a consent obtained during the stress of labor might be inadequate for that reason. Each court cited three common factors that supported its finding of informed consent: the information given to the patients, the lack of objection by the patients, and the cooperation given by the patients during performance of the procedures.

In summary, it seems reasonable for the patient to provide her signature as evidence of her consent, if her condition permits. This can be included on a separate anesthesia consent form or as part of a consent form for all obstetric care, including anesthesia. A signed consent form is not necessary, but it should be standard practice for the anesthesiologist to explain the intended procedure, risks, and alternatives and to document this discussion in the medical record. (Editor's note: At the University of Alabama at Birmingham Hospital, we do *not* obtain separate, written consent before the administration of anesthesia for labor or cesarean section.)

REFUSAL OF CARE

Documentation

Competent adult patients may refuse medical treatment, including life-saving care.[24] Health care providers generally determine whether a patient is capable of making medical treatment choices (*vide supra*). In theory, the health care providers' clinical judgment about a patient's capacity to provide informed consent is the same regardless of whether the patient approves or disapproves the treatment plan. However, in practice, these situations often are handled differently. When a patient consents to the recommended medical treatment, there typically is minimal scrutiny of his or her decision-making capacity. However, when a patient refuses potentially life-saving treatment, a higher level of scrutiny is given to the patient's ability to understand and make a choice of nontreatment.

Determination of a patient's capacity to give informed consent typically is a clinical judgment. However, state law usually provides some definitions. For example, Washington law recognizes that a person may be incompetent and unable to give consent because of "mental illness, developmental disability, senility, habitual drunkenness, excessive use of drugs, or other mental incapacity."[44]

If a patient refuses potentially life-saving treatment, the health care providers should carefully assess the patient's capacity to provide informed consent. It may be advisable to obtain a psychiatric consultation as part of this clinical determination. It is important to document the determination of capacity and the objective facts supporting the decision. If a patient is deemed able to provide consent, he or she is able to either choose the recommended treatment plan or reject all care. Institutional policies may require the patient (or health care provider if the patient refuses) to sign an "Against Medical Advice" form for a non-medically approved discharge. If a patient is deemed unable to consent, the health care providers should obtain consent from a legally authorized surrogate decision-maker on the patient's behalf. If an incompetent patient needs emergency medical care, it may be provided consistent with an "emergency exception" *(vide supra)*.

Pregnant Patients

Additional concerns may arise when pregnant patients refuse recommended medical treatment, especially during late pregnancy, when the fetus is deemed viable. These concerns involve both ethical and medicolegal issues. Medical ethicists have debated whether a one-patient or two-patient model is more appropriate when treating pregnant women.[45-47] Likewise, case law reflects a lack of unanimity as to how to approach situations in which a woman refuses to consent to medically indicated life-saving treatment on behalf of herself and/or her unborn child.

AMERICAN COLLEGE OF OBSTETRICIANS AND GYNECOLOGISTS GUIDELINES

In 1999, the American College of Obstetricians and Gynecologists (ACOG) Committee on Ethics issued an opinion regarding patient choice and the maternal-fetal relationship.[48] The ACOG recognized that the maternal-fetal relationship is unique and requires balance between maternal health and autonomy and fetal needs. The ACOG[48] stated, "Every reasonable effort should be made to protect the fetus, but the pregnant woman's autonomy should be respected."

Difficulties arise when a woman appears to resist following medical advice that is intended to benefit her health or the health of her fetus. Within the context of limited medical knowledge and fallibility of judgment, the ACOG[48] recommends that great care be exercised to "present a balanced evaluation of expected outcomes for both parties." If needed, family members, friends, and other caregivers as well as other institutional resources may be enlisted to assist in clarification. Medical ethicists and practitioners agree that clear communication and patient education represent the best means to address maternal-fetal conflict.[46,48,49] Failing resolution, the ACOG[48] outlines three options: (1) respect the patient's autonomy and not proceed with the recommended intervention regardless of the consequences, (2) offer the patient the option of obtaining medical care from another individual before conditions become emergent, and (3) request that the court issue an order to permit the recommended treatment.

When contemplating this last option, the ACOG[48] defines four requisite conditions: (1) "there is a high probability of serious harm to the fetus in respecting the patient's decision"; (2) "there is a high probability that the recommended treatment will prevent or substantially reduce harm to the fetus"; (3) "there are no comparably effective, less intrusive options to prevent harm to the fetus"; and (4) "there is a high probability that the recommended treatment [will] also benefit the pregnant woman or that the risks to the pregnant woman are relatively small."

The ACOG[48] opinion assumes competency and informed consent. Thus, if a pregnant patient is believed to be incompetent and incapable of providing informed consent, the health care providers may not be required to respect the patient's refusal of care. Moreover, if the patient is deemed incompetent and/or a medical emergency exists, care may be provided with consent from a legally authorized surrogate decision-maker or as an "emergency exception" *(vide supra)*.

LEGAL APPROACHES

Conflicts regarding maternal versus fetal rights have resulted in inconsistent court decisions. In some cases the appellate courts have affirmed court orders allowing health care providers to provide medically indicated treatment despite the objections of competent pregnant women. The courts justified these decisions based on the state's interests in protecting the health and welfare of both the mother and the viable unborn child. Examples have involved patients who refused blood transfusion on religious grounds. In some cases, the courts have allowed cesarean delivery despite the objection of a competent patient. Critics of such intervention argue that coercing a pregnant woman to protect her unborn child violates a woman's rights to privacy, bodily autonomy, and equal protection.[50-53] Nonetheless, some courts have placed limits on the rights of pregnant women to refuse treatment.[54-56] The federal courts specifically addressed this issue in the 1990 landmark case, *In re: A.C.*[57]

Angela Carder was a 26-year-old married woman who had had cancer since age 13. At 25 weeks' gestation, she was admitted to George Washington University Hospital, where a massive tumor was found in her lung. Her physicians determined that she would die within a short time. Her husband, her mother, and her physician agreed with her expressed wishes to be kept comfortable during her dying process. Ultimately, the hospital sought judicial review of this course of action. The hospital asked whether a surgical delivery should be authorized to save the potentially viable fetus. The situation was presented to a judge who authorized an emergency cesarean section without first ascertaining (using the principle of substituted judgment) the patient's wishes. Sadly, a cesarean section was performed without full consideration of the patient's wishes, the infant died approximately 2 hours after delivery, and the mother died 2 days later.

This case spawned extensive debate as to whether coercive intervention to protect the fetus is ever morally and legally justifiable.[58,59] With the assistance of the American Civil Liberties Union, Angela's parents sued the hospital, two administrators, and 33 physicians for claims including battery, false imprisonment, discrimination, and medical malpractice. These civil lawsuits were settled after several years of litigation and, as part of this process, the hospital adopted a written policy regarding decision-making for pregnant patients.[46] The court later reversed its initial decision authorizing the surgical delivery and ultimately issued an opinion setting forth the legal principles that should govern the doctor-pregnant patient relationship. The court stated: "In virtually all cases the question of what is to be done is to be decided by the patient—the pregnant woman—on behalf of herself and the fetus. If the patient is incompetent . . . her decision must be ascertained through substituted judgment."[57] In affirming that the patient's wishes, once ascertained, must be followed in "virtually all cases" unless there are "truly extraordinary or compelling reasons to override them," the court did not foreclose the possibility of exceptions to this rule. Typically, these have occurred in fact situations involving "minimally invasive" treatments.[57]

In summary, two approaches are available to the practitioner when dealing with maternal-fetal conflict. One approach is to honor a competent pregnant patient's refusal of care. The other approach (which appears least favored by both contemporary medical ethicists and the ACOG) is to seek judicial review authorizing treatment to override a competent pregnant patient's refusal of care.[60]

In honoring a competent patient's desires to refuse treatment, the health care providers should carefully document the woman's competency and ability to provide informed consent. Every attempt should be made to counsel her to follow the treatment recommendations. Documentation should include how, when, and what information was provided to the patient and the patient's husband and family about the significant risks to both the patient and the unborn child if the recommended care is not provided. If time permits, the treatment options should be reevaluated with the patient at frequent intervals, with detailed documentation in the patient's medical record. Additionally, legal counsel for the health care providers and medical facility may wish to prepare an "assumption of risk" form for the patient (and, if possible, her husband) to sign. This represents another level of documentation (beyond the detailed notes in the patient's medical records) demonstrating that the patient was fully informed about the risks associated with her refusal of treatment and that she voluntarily elected to accept those risks. However, such a release signed by the parents may not protect the physician and medical facility from a claim brought on behalf of the child who suffers an injury as a result of nonintervention. In some cases the court has found that physicians have a duty to provide care to the unborn child.[61,62]

Assumption of the risk does not release a health care provider from his or her obligations to provide treatment within the accepted standard of care. For example, in *Shorter v. Drury*, a case involving a refusal of blood transfusion because of religious preferences, the court upheld the validity of an "assumption of risk" (i.e., release) form that relieved the physician from liability for compliance with the patient's refusal of blood transfusions before or after surgery but nonetheless held him partially responsible for her death because of his negligent performance of the surgery.[63]

Before deciding whether to seek court review, health care providers should identify what issue(s) they want the court to resolve. Is it whether the pregnant patient is competent? Is it whether there is a superior state interest in preserving the life of the viable fetus and/or the pregnant woman despite the (competent) patient's desire to refuse recommended care? Health care providers also should consider whether a court is the proper forum for resolving those issues or whether another forum, such as an institutional ethics committee, may be a better choice. If a patient care dilemma is put before a judge, the health care providers give up a large amount of control over the disposition of the case. Nonetheless, if a patient's competency is at issue and there is adequate time, court review to settle the patient's competency may be beneficial and is supported by both the ACOG guidelines and the *In re: A.C.* decision. It is beneficial to obtain authorization for the provision of medically recommended care without waiting until the health care providers believe it has become an emergency. (Note: For mentally ill patients, a referral to mental health authorities may be necessary to obtain authorization to keep the woman hospitalized.) If the patient is deemed incompetent, the court may appoint a surrogate decision-maker or instead authorize directly (by court order) the provision of medically indicated care.

Several years ago, the University of Washington obtained a court order authorizing a recommended cesarean section for a mentally ill woman who was unable to provide consent and who was estranged from her family, who were her legally authorized surrogate decision-makers. This type of judicial resolution differs from a request for a court order to compel treatment over the objections of a competent patient. The ability of a competent patient to reject even potentially life-saving treatment on behalf of herself and her fetus is supported by both the ACOG opinion and the most recent judicial reasoning.

LIABILITY PROFILES IN OBSTETRIC ANESTHESIA: THE ASA CLOSED-CLAIMS PROJECT

In 1985 the ASA Committee on Professional Liability began an ongoing study of insurance company liability files involving anesthesiologists. Cases that are closed (i.e., no longer active) are reviewed by practicing anesthesiologists, abstracted, double-checked by the ASA Closed-Claims Committee, and entered into a computer database. In 1991 the first analysis of obstetric anesthesia cases was published, based on a total database of 1541 files.[64] Another comprehensive analysis of the obstetric anesthesia cases was published in 1996 when the database contained 3533 files.[65] As of June 2003, some 5803 files (excluding those for dental injuries) from over 35 insurance companies from across the country have been reviewed and entered into the ASA Closed-Claims Project database. The analysis reported in this chapter has not been published elsewhere and focuses specifically on the 706 obstetric files in the ASA Closed-Claims database.

It is important to recognize the limitations of this kind of study. A closed-claims study cannot determine the incidence of a complication, for a number of reasons. First, the denominator is unknown. That is to say, neither the total number of anesthetics in each category given each year nor the actual number of injuries per year is known. Second, not all injuries result in a claim of malpractice, and the anesthesiologist may not be named in a claim resulting from an anesthesia-related injury. This latter category may comprise a significant population of patients, which may make the relationship between cause and injury impossible to construct.[66] Conversely, anesthesiologists may be named in claims in which there was no anesthesia-related adverse event.

The files that have been reviewed are not a random sample of such data. However, given the large number of participating insurance carriers, they most likely are broadly representative of liability files involving obstetric anesthesia care in the United States.

Despite the significant limitations of closed-claims studies, such efforts do provide information that cannot be obtained in other ways. For example, files involving obstetric anesthesia care can be compared with those from other types of anesthesia practice to determine whether different patterns of injury and outcome emerge. We can ask such questions as: What injuries are most common in obstetric anesthesia files? What is the relationship between the type of anesthesia and the presumed injury? What are the precipitating events that lead to the injuries? How do payment rates compare between obstetric and nonobstetric claims?

Approximately 12% of the 5803 files in the ASA Closed-Claims database involve anesthesia care for patients undergoing vaginal delivery or cesarean section. Of these obstetric cases, 67% involve cesarean section. The anesthesia workforce survey conducted in 1981 and again in 1992 revealed a significant increase in the proportion of cesarean sections performed under regional anesthesia and a corresponding decrease in those performed with general anesthesia.[67,68] An analysis of the ASA Closed-Claims database illustrates a similar trend in the claims for cases involving regional and general anesthesia for cesarean delivery (Figure 29-1). Together, the parallel trends between the ASA Closed-Claims database and the workforce survey suggest that no anesthetic technique for cesarean section is inherently more (or less) likely to result in a malpractice suit.

Anesthesia-Related Injuries

Table 29-1 lists all injuries or complications that had a frequency of 5% or greater in the obstetric files, as well as the type of anesthesia that resulted in the injury. **Maternal death** and **neonatal brain damage** were the most common injuries. A significantly greater proportion of the maternal deaths involved general anesthesia. Since the 1970s the proportion of maternal deaths in the closed claims involving regional anesthesia has been declining while the proportion of deaths involving general anesthesia has remained relatively constant (FW Cheney, personal communication). As the number of women receiving general anesthesia for cesarean section decreases, this group of patients may be disproportionately represented by the highest risk patients.[69]

The reports of neonatal brain damage also varied according to the type of anesthesia, with a higher incidence of claims associated with general anesthesia. The claims involving

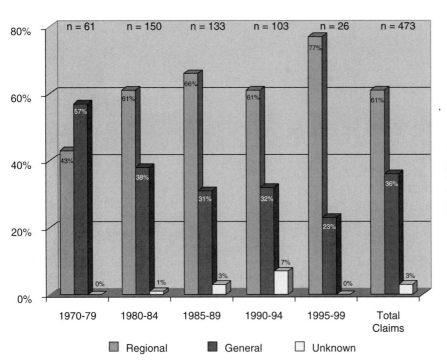

FIGURE 29-1. The percentage of closed-claims files in which the anesthetic technique for cesarean section was either regional, general, or unknown. Data are shown as the percentage of the total number of claims for the years indicated. (From ASA Closed-Claims Project database, $n = 5803$, June, 2003.)

TABLE 29-1	MOST COMMON INJURIES IN THE OBSTETRIC ANESTHESIA FILES				
	Obstetric files ($n = 706$)	Regional anesthesia ($n = 488$)	General anesthesia ($n = 193$)	Cesarean section ($n = 473$)	Vaginal delivery ($n = 232$)
Maternal death	17% (117)	9% (43)*	37% (71)	21% (100)*	7% (17)
Neonatal brain damage	18% (124)	15% (71)*	24% (46)	18% (86)	16% (38)
Headache	14% (99)	19% (94)*	2% (3)	9% (45)*	23% (54)
Maternal nerve damage	14% (96)	18% (90)*	3% (5)	12% (55)	18% (41)
Pain during anesthesia	8% (53)	10% (48)*	2% (3)	10% (47)*	3% (6)
Back pain	10% (69)	14% (69)*	0% (0)	6% (29)	17% (40)
Maternal brain damage	7% (50)	6% (28)	9% (18)	8% (40)	4% (10)
Emotional distress	8% (53)	8% (40)	7% (13)	8% (38)	6% (15)
Neonatal death	6% (44)	5% (24)	8% (15)	7% (33)	5% (11)
Aspiration pneumonitis	4% (25)	1% (4)*	11% (21)	4% (21)	2% (4)

The most common injuries in the obstetric group of files are shown in order of decreasing frequency. Percentages are based on the total files in each group. Some files indicated more than one injury and are represented more than once. Files involving brain damage include only patients who were alive when the file was closed. In some files the type of anesthetic was not recorded; thus the n for the anesthesia files equals 681 rather than 706. (From ASA Closed-Claims Project database, $n = 5803$, June, 2003.)
* $P \leq 0.05$.

newborn injury presented a particular problem (i.e., determining whether a causal link existed between the anesthetic care and the injury to the newborn). Anesthesiologist reviewers identified a causal relationship between anesthetic care (negligent or otherwise) and adverse outcome in only 25% of newborn brain-injury claims and 23% of newborn deaths. By comparison, a causal relationship was thought probable between anesthesia and injury in 65% of all obstetric files and 67% of all nonobstetric files. (Again, this ignores issues related to negligence or standard of care.) This disparity suggests that anesthesiologists might be more likely to be named unfairly in claims involving newborn injury than in claims involving other types of injury. The payment rate was 43% in the files involving neonatal brain injury and 34% in those involving neonatal death. This was lower than the rate in all obstetric (46%) and nonobstetric (54%) liability files. It appeared that, to some extent, the legal system and insurance industry are able to identify unjust claims involving newborn injury.

Some injuries (e.g., headache, pain during anesthesia, back pain) were almost exclusively associated with regional anesthetic techniques. Most files involving pain during anesthesia were associated with cesarean delivery (see Table 29-1). This indicates that inadequate analgesia for labor and vaginal delivery is rarely a source of liability risk. However, women expect to have satisfactory anesthesia during cesarean section, as do patients undergoing other types of surgery. It also is interesting to note that headache and back pain are relatively more common in the files involving vaginal delivery. This may, in part, be a result of factors unique to labor and vaginal delivery (e.g., back strain from assumption of unnatural positions during anesthesia, bearing down during the second stage).[70,71]

Table 29-2 depicts the most common injuries identified after eliminating those involving only the newborn. This allows comparison of the profiles of maternal injury with those among the nonobstetric population. The most striking finding is that the maternal files contain a much higher proportion of relatively minor injuries such as headache, pain during anesthesia, back pain, and emotional distress (47%) than do the nonobstetric files (9%). Obstetric patients may be at greater risk for some of these complications. For example, the popularity of regional anesthetic techniques in obstetrics combined with the greater risk of postdural puncture headache in young females may account for the greater number of headache claims in the obstetric group. Pain during anesthesia almost always is associated with cesarean section conducted with regional anesthesia. These claims may have resulted from a reluctance by the anesthesiologist to convert to general anesthesia because of the risk of aspiration. In some cases claims may have resulted from other factors, such as unrealistic expectations or general dissatisfaction with the care provided.

Precipitating Events Leading to Injuries

Perhaps even more important than the injuries and complications that may result in claims are the precipitating events that lead to the injuries (Table 29-3). Critical events involving the respiratory system are the most common events in both the obstetric and nonobstetric populations. The literature supports the observations that difficult tracheal intubation and pulmonary aspiration are more likely in pregnant than in nonpregnant patients undergoing anesthesia.[72,73] Difficult intubation was the precipitating event in 38 (5%) of the

TABLE 29-2	MATERNAL INJURIES COMPARED WITH SIMILAR INJURIES IN NONOBSTETRIC FILES	
	Maternal injury files (*n* = 583)	Nonobstetric files (*n* = 5097)
Maternal/patient death	20% (117)*	32% (1608)
Headache	17% (99)*	2% (97)
Maternal/patient nerve damage	16% (96)*	19% (945)
Pain during anesthesia	9% (53)*	1% (45)
Back pain	12% (68)*	2% (95)
Maternal/patient brain damage	9% (50)*	12% (627)
Emotional distress	9% (53)*	4% (192)
Aspiration pneumonitis	4% (25)	2% (121)

The most common maternal injuries in the obstetric anesthesia files are shown in order of decreasing frequency. Percentages are based on the total files in each group. Some files, especially those with a fatal outcome, had more than one injury and are represented more than once. Cases involving brain damage include only patients who were alive when the file was closed. (From ASA Closed-Claims Project database, *n* = 5803, June, 2003.)
* $P \leq 0.05$.

claims and pulmonary aspiration was the precipitating event in 19 (3%) of the claims. General anesthesia was the primary anesthetic technique in a majority (> 80%) of these cases, despite general anesthesia being used in only 28% of the obstetric claims. In half of the cases aspiration occurred during difficult endotracheal intubation or following an esophageal intubation. In several cases general anesthesia was given by mask, and in three cases aspiration was noted to have occurred during the induction of anesthesia without cricoid pressure. Two cases of aspiration associated with regional anesthesia occurred during resuscitation and intubation efforts in patients with high spinal anesthesia. In two other cases, aspiration occurred during successful regional anesthesia. In one case heavy sedation was implicated; in the other, the patient apparently aspirated while vomiting after delivery of the infant.

Other reports have suggested that difficult intubation and pulmonary aspiration are the leading causes of anesthesia-related maternal mortality[69,73,74] (see Chapters 30 and 31). A survey of members of the Society for Obstetric Anesthesia and Perinatology (SOAP) found that pulmonary aspiration typically is associated with difficult intubation.[75] Together, these data reemphasize the need to consider all obstetric patients as having a full stomach. These data also reinforce the need to have appropriate protocols and equipment immediately available for the management of patients in whom tracheal intubation proves difficult.

Obesity increases the risk for both obstetric[76,77] and anesthetic[73,78,79] complications in pregnant women (see Chapter 49). In the ASA Closed-Claims Study, damaging events related to the respiratory system were significantly more common among the claims involving obese parturients (20%) than among the claims involving nonobese parturients (9%) ($P < 0.05$). However, other injuries were not significantly different when obese and nonobese parturients were compared.[65]

A total of 69 files (compared with 34 in the previous report in 1998) describe the occurrence of convulsions. Because the data are now collected in a different format, a comparative analysis of these data is not possible. In the previous analysis, maternal convulsions represented the single most common

TABLE 29-3   MOST COMMON PRECIPITATING EVENTS IN THE OBSTETRIC ANESTHESIA FILES

	Nonobstetric files (n = 5097)	Obstetric files (n = 706)	Obstetric regional anesthesia (n = 488)	Obstetric general anesthesia (n = 193)
Respiratory system	25% (1284)*	13% (92)	2% (11)*	41% (80)
Difficult intubation	6% (304)	5% (38)	< 0.5% (1)*	19% (37)
Aspiration	2% (109)	3% (19)	< 0.5% (1)*	9% (18)
Esophageal intubation	4% (195)*	1% (9)	0% (0)*	5% (9)
Inadequate ventilation/oxygenation	6% (321)*	1% (10)	1% (4)	3% (5)
Bronchospasm	1% (52)	1% (7)	< 0.5% (2)	3% (5)
Premature extubation	2% (90)	1% (4)	0% (0)	2% (4)
Airway obstruction	2% (110)*	< 0.5% (3)	< 0.5% (2)	1% (1)
Inadequate Fio_2	< 0.5% (5)	< 0.5% (2)	< 0.5% (1)	1% (1)
Convulsions	1% (69)*	6% (42)	7% (32)	4% (8)
Equipment problems	11% (551)*	6% (43)	8% (37)*	3% (6)
Cardiovascular system	13% (680)	11% (78)	13% (61)*	6% (12)
Wrong drug/dose	4% (193)	2% (16)	2% (8)	4% (7)

The most common damaging events in the obstetric files are illustrated in order of decreasing frequency. Percentages are based on the total files in each group. Specific precipitating events were not identified in all cases. Some files indicated more than one damaging event, but only the most significant event is listed. Statistical comparisons are made between obstetric and equivalent nonobstetric files as well as between obstetric regional and obstetric general anesthetics. (From ASA Closed-Claims Project database, n = 5803, June, 2003.)
* $P \leq 0.05$.

damaging event in the obstetric files. Among those 34 files, five cases were not associated with epidural anesthesia and appeared to signal eclampsia. Of the remaining 29, all were associated with epidural anesthesia, and at least 22 of these appeared to result from systemic local anesthetic toxicity. A test dose was given in 13 of these 22 cases, but the medical record documented the use of epinephrine in only 3 of these cases. In the remaining nine files there was no documentation of *any* test dose. In files in which convulsions were listed as the primary damaging event, the adverse outcome was neurologic injury or death to the mother, newborn, or both in 74% of the cases.

Since 1984 there has been a marked decrease in the number of claims involving convulsions. This may be a result of a greater awareness of the problems of local anesthetic toxicity in parturients, which became apparent in the early 1980s. Clearly the quality of obstetric anesthesia care (including the use of appropriate monitoring and resuscitation equipment) has improved in the past two decades. The use of an effective test dose, the incremental injection of the therapeutic dose of local anesthetic, and the proscription against the epidural injection of 0.75% bupivacaine in pregnant women have undoubtedly contributed to a reduction in the risk of serious adverse outcomes associated with epidural anesthesia in obstetric patients.

Some obstetric patients are reluctant to accept regional anesthesia because of the fear of nerve injury. Because such injuries are very rare, anesthesiologists often minimize the risks of neurologic injury. However, nerve injury was the third most common injury among the maternal injury claims. In 1998 a panel of anesthesiologists reviewed each of the cases of nerve injury associated with epidural or spinal anesthesia to gain more insight into the likely etiology of these injuries.[80] The panel judged that 21 of 38 (55%) of these maternal nerve injuries were direct complications of the regional block procedure. The panel also attempted to determine a likely mechanism of injury (Table 29-4). A surprising finding was that most of the cases of nerve injury appeared to result from

TABLE 29-4   CAUSES OF REGIONAL ANESTHESIA-RELATED MATERNAL NERVE INJURIES

Likely etiology	% (n = 21)
Needle or catheter trauma	52% (11)
Neurotoxicity	19% (4)
Ischemia (e.g., abscess, hematoma, hypotension, vascular insufficiency)	14% (3)
Other identified causes	10% (2)
Undetermined	5% (1)

A panel of five anesthesiologists independently reviewed all maternal nerve injury closed-claims files in which epidural or spinal anesthesia was used (n = 38). In 21 (55%) of these cases, the injury was judged to be a result of the regional block procedure. For those 21 cases, the likely mechanism of injury is indicated in the table. (From ASA Closed Claims Project database, n = 3533.)
Modified from Chadwick HS. An analysis of obstetric anesthesia cases from the American Society of Anesthesiologists Closed-Claims Project database. Int J Obstet Anesth 1996; 5:258-63.

direct trauma to neural tissue by the needle or catheter. Neurotoxicity and ischemic injury from epidural abscess, hypotension, or vascular insufficiency were less common. Of interest, there were no cases of epidural hematoma among the maternal injury claims.

Payments

Obstetrics and anesthesiology are specialties with high medicolegal risk. Thus it seems logical that obstetric anesthesia is a subspecialty with especially high risk. This belief is reinforced by well-publicized cases involving huge monetary awards. However, the ASA Closed-Claims Project provides a somewhat different perspective. For the purposes of this discussion, payments are considered to be any expenditure by the insurance carrier in the form of a settlement or award. Obstetric files constitute 12% of the ASA Closed-Claims database. Similarly, the obstetric files account for 10% of the total number of payments made and 14% of the total dollars expended in payments. Clearly, the payments for obstetric claims were not disproportionately frequent or large. Table 29-5 provides additional payment information. For cases in which payments were made, the median payment was greater in the obstetric group. This is not surprising, considering that there are two patients at risk in obstetric anesthesia and both the mother and her infant are younger than the average age of patients in the nonobstetric files. Although the obstetric files contained a lower proportion of deaths (either maternal or newborn), there was a greater proportion of brain injuries (either maternal or newborn) as compared with the nonobstetric files. Such injuries typically result in higher payments for projected lifelong care requirements.

Lessons Learned

The obstetric anesthesia files reveal a risk profile that differs from that of the nonobstetric anesthesia files. To a large extent the findings support the commonly held beliefs regarding risk areas in obstetric anesthesia. Anesthesiologists frequently are named in lawsuits involving "bad baby" outcomes. Reassuringly, the proportion of these cases that result in payments does not seem excessive. Problems involving airway management, especially difficult intubation and pulmonary aspiration, are disproportionately represented in the obstetric files. One of the major causes of severe adverse outcomes with regional anesthesia is systemic local anesthetic toxicity. Fortunately evidence suggests that the incidence of this problem is declining. The data suggest that we need to continue our efforts to reduce the known causes of major anesthetic complications.

Perhaps the most surprising finding is the large proportion of relatively minor injuries in the obstetric files. This is in marked contrast to the nonobstetric files and suggests that efforts to reduce the incidence of major injuries will not solve the medical malpractice problem in obstetric anesthesia. Clearly factors other than major injury must motivate patients to bring a claim. It is overly simplistic to equate lawsuits with injury. A 1991 study found that the proportion of patients harmed by negligent care who actually file a claim is only 2%.[16] However, a lawsuit does not occur unless someone perceives that he or she or a loved one has been wronged. One of the unique advantages of closed-claims studies is that they reflect the consumer perspective.

To some extent the large proportion of relatively minor injuries in the obstetric files may reflect a greater incidence of such problems among obstetric patients. However, it is clear that many of these patients were unhappy with the care provided and believed that they had been ignored, mistreated, or assaulted. It has been suggested that malpractice litigation serves the purposes not only of reparation of injury and deterrence of substandard care but also of emotional vindication.[81,82] Anesthesia care providers should give attention to conducting themselves in such a manner that patients will not be motivated to bring suit for an unexpected outcome.[83] The importance of establishing good rapport with patients cannot be overemphasized. Whenever possible anesthesiologists should involve themselves in the prenatal education process. A careful preanesthetic evaluation is very important and should occur as early in labor as possible. Special care should be taken to provide patients with realistic expectations and knowledge of potential major and minor risks associated with anesthetic procedures.

PROFESSIONAL PRACTICE STANDARDS

One beneficial effect of closed-claims analysis has been the greater attention to steps to minimize the occurrence of severe adverse outcomes. Based on an analysis of malpractice claims in 1985, the Harvard University-affiliated medical institutions adopted a set of minimal monitoring standards within their system. Since that time the malpractice losses (normalized for the number of anesthetics given) have declined by more than 50%.[84] In 1986 the ASA became the first professional medical society to promulgate professional standards of care. The introduction of the ASA "Standards for Basic Intra-Operative Monitoring" was accompanied by a decrease in the number of anesthesia-related liability claims. Although it is difficult to prove a cause-and-effect relationship between the introduction of these standards and fewer claims and payments, the arguments seem compelling.[84] Improved monitoring, especially the greater use of pulse oximetry and capnography, has undoubtedly contributed to the decrease in severe complications and associated large awards.[85,86]

The ASA also has directed its efforts at improving obstetric anesthesia care in this country through a variety of position statements. In 1986 the ASA House of Delegates and the ACOG approved a joint statement entitled "Optimal Goals for Anesthesia Care in Obstetrics." This policy-oriented document recognized the need for (1) appropriately trained physicians to

TABLE 29-5	PAYMENT DATA			
	Nonobstetric files (n = 5097)	Obstetric files (n = 706)	Obstetric regional anesthesia (n = 488)	Obstetric general anesthesia (n = 193)
No payment	36% (1850)*	44% (314)	50% (243)*	31% (60)
Payments made	54% (2758)*	46% (323)	39% (190)*	63% (121)
Median payment	$100,000†	$150,000	$75,000†	$345,000
Range	$15 to $23,200,000	$420 to $7,000,000	$420 to $6,800,000	$750 to $7,000,000

Payment frequency and dollar amounts (not adjusted for inflation) are illustrated. Percentages are based on the total number of files in each group and do not equal 100% because of missing data. Statistical comparisons are made between payment distributions for obstetric and nonobstetric claims and between payment distributions for cases involving obstetric regional and obstetric general anesthetics. Claims with no payments were excluded from calculations of median payment and range. (From ASA Closed-Claims Project database, n = 5803, June, 2003.)
* $P \leq 0.05$.
† $P \leq 0.01$.

provide anesthesia care when necessary, (2) a qualified obstetrician to be readily available during the administration of anesthesia, and (3) equipment, facilities, and support personnel for labor and delivery units equal to that provided in the surgical suite. The document served as the basis for the ASA "Standards for Conduction Anesthesia in Obstetrics," which was approved by the ASA House of Delegates in 1988. Unfortunately, unlike the widely acclaimed "Standards for Basic Intra-Operative Monitoring," these obstetric anesthesia practice standards generated immediate and widespread controversy. In part, this was because they had implications with regard to nursing, obstetric, and pediatric practices and were considered too restrictive and too difficult to meet, especially for smaller or rural obstetric facilities. Consequently, in 1991 the document was revised and renamed "Guidelines for Regional Anesthesia in Obstetrics" and was last amended in 2000 (see Appendix A on p. 951).

In October 1998, the ASA House of Delegates approved a document developed by the ASA Task Force on Obstetrical Anesthesia. This document, titled "Practice Guidelines for Obstetrical Anesthesia," is more clinically oriented than the aforementioned guidelines (see Appendix B on p. 953). It synthesizes a large body of published studies "to enhance the quality of anesthesia care for obstetric patients, reduce the incidence and severity of anesthesia-related complications, and increase patient satisfaction." The document provides analytic assessments of specific anesthetic techniques and practices, along with general recommendations. It is unclear to what extent these practice guidelines will affect the quality of care or the liability profiles in obstetric anesthesia practice. These practice guidelines are now amplified by an updated version of "Optimal Goals for Anesthesia Care in Obstetrics," another joint statement from the ASA and the ACOG (see Appendix C on p. 959).

Practice guidelines suggest a standard of care and are based on expert opinion. As such they often are used as evidence in cases of medical malpractice. Such documents can be used for exculpatory purposes (i.e., to exonerate a defendant physician) or as inculpatory evidence (i.e., to implicate a defendant physician). A two-part study surveyed 960 randomly selected malpractice attorneys and 259 open and closed claims from two malpractice insurance companies.[87] The claims were opened during a 2-year period (1990 to 1992) and included all claims involving obstetric and anesthetic cases. Practice guidelines played a pivotal role in 17 cases. In 12 cases they were used as inculpatory evidence and in 4 as exculpatory evidence. (In one case the use of practice guidelines could not be classified.) Similarly, the surveyed attorneys responded that guidelines were used to implicate malpractice more than twice as often as they were used to defend against a claim of malpractice (54% versus 23%). The ACOG guidelines were used most frequently in these claims but the ASA guidelines rarely were used. The authors speculated that the simplicity and clarity of the ASA guidelines may make compliance easier. Clearly, practice guidelines may act as a double-edged sword in medical litigation. Nonetheless, guidelines may reduce litigation expenses by dissuading plaintiffs' attorneys from pursuing cases in which guidelines have been met or by encouraging early settlement by the defense in cases in which guidelines were not followed without good reason.

POTENTIAL RISK MANAGEMENT PROBLEM AREAS

Obstetric anesthesia often is an unpredictable, difficult, and high-stress environment for the anesthesiologist. Compared with the operating room environment, the typical obstetric service is less familiar and more chaotic. The role and responsibility of the anesthesiologist is less clearly defined. Anesthesia services may be urgently requested in a situation in which there is little information available about the patient and the patient is unable or unwilling to answer questions. Laboring women typically are not sedated and calm when they request regional anesthesia. Rather, women in active labor may be uncooperative and even combative during the administration of regional anesthesia. The anesthesiologist may need to provide care for multiple patients simultaneously and may need to entrust some monitoring responsibilities to nurses. In some situations the choice of anesthesia may be dictated by others, and anesthesiologists may feel that they are little more than technicians. Perhaps it is not surprising that many anesthesia care providers are uncomfortable in that environment and prefer to minimize their liability and discomfort by limiting their time in obstetrics.

Unique to obstetric anesthesia is the presence of the patient's husband, boyfriend, or other support person during anesthesia care. In the past it was considered a privilege for a husband or relative to be present during a cesarean section, and often there were preconditions such as documentation of attendance at prenatal classes. Today, in many obstetric centers, it is taken for granted that one or more support persons will be present for virtually any type of delivery. Undoubtedly, this trend has resulted in part from a sincere desire to facilitate a more family-centered experience. A second motivation may be to attract patients in a competitive, market-oriented environment.

We are not aware of specific case law regarding the issues involving support persons. However, the topic does raise a number of risk management questions. What are the parturient's rights with regard to having support personnel present during labor and delivery? What are the rights of the institution and health care providers? The presence of a support person often helps reassure and calm the parturient, but this is not always true. In some cases the presence of a support person can adversely affect patient care. Melzack[88] found that women have higher pain scores during labor when the husband is present. Many anesthesiologists are not accustomed to having lay observers present during anesthesia procedures. Their presence can distract the anesthesiologist's attention and adversely affect judgment and performance. It is helpful, especially in obstetrics, for the anesthesiologist to develop a close physician-patient relationship. The presence of a support person often distracts the patient's attention away from the conversation and activities of the anesthesiologist. In some cases this is helpful, but in others, that distraction interferes with the provision of anesthesia care.

The support person also may be at risk for unanticipated injury.[89] We are aware of a number of instances in which a father suffered an injury as a consequence of a vasovagal episode. In one case the father dropped the newborn infant on the floor as he lost consciousness. Although there was no legal action in any of these cases, the potential liability issues are self-evident.

In some cases, support persons may request that they be present during the delivery even when the patient receives general anesthesia. At the University of Washington, we do not allow support persons in the operating room during administration of general anesthesia because we believe that the possibility for complications is ever present. Even under the best of circumstances, the presence of such a person makes it more difficult for the anesthesiologist to give full attention to the patient. Routine anesthesia practices and procedures during general anesthesia may be frightening and misunderstood by laypersons. No matter how well intentioned and well prepared, the sight of a loved one who is unresponsive, intubated, and mechanically ventilated can be traumatic emotionally.

(Editor's note: At the University of Alabama at Birmingham Hospital, we do *not* allow a support person to be present during the induction of general anesthesia. In selected cases, we allow the support person to enter the operating room after intubation, provided the patient is stable and provided we do not anticipate any maternal complications. The support person sits beyond the foot of the operating table and is unable to see the face of the patient. The circulating nurse assumes responsibility for the support person. The support person leaves the operating room when the pediatrician exits with the infant.)

Physicians and hospitals also should consider policies regarding the use of audio/video equipment in the delivery room. Clearly all patients have a right to refuse to be photographed, filmed, or videotaped. However, a woman often wants a photographic record or videotape of events surrounding her delivery. Such a record can provide dramatic documentation of unfortunate interactions or suboptimal medical care. Courts typically allow videotapes to be entered into evidence and permit videotapes to be edited reasonably.[90] The visual impact of delivery room events can have a profound impact on a jury, regardless of whether the videotape has been edited to the advantage of the plaintiff. After the presentation of such evidence, it may be difficult to convince a jury of the appropriateness of treatment.

A survey of 35 members of the American College of Legal Medicine identified nine cases in which an obstetric videotape was used as evidence.[90] In response to such cases, some hospitals have instituted policies to limit the use of video equipment in their labor and delivery suites. Such policies may antagonize patients and prompt them to seek care elsewhere. A balanced approach may be the best solution (i.e., it may be reasonable to allow use of video equipment but to establish clear, fair, and unambiguous policies regarding its use). The policies must be understood by all members of the staff and should be made known to patients and their families, preferably before the patient is admitted to the hospital. Prenatal classes can serve as a means to disseminate such information. One approach is to have informational material and/or specific consent forms for patients and their families. Another option is to combine such policy statements with a "hold harmless" waiver for the support person (see Appendix at the end of this chapter). Although none of these measures can eliminate the potential liability risks associated with these issues, they may serve to educate patients and their families about their rights and about hospital policies and procedures.

KEY POINTS

- Altered maternal physiology during pregnancy and labor, the existence of two patients with differing needs, and the fact that labor and delivery are viewed as normal processes all challenge the anesthesiologist to provide a service that is beneficial

to the woman, safe for the mother and fetus, and one that does not impede or disrupt the process of labor and delivery.
- Honest, caring, and comprehensive discussion with the patient before the administration of anesthesia meets legal and ethical standards, improves the image of the anesthesiologist, and reduces the likelihood of dissatisfaction and possible litigation after unanticipated complications.
- Refusal of care by pregnant patients may raise unique legal and ethical concerns. In such situations, the woman's competency or ability to make an informed medical decision may be an issue. When the patient is competent, the health care providers should attempt to resolve treatment conflicts through additional patient education and discussion. Rarely, it may be advisable to seek a court order to resolve competency and/or medical treatment issues.
- Critical events involving the respiratory system were the most common precipitating events leading to adverse outcome in both the obstetric and nonobstetric ASA Closed-Claim files. Failed intubation and pulmonary aspiration are more common during administration of general anesthesia in pregnant women than in nonpregnant women.
- Maternal closed-claim files include a much higher proportion of relatively minor injuries (e.g., headache, pain during anesthesia, back pain, emotional distress) than do nonobstetric files.
- The careful use of a test dose, the incremental injection of a local anesthetic agent, and the avoidance of 0.75% bupivacaine appear to have reduced the incidence of maternal convulsions during the administration of epidural anesthesia.
- The relief of pain, maintenance of maternal and fetal homeostasis, and participation in and contribution toward a joyous event constitute the rewards of obstetric anesthesia practice.

REFERENCES

1. Furrow BR, Greaney TL. Liability and Quality Issues in Health Care, 4th ed. St. Paul, West Publishing Co., 2001: 139-48.
2. Rev. Code Wash. (ARCW) § 7.70.030 (Lexis 2003).
3. Rev. Code Wash. (ARCW) § 7.70.040 (Lexis 2003).
4. *Miller v. Jacoby.* 145 Wash. 2d 65, 33 P.3d 68 (2001).
5. Furrow BR, Greaney TL. Liability and Quality Issues in Health Care, 4th ed. St. Paul, West Publishing Co., 2001: 163-6.
6. *Brown v. Dahl.* 41 Wash. App. 565, 705 P.2d 781 (1985).
7. Cheney FW, Perioperative Ulnar Nerve Injury: A Continuing Medical and Liability Problem. ASA Newsletter, Volume 62, May 3, 2003.
8. Beauchamp TL, Childress JF. Principles of Biomedical Ethics, 5th ed. New York, Oxford University Press, 2001: 57-112.
9. *Degel v. Buty.* 108 Wash. App. 126, 29 P.3d 768 (2001).
10. Berg JW, Appelbaum PS, Lidz CW, Parker LS. Informed Consent: Legal Theory and Clinical Practice, 2nd ed. New York, Oxford University Press, 2001: 41-74.
11. *Ruffer v. St. Cabrini Hospital*, 56 Wash. App. 625, 784 P.2d 1288, (1990), *cert. denied*, 114 Wash. 2d 1023 (1990).
12. *Mason v. Ellsworth*, 3 Wash. App. 298, 474 P.2d 909 (1970).
13. *Villanueva v. Harrington*, 80 Wash. App. 36, 906 P.2d 374 (1995).
14. *Barth v. Rock*, 36 Wn. App. 400, 674 P.2d 1265 (1984), *rev. denied*, 101 Wn.2d 1014 (1984).

15. *Rev. Code Wash.* (ARCW) § 7.70.050 (Lexis 2003).
16. *Roe v Wade*, 410 U.S. 113, 93 S. Ct. 705, 35 L. Ed. 2d 147 (1973).
17. *Woe v. Coumo*, 729 F.2d 96 (2nd Cir 1984).
18. Kinney ED. The brave new world of medical standards of care. J Law Med Eth 2001; 29:323-34.
19. Fla. Stat. ch. 408.02(1998); Ky. Rev. Stat. Ann. § 342.035 (Michie 1997); Me. Rev. Stat. Ann. tit. 24 §§ 2971-2979 (West Supp 2000); Md. Code Ann., Health–Gen. I § 19-1602 (2000).
20. Localio AR, Lawthers AG, Brennan TA, et al. Relation between malpractice claims and adverse events due to negligence. Results of the Harvard Medical Practice Study III. N Engl J Med 1991; 325:245-51.
21. Ostrom B, Rottman D, Hanson R. What are tort awards really like? The untold story from the state courts. Law and Policy 1992; 14:77-81.
22. *Rev. Code Wash.* (ARCW) § 7.70.100 (Lexis 2003).
23. *Rev. Code Wash.* (ARCW) § 7.70.060 (Lexis 2003).
24. Rosovsky FA. Consent to Treatment: A Practical Guide, 3rd ed. Gaithersburg, Aspen, 2001.
25. Moore RA, DiBlasio WJ, Amini SB, Amini SB. Anesthesia informed consent in New Jersey (abstract). Anesthesiology 1986; 65:A468.
26. ECRI. Overview of anesthesia liability. Healthcare Risk Control 1996; 4:2-6.
27. *Funke v. Fieldman*, 212 Kan. 524, 512 P.2d 539 (1973).
28. American Society of Anesthesiologists. Documentation of Anesthesia Care. Park Ridge, IL, October 12, 1988.
29. *Rev. Code Wash.* (ARCW) § 7.70.065 (Lexis 2003).
30. Holder AR. Minors' rights to consent to medical care. JAMA 1987; 257:3400-2.
31. *Rev. Code Wash.* (ARCW) § 70.24.110 (Lexis 2003).
32. *Rev. Code Wash.* (ARCW) § 71.34.030 (Lexis 2003).
33. *Rev. Code Wash.* (ARCW) § 70.96A.095 (Lexis 2003).
34. *Rev. Code Wash.* (ARCW) § 26.28.010 (Lexis 2003).
35. *State v. Koome*, 84 Wash.2d 901, 530 P.2d 260 (1975).
36. Katz KD. The Pregnant Child's Right to Self-Determination. 62 Alb. L. Rev. 1119, 1145 (1999).
37. Annas GJ. The Rights of Patients: The Basic ACLU Guide to Patient Rights, 2nd ed. Carbondale, Southern Illinois University Press, 1992: 110-14.
38. Hawkins LA. Living will statutes: A minor oversight. Virginia Law Rev 1992; 78:1581-615.
39. Bush DJ. A comparison of informed consent for obstetric anaesthesia in the USA and the UK. Internat J Obstet Anesth 1995; 4:1-6.
40. Pattee C, Ballantyne M, Milne B. Epidural analgesia for labour and delivery: Informed consent issues. Can J Anaesth 1997; 44:918-23.
41. Grice SC, Eisenach JC, Dewan DM, Robinson ML. Evaluation of informed consent for anesthesia for labor and delivery (abstract). Anesthesiology 1988; 69:A664.
42. Clark SK, Leighton BL, Seltzer JL. A risk-specific anesthesia consent form may hinder the informed consent process. J Clin Anesth 1991; 3:11-3.
43. Knapp RM. Legal view of informed consent for anesthesia during labor (letter). Anesthesiology 1990; 72:211.
44. *Rev. Code Wash.* (ARCW) § 11.88.010 (Lexis 2003).
45. Mattingly SS. The maternal-fetal dyad: Exploring the two patient obstetric model. Hastings Center Report 1992; 22:13-8.
46. Mishkin DB, Povar GJ. Decision making with pregnant patients: A policy born of experience. Joint Comm J Qual Improv 1993; 19:291-302.
47. Rosner F, Bennett AJ, Cassell EJ, et al. Fetal therapy and surgery: Fetal rights versus maternal obligations. NY State J Med 1989; 89:80-4.
48. American College of Obstetricians and Gynecologists Committee on Ethics. Patient Choice and the Maternal-Fetal Relationship. ACOG Committee Opinion No. 214, April 1999.
49. Mathieu D. Preventing Prenatal Harm: Should the State Intervene? Boston, Kluwer Academic Publishers, 1991: 94-6.
50. Steinbock B. The relevance of illegality. Hastings Center Report 1992; 22:19-22.
51. Gallagher J. Prenatal invasions and interventions: What's wrong with fetal rights. Harvard Women's Law J 1987; 10:4-7.
52. Johnsen DE. The creation of fetal rights: Conflicts with women's constitutional rights to liberty, privacy and equal protection. Yale Law J 1986; 95:599-625.
53. Rhoden NK. The judge in the delivery room: The emergence of court-ordered cesareans. California Law Rev 1986; 74:1986-9.
54. *Jefferson v. Griffin Spalding County Hosp.*, 247 Ga. 85, 274 S.E.2d 457 (1981).
55. *Raleigh Fitkin-Paul Morgan Memorial Hosp. v. Anderson*, 42 N.J. 421, 201 A.2d, *cert. denied*, 377 U.S. 985 (1964).
56. *Crouse Irving Memorial Hosp. v. Paddock*, 485 N.Y.S.2d 443 (Sup. Ct. 1985).
57. *In re: A.C.*, 573 A.2d 1235, 1237 (D.C. App. 1990).
58. Annas GJ. The Rights of Patients: The Basic ACLU Guide to Patient Rights, 2nd ed. Carbondale, Southern Illinois University Press, 1992: 127-30.
59. Neale H. Mother's rights prevail: *In re: A.C.* and the status of forced obstetrical intervention in the District of Columbia. J Health Hosp Law 1990; 23:208-13, 24.
60. Jonsen AR, Siegler M, Winslade WJ. Clinical Ethics, 3rd ed. New York, McGraw-Hill, Inc., 1992: 177-78.
61. *Moen v. Hanson*, 85 Wash.2d 597, 537 P.2d 266 (1975).
62. *Harbeson v. Parke-Davis, Inc.*, 98 Wash.2d 460, 656 P.2d 483 (1983).
63. *Shorter v. Drury*, 103 Wash.2d, 695 P.2d 116 (1985).
64. Chadwick HS, Posner K, Caplan RA, et al. A comparison of obstetric and nonobstetric anesthesia malpractice claims. Anesthesiology 1991; 74:242-9.
65. Chadwick HS. An analysis of obstetric anesthesia cases from the American Society of Anesthesiologists closed-claims project database. Int J Obstet Anesth 1996; 5:258-63.
66. Edbril SD, Lagasse RS. Relationship between malpractice litigation and human errors. Anesthesiology 1999; 91:848-55.
67. Gibbs CP, Krischer J, Peckham BM, et al. Obstetric anesthesia: A national survey. Anesthesiology 1986; 65:298-306.
68. Hawkins JL, Gibbs CP, Orleans M, et al. Obstetric anesthesia work force survey, 1981 versus 1992. Anesthesiology 1997; 87:135-43.
69. Hawkins JL, Koonin LM, Palmer SK, Gibbs CP. Anesthesia-related deaths during obstetric delivery in the United States, 1979-1990. Anesthesiology 1997; 86:277-84.
70. Okell RW, Sprigge JS. Unintentional dural puncture. A survey of recognition and management. Anaesthesia 1987; 42:1110-3.
71. MacArthur C, Lewis M, Knox EC, Crawford JS. Epidural anaesthesia and long term backache after childbirth. Br Med J 1990; 301:9-12.
72. Sreide E, Bjrnestad E, Steen PA. An audit of perioperative aspiration pneumonitis in gynecological and obstetric patients. Acta Anaesthesiol Scand 1996; 40:14-9.
73. Glassenberg R. General anesthesia and maternal mortality. Semin Perinatol 1991; 15:386-96.
74. Hibbard BM, Anderson MM, O Drife J, et al., editors. Report on Confidential Enquiries into Maternal Deaths in the United Kingdom, 1991-1993. London, HMSO, 1996: 51.
75. Gibbs CP, Rolbin SH, Norman P. Cause and prevention of maternal aspiration. Anesthesiology 1984; 61:112-3.
76. Garbaciak JAJ, Richter M, Miller S, Barton JJ. Maternal weight and pregnancy complications. Am J Obstet Gynecol 1985; 152:238-45.
77. Kliegman RM, Gross T. Perinatal problems of the obese mother and her infant. Obstet Gynecol 1985; 66:299-306.
78. Endler GC, Mariona FG, Sokol RJ, Stevenson LB. Anesthesia-related maternal mortality in Michigan, 1972 to 1984. Am J Obstet Gynecol 1988; 159:187-93.
79. Rocke DA, Murray WB, Rout CC, Gouws E. Relative risk analysis of factors associated with difficult intubation in obstetric anesthesia. Anesthesiology 1992; 77:67-73.
80. Chadwick HS, Gunn HC, Ross BK, et al. Nerve injury and regional anesthesia in obstetrics: A review of the ASA Closed Claims Project database (abstract). Anesthesiology 1995; 83:A951.
81. Meyers AR. "Lumping it": The hidden denominator of the medical malpractice crisis. Am J Public Health 1987; 77:1544-8.
82. Hickson GB, Clayton EW, Githens PB, Sloan FA. Factors that prompted families to file medical malpractice claims following perinatal injuries. JAMA 1992; 267:1359-63.
83. Palmer SK, Gibbs CP. Risk management in obstetric anesthesia. Int Anesthesiol Clin 1989; 27:188-99.
84. Holzer JF. The advent of clinical standards for professional liability. Qual Rev Bull 1990; 16:71-9.
85. Eichhorn JH. Prevention of intraoperative anesthesia accidents and related severe injury through safety monitoring. Anesthesiology 1989; 70:572-7.
86. Tinker JH, Dull DL, Caplan RA, et al. Role of monitoring devices in prevention of anesthetic mishaps: A closed claims analysis. Anesthesiology 1989; 71:541-6.
87. Hyams AL, Brandenburg JA, Lipsitz SR, et al. Practice guidelines and malpractice litigation: A two way street. Ann Intern Med 1995; 122:450-5.
88. Melzack R. The myth of painless childbirth (The John J. Bonica Lecture). Pain 1984; 19:321-37.
89. DeVore JS. Paternal fractured skull as a complication of obstetric anesthesia (letter) · Anesthesiology 1978; 48:386.
90. Eitel DR, Yankowitz J, Ely JW. Legal implications of birth videos. J Fam Pract 1998; 46:251-6.

Appendix

Sample Permit for Presence of a Support Person During Cesarean Section

The Medical Center allows the presence of one support person in the operating room for patients undergoing a cesarean section under regional anesthesia (spinal or epidural). The purpose of allowing the support person to be present is to provide comfort and emotional support to the mother during her operation.

The following rules apply for the support person:

1. The support person must wear a jump suit, surgical cap, shoe covers, and a face mask while in the operating room. The support person should leave any personal possessions with others because the Medical Center cannot be responsible for the loss or damage of personal items.
2. The support person will be taken to the operating room by a member of the nursing staff. This typically occurs after regional anesthesia has been established successfully.
3. The support person will be provided with a seat at the head of the operating table. In order for the operating room to function smoothly, the support person must remain at the head of the operating table.
4. If there are any unforeseen circumstances that arise during the operation, such as the need to induce general anesthesia, the support person must leave the operating room when asked to do so. This is done so that the mother's and infant's care are the only focus of attention for the care providers.
5. The support person typically may take photographs or make audio/video recordings of events surrounding the birth of the infant. If the medical or nursing staff request that such recordings be discontinued, the support person must agree to do so immediately. Hospital staff may not be photographed or recorded without their consent.

Patient and Support Person's Statement:

I,_____ wish to have _____ present in the operating room with me during my cesarean section. We have received the necessary instructions regarding his/her participation as outlined above.

My support person and I participate willingly in this process and agree to hold harmless the Medical Center and its staff for any adverse effects that may result from his/her attendance.

Signature of patient:_____
Date/Time:_____
Signature of support person:_____
Date/Time:_____
Witness:_____ Date/Time:_____

Chapter 30
Aspiration: Risk, Prophylaxis, and Treatment
Geraldine M. O'Sullivan, M.D., FRCA · Thomas S. Guyton, M.D.

HISTORY

Sir James Simpson first suggested aspiration as a cause of death during anesthesia. Hannah Greener, a 15-year-old given chloroform for a toenail extraction, became cyanotic and "sputtered" during the anesthetic. She then developed a "rattling in her throat" and soon expired. Her physician administered water and brandy by mouth. Simpson[1] contended that it was the aspiration of water and brandy and not the adverse effects from the chloroform that caused her death.

In 1940 a Californian obstetrician published a report of 15 cases of aspiration, 14 of which occurred in mothers receiving inhalation anesthesia for a vaginal or cesarean delivery.[2] Among the 14 obstetric cases, 5 mothers died. Subsequently Curtis Mendelson's landmark paper described the syndrome that now bears his name, *Mendelson's syndrome.*[3] His paper included a series of animal experiments that clearly described the clinical course and pathology of pulmonary acid aspiration. In the same paper, Mendelson also audited 44,016 deliveries at the New York Lying-In Hospital between 1932 and 1945. He identified 66 (0.15%) cases of aspiration, and in 45 of these cases the aspirated material was recorded; 40 mothers aspirated liquid and the remaining 5 aspirated solid food. Of significance, yet not often reported, is the fact that no mother died from acid aspiration while two mothers died from asphyxiation caused by the aspiration of solid food. Mendelson therefore advocated (1) the withholding of food during labor, (2) the greater use of regional anesthesia, (3) the administration of antacids, (4) emptying the stomach before administration of general anesthesia, and (5) the competent administration of general anesthesia. This advice became the foundation of obstetric anesthetic practice during subsequent decades.

INCIDENCE, MORBIDITY, AND MORTALITY

Anesthesia-related maternal mortality has declined significantly in recent years (Figure 30-1), and the more widespread use of regional anesthesia has probably played a significant role in this reduction. Unfortunately, airway problems associated with the use of general anesthesia now represent the most common cause of anesthesia-related maternal death.[4] This may be related to the more frequent administration of general anesthesia—often under emergency conditions—in high-risk parturients. Unfortunately, the overall decline in the use of general anesthesia in obstetric practice has implications for both training and skill maintenance in airway management in obstetric patients.

The reported incidence of aspiration pneumonitis varies depending on the criteria used for making the diagnosis. Comparisons within the same study allow the estimation of the relative risk of aspiration in pregnant versus nonpregnant patients. Olsson et al.[5] reported an overall incidence of aspiration of 1 in 2131 in the general population and 1 in 661 in patients undergoing cesarean section (i.e., a threefold increase in aspiration risk during pregnancy). In two more recent surveys relating to aspiration,[6,7] one a retrospective review of 172,334 consecutive patients undergoing general anesthesia and the other a review of 133 cases of aspiration from the Australian Anaesthetic Incident Monitoring Study (AIMS), there were no cases of pulmonary aspiration in mothers undergoing either elective or emergency cesarean section. However, in both studies, emergency surgery was a significant predisposing factor for aspiration; this is especially relevant for obstetric anesthesia practice, given that most obstetric surgical procedures are performed as emergencies. The Australian study also implicated obesity as a significant risk factor for aspiration;

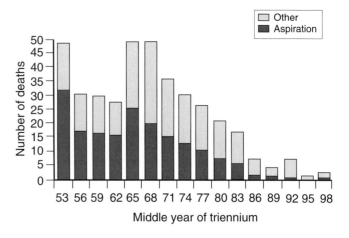

FIGURE 30-1. Maternal mortality from anesthesia and pulmonary aspiration, 1952-1999. (Compiled from the *Report on Confidential Enquiries into Maternal Death in the United Kingdom.*[9])

others have noted that obesity is associated with an increased risk of maternal mortality.[8]

Morbidity and mortality associated with aspiration will vary depending on the physical status of the patient, the type of aspirate, therapy, and the criteria used for making the diagnosis. Data from the *Report on Confidential Enquiries into Maternal Deaths in the United Kingdom* indicate that death from pulmonary aspiration in obstetrics is now rare (Figure 30-1).[9] In the last five reports that cover the period 1985-1999, there were five maternal deaths from aspiration. The denominator used by the *Confidential Enquiries* is the total number of maternities resulting in a live birth. Although the number of anesthetics administered to mothers during this 15-year period is unknown, there were 11,265,533 maternities, indicating that the mortality from aspiration was less than 1 in 2 million maternities. However, mortality statistics are a poor predictor of maternal *morbidity,* and several studies indicate that perioperative aspiration is associated with significant morbidity in obstetric patients.[10,11]

GASTROESOPHAGEAL ANATOMY AND PHYSIOLOGY

Esophagus

In the adult, the esophagus measures approximately 25 cm in length; the esophagogastric junction is approximately 40 cm from the incisor teeth. In humans the proximal one third of the esophagus is composed of striated muscle, while the distal end contains only smooth muscle. At both ends there are muscular sphincters that are normally closed. The cricopharyngeal or upper esophageal sphincter prevents the entry of air into the esophagus during respiration, while the gastroesophageal or lower esophageal sphincter prevents the reflux of gastric contents. The lower esophageal sphincter is characterized anatomically and manometrically as a 3-cm zone of specialized muscle that maintains a tonic activity. The end-expiratory pressure in the sphincter is 8 to 20 mm Hg above the end-expiratory gastric pressure. The lower esophageal sphincter is kept in place by the phreno-esophageal ligament, which is inserted into the esophagus approximately 3 cm above the diaphragmatic opening (Figure 30-2). The lower esophageal sphincter is not always closed but shows transient relaxations.[12] These relaxations account for the gastroesophageal reflux that occurs in normal subjects.

Gastrointestinal Motility

Differences in fasting and fed patterns of gut motility are now firmly established. During fasting, the main component of peristalsis is the migrating motor complex (MMC).[13] Each cycle of the MMC is composed of four phases. Phase I has little or no electrical spike activity and thus no measurable contractions; phase II has intermittent spike activity; phase III has spikes of large amplitude and is associated with strong contractile activity; and phase IV is a brief period of intermittent activity leading back to phase I. In humans the duration of each cycle of the MMC is approximately 90 to 120 minutes. The MMC appears first in the lower esophageal sphincter and stomach and then in the duodenum from where it migrates to the terminal ileum, at which time a new cycle begins in the lower esophageal sphincter and the stomach. The phase of the MMC at the time of administration of certain drugs can affect absorption and thereby the onset of therapeutic effect.[14] Eating abolishes the MMC and induces a pattern of intermittent spike activity that appears similar to phase II. The duration of the fed pattern is determined both by the calorie content and the type of nutrients in the meal.

The stomach, through the processes of receptive relaxation and gastric accommodation, can accept 1.0 to 1.5 L of food before intragastric pressure begins to increase. The contraction waves that propel food into the small intestine begin in the antrum, and the pylorus closes midway through the contraction wave.[15] Fluid first moves through the pyloric valve; fluid subsequently hits a closed pylorus and moves retrograde toward the body of the stomach. The jet of fluid that exits the pylorus primarily contains liquid and fine particles. Large particles lag behind and are hit by the retrograde flow of fluid. This motion breaks up the larger particles. Thus the way that individual components of a meal pass through the stomach depends on the size of the particles and the viscosity of the suspension. Fluids and small particles exit the stomach faster than larger particles.[15] The outlet of the stomach—the pylorus—takes advantage of both its chronic tone and anatomic position to limit outflow. The pylorus is higher than the most dependent portion of the stomach in both the supine and standing positions.[15]

Gastric Secretion

In one day, the stomach produces as much as 1500 mL of highly acidic fluid containing the proteolytic enzyme

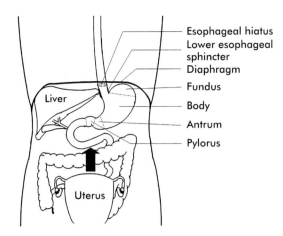

FIGURE 30-2. The stomach and its relationship to the diaphragm. The stomach consists of a fundus, body, antrum, and pylorus. The lower esophageal sphincter depends on chronic contraction in circular muscle fibers, the wrapping of the esophagus by the crus of the diaphragm at the esophageal hiatus, and the length of the esophagus exposed to intraabdominal pressure. The term uterus may encroach on the stomach and alter the effectiveness of the lower esophageal sphincter.

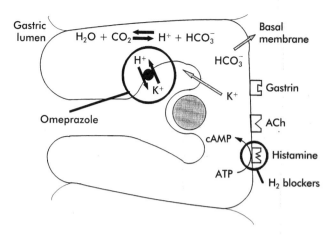

FIGURE 30-3. The oxyntic cell produces hydrogen ions that are secreted into the gastric lumen and bicarbonate ions that are secreted into the blood stream. H_2-receptor antagonists (e.g., cimetidine, ranitidine) and proton pump inhibitors act on the oxyntic cell to reduce gastric acid secretion. Omeprazole blocks the active transport of the hydrogen ions into the gastric lumen. H_2-receptor antagonists block the histamine receptor on the basal membrane to decrease hydrogen ion production in the oxyntic cell.

pepsin.[16] Normal individuals can produce a peak acid output of 38 mmol/hr.[17] Acid is secreted at a low rate even when the stomach is empty. The basal rate is approximately 10% of the maximum rate.[17,18] However, the rate of gastric acid secretion is not constant even when the stomach is empty. Rather, gastric acid secretion shows a diurnal variation; it is lowest in the morning and highest in the evening.

The stomach lining has two types of glands: pyloric glands and oxyntic glands. The **pyloric** glands contain chief cells, which secrete pepsinogen, the precursor for pepsin. The **oxyntic** glands contain the oxyntic cells, which secrete hydrochloric acid. Water molecules and carbon dioxide in the oxyntic cells combine to form carbonic acid, which dissociates into hydrogen ions and bicarbonate. The bicarbonate leaves the cell for the bloodstream, and the hydrogen ions are actively exchanged for the potassium ions in the canaliculi connecting with the lumen of the oxyntic gland. The oxyntic cell secretions may have a hydrochloric acid concentration of as much as 160 mmol/L (pH of 0.8).[16] Proton pump inhibitors block the hydrogen ion pump on the canaliculi to decrease acid production.[19]

The pylorus contains cells known as G cells, which secrete **gastrin** into the bloodstream when stimulated by the vagus nerve, stomach distention, tactile stimuli, and chemical stimuli (e.g., amino acids, certain peptides). Gastrin combines with gastrin receptors on the oxyntic cell to stimulate the secretion of hydrochloric acid. **Acetylcholine** binds to muscarinic (M_1) receptors on the oxyntic cell to cause an increase in intracellular calcium ions, which results in hydrochloric acid secretion. **Histamine** potentiates the effects of both acetylcholine and gastrin by combining with H_2-receptors on the oxyntic cell to increase intracellular cyclic adenosine monophosphate (cAMP) and cause a dramatic increase in the production of acid.[16] H_2-blocking agents (e.g., cimetidine, ranitidine) prevent histamine's potentiation of acid production (Figure 30-3).

Ingestion of Food

When a meal is eaten, the mechanisms that control the secretion of gastric juice and the motility and emptying of the stomach interact in a complex manner to coordinate the functions of the stomach. The response to eating is divided into three phases: cephalic, gastric, and intestinal. Chewing, tasting, and smelling cause an increase in vagal stimulation of the stomach, which results in an increase in gastric acid production. This represents the **cephalic** phase of digestion.[16] In this phase, gastric acid output increases to a level that is approximately 55% of peak acid output.[20] The **gastric** phase begins with the release of gastrin. Gastric acid secretion depends on antral distention, vagal activity, gastrin concentrations, and the composition of the meal.[16,18,21] Gastric acid secretion during a mixed composition meal increases to a level that is approximately 80% of peak acid output.[20] The **intestinal** phase begins with the movement of food into the small intestine and is largely inhibitory. Hormones (e.g., gastrin, cholecystokinin, secretin) and an enterogastric reflex further modulate gastric acid secretion and motility depending on the composition and volume of the food in the duodenum.[16] The inhibition of gastric emptying by food in the duodenum enables the duodenal contents to be processed before more material enters it from the stomach.

After the ingestion of a meal, gastric emptying depends on (1) pre-meal volume, (2) volume ingested, (3) composition of the meal, (4) size of the solids, (5) the amount of gastric secretion, (6) the physical characteristics of the stomach contents entering the duodenum, and (7) patient position.[16,18,22,23] A mixture of solids and liquids passes through the stomach much more slowly than liquids alone. Gastric emptying of a meal is slowed by high lipid content, high caloric load, and large particle size.[18,24,25] Thus, predicting an exact time for the passage of liquids and solids through the stomach is very difficult. For non-nutrient liquids (e.g., normal saline), the gastric volume decreases exponentially with respect to time.[22] In one study,[23] 90% of a 150-mL saline meal given to fasting adults in the sitting position passed through the stomach in a median time of 14 minutes. However, the median time for gastric emptying increased to 28 minutes in the left lateral position. In another study, 100% of a 500-mL saline meal given to fasting adults passed through the stomach within 2 hours, as determined by a polyethylene glycol marker.[18] However, at the end of 2 hours, the mean residual gastric volume was 46 mL. The saline meal caused an increase in gastric acid production that was 30% of maximum acid output.[18] This study demonstrates that the volume of the gastric secretions and saliva produced in response to the test meal and the volume of the test meal itself must be considered. For example, the patient described in Figure 30-4 responded to the test meal by secreting 800 mL of gastric juice, and consequently the volume in the stomach remained high for almost 2 hours despite early, rapid emptying.[26]

Effects of Pregnancy on Gastric Function

Gastroesophageal reflux, resulting in heartburn, is a common complication of late pregnancy. Pregnancy compromises the integrity of the lower esophageal sphincter. It alters the anatomic relationship of the esophagus to the diaphragm and stomach, increases intragastric pressure, and in some women limits the ability of the lower esophageal sphincter to increase its tone.[27-30] Progesterone, which relaxes smooth muscle, probably accounts for the inability of the lower esophageal sphincter to increase its tone.[31]

Serial studies assessing **gastric acidity** during pregnancy have proved difficult to perform because pregnant women do not usually wish to repeatedly swallow nasogastric tubes for research purposes. However, in the most comprehensive study of gastric acid secretion during pregnancy,[32] basal and histamine-augmented gastric secretion were measured in 10 controls and 30 pregnant women equally distributed throughout the three trimesters of pregnancy. No significant differences in basal gastric acid secretion were seen between the pregnant and the nonpregnant women. However, when the mothers were divided into groups according to gestation, the mean rate of gastric acid secretion was reduced during the second trimester. The maximal response to histamine was significantly depressed in the first and second trimester when compared with the response in nonpregnant women and women in the third trimester of pregnancy.[32]

Measuring **gastric emptying** during pregnancy and labor presents technical and ethical challenges, and again a variety of techniques have been used.[33-38] Pregnancy does not significantly alter the rate of gastric emptying.[33] Gastric emptying appears to be normal in early labor but becomes delayed as labor advances.[35,36] The cause of this delay in gastric emptying during advanced labor is unclear. Pain is known to delay gastric emptying, but even when labor pain is abolished with epidural analgesia with local anesthetics alone, the delay still occurs.[36] Parenteral opioids *significantly delay* gastric emptying, as do bolus doses of epidural and intrathecal opioids.[35,39-41] Continuous epidural infusion of low-dose local anesthetic with fentanyl does not delay gastric emptying until the total dose of fentanyl exceeds 100 μg.[42]

A recent study noted that gastric emptying is not delayed in healthy, non-obese term parturients who ingest 300 mL of water after an overnight fast.[43]

Plasma concentrations of the gastrointestinal hormone motilin are decreased during pregnancy.[44] Studies have shown either no change[28,30,45] or an increase[46] in the plasma concentrations of gastrin.

RISK FACTORS FOR ASPIRATION PNEUMONITIS

Mendelson[3] divided aspiration pneumonitis into two types: liquid and solid. Mendelson recognized that liquid aspiration

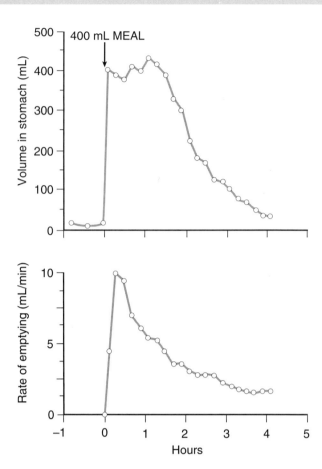

FIGURE 30-4. Volume of gastric contents and rate of gastric emptying in a subject eating a 400 mL-meal of steak, bread and vanilla ice cream. (From Malagelada JR, Longstreth GF, Summerskill WHJ et al. Measurements of gastric functions during digestion of ordinary solid meals in man. Gastroenterology 1976; 70:203-10.)

was more severe clinically and pathologically when the aspirated liquid was highly acidic. His observations are complemented by other observations[47-56] that allow us to speculate that the morbidity and mortality of aspiration depends on three variables: (1) the chemical nature of the aspirate, (2) the physical nature of the aspirate, and (3) the volume of the aspirate. Aspirates with a pH less than 2.5 cause an ongoing granulocytic reaction beyond the acute phase.[50] Aspiration of particulate material can cause a clinical picture of equal or greater severity than that caused by the aspiration of acidic liquid.[54] Aspiration of small volumes of neutral liquid results in a very low rate of mortality. However, aspiration of large volumes of neutral liquid results in a high mortality rate, presumably as a result of the disruption of surfactant by a large volume of liquid or from a mechanism similar to that seen in "near drowning."[56]

Historically, anesthesiologists have considered a nonparticulate gastric fluid with a pH less than 2.5 and a gastric volume greater than 25 mL (i.e., 0.4 mL/kg) as risk factors for aspiration pneumonitis.[47,53,55] The American Society of Anesthesiologists (ASA) Task Force on Preoperative Fasting found that no human studies have directly addressed the relationship between preoperative fasting, gastric acidity, or gastric volume and the risk of pulmonary aspiration during anesthesia.[57] A reasonable scientific basis appears to exist for the use of a gastric pH of less than 2.5 as a risk factor. In animal experiments, the risk of aspiration pneumonitis clearly

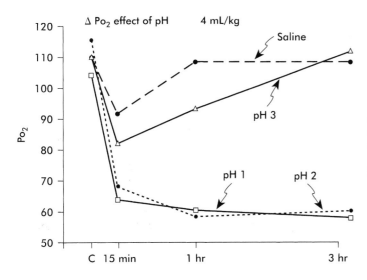

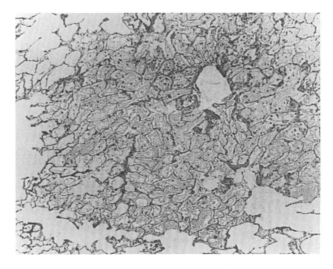

FIGURE 30-5. Relationship between acidity and PaO$_2$. In this study, 4 mL/kg of fluid of varying pH was instilled into the tracheas of dogs. The severity of the hypoxemia correlated with the pH of the aspirate. A maximal decrease in PaO$_2$ occurred with aspirates with a pH of less than 2.5. *C,* Control. (From Awe WC, Fletcher WS, Jacob SW. The pathophysiology of aspiration pneumonitis. Surgery 1966; 60:232-9.)

increases with decreasing pH of the tracheal aspirate.[47,56] Awe et al.[47] illustrated this concept in their graph of PaO$_2$ versus time for aspirates of varying pH (Figure 30-5).

Animal studies clearly demonstrate that increasing the volume of the tracheal aspirate increases the risk of aspiration pneumonitis.[56] The dogma that a gastric volume greater than 25 mL places a patient at risk emanated from a single Rhesus monkey study in which 0.4 mL/kg of an acidic liquid was administered into the right mainstem bronchus.[55] The authors assumed that all the gastric contents would be aspirated. Subsequently, Raidoo et al.[58] demonstrated variability in the response of juvenile monkeys to different volumes of an acidic tracheal aspirate. Mortality was seen with aspirate volumes of 0.8 and 1.0 mL/kg, but not with volumes of 0.4 and 0.6 mL/kg. Likewise, Plourde and Hardy[59] refuted the assumption that all the gastric contents would be aspirated and demonstrated that gastric volumes of 0.4 mL/kg did not increase the risk of aspiration. Hence the gastric volume that places a patient at risk for aspiration pneumonitis cannot be determined.

However, a reasonable goal of any prophylactic therapy would be a gastric pH greater than 2.5 and a gastric volume as low as possible.

PATHOPHYSIOLOGY

Aspiration of acidic liquid injures the alveolar epithelium and results in an alveolar exudate composed of edema, albumin, fibrin, cellular debris, and red blood cells[3,50,53,54] (Figure 30-6). The phospholipid and apoprotein composition of the surfactant changes and exerts a negative effect on the surface active properties of the surfactant.[60] This leads to (1) a decrease in pulmonary compliance, (2) an increase in alveolar water content, (3) a loss of lung volume, and (4) intrapulmonary shunting of blood. The pulmonary edema and shunting result in hypoxemia, and the cellular debris and bronchial denuding result in bronchial obstruction. The lung injury causes alveolar macrophages to secrete cytokines, interleukin-1, -6, -8, and -10 (IL-1, 6, 8, and 10) and tumor necrosis factor-alpha (TNF-α).[61] After several hours, these factors lead to the chemotaxis, accumulation, and activation of neutrophils in the alveolar exudate. The neutrophils release oxidants, proteases, leukotrienes, and other proinflammatory molecules.[61] Amplification of these inflammatory processes may result in the development of acute lung injury or acute respiratory distress syndrome (ARDS).[61,62]

FIGURE 30-6. Liquid acid aspiration causes the production of an alveolar exudate consisting of edema, fibrin, hemorrhage, and neutrophils. Lung architecture remains intact. (From Gibbs CP, Modell JH. Pulmonary aspiration of gastric contents: Pathophysiology, prevention, and management. In Miller RD, editor. Anesthesia, 4th ed. New York, Churchill Livingstone, 1994; 1446.)

After the acute period described above, the process resolves by the proliferation and differentiation of surviving type II pneumocytes into the alveolar epithelial cells.[61,62] The type II pneumocytes actively transport sodium out of the alveolus, and water follows passively. Soluble proteins are removed by paracellular diffusion and endocytosis. Neutrophils are removed by programmed cell death and subsequent phagocytosis by macrophages. Macrophages remove insoluble proteins and neutrophils by phagocytosis. Type II pneumocytes gradually restore the normal composition of the surfactant. In a subset of patients with ARDS, the injury progresses to a fibrosing alveolitis—an accumulation of mesechymal cells, their products, and new blood vessels.

Aspiration of neutral, nonparticulate liquid results in an alveolar exudate with minimal damage to the alveolus (Figure 30-7). Bronchospasm and disruption of surfactant likely account for a slight decrease in PaO$_2$ and an increase in shunting.[50] Aspiration of large solid particles may cause atelectasis by obstructing large airways.[3] Aspiration of smaller

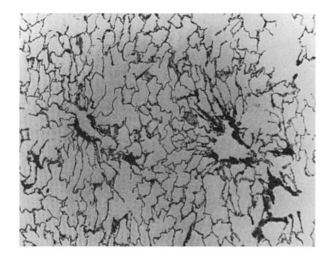

FIGURE 30-7. After normal saline aspiration, the lung has essentially normal lung histology with little alveolar exudate and no hemorrhage. (From Gibbs CP, Modell JH. Pulmonary aspiration of gastric contents: Pathophysiology, prevention, and management. In Miller RD, editor. Anesthesia, 4th ed. New York, Churchill Livingstone, 1994; 1445.)

particulate matter causes an exudative neutrophilic response at the level of the bronchioles and alveolar ducts. The extent of hypoxemia and the clinical picture are similar to those following the aspiration of acidic liquid.[50,51,54]

CLINICAL COURSE

In most cases of aspiration during anesthesia, the anesthesiologist will witness regurgitation of gastric contents into the hypopharynx.[3] Patients who aspirate while breathing spontaneously will have a brief period of breath holding followed by tachypnea, tachycardia, and a slight respiratory acidosis. Significant aspiration always results in some degree of hypoxemia caused by increased shunting, and bronchospasm often occurs. Severe hypoxemia may cause hypotension (which results from a decrease in cardiac index), an increase in central venous and pulmonary capillary wedge pressures, and an increase in pulmonary vascular resistance.[47,54] With severe lung injury and a massive transfer of plasma from the intravascular space to the alveoli, shock ensues, which is accompanied by a decrease in central venous and pulmonary capillary wedge pressures. After aspiration of saline solution (pH of 5.9), PaO_2 returns to normal within 24 hours, but aspiration of acidic liquid results in a longer duration of hypoxemia.[63]

Approximately 85% to 90% of patients who aspirate gastric contents will develop an abnormality on chest radiographs.[49,64] Because these chest radiographic findings may lag behind clinical signs by as much as 12 to 24 hours, the initial radiograph may appear normal.[64] In mild cases, patches of alveolar infiltrate in dependent portions of the lung occur. The right lower lobe is the most common site for aspiration pneumonitis because of the wider and more vertical nature of the right mainstem bronchus. Severe aspiration results in diffuse bilateral infiltrates without signs of heart failure (e.g., engorged pulmonary vasculature, enlarged cardiac silhouette).

TREATMENT

Rigid Bronchoscopy and Lavage

Rigid bronchoscopy may be required to remove large food particles that cause airway obstruction. Aspirated liquid is rapidly absorbed by the lung and only poorly buffered by saliva. Attempts to lavage the lung with saline or bicarbonate will not decrease the parenchymal damage caused by acid aspiration, and lavage can worsen preexisting hypoxemia.[63,65]

Steroids and Antiinflammatory Agents

Despite the inflammatory processes present, clinical trials of glucocorticoids and antiinflammatory agents such as ibuprofen, ketoconazole, and lisofylline have shown no benefit in the treatment of ARDS in large clinical trials.[62,66] High concentrations of macrophage inhibitory factor in the alveolar fluid is one possible explanation for this lack of response to glucocorticoids and antiinflammatory agents. Macrophage inhibitory factor amplifies the production of interleukin-8 and tumor necrosis factor and can override the glucocorticoid-mediated inhibition of cytokine secretion.[62] On a positive note, Meduri et al.[67] proposed that prolonged methylprednisolone treatment could reduce signs of systemic inflammation in patients with unresolving ARDS. The potential for prolonged methylprednisolone treatment to rescue ARDS patients in the fibrosing alveolitis stage is being examined in a phase III trial.

Treatment of Hypoxemia

Exudation of fluid into the alveoli, decreased surface activity of surfactant, and atelectasis all result in intrapulmonary shunting and hypoxemia. The administration of continuous positive airway pressure (CPAP) to patients who are breathing spontaneously, or the use of positive end-expiratory pressure (PEEP) in patients who are undergoing mechanical ventilation, restores functional residual capacity, reduces pulmonary shunting, and reverses hypoxemia. The majority of practitioners adjust the level of PEEP to achieve oxygenation goals.[68] However, either CPAP or PEEP may reduce both cardiac output and oxygen delivery and alter regional blood flow. Evidence suggests that prophylactic PEEP does not provide any benefit.[62]

The most recent improvement in the treatment of ARDS is a change in ventilator management. In a recent ARDS Network clinical trial, investigators achieved a 22% decrease in mortality (i.e., from 40% to 31%) by reducing the tidal volume to 6 mL/kg of ideal body weight and limiting plateau pressure to 30 cm H_2O or less.[69] The low tidal volume group had significantly lower plasma interleukin-6 levels than the group that received the more traditional tidal volume of 12 mL/kg. The greater activation of inflammatory processes in the larger tidal volume group is thought to be a result of either stretch injury or injury caused by opening and closing alveoli in atelectatic lung tissue.[69] Hypothetically, higher levels of PEEP may exert a protective effect by keeping the alveolus open throughout the ventilatory cycle. The optimal level of PEEP and other modes of ventilation are currently being studied.[68]

Prophylactic Antibiotics

Prophylactic antibiotics are not efficacious and may lead to the development of infection with resistant organisms. Infection is not a component of acute pulmonary injury.[50,51] Antibiotics should be administered only in the presence of clinical findings that suggest infection (e.g., fever, worsening infiltrates on chest radiographs, leukocytosis, positive Gram stain of sputum, clinical deterioration). Empiric therapy of secondary bacterial infections should be broad spectrum. Common organisms found include *Streptococcus pneumoniae*, *Staphylococcus aureus*, *Haemophilus influenzae*, and gram-negative organisms such as Enterobacteriaceae and *Pseudomonas aeruginosa*.[70] Anaerobes are no longer thought to be present in the majority of cases.[70] Tracheal sputum samples may be insufficient to identify the bacterial pathogen, and bronchoscopy utilizing protected specimen brushes may be necessary.[70] After identification of pathogens and their sensitivities to antibiotics, pharmacologic therapy should be altered to treat specific pathogens.

Other Therapeutic Trends

Other therapeutic trends may be associated with the reduction in mortality from ARDS.[62] The most appropriate intravascular volume is now considered to be the lowest level that supports normal acid-base status and renal function. To minimize the risk of sepsis, central venous catheters and other invasive hemodynamic monitors are used only when necessary. Enteral feeding is preferred when possible. Infections are treated utilizing antibiotics specific to the bacterial pathogen. Prophylaxis for gastrointestinal bleeding and thromboembolic events is recommended.

An ARDS Network of clinical sites has been established to investigate different modes of mechanical ventilation, new pharmacologic therapy (i.e., nitric oxide, surfactant, anti-inflammatory agents) and changes in supportive care.[62] Ongoing phase III clinical trials will likely alter our approach to the patient with ARDS.

PROPHYLAXIS

Pregnant women undergoing cesarean section or other surgical procedures are at increased risk for aspiration pneumonitis and should receive pharmacologic prophylaxis. The risk of failed intubation is three to eleven times greater in pregnant patients than in nonpregnant patients.[71-73] Airway edema, breast enlargement, and the high rate of emergency surgery all contribute to the risk of failed intubation in pregnant women (see Chapter 31). Aspiration pneumonitis is associated with difficult or failed intubation during the induction of general anesthesia. In a survey conducted by the Society for Obstetric Anesthesia and Perinatology, difficult or failed intubation occurred in 14 of 19 cases of aspiration associated with intubation.[74] Warner et al.[6] documented that the risk of aspiration is almost as great during emergence as during induction. Thus the prophylactic regimen must provide protection during both induction of—and emergence from—general anesthesia.

Because the incidence of aspiration pneumonitis is low, the efficacy of prophylactic regimens is measured by their ability to alter gastric pH and volume. Approximately 30% to 43% of pregnant women have a fasting gastric volume greater than 25 mL and a gastric fluid pH less than 2.5.[75-77] However, the percentage of term pregnant patients at risk may not differ from that for patients undergoing elective abortion, postpartum sterilization, or gynecologic surgery (Table 30-1).[77-79] Gastric volume and acidity at term gestation are similar to gastric volume and acidity during early pregnancy, during the postpartum period, and in nonpregnant patients.[75-83] Decreased lower esophageal sphincter tone and an increased risk of difficult intubation are the primary factors that

TABLE 30-1	PERCENTAGE OF POPULATION AT RISK FOR ASPIRATION		
	pH < 2.5 (%)	Volume > 25 mL (%)	pH < 2.5 and volume > 25 mL (%)
Pregnant[75-77]	57-80	51-54	31-43
Nonpregnant[77-79]	75-95	45-67	45-60
Postpartum[78-80]	54-93	61	60
Children[81,82]	93-100	64-78	64-77
Obese, nonpregnant[83]	88	86	75

increase the risk of aspiration during pregnancy and immediately postpartum.

Preoperative Oral Fluid Administration

Multiple studies have described no increase in gastric volume or acidity after the oral administration of 150 mL of fluid (e.g., coffee, tea, water, other clear liquids, orange juice) in nonpregnant adults 2 hours before elective surgery.[84,85] All of these patients fasted overnight and should have had a low gastric volume when the test meal was given. Similarly, other studies have demonstrated that unrestricted intake of clear fluids up to 2 hours before anesthesia has no ill effect on gastric volume and pH in pediatric patients.[84] However, ingestion of milk and orange juice containing pulp increases gastric volume.[84] Lewis and Crawford[86] noted that in patients undergoing elective cesarean section, a meal of both tea and toast 2 to 4 hours preoperatively resulted in an increased gastric volume and a decreased gastric pH when compared with a control group of patients. Consumption of tea *without* toast resulted in an increase in gastric volume, but it did not alter gastric pH. Particulate material was aspirated from the stomachs of 2 of the 11 patients who consumed both tea and toast. The authors did not state the volume of tea consumed by these patients.

Also, gastric emptying is not delayed in healthy, non-obese term parturients who ingest 300 mL of water after an overnight fast.[43] This suggests that the guidelines outlined by the ASA Task Force on Preoperative Fasting[57] could be applied to healthy pregnant women presenting for elective surgery. However, larger studies are required to confirm this hypothesis.

Choice of Anesthesia

The Obstetric Anesthesia Work Force Survey reported that the use of regional anesthesia for cesarean section increased from approximately 55% of cesarean sections performed in 1981 to approximately 84% of cesarean sections performed in 1992.[87] A review performed at a large tertiary care obstetric facility showed that from 1990 to 1995 the use of general anesthesia for cesarean section decreased from 7.2% to 3.6% of cases. The yearly incidence of difficult intubation ranged from 1.3% to 16.3%, with one maternal death as a result of failed intubation.[88] The National Sentinel Caesarean Section Audit,[89] commissioned by the government of the United Kingdom in response to concern about the rising cesarean section rate, was performed in England and Wales between May 1, 2001, and July 31, 2001. It showed that 77% of emergency and 91% of elective cesarean sections were performed under regional anesthesia. The increased use of regional anesthesia for operative obstetrics has resulted in part from the increased use of epidural analgesia during labor. An additional reason for the decreased use of general anesthesia is the perception that administration of regional anesthesia reduces the risk of failed intubation and aspiration. Hawkins et al.[4] reported 67 maternal deaths that resulted from complications of general anesthesia and 33 maternal deaths that resulted from complications of regional anesthesia in the United States for the years 1979 to 1990. Approximately 73% of general anesthesia-related maternal deaths resulted from airway problems, primarily failed intubation and/or aspiration. In contrast, deaths from regional anesthesia began to decline in the mid-80s, coincident with the withdrawal of 0.75% bupivacaine and probably caused by the increasing awareness of local anesthetic toxicity and the more consistent use of the epidural test dose.[4,8] For the years 1985 to 1990, Hawkins et al.[4] estimated that the risk of maternal death was 16.7 times *greater* with general anesthesia than with regional anesthesia for cesarean section. Assessment of these data should be tempered by the recognition that general anesthesia often is reserved for pregnant patients at greater risk for complications from anesthesia. For example, the general anesthesia group undoubtedly included a disproportionate number of women who required emergency cesarean section for maternal and/or fetal indications (e.g., uterine rupture, placental abruption). The triennial *Report on Confidential Enquiries into Maternal Deaths in the United Kingdom*[9] also suggests that regional anesthesia is safer than general anesthesia for cesarean section.

Antacids

The ASA Task Force on Preoperative Fasting found that antacids were efficacious in raising gastric pH but not in reducing gastric volume.[57] A nonparticulate antacid (e.g., 0.3 M sodium citrate, Bicitra, Alka-Seltzer Effervescent) is preferred.[90-93] The efficacy of sodium citrate depends on gastric volume and acidity.[94] A total of 30 mL of sodium citrate neutralizes 255 mL of hydrochloric acid with a pH of 1.0. The effective duration of action of sodium citrate is variable and depends on the rate of gastric emptying.[92,93] One of us (GMO) used radiotelemetry pH pills to perform noninvasive assessments of the efficacy of sodium citrate in pregnant women.[92,93] After the administration of 15 mL of sodium citrate to women in the third trimester of pregnancy, the time that the pH remained greater than 3.0 was less than 30 minutes.[92] When the same study was repeated in laboring women, the duration of time that the pH remained greater than 3.0 was 57 minutes in those who had received no analgesia and 166 minutes in those who had received meperidine.[93]

The ASA Task Force also concluded that pulmonary aspiration of particulate antacids (e.g., magnesium trisilicate) entails a higher risk of aspiration pneumonitis than aspiration of nonparticulate antacids.[57] Gibbs et al.[63] demonstrated that aspiration of a magnesium hydroxide-aluminum hydroxide antacid caused pulmonary shunting and hypoxemia similar in magnitude to that caused by acid aspiration and greater than that caused by saline or alkalinized saline. A neutrophilic, exudative foreign body reaction surrounded the antacid particles in the lung.[63] Likewise, Eyler et al.[95] observed that aspiration of a particulate antacid caused significantly greater hypoxemia and more parenchymal exudates than aspiration of sodium citrate.

H$_2$-Receptor Antagonists

The ASA Task Force concluded that H$_2$-receptor blockers are efficacious in reducing gastric acidity and volume.[57] H$_2$-receptor antagonists block histamine receptors on the oxyntic cell and thus decrease gastric acid production. This results in a slight reduction in gastric volume in the fasting patient.[96] When given intravenously, an H$_2$-receptor antagonist begins to take effect in as little as 30 minutes, but 60 to 90 minutes are required for maximal effect.[96,98] After oral administration, gastric pH is greater than 2.5 in approximately 60% of patients at 60 minutes and in 90% at 90 minutes.[96-98] The duration of action is sufficiently long to cover emergence from general anesthesia for a cesarean section.

Cimetidine (given in doses of 200 and 400 mg intravenously, intramuscularly, or orally) reduces gastric acidity within 60 to 90 minutes.[96-98] Therapeutic plasma concentrations are sustained for approximately 4 hours. Cimetidine may decrease the rate of plasma clearance of certain drugs, including some local anesthetics (e.g., lidocaine) by binding to the cytochrome P450 system in the hepatocyte and by decreasing hepatic blood flow.[99] Feely et al.[100] observed that chronic administration of cimetidine results in increased plasma lidocaine concentrations and an increased risk of toxicity during intravenous infusion of lidocaine. Cimetidine crosses the placenta, but it does not appear to have harmful effects.[101] Because of case reports of sinus arrest and arrhythmias with rapid intravenous administration,[102] intravenous administration of cimetidine has little benefit over oral administration.

Ranitidine is a substituted amino-alkyl furan derivative. Most studies have evaluated the administration of 50 to 100 mg of ranitidine administered intravenously or intramuscularly or 150 mg administered orally.[103-106] These studies have noted that the administration of ranitidine results in a gastric pH greater than 2.5 within 1 hour.[103-106] Therapeutic concentrations of ranitidine are sustained for approximately 8 hours. Ranitidine does not have any major interaction with the cytochrome P450 system,[107] and it does not alter plasma local anesthetic concentrations after epidural administration of lidocaine or bupivacaine.[108]

Nizatidine[109] (given in doses of 150 to 300 mg orally) and **famotidine** (given in doses of 20 to 40 mg orally or intravenously[109,110]) are newer, alternative H$_2$-receptor antagonists. Both have a duration of action of greater than 10 hours and do not interfere with the metabolism of other drugs by the cytochrome P450 system.[109,110]

Proton Pump Inhibitors

Omeprazole (20 to 40 mg orally) and **lansoprazole** (15 to 30 mg orally) are substituted benzimidazoles that inhibit the hydrogen ion pump on the gastric surface of the oxyntic cell.[19,111-114] Theoretical advantages of proton pump inhibitors include a long duration of action, little toxicity, and the potential for low maternal and fetal blood concentrations at the time of delivery. The ASA Task Force on Preoperative Fasting concluded that existing studies support the efficacy of raising gastric pH to a level greater than 2.5.[57] The efficacy of prophylaxis when using a proton pump inhibitor is similar to that achieved with an H$_2$-receptor antagonist. A two-dose regimen with an oral dose at bedtime and on the morning of surgery is preferred by some investigators for prophylaxis in patients undergoing elective cesarean section.[110] Published studies have reported no adverse effects on the fetus and neonate.[112]

Esomeprazole (20 to 40 mg orally), **pantoprazole** (40 mg orally or intravenously), and **rabeprazole** (20 mg orally) are newer, alternative proton pump inhibitors.[115-117] However, their efficacy and safety profiles have not been established in obstetric practice.

Metoclopramide

Metoclopramide is a procainamide derivative that is a cholinergic agonist peripherally and a dopamine receptor antagonist centrally. A 10-mg intravenous dose of metoclopramide increases lower esophageal sphincter tone and reduces gastric volume by increasing gastric peristalsis. Metoclopramide can have a significant effect on gastric volume in as little as 15 minutes.[118] Prior administration of atropine or an opioid antagonizes the effect of metoclopramide.[119] Extrapyramidal effects represent the major side effects of metoclopramide. Metoclopramide crosses the placenta, but studies have reported no significant effects on the fetus or neonate.[120]

Sellick Maneuver

Sellick demonstrated that the occlusion of the esophagus by cricoid pressure in cadavers prevented flow of barium from the stomach to the pharynx. He also reported that he had successfully used this maneuver in 26 cases to prevent the passive regurgitation of gastric contents into the airway.[121] During the induction of anesthesia, a trained assistant should place the thumb and middle finger on either side of the cricoid cartilage and apply firm downward pressure to the cricoid cartilage with the middle finger. The head should be fully extended; it may help if the assistant places the left hand behind the mother's neck, so that the cervical vertebrae and esophagus are brought forward, making it easier to occlude the latter. Proper application of cricoid pressure results in occlusion of the proximal esophagus even up to esophageal pressures of 100 cm H_2O. Cricoid pressure is maintained until the endotracheal tube position is confirmed and the endotracheal tube cuff is inflated. There is no need to remove an oral or nasogastric tube before induction of anesthesia. Although cricoid pressure would appear to be a relatively simple maneuver, no randomized controlled trial has ever been conducted to assess its efficacy.[122] On the negative side, the misapplication of cricoid pressure can cause difficulties with intubation.

RECOMMENDATIONS FOR CESAREAN SECTION

When possible, all mothers should be actively encouraged to have regional anesthesia for cesarean section. Mothers with a potentially difficult airway, who require general anesthesia, should have an awake fiberoptic intubation. For **elective cesarean section,** a suitable antacid regimen may include the oral administration of an H_2-receptor antagonist (e.g., 300 mg cimetidine, 150 mg ranitidine, or 20 mg famotidine) or a proton pump inhibitor (omeprazole 40 mg) at bedtime and again 60 to 90 minutes before the induction of anesthesia. (The patient may take the preoperative dose with water.) Some practitioners also give metoclopramide 10 mg orally at the same time as the H_2-receptor antagonist or intravenously at least 15 minutes before the induction of anesthesia. Administration of metoclopramide not only increases lower esophageal sphincter tone and accelerates gastric emptying but also decreases the

incidence of nausea and vomiting during the administration of regional anesthesia for cesarean section.[123]

For **emergency cesarean section under general anesthesia,** 30 mL of sodium citrate should be administered just after transfer of the patient to the operating room. This timing is important because sodium citrate has a relatively short duration of action, except in those mothers in whom gastric emptying has been delayed by the administration of opioid. In addition, 10 mg of metoclopramide and 50 mg of ranitidine should be given intravenously when time allows. Administration of the latter two drugs may not result in decreased gastric volume or acidity at the time of intubation, but will decrease the risk of aspiration at the time of extubation. Some units administer a H_2-receptor antagonist every 6 hours during labor to all mothers considered to be at risk of an operative delivery.

While obstetric anesthesiologists will and should continue to use antacids, H_2-receptor antagonists, proton pump inhibitors, and/or prokinetic agents in obstetric patients, their use has never been shown scientifically to decrease the incidence of aspiration.

ORAL INTAKE DURING LABOR

Women in the third trimester of pregnancy exhibit a state of "accelerated starvation" if denied food and drink.[124] Fasting results in the production of ketones, primarily beta-hydroxybutyrate and acetoacetic acid and the non-esterified fatty acids from which they are derived. These changes are exacerbated by the metabolic demands of labor and delivery. Consequently some obstetricians and nurse midwives have suggested that hospitals and physicians should liberalize oral intake during labor.[125-127] It is argued that allowing mothers to eat and drink during labor will prevent ketosis and dehydration and may thereby improve obstetric outcome.

A randomized controlled trial of the effect of increased intravenous hydration during labor (i.e., Ringer's lactate solution, 125 mL/hr versus 250 mL/hr) showed that the incidence of labor lasting more than 12 hours was significantly higher in the 125 mL/hr group.[128] The primary finding of this study is that prevention of dehydration during labor is beneficial. However, given that large volumes of intravenous fluids are potentially harmful to the mother, it could be argued that hydration should be maintained by the oral route and that the volume consumed should be dictated by maternal thirst.

A prospective randomized study examined the effect of a light diet on the maternal metabolic profile, the residual gastric volume, and the outcome of labor.[129] Women presenting at term in early uncomplicated labor were stratified by parity and randomized to receive either a light diet or water only. The results demonstrated that mothers who consumed a light diet did not show the rise in beta-hydroxybutyrate and non-esterified acids seen in the starved mothers. However, the gastric volumes as measured by ultrasonography were significantly larger in those who had eaten, as were both the incidence of vomiting and the volume of the vomitus. Thus mothers who consume a light diet during labor are at risk of aspiration should general anesthesia be required.

This same study design was repeated in another group of mothers, but *isotonic* "sport drinks" were administered instead of solid food.[130] It was found that isotonic "sport drinks" reduced ketosis without increasing intragastric volume, and the incidence of vomiting and the volume of the vomitus were similar in the two groups. No difference in labor outcome was seen in either study, but the numbers were too small to allow statistical evaluation of obstetric outcome. Consequently a study evaluating the effect of feeding in labor on obstetric outcome is currently in progress, and its conclusions could force a further re-evaluation of labor ward practice.

Maternal death from Mendelson's syndrome is now extremely rare, and its decline probably owes more to the widespread use of regional anesthesia than to *nil per os* (NPO) policies. Thus rigid NPO policies are no longer appropriate on the labor and delivery suite, and mothers should be allowed to alleviate thirst during labor by consuming water and ice chips.[131] Evidence also suggests that isotonic "sport drinks" are a suitable alternative to water, with the potential additional benefit of providing a calorie intake. However, in some high-risk pregnancies it will remain appropriate to achieve hydration by the intravenous route, and such mothers must be managed on a case-by case-basis. Current evidence suggests that solid or semi-solid meals should be avoided once a mother is in active labor or has received opioid-containing analgesics.

KEY POINTS

- Airway problems associated with the use of general anesthesia now represent the most common cause of anesthesia-related maternal deaths.
- Decreased lower esophageal sphincter tone and an increased risk of difficult intubation are the primary factors that increase the risk of aspiration during pregnancy and immediately postpartum.
- Although pulmonary aspiration of gastric contents is rare in contemporary obstetric anesthesia practice, many cases of fatal aspiration occur during difficult or failed intubation at cesarean section.
- The most effective way to decrease the risk of aspiration is to avoid the administration of general anesthesia.
- The mother undergoing elective cesarean section should fast from solid food, as recommended by the ASA Task Force on Preoperative Fasting. Preoperative prophylaxis should include an H_2-receptor antagonist or a proton pump inhibitor.
- Administration of a clear antacid effectively increases gastric pH and is mandatory prior to a cesarean section performed under general anesthesia. A clear antacid is preferred because aspiration of a particulate antacid results in pulmonary parenchymal damage similar to that which occurs after the aspiration of gastric acid.
- Hypoxemia is the hallmark of aspiration pneumonitis. Mechanical ventilation with PEEP is the most effective treatment for severe hypoxemia.
- The oral intake of clear fluids may be allowed during labor in uncomplicated parturients.

REFERENCES

1. Simpson JY. Remarks on the alleged case of death from the action of chloroform. Lancet 1848; 1:175.
2. Hall CC. Aspiration pneumonitis. An obstetric hazard. JAMA 1940; 114: 728-33
3. Mendelson CL. The aspiration of stomach contents into the lungs during obstetric anesthesia. Am J Obstet Gynecol 1946; 52:191-205.
4. Hawkins JL, Koonin LM, Palmer SK, Gibbs CP. Anesthesia-related deaths during obstetric delivery in the United States, 1979-1990. Anesthesiology 1997; 86: 277-84.
5. Olsson GL, Hallen B, Hambraeus-Jonzon K. Aspiration during anaesthesia: A computer-aided study of 185,358 anaesthetics. Acta Anaesthesiol Scand 1986; 30:84-92.
6. Warner MA, Warner ME, Weber JG. Clinical significance of pulmonary aspiration during the perioperative period. Anesthesiology 1993; 78: 56-62.
7. Kluger MT, Short TG. Aspiration during anaesthesia: a review of 133 cases from the Australian Anaesthetic Incident Monitoring Study (AIMS). Anaesthesia 1999; 54:19-26.
8. Chestnut DH. Anesthesia and maternal mortality (editorial). Anesthesiology 1997; 86:273-5.
9. Lewis G, Drife J. Report on Confidential Enquiries into Maternal Deaths in the United Kingdom, 1997-1999. London, HMSO, 2001.
10. Soreide E, Bjornestad E, Steen PA. An audit of perioperative aspiration pneumonitis in gynaecological and obstetric patients. Acta Anaesthesiol Scand 1996; 40:14-9.
11. Catanzarite V, Willms D, Wong D, et al. Acute respiratory distress syndrome in pregnancy and the puerperium: causes, courses and outcome. Obstet Gynecol 2001; 97:760-4.
12. Dodds WJ, Dent J, Hogan WJ et al. Mechanisms of gastroesophageal reflux in patients with reflux esophagitis. NEJM 1982; 307:1547-52.
13. Code CF, Marlett JA. The interdigestive myo-electric complex of the stomach and small bowel of dogs. J Physiol (Lond) 1975; 246: 289-309.
14. Schurizek BA, Kraglund K, Andreasen F, et al. Gastrointestinal motility and gastric pH and emptying following ingestion of diazepam. Br J Anaesth 1988; 61:712-9.
15. Meyer JH. Motility of the stomach and gastroduodenal junction. In Johnson LR, editor. Physiology of the Gastrointestinal Tract. New York, Raven Press, 1987: 613-29.
16. Brooks FP. Physiology of the stomach. In Berk JE, editor. Gastroenterology. Philadelphia, WB Saunders, 1985: 874-940.
17. Feldman M, Richardson CT. Total 24-hour gastric acid secretion in patients with duodenal ulcer: Comparison with normal subjects and effects of cimetidine and parietal cell vagotomy. Gastroenterology 1986; 90:540-4.
18. Richardson CT, Walsh JH, Hicks MI, et al. Studies on the mechanisms of food-stimulated gastric acid secretion in normal human subjects. J Clin Invest 1976; 58:623-31.
19. Ewart MC, Yau G, Gin T, et al. A comparison of the effects of omeprazole and ranitidine on gastric secretion in women undergoing elective caesarean section. Anaesthesia 1990; 45:527-30.
20. Mayer G, Arnold R, Feurle G, et al. Influence of feeding and sham feeding upon serum gastrin and gastric acid secretion in control subjects and duodenal ulcer patients. Scand J Gastroenterol 1974; 9:703-10.
21. Bergegardh S, Olbe L. Gastric acid response to antrum distention in man. Scand J Gastroenterol 1975; 10:171-6.
22. Hunt JN, MacDonald I. The influence of volume on gastric emptying. J Physiol (London) 1954; 126:459-74.
23. Anvari M, Horowitz M, Fraser R, et al. Effect of posture on gastric emptying of nonnutrient liquid and antropyloroduodenal motility. Am J Physiol 1995; 268:G868-71.
24. Jian R, Vigneron N, Najean Y, et al. Gastric emptying and intragastric distribution of lipids in man: New scintigraphic method of study. Dig Dis Sci 1982; 27:705-11.
25. Collins PJ, Horowitz M, Maddox A, et al. Effects of increasing solid component size of a mixed solid/liquid meal on solid and liquid gastric emptying. Am J Physiol 1996; 271:G549-54.
26. Malagelada JR, Longstreth GF, Summerskill WHJ et al. Measurements of gastric functions during digestion of ordinary solid meals in man. Gastroenterology 1976; 70:203-10.
27. Lind JF, Smith AM, McIver DK, et al. Heartburn in pregnancy: A manometric study. Can Med Assoc J 1968; 98:571-4.
28. Hey VMF, Cowley DJ, Ganguli PC, et al, Gastro-oesophageal reflux in late pregnancy Anaesthesia 1977; 32:372-7.
29. Vanner Rg, Goodman NW. Gastro-oesophageal reflux in pregnancy at term and after delivery. Anaesthesia 1989; 44:808-11.

30. Van Thiel DH, Gavaler JS, Joshi SN, et al. Heartburn of pregnancy. Gastroenterology 1977; 72:666-8.

31. Van Thiel DH, Gavaler JS, Stremple J. Lower esophageal sphincter pressure in women using sequential oral contraceptives. Gastroenterology 1976; 71:232-4.

32. Murray FA, Erskine JP, Fielding J. Gastric secretion in pregnancy. Br J Obstet Gynaecol 1957; 64:373-81.

33. Davison JS, Davison MC, Hay DM. Gastric emptying in late pregnancy. Br J Obstet Gynaecol 1970;77:37-41.

34. La Salvia LA, Steffen EA. Delayed gastric emptying in labor. Am J Obstet Gynecol 1950; 59:1075-81.

35. Nimmo WS, Wilson J, Prescott LF. Narcotic analgesics and delayed gastric emptying during labour. Lancet 1975; 1:890-3.

36. Nimmo WS, Wilson J, Prescott LF. Further studies of gastric emptying during labour. Anaesthesia 1977; 32:100-1.

37. O'Sullivan G, Sutton AJ, Thompson SA, et al. Noninvasive measurement of gastric emptying in obstetric patients. Anesth Analg 1987; 66:505-9.

38. Carp H, Jayaram A, Stoll M. Ultrasound examination of the stomach contents of parturients. Anesth Analg 1992; 74:683-7.

39. Wright PM, Allen RW, Moore J, et al. Gastric emptying during lumbar extradural analgesia in labour: Effect of fentanyl supplementation. Br J Anaesth 1992; 68:248-51.

40. Geddes SM, Thorburn J, Logan RW. Gastric emptying following caesarean section and the effect of epidural fentanyl. Anaesthesia 1991; 46:1016-8.

41. Kelly MC, Carabine UA, Hill DA, Mirakhur RK. A comparison of the effect of intrathecal and extradural fentanyl on gastric emptying in laboring women. Anesth Analg 1997; 85:834-8.

42. Porter JS, Bonello E, Reynolds F. The influence of epidural administration of fentanyl infusion on gastric emptying in labour. Anaesthesia 1997;52:1151-6.

43. Wong CA, Loffredi M, Ganchiff JN, et al. Gastric emptying of water in term pregnancy. Anesthesiology 2002; 96:1395-1400.

44. Christofides ND, Ghatei MA, Bloom SR, et al. Decreased plasma motilin concentrations in pregnancy. Br Med J 1982; 285:1453.

45. O'Sullivan G, Sear JW, Bullingham RES et al. The effect of magnesium trisilicate mixture, metoclopramide and ranitidine on gastric pH, volume and serum gastrin Anaesthesia 1985; 40:246-53.

46. Attia RR, Ebeid AM, Fischer JE, et al. Maternal fetal and placental gastrin concentrations. Anaesthesia 1982; 37:18.

47. Awe WC, Fletcher WS, Jacob SW. The pathophysiology of aspiration pneumonitis. Surgery 1966; 60:232-9.

48. Cameron JL, Mitchell WH, Zuidema GD. Aspiration pneumonia: Clinical outcome following documented aspiration. Arch Surg 1973; 106:49-52.

49. LeFrock JL, Clark TS, Davies B, Klainer AS. Aspiration pneumonia: A ten-year review. Am Surg 1979; 45:305-13.

50. Teabeaut JR. Aspiration of gastric contents: An experimental study. Am J Pathology 1951; 28:51-67.

51. Hamelberg W, Bosomworth PP. Aspiration pneumonitis: Experimental studies and clinical observations. Anesth Analg 1964; 43:669-77.

52. Exarhos ND, Logan WD, Abbott OA, et al. The importance of pH and volume in tracheobronchial aspiration. Dis Chest 1965; 47:167-9.

53. Roberts RB, Shirley MA. Reducing the risk of acid aspiration during cesarean section. Anesth Analg 1974; 53:859-68.

54. Schwartz DJ, Wynne JW, Gibbs CP, et al. The pulmonary consequences of aspiration of gastric contents at pH values greater than 2.5. Am Rev Respir Dis 1980; 121:119-26.

55. Roberts RB, Shirley MA. Antacid therapy in obstetrics (letter). Anesthesiology 1980; 53:83.

56. James CF, Modell JH, Gibbs CP, et al. Pulmonary aspiration: Effects of volume and pH in the rat. Anesth Analg 1984; 63:665-8.

57. The American Society of Anesthesiologist Task Force on Preoperative Fasting. Practice guidelines for preoperative fasting and the use of pharmacologic agents to reduce the risk of pulmonary aspiration: Application to healthy patients undergoing elective procedures. Anesthesiology 1999; 90:896-905.

58. Raidoo DM, Rocke DA, Brock-Utne JG, et al. Critical volume for pulmonary acid aspiration: reappraisal in a primate model. Br J Anaesth 1990; 65:248-50.

59. Plourde G, Hardy JF. Aspiration pneumonia: Assessing the risk of regurgitation in the cat. Can Anaesth Soc J 1986; 33:345-8.

60. Gunther A, Ruppert C, Schmidt R, et al. Surfactant alteration and replacement in acute respiratory distress syndrome. Respir Res 2001; 2:353-64.

61. Ware LB, Matthay MA. The acute respiratory distress syndrome. N Engl J Med 2000; 342:1334-49.

62. Matthay MA. Conference summary: acute lung injury. Chest 1999; 116:119-26S.

63. Gibbs CP, Schwartz DJ, Wynne JW, et al. Antacid pulmonary aspiration in the dog. Anesthesiology 1979; 51:380-5.

64. Landay MJ, Christensen EE, Bynum LJ. Pulmonary manifestations of acute aspiration of gastric contents. AJR Am J Roentgenol 1978; 131:587-92.

65. Wynne JW, Modell JH. Respiratory aspiration of stomach contents. Ann Intern Med 1977; 87: 466-74.

66. Bernard GR, Luce JM, Sprung CL, et al. High-dose corticosteroids in patients with the adult respiratory distress syndrome. N Engl J Med 1987; 317:1565-70.

67. Meduri GU, Tolley EA, Chrousos GP, et al. Prolonged methylprednisolone treatment suppresses systemic inflammation in patients with unresolving acute respiratory distress syndrome. Am J Respir Crit Care Med 2002; 165:983-91.

68. Thompson BT, Hayden D, Matthay MA, et al. Clinicians' approaches to mechanical ventilation in acute lung injury and ARDS. Chest 2001; 120:1622-7.

69. The Acute Respiratory Distress Syndrome Network. Ventilation with lower tidal volumes as compared with traditional tidal volumes for acute lung injury and the acute respiratory distress syndrome. N Engl J Med 2000; 342:1301-8.

70. Marik PE. Aspiration pneumonitis and aspiration pneumonia. N Engl J Med 2001; 344:665-71.

71. Lyons G. Failed intubation: Six years' experience in a teaching maternity unit. Anaesthesia 1985; 40:759-62.

72. Samsoon GL, Young JR. Difficult tracheal intubation: A retrospective study. Anaesthesia 1987; 42:487-90.

73. Rocke DA, Murray WB, Rout CC, et al. Relative risk analysis of factors associated with difficult intubation in obstetric anesthesia. Anesthesiology 1992; 77:67-73.

74. Gibbs CP, Rolbin SH, Norman P. Cause and prevention of maternal aspiration (letter). Anesthesiology 1984; 61:111-2.

75. Cohen SE, Jasson J, Talafre ML, et al. Does metoclopramide decrease the volume of gastric contents in patients undergoing cesarean section? Anesthesiology 1984; 61:604-7.

76. McCaughey W, Howe JP, Moore J, et al. Cimetidine in elective caesarean section: Effect on gastric acidity. Anaesthesia 1981; 36:167-72.

77. Wyner J, Cohen SE. Gastric volume in early pregnancy: Effect of metoclopramide. Anesthesiology 1982; 57:209-12.

78. Blouw R, Scatliff J, Craig DB, et al. Gastric volume and pH in postpartum patients. Anesthesiology 1976; 45:456-7.

79. James CF, Gibbs CP, Banner T. Postpartum perioperative risk of aspiration pneumonia. Anesthesiology 1984; 61:756-9.

80. Rennie AL, Richard JA, Milne MK, et al. Postpartum sterilization: An anaesthetic hazard? Anaesthesia 1979; 34:267-9.

81. Cote CJ, Goudsouzian NG, Liu LM, et al. Assessment of risk factors related to the acid aspiration syndrome in pediatric patients: Gastric pH and residual volume. Anesthesiology 1982; 56:70-2.

82. Goudsouzian N, Cote CJ, Liu LM, et al. The dose-response effects of oral cimetidine on gastric pH and volume in children. Anesthesiology 1981; 55:533-6.

83. Vaughan RW, Bauer S, Wise L. Volume and pH of gastric juice in obese patients. Anesthesiology 1975; 43:686-9.

84. Kallar SK, Everett LL. Potential risks and preventive measures for pulmonary aspiration: New concepts in preoperative fasting guidelines. Anesth Analg 1993; 77:171-82.

85. Agarwal A, Chari P, Singh H. Fluid deprivation before operation: The effect of a small drink. Anaesthesia 1989; 44:632-4.

86. Lewis M, Crawford JS. Can one risk fasting the obstetric patient for less than 4 hours? Br J Anaesth 1987; 59:312-4.

87. Hawkins JL, Gibbs CP, Orleans M, et al. Obstetric anesthesia work force survey, 1981 versus 1992. Anesthesiology 1997; 87:135-43.

88. Tsen LC, Pitner R, Camann WR. General anesthesia for cesarean section at a tertiary care hospital 1990-1995: Indications and implications. Internat J Obstet Anesth 1998; 7:147-52.

89. May AE, Yentis SM. Up, up and away: watching the caesarean section rate rise. Anaesthesia 2002; 57:317-8.

90. Gibbs CP, Spohr L, Schmidt D. The effectiveness of sodium citrate as an antacid. Anesthesiology 1982; 57:44-6.

91. Chen CT, Toung TJ, Haupt HM, et al. Evaluation of the efficacy of Alka-Seltzer Effervescent in gastric acid neutralization. Anesth Analg 1984; 63:325-9.

92. O'Sullivan GM, Bullingham RES. The assessment of gastric acidity and antacid effect in pregnant women by a noninvasive radiotelemetry technique. Br J Obstet Gynaecol 1984; 91:973-8.

93. O'Sullivan GM, Bullingham RES. Noninvasive assessment of antacid effect during labor. Anesth Analg 1985; 64:95-100.

94. Gillett GB, Watson JD, Langford RM. Prophylaxis against acid aspiration syndrome in obstetric practice (letter). Anesthesiology 1984; 60:525.

95. Eyler SW, Cullen BF, Murphy ME, et al. Antacid aspiration in rabbits: A comparison of Mylanta and Bicitra. Anesth Analg 1982; 61:288-92.

96. Coombs DW, Hooper D, Colton T. Acid-aspiration prophylaxis by use of preoperative oral administration of cimetidine. Anesthesiology 1979; 51:352-6.

97. Johnston JR, McCaughey W, Moore J, et al. Cimetidine as an oral antacid before elective Caesarean section. Anaesthesia 1982; 37:26-32.

98. Manchikanti L, Kraus JW, Edds SP. Cimetidine and related drugs in anesthesia. Anesth Analg 1982; 61:595-608.

99. Somogyi A, Gugler R. Drug interactions with cimetidine. Clin Pharmacokinet 1982; 7:23-41.

100. Feely J, Wilkinson GR, McAllister CB, et al. Increased toxicity and reduced clearance of lidocaine by cimetidine. Ann Intern Med 1982; 96:592-4.

101. Howe JP, McGowan WA, Moore J, et al. The placental transfer of cimetidine. Anaesthesia 1981; 36:371-5.

102. Lineberger AS, Sprague DH, Battaglini JW. Sinus arrest associated with cimetidine. Anesth Analg 1985; 64:554-6.

103. Dammann HG, Muller P, Simon B. Parenteral ranitidine: onset and duration of action. Br J Anaesth 1982; 54:1235-6.

104. Francis RN, Kwik RS. Oral ranitidine for prophylaxis against Mendelson's syndrome. Anesth Analg 1982; 61:130-2.

105. Maile CJ, Francis RN. Pre-operative ranitidine. Effect of a single intravenous dose on pH and volume of gastric aspirate. Anaesthesia 1983; 38:324-6.

106. Brock-Utne JG, Downing JW, Humphrey D. Effect of ranitidine given before atropine sulphate on lower oesophageal sphincter tone. Anaesth Intensive Care 1984; 12:140-2.

107. Kirch W, Hoensch H, Janisch HD. Interactions and non-interactions with ranitidine. Clin Pharmacokinet 1984; 9:493-510.

108. Dailey PA, Hughes SC, Rosen MA, et al. Effect of cimetidine and ranitidine on lidocaine concentrations during epidural anesthesia for cesarean section. Anesthesiology 1988; 69:1013-7.

109. Pattichis K, Louca LL. Histamine, histamine H2-receptor antagonists, gastric acid secretion and ulcers: an overview. Drug Metabol Drug Interact 1995; 12:1-36.

110. Howden CW, Tytgat GN. The tolerability and safety profile of famotidine. Clin Ther 1996; 18:36-54.

111. Ng A, Smith G. Gastroesophageal reflux and aspiration of gastric contents in anesthetic practice. Anesth Analg 2001; 93:494-513.

112. Yau G, Kan AF, Gin T, et al. A comparison of omeprazole and ranitidine for prophylaxis against aspiration pneumonitis in emergency caesarean section. Anaesthesia. 1992; 47:101-4.

113. Blum RA, Shi H, Karol MD, et al. The comparative effects of lansoprazole, omeprazole, and ranitidine in suppressing gastric acid secretion. Clin Ther 1997; 19:1013-23.

114. Levack ID, Bowie RA, Braid DP, et al. Comparison of the effect of two dose schedules of oral omeprazole with oral ranitidine on gastric aspirate pH and volume in patients undergoing elective surgery. Br J Anaesth 1996; 76:567-9.

115. Kale-Pradhan PB, Landry HK, Sypula WT. Esomeprazole for acid peptic disorders. Ann Pharmacother 2002; 36:655-63.

116. Cheer SM, Prakash A, Faulds D, et al. Pantoprazole: an update of its pharmacological properties and therapeutic use in the management of Acid-related disorders. Drugs 2003; 63:101-33.

117. Carswell CI, Goa KL. Rabeprazole: an update of its use in acid-related disorders. Drugs 2001; 61:2327-56.

118. Cohen SE, Jasson J, Talafre ML, et al. Does metoclopramide decrease the volume of gastric contents in patients undergoing cesarean section? Anesthesiology 1984; 61:604-7.

119. Hey VM, Ostick DG, Mazumder JK, et al. Pethidine, metoclopramide and the gastro-oesophageal sphincter. A study in healthy volunteers. Anaesthesia 1981; 36:173-6.

120. Bylsma-Howell M, Riggs KW, McMorland GH, et al. Placental transport of metoclopramide: assessment of maternal and neonatal effects. Can Anaesth Soc J 1983; 30:487-92.

121. Sellick BA. Cricoid pressure to control regurgitation of stomach contents during induction of anaesthesia. Lancet 1961; 1:404-6.

122. Maltby JR, Beriault MT. Science, pseudoscience and Sellick. Can J Anesth 2002; 49:443-6.

123. Lussos SA, Bader AM, Thornhill ML, Datta S. The antiemetic efficacy and safety of prophylactic metoclopramide for elective cesarean section delivery during spinal anesthesia. Reg Anesth 1992; 17:126-30.

124. Metzger BE, Vileisis RA, Ramikar V et al. `Accelerated starvation' and the skipped breakfast in late normal pregnancy. Lancet 1982; 1: 588-92.

125. Elkington KW. At the water's edge: Where obstetrics and anesthesia meet. Obstet Gynecol 1991; 77:304-8.

126. O'Sullivan G, Shennan A. Labour – a gastronomic experience! Internat J Obstet Anesth 2002; 11:1-3.

127. Shipp TD, Repke JT. Normal labor and delivery. In Intrapartum Obstetrics. Repke JT, editor. Churchill Livingstone, 1996: 67-108.

128. Garite TJ, Weeks J, Peters-Phair K et al. A randomized control trial of the effect of increased intravenous hydration the course of labor in nulliparous women. Am J Obstet Gynecol 2000; 183: 1544-8.

129. Scrutton MJl. Metcalfe GA. Lowy C et al. Eating in labour. Anaesthesia 1999; 54:329-34.

130. Kubli M Scrutton MJ, Seed PT et al. An evaluation of isotonic "sport drinks" during labor. Anesth Analg 2002; 94: 404-8.

131. American Society of Anesthesiologists Task Force on Obstetrical Anesthesia. Practice guidelines for obstetrical anesthesia. Anesthesiology 1999; 90:600-11.

Chapter 31

The Difficult Airway: Risk, Prophylaxis, and Management

Krzysztof M. Kuczkowski, M.D. ·
Laurence S. Reisner, M.D. · Jonathan L. Benumof, M.D.

RISK

One of the principal responsibilities of an anesthesiologist is to maintain an adequate airway for effective gas exchange. The inability to maintain a patent airway can result in brain damage or death. In the United States, more than 85% of all malpractice claims for adverse respiratory events during anesthesia involve a brain-damaged or dead patient.[1] It has been estimated that the inability to manage a difficult airway successfully is responsible for as many as 30% of anesthesia-related deaths in the United States.[2,3] In the United Kingdom, one in three anesthesia-related deaths is a direct result of the inability to intubate the trachea.[4] These data apply to nonobstetric surgical patients, in whom the incidence of failed intubation is approximately 1 in 2330.[5] The incidence of failed intubation is approximately eight times higher in the obstetric population, with an estimated occurrence of 1 in 280.[6]

Maternal Morbidity and Mortality

The first reported death after chloroform anesthesia in Great Britain occurred in 1848.[7] In a commentary on this case, Sir James Young Simpson stated: "If we can induce anaesthesia without the absence of consciousness which is found in the state of general anaesthesia, many would still regard it as a greater advance." Widespread use of regional anesthesia in obstetric patients was not established until a century later. Today, the administration of regional anesthesia has transformed the practice of obstetrics and obstetric anesthesia.

During the last four decades, anesthesia-related maternal mortality has decreased dramatically but to a lesser degree than overall maternal mortality.[7-12] Great Britain has an exemplary system for the review of maternal deaths. Since 1952, the *Report on Confidential Enquiries into Maternal Deaths* has been published every 3 years.[7-12] Anesthesia-related complications represented the third most common cause of maternal death (after hypertension and pulmonary embolism) between 1952 and 1984 and accounted for approximately 12.6% of all direct maternal deaths.[4] The reports for the years 1985 to 1999 included data for the four countries that comprise the United Kingdom (England, Wales, Scotland, and Northern Ireland).[8-12] In 1985-1987, anesthesia-related deaths accounted for 4.4% of direct maternal deaths. Of the eight deaths attributed to anesthesia, five resulted from a misplaced endotracheal tube (ETT), one from a kinked ETT, one from pulmonary aspiration of gastric contents, and one from high epidural blockade in a woman with aortic insufficiency (Table 31-1).

In the United States, the current overall maternal mortality rate is approximately 9.2 per 100,000 live births.[13] Anesthesia-related maternal mortality in the United States has declined from 4.3 per million live births (1979 to 1981) to 1.7 per million live births (1988 to 1990), and this represents 3.2% of all maternal deaths during the surveillance period.[14] The majority of these deaths occurred during cesarean section, and 49% were caused by airway difficulties. General anesthesia was administered to 67 of the 129 patients who died, and the causes of death were determined to be aspiration (33%), induction/intubation problems (22%), inadequate ventilation (15%), respiratory failure (3%), cardiac arrest during anesthesia (22%), and unknown (5%).[14] Anesthesia continues to be a worrisome cause of maternal mortality, and difficulty with the airway and ventilation remains a primary concern.

Contemporary obstetric anesthesia practice mandates the vigilance of a trained anesthetist who has a thorough knowledge of the anatomy, physiology, and pharmacologic responses peculiar to the parturient. Further, anesthesiologists should be familiar with the American Society of Anesthesiologists (ASA) Practice Guidelines for Management of the Difficult Airway,[15-17] which serves as a foundation for this chapter's discussion of the difficult airway in the parturient (Figure 31-1).

Definition and Classification of the Difficult Airway

There are two common methods of maintaining a patent airway. The first method is by mask ventilation. Inspired gas is delivered to a patient's face by a sealed mask on the face while

TABLE 31-1   MATERNAL DEATHS DIRECTLY ATTRIBUTABLE TO ANESTHESIA

Cause	1973–75	1976–78	1985–87	1988–90	1991–93	1994–96	1997–99
Inhalation of stomach contents during induction of anesthesia	9	4	1	1	0	0	1
Inhalation of stomach contents during difficult intubation	4	7	0	1	0	0	0
Hypoxia due to esophageal/failed intubation	3	9	6	1	0	0	0
Misuse of drugs	4	3	0	0	0	0	0
Accidents with apparatus	2	2	0	0	0	0	0
Subarachnoid injection of anesthetic during attempted epidural block/high spinal	2	1	0	0	0	0	1
Miscellaneous causes*	7	4	1	2	8	1	1
Total	31	30	8	5	8	1	3

*Miscellaneous causes included allergic reaction, inadequate reversal of muscle relaxant, intravenous overload, postoperative asphyxial episode, and mismanagement of epidural block in a patient with cardiac disease. The one death in the 1994-96 report appears in the "miscellaneous" category because it exhibited features of excessive drug dosage, inappropriate management of regional block, misuse of drugs, and "unconventional" resuscitation. The "miscellaneous" category death from the 1997-99 report resulted from multiple problems, including failure to crossmatch blood in a timely manner, volume overload and pulmonary edema, loss of the airway during an attempt to change the tracheostomy tube in the ICU, and subsequent barotruma during attempted jet ventilation.
Data from Confidential Enquiries Into Maternal Deaths in England and Wales reports 1973–1975, 1976–1978, 1985–1987, 1988–1990, 1991–1993, 1994–1996, and 1997–1999.[7-12]
Adapted from Hawkins JL, Bassell GM, Marx GF. Anesthesia-related maternal mortality. In Hughes SC, Levinson G, Rosen MA. Shnider and Levinson's Anesthesia for Obstetrics, 4th ed. Philadelphia, Lippincott Williams & Wilkins, 2002: 432.

patency from the face to the vocal cords is maintained, with or without external jaw thrust maneuvers and/or internal upper airway devices. The second method consists of passing a tube from the outside environment to a point below the vocal cords to keep the airway open to inspired gases (i.e., endotracheal intubation).

The level of difficulty in maintaining **mask ventilation** can range from zero to infinite (Figure 31-2). During mask ventilation, a zero degree of difficulty means that no external effort or internal airway device is needed to maintain airway patency. An infinite degree of difficulty means that despite maximal external efforts and full use of oropharyngeal and nasopharyngeal airways, maintaining a patent airway is impossible. The degree of difficulty with mask ventilation can change at any time in a given patient.

Similarly, the degree of difficulty with **endotracheal intubation** under direct vision can range from zero to infinite (Figure 31-2). Cormack and Lehane[18] classified difficult intubation into four grades according to the view obtained with direct laryngoscopy with a MacIntosh blade (Figure 31-3):

Grade I: The entire laryngeal aperture is visible; there is no difficulty with intubation.

Grade II: The posterior portion of the aperture is visualized; there is slight difficulty with intubation. Typically the arytenoids, if not the vocal cords, can be brought into view with external laryngeal pressure (e.g., over the thyroid cartilage).[19]

Grade III: Only the epiglottis is visualized; there may be severe difficulty with intubation. External laryngeal pressure may bring the arytenoid cartilages into view.

Grade IV: Only the soft palate is visualized; intubation is extremely difficult or impossible except by special techniques.

An infinitely difficult intubation means that the trachea cannot be intubated under direct vision despite optimal head and neck positioning, forceful anterior elevation of the laryngoscope blade, use of different laryngoscope blades, multiple attempts by multiple laryngoscopists, external displacement of the larynx in a posterior and cephalad direction, and full paralysis. The severity of difficulty with tracheal intubation may be independent of the degree of difficulty with mask ventilation and can increase progressively, especially after multiple attempts at intubation.

Incidence of the Difficult Airway

Table 31-2 summarizes the incidence of airway difficulty in the nonpregnant population. A grade II or III laryngoscopic view occurs in 1% to 18% of the population and may require multiple attempts and blades to achieve successful endotracheal intubation.[18,20-24] A definite grade III laryngoscopic view occurs in 1% to 4% of the population.[5] The incidence of a severe grade III or grade IV laryngoscopic view (with subsequent failed endotracheal intubation) ranges from 0.05% to 0.35% of the population.[5,6,18,25-27] The high end of this range applies to the obstetric population. Often-quoted reasons for difficult intubation in pregnant women include the presence of enlarged breasts and pharyngolaryngeal edema, as well as reduced time available for airway instrumentation resulting from reduced functional residual capacity (FRC). There are no published data regarding the incidence of difficulty with mask ventilation in pregnant women. The incidence of both failed endotracheal intubation and mask ventilation (which often results in brain damage or death) ranges from 0.0001% to 0.02% of the population.[2,3,28]

A correlation exists between the difficulty in maintaining an airway and (1) the use of physical force, (2) the number of attempts at endotracheal intubation, and (3) the incidence of complications. The incidence of relatively minor complications (e.g., lacerations and bruises of the lip and posterior pharynx) during direct laryngoscopy and intubation in patients with a normal airway is approximately 5%.[29] When difficulty with intubation is anticipated, the incidence of minor trauma to the upper airway increases to 17%.[29] In patients in whom tracheal intubation is difficult

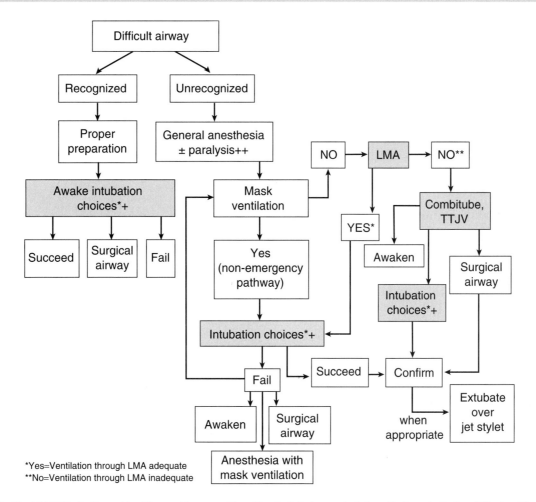

FIGURE 31-1. The ASA Difficult Airway Algorithm. +, Always *consider* calling for help (e.g., technical, medical, surgical) when difficulty with mask ventilation and/or tracheal intubation is encountered; ++, Consider the need to preserve spontaneous ventilation; *, Nonsurgical tracheal intubation choices consist of laryngoscopy with a rigid laryngoscope blade (many types), blind orotracheal or nasotracheal technique, fiberoptic/stylet technique, retrograde technique, illuminating stylet, rigid bronchoscope, and percutaneous dilational tracheal entry. See reference 2 below for a complete discussion of these intubation choices. (From [1] Benumof JL. Management of the difficult airway. Anesthesiology 1991; 75:1087-110; [2] Practice guidelines for management of the difficult airway. An updated report by the American Society of Anesthesiologists Task Force on Management of the Difficult Airway. Anesthesiology 2003; 98:1269-77; [3] Benumof JL. The laryngeal mask airway and the American Society of Anesthesiologists Difficult Airway Algorithm. Anesthesiology 1996; 84:686-99.)

(i.e., intubation requires multiple attempts but eventually is successful), the incidence of upper airway complications increases to 63%.[29] The inability to maintain an adequate airway results in an increased incidence of very severe complications, including brain damage and death.

AIRWAY ASSESSMENT

Multivariable Prediction/Assessment of Airway Difficulty

Most airway catastrophes occur when airway difficulty is not recognized before the induction of anesthesia.[30-34] An estimated 90% of cases of difficult intubation should be anticipated,[32] but one prospective study of 1200 patients found that only 22 (51%) of 43 difficult intubations were anticipated.[35] Therefore it is evident that unexpected airway difficulties commonly occur. Conversely, some predicted difficult airways are easy to manage.

Frerk[36] prospectively evaluated the combination of Mallampati classification (*vide infra*) plus assessment of thyromental distance in 244 patients; the authors found a 98% specificity and 80% sensitivity, respectively. Lewis et al.[37] combined the thyromental distance and the Mallampati clas-

sification into a statistical formula called the Performance Index. The Performance Index establishes a threshold that, depending on the incidence of difficult intubation in the specific clinical practice, can be used to predict the ratio of unexpected difficult intubations to "false alarms."

Other investigators have examined combinations of more than two predictors of a difficult airway. Wilson et al.[38] examined combinations of five risk factors, including weight, head and neck movement, jaw movement, receding mandible, and buck teeth (i.e., the Wilson Risk Sum). The authors assigned one of three levels of severity for each risk factor, and they created a predictive index that allowed detection of 75% of difficult laryngoscopies at a cost of falsely identifying 12% of the "not difficult" laryngoscopies.[38] Oates et al.[39] subsequently compared the Wilson Risk Sum with the Mallampati classification and found the former to be slightly superior.

Bellhouse and Dore[2] examined radiographic measurements in 19 patients with a known difficult airway and compared these with measurements in 14 patients with a known easy airway. Subsequently, the authors looked for clinical parameters that would correspond to the radiographic predictors that distinguished between these two patient groups, and they identified three suggestive clinical measures: Mallampati classification III or IV, limited atlantooccipital joint mobility, and receding chin. Rocke et al.[40] evaluated nine risk factors in 1500 obstetric patients and found that four of the nine factors (i.e., Mallampati classification, short neck, receding mandible, protruding maxillary incisors) were predictive of a difficult intubation (Table 31-3). Tse et al.[41] evaluated 471 patients and assessed combinations of three variables including the Mallampati classification, head exten-

sion, and the thyromental distance. The authors concluded that the combination of these tests improved the specificity of difficult airway prediction, at a great cost in sensitivity. El-Ganzouri et al.[42] reported a prospective analysis of 10,507 consecutive patients presenting for surgery under general anesthesia. A multivariate model for stratifying the risk of difficult intubation was developed from seven crite-

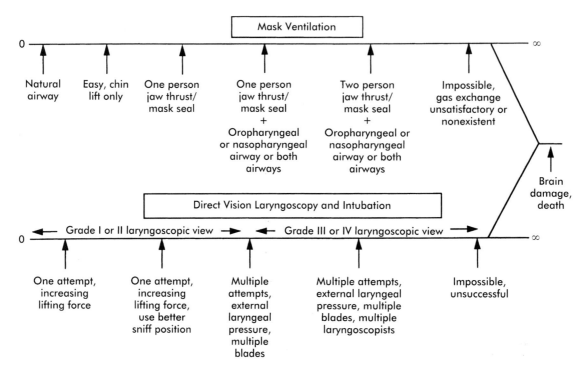

FIGURE 31-2. Definition of different degrees of a difficult airway. Airway refers to either mask ventilation or endotracheal intubation by direct vision laryngoscopy. The degree of difficulty can range from zero (extremely easy) to infinite (impossible). When both mask ventilation and direct vision laryngoscopy are impossible and no other maneuver is successful, brain damage or death will ensue. Between these extremes are several well-defined, commonly encountered degrees of difficulty. The grade of laryngoscopic view is represented as an approximate continuum above the discrete progressive indices of laryngoscopic difficulty (see Figure 31-3). (From Benumof JL. Management of the difficult airway. Anesthesiology 1991; 75:1087-110.)

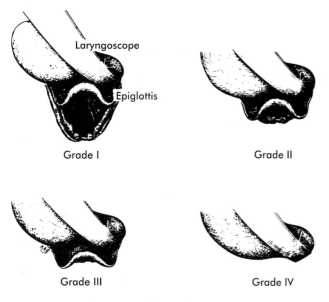

FIGURE 31-3. The four grades of laryngoscopic view as defined by Cormack and Lehane.[18] Grade I is visualization of the entire laryngeal aperture. Grade II is visualization of just the posterior portion of the laryngeal aperture. Grade III is visualization of only the epiglottis. Grade IV is visualization of only the soft palate. (From Cormack RS, Lehane J. Difficult tracheal intubation in obstetrics. Anaesthesia 1984; 39:1105-11.)

TABLE 31-2	INCIDENCE OF DIFFICULT INTUBATION ACCORDING TO DEGREE OF DIFFICULTY[2-6,18,20-28]	
	Range of incidence	
Degree of difficulty with intubation	**Per 10,000**	**%**
Endotracheal intubation successful but multiple attempts and/or blades may be required; probable grade II or III	100-1800	1-18
Endotracheal intubation successful but multiple attempts and/or blades and/or laryngoscopists required; grade III	100-400	1-4
Endotracheal intubation not successful; grade III or IV	5-35	0.05-0.35
Cannot ventilate by mask plus cannot intubate; transtracheal jet ventilation, tracheostomy, brain damage, or death	0.01-2.0	0.0001-0.02

ria, including mouth opening, thyromental distance, the Mallampati classification, neck movement, ability to protrude the mandible, body weight, and a history of difficult intubation.

TABLE 31-3	RELATIVE RISK FACTORS ASSOCIATED WITH DIFFICULT TRACHEAL INTUBATION COMPARED WITH A RISK OF 1.0 FOR PATIENTS WITH AN UNCOMPLICATED MALLAMPATI CLASS I AIRWAY

Risk factors	Relative risk (95% confidence intervals)
Mallampati class	
II	3.23 (1.70-6.13)
III	7.58 (4.07-14.12)
IV	11.30 (5.03-25.38)
Short neck	5.01 (2.40-10.45)
Receding mandible	9.71 (1.91-49.32)
Protruding maxillary incisors	8.0 (1.50-42.50)

From Rocke DA, Murray WB, Rout CC, Gouws E. Relative risk analysis of factors associated with difficult intubation in obstetric anesthesia. Anesthesiology 1992; 77:67-73.

Certain conditions allow easy recognition of a difficult airway: (1) congenital facial and upper airway deformities, (2) maxillofacial and airway trauma, (3) airway tumors and abscesses, (4) an immobile cervical spine, (5) fibrosis of the face and neck from burns or radiation exposure, (6) surgically induced deformities, and (7) selected systemic diseases.[30,43-46] In addition, certain facial characteristics contribute to increased difficulty in establishing adequate mask ventilation: (1) a thick beard, (2) massive jaw, (3) lack of teeth, (4) extreme skin sensitivity to friction (e.g., burns, skin grafts, epidermolysis bullosa), and (5) the presence of large facial dressings. These conditions are obvious and easy to recognize before the induction of anesthesia. They have contributed little to anesthesia-related airway catastrophes such as brain damage or death.[5,29-34]

Other causes of airway difficulty may be subtle and may require careful examination of the patient. Table 31-4 lists the essential airway examinations, the minimal acceptable/desirable findings, and the significance of each airway examination. This information is included in the revised ASA Practice Guidelines for Management of the Difficult Airway, which was approved by the ASA House of Delegates in October, 2002.[15] The preoperative airway evaluation outlined in Table 31-4 requires no equipment, is entirely noninvasive, and should take less than 1 minute to perform. The examination first

TABLE 31-4	PREOPERATIVE AIRWAY EXAMINATION, MINIMAL ACCEPTABLE/DESIRABLE VALUES/ENDPOINTS, AND SIGNIFICANCE OF THE AIRWAY EXAMINATION

Preoperative airway examination	Minimal acceptable values/endpoints	Significance of the airway examination
1. Length of incisors	Qualitative/relative	Long incisors unalign the oral axis from the pharyngeal axis (creates a sharper angle between the two axes).
2. Involuntary anterior overriding of maxillary teeth on the mandibular teeth	No overriding of maxillary teeth on the mandibular teeth	Same as long incisors.
3. Voluntary protrusion of the mandibular teeth anterior to the maxillary teeth	Anterior protrusion of the mandibular teeth relative to the maxillary teeth	Test of TMJ function; a positive result means that a good view of the larynx with conventional laryngoscopy is likely.
4. Inter-incisor distance	> 3 cm	A positive result (> 3 cm) means that the 2-cm deep flange on a Macintosh blade can be easily inserted without hitting the teeth.
5. Oropharyngeal class	≤ Class II	A positive result (≤ Class II) means that the tongue is reasonably small in relation to the size of the oropharyngeal cavity and will be relatively easy to retract out of the line of sight.
6. Configuration of the palate	Should not appear very narrow and/or highly arched	A narrow palate decreases the oropharyngeal volume and the ability to continue to visualize the larynx when both the laryngoscope and endotracheal tube are in the mouth.
7. Mandibular space length (thyromental distance)	≥ 5 cm or ≥ 3 ordinary-sized fingerbreadths	A positive result means that the larynx is reasonably posterior relative to the other upper airway structures, resulting in a favorable line of sight.
8. Mandibular space compliance	Qualitative palpation of normal resilience/softness	A laryngoscope retracts the tongue into the mandibular space. The compliance of the mandibular space determines the ability of the mandibular space to accept the tongue and create a favorable line of sight.
9. Length of neck	Qualitative. A quantitative index is not yet available.	A short neck decreases the ability to align the upper airway axes.
10. Thickness of neck	Qualitative. A quantitative index is not yet available.	A thick neck decreases the ability to align the upper airway axes.
11. Range of motion of head and neck	Neck flexed 35° on the chest, and head extended 80° on the neck (i.e., the sniffing position)	The sniffing position aligns the oral, pharyngeal, and laryngeal axes to create a favorable line of sight.

focuses on the teeth (steps 1 through 4) and then sequentially focuses on the inside of the mouth (steps 5 and 6), the mandibular space (steps 7 and 8), and finally the neck (steps 9 through 11). None of the 11 examinations in Table 31-4 should be considered a fail-safe predictor of intubation difficulty. Typically it is the combination or integration of findings that determines the index of suspicion of airway difficulty; only occasionally is one airway assessment parameter so abnormal that it alone results in the diagnosis of a difficult airway.

Three of the examinations listed in Table 31-4 have received a great deal of attention in recent years and thus deserve further discussion.

RELATIVE TONGUE/PHARYNGEAL SIZE

Mallampati et al.[21] described a test that evaluates the size of the tongue relative to the size of the oropharyngeal cavity. The airway is classified according to the pharyngeal structures visualized when the patient opens her mouth. The test is performed with the patient sitting upright and the head in the neutral position. The patient opens her mouth as wide as possible and protrudes the tongue as far as possible without phonation. The observer then classifies the airway according to the pharyngeal structures seen (Figure 31-4). The classification is as follows:

Class I: The soft palate, fauces, uvula, and anterior and posterior tonsillar pillars can be seen.

Class II: The soft palate, fauces, and uvula can be seen.

Class III: The soft palate and base of the uvula can be seen.

Class IV: The soft palate is not visible at all.

A significant correlation has been noted between the ability to visualize pharyngeal structures and the ease of laryngoscopy.[5,21] Specifically, 99% to 100% of patients with a class I airway have a grade I laryngoscopic view.[5,21,47] Conversely, the laryngoscopic view is grade III or IV in 100% of patients with a class IV airway.[21,48] This positive correlation between the extremes of tongue size and difficult intubation has led some obstetric anesthesiologists to encourage the early use of epidural analgesia in patients with a class III or IV airway to avoid general anesthesia and probable difficult intubation if a cesarean section should be necessary.[5] However, patients with an intermediate airway classification (e.g., II or III) have a relatively uniform distribution of grades of laryngoscopic view (I to IV).[21,46] In addition, use of the Mallampati classification has sig-

nificant false-negative[49,50] and false-positive rates[47] for the following reasons: (1) the test is performed incorrectly with the patient in the supine position; (2) phonation is encouraged (e.g., saying "ah") during the test, which falsely improves the view; (3) the patient may arch her tongue, which obscures the uvula; and (4) interobserver variability occurs.[49] Therefore this test cannot be used alone to predict intubation difficulty and must be used in combination with other predictors of airway difficulty.

ATLANTOOCCIPITAL JOINT EXTENSION

When the neck is moderately flexed (e.g., 25 to 35 degrees) on the chest and the atlantooccipital joint is well extended (head extended on the neck), the oral, pharyngeal, and laryngeal axes are brought more closely into a straight line. This is commonly known as the *sniffing* or *Magill position*.[51-53] With the patient in a proper sniffing position, the view of the larynx is less obscured by the tongue. This results in less need for strenuous effort to displace the tongue anteriorly. For a normal atlantooccipital joint, 80 degrees of extension is possible.[54] A proper evaluation of maximal atlantooccipital joint extension consists of having the patient sit straight and face forward with the head held erect. In this position, the occlusal surface of the teeth is horizontal and parallel to the floor. With the patient extending the atlantooccipital joint as much as possible, the observer estimates the angle traversed by the occlusal surface of the upper teeth (Figure 31-5). In addition, a goniometer can be used for greater accuracy. A reduction in atlantooccipital joint extension can be expressed as a fraction of normal and is graded accordingly (Table 31-5). With complete atlantooccipital joint immobility, an attempt to extend the neck will push the convexity of the cervical spine anteriorly, which displaces the larynx and compromises the view at laryngoscopy.[55-57]

MANDIBULAR SPACE

The mandibular space anterior to the larynx determines how easily the laryngeal axis will fall into line with the pharyngeal axis when the atlantooccipital joint is fully extended. This space is easy to measure, either with a ruler or by the number of fingerbreadths, and it is expressed as the thyromental or

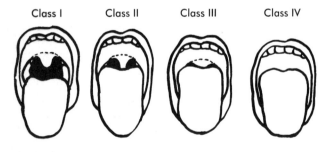

FIGURE 31-4. Classification of the upper airway in terms of the size of the tongue and the pharyngeal structures that are visible with the mouth open. In class I patients, the soft palate, fauces, uvula, and anterior and posterior tonsillar pillars can be seen. In class II patients, all of the above can be seen except the tonsillar pillars, which are hidden by the tongue. In class III patients, only the soft palate and the base of the uvula can be seen. In class IV patients, not even the uvula can be visualized. (From Mallampati SR, Gatt SP, Gugino LD, et al. A clinical sign to predict difficult tracheal intubation: A prospective study. Can J Anaesth 1985; 32:429-34.)

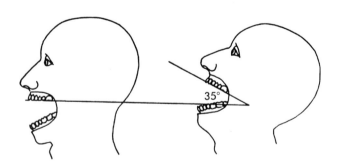

FIGURE 31-5. Clinical method for quantitating atlantooccipital joint extension. When the head is held erect and faces forward, the plane of the occlusal surface of the upper teeth is horizontal and parallel to the floor. When the atlantooccipital joint is extended, the occlusal surface of the upper teeth form an angle with the plane parallel to the floor. The angle between the erect and the extended planes of the occlusal surface of the upper teeth quantitates the degree of atlantooccipital joint extension. A normal person can produce 35 degrees of atlantooccipital joint extension. (From Bellhouse CP, Dore C. Criteria for estimating likelihood of difficulty of endotracheal intubation with Mac-Intosh laryngoscope. Anaesth Intensive Care 1988; 16:329-37.)

hyomental distance and the horizontal length of the mandible. If this distance is very short, the angle of the laryngeal axis and the pharyngeal axis is more acute, so with full atlantooccipital joint extension, it is more difficult to bring these two axes into alignment. There is an inverse correlation between the Mallampati numerical classification and both the thyromental distance and the horizontal length of the mandible.[47,58] With a thyromental distance of 6 cm and a horizontal length of the mandible greater than 9 cm, there is a low tongue/pharyngeal size classification, and visualization of the vocal cords is relatively easy during direct laryngoscopy.[30,47,58]

The combination of tongue/pharyngeal size class and thyromental distance is a good two-variable predictor of difficult intubation. During direct laryngoscopy, difficulty visualizing the vocal cords may occur if the vocal cords, upper teeth, and tongue are displaced in the direction depicted by the arrows in Figure 31-6. Figure 31-7 illustrates a schematic view of the mandible, the plane of the line of vision to the vocal cords, the mandibular space, and the position of the larynx. The boundaries of the mandibular space are the plane of the line of vision and the mandibular arch in front of this plane.[2] If the mandibular space is large, the larynx lies relatively posterior and the tongue can be easily compressed into this space so that with direct laryngoscopy, the larynx is visualized easily.

When the mandibular space is small, the larynx lies relatively anterior, and the tongue must be pulled forward maximally and compressed into a smaller compartment to view the larynx. One also can see from Figure 31-7 how the ability to bring the mandibular teeth anterior to the maxillary teeth aids in visualizing the larynx (see also Table 31-4, step 3).

Although these three tests are useful, it is important for the practitioner to do all 11 examinations listed in Table 31-4, integrate and synthesize the findings, and make an airway management plan based on *all* of the findings.

Several studies have evaluated the use of radiographic measurements to diagnose a difficult airway,[2,55,56,59] but the only measurements that were determined to be useful were related to tongue/pharyngeal size, atlantooccipital joint extension, and anterior mandibular space. Further, there was no consensus as to which measurements were most valuable. Therefore no single radiographic measurement can be used to determine the ease of intubation. Perhaps a combination of radiographic measurements would be a much more powerful predictive tool.[60]

Physiologic/Anatomic Changes Associated with Pregnancy

Several physiologic and anatomic factors place the parturient at increased risk for difficult intubation (Box 31-1).

PHARYNGOLARYNGEAL EDEMA

Vascular engorgement of the respiratory tract during pregnancy leads to edema of the nasal and oral pharynx, larynx and trachea.[61-64] These physiologic changes often cause difficulty with nasal breathing, an increased incidence of nasal

TABLE 31-5	GRADING OF THE REDUCTION IN ATLANTOOCCIPITAL JOINT EXTENSION
Grade	**Reduction of atlantooccipital joint extension***
1 (no appreciable reduction of extension)	None
2 (approximately one-third reduction)	One third
3 (approximately two-thirds reduction)	Two thirds
4 (no appreciable extension)	Complete

*Normal atlantooccipital joint extension is approximately 35 degrees.
From Bellhouse CP, Doré C. Criteria for establishing likelihood of difficulty of endotracheal intubation with MacIntosh laryngoscope. Anaesth Intensive Care 1988; 16:329-37.

Box 31-1 RISK FACTORS FOR INTUBATION AND HYPOXEMIA SPECIFIC TO THE PREGNANT WOMAN

- Pharyngolaryngeal edema
- Weight gain
- Increased breast size
- Full dentition
- Rapid onset of hypoxemia during apnea as a result of decreased functional residual capacity, decreased cardiac output secondary to aortocaval compression, and increased oxygen consumption

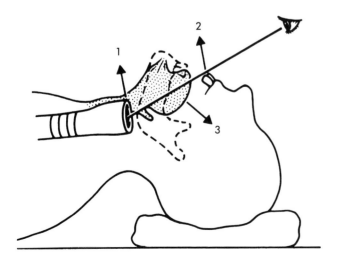

FIGURE 31-6. The direct line of sight to the vocal cords may be blocked by (1) a relatively anterior larynx, (2) prominent upper incisors, (3) and a large and posteriorly located tongue. (From Cormack RS, Lehane J. Difficult tracheal intubation in obstetrics. Anaesthesia 1984; 39:1105-11.)

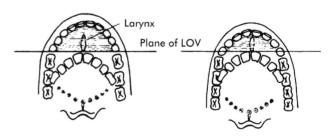

FIGURE 31-7. The mandibular space. If the line of vision *(LOV)* to the larynx depicted in Figure 31-6 were made perfectly horizontal and the observer was standing behind the top of the patient's head, the most posterior structure along the line of vision would be the upper teeth, the most anterior structure would be the lower incisors, and the tongue and larynx would be between the upper and lower incisors. The mandibular space *(shaded area)* is the area bounded by the plane of the line of vision and the part of the mandibular arch in front of this plane. (From Bellhouse CP, Doré C. Criteria for estimating likelihood of difficulty of endotracheal intubation with MacIntosh laryngoscope. Anaesth Intensive Care 1988; 16:329-37.)

bleeding, and voice changes. These changes in the nasal mucosa may also result in bleeding at the time of airway manipulation or nasogastric tube placement.

Laryngeal edema may be exacerbated by concurrent upper respiratory tract infection, preeclampsia, and/or prolonged, strenuous bearing-down efforts during the second stage of labor. Laryngeal edema may inhibit the passage of a standard-sized endotracheal tube—despite adequate vocal cord visualization at laryngoscopy—and thus require placement of a smaller-sized endotracheal tube. Further, tongue enlargement may make it difficult to displace the tongue into the mandibular space during direct laryngoscopy.[65]

WEIGHT GAIN

Another factor that increases the likelihood of difficult intubation is a significant amount of weight gain during pregnancy. It is not uncommon for the parturient to gain 20 kg or more during pregnancy. Weight gain and uterine enlargement leads to a decreased FRC, which hastens the onset of hypoxemia during periods of hypoventilation or apnea.[66] Weight gain likely increases the risk of pulmonary aspiration of gastric contents. A high body mass index (BMI) has been associated with an increased risk of airway management problems, including difficult intubation.[67] In addition, parturients with a high BMI are at increased risk for cesarean section (see Chapter 49). Therefore some obstetric anesthesiologists recommend the early administration of epidural anesthesia in patients with excessive weight gain or obesity.

ENLARGED BREASTS

Pregnancy results in a significant increase in breast size. In the supine position the enlarged breasts tend to fall back against the neck, which can interfere with insertion of the laryngoscope and subsequent intubation. Proposed solutions to overcome this problem include (1) use of a short-handled laryngoscope, (2) use of a pediatric laryngoscope handle (rather than an adult-length handle) and attachment of a normal-sized adult laryngoscope blade,[68,69] (3) taping the breasts laterally and caudad, (4) directing the handle of the laryngoscope laterally (distal end of the handle pointing to the right shoulder) when the laryngoscope blade is first inserted into the mouth, and (5) separation of the laryngoscope blade from the handle and placement of the blade in the mouth, followed by reattachment of the blade to the handle. In addition, placing the patient in the sniffing position helps keep the laryngoscope handle away from the breasts. It may be necessary to place several blankets under the shoulders (as well as the neck and occiput) to achieve the proper position.

FULL DENTITION

Most pregnant women are young, and typically they have full dentition. Protruding or "buck" teeth can further complicate intubation by interfering with the direct line of sight to the vocal cords.

RAPID ARTERIAL OXYGEN DESATURATION DURING APNEA

Increased maternal metabolic requirements combined with fetal metabolic needs result in increased maternal oxygen consumption. Painful uterine contractions during labor further increase maternal oxygen consumption. In addition, the gravid uterus pushes up on the diaphragm, which results in a 15% to 20% decrease in expiratory reserve volume (ERV) and FRC. The decrease in FRC can result in airway closure and an increased alveolar-arterial oxygen gradient during normal tidal respiration.

In the supine position, the gravid uterus also compresses the inferior vena cava. This results in decreased venous return, cardiac output, and uterine blood flow. The decrease in cardiac output, combined with an increase in oxygen consumption, results in a decrease in mixed venous oxygen content, with a further decrease in PaO_2 and SaO_2. In 15% of patients near term, the supine position results in signs of shock, including hypotension, pallor, sweating, nausea, vomiting, and changes in cerebration (i.e., supine hypotension syndrome). Inferior vena cava compression results in pooling of venous blood and increased uterine and lower extremity venous pressures. Increased uterine venous pressure also results in decreased uterine blood flow (uterine perfusion pressure = uterine artery pressure [which is decreased secondary to a decrease in cardiac output] – uterine venous pressure [which is increased with aortocaval compression]). Therefore the supine position should be avoided in pregnant women at term.

Collectively, these factors predispose pregnant women to more rapid arterial oxygen desaturation and hypoxemia during periods of hypoventilation or apnea. Denitrogenation with the administration of 100% oxygen is mandatory before rapid-sequence induction of general anesthesia. Nevertheless, computer modeling of arterial oxyhemoglobin desaturation versus time in fully preoxygenated patients shows that the rate of desaturation in obese patients and moderately ill patients is greatly increased compared with that of a perfectly normal person (Figure 31-8). In fact, the supine term pregnant patient may be considered to have the oxygenation difficulties of obesity (i.e., decreased FRC) as well as increased oxygen consumption. Therefore the rate of desaturation may be a multiple of two individual rates. Certainly, the period of apnea that could be survived is far less than the duration of action of 1 mg/kg of succinylcholine.[70]

Summary

Although the use of general anesthesia in obstetric patients has declined, it may still be required in selected cases. Thus it is essential for the anesthesiologist to perform a proper preanesthetic evaluation and identify the factors predictive of difficult intubation (vide supra). Although several authors have attempted to quantitate the contribution of a combination of specific risk factors to airway management difficulty in pregnant women, no single specific multivariable assessment plan has been widely accepted.[40] Thus we join the ASA in recommending that all 11 risk factors listed in Table 31-4 be assessed and that a judgment of airway difficulty be based on integration of all 11 factors.

PROPHYLAXIS

Regional Versus General Anesthesia

The recent decline in maternal mortality during the administration of regional anesthesia may be attributed to the recognition of four factors: (1) decreased doses of local anesthetic agents are required for spinal anesthesia in pregnant women; (2) it is important to give a test dose and incremental boluses of the therapeutic dose of the local anesthetic agent during administration of epidural anesthesia; (3) it is essential to avoid aortocaval compression; and (4) safety is enhanced by prevention or prompt treatment of hypotension.

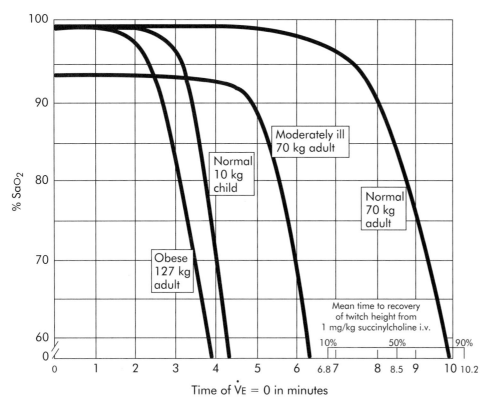

FIGURE 31-8. Time to hemoglobin desaturation (initial $F_{A_{O_2}} = 0.87$). Sa_{O_2} *versus* time of apnea for various types of patients. The physiologic characteristics of these patients can be obtained from the authors on request. (The Sa_{O_2} *versus* time curves, produced by a computer apnea model, and the mean times to recovery from 1 mg/kg of succinylcholine *[lower righthand corner]* are taken from Benumof JL, Dagg R, Benumof R. Critical hemoglobin desaturation will occur before return to an unparalyzed state following 1 mg/kg intravenous succinylcholine. Anesthesiology 1997; 87:979-82.)

The leading cause of maternal mortality during the administration of general anesthesia in both the United States and the United Kingdom is failure to intubate the trachea successfully. Most airway catastrophes have occurred when potential difficulty with the airway was not identified before the induction of anesthesia.[5,28-31,33,34] Ideally, the anesthesia care provider should evaluate the airway of each parturient shortly after admission by using the 11 quick, simple, and easy-to-perform tests discussed earlier (Table 31-4). Performance of these tests should identify patients in whom difficult intubation can be predicted. In such patients, it seems prudent to avoid general anesthesia by encouraging the use of regional anesthesia for elective cesarean section. (Alternatively, awake intubation may be performed before induction of general anesthesia.) During labor, it seems prudent to encourage prophylactic administration of epidural anesthesia, which can be extended for emergency cesarean section.

In addition, administration of epidural or spinal anesthesia de novo for emergency cesarean section (provided there is no dire maternal or fetal distress) reduces the need for urgent administration of general anesthesia. Unfortunately, regional anesthesia may not always provide adequate intraoperative anesthesia. Further, in some patients, either maternal or fetal distress (e.g., placental abruption, uterine rupture, maternal hemorrhage, coagulopathy) contraindicates the administration of regional anesthesia. In these cases, urgency may limit the anesthesiologist's opportunity to perform a complete assessment of the airway. Such circumstances prompt anxiety regarding the well-being of both the mother and baby and represent some of the most stressful situations in clinical anesthesia.

During the administration of regional anesthesia, the anesthesiologist must be fully prepared for the emergency administration of general anesthesia. Preparation includes the development of a well-formulated plan for (1) management of inadequate regional anesthesia, (2) emergency induction of general anesthesia, and (3) management of unexpected cases of difficult or failed intubation and ventilation.

Preparation for General Anesthesia

AIRWAY SUPPLIES

The ASA Difficult Airway Algorithm lists the equipment that should be included in a difficult airway cart.[15] In addition to the standard MacIntosh and Miller laryngoscope blades, alternative intubating devices should be available in case direct laryngoscopy results in a failed intubation (e.g., laryngeal mask airway [LMA], Combitube, equipment for transtracheal jet ventilation [TTJV]) (Box 31-2). Finally, an experienced aide should be in constant attendance to provide cricoid/external laryngeal pressure, to hand items (e.g., suction catheters, airways, endotracheal tubes) to the laryngoscopist, and to administer the appropriate drugs as indicated.

POSITIONING

Optimal positioning of both the table and patient facilitates successful intubation. The operating room table should be adjusted to the level of the laryngoscopist's intercostal margin, and the table surface should be fixed in place (i.e., rolling parts locked). It is essential to place the patient in the correct position for laryngoscopy before the induction of general anesthesia. Successful direct laryngoscopy requires alignment of the oral, pharyngeal, and laryngeal axes so that the passageway from the incisors to the glottis approximates a straight line (Figures 31-9 and 31-10). First, the neck must be flexed on the chest by elevating the head approximately 10 cm to bring the laryngeal axis in line with the pharyngeal axis. In the nonobese, nonpregnant patient, the shoulders remain on the table. In contrast, in an obese or pregnant patient, appropriate neck flexion is facilitated by placing several pads or blankets under the shoulders and upper back, thereby flattening the kyphotic curvature in the thoracic spine. The head also must be extended on the neck (i.e., extension of the atlantooccipital joint) to bring the oral axis in line with both the pharyngeal and laryngeal axes. This position is known as the *Magill* or *sniffing position.* In this position, patency of the airway is maximized. If the head is put in full extension without elevation of the occiput, the lips-to-glottis distance increases secondary to malalignment of the oral axis with the pharyngeal and laryngeal axes. This position rotates the larynx anteriorly and may necessitate leverage on the maxillary teeth or gums to visualize the larynx during laryngoscopy.

It also is essential to avoid aortocaval compression during the administration of general anesthesia. Assumption of the supine position predisposes the patient to aortocaval compression by the gravid uterus, which results in decreased venous return and cardiac output. Left uterine displacement minimizes the decrease in cardiac output in almost all patients. This is easily achieved by tilting the operating room table 15 degrees to the left or placing a wedge cushion under the right buttock. In our institution, we place an inflatable genitourinary irrigation bag beneath the right buttock (under the operating table pad) to elevate the right buttock and lower trunk approximately 10 to 15 cm. These measures reduce aortocaval compression and help preserve cardiac output and uteroplacental blood flow.

DENITROGENATION (PREOXYGENATION)

A period of time must pass between the onset of apnea and the initiation of positive-pressure ventilation by means of the endotracheal tube. During this time, the body's continuing requirements for oxygen are supplied from the FRC. The duration of this period is directly proportional to the degree of difficulty of exposure of the larynx and is inversely proportional to the skill of the laryngoscopist. Denitrogenation with 100% oxygen is always indicated because even skilled laryngoscopists may require a minute or longer for laryngoscopy and intubation. This is especially important for the pregnant

patient, who is at increased risk for hypoxemia during the induction of general anesthesia.

Various techniques have been advocated for denitrogenating the FRC and thereby delaying the onset of hypoxemia (defined as an Sao_2 less than 90%). Historically, most anesthesiologists have advocated 3 to 5 minutes of preoxygenation.[71,72] Denitrogenation of the lungs is more than 95% complete in 3 minutes or less in patients breathing through a circle system with a fresh gas flow of 4 L/min or more. Others have demonstrated comparable increases in Pao_2 (used as a surrogate for efficacy of preoxygenation) with either 5 minutes of normal tidal ventilation or four "maximally deep breaths" in awake patients *(vide infra).*[73,74] In general, if the tidal volume is large and the respiratory rate is high (i.e., the patient has a high minute ventilation), the duration of preoxygenation need be only 1 minute[75]; however, if the tidal volume is small or the respiratory rate is slow (i.e., a low minute ventilation), the duration of preoxygenation should be 3 minutes.[76] When time is of the essence, instructing the patient to take four vital-capacity breaths is an acceptable, rapid method of preoxygenation.[73,74]

More recent studies have provided a better understanding of the preoxygenation process. Three studies have shown that there is no significant difference between the Pao_2 achieved with the "3 to 5 minutes of normal tidal volume ventilation with $F_1O_2 = 1.0$" method of preoxygenation, termed the traditional (T) method, compared with the "four maximally deep breaths in 30 seconds" (4DB/30 sec) method.[74-76] Norris and Dewan[75] observed that 3 minutes of preoxygenation and the 4-breath preoxygenation technique resulted in similar measurements of Pao_2 in pregnant women undergoing rapid-sequence induction of general anesthesia for cesarean section. The similarity in Pao_2 (used as a surrogate for rate of desaturation) between the T and 4DB/30 sec methods of preoxygenation has led to the erroneous, superficial conclusion that the 4DB/30 sec method provides the same amount of preoxygenation as the T method.[77]

Box 31-2 MINIMUM RECOMMENDED EQUIPMENT FOR TRACHEAL INTUBATION

PREOXYGENATION AND VENTILATION

- Oxygen source turned on and attached to a self-inflating ventilation bag
- Small, medium, and large anesthesia masks
- Small, medium, and large oropharyngeal and nasopharyngeal airways
- Tongue depressors

PREPARATION OF THE ENDOTRACHEAL TUBE

- Small, medium, and large orotracheal tubes (5.0-7.0 mm)
- Small, medium, and large nasotracheal tubes (5.0-7.0 mm)
- Malleable stylet
- 10-mL syringe
- 4% lidocaine jelly and ointment

ANESTHESIA

- Intravenous anesthetics and muscle relaxants
- Syringes and needles
- Atomizer, topical anesthetics, and vasoconstrictors

LARYNGOSCOPY

- Suction apparatus turned on and a metal or hard plastic suction catheter attached

- Towels or blankets to place the patient's head in the sniffing position
- Magill forceps
- No. 3 and No. 4 Miller blades with functioning light source
- No. 3 and No. 4 MacIntosh blades with functioning light source
- Access to fiberoptic bronchoscope

UNEXPECTED DIFFICULT AIRWAY

- At least one device suitable for emergency nonsurgical oxygenation and ventilation (e.g., laryngeal mask airway, esophageal-tracheal Combitube, equipment for transtracheal jet ventilation)
- Equipment suitable for emergency surgical airway access

DETERMINATION OF ENDOTRACHEAL TUBE LOCATION

- Stethoscope
- End-tidal CO_2 monitor
- Pulse oximeter

FIXATION OF THE ENDOTRACHEAL TUBE

- Tincture of benzoin
- Adhesive and umbilical tape

Three studies have clearly shown that patients preoxygenated with the 4DB/30 sec method desaturate faster than patients preoxygenated with the T method.[78-80] Patients will reach $SpO_2 < 90\%$ (from $SpO_2 = 100\%$) 100 to 200 seconds faster during apnea after the use of the 4DB/30 sec method than with the use of the T method. The primary reason patients preoxygenated with the 4DB/30 sec method desaturate faster is that the tissue and venous compartments need more than 30 seconds to fill with oxygen; these compartments have the capacity of holding approximately 1500 mL of additional oxygen above the amount that can be brought into the body in 30 seconds.[81] The extra oxygen stored in the tissues and venous blood easily explains the different rate of desaturation between the 4DB/30 sec method and the T method.

ASPIRATION PROPHYLAXIS

Various anatomic, physiologic, and pharmacologic factors increase the risk of aspiration in pregnant women. Anesthesiologists should consider every parturient to be at risk for aspiration of gastric contents during induction of general anesthesia (see Chapters 2 and 30). Further, pulmonary aspiration of gastric contents often complicates cases of difficult or failed intubation in obstetric patients. All pregnant women who require anesthesia for cesarean section should receive pharmacologic prophylaxis.

Pharmacologic prophylaxis usually consists of intravenous administration of an H_2-receptor antagonist and metoclopramide combined with oral administration of a clear, nonparticulate antacid before induction of anesthesia. Pharmacologic prophylaxis is only one component in the prevention of acid aspiration. Aspiration prophylaxis includes rapid-sequence induction of general anesthesia, followed by expeditious intubation with a cuffed endotracheal tube. A typical rapid-sequence induction includes denitrogenation with 100% oxygen, application of cricoid pressure, and intravenous administration of a hypnotic agent (e.g., thiopental 4 mg/kg or propofol 2 to 3 mg/kg) and succinylcholine (1.0 to 1.5 mg/kg). Prior administration of a defasciculating dose of a nondepolarizing muscle relaxant is an acceptable option that is used by a minority of obstetric anesthesiologists.

Thorough denitrogenation minimizes the development of hypoxemia during the period of apnea before insertion of the endotracheal tube. Direct laryngoscopy typically can be performed approximately 60 seconds after the administration of succinylcholine. Positive-pressure ventilation is best avoided before intubation to prevent inflation of the stomach, which predisposes the patient to regurgitation of gastric contents. It is best to await the onset of complete muscle relaxation before performing laryngoscopy. Use of a nerve stimulator allows the anesthesiologist to identify the onset of adequate paralysis. Rarely, administration of succinylcholine is contraindicated (e.g., malignant hyperthermia). In such cases, the anesthesiologist can substitute a large dose of a nondepolarizing muscle relaxant (e.g., rocuronium 0.9 to 1.2 mg/kg) (see Chapters 25 and 46). Other nondepolarizing muscle relaxants may have an onset that is acceptable for laryngoscopy and intubation when used in a dose three to four times the ED_{95} (the effective dose that produces the desired effect in 95% of the population).

Posterior pressure on the cricoid cartilage (cricoid pressure, also known as the Sellick maneuver) results in temporary occlusion of the upper end of the esophagus because the esophagus is compressed between the body of the fifth cervical vertebra and the posterior part of the cricoid cartilage.[82] Before induction of anesthesia, the assistant uses one hand to identify the cricoid ring and one or two fingers to apply firm backward pressure on the cricoid cartilage. The assistant should use the other hand to provide posterior support of the neck, which facilitates extension of the atlantooccipital joint. As soon as the patient loses consciousness, the assistant should apply and maintain firm posterior pressure. Application of cricoid pressure is used throughout the entire induction period until the endotracheal tube cuff is inflated

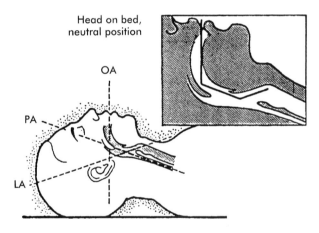

FIGURE 31-9. The alignment of the oral axis *(OA)*, pharyngeal axis *(PA)*, and laryngeal axis *(LA)* is shown. With the head in the neutral position, there is a marked degree of nonalignment of the OA, PA, and LA. (From Benumof JL. Conventional [laryngoscopic] orotracheal and nasotracheal intubation [single-lumen type]. In Benumof JL, editor. Clinical Procedures in Anesthesia and Intensive Care. Philadelphia, JB Lippincott, 1991:115-48.)

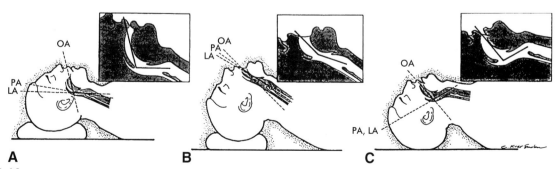

FIGURE 31-10. As the head position changes from neutral, the continuity of the oral axis *(OA)*, pharyngeal axis *(PA)*, and laryngeal axis *(LA)* changes within the upper airway. **A,** The head is resting on a large pad that flexes the neck on the chest and aligns the LA with the PA (the neutral position). **B,** The head is resting on a pad (which flexes the neck on the chest) and concomitant extension of the head on the neck can be seen, which brings all three axes into alignment (the sniffing position). **C,** Extension of the head on the neck without concomitant elevation of the head on a pad. This results in nonalignment of the PA and LA with the OA. (From Benumof JL. Conventional [laryngoscopic] orotracheal and nasotracheal intubation [single-lumen type]. In Benumof JL, editor. Clinical Procedures in Anesthesia and Intensive Care. Philadelphia, JB Lippincott, 1991: 115-48.)

and the anesthesiologist has confirmed that the endotracheal tube is positioned within the trachea. In cases of difficult or failed intubation, the assistant should maintain cricoid pressure while the anesthetist performs mask ventilation.

Unfortunately, this maneuver is not infallible, even in trained hands.[83] Application of cricoid pressure may result in complete airway obstruction in a patient with an undiagnosed supraglottic mass[84] or an undiagnosed traumatic injury to the larynx.[85] The following conditions contraindicate the application of cricoid pressure: (1) suspected airway trauma,[86] (2) active vomiting, (3) an unstable cervical spine fracture, (4) a sharp intraesophageal foreign body, and (5) the presence of Zenker's diverticulum.

FAILED REGIONAL ANESTHESIA

Neither spinal nor epidural anesthesia uniformly provides adequate intraoperative anesthesia for cesarean section. When regional anesthesia fails, the options include performance of a second regional anesthetic procedure and administration of general anesthesia. The anesthesiologist always should consider the potential for failure of regional anesthesia and be prepared to administer general anesthesia. The extent of patient preparation for general anesthesia depends on the amount of concern elicited by the preoperative airway examination. Presumably, if time permitted administration of regional anesthesia, a thorough airway evaluation should have been performed first.

Airway management should not present a problem for a patient with a Mallampati class I airway with full range of motion of the neck and an adequate anterior mandibular space. For these patients, appropriate preparation consists of the precautions outlined earlier: (1) pharmacologic aspiration prophylaxis, which should include at least the administration of a clear, nonparticulate antacid (e.g., 30 mL of 0.3 M sodium citrate); (2) immediate availability of adequate airway supplies; (3) placement of the patient in the proper sniffing position; (4) administration of supplemental oxygen, with the ability to rapidly convert to the administration of 100% oxygen by means of a sealed face mask; and (5) the presence of an assistant who can apply cricoid pressure if necessary.

If the preanesthetic evaluation suggests that the patient may have a difficult airway, the anesthesiologist should take additional precautions even though regional anesthesia may have been selected as the primary anesthetic technique. In other words, the anesthesiologist always should have a backup plan. The amount of preparation will vary depending on the anesthesiologist's level of concern regarding the ability to manage the airway effectively and experience with alternative airway management techniques.

Using the extreme as an example, let us assume that the preoperative airway evaluation reveals a short, obese parturient with a Mallampati class IV airway, limited neck extension, and a short hyomental distance. It should be assumed that this patient will be difficult if not impossible to intubate and perhaps impossible to ventilate by mask. If there is evidence that regional anesthesia is inadequate in this patient, preparatory steps might include: (1) topicalization of the nasal airway and gradual dilation of the nasal passages with nasal airway trumpets (to assist with mask ventilation or blind nasal or fiberoptic intubation), (2) location and infiltration of the cricothyroid membrane with a local anesthetic agent (to facilitate rapid institution of transtracheal jet ventilation), or (3) actual insertion of a transtracheal jet ventilation catheter. The extent to which a patient with a potentially difficult airway is prepared prophy-

lactically for general anesthesia depends on the anesthesiologist's level of concern regarding the ability to maintain airway patency and adequate gas exchange.

MANAGEMENT

The Recognized Difficult Airway

A subset of patients have certain anatomic features that should indicate that endotracheal intubation via conventional means is very likely to be difficult if not impossible. Certain anatomic features (e.g., very large breasts and heavy chest wall, large tongue, no teeth and sunken cheeks, fixed position of the head and neck, massive jaw, upper airway mass) may also render mask ventilation difficult or impossible. If there is any doubt regarding the ability to maintain airway patency during general anesthesia, alternative methods of anesthesia should be considered. Options include the use of regional anesthesia, local infiltration anesthesia, or if there is adequate time, an awake intubation followed by induction of general anesthesia (Figure 31-1).

REGIONAL ANESTHESIA

Regional anesthesia is the best choice for cesarean section in most cases of anticipated difficulty with endotracheal intubation. Either spinal or epidural anesthesia is acceptable providing there is no contraindication (see Chapters 11 and 25). Both techniques allow the mother to be awake and minimize the potential for acid aspiration. However, the anesthesiologist should understand that regional anesthesia itself does not solve the problem of a difficult airway and should anticipate potential complications (e.g., failed anesthesia, total spinal anesthesia) and be fully prepared (both mentally and technically) to administer general anesthesia.

Nausea and vomiting is a common complication during the administration of regional anesthesia for cesarean section. In addition, in the event of a failed block, general anesthesia may be required. Therefore all patients should receive pharmacologic prophylaxis against acid aspiration. All patients also should receive supplemental oxygen during the administration of spinal or epidural anesthesia for cesarean section. The increased maternal fractional inspired oxygen concentration (FiO_2) increases fetal oxygenation.[87]

LOCAL ANESTHESIA

If a patient with a difficult airway requires urgent cesarean section and if there is a contraindication to the use of spinal or epidural anesthesia, local anesthetic infiltration can be used as the *primary* anesthetic technique (see Chapter 25).[88-90] However, local anesthetic infiltration is a technique rarely used today for cesarean section in developed countries. It is more often used in undeveloped countries with an inadequate number of experienced anesthesia providers and/or limited anesthesia equipment and supplies. This technique requires a limited amount of skill. It can provide reasonable anesthesia, provided the obstetrician gives adequate attention to detail, administers an adequate volume of local anesthetic agent, and allows time for the local anesthetic agent to take effect (see Chapter 25).

Advantages of local anesthetic infiltration include the following: (1) the obstetrician does not need to wait for a skilled anesthesia care provider to arrive and perform awake endotracheal intubation; (2) the patient remains awake, and protective airway reflexes are maintained; (3) significant hemodynamic changes do not occur, provided the obstetrician does not exceed the maximum safe dose of the local anesthetic agent; and (4) the risks of neuromuscular blockade and residual paralysis are avoided. A large volume (e.g., 80 to 100 mL) of a dilute solution of local anesthetic agent (e.g., 0.5% lidocaine) often is required.[88-90] Of course, administration of such a large volume of local anesthetic agent entails a risk of local anesthetic systemic toxicity. Ideally, a skilled anesthesia care provider is present to supervise and monitor the infiltration of the local anesthetic agent. Appropriate airway equipment and resuscitation drugs should be immediately available in case maternal resuscitation or general anesthesia is required.

AWAKE INTUBATION FOLLOWED BY GENERAL ANESTHESIA

When the anesthesiologist anticipates that management of the airway will be difficult, a very safe option is to secure the airway with an endotracheal tube while the patient remains awake. Although awake intubation can be somewhat time consuming, there are several compelling reasons to perform the procedure in a patient with a recognized difficult airway: (1) the natural airway is better maintained in an awake patient; (2) the presence of normal muscle tone helps maintain the natural separation of the upper airway structures, which facilitates the identification of anatomic landmarks; and (3) induction of general anesthesia and muscle paralysis results in anterior movement of the larynx, which makes it more difficult to visualize the larynx during direct laryngoscopy.[91]

Successful awake endotracheal intubation requires proper preparation of the patient. Ideal preparation results in a quiet and cooperative patient and a larynx that is nonreactive to physical stimuli. The first step is psychological preparation. The patient who knows what is going to happen typically is more receptive and cooperative. Minimal monitoring should include the use of an automated blood pressure cuff, pulse oximetry, and an electrocardiogram (ECG). Supplemental oxygen should be administered at all times during the procedure.

Administration of an anticholinergic drying agent (e.g., glycopyrrolate) allows better application of local anesthetic spray to the airway mucosa, improves visualization, and inhibits vagal reflexes. Glycopyrrolate is poorly transferred across the placenta, and its maternal administration does not result in a detectable fetal hemodynamic response (see Chapter 4).

Judicious use of intravenous sedation helps relieve anxiety, increases the pain threshold in an awake patient, and facilitates patient tolerance and acceptance of the entire awake intubation process. It is essential to titrate analgesic and sedative drugs carefully so that the patient remains rational, alert, and able to respond to commands in a clear and unambiguous manner. Respiratory depression and aspiration of stomach contents during the application of a local anesthetic agent are much less likely to occur if the patient remains awake and alert. In addition, avoidance of heavy sedation minimizes the risk of neonatal depression. Midazolam is the benzodiazepine recommended for this purpose. The fetal/maternal concentration ratio is approximately 0.76 at 20 minutes after maternal administration; however, the ratio falls rapidly.

Topical anesthesia is the primary anesthetic technique for awake intubation. In some patients, topical anesthesia is the only anesthetic needed, provided sufficient time is allowed to anesthetize all portions of the airway adequately. If the nasal route is chosen, the nasal mucosa also should be sprayed with a vasoconstrictor and the nasal passage should be dilated with a progressively larger series of soft nasopharyngeal airways that are liberally coated with lidocaine ointment. The pressure receptors that elicit the gag reflex at the root of the tongue are submucosal in location. Therefore, topical anesthesia may not uniformly provide adequate blockade of these pressure receptors, and bilateral blockade of the lingual branch of the glossopharyngeal nerve (i.e., cranial nerve IX) may be required.[92,93] However, some have recently questioned the efficiency of this block plus topicalization as compared with topical anesthesia alone for awake laryngoscopy.[94]

Blockade of the internal branch of the superior laryngeal nerve represents a second upper airway nerve block that is a helpful supplement to the use of topical anesthesia and blockade of the lingual branch of the glossopharyngeal nerve. This block consists of application of a local anesthetic agent superficial or deep to the thyrohyoid membrane between the superior lateral cornu of the thyroid cartilage and the inferior lateral margin of the cornu of the hyoid bone. (The nerve pierces the membrane at this point and can be blocked on either side of the membrane.[95,96]) This block, performed in conjunction with a lingual nerve block, often allows direct laryngoscopy with a Miller blade.

Transtracheal administration of a local anesthetic agent (administered through the cricothyroid membrane) also may be performed easily. Unfortunately, this technique is associated with a low but serious risk of bleeding from disruption of an aberrant thyroid vessel.[3] This block is typically unnecessary if topical anesthesia has been applied properly.

There is some controversy as to the appropriate use and extent of local anesthesia for awake intubation in a patient with a presumed full stomach. In theory, blockade of the superior laryngeal nerve may allow food and water to enter the trachea during deglutition.[95] Some anesthesiologists have recommended that airway anesthesia be limited to the transtracheal injection of local anesthetic in patients with a full stomach.[97] However, Cooper and Watson[96] reported no complications with the use of topical cocaine spray combined with lingual and superior laryngeal nerve blocks to facilitate awake intubation in patients with a full stomach. Subsequently, Duncan[98] used topical anesthesia from the tongue to the trachea; none of these patients vomited or aspirated.

In our experience, the key to avoiding aspiration is avoidance of oversedation. There is a low risk of aspiration of gastric contents in an awake, alert, and rational patient, regardless of the extent of topical anesthesia. Lower esophageal sphincter tone is maintained if the patient is not oversedated. Also, in the event of impending vomiting, an awake patient can help turn her head and body to the side, open her mouth for suctioning, delay the next inhalation, and produce a cough (provided the trachea is not completely anesthetized).[30,99,100]

Management priorities must be established for the parturient with a difficult airway; obviously, successful tracheal intubation should be the first priority, and it is absolutely essential that the patient's airway be anesthetized adequately. The risk of aspiration in a well-anesthetized but awake patient can be further minimized by intravenous administration of an H_2-receptor antagonist and metoclopramide and oral administration of a nonparticulate antacid before the procedure is begun.

Once the upper airway has been anesthetized adequately, there are numerous ways to intubate the trachea. The choice of technique depends on several factors, including the skill and experience of the laryngoscopist and the urgency of cesarean section.

Direct Laryngoscopy

Of all intubation techniques, direct laryngoscopy results in the most noxious stimulation for the patient. Thus it requires the best patient preparation. However, most well-prepared patients easily tolerate direct laryngoscopy.

If the larynx is poorly visualized with direct laryngoscopy, several aids may be used to facilitate intubation. The Eschmann malleable stylet (a gum elastic bougie) is a guiding stylet that is placed blindly around the epiglottis and into the trachea. After the stylet is placed in the trachea, the endotracheal tube is threaded over the stylet and the stylet is removed. Cahen[101] has recommended use of a laryngotracheal anesthesia (LTA) cannula for this purpose. The tip of the LTA cannula is inserted through the Murphy eye at the tip of a well-lubricated endotracheal tube. Direct laryngoscopy is performed, and the tip of the LTA cannula is inserted through the vocal cords. The endotracheal tube subsequently is advanced over the LTA cannula into the trachea, and the cannula is removed. With either of these techniques, orientation of the Murphy eye at the 12 o'clock position facilitates the passage of the endotracheal tube over the stylet into the trachea.[101-103]

Blind Nasal Intubation

Blind nasal intubation is much less stimulating than direct laryngoscopy, and it may be worth a try in patients who are breathing spontaneously. If attempted, a small (6.0 to 6.5 mm) endotracheal tube should be used. Unfortunately, pregnant women have hyperemic nasal mucosae. Instrumentation of the nose entails the risk of nasal and nasopharyngeal bleeding. Such bleeding can be substantial in pregnant women and can compromise subsequent efforts at direct or fiberoptic laryngoscopy.

Fiberoptic Laryngoscopy

The flexible fiberoptic bronchoscope/laryngoscope is an extremely useful aid to awake intubation in the parturient with a known difficult airway.[104-106] Fiberoptic laryngoscopy is less stimulating than direct laryngoscopy and can be performed either orally or nasally. (However, nasal trauma in the parturient may cause significant nasal bleeding.) The major impediments to success with the fiberoptic bronchoscope are significant amounts of blood or secretions and lack of patient preparation and cooperation. The fiberoptic bronchoscope can suction only small amounts of secretions. Insufflation of oxygen through the suction port can blow secretions away from the tip of the bronchoscope, serve as a defogging mechanism, and provide supplemental oxygen. Immersion of the tip of the bronchoscope into warm saline (or anti-fog solution) before insertion into the patient also decreases the amount of fogging. If oxygen is insufflated through the suction port, one must be careful not to allow the tip of the fiberoptic bronchoscope to enter the esophagus (i.e., avoid esophagogastric barotrauma).

Extension of the cervical spine represents the optimal position for the performance of fiberoptic laryngoscopy. Extension tilts the larynx anteriorly and lifts the epiglottis off the posterior pharyngeal wall.[56] Numerous devices are available to facilitate fiberoptic intubation. The oral fiberoptic intubation guides[104,105,107-109] are rigid, hollow oropharyngeal conduits that are designed to bring the tip of the fiberoptic bronchoscope close to the laryngeal aperture without requiring much endoscopic skill. For nasotracheal intubations, the conduit is a nasotracheal tube advanced into the oropharynx; when the 15-cm mark of the nasotracheal tube is at the nares

of the average adult, the tip of the tube typically is 1 to 2 cm proximal to the epiglottis. With this distance, there is adequate room to manipulate the fiberoptic bronchoscope into the trachea.

An appropriately sized, well-lubricated endotracheal tube (ETT) is placed on the bronchoscope before its insertion. Once the fiberoptic bronchoscope is passed into the trachea, the ETT is threaded off the fiberoptic bronchoscope, the bronchoscope is withdrawn, the ETT adaptor is reattached, and the ETT is connected to the breathing circuit. Even with the fiberoptic bronchoscope in the correct position, the ETT may not always follow easily into the trachea for one of the following reasons[109]:

1. A large, stiff ETT may displace the thin fiberoptic bronchoscope into the esophagus if the ETT is aligned posteriorly.
2. The right arytenoid or right vocal cord may obstruct the ETT as it is passed off the fiberoptic bronchoscope. This problem is corrected by withdrawing the tube slightly and then rotating it 90 degrees counterclockwise so that the bevel tip and Murphy eye are at the 12 o'clock position.
3. If the fiberoptic bronchoscope exits the ETT by means of the Murphy eye, the fiberoptic bronchoscope may enter the trachea, but it is impossible to slide the ETT off the fiberoptic bronchoscope into the trachea.

After the ETT has been passed over the fiberoptic bronchoscope and into the trachea, the distance between the carina and the tip of the ETT should be noted to ensure proper positioning of the tube.

Retrograde Intubation

Retrograde intubation techniques have been used for several decades with good success,[111,112] especially in patients with maxillofacial trauma.[113] Although this technique has been of value in the management of the difficult airway, it has been used infrequently in the obstetric situation but might prove of benefit if the patient has a restricted mouth opening or a facial deformity and an elective general anesthetic technique is planned. After proper preparation of the patient (including topical anesthesia of the airway and nerve blocks), infiltration of a local anesthetic agent is performed over the cricothyroid membrane, and the cricothyroid membrane is punctured with a thin-wall needle aligned with the airway and directed 30 degrees cephalad from the perpendicular. The tracheal lumen is identified by aspirating air, and a long, thin wire is passed through the needle until it emerges from the mouth or nose. This wire subsequently serves as a guide for an ETT that is passed over it, as the wire is pulled taut. If the wire is long enough and of proper diameter, it may be passed through the suction channel of a fiberoptic bronchoscope and thereby guide the bronchoscope (with the ETT jacketed on the bronchoscope) into the trachea; this latter method is almost fail-safe.

The Bullard Laryngoscope

The Bullard laryngoscope (Circon ACMI, Stamford, CT) functions as an indirect rigid fiberoptic laryngoscope. A fiberoptic bundle is positioned along the length of the posterior aspect of the blade (down to the distal tip), which gives the endoscopist a view at the end of the blade. Some have reported that this laryngoscope makes visualization of the larynx much easier.[114,115] Because visualization of the larynx is based on the presence of a fiberoptic bundle at the tip of the blade, positioning of the head in the usual sniffing position is unnecessary; this is advantageous when manipulation of the head is contraindicated (e.g., cervical spine fracture). Intubation with this laryngoscope is accomplished more easily with the new intubating stylet, which correctly aligns the ETT with the laryngeal aperture. A considerable amount of practice is necessary to become skilled in the use of this laryngoscope, as is true for the other types of new blades. There is one published report of use of the Bullard laryngoscope for emergency airway management in a morbidly obese parturient.[116]

Illuminating Intubating Stylet

A malleable, illuminating intubating stylet (also known as a *lightwand*) differs from all other intubating techniques. Entry into the trachea is signaled by a jack-o'-lantern effect observed externally in the anterior neck. This signal should not appear if the lighted stylet is located elsewhere. With correct placement of the illuminating stylet, transillumination appears abruptly as the light bulb passes around the base of the tongue and the epiglottis, just superior to the thyroid cartilage. When the light and the ETT enter the larynx itself, a jack-o'-lantern effect is produced, which is quite prominent if the room is completely darkened.[117] As the ETT is advanced into the trachea, the light in the neck may seem to separate, forming an expanding dumbbell shape as the ETT enters the thorax. The usual steps to confirm end-tidal CO_2 and bilateral gas exchange through the ETT subsequently should be taken.

The illuminating stylet has been found to be just as efficient as direct laryngoscopy in cases of routine intubation[118] and in cases of difficult intubation in adults.[119,120] Application of cricoid pressure and the use of a nasogastric tube do not decrease the rate of success for this technique.[119] Thus this technique may be a useful backup intubation device when direct laryngoscopy has failed. False-positive or false-negative results may occur in patients at the extremes of physical habitus. For example, false-positive results may occur in patients who are very thin or young. Conversely, false-negative results may occur in patients who are morbidly obese or who have a thick neck. Moreover, anything that might interfere with transmission of light from the neck will decrease the effectiveness of this technique. Such interference might occur with any of the following conditions: (1) anterior neck scarring, (2) flexion contractions, (3) excess cervical adipose tissue, (4) a cervical mass, (5) a bulb that is covered with blood or secretions, and (6) inability to darken the room lights.

The best commercially available illuminating stylet is the Trachlight (Sheridan, Inc.), because it emits light that covers 360 degrees, which most importantly includes the anterior direction.

The Unrecognized Difficult Airway

Ideally, a skilled anesthesia care provider will perform a complete, preanesthetic airway evaluation in every laboring parturient (Table 31-4). In some cases (e.g., dire fetal distress), the obstetrician will ask the anesthesiologist to administer anesthesia as rapidly as possible. However, even in an emergency situation, there should be time to perform an airway examination. In other instances, maternal conditions (e.g., hemorrhage, coagulopathy) may contraindicate the administration of regional anesthesia. In most of these cases, the anesthesiologist will opt for rapid-sequence induction of general anesthesia. In the event that intubation is not successful, the anesthesiologist should have a well-formulated plan in mind, and the appropriate equipment and supplies should be immediately available to implement that plan.

The availability of equipment for the management of airway emergencies is associated with a reduced incidence of maternal complications.[120] The ASA recommends that labor and delivery units have both equipment and personnel readily available to manage airway emergencies. Basic airway management equipment should be immediately available during the provision of regional anesthesia. In addition, portable equipment for difficult airway management should be readily available in the operative area of labor and delivery units.[120] Figure 31-11 includes the algorithm that details emergency airway management, with special reference to the presence or absence of fetal distress.

The first step is to prepare the parturient with a "full stomach" for rapid-sequence induction of general anesthesia. Several treatments can be used to decrease the risk of damage from aspiration of stomach contents. First, the pH of gastric fluid should be increased. Every patient should receive 30 mL of a clear, nonparticulate antacid (e.g., 0.3 M sodium citrate). If time permits, an H_2-receptor antagonist can be given intravenously. Second, gastric emptying should be accelerated. Metoclopramide 10 mg may be administered intravenously. An orogastric or a nasogastric tube also may be placed to decompress the stomach. (We prefer to remove the orogastric or nasogastric tube before the induction of anesthesia to preserve the function of the lower esophageal sphincter.) Third, induction of anesthesia is performed in a rapid-sequence fashion. Fourth, an assistant applies cricoid pressure immediately before the induction of anesthesia, and cricoid pressure is maintained until the endotracheal tube has been placed within the trachea, the cuff is inflated, and the position is confirmed by detection of end-tidal CO_2.

If the anesthesiologist is confronted with an unexpected difficult intubation, it is important to take inventory of what has been tried and what other manipulations can be tried in accordance with fetal well-being, hemodynamic stability, and the respiratory status of the patient. For example, if there is no fetal distress, the patient is hemodynamically stable, there is adequate gas exchange by mask, and only one anesthesiologist has attempted intubation with one type of blade, time permits optimization of the chances of successful intubation (Box 31-3). This should include (1) repositioning the patient into a better (e.g., sniffing) position, (2) applying external laryngeal manipulation (e.g., over the thyroid cartilage), (3) using a different laryngoscope blade (i.e., different length and/or type), and (4) having another anesthetist attempt intubation. An optimal attempt at intubation should be achieved by the third or fourth attempt. With respect to mask ventilation, if only one hand has manipulated the jaw (unilateral jaw thrust) and held the mask seal (unilateral mask seal) and no oropharyngeal or nasopharyngeal airways have been used, then it is appropriate to place an oropharyngeal and/or nasopharyngeal airway and institute a two- or three-handed bilateral jaw thrust/mask seal (requiring two persons) mask ventilation effort (Box 31-4). However, if the patient is hypotensive and hypoxemic, with clusters of multifocal premature ventricular contractions (PVCs), the patient's clinical status mandates aggressive airway control, regardless of how many attempts at intubation have been made.

THE PATIENT WHO CANNOT BE INTUBATED BUT CAN BE VENTILATED BY MASK WITH NO FETAL DISTRESS

When the anesthesiologist is unable to intubate the trachea of an anesthetized patient, it is essential to try to maintain gas exchange by mask ventilation between intubation attempts.

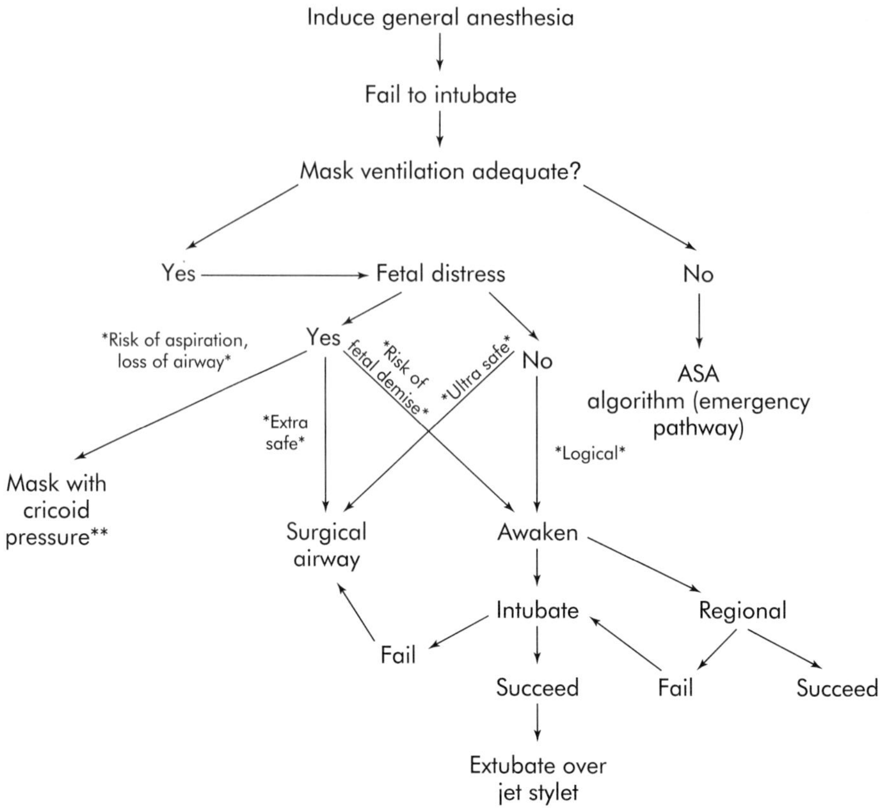

FIGURE 31-11. Supplement to the difficult airway management algorithm, with special reference to the presence or absence of fetal distress. This algorithm includes options in the management of a recognized difficult airway in an uncooperative patient or in a cooperative patient with dire fetal distress.
*Denotes implications of this choice.
**Conventional face mask or laryngeal mask airway.

Box 31-3 DEFINITION OF OPTIMAL INTUBATION ATTEMPT
1. Reasonably experienced laryngoscopist
2. No significant muscle tone
3. Optimal sniff position
4. Optimal external laryngeal pressure
5. Change length of blade once
6. Change type of blade once

Box 31-4 DEFINITION OF OPTIMAL ATTEMPT AT MASK VENTILATION
1. Two-person additive/synergistic effort → optimal jaw thrust + mask seal
2. Big oropharyngeal airway
3. Big bilateral nasopharyngeal airways

During positive-pressure mask ventilation, maintenance of cricoid pressure is mandatory. All the intubation techniques previously described for the awake patient can be used in the unconscious patient, without modification. However, with every intubation attempt, the amount of laryngeal edema and bleeding is likely to increase. Therefore, if no new atraumatic manipulation can be tried quickly (e.g., better sniffing position, application of external laryngeal pressure, new laryngoscope blade, new technique, more experienced laryngoscopist [Box 31-3]) and ventilation by mask is still possible, it is prudent to cease attempts to intubate the trachea and either awaken the patient or perform a cricothyrotomy or tracheostomy (Figure 31-11). If the patient is awakened, assisted mask ventilation should continue while an assistant maintains cricoid pressure. Subsequent to awakening the patient,

options include awake intubation, regional anesthesia, and local infiltration anesthesia. Establishment of a surgical airway is an acceptable alternative because emergence may be accompanied by progressive difficulty with adequate mask ventilation (e.g., secondary to increased secretions, edema, or airway reactivity). The ASA Closed-Claims Study has noted that death after failed intubation may be a result of failure to effectively ventilate the patient by face-mask.[121]

THE PATIENT WHO CANNOT BE INTUBATED BUT CAN BE VENTILATED BY MASK WITH FETAL DISTRESS PRESENT

In the presence of fetal distress, management decisions are more problematic. The first option is to awaken the patient. This conservative yet difficult decision most likely will preserve the mother's life, but it may result in the demise of the fetus. The second option is to perform a cricothyrotomy or tracheostomy before the ability to ventilate the lungs by means of a mask is lost. The third option is to continue anesthesia by mask ventilation while an assistant maintains cricoid pressure (i.e., the "failed intubation drill"). The use of the LMA is tempting in this situation as it frees the anesthetist's hands, but the hazards of failed insertion and maternal oxyhemoglobin desaturation during insertion must be carefully considered. Moreover, the LMA does not guarantee effective protection from aspiration.

Failed Intubation Drill

Tunstall[122] proposed a failed intubation drill, which was later revised by Rosen[123] and is now common practice in the United Kingdom. The objective of the failed intubation drill is to achieve spontaneous ventilation and oxygenation by mask, without aspiration. The sequence of events in this drill is as follows[122,123]:

1. Maintain cricoid pressure.
2. Place the patient in a complete left lateral position with the head down. Postpone use of the left lateral position if ventilation is difficult.
3. Maintain oxygenation by intermittent positive-pressure ventilation with 100% oxygen. If difficulty occurs, try a different position, place an oropharyngeal airway, and try two-person mask ventilation (i.e., bilateral jaw thrust and mask seal). Aspirate the pharynx as required.
4. For persistent airway obstruction, release cricoid pressure. Current recommendations are to release cricoid pressure only when the patient is in the full left lateral position with the head down, an esophageal obturator is in place, or spontaneous ventilation is well established (awake or under general anesthesia).
5. If ventilation and oxygenation are easy, ventilate with oxygen, nitrous oxide, and a volatile halogenated agent. Establish surgical anesthesia with face-mask ventilation. Allow a resumption of spontaneous ventilation.
6. Pass a 33- to 36-Fr gastric tube through the mouth, aspirate the gastric contents, and instill a nonparticulate antacid. Withdraw the tube and suction the oropharynx during withdrawal. (Avoid passage of a gastric tube if it is likely to stimulate vomiting from active reflexes.)
7. Level the table and place the patient supine with left uterine displacement. Allow the surgery to continue with inhalation anesthesia with a face-mask. An experienced pediatrician should be present at delivery.

A great limitation of the failed intubation is that it does not address what to do if mask ventilation (either with spontaneous or positive-pressure ventilation) is inadequate.

Spontaneous Versus Controlled Ventilation

When the decision is made to proceed with general anesthesia by mask, the anesthesiologist must decide whether to allow the patient to breathe spontaneously or to control ventilation by maintaining muscle relaxation. In the failed intubation drill, ventilation is controlled initially and is followed by the resumption of spontaneous ventilation. Unfortunately, an absence of muscle relaxation may complicate attempts to proceed with surgery and may result in a difficult, traumatic delivery of the fetus. Maintenance of muscle relaxation may facilitate not only operative delivery but also positive-pressure ventilation by mask. On the other hand, if muscle relaxation is maintained, the options of allowing the patient to resume spontaneous ventilation and to awaken are lost. Muscle relaxation and immobility can be achieved through deep inhalational anesthesia, but at this depth of anesthesia, spontaneous ventilation is unlikely to result in adequate ventilation and oxygenation, especially in a parturient in the Trendelenburg position (which results in increased pressure on the diaphragm). Deep inhalational anesthesia also may further depress the fetus and decrease uterine tone, which may result in uterine atony and excessive blood loss after delivery.

Management of Regurgitation in the Anesthetized Patient

The failed intubation drill most likely will result in expeditious delivery of the fetus. However, it entails a substantial risk of aspiration of gastric contents and complete loss of the airway, both of which are associated with a significant risk of maternal mortality. If regurgitation or vomiting occurs during attempted endotracheal intubation or during mask ventilation in an anesthetized patient, there are several therapeutic

steps that must be initiated immediately. First, the patient is placed in the Trendelenburg position, and the head and body are turned to the left. Second, the mouth and pharynx are suctioned with a large-bore catheter. If the ETT was passed into the esophagus, it should be left there; the ETT may decompress the stomach and perhaps guide (by negative example) future intubation attempts. A disadvantage of leaving an ETT in the esophagus is that it may be more difficult to obtain a satisfactory mask seal.

Once the airway is secured in a patient with presumed aspiration, standard therapy consists of suctioning, followed by mechanical ventilation with positive end-expiratory pressure (see Chapter 30).

THE PATIENT WHO CANNOT BE INTUBATED OR VENTILATED BY MASK

Included in the failed intubation drill is the following option: "if oxygenation is difficult, allow suxamethonium to wear off and let the patient wake up," bearing in mind that "the airway may be difficult to maintain."[123] Often quoted reasons for difficult intubation and/or ventilation during pregnancy include the presence of enlarged breasts, pharyngolaryngeal edema, and reduced time available for airway instrumentation resulting from reduced FRC.[124,125]

Successful management of a difficult airway often takes several minutes. Figure 31-8 shows arterial oxygen saturation-versus-time curves for various patients who initially were fully oxygenated. For the patient who cannot be intubated or ventilated by mask there are four rescue options: (1) insertion of an esophageal-tracheal Combitube, (2) insertion of a laryngeal mask airway (LMA), (3) institution of TTJV, and (4) emergent cricothyrotomy or tracheostomy.

The Combitube

The esophageal-tracheal Combitube (ETC) (Sheridan Catheter Corporation, Argyle, NY) is a plastic, twin-lumen tube with an outer diameter of 13 mm (Figure 31-12). One lumen resembles an ETT, and the other lumen has the distal end closed. A 100-mL proximal pharyngeal balloon is located on the ETC, so that when the ETC is properly positioned, the pharyngeal balloon will fill the space between the base of the tongue and the soft palate. The inflated proximal balloon serves to seal the oral and nasal cavities. Just distal to the pharyngeal balloon but proximal to the level of the larynx are perforations in the esophageal lumen. A smaller, 15-mL distal cuff (similar to an ETT cuff) serves to seal either the esophagus or trachea when inflated. The ETC is inserted with or without the aid of a laryngoscope (we recommend the use of a laryngoscope), but it is not necessary to visualize the larynx. (In the usual clinical context, the larynx cannot be visualized). Almost certainly the ETC will enter the esophagus, and the patient can be ventilated by means of the esophageal lumen perforations. If the ETC enters the trachea, the patient can be ventilated directly through the tracheal lumen. In terms of ability to ventilate the patient, it does not matter whether the ETC enters the trachea or the esophagus.[126]

In most reports the ETC provided adequate ventilation within 15 to 30 seconds of insertion. The ETC allows adequate ventilation while preventing aspiration of gastric contents. Use of the ETC has resulted in adequate ventilation and oxygenation under diverse clinical conditions (e.g., failed intubation during surgery, cardiopulmonary resuscitation, respiratory failure in the intensive care unit).[127] In the esophageal position, the unused tracheal lumen can be connected to a suction device to aspirate gastric fluids. There is one published report documenting the use of the ETC in a parturient undergoing cesarean section.[128] Of interest, Tunstall and Geddes[129] described the successful use of the esophageal gastric tube airway (which was a forerunner of the ETC) following failed intubation at emergency cesarean section.

The Laryngeal Mask Airway: Use as an Airway

The laryngeal mask airway (LMA) is now a recognized part of the ASA Difficult Airway Algorithm and should be a part of every obstetric anesthesiologist's armamentarium for managing the difficult airway.[130-133]

One of the reasons the LMA works well as a routine airway is that exact positioning is not critical for establishing a clinically acceptable airway. The typical fit of the LMA around the larynx, as assessed by using flexible fiberoptic endoscopy, radiologic investigation, and magnetic resonance imaging, is somewhat variable.[17] Nevertheless, in 94% to 99% of adult and pediatric patients, there is no difficulty with ventilation and the airway is ultimately judged to be clinically acceptable (although proper position may require two insertion attempts). Indeed, Han et al.[133] prospectively studied the use of the LMA in 1067 consecutive ASA I-II patients who chose general anesthesia for elective cesarean section. The authors concluded that the LMA is effective and probably safe for elective cesarean section in selected healthy patients when managed by experienced LMA users.[133] Because the LMA works well as a routine airway/ventilatory device in most patients,

it is not surprising that the LMA has been found to be a life-saving emergency airway/ventilatory device in obstetric patients undergoing emergency cesarean section who could not be ventilated with a conventional mask and whose trachea could not be intubated by conventional techniques.[134-138]

Nevertheless, the routine use of the LMA for airway management can be associated with a number of problems. These problems include: (1) clinically unacceptable nonpatent airway, (2) the requirement for multiple insertion attempts in a small percentage of patients, (3) aspiration of gastric contents, and (4) suboptimal positive-pressure ventilation. The exact incidence of each of these problems must, to some extent, depend on the insertion technique and skill of the operator. Inadequate anesthesia may cause all of these problems, and therefore a basic requirement for the safe use of the LMA is an adequate depth of anesthesia.[17] The most serious problem is that in 0.4% to 0.6% of anatomically normal patients, placement of the LMA is inadequate clinically because of backfolding of the distal cuff, occlusion of the glottis by the distal cuff, complete backfolding of the epiglottis, or 90- to 180-degree rotation of the mask around the long axis.[17] However, in view of such a small incidence of failure, it is logical to quickly use the LMA as a first-try rescue option for the cannot-intubate, cannot-ventilate situation. The major contraindication to the use of the LMA is the presence of local pathology in the pharynx or larynx, which precludes a reasonable chance of proper placement and function. If insertion of an LMA or an ETC does not quickly result in effective gas exchange, then either TTJV should be instituted or a surgical airway should be created immediately *(vide infra)*.[15-17]

The ProSeal™ laryngeal mask airway (PLMA) is a new laryngeal mask device with a modified cuff and a drainage tube designed to isolate the airway from the digestive tract.[139] The design should also improve the seal around the glottis. Evans et al.[139] assessed insertion characteristics, airway seal pressures, hemodynamic response to insertion, ease of gastric tube placement, gastric insufflation, and postoperative discomfort associated with the use of PLMA in 300 anesthetized adults. The authors concluded that the PLMA is a reliable airway-management device that can give an effective glottic seal in both paralyzed and non-paralyzed patients. The device allowed the easy passage of a gastric tube, caused a minimal hemodynamic response to insertion, and resulted in an acceptable incidence of sore throat.[139] Cook et al.[140] conducted a randomized, crossover comparison study of the PLMA with the classic LMA in 180 non-paralyzed anesthetized patients and concluded that the PLMA allowed positive-pressure ventilation more reliably than the classic LMA. The PLMA's ability to allow positive-pressure ventilation more reliably than the classic LMA and to permit decompression of the stomach might have some advantages in obstetric anesthesia practice.

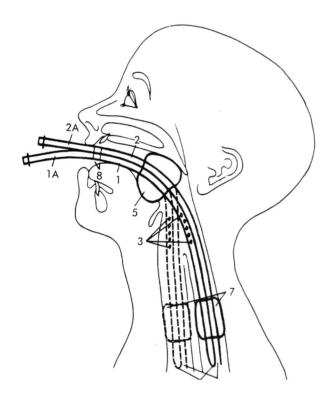

FIGURE 31-12. Sagittal section of the esophageal-tracheal Combitube (ETC) in esophageal *(continuous lines)* and tracheal *(dotted lines)* position. *1,* "Esophageal" lumen; *1A,* longer, blue connector leading to lumen 1; *2,* "tracheal" lumen; *2A,* shorter, clear connector leading to lumen 2; *3,* perforations of lumen 1; *4,* distal blocked end of lumen 1; *5,* pharyngeal balloon; *6,* distal open end of lumen 2; *7,* distal cuff (for sealing of either the esophagus or the trachea); *8,* printed rings indicating depth of insertion. (From Frass M, Rodler S, Frenzer R, et al. Esophageal tracheal Combitube, endotracheal airway, and mask: Comparison of ventilatory pressure curves. J Trauma 1989; 29:1476-9.)

The Laryngeal Mask Airway: Use as a Conduit for Tracheal Intubation

Numerous reports have described the use of the LMA as an airway conduit for either the blind passage of an endotracheal tube (the intubating or Fastrach™ LMA)[141-146] or for the passage of a flexible fiberoptic bronchoscope (classic LMA).[17] The intubating laryngeal mask airway (ILMA) or Fastrach™ LMA was introduced into clinical practice in 1997 after performance of clinical trials involving 1110 patients.[141] The ILMA, like the conventional LMA, allows effective ventilation but also functions as a conduit for the blind passage of an endotracheal tube.[142] The ILMA is designed to accept an ETT as large as 8.0 mm in diameter.[142] To reduce the risk of airway trauma associated with the use of blind intubation techniques, a special silicone ETT has been developed for use with the ILMA.[146] Size selection for the ILMA is the same as for the standard LMA. Fiberoptic intubation through the ILMA is significantly hampered by the presence of a bar that directs the epiglottis anteriorly.

The most worrisome complication of using the ILMA (or any LMA) in the obstetric patient is aspiration of gastric contents. Because the obstetric patient is considered to have a full stomach, cricoid pressure should ordinarily be used when passing any LMA. However, cricoid pressure may prevent the ILMA (or any LMA) from seating properly in the hypopharynx.[142]

When cricoid pressure is applied before the LMA is placed, the pressure prevents the tip of the LMA from fully occupying the 3.5-cm length of the hypopharynx behind both the arytenoid and cricoid cartilages. (Compare panels 3 and 4 of Figure 31-13.) Thus, with cricoid pressure, the LMA may be wedged in the hypopharynx, but it can occupy only the 1.5 cm of the hypopharynx behind the arytenoid cartilages and is therefore 2 cm more proximal than usual. Variable obstruction to the passage of the LMA by cricoid pressure may explain why the concomitant use of cricoid pressure has resulted in widely variable success rates in simple insertion of the LMA from a low of 15% to a high of 90%.[17] In addition, the wedging into and subsequent full inflation of the LMA cuff in the hypopharynx that has been constricted by the application of cricoid pressure causes the plane of the laryngeal aperture to tilt approximately 40 degrees anteriorly around the fulcrum of the inflated LMA cuff. It seems likely that it would be more difficult for a blindly inserted intubating device to enter an aperture that is in a plane 40 degrees off the perpendicular to the insertion pathway than an aperture that is in the plane perpendicular to the insertion pathway.

The placement of an LMA in the obstetric patient who can be ventilated by face-mask while cricoid pressure is being continuously applied would have little benefit and might induce vomiting and aspiration.[147-150] A reasonable alternative between the competing concerns of continuously maintaining cricoid pressure in a patient at risk for aspiration and failure to properly insert the LMA during cricoid pressure is to momentarily release cricoid pressure as the distal tip of the LMA reaches the hypopharynx[150]; this maximizes the chance of correct LMA placement while minimizing the risk of aspiration. Once the LMA is in situ, it probably does not interfere with the efficacy of cricoid pressure.[151]

Passage of a fiberoptic bronchoscope through a standard LMA has a greater chance of success and is nearly 100% successful in most series.[17] A 6-mm internal diameter (ID) cuffed ETT (a nasal RAE tube [Mallinckrodt, St. Louis, MO] is most suitable because of adequate length and widespread availability) may be passed over the fiberoptic bronchoscope and through the shaft of LMA sizes 3 and 4, and a 7-mm ID cuffed ETT may be passed over the fiberoptic bronchoscope and through the shaft of a size 5 LMA. If a larger ETT is desired, the LMA and the 6- or 7-mm ID cuffed ETT may be exchanged for a larger ETT over a jet stylet.[16] The lungs can be continuously ventilated around the fiberoptic bronchoscope but within the ETT by passing the fiberoptic bronchoscope through the self-sealing diaphragm of a bronchoscopy elbow adaptor; the distal and proximal ends of the bronchoscopy elbow adaptor are connected to the ETT and the ventilatory apparatus, respectively. Figure 31-14 illustrates the use of the bronchoscopy elbow adaptor and the LMA for the continuous ventilation fiberoptic intubation method for both a nasal RAE and standard 6-mm ETT. When a 4-mm OD fiberoptic bronchoscope is combined with a 6-mm ID ETT, the space available for ventilation around the fiberoptic bronchoscope is equivalent to that available with a 4.5-mm ID ETT.

Transtracheal Jet Ventilation

Percutaneous insertion of a large-gauge intravenous catheter through the cricothyroid membrane is simple, quick, and relatively safe in most patients. Jet ventilation through the catheter (called transtracheal jet ventilation or TTJV) is an effective rescue method of ventilation in desperate, cannot-intubate or cannot-ventilate-by-mask situations.[152] Compared with emergency surgical cricothyrotomy or tracheostomy, establishment of percutaneous TTJV is usually quicker, simpler, and more efficacious. In other words, most anesthesiologists can insert a needle into the trachea and aspirate air faster than anyone can cut through the cricothyroid membrane,

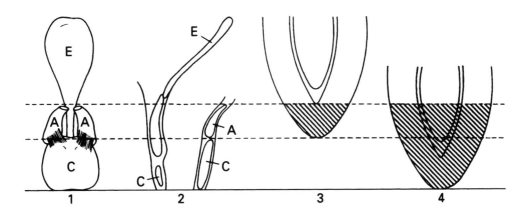

FIGURE 31-13. The level of the distal part of the LMA. The hatched area indicates the distal part of the LMA that occupies the hypopharynx. *1*, Posterior view of the larynx; *2*, lateral view of the larynx; *3*, position of the tip of the LMA when cricoid pressure is applied. When cricoid pressure is applied before placement, the LMA, in theory, might be wedged in the hypopharynx but is more likely to occupy the space behind the arytenoid cartilages. The LMA is positioned at least 2 cm more proximal than usual. *4*, Position of the LMA when no cricoid pressure is applied. When the LMA is placed correctly, the distal tip is at the distal end of C5 (fifth cervical vertebra), and the distal part of the LMA should fully occupy the hypopharynx and the pharyngeal space behind both the arytenoid and cricoid cartilages. *E*, epiglottis; *A*, arytenoid cartilages; *C*, cricoid cartilage. (Reproduced with permission from Asai T, Barclay K, Power I, et al. Cricoid pressure and the LMA: Efficacy and interpretation (letter). Br J Anaesth 1994; 73:863-5.)

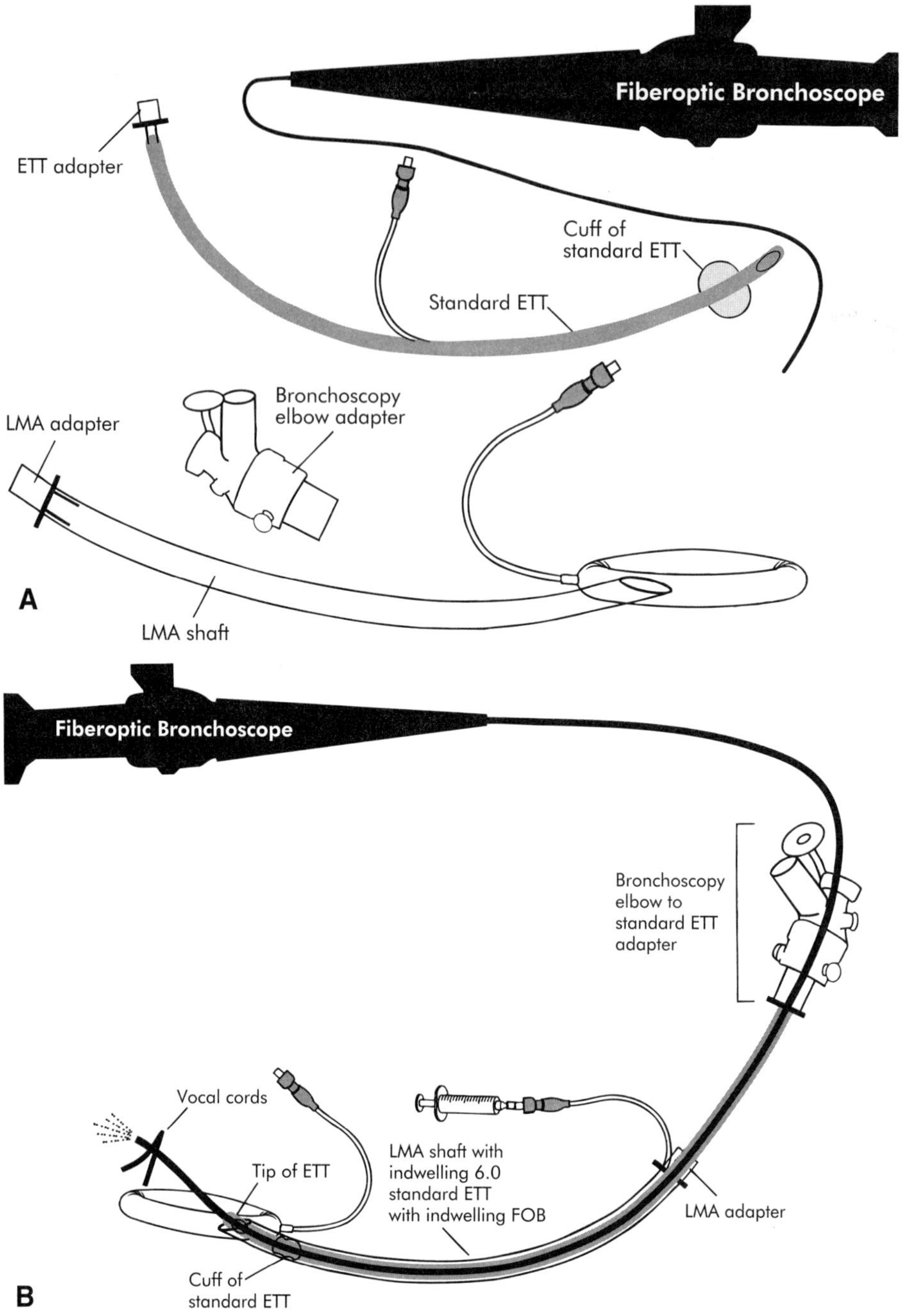

FIGURE 31-14. Schematic diagram showing that a patient can be continuously ventilated during fiberoptic tracheal intubation using the LMA as a conduit for both the endotracheal tube *(ETT)* and the fiberoptic bronchoscope *(FOB).* In panels A and B the ETT is a standard 28-cm long tube. *Panel A,* Components of the continuous ventilation system. *Panel B,* By passing the tip of a cuffed 6-mm ID endotracheal tube to the level of the grille on the LMA and a 4-mm OD FOB through the self-sealing diaphragm of a bronchoscopy elbow adaptor, ventilation can occur around the FOB but within the lumen of the ETT; the deflated cuff of the ETT inside the shaft of the LMA makes an airtight seal and permits positive-pressure ventilation.

spread the cricothyroid membrane with a hemostat, insert a conventional ETT through the hole of the membrane, and then inflate the cuff—even if all of these surgical steps proceed smoothly. Numerous reports have documented the use of TTJV to prevent life-threatening gas exchange problems in patients who are difficult to ventilate or intubate during general anesthesia.[3,153,154] This technique permits continuous, uninterrupted oxygenation and ventilation while allowing unhurried access to secure the patient's airway.

The method of insertion of the intravenous catheter through the cricothyroid membrane is as follows. First, the cricothyroid membrane is palpated with the neck of the patient extended (Figure 31-15). Subsequently a 14- or 16-gauge intravenous catheter is used to puncture the cricothyroid membrane with the needle pointed 30 degrees caudad from the perpendicular. A 20-mL syringe is then attached to the catheter, and aspiration of air confirms its transtracheal loca-

tion. (Use of a smaller syringe may result in removal of the plunger from the syringe barrel with vigorous aspiration; thus we recommend the use of a 20-mL syringe.) The needle stylet is withdrawn (at least partially), and the catheter is advanced into the trachea until the hub of the catheter is at the skin line. The TTJV catheter should always be reaspirated to reconfirm intratracheal lumen location. The hub of the TTJV catheter is subsequently connected to a TTJV system. A designated individual should be responsible for holding the hub of the TTJV catheter secure to the skin. During TTJV, it is important to maintain the natural airway by using bilateral jaw thrust and oropharyngeal and nasopharyngeal airways to allow for the exhalation of inspired gas and to prevent air trapping and lung hyperinflation.

To achieve adequate oxygenation and ventilation, the TTJV system must have a sufficient high-pressure oxygen source (approximately 20-50 psi) that can drive oxygen

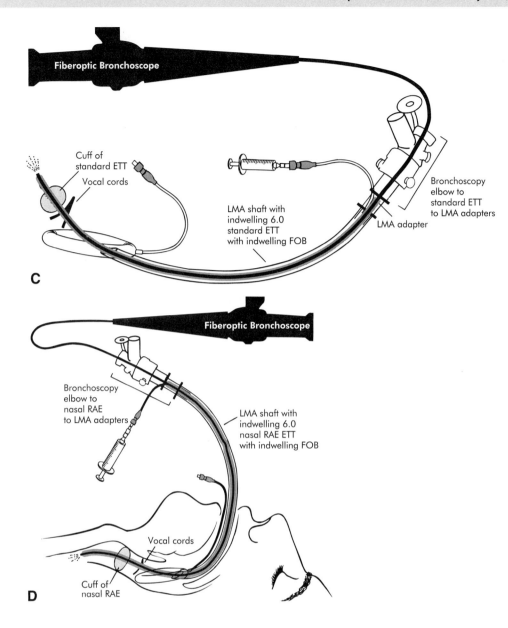

FIGURE 31-14, cont'd *Panel C*, Once the FOB is passed well into the trachea, the 6-mm ID ETT is pushed over the FOB into the trachea until the adaptor of the ETT is near the adaptor of the LMA (nasal RAE tube) or is flush up against the adaptor of the LMA (standard ETT). The preformed curvature of the nasal RAE tube presents no problem with insertion if the outside of the tube is adequately lubricated. *Panel D*, Schematic of Panel C with superimposed upper airway anatomy.

through noncompliant tubing and the relatively small TTJV catheter.[155,156] Use of central wall pressure requires down-regulation of the pressure to avoid barotrauma.[157] Commercially manufactured systems, which include a 0-50 psi in-line regulator, should be used. Reducing the pressure to 20-30 psi still allows these power sources to provide adequate tidal volumes (V_T) and minute ventilation (V_E) through 14- to 20-gauge catheters at lung compliances that range from normal (100 mL/cm H_2O) to noncompliant (30 mL/cm H_2O).[155] The actual minute ventilations achieved through 14-, 16-, 18-, and 20-gauge catheters with a 50-psi oxygen source at an inspiratory-to-expiratory (I:E) ratio of 1:1 (unit of time = 1 sec), with lung compliances of 30 and 50 mL/cm H_2O, are presented in Table 31-6. The smallest V_E of 12 L/min through a 20-gauge catheter at a lung compliance of 30 mL/cm H_2O still allows partial if not total ventilatory support in the majority of clinical situations. Box 31-5 summarizes the most important clinical considerations to minimize the risk of barotrauma (e.g., subcutaneous air, pneumomediastinum, pneumothorax) during TTJV.

Percutaneous or Open Surgical Cricothyrotomy and Tracheostomy

Performance of a hurried, open surgical cricothyrotomy or tracheostomy under suboptimal conditions is questionable and may be dangerous. Some physicians advocate percutaneous surgical cricothyrotomy or tracheostomy as an alternative to open surgical cricothyrotomy or tracheostomy. These physicians argue that percutaneous surgical cricothyrotomy is just as safe, quick, and easy to perform as percutaneous needle cricothyrotomy and TTJV.[158] Toye and Weinstein[159] first described percutaneous tracheostomy (and cricothyrotomy) in 1969. The technique evolved from the premise that the percutaneous technique allows a functional airway to be obtained more rapidly than the standard tracheostomy dissection method. Several techniques have been described. These techniques typically include insertion of a needle into the trachea and subsequent dilation of the needle track to accommodate a functional airway. Recently, several kits have become commercially available.[160-162] A thorough review and comparison of the presently available percutaneous cricothyrotomy and tracheostomy kits/procedures has recently been published.[163]

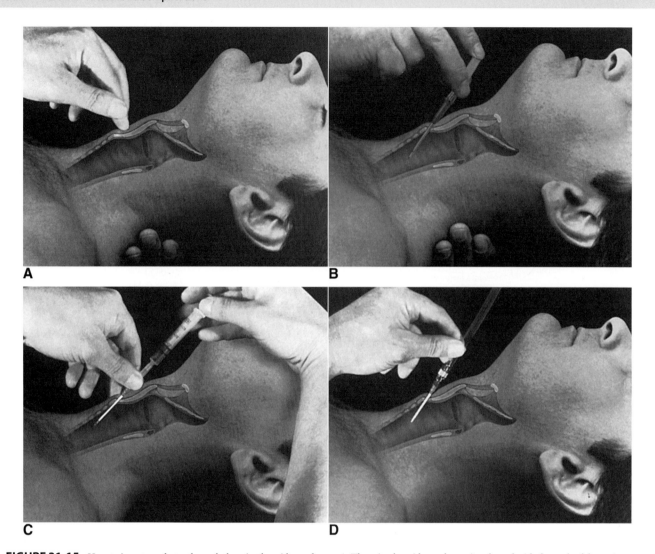

FIGURE 31-15. How to insert a catheter through the cricothyroid membrane. **A,** The cricothyroid membrane is palpated with the neck of the patient extended. **B,** A 14- or 16-gauge intravenous catheter is used to puncture the cricothyroid membrane 30 degrees caudad from the perpendicular. **C,** A 20-mL syringe is connected to the catheter, and its transtracheal location is verified by aspiration of air. **D,** The needle stylet is withdrawn (at least partially), the catheter is advanced into the trachea until the hub of the catheter is at the skin line, and the hub of the intravenous catheter is connected to a transtracheal jet ventilation system. (From Benumof JL, Shroff PK, Skerman JH. Transtracheal ventilation. In Benumof JL, editor. Clinical Procedures in Anesthesia and Intensive Care. Philadelphia, JB Lippincott, 1991: 195-209.)

TABLE 31-6	MINUTE VENTILATION (L/MIN) I:E = 1:1, USING 50 psi POWER SOURCE	
IV catheter	**C_{set} = 50 (mL/cm H_2O)**	**C_{set} = 30 (mL/cm H_2O)**
20 gauge	15.6	12.0
18 gauge	25.2	21.6
16 gauge	33.0	28.8
14 gauge	54.0	49.8

I:E, Inspiratory to expiratory ratio in 1 sec; *C_{set},* set compliance of mechanical lung model.
From Gaughan S, Benumof JL, Ozaki G. Comparison of a low-flow and high-flow regulator in a variable compliance lung model. Anesthesiology 1992; 77:189-99.

There is some question as to who should perform percutaneous and open cricothyrotomy and tracheostomy. Most surgeons should be able to perform this operation, but it is unclear whether anesthesiologists, who are already skilled in vascular access with the Seldinger technique, should be trained to perform percutaneous tracheostomy. The same considerations apply to open (e.g., scalpel) cricothyrotomy, which should be considered the failed-airway resuscitation maneuver of last resort. Surgical assistance always should be summoned or available if these procedures are performed by nonsurgeons. The call for surgical assistance must occur early in the management of the difficult airway so that assistance will be available at the appropriate time.

Extubation of the Patient with a Difficult Airway

If intubation was difficult, reintubation of an extubated patient is likely to be as difficult if not more so. Such a situation often is approached with much trepidation. Lengthy operative procedures or procedures that affect pulmonary and airway function further complicate management. The ideal method of extubation permits a controlled, gradual, reversible withdrawal of the ETT from the airway. Extubation over an airway exchange catheter (AEC) or a jet stylet (JS) approximates the ideal method.

Box 31-5 THE MOST IMPORTANT CONSIDERATIONS FOR MINIMIZING THE RISK OF BAROTRAUMA DURING TRANSTRACHEAL JET VENTILATION (TTJV)

Clinical considerations for minimizing barotrauma	Rationale
1. The last maneuver before first TTJV should be reaspiration/reconfirmation of free flow of air through the catheter	1. Assure placement of catheter in tracheal lumen after initial identification of tracheal lumen.
2. Use a preassembled commercially made system that has an additional in-line pressure regulator (0-50 psi).	2. Obtain the quality assurance that is associated with a commercial product and the ability to down-regulate standard wall gas pressure to a lower level (see #3).
3. Preset additional in-line regulator at 25-30 psi. Setting can be increased incrementally by 5-10 psi at a time if necessary.	3. Minimize risk of barotrauma, and with 14-16g catheter, maintain efficacy.
4. Use 0.5-second inspiratory time.	4. Minimize risk of barotrauma, and with 14-16g catheter, maintain efficacy.
5. Maintain maximal upper airway patency by *continuously* maintaining bilateral jaw thrust and by placing oropharyngeal and nasopharyngeal airways.	5. Exhalation *only* occurs through a patent upper airway.

GENERAL ROUTINE MEASURES

Several routine measures should be undertaken before extubation is performed in any patient. All relevant catheters (e.g., ETT, nasogastric tube) and orifices (mouth, pharynx, nose) should be suctioned thoroughly. Inadequate clearing of secretions can result in laryngeal spasm after extubation. After adequate suctioning, the patient should receive 100% oxygen for 2 to 5 minutes to ensure adequate denitrogenation and oxygenation. Just before extubation, the patient is given a large, sustained inflation. While the lungs are at or near total capacity, the ETT cuff is deflated while the anesthetist simultaneously pulls the tube. This sequence of events elicits a forceful cough secondary to the high expiratory flow that is generated by the elastic recoil of the lungs from total lung capacity. Coughing aids in clearing the airway and vocal cords of secretions, which reduces the incidence of postextubation laryngospasm and breath holding.

PREDICTING SAFE EXTUBATION

Airway management problems are predictable in patients with upper airway obstruction or edema secondary to trauma or surgery. A life-threatening situation could arise when these patients are extubated, especially if the jaws are immobilized. Demling et al.[164] prospectively evaluated 700 consecutive, intubated surgical patients to identify predictors of extubation failure. They found no clearly identifiable factors that contribute to extubation difficulty. Others have found that the presence of a leak around the ETT cuff is a useful if not universal predictor of successful extubation.[165] Perhaps the best study on the "leak test" for extubation involved 72 spontaneously breathing patients with a known history of upper airway obstruction in the intensive care unit.[166] The ETT cuff was deflated, and the ETT was occluded. If a peritubular cuff leak was detected during spontaneous ventilation, the ETT was removed. If no peritubular leak was detected with occlusion of the ETT, extubation was performed over a fiberoptic bronchoscope or bougie to facilitate reintubation, if necessary. Among the 62 patients extubated with a cuff leak, 2 required reintubation and 5 required tracheostomy secondary to repeated failures at extubation trials. Among the 10 patients without a cuff leak, 3 required reintubation and eventual tracheostomy. The authors concluded that although the presence of a cuff leak demonstrates that extubation is likely to be successful, a failed leak test does not indicate that extubation will fail automatically. They recommended that patients with no cuff leak should be extubated only in the presence of experienced personnel who are "able to effect an often difficult reintubation."

USE OF AN AIRWAY EXCHANGE CATHETER OR JET STYLET FOR EXTUBATION

The concept and use of an airway exchange catheter (AEC) as an additional safety measure during extubation of the trachea in patients in whom subsequent ventilation and/or reintubation of the trachea may be difficult has been described.[167] An AEC is a long, small ID, hollow, semi-rigid catheter that is inserted through an in situ ETT before extubation. After the ETT is withdrawn over the AEC, the AEC can serve multiple functions: (1) it can be a conduit to administer oxygen by either insufflation or manual or jet ventilation (which in turn provides time to use alternative airway management strategies); (2) it allows intermittent measurement of PET_{CO_2} from the trachea; and (3) it may serve as a stylet for reintubation. Because the reintubation rate is as high as 19% in extubated surgical ICU patients, the airway management capabilities provided by an AEC are extremely important and are well recognized by the ASA.[167] Many types of AECs have been used; however, the most widely used are the multiple-sized, appropriately adapted, centimeter depth-marked, commercial ones made by Cook Critical Care (Bloomington, IN), Sheridan Catheter Corporation (Argyle, NY), and CardioMed Supplies (Gormley, Ontario, Canada).

Before extubation, the size and type of AEC and the size of the reintubation ETT must be chosen. A relatively large-diameter AEC has important advantages, such as the best chance of reintubation success and ease of intraluminal manual or jet ventilation. Conversely, a relatively small-diameter AEC has important advantages such as ease of spontaneous ventilation around the AEC and reintubation capnography through the annular space that surrounds the AEC. The advantages and disadvantages of the size of the reintubation ETT are opposite to those of the size of the AEC. If there is any question at all, the fit of the specific anticipated reintubation ETT over the specific AEC should be tested in vitro before using the AEC. (The AEC manufacturer's instructions are incorrect for some ETTs.)

The AEC should never be inserted against a resistance. Although the tips of the commercially made AECs are somewhat rounded and blunt, perforations of the tracheobronchial tree have occurred.[167]

During insertion into the in situ ETT, one always must be cognizant of the depth of insertion. Excessive depth of insertion (e.g., beyond the tip of the ETT or greater than 26 cm for an orotracheal AEC in a normal-sized adult) increases the risk of tracheobronchial tree perforation and barotrauma with jet ventilation. If the tip of the in situ ETT has adequate tracheal depth (e.g., mid-trachea or 23 cm), a prudent rule to follow is to simply align the centimeter markings on the AEC with the centimeter markings on the ETT. Keeping the tip of the AEC just within the tip of the ETT prevents direct trauma to the tracheal mucosa and assures a supracarinal location (and minimizes the danger of barotrauma from unilateral or unilobar jet ventilation).

Sensible use of extubation AEC adjuncts can increase and/or prolong the efficacy of the AEC-aided extubation. These adjuncts consist of administration of intraluminal AEC humidified oxygen, face-mask FiO_2 supplementation, nebulization of racemic epinephrine (presumably to decrease mucosal edema), administration of Heliox, maintenance of nothing-by-mouth status, and immobilization and clear labeling of the AEC. Adequate tolerance of the AEC should allow administration of all respiratory care therapies that could be given to a fully extubated patient, including chest physiotherapy, suctioning, administration of bronchodilators, and analgesic/sedative therapy.

A jet ventilator should be immediately available as an alternative plan, especially in cases of known difficult intubation, and the jet ventilator should be pre-set at 25 psi with the use of an additional in-line regulator. For even the smallest-sized commercially available AECs, a 1-second inspiratory time at 25 psi with an FiO_2 near 1.0 (air entrainment is minimal with a long catheter in the trachea) provides at least partial life-sustaining ventilatory support.[156,168] For the medium- and large-sized AEC, a $1/2$ second inspiratory time at 25 psi provides total ventilatory support.[156,168] Use of a jet ventilator with an additional in-line regulator allows for breath-by-breath increases in tidal volume if necessary. With the medium- and large-sized AECs, the greatest danger is the administration of too large a tidal volume (because of too great a psi and/or inspiratory time) resulting in barotrauma. Use of an initial 25 psi minimizes this risk. In view of the fact that even experienced users of AECs can have an 11% incidence of barotrauma when the AEC is used with 50-psi jet ventilation,[169] the precautions of low psi, short inspiratory time, long expiratory time, and avoidance of excessive depth of insertion are very important measures to prevent barotrauma. In addition, the upper airway should be maximally patent by putting the patient in an optimal "sniff" position (i.e., neck slightly flexed on chest, head extended on the neck at the atlantooccipital joint), by use of bilateral jaw thrust and oropharyngeal and nasopharyngeal airways (i.e., the same maneuvers used for difficult mask ventilation; see Box 31-3), and by avoiding jet ventilation during phonation.

If reintubation is necessary, a laryngoscope should be used, if possible, to facilitate passage of the ETT over the AEC. In appropriate hands, there is very little risk with laryngoscopy and the potential benefit is great. When the tip of an ETT fails to pass the laryngeal inlet, it typically is because the tip of the ETT has engaged the right vocal cord or arytenoid; the correct maneuver is a 90-degree counterclockwise rotation of the ETT (which rotates the tip from a 3 o'clock position to a 12 o'clock position). The risk of an ETT failing to pass the laryngeal inlet is minimized by using a relatively small ETT and a relatively large AEC.

Finally, if the combination of AEC and ETT creates a sufficiently large annular space between them, the annular

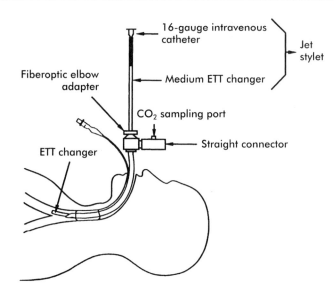

FIGURE 31-16. Method for preserving the intratracheal location of the tracheal tube exchanger during confirmation of intratracheal placement of a tracheal tube. The tracheal tube exchanger is passed through a self-sealing diaphragm in a fiberoptic elbow adapter. With this method, positive-pressure ventilation and carbon dioxide sampling may occur around the tracheal tube exchanger but within the endotracheal tube. *ETT*, Endotracheal tube. (From Goskowicz R, Gaughan S, Benumof JL, Ozaki G. It is not necessary to remove a jet stylet in order to determine tracheal tube location: Case report. J Clin Anesth 1992; 4:42-4.)

space can be used for capnographic and clinical confirmation that tracheal reintubation has in fact occurred.[170] This can be accomplished by passing the AEC out the self-sealing diaphragm of a bronchoscopy elbow and ventilating around the AEC but within the lumen of the ETT (Figure 31-16).[170] The great benefit of this procedure is that removal of the AEC is unnecessary (and the known intratracheal location of the AEC is not forfeited) to find out whether tracheal reintubation has occurred.

KEY POINTS

- Careful preanesthetic evaluation should identify the majority of difficult airways. The evaluation should include all 11 tests outlined in Table 31-4, with an emphasis on the assessment of tongue versus pharyngeal size, atlantooccipital joint extension, mandibular space, neck length and musculature, dental and palatal configuration, and facial and oral edema if present.
- If the airway is recognized to be difficult and the clinical situation is not urgent, the patient should be intubated awake (followed by general anesthesia), or she should receive regional anesthesia (preferably established early in labor).
- After induction of general anesthesia, if a patient cannot be intubated by any means but can be ventilated by face-mask or LMA and there is no fetal distress or maternal emergency, the anesthesiologist can either awaken the patient (which should be followed by either awake intubation or administration of regional anesthesia) or establish a surgical airway.

- After induction of general anesthesia, if a patient cannot be intubated by any means but can be ventilated by face-mask or LMA and severe fetal distress or maternal emergency is present, the anesthesiologist can awaken the patient (which should be followed by either awake intubation or administration of regional or local anesthesia), administer general anesthesia by means of face-mask or LMA ventilation while an assistant maintains cricoid pressure, or establish a surgical airway.
- After induction of general anesthesia, if a patient cannot be intubated or ventilated by mask, the anesthesiologist must choose an alternative means of maintaining ventilation and oxygenation such as use of the LMA, institution of TTJV, use of the Combitube, or establishment of a surgical airway.
- Extubation over an airway exchange catheter is the optimal method of extubating a patient with a known difficult airway.

REFERENCES

1. Caplan RA, Posner KL, Ward RJ, Chaney SW. Adverse respiratory events in anesthesia: A closed claims analysis. Anesthesiology 1990; 72:828-33.
2. Bellhouse CP, Doré C. Criteria for estimating likelihood of difficulty of endotracheal intubation with MacIntosh laryngoscope. Anaesth Intensive Care 1988; 16:329-37.
3. Benumof JL, Scheller MS. The importance of transtracheal jet ventilation in the management of difficult airway. Anesthesiology 1989; 71:769-78.
4. Buck N, Devlon HB, Lun JN. The Report of a Confidential Enquiry into Perioperative Deaths. London, The Nuffield Prevential Hospital Trust, 1987.
5. Samsoon JLP, Young RJB. Difficult tracheal intubation: A retrospective study. Anaesthesia 1987; 42:487-90.
6. Lyons G. Failed intubation: Six year's experience in a teaching maternity unit. Anaesthesia 1985; 40:759-62.
7. Reports on Confidential Enquires into Maternal Deaths in England and Wales 1952-1954 to 1976-1978 [Triennial Series]. London, HMSO, 1982.
8. Abrams ME, Metters JS, Tindall VR, et al. Report on Confidential Enquiries into Maternal Deaths in the United Kingdom 1985-1987. London, HMSO, 1991.
9. Hibbard BM, Anderson MM, Drife JO, et al. Report on Confidential Enquiries into Maternal Deaths in the United Kingdom 1988-1990. London, HMSO, 1994.
10. Hibbard BM, Anderson MM, Drife JO, et al. Report on Confidential Enquiries into Maternal Deaths in the United Kingdom 1991-1993. London, HMSO, 1996.
11. Lewis G, Drife J, Botting B, et al. Why Mothers Die: Report on Confidential Enquiries into Maternal Deaths in the United Kingdom 1994-1996. London, TSO, 1998.
12. Lewis G, Drife J, Botting B, et al. Why Mothers Die 1997-1999: The Confidential Enquiries into Maternal Deaths in the United Kingdom. London, RCOG Press, 2001.
13. Koonin LM, MacKay AP, Berg CJ, et al. Pregnancy-related mortality surveillance: United States. 1987-1990. MMWR CDC Surveill Summ 1997; 46:17-36.
14. Hawkins JL, Koonin LM, Palmer SK, Gibbs CP. Anesthesia-related deaths during obstetric delivery in the United States, 1979-1990. Anesthesiology 1997; 86: 277-84.
15. American Society of Anesthesiologists. Practice guidelines for management of the difficult airway: An updated report by the American Society of Anesthesiologists Task Force on Management of the Difficult Airway. Anesthesiology 2003; 98:1269-77.
16. Benumof JL. Management of the difficult airway. Anesthesiology 1991; 75:1087-110.
17. Benumof JL. The laryngeal mask airway and the American Society of Anesthesiologists Difficult Airway Algorithm. Anesthesiology 1996; 84:686-99.
18. Cormack RS, Lehane J. Difficult tracheal intubation in obstetrics. Anaesthesia 1984; 39:1105-11.
19. Benumof JL, Cooper SD. Quantitative improvement in laryngoscopic view by optimal external laryngeal manipulation. J Clin Anesth 1996; 8:136-40.
20. Aro L, Takki S, Aromaa U. Technique for difficult intubation. Br J Anaesth 1971; 43:1081-3.
21. Mallampati SR, Gatt SP, Gugino LD, et al. A clinical sign to predict difficult tracheal intubation: A prospective study. Can J Anaesth 1985; 32:429-34.
22. Phillips OC, Dureksen RL. Endotracheal intubation: A new blade for direct laryngoscopy. Anesth Analg 1973; 52:691-8.
23. Finucane BT, Santora AH. Difficult intubation. In Finucane BT, Santora AH, editors. Principles of Airway Management. Philadelphia, FA Davis, 1988:147.
24. Deller A, Schreiber MN, Gromer J, Ahnefeld FW. Difficult intubation: Incidence and predictability: A prospective study of 8,284 adult patients (abstract). Anesthesiology 1990; 73:A1054.
25. Bellhouse CP. An angulated laryngoscope for routine and difficult tracheal intubation. Anesthesiology 1988; 69:126-9.
26. Lyons G, MacDonald R. Difficult intubation in obstetrics (letter). Anaesthesia 1985; 40:1016.
27. Glassenburg R, Vaisrub N, Albright G. The incidence of failed intubation in obstetrics: Is there an irreducible minimum? (abstract). Anesthesiology 1990; 73:A1061.
28. Tunstall ME. Failed tracheal intubation in the parturient (editorial). Can J Anaesth 1989; 36:611-3.
29. Hirsch IA, Reagan JO, Sullivan N. Complications of direct laryngoscopy: A prospective analysis. Anesthesiol Rev 1990; 17:34-40.
30. King TA, Adams AP. Failed tracheal intubation. Br J Anaesth 1990; 65:400-14.
31. Finucane BT. Evaluation of the airway prior to intubation. In Finucane BT, Santora AH, editors. Principles of Airway Management. Philadelphia, FA Davis, 1988:69-83.
32. Sia RL, Eden ET. How to avoid problems when using the fiberoptic bronchoscope for difficult intubations (letter). Anaesthesia 1988; 36:74-5.
33. Norton ML, Wilton H, Brown A. The difficult airway clinic. Anesthesiol Rev 1988; 25:25-8.
34. American Society of Anesthesiologists Committee on Professional Liability. Personal communication. March 1990.
35. Latto IP, Rosen M. Management of difficult intubation. In Latto IP, Rosen M, editors. Difficulties in Tracheal Intubation. London, Bailliere Tindall, 1985:99-141.
36. Frerk CM. Predicting difficult intubation. Anaesthesia 1991; 46: 1005-8.
37. Lewis M, Keramati S, Benumof JL, et al. What is the best way to determine oropharyngeal classification and mandibular space length to predict difficult laryngoscopy? Anesthesiology 1994; 81: 69-75.
38. Wilson ME, Spiegelhalter D, Robertosn JA, et al. Predicting difficult intubation. Br J Anaesth 1988; 61: 211-6.
39. Oates JD, Macleod AD, Oates PD, et al. Comparison of two methods for predicting difficult intubation. Br J Anaesth 1991; 66: 305-9.
40. Rocke DA, Murray WB, Rout CC, Gouws E. Relative risk analysis of factors associated with difficult intubation in obstetric anesthesia. Anesthesiology 1992; 77:67-73.
41. Tse JC, Rimm EB, Hussain A. Predicting difficult endotracheal intubation in surgical patients scheduled for general anesthesia: A prospective blind study. Anesth Analg 1995; 81: 254-8.
42. El-Ganzouri AR, McCarthy RJ, Tuman KJ, et al. Prospective airway assessment: Predictive value of a multivariate risk index. Anesth Analg 1996; 82: 1197-204.
43. McIntyre JRW. The difficult intubation. Can J Anaesth 1987; 34:204-13.
44. Latto IP, Rosen M. Intubation procedures and causes of difficult intubation. In Latto IP, Rosen M, editors. Difficulties in Tracheal Intubation. London, Bailliere Tindall, 1985:76-89.
45. Stewart DJ. Anesthetic Implications of Syndromes and Unusual Disorders (Appendix I). Manual of Pediatric Anesthesia, 2nd ed. New York, Churchill Livingstone, 1985:289-343.
46. Jones AEP, Pelton DA. An index of syndromes and their anesthetic implications. Can Anaesth Soc J 1976; 23:207-26.
47. Cohen SM, Zaurito CE, Segil LJ. Oral exam to predict difficult intubations: A large prospective study (abstract). Anesthesiology 1989; 71:A937.
48. Mathew M, Hanna LS, Aldrete JA. Preoperative indices to anticipate a difficult tracheal intubation. Anesth Analg 1989; 68:S187.
49. Wilson ME, John R. Problems with the Mallampati sign. Anaesthesia 1990; 45:486-7.
50. Charters P, Perera S, Horton A. Visibility of pharyngeal structures as a predictor of difficult intubation (letter). Anaesthesia 1987; 42:1115.

51. Horton WA, Fahy L, Charters P. Defining a standard intubation position using "angle finder." Br J Anaesth 1989; 62:6-12.
52. McGill IW. Technique in endotracheal anaesthesia. Br Med J 1930; 2:817-20.
53. Salem MR, Methrubhutham M, Bennett EJ. Difficult intubation. N Engl J Med 1976; 295:879-81.
54. Brechner VL. Unusual problems in the management of airways. I. Flexion-extension mobility of the cervical spine. Anesth Analg 1968; 47:362-73.
55. White A, Kander PL. Anatomical factors in difficult direct laryngoscopy. Br J Anaesth 1975; 47:488.
56. Nichol HL, Zuck B. Difficult laryngoscopy: The "anterior" larynx and the atlanto-occipital gap. Br J Anaesth 1983; 55:141-4.
57. Roberts JT, Ali HH, Shorten GD, Gorback MS. Why cervical flexion facilitates laryngoscopy with a MacIntosh laryngoscope but hinders it with a flexible fiberscope (abstract). Anesthesiology 1990; 73:A1012.
58. Patil VU, Stehling LC, Zauder HL. Techniques of Endotracheal Intubation. Fiberoptic Endocopy in Anaesthesia. Chicago, Year Book, 1983:79.
59. Cass NM, James NR, Lines V. Difficult direct laryngoscopy complicating intubation for anaesthesia. Br Med J 1956; 1:488-9.
60. Van der Linde JC, Revelopa JA, Steenkamp ED. Anatomical factors relating to difficult intubation. S Afr Med J 1983; 63:976-7.
61. Jouppila R, Jouppila P, Hollman A. Laryngeal oedema as an obstetric anaesthesia complication. Acta Anaesth Scand 1980; 24:97.
62. Keeri-Szanto M. Laryngeal oedema complicating obstetric anaesthesia, yet another case. Anaesthesia 1978; 33:272.
63. Brocke-Utne JG, Downing AJW, Seedat I. Laryngeal oedema associated with pre-eclamptic toxemia. Anaesthesia 1977; 32:556.
64. McKenzie AI. Laryngeal oedema complicating obstetric anesthesia: Three cases. Anaesthesia 1978; 33:271.
65. Boliston TA. Difficult tracheal intubation in obstetrics. Anaesthesia 1985; 40:389.
66. Archer GW, Marx GF. Arterial oxygen tension during apnoea in parturient women. Br J Anaesth 1974; 46:358-60.
67. Dupont X, Hamza J, Jullien P, Narchi P. Risk factors associated with difficult airway in normotensive parturients (abstract). Anesthesiology 1990; 73:A999.
68. Datta S, Briwa J. Modified laryngoscope for endotracheal intubation in obese patients (letter). Anesth Analg 1981; 60:120-1.
69. Kay NH. Mammomegaly and intubation. Anaesthesia 1982; 37:221.
70. Benumof JL, Dagg R, Benumof R. Critical arterial hemoglobin desaturation will occur before return to an unparalyzed state following 1 mg/kg intravenous succinylcholine. Anesthesiology 1997; 87:979-82.
71. Dillon JB, Darsie ML. Oxygen for acute respiratory depression due to administration of thiopental sodium. JAMA 1955; 159:1114-6.
72. Hamilton WK, Eastwood DW. A study of denitrogenation with some inhalation anesthetic systems. Anesthesiology 1955; 16:861-7.
73. Gold MI, Muravchick S. Arterial oxygenation during laryngoscopy and intubation. Anesth Analg 1981; 60:316-8.
74. Gold MI, Duarte I, Muravchick S. Arterial oxygenation in conscious patients after 5 minutes and after 30 seconds of oxygen breathing. Anesth Analg 1981; 60:313-5.
75. Norris MC, Dewan DM. Preoxygenation for cesarean section: A comparison of two techniques. Anesthesiology 1985; 62:827-9.
76. Goldberg ME, Norris MC, Laryani GE, et al. Preoxygenation in the morbidly obese: A comparison of two techniques. Anesth Analg 1989; 68:520-2.
77. Benumof JL. Preoxygenation. Anesthesiology 1999; 91: 603-5.
78. Gambee AM, Hertzka RE, Fisher DM. Preoxygenation techniques: Comparison of 3 minutes and 4 breaths. Anesth Analg 1987; 66:468-70.
79. Valentine SJ, Marjot R, Monk CR. Preoxygenation in the elderly: A comparison between the four-maximal-breath and three-minute techniques. Anesth Analg 1990; 71: 516-9.
80. McCarthy G, Elliott P, Mirakhur K, et al. A comparison of different preoxygenation techniques in the elderly. Anaesthesia 1991; 46: 824-7.
81. Campbell IT, Beatty PCW. Monitoring preoxygenation. Br J Anaesth 1994; 72: 3-4.
82. Sellick BA. Cricoid pressure to control regurgitation of stomach contents prior to induction of anaesthesia. Lancet 1961; 2:404-6.
83. Howells TH, Chamney AR, Wraight WJ, Simons RS. The application of cricoid pressure: An assessment and a survey of its practice. Anaesthesia 1983; 38: 457-60.
84. Georgescu A, Miller JN, Lecklither ML. The Sellick maneuver causing complete airway obstruction. Anesth Analg 1992; 74:457-9.
85. Shorten GD, Alfille PH, Gliklich RE. Airway obstruction following application of cricoid pressure. J Clin Anesth 1991; 3:403-5.
86. Cicala RS, Kudsska, Butts A. Initial evaluation and management of upper airway injuries in trauma patients. J Clin Anesth 1991; 3:91-8.
87. Ramanthan S, Gandhi S, Arismendy J, et al. Oxygen transfer from mother to fetus during cesarean section under epidural anesthesia. Anesth Analg 1982; 61:576-81.
88. Bonica JJ. Local-regional analgesia for abdominal delivery. In Bonica JJ, editor. Obstetric Analgesia and Anesthesia. Philadelphia, FA Davis, 1967:527-38.
89. Moir DD. Local anaesthetic technique in obstetrics. Br J Anaesth 1986; 58:747-59.
90. Cooper MG, Feeney EM, Joseph M, McGuinness JJ. Local anaesthetic infiltration for caesarean section. Anaesth Intensive Care 1989; 17:198-201.
91. Sivarajan M, Fink RB. The position and the state of the larynx during general anesthesia and muscle paralysis. Anesthesiology 1990; 72:439-42.
92. Brown DL. Glossopharyngeal nerve block. In Brown DL, editor. Atlas of Regional Anesthesia Philadelphia, WB Saunders, 1992: 187-92.
93. Sanchez A, Trivedi NS, Morrison DE. Preparation of the patient for awake intubation. In Benumof JL, editor. Airway Management: Principles and Practice. St. Louis, Mosby-Year Book, 1996: 172-4.
94. Sitzman TB, Rich GF, Rockwell JJ, et al. Local anesthetic administration for awake direct laryngoscopy. Anesthesiology 1997; 86: 34-40.
95. Gotta AW, Sullivan KCA. Anaesthesia of the upper airway using topical anaesthetic and superior laryngeal nerve block. Br J Anaesth 1983; 53:1055-7.
96. Cooper M, Watson RL. An improved regional anesthetic technique for perioral endoscopy. Anesthesiology 1975; 42:273-4.
97. Walts LP. Anesthesia of larynx in patients with full stomach. JAMA 1965; 192:705.
98. Duncan JT. Intubation of the trachea in the conscious patient. Br J Anaesth 1977; 49:619-23.
99. Kopriva CJ, Eltringham RJ, Siebert PE. A comparison of the effects of Innovar and topical spray on the laryngeal closure reflex. Anesthesiology 1974; 40:596-8.
100. Ovassapian A, Krejcie TC, Yelich SJ, Dykes MHM. Awake fiberoptic intubation in the patient at high risk of aspiration. Br J Anaesth 1989; 62:13-6.
101. Cahen CR. An aid in cases of difficult tracheal intubation (letter). Anesthesiology 1991; 74:197.
102. Dogra S, Falconer R, Latto IP. Successful difficult intubation: Tracheal tube placement over a gum-elastic bougie. Anaesthesia 1990; 45: 774-6.
103. Schwartz KD, Johnson C, Roberts J. A maneuver to facilitate flexible fiberoptic intubation. Anesthesiology 1989; 71:470-1.
104. Williams RT, Maltby JR. Airway intubator (letter). Anesth Analg 1982; 61:309.
105. Rogers S, Benumof JL. New and easy fiberoptic endoscopy-aided tracheal intubation. Anesthesiology 1983; 59:569-72.
106. Ovassapian A. Fiberoptic Airway Endoscopy in Anesthesia and Critical Care. New York, Raven Press, 1990.
107. Berman RA. A method for blind oral intubation of the trachea or the esophagus. Anesth Analg 1977; 56:866-7.
108. Patil V, Stehling LC, Zauder HL, Koch JP. Mechanical aids for fiberoptic endoscopy. Anesthesiology 1982; 57:69-70.
109. Ovassapian A, Dykes MHM. The role of fiberoptic endoscopy for airway management. Semin Anesth 1987; 6:93-104.
110. Nichols KP, Zornow MH. A potential complication of fiberoptic intubation. Anesthesiology 1989; 70:562-3.
111. Butler FS, Circillo AA. Retrograde tracheal intubation. Anesth Analg 1960; 39:333.
112. Sanchez A., Pellares V. Retrograde intubation technique. In Benumof JL, editor. Airway Management: Principles and Practice. Mosby, St. Louis 1996; 320-341.
113. Barriot P, Riou B. Retrograde technique for tracheal intubation in trauma patients. Crit Care Med 1988; 16:712-3.
114. Saunders PA, Geisecke AH. Clinical assessment of the adult Bullard laryngoscope. Can J Anaesth 1989; 36:S118-9.
115. Borland LM, Casselbrandt M. The Bullard laryngoscope: A new indirect oral laryngoscope (pediatric version). Anesth Analg 1990; 70:105-8.
116. Cohn AI, Hart RT, McGraw SR, et al. The Bullard laryngoscope for emergency airway management in a morbidly obese parturient. Anesth Analg 1995; 81: 872-3.
117. Mehta S. Transtracheal illumination for optimal tracheal tube placement: A clinical study. Anaesthesia 1989; 44:970-1.
118. Ellis DG, Jakymec A, Kaplan RM, et al. Guided orotracheal intubation in the operating room using a lighted stylet: A comparison with direct laryngoscopic technique. Anesthesiology 1986; 64:823-6.
119. Hung OR, Stewart RD. Illuminating Stylet (Lightwand). In Benumof JL, editor. Airway Management: Principles and Practice. Mosby, St. Louis 1996; 342-52.

120. American Society of Anesthesiologists Task Force on Obstetrical Anesthesia. Practice Guidelines for Obstetrical Anesthesia. Anesthesiology 1999; 90:600-11.

121. Caplan R, Benumof JL, Berry FA, et al. Practice guidelines for management of the difficult airway: A report of the ASA Task Force on Management of the Difficult Airway. Anesthesiology 1993; 78: 597-602.

122. Tunstall ME. Anaesthesia for obstetric operations. Clin Obstet Gynaecol 1980; 7:665-94.

123. Rosen M. Difficult and failed intubation in obstetrics. In Latto IP, Rosen M, editors. Difficulties in Tracheal Intubation. London, Balliere Tindall, 1987:152-5.

124. Crosby ET. The difficult airway in obstetric anesthesia. In Benumof JL, editor. Airway Management: Principles and Practice. Mosby, St. Louis 1996; 638-65.

125. Ezri T, Szmuk P, Evron S, et al. Difficult airway in obstetric anesthesia: A review. Obstet Gynecol Surv 2001; 56: 631-41.

126. Bishop MJ, Kharasch ED. Is the Combitube™ a useful emergency airway device for anesthesiologists? Anesth Analg 1998; 86:1141-2.

127. Frass M. The Combitube: Esophageal/Tracheal Double Lumen Airway. In Benumof JL (ed.) Airway Management: Principles and Practice. Mosby, St. Louis 1996; 444-454.

128. Wissler RN. The esophageal-tracheal Combitube. Anesthesiol Rev 1993; 20:147-52.

129. Tunstall ME, Geddes C. Failed intubation in obstetric anesthesia: An indication for use of the esophageal gastric tube airway. Br J Anaesth 1984; 56: 659-61.

130. Benumof JL. Laryngeal mask airway and the ASA Difficult Airway Algorithm. Anesthesiology 1996; 84: 686-99.

131. Preston R. The evolving role of the laryngeal mask airway in obstetrics. Can J Anesth 2001; 48: 1061-5.

132. Joshi GP, Smith I, White PF. Laryngeal mask airway. In Benumof JL, editor. Airway Management: Principles and Practice. Mosby, St. Louis 1996; 353-73.

133. Han TH, Brimacombe J, Lee EJ, et al. The laryngeal mask airway is effective (and probably safe) in selected healthy parturients for elective cesarean section: A prospective study of 1067 cases. Can J Anesth 2001; 48: 1117-21.

134. DeMello WF, Kocan M. The laryngeal mask in failed intubation. Anaesthesia 1990; 45:689-90.

135. McClune S, Regan M, Moore J. Laryngeal mask airway for Caesarean section. Anaesthesia 1990; 45:227-8.

136. Priscu V, Priscu L, Sonker D. Laryngeal mask for failed intubation in emergency Cesarean section. Can J Anaesth 1992; 39:893.

137. Stoney J. The laryngeal mask for failed intubation at cesarean section. Anaesth Intensive Care 1992; 20:118-9.

138. Awan R, Nolan JP, Cook TM. Use of ProSeal™ laryngeal mask airway for airway maintenance during emergency caesarean section after failed tracheal intubation. Br J Anaesth 2004; 92:144-6.

139. Evans NR, Gardner SV, James MF, et al. The Proseal laryngeal mask: Results of a descriptive trial with experience of 300 cases. Br J Anaesth 2002; 88: 534-39.

140. Cook TM, Nolan JP, Verghese C, et al. Randomized crossover comparison of the proseal with the classic laryngeal mask airway in unparalysed anaesthetized patients. Br J Anaesth 2002; 88: 527-33.

141. Caponas G. Intubating laryngeal mask airway. Anaesth Intensive Care 2002; 30:551-69.

142. Reardon RF, Martel M. The intubating laryngeal mask airway: Suggestions for use in the emergency department. Acad Emerg Med 2001; 8: 833-38.

143. van Vlymen JM, Coloma M, Tongier WK, et al. Use of the intubating laryngeal mask airway: Are muscle relaxants necessary? Anesthesiology 2000; 93:340-5.

144. Kihara S, Yaguchi Y, Brimacombe J, et al. Intubating laryngeal mask airway size selection: A randomized triple crossover study in paralyzed, anesthetized male and female adult patients. Anesth Analg 2002; 94:1023-7.

145. Dimitriou V, Voyagis GS, Brimacombe JR. Flexible lightwand-guided tracheal intubation with the intubating laryngeal mask Fastrach™ in adults after unpredicted failed laryngoscope-guided tracheal intubation. Anesthesiology 2002; 96:296-9.

146. Ferson DZ, Rosenblatt WH, Johansen MJ, et al. Use of the intubating LMA-Fastrach™ in 254 patients with difficult-to-manage airways. Anesthesiology 2001; 95:1175-81.

147. Levy DM. LMA for failed intubation. Can J Anaesth 1993; 40:801-2.

148. King TA, Adam AP. Failed tracheal intubation. Br J Anaesth 1991; 65:400-14.

149. Asai T, Appadurai I. LMA for failed intubation. Can J Anaesth 1993; 40:802-3.

150. Brimacombe J, Berry A. LMA for failed intubation. Can J Anaesth 1993; 41:802-3.

151. Strang TI: Does the laryngeal mask airway compromise cricoid pressure? Anaesthesia 1992; 47:829-31.

152. Benumof JL. Transtracheal jet ventilation via percutaneous catheter and high-pressure source. In Benumof JL, editor. Airway Management: Principles and Practice. Mosby, St. Louis 1996; 455-76.

153. McLellan I, Gordon P, Khawaja S, et al. Percutaneous transtracheal high frequency jet ventilation as an aid to difficult intubation. Can Anaesth Soc J 1988; 35:404-5.

154. Baraka A. Transtracheal jet ventilation during fiberoptic intubation under general anesthesia. Anesth Analg 1986; 65:1091-2.

155. Gaughan S, Benumof JL, Ozaki G. Comparison of a low flow and high flow regulator in a variable compliance lung model. Anesthesiology 1992; 77:189-99.

156. Gaughan S, Benumof JL, Ozaki G. Can an anesthesia machine flush valve provide for effective jet ventilation? Anesth Analg 1993; 76:800-8.

157. Benumof JL. Additional safety methods when changing an endotracheal tube (letter). Anesthesiology 1991; 75:920-1.

158. Tighe SQM. Failed tracheal intubation (letter). Anaesthesia 1992; 47:356.

159. Toye FJ, Weinstein JD. A percutaneous tracheostomy device. Surgery 1969; 65:384-9.

160. Ciaglia P, Firsching R, Syniec C. Elective percutaneous dilatational tracheostomy. Chest 1985; 87:715-9.

161. Schachner A, Ovil Y, Sidi J, et al. Percutaneous tracheostomy: A new method. Crit Care Med 1989; 17:1052-6.

162. Schachner A, Ovil Y, Sidi J, et al. Rapid percutaneous tracheostomy. Chest 1990; 98:1266-70.

163. Melker RJ, Florete OG. Percutaneous dilational cricothyrotomy and tracheostomy. In Benumof JL, editor. Airway Management: Principles and Practice. Mosby, St. Louis 1996; 484-512.

164. Demling RH, Read T, Lind LJ, Flanagan HL. Incidence and mortality of extubation failure in surgical intensive care patients. Crit Care Med 1988; 16:573-7.

165. Adderly RJ, Mullins GC. When to extubate the croup patient: The "leak" test. Can J Anaesth 1987; 34:304-6.

166. Fisher M, Raper RF. The "cuff-leak" test for extubation. Anaesthesia 1992; 47:10-2.

167. Benumof JL. Airway exchange catheters for safe extubation: The clinical and scientific details that make the concept work. Chest 1997; 111:1483-6.

168. Gaughan SD, Benumof JL, Ozaki GT. Quantification of the jet function of a jet stylet. Anesth Analg 1992; 74:580-5.

169. Cooper RM, Cohen DR. The use of an endotracheal ventilation catheter for jet ventilation during difficult intubation. Can J Anaesth 1994; 41:1196-9.

170. Takata M, Benumof JL, Ozaki G. Confirmation of endotracheal intubation over a jet stylet. Anesth Analg 1995; 80:800-5.

Chapter 32
Postpartum Headache

Sally K. Weeks, M.B., B.S., FRCA

Postdural puncture headache (PDPH) during the postpartum period is usually a complication of an anesthetic intervention. A patient with PDPH experiences an exacerbation of symptoms when she moves from the horizontal to the upright position. This does not occur with other forms of postpartum headache with the exception of pneumocephalus.

Physicians and nurses should be aware that dural puncture is only one of many causes of postpartum headache (Box 32-1). Difficult diagnostic problems require the opinion of a neurologist. The purpose of this chapter is to discuss the differential diagnosis of postpartum headache and PDPH in detail.

DIFFERENTIAL DIAGNOSIS OF POSTPARTUM HEADACHE

Nonspecific Headache

After delivery, women frequently suffer from headache that is unrelated to anesthesia. Benhamou et al.[1] determined the incidence of headache during the first postpartum week. Headache was reported by 12% of 1058 patients who had epidural anesthesia without dural puncture and by 15% of 140 patients who delivered without epidural anesthesia. A history of migraine and preeclampsia were risk factors for the development of postpartum headache. The postpartum period is always a challenge and seldom is a time for relaxation (Box 32-2). It is not surprising that headache is a common complaint during this time.

Migraine

Migraine occurs in 10% to 20% of the population and is three times more common in women than in men. Visual disturbances predominate during the prodromal stage. The subsequent throbbing headache often is unilateral and is accompanied by nausea, vomiting, and occasional focal neurologic symptoms. Pregnancy has an ameliorating effect on migraine in the majority of sufferers but headache may recur soon after delivery.[2] It is rare for migraine to present for the first time during the postpartum period.

Hypertension

Eclampsia is a form of hypertensive encephalopathy that includes headache, visual disturbances, nausea, vomiting, seizures, stupor and sometimes coma. Seizures may occur even when hypertension is not severe. Headache always is a serious premonitory sign. Other hypertensive disorders, with or without superimposed preeclampsia, also may cause postpartum headache and lead to encephalopathy.

Brain Tumor

Headache that is dull rather than throbbing in character may be an early symptom of a brain tumor. Nausea, vomiting, seizures, and focal signs may occur. Neurologic examination may reveal evidence of increased intracranial pressure (ICP) and other abnormalities. Alfery et al.[3] reported one case of a brain tumor that was diagnosed during the postpartum period in a woman who also showed features of PDPH.

Subdural Hematoma

In rare instances, dural puncture is associated with the subsequent development of a subdural hematoma, which typically is preceded by symptoms of PDPH.[4-6] Dural puncture results in leakage of cerebrospinal fluid (CSF) and decreased ICP. Presumably, decreased ICP causes stress on cerebral vessels, which may precipitate bleeding. Neurologic signs of subdural hematoma are variable but include evidence of increased ICP (e.g., headache, somnolence, vomiting, confusion) and focal abnormalities. Radiologic studies confirm the diagnosis, and surgical evacuation of the hematoma may be necessary.

Subarachnoid Hemorrhage

Rupture of a cerebral aneurysm or arteriovenous malformation produces sudden, severe headache, predominantly in the occipital region.[7] Other signs and symptoms include vomiting, neck stiffness and a decreased level of consciousness or coma. Focal signs may be present. The diagnosis is made primarily with scanning techniques, and surgery may be needed.

Cortical Vein Thrombosis

Cerebral cortical vein thrombosis may cause severe headache, focal signs, seizures, and coma. ICP is increased and CSF absorption in the arachnoid villi is impaired. Cerebral infarction may ensue. Postpartum patients appear to be especially susceptible to this condition. Risk factors during pregnancy and the puerperium include venous stasis, hypercoagulability, and damage to the venous endothelium. Diagnosis is best confirmed by magnetic resonance imaging (MRI). There are several published reports of cortical vein thrombosis in patients with presumed PDPH,[8-11] and distinguishing between the two conditions can be very difficult. Gewirtz et al.[11] have proposed that cortical vein thrombosis be excluded before the administration of a blood patch in a patient with intense throbbing headache accompanied by sweating, nausea, and vomiting. Treatment of cortical vein thrombosis largely is symptomatic, with the aim of preventing seizures. Although anticoagulation may prevent an extension of the thrombus, it also may predispose the patient to hemorrhagic brain infarction.

Cerebral Infarction/Ischemia

Nicol and Millns[12] reported the development of an acute cerebellar infarct that caused a severe *non*postural headache in a postpartum patient. This woman had received uncomplicated epidural anesthesia during labor followed by general anesthesia for urgent cesarean section. Mercieri et al.[13] described the occurrence of cerebral ischemia after unintentional dural puncture during labor. Two epidural blood patches were performed to treat severe postural headache—7 hours postpartum and on the second postpartum day, respectively. Mental confusion and agitation followed the second blood patch, but CT and MRI were normal. Generalized seizures, accompanied by right hemiparesis and visual disturbances, occurred on the ninth postpartum day. Transcranial Doppler ultrasonography demonstrated spasm of the left middle cerebral artery. Motor symptoms slowly resolved but hemianopsia persisted 1 year later.

Pseudotumor Cerebri/Benign Intracranial Hypertension

Pseudotumor cerebri (i.e., increased ICP in the absence of a mass lesion) may cause headache and visual disturbances. It occurs most frequently in young obese women and is associated with a variety of endocrine disorders and the administration of certain drugs. The diagnosis largely is one of exclusion (see Chapter 48).

Sinusitis

Headache caused by inflamed paranasal sinuses is associated with purulent nasal discharge and occasionally fever. Pain may be unilateral or bilateral depending on the extent of the disease, and the skin over the affected sinus may be tender. Frontal sinus infection causes headache in the frontal region. Ethmoidal and sphenoidal sinus infections cause periorbital pain, and maxillary sinus infection may cause diffuse facial discomfort. The sinuses fill overnight, and pain typically is worse on awakening. Pain improves in the upright position, which assists drainage.

Meningitis

The severe headache of meningitis is accompanied by fever, nuchal rigidity, and positive Kernig and Brudzinski signs. Lethargy, confusion, vomiting, seizures and a skin rash also may occur. The diagnosis is confirmed by examination of the CSF.

Pneumocephalus

The subdural or subarachnoid injection of air used for identification of the epidural space may be associated with the sudden onset of severe headache, sometimes accompanied by neck pain, back pain, or changes in mental status.[14-16] Symptoms may be worse in the sitting position and may be relieved by lying down. Radiologic studies confirm the presence of intracranial air. Headache typically disappears after a few hours, and denitrogenation with a high concentration of inspired oxygen should assist recovery.

Caffeine Withdrawal

The withdrawal of caffeine from regular moderate consumers may lead to headache, increased fatigue, and anxiety. Caffeine withdrawal may be the cause of postoperative headache. Although it has not been confirmed as a cause of postpartum headache, the diagnosis should be considered.

Lactation Headache

Askmark and Lundberg[17] reported episodes of intense headache during periods of breast-feeding in a woman known to suffer from migraine. Headache was associated with an increased plasma vasopressin concentration.

POSTDURAL PUNCTURE HEADACHE (PDPH)

Symptoms

Patients typically feel pain in the frontal and occipital regions. Pain often radiates to the neck, which may be stiff. Some women have a mild headache that permits full ambulation. In others, pain is severe and incapacitating. Symptoms are worse in the upright position and are relieved to some extent in the horizontal position. The diagnosis should be questioned in the absence of a postural contribution to symptoms. Abdominal compression may relieve pain in some patients.

In a prospective study of 75 nonobstetric patients with PDPH, Lybecker et al.[18] noted the following incidence of symptoms: nausea 60%, vomiting 24%, neck stiffness 43%, ocular (photophobia, diplopia, difficulty in accommodation) 13%, and auditory (hearing loss, hyperacusis, tinnitus) 12%.

Cranial nerve palsy occurs occasionally. The sixth cranial nerve is most susceptible to traction during its long intracranial course.

Shearer et al.[19] reported postpartum seizures in eight women with severe PDPH and with no convincing evidence of preexisting hypertension. Cerebral vasospasm was thought to be the etiologic factor. Vercauteren et al.[20] described a woman who had received epidural analgesia and developed postpartum seizures with a severe headache. The CSF was blood-stained, but a CT scan showed no source of hemorrhage. This patient improved dramatically after the performance of a blood patch.

Onset and Duration

Headache typically occurs on the first or second day after dural puncture. Most headaches last less than a week. Tohmo et al.[21] sent questionnaires to 325 patients during the first year after diagnostic lumbar puncture. Daily activities were curtailed by PDPH in 7% of subjects for more than 1 week and in one patient for 30 days. There are rare reports of symptoms lasting for months or even years.[22]

Pathophysiology

The German surgeon August Bier pioneered work on spinal anesthesia with cocaine. In 1899 he published his results in a report that is fascinating to modern eyes.[23] He and an assistant performed spinal anesthesia on each other. In Bier's case CSF flowed before the injection of the local anesthetic agent but anesthesia was ineffective. His assistant developed excellent anesthesia, which subsequently was tested by a burning cigar and strong blows to the shin with an iron hammer. Both later developed severe PDPH. The assistant forced himself to work the next day but Bier stayed in bed for 9 days. Bier is credited with the first description of PDPH and he surmised that it might be caused by CSF loss. Today there is no doubt that leakage of CSF initiates the syndrome. Kunkle et al.[24] consistently produced PDPH by draining 20 mL of CSF from volunteers. Symptoms were relieved immediately by subarachnoid injection of saline to restore initial CSF pressure.

Total CSF volume is estimated to be 150 mL, and the production rate is approximately 0.35 mL/min. The rate of CSF leakage through a dural hole may exceed the rate of CSF production. If this occurs, low CSF pressure will result in a loss of the cushion effect provided by intracranial fluid. Some of the pain of PDPH is thought to result from traction on pain-sensitive structures within the cranium, especially when the patient assumes the upright position.

Descent of intracranial elements also may occur. One man who developed severe PDPH after spinal anesthesia subsequently became stuporous.[25] Eventually brain death was diagnosed and herniation of the uncus against the tentorium was seen at autopsy. Hullander et al.[26] reported a case of Chiari I malformation (i.e., displacement of the cerebellar tonsils through the foramen magnum) in association with PDPH. Although this could have been congenital, the condition also may have been acquired as a consequence of low CSF pressure.

Grant et al.[27] used MRI to demonstrate a significant reduction in intracranial CSF volume after lumbar puncture. They noted a trend toward a relationship between the degree of reduction of CSF volume and the incidence of PDPH. No measurable change in the position of the cerebellar tonsils occurred. Panullo et al.[28] studied cranial MRI images in seven patients with postural headache attributed to intracranial hypotension. Symptoms had occurred after lumbar puncture in three of these subjects. The investigators identified meningeal enhancement in all seven patients and descent of the brain in six. These findings improved or resolved when headache disappeared.

Iqbal et al.[29] used lumbar MRI to examine CSF leakage 8 to 36 hours after lumbar puncture in 11 patients. The estimated volume of fluid leak varied widely (1 to 460 mL) and the volume of leak did not correlate with the development of PDPH. One patient who developed PDPH still had demonstrable CSF leakage 4 days after headache had resolved.

Schabel et al.[30] described a patient without headache who developed severe bilateral forearm pains after dural puncture. The arm pains were present only in the upright position and were completely relieved by epidural blood patch. The authors concluded that the symptoms were caused by traction on cervical nerve roots as a result of low CSF pressure. Severe interscapular pain with postural exacerbation has also occurred after lumbar puncture and was relieved by epidural blood patch.[31]

The pain of PDPH may be caused, in part, by an increase in cerebral blood flow as a consequence of low CSF pressure. This phenomenon has been observed in animals.[32,33] The inverse relationship between intracranial blood volume and CSF volume reflects the body's effort to maintain a constant intracranial volume.[34] The lumbar CSF compartment is a dynamic structure and acts as a reservoir for intracranial CSF volume adjustment.[35] The beneficial effect of the cerebral vasoconstrictor drugs (e.g., caffeine, theophylline) supports a vascular etiology for PDPH pain.

In the past, the belief that PDPH could have a psychologic component has led some physicians to suggest that the patient should not be warned about this complication. Vandam and Dripps[36] did not find a decreased incidence of PDPH in patients who unknowingly received spinal anesthesia during general anesthesia. In my opinion, psychologic factors do not affect the onset or incidence of PDPH, but they may affect the patient's response to PDPH.

Epidemiology

In a classic study of 10,098 spinal anesthetics published in 1956, Vandam and Dripps[36] noted that three patient factors influenced the incidence of PDPH: age, gender, and pregnancy.

AGE

Many clinical studies support the observation that PDPH is uncommon in patients older than 60 years of age and is most common in patients who are less than 40 years of age. In the elderly, the dura may be inelastic and less likely to gape. CSF leakage may be impeded by adhesions and calcification. The cerebrovascular system also may be less reactive in older patients. Further, this group is less active physically and older patients may be less likely to complain. It is possible that diligent questioning would reveal a higher incidence of PDPH in the elderly. Harrison and Langham[37] reported a 24% incidence of PDPH in a group of urology patients with a mean age of 71 years.

GENDER

Vandam and Dripps[36] observed a twofold increase in the incidence of PDPH in women (14% in women versus 7% in men). How can this be explained? Migraine occurs predominantly in females and is influenced by hormonal changes. Further, migraine results from changes in cerebral blood flow. The observed gender difference in the incidence of PDPH supports a cerebrovascular contribution to the symptomatology. Women may have enhanced vascular reactivity, or perhaps changes in cerebral blood flow are more likely to produce pain in women than in men. Some authors have even suggested that women are more likely to voice complaints than men!

More recent studies also support the concept that women are more susceptible to PDPH than men. A notable exception is the large prospective study by Lybecker et al,[38] which failed to show a gender difference.

PREGNANCY

Vandam and Dripps[36] also observed that the highest incidence of PDPH (22%) occurred after vaginal delivery. Migraine typically improves during pregnancy but may relapse soon after delivery. The cerebrovascular system appears to be especially reactive at a time when large hormonal changes are occurring in postpartum women. The reduction of intraabdominal pressure after delivery may reduce epidural pressure and encourage CSF leakage. Expulsive efforts in the second stage also would be expected to increase CSF leakage. This has prompted some physicians to restrict maternal pushing after dural puncture and to use forceps to shorten the second stage of labor. Stride and Cooper[39] reviewed 20 years of experience at the Birmingham Maternity Hospital. The use of prophylactic forceps did not affect the incidence of PDPH in those women who had sustained an unintentional dural puncture. In contrast, in a retrospective review of the records of laboring women who had experienced unintentional dural puncture, Angle et al.[40] found that those allowed to push were more likely to develop PDPH and to require epidural blood patch.

The concept that pregnancy is a risk factor for PDPH is not supported by contemporary practice. After spinal anesthesia, the incidence of PDPH in the parturient currently is similar to that reported in young men and nonpregnant women.

EFFECT OF HISTORY OF PREVIOUS PDPH

A history of PDPH after previous spinal anesthesia predisposes patients to the development of PDPH with another spinal anesthetic.[38,41]

EFFECT OF MULTIPLE DURAL PUNCTURES

Seeberger et al.[42] found that multiple dural punctures significantly increased the risk of PDPH.

CONTINUOUS SPINAL ANESTHESIA

Denny et al.[43] found a low incidence of PDPH after continuous spinal anesthesia in nonobstetric patients (mean age 63 years). They speculated that the presence of a spinal catheter caused an inflammatory response that promoted dural closure. Experience with prolonged spinal catheterization in obstetric patients has produced conflicting results.[44-46] Russell and Laishley[47] have debated the value of intrathecal catheterization after unintentional dural puncture.

COMBINED SPINAL EPIDURAL (CSE) ANESTHESIA

The CSE technique is widely used today for labor analgesia and, to a lesser extent, for cesarean section. Intuitively, it seems that the incidence of PDPH should be identical to that after single-shot spinal anesthesia with the same needle. However, it is possible that the CSE technique may lead to a lower incidence of PDPH than expected. Initial placement of the epidural needle facilitates precise dural puncture, and the subsequent increase in epidural space pressure after the epidural injection of local anesthetic may decrease CSF leakage. If the anesthesiologist is in doubt about correct epidural needle placement, a needle-through-needle dural puncture might resolve the issue and prevent dural puncture with a large-gauge epidural needle.[48] In vitro studies have shown that it is very difficult to force an epidural catheter through a dural hole made by a small-gauge needle.[49] It certainly is possible to achieve very low rates of PDPH with the CSE technique. Cox et al.[50] retrospectively reviewed records for more than 6000 obstetric patients who had CSE analgesia with a 27-gauge Whitacre needle. Among patients who had no more than two dural punctures, the incidence of PDPH was 0.13%.

MORBID OBESITY

Some evidence suggests that morbidly obese patients are less susceptible to PDPH.[51] Perhaps the increased intraabdominal pressure associated with obesity is transmitted to the epidural space and reduces CSF leakage.

Treatment

Early treatment of PDPH is indicated. Not only does this avert the vicious cycle of immobility, weakness, and depression, but it also may help prevent the rare case of subdural hematoma or cranial nerve palsy in patients with persistent PDPH.

PSYCHOLOGIC SUPPORT

The patient is aware that PDPH is an iatrogenic problem, and she may be angry and resentful as well as depressed and tearful. Headache makes it more difficult to care for the baby and to interact with other family members. Severe PDPH may delay discharge from the hospital and have economic consequences. Unlike patients who have PDPH after nonobstetric surgery, these patients typically are healthy and do not expect to feel ill. Two patients have eloquently described their own miserable experiences with postpartum PDPH.[52,53] Not surprisingly, a retrospective study of 43 obstetric patients with PDPH showed that this complication leads to a negative attitude toward epidural anesthesia.[54]

It is essential to visit the patient at least once daily to explain symptoms and prognosis, give support, and offer therapeutic options. If feasible, the patient's partner should attend these discussions. Nurses should help the patient as much as possible, especially with breast-feeding, which can be done in the lateral horizontal position.

The anesthesiologist and nurse should write detailed notes in the patient's record. After discharge, notes describing any follow-up telephone conversations should also be filed. Headache associated with regional anesthesia was the third most common reason for litigation in the obstetric anesthesia database of the American Society of Anesthesiologists (ASA) Closed-Claims Study.[55] Only maternal death and newborn brain damage were more common reasons for litigation. This should dispel any notion that postpartum PDPH is a trivial complaint.

POSTURE

The diagnosis of PDPH requires demonstration of a postural component. At least partial relief should occur when the patient assumes the horizontal position. The prone position relieves PDPH in some patients, presumably because increased intraabdominal pressure results in an increase in CSF pressure. Unfortunately, this position is not comfortable for many patients, especially those who delivered by cesarean section.

HYDRATION

Enhanced oral hydration remains a popular therapy for PDPH,[56] but there is no evidence that vigorous hydration has any therapeutic benefit in a patient with normal fluid intake. However, no patient with PDPH should be allowed to become dehydrated.

ABDOMINAL BINDER

A tight abdominal binder causes increased intraabdominal pressure, which may result in an increase in CSF pressure. This method of treatment has never undergone proper assessment but is still favored by some physicians.[56]

DRUGS

In the past, a variety of drugs have been used to treat PDPH, including steroids, vasopressin, alcohol, and ergotamine. A safe and effective oral drug therapy for PDPH would be very useful, even if relief is transient. Blood patch is not appropriate or effective in all patients.

Caffeine has been used to treat PDPH for many years, and Sechzer and Abel[57] have assessed its value in a randomized double-blind trial. Patients who received caffeine sodium benzoate 500 mg intravenously had better relief of PDPH than patients who received a placebo. The headache did not return after one or two doses of caffeine in 70% of patients. Camann et al.[58] observed that oral caffeine 300 mg was superior to a placebo for the relief of PDPH. Both studies showed that the beneficial effect of caffeine may be only transient. The caffeine content of a 150-mL cup of drip coffee is approximately 150 mg.[58]

Caffeine is a cerebral vasoconstrictor,[59] and one study has demonstrated a reduction of cerebral blood flow after intravenous administration of caffeine sodium benzoate for the treatment of PDPH.[60] Caffeine also is a potent central nervous system (CNS) stimulant. There are published case reports of seizures after intravenous administration of caffeine for the treatment of PDPH in postpartum patients.[61,62] Bolton et al.[62] described a seizure shortly after combined blood patch and intravenous caffeine therapy. Paech[63] reported seizures in a patient who had received oral caffeine (1000 mg during a 23-hour period). Transient atrial fibrillation complicated intravenous caffeine therapy for PDPH in a 71-year-old man.[64]

Caffeine appears in breast milk in very small amounts.[65] To my knowledge, there are no reports of adverse effects on the infant after maternal administration of one or two doses of caffeine for the treatment of PDPH. The risk:benefit ratio to mother and baby of multiple doses of caffeine has not been addressed. Until such studies are available it seems wise to restrict the prescription of oral caffeine to 600 mg in 24 hours, given as 300-mg doses at least 8 hours apart. Long-term caffeine therapy cannot be recommended.

Another methylxanthine, **theophylline**, also is a cerebral vasoconstrictor and is available in long-acting preparations. Some physicians have found that oral theophylline is more effective than placebo in the treatment of PDPH, but it has not become a popular therapy.

Sumatriptan is a serotonin agonist that affects predominantly type 1-D receptors. It has cerebral vasoconstrictor properties and is used in the treatment of migraine. This drug is expensive and is given by subcutaneous injection. Side effects include pain at the injection site and, uncommonly, chest tightness. Sumatriptan may promote coronary artery vasospasm and should not be used in those with Prinzmetal angina or known coronary artery disease. Carp et al.[66] reported the administration of sumatriptan 6 mg to six patients with PDPH, with complete resolution of headache in four. Others have concluded that sumatriptan may alleviate PDPH.[67,68] Connelly et al.[69] studied 10 patients with severe PDPH scheduled for epidural blood patch, who first received either sumatriptan 6 mg or placebo. After 1 hour only one patient in each group had significant relief, and the authors concluded that sumatriptan was of no value.

Kshatri and Foster[70] described a curative response to **adrenocorticotropic hormone (ACTH)** in two patients with PDPH. The dose used was 1.5 units/kg in 250 mL of normal saline, infused intravenously over 30 minutes. Gupta and Agrawal[71] assessed the effect of ACTH 60 units intramuscularly in 48 patients with PDPH. Complete and permanent relief was obtained in 40 patients, without any side effects. Carter and Pasupuleti[72] described the management of a patient with intractable PDPH who had already received three epidural blood patches. An infusion of **cosyntropin** 0.5 mg in 1L Ringer's lactate was infused over 8 hours, and the headache was completely and permanently relieved. Cosyntropin is a synthetic form of ACTH, and its side effects are restricted to glucocorticoid stimulation and rare hypersensitivity. Mood elevation, antiinflammatory effects, increased endorphin levels, and augmented intravascular volume are postulated as possible modes of action in the relief of headache with ACTH. Oliver and White[73] described three patients who experienced PDPH after administration of epidural analgesia during labor and who subsequently developed seizures. All had received two or three doses of ACTH (Synacthen 1 mg intramuscularly), and one had also received sumatriptan. No epidural blood patches were performed. CT scans showed or suggested infarction in two of these subjects. The authors stated that before the occurrence of these three cases, ACTH had been used regularly to treat PDPH in their institution, but that subsequently they had discontinued the administration of ACTH as a therapy for PDPH. No conclusion can be drawn about the possible contribution of ACTH therapy to the observed seizure activity. Proper prospective evaluation of the value of ACTH in the treatment of PDPH is required.

EPIDURAL MORPHINE

Eldor et al.[74] reported that epidural morphine helps relieve the symptoms of PDPH. However, caution is advised. In the presence of a dural hole, a local anesthetic agent injected epidurally may result in a more extensive block than anticipated. In a similar manner, epidural morphine might pass more readily into the CSF in a patient with a large hole in the dura.

EPIDURAL SALINE

Usubiaga et al.[75] demonstrated that epidural saline could relieve PDPH. They observed that injection of 10 to 20 mL of saline resulted in an immediate increase in both lumbar epidural and CSF pressures. A greater increase in CSF pressure than epidural pressure was observed. Both pressures returned to baseline measurements within 7 to 10 minutes. They concluded that the transient tamponade from increased epidural pressure could not account for the relief of headache. In a similar study in rats, Kroin et al.[76] have confirmed Usubiaga's findings with bolus epidural injections of saline. These authors also studied the effect of an epidural saline infusion. During infusion a sustained rise in CSF pressure was seen, but CSF pressure rapidly returned to baseline when the infusion was stopped. It is believed that the immediate relief of headache with a saline bolus results from transmission of increased lumbar CSF pressure to the brain, which decreases intracranial traction and causes reflex cerebral vasoconstriction.

Bolus epidural saline is less effective therapy for PDPH than blood patch, and the benefit typically is transient.[77] Some anesthesiologists have reported the successful use of prolonged (e.g., 24 hours) epidural saline infusion for the treatment of persistent PDPH in patients with a failed blood patch.[78,79] The rate of infusion (15 to 20 mL/hr) was limited by the onset of pain in the back, legs, and eyes.

EPIDURAL BLOOD PATCH

In 1960 Gormley[80] introduced autologous epidural blood patch into clinical practice. He reported relief of headache after epidural administration of only 2 to 3 mL of blood. Subsequently, DiGiovanni and Dunbar[81] reported an immediate and permanent cure of PDPH in 41 of 45 patients who received 10 mL of epidural blood. Their success led to the widespread adoption of this technique for the relief of PDPH.

The optimum volume of injected blood remains controversial. Crawford[82] obtained better results with 20 mL of blood than with the smaller volumes used by Gormley and DiGiovanni.[80,81]

Szeinfeld et al.[83] used a gamma camera to observe the epidural spread of technetium-labeled red blood cells during and after epidural blood patch. They injected blood until pain occurred in the back, buttocks, or legs. The mean ± SD volume injected was 14.8 ± 1.7 mL of blood, and the mean ± SD spread was 9.0 ± 2.0 spinal segments (Figure 32-1). Blood spread more readily in the cephalad than in the caudad direc-

tion. Blood patch relieved headache in all 10 patients. The investigators concluded that 12 to 15 mL of blood should be sufficient for blood patch in most patients. Taivenen et al.[84] found that injection of a "height-adjusted" volume of blood (minimum of 10 mL to a maximum of 15 mL) conferred no advantage over a standard 10-mL injection.

Beards et al.[85] performed MRI studies after performance of blood patch (18 to 20 mL) in five patients (Figures 32-2 and 32-3). They noted that the injected blood spread over three to five segments in a predominantly cephalad direction. All patients had an extensive hematoma in subcutaneous fat, and some also had displacement of nerve roots and/or evidence of intrathecal blood. A thick layer of mature clot had formed by 7 hours, but this had broken up into smaller clots by 18 hours. These findings may help to explain the back pain and occasional nerve root pain that occur after blood patch. Vakharia et al.[86] also performed MRI studies after blood patch. They noted compression of the thecal sac and a mean spread of 4.6 segments after the injection of 20 mL of blood (Figures 32-4 and 32-5).

Djurhuus et al.[87] employed CT epidurography in four patients immediately and 24 hours after an 18-mL blood patch. Initial images showed adherence of clot to the dura in three patients, as well as dural compression in two patients, but there was no evidence of compression at 24 hours.

Subsequent studies have not confirmed initial reports that epidural blood patch results in at least 90% permanent cure of PDPH. Lack of proper follow-up probably accounts for the higher success rates noted in earlier reports. Taivainen et al.[84] found that although immediate relief was reported in 88% to 96% of patients, a permanent cure was achieved in only 61%. Safa-Tisseront et al.[88] reviewed the experience with blood patch at their institution over a 12-year period. The 504 patients studied were a heterogenous group and included 78 parturients. Complete relief of PDPH was obtained in 75%, partial relief in 18%, and treatment failed in 7% of patients. The authors noted a significant increase in the failure rate of blood patch after large-gauge needle puncture of the dura.

In populations limited to obstetric patients, the published success rates of epidural blood patch have been even less

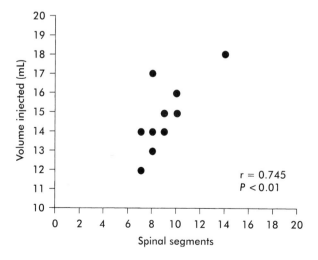

FIGURE 32-1. Correlation between milliliters of injected blood and number of spinal segments of blood-spread. (Modified from Szeinfeld M, Ihmeidan IH, Moser MM, et al. Epidural blood patch: Evaluation of the volume and spread of blood injected into the epidural space. Anesthesiology 1986; 64:820-2.)

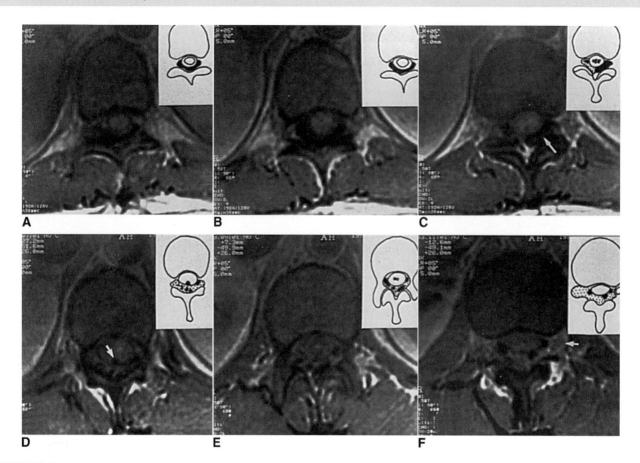

FIGURE 32-2. A-F, A series of six axial T1 weighted GE images, demonstrating the distribution of blood within the epidural space in a patient 3 hours after injection. The inset on each image shows the distribution of blood as derived from both T1 and sagittal Short Tau Inversion Recovery (STIR) images. Images are equidistantly spaced between T10 (**A**) and L3 (**F**). The arrow on **C** indicates a clot extending out through the left neural outlet foramen. In **D**, the arrow indicates a small focus of clot lying within and adherent to the thecal sac. The arrow in **F** indicates the dorsal root ganglion displaced downwards and anteriorly by the epidural clot. (From Beards SC, Jackson A, Griffiths AG, Horsman EL. Magnetic resonance imaging of extradural blood patches: Appearances from 30 min to 18 H. Br J Anaesth 1993; 71:182-8.)

encouraging. Stride and Cooper[39] noted 64% complete and permanent relief of headache after one blood patch. Banks et al.[89] concluded that the first blood patch resulted in permanent relief of PDPH in 43% of parturients. Williams et al.[90] presented especially disappointing results; only 33% of their patients obtained complete and permanent relief from the first blood patch. The authors suggested that this high failure rate might be related, in part, to their frequent performance of blood patch within 24 hours of dural puncture.

Using a goat model, DiGiovanni et al.[91] examined the microscopic appearance of the dura as long as 6 months after dural puncture. Some study animals received a 2-mL blood patch in addition to dural puncture. The authors concluded that the blood patch acted as a gelatinous tampon that produced no harmful tissue reaction.

Relief of PDPH after blood patch is often rapid, but CSF volume is not restored immediately. There must be another explanation for the immediate relief of headache. Carrie[92] hypothesized that epidural injection of blood increases increased lumbar CSF pressure, which restores intracranial CSF pressure and results in decreased symptoms. Increased CSF pressure also may result in reflex cerebral vasoconstriction. Coombs and Hooper[93] demonstrated that epidural blood patch resulted in a threefold increase in lumbar CSF pressure. Further, they noted that 15 minutes later, lumbar CSF pressure was sustained at greater than 70% of the peak pressure observed after the injection of blood. Kroin et al.[76]

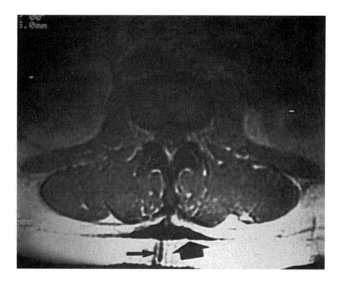

FIGURE 32-3. Axial T1 image after blood patch in a patient, showing blood spread into the subcutaneous fat (*large arrow;* blood appears dark) at the level of the needle track (*small arrow*). (From Beards SC, Jackson A, Griffiths AG, Horsman EL. Magnetic resonance imaging of extradural blood patches: Appearances from 30 min to 18 H. Br J Anaesth 1993; 71:182-8.)

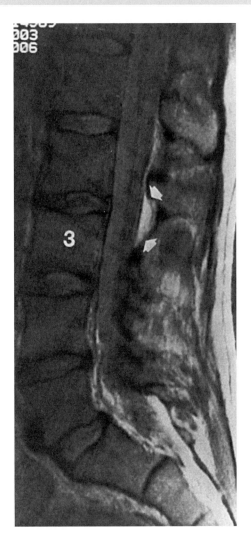

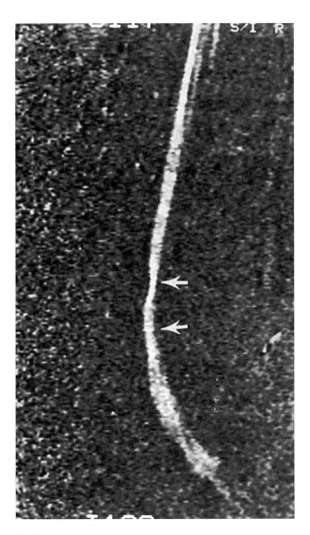

FIGURE 32-4. Pre-blood patch (sagittal spin proton echo density). The dural puncture has been performed at L2-3, and local static fluid collection (*arrows*) affirms this. (From Vakharia SB, Thomas PS, Rosenbaum AE, et al. Magnetic resonance imaging of cerebrospinal fluid leak and tamponade effect of blood patch in postdural puncture headache. Anesth Analg 1997; 84:585-90.)

FIGURE 32-5. Post-blood patch CSF flow study in systole shows the long length of the compression of the thecal sac posteriorly (*arrows*). (From Vakharia SB, Thomas PS, Rosenbaum AE, et al. Magnetic resonance imaging of cerebrospinal fluid leak and tamponade effect of blood patch in postdural puncture headache. Anesth Analg 1997; 84:585-90.)

observed that epidural injection of blood in rats caused a sustained increase in CSF pressure throughout a 4-hour study period.

In a Cochrane Review, Sudlow and Warlow[94] assessed the value of blood patch for prevention and treatment of PDPH. They noted a striking lack of reliable scientific data for analysis. Only one small randomized trial of the therapeutic use of blood patch was eligible for review.[95] That study showed that a true blood patch is more effective than a sham patch. Sudlow and Warlow[94] concluded that properly conducted randomized trials are needed before conclusions can be drawn about the value and safety of blood patch. Meanwhile, they suggested that epidural blood patch be reserved for exceptional cases. While I agree that far more work needs to be done, few anesthesiologists would be willing to abandon epidural blood patch for the treatment of severe PDPH. This treatment, while not perfect, often dramatically relieves this debilitating condition, and at present we have little else to offer.

Blood patch also has been used successfully for the treatment of hearing loss,[96] durocutaneous fistula,[97] and postural

arm[30] and thoracic[31] pain after dural puncture; spontaneous intracranial hypotension[98]; and CSF leak after spinal surgery.[99]

Risks of Blood Patch

Conventional wisdom holds that the patient should be afebrile at the time of blood patch. Many anesthesiologists believe that it is wise to avoid the epidural injection of blood in the presence of systemic infection. Meningitis[100,101] and acute severe aseptic meningeal irritation[102] have occurred after blood patch.

After conservative measures have failed, the optimal way of treating a febrile patient with severe, persistent PDPH is controversial. Epidural infusion of saline involves the use of an indwelling epidural catheter for many hours, which also may be undesirable in a febrile patient. Dextran-40 may be an alternative choice for patch in febrile patients, but further experience is needed in healthy patients before this technique can be recommended. The presence of high fever and/or other evidence of sepsis contraindicates the performance of blood patch. However, I do not believe that a low-grade fever of known etiology is an absolute contraindication to epidural blood patch, provided the patient is receiving appropriate antibiotic therapy. Management should be individualized, and the known benefits of blood patch should be weighed against the unknown risk of infection.

Bucklin et al.[103] reported the conservative management of a woman with acute leukemia and PDPH. The authors discussed the therapeutic options in this immunocompromised patient.

The risk of epidural blood patch in the presence of HIV infection has been debated.[104] There are published cases of the successful use of blood patch, without sequelae, in patients with AIDS or who are HIV-positive.[105,106]

Abouleish et al.[107] reported the results of the long-term evaluation of 118 patients who had received an epidural blood patch. They observed that back pain was the most common complication. Back pain occurred during the first 48 hours in 35% of patients and persisted in 16% of patients, with a mean duration of 27 days. These investigators also noted some cases of neck pain, lower extremity radicular pain, and transient temperature elevation. Others have reported cases of transient but severe nerve root irritation[108,109] and seventh cranial nerve palsy[110] after blood patch. There have been two reports of spinal subdural hematoma after the use of an unusual technique for blood patch.[111,112] (Dural puncture was performed and the needle subsequently withdrawn until CSF no longer flowed. Blood was then injected.) A similar method produced lumbosacral meningismus with serious sequelae in another patient.[113] This technique cannot be recommended for routine practice. However, Shantha and Bisese[114] reported the deliberate, uncomplicated subdural injection of blood under radiographic guidance in one patient who had received two unsuccessful blood patches. Incapacitating back pain, which eventually resolved, has been reported after blood patch.[115-117]

Acute mental deterioration after blood patch should be considered as evidence of possible intracranial pathology (e.g., increased ICP) and investigated immediately.[13,118,119]

Blood patch has been temporally associated with seizures and a subsequent diagnosis of late-onset eclampsia.[120,121] Woodward et al.[122] noted immediate and severe exacerbation of headache, as well as neck and shoulder symptoms, after a blood patch. These symptoms responded to analgesic therapy.

Dunbar and Katz[123] described three patients with PDPH and cranial nerve palsies who were treated with blood patch. The palsies failed to resolve for several months after treatment. They suggested that earlier use of blood patch in the treatment of PDPH might have avoided the development of this serious complication.

Ong et al.[124] found that a history of wet tap decreased the success of future epidural anesthesia, but this was not confirmed by Blanche et al.[125] In both of these retrospective studies, a history of blood patch had no apparent effect on the quality of subsequent epidural anesthesia. In a retrospective study, Hebl et al.[126] examined this issue using matched controls. They concluded that future epidural analgesia was not impaired after dural puncture, with or without blood patch. Loughrey et al.[127] described a patient who experienced PDPH after diagnostic lumbar puncture at term gestation. Blood patch was performed and headache was relieved, but 6 hours later urgent cesarean section was required. Spinal anesthesia was administered via the same intervertebral space as the blood patch. The anesthetic course and postoperative period were uneventful, and the patient had no recurrence of headache.

Serious problems after blood patch are rare and typically appear in association with an unusual technique or steroid injection. However, Diaz[128] has described a woman who developed permanent paraparesis and cauda equina syndrome after epidural blood patch for PDPH. Thirty ml of blood were injected slowly and without symptoms. After treatment low back pain and leg pain developed, and later the patient also developed incontinence. Twelve days after the patch a subdural hematoma at L2-L4 was diagnosed and surgically treated. Six months later the patient still had marked symptoms. This case report is alarming. Although a larger volume of blood than usual was injected, the technique appears to have been within normal practice standards.

Apart from these reports of rare problems, epidural blood patch has a good track record. It may be repeated, perhaps with a larger volume of blood, if the initial patch fails to relieve pain. Often the second patch is successful. The diagnosis should be reconsidered if headache persists after two failed blood patches. A neurology consultation is desirable when a PDPH fails to respond to two blood patches and should definitely be requested if there is any doubt about the diagnosis.

Technique for Blood Patch

The anesthesiologist must provide a thorough explanation of the risks and benefits. The patient should give written consent to the procedure, which can be accomplished on an outpatient basis if necessary. Transient bradycardia was observed in 10 patients after blood patch, and some anesthesiologists may choose to establish intravenous access and monitor the ECG in selected patients.[129] The lateral position is more comfortable than the sitting position in patients with severe headache. If the anesthesiologist is uncertain as to the location of the dural puncture, the more caudad interspace should be chosen. The anesthesiologist identifies the epidural space in the usual manner. Using meticulous sterile technique, an assistant then withdraws 15 to 20 mL of blood. This blood is injected slowly, but the injection is terminated if pain occurs. Blood patch has been used in a Jehovah's Witness with a technique designed to keep blood in continuity with the circulation.[130]

Occasionally a few drops of CSF are encountered on entering the epidural space, which may lead to doubt about correct needle placement.[131] In this situation a small test dose of a local anesthetic agent should be administered, sufficient to cause a rapid onset of spinal anesthesia. If no block results, blood patch can be performed.

After the procedure the patient should rest quietly in the horizontal position for 1 to 2 hours.[132] Subsequently the patient may resume ambulation, but she should avoid vigorous physical activity for several days. It would be wise for the patient to avoid the Valsalva maneuver and heavy lifting. A stool softener should be prescribed.

DEXTRAN PATCH

Barrios-Alarcon et al.[133] reported that epidural administration of 20 to 30 mL of dextran-40 is as effective and safe as blood patch for the relief of PDPH. In their series of 56 patients, all headaches were relieved permanently. Relief occurred within 2 hours in the majority of patients. The only side effect was a transient discomfort or burning sensation at the time of injection in six patients. Others also have had success with this method.[134] Some physicians have treated intractable PDPH successfully by performing a dextran-40 patch followed by epidural infusion of dextran at 3 mL/hour.[135,136] The duration of infusion was 12 hours in Reynvoet's patient[136] but was not specified by Aldrete.[135]

Lander and Korbon[137] reported (in abstract form) a study of three groups of sheep subjected to dural puncture. The first group received epidural blood patch, the second a dextran-40 patch, and the third no treatment. They examined the microscopic appearance of the dura at 24 and 48 hours and at 7 and 30 days after the puncture. Vigorous fibroblastic activity was observed in the blood-patch group. In contrast, the dura from animals in the other two groups appeared normal.

Additional information on the neurologic effects of dextran is needed before it can be widely adopted for patching. From MRI studies of blood patch we can anticipate that some dextran will enter the subarachnoid space. The small but definite risk of anaphylaxis after the injection of dextran also must be considered.

FIBRIN GLUE FOR PATCH

Fibrin glue is prepared from human pooled plasma and, among other uses, it is employed to repair dural leaks during surgery.[138] When injected it forms a firm, nonretractable fibrin clot. Epidural injection of fibrin glue in rats produces a sustained rise in CSF pressure comparable to the increase that occurs after injection of blood.[76] An epidural fibrin glue patch has been used successfully to treat recurrent PDPH,[139] spontaneous intracranial hypotension,[140] and CSF leak after long-term intrathecal catheterization.[141] In the future, fibrin glue may have a role in patients with intractable PDPH, but today it is certainly not to be recommended for routine use.

SURGERY

There are rare reports of curative surgical closure of a dural rent for intractable PDPH. In one case, the interval between dural puncture and surgery was 5 years.[22]

SUMMARY OF TREATMENT

Patients with PDPH should rest in the horizontal position and receive psychologic support. Mild headache often responds to oral analgesics and/or caffeine. If headache is severe, the physician may either try caffeine or proceed directly to blood patch. The optimal timing for blood patching has never been studied adequately, but some anesthesiologists have an *impression* that a blood patch done within the first 24 hours of dural puncture is more likely to fail. Perhaps this is because the large CSF leak displaces the clot. Alternatively, early-onset PDPH (often resulting from dural puncture with a large-gauge needle) is likely to be more severe and more difficult to treat. A second blood patch can be performed if the first patch fails. If the second blood patch fails, alternative diagnoses should be excluded before the performance of a third patch or a trial of other therapies.

Prevention of PDPH

POSTURE

Studies consistently have shown that 24 hours of prophylactic bed rest does *not* decrease the incidence or severity of PDPH after inpatient spinal anesthesia[142,143] or diagnostic lumbar puncture.[144] Other postural maneuvers during the immediate postdural puncture period (e.g., adoption of the head-down or prone position) also are not helpful. In a Cochrane Review, Sudlow and Warlow[145] have made the same conclusion. It is important to encourage early ambulation during the puerperium. Pregnant women are hypercoagulable and are at

increased risk for deep vein thrombosis and pulmonary embolism (see Chapter 38).

Outpatient surgery patients typically are discharged early and may be remarkably active for prolonged periods soon after spinal anesthesia dissipates. Compared with gentle mobilization in a hospital room, this vigorous activity could possibly provoke PDPH. A high incidence of PDPH has been reported with the use of fine-gauge needles in young patients undergoing outpatient surgery.[146,147] It is conceivable, but as yet unproven, that there may be benefits to resting quietly and limiting activity on the day of surgery.

HYDRATION

Many physicians continue to encourage patients to drink copious volumes of fluid after dural puncture[56] in the belief that excess hydration will increase CSF production. The rate of CSF formation is thought to be relatively constant, but data in humans are limited.[148] A Cochrane Review found insufficient evidence to support or refute the beneficial effect of prophylactic supplemental hydration.[145] I know of no clinically useful method of increasing CSF production and recommend maintenance of normal hydration.

ABDOMINAL BINDER

Some physicians have recommended the use of a tight abdominal binder to prevent PDPH, but it is seldom used today.

INTRASPINAL OPIOIDS

In a randomized trial of spinal anesthesia with bupivacaine, Abboud et al.[149] showed that the addition of morphine 0.2 mg offered no protection against PDPH. Eldor and Guedj[150] reported that 3 to 4 mg of epidural morphine, given once after spinal anesthesia and repeated 14 hours later, did not prevent PDPH. Devcic et al.[151] found that the addition of intrathecal fentanyl to bupivacaine did not reduce the incidence of PDPH.

PROPHYLACTIC EPIDURAL SALINE

In an uncontrolled study, Craft et al.[152] found that two boluses of epidural saline through a catheter were highly effective in reducing the incidence of PDPH after inadvertent dural puncture. This work has not been confirmed. Shah[153] studied 17 patients who received an epidural saline infusion (at a rate of approximately 40 mL/hr) for 24 to 36 hours after unintentional dural puncture. Four patients complained of severe interscapular pain, which resolved when the infusion rate was reduced. Severe PDPH developed in 47% of patients after the infusion was stopped. In the retrospective survey by Stride and Cooper,[39] prophylactic epidural infusion of crystalloid had no effect on the overall incidence of PDPH but did reduce the severity of symptoms. Despite these discouraging results, prophylactic epidural saline infusions continue to be popular in some centers. All residual local anesthetic effects should disappear before an epidural saline infusion is started.

PROPHYLACTIC INTRATHECAL SALINE

Charsley and Abram[154] reported a nonrandomized, controlled study of patients who experienced unintentional dural puncture. Immediate injection of 10 mL of normal saline before needle withdrawal reduced the subsequent incidence of headache and the need for blood patch. Kuczkowski and Benumof[155] treated seven laboring patients—who experienced unintentional dural puncture—with reinjection of lost

CSF, intrathecal catheterization, and injection of 3 to 5 mL of normal saline. This was followed by maintenance of continuous spinal analgesia, and the intrathecal catheter was left in place for 12 to 20 hours. Only one patient developed PDPH, but no conclusion can be drawn regarding the contribution of intrathecal saline to this result. The intrathecal injection of saline after unintentional dural puncture deserves further study.

PROPHYLACTIC BLOOD PATCH

DiGiovanni and Dunbar[81] first suggested that prophylactic epidural blood patch might help prevent PDPH, but early studies were disappointing. However, treatments were not randomly assigned, and the amount of blood injected was sometimes smaller than that recommended today. Colonna-Romano and Shapiro[156] have reevaluated the use of prophylactic blood patch. They studied patients who suffered unintentional dural puncture and in whom an epidural catheter was placed correctly at an alternative interspace. After either vaginal or cesarean delivery, they randomized these patients to receive either a prophylactic blood patch (15 mL of blood administered through the catheter) or no treatment. The incidence of PDPH was 21% in the blood-patch group versus 80% in the control group. Others have reported similar results.[157-159] However, a Cochrane Review found insufficient scientific evidence to recommend the use of prophylactic blood patch.[94]

Because unintentional dural puncture with a 16- or 18-gauge epidural needle results in a 70% to 80% incidence of PDPH, some anesthesiologists believe that prophylactic blood patch is always justified. Others argue that a significant number of patients will receive unnecessary treatment and that blood patch is not devoid of complications. Some anesthesiologists call attention to the potential for epidural catheters to become contaminated after prolonged use. The injection of blood through a nonsterile catheter could increase the risk of infection when compared with injection through an epidural needle placed *de novo*. Prophylactic blood patch is gaining in popularity and is performed in 25% of the North American academic centers surveyed by Berger et al.[56] The economic impact of prolonged hospitalization for PDPH may be partly responsible for the increased popularity of this technique.

For several reasons a prophylactic blood patch should not be performed until all evidence of local anesthetic block has disappeared. First, the patient should have full return of sensation because the occurrence of pain is a signal to stop the injection of blood. Second, evidence suggests that lidocaine may inhibit coagulation.[160] Third, Leivers[161] reported a case of total spinal anesthesia after the epidural injection of 15 mL of blood before epidural anesthesia had regressed. The patient made an uneventful recovery. He speculated that residual lidocaine in the lumbar CSF was transferred to the brain as a consequence of an increase in lumbar CSF pressure produced by the patch. (Editor's note: I have observed one case of transient, total blindness after the rapid, bolus injection of 30 mL of epidural saline after vaginal delivery in a patient who had experienced unintentional dural puncture during labor. The blindness resolved after approximately 15 to 20 minutes, and subsequent ophthalmologic and neurologic examinations were normal. The etiology of the transient blindness was unclear. Nonetheless, it seems prudent to delay administration of prophylactic epidural saline or blood patch until the block has regressed and to avoid rapid epidural administration of blood or saline at any time.)

It is extremely important to avoid the intrathecal injection of blood. Aldrete and Brown[162] reported a case of intrathecal hematoma and arachnoiditis with prolonged neurologic sequelae after prophylactic blood patch. Twenty milliliters of blood were injected through an epidural catheter that in retrospect had been positioned in the subarachnoid space. There was considerable resistance to injection of the blood, and severe lower back pain with tinnitus accompanied the procedure.

Waters et al.[163] described their management of nine patients in whom postoperative epidural analgesia was planned but who sustained unintentional preoperative dural puncture. An epidural catheter was subsequently placed at a different interspace, and immediate prophylactic blood patch was performed through the catheter. General anesthesia was then administered for surgery, and bupivacaine and fentanyl were given through the epidural catheter for postoperative analgesia. Satisfactory pain relief was obtained and only one mild PDPH occurred. In spite of this report, I remain concerned that any adverse effects of blood patch could be masked by general anesthesia and subsequent epidural infusion of local anesthetic.

PROPHYLACTIC DEXTRAN PATCH

Salvador et al.[164] reported the prophylactic epidural injection of 20 mL of dextran-40 in 17 patients (mean age of 26 years) who had experienced unintentional dural puncture with a 17- or 18-gauge needle. None of these patients experienced PDPH.

MODIFICATIONS OF REGIONAL ANESTHETIC TECHNIQUE

Many technical factors influence the incidence of PDPH.

Needle Size

With the Quincke needle, the incidence and severity of PDPH are directly related to the size of the needle used.[165] A similar relationship may exist with pencil-point needles.[166] When needles smaller than 27-gauge are used, the incidence of PDPH is very low, but technical problems with needle insertion and failure to produce adequate anesthesia are more common.[167,168] Locating the epidural space before insertion of the spinal needle may improve the rate of success with these fine-gauge needles. The experience of the anesthesia provider is another important factor.[169]

Needle Design

In the past, the beveled Quincke needle (Figure 32-6) has been the most widely used needle for dural puncture for both diagnostic and anesthetic purposes. If this needle is used for spinal anesthesia in the parturient, the incidence of PDPH appears to be lower with a 27-gauge needle than with 25- and 26-gauge needles.[170,171] The 27-gauge Quincke needle is easy to use and the bevel should be inserted parallel to the long axis of the spine.[172]

In 1951, Hart and Whitacre[173] introduced a solid-tipped, pencil-point spinal needle with a lateral injection port, which is now known as the Whitacre design (see Figure 32-6). They believed that their new needle would stretch and separate rather than cut the dural fibers and result in a lower incidence of PDPH. Both 25- and 27-gauge Whitacre needles currently are very popular, and studies have confirmed the anticipated low incidence of PDPH.[170,174,175] A randomized comparison of 27-gauge Quincke and pencil-point needles revealed a significantly lower incidence of PDPH in the pencil-point group.[176] Some evidence *in vitro* suggests that fluid leak through a dural hole is lower with pencil-point than with beveled needles.[177] Deviation of the needle from the midline also may occur less frequently with the pencil-point design.[178]

In 1987 Sprotte et al.[179] reported experience with the use of a new needle that was designed to reduce the risk of neural and dural trauma (see Figure 32-6). They reported a 0.02% incidence of PDPH in a heterogeneous patient population. The Sprotte needle has a solid ogival tip and a longer side-port than the Whitacre needle. Earlier concerns that the long side-port might lead to an increased failure rate of spinal anesthesia have not been confirmed in clinical practice. Cesarini et al.[171] performed a randomized trial of 24-gauge Sprotte and 25-gauge Quincke needles in patients receiving spinal anesthesia for cesarean section. There were no cases of PDPH in the Sprotte group but a 14.5% incidence of PDPH in the Quincke group. Ross et al.[180] confirmed a significantly lower incidence of PDPH with the 24-gauge Sprotte needle compared with 25- and 26-gauge Quincke needles in obstetric patients.

A modification of the Quincke needle has been made available. Known as the Atraucan needle, it has a cutting point and a double bevel, which are intended to cut a small dural hole and then dilate it (see Figure 32-6).[181] Clinical experience with the Atraucan needle has been generally good,[182] but one study noted an increased need for blood patch compared with the use of a pencil-point needle.[183]

The current popularity of spinal anesthesia in obstetric patients largely is a result of new needle technology. Refinements of needle gauge and design have led to a reduction in the incidence of PDPH (Table 32-1). Which needle should be chosen for spinal anesthesia? In a meta-analysis, Halpern and Preston[184] concluded that (1) a non-cutting needle should be used for patients at high risk for PDPH, and (2) the smallest gauge needle available should be used for all patients. There are times when urgency or body habitus will dictate the use of a larger needle, but there is seldom justification for using a Quincke needle larger than 27-gauge.

Manufacturers throughout the world are now marketing high quality needles of the pencil-point type, sometimes with design variations. The anesthesiologist should gain experience with one needle and examine the associated technical failure rate and incidence of PDPH. If results are unsatisfactory, another needle should be chosen. Every effort should be made to use a needle associated with a low incidence of PDPH. The additional cost is entirely justified if it prevents this debilitating symptom that interferes with everyday life and may delay return to normal activity for a prolonged period.

Direction of Bevel of Quincke Needle

An early study by Franksson and Gordh[185] demonstrated that orientation of the bevel of a Quincke spinal needle parallel to the long axis of the spine produced less dural trauma than occurred when the bevel was inserted perpendicularly. These investigators thought that the dural fibers were predominantly longitudinal in direction. Electron microscopy has revealed that the dural structure is far more complex than originally was supposed. Fink and Walker[186] noted that the dura consists of multidirectional interlacing collagen fibers and both transverse and longitudinal elastic fibers. However, they suggested that the insertion of the needle with the bevel parallel to the long axis of the spine most likely results in less tension on the dural hole. Patin et al.[187] studied specimens of human and canine lumbar dura mater and concluded that "the lumbar dura is a longitudinally oriented structure." On the other hand, a study by Reina et al.[188] demonstrated no evidence of longitudinal parallel fibers in the dura. Rather, they found the dura to be oriented concentrically in well-defined layers.

In vitro studies of bevel orientation and fluid leak have provided conflicting results.[189,190] Dittmann et al.[191] noted that after puncture, the microscopic appearance of the dura resembled a tin-can lid. This could act like a flap and reduce the leakage of CSF. Despite confusing anatomic evidence, clinical experience strongly supports insertion of the Quincke needle with the bevel parallel to the long axis of the spine. Studies have confirmed that this maneuver reduces the incidence of PDPH after diagnostic lumbar puncture[192] and spinal anesthesia.[38,193] The influence of the orientation of the bevel remains important with the 27-gauge needle.[172]

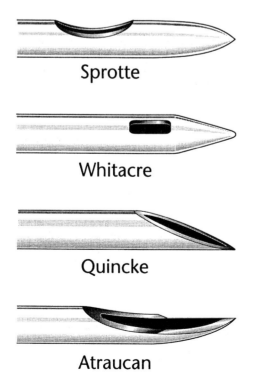

FIGURE 32-6. Spinal needle tip design (not to scale).

TABLE 32-1	PDPH: EXPERIENCE AT BRIGHAM AND WOMEN'S HOSPITAL		
Year	Needle	Number of patients	PDPH (%)
1987-88	26Q	1072	5.6
1988-89	26Q	1024	4.7
1989-90	26Q	152	5.9
	27Q	779	2.7
	25W	64	0
	27Q	81	1.2
1990-91	25W	936	1.2

Q, Quincke; W, Whitacre.
Modified from Lambert DH, Hurley RJ, Hertwig L, et al. Role of needle gauge and tip configuration in the production of lumbar puncture headache. Reg Anesth 1997; 22:66-72.

Direction of Bevel of Tuohy Needle

Norris et al.[194] examined two groups of women who received epidural anesthesia with a Tuohy needle. In one group the bevel was kept perpendicular to the long axis of the spine. In the other group the needle entered the epidural space with the bevel parallel to the long axis and the needle was then rotated 90 degrees before insertion of the catheter. The authors observed a decreased incidence of PDPH in the latter group. However, some anesthesiologists argue that rotation of the needle within the epidural space may increase the risk of inadvertent dural puncture. Richardson and Wissler[195] randomized laboring patients to a cephalad or lateral orientation of the Tuohy bevel during epidural needle insertion. The needle was not rotated before insertion of the epidural catheter. There was no difference in dural puncture rates, but catheter insertion was easier with a cephalad orientation of the bevel. Lewis et al.[196] demonstrated that more force was required to puncture the dura *in vitro* if an epidural needle was inserted perpendicular to the dural fibers rather than parallel.

Midline or Paramedian Approach

At least one *in vitro* study suggests that insertion of the needle at an acute angle results in decreased leakage of CSF.[190] Hatfalvi[197] reported no cases of PDPH in a retrospective survey of 4465 spinal anesthetics. The author used a paramedian approach with a 20-gauge Quincke needle, and the skin was punctured 3 cm from the midline. He suggested that tangential puncture, at approximately 35 degrees with the bevel facing the dura, creates a dural flap and prevents PDPH.

Using a rigid paper cylinder model of the dura, Kempen and Mocek[198] studied median and paramedian punctures with a 22-gauge Quincke needle in different orientations. With median punctures, all entry and exit holes were of uniform size regardless of bevel orientation, and no flaps were seen. After paramedian punctures, flaps formed when the needle bevel faced the cylinder surface with a near-tangential angle of perforation.

As yet no convincing clinical evidence suggests that the paramedian approach consistently protects against PDPH. However, it certainly is possible that the angle and site of dural perforation could influence the incidence of PDPH.

Needle Tip Damage

It is conceivable that a damaged needle tip might increase dural trauma and predispose a patient to PDPH. Puolakka et al.[199] performed a randomized study of 400 spinal anesthetics, comparing 27-gauge pencil-point and Quincke needles. Each needle was examined with a microscope after use. None of the pencil-point needles were damaged, but 13% to 14% of the Quincke needles were blunt, bent, or hooked. However, the occurrence of PDPH did not correlate with needle damage.

Method of Locating the Epidural Space: Air or Saline

The method of locating the epidural space may influence the incidence of PDPH, and this issue has been debated by Russell and Douglas.[200] In Great Britain the loss-of-resistance-to-saline technique has been widely adopted in the belief that it is associated with a lower incidence of unintentional dural puncture and PDPH than the use of air. The use of air for loss of resistance certainly increases the risk of pneumocephalus.

Reinsertion of the Stylet after Lumbar Puncture

Strupp and Brandt[201] reported that reinsertion of the stylet prior to withdrawal of a 21-gauge Sprotte needle used for diagnostic lumbar puncture significantly reduced the incidence of PDPH. Perhaps the dural tear is reconfigured by this maneuver, which deserves further evaluation.

Choice of Local Anesthetic Drug for Spinal Anesthesia

Naulty et al.[202] reported that the use of bupivacaine-glucose or lidocaine-glucose for spinal anesthesia was associated with a higher incidence of PDPH than tetracaine-procaine. They postulated that osmotic, cerebral irritant, and/or cerebrovascular effects could be responsible for these findings.

Air Travel

There have been several reports of recurrence of PDPH during air travel.[203-205] Presumably, these recurrences were precipitated by decreased atmospheric pressure changing the gradient between the subarachnoid and the epidural space.

CONCLUDING CAUTIONARY REMARKS

We continue to lack much important information about PDPH. A large, detailed prospective study of PDPH, with and without blood patch, with a follow-up period of 1 year, is needed in obstetric patients. What are the long-term effects of both PDPH and blood patch? How common are residual back pain, neurologic symptoms, auditory/visual symptoms, and interference with everyday life? Answers to these questions are needed to give our patients reliable information, a sound basis for informed consent, and the best possible care.

KEY POINTS

- Dural puncture is only one of many causes of postpartum headache.
- A patient with PDPH experiences an exacerbation of symptoms when she moves from the horizontal to the upright position.
- After dural puncture, leakage of CSF produces decreased ICP, traction on pain-sensitive intracranial structures, and cerebral vasodilation.
- The initial therapy for PDPH includes psychologic support, bed rest in the horizontal position, and oral analgesics. Although dehydration should be avoided, no evidence suggests that vigorous hydration has any prophylactic or therapeutic benefit.
- Intravenous or oral caffeine ameliorates the symptoms of PDPH in some patients.
- The first epidural blood patch often results in permanent relief of PDPH. A second blood patch may be performed—and typically is successful—if the first patch fails. If the second blood patch fails, alternative diagnoses should be excluded before the performance of a third patch or a trial of other therapies.

REFERENCES

1. Benhamou D, Hamza J, Ducot B. Postpartum headache after epidural analgesia without dural puncture. Internat J Obstet Anesth 1995; 4: 17-20.
2. Silberstein SD. Migraine and pregnancy. J Soc Obstet Gynaecol Can 2000; 22:700-7.
3. Alfery DD, Marsh ML, Shapiro HM. Postspinal headache or intracranial tumor after obstetric anesthesia. Anesthesiology 1979; 51:92-4.
4. Kardash K, Morrow F, Béïque F. Seizures after epidural blood patch with undiagnosed subdural hematoma. Reg Anesth Pain Med 2002; 27:433-6.
5. Vaughan DJA, Stirrup CA, Robinson PN. Cranial subdural haematoma associated with dural puncture in labour. Br J Anaesth 2000; 84:518-20.
6. Davies JM, Murphy A, Smith M, et al. Subdural haematoma after dural puncture headache treated by epidural blood patch. Br J Anaesth 2001; 86:720-3.
7. Eggert SM, Eggers KA. Subarachnoid haemorrhage following spinal anaesthesia in an obstetric patient. Br J Anaesth 2001; 86:442-4.
8. Aidi S, Chaunu M-P, Biousse V, et al. Changing pattern of headache pointing to cerebral venous thrombosis after lumbar puncture and intravenous high-dose corticosteroids. Headache 1999; 39:559-64.
9. Borum SE, Naul LG, McLeskey CH. Postpartum dural venous sinus thrombosis after postdural puncture headache and epidural blood patch. Anesthesiology 1997; 86:487-90.
10. Stocks GM, Wooler DJA, Young JM, et al. Postpartum headache after epidural blood patch: Investigation and diagnosis. Br J Anaesth 2000; 84:407-10.
11. Gewirtz EC, Costin M, Marx GF. Cortical vein thrombosis may mimic postdural puncture headache. Reg Anesth 1987; 12:188-90.
12. Nicol GLJ, Millns JP. Cerebellar infarction as a cause of post-partum headache. Int J Obstet Anesth 2002; 11:306-9.
13. Mercieri M, Mercieri A, Paolini S, et al. Postpartum cerebral ischaemia after accidental dural puncture and epidural blood patch. Br J Anaesth 2003; 90:98-100.
14. Saberski LR, Kondamuri S, Osinubi OYO. Identification of the epidural space: Is loss of resistance to air a safe technique? A review of the complications related to the use of air. Reg Anesth 1997; 22:3-15.
15. Laviola S, Kirvelä M, Spoto M-R, et al. Pneumocephalus with intense headache and unilateral pupillary dilatation after accidental dural puncture during epidural anesthesia for cesarean section. Anesth Analg 1999; 88:582-3.
16. Sherer DM, Onyeije CI, Yun E. Pneumocephalus following inadvertent intrathecal puncture during epidural anesthesia: A case report and review of the literature. J Matern-Fetal Med 1999; 8:138-40.
17. Askmark H, Lundberg PO. Lactation headache: A new form of headache? Cephalalgia 1989; 9:119-22.
18. Lybecker H, Djernes M, Schmidt JF. Postdural puncture headache (PDPH): Onset, duration, severity, and associated symptoms. An analysis of 75 consecutive patients with PDPH. Acta Anaesthesiol Scand 1995; 39:605-12.
19. Shearer VE, Jhaveri HS, Cunningham FG. Puerperal seizures after postdural puncture headache. Obstet Gynecol 1995; 85:255-60.
20. Vercauteren MP, Vundelinckx GJ, Hanegreefs GH. Postpartum headache, seizures and bloodstained CSF: A possible complication of dural puncture? Intensive Care Med 1988; 14:176-7.
21. Tohmo H, Vuorinen E, Muuronen A. Prolonged impairment in activities of daily living due to postdural puncture headache after diagnostic lumbar puncture. Anaesthesia 1998; 53:296-307.
22. Harrington H, Tyler HR, Welch K. Surgical treatment of post-lumbar puncture dural CSF leak causing chronic headache. J Neurosurg 1982; 57:703-7.
23. Bier A. Versucheüber cocainisirung des rückenmarkes. Dtsch Zeitschr Chir 1899; 51:361-9.
24. Kunkle EC, Ray BS, Wolff HG. Experimental studies on headache: Analysis of the headache associated with changes in intracranial pressure. Arch Neurol Psychiatr 1943; 49:323-58.
25. Eerola M, Kaukinen L, Kaukinen S. Fatal brain lesion following spinal anaesthesia. Acta Anesthesiol Scand 1981; 25:115-6.
26. Hullander RM, Bogard TD, Leivers D, et al. Chiari I malformation presenting as recurrent spinal headache. Anesth Analg 1992; 75:1025-6.
27. Grant R, Condon B, Hart I, et al. Changes in intracranial CSF volume after lumbar puncture and their relationship to post-LP headache. J Neurol Neurosurg Psychiatr 1991; 54:440-2.
28. Pannullo SC, Reich JB, Krol G, et al. MRI changes in intracranial hypotension. Neurology 1993; 43:919-26.
29. Iqbal J, Davis LE, Orrison WW. An MRI study of lumbar puncture headaches. Headache 1995; 35:420-2.
30. Schabel JE, Wang ED, Glass PSA. Arm pain as an unusual presentation of postdural puncture intracranial hypotension. Anesth Analg 2000; 91:910-2.
31. Errando CL, Peiró CM. Postdural puncture upper back pain as an atypical presentation of postdural puncture symptoms. Anesthesiology 2002; 96:1019-20.
32. Hattingh J, McCalden TA. Cerebrovascular effects of cerebrospinal fluid removal. S Afr Med J 1978; 54:780-1.
33. Boezaart AP. Effects of cerebrospinal fluid loss and epidural blood patch on cerebral blood flow in swine. Reg Anesth Pain Med 2001; 26:401-6.
34. Grant R, Condon B, Patterson J, et al. Changes in cranial CSF volume during hypercapnia and hypocapnia. J Neurol Neurosurg Psychiatr 1989; 52:218-22.
35. Martins AN, Wiley JK, Myers PW. Dynamics of the cerebrospinal fluid and the spinal dura mater. J Neurol Neurosurg Psychiatr 1972; 35: 468-73.
36. Vandam LD, Dripps RD. Long-term follow-up of patients who received 10,098 spinal anesthetics. JAMA 1956; 161:586-91.
37. Harrison DA, Langham BT. Spinal anaesthesia for urological surgery: A survey of failure rate, postdural puncture headache and patient satisfaction. Anaesthesia 1992; 47:902-3.
38. Lybecker H, Møller JT, May O, et al. Incidence and prediction of postdural puncture headache: A prospective study of 1,021 spinal anesthesias. Anesth Analg 1990; 70:389-94.
39. Stride PC, Cooper PC. Dural taps revisited. A 20-year survey from Birmingham Maternity Hospital. Anaesthesia 1993; 48:247-55.
40. Angle P, Thompson D, Halpern S, et al. Second stage pushing correlates with headache after unintentional dural puncture in parturients. Can J Anesth 1999; 46:861-6.
41. Poukkula E. The problem of post-spinal headache. Ann Chir Gynaecol 1984; 73:139-42.
42. Seeberger MD, Kaufmann M, Staender S, et al. Repeated dural punctures increase the incidence of postdural puncture headache. Anesth Analg 1996; 82:302-5.
43. Denny N, Masters R, Pearson D, et al. Postdural puncture headache after continuous spinal anesthesia. Anesth Analg 1987; 66:791-4.
44. Cohen S, Amar D, Pantuck EJ, et al. Decreased incidence of headache after accidental dural puncture in caesarean delivery patients receiving continuous postoperative intrathecal analgesia. Acta Anaesthesiol Scand 1994; 38:716-8.
45. Rutter SV, Shields F, Broadbent CR, et al. Management of accidental dural puncture in labour with intrathecal catheters: An analysis of 10 years' experience. Int J Obstet Anesth 2001; 10:177-81.
46. Norris MC, Leighton BL. Continuous spinal anesthesia after unintentional dural puncture in parturients. Reg Anesth 1990; 15:285-7.
47. Russell I, Laishley R. Controversies: In the event of accidental dural puncture by an epidural needle in labour, the catheter should be passed into the subarachnoid space. Int J Obstet Anesth 2002; 11:23-7.
48. Norris MC, Grieco WM, Borkowski, M, et al. Complications of labor analgesia: Epidural versus combined spinal epidural techniques. Anesth Analg 1994; 79:529-37.
49. Rawal N, Van Zundert A, Holmström B, Crowhurst JA. Combined spinal-epidural technique. Reg Anesth 1997; 22:406-23.
50. Cox M, Lawton G, Gowrie-Mohan S, et al. Ambulatory extradural analgesia (letter). Br J Anaesth 1995; 75:114.
51. Faure E, Moreno R, Thisted R. Incidence of postdural puncture headache in morbidly obese parturients (letter). Reg Anesth 1994; 19:361-3.
52. Magides AD. A personal view of post-dural puncture headache (letter). Anaesthesia 1991; 46:694.
53. Weir EC. The sharp end of the dural puncture. BMJ 2000; 320:127.
54. Costigan SN, Sprigge JS. Dural puncture: The patients' perspective. A patient survey of cases at a DGH maternity unit 1983-1993. Acta Anaesthesiol Scand 1996; 40:710-4.
55. Chadwick HS. An analysis of obstetric anesthesia cases from the American Society of Anesthesiologists closed claims project database. Internat J Obstet Anesth 1996; 5:258-63.
56. Berger CW, Crosby ET, Grodecki W. North American survey of the management of dural puncture occurring during labour epidural analgesia. Can J Anaesth 1998; 45:110-14.
57. Sechzer PH, Abel L. Post-spinal anesthesia headache treated with caffeine. Evaluation with demand method. Part I. Curr Therap Res 1978; 24:307-12.
58. Camann WR, Murray RS, Mushlin PS, et al. Effects of oral caffeine on postdural puncture headache: A double-blind, placebo-controlled trial. Anesth Analg 1990; 70:181-4.
59. Mathew RJ, Wilson WH. Caffeine induced changes in cerebral circulation. Stroke 1985; 16:814-7.

60. Dodd JE, Efird RC, Rauck RL. Cerebral blood flow changes with caffeine therapy for postdural headaches (abstract). Anesthesiology 1989; 71:A679.

61. Cohen SM, Laurito CE, Curran MJ. Grand mal seizure in a postpartum patient following intravenous infusion of caffeine sodium benzoate to treat persistent headache. J Clin Anesth 1992; 4:48-51.

62. Bolton VE, Leicht CH, Scanlon TS. Postpartum seizure after epidural blood patch and intravenous caffeine sodium benzoate. Anesthesiology 1989; 70:146-9.

63. Paech M. Unexpected postpartum seizures associated with post-dural puncture headache treated with caffeine. Internat J Obstet Anesth 1996; 5:43-6.

64. McSwiney M, Phillips J. Post dural puncture headache. Acta Anaesthesiol Scand 1995; 39:990-5.

65. Ryu JE. Effect of maternal caffeine consumption on heart rate and sleep time of breast-fed infants. Dev Pharmacol Ther 1985; 8:355-63.

66. Carp H, Singh PJ, Vadhera R, et al. Effects of the serotonin-receptor agonist sumatriptan on postdural puncture headache: Report of six cases. Anesth Analg 1994; 79:180-2.

67. Hodgson C, Roitberg-Henry A. The use of sumatriptan in the treatment of postdural puncture headache (letter). Anaesthesia 1997; 52:808.

68. Rohmer C, Le Bourlot G. Céphalées après rachianesthesieésie traitées par le sumatriptan (letter). Ann Fr Anesth Réanim 1995; 14:237.

69. Connelly NR, Parker RK, Rahimi A, et al. Sumatriptan in patients with postdural puncture headache. Headache 2000; 40:316-9.

70. Kshatri AM, Foster PA. Adrenocorticotropic hormone infusion as a novel treatment for postdural puncture headache. Reg Anesth 1997; 22:432-4.

71. Gupta S, Agrawal A. Postdural puncture headache and ACTH (letter). J Clin Anesth 1997; 9:258.

72. Carter BL, Pasupuleti R. Use of intravenous cosyntropin in the treatment of postdural puncture headache. Anesthesiology 2000; 92:272-4.

73. Oliver CD, White SA. Unexplained fitting in three parturients suffering from postdural puncture headache. Br J Anaesth 2002; 89:782-5.

74. Eldor J, Guedj P, Cotev S. Epidural morphine injections for the treatment of postspinal headache (letter). Can J Anaesth 1990; 37:710-1.

75. Usubiaga JE, Subiaga LE, Brea LM, et al. Effect of saline injections on epidural and subarachnoid space pressures and relation to postspinal anesthesia headache. Anesth Analg 1967; 46:293-6.

76. Kroin JS, Nagalla SKS, Buvanendran A, et al. The mechanisms of intracranial pressure modulation by epidural blood and other injectates in a postdural puncture rat model. Anesth Analg 2002; 95:423-9.

77. Bart AJ, Wheeler AS. Comparison of epidural saline placement and epidural blood placement in the treatment of post-lumbar-puncture headache. Anesthesiology 1978; 48:221-3.

78. Stevens RA, Jorgensen N. Successful treatment of dural puncture headache with epidural saline infusion after failure of epidural blood patch. Acta Anaesthesiol Scand 1988; 32:429-31.

79. Baysinger CL, Menk EJ, Harte E, et al. The successful treatment of dural puncture headache after failed epidural blood patch. Anesth Analg 1986; 65:1242-4.

80. Gormley JB. Treatment of postspinal headache. Anesthesiology 1960; 21:565-6.

81. DiGiovanni AJ, Dunbar BS. Epidural injections of autologous blood for postlumbar-puncture headache. Anesth Analg 1970; 49:268-71.

82. Crawford JS. Experiences with epidural blood patch. Anaesthesia 1980; 35:513-5.

83. Szeinfeld M, Ihmeidan IH, Moser MM, et al. Epidural blood patch: Evaluation of the volume and spread of blood injected into the epidural space. Anesthesiology 1986; 64:820-2.

84. Taivainen T, Pitkänen M, Tuominen M, et al. Efficacy of epidural blood patch for postdural puncture headache. Acta Anaesthesiol Scand 1993; 37:702-5.

85. Beards SC, Jackson A, Griffiths AG, et al. Magnetic resonance imaging of extradural blood patches: Appearances from 30 min to 18 H. Br J Anaesth 1993; 71:182-8.

86. Vakharia SB, Thomas PS, Rosenbaum AE, et al. Magnetic resonance imaging of cerebrospinal fluid leak and tamponade effect of blood patch in postdural puncture headache. Anesth Analg 1997; 84:585-90.

87. Djurhuus H, Rasmussen M, Jensen EH. Epidural blood patch illustrated by CT-epidurography. Acta Anaesthesiol Scand 1995; 39:613-7.

88. Safa-Tisseront V, Thormann F, Malassiné, et al. Effectiveness of epidural blood patch in the management of post-dural puncture headache. Anesthesiology 2001; 95:334-9.

89. Banks S, Paech M, Gurrin L. An audit of epidural blood patch after accidental dural puncture with a Tuohy needle in obstetric patients. Int J Obstet Anesth 2001; 10:172-6.

90. Williams EJ, Beaulieu P, Fawcett WJ, et al. Efficacy of epidural blood patch in the obstetric population. Internat J Obstet Anesth 1999; 8: 105-9.

91. DiGiovanni AJ, Galbert MW, Wahle WM. Epidural injection of autologous blood for postlumbar-puncture headache. II. Additional clinical experiences and laboratory investigation. Anesth Analg 1972; 51: 226-32.

92. Carrie LE. Epidural blood patch: Why the rapid response? (letter). Anesth Analg 1991; 72:129-30.

93. Coombs DW, Hooper D. Subarachnoid pressure with epidural blood patch. Reg Anesth 1979; 4:3-6.

94. Sudlow C, Warlow C. Epidural blood patching for preventing and treating post-dural puncture headache (Cochrane Review). In: The Cochrane Library, Issue 4, 2002. Oxford: Update Software.

95. Seebacher J, Ribeiro V, LeGuillou JL, et al. Epidural blood patch in the treatment of post-dural puncture headache: A double blind study. Headache 1989; 29:630-2.

96. Lybecker H, Andersen T. Repetitive hearing loss following dural puncture treated with autologous epidural blood patch. Acta Anaesthesiol Scand 1995; 39:987-9.

97. Longmire S, Joyce TH. Treatment of a duro-cutaneous fistula secondary to attempted epidural anesthesia with an epidural autologous blood patch. Anesthesiology 1984; 60:63-4.

98. Sencakova D, Mokri B, McClelland RL. The efficacy of epidural blood patch in spontaneous CSF leaks. Neurology 2001; 57:1921-3.

99. Elbiaadi-Aziz N, Benzon HT, Russell EJ, et al. Cerebrospinal fluid leak treated by aspiration and epidural blood patch under computed tomography guidance. Reg Anesth Pain Med 2001; 26:363-7.

100. Harding SA, Collis RE, Morgan BM. Meningitis after combined spinal-extradural anaesthesia in obstetrics. Br J Anaesth 1994; 73:545-7.

101. Berga S, Trierweiler MW. Bacterial meningitis following epidural anesthesia for vaginal delivery: A case report. Obstet Gynecol 1989; 74:437-9.

102. Oh J, Camann W. Severe, acute meningeal irritative reaction after epidural blood patch. Anesth Analg 1998; 87:1139-40.

103. Bucklin BA, Tinker JH, Smith CV. Clinical dilemma: A patient with postdural puncture headache and acute leukemia. Anesth Analg 1999; 88:166-7.

104. Newman P, Carrington D, Clarke J, et al. Debate. Epidural blood patch is contraindicated in HIV-positive patients. Int J Obstet Anesth 1994; 3:167-9.

105. Tom DJ, Gulevich SJ, Shapiro HM, et al. Epidural blood patch in the HIV-positive patient. Anesthesiology 1992; 76:943-7.

106. Parris WC. Post-dural puncture headache and epidural blood patch in an AIDS patient (letter). J Clin Anesth 1997; 9:87-8.

107. Abouleish E, de la Vega S, Blendinger I, et al. Long-term follow-up of epidural blood patch. Anesth Analg 1975; 54:459-63.

108. Cornwall RD, Dolan WM. Radicular back pain following lumbar epidural blood patch. Anesthesiology 1975; 43:692-3.

109. Shantha TR, McWhirter WR, Dunbar RW. Complications following epidural blood patch for postlumbar-puncture headache. Anesth Analg 1973; 52:67-72.

110. Lowe DM, McCullough AM. 7th nerve palsy after extradural blood patch. Br J Anaesth 1990; 65:721-2.

111. Reynolds AF, Hameroff SR, Blitt CD, et al. Spinal subdural epiarachnoid hematoma: A complication of a novel epidural blood patch technique. Anesth Analg 1980; 59:702-3.

112. Tekkök IH, Carter DA, Brinker R. Spinal subdural haematoma as a complication of immediate epidural blood patch. Can J Anaesth 1996; 43:306-9.

113. Wilkinson HA. Lumbosacral meningismus complicating subdural injection of blood patch. J Neurosurg 1980; 52:849-51.

114. Shantha TR, Bisese J. Subdural blood patch for spinal headache (letter). N Engl J Med 1991; 325:1252-3.

115. Gregg R, Gravenstein N. Low back pain following epidural blood patch. J Clin Anesth 1992; 4:413-8.

116. Seeberger M, Urwyler A. Lumbovertebral syndrome after extradural blood patch. Br J Anaesth 1992; 69:414-6.

117. Palmer JHM, Wilson DW, Brown CM. Lumbovertebral syndrome after repeat extradural blood patch. Br J Anaesth 1997; 78:334-6.

118. Sperry RJ, Gartrell A, Johnson JO. Epidural blood patch can cause acute neurologic deterioration. Anesthesiology 1995; 82:303-5.

119. Beers RA, Cambareri JJ, Rodziewicz GS. Acute deterioration of mental status following epidural blood patch. Anesth Analg 1993; 76:1147-9.

120. Frison LM, Dorsey DL. Epidural blood patch and late postpartum eclampsia. Anesth Analg 1996; 82:666-8.

121. Marfurt D, Lyrer P, Rüttimann U, et al. Recurrent post-partum seizures after epidural blood patch. Br J Anaesth 2002; 90:247-50.

122. Woodward WM, Levy DM, Dixon AM. Exacerbation of post-dural puncture headache after epidural blood patch. Can J Anaesth 1994; 41:628-31.

123. Dunbar SA, Katz NP. Failure of delayed epidural blood patching to correct persistent cranial nerve palsies. Anesth Analg 1994; 79:806-7.

124. Ong BY, Graham CR, Ringaert KR, et al. Impaired epidural analgesia after dural puncture with and without subsequent blood patch. Anesth Analg 1990; 70:76-9.

125. Blanche R, Eisenach JC, Tuttle R, et al. Previous wet tap does not reduce success rate of labor epidural analgesia. Anesth Analg 1994; 79:291-4.

126. Hebl JR, Horlocker TT, Chantigian RC, et al. Epidural anesthesia and analgesia are not impaired after dural puncture with or without epidural blood patch. Anesth Analg 1999; 89:390-4.

127. Loughrey JPR, Eappen S, Tsen LC. Spinal anesthesia for cesarean delivery shortly after an epidural blood patch. Anesth Analg 2003; 96:545-7.

128. Diaz JH. Permanent paraparesis and cauda equina syndrome after epidural blood patch for postdural puncture headache. Anesthesiology 2002; 96:1515-7.

129. Andrews PJD, Ackerman WE, Juneja M, et al. Transient bradycardia associated with extradural blood patch after inadvertent dural puncture in parturients. Br J Anaesth 1992; 69:401-3.

130. Brimacombe J, Clarke G, Craig L. Epidural blood patch in the Jehovah's Witness (letter). Anaesth Intens Care 1994; 22:319.

131. Cucchiara RF, Wedel DJ. Finding cerebrospinal fluid during epidural blood patch: How to proceed. Anesth Analg 1984; 63:1121-3.

132. Martin R, Jourdain S, Clairoux M, et al. Duration of decubitus position after epidural blood patch. Can J Anaesth 1994; 41:23-5.

133. Barrios-Alarcon J, Aldrete JA, Paragas-Tapia D. Relief of post-lumbar puncture headache with epidural dextran 40: A preliminary report. Reg Anesth 1989; 14:78-80.

134. Stevens DS, Peeters-Asdourian C. Treatment of postdural puncture headache with 'Epidural Dextran Patch' (letter). Reg Anesth 1993; 18:324-5.

135. Aldrete JA. Persistent post-dural-puncture headache treated with epidural infusion of Dextran. Headache 1994; 34:265-7.

136. Reynvoet MEJ, Cosaert PAJM, Desmet MFR, et al. Epidural dextran 40 patch for postdural puncture headache. Anaesthesia 1997; 52:886-8.

137. Lander CJ, Korbon GA. Histopathologic consequences of epidural blood patch and epidurally administered Dextran 40 (abstract). Anesthesiology 1988; 69:A410.

138. Jackson MR. Fibrin sealants in surgical practice: An overview. Am J Surg 2001; 182:1-7S.

139. Crul BJP, Gerritse BM, van Dongen RTM, et al. Epidural fibrin glue injection stops persistent postdural puncture headache. Anesthesiology 1999; 91:576-7.

140. Kamada M, Fujita Y, Ishii R, et al. Spontaneous intracranial hypotension successfully treated by epidural patching with fibrin glue. Headache 2000; 40:844-7.

141. Gerritse BM, van Dongen RTM, Crul BJP. Epidural fibrin glue injection stops persistent cerebrospinal fluid leak during long-term intrathecal catheterization. Anesth Analg 1997; 84:1140-1.

142. Cook PT, Davies MJ, Beavis RE. Bed rest and postlumbar puncture headache. Anaesthesia 1989; 44:389-91.

143. Thornberry EA, Thomas TA. Posture and post-spinal headache: A controlled trial in 80 obstetric patients. Br J Anaesth 1988; 60:195-7.

144. Carbaat PAT, van Crevel H. Lumbar puncture headache: Controlled study on the preventive effect of 24 hours' bed rest. Lancet 1981; ii: 1133-5.

145. Sudlow C, Warlow C. Posture and fluids for preventing post-dural puncture headache (Cochrane Review). In: The Cochrane Library, Issue 4, 2002. Oxford: Update Software.

146. Despond O, Meuret P, Hemmings G. Postdural puncture headache after spinal anaesthesia in young orthopaedic outpatients using 27-g needles. Can J Anaesth 1998; 45:1106-9.

147. Kang SB, Goodnough DE, Lee YK, et al. Comparison of 26- and 27-g needles for spinal anesthesia for ambulatory surgical patients. Anesthesiology 1992; 76:734-8.

148. Fishman RA. Cerebrospinal Fluid in Diseases of the Nervous System, 2nd ed. Philadelphia, WB Saunders, 1992:23-42.

149. Abboud TK, Miller H, Afrasiabi A, et al. Effect of subarachnoid morphine on the incidence of spinal headache. Reg Anesth 1992; 17:34-6.

150. Eldor J, Guedj P. Epidural morphine for prophylaxis of post dural puncture headache in parturients (letter). Reg Anesth 1992; 17:112.

151. Devcic A, Sprung J, Patel S, et al. PDPH in obstetric anesthesia: Comparison of 24-gauge Sprotte and 25-gauge Quincke needles and effect of subarachnoid administration of fentanyl. Reg Anesth 1993; 18:222-5.

152. Craft JB, Epstein BS, Coakley CS. Prophylaxis of dural-puncture headache with epidural saline. Anesth Analg 1973; 52:228-31.

153. Shah JL. Epidural pressure during infusion of saline in the parturient. Int J Obstet Anesth 1993; 2:190-2.

154. Charsley MM, Abram SE. The injection of intrathecal normal saline reduces the severity of postdural puncture headache. Reg Anesth Pain Med 2001; 26:301-5.

155. Kuczkowski KM, Benumof JL. Decrease in the incidence of post-dural puncture headache: Maintaining CSF volume. Acta Anaesthesiol Scand 2003; 47:98-100.

156. Colonna-Romano P, Shapiro BE. Unintentional dural puncture and prophylactic epidural blood patch in obstetrics. Anesth Analg 1989; 69:522-3.

157. Ackerman WE, Juneja MM, Kaczorowski DM. Prophylactic epidural blood patch for the prevention of postdural puncture headache in the parturient. Anesthesiol Rev 1990; 17:45-9.

158. Quaynor H, Corbey M. Extradural blood patch: Why delay? Br J Anaesth 1985; 57:538-40.

159. Cheek TG, Banner R, Sauter J, et al. Prophylactic extradural blood patch is effective. Br J Anaesth 1988; 61:340-2.

160. Tobias MD, Pilla MA, Rogers C, et al. Lidocaine inhibits blood coagulation: Implications for epidural blood patch. Anesth Analg 1996; 82:766-9.

161. Leivers D. Total spinal anesthesia following early prophylactic epidural blood patch. Anesthesiology 1990; 73:1287-9.

162. Aldrete JA, Brown TL. Intrathecal hematoma and arachnoiditis after prophylactic blood patch through a catheter (letter). Anesth Analg 1997; 84:233-4.

163. Waters JH, Sabharwal V, Grass JA. Prophylactic blood patch performed prior to continuous epidural analgesia. J Clin Anesth 2000; 12:558-60.

164. Salvador L, Carrero E, Castillo J, et al. Prevention of post dural puncture headache with epidural-administered Dextran 40 (letter). Reg Anesth 1992; 17:357-8.

165. Tourtellotte WW, Henderson WG, Tucker RP, et al. A randomized, double-blind clinical trial comparing the 22 versus 26 gauge needle in the production of the post-lumbar puncture syndrome in normal individuals. Headache 1972; 12:73-8.

166. Landau R, Ciliberto CF, Goodman SR, et al. Complications with 25-gauge and 27-gauge Whitacre needles during combined spinal-epidural analgesia in labor. Internat J Obstet Anesth 2001; 10:168-71.

167. Flaatten NH, Rodt SÅ, Vamnes J, et al. Postdural puncture headache: A comparison between 26- and 29-gauge needles in young patients. Anaesthesia 1989; 44:147-9.

168. Lesser P, Bembridge M, Lyons G, et al. An evaluation of a 30-gauge needle for spinal anaesthesia for Caesarean section. Anaesthesia 1990; 45:767-8.

169. Tarkkila P, Huhtala J, Salminen U. Difficulties in spinal needle use. Anaesthesia 1994; 49:723-5.

170. Lambert DH, Hurley RJ, Hertwig L, et al. Role of needle gauge and tip configuration in the production of lumbar puncture headache. Reg Anesth 1997; 22:66-72.

171. Cesarini M, Torrielli R, Lahaye F, et al. Sprotte needle for intrathecal anaesthesia for caesarean section: Incidence of postdural puncture headache. Anaesthesia 1990; 45:656-8.

172. Flaatten H, Thorsen T, Askeland B, et al. Puncture technique and postural postdural puncture headache. A randomised, double-blind study comparing transverse and parallel puncture. Acta Anaesthesiol Scand 1998; 42:1209-14.

173. Hart JR, Whitacre RJ. Pencil-point needle in prevention of postspinal headache. JAMA 1951; 147:657-8.

174. Corbey MP, Bach AB, Lech K, et al. Grading of severity of postdural puncture headache after 27-gauge Quincke and Whitacre needles. Acta Anaesthesiol Scand 1997; 41:779-84.

175. Douglas MJ, Ward ME, Campbell DC, et al. Factors involved in the incidence of post-dural puncture headache with the 25 gauge Whitacre needle for obstetric anesthesia. Int J Obstet Anesth 1997; 6:220-3.

176. Flaatten H, Felthaus J, Kuwelker M, et al. Postural post-dural puncture headache. A prospective randomised study and a meta-analysis comparing two different 0.40 mm O.D. (27 g) spinal needles. Acta Anaesthesiol Scand 2000; 44:643-7.

177. Westbrook JL, Uncles DR, Sitzman BT, et al. Comparison of the force required for dural puncture with different spinal needles and subsequent leakage of cerebrospinal fluid. Anesth Analg 1994; 79:769-72.

178. Sitzman BT, Uncles DR. The effects of needle type, gauge, and tip bend on spinal needle deflection. Anesth Analg 1996; 82:297-301.

179. Sprotte G, Schedel R, Pajunk H, et al. An atraumatic needle for single-shot regional anesthesia. Reg Anaesth 1987; 10:104-8.

180. Ross BK, Chadwick HS, Mancuso JJ, et al. Sprotte needle for obstetric anesthesia: Decreased incidence of post-dural puncture headache. Reg Anesth 1992; 17:29-33.

181. Sharma SK, Gambling DR, Joshi GP, et al. Comparison of 26-gauge Atraucan (Rx) and 25-gauge Whitacre needles: Insertion characteristics and complications. Can J Anaesth 1995; 42:706-10.

182. Pan PH, Fragneto R, Moore C, et al. The incidence of failed spinal anesthesia, postdural puncture headache and backache is similar with Atraucan and Whitacre spinal needles. (letter). Can J Anesth 2002; 49:636.

183. Vallejo MC, Mandell GL, Sabo DP, et al. Postdural puncture headache: A randomized comparison of five spinal needles in obstetric patients. Anesth Analg 2000; 91:916-20.

184. Halpern S, Preston R. Postdural puncture headache and spinal needle design: Metaanalyses. Anesthesiology 1994; 81:1376-83.

185. Franksson C, Gordh T. Headache after spinal anesthesia and a technique for lessening its frequency. Acta Chir Scand 1946; 94:443-54.

186. Fink BR, Walker S. Orientation of fibers in human dorsal lumbar dura mater in relation to lumbar puncture. Anesth Analg 1989; 69:768-72.

187. Patin DJ, Eckstein EC, Harum K. et al. Anatomic and biomechanical properties of human lumbar dura mater. Anesth Analg 1993; 76:535-40.

188. Reina MA, Dittmann M, Garcia AL, et al. New perspectives in the microscopic structure of human dura mater in the dorsolumbar region. Reg Anesth 1997; 22:161-6.

189. Cruickshank RH, Hopkinson JM. Fluid flow through dural puncture sites: An in vitro comparison of needle point types. Anaesthesia 1989; 44:415-8.

190. Ready LB, Cuplin S, Haschke RH, et al. Spinal needle determinants of rate of transdural fluid leak. Anesth Analg 1989; 69:457-60.

191. Dittmann M, Schäfer H-G, Ulrich J, et al. Anatomical reevaluation of lumbar dura mater with regard to postspinal headache: Effect of dural puncture. Anaesthesia 1988; 43:635-7.

192. Mihic DN. Postspinal headache and relationship of needle bevel to longitudinal dural fibers. Reg Anesth 1985; 10:76-81.

193. Tarkkila PJ, Heine H, Tervo R-R. Comparison of Sprotte and Quincke needles with respect to post dural puncture headache and backache. Reg Anesth 1992; 17:283-7.

194. Norris MC, Leighton BL, DeSimone CA. Needle bevel direction and headache after inadvertent dural puncture. Anesthesiology 1989; 70:729-31.

195. Richardson MG, Wissler RN. The effects of needle bevel orientation during epidural catheter insertion in laboring parturients. Anesth Analg 1999; 88:352-6.

196. Lewis MC, Lafferty JP, Sacks MS, et al. How much work is required to puncture dura with Tuohy needles? Br J Anaesth 2000; 85:238-41.

197. Hatfalvi BI. Postulated mechanisms for postdural puncture headache and review of laboratory models: Clinical experience. Reg Anesth 1995; 20:329-36.

198. Kempen PM, Mocek CK. Bevel direction, dura geometry, and hole size in membrane puncture. Laboratory report. Reg Anesth 1997; 22:267-72.

199. Puolakka R, Jokinen M, Pitkänen MT, et al. Comparison of postanesthetic sequelae after clinical use of 27-gauge cutting and noncutting spinal needles. Reg Anesth 1997; 22:521-6.

200. Russell R, Douglas J. Controversies: Loss of resistance to saline is better than air for obstetric epidurals. Internat J Obstet Anesth 2001; 10:302-6.

201. Strupp M, Brandt T. Should one reinsert the stylet during lumbar puncture? (letter). N Engl J Med 1997; 336:1190.

202. Naulty JS, Hertwig L, Hunt CO, et al. Influence of local anesthetic solution on postdural puncture headache. Anesthesiology 1990; 72:450-4.

203. Vacanti JJ. Post-spinal headache and air travel (letter). Anesthesiology 1972; 37:358-9.

204. Panadero A, Bravo P, Garcia-Pedrajas F. Postdural puncture headache and air travel after spinal anesthesia with a 24-gauge Sprotte needle (letter). Reg Anesth 1995; 20:463-4.

205. Mulroy MF. Spinal headache and air travel (letter). Anesthesiology 1979; 51:479.

Chapter 33

Neurologic Complications of Pregnancy and Regional Anesthesia

Felicity Reynolds, M.B., B.S., M.D., FRCA, FRCOG ad eundem · Philip R. Bromage, M.B., B.S., FRCA, FRCPC

Neurologic complications of childbirth may be associated with regional analgesia and anesthesia, or they may arise from some other cause that is either related to childbirth itself or is coincidental. Complications associated with regional anesthesia may be immediate (e.g., motor block, unexpectedly high or prolonged block, seizures following unintentional intravenous injection of local anesthetic), or they may be prolonged or delayed. Immediate complications are described in Chapter 21; this chapter includes a discussion of prolonged or delayed neurologic complications.

Although neurologic disorders following childbirth are more likely to have obstetric than anesthetic causes, all too often it is the regional anesthetic technique that receives the blame. For example, Turbridy and Redmond[1] described seven women referred with neurologic symptoms, *all* of which had been attributed to epidural analgesia. These seven women suffered respectively from brachial neuritis (1), peroneal neuropathy (2), femoral neuropathy (1), neck strain (1), and leg symptoms for which there was no obvious physical cause (2). When a postpartum palsy occurs, a careful history and neurologic examination, together with modern diagnostic aids such as electromyography (EMG), nerve conduction studies, and imaging techniques, should make it possible to localize the lesion and differentiate intrinsic maternal causes from medical misadventure. Accurate and prompt diagnosis is essential. Much can be done at the bedside. Figure 33-1 illustrates how very different is the cutaneous distribution of a peripheral nerve from that of a nerve root. Figure 33-2 may also help the physician assess whether a pattern of deficit in leg movements can be attributed to a root lesion.

THE INCIDENCE OF NEUROLOGIC SEQUELAE

Patients frequently ask obstetricians and anesthesiologists about the incidence of complications of neuraxial anesthesia, but such a question is difficult to answer, for at least two rea-

sons: (1) accurate data are lacking, and (2) the incidence of problems varies widely, depending on the skill and training of the practitioners. Some old surveys may be based on accurate local records, but the data relate to a time when practices, equipment, and local anesthetic drugs were less safe and sophisticated than they are today. The incidence of rare complications can no longer be estimated accurately on a local basis.

Nevertheless, anesthesiologists have a duty to inform patients appropriately of the risks associated with a proposed procedure, and some reliance must be placed on surveys to provide this information.

Obstetric Surveys

Between 1935 and 1965 the reported incidence of neurologic deficits in obstetric patients ranged from 1 in 2100 to 1 in 6400.[2-5] During this period, long labor and difficult rotational forceps delivery were commonplace, but neuraxial anesthetic intervention was relatively unusual. Subsequently many surveys have attempted to assess the incidence of neurologic complications of regional anesthesia, but they have many sources of error (Box 33-1). Not only may the individuals recording the complications fail to distinguish obstetric from anesthetic causes, but also they may overlook minor neurologic disorders already present in the childbearing population (e.g., among patients with diabetes). Thus it would be necessary to survey both ante- and post-partum neurologic status in a very large number of women to detect genuine obstetric and anesthetic injuries that arise *de novo* during childbirth.

A number of surveys of varying quality have been conducted in obstetric populations; the more recent are listed in Table 33-1. Earlier surveys often lacked diagnostic precision, while all those up to 1999 have been ably reviewed by Loo et al.[6] Ong et al.[7] performed a thorough survey of

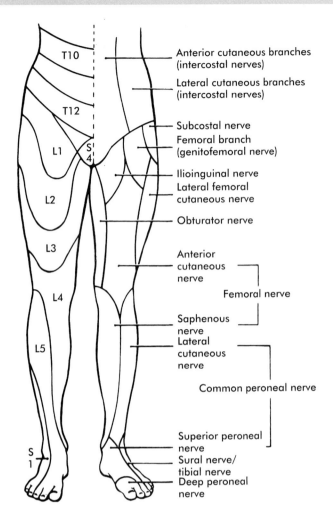

FIGURE 33-1. The segmental *(right leg)* and peripheral *(left leg)* sensory nerve distributions useful in distinguishing central from peripheral nerve injury. (From Redick LF. Maternal perinatal nerve palsies. Postgrad Obstet Gynecol 1992; 12:1-6.)

postpartum neurologic deficits, in which they reviewed the charts of 23,827 women delivering in Winnipeg over a 9-year period, and interviewed all those receiving anesthesia. All neurologic deficits in this series were transient, none lasting more than 72 hours. The incidence of neurologic symptoms was similar after epidural and general anesthesia, but neurologic deficits were more likely to be detected in women who received any form of anesthesia than in women who received no anesthesia. This is not surprising since only those women who had received anesthesia were interviewed. Indeed, the survey identified 45 cases of neurologic deficit, of which only 10 had been noted in the hospital record, which suggests that many disorders may have been missed in the patients who did not receive anesthesia. Moreover, modern statistical methods (e.g., logistic regression) were not used to tease out the influence of prolonged labor and traumatic delivery, which the authors noted as possible causative factors.

In a large retrospective survey of long-term symptoms, women who delivered in one hospital in Birmingham, United Kingdom, were asked to recall events 2 to 9 years after delivery.[8] The two main problems with this survey were a response rate of only 39% (i.e., 11,701 responses from 30,096 eligible women) and the fact that all those and *only* those women who received epidural analgesia were interviewed intensively about their symptoms in the immediate postpartum period, thereby enhancing subsequent recall in this subset of the population. Logistic regression analysis demonstrated a link between epidural analgesia and many symptoms, including tingling and numbness. However, these symptoms were much more common in the arms than in the legs, calling into question any causative link. No major neurologic sequelae were detected.

A retrospective British survey of over 500,000 epidural procedures administered between 1982 and 1986 detected a number of serious sequelae, including one epidural abscess, one hematoma, and one anterior spinal artery syndrome, but many of the diagnoses were only presumptive.[9] This retrospective survey probably failed to detect many minor lesions, but it was followed by a smaller prospective one,[10] which included some spinal anesthetics and involved a non-randomized, self-selected group of respondents. The authors found no major neurologic disorders but a more believable number of mononeuropathies. Both of these studies overlooked the need for a control group of patients who did not receive a neuraxial block.

The study by Holdcroft et al.[11] did not fall into this trap; their denominator included all 48,066 women who delivered in one region over a year, and every effort was made to detect neurologic symptoms in the community.[11] However, the pitfall in this study was that there was no way to assess detection or response rate, since the women themselves were not sent questionnaires. Rather, health professionals were asked to report cases, which were then vetted to exclude groundless complaints. The authors judged that only one case of paresthesia, without physical signs, could be attributed to epidural analgesia, and none could be attributed to spinal anesthesia. Peripheral nerve damage was more common. The most serious was one case of foot drop in a woman who had spontaneous delivery of a large baby with only inhalational analgesia.

With the increased popularity of spinal anesthesia, concern at growing numbers of reports of paresthesias and possible root trauma led Holloway et al.[12] to conduct a retrospective national survey of spinal and combined spinal-epidural (CSE) anesthesia in the 1990s. The Quincke-type needle was already too rarely used to allow any comparison with pencil-point needles, but no difference in frequency of neuropathy was detected between Whitacre and Sprotte needles or between single-shot spinal and CSE techniques. Imprecise diagnoses made it difficult to sort anesthetic from coincidental causes, but after eliminating obvious obstetric or peripheral nerve palsies while otherwise erring on the pessimistic side, the incidence of neurologic sequelae was approximately 1 in 1000, with two cases of conus damage and the rest minor root palsies.

Two reports of painstaking local audit of immediate postpartum symptoms provide somewhat contrasting findings. One report from Paech et al.[13] in Perth, Australia, involved a prospective recording of complications in 10,995 women receiving epidural analgesia, but regrettably no controls. The authors detected only a single case of mononeuropathy, while no peripheral nerve deficits were mentioned. The second report came from Leeds, United Kingdom, where 3991 women delivered in 1 year; 21 women presenting with symptoms after neuraxial blockade were matched with 21 asymptomatic controls who had also received neuraxial blockade and 21 who had not.[14] Only one woman who had not had a regional block presented with symptoms, and she was found to have a foot drop after vacuum extraction delivery. Typical peripheral neuropathies occurred among those delivering

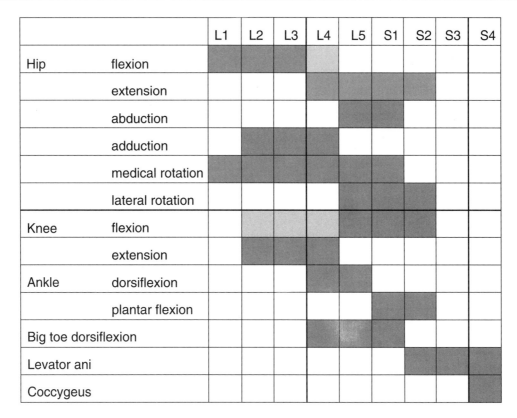

		L1	L2	L3	L4	L5	S1	S2	S3	S4
Hip	flexion	■	■	■	■					
	extension				■	■	■			
	abduction					■	■			
	adduction		■	■	■					
	medical rotation	■	■	■		■	■			
	lateral rotation					■	■	■		
Knee	flexion		■	■		■	■	■		
	extension			■	■	■				
Ankle	dorsiflexion				■	■				
	plantar flexion						■	■		
Big toe dorsiflexion					■	■				
Levator ani								■	■	■
Coccygeus										■

FIGURE 33-2. The spinal segments involved in the movements of joints in the leg. (From Russell R. Assessment of motor blockade during epidural analgesia in labour. Int J Obstet Anesth 1992; 4:230-4.)

vaginally; sacral numbness was most commonly detected after cesarean section. All changes were transient, and none could be attributed to regional anesthesia. Little wrong could be detected among the 21 uncomplaining control women who had had anesthetic intervention. In contrast, similar neurologic deficits were detected among the randomly selected, uncomplaining 21 controls with no anesthetic intervention when compared with women who presented with symptoms following regional blockade. This important finding demonstrates how very frequently minor neurologic deficits are to be found postpartum if sought, but those women who have not had anesthetic intervention tend to make no fuss about them. These two studies also suggest that women from Perth, Western Australia, may well complain less than those from Leeds, United Kingdom.

A prospective survey among 6057 women delivering in 1 year in Chicago revealed an incidence of lower limb nerve injuries of approximately 1%: 24 lateral femoral cutaneous nerve, 22 femoral nerve, 3 peroneal nerve, 3 lumbosacral plexus, 2 sciatic nerve, 3 obturator nerve, and 5 radicular injuries.[15] Significant risk factors identified by logistic regression included a prolonged second stage and nulliparity but not regional anesthesia.

The conclusions that can be drawn from these obstetric surveys are that the frequency of neurologic sequelae depends on how hard you seek them. The risk of transient mild deficits after childbirth may be very high. (Dar et al.[14] detected at least 5 cases among 22 women, 21 of whom were randomly selected, who had not received anesthetic intervention). A true figure for anesthetic complications cannot possibly be calculated even from accurate surveys, as the diagnosis is rarely firm, severity and duration are not defined, and skills vary. Moreover, these studies illustrate the bias that is created

Box 33-1 SOURCES OF INACCURACY IN SURVEYS OF NEUROLOGIC SEQUELAE OF REGIONAL ANESTHESIA

- Poor response rate
- Positive reporting bias
- Inclusion of non-neurologic conditions such as backache
- Absence of controls (i.e., patients who did not receive regional anesthesia)
- Greater attention given to those given neuraxial anesthesia
- Failure to consider possibility of preexisting neurologic lesion
- Poor localization of the lesion
- Inadequate investigation and lack of accurate diagnosis
- Inaccurate counting of numerator and denominator
- Cases arising in the community may be missed
- Small local surveys lack power to assess incidence of severe disorders with accuracy
- Older surveys relate to outdated practices

when we pay more attention postpartum to patients who have received neuraxial blockade than to those who have not.

Nonobstetric Surveys

Modern surveys of neurologic complications of spinal and epidural anesthesia among nonobstetric populations may yield more reliable results, but may still lack sensitivity to detect all potential problems and are commonly conducted in a relatively elderly and sick population. In a follow-up study from Sweden of 8501 spinal and 9232 epidural anesthetics, Dahlgren et al.[16] calculated a risk of permanent neurologic injury of between 1/2834 and 1/4251 spinal anesthetics and of 1/923 to1/3077 epidural anesthetics.[16] Epidural patients were

TABLE 33-1 SURVEYS OF NEUROLOGIC COMPLICATIONS OF CHILDBIRTH AND OF NEURAXIAL BLOCKS IN OBSTETRIC PATIENTS

Author	Type of study	Population	Numbers of neurologic deficits (risk ratio)
Ong et al. 1987[7]	Chart review of all patients; interview of those receiving anesthesia in one center in 1975-83	23,827 deliveries 　12,964 no analgesia or inhalational 　9403 epidural procedures 　1460 general anesthetics and other	45 (1/530) all transient 　5 (1/2593) 　34 (1/277) 　6 (1/243)
Scott & Hibbard 1990[9]	Retrospective multicenter review 1982-6	505,000 epidural procedures	47 (1/10,745) 　1 anterior spinal artery syndrome, 　1 epidural abscess, 1 epidural hematoma (?), 　38 mononeuropathies, 5 cranial nerve 　palsies, 1 subdural hematoma
MacArthur et al. 1992[8]	Questionnaire sent in 1987 to mothers delivering in one center, 1978-85	11,701 women (39%) who responded 　4766 epidural procedures 　6935 no epidural procedures	Tingling/paresthesia 　143 upper limb, 23 lower limb 　150 upper limb, 3 lower limb
Scott & Tunstall 1995[10]	Prospective multicenter review 1990-1	108,133 epidural procedures 14,856 spinal anesthetics	38 (1/2846) 8 (1/1857) 　1 foot drop, 45 mononeuropathies
Holdcroft et al. 1995[11]	Regional community and hospital-based trawl 1991-2	48,066 deliveries 　34,430 no neuraxial block 　13,007 epidural procedures	10 new neurologic complications (1/4807) 　1 foot drop, 1 cervical nerve lesion 　　(1/17,215) 　1 paresthesia of nerve root distribution 　　(1/13,007) 　Disorders unrelated to anesthesia: 　2 cranial nerve palsies, 1 hypotensive cord 　damage, 5 peripheral nerve lesions (overall 　1/1626)
Paech et al. 1998[13]	Prospective local audit 1989-94	629 spinal anesthetics 10,995 epidural procedures	0 1 traumatic mononeuropathy (1/10,995)
Holloway et al. 2000[12]	Retrospective multicenter trawl, elastic time frame	29,698 spinal anesthetics 12,254 combined spinal-epidural blocks	4 peripheral nerve damage, 10 ?root damage, 　1 conus damage, 22 uncertain; 　(overall incidence ?1/986) 5 peripheral nerve damage, 6 root damage, 　1 meningitis, 1 conus damage, 6 uncertain; 　overall incidence (?1/901)
Dar et al. 2002[14]	Prospective local audit of immediate symptoms 1998-9	1376 vaginal deliveries without anesthesia (random sample of 22 examined) 2615 regional blocks (all followed up) 1782 vaginal deliveries 833 cesarean sections	4 peripheral neuropathy, 1 foot drop, 2 vague (1/3) 21 had neurologic symptoms 7 peripheral neuropathies, 1 foot drop, 3 vague (1/162) 8 numb areas, 2 vague (1/83)

not without risk factors for hematoma and ischemia. In a Finnish study of insurance claims, the risk of serious damage was estimated as 1/22,222 for spinal anesthesia and 1/19,231 for epidural anesthesia.[17] Horlocker et al.[18] retrospectively reviewed complications among 4767 consecutive spinal anesthetics (mean age of the patients was 65 years); the authors detected six cases of persistent paresthesia and two of infection (one disc, one paraspinal), an incidence of 1/600. In a prospective multicenter survey in France that included 40,640 spinal and 30,413 epidural anesthetics, the risk of neurologic injury appeared to be 1/1693 for spinal anesthesia (including five cases of cauda equina syndrome) and 1/5069 for epidural anesthesia (including one case of paraplegia following an episode of hypotension).[19] A more recent report from the same team found only transient neurologic sequelae among 158,083 regional anesthetic procedures.[20] The range of incidences that have been reported is therefore 0.45 to 17 per 10,000 for spinal anesthesia and 0.52 to 10.8 per 10,000 for epidural anesthesia. It is clear that the reported risk of neurologic problems varies greatly with the patient population, local

practice and skill, completeness of detection, and inclusion criteria. To put any firm figure on it would be meaningless.

PERIPHERAL NERVE PALSIES

Anecdotal case reports and small retrospective studies published since 1838 confirm that, before the days of interventional obstetrics, neuropathies following vaginal birth were relatively common. In contemporary obstetric practice, cesarean section is usually preferred to prolonged labor and difficult high- or mid-forceps delivery, and we thereby expect to minimize the occurrence of traumatic and compressive lesions within the pelvis. Nevertheless, sporadic cases still occur, from a variety of causes. Recent surveys have detected cases of foot drop that followed delivery of a large baby,[10-12,14] often without any anesthetic intervention. An abnormal presentation such as transverse lie, a persistent occiput posterior position, fetal macrosomia, and/or difficult instrumental delivery typically presage such a neuropathy. The patient may recall "a stab of searing pain and a painful muscle spasm . . .

during labor, with the subsequent palsy in the same limb."[21] Such pain can penetrate a working epidural block. When this disorder is bilateral, it may be mistaken for an intraspinal lesion but more probably relates to a lesion of the lumbosacral plexus or the obturator nerve.

Prolonged use of the lithotomy position is the only significant factor in the etiology of femoral, sciatic, obturator, and peroneal nerve palsies following gynecologic surgery[22] and may presumably also contribute to their occurrence in obstetrics.

Compression of the Lumbosacral Trunk

Compression of the lumbosacral trunk (L4/5) is probably the most common cause of postpartum foot drop. In addition to weakness predominantly affecting ankle *dorsi*flexion, compression of the lumbosacral trunk produces sensory disturbance mainly involving the L5 dermatome (see Figure 33-1). Such palsy most often results from some degree of cephalopelvic disproportion and is therefore typically seen following prolonged labor and difficult vaginal delivery.[2-5] The fetal head—usually the brow—may compress the lumbosacral trunk as it crosses the pelvic brim and descends in front of the ala of the sacrum (Figure 33-3).

Obturator Nerve Palsy

The obturator nerve is susceptible to compressive injury as it crosses the brim of the pelvis or within the obturator canal (see Figure 33-3). The mother may complain of pain when the damage occurs, followed by weakness of hip adduction and internal rotation, with sensory disturbance over the upper inner thigh (see Figure 33-1). Cases are rarely reported among parturients, although three were detected when sought prospectively by Wong et al.[15] As the nerve would appear to be in a vulnerable position, it may be that the correct diagnosis is often missed.

Femoral Nerve Palsy

Femoral nerve palsy is more frequently diagnosed.[15] Dar et al.[14] detected five cases in their small population, albeit the symptoms were transient. The femoral nerve may be damaged during pelvic surgery,[23] but more important, it is vulnerable to stretching injury as it passes beneath the inguinal ligament. Damage may result from prolonged flexion, abduction, and external rotation of the hips during the second stage of labor, and also following procedures conducted in an excessive lithotomy position. Therefore the hips should never remain flexed continuously during the second stage of labor. In a true femoral neuropathy, the nerve supply to the ilio-psoas muscles is spared, so that some hip flexion is still possible. The patient with a femoral neuropathy may walk satisfactorily on a level surface but may be unable to climb stairs, while the patellar reflex is diminished or absent.

Meralgia Paresthetica

Meralgia paresthetica is a neuropathy of the lateral femoral cutaneous nerve, a purely sensory nerve also known as the lateral cutaneous nerve of the thigh. First described over 100 years ago, meralgia paresthetica is probably the most frequently encountered neuropathy in any survey related to childbirth.[12,14,15] It may arise both during pregnancy, typically about 30 weeks' gestation, and *intra*partum, in association with rising intraabdominal pressure. It may recur during successive pregnancies. The most likely cause is entrapment of the nerve as it passes round the anterior superior iliac spine beneath the inguinal ligament,[24] where its vulnerability is increased by a large intraabdominal mass or by retractors used during pelvic surgery. The compressive effect of edema may contribute, as with the increased incidence during pregnancy of carpal tunnel syndrome and possibly Bell's palsy.[25] The presentation in meralgia paresthetica is one of numbness, tingling, burning, or other paresthesias affecting the anterolateral aspect of the thigh. The distribution is quite unlike that of a root lesion, yet the disturbance will commonly be attributed to neuraxial blockade by those ignorant of neuroanatomy. The condition can be expected to resolve following childbirth, but the pain may also be relieved by local infiltration analgesia.

Sciatic Nerve Palsy

Sciatic nerve palsy is not commonly mentioned in surveys or generally recognized as a complication of childbirth, but this may be because it is mistaken for a lesion of the lumbosacral

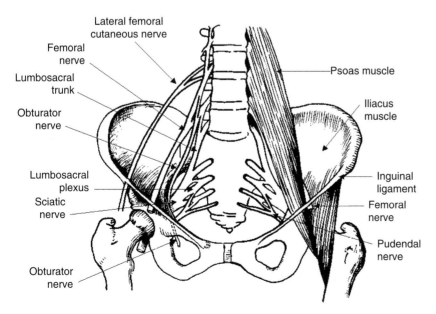

FIGURE 33-3. The lumbosacral trunk (L4/5) and obturator nerve (L2/3/4) are vulnerable to pressure as they cross the pelvic brim, in cases of cephalopelvic disproportion. The femoral (L2/3/4) and lateral femoral cutaneous (L2/3) nerves are vulnerable, especially in the lithotomy position, where they pass beneath the inguinal ligament. (Adapted from Cole JT. Maternal obstetric paralysis. Am J Obstet Gynecol 1946; 52:374.)

trunk. Although it was first described in 1944,[26] it was overlooked until 1996, when it was described in two parturients who had *not* undergone vaginal delivery.[27] One woman, who had a breech presentation, was thin and was kept sitting in one position while her leg numbness was wrongly attributed to epidural blockade. The other woman was obese, with a high station of the fetal head, and she suffered a period of hypotension during preparation for elective cesarean section under epidural anesthesia. Both women experienced (1) loss of sensation, with subsequent dysesthesia, below the knee, with sparing of the medial side; and also (2) an absence of movement below the knee, which recovered more quickly than the sensory changes. Both had intact posterior cutaneous nerve and gluteal function, which implies that the damage had occurred distal to the lumbosacral plexus, where the gluteal nerves branch off from the sciatic nerve (Figure 33-4). Had they undergone vaginal delivery, and had they had less conscientious evaluation, their lesions probably would have been attributed to root or plexus damage. Subsequently three cases have been detected by Wong et al.,[15] and two more cases of sciatic nerve damage have been described in women who had cesarean section without hypotension, and in whom compression of the sciatic nerve by a hip wedge was implicated.[28,29] Despite the peripheral location of the lesions, regional anesthesia cannot be entirely exonerated, as the symptoms of nerve compression, which otherwise would have prompted a change of position, were overlooked or wrongly attributed to the block.

Peroneal Nerve Palsy

Peroneal nerve palsy has been described in association with regional anesthesia and the lithotomy position. Again, signs of nerve compression may go unnoticed in the presence of regional blockade. Improper and/or prolonged positioning in stirrups, or compression of the lateral side of the knee against any hard object, may result in damage to the common peroneal nerve as it winds round the neck of the fibula. When the peroneal nerve is damaged in this position, foot drop may be profound, but plantar flexion and inversion at the ankle are preserved, unlike that with an L4/5 lesion.[30] Sensory impairment spares the lateral border of the foot, which distinguishes it from sciatic nerve palsy.

Anesthesia providers cannot be wholly absolved from responsibility for peripheral neuropathies, and adverse factors can be minimized by attention to simple rules (Box 33-2). One group of patients—those with a hereditary liability to pressure palsy—require particular attention. In these women, even relatively brief periods of immobility or pressure on any one site must be avoided.[31]

POSTPARTUM BLADDER DISTURBANCE

There are several mechanisms by which bladder function may be disturbed postpartum (Figure 33-5). It is true that, in theory, neuraxial blockade may (1) provoke the need for catheterization with consequent possibility of infection, (2) allow bladder distention to go undetected, and (3) on very rare occasions, be associated with cauda equina syndrome *(vide infra)*. Therefore it cannot be totally absolved from blame. However, several studies of bladder function have found no association[32,33] or only a weak correlation[34] between epidural analgesia and an increased residual volume in the immediate postpartum period. In contrast, a prolonged second stage of labor,[33] instrumental delivery, and perineal damage[34] have been identified as far more significant factors. Not surprisingly, in the large survey of long-term symptoms following childbirth conducted in Birmingham, England, no association was found between epidural analgesia and stress incontinence or urinary frequency.[35] By far the most common cause of disturbed bladder function appears to be non-neurologic. Nevertheless it must be part of our responsibility to ensure that the bladder does not become over-distended either intra- or post-partum.

CENTRAL LESIONS

Lesions of the central nervous system following childbirth have complex etiologies (Figure 33-6). In broad categories,

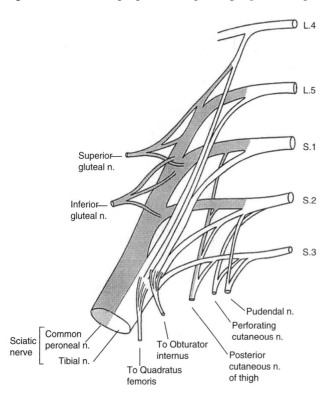

FIGURE 33-4. The lumbosacral plexus, showing the dorsal divisions of the spinal nerves shaded. (From Silva M, Mallinson C, Reynolds F. Sciatic nerve palsy following childbirth. Anaesthesia 1996; 51:1144-8.)

Labels in figure: L.4, L.5, S.1, S.2, S.3, Superior gluteal n., Inferior gluteal n., Sciatic nerve, Common peroneal n., Tibial n., To Quadratus femoris, To Obturator internus, Pudendal n., Perforating cutaneous n., Posterior cutaneous n. of thigh

---

Box 33-2 SAFEGUARDS TO MINIMIZE PERIPHERAL NERVE COMPRESSION

- Be watchful for the possibility of nerve compression under regional blockade.
- Avoid prolonged use of the lithotomy position, or else ensure that hip flexion and abduction are reduced to a minimum.
- Avoid prolonged positioning that may cause compression of the sciatic or peroneal nerve.
- Ensure that a hip wedge is placed under the bony pelvis rather than the buttock.
- Use low-dose local anesthetic/opioid combinations during labor to minimize numbness and allow maximum mobility.
- Use opioid only for postoperative analgesia, for the same reasons.
- Ensure that those caring for women receiving low-dose solutions understand that numbness or weakness should not occur; hence such symptoms should prompt a change of position.

the etiologies may be considered to be **traumatic** (to nervous tissue, meninges, or blood vessel), **infective, ischemic,** or **chemical** (to nervous tissue or meninges). Most of the serious sequelae are remarkably rare.

Neurologic Sequelae of Unintentional Dural Puncture

The subject of postdural puncture headache (PDPH) is discussed in Chapter 32. There are several other causes of

severe postpartum headache, some of which have serious neurologic implications. Postpartum headache requires *diagnosis* first and foremost, followed by treatment that is curative rather than palliative. Cortical vein and venous sinus thrombosis are more common than expected because of the hypercoagulable state of the blood postpartum.[36-38] Headaches caused by meningitis, venous sinus thrombosis, hypertensive encephalopathy, and subdural hematoma have also caused difficulty in diagnosis because they may occur following epidural top-up injection, unintentional dural

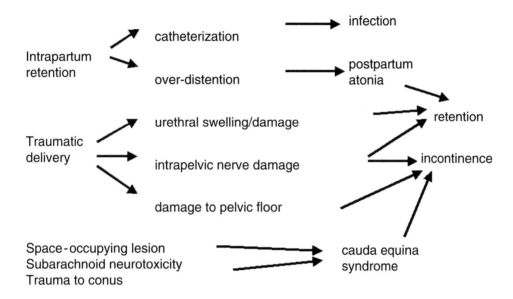

FIGURE 33-5. Mechanisms by which bladder function may be disturbed following parturition.

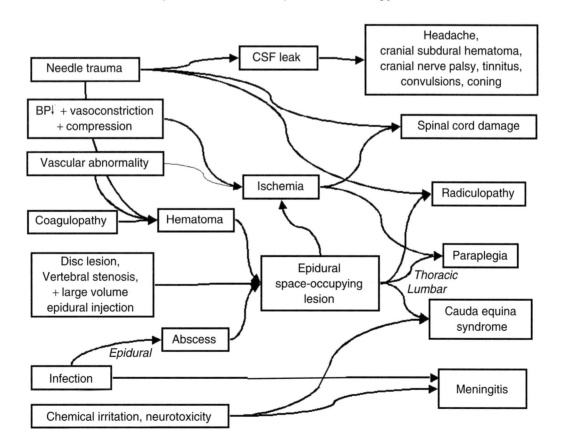

FIGURE 33-6. Mechanisms by which lesions of the central nervous system may arise in parturients.

puncture, or administration of an epidural blood patch.[36-39] Seizures may occur in patients with eclampsia, hypertensive encephalopathy, meningitis, or pneumocephalus but may also follow dural puncture or performance of epidural blood patch.[38,40-44]

It is commonly assumed that headache following dural puncture will resolve spontaneously over time, but unfortunately a dural leak can persist and occasionally may have more serious consequences. Although serious problems are more likely to result from unintentional dural puncture with a large epidural needle and a neglected headache, they may occasionally follow deliberate dural puncture with a small-gauge spinal needle.

CRANIAL NERVE PALSY

Because of its long course within the cranium, the abducent nerve is the most susceptible to damage by loss of cerebrospinal fluid (CSF). Abducent nerve palsy may follow unintentional dural puncture with an epidural needle, and recovery may be delayed even after performance of epidural blood patch.[45,46] Although uncommon following dural puncture with a small-gauge or atraumatic spinal needle, it has been reported following CSE blockade, although this may have resulted from undetected dural damage by the Tuohy needle.[47] Facial nerve palsy[46,48-50] may require weeks to recover. Cranial nerve VIII dysfunction[46,51,52] requires prompt performance of epidural blood patch; otherwise the patient is at risk for permanent tinnitus. Visual field defects have been reported and may also become permanent.[42,53,54] Trigeminal nerve disturbance is usually a transient effect from a high block.[6]

CRANIAL SUBDURAL HEMATOMA

More seriously, reduced CSF pressure may cause rupture of bridge meningeal veins[55] and result in cranial subdural hematoma,[39,56,57] which is reported with surprising frequency. Loo et al.[6] identified eight cases, while more have been reported since.[56-59] Although commonly believed to result only from neglect of a dural puncture with a large needle[60] or a cutting spinal needle,[56,57] subdural hematoma requiring craniotomy has been reported after puncture with a small-gauge, atraumatic needle[61] and after an unintentional dural puncture that had been correctly treated by epidural blood patch (Figure 33-7).[58] Whenever headache persists after dural puncture, despite performance of epidural blood patch, and if accompanied by altered consciousness, seizures, or other focal neurologic findings,[59] MRI is warranted to exclude subdural hematoma, which may be fatal without urgent surgery.[62] Neglected CSF leak has also been known to induce medullary and tentorial coning.[60]

One case of cranial *epi*dural hematoma arose after spinal anesthesia for removal of the placenta; this occurred following a seizure, which turned out to be epileptic.[63] Nothing is as it seems: the seizure was not eclamptic, and the hematoma was not a result of the spinal anesthetic.

Trauma to Nerve Roots and the Spinal Cord

Insertion of a spinal needle or epidural catheter is not infrequently accompanied by paresthesias that are more or less painful. While a flexible catheter is unlikely to do lasting

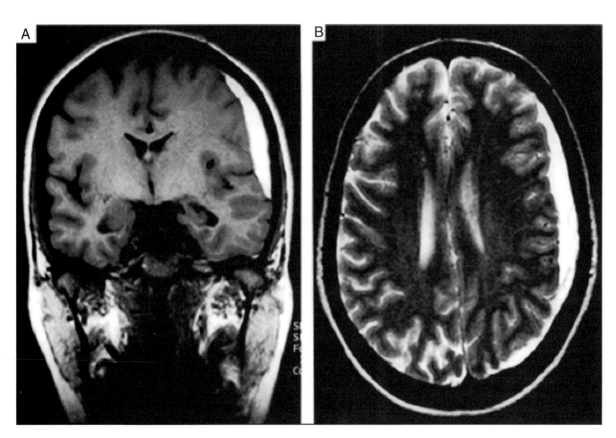

FIGURE 33-7. MRI of cranial subdural hematoma. (From *Davies JM, Murphy A, Smith M, O'Sullivan G*. Subdural haematoma after dural puncture headache treated by epidural blood patch. Br J Anaesth 2001; 86:720-3.)

damage to a nerve root in the epidural space, nerve roots in the subarachnoid space are more vulnerable.

TRAUMA ASSOCIATED WITH ATTEMPTED EPIDURAL CATHETER INSERTION

Epidural catheters may injure nerve roots either because they are inappropriately rigid[64] or because an undue length is threaded and ensnares a root.[65] A catheter seemingly threaded into the epidural space may lodge in an intervertebral foramen or even pass into the paravertebral space. In rare instances the epidural catheter and the artery of Adamkiewicz (entering the spinal canal between T9 and L3) may share the same foramen. If the epidural catheter is sufficiently stiff to compress the artery within the unyielding foramen, the blood supply to the lumbosacral enlargement of the spinal cord may be impaired, resulting in ischemia of the anterior two-thirds of the lower spinal cord, with resulting motor paralysis and loss of pain and temperature sensation but sparing of posterior column function. Clinical reports indicate that the condition resolves rapidly and completely if the catheter is withdrawn before permanent damage has occurred.[66,67]

Injury to the spinal cord may result from attempted identification of the epidural space in the presence of an undetected spina bifida occulta or a tethered cord,[68,69] or as a result of an unsteady grip or intermittent advancement of the epidural needle. Insertion of a thoracic epidural catheter and/or performance of procedures in anesthetized patients greatly increase the risk of spinal cord damage.[70,71] Catastrophic injury may arise with injection of fluid into the substance of the spinal cord.[71,72]

TRAUMA ASSOCIATED WITH SPINAL ANESTHESIA

A single insertion of a spinal needle below the level of the spinal cord sometimes causes brief, radiating pain or paresthesias without lasting symptoms or visible evidence on MRI. Nevertheless, such paresthesias significantly increase the likelihood of persistent symptoms in the same dermatomal distribution.[18]

Prolonged symptoms involving more than one spinal segment imply damage to the spinal cord itself. The unconscious patient, a high approach to the subarachnoid space, and injection into the substance of the spinal cord are all known dangers. Damage to the terminal portion of the cord (the conus medullaris) *without* intracord injection has also been reported in healthy conscious parturients receiving spinal or CSE anesthesia when using pencil-point needles in the lumbar region.[73-75] Typically the patient complains of pain on needle insertion, before any fluid is injected, often followed by the normal appearance of CSF from the needle hub, easy injection of the local anesthetic agent, and a normal spread of block. On recovery, there is unilateral numbness, which is succeeded by pain and paresthesias of L5/S1 distribution and foot drop, and in some cases urinary symptoms; sensory symptoms may last for months or years. The MRI appearance is one of a small syrinx or hemorrhage within the conus at the level of the body of T12 on the same side as the pain on insertion and subsequent leg symptoms (Figure 33-8).[74] In the majority of such cases, the anesthesiologist believed the interspace selected was L2-3. In one patient who subsequently died from other causes, hematomyelia was confirmed at autopsy.[76]

Why do these cases occur? Although unconfirmed by any prospective study, it has been argued that so-called atraumatic needles may be more prone to produce lasting neurologic damage since, being less sharp than cutting needles, they require greater force for insertion and must be advanced further before the hole is within the subarachnoid space.[77] Also, it is apparent that the tip may enter the spinal cord while the

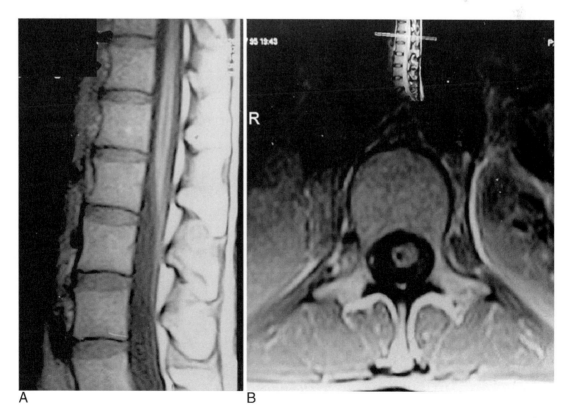

A   B

FIGURE 33-8. MRI of conus lesion. (First reproduced in Reynolds F. Damage to the conus medullaris following spinal anaesthesia. Anaesthesia 2001; 56:238-47.)

aperture remains within the subarachnoid space. Moreover, choice of a puncture site below the termination of the spinal cord is subject to error for the following reasons[78]:

1. The vertebral level of the termination of the cord varies between the bodies of T12 and L3 (Figure 33-9),[79,80] and is *lower in women* than in men.[81]
2. A standard method of identifying lumbar interspaces is to use Tuffier's line (i.e., the line joining the two iliac crests). When the parturient is in the lateral position, it is common practice to use half of Tuffier's line by dropping a perpendicular from the iliac crest to the lumbar spine. This is less accurate than palpation of both iliac crests,[82] particularly in obese or pregnant women, in whom the pelvis may be tilted in the lateral position (Figure 33-10).
3. Even when accurately assessed, Tuffier's line is an inconstant landmark.[83] Although typically at the L4 spinous process or L4-5 interspace, the line may be as high (cephalad) as the L2-3 interspace, and as low (caudad) as the L5-S1 interspace.

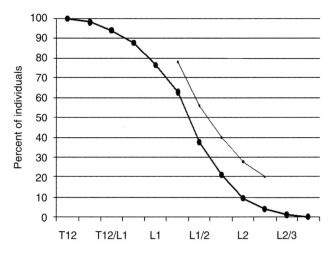

FIGURE 33-9. Variation in the level of the tip of the conus medullaris assessed by MRI of the lumbar spine among 504 consecutive adults. The unlabelled data points represent locations intermediate between the middle of each vertebra and the adjacent disc. (Cumulative data for the complete line are derived from Saifuddin A, Burnett SJ, White J. The variation of position of the conus medullaris in an adult population. A magnetic resonance imaging study. Spine 1998; 23: 1452-6. The data for the partial line are derived from Reimann AF, Anson BJ. Vertebral level of termination of the spinal cord with report of a case of sacral cord. *Anatomical Record* 1944; 88:127-38.)

4. Other approaches to identification of the interspace, such as counting down from C7 or finding the vertebra that is attached to the twelfth rib, are tedious and of little help in obese patients.

Not surprisingly, error in identification of lumbar interspaces is commonplace. Van Gessell et al.[84] demonstrated that 59% of dural punctures were performed one or two spaces higher than assumed, while a group of experienced Oxford anesthetists identified lumbar interspaces that were found by MRI to be one to four segments higher than assumed in 68% of cases (Figure 33-11).[85] Observers were more likely to agree with one another than with the MRI scan. Clinical anesthesiologists, who rarely use radiologic verification, have little opportunity for feedback to improve their skill in this respect.

Medical students and interns are usually instructed to select the L4-5 interspace, or thereabouts, for diagnostic lumbar puncture, but anesthesiologists are often more liberal in their approach. Given the inaccuracy of identification of lumbar interspaces, and the variability of the position of the conus, it is both logical and prudent that anesthesia providers insert a spinal needle *below* the spinous process of L3, or at least into a *lower* lumbar interspace, especially in women. Box 33-3 includes a summary of problems and precautions.

Space-Occupying Lesions of the Spinal Canal

Space-occupying lesions of the spinal canal include epidural hematoma, epidural abscess, and intraspinal tumors, any of which—within the rigid confines of the spinal canal—can cause dangerous compression of nervous tissue and its blood supply, necessitating urgent laminectomy. Preexisting vertebral stenosis or lumbar disc protrusion may exacerbate the compression, or mimic a space-occupying lesion, when a large volume is injected into the epidural space.[86-88] The neurologic deficits that arise from these lesions depend on their height; lower thoracic lesions are associated with leg weakness or paraplegia, and lumbar lesions are associated with cauda equina syndrome. Back pain is a common feature of all these lesions.

Although these are rare events that may be seen only a few times in a professional career, delayed recognition and treatment may result in a catastrophic outcome for the patient and grave medicolegal implications for the anesthesiologist. All compressive lesions may make their first appearance after

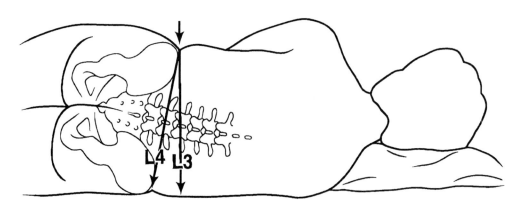

FIGURE 33-10. Error that may arise if Tuffier's line is judged in a pregnant patient in the lateral position, by dropping a perpendicular from the uppermost iliac crest rather than drawing the line through both crests. In pregnant patients at term, the hips may have a greater width than the shoulders. The resulting cephalad pelvic tilt may lead to an error in a cephalad direction.

childbirth or surgery, with or without a history of regional anesthesia.

SPINAL HEMATOMA

Intraspinal hematomas may be epidural or subdural. The clinical presentation depends on the size and site of the lesion and includes back pain (sometimes radiating to the legs), leg weakness, and urinary retention or incontinence.

Most **epidural hematomas** that cause neurologic damage typically occur in elderly patients with diffuse arterial disease and are very rare in obstetric patients, despite the engorgement of the epidural veins that occurs during pregnancy. One case was detected in a retrospective survey of 505,000 obstetric epidural blocks.[9] Three prospective surveys that included 182,000 obstetric blocks identified no cases,[10,11,13] although Loo et al.[6] identified three published cases of epidural hematoma in the *absence* of regional anesthesia in obstetric patients. One estimate of the incidence of spinal hematoma in the general population was approximately 1:150,000 with epidural anesthesia and 1:220,000 with spinal anesthesia.[89] In a prospective, follow-up study, Dahlgren et al.[16] reported one case of epidural hematoma (in a patient with no risk factors) among 8501 spinal anesthetics, and three cases (all in patients with risk factors) among 9232 epidural anesthetics for surgery.[16] However, in two prospective surveys of 229,136 epidural and spinal procedures in surgical patients in France—where anticoagulation is regarded as an absolute contraindication to regional anesthesia—no cases of spinal hematoma were found.[19,20] Similarly, there were none in an overview of surveys that covered 324,291 epidural and spinal anesthetics among a variety of patients, of whom 18% were obstetric, despite evidence of vessel trauma in 25% of patients.[90]

It appears that not only vessel damage but also coagulopathy is required to produce a hematoma large enough to cause a neurologic deficit. In the performance of an epidural blood patch, 20 mL of blood is commonly injected with impunity. Risk factors identified from comprehensive reviews of case reports include: (1) difficult or traumatic epidural needle/catheter placement, (2) coagulopathy or therapeutic anticoagulation, and (3) spinal deformity.[90,91] Vascular abnormality is also a theoretical risk factor.[92] Red blood cells have been noted in as many as 38% of CSF samples obtained during administration of spinal anesthesia,[93] while antiplatelet therapy increases the incidence of blood-tinged CSF,[94] but not of neurologic dysfunction following regional anesthesia.[95]

Although care is taken in obstetric patients to avoid neuraxial block in the presence of coagulopathy, epidural catheters have been placed with impunity in parturients with thrombocytopenia.[96-98] However, the frequency of vessel trauma among these patients was not regularly recorded. One important factor in minimizing the occurrence of spinal hematoma in parturients may be the normally hypercoagulable status of their blood. Further, neurologic deficits may be rare because of the ease with which a large volume of anticoagulated blood may flow out of the unrestricting intervertebral foramina in young patients.

Apart from the case detected retrospectively by Scott and Hibbard,[9] the only case report of *authenticated* epidural hematoma with neurologic sequelae in a parturient occurred in association with coagulopathy resulting from cholestasis.[99] Coagulation status was not investigated before insertion of the epidural catheter. A small epidural hematoma was found on MRI in a parturient with neurofibromatosis who developed urinary incontinence after dural puncture, but the disorder resolved spontaneously.[100] A preeclamptic patient with thrombocytopenia suffered a persistent lower limb deficit

---

Box 33-3 POINTS TO REMEMBER IN ORDER TO AVOID DAMAGE TO THE CONUS DURING INSERTION OF A SPINAL NEEDLE

- The conus reaches L2 in 43% of women but in only 27% of men.
- From the L1-2 interspace the needle tip may reach the conus in approximately 60% of individuals.
- Tuffier's line, even using both iliac crests, is not wholly accurate.
- The space chosen is usually higher than supposed.
- The spinal needle should not knowingly be inserted above the L3 spinous process.
- Non-cutting spinal needles have at least 1 mm of "blind tip" beyond the aperture.
- Spinal needles must be inserted with gentleness and control.
- The procedure should be abandoned if the patient is unable to cooperate.
- Aspiration (loss of resistance to negative pressure) should be used to help ensure immediate detection of entry into the subarachnoid space.

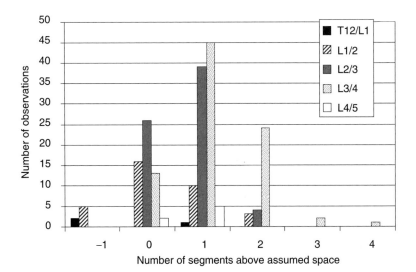

FIGURE 33-11. Identification of lumbar interspaces by Oxford anaesthetists. The horizontal axis shows the position of the actual interspace, identified by MRI, relative to the assumed space, in 200 observations. (Data from Broadbent C R, Maxwell W B, Ferrie R, et al. Ability of anaesthetists to identify a marked lumbar interspace. Anaesthesia 2000; 55: 1122-6.)

after a traumatic epidural catheter insertion using the loss-of-resistance-to-air technique.[101] Laminectomy revealed multiple bubbles but a blood clot of only 4 mL, the exact site of which was not stated.

Spinal **subdural hematoma** has been reported not only in surgical[102-104] but also in obstetric patients, one in association with an ependymoma,[105] and another in a woman with preeclampsia.[106] Dural puncture is a prerequisite for subdural hematoma, but coagulopathy may not be, because a smaller volume of blood within the restricted confines of the subdural space may compress adjacent nerve roots more readily than in the capacious epidural space.

The dangers of regional anesthesia in the presence of coagulopathy and anticoagulant treatment are discussed in Chapter 42. Under these circumstances it is an essential responsibility of the anesthesiologist to examine the lower limbs after delivery, to confirm and document that normal motor and sensory function have returned, and to request subsequent checks by the nursing staff. Physicians and nurses should remain vigilant for evidence of intraspinal bleeding. Severe back pain, a significant delay in normal recovery, or deterioration of lower limb or bladder function should signal the need for emergency imaging of the spine and appropriate neurologic intervention if intraspinal compression is confirmed by MRI.

EPIDURAL ABSCESS

Incidence

Epidural abscess, though rare, is more frequently reported than epidural hematoma, especially in obstetric patients. There was one case noted in the retrospective survey of 505,000 obstetric epidural blocks[9] and none in three prospective surveys.[10,11,13] This may appear similar to the incidence of hematoma, until one considers that in their literature search, Loo et al.[6] found 13 genuine cases in obstetric patients alone, 8 following epidural anesthesia (including one CSE) and 5 arising spontaneously,[6] while more have been reported since.[107,108] Some published case reports have included retrospective assessments of incidence,[109,110] but these cannot be regarded as accurate since they start with a positive reporting bias. In a national, 1-year prospective survey of 17,372

epidural anesthetics given for a variety of procedures in 46 departments in Denmark, nine epidural abscesses were found in eight different institutions, giving an incidence of 1:1930.[111] Catheters had been in situ for 3 to 31 days, the patients were elderly, eight of them were immunocompromised, and six were receiving thromboprophylaxis. This is the sort of survey that produces meaningful data and should have prompted a change in anesthetic practice, although it may not be directly applicable to obstetrics.

Risk factors for obstetric patients are outlined in Table 33-2. An epidural abscess typically follows prolonged epidural catheterization, reportedly between 1 and 4 days in obstetric cases.[107,109,112,113] The shortest recorded period of catheterization that was followed by epidural abscess was 6.5 hours, which occurred in a patient with evidence of venous trauma during placement of the epidural catheter.[114] Other factors may be epidural administration of opioid without local anesthetic,[107,108,112] traumatic or difficult insertion of the catheter,[112] and diabetes or immunosuppression from any cause.[111] Among surgical patients, inflammation at the epidural catheter entry point has been found to be increased in frequency when there is wound infection elsewhere in the body.[115,116] Although none of these factors by itself is an absolute contraindication to regional blockade, prolonged catheterization is best avoided in the presence of other risks.

Clinical presentation

The onset typically occurs 4 to 10 days after removal of the epidural catheter. Severe backache (with local tenderness) and fever, with or without radiating or root pain, are the presenting features. Inspection often reveals an inflamed catheter entry point with some fluid leak, and hematology screen typically reveals a leukocytosis. Such findings should prompt MRI, which may allow early diagnosis before the onset of neurologic changes (Figure 33-12).[117] Neck stiffness, headache, sensory and motor deficits in the legs, and bladder complications are common neurologic features. Diagnostic lumbar puncture is contraindicated.

Management

As with spinal hematoma, once neurologic signs are present, early diagnosis with prompt laminectomy is essential to

TABLE 33-2	POSSIBLE ETIOLOGIC FACTORS FOR EPIDURAL ABSCESS AND MENINGITIS	
	Epidural abscess	**Meningitis**
Entry point	• Through the catheter or along its track	• Blood, via the dural puncture
Usual causative organism	• Staphylococcus aureus	• Viridans type streptococcus
Possible source of infection	• Patient's skin, tracking along the catheter entry point	• Operator's mouth
	• Epidural equipment contaminated by operator's skin	• Talking without a mask
	• Body fluids in the bed	• Blood borne
	• Injectate without local anesthetic	• Vagina
Risk factors	• Prolonged catheterization	• Dural puncture ± epidural catheterization
	• Poor aseptic technique	• No face mask
	• Multiple attempts at insertion	• Vaginal delivery
	• Epidural hematoma	• Manual removal of the placenta
	• No bacterial filter	• Vaginal infection
	• Lying in a wet, contaminated bed	• Bacteremia
	• Polyurethane occlusive dressing	• Epidural blood patch
	• Absence of antimicrobial local anaesthetic	• Immunocompromise?
	• Immunocompromise: steroids, diabetes, AIDS	• No bacterial filter if epidural catheter used

recovery. The prognosis is improved if the abscess is evacuated before neurologic signs develop. In the presence of mild symptoms without neurologic changes, successful conservative treatment with antibiotics has been reported,[118] but emergency surgical drainage is the more secure option. Successful percutaneous needle drainage of epidural abscesses has also been reported,[119] although emergency laminectomy is the preferred treatment to ensure that all loculations are drained under direct vision. Prompt identification of the infectious organism(s) and discriminative antibiotic therapy are mandatory. Antibiotic treatment should be continued for 2 to 4 weeks.[117]

Etiology

It is inappropriate to bracket epidural abscess with meningitis, as both the etiology and the causative organisms are dissimilar (Table 33-2). *Staphylococcus aureus* is most commonly the causative organism in epidural abscess, and the skin would appear to be the most likely source of infection.[6] The few reported cases of epidural abscess caused by β-hemolytic streptococci[120,121] were not always associated with epidural blockade and therefore more probably stemmed from vaginal infection and hematogenous spread.

The skin is commonly colonized by *Staphylococcus epidermidis* and other weakly pathogenic bacteria, and occasionally by *Staphylococcus aureus*. The highest concentration of colonies is found in the hair follicles,[122] where they may be protected from briefly applied disinfectants. Infectious organisms from the skin can reach deeper tissue planes via needle tracks and implanted epidural catheters to create localized abscesses in the paraspinal or epidural spaces. Despite all aseptic precautions, some degree of detectable bacterial colonization of the epidural catheter is very common, but host defenses are normally robust. When infection containment breaks down, the process of epidural abscess formation begins, and expansion of the abscess and local vasculitis within the rigid confines of the spinal canal combine to cause ischemia of the underlying spinal cord or cauda equina, which results in paraplegia and sphincter disturbance.

The potential for the parturient's bed to be contaminated with amniotic fluid and excrement has prompted the use of occlusive dressings, but these may themselves be an infection risk.[109] Most local anesthetics, such as racemic bupivacaine and lidocaine, have an antibacterial effect in concentrations administered for regional anesthesia, although the antibacterial effect of the pure L-isomers levobupivacaine and ropivacaine is weaker.[123-126]

Paraspinal abscess[127,128] has been reported following epidural analgesia, and **discitis**[129] has been reported following spinal blockade in obstetric patients. Both are associated with back pain and signs of inflammation but without neurologic changes.

Meningitis

INCIDENCE

Meningitis was suspected in two cases in the prospective survey by Scott and Tunstall[10] of 108,133 epidural anesthetics and 14,865 spinal anesthetics, although which group they fell into was not stated. No case of meningitis was reported among the other surveys of epidural blockade summarized in Table 33-1, but one case was identified in the survey of spinal and CSE anesthesia (1:42,000 procedures).[12] A French survey identified three cases (1:100,000) among obstetric epidural procedures,[130] while a retrospective review of surgical patients in one hospital in Brazil found three cases among 38,128 spinal anesthetics (1:12,709) and none among 12,822 patients receiving other types of anesthesia.[131] Meningitis is probably the most common serious neurologic complication of neuraxial analgesia in labor. Loo et al.[6] found published reports of at least 20 cases in obstetric patients,[132-144] and there are others.[145-149]

ETIOLOGY

Risk factors and sources of infection are summarized in Table 33-2. It is recognized that the vagina may be colonized by streptococci, usually of the viridans type or occasionally beta-hemolytic, and that vaginal delivery is commonly followed by mild bacteremia. In normal circumstances the blood-brain barrier (i.e., the endothelial lining of the capillaries, which are continuous, with tight junctions and no pinocytotic vesicles) protects the central nervous system against weakly pathogenic bacteria in the blood stream. The dura mater should not be confused with the blood-brain barrier, but dural puncture may be associated with vascular trauma,[93] which allows blood to enter the CSF. The Brazilian survey tends to confirm that dural puncture is an important risk factor for meningitis.[131] Among the 26 published cases of puerperal meningitis for which details are available (Table 33-3), 20 followed known dural puncture, and streptococci of the viridans type were usually implicated. Blood-borne infection from the vagina would appear to be the common factor.

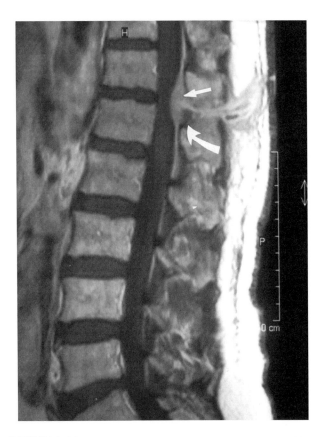

FIGURE 33-12. Mid-sagittal T1-weighted MRI of the lumbar and lower thoracic region, after intravenous gadolinium DTPA. Note the dorsal epidural mass at T12-L1 (arrow) convex anteriorly but not compressing the conus. Normal epidural fat is flat anteriorly. (From Royakkers AANM, Willigers H, van der Ven AJ, et al. Catheter-related epidural abscesses: Don't wait for neurological deficits. Acta Anaesthesiol Scand 2002; 46: 611-5.)

In three of the six cases following apparently uncomplicated labor epidural analgesia, hematogenous spread from vaginal infection (in two cases with group B streptococcus[139,142]) was implicated, while absence of a bacterial filter with an indwelling epidural catheter[135] must have been an additional risk factor. In the fourth case, Coxsackie B virus infection was diagnosed,[146] suggesting that the meningitis could have been coincidental and unrelated to the epidural anesthetic. The fifth case was associated with low-grade inflammation at the epidural catheter entry site and was probably best classified as a streptococcal epidural abscess that did not quite mature.[135] The sixth case was possibly viral and was tragically fatal.[147]

The most striking feature of the 20 cases associated with dural puncture was that 18 followed analgesia for labor (Table 33-3). This is remarkable, given that spinal anesthesia is far more commonly used for cesarean section. Thus labor, with its potential for vaginal trauma, is clearly an important risk factor for meningitis. One of the two cases that followed cesarean section was associated with genital herpes infection.[138] In the other case, no organism was isolated, but the meningitis was thought to be coincidental.[145] To prove this would depend on positive identification; naturally-acquired meningitis is caused by a different spectrum of organisms.

Community-acquired meningitis is caused by *Neisseria meningitidis, Streptococcus pneumoniae,* or *Haemophilus influenzae,* whereas streptococci of the viridans type (*salivarius, sanguis, uberis*) are most commonly implicated in meningitis following dural puncture. Such organisms are rarely found in the skin but rather in the vagina and nasal passages. Case reports seldom mention a face mask, and then only to admit that the anesthesiologist did not wear one. In the single case involving *Staphylococcus epidermidis* infection following CSE anesthesia,[141] the source was presumably the skin, via the epidural catheter track. Pseudomonas meningitis has been reported from contaminated saline used to rinse the spinal needle stylet.[134] In several cases no organisms have been grown,[132,133,141] and chemical contamination has been blamed. Such cases, however, often have other features of bacterial meningitis, and nowadays it may be possible to identify the causative organism from dead fragments by using the polymerase chain reaction.[148]

Bacteremia has been detected in approximately 8% of women with chorioamnionitis,[150] but two small studies found no evidence of spinal infection among 12 women with bacteremia who received epidural blockade without antibiotic treatment.[151,152] Such negative findings, although reassuring, are not conclusive, and do *not* pertain to spinal anesthesia.

Human immunodeficiency virus (HIV) infection and AIDS should not, however, be regarded as contraindications to regional analgesia, in view of the early presence of the HIV within the central nervous system.[153]

Manual removal of the placenta is a postulated risk factor for meningitis, and one such case has been reported,[137] although, given the popularity of spinal anesthesia for this procedure, one would perhaps expect a greater frequency. Performance of epidural blood patch in the presence of systemic infection is also a theoretical risk for both meningitis and abscess, but any additional risk in HIV-positive patients has been denied.[154] It has been postulated that use of the CSE technique, with the presence of a foreign body next to a dural hole, may increase the risk of meningitis, especially if epidural catheterization is prolonged.

Does uncomplicated epidural catheterization itself increase the risk of puerperal meningitis? Although epidural analgesia is used more commonly than spinal analgesia in labor, the number of case reports of meningitis following spinal analgesia far outweigh the number following epidural analgesia. Is epidural analgesia purely coincidental then? If that were so, one would expect meningitis to be reported following vaginal delivery without regional blockade. A Medline search dating back to 1970 combining *meningitis* with *puerperium* or *labor* or *labor and delivery* found mention of neonatal meningitis but no reports of maternal meningitis *without* regional anesthesia. In one survey from Iowa, among 73 women with beta-hemolytic streptococcal infections in the puerperium, the only one who suffered meningitis had had low spinal anesthesia.[155] Women with other types of streptococcal infection were not investigated. A search of 30 years of maternal mortality reports from the United Kingdom (with more than 20 million births) revealed (1) fulminating streptococcal septicemia without overt meningitis as a repeated cause of death; (2) one case of *E. coli* meningitis in the 1979-1981 report; and (3) one case of pneumococcal meningitis in mid-pregnancy, one case of group A streptococcal meningitis in a patient with spina bifida, and one case of purulent meningitis after spinal anesthesia for cesarean section in a sick patient in the 1997-1999 report. It would appear that vaginal delivery, even with genital tract sepsis, but without neuraxial anesthesia, is *not* a potent risk factor for meningitis, unless meningitis is regarded as a chance finding and therefore never reported. Therefore a causative relationship between epidural catheterization and meningitis after vaginal delivery cannot be excluded and may be attributed to silent dural puncture, which is known to occur even with apparently uncomplicated epidural catheter insertion.

TABLE 33-3	CASE REPORTS OF MENINGITIS AMONG OBSTETRIC PATIENTS				
	Labor			**Cesarean section**	
	Number of cases	**References**		**Number of cases**	**References**
Spinal	11	132, 133, 134, 137, 140, 210		2	138, 145
Combined spinal-epidural	5	141, 143, 144, 148, 149			
Unintentional dural puncture	2	41, 136			
"Uncomplicated" epidural	5	135, 139, 142, 146, 147		1	135
Total	*23*			*3*	

CLINICAL PRESENTATION AND MANAGEMENT

Fever, headache, photophobia, nausea, vomiting, and neck stiffness are typical symptoms, and when they are accompanied by confusion, drowsiness, and a positive Kernig's sign (i.e., inability to straighten the knee when the hip is flexed), meningitis should be strongly suspected. The onset may be 12 hours to a few days after delivery. Diagnostic lumbar puncture reveals increased CSF pressure, and an elevated protein and white blood cell count (mainly polymorphs in patients with bacterial meningitis), but a CSF glucose concentration that is lower than that in the blood. Culture may be negative if antibiotics have been given, but if positive, swab of the vagina usually reveals similar organisms. Treatment with an appropriate antibiotic must be vigorous and should not await the microbiology results. This usually leads to full recovery.[6] Third-generation cephalosporins have been recommended as a first-line treatment,[131] which can be adjusted according to results of culture and sensitivity.

Prevention of Intraspinal Infection Following Regional Anesthesia

Measures to prevent intraspinal infection are summarized in Box 33-4. Means of preventing meningitis and epidural abscess are not identical, since abscess usually follows epidural catheterization and is mainly caused by *Staphylococcus aureus*, which enters via the skin, whereas meningitis classically follows dural puncture, arises from vaginal or nasal organisms, may be blood-borne, and is usually caused by a streptococcus and never by *Staphylococcus aureus*.[6]

Sterile precautions that should be routine are not well described in many texts, few are supported by good evidence, and most are matters of local and individual habit.

THE FACE MASK

Oddly enough, when sterile procedures are described, the mask—if worn—is always mentioned last, whereas it must of course be donned *first*, before starting to clean the hands. This slip of the pen is consistent with the constant forgetfulness of those performing neuraxial blocks. Several surveys[131,156] indicate a widespread neglect of surgical masks as an essential element of infection control during the administration of neuraxial blockade. Meanwhile, case reports of intraspinal infection may state that the procedure was performed "under full aseptic precautions" when, in fact, the anesthesiologist did not wear a surgical mask.[136,139,140] In one case report the authors stated that the face mask "is of doubtful value,"[139] but "of doubtful value" does not mean that it is harmful. Such a departure from established surgical technique would seem unwise, both as a denial of an available aseptic precaution and as a serious weakening of defense against any subsequent lawsuit arising from intraspinal infection from whatever cause.

The effect of wearing a face mask in the prevention of such rare infective complications cannot readily be ascertained by a randomized controlled trial. Nevertheless, it has not been difficult to demonstrate the obvious value of face masks in reducing the dispersion of bacteria from the mouth and nose,[157,158] which is of acknowledged importance in the causation of iatrogenic meningitis. Face masks must surely be mandatory in the administration of spinal anesthesia, and because of the possibility of accidental dural puncture, face masks should also be mandatory during insertion of an epidural catheter. However, masks must be of good quality, preferably fiberglass and not simply woven linen or paper, and changed between each case.[131]

THE STERILE GOWN

Though undeniably part of "full aseptic precautions" as employed by a surgeon, a sterile gown is rarely worn for spinal needle placement. When inserting an epidural catheter, a gown is commonly worn in the United Kingdom, unlike the typical practice in the United States and France.[159] The value of wearing a gown is not supported by good evidence, but it can only be safer than not doing so. When a catheter is being inserted by a novice who is not wearing a gown, it may inadvertently come into contact with the skin of the upper arm or the unsterile clothing on the body. This may facilitate entry—via the catheter—of skin organisms, which are causative of epidural abscess.

STERILIZING THE SKIN

Evidence from laboratory studies shows that chlorhexidine in 80% ethanol kills both skin flora and *Staphylococcus aureus* far more quickly and completely than does povidone iodine or aqueous chlorhexidine gluconate,[122,160] which suggests that it is the alcohol that is the important factor, though its effect is brief. Moreover, open bottles of povidone iodine may be contaminated with various bacterial rods and skin flora,[161] attesting to its feeble antibacterial effect. A skin disinfectant preparation in which the iodine is present as an iodophor (a combination with a surfactant) plus isopropyl alcohol (DuraPrep™) has a prolonged effect and greatly reduces the colonization of skin and epidural catheter tips removed after labor.[162]

MAINTAINING STERILITY OF THE EPIDURAL CATHETER, ITS CONTENTS, AND THE ENTRY POINT

The entry point of the epidural catheter clearly needs to be protected from contamination. For prolonged analgesia with any sort of reservoir, racemic bupivacaine may be safer than

---

Box 33-4 PREVENTION OF INFECTION FOLLOWING REGIONAL ANESTHESIA

- Avoid dural puncture:
  - During labor, unless strongly indicated.
  - In the presence of known genital tract infection.
  - In the presence of systemic infection.
- In the presence of systemic infection, use an epidural technique and give a prophylactic antibiotic.
- Wear an effective mask that is changed between each patient.
- Wash hands, either with surgical scrub or alcohol wash.
- In the United Kingdom, a gown is worn for epidural catheter insertion.
- Don powder-free gloves in a sterile manner.
- Spray or paint the patient's skin twice with an alcohol preparation, allowing the skin to dry after each application.
- Make sure the area is securely draped.
- Avoid contaminating any equipment that is used in the procedure, and avoid touching any parts of the equipment that will enter the patient.
- Use a bacterial filter with an indwelling epidural or spinal catheter.
- Do not leave an epidural catheter *in situ* after delivery:
  - If the dura has been punctured during labor.
  - If there were multiple attempts at insertion.
  - If there is any evidence of sepsis.
  - If there is likely to be immunosuppression for any reason.

opioid alone or the pure L-isomers of local anesthetics, either of which may permit bacterial growth in the solution. Also, it seems logical to attach a bacterial filter during prolonged use of an epidural catheter. Prolonged catheterization is best avoided after dural puncture, whether unintentional or deliberate, and when sepsis or immunocompromise is present or suspected.

Vascular Disorders

ISCHEMIC INJURY TO THE SPINAL CORD

Ischemic injury is seen typically in elderly patients given epidural or spinal anesthesia, often with epinephrine, or indeed general anesthesia, with accompanying hypotension. It is rare in the obstetric population, in whom arterial disease is unusual and hypotension is treated aggressively. In their retrospective survey of 505,000 epidural blocks in obstetric patients, Scott and Hibbard[9] reported two patients who developed irreversible lesions of the spinal cord. One suffered a quadriplegia following thrombosis of a cervical hemangioma 10 days postpartum. In the second patient, paraplegia occurred 12 hours after full recovery from her epidural anesthetic, with a clinical picture of anterior spinal artery syndrome. In neither case was epidural blockade thought to be directly implicated. Anterior spinal artery syndrome has also been described in a diabetic parturient with scleredema[163] and in another with systemic lupus erythematosus.[164] Clearly, vascular disease and malformations must be risk factors for spinal cord damage,[92] and should be respected as such. One report outlined a cluster of accidents, in which a parous woman received epidural analgesia with lidocaine, then bupivacaine with epinephrine, followed by 2-chloroprocaine, when she required urgent cesarean section. A period of hypotension occurred when she was transferred to the operating room; this was associated with blood loss from a ruptured uterus, while placenta previa was also present. Typical irreversible anterior spinal artery syndrome followed.[165] Hypotension due to blood loss is likely to cause a greater degree of ischemia than that due to vasodilation, and the use of epinephrine may have contributed to the risk.

ETIOLOGY

The spinal cord, like the brain, can suffer ischemic injury from inadequate perfusion because of arterial disease or severe hypotension. The blood supply to the spinal cord depends on a single anterior and bilateral posterior spinal arteries, which arise from the Circle of Willis and receive reinforcements during their descent. The posterior spinal arteries receive regular contributions from radicular arteries, but the single anterior spinal artery, which supplies the anterior two-thirds of the spinal cord, receives only sporadic reinforcements. Anterior spinal artery syndrome may result from arterial compression or hypotension and is characterized by a predominantly motor deficit, with or without loss of pain and temperature sensation, but with sparing of vibration and joint sensations, which are transmitted in the posterior columns. Pressure from spinal stenosis, intraspinal tumors, or collagen deposits (e.g., in patients with scleredema[163,164]) may increase CSF pressure or spinal venous pressure and result in inadequate spinal cord capillary flow.

The major supply to the lumbar enlargement of the spinal cord is the artery of Adamkiewicz (arteria magna), a unilateral structure that typically arises from the lower thoracic or upper lumbar portion of the aorta between T9 and L2. However, in 1962, Lazorthes et al.[166] demonstrated a dual blood supply to the termination of the cord. A secondary source ascends from the internal iliac arteries by means of the iliolumbar and lateral sacral arteries. The two sources meet in an anastomosis surrounding the conus medullaris. In 85% of the population, the major supply comes from above, while the iliac contribution is relatively unimportant. In the remaining 15% the arteria magna arises from the upper half of the descending aorta (average level T5); in these people, the ascending iliac contribution assumes a greater role in maintaining the vitality of the conus medullaris. These ascending arteries lie close to the lumbosacral trunk. Therefore the fetal head may cause obstruction to arterial flow, or obstetric instrumentation may cause arterial injury. On the basis of this evidence, approximately 15% of pregnant women who undergo obstructed labor and/or traumatic delivery may be at risk of permanent neurologic damage resulting from insufficient arterial perfusion of the cord rather than the transient injury associated with trauma to the lumbosacral trunk. These anatomic studies received clinical support in a report from University College Hospital in Ibadan, Nigeria.[167] A total of 34 women with postpartum palsy were identified between 1966 and 1976, of whom 29 (85%) made a partial or complete recovery, and 5 (15%) suffered permanent spastic paraparesis. None had received regional anesthesia. These proportions fit nicely with Lazorthes' anatomic findings. However, infarct of the conus medullaris, which would be expected following such impairment of blood supply, usually resembles cauda equina syndrome[168] rather than a more extensive paraplegia.

SPINAL VASCULAR MALFORMATIONS

Spinal arteriovenous malformations (AVM) were difficult to detect before the development of MRI. Some cases of paraplegia attributed to anterior spinal artery syndrome secondary to arterial hypotension may have resulted from modest arterial hypotension and increased spinal venous pressure from a preexisting AVM. Although vascular malformations are an obvious cause for concern to the obstetric anesthesiologist,[169] reports of neurologic disorders associated with regional anesthesia in affected parturients do not abound.

Approximately 20% of patients with a cutaneous arteriovenous abnormality have a spinal AVM of the same spinal segment.[170] Small arterial feeders from a segmental intercostal artery feed into dilated serpiginous epidural veins that may extend over many segments of the spinal canal.[171,172] Occult angiomas may become symptomatic during late pregnancy or postpartum because of vasodilation from increased estrogen concentrations and increased spinal venous pressure. When this occurs, capillary flow is reduced within the affected region of the spinal cord, and outside the cord epidural veins may become distended and tortuous over many segments. Transient or permanent paraplegia may follow.[171,172]

Anesthesiologists should take account of the potential hazards associated with such disorders. Preanesthetic examination should therefore include inspection of the back for cutaneous angiomata or macular areas of skin discoloration, which may suggest the presence of an underlying spinal angioma at the same segmental level. Because spinal cord capillary flow is handicapped in the drainage area of an AVM, systemic arterial pressure should be maintained close to normal throughout the peripartum period, regardless of the anesthetic technique.

Chemical Injury

THE EPIDURAL SPACE

The epidural space is remarkably tolerant of foreign and potentially neurotoxic substances because of two protective factors. First, vascular uptake and outward flow via the intervertebral foramina remove a large proportion of drugs deposited in the epidural space. Second, nerve roots within the epidural space are protected by a cuff of dura and arachnoid. Severe neuraxial damage occurs only when these defenses are overwhelmed either by gross overdose or by unintentional contamination of the subarachnoid space. Occult dural puncture may occur more frequently than we think.[173] Therefore it is reasonable to suppose that some patients may be at increased risk after unintentional administration of a potentially neurotoxic substance such as traces of alcohol, anti-oxidant, or preservative.

There are many case reports of unintentional epidural injection of the wrong substance, including the following:

1. *Thiopental.* This has occurred from the use of an unlabeled syringe or failure to check the label. Vascular uptake leads to transient somnolence or light anesthesia, but no permanent sequelae have been reported.

2. *Ephedrine.* This was followed by bouts of severe hypertension.

3. *Potassium chloride.* At least four well-documented cases have been reported. Three were associated with look-alike vials and a failure to distinguish between 15% KCl and 0.9% NaCl as diluents for epidural injections. All three patients had profound motor and sensory block with pain or depolarizing spasms. Two patients recovered in 6 to 9 hours without any sequelae. The third patient, who received the largest epidural dose (15 mL of 11.25% KCl), remained permanently paraplegic.[174] A fourth patient got out of bed and accidentally disconnected his central venous and epidural catheters. The catheters were mistakenly crossed on reconnection, allowing 15 to 20 mmol of KCl to enter the epidural space. Profound motor and sensory block followed but lasted only a few hours.[175]

4. *Other potentially noxious substances.* Paraldehyde is believed to have been the cause of an incident that occurred during administration of epidural analgesia for labor, which resulted in permanent painful quadriplegia and the largest monetary award for damages in Great Britain at that time.[176] Unintentional misconnections of intravenous and epidural infusion systems have led to large-volume epidural infusion of potentially harmful substances, including total parenteral nutrition solutions with a high osmolality[177] and ranitidine in a phenol-containing solution.[178] No neurologic sequelae were reported, but the potential for an adverse outcome would seem high.

In summary, the epidural space is remarkably forgiving of such errors, and appears merely to be an exotic means of systemic administration. Nevertheless, vigilance to avoid such errors is mandatory, as harm may arise, for which there can be no defense.

THE SUBARACHNOID SPACE

The subarachnoid space, with its direct communication to intracranial structures, is a far more dangerous site than the epidural space for inadvertent errors. Intrathecal potassium does not merely maim, it can kill.[179] Irritant solutions may also cause arachnoiditis (vide infra).

Nerve roots within the subarachnoid space are highly vulnerable to chemical damage, particularly the sacral roots, which possess very thin sheaths. Therefore neurotoxicity associated with intrathecal injection classically produces **cauda equina syndrome**. Such damage has long been reported among surgical patients given spinal anesthesia, but the incidence cannot be determined, since practice varies in the deliberate administration of potentially neurotoxic substances.

For example, in 1937, 14 cases of severe cauda equina syndrome were reported following spinal anesthesia using hyperbaric "duracaine," a mixture—in 15% *ethanol*—of procaine, glycerin, and gliadin or gum acacia, which presumably was added in an attempt to prolong the action of procaine.[180] As hyperbaric dibucaine was available at that time, it is hard to understand why it was thought necessary to administer adulterated procaine. In the 1940s and 1950s the light spinal technique with 10 mL of hypo-osmolar dibucaine was associated with paraplegia,[181] but whether this resulted from disturbance of the intrathecal milieu or contamination with phenol was argued.

More recently, numerous cases of cauda equina syndrome have occurred in association with intrathecal injection of less obviously noxious spinal agents. Cases have followed continuous or single-shot spinal anesthesia, usually with 5% hyperbaric lidocaine but also with tetracaine or dibucaine.[19,182-184] Cases have also followed unintentional intrathecal administration of 2% lidocaine intended for the epidural space.[185,186]

Various risk factors for neurotoxic damage have been identified (Box 33-5), but also there is ample evidence to suppose that this danger is not present if hyperbaric or isobaric bupivacaine is used. In their surveys of spinal anesthesia in France, Auroy et al.[19,20] noted that the incidence of deficits that were not associated with painful insertion (i.e., were not due to trauma) was seven-fold higher with lidocaine than with bupivacaine.[19,20] Loo and Irestedt[187] reported six cases of cauda equina syndrome following spinal anesthesia with 5% lidocaine (five of which were single-shot injections) and none with bupivacaine. They estimated that the incidence was 1:25,600 spinal anesthetics with lidocaine and 0:440,000 with bupivacaine. In all these cases, other causes of neurologic deficit—trauma, ischemia, infection, compression, contamination, and adverse positioning—had all been excluded.

Drasner,[188] who suggests that spinal lidocaine may have a vanishing therapeutic index, has recommended that the dose of spinal lidocaine should be limited to 60 mg and the concentration no higher than 2.5% and that epinephrine should not be added. Meanwhile, the only preparation available for spinal anesthesia in the United Kingdom is hyperbaric bupivacaine, and in 2002 hyperbaric lidocaine was also withdrawn in Australia. Parturients appear to remain remarkably free of this dreadful condition, but it is perhaps preferable not to continue to put that theory to the test.

Box 33-5 RISK FACTORS FOR CHEMICAL DAMAGE TO THE CAUDA EQUINA

- Poor spread of local anesthetic:
  - Failure of the block, need for repeat injection
  - Fine gauge or pencil-point needle
  - Microspinal catheters
  - Continuous infusion
  - Hyperbaric solution
  - Lithotomy position
- Unintentional injection of a large volume intended for the epidural space
- Incorrect formulation, with unsuitable preservative or anti-oxidant
- Intrathecal **lidocaine**, particularly the 5% solution (tetracaine or dibucaine?)

Conus damage and cauda equina syndrome may appear similar. Although conus damage may involve upper motor neuron signs, these are not always present, and both conditions may have unilateral or bilateral features.[74,168] However, the causation is different. Whereas conus damage may result from ischemia or trauma, cauda equina syndrome typically results from compression within the lumbar spinal canal or from chemical damage.

TRANSIENT NEUROLOGIC SYNDROME (OR TRANSIENT RADICULAR IRRITATION)

Although this condition is not associated with any detectable neurologic deficit, the distribution of the pain that is suffered—in the back, buttocks and thighs—mirrors the distribution of nerve damage in cauda equina syndrome sufficiently to support the theory that the nerves are indeed irritated by a noxious intrathecal injection. Moreover, the risk factors appear to be similar (Box 33-5), although it has occurred after 2% as well as 5% lidocaine,[189,190] and early mobility has been proposed as an additional risk factor.[191] Its incidence varies greatly between studies,[192-198] but the preponderance of evidence suggests that bupivacaine is relatively blameless (Figure 33-13), while mepivacaine would appear to be as noxious as lidocaine.[199,200] Two large studies suggested that parturients did not experience transient neurologic symptoms,[201,202] while a third found an incidence of 8.8% among women having cesarean section under spinal anesthesia with hyperbaric bupivacaine,[203] and a number of individual cases have been reported.[204,205] One study reported the occurrence of transient neurologic symptoms among women undergoing postpartum tubal ligation with either spinal lidocaine or bupivacaine.[206] The authors speculated that these symptoms may be related, in part, to musculoskeletal strain.

ARACHNOIDITIS

While this diagnosis has been invoked by some individuals with vague symptoms and a desire to sue, true arachnoiditis is a disastrous condition, often with a much delayed onset of permanent paraplegia. Among parturients, chronic adhesive arachnoiditis of chemical origin has arisen after unintentional intrathecal injection of a large dose of 2-chloroprocaine with anti-oxidant and preservative intended for the epidural space,[207] while seven cases were described in a single report from Miami following epidural analgesia for childbirth with 2% lidocaine, probably with preservative.[208] Six cases were reported among Italian surgical patients following what were regarded as standard epidural anesthetics with bupivacaine and/or mepivacaine, usually with epinephrine.[209] The local anesthetic agents used, however, were obtained from multidose vials containing parabens as preservative, while glass syringes that had been washed in detergent were used for loss of resistance. In earlier publications it is not always possible to distinguish the cause of paraplegia, but arachnoiditis appears to crop up in clusters, when there may be some shortcomings in anesthetic practice or aseptic technique.

RISK MANAGEMENT

In an ideal world all truly high-risk women would be referred to the obstetric anesthesia clinic during pregnancy, so that anesthesia providers could obtain a thorough history, perform a careful examination, investigate further as needed, and plan the anesthetic strategy. We can but strive towards these ideals. The recommended points to explore in the history and physical examination are summarized in Boxes 33-6 and 33-7.

In addition to minimizing risk by adopting good and safe practices, vigilance must be extended postpartum to detect, diagnose, and treat any disorders that may arise. Early hospital discharge presents a problem in the detection of PDPH or

---

Box 33-6 POINTS TO REMEMBER IN THE PREANESTHETIC HISTORY

- Allergies or recreational drugs?
- Diabetes or cardiovascular disorder?
- Previous spinal or epidural anesthetics? What was the outcome?
- Preexisting neurologic signs or symptoms (e.g., sciatica, leg weakness)?
- Skeletal abnormality or back surgery?
- History of trauma or automobile accident, and if so, is it under litigation?
- Anticoagulant medication?
- Recent history of bleeding gums after dental hygiene (common in late pregnancy and not relevant as an isolated sign) or bruising of the ankles?
- Recent infection, including vaginal infection?
- Possibility of immunocompromise?

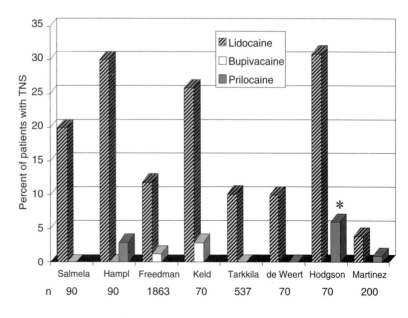

FIGURE 33-13. Proportions of patients reporting transient neurologic symptoms after spinal anesthesia. The trials selected are those in which lidocaine was compared with bupivacaine and/or prilocaine (or * procaine in the study by Hodgson et al.). Note the pale areas on the floor of the chart denoting zero values. The total numbers in the trials are shown below the chart. (Data from references 190, 192-198.)

space-occupying lesions, both of which require assessment and treatment, the latter on an urgent basis. It is important that those caring for women postpartum and responsible for their discharge are educated to look for signs of trouble and that women once home know how to recognize possible postanesthesia symptoms and how to contact an anesthesiologist if they experience them.

Diagnosis of Possible Neurologic Injury

A careful history and neurologic examination form the foundation on which other tests rest. Using simple clinical examination, coupled with a knowledge of basic neuroanatomy outlined in this chapter, it is usually possible to distinguish peripheral from central lesions. The anesthesiologist's preanesthetic history and physical examination may reveal some helpful clues, and any preexisting signs or deficits documented in the record will narrow the search or even provide an immediate answer. The history and physical examination should seek answers to these specific questions:

1. Is the lesion real or imagined?
2. Where is the lesion?
3. What is the nature of the lesion?
4. What is the cause of the lesion? Is it intrinsic, iatrogenic, or both?

The basic physical examination outlined in Box 33-7 should be repeated and the results should be compared with the preanesthetic findings. Fever and leukocytosis indicate an infective cause. Severe back pain and localized tenderness suggest epidural abscess, and pain radiating to the legs or buttocks is a late and urgent sign of cord or cauda equina compression. Headache with or without neck stiffness suggests meningitis but may also be present in severe PDPH.

Recent advances in imaging techniques have revolutionized the speed and precision with which intraspinal lesions can be identified. MRI has supplanted radiographic studies, and gadolinium enhancement further improves its sensitivity. The specificity is still imperfect in certain instances because MRI cannot distinguish clearly between blood and other fluid, although the distinction can usually be made on other grounds. Rarely, viral or other community-acquired infections may coincide with pregnancy and childbirth and cause a meningitis that presents diagnostic difficulty. In these cases, MRI with gadolinium enhancement shows swelling of the cord and punctate areas of increased density, reflecting inflammatory cell infiltrates. Arteriovenous malformations of the cord or dura also may be visible, and the enlarged veins draining them may be seen as serpiginous signal voids.

KEY POINTS

- Maternal obstetric palsy may arise from: (1) the process of childbirth, (2) pre-existing maternal pathology that predisposes to peripartum palsy, (3) coincidental pathology, and/or (4) neurologic injury directly attributable to anesthesia.
- Postpartum neurologic deficit is less likely to have anesthetic than other causes. Transient postpartum peripheral palsy is extremely common. Nevertheless, there is a widespread tendency to attribute every neurologic deficit to regional anesthesia.
- Careful examination and a knowledge of anatomy can usually suggest whether the lesion is central or peripheral.
- Meticulous technique, vigilance, and frequent observation of the patient are keystones to avoiding complications.
- A face mask should be worn and a proper sterile technique should be maintained when performing a neuraxial block.
- Good epidural needle insertion technique should minimize the risk of unintentional dural puncture, and postdural puncture headache, should it occur, must never be neglected.
- It is wise to avoid risking damage to the spinal cord by choosing a lower lumbar interspace for spinal needle insertion.
- Dural puncture during labor should be avoided in the presence of systemic or vaginal infection.
- Mistakes in drug administration may be avoided by obsessively careful reading of drug labels.
- It is crucial to be alert to the possibility of nerve compression that may be unnoticed under regional anesthesia.
- The results of examination and the details of all anesthetic procedures should be documented carefully.
- Rapid diagnosis and treatment are essential to successful outcome if neurologic complications should develop. Compressive intraspinal lesions require urgent laminectomy within 6 to 12 hours of the onset of symptoms.
- Early hospital discharge creates the need for a safety net to detect neurologic complications arising after the return home. Patients should be adequately informed about the presenting symptoms of the rare but potentially catastrophic complications of spinal and epidural anesthesia.

Box 33-7 PREANESTHETIC EXAMINATION

- Consider ease of intubation: mouth opening, teeth and neck.
- Examine the lower limbs:
  - If there is a question of a neurologic disorder, examine sensation to pin-prick or ice over the lateral surfaces of the lower leg and foot, and vibration sense using a tuning fork.
  - Knee and ankle tendon reflexes and Babinski reflex
  - Motor power of hips, knees, and ankles
- Examine the back for:
  - Signs of infection (any pustules to be avoided)
  - Nevi, suggesting a possible metameric AVM
  - Midline hair tuft or fat pad, suggesting some degree of dysraphism (e.g., spina bifida occulta)
  - Scoliosis
  - If the back looks technically difficult, as in severe scoliosis, is there an easily palpable sacral hiatus as an alternative to the lumbar epidural space?
- Look for signs of bleeding tendency.
- Document the history and physical examination, and note any abnormalities and any treatment decisions related to those abnormalities. Document any differences of opinion with other consultants in the case. In cases where an anesthetic is administered despite the presence of a relative contraindication, document the reasons for your decision.

REFERENCES

1. Turbridy N, Redmond JMT. Neurological symptoms attributed to epidural analgesia in labour: an observational study of seven cases. Br J Obstet Gynaecol 1996; 103:832-3.

2. Tillman AJB. Traumatic neuritis in the puerperium. Am J Obstet Gynecol 1935; 29:660-6.

3. Chalmers JA. Traumatic neuritis of the puerperium. J Obstet Gynaecol Br Emp 1949; 56:205-16.

4. Hill EC. Maternal obstetric paralysis. Am J Obstet Gynecol 1962; 83:1452-60.

5. Murray RR. Maternal obstetric paralysis. Am J Obstet Gynecol 1964; 88:399-403.

6. Loo CC, Dahlgren G, Irestedt L. Neurological complications in obstetric regional anaesthesia. Int J Obstet Anesth 2000; 9:99-124.

7. Ong BY, Cohen MM, Esmail A, Cumming M, Kozody R, Palahniuk RJ. Paresthesias and motor dysfunction after labor and delivery. Anesth Analg 1987; 66:18-22.

8. MacArthur C, Lewis M, Knox EG. Investigation of long term problems after obstetric epidural anaesthesia. BMJ 1992; 304:1279-82.

9. Scott DB, Hibbard BM. Serious non fatal complications associated with extradural block in obstetric practice. Br J Anaesth 1990:64:537-41.

10. Scott DB, Tunstall ME. Serious complications associated with epidural/spinal blockade. Int J Obstet Anesth 1995; 4:133-9.

11. Holdcroft A, Gibberd FB, Hargrove RL, Hawkins DF, Dellaportas CI. Neurological problems associated with pregnancy. Br J Anaesth 1995; 75:522-6.

12. Holloway J, Seed PT, O'Sullivan G, Reynolds F. Paraesthesiae and nerve damage following combined spinal epidural and spinal anaesthesia. Int J Obstet Anesth 2000; 9:151-5.

13. Paech MJ, Godkin R, Webster S. Complications of obstetric epidural analgesia and anaesthesia: a prospective analysis of 10995 cases. Int J Obstet Anaesth 1998; 7:5-11.

14. Dar AQ, Robinson APC, Lyons G. postpartum neurological symptoms following regional blockade: a prospective study with case controls. Int J Obstet Anesth 2002; 11:85-90.

15. Wong CA, Scavone BM, Dugan S et al. Incidence of postpartum lumbosacral spine and lower extremity nerve injuries. Obstet Gynecol 2003; 101:279-88.

16. Dahlgren N, Tornebradt K. Neurological complications after anaesthesia. A follow-up of 18,000 spinal and epidural anaesthetics performed over three years. Acta Anaesthesiol Scand 1995; 39:872-80.

17. Aromaa U, Lahdensuu M, Cozanitis DA. Severe complications associated with epidural and spinal anaesthesia in Finland 1987-1993. A study based on patient insurance claims. Acta Anaesthesiol Scand 1997; 41:445-52.

18. Horlocker TT, McGregor DG, Matsushige DK, Schroeder DR, Besse JA. A retrospective review of 4767 consecutive spinal anesthetics: central nervous system complications. Anesth Analg 1997; 84:578-84.

19. Auroy Y, Narchi P, Messiah A, et al. Serious complications related to regional anesthesia: Results of a prospective survey in France. Anesthesiology 1997; 87:479-86.

20. Auroy Y, Benhamou D, Bargues L, et al. Major complications of regional anesthesia in France: The SOS regional anesthesia hotline service. Anesthesiology 2002; 97:1274-80.

21. Donaldson JO. Neurology of Pregnancy, 2nd ed. Philadelphia, WB Saunders, 1989.

22. Warner MA, Warner DO, Harper M, Schroeder DR, Maxson PM. Lower extremity neuropathies associated with lithotomy positions. Anesthesiology 2000; 93:938-42.

23. Chan JK, Manetta A. Prevention of femoral nerve injuries in gynecologic surgery. Am J Obstet Gynecol 2002; 186:1-7.

24. Van Diver T, Camann W. Meralgia paresthetica in the parturient. Int J Obstet Anesth 1995; 4:109-12.

25. Farrar D, Raoof N. Bell's palsy, childbirth and epidural analgesia. Int J Obstet Anesth 2001; 10:68-70.

26. O'Connell JEA. Maternal obstetrical paralysis. Surg Gynecol Obstet 1944; 79:374-82.

27. Silva M, Mallinson C, Reynolds F. Sciatic nerve palsy following childbirth. Anaesthesia 1996; 51:1144-8.

28. Umo-Etuk J, Yentis SM. Sciatic nerve injury and caesarean section (letter). Anaesthesia 1997; 52:605-6.

29. Roy S, Levine AB, Herbison GJ, Jacobs SR. Intraoperative positioning during cesarean as a cause of sciatic neuropathy. Obstet Gynecol 2002; 99:652-3.

30. Cohen DE, Van Duker B, Siegel S, Keon TP. Common peroneal nerve palsy associated with epidural analgesia. Anesth Analg 1993; 76:429-31.

31. Lepski GR, Alderson JD. Epidural analgesia in labour for a patient with hereditary neuropathy with liability to pressure palsy. Int J Obstet Anesth 2001; 10:198-201.

32. Weissman A, Grisaru D, Shenhav M, et al. Postpartum surveillance of urinary retention by ultrasonography: the effect of epidural analgesia. Ultrasound Obstet Gynecol 1995; 6:130-4.

33. Chien PFW, Khan KS, Agustsson P, et al. The determinants of residual bladder volume following spontaneous vaginal delivery. J Obstet Gynecol 1996; 16:146-50.

34. Liang C-C, Wong S-Y, Tsay P-T, et al. The effect of epidural analgesia on postpartum urinary retention in women who deliver vaginally. Int J Obstet Anesth 2002; 11:164-9.

35. MacArthur C, Lewis M, Knox EG. Health after childbirth. London: HMSO, 1991.

36. Borum SE, Naul LG, McLeskey CH. Postpartum dural venous sinus thrombosis after postdural puncture headache and epidural blood patch. Anesthesiology 1997; 86:487-90.

37. Ravindran RS, Zandstra GC, Viegas OJ. Postpartum headache following regional analgesia: A symptom of cerebral venous thrombosis. Can J Anaesth 1989; 36:705-7.

38. Ariola SE, Russo TO, Marx GF. Postdural puncture headache or incipient eclampsia? Int J Obstet Anesth 1991; 1:33-4.

39. Diemunsch P, Balabaud VP, Petiau Cet al. Bilateral subdural hematoma following epidural anesthesia. Can J Anaesth 1998; 45:328-31.

40. Shah JL. Severe headache following an epidural top-up. Int J Obstet Anesth 1991; 1:29-31.

41. Sansome AJT, Barnes GR, Barrett RF. An unusual presentation of meningitis as a consequence of inadvertent dural puncture. Int J Obstet Anesth 1991; 1:35-7.

42. Shearer VE, Jhaveri HS, Cunningham FG. Puerperal seizures after post dural puncture headache. Obstet Gynecol 1995; 85:225-60.

43. Rodrigo P. Garcia JM. Ailagas J. [General convulsive crisis related to pneumocephalus after inadvertant dural puncture in an obstetric patient]. Revista Espanola de Anestesiologia y Reanimacion 1997; 44:247-9.

44. Oliver CD, White SA. Unexplained fitting in three parturients suffering from postdural puncture headache. Br J Anaesth 2002; 89:782-5.

45. Heyman HJ, Salem MR, Klimov I. Persistent sixth cranial nerve paresis following blood patch for postdural puncture headache. Anesth Analg 1982; 61:948-9.

46. Dunbar SA, Katz, NP. Failure of delayed epidural blood patching to correct persistent cranial nerve palsies. Anesth Analg 1994; 79:806-7.

47. Chohan U, Khan M, Saeed-uz-zafar: Abducent nerve palsy in a parturient with a 25-gauge Sprotte needle. Int J Obstet Anesth 2003; 12:235-6.

48. Lowe DM, McCullough AM. 7th nerve palsy after extradural blood patch. Br J Anaesth 1990; 65:721-2.

49. Perez M, Olmos M, Garrido FJ. Facial nerve paralysis after epidural blood patch. Reg Anesth 1993; 18:196-8.

50. Carrero EJ, Agusti M, Fabregas N, et al. Unilateral trigeminal and facial nerve palsies associated with epidural analgesia in labour. Can J Anaesth 1998; 45:893-7.

51. Martin-Hirsch DP, Martin-Hirsch PL. Vestibulocochlear dysfunction following epidural anaesthesia in labour. Br J Clin Pract 1994; 48:340-1.

52. Viale M, Narchi P. Veyrac P. Benhamou D. Chronic tinnitus and hearing loss caused by cerebrospinal fluid leak treated with success with peridural blood patch. Apropos of 2 cases. Annales d'Oto-Laryngologie et de Chirurgie Cervico-Faciale1996; 113:175-7.

53. Weitz SR. Drasner K. Spontaneous intracranial hypotension: a series. Anesthesiology 1996; 85:923-5.

54. Beck CE. Rizk NW. Kiger LT. Spencer D. Hill L. Adler JR. Intracranial hypotension presenting with severe encephalopathy. Case report. J Neurosurg 1998; 8:470-3.

55. Spencer HC. Post dural puncture headache: What matters in technique. Reg Anesth Pain Med 1998; 23:374-9.

56. Akpek EA, Karaaslan D, Erol E, Caner H, Kayhan Z. Chronic subdural haematoma following caesarean section under spinal anaesthesia. Anaesth Intensive Care 1999; 27:206-8.

57. Achyra R, Chhabra SS, Ratra M, Sehgal AD. Cranial subdural haematoma after spinal anaesthesia. Br J Anaesth 2001; 86:893-5.

58. Davies JM, Murphy A, Smith M, O'Sullivan G. Subdural haematoma after dural puncture headache treated by epidural blood patch. Br J Anaesth 2001; 86:720-3.

59. Kardash K, Morrow F, Béïque F. Seizures after epidural blood patch with undiagnosed subdural hematoma. Reg Anesth Pain Med 2002; 27:433-6.

60. Reynolds F. Dural puncture and headache. Avoid the first but treat the second. BMJ 1993; 306:874-6.

61. Cantais E, Behamou D, Petit D, Palmier B. Acute subdural hematoma following spinal anesthesia with a very small spinal needle. Anesthesiology 2000; 93:1354-5.

62. Edelman JD, Wingard DW. Subdural hematoma after lumbar puncture. Anesthesiology 1980; 52:166-7.

63. Ayorinde BT, Mushambi M. Extradural haematoma in a patient following manual removal of the placenta under spinal anaesthesia: was the spinal to blame? Int J Obstet Anesth 2002; 11:216-8.

64. Yoshii WY, Rottman RL, Rosenblatt RM et al. Epidural catheter induced traumatic radiculopathy in obstetrics: one center's experience. Reg Anesth 1994; 19:132-5.

65. Loo CC, Cheong KF. Monoplegia following obstetric epidural anaesthesia. Ann Acad Med Singapore 1997; 26:232-4.

66. Richardson J, Bedder M. Transient anterior spinal cord syndrome with continuous postoperative epidural analgesia. Anesthesiology 1990; 72:764-6.

67. Ben-David B, Vaida S, Collins G, et al. Transient paraplegia secondary to an epidural catheter. Anesth Analg 1994; 79:598-600.

68. Warder DE, Oakes WJ. Tethered cord syndrome: the low-lying and normally positioned conus. Neurosurgery 1994; 34:597-600.

69. Reynolds F. Litigation in obstetric regional anaesthesia. In: Highlights in Pain Therapy and Regional Anaesthesia V. Editor A Van Zurdert. Barcelona: Publicidad Permanyer, 1996:39-43.

70. Bromage PR, Benumof JL. Paraplegia following intracord injection during attempted epidural anesthesia under general anesthesia. Reg Anesth 1998; 23:104-7.

71. Mayall MF, Calder I. Spinal cord injury following an attempted thoracic epidural. Anaesthesia 1999; 54:987-8.

72. Katz N, Hurley R. Epidural anaesthesia complicated by fluid collection within the spinal cord. Anesth Analg 1993; 77:1064-5

73. Rajakulendran Y, Rahman S, Venkat N. Long-term neurological complication following traumatic damage to the spinal cord with a 25 gauge Whitacre spinal needle. Int J Obstet Anesth 1999; 8:62–6.

74. Reynolds F. Damage to the conus medullaris following spinal anaesthesia. Anaesthesia 2001; 56:238-47.

75. Parry H. Spinal cord damage (letter). Anaesthesia 2001; 56:290.

76. Greaves JD. Serious spinal cord injury due to haematomyelia caused by spinal anaesthesia in a patient treated with low-dose heparin. Anaesthesia 1997; 52:150-4.

77. Collier CB, Turner MA. Are pencil point needles safe for subarachnoid block? (letter) Anaesthesia 1998; 53:411-2.

78. Reynolds F. Logic in the safe practice of spinal anaesthesia (Editorial). Anaesthesia 2000; 55:1045-6.

79. Reimann AF, Anson BJ. Vertebral level of termination of the spinal cord with report of a case of sacral cord. Anatomical Record 1944; 88:127–38.

80. Saifuddin A, Burnett SJ, White J. The variation of position of the conus medullaris in an adult population. A magnetic resonance imaging study. Spine 1998; 23:1452-6.

81. Thomson A. Fifth annual report of the committee of collective investigation of the Anatomical Society of Great Britain and Ireland for the year 1893-94. J Anat Physiol 1894; 29:35-60.

82. Ievins FA. Accuracy of placement of extradural needles in the L_{3-4} interspace: comparison of two methods of identifying L4. Br J Anaesth 1991; 66:381-2.

83. Render CA. The reproducibility of the iliac crest as a marker of lumbar spine level. Anaesthesia 1996; 51:1070-1.

84. Van Gessel EF, Forster A, Gamulin Z. Continuous spinal anesthesia: where do spinal catheters go? Anesth Analg 1993; 76:1004-7.

85. Broadbent C R, Maxwell W B, Ferrie R, et al. Ability of anaesthetists to identify a marked lumbar interspace. Anaesthesia 2000; 55:1122-6.

86. Forster MR, Nimmo GR, Brown AG. Case report: Prolapsed intervertebral disc after epidural analgesia in labour. Anaesthesia 1996; 51:773-5.

87. Chaudhari LS, Kop BP, Dhruva AJ. Paraplegia and epidural analgesia. Anaesthesia 1978; 33:722-5.

88. Ballin NC. Paraplegia following epidural analgesia. Anaesthesia 1981; 36:952-3.

89. Haljamae H. Thromboprophylaxis, coagulation disorders, and regional anaesthesia. Acta Anaesthesiol Scand 1996; 40:1024-40.

90. Vandermeulen EP, Van Aken H, Vermylen J. Anticoagulants and spinal-epidural anesthesia. Anesth Analg 1994;79:1165-77.

91. Wulf H. Epidural anaesthesia and spinal haematoma. Can J Anaesth 1996; 43:1260-71.

92. Horlocker TT. Low molecular weight heparin and neuraxial anesthesia. Thromb Res 2001; 101:V141-54.

93. Knowles PR, Randall NP, Lockhart AS. Vascular trauma associated with routine spinal anaesthesia. Anaesthesia 1999;54:647-50.

94. Horlocker TT, Wedel DJ, Offord KP. Does preoperative antiplatelet therapy increase the risk of hemorrhagic complications associated with regional anesthesia? Anesth Analg 1990; 70:631-4.

95. Horlocker TT, Wedel DJ, Schroder DR, et al. Preoperative antiplatelet therapy does not increase the risk of spinal hematoma associated with regional anesthesia. Anesth Analg 1995; 80:303-9.

96. Rasmus KT, Rottman RL. Kotelko DM. Wright WC. Stone JJ. Rosenblatt RM. Unrecognized thrombocytopenia and regional anesthesia in parturients: a retrospective review. Obstet Gynecology 1989; 73:943-6.

97. Hew-Wing P, Rolbin SH, Hew E, Amato D. Epidural anaesthesia and thrombocytopenia. Anaesthesia 1989; 44:775-7.

98. Beilin Y, Zahn J, Comerford M. Safe epidural analgesia in thirty parturients with platelet counts between 69,000 and 98,000 mm^{-3}. Anesth Analg 1997; 85:385-8.

99. Yarnell RW, D'Alton ME. Epidural hematoma complicating cholestasis of pregnancy. Curr Opin Obstet Gynecol 1996; 8:239-42.

100. Esler MD, Durbridge J, Kirby S. Epidural haematoma after dural puncture in a parturient with neurofibromatosis. Br J Anaesth 2001; 87:932-4.

101. Yuen TST, Kua JSW, Tan IKS. Spinal haematoma following epidural anaesthesia in a patient with eclampsia. Anaesthesia 1999; 54:350-71.

102. Brougher RJ, Ramage D. Spinal subdural haematoma following combined spinal-epidural anaesthesia. Anaesth Intensive Care 1995; 23: 111-3.

103. Pryle BJ, Carter JA, Cadoux-Hudson T. Delayed paraplegia following spinal anaesthesia. Anaesthesia 1996; 51:263-5.

104. Pedraza Gutierrez S, Coll Masfarre S, Castano Duque CH, et al. Hyperacute spinal subdural haematoma as a complication of lumbar spinal anaesthesia: MRI. Neuroradiology 1999; 41:910-4.

105. Roscoe MWA, Barrington TW. Acute spinal subdural hematoma: a case report and review of literature. Spine 1984; 9:672-5.

106. Lao TT, Halpern SH, MacDonald D, Huh C. Spinal subdural haematoma in a parturient after attempted epidural anaesthesia. Can J Anaesth 1993; 40:340-5.

107. Collier CB, Gatt SP. Epidural abscess in an obstetric patient. Anaesth Intensive Care 1999; 27:662-6.

108. Rathmell JP, Garahan MB, Alsofrom GF. Epidural abscess following epidural analgesia. Reg Anesth Pain Med 2000; 25:79-82.

109. Kindler C, Seeberger M, Siegmund M, Schneider M. Extradural abscess complicating lumbar extradural anaesthesia and analgesia in an obstetric patient. Acta Anaesthesiol Scand 1996; 40:858-61.

110. Phillips JMG, Stedeford JC, Hartsilver E, Roberts C. Epidural abscess complicating inertion of epidural catheters. Br J Anaesth 2002; 89: 778-82.

111. Wang LP, Hauerberg J, Schmidt JF. Incidence of spinal epidural abscess after epidural analgesia: a national 1-year survey. Anesthesiology 1999; 91:1928-36.

112. Ngan Kee WD, Jones MR, Thomas P, Worth RJ. Extradural abscess complicating extradural anaesthesia for caesarean section. Br J Anaesth 1992; 69:647-52.

113. Borum SE, McLeskey CH, Williamson JB, Harris FS, Knight AB. Epidural abscess after obstetric epidural analgesia. Anesthesiology 1995; 82:1523-6.

114. Dhillon AR, Russell IF. Epidural abscess in association with obstetric analgesia. Int J Obstet Anesth 1998;6:118-21.

115. Jakobsen KB, Christensen MK, Carlsson PS. Extradural anaesthesia for repeated surgical treatment in the presence of infection. Br J Anaesth 1995; 75:536-40.

116. Bengtsson M, Nettelblad H, Sjoberg F. Extradural catheter-related infections in patients with infected cutaneous wounds. Br J Anaesth 1997; 79:668-70.

117. Royakkkers AANM, Willigers H, van der Ven AJ, Durieux M, van Kleef M. Catheter-related epidural abscesses -don't wait for neurological deficits. Acta Anaesthesiol Scand 2002; 46:611-5.

118. Dysart RH, Balakrishnan V. Conservative management of extradural abscess complicating spinal-extradural anaesthesia for caesarean section. Br J Anaesth 1997; 78:591-3.

119. Tabo E, Ohkuma Y, Kimura S, et al. Successful percutaneous drainage of epidural abscess with epidural needle and catheter. Anesthesiology 1994; 80:1393-5.

120. Jenkin G, Woolley IJ, Brown GV, Richards MJ. Post partum epidural abscess due to group B Streptococcus. Clin Infect Dis 1997; 25:1249.

121. Crawford JS. Pathology in the extradural space. Br J Anaesth 1975; 47:412-5.

122. Sato S, Sakuragi T, Dan K. Human skin flora as a potential source of epidural abscess. Anesthesiology 1996; 85:1276-82.

123. Zaidi S, Healy TEJ. A comparison of the antibacterial properties of six local analgesic agents. Anaesthesia 1977; 32:69-70.

124. Pere P, Lindgren L, Vaara M. Poor antibacterial effect of ropivacaine: comparison with bupivacaine. Anesthesiology 1999; 91:884-6.

125. Hodson M, Gajraj R, Scott NB. A comparison of the antimicrobial activity of levobupivacaine vs bupivacaine: an in vitro study with bacteria implicated in epidural infection. Anaesthesia 1999; 54:699-702.

126. Goodman EJ, Jacobs MR, Bajaksouzian S et al. Clinically significant concentrations of local anesthetics inhibit Staphylococcus aureus in vitro. Int J Obstet Anesth 2002; 11:95-9.

127. Hill JS, Hughes EW, Robertson PA. A Staphylococcus aureus paraspinal abscess associated with epidural analgesia in labour. Anaesthesia 2001; 56:871-8.

128. Raj V, Foy J. Paraspinal abscess associated with epidural in labour. Anaesth Intensive Care 1998; 26:424-6.

129. Bajwa ZH, Ho C, Grush A, et al. Discitis associated with pregnancy and spinal anesthesia. Anesth Analg 2002; 94:415-6.

130. Palot M, Visseaux H, Botmans C, Pire JC. [Epidemiology of complications of obstetrical epidural analgesia.] Cah Anesthesiol 1984; 42:229-33.

131. Videira RLR, Ruiz-Neto PP, Neto MB. Post spinal meninigitis and sepsis. Acta Anaesthesiol Scand 2002; 46:639-46.

132. Gibbons RB. Chemical meningitis following spinal anesthesia. JAMA 1969; 210:900-2.

133. Phillips OC. Aseptic meningitis following spinal anesthesia. Anesth Analg 1970; 49:866-71.

134. Corbett JJ, Rosenstein BJ. Pseudomonas meningitis related to spinal anesthesia. Report of three cases with a common source of infection. Neurology 1971; 21:946-50.

135. Ready LB, Helfer D. Bacterial meningitis in parturients after epidural anesthesia. Anesthesiology 1989; 71:988-90.

136. Berga S, Trierweiler MW. Bacterial meningitis following epidural anesthesia for vaginal delivery: A case report. Obstet Gynecol 1989; 74:437-9.

137. Roberts SP, Petts HV. Meningitis after obstetric anaesthesia. Anaesthesia 1990; 45:376-7.

138. Lee JJ, Parry H. Bacterial meningitis following spinal anaesthesia for caesarean section. Br J Anaesth 1991; 66:383-6.

139. Davis L, Hargreaves C, Robinson PN. Postpartum meningitis. Anaesthesia 1993; 48:788-9.

140. Newton JA, Lesnik IK, Kennedy CA. Streptococcus salivarius meningitis following spinal anesthesia. Clin Infect Dis 1994; 18:840-1.

141. Harding SA, Collis RE, Morgan BM. Meningitis after combined spinal-extradural anaesthesia in obstetrics. Br J Anaesth 1994; 73:545-7.

142. Goldstein MJ, Parker RL, Dewan DM. Status epilepticus amauroticus secondary to meningitis as a cause of postpartum cortical blindness. Reg Anesth 1996; 21:595-8.

143. Cascio M, Heath G. Meningitis following a combined spinal-epidural technique in a labouring term parturient. Can J Anaesth 1996; 43: 399-402.

144. Bouhemad B, Dounas M, Mercier FJ, Benhamou D. Bacterial meningitis following combined spinal-epidural analgesia for labour. Anaesthesia 1998; 53:292-5.

145. Donnelly T, Koper M, Mallaiah S. Meningitis following spinal anaesthesia: A coincidental infection? Int J Obstet Anesth 1998; 7:170-2.

146. Neumark J, Feichtinger W, Gassner A. Epidural block in obstetrics followed by aseptic meningitis. Anesthesiology 1980; 52:518-9.

147. Choy JC. Mortality from peripartum meningitis. Anaesth Intensive Care 2000; 28:328-30.

148. Pinder AJ, Dresner M. Meningococcal meningitis after combined spinal-epidural analgesia. Int J Obstet Anesth 2003; 12:183-7.

149. Stallard N, Barry P. Another complication of the combined extradural-subarachnoid technique. Br J Anaesth 1995; 75:370-1.

150. Gibbs RS, Castillo MS, Rodgers PJ. Management of acute chorioamnionitis. Am J Obstet Gynecol 1980; 136:709-13.

151. Bader AM, Gilbertson L, Kirz L, Datta S. Regional anesthesia in women with chorioamnionitis. Reg Anesth 1992; 17:84-6.

152. Goodman EJ, DeHorta E, Taguiam JM. Safety of spinal and epidural anesthesia in parturients with chorioamnionitis. Reg Anesth 1996; 21:436-41.

153. Gershon RY, Manning-Williams D. Anesthesia and the HIV-infected parturient: A retrospective study. Int J Obstet Anesth 1997; 6:76-81.

154. Shapiro HM. Opposer: Epidural blood patch is contraindicated in HIV-positive patients. Int J Obstet Anesth 1994; 3:168-9.

155. White CA. Koontz FP. Hemolytic streptococcus infections in postpartum patients. Obstet Gynecol 1973; 41:27-32.

156. Panikkar KK, Yentis SM. Wearing of masks for obstetrical regional anaesthesia. A postal survey. Anaesthesia 1996; 51:398-400.

157. Phillips BJ, Fergusson S, Armstrong P, Wildsmith JAW. Surgical facemasks are effective in reducing bacterial contamination caused by dispersal from the upper airway. Br J Anaesth 1992; 69:407-8.

158. McLure HA, Talboys CA, Yentis SM, Azadian BS. Surgical face masks and downward dispersal of bacteria. Anaesthesia 1998; 53:624-6.

159. Benhamou D, Mercier FJ, Dounas M. Hospital policy for prevention of infection after neuraxial blocks in obstetrics. Int J Obstet Anesth 2002; 11:265-9.

160. Sakuragi T, Yanagisawa K, Dan K. Bactericidal activity of skin disinfectants on methicillin-resistant Staphylococcus aureus. Anesth Analg 1995; 81:555-8.

161. Birnbach DJ, Stein DJ, Murray O, et al. Povidone iodine and skin disinfection before initiation of epidural anesthesia. Anesthesiology 1998; 88:668-72.

162. Birnbach DJ, Meadows W, Stein DJ, et al. Comparison of povidone iodine and DuraPrep, an iodophor-in-isopropyl alcohol solution, for skin disinfection prior to epidural catheter insertion in parturients. Anesthesiology 2003; 98:164-9.

163. Eastwood DW. Anterior spinal artery syndrome after epidural anesthesia in a pregnant diabetic patient with scleredema. Anesth Analg 1991; 73:90-1.

164. Dell'Isola B, Vidailhet M, Gatfosse M, et al. Recovery of anterior spinal artery syndrome in a patient with systemic lupus erythematosus and antiphospholipid antibodies. Br J Rheumatol 1991; 30:314-5.

165. Ackerman WE, Juneja MM, Knapp RK. Maternal paraparesis after epidural anesthesia and cesarean section. South Med J 1990; 83:695-7.

166. Lazorthes G, Poulhes J, Bastide G, et al. La vascularization de la moelle epiniere (etude anatomique et physiologique). Rev Neurol 1962; 106:535-7.

167. Bademosi O, Osuntokun BO, Van der Werd JH, et al. Obstetric neuropraxia in the Nigerian African. Internat J Gynaecol Obstet 1980; 17:611-4.

168. Anderson NE. Willoughby EW. Infarction of the conus medullaris. Ann Neurol 1987; 21:470-4.

169. Ong BY. Littleford J. Segstro R. Paetkau D. Sutton I. Spinal anaesthesia for Caesarean section in a patient with a cervical arteriovenous malformation. Can J Anaesth 1996; 43:1052-8.

170. Doppman JL, Wirth FP, Di Chiro G, Ommaya AK. Value of cutaneous angiomas in the arteriographic localization of spinal cord arteriovenous malformations. N Engl J Med 1969; 281:1440-4.

171. Hirsch NP, Child CS, Wijetilleka SA. Paraplegia caused by spinal angioma: Possible association with epidural analgesia. Anesth Analg 1985; 64:937-40.

172. Liu C-L, Yang D-J. Paraplegia due to vertebral hemangioma during pregnancy: A case report. Spine 1988; 13:107-8.

173. Lubenow T, Keh-Wong E, Kristof K, et al. Inadvertent subdural injection: A complication of an epidural block. Anesth Analg 1988; 67: 175-9.

174. Shanker KB, Palkar NV, Nishkala R. Paraplegia following epidural potassium chloride. Anaesthesia 1985; 40:45-7.

175. Lin D, Becker K, Shapiro HM. Neurologic changes following epidural injection of potassium chloride and diazepam: A case report with laboratory correlations. Anesthesiology 1986; 65:210-2.

176. Brahams D. Record award of personal injuries sustained as a result of negligent administration of epidural anaesthesia. Lancet 1982; 1:159.

177. Patel PC, Sharif AMY, Farnando PUE. Accidental infusion of total parenteral nutrition solution through an epidural catheter. Anaesthesia 1984; 39:383-4.

178. McGuinness JP, Cantees KK. Epidural injection of a phenol-containing ranitidine preparation. Anesthesiology 1990; 73:553-5.

179. Meel B. Inadvertent intrathecal administration of potassium chloride during routine spinal anaesthesia: case report. Am J Forensic Med Path 1998; 19:255-7.

180. Ferguson FR, Watkins KH. Paralysis of the bladder and associated neurological sequelae of spinal anaesthesia (cauda equina syndrome). Br J Surg 1937; 25:735-52.

181. Kennedy F, Effron A, Perry G. The grave spinal cord paralysis caused by spinal anaesthesia. Surg Gynecol Obstet 1950; 91:385-98.

182. Rigler ML, Drasner K, Krejchie TC, et al. Cauda equina syndrome after continuous spinal anesthesia. Anesth Analg 1991; 72:275-281.

183. Snyder R, Hui G, Flugstad P, Viarengo C. More cases of possible neurotoxicity associated with single subarachnoid injections of 5% hyperbaric lidocaine. Anesth Analg 1994; 78:411

184. Yamauchi Y, Nomoto Y. Irreversible damage to the cauda equina following repeated intrathecal injection of hyperbaric dibucaine. J Anesth 2002; 16:176-8.

185. Cheng ACK. Intended epidural anesthesia as possible cause of cauda equina syndrome. Anesth Analg 1994; 78:157-9.

186. Drasner K, Rigler ML, Sessler DI, Stoller ML. Cauda equina syndrome following intended epidural anesthesia. Anesth Analg 1992; 77:582-5.

187. Loo CC, Irestedt L. Cauda equina syndrome after spinal anaesthesia with hyperbaric 5% lidocaine: a review of six cases of cauda equina syndrome reported to the Swedish Pharmaceutical Insurance 1993-1997. Acta Anaesthesiol Scand 1999; 43:371-9.

188. Drasner K. Local anesthetic neurotoxicity: Clinical injury and strategies that may minimize risk. Reg Anesth Pain Med 2002; 27:576-80.

189. Fenerty J, Sonner J, Sakura S, Drasner K. Transient radicular pain following spinal anesthesia: Review of the literature and report of a case involving 2% lignocaine. Int J Obstet Anesth 1996; 5:32-5.

190. Hampl KF, Heinzmann-Wiedmer S, Luginbuehl I, Harms C, Seeberger M, Schneider MC, Drasner K. Transient neurologic syndrome after spinal anesthesia: a lower incidence with prilocaine and bupivacaine than with lidocaine. Anesthesiology 1998; 88:629-33.

191. Lindh A, Andersson AS, Westman L. Is transient lumbar pain after spinal anaesthesia with lidocaine influenced by early mobilisation? Acta Anaesthesiol Scand 2001; 45:290-3.

192. Salmela L, Aromaa U. Transient radicular irritation after spinal anesthesia induced with hyperbaric solutions of cerebrospinal fluid-diluted lidocaine 50 mg/ml or mepivacaine 40 mg/mL or bupivacaine 5 mg/mL. Acta Anaesthesiol Scand 1998; 42:765-9.

193. Freedman JM, Li DK, Drasner K, et al. Transient neurologic symptoms after spinal anesthesia: An epidemiologic study Anesthesiology 1998; 89:633-41.

194. Keld DB, Hein L, Dalgaard M et al. The incidence of transient neurologic symptoms (TNS) after spinal anaesthesia in patients undergoing surgery in the supine position. Hyperbaric lidocaine 5% versus hyperbaric bupivacaine 0.5%. Acta Anaesthesiol Scand 2000; 44:285-90.

195. Tarkkila P, Huhtala J, Tuominen M. Transient radicular irritation after spinal anaesthesia with hyperbaric 5% lidocaine. Br J Anaesth 1995; 74:328-9.

196. de Weert K, Traksel M, Gielen M, et al. The incidence of transient neurological symptoms after spinal anaesthesia with lidocaine compared to prilocaine. Anaesthesia 2000; 55:1020-4.

197. Hodgson PS, Liu SS, Batra MS, et al. Procaine compared with lidocaine for incidence of transient neurologic symptoms. Reg Anesth Pain Med 2000; 25:215-7.

198. Martinez-Bourio R, Arzuaga M, Quintana JM et al. Incidence of transient neurologic symptoms after hyperbaric subarachnoid anesthesia with 5% lidocaine and 5% prilocaine. Anesthesiology 1998; 88:624-8.

199. Hiller A, Rosenberg PH. Transient neurological symptoms after spinal anaesthesia with 4% mepivacaine and 0.5% bupivacaine. Br J Anaesth 1997; 79:301-5.

200. Errando CL. Transient neurologic syndrome, transient radicular irritation, or postspinal musculoskeletal symptoms: Are we describing the same "syndrome" in all patients? Reg Anesth Pain Med 2001; 26: 178-80.

201. Wong CA, Slavenas P. The incidence of transient radicular irritation after spinal anesthesia in obstetric patients. Reg Anesth Pain Med 1999; 24:55-8.

202. Aouad MT, Siddik SS, Jalbout MI et al. Does pregnancy protect against itrathecal lidocaine-induced transient neurologic symptoms? Anesth Analg 2001;92:401-4.

203. Rorarius M, Suominen P, Haanpaa M, et al. Neurologic sequelae after caesarean section. Acta Anaesth Scand 2001; 45:34-41.

204. Newman LM, Iyer NR, Tuman KJ. Transient radicular irritation after hyperbaric lidocaine spinal anesthesia in parturients. Int J Obstet Anesth 1997; 6:132-4.

205. Sakura S, Toyota K, Doi K, Saito Y. Recurrent neurological symptoms in a patient following repeat combined spinal and epidural anaesthesia. Br J Anaesth 2002; 89:141-3.

206. Philips J, Sharma SK, Vijaya NR, et al. Transient neurologic symptoms after spinal anesthesia with lidocaine in obstetric patients. Anesth Analg 2001; 92:405-9.

207. Reisner LS, Hochman BN, Plumer MH. Persistent neurologic deficit and adhesive arachnoiditis following intrathecal 2-chloroprocaine injection. Anesth Analg 1980; 59:452-4.

208. Sklar EM, Quencer RM, Green BA, et al. Complications of epidural anesthesia: MR appearance of abnormalities. Radiology 1991; 181:549-54.

209. Sgchirlanzoni A, Marazzi R, Pareyson D, et al. Epidural anaesthesia and spinal arachnoiditis. Anaesthesia 1989; 44:317-21.

210. Lurie S, Feinstein M, Heifetz C, Mamet Y. Iatrogenic bacterial meningitis after spinal anesthesia for pain relief in labor. J Clin Anesth 1999; 11:438-9.

Part IX
Obstetric Complications

The philosophy of obstetric management changed in the early decades of the twentieth century, and this had a profound effect on the use of obstetric anesthesia. Until 1900, obstetricians considered childbirth a physiologic process, best left to proceed without interference by physician or midwife. They criticized "meddlesome practices" for normal deliveries. Then a new generation of obstetricians, concerned about the high rate of complications associated with routine deliveries, began to advocate more active management of childbirth. They envisioned the practice of obstetrics as a form of preventive medicine. Leaders of this movement, such as Joseph DeLee of Chicago, became strong advocates for the routine use of episiotomy, forceps delivery, and manual removal of the placenta. Of course, these measures also necessitated greater use of anesthesia.[1]

DeLee acknowledged that his methods "interferes much with Nature's process," but he felt justified. With conservative management, he said, a dismal outcome was so common that he "often wondered whether Nature did not deliberately intend women should be used up in the process of reproduction, in a manner analogous to that of the salmon, which dies after spawning. Perhaps laceration, prolapse and all the evils are, in fact, natural to labor and therefore normal. . . . If you adopt this view, I have no ground to stand on, but, if you believe that a woman after delivery should be as healthy, as well as anatomically perfect as she was before, and that the child should be undamaged, then you will have to agree with me that labor is pathogenic, because experience has proved such ideal results exceedingly rare."[2] Other physicians agreed with DeLee. Austin Flint asked how a "process that kills thousands of women each year, leaves a quarter of all cases more or less invalidate, is attended by severe pain and tearing of tissues, and kills three to seven percent of all babies, can be called a normal or physiologic function?"[3]

The change in the philosophy of obstetric management was further stimulated by early feminists. In the United States, but especially in Great Britain, feminists formed a coalition with obstetricians to improve teaching, build new facilities, and fund better care for women in hospitals. They also demanded better anesthesia coverage, and even funded research to develop new anesthetic techniques. In response to this movement, physicians developed many new techniques for laboring patients. Many of the anesthetic methods now favored for normal deliveries are a direct outgrowth of public support for innovation and improvement that began during this time.

Donald Caton, M.D.

REFERENCES

1. Leavitt W. Joseph B. DeLee and the practice of preventive obstetrics. Am J Public Health 1988; 78:1353-9.
2. DeLee JB. The prophylactic forceps operation. Am J Obstet Gynecol 1920; 1:34-44.
3. Flint A. Responsibility of the medical profession in further reducing maternal mortality. Am J Obstet Gynecol 1925; 19:864-6.

Chapter 34
Preterm Labor and Delivery

Holly A. Muir, M.D., FRCPC · David H. Chestnut, M.D.

Despite improved antenatal care, the incidence of preterm delivery in the United States has increased from 9.5% in 1982 to just over 11% in 1999.[1] Preterm delivery accounts for 69% to 83% of neonatal deaths in the United States.[2] The high incidence of preterm delivery is a major reason the United States ranked 23rd in the world in infant mortality in 1988, behind most other developed nations and on a par with some third-world countries.[3] For example, France reports a preterm delivery rate of 5.6% and Germany claims a rate of 4%. In *Healthy People 2010*, the United States Department of Health and Social Services has acknowledged the magnitude of this problem and has announced its desire to reduce the incidence to 7.6% or less over the next decade.[4] Current research is focusing on the following: (1) determination of the causes of preterm labor, (2) early identification of women at risk for preterm labor, and (3) optimal recognition and treatment of preterm labor.[5,6]

DEFINITIONS

A preterm infant is defined as one delivered between 20 and 37 weeks after the first day of the last menstrual period (i.e., at least 3 weeks before the expected date of term delivery).[7] Gestational age often is unknown or difficult to determine in neonates that are small in size. Some of these infants are small for gestational age (SGA) rather than preterm. An infant who weighs less than 2500 g at birth is considered a low birth weight (LBW) infant, regardless of gestational age. Likewise, an infant who weighs less than 1500 g at birth is considered a very low birth weight (VLBW) infant.

NEONATAL MORTALITY

The survival rate among neonates increases as the birth weight or gestational age increases[8] (Tables 34-1 and 34-2;

Figure 34-1). During the past two decades, there has been a significant improvement in the survival rate in every VLBW subgroup, with the greatest improvement occurring in the subgroup with a birth weight of 750 to 1000 g.[9] Infants with a birth weight of less than 750 g continue to have a high mortality rate. However, there is great inter-center variation in neonatal survival for this group, with a range of 12% to 72% reported by different investigators between 1978 and 1985.[9]

The rate of neonatal survival now exceeds 90% for infants born after 30 weeks' gestation, and a neonatal survival rate near 100% can be expected for infants born after 32 weeks' gestation. Greater attention is now given to infants born before 32 weeks' gestation. These represent approximately 1% to 2% of all deliveries and 30% to 40% of all preterm deliveries. However, this cohort of patients includes 60% of all cases of perinatal mortality and 50% of cases of long-term neurologic morbidity.[10]

A recent retrospective cohort study assessed the survival and cost of pregnancies delivered at 24 to 26 weeks' gestation.[11] Neonatal survival was 43%, 74%, and 83% at 24, 25, and 26 weeks' gestation, respectively. In this cohort, the majority of women received antenatal steroids, and the majority of neonates received exogenous surfactant. This study suggested that the greatest gain in survival is achieved by prolonging gestation beyond 24 weeks' gestation. A delay in delivery of even 1 week results in significantly better outcome and reduced cost.

NEONATAL MORBIDITY

Approximately 90% of preterm births occur between 30 and 36 weeks' gestation. Morbidity is the primary concern at this gestational age. A significant reduction in morbidity from respiratory distress syndrome (RDS) occurs by extending an otherwise uncomplicated pregnancy until 36 weeks' gestation.

TABLE 34-1	NEONATAL SURVIVAL ACCORDING TO BIRTH WEIGHT*	
Birth weight (g)	Survival (%)	Improvement in survival per 100-g increase in birth weight (%)
450	0.0	0.0
550	12.1	12.1
650	15.4	3.3
750	43.9	28.5
850	72.5	28.6
950	77.6	5.1
1050	82.0	4.4
1150	85.7	3.7
1250	88.7	3.0
1350	91.2	2.5
1450	93.1	1.9
1550	94.7	1.6
1650	95.9	1.2
1750	96.9	1.0
1850	97.6	0.7
1950	98.2	0.6
2050	98.6	0.4
2150	98.9	0.3
2250	99.2	0.3
2350	99.4	0.2
2450	99.5	0.1

*Predicted survival at midpoint of 100-g birth weight categories and increase in survival to be attained by a 100-g increase above that birth weight derived from logistic regression equation.
From Copper RL, Goldenberg RL, Creasy RK, et al. A multicenter study of preterm birth weight and gestational age-specific neonatal mortality. Am J Obstet Gynecol 1993; 168:78-84.

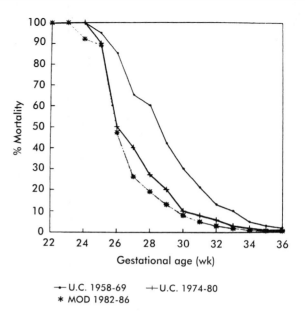

FIGURE 34-1. Percent neonatal mortality at 50th percentile birth weight for gestational age. *MOD*, Multicenter study group; *U.C.*, University of Colorado. (From Copper RL, Goldenberg RL, Creasy RK, et al. A multicenter study of preterm birth weight and gestational age-specific neonatal mortality. Am J Obstet Gynecol 1993; 168:78-84.)

TABLE 34-2	NEONATAL SURVIVAL BY GESTATIONAL AGE AND IMPROVEMENT IN SURVIVAL BY WEEK	
Gestational age (wk)	Approximate survival (%)	Approximate improvement in survival per week (%)
21	0	—
22	Rare	—
23	25	25
24	50	25
25	70	20
26	80	10
27	86	6
28	91	5
29	94	3
30	95	1
31	96	1
32	97	1
33	98	1
34	99	1
35	99+	< 1
36	99+	< 1

From Goldenberg RL. The management of preterm labor. Obstet Gynecol 2002; 100:1020-37.

The incidence of high grade (III or IV) intraventricular hemorrhage (IVH) diminishes rapidly after 27 weeks' gestation, and grade III or IV hemorrhages are very rare after 32 weeks' gestation. Likewise, neonatal morbidity from patent ductus arteriosus and necrotizing enterocolitis decreases significantly after 32 weeks' gestation.[2]

The economic costs of surviving preterm infants (especially VLBW infants) can be enormous. In 1986, Hack and Fanaroff[12] reported that the mean length of hospital stay for infants who weighed 500 to 750 g at birth and who survived was 137 days (range of 71 to 221 days), and the mean cost of care per infant was $158,800 (range of $72,110 to $524,110). Approximately 33% of these infants had significant neurodevelopmental handicaps. Ehrenhaft et al.[9] reviewed the studies of morbidity published between 1975 and 1985; they observed major handicaps at 1 or 2 years of age in 26% of surviving infants with a birth weight of less than 800 g, in 17% of survivors with a birth weight between 750 and 1000 g, and in 11% of survivors with a birth weight between 1000 and 1500 g. (Major handicaps included severe mental retardation, cerebral palsy of significant degree, major seizure disorders, blindness, and severe hearing defects.) In addition, a higher incidence of moderate handicaps (intelligence or developmental quotient between 70 and 80) and mild handicaps (behavioral, learning, and language disorders) occurs among VLBW infants than among normal birth weight infants.[13] In the study by Kilpatrick et al.,[11] the total hospital cost for the 29 nonsurviving infants was $1,460,000, and the total cost for the 94 surviving infants was $16,900,000. The cost per day for the surviving infants was $294,749, $181,062, and $166,215 for those delivered at 24, 25, and 26 weeks' gestation, respectively.[11]

Piecuch et al.[14] reported data for a cohort of 138 nonanomalous infants delivered between 24 and 26 weeks' gestation between 1990 and 1994. The incidence of cerebral palsy did not differ significantly among the three groups (11%, 20%, and 11% at 24, 25, and 26 weeks' gestation, respectively). However, the incidence of normal cognitive outcome was associated with gestational age at birth

(28%, 47%, and 71% at 24, 25, and 26 weeks' gestation, respectively).

A recent report from the EPICure Study Group assessed the association between extreme preterm delivery and long-term physical and mental disability in a cohort of infants delivered between 22 and 25 weeks' gestation. The authors noted rates of severe disability of 54%, 52%, and 45% among infants delivered at 23, 24, and 25 weeks' gestation, respectively.[15] The incidence of cerebral palsy is 40 times higher in infants born with a birth weight less than 750 g than in term infants.[16]

PRETERM LABOR

Risk Factors

Box 34-1 lists factors associated with preterm labor.[6,7,17] These associations do not necessarily indicate cause-and-effect relationships. Significant risk factors include a history of previous preterm delivery, black race (irrespective of socioeconomic status), and multiple gestation. One of the most consistent risk factors is a history of previous preterm delivery. This suggests a genetic contribution to the etiology of this condition.

In many cases, the cause of preterm labor is unclear. As we develop a greater understanding of the mechanism(s) for the initiation of labor at term, we should develop a better understanding of the various etiologies of preterm labor. Some investigators have speculated that an "up regulation of oxytocin receptors" may initiate preterm labor.[18] Consequently, some studies have evaluated oxytocin antagonists as tocolytic agents (vide infra). Prostaglandins are potent stimulants of uterine contractility. They are produced throughout pregnancy by the amnion and decidua and are destroyed by the chorion. Loss of chorionic prostaglandin dehydrogenase activity may be a significant factor in the initiation of preterm labor.[19] Cytokines also may promote the production of oxytocin and corticotropin releasing hormone (CRH) in the decidua. CRH is synthesized by the placenta and is found in increased concentrations both at term and in patients with preterm labor. CRH not only stimulates prostaglandin production, but also it may act synergistically with oxytocin to cause uterine contractions.[20] Investigators have also evaluated the role of nitric oxide as a uterine relaxant.[21]

Certain infections are more consistently associated with preterm labor, such as untreated syphilis and *Neisseria gonorrhoeae*, asymptomatic group B streptococcal bacteriuria, and untreated acute pyelonephritis. Other cervicovaginal microorganisms and infections have been implicated in preterm delivery.[22] Approximately 50% of preterm deliveries occur in women with no apparent risk factors. Subclinical infection may precipitate preterm labor in some of these cases.[22,23] Investigators have found positive amniotic fluid cultures[24] and products of infection (e.g., C-reactive protein[25]) in some patients who present with preterm labor. Studies of prostaglandins, their metabolites, and cytokines suggest a biochemical mechanism for preterm labor in the presence of infection.

Empiric trials of antibiotic therapy have produced conflicting results in patients with intact membranes.[26] The results of a large multicenter randomized controlled trial (ORACLE II) did not support the use of prophylactic antibiotic therapy in the management of preterm labor in patients with intact membranes.[27] However, a meta-analysis suggested that prophylactic antibiotics may result in a modest prolongation

---

Box 34-1 FACTORS ASSOCIATED WITH PRETERM LABOR

MATERNAL

History of preterm delivery
History of diethylstilbestrol exposure
History of second-trimester abortion
Young age (< 18 years old)
Low socioeconomic status
Acute or chronic systemic disease
Trauma
Abdominal surgery during pregnancy
Difficult work
Infection (genital, urinary tract)
Pyelonephritis
Smoking
Drug use

UTERINE

Overdistention of cavity (e.g., multiple gestation, polyhydramnios)
Abnormal cavity (e.g., uterine anomaly, fibroids)
Foreign body (e.g., intrauterine device)

CERVICAL

Incompetence
Trauma

FETOPLACENTAL

Faulty placentation (e.g., placenta previa, placental abruption)
Genetic abnormality
Fetal death

MEMBRANES

Premature rupture
Infection

IATROGENIC

Modified from Chestnut DH. Anesthesia for preterm labor and delivery. In Hood D, guest editor. Anesthesia in Obstetrics and Gynecology: Problems in Anesthesia. Philadelphia, JP Lippincott, 1989: 32-44.

---

of pregnancy (i.e., approximately 0.60 week) in this patient population.[28]

In contrast, a meta-analysis of randomized clinical trials concluded that antimicrobial therapy prolongs pregnancy and reduces both maternal and neonatal morbidity in patients with preterm, premature rupture of membranes (preterm PROM).[29] These findings were confirmed by the ORACLE I randomized trial, which demonstrated a prolongation of pregnancy and improved neonatal outcome in women treated with erythromycin after preterm PROM.[30]

As many as 20% to 25% of all preterm deliveries do not follow preterm labor. The obstetrician may perform elective delivery for maternal or fetal indications such as severe preeclampsia or nonreassuring fetal heart rate (FHR) patterns. Unfortunately, some cases of RDS are iatrogenic. That is, the obstetrician may unnecessarily perform an elective repeat cesarean section in a preterm patient.

In the past two decades we have witnessed a significant increase in the incidence of multiple gestation (i.e., 18.9 per 1000 live births in 1980 versus 26.9 per 1000 in 1997).[31] This is likely a result of the significant increase in the use of assisted reproductive techniques (ART). Multiple gestations account for 12% to 27% of all preterm births. ART pregnancies are also associated with a substantial increase in risk of preterm delivery, even for singleton pregnancies.[32]

Prevention Programs

Prevention of preterm labor and delivery includes efforts to prevent the initiation of labor. Preterm birth-prevention programs typically include (1) initial assessment of patient risk, (2) intensive patient education, (3) weekly or biweekly clinic visits and cervical examinations, and (4) ready telephone access to health-care providers. Herron et al.[33] reported that their preterm birth-prevention program significantly reduced the incidence of preterm births in a population of middle-class women in San Francisco. Other, similar programs have not significantly decreased the preterm birth rate.[34-36] The latter programs were applied to different populations of women, including predominantly white women in northern California,[34] indigent black women in Alabama,[35] and inner-city black-women in Philadelphia.[36] Analyses of four larger preterm birth-prevention programs have reached different conclusions regarding the benefit of these programs. Two studies (one a multicenter randomized trial) found that their prevention programs resulted in a lower rate of preterm delivery.[37,38] In contrast, in another multicenter, randomized trial, the Collaborative Group on Preterm Birth Prevention demonstrated no consistent benefit for the intervention group.[39] Likewise, Dyson et al.[40] recently found no benefit to daily patient contact and home uterine activity monitoring (HUAM) in a study of 2442 high-risk patients.

The role of HUAM is less controversial.[41,42] Despite gaining limited approval from the Food and Drug Administration (FDA), the American College of Obstetricians and Gynecologists (ACOG) has stated that "there is no demonstrated role for HUAM in the prevention of preterm birth," and that "data are insufficient to support a benefit from HUAM in preventing preterm birth."[23]

Diagnosis

Often it is difficult to determine whether a woman is in early preterm labor or in false labor. Criteria for the diagnosis of preterm labor include (1) gestational age between 20 and 37 weeks, (2) at least four documented uterine contractions in 20 minutes or eight in 60 minutes, and (3) documented change in cervical dilation or effacement, cervical dilation of 2 cm, *or* cervical effacement of 80%.[2] Several investigators have noted the predictive value of fetal breathing movements (as seen during real-time ultrasonography) in the diagnosis of preterm labor in parturients with intact membranes. They observed that preterm patients with contractions and fetal breathing movements were not likely to progress into active labor and that the pregnancy typically continued for at least another week.[43,44] In those patients with absent fetal breathing movements, delivery was more likely to occur within 48 hours.

Recent studies have helped identify biochemical markers that may predict preterm labor and delivery. The most studied marker is fetal fibronectin, a glycoprotein found in the extracellular matrix. When found in the vagina or cervix, fibronectin may be a marker of choriodecidual disruption. Fetal fibronectin is normally absent from vaginal secretions from 20 weeks' gestation until near term. Detection of elevated fetal fibronectin levels is associated with an increased risk of preterm delivery. If fibronectin is absent (i.e., a negative test), the risk of preterm delivery within 1 or 2 weeks is less than 1%.[45]

Another potential biochemical marker is salivary estriol. In humans an increase in the maternal estriol level occurs before parturition. The increased serum levels are reflected in salivary levels. A surge in estriol occurs in women without symptoms of labor approximately 3 weeks before delivery. As with fetal fibronectin, the primary value of this test is its negative predictive value. In studies of both asymptomatic and symptomatic patients, the negative predictive value of this test is consistently greater than 90%. However, its application is limited because bedside testing is not available, and results are not available for 24 hours.[46] The ACOG has noted that the test carries a high percentage of false-positive results, and that its use could add significantly to the cost of prenatal care, especially if it is used in a low-risk population.[23]

Assessment and Therapy

Initial assessment and therapy includes physical examination, intravenous hydration, bed rest, FHR monitoring, and ultrasonographic evaluation. Maternal physical examination may include a sterile speculum examination to exclude preterm PROM. In many women, uterine contractions cease with bed rest alone. In the past, clinicians assumed that intravenous hydration was a necessary component of therapy. However, Helfgott et al.[47] demonstrated that bed rest alone is responsible for stopping the labor, and that hydration is not an essential component.

Ultrasonographic evaluation is noninvasive and can be performed on admission to estimate gestational age and fetal weight. If necessary, amniocentesis can be performed to determine fetal pulmonary maturity and to look for evidence of infection.

Once the diagnosis of preterm labor is established, the obstetrician must decide whether to begin tocolytic therapy. Criteria for the use of tocolytic therapy include (1) gestational age between 20 and 34 weeks, (2) fetal weight less than 2500 g, and (3) absence of fetal distress. The potential benefits of delaying delivery of the preterm infant (i.e., decreased neonatal morbidity and mortality) must be weighed against the maternal and fetal risks (i.e., maternal and/or fetal sepsis, maternal side effects of tocolytic drugs, further compromise of a distressed fetus). Box 34-2 lists contraindications to the

---

Box 34-2 CONTRAINDICATIONS TO INHIBITION OF PRETERM LABOR

CONTRAINDICATIONS TO LONG-TERM INHIBITION

Fetal death
Fetal anomalies incompatible with life
Fetal distress that warrants immediate delivery
Chorioamnionitis/fever of unknown origin
Severe hemorrhage
Severe chronic and/or pregnancy-induced hypertension

RELATIVE CONTRAINDICATIONS TO LONG-TERM INHIBITION

Cervical dilation > 4 cm
Ruptured membranes
SGA fetus
Maternal cardiac disease

inhibition of labor. In recent years, conditions once considered relative contraindications to tocolysis no longer prevent clinicians from initiating tocolytic therapy.

The benefits of glucocorticoid administration before preterm delivery have been clearly demonstrated in large clinical trials. These benefits often outweigh the potential risks of tocolytic therapy. The National Institute of Child Health and Human Development (NICHD) Neonatal Research Network evaluated outcome for 11,718 preterm infants delivered after antenatal corticosteroid administration between 1988 and 1992. Antenatal steroid treatment significantly reduced the incidence of RDS, IVH, and neonatal death in all subgroups of the population studied (including male and female infants, black and white infants, and infants delivered before 30 weeks' gestation).[48] The reduction in neonatal morbidity and mortality from antenatal steroids is additive to the reduction observed with the use of surfactant alone.[49]

While there is little controversy regarding the efficacy of a single course of antenatal steroids, there remains debate over the use of multiple courses of corticosteroids for women who remain undelivered 7 days after the initial dose of steroids. A recent review[50] and an NIH consensus panel statement[51] did not recommend multiple courses of steroids; however, both documents cited some evidence of possible benefit. They also identified possible risks, including an increased incidence of neonatal infection and potentially deleterious effects on neuronal and organ growth.[50,51]

In some cases, there are benefits to a short course of tocolytic therapy, even if the patient delivers shortly thereafter. For example, tocolytic therapy may facilitate transport of the patient from a small, community hospital to a tertiary care facility that can provide optimal care for the preterm neonate. Moreover, a short course of tocolytic therapy may delay delivery for 24 to 48 hours, which allows administration of a glucocorticoid to accelerate fetal lung maturity. Finally, obstetricians may give a single bolus dose of a tocolytic agent to facilitate fetal resuscitation in utero in cases of fetal distress.

Controversy continues regarding the use of tocolytic therapy in patients with preterm PROM. Historically, obstetricians have worried that tocolytic therapy might increase the risk of maternal and/or fetal infection in these patients. It also seems logical that tocolytic therapy is less effective in patients with preterm PROM. Prospective, randomized studies have observed that tocolytic therapy did not improve neonatal outcome when compared with conservative expectant management in patients with preterm PROM.[52] However, Weiner et al.[53] suggested that tocolytic therapy may have some benefit in patients with preterm PROM before 28 weeks' gestation.

The cost-effectiveness of tocolytic therapy has been questioned. However, in 1984, Korenbrot et al.[54] reported that the combined maternal and neonatal medical costs were less when tocolysis was used between 26 and 34 weeks' gestation than when no tocolytic therapy was given. However, a recent meta-analysis concluded that tocolytic therapy is not associated with improved perinatal or neonatal outcome.[55]

SELECTION OF TOCOLYTIC AGENT

Once the obstetrician has decided to begin tocolytic therapy, an appropriate agent must be selected (Box 34-3). (Each specific class of tocolytic agent is discussed in detail later in this chapter.) A number of tocolytic agents have passed in and out of favor, some because of intolerable side effects and others after the scientific community reviewed their efficacy. Ethanol

is an example of a tocolytic agent that has been abandoned because of intolerable side effects.

PHYSIOLOGY OF UTERINE CONTRACTIONS

The contractile elements in myometrial smooth muscle consist of thick (myosin) and thin (actin) filaments that interact and slide past one another, generating the contractile force for uterine contractions. The myometrium has pacemaker cells with spontaneous contractile ability, which spread activity throughout the rest of the uterus by means of gap junctions between myometrial cells. Myometrial contractions are preceded by a rise in intracellular calcium concentration through the influx of calcium across the sarcolemma and/or release from internal stores such as the sarcoplasmic reticulum. Hormones and neurotransmitters may play a role in the regulation of uterine activity by causing agonist-induced entry of calcium or other ions by means of receptor-operated channels and the release of calcium from internal stores.[56]

The rise in intracellular calcium results in the formation of a complex between calcium and calmodulin (a regulatory enzyme), which activates myosin light-chain kinase (MLCK). Activated MLCK then phosphorylates the light-chain subunit of myosin, allowing actin to bind to myosin and activate myosin adenosine triphosphatase (ATPase). Adenosine triphosphate (ATP) is then hydrolyzed, and muscle shortening or contraction results. Relaxation of smooth muscle results from a reduction in the intracellular calcium concentration and/or dephosphorylation of the myosin light chain by myosin light-chain phosphatase. Increases in intracellular cyclic adenosine monophosphate (cAMP) also can result in muscle relaxation by two mechanisms: (1) by activating a cAMP-dependent protein kinase, which decreases the activity of MLCK, and (2) by lowering the intracellular calcium concentration.

The control of labor and the processes for signaling its onset are complex. During pregnancy, the uterus remains in a state of functional quiescence as a result of the activity of various inhibitors, including progesterone, prostacyclin, relaxin, nitric oxide, parathyroid hormone-related peptide, CRH, human placental lactogen, calcium gene-related peptide, adrenomedullin, and vasoactive intestinal peptide. Before term the uterus goes through an activation phase in response to uterotropins, including estrogen. This activation phase is characterized by (1) increased expression of a series of contraction-associated proteins (including myometrial receptors for prostaglandins and oxytocin), (2) activation of certain ion channels, and (3) an increase in connexin-43. Once activated the uterus can be stimulated to contract by the action of uterotonins such as oxytocin and prostaglandins E_2 and $F_{2\text{-alpha}}$. A parturition cascade likely removes the mechanisms that have maintained uterine quiescence and recruits factors that promote uterine activity.

Box 34-3 PHARMACOLOGIC AGENTS USED FOR TOCOLYTIC THERAPY

Beta-adrenergic agonists
   Ritodrine
   Terbutaline
Magnesium sulfate
Prostaglandin synthetase inhibitors
   Indomethacin
Calcium entry-blocking agents
   Nifedipine

Once the uterus has been "activated," endocrine, paracrine, and autocrine factors from the fetoplacental unit initiate a change in the pattern of uterine activity from irregular to regular contractions. Evidence from animal models suggests that the fetus may coordinate this change in activity through (1) its influence on the production of placental steroid hormones, (2) mechanical distention of the uterus, and (3) secretion of neurohypophyseal hormones and other stimulators of prostaglandin synthesis. The final common pathway for labor in all species appears to be the activation of the fetal hypothalamic-pituitary-adrenal axis.[57]

Preterm labor may result from a loss of inhibitory factors on uterine quiescence, or it may represent a short-circuiting of the normal parturition cascade through the overproduction of a critical factor. As our understanding of the physiology of uterine activity increases, our approach to both predicting and treating preterm labor will become more focused. Multimodal therapy may become a standard, given that recent evidence suggests that labor is initiated by the interaction of multiple factors.

EFFICACY OF TOCOLYTIC THERAPY

Prospective, randomized studies have provided conflicting results regarding the efficacy of tocolytic therapy.[55,58-65] These studies typically have noted a high rate of success with placebo, which likely reflects an incorrect diagnosis of preterm labor in some patients.

Ritodrine remains the only drug approved by the FDA for tocolytic therapy. Several investigators have raised questions regarding the efficacy of ritodrine in the treatment of preterm labor.[55,58,59,65,66] Studies of the efficacy of **terbutaline** have also produced conflicting results.[60,61] King et al.[65] performed a meta-analysis of 16 controlled studies in which tocolytic agents, primarily ritodrine, were evaluated. Beta-adrenergic agents delayed delivery for 24 to 48 hours but did not significantly decrease perinatal mortality or morbidity from respiratory distress.[65] The Canadian Preterm Labor Investigators Group[59] studied 708 women with preterm labor in a randomized, controlled, multicenter study that compared the effects of ritodrine and placebo for treatment of preterm labor. There was no difference between the two groups in the following outcome measures: (1) incidence of delivery before 37 weeks' gestation, (2) proportion of infants with a birth weight less than 2500 g, (3) incidence of perinatal mortality, and (4) neonatal morbidity. The investigators *did* observe a significant decrease in the rate of delivery within 24 hours and within 48 hours in the ritodrine group. However, the authors stated that "this immediate effect has not led to clinically important reductions in the rates of preterm delivery or low birth weight."[59] The Canadian study has been criticized for its study design, particularly its definition of preterm labor and its inclusion of women with ruptured membranes, twin gestation, and concurrent use of glucocorticoids.[67] A recent meta-analysis confirmed that tocolytic therapy decreased the risk of delivery within 7 days, but did not improve perinatal outcome.[55]

Several clinical studies have reported the efficacy of prostaglandin synthetase inhibitors such as **indomethacin** for tocolysis.[62,63] Other studies have evaluated the efficacy of calcium entry-blocking agents such as **nifedipine**.[64,68,69] The calcium entry-blocking agents have a reduced side-effect profile when compared with the beta-adrenergic agonists, and some investigators have suggested that nifedipine should be a first-line therapy in the treatment of preterm labor.[69]

THE PRETERM INFANT

Physiology

The healthy term fetus tolerates the stress of labor and delivery well. The preterm fetus (especially if it is less than 30 weeks' gestation or has a weight of less than 1500 g) is physiologically less well adapted to this stress.[70] Some (but not all) studies suggest that the incidence of intrapartum acidosis and asphyxia is greater in the preterm fetus than in the mature fetus.[71] The preterm fetus has a decreased hemoglobin concentration and a decreased oxygen-carrying capacity.[70] Of interest, these characteristics do not result in an increased risk of intrapartum fetal neurologic injury.

There is a higher incidence of IVH in the preterm infant, particularly in the fetus with a gestational age of less than 35 weeks.[72] Factors that contribute to the development of IVH in preterm fetuses include (1) poor tissue support surrounding the germinal matrix blood vessels, (2) a disproportionately higher amount of total cerebral blood flow to the periventricular circulation, and (3) impaired autoregulation of cerebral blood flow, which makes blood flow to the periventricular area extremely sensitive to fluctuations in arterial blood pressure. Hypoxia-induced damage to the periventricular capillaries also increases susceptibility to IVH.[73] In addition, the preterm fetus has a relative deficiency of clotting factors, which can be exacerbated by the presence of asphyxia.[70] These limitations increase the risk of hemorrhage if there is stretching and tearing of subependymal vessels from molding of the fetal head during labor and delivery.

Method of Delivery

The ideal method of delivery for the preterm infant (especially the VLBW infant) remains controversial. Some studies suggest that the preterm fetus is at higher risk for acidosis during labor and delivery,[71] and the preterm infant is at higher risk for IVH. Therefore obstetric management includes FHR monitoring and efforts to minimize trauma during delivery.

The cesarean section rate for delivery of infants with a birth weight of less than 1500 g has increased in the United States and other countries.[74-77] Some reports have claimed decreased neonatal mortality with the liberal use of cesarean section for preterm infants,[78-83] and others have found no advantage of cesarean section over vaginal delivery.[75,77,84-86] However, most of these studies were retrospective and not well controlled. Malloy et al.[75] analyzed birth and death certificate information from Missouri for the years 1980 to 1984. The cesarean section rate for VLBW infants (500 to 1499 g) increased from 24% to 44%. During the same time period, the cesarean section rate for infants weighing 1500 to 2499 g increased from 21% to 26%, and the rate for infants weighing 2500 g or more increased from 14% to 18%. The first-day death rates were significantly higher among the smallest infants (weighing 500 to 749 g) that were delivered vaginally when compared with those delivered by cesarean section (59% and 33%, respectively). However, the mortality rates for the two methods of delivery for these infants did *not* differ after the first 6 days of life. There was no association between the method of delivery and first-day death rates for infants that weighed between 750 and 1500 g. The authors concluded that the use of cesarean section did not improve overall survival for VLBW infants. Malloy et al.[86] later reviewed the incidence of IVH and neonatal mortality in 1765 VLBW infants admitted to seven neonatal intensive care units between 1987 and 1988. After adjusting for gestational age and other maternal and fetal factors, they concluded that cesarean delivery did not lower the risk of either mortality or IVH for infants who weighed less than 1500 g at birth.

Among infants with a birth weight of 751 to 1000 g, Barrett et al.[84] reported no difference in neonatal morbidity or mortality between those delivered vaginally and those delivered by cesarean section. Infants with a birth weight of 501 to 1000 g who were delivered in the absence of labor had a significantly lower mortality rate than those who were delivered after the onset of labor. The authors hypothesized that "the circumstances dictating delivery without the occurrence of labor, rather than the occurrence of labor itself, caused the improved outcome in neonates delivered without labor occurring." Anderson et al.[85] noted an increased incidence of IVH in the first hour after delivery among infants with a birth weight of less than 1750 g if their mothers experienced the active phase of labor, regardless of the method of delivery. The authors suggested that regardless of the method of delivery, infants whose mothers enter the active phase of labor are more likely to have more severe grades of IVH.

Most obstetricians perform cesarean section for the delivery of VLBW fetuses with a breech presentation. Similarly, cesarean delivery has been recommended for LBW twins in whom twin A has a nonvertex presentation, although there are no prospective, controlled studies to support this practice.[87] Head entrapment behind an incompletely dilated cervix is more common in preterm fetuses with a breech presentation because the head is somewhat larger than the wedge formed by the buttocks and thighs. Several studies have noted that vaginal delivery of VLBW fetuses with a breech presentation resulted in a higher rate of neonatal mortality.[78-83] In contrast, Kitchen et al.[88] adjusted for other risk factors and found no difference in survival between preterm fetuses (with a breech presentation at 24 to 28 weeks' gestation) delivered vaginally and those delivered by cesarean section. To date, no prospective, randomized studies have confirmed that cesarean section results in better outcome than vaginal delivery for the preterm fetus with a breech presentation. However, the frequency of planned vaginal delivery of a singleton fetus with a breech presentation (either preterm or at term) has markedly declined in the United States (see Chapter 35).

The survival rate remains low for infants with a birth weight of 500 to 750 g. In these cases, obstetricians must decide whether they will recommend cesarean delivery in cases of fetal distress or breech presentation. The obstetrician often asks a neonatologist to speak with the patient about the infant's risk of morbidity and mortality so that the patient can make an informed decision regarding the method of delivery.

Ethical Issues

The antenatal administration of corticosteroids, the application of advanced ventilation techniques, the use of neonatal surfactant therapy, and the use of extracorporeal membrane oxygenation (ECMO) have reduced mortality and morbidity for preterm neonates. A clear association exists between the likelihood of survival and advanced gestational age; however, the relationship is more difficult to define at the lower extremes of extrauterine viability. Further, questions remain regarding the risk of long-term morbidity for these infants. These uncertainties often lead to controversy regarding the decision to resuscitate (or not resuscitate) a preterm infant. Obstetricians tend to be more pessimistic than neonatologists regarding the prognosis for these infants. Obstetricians may underestimate survival rates for neonates born between 23 and 29 weeks' gestation by as much as 25% to 30%.[89] This situation is further complicated by the lack of precision in estimation of gestational age and birth weight,[90] as well as concerns for long-term neurologic and neurodevelopmental abnormalities in infants with a birth weight less than 1000 g.[91]

Parents, obstetricians, and neonatologists must be involved in the decision-making process. For an infant of 25 weeks' gestation or greater, with no known anomalies, the decision to offer full resuscitation and support is typically straightforward. Controversy and conflict may arise when making decisions regarding infants born at 22 to 24 weeks' gestation. Many ethicists recommend assessment of the "best interests" of the patient. However, it is often difficult to define the "best interests" of the patient in these situations. Some even argue (incorrectly in our view) that VLBW infants should not be granted personhood because they lack advanced brain function. Other questions relate to the extent of acceptable pain and suffering for these newborn infants, as well as the definition of an "acceptable" outcome. However, most ethicists agree that it is preferable to withdraw therapy, when appropriate, rather than withhold it.

Anesthesiologists may find themselves in the middle of these ethical dilemmas if they are practicing in a location wherein the anesthesiologist is responsible for neonatal resuscitation. Unfortunately no firm guidelines exist. However, some basic principles can be applied. First, the parents have a critical role in the decision-making process. Second, it is difficult to make decisions about withholding therapy without adequate data. Third, discussion of these issues should be done *before* delivery, not in the moment of crisis. Neither the American Academy of Pediatrics (AAP) nor the ACOG have made specific recommendations for neonatal resuscitation based on gestational age. However, the Canadian Paediatric Society and the Society of Obstetricians and Gynaecologists of Canada have issued relatively specific recommendations.[92] At 22 to 23 weeks' gestation, they suggest that resuscitation efforts be initiated only if uncertainty of gestational age exists *or* if fully informed parents request that resuscitation be performed. At 23 to 24 weeks' gestation, resuscitation can be offered as long as parents are informed of the need to reassess this decision at critical intervals and possibly withdraw therapy. At 25 weeks' gestation they recommend full resuscitation, in the absence of fatal anomalies.[92]

Extremes of prematurity (less than 23 weeks' confirmed gestation) and severe congenital anomalies incompatable with life (e.g., anencephaly) are examples of circumstances when noninitiation of resuscitation is considered appropriate. Revised neonatal resuscitation guidelines address the ethical issues of noninitiation or discontinuation of resuscitation in the delivery room.[93] In some cases, a trial of therapy may be appropriate, but this does not always mandate continued support.

Fetal Heart Rate Monitoring

Most obstetricians use continuous electronic FHR monitoring once preterm labor becomes established. Preterm gestation may complicate the interpretation of FHR patterns. Preterm fetuses may have decreased variability, and the baseline FHR is higher in preterm fetuses (especially less than 34 weeks' gestation) than in term fetuses.[94] The presence of chorioamnionitis or the use of beta-adrenergic receptor agonists also can confound the interpretation of the FHR tracing.

The value of continuous electronic FHR monitoring versus intermittent auscultation of the FHR remains controversial. Luthy et al.[95] performed a randomized trial that compared continuous electronic FHR monitoring (with selective fetal blood gas sampling) versus periodic auscultation of the FHR during preterm labor in women with a fetus that weighed between 700 and 1750 g. There was no significant difference between groups in the incidence of cesarean section, low 5-minute Apgar scores, intrapartum acidosis, intracranial hemorrhage, and perinatal death. At 18 months of age, the incidence of cerebral palsy was significantly higher in the electronic FHR group than in the intermittent auscultation group (20% versus 8%, respectively).[96]

ANESTHETIC MANAGEMENT

Anesthesiologists often participate in the care of preterm parturients. Many of these women request epidural analgesia for labor and vaginal delivery. These patients also have a higher incidence of cesarean section, often in situations of fetal distress, which necessitates urgent administration of anesthesia.

Conventional wisdom holds that the preterm fetus is more vulnerable than the term fetus to the depressant effects of analgesic and anesthetic drugs for the following reasons: (1) decreased protein available for drug binding and decreased protein-drug affinity by the protein that is present; (2) higher levels of bilirubin, which may compete with the drug for protein binding; (3) greater drug access to the central nervous system (CNS) because of the presence of an incomplete blood-brain barrier; (4) decreased ability to metabolize and excrete drugs; and (5) a higher incidence of acidosis during labor and delivery.[71-73,97,98] However, few controlled studies have documented the maternal and fetal pharmacokinetics and pharmacodynamics of anesthetic agents throughout gestation. The preterm fetus may be less vulnerable to the depressant effects of local anesthetics than originally thought. The human fetal liver cytochrome P-450 system is present as early as the fourteenth week of gestation and has the capability to oxidize several drugs.[99-101]

Teramo et al.[102] noted that the amount of lidocaine necessary to produce seizure activity in preterm sheep fetuses was greater than that required in older fetuses. They also observed that the cardiovascular response to lidocaine (i.e., increases in blood pressure and heart rate) was less severe in fetuses with a younger gestational age. Pedersen et al.[103] evaluated the effects of gestational age on the pharmacokinetics and pharmacodynamics of lidocaine in gravid ewes and fetal lambs. They studied two groups of animals: *preterm* (119 ± 1 days' gestation or 0.8 of term pregnancy) and *near-term* (138 ± 1 days' gestation or 0.95 of term pregnancy). They administered an intravenous infusion of lidocaine to obtain a maternal steady-state plasma concentration of 2 μg/mL. Transplacental transfer of lidocaine did not adversely affect fetal cardiac output, organ blood flow, or blood gas and acid-base measurements in either group. Tissue uptake of lidocaine was similar in the two groups of fetal lambs, except that it was greater in the lungs and liver of the term fetuses. They concluded that there was no significant difference in the pharmacokinetics and pharmacodynamics of lidocaine between the two gestational ages studied.[103]

Smedstad et al.[104] also concluded that there was no difference in fetal blood pressure, heart rate, or blood gas measurements in response to maternal intravenous infusion of lidocaine or bupivacaine in early preterm (119 days' gestation) fetal lambs compared with late preterm (132 days' gestation) fetal lambs. In addition, the plasma concentrations of bupivacaine and lidocaine and the fetal:maternal ratios of both drugs were similar in the two groups of fetuses.

None of these studies evaluated the effects of anesthetic agents on the acidotic preterm fetus. Acidotic preterm fetuses are at increased risk for an adverse response to analgesic and anesthetic drugs administered to the mother. Asphyxia increases these risks by causing the following changes in the fetal environment: (1) reduced plasma protein-binding capacity (which increases the proportion of free drug available)[105-107]; (2) increased maternal-fetal hydrogen ion difference, which causes "ion trapping" of weak bases (e.g., amide local anesthetics, opioids) on the fetal side of the circulation[108,109]; (3) increased blood-brain permeability[110-112]; and (4) enhanced susceptibility to the myocardial depressant effects of local anesthetics.[113-118]

Morishima et al.[118] subjected a group of preterm fetal lambs (0.8 of timed gestation) to asphyxia by causing partial occlusion of the umbilical cord. They subsequently administered either lidocaine or saline-control intravenously to the gravid ewes for 180 minutes. The maternal and fetal steady-state plasma lidocaine concentrations were 2.32 ± 0.12 and 1.23 ± 0.17 μg/mL, respectively. (These concentrations are similar to those that occur during epidural anesthesia in humans.) Umbilical cord occlusion resulted in the typical fetal compensatory response to hypoxia (i.e., decreased FHR and increased blood flow to the fetal brain, heart, and adrenal glands). Maternal administration of saline-control did not result in additional deterioration of the fetus. However, maternal administration of lidocaine resulted in a significant increase in $PaCO_2$, and decreases in pH, mean arterial pressure (MAP), and blood flow to the brain, myocardium, and adrenal glands. Thus lidocaine attenuated the normal fetal compensatory response to asphyxia. In an earlier study,[119] these same investigators observed that lidocaine did not affect the fetal compensatory response to asphyxia in term fetuses. The authors concluded that "the immature fetus loses its cardiovascular adaptation to asphyxia when exposed to clinically acceptable plasma concentrations of lidocaine obtained transplacentally from the mother." Limitations of this study include a failure to compare the fetal response to lidocaine versus the response to other anesthetic, analgesic, or sedative drugs and consideration of only the effects of a steady-state concentration of lidocaine in the presence of asphyxia. That is, the investigators did not evaluate the potential benefits derived from epidural anesthesia, such as the decreased maternal concentrations of catecholamines and the ability of epidural anesthesia to facilitate a controlled, atraumatic delivery of the preterm infant.

Bupivacaine has a low fetal:maternal plasma concentration ratio because of its relatively high (96%) maternal protein binding; therefore the potential for fetal toxicity seems minimal.[98] Studies of the effects of bupivacaine on the compensatory response to asphyxia in the preterm fetal lamb have demonstrated results similar to those seen with lidocaine. Santos et al.[120] observed that bupivacaine abolished the compensatory increase in blood flow to vital organs in asphyxiated preterm fetal lambs. However, bupivacaine did not affect fetal heart rate, blood pressure, or acid-base measurements. The authors suggested that these changes were less severe than those seen with lidocaine in their earlier study.[118,120]

Ropivacaine and bupivacaine have almost identical dissociation constants (pK_B of 8.0 and 8.2, respectively), but ropivacaine's protein binding is slightly less than that for bupivacaine (92% versus 96%, respectively), and it is substantially less lipid-soluble than bupivacaine.[121] These differences may affect maternal and fetal free plasma concentrations of drug. Investigators have documented higher maternal and fetal plasma concentrations with ropivacaine than with bupivacaine.[122,123] Studies suggest that ropivacaine is less cardiotoxic than bupivacaine. However, no study has evaluated the effect of ropivacaine on the fetal compensatory response to hypoxia.

2-Chloroprocaine also is a good choice of local anesthetic in preterm patients because it is rapidly metabolized in both the maternal and fetal plasma.[124] Further, placental transfer of 2-chloroprocaine is not increased by fetal acidosis.[125]

Vaginal Delivery

Specific anesthetic requirements for vaginal delivery of the preterm infant include the following: (1) inhibition of inappropriate expulsive efforts before complete cervical dilation, especially with a breech presentation; (2) avoidance of precipitous delivery, which can result in rapid decompression of the fetal head and increase the risk of intracranial hemorrhage; and (3) provision of a relaxed pelvic floor and perineum to facilitate a smooth, controlled delivery of the infant's head, which is especially important with a breech delivery. Many obstetricians perform an episiotomy to facilitate an atraumatic delivery of the infant's head. Some disagreement remains regarding the wisdom of elective forceps delivery of the preterm infant. Although the use of forceps shortens the second stage of labor, misplacement of excessive force may fracture the immature fetal skull or tentorium.[97]

Neither pudendal nerve block nor local infiltration of the perineum provides profound relaxation of the levator ani and bulbocavernosus muscles. Continuous lumbar epidural anesthesia is the technique of choice during labor and vaginal delivery. If delivery appears imminent, a low level of spinal anesthesia may be a good choice. Epidural anesthesia also decreases the likelihood of premature maternal expulsive efforts and precipitous delivery of the vulnerable, preterm fetal head. In cases of preterm fetal breech presentation, it is essential that the mother not push the breech through a partially dilated cervix.

Epidural anesthesia decreases maternal concentrations of catecholamines, and in some patients, it may improve uteroplacental perfusion in the absence of hypotension.[126] No prospective, controlled studies have evaluated the effect of epidural anesthesia on outcome for the preterm fetus. Two retrospective studies compared outcome for preterm infants whose mothers received anesthesia versus infants whose mothers received no anesthesia.[127,128] One multicenter study[127] reported that the perinatal death rate for preterm infants was 446 per 1000 when no anesthesia was given, compared with 157 per 1000 when regional anesthesia was used. Wright et al.[128] reviewed the outcome of neonates delivered between 25 and 36 weeks' gestation over a 10-year period. They included only those patients with a singleton fetus and a vertex presentation with no congenital anomalies. The infants were divided into groups according to gestational age as well as type of anesthesia (e.g., spinal or epidural anesthesia versus pudendal nerve block, local infiltration, or no anesthesia).

The authors found no significant difference between the two groups in umbilical cord blood gas and acid-base measurements, Apgar scores, or time to sustained respiration. There was a tendency toward more vigorous neonates and decreased neonatal morbidity and mortality after administration of regional anesthesia in patients delivered between 25 and 28 weeks' gestation, but the differences were not statistically significant. The authors concluded that "the use of major regional anesthesia for labor and vaginal delivery of the preterm infant is safe with respect to the clinical and biochemical condition of the neonate at birth." Further, for reasons cited earlier, many obstetricians consider the use of regional anesthesia to be an essential component of an optimal preterm delivery.

The timing of the administration of epidural analgesia in preterm parturients may be problematic for several reasons. First, preterm women often have a prolonged latent phase of labor because of the administration of tocolytic agents for several hours or days. Second, when tocolysis fails, the patient may be in advanced labor, and delivery may be imminent. Third, a cervical dilation of only 6 or 7 cm (rather than 10 cm) may be sufficient to allow delivery of the small preterm fetus. We recommend early placement of an epidural catheter in patients at high risk for failed tocolysis. In some cases, it may be appropriate to establish epidural analgesia while the obstetrician continues the efforts to stop labor. In these cases, preterm labor may cease after administration of epidural analgesia, and the anesthesiologist may allow analgesia to regress.[129] Rarely, the anesthesiologist may even remove the catheter in an undelivered patient whose labor has stopped. We do not consider epidural analgesia to be a primary means of tocolysis. However, we consider it preferable to have an occasional patient cease preterm labor after administration of epidural analgesia than to have too many patients deliver precipitously without adequate anesthesia. Moreover, early induction of epidural analgesia facilitates the use of regional anesthesia for emergency cesarean section. Although the obstetrician may attempt tocolysis, there is a high likelihood that tocolysis will fail and that the patient will require emergency cesarean section.

Combined spinal-epidural (CSE) analgesia has gained popularity in recent years. For preterm patients, the advantages of CSE analgesia include its rapid onset and a reduction in the total dose of drug(s) needed to provide analgesia.[130,131] However, these advantages should be weighed against the disadvantages of CSE analgesia. Some studies suggest that there is an increased incidence of fetal bradycardia after intrathecal opioid administration. This bradycardia does not seem to have an adverse effect on term fetuses,[132] but no study has evaluated outcome in preterm fetuses. Further, when using the CSE technique, there is a delay in confirmation of placement of the epidural catheter. This may be disadvantageous if urgent cesarean section is necessary before the location (and function) of the epidural catheter have been confirmed. Finally, some investigators have expressed concern that CSE analgesia is associated with an increased incidence of meningitis.[133,134] Recently published reports of meningitis following CSE analgesia may represent publication bias resulting from the identification of complications associated with a relatively new technique. Nonetheless, given the association between infection (e.g., chorioamnionitis) and preterm labor, some anesthesiologists worry that use of the CSE technique may result in an increased risk of meningitis in preterm patients. At present, this represents speculation.

Cesarean Section

Administration of general anesthesia is similar to that for patients at term (see Chapter 25). Most of the anesthetic agents that are used for induction and maintenance of general anesthesia cross the placenta and may further depress the already compromised preterm infant. If cesarean delivery is necessary, conventional wisdom holds that it is preferable to give either epidural anesthesia or spinal anesthesia to avoid the depressant effects of these agents. However, some cases of dire maternal or fetal distress require the administration of general anesthesia. Some investigators also have suggested that general anesthetic agents may protect the immature, preterm fetal brain (see Chapter 9). In a study of anesthesia for elective cesarean section at term, Hodgson and Wauchob[135] observed that infants exposed to spinal anesthesia were in better condition at delivery than those exposed to general anesthesia. Similarly, Rolbin et al.[136] observed that preterm infants exposed to epidural anesthesia for cesarean section had higher 1- and 5-minute Apgar scores than similar infants exposed to general anesthesia. Maternal administration of supplemental oxygen is essential, regardless of the choice of anesthetic technique.[137]

INTERACTIONS BETWEEN TOCOLYTIC THERAPY AND ANESTHESIA

Indications for Anesthesia During and After Tocolytic Therapy

There are at least three situations in which obstetric patients require anesthesia during or after tocolytic therapy. First, failure of tocolysis often occurs. In this case, the patient may desire pain relief during labor and vaginal delivery. Other patients require anesthesia for cesarean section. Second, some obstetricians give a tocolytic agent before and during the performance of cervical cerclage. Third, some obstetricians advocate the bolus injection of a tocolytic agent to facilitate fetal resuscitation in cases of fetal distress. Uteroplacental perfusion occurs during uterine diastole. Therefore relaxation of the uterus should result in improved uteroplacental perfusion.

Beta-Adrenergic Agents

Ritodrine and terbutaline are commonly used beta-adrenergic tocolytic agents. These agents may delay delivery for 24 to 48 hours, which allows administration of a glucocorticoid to accelerate fetal lung maturity. However, studies suggest that these agents do not result in a substantial prolongation of pregnancy.[55,59,138]

All beta-adrenergic tocolytic drugs have both beta$_1$- and beta$_2$-receptor effects but in different proportions. Beta$_2$ receptors are found in smooth muscle (uterus, blood vessels, bronchi, intestine, detrusor, and spleen capsule), adipose tissue, liver, skeletal muscle, pancreas, and salivary glands. Ritodrine and terbutaline are relatively selective for beta$_2$ receptors; stimulation of these receptors in the myometrium results in relaxation of uterine smooth muscle. Unfortunately, other undesired beta$_2$ effects (vasodilation, glycogenolysis) and beta$_1$ effects still occur. Beta$_1$ receptors are located predominantly in the heart and adipose tissue. Beta$_1$-receptor stimulation causes clinically significant cardiovascular side effects, such as increased maternal heart rate and cardiac output.[139]

MECHANISM OF ACTION

Beta-adrenergic agents interact with beta$_2$-receptor sites on the outer membrane of uterine myometrial cells, activating the enzyme adenyl cyclase. This enzyme catalyzes the conversion of ATP to cAMP, causing an increase in the intracellular concentration of cAMP. The increased cAMP decreases the available intracellular concentration of calcium and inhibits MLCK activity. This decreases the interaction between actin and myosin and results in myometrial relaxation.[140]

TREATMENT REGIMEN

Before beginning tocolytic therapy with a beta-adrenergic agent, the obstetrician should determine baseline maternal vital signs and weight and should exclude significant cardiovascular or pulmonary disease. In the past, some physicians recommended the performance of a baseline electrocardiogram (ECG).[141,142] Although it seems prudent to avoid beta-adrenergic therapy in a patient with cardiovascular disease, a screening ECG rarely affects management. Many obstetricians no longer obtain a baseline ECG before giving beta-adrenergic tocolytic therapy in healthy preterm patients.

These agents may be administered intravenously, subcutaneously, or orally. Initial studies suggested that long-term therapy with an oral agent was a successful strategy for preventing recurrence of preterm labor.[143,144] However a meta-analysis did not confirm any benefit from this strategy with either terbutaline or ritodrine.[145]

If uterine activity persists, the obstetrician may substitute an alternative tocolytic agent for the beta-adrenergic agonist. Prolonged administration of a beta-adrenergic tocolytic agent is ineffective, in part because prolonged administration results in down-regulation (or desensitization) of the myometrial beta$_2$ receptors.[146-150]

Terbutaline can be administered subcutaneously by a portable infusion pump, which allows administration of a continuous low-dose basal infusion with intermittent bolus doses.[151] In theory, this low-dose/intermittent bolus therapy might prevent or delay desensitization of the myometrial beta$_2$ receptors, which occurs with prolonged exposure to beta-adrenergic agents.[150] However, randomized double-blind clinical trials have not shown any reduction in the rate of preterm delivery with subcutaneous terbutaline pump infusion.[152] In 1997 the FDA issued a statement regarding the lack of efficacy of the subcutaneous terbutaline pump, and it also noted that this treatment modality is potentially dangerous.[153]

SIDE EFFECTS

The administration of beta-adrenergic tocolytic therapy may result in troublesome maternal side effects, including hypotension; tachycardia, with or without cardiac arrhythmias and myocardial ischemia; pulmonary edema; hyperglycemia; and hypokalemia.[140] The incidence of these side effects is unclear. Earlier studies reported an incidence of 2% to 9%.[154,155] However, Perry et al.[156] performed a retrospective review of outcome for 8709 patients who had received a low-dose, continuous infusion of terbutaline. They noted adverse cardiopulmonary effects in only 47 of 8709 patients, an incidence of 0.54%.[156]

Hypotension and Tachycardia

The frequency and severity of cardiovascular side effects are dose related and can be minimized by limiting the dose of the beta-adrenergic agent. Stimulation of the beta$_1$ receptors on the myocardium results in direct inotropic and chronotropic effects.[142,157] To a lesser degree, stimulation of beta$_2$-receptor sites in the vascular beds causes vasodilation, diastolic hypotension, and a reflex compensatory increase in heart rate, stroke volume, and cardiac output.[157] Palpitations and chest pain or tightness are common complaints during ritodrine therapy. Cardiac arrhythmias, primarily supraventricular tachycardia, have been reported.[141,142,144,158,159] There have been several reports of myocardial ischemia in patients receiving beta-adrenergic therapy; ischemia may result from an increase in myocardial oxygen demand because of the inotropic and chronotropic effects of the drug.[141,142,160] ECG changes such as ST-segment depression and T-wave flattening or inversion may occur; these changes typically resolve after the discontinuation of beta-adrenergic therapy.[161-164] It is unclear whether these ECG changes represent myocardial ischemia. In asymptomatic patients, these changes may result from ritodrine-induced tachycardia or hypokalemia.[165,166]

Pulmonary Edema

Pulmonary edema is a life-threatening complication of beta-adrenergic tocolytic therapy. Earlier reports estimated that pulmonary edema occurred in as many as 5% of patients who received beta-adrenergic tocolytic therapy.[159] More recent studies suggest a lesser incidence of pulmonary edema during beta-adrenergic therapy.[59,156] Perhaps heightened awareness of the relationship between excessive beta-adrenergic therapy and pulmonary edema has led to a reduction in the incidence of this serious complication.[167]

In several case reports, pulmonary edema developed within 24 to 72 hours after the start of beta-adrenergic therapy.[154,168-170] Earlier reports suggested an association between the concurrent use of glucocorticoids (e.g., dexamethasone, betamethasone) and the development of pulmonary edema in patients receiving beta-adrenergic therapy.[154,169] However, these steroids have little mineralocorticoid activity, and pulmonary edema has occurred in patients who did not receive a glucocorticoid. Philipsen et al.[171] concluded that glucocorticoid therapy is not a risk factor for the development of pulmonary edema during ritodrine therapy.

The underlying mechanism for the development of pulmonary edema during beta-adrenergic therapy remains unclear. Some investigators have speculated that beta-adrenergic therapy precipitates myocardial failure, and others have suggested that the pulmonary edema is noncardiogenic (i.e., increased pulmonary vascular permeability).[141,154] Several studies have found no evidence of myocardial failure in patients receiving beta-adrenergic therapy.[172,173]

Plasma volume expansion leading to volume overload during beta-adrenergic therapy also has been proposed as the principal mechanism for pulmonary edema.[174] Fluid overload during beta-adrenergic therapy may occur as a result of intravenous overhydration and/or as a result of fluid and sodium retention secondary to increased renin and antidiuretic hormone activity from beta-adrenergic receptor stimulation.[174-176]

Kleinman et al.[139] studied the circulatory and renal effects of ritodrine infusion with three different types of intravenous hydration in gravid ewes. The authors evaluated the possible contribution of these effects to the development of pulmonary edema. They demonstrated that ritodrine infusion produced a significant increase in maternal heart rate and cardiac output and a decrease in systemic vascular resistance (SVR). Pulmonary artery and pulmonary capillary wedge pressures (PCWP) also tended to increase during ritodrine infusion, but the increase was not statistically significant. The

circulatory effects during ritodrine infusion were similar for the three types of intravenous hydration: (1) maintenance infusion of normal saline (NS) at a rate of 125 mL/hr, (2) 1 L bolus of NS followed by infusion of NS at a rate of 250 mL/hr, and (3) 1 L bolus of 5% dextrose in water (D5W) followed by infusion of D5W at a rate of 250 mL/hr. The authors noted an antidiuretic and antinatriuretic effect during ritodrine infusion, irrespective of the type of intravenous fluid used. These renal effects seemed related to increased renal reabsorption in the animals receiving the NS solutions; however, in the animals receiving D5W, the antidiuresis appeared to be related to increased antidiuretic hormone secretion. The amount of fluid retained was significantly greater when ritodrine was infused with NS than when it was infused with D5W. The authors suggested that the central hemodynamic effects of beta-adrenergic receptor stimulation place an added overload on the circulatory system during pregnancy (which is already associated with increased cardiac output and plasma volume). In addition, they suggested that the antidiuretic and antinatriuretic effects from beta-adrenergic therapy lead to fluid retention and further circulatory overload. The result is enhancement of fluid diffusion from the pulmonary vasculature to the pulmonary interstitium.

Other investigators have noted that concurrent administration of an intravenous saline solution with a beta-adrenergic agent may increase the risk of developing pulmonary edema. Philipsen et al.[171] compared the effects of glucose and saline solutions on fluid retention in patients receiving ritodrine therapy. Intravenous infusion of isotonic sodium chloride caused retention of more fluid than infusion of glucose solution, and patients in the saline group were more likely to develop pulmonary congestion that required treatment. Studies of pregnant baboons receiving intravenous Ringer's lactate solution demonstrated more fluid and sodium retention when ritodrine was administered than when Ringer's lactate solution was given alone.[177,178] Colloid oncotic pressure decreased during volume infusion in both groups. However, the ritodrine-treated group had a colloid oncotic pressure-to-pulmonary artery pressure gradient that favored net movement of water from the pulmonary vasculature to the pulmonary interstitium.

Normal-to-low PCWPs have been reported in patients who developed pulmonary edema during beta-adrenergic therapy.[179] This suggests a noncardiogenic mechanism (i.e., increased pulmonary vascular permeability) for the development of pulmonary edema in these patients. Women with preterm labor and concurrent infection may be at increased risk for developing pulmonary edema during beta-adrenergic tocolysis.[142,155] Infection may increase pulmonary vascular permeability through the release of endotoxin and may result in noncardiogenic pulmonary edema.[180] A case report detailed the hemodynamic measurements in such a case. A woman who had received long-term beta-adrenergic therapy presented for preterm delivery. She was febrile, which was thought to be a result of bacteremia after amniocentesis. She received general anesthesia for cesarean section, and despite a negative fluid balance, she subsequently developed pulmonary edema. She had a central venous pressure of 8 and a PCWP of 11, but she had a decreased cardiac index (2.35 L/min/m^2), and she demonstrated a sluggish response to infusions of both dopamine and dobutamine. The authors hypothesized that she had increased pulmonary vascular permeability, most likely as a result of the infection. Further, they speculated that her decreased cardiac index and her sluggish response to inotropic support resulted from the desensitization of her beta-adrenergic receptors.[181]

Regardless of the etiology, the hypoxemia that accompanies beta-adrenergic-related pulmonary edema may seem disproportionate to the degree of edema noted with a chest radiograph. Conover et al.[182] demonstrated that ritodrine significantly inhibits hypoxic pulmonary vasoconstriction in dogs. This inhibition of hypoxic pulmonary vasoconstriction may worsen the hypoxemia that accompanies pulmonary edema during beta-adrenergic therapy.

Total intake and output, daily weights, and serial hematocrit determinations should be monitored carefully during beta-adrenergic therapy. The choice of intravenous fluid may influence the degree of fluid retention and the development of metabolic changes.[183] Isotonic solutions (e.g., NS) increase the severity of sodium and fluid retention, and dextrose-containing solutions increase the likelihood of hyperglycemia and hypokalemia. One option is to give the beta-adrenergic agent with a solution of 0.45 sodium chloride *without* dextrose. It seems reasonable to limit total fluid intake to 1.5 to 2.5 L/24 hr.

Limiting the dose of the beta-adrenergic agent also should lessen the risk of pulmonary edema. Little tocolytic efficacy is gained by administering more beta-adrenergic agent than that necessary to increase maternal heart rate by 20% to 30%. Patients receiving beta-adrenergic tocolysis should be monitored closely for signs of pulmonary edema. Pulse oximetry facilitates detection of early changes in oxygenation in patients receiving beta-adrenergic tocolysis.

If pulmonary edema develops, the beta-adrenergic agent should be discontinued immediately, supplemental oxygen should be administered, fluids should be restricted, and a diuretic agent should be administered. Most patients respond to these simple measures. Rarely, patients with severe, persistent hypoxemia require invasive hemodynamic monitoring, endotracheal intubation, and mechanical ventilation. Pisani and Rosenow[179] reviewed 58 published cases of pulmonary edema associated with beta-adrenergic tocolytic therapy. Only 4 of the 58 patients required intubation and mechanical ventilation. A recent case report documented the successful use of a tight-fitting face mask to deliver continuous positive airway pressure (CPAP), thus avoiding the need for intubation in a preterm patient with pulmonary edema associated with beta-adrenergic tocolytic therapy.[184]

Hyperglycemia

Plasma glucose levels increase rapidly after the initiation of beta-adrenergic therapy.[141,185-187] Insulin release occurs before the rise in glucose levels and parallels the level of hyperglycemia. This initial insulin release most likely is mediated by direct beta-adrenergic receptor stimulation of the maternal pancreas.[187] Glucose levels return to baseline within 24 hours of initiating therapy, and supplemental insulin typically is not necessary in nondiabetic patients.[188] The use of a beta-adrenergic agent in insulin-dependent diabetic patients is controversial.[141,189] Hyperglycemia and ketoacidosis typically can be avoided with careful monitoring of serum glucose concentrations and concurrent intravenous insulin infusion.[189]

Hypokalemia

Hypokalemia most likely results from insulin-mediated transport of potassium and glucose from the extracellular space to the intracellular space. Urinary excretion of potassium is not increased; therefore total body potassium levels remain the same.[141] Correction therefore is not necessary. Serum potassium concentrations typically return to normal within 24 hours of starting beta-adrenergic therapy, and no adverse effects associated with hypokalemia have been reported.[141,185,190]

Hyperkalemia

Recently two reports have documented a rebound hyperkalemia after treatment with ritodrine.[191,192] In one report six patients had rebound hyperkalemia that was noted 60 to 150 minutes after cessation of ritodrine treatment. All six patients had received supplemental potassium for treatment of hypokalemia, prior to discontinuation of the ritodrine. All patients received general anesthesia for emergency cesarean delivery, for which thiopental and vecuronium were used during induction. The peak potassium levels ranged from 6.8 to 7.9 mmol/L and were associated with ECG changes (peaked T waves).[191] In another report, hyperkalemia was observed after succinylcholine administration in three patients who had received prolonged treatment with both magnesium sulfate and ritodrine, and who also had been subjected to prolonged immobilization for treatment of preterm labor.[192] Thus, anesthesiologists should exercise caution when giving general anesthesia immediately after cessation of ritodrine therapy. The anesthesiologist should watch for signs of hyperkalemia, especially if the patient received supplemental potassium for treatment of hypokalemia during beta-adrenergic therapy.

Other Maternal Side Effects

Other infrequent maternal side effects reported with the use of beta-adrenergic agents include elevations in serum transaminase levels,[193] paralytic ileus,[194] cerebral vasospasm in patients with a previous history of migraine syndrome,[195] and respiratory arrest caused by increased muscle weakness in a patient with myasthenia gravis.[196]

Fetal Side Effects

Placental transfer of beta-adrenergic agents is rapid. An increased FHR, which is presumed to be a result of direct stimulation of fetal myocardial beta$_1$ receptors, may be seen. Neonatal hypoglycemia may occur as a result of maternal hyperglycemia and hyperinsulinemia.[197] Some physicians have suggested that the use of beta-adrenergic agents may be associated with a higher incidence of neonatal IVH[198,199]; however, this observation has not been confirmed in other studies.[59,200] There are few reports of the long-term fetal effects of beta-adrenergic agents, and most of these studies are retrospective, but they have failed to demonstrate any long-term, adverse fetal effects.[200-202] Some studies have demonstrated transient echocardiographic evidence of decreased fetal myocardial contractility after prolonged beta-adrenergic tocolysis.[203,204] However, after an extensive review of this subject, Kast and Hermer[205] concluded that beta-adrenergic tocolysis has no long-term, adverse effect on the fetal and neonatal heart.

ANESTHETIC MANAGEMENT

Kuhnert et al.[206] observed that the distribution phase and equilibrium phase half-lives for ritodrine in pregnant women are 32 ± 20 minutes and 17 ± 10 hours, respectively. The cardiovascular effects of the beta-adrenergic agents persist for 60 to 90 minutes after their discontinuation.[139,207] It would seem ideal to delay administration of anesthesia until maternal tachycardia subsides. However, advanced labor, an abnormal presentation, and/or fetal distress often require emergency administration of anesthesia.

Published reports of anesthetic management after administration of a beta-adrenergic agent are scarce.[208-215] Ravindran et al.[211] reported one case each of intraoperative pulmonary edema, sinus tachycardia, and ventricular arrhythmia during general anesthesia in patients who had received terbutaline therapy immediately before or 15 minutes after the induction of anesthesia. They recommended that induction of general anesthesia be delayed at least 10 minutes after discontinuation of the beta-adrenergic agent.

Shin and Kim[214] retrospectively observed that maternal hypotension was more common when induction of anesthesia occurred within 30 minutes of the discontinuation of ritodrine compared with a delay of more than 30 minutes. In contrast, Ueyama et al.[215] prospectively assessed outcome for women who received spinal anesthesia for cesarean section within 30 minutes of discontinuation of ritodrine, with or without prophylactic intravenous ephedrine. They also studied two other groups of patients—laboring patients who had *not* received ritodrine and nonlaboring patients undergoing elective cesarean section. Among the patients who did not receive prophylactic ephedrine, hypotension occurred more frequently in the ritodrine (44%) and the nonlaboring patients (40%) than in the laboring, no-ritodrine patients (10%). Among the patients who received prophylactic ephedrine, the incidence of hypotension was similar in the ritodrine (12%) and the laboring, no-ritodrine patients (6%), but less than that in the nonlaboring patients (30%). This study provides support for the use of regional anesthesia in patients who have recently received ritodrine. Further, the authors concluded that prophylactic ephedrine was more effective in ritodrine-treated patients than in nonlaboring patients or in laboring patients who had not received ritodrine.

Chestnut et al.[216] performed a controlled study to determine whether prior administration of ritodrine worsens maternal hypotension during epidural anesthesia in gravid ewes. Ritodrine was infused intravenously for 2 hours and then discontinued, followed by administration of a 500-mL intravenous bolus of NS. Lidocaine (without epinephrine) or NS was administered epidurally 15 minutes later. A third group of animals received an intravenous infusion of NS followed by epidural lidocaine. There was no significant difference in maternal MAP or uterine blood flow during administration of epidural anesthesia in the ritodrine-lidocaine and saline-lidocaine groups (Figure 34-2). Maternal cardiac output remained above baseline during administration of epidural anesthesia in the ritodrine-lidocaine group. The authors concluded that prior administration of ritodrine did not worsen maternal hypotension during epidural lidocaine anesthesia in gravid ewes. The authors suggested that "the inotropic and chronotropic activity of ritodrine helped maintain maternal cardiac output and uterine blood flow during epidural anesthesia."[216]

A delay of 15 minutes often results in sufficient slowing of the maternal heart rate to allow slow induction of epidural anesthesia. When time allows, slow induction of epidural anesthesia seems preferable to single-shot spinal anesthesia. The slow onset allows the mother to compensate for the sympathectomy and allows the anesthesiologist to give crystalloid as needed. However, the study by Ueyama et al.[215] supports the administration of spinal anesthesia in these patients. Further, if vaginal delivery is imminent, a low level of spinal anesthesia is preferred in patients without preexisting epidural analgesia.

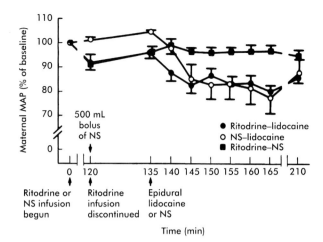

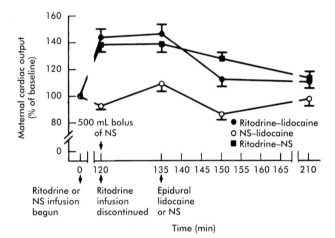

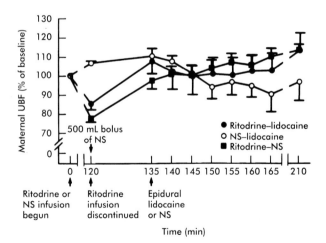

FIGURE 34-2. Response over time of maternal mean arterial pressure *(MAP)*, cardiac output, and uterine blood flow *(UBF)* after intravenous infusion of either ritodrine 0.004 mg/kg/min or normal saline *(NS)*-control for 120 min, followed by a 500-mL intravenous bolus of NS over 15 min, and then epidural injection of lidocaine or NS-control in gravid ewes. (From Chestnut DH, Pollack KL, Thompson CS, et al. Does ritodrine worsen maternal hypotension during epidural anesthesia in gravid ewes? Anesthesiology 1990; 72:315-21.)

Patients receiving beta-adrenergic therapy are at risk for developing pulmonary edema *(vide supra)*. Therefore aggressive hydration should be avoided before and during the induction of anesthesia in these patients. We first administer a modest fluid bolus (e.g., 250 to 500 mL of Ringer's lactate) and then slowly induce epidural anesthesia. Additional intravenous crystalloid and a vasopressor can be safely administered to maintain normal maternal blood pressure.[215]

Ephedrine, a mixed alpha- and beta-adrenergic agonist, has been the vasopressor of choice for treatment of hypotension in obstetric practice because of its protective effect on uterine blood flow (UBF) in gravid ewes.[217,218] Historically, anesthesiologists have believed that ephedrine's beta-receptor activity increases cardiac output, which compensates for its alpha-receptor mediated uterine vasoconstriction. Chestnut et al.[219,220] hypothesized that in a patient already receiving a beta-adrenergic agonist, any vasopressor effect from ephedrine should result from alpha-receptor stimulation. The accompanying uterine vasoconstriction subsequently would result in decreased UBF. However, ephedrine restored uterine blood flow velocity (UBFV) during hemorrhagic hypotension in gravid guinea pigs subjected to terbutaline infusion (Figure 34-3).[219] In a subsequent study,[220] ephedrine preserved UBFV during ritodrine infusion in normovolemic gravid guinea pigs (Figure 34-4). Both epinephrine and phenylephrine decreased UBFV, whereas mephentermine resulted in an intermediate response. These studies suggest that ephedrine does not depend solely on beta-adrenergic stimulation to increase cardiac output. Ramanathan et al.[221] observed that ephedrine increases cardiac preload in pregnant women to a greater degree than it increases afterload. Others have concluded that ephedrine produces more venoconstriction than arterial constriction.[222] This results in improved venous return and increased cardiac output.

Tong and Eisenach[223] evaluated the effects of ephedrine and metaraminol on the uterine and femoral vessels of gravid and nongravid ewes *in vitro*. Uterine but not systemic arteries became less responsive to both ephedrine and methoxamine during pregnancy, and constriction was reduced more in uterine vessels in response to ephedrine than in response to metaraminol, an alpha-adrenergic agonist. Constriction to both agents was abolished by phentolamine. The authors suggested that "both ephedrine and metaraminol constrict uterine and systemic vessels by actions on alpha-adrenoceptors" and that "ephedrine may spare uterine perfusion during pregnancy due to more selective constriction of systemic vessels than that caused by metaraminol."[223] This study also suggests that ephedrine's protective effects on UBF do not depend solely on beta-adrenergic stimulation. (See Chapter 3 for a discussion of the role of nitric oxide in ephedrine's protective effects on UBF.)

McGrath et al.[224] evaluated the use of ephedrine and phenylephrine for the treatment of hypotension during ritodrine infusion and epidural anesthesia in gravid ewes. Ephedrine restored UBF, whereas phenylephrine resulted in a significant decrease in UBF and an increase in uterine vascular resistance.

Caution should be exercised when extrapolating animal studies to humans. However, these laboratory studies,[219,220,223,224] as well as the clinical study by Ueyama et al.,[215] suggest that ephedrine remains a satisfactory choice of vasopressor in patients who have recently received beta-adrenergic therapy. Some anesthesiologists worry that ephedrine will worsen tachycardia in patients who have recently received beta-adrenergic tocolytic therapy. However, in our experience, the heart rate typically decreases when a dose of ephedrine sufficient to restore blood pressure is given to these patients. One report described a patient in whom ventricular

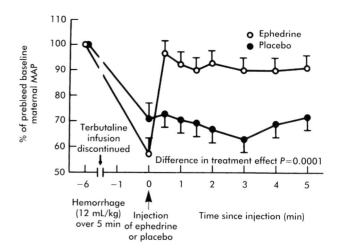

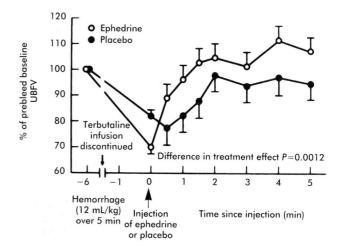

FIGURE 34-3. Response over time of maternal mean arterial pressure *(MAP)* and uterine artery blood flow velocity *(UBFV)* after hemorrhage and intravenous administration of ephedrine, 1.0 mg/kg, or placebo (saline, 0.2 mL) in gravid guinea pigs. All values are expressed as mean (± SEM) percent of the prebleed baseline. (From Chestnut DH, Weiner CP, Wang JP, et al. The effect of ephedrine upon uterine artery blood flow velocity in the pregnant guinea pig subjected to terbutaline infusion and acute hemorrhage. Anesthesiology 1987; 66:508-12.)

tachycardia and fibrillation developed after she received ephedrine for treatment of hypotension during epidural anesthesia for cesarean section.[212] The incident occurred 30 minutes after discontinuation of the ritodrine infusion.

Alternatively, small doses of phenylephrine can be administered if there is concern that ephedrine may worsen maternal tachycardia or precipitate arrhythmia. Small doses of phenylephrine are safe and effective for the treatment of hypotension in healthy, term parturients receiving regional anesthesia for elective cesarean section.[225-227] A randomized clinical trial comparing ephedrine, phenylephrine, and a combination of phenylephrine and ephedrine surprisingly noted a higher incidence of fetal acidosis in infants whose mothers had received ephedrine during administration of spinal anesthesia for elective cesarean section.[227] The authors speculated that "increased fetal metabolic rate, secondary to ephedrine-induced beta-adrenergic stimulation, was the most likely mechanism for the increased incidence of fetal acidosis in the ephedrine group."[227]

If general anesthesia is required in a patient who has recently received beta-adrenergic tocolysis, agents that might exacerbate maternal tachycardia (e.g., atropine, glycopyrro-

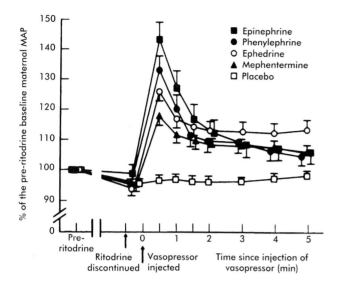

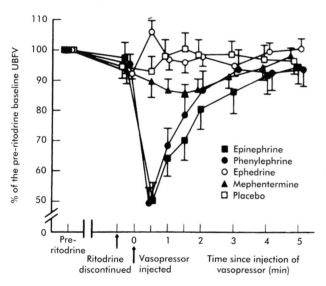

FIGURE 34-4. Response over time of maternal mean arterial pressure *(MAP)* and uterine artery blood flow velocity *(UBFV)* after intravenous infusion of ritodrine and subsequent injection of epinephrine (0.001 mg/kg), phenylephrine (0.01 mg/kg), mephentermine (1.0 mg/kg), ephedrine (1.0 mg/kg), or placebo (saline, 0.02 mL) in gravid guinea pigs. All values are expressed as mean (± SEM) percent of the pre-ritodrine baseline for that vasopressor. (From Chestnut DH, Ostman LG, Weiner CP, et al. The effect of vasopressor agents upon uterine artery blood flow velocity in the gravid guinea pig subjected to ritodrine infusion. Anesthesiology 1988; 68:363-6.)

late, pancuronium) should be avoided. Residual maternal tachycardia may make it more difficult to assess volume status and depth of anesthesia. Halothane—which sensitizes the myocardium to catecholamine-induced arrhythmias—should *not* be used. Hyperventilation should be avoided, as it may exacerbate hypokalemia and potentiate the hyperpolarization of the cell membrane. From et al.[228] reported that terbutaline pretreatment shortened the onset time and recovery of succinylcholine-induced neuromuscular blockade in nonpregnant patients. It seems prudent to monitor neuromuscular function with a peripheral nerve stimulator during general anesthesia.

Obstetricians continue to question the efficacy of beta-adrenergic tocolytic therapy. Nonetheless, anesthesiologists are likely to continue to encounter patients who require urgent administration of anesthesia shortly after administration of a beta-adrenergic tocolytic agent.[229]

Magnesium Sulfate

Obstetricians have gained extensive experience with the use of magnesium sulfate for seizure prophylaxis in preeclamptic women. In 1959, Hall et al.[230] first reported that hypermagnesemia prolonged the duration of labor in patients with preeclampsia. Subsequently, other studies have suggested that magnesium sulfate decreases uterine activity during labor.[231-234]

However, there is little scientific evidence of the efficacy of magnesium sulfate for tocolysis. Few studies of magnesium sulfate have used a randomized, placebo-controlled study design. In a prospective, randomized study, Cox et al.[235] showed that magnesium sulfate therapy did not prolong gestation or improve neonatal outcome, when compared with no therapy. A recent meta-analysis indicated that tocolytic therapy with beta-adrenergic agents, indomethacin, atosiban, and/or ethanol—but *not* magnesium sulfate—was associated with a significant prolongation of pregnancy. However, this prolongation was not associated with improved perinatal or neonatal outcome.[55]

MECHANISM OF ACTION

Extracellular magnesium affects uptake, binding, and distribution of cellular calcium in vascular smooth muscle.[236] Magnesium competes with calcium for low-affinity calcium binding sites on the outside of the sarcoplasmic reticulum membrane and prevents the increase in free intracellular calcium concentration. This inhibits MLCK activity and prevents the interaction of actin and myosin that is necessary for contraction.[237] Magnesium ions may increase the intracellular levels of cAMP, which also inhibits light-chain kinase activity and actin-myosin interaction.[236]

Hypermagnesemia results in abnormal neuromuscular function. Magnesium also decreases the release of acetylcholine at the neuromuscular junction and the sensitivity of the end plate to acetylcholine.

TREATMENT REGIMEN

An intravenous loading dose of 4 g is administered over 15 to 20 minutes, followed by a continuous infusion of 1 to 4 g/hr. Serum concentrations of 5.0 to 7.0 mg/dL typically are necessary for the inhibition of uterine activity. Once tocolysis is successful, the obstetrician may continue magnesium sulfate therapy at a lower maintenance rate or may discontinue magnesium sulfate in favor of an oral agent such as indomethacin or nifedipine.

SIDE EFFECTS

Most studies have reported that magnesium sulfate results in less frequent and severe cardiovascular side effects in unstressed patients than the beta-adrenergic tocolytic agents.[231,232,234] Nonetheless, magnesium sulfate may result in side effects similar to those that occur during beta-adrenergic tocolytic therapy. Chest pain and tightness, palpitations, nausea, transient hypotension, blurred vision, sedation, and pulmonary edema have been reported.[232-234,238] The occurrence of pulmonary edema during magnesium sulfate therapy demonstrates that pulmonary edema is not a unique complication of beta-adrenergic tocolytic therapy. The etiology of magnesium-induced pulmonary edema remains unclear. A prospective analysis of 294 patients receiving magnesium sulfate for treatment of either preterm labor or preeclampsia suggested an association between low colloid osmotic pressure and the development of pulmonary edema.[239] However, the authors did not demonstrate a causal relationship between hypermagnesemia and the development of low colloid osmotic pressure. In all likelihood the pulmonary edema in these patients was precipitated by fluid overload.

One study suggested that the co-administration of both magnesium sulfate and ritodrine results in a greater incidence of serious side effects (e.g., chest pain with or without ECG changes, adult RDS) than the administration of ritodrine alone.[240]

Magnesium is eliminated almost entirely by renal excretion. Therefore patients with abnormal renal function should be monitored carefully. The loss of deep tendon reflexes occurs at serum magnesium concentrations of 8 to 10 mg/dL. Respiratory depression occurs at concentrations of 10 to 15 mg/dL, and above this level, cardiac conduction defects (e.g., widened QRS complex, increased P-R interval) and cardiac arrest can occur. As long as deep tendon reflexes are present, the more serious side effects typically are avoided. Fortunately, most patients who are candidates for tocolytic therapy have normal renal function. Therefore magnesium toxicity occurs less frequently during tocolytic therapy than during the administration of magnesium sulfate for seizure prophylaxis in preeclamptic women.

In preeclamptic women, bolus administration of magnesium sulfate results in a decrease in SVR and an increase in cardiac index, which persists for as long as 4 hours. However, bolus administration of magnesium sulfate typically results in only transient decreases in SVR and MAP in patients with preterm labor.[241] Benedetti[141,142] suggested that magnesium sulfate is a safe alternative tocolytic agent to beta-adrenergic agents in patients at risk for bleeding (e.g., placenta previa). Thus, many clinicians consider magnesium sulfate to be the tocolytic drug of choice in patients at high risk for hemorrhage.

However, Chestnut et al.[242] demonstrated that magnesium sulfate but not ritodrine worsened maternal hypotension during hemorrhage in gravid ewes (Figure 34-5). The authors speculated that magnesium attenuated the compensatory response to hemorrhage and that ritodrine's inotropic and chronotropic activity helped maintain maternal cardiac output and MAP during hemorrhage. Subsequently, Reynolds et al.[243] evaluated the effects of hypermagnesemia on the compensatory circulatory response to maternal hemorrhage and hypotension in fetal lambs. Hypermagnesemia attenuated the compensatory increase in fetal cerebral blood flow and resulted in an increased incidence of fetal death.

Others have expressed concern regarding the potential adverse fetal and neonatal effects of magnesium sulfate, including a possible increase in perinatal mortality[244,245] (see Chapter 10). The debate began in 1995 with the publication of a retrospective analysis that suggested a lower prevalence of cerebral palsy when mothers who delivered a newborn of 1500 g or less were treated antenatally with magnesium sulfate (either for tocolysis or seizure prophylaxis).[246] This report was criticized for inclusion of patients in whom the indication for magnesium sulfate therapy was *either* tocolysis *or* seizure prophylaxis, as it was suggested that preeclampsia may provide some neuroprotective effect. This was followed by a prospective study, which was halted because of an apparent increase in total pediatric mortality in the magnesium sulfate group.[247] Subsequently, a retrospective case-control study suggested that antenatal exposure to a high tocolytic dose of magnesium sulfate (i.e., 48 g or more) was associated with a significant increase in perinatal mortality among neonates weighing 700 to 1249 g at delivery.[248] Given these findings—combined with

the questionable tocolytic efficacy of magnesium sulfate—this group of investigators recommended reconsideration of the use of magnesium sulfate as a first-line tocolytic agent.[248] In response, a large retrospective analysis of data for 12,876 deliveries from 100 tertiary care centers did not identify any evidence of increased mortality in the neonates exposed to magnesium sulfate. These investigators emphatically concluded that antenatal magnesium exposure is not associated with a higher risk of perinatal death.[249] Unfortunately this retrospective analysis did not address the incidence of cerebral palsy.

ANESTHETIC MANAGEMENT

Suresh and Lawson[250] suggested that magnesium sulfate should be discontinued before the administration of epidural anesthesia "because magnesium can increase the likelihood of hypotension through its generalized vasodilating properties." Vincent et al.[251] observed that magnesium sulfate decreased

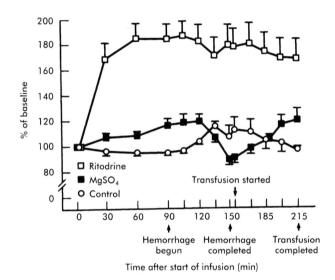

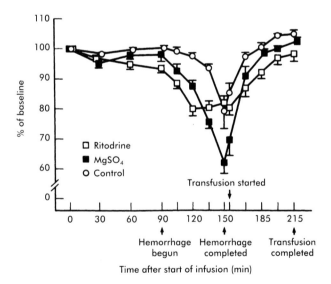

FIGURE 34-5. Response over time of maternal mean arterial pressure *(MAP)* and maternal heart rate *(HR)* during intravenous infusion of ritodrine (0.004 mg/kg/min), magnesium sulfate (MgSO₄, 4 g/hr), or saline-control and maternal hemorrhage in gravid ewes. All values are expressed as mean (± SEM) percent of baseline. (From Chestnut DH, Thompson CS, McLaughlin GL, Weiner CP. Does the intravenous infusion of ritodrine or magnesium sulfate alter the hemodynamic response to hemorrhage in gravid ewes? Am J Obstet Gynecol 1988; 159:1467-73.)

maternal blood pressure but not UBF or fetal oxygenation during epidural lidocaine anesthesia in gravid ewes (Figure 34-6). This study suggests that hypermagnesemia may increase the likelihood of modest hypotension during regional anesthesia in normotensive parturients. Recent studies have suggested that spinal anesthesia can be safely administered in preeclamptic women who are receiving magnesium sulfate for seizure prophylaxis (see Chapter 44). Although those data may not be applicable to normotensive patients, it is our experience that spinal anesthesia can be safely administered to preterm parturients who require urgent cesarean section after failed tocolytic therapy.

Magnesium sulfate alters the maternal hemodynamic response to endogenous and exogenous vasopressor agents.[242,251,252] Sipes et al.[252] observed that magnesium sulfate did not affect the action of phenylephrine on SVR but instead attenuated

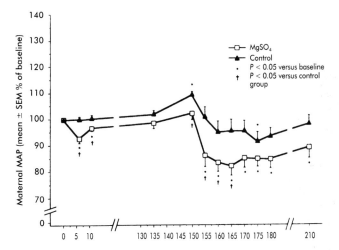

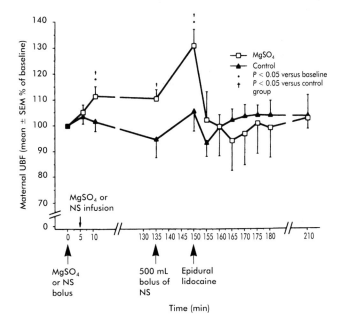

FIGURE 34-6. Response over time of maternal mean arterial pressure *(MAP)* and uterine blood flow *(UBF)* after an intravenous bolus of magnesium sulfate (MgSO₄, 4 g) or normal saline (NS), followed by an infusion of MgSO₄ (4 g/hr) or saline-control in gravid ewes. Subsequently, a 500-mL intravenous bolus of NS was given over 15 min, followed by epidural administration of 2% lidocaine. All values are expressed as mean (± SEM) percent of baseline. (From Vincent RD, Chestnut DH, Sipes SL, et al. Magnesium sulfate decreases maternal blood pressure but not uterine blood flow during epidural anesthesia in gravid ewes. Anesthesiology 1991; 74:77-82.)

the increase in uterine vascular resistance and the decrease in UBF during phenylephrine infusion in gravid ewes. They hypothesized that hypermagnesemia might alter the uterine vascular response to ephedrine or phenylephrine during epidural anesthesia-induced hypotension. However, in a later study[253] the same authors observed that ephedrine restored UBF and did not alter uterine vascular resistance during epidural anesthesia in hypermagnesemic gravid ewes. In contrast, phenylephrine did not restore UBF and markedly increased uterine vascular resistance during epidural anesthesia (Figure 34-7). Moreover, ephedrine but not phenylephrine maintained fetal pH and fetal oxygenation during treatment of hypotension. Therefore, even in the presence of hypermagnesemia (which may have provided partial protection of UBF during phenylephrine infusion), phenylephrine increased uterine vascular resistance and did not maintain fetal pH during epidural anesthesia-induced hypotension. This study suggests that ephedrine is preferred to phenylephrine for treatment of hypotension during regional anesthesia in hypermagnesemic patients.

Magnesium sulfate also results in abnormal neuromuscular function. Magnesium attenuates the release of acetylcholine at the neuromuscular junction, reduces the sensitivity of the endplate to acetylcholine, and decreases the excitability of the muscle membrane. Ramanathan et al.[254] reported that neuromuscular transmission was abnormal in unanesthetized preeclamptic women receiving magnesium sulfate and that the intensity of the abnormality correlated with increased serum magnesium levels. Magnesium sulfate potentiates the action of both depolarizing and nondepolarizing muscle relaxants.[255,256] A defasciculating dose of a nondepolarizing muscle relaxant should not be given before administration of succinylcholine in hypermagnesemic women. A standard intubating dose of muscle relaxant (e.g., succinylcholine 1 mg/kg) should be used because the extent of potentiation by magnesium sulfate is variable.[257,258] However, a reduced dose of a nondepolarizing muscle relaxant should be administered during the maintenance of anesthesia. We have observed that patients who have received prolonged magnesium sulfate therapy are especially sensitive to nondepolarizing muscle relaxants. Neuromuscular blockade should be monitored with a peripheral nerve stimulator.

Parturients receiving magnesium sulfate often appear sedated. Thompson et al.[259] evaluated the anesthetic effects of magnesium sulfate and ritodrine on the minimum alveolar concentration (MAC) of halothane in pregnant and nonpregnant rats. They reported a 20% decrease in MAC with serum magnesium levels of 7 to 11 mg/dL. Koinig et al.[260] recently assessed the analgesic effect of perioperative magnesium sulfate administration in nonpregnant patients undergoing arthroscopic knee surgery. Magnesium sulfate reduced both intraoperative and postoperative analgesic requirements (i.e., fentanyl consumption).

Magnesium may have a modest effect on platelet function, most likely because of its ability to antagonize the effects of calcium, which is necessary for platelet aggregation. Thus concern has been raised about magnesium's potential effect on hemostasis. Fuentes et al.[261] noted that infusion of magnesium sulfate resulted in a modest prolongation of the bleeding time (i.e., from 5.7 ± 1.7 to 6.8 ± 2.1 minutes) in 24 pregnant women. Although this change was statistically significant, most physicians would conclude that the magnitude of the change is of little if any clinical significance. However, three of the patients had a bleeding time of 10.5 to 11.5 minutes, and

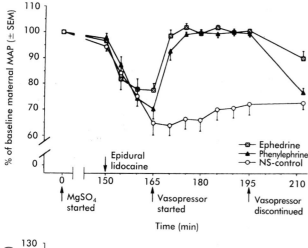

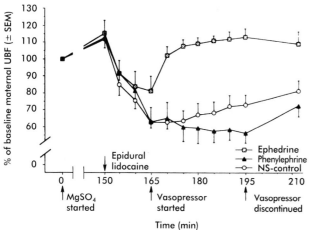

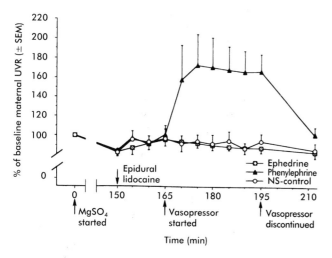

FIGURE 34-7. Response over time of maternal mean arterial pressure *(MAP)*, maternal uterine blood flow *(UBF)*, and maternal uterine vascular resistance *(UVR)* after an intravenous bolus of magnesium sulfate (MgSO₄, 4 g), followed by an infusion of MgSO₄ (4 g/hr), followed by epidural administration of 2% lidocaine to achieve a thoracic level of anesthesia in gravid ewes. Subsequently, an intravenous infusion of ephedrine, phenylephrine, or normal saline-control was administered for 30 min, with the ephedrine or phenylephrine infusion rate adjusted to maintain maternal MAP at the baseline level. All values are expressed as mean (± SEM) percent of baseline. (From Sipes SL, Chestnut DH, Vincent RD, et al. Which vasopressor should be used to treat hypotension during magnesium sulfate infusion and epidural anesthesia? Anesthesiology 1992; 77:101-8.)

the authors suggested that this may be clinically relevant. However, it is unclear that a modest prolongation of the bleeding time predicts an increased risk of bleeding in the epidural space or elsewhere in the body (see Chapter 42). Regional anesthesia has a long history of safety in preeclamptic women receiving magnesium sulfate for seizure prophylaxis. Few experienced obstetric anesthesiologists would be concerned about a possible modest prolongation of the bleeding time resulting from magnesium sulfate therapy.

Prostaglandin Synthetase Inhibitors

Prostaglandin synthetase inhibitors are effective tocolytic agents, alone or with another agent.[62,63,262-267] These drugs are easily administered orally or rectally and are well tolerated by the mother. **Indomethacin** is the prototype prostaglandin synthetase inhibitor used for tocolysis. Both **sulindac** and **ketorolac** have also been evaluated and found to be effective. Both of these agents are significantly more expensive than indomethacin. Ketorolac may offer the advantage of intravenous administration.[264] Sulindac is reported to have fewer fetal side effects because it crosses the placenta less readily and possibly because of its more complex metabolism.[267]

MECHANISM OF ACTION

Prostaglandin synthetase inhibitors inhibit cyclooxygenase and thus prevent the synthesis of prostaglandins from the precursor, arachidonic acid. Prostaglandins E₂ and F₂-alpha play an important role in the stimulus of uterine contractions. During parturition, blood and amniotic fluid prostaglandin concentrations increase.[268,269] Increased concentrations of prostaglandin metabolites have been measured in patients who present with preterm labor.[17,270]

TREATMENT REGIMEN

A 50-mg oral or rectal dose of indomethacin is followed by oral administration of 25 mg every 4 to 6 hours. Indomethacin readily crosses the placenta and appears in the fetal blood within 15 minutes.[271] The half-life of indomethacin in nonpregnant adults is approximately 2.2 hours. In contrast, the half-life of indomethacin in the fetus is 11 to 15 hours and is prolonged to 19 hours in neonates delivered before 32 weeks' gestation.[271]

SIDE EFFECTS

Maternal side effects from indomethacin are minimal when it is used for tocolytic therapy. Indomethacin does not alter maternal heart rate or blood pressure. The most common complaints are nausea and heartburn.[262,271] Inhibition of cyclooxygenase results in decreased production of thromboxane A₂ and abnormal platelet aggregation. Aspirin permanently inhibits cyclooxygenase; therefore platelet aggregation is abnormal for the lifetime (7 to 10 days) of the exposed platelets. In contrast, indomethacin and most other prostaglandin synthetase inhibitors *reversibly* inhibit cyclooxygenase; thus their effect on platelet function is only transient.[272]

Maternal administration of a prostaglandin synthetase inhibitor may cause premature closure of the ductus arteriosus in utero and result in persistent fetal circulation after delivery. Indomethacin often is used to promote closure of the ductus arteriosus in the preterm neonate.[271] Moise et al.[273] used fetal echocardiography to evaluate the fetal response to short-term (less than 72 hours) indomethacin therapy. They observed evidence of transient ductal constriction in 7 of

14 fetuses between 26 and 31 weeks' gestation. Tricuspid regurgitation also was noted in three fetuses. There was no statistically significant difference between the mean gestational age of the fetuses with ductal constriction and that of those without constriction (29.3 and 28.4 weeks, respectively). However, these changes reversed within 24 hours of discontinuing indomethacin.

Some animal and clinical studies suggest that indomethacin is less likely to cause in utero closure of the ductus arteriosus at earlier gestational ages.[274-278] Niebyl and Witter[276] observed that adverse neonatal effects (including closure of the ductus arteriosus) are unlikely if indomethacin is used in short courses (e.g., 24 to 48 hours), is restricted to patients less than 34 weeks' gestation, and is stopped at an appropriate interval before delivery. Moise[277] retrospectively analyzed fetal echocardiograms performed in 44 patients with preterm labor or polyhydramnios who were treated with indomethacin. The frequency of ductal constriction was relatively low (approximately 5% to 10%) until 32 weeks' gestation, when it increased to approximately 50%. Similarly, Vermillion et al.[278] observed that indomethacin results in a "dramatic increase in the incidence of ductal constriction . . . after 31 weeks' gestation." However, they noted that indomethacin tocolysis may result in reversible constriction of the ductus arteriosus at any gestational age. Moise[277] suggested that the use of indomethacin should be restricted to gestational ages of less than 32 weeks.

Long-term indomethacin administration may result in oligohydramnios secondary to decreased fetal urine excretion.[279] Kirshon et al.[280] noted decreased fetal urine output after short-term maternal administration of indomethacin for tocolytic therapy. Kirshon et al.[281] also reported decreased fetal urine output resulting in oligohydramnios in six preterm fetuses whose mothers received long-term (15 to 28 days) indomethacin therapy. Amniotic fluid volume reaccumulated within 1 week after the discontinuation of indomethacin. Indomethacin may be used to treat polyhydramnios in selected cases. One mechanism that has been proposed to explain the decrease in fetal urine output is enhanced antidiuretic hormone effect after prostaglandin synthesis inhibition.[282] Wurtzel[283] evaluated renal function during the first 10 postnatal days in 14 preterm infants exposed to indomethacin in utero and in 10 control infants. Long-term maternal administration of indomethacin did not significantly alter neonatal renal function when compared with control infants.

Investigators have expressed concern over the risk of other neonatal complications after antenatal exposure to indomethacin. Norton et al.[284] evaluated 57 neonates delivered at or before 30 weeks' gestation, who were exposed to indomethacin for treatment of preterm labor. They found a significant increase in the incidence of necrotizing enterocolitis, intracranial hemorrhage (grades II to IV), and patent ductus arteriosus requiring surgical ligation.[284]

Mayer et al.[285] specifically attempted to determine whether antenatal exposure to indomethacin increases the risk of neonatal necrotizing enterocolitis. In a retrospective analysis of 56 neonates exposed to indomethacin, they found that exposure to indomethacin of at least 48 hours' duration—and occurring within 24 hours of delivery—was associated with a significant increase in the incidence of necrotizing enterocolitis in LBW neonates. In contrast, in a larger study of 140 indomethacin-exposed neonates, Pietrantoni et al.[286] did not find an increased incidence of IVH among 140 indomethacin-

exposed neonates. Further, a multicenter trial suggested that low-dose indomethacin therapy may actually prevent neonatal IVH.[287]

Two recent studies likewise did not detect an increased incidence of neonatal complications after exposure to indomethacin.[288,289] In both studies the duration of exposure was less than 72 hours, and the exposure occurred before 32 weeks' gestation. Thus the current recommendations for use of these agents are to limit the course of therapy to less than 72 hours and to use them only before 32 weeks' gestation. This approach may delay delivery and allow maternal administration of corticosteroids to accelerate fetal lung maturity.

ANESTHETIC MANAGEMENT

The effects of indomethacin on platelet function are transient. In the past, some anesthesiologists obtained a bleeding time measurement in patients who had recently received a prostaglandin synthetase inhibitor for tocolysis. Lunt et al.[290] demonstrated a prolongation of the bleeding time (i.e., from 4.5 ± 1.6 to 8.8 ± 3.5 minutes) in 20 women who had received indomethacin for tocolysis. No patient had a hemorrhagic complication attributed to indomethacin, which the authors attributed to the significant time interval between indomethacin administration and delivery. They recommended that a bleeding time measurement be obtained in women who labor or require operative delivery after receiving indomethacin for tocolysis.

In contrast, Rogers and Levin[291] performed a critical appraisal of the bleeding time measurement. They concluded that there is little evidence that the bleeding time measurement predicts the risk of hemorrhage elsewhere in the body. Several large studies have demonstrated the safety of epidural and spinal anesthesia in patients receiving low-dose aspirin or one of a variety of nonsteroidal antiinflammatory drugs (NSAIDs).[292-294]

There are few published reports of epidural hematoma after regional anesthesia in patients who were receiving a prostaglandin synthetase inhibitor. One report described a cervical epidural hematoma after steroid injection into the cervical epidural space of a patient who had been taking indomethacin.[295] (This patient had received seven epidural steroid injections during a 2-year period.) We are unaware of any published case of epidural hematoma after the administration of epidural anesthesia in an obstetric patient who had recently received a prostaglandin synthetase inhibitor. There is no indication for a bleeding time measurement or other measure of coagulation before administration of regional anesthesia in a patient whose only risk factor is recent ingestion of a prostaglandin synthetase inhibitor.

Calcium Entry-Blocking Agents

Calcium entry-blocking drugs are capable of inhibiting uterine contractions. Among these drugs, **nifedipine** has undergone the most extensive evaluation as a tocolytic agent. Nifedipine has fewer effects on cardiac conduction, more specific effects on myometrial contractility, and less effect on serum electrolytes than the other calcium entry-blocking drugs. Maternal side effects are typically mild (e.g., facial flushing, transient increase in heart rate).[296] In a multi-center randomized trial, Papatsonis et al.[297] found that nifedipine administration had greater efficacy, resulted in fewer maternal side effects, and was followed by fewer admissions to the neonatal intensive care unit, when compared to ritodrine administration. In contrast, in another prospective randomized trial, Kupferminc et al.[298] found nifedipine's efficacy to be similar to that of ritodrine. The authors observed significantly fewer maternal side effects in the nifedipine group, but they demonstrated no difference in neonatal outcome. A meta-analysis of randomized comparisons of nifedipine versus beta-adrenergic agonists concluded that nifedipine was more effective than ritodrine in delaying delivery at least 48 hours, was more likely to result in a prolongation of pregnancy beyond 34 weeks' gestation, was associated with fewer side effects, and was associated with better neonatal outcome (i.e., fewer cases of neonatal RDS).[299]

These conclusions are reassuring, given that some animal studies have demonstrated adverse fetal effects. Several studies have noted that nifedipine or **nicardipine** decreases UBF and results in fetal hypoxemia and acidosis in laboratory animals.[300-302] Blea et al.[302] demonstrated that maternal infusion of nifedipine is associated with hypoxia and acidosis in fetal lambs, despite the fact that nifedipine results in little change in maternal blood pressure or uteroplacental perfusion. The authors noted that "the deterioration of fetal blood gases is out of proportion to the transient decreases in uteroplacental blood flow and demonstrates that another mechanism for this fetal acidosis and hypoxia exists during nifedipine infusion."[302]

Two clinical studies have suggested that short-term administration of nifedipine does not adversely affect the uteroplacental or fetal circulation.[303,304] Likewise, a retrospective study noted that neonates exposed to nifedipine had normal umbilical cord blood gas and pH measurements at delivery.[305]

Two recent reviews confirmed both the efficacy and favorable side-effect profile of calcium entry-blocking agents in the management of preterm labor.[306,307] Many obstetricians have suggested that these agents should become first-line therapy in the treatment of pretem labor.

MECHANISM OF ACTION

Calcium entry-blocking drugs act by blocking the aqueous voltage-dependent cell membrane channels that are selective for calcium. They also act by preventing calcium release from the sarcoplasmic reticulum. The net result is a decrease in available intracellular calcium, which inhibits MLCK activity. This results in decreased actin-myosin interaction, which results in relaxation of smooth muscle (including myometrial smooth muscle).[308,309]

TREATMENT REGIMEN

Nifedipine can be administered orally or sublingually. Initially, it may be administered sublingually. The dose may be repeated as needed every hour, up to a maximum dose of 40 mg. The typical oral dose is 10 to 20 mg every 4 to 6 hours.

ANESTHETIC MANAGEMENT

Although nifedipine has fewer effects on cardiac conduction than some of the other calcium-entry blocking agents, it has the potential to cause vasodilation, hypotension, myocardial depression, and conduction defects when used in combination with one of the volatile halogenated anesthetic agents.[310] One report noted that administration of both nifedipine and magnesium sulfate caused neuromuscular blockade in a preeclamptic patient at 28 weeks' gestation.[311] Thus the anesthesiologist should exercise caution when giving a muscle relaxant to a patient who has received these two drugs.

Postpartum hemorrhage may result from postpartum uterine atony that is unresponsive to oxytocin and prostaglandin $F_{2\text{-alpha}}$.[312] It seems prudent to establish large-bore intravenous access in these patients and to ensure the ready availability of blood products.

Oxytocin Antagonists

In recent years, investigators have made significant progress in advancing our understanding of the molecular mechanisms involved in the initiation of labor. As a result, new agents have been developed and evaluated for the treatment of preterm labor.

Atosiban (1-deamino-2-D-tyr-[OEt]-4-thr-8-orn-vasotocin/oxytocin) is an oxytocin antagonist that is undergoing evaluation for use as a tocolytic agent.[313-319] Atosiban is a competitive inhibitor of oxytocin that binds to both myometrial and decidual receptors. It does not alter the subsequent sensitivity of the myometrium to oxytocin.[320] Clinically this represents a major advantage and should reduce the risk of postpartum uterine atony and hemorrhage. Phase II and III studies have shown that atosiban is an effective tocolytic agent. It appears to have major advantages over other agents in that it results in few maternal side effects, undergoes minimal placental transfer, causes no adverse fetal effects, and does not increase maternal blood loss at delivery.[314,316] In a direct comparison with beta-adrenergic agonists, atosiban compares favorably in terms of obtaining and maintaining uterine quiescence.[317-319]

There are no data on the interaction between atosiban and anesthetic agents. However, given the hemodynamic profile of this agent, one would not expect significant interactions. At publication this agent was in widespread clinical use in Europe. However, the FDA has not yet approved its use in the United States.

INVESTIGATIONAL TOCOLYTIC AGENTS

Nitric Oxide Donors

For several years, anesthesiologists have used **nitroglycerin** in situations in which a rapid onset of profound uterine relaxation is desired (e.g., uterine hyperstimulation, fetal head entrapment, internal version and extraction of the second twin, uterine inversion, retained placenta).[321] Nitroglycerin acts as a **nitric oxide** donor. In 1992 the journal *Science* hailed nitric oxide as the molecule of the year, and in 1998 Murad, Furchgott, and Ingnarro received the Nobel prize for their discoveries involving this molecule.[322]

Nitric oxide is a potent smooth muscle relaxant. This effect is mediated, in part, by activation of guanylate cyclase, which results in an increase in intracellular cyclic guanosine monophosphate (cGMP). The increased cGMP activates cGMP-dependent protein kinase, which inhibits the influx of Ca^{2+} from the extracellular space and the release of Ca^{2+} from intracellular stores. The protein kinase also activates the Ca^{2+} pump, thereby increasing Ca^{2+} extrusion across the plasma membrane and Ca^{2+} reuptake by the sarcoplasmic reticulum.[322] Nitric oxide can also relax human myometrium by other pathways such as direct activation of Ca^{2+}-activated K^+ channels.[322-324] Nitric oxide may be responsible for the normal vascular adaptation to pregnancy, and disturbances in this system may lead to preeclampsia (see Chapter 44).

Nitric oxide is synthesized from L-arginine by nitric oxide synthase (NOS). The constitutive isoforms of NOS found in endothelial cells and neurons are dependent on Ca^{2+} for their activity. The inducible forms (iNOS) are Ca^{2+}-independent, can synthesize nitric oxide at very high rates, and are present in the myometrium and placenta.[322] The ability of the myometrium to synthesize nitric oxide—as well as its sensitivity to nitric oxide—varies during and after pregnancy, labor, and delivery. For example, evidence suggests "a reduced production of, and sensitivity to, nitric oxide within the myometrium during labor when compared to late gestation."[324] Nitric oxide of placental origin may play a role in maintaining uterine quiescence, and placental nitric oxide activity decreases near term. A down-regulation of uteroplacental nitric oxide activity may initiate labor.

Uterine sensitivity to nitric oxide is much lower than seen with vascular tissues. Thus large amounts of nitric oxide would be required to inhibit uterine contractions. At these doses, one might expect to see significant hemodynamic side effects. Studies in laboring sheep have demonstrated that nitroglycerin effectively inhibits spontaneous uterine contractions and results in a modest reduction in maternal MAP, without causing an adverse effect on fetal circulation or blood gas and pH measurements.[325,326] These investigators suggested that "intravenous nitroglycerin has an excellent margin of safety and possibly could be used as a uterine tocolytic agent."[326] However, a recent study observed that sublingual administration of nitroglycerin (three doses of 800 µg, administered 10 minutes apart) did not reduce uterine activity or tone in healthy laboring women at term, despite reducing maternal MAP approximately 20%.[327]

Few clinical studies have evaluated the use of nitroglycerin for tocolysis in preterm patients. Lees et al.[21] administered glyceryl trinitrate (nitroglycerin) patches to 13 patients in preterm labor, and noted that this therapy was both well-tolerated and effective in prolonging pregnancy. However, in a randomized study, El-Sayed et al.[328] observed more "tocolytic failures" with nitroglycerin than with magnesium sulfate. Moreover, persistent hypotension occurred in 4 (25%) of 16 patients who received nitroglycerin.

A recent publication from a multicenter, international study group randomizing patients to glyceryl trinitrate patches or beta-adrenergic receptor therapy found no difference in efficacy between the two agents.[329] The method of delivery of the nitric oxide donor may be critical. Some of the studies with favorable results utilized a glyceryl trinitrate patch, Deponit, which may have more favorable delivery kinetics.[21,322] This formulation is not available in the United States.

COX-2 Inhibitors

Prostaglandins and nitric oxide are intimately involved with cervical ripening. Cyclooxygenase (COX) and NOS are present in the cervix during pregnancy. During labor, increased amounts of COX-2 and iNOS are found in the cervix. In animal models, administration of a COX-2 inhibitor was effective in delaying the onset of labor.[330] Initial studies in humans demonstrated encouraging results with the use of **nimesulide** (a selective COX-2 inhibitor) for the treatment of preterm labor. As occurs with the other NSAIDs, oligohydramnios occurred in approximately 30% of patients. More disturbing have been the reports of neonatal renal failure with the use of this agent.[331]

KEY POINTS

- Despite improved antenatal care, the incidence of preterm delivery in the United States has not decreased and remains greater than 11%.
- Short-term tocolytic therapy may (1) facilitate transfer of the patient from a small community hospital to a tertiary care facility, (2) delay delivery to allow maternal administration of a glucocorticoid to accelerate fetal lung maturity, and (3) facilitate fetal resuscitation in utero in cases of fetal distress.
- Ritodrine is the only drug specifically approved by the FDA for tocolysis. However, other drugs (e.g., terbutaline, magnesium sulfate, nifedipine, indomethacin) are widely used in the United States.
- During labor and delivery the preterm fetus is at greater risk for acidosis and has a higher incidence of intracranial hemorrhage.
- Specific anesthetic requirements for vaginal delivery of the preterm infant include (1) inhibition of inappropriate maternal expulsive efforts before complete cervical dilation, especially in patients with a breech presentation; (2) prevention of precipitous delivery, which can result in rapid decompression of the fetal head and increase the risk of intracranial hemorrhage; and (3) provision of a relaxed pelvic floor and perineum to facilitate a smooth, controlled delivery of the more vulnerable, preterm fetal head.
- Side effects of beta-adrenergic tocolytic therapy include (1) hypotension; (2) tachycardia, with or without cardiac arrhythmias and myocardial ischemia; (3) pulmonary edema; (4) hyperglycemia; and (5) hypokalemia. Pulmonary edema is the most serious complication, and it may be life threatening. Hyperglycemia is problematic in diabetic patients. Hypokalemia rarely is a problem clinically.
- Prior administration of a beta-adrenergic tocolytic agent does not contraindicate the administration of regional anesthesia.
- Prostaglandin synthetase inhibitors reversibly inhibit cyclooxygenase, which results in a transient effect on platelet function. However, their use does not necessitate the assessment of coagulation status before administration of regional anesthesia in a patient whose only risk factor is recent ingestion of a prostaglandin synthetase inhibitor.
- Studies of new agents for the treatment of preterm labor are in progress. Advancement in the understanding of the physiology of labor will help with future directions for therapy. The ideal therapy will likely target multiple mechanisms involved in the physiology of labor and will have minimal adverse effects on the mother and fetus.

REFERENCES

1. Goldenberg RL. The management of preterm labor. Obstet Gynecol 2002; 100:1020-37.
2. Creasy RK. Preterm birth prevention: Where are we? Am J Obstet Gynecol 1993; 168:1223-30.
3. National Center for Health Statistics. Health, United States, 1991. Hyattsville, Md, US Department of Health and Human Services, Public Health Service, CDC, 1992; DHHS pub no. (PHS)92-1232.
4. United States Department of Health and Social Services. Healthy People 2010. Washington:US Department of Health and Social Services, 2000.
5. Keirse MJ. New perspectives for the effective treatment of preterm labor. Am J Obstet Gynecol 1995; 173:618-28.
6. Goldenberg RL, Rouse DJ. Prevention of premature birth. N Engl J Med 1998; 339:313-20.
7. American College of Obstetrics and Gynecologists. Management of preterm labor. ACOG Practice Bulletin No. 43, May 2003 (Obstet Gynecol 2003; 101:1039-47).
8. Copper RL, Goldenberg RL, Creasy RK, et al. A multicenter study of preterm birth weight and gestational age-specific neonatal mortality. Am J Obstet Gynecol 1993; 168:78-84.
9. Ehrenhaft PM, Wagner JL, Herdman RC. Changing prognosis for very low birth weight infants. Obstet Gynecol 1989; 74:528-35.
10. Hack M, Fanaroff AA. Outcomes of children of extremely low birthweight and gestational age in the 1990's. Early Hum Dev 1999; 53:193-218.
11. Kilpatrick SJ, Schlueter MA, Piecuch R, et al. Outcome of infants born at 24-26 weeks gestation. I. Survival and outcome. Obstet Gynecol 1997; 90:803-8.
12. Hack M, Fanaroff AA. Special report: Changes in the delivery room care of the extremely small infant (<750 g): Effects on morbidity and outcome. N Engl J Med 1986; 314:660-4.
13. Robertson PA, Sniderman SH, Laros RK, et al. Neonatal morbidity according to gestational age and birth weight from five tertiary care centers in the United States, 1983 through 1986. Am J Obstet Gynecol 1992; 166:1629-45.
14. Piecuch RE, Leonard CH, Cooper BA, et al. Outcome of infants born at 24-26 weeks gestation. II. Neurodevelopmental outcome. Obstet Gynecol 1997; 90:809-14.
15. Wood NS, Marlow N, Costeloe K, et al. Neurological and developmental disability after extremely preterm birth. N Engl J Med 2000; 343:378-84.
16. Hack M, Taylor HG, Klein N, et al. School age outcomes in children with birth weights under 750 gm. N Engl J Med 1994; 331:753-9.
17. Pschirrer ER, Monga M. Risk factors for preterm labor. Clin Obstet Gynecol 2000; 43:727-34.
18. Pregnancy and Perinatology Branch, Center for Research for Mothers and Children, National Institute of Child Health and Human Development: Report to the National Advisory Child Health and Human Development Council 1987; 9.
19. Challis JR, Mitchell MD. Basic mechanisms of preterm labour. Res Clin Forum 1994; 16:39-58.
20. Quatero HWP, Noort WA, Fry CH, Keirse MJNC. Role of prostaglandins and leukotrenes in the synergistic effect of oxytocin and corticotropin releasing factor (CRF) in the contraction force in human gestational myometrium. Prostaglandins 1991; 42:137-50.
21. Lees C, Campbell S, Jauniaux E, et al. Arrest of preterm labor and prolongation of gestation with glyceryl trinitrate, a nitric oxide donor. Lancet 1994; 343:1325-6.
22. Gibbs RS, Romero R, Hillier SL, et al. A review of premature birth and subclinical infection. Am J Obstet Gynecol 1992; 166:1515-28.
23. American College of Obstetricians and Gynecologists. Assessment of risk factors for preterm birth. ACOG Practice Bulletin No. 31, October 2001.
24. Romero R, Sirtori M, Oyarzun E, et al. Infection and labor. V. Prevalence, microbiology, and clinical significance of intraamniotic infection in women with preterm labor and intact membranes. Am J Obstet Gynecol 1989; 161:817-24.
25. Potkul RK, Moawad AH, Ponto KL. The association of subclinical infection with preterm labor: The role of C-reactive protein. Am J Obstet Gynecol 1985; 153:642-5.
26. Kirschbaum T. Antibiotics in the treatment of preterm labor. Am J Obstet Gynecol 1993; 168:1239-46.
27. Kenyon SL, Taylor DJ, Tarrow-Mordi W. Broad spectrum antibiotics for spontaneous preterm labour: The ORACLE II randomized trial. Lancet 2001; 357:989-94.
28. Thorp JM, Hartmann KE, Berkman ND, et al. Antibotic therapy for treatment of preterm labor: A review of the evidence. Am J Obstet Gynecol 2002; 186:587-92.
29. Mercer BM, Arheart KL. Antimicrobial therapy in expectant management of preterm premature rupture of the membranes. Lancet 1995; 346:1271-9.
30. Kenyon SL, Taylor DJ, Tarrow-Mordi W. Broad spectrum antibiotics for preterm, prelabour rupture of fetal membranes: The ORACLE I randomized trial. Lancet 2001; 357:979-88.
31. Ventura SJ, Martin JA, Curtin SC, Mathews TJ. Births: Final data for 1997. National vital statistics report, vol 47, No 18. Hyattsville: National Center for Health Statistics, 1999.
32. Perri T, Chen R, Yoeli R, et al. Are singleton pregnancies at risk of prematurity? J Assist Reprod Genet 2001; 18:245-9.
33. Herron MA, Katz M, Creasy RK. Evaluation of a preterm birth prevention program: Preliminary report. Obstet Gynecol 1982; 59:452-6.
34. Konte JM, Creasy RK, Laros RK. California North Coast preterm birth prevention project. Obstet Gynecol 1988; 71:727-30.
35. Goldenberg RL, Davis RO, Copper RL, et al. The Alabama preterm birth prevention project. Obstet Gynecol 1990; 75:933-9.
36. Main DM, Richardson DK, Hadley CB, Gabbe SG. Controlled trial of a preterm labor detection program: Efficacy and costs. Obstet Gynecol 1989; 74:873-7.
37. Fangman JJ, Mark PM, Pratt L, et al. Prematurity prevention programs: An analysis of successes and failures. Am J Obstet Gynecol 1994; 170:744-50.
38. Corwin MJ, Mou SM, Sunderji SG, et al. Multicentre randomized clinical trial of home uterine activity monitoring: Pregnancy outcomes for all women randomized. Am J Obstet Gynecol 1996; 175:1281-5.
39. Collaborative Group on Preterm Birth Prevention. Multicenter randomized, controlled trial of a preterm birth prevention program. Am J Obstet Gynecol 1993; 169:352-66.
40. Dyson DC, Danbe KH, Bamber JA, et al. Monitoring women at risk for preterm labor. N Engl J Med 1998; 338:15-9.
41. Mou SM, Sunderji SG, Gall S, et al. Multicenter randomized clinical trial of home uterine activity monitoring for detection of preterm labor. Am J Obstet Gynecol 1991; 165:858-66.
42. Sachs BP, Hellerstein S, Freeman R, et al. Home monitoring of uterine activity: Does it prevent prematurity? N Engl J Med 1991; 325:1374-7.
43. Castle BM, Turnbull AC. The presence or absence of fetal breathing movements predicts the outcome of preterm labour. Lancet 1983; 2:471-3.
44. Schreyer P, Caspi E, Natan NB, et al. The predictive value of fetal breathing movement and Bishop score in the diagnosis of "true" preterm labor. Am J Obstet Gynecol 1989; 161:886-9.
45. Peaceman AM, Andrews WW, Thorp JM, et al. Fetal fibronectin as a predictor of preterm birth in patients with symptoms: A multicenter trial. Am J Obstet Gynecol 1997; 177:13-8.
46. Hayashi RH, Mozurekewich EL. How to diagnose preterm labor: A clinical dilemma. Clin Obstet Gynecol, 2000; 43:768-77.
47. Helfgott AW, Willis DC, Blanco JD. Is hydration and sedation beneficial in the treatment of threatened preterm labor? A preliminary report. J Matern Fet Med 1994; 3:37-42.
48. Wright LL, Verter J, Younes N, et al. Antenatal corticosteroid administration and neonatal outcome in very low birth weight infants: The NICHD Neonatal Research Network. Am J Obstet Gynecol 1995; 173:269-74.
49. Andrews EB, Marcucci G, White A, Long W. Associations between use of antenatal corticosteroids and neonatal outcomes within the Exosurf Neonatal Treatment Investigational New Drug Program. Am J Obstet Gynecol 1995; 173:290-5.
50. Murphy K, Aghajafari F, Hannah M. Antenatal corticosteriods for preterm birth. Sem Perinatol 2001; 25:341-7.
51. National Institutes of Health Consensus Development Panel. Antenatal corticosteroids revisited: Repeated courses. National Institutes of Health Consensus Development Conference Statement, August 17-18, 2000 (Obstet Gynecol 2001; 98:144-150).
52. Garite TJ, Keegan KA, Freeman RK, Nageotte MP. A randomized trial of ritodrine tocolysis versus expectant management in patients with premature rupture of membranes at 25 to 30 weeks of gestation. Am J Obstet Gynecol 1987; 157:388-93.
53. Weiner CP, Renk K, Klugman M. The therapeutic efficacy and cost-effectiveness of aggressive tocolysis for premature labor associated with premature rupture of the membranes. Am J Obstet Gynecol 1988; 159:216-22.
54. Korenbrot CC, Aalto LH, Laros RK. The cost effectiveness of stopping preterm labor with beta-adrenergic treatment. N Engl J Med 1984; 310:691-6.
55. Gyetvai K, Hannah M, Hodnett ED, Ohlsson A. Tocolytics for preterm labor: A systematic review. Obstet Gynecol 1999; 94:869-77.
56. Wray S. Uterine contraction and physiological mechanisms of modulation. Am J Physiol 1993; 264:C1-18.
57. Norwitz ER, Robinson JN, Challis JRG. The control of labor. N Engl J Med 1999; 341:660-6.

58. Leveno KJ, Klein VR, Guzick DS, et al. Single-centre randomized trial of ritodrine hydrochloride for preterm labour. Lancet 1986; 1:1293-6.

59. The Canadian Preterm Labor Investigators Group. Treatment of preterm labor with the beta-adrenergic agonist ritodrine. N Engl J Med 1992; 327:308-12.

60. Howard TE, Killam AP, Penney LL, Daniell WC. A double-blind randomized study of terbutaline in premature labor. Mil Med 1982; 147:305-7.

61. Cotton DB, Strassner HT, Hill LM, et al. Comparison of magnesium sulfate, terbutaline and placebo for inhibition of preterm labor. J Reprod Med 1984; 29:92-7.

62. Niebyl JR, Blake DA, White RD, et al. The inhibition of preterm labor with indomethacin. Am J Obstet Gynecol 1980; 136:1014-9.

63. Zuckerman H, Shalev E, Gilad G, Katzuni E. Further studies of inhibition of preterm labor with indomethacin. Part II. Double-blind study. J Perinat Med 1984; 12:25-9.

64. Read MD, Welby DE. The use of calcium antagonist (nifedipine) to suppress preterm labour. Br J Obstet Gynaecol 1986; 93:933-7.

65. King JF, Grant AM, Keirse M, Chalmers I. Beta-mimetics in preterm labour: An overview of the randomized controlled trials. Br J Obstet Gynaecol 1988; 95:211-22.

66. Leveno KJ, Little BB, Cunningham FG. The national impact of ritodrine hydrochloride for inhibition of preterm labor. Obstet Gynecol 1990; 76:12-5.

67. Ledger WJ. Treatment of preterm labor with beta-adrenergic agonist ritodrine (letter). N Engl J Med 1992; 327:1758-9.

68. Ferguson JE, Dyson DC, Schutz T, Stevenson DK. A comparison of tocolysis with nifedipine or ritodrine: Analysis of efficacy and maternal, fetal, and neonatal outcome. Am J Obstet Gynecol 1990; 163: 105-11.

69. Tatsaris V, Papatsonis D, Goffinet F, et al. Tocolysis with nifedipine or beta-adrenergic agonists: A meta-analysis. Obstet Gynecol 2001; 97: 840-7.

70. Bowes WA. Delivery of the very low birth weight infant. Clin Perinatol 1981; 8:183-95.

71. Low JA, Wood SL, Killen HL, et al. Intrapartum asphyxia in the preterm fetus < 2000 gm. Am J Obstet Gynecol 1990; 162:378-82.

72. Ahmann PA, Lazzara A, Dykes FD, et al. Intraventricular hemorrhage in the high-risk preterm infant: Incidence and outcome. Ann Neurol 1980; 7:118-24.

73. Volpe JJ. Neonatal intraventricular hemorrhage. N Engl J Med 1981; 304:886-91.

74. Williams RL, Chen PM. Identifying the sources of the recent decline in perinatal mortality rates in California. N Engl J Med 1982; 306:207-14.

75. Malloy MH, Rhoads GG, Schramm W, Land G. Increasing cesarean section rates in very low birth weight infants: Effect on outcome. JAMA 1989; 262:1475-8.

76. Thiery M, Derom R, Buekens P. Frequency of cesarean deliveries in Belgium. Biol Neonate 1989; 55:90-6.

77. Lumley J, Kitchen WH, Roy ND, et al. Methods of delivery and resuscitation of very-low-birth weight infants in Victoria: 1982-1985. Med J Aust 1990; 152:1436.

78. Smith ML, Spencer SA, Hull D. Mode of delivery and survival in babies weighing less than 2000 g at birth. Br Med J 1980; 281:1118-9.

79. Goldenberg RL, Nelson KG. The premature breech. Am J Obstet Gynecol 1977; 127:240-4.

80. Ingemarsson I, Westgren M, Svenningsen NW. Long-term follow-up of preterm infants in breech presentation delivered by ceasarean section. Lancet 1978; 2:172-5.

81. Sachs BP, McCarthy BJ, Rubin G, et al. Cesarean section: Risk and benefits for mother and fetus. JAMA 1983; 250:2157-9.

82. Duenhoelter JH, Wells CE, Reisch JS, et al. A paired controlled study of vaginal and abdominal delivery of the low birth weight breech fetus. Obstet Gynecol 1979; 54:310-3.

83. Main DM, Main EK, Maurer MM. Cesarean section versus vaginal delivery for the breech fetus weighing less than 1500 grams. Am J Obstet Gynecol 1983; 146:580-4.

84. Barrett JM, Boehm FH, Vaughn WK. The effect of type of delivery on neonatal outcome in singleton infants of birth weight of 1000 g or less. JAMA 1983; 250:625-9.

85. Anderson GD, Bada HS, Sibai BM, et al. The relationship between labor and route of delivery in the preterm infant. Am J Obstet Gynecol 1988; 158:1382-90.

86. Malloy MH, Onstad L, Wright E, et al. The effect of cesarean delivery on birth outcome in very low birth weight infants. Obstet Gynecol 1991; 77:498-503.

87. Chervenak FA, Johnson RE, Youcha S, et al. Intrapartum management of twin gestation. Obstet Gynecol 1985; 65:119-24.

88. Kitchen W, Ford GW, Doyle LW, et al. Cesarean section or vaginal delivery at 24 to 28 weeks gestation: Comparison of survival and neonatal and two-year morbidity. Obstet Gynecol 1985; 66:149-57.

89. Boyle RJ, Kattwinkel J. Ethical issues surrounding resuscitation. Clin Perinatol 1999; 26:779-92.

90. Hack M, Friedman H, Fanaroff AA. Outcomes of extremely low birth weight infants. Pediatrics 1998; 98:931-7.

91. Piecuch RE, Leonard CH, Cooper BA et al. Outcome of extremely low birth weight infants (500-999 grams) over a 12 year period. Pediatrics 1997; 100:633-9.

92. Canadian Paediatric Society Fetus and Newborn Committee, and Society of Obstetricians and Gynaecologists of Canada Maternal-Fetal Medicine Committee. Management of the woman with threatened birth of an infant of extremely low gestational age. Can Med Assoc J 1994; 151:547-53.

93. Niermeyer S (editor), Kattwinkel J, Van Reempts P, et al. International Guidelines for Neonatal Resuscitation: An Excerpt from the Guidelines 2000 for Cardiopulmonary Resuscitation and Emergency Cardiovascular Care: International Consensus on Science. Pediatrics 2000; 106:E29:1-16.

94. Westgren M, Holmquist P, Svenningsen NW, Ingemarsson I. Intrapartum fetal monitoring in preterm deliveries: Prospective study. Obstet Gynecol 1982; 60:99-106.

95. Luthy DA, Shy KK, van Belle G, et al. A randomized trial of electronic fetal monitoring in preterm labor. Obstet Gynecol 1987; 69:687-95.

96. Shy KK, Luthy DA, Bennett FC, et al. Effects of electronic fetal-heart-rate monitoring, as compared with periodic auscultation, on the neurologic development of premature infants. N Engl J Med 1990; 322:588-93.

97. Chestnut DH, Dailey PA. Anesthesia for preterm labor and delivery. In Shnider SM, Levinson G, editors. Anesthesia for Obstetrics, 3rd ed. Baltimore, Williams & Wilkins, 1993: 354-64.

98. Thomas J, Long G, Moore G, Morgan D. Plasma protein binding and placental transfer of bupivacaine. Clin Pharmacol Ther 1976; 19:426-34.

99. Rane A, Sjoqvist F, Orrenius S. Cytochrome P-450 in human fetal liver microsomes. Chem Biol Interact 1971; 3:305.

100. Pelkonen O, Vorne M, Arvela P, et al. Drug metabolizing enzymes in human foetal liver and placenta in early pregnancy (abstract). Scand J Clin Lab Invest (Suppl) 1971; 27(S116):7.

101. Rane A, Sjoqvist F, Orrenius S. Drugs and fetal metabolism. Clin Pharmacol Ther 1973; 14:666-72.

102. Teramo K, Benowitz N, Heymann MA, Rudolph AM. Gestational differences in lidocaine toxicity in the fetal lamb. Anesthesiology 1976; 44:133-8.

103. Pedersen H, Santos AC, Morishima HO, et al. Does gestational age affect the pharmacokinetics and pharmacodynamics of lidocaine in mother and fetus? Anesthesiology 1988; 68:367-72.

104. Smedstad KG, Morison DH, Harris WH, Pascoe P. Placental transfer of local anesthetic in the premature sheep fetus. Int J Obstet Anesth 1993; 2:34-8.

105. Tucker GT, Mather LE. Pharmacokinetics of local anaesthetic agents. Br J Anaesth 1975; 47:213-24.

106. Tucker GT. Plasma binding and disposition of local anesthetics. Int Anesthesiol Clin 1975; 13:33-59.

107. Shnider SM, Way EL. Plasma levels of lidocaine (Xylocaine) in mother and newborn following obstetrical conduction anesthesia: Clinical applications. Anesthesiology 1968; 29:951-8.

108. Brown WU, Bell GC, Alper MH. Acidosis, local anesthetics, and the newborn. Obstet Gynecol 1976; 48:27-30.

109. Biehl D, Shnider SM, Levinson G, Callender K. Placental transfer of lidocaine: Effects of fetal acidosis. Anesthesiology 1978; 48:409-12.

110. Lending M, Slobody LB, Mestern J. Effect of hyperoxia, hypercapnia and hypoxia on blood-cerebrospinal fluid barrier. Am J Physiol 1961; 200:959-62.

111. Evans CAN, Reynolds JM, Reynolds ML, Saunders NR. The effect of hypercapnia and hypoxia on a blood-brain barrier mechanism in foetal and newborn sheep. J Physiol 1976; 255:701-14.

112. Ritter DA, Kenny JD, Norton HJ, Rudolph AJ. A prospective study of free bilirubin and other risk factors in the development of kernicterus in premature infants. Pediatrics 1982; 69:260-6.

113. Asling JH, Shnider SM, Margolis AJ, et al. Paracervical block anesthesia in obstetrics. II. Etiology of fetal bradycardia following paracervical block anesthesia. Am J Obstet Gynecol 1970; 107:626-34.

114. Rosefsky JB, Petersiel ME. Perinatal deaths associated with mepivacaine paracervical block anesthesia in labor. N Engl J Med 1968; 278:530-3.

115. Anderson KE, Gennser G, Nilsson E. Influence of mepivacaine on isolated human foetal hearts at normal and low pH. Acta Physiol Scand (suppl) 1970; 353:34-47.

116. Morishima HO, Heymann MA, Rudolph AM, et al. Transfer of lidocaine across the sheep placenta to the fetus: Hemodynamic and acid-base responses of the fetal lamb. Am J Obstet Gynecol 1975; 122:581-8.

117. Thigpen JW, Kotelko DM, Shnider SM, et al. Bupivacaine cardiotoxicity in hypoxic-acidotic sheep (abstract). Anesthesiology 1983; 59:A204.

118. Morishima HO, Pedersen H, Santos AC, et al. Adverse effects of maternally administered lidocaine on the asphyxiated preterm fetal lamb. Anesthesiology 1989; 71:110-5.

119. Morishima HO, Santos AC, Pedersen H, et al. Effect of lidocaine on the asphyxial responses in the mature fetal lamb. Anesthesiology 1987; 66:502-7.

120. Santos AC, Yun EM, Bobby PD, et al. The effects of bupivacaine, 1-nitro-1-arginine-methyl ester, and phenylephrine on cardiovascular adaptations to asphyxia in the preterm fetal lamb. Anesth Analg 1997; 85:1299-306.

121. Arthur GR, Feldman HS, Covino BG. Comparative pharmacokinetics of bupivacaine and ropivacaine, a new amide local anesthetic. Anesth Analg 1988; 67:1053-8.

122. Datta S, Camann W, Bader A, VanderBurgh L. Clinical effects and maternal and fetal plasma concentrations of epidural ropivacaine versus bupivacaine for cesarean section. Anesthesiology 1995; 82:1346-52.

123. Ala-kokko TI, Alahuhta S, Jouppila P, et al. Feto-maternal distribution of ropivacaine and bupivacaine after epidural administration for cesarean section. Internat J Obstet Anesth 1997; 6:147-52.

124. Kuhnert BR, Kuhnert PM, Reese ALP, et al. Maternal and neonatal elimination of CABA after epidural anesthesia with 2-chloroprocaine during partuition. Anesth Analg 1983; 62:1089-94.

125. Philipson EH, Kuhnert BR, Syracuse CD. Fetal acidosis, 2-chloroprocaine, and epidural anesthesia for cesarean section. Am J Obstet Gynecol 1985; 151:322-4.

126. Hollmen AI, Jouppila R, Jouppila P, et al. Effect of extradural analgesia using bupivacaine and 2-chloroprocaine on intervillous blood flow during normal labor. Br J Anaesth 1982; 54:837-41.

127. Ontario Perinatal Mortality Study Committee. Second Report of the Perinatal Mortality Study in Ten University Teaching Hospitals. Three reports. Department of Health, Toronto, 1967, Sec 1, 1961, Suppl. to 2nd Report, Tables 108-24.

128. Wright RG, Shnider SM, Thirion A-V, et al. Regional anesthesia for preterm labor and vaginal delivery: Effects on the fetus and neonate (abstract). Anesthesiology 1988; 69:A654.

129. Melsen NC, Noreng MF. Epidural blockade in the treatment of preterm labour. Anaesthesia 1988; 43:126-7.

130. Norris MC, Arkoosh VA. Spinal opioid analgesia for labor. Internat Clin Anesth 1997; 2:69-80.

131. Gamlin FMC, Lyons C. Spinal analgesia in labour. Internat J Obstet Anesth 1997; 2:161-72.

132. Albright GA, Forster RM. Does combined spinal-epidural analgesia with subarachnoid sufentanil increase the incidence of emergency cesarean delivery? Reg Anesth 1997; 22:400-5.

133. Harding SA, Collis RE, Morgan BM. Meningitis after combined spinal-extradural anaesthesia in obstetrics. Br J Anaesth 1994; 73:545-7.

134. Burke D, Wildsmith JAW. Meningitis after spinal anaesthesia. Br J Anaesth 1997; 78:635-6.

135. Hodgson CA, Wauchob TD. A comparison of spinal and general anaesthesia for elective caesarean section: Effect on neonatal condition at birth. Internat J Obstet Anesth 1994; 3:25-30.

136. Rolbin SH, Cohen MM, Levinton CM, et al. The premature infant: Anesthesia for cesarean delivery. Anesth Analg 1994; 78:912-7.

137. Bassell GM, Marx GF. Optimization of fetal oxygenation. Internat J Obstet Anesth 1995; 4:238-43.

138. Lamant RF. The contemporary use of β-agonists. Br J Obstet Gynaecol 1993; 100:890-2.

139. Kleinman G, Nuwayhid B, Rudelstorfer R, et al. Circulatory and renal effects of β-adrenergic-receptor stimulation in pregnant sheep. Am J Obstet Gynecol 1984; 149:865-74.

140. Roberts JM. Current understanding in pharmacologic mechanisms in the prevention of preterm birth. Clin Obstet Gynecol 1984; 27:592-605.

141. Benedetti TJ. Maternal complications of parenteral β-sympathomimetic therapy for premature labor. Am J Obstet Gynecol 1983; 145:1-6.

142. Benedetti TJ. Life-threatening complications of beta-mimetic therapy for preterm labor inhibition. Clin Perinatol 1986; 13:843-52.

143. Rust OA, Bofill JA, Arriola RM, et al. The clinical efficacy of oral tocolytic therapy. Am J Obstet Gynecol 1996; 175:838-42.

144. Caritis SN, Toig G, Heddinger LA, et al. A double-blind study comparing ritodrine and terbutaline in the treatment of preterm labor. Am J Obstet Gynecol 1984; 150:7-14.

145. Macones GA, Berlin M, Berlin J. Efficacy of oral beta-agonist maintenance therapy in preterm labor: A meta-analysis. Obstet Gynecol 1995; 85:313-7

146. Berg G, Andersson RGG, Ryden G. β-adrenergic receptors in human myometrium during pregnancy: Changes in the number of receptors after beta-mimetic treatment. Am J Obstet Gynecol 1985; 151:392-6.

147. Harden TK. Agonist-induced desensitization of the beta-adrenergic receptor-linked adenylate cyclase. Pharm Reviews 1983; 35:5-32.

148. Ryden G, Rolf G, Andersson G, Berg G, et al. Is the relaxing effect of β-adrenergic agonists on the human myometrium only transitory? Acta Obstet Gynecol Scand (suppl) 1982; 108:47-51.

149. Wolfe BB, Harden TK, Molinoff PB. In vitro study of the β-adrenergic receptors. Ann Rev Pharmacol Toxicol 1977; 17:575-604.

150. Casper RF, Lye SJ. Myometrial desensitization to continuous but not to intermittent β-adrenergic agonist infusion in the sheep. Am J Obstet Gynecol 1986; 154:301-5.

151. Lam F, Gill P, Smith M, et al. Use of the subcutaneous terbutaline pump for long-term tocolysis. Obstet Gynecol 1988; 72:810-3.

152. Guin DA, Goepfert AR, Owen J, et al. Terbutaline pump maintenance therapy for prevention of preterm delivery: A double-blind trial. Am J Obstet Gynecol.1998; 179:874-8.

153. Higby K, Suiter CR. A risk-benefit assessment of therapies for premature labour. Drug Safety 1999; 21:35-56.

154. Benedetti TJ, Hargrove JC, Rosene KA. Maternal pulmonary edema during premature labor inhibition. Obstet Gynecol 1982; 59:33-7S.

155. Hatjis CG, Swain M. Systemic tocolysis for premature labor is associated with an increased incidence of pulmonary edema in the presence of maternal infection. Am J Obstet Gynecol 1988; 159:723-8.

156. Perry KG, Morrison JC, Rust OA, et al. Incidence of adverse cardiopulmonary effects with low-dose continuous terbutaline infusion. Am J Obstet Gynecol 1995; 173:1273-7.

157. Hosenpud JD, Morton MJ, O'Grady JP. Cardiac stimulation during ritodrine hydrochloride tocolytic therapy. Obstet Gynecol 1983; 62:52-8.

158. Kjer JJ, Pedersen KH. Persistent supraventricular tachycardia following infusion with ritodrine hydrochloride. Acta Obstet Gynecol Scand 1982; 61:281-2.

159. Katz M, Robertson PA, Creasy RK. Cardiovascular complications associated with terbutaline treatment for preterm labor. Am J Obstet Gynecol 1981; 139:605-8.

160. Bieniarz J, Ivankovich A, Scommegna A. Cardiac output during ritodrine treatment in premature labor. Am J Obstet Gynecol 1974; 118:910-20.

161. Michalak D, Klein V, Marquette GP. Myocardial ischemia: A complication of ritodrine tocolysis. Am J Obstet Gynecol 1983; 146:861-2.

162. Ron-el R, Caspi E, Herman A, et al. Unexpected cardiac pathology in pregnant women treated with beta-adrenergic agents (ritodrine). Obstet Gynecol 1983; 61:10-2S.

163. Tye K-H, Desser KB, Benchimol A. Angina pectoris associated with use of terbutaline for premature labor. JAMA 1980; 244:692-3.

164. Ying Y-K, Tejani NA. Angina pectoris as a complication of ritodrine hydrochloride therapy in premature labor. Obstet Gynecol 1982; 60:385-8.

165. Hendricks SK, Keroes J, Katz M. Electrocardiographic changes associated with ritodrine-induced maternal tachycardia and hypokalemia. Am J Obstet Gynecol 1986; 154:921-3.

166. Faidley CK, Dix PM, Morgan MA, Schechter E. Electrocardiographic abnormalities during ritodrine administration. South Med J 1990; 83:503-6.

167. Caritis SN, Venkataramanan R, Darby MJ, et al. Pharmacokinetics of ritodrine administered intravenously: Recommendations for changes in the current regimen. Am J Obstet Gynecol 1990; 162:429-37.

168. Stubblefield PG. Pulmonary edema occurring after therapy with dexamethasone and terbutaline for premature labor: A case report. Am J Obstet Gynecol 1978; 132:341-2.

169. Jacobs MM, Knight AB, Arias F. Maternal pulmonary edema resulting from betamimetic and glucocorticoid therapy. Obstet Gynecol 1980; 56:56-9.

170. Tinga DJ, Aarnoudse JG. Post-partum pulmonary oedema associated with preventive therapy for premature labor (letter). Lancet 1979; 1:1026.

171. Philipsen T, Eriksen PS, Lynggard F. Pulmonary edema following ritodrine-saline infusion in premature labor. Obstet Gynecol 1981; 58:304-8.

172. Finley J, Katz M, Rojas-Perez M, et al. Cardiovascular consequences of β-agonist tocolysis: An echocardiographic study. Obstet Gynecol 1984; 64:787-91.

173. Wagner JM, Morton MJ, Johnson KA, et al. Terbutaline and maternal cardiac function. JAMA 1981; 246:2697-701.

174. Armson BA, Samuels P, Miller F, et al. Evaluation of maternal fluid dynamics during tocolytic therapy with ritodrine hydrochloride and magnesium sulfate. Am J Obstet Gynecol 1992; 167:758-65.

175. Schrier RW, Lieberman R, Ufferman RC. Mechanism of antidiuretic effect of beta-adrenergic stimulation. J Clin Invest 1972; 51:97-111.

176. Grospietsch G, Fenske M, Girndt J, et al. The renin-angiotensin-aldosterone system, antidiuretic hormone levels and water balance under tocolytic therapy with fenoterol and verapamil. Int J Gynaecol Obstet 1980; 17:590-5.

177. Hauth JC, Hankins GD, Kuehl TJ, Pierson WP. Ritodrine hydrochloride infusion in pregnant baboons. I. Biophysical effects. Am J Obstet Gynecol 1983; 146:916-24.

178. Hankins GD, Hauth JC, Kuehl TJ, et al. Ritodrine hydrochloride infusion in pregnant baboons. II. Sodium and water compartment alterations. Am J Obstet Gynecol 1983; 147:254-9.

179. Pisani RJ, Rosenow EC. Pulmonary edema associated with tocolytic therapy. Ann Intern Med 1989; 110:714-8.

180. Gabel JC, Drake RE. Effects of endotoxin on lung fluid balance in unanesthetized sheep. J Appl Physiol 1984; 56:489-94.

181. Tatara T, Morisaki H, Shimada M, et al. Pulmonary edema after long-term adrenergic therapy and cesarean section. Anesth Analg 1995; 81:417-8.

182. Conover WB, Benumof JL, Key TC. Ritodrine inhibition of hypoxic pulmonary vasoconstriction. Am J Obstet Gynecol 1983; 146:652-6.

183. Perkins RP, Varela-Gittings F, Dunn TS, et al. The influence of intravenous solution content on ritodrine-induced metabolic changes. Obstet Gynecol 1987; 70:892-5.

184. Chapelle A, Benoit S, Bouregba M, et al. The treatment of severe pulmonary edema induced by beta-adrenergic agonist tocolytic therapy with continuous positive airway pressure delivered by facemask. Anesth Analg 2002; 94:1593-4.

185. Cano A, Tovar I, Parilla JJ, et al. Metabolic disturbances during intravenous use of ritodrine: Increased insulin levels and hypokalemia. Obstet Gynecol 1985; 65:356-60.

186. Spellacy WN, Cruz AC, Buhi WC, Birk SA. The acute effects of ritodrine infusion on maternal metabolism: Measurements of levels of glucose, insulin, glucagon, triglycerides, cholesterol, placental lactogen, and chorionic gonadotropin. Am J Obstet Gynecol 1978; 131:637-42.

187. Cotton DB, Strassner HT, Lipson LG, Goldstein DA. The effects of terbutaline on acid base, serum electrolytes, and glucose homeostasis during the management of preterm labor. Am J Obstet Gynecol 1981; 141:617-24.

188. Young DC, Toofanian A, Leveno KJ. Potassium and glucose concentrations without treatment during ritodrine tocolysis. Am J Obstet Gynecol 1983; 145:105-6.

189. Miodovnik M, Peros N, Holroyde JC, Siddiqi TA. Treatment of premature labor in insulin-dependent diabetic women. Obstet Gynecol 1985; 65:621-7.

190. Moravec MA, Hurlbert BJ. Hypokalemia associated with terbutaline administration in obstetrical patients. Anesth Analg 1980; 59:917-20.

191. Katani N, Kushikata T, Hashimoto H, et al. Rebound perioperative hyperkalemia in six patients after cessation of ritodrine for premature labor. Anesth Analg 2001; 93:709-11.

192. Sato K, Nishiwaki K, Kuno N, et al. Unexpected hyperkalemia following succinylcholine administration in prolonged immobilized parturients treated with magnesium and ritodrine. Anesthesiology 2000; 93:1539-41.

193. Lotgering FK, Lind J, Huikeshoven FJM, Wallenburg HCS. Elevated serum transaminase levels during ritodrine administration. Am J Obstet Gynecol 1986; 155:390-2.

194. Nair GV, Ghosh AK, Lewis BV. Bowel distention during treatment of premature labor with beta-receptor agonists (letter). Lancet 1976; 1:907.

195. Rosene KA, Featherstone HJ, Benedetti TJ. Cerebral ischemia associated with parenteral terbutaline use in pregnant migraine patients. Am J Obstet Gynecol 1982; 143:405-7.

196. Catanzarite VA, McHargue AM, Sandberg EC, Dyson DC. Respiratory arrest during therapy for premature labor in a patient with myasthenia gravis. Obstet Gynecol 1984; 64:819-22.

197. Epstein MF, Nicholls E, Stubblefield PG. Neonatal hypoglycemia after beta-sympathomimetic tocolytic therapy. J Pediatr 1979; 94:449-53.

198. Pranikoff J, Helmchen R, Evertson L. Tocolytic therapy and intraventricular hemorrhage in the neonate (abstract). Am J Obstet Gynecol 1991; 164:511A.

199. Groome LJ, Goldenberg RL, Cliver SP, et al. Neonatal periventricular-intraventricular hemorrhage after maternal beta-sympathomimetic tocolysis. Am J Obstet Gynecol 1992; 167:873-9.

200. Laros RK, Kitterman JA, Heilbron DC, et al. Outcome of very-low-birth weight infants exposed to β-sympathomimetics in utero. Am J Obstet Gynecol 1991; 164:1657-65.

201. Freysz H, Willard D, Lehr A, et al. A long-term evaluation of infants who received a beta-mimetic drug while in utero. J Perinat Med 1977; 5:94-9.

202. Hadders-Algra M, Touwen BCL, Huisjes HJ. Long-term follow-up of children prenatally exposed to ritodrine. Br J Obstet Gynaecol 1986; 93:156-61.

203. Nuchpuckdee P, Brodsky N, Porat R, et al. Ventricular septal thickness and cardiac function in neonates after in utero ritodrine exposure. J Pediatr 1986; 109:687-91.

204. Friedman DM, Blackstone J, Young BK et al. Fetal cardiac effects of oral ritodrine tocolysis. Am J Perinatol 1994; 11:109-12.

205. Kast A, Hermer M. Beta-adrenoceptor tocolysis and effects on the heart of fetus and neonate: A review. J Perinat Med 1993; 21:97-106.

206. Kuhnert BR, Gross TL, Kuhnert PM, et al. Ritodrine pharmacokinetics. Clin Pharmacol Ther 1986; 40:656-64.

207. Barden TP. Effect of ritodrine on human uterine motility and cardiovascular responses in term labor and the early postpartum state. Am J Obstet Gynecol 1972; 112:645-52.

208. Knight RJ. Labour retarded with β-agonist drugs: A therapeutic problem in emergency anesthesia. Anaesthesia 1977; 32:639-41.

209. Schoenfeld A, Joel-Cohen SJ, Duparc H, Levy E. Emergency obstetric anaesthesia and the use of 2-sympathomimetic drugs. Br J Anaesth 1978; 50:969-71.

210. Crowhurst JA. Salbutamol, obstetrics and anaesthesia: A review and case discussion. Anaesth Intensive Care 1980; 8:39-43.

211. Ravindran R, Viegas OJ, Padilla LM, LaBlonde P. Anesthetic considerations in pregnant patients receiving terbutaline therapy. Anesth Analg 1980; 59:391-2.

212. Shin YK, Kim YD. Ventricular tachyarrhythmias during cesarean section after ritodrine therapy: Interaction with anesthetics. South Med J 1988; 81:528-30.

213. Suppan P. Tocolysis and anaesthesia for caesarean section (letter). Br J Anaesth 1982; 54:1007.

214. Shin YK, Kim YD. Anesthetic considerations in patients receiving ritodrine therapy for preterm labor (abstract). Anesth Analg 1986; 65:S140.

215. Ueyama H, Tashiro C, Kinouchi K, et al. Ritodrine prior to spinal anesthesia for Cesarean section (abstract). Anesthesiology 1993; 79:A996.

216. Chestnut DH, Pollack KL, Thompson CS, et al. Does ritodrine worsen maternal hypotension during epidural anesthesia in gravid ewes? Anesthesiology 1990; 72:315-21.

217. James FM, Greiss FC, Kemp RA. An evaluation of vasopressor therapy for maternal hypotension during spinal anesthesia. Anesthesiology 1970; 33:25-34.

218. Ralston DH, Shnider SM, deLorimier AA. Effects of equipotent ephedrine, metaraminol, mephentermine, and methoxamine on uterine blood flow in the pregnant ewe. Anesthesiology 1974; 40:354-70.

219. Chestnut DH, Weiner CP, Wang JP, et al. The effect of ephedrine upon uterine artery blood flow velocity in the pregnant guinea pig subjected to terbutaline infusion and acute hemorrhage. Anesthesiology 1987; 66:508-12.

220. Chestnut DH, Ostman LG, Weiner CP, et al. The effect of vasopressor agents upon uterine artery blood flow velocity in the gravid guinea pig subjected to ritodrine infusion. Anesthesiology 1988; 68:363-6.

221. Ramanathan S, Grant G, Turndorf H. Cardiac preload changes with ephedrine therapy for hypotension in obstetrical patients (abstract). Anesth Analg 1986; 65:S125.

222. Lawson NW, Wallfisch HK. Cardiovascular pharmacology: A new look at the "pressors." In Stoelting RK, Barash PG, Gallagher TJ, editors. Advances in Anesthesia. Chicago, Year Book, 1986: 195-270.

223. Tong C, Eisenach JC. The vascular mechanism of ephedrine's beneficial effect on uterine perfusion during pregnancy. Anesthesiology 1992; 76:792-8.

224. McGrath J, Chestnut D, Vincent R, et al. Ephedrine remains the vasopressor of choice for treatment of hypotension during ritodrine infusion and epidural anesthesia. Anesthesiology 1994; 80:1073-81.

225. Moran DH, Perillo M, LaPorta RF, et al. Phenylephrine in the prevention of hypotension following spinal anesthesia for cesarean section. J Clin Anesth 1991; 3:301-5.

226. Alahuhta S, Adas R, Adanen J, Jouppila P, et al. Ephedrine and phenylephrine for avoiding maternal hypotension due to spinal anaesthesia for caesarean section. Int J Obstet Anesth 1992; 1:129-34.

227. Cooper DW, Carpenter M, Mowbray P, et al. Fetal and neonatal effects of phenylephrine and ephedrine during spinal anesthesia for cesarean delivery. Anesthesiology 2002; 97:1582-90.

228. From RP, Slater RM, Sum-Ping ST, et al. Onset and recovery of succinylcholine induced neuromuscular blockade in patients receiving terbutaline (abstract). Anesthesiology 1989; 71:A885.

229. Rodgers SJ, Morgan M. Tocolysis, B2 agonists and anesthesia. Anaesthesia 1994; 49:185-7.
230. Hall DG, McGaughey HS, Corey EL, Thornton WN. The effects of magnesium therapy on the duration of labor. Am J Obstet Gynecol 1959; 78:27-32.
231. Beall MG, Edgar BW, Paul RH, Smith-Wallace T. A comparison of ritodrine, terbutaline, and magnesium sulfate for the suppression of preterm labor. Am J Obstet Gynecol 1985; 153:854-9.
232. Hollander DI, Nagey DA, Pupkin MJ. Magnesium sulfate and ritodrine hydrochloride: A randomized comparison. Am J Obstet Gynecol 1987; 156:631-7.
233. Wilkins IA, Lynch L, Mehalek KE, et al. Efficacy and side effects of magnesium sulfate and ritodrine as tocolytic agents. Am J Obstet Gynecol 1988; 159:685-9.
234. Chau AC, Gabert HA, Miller JM Jr. A prospective comparison of terbutaline and magnesium for tocolysis. Obstet Gynecol 1992; 80:847-51.
235. Cox SM, Sherman ML, Levino KS. Randomized investigation of magnesium sulfate for prevention of preterm birth. Am J Obstet Gynecol 1990; 163:767-72.
236. Altura BM, Altura BT. Magnesium ions and contraction of vascular smooth muscles: Relationship to some vascular diseases. Fed Proc 1981; 40:2672-9.
237. Iseri LT, French JH. Magnesium: Nature's physiologic calcium blocker. Am Heart J 1984; 108:188-93.
238. Elliott JP, O'Keefe DF, Greenberg P, Freeman RK. Pulmonary edema associated with magnesium sulfate and betamethasone administration. Am J Obstet Gynecol 1979; 134:717-9.
239. Yeast JD, Halberstadt C, Meyer BA, et al. The risk of pulmonary edema and colloid osmotic pressure changes during magnesium sulfate infusion. Am J Obstet Gynecol 1993; 169:1566-71.
240. Ferguson JE, Hensleigh PA, Kredenster D. Adjunctive use of magnesium sulfate with ritodrine for preterm labor tocolysis. Am J Obstet Gynecol 1984; 148:166-71.
241. Scardo JA, Hogg BB, Newman RB. Favourable hemodynamic effects of magnesium sulfate in preeclampsia. Am J Obstet Gynecol 1995; 173:1249-53.
242. Chestnut DH, Thompson CS, McLaughlin GL, Weiner CP. Does the intravenous infusion of ritodrine or magnesium sulfate alter the hemodynamic response to hemorrhage in gravid ewes? Am J Obstet Gynecol 1988; 159:1467-73.
243. Reynolds JD, Chestnut DH, Dexter F, et al. Magnesium sulfate adversely affects fetal lamb survival and blocks fetal cerebral blood flow response during maternal hemorrhage. Anesth Analg 1996; 83:493-9.
244. Mittendorf R, Pryde P, Khoshnood B, Lee KS. If tocolytic magnesium sulfate is associated with excess total pediatric mortality, what is its impact? Obstet Gynecol 1998; 92:308-11.
245. Grether JK, Hoogstrate J, Selvin S, Nelson KB. Magnesium sulfate tocolysis and risk of neonatal death. Am J Obstet Gynecol 1998; 178:1-6.
246. Nelson KB, Grether JK. Can magnesium sulfate reduce the risk of cerebral palsy in very low birth weight infants? Pediatrics 1995; 95:263-9.
247. Mittendorf R, Covert R, Boman J, et al. Is tocolytic magnesium sulphate associated with increased total paediatric mortality? Lancet 1997; 350:1517-8.
248. Scudiero R, Khoshnood B, Pryde PG, et al. Perinatal death and tocolytic magnesium sulfate. Obstet Gynecol 2000; 96:178-82.
249. Farkouh LJ, Thorp JA, Jones PG, et al. Antenatal magnesium exposure and neonatal demise. Am J Obstet Gynecol 2001; 185:869-72.
250. Suresh MS, Lawson NW. Anesthesia for parturients with toxemia of pregnancy. In Datta SJ, Ostheimer GW, editors. Common Problems in Obstetric Anesthesia. Chicago, Year Book, 1987: 332-47.
251. Vincent RD, Chestnut DH, Sipes SL, et al. Magnesium sulfate decreases maternal blood pressure but not uterine blood flow during epidural anesthesia in gravid ewes. Anesthesiology 1991; 74:77-82.
252. Sipes SL, Chestnut DH, Vincent RD, et al. Does magnesium sulfate alter the maternal cardiovascular response to vasopressor agents in gravid ewes? Anesthesiology 1991; 75:1010-8.
253. Sipes SL, Chestnut DH, Vincent RD, et al. Which vasopressor should be used to treat hypotension during magnesium sulfate infusion and epidural anesthesia? Anesthesiology 1992; 77:101-8.
254. Ramanathan J, Sibai BM, Pillai R, Angel JJ. Neuromuscular transmission studies in preeclamptic women receiving magnesium sulfate. Am J Obstet Gynecol 1988; 158:40-6.
255. DeVore JS, Asrani R. Magnesium sulfate prevents succinylcholine induced fasciculations in toxemic parturients. Anesthesiology 1980; 52:76-7.
256. Morris R, Giesecke AH. Potentiation of muscle relaxants by magnesium sulfate therapy in toxemia of pregnancy. South Med J 1968; 61:25-8.
257. Kambam JR, Perry SM, Entman S, et al. Effect of magnesium on plasma cholinesterase activity. Am J Obstet Gynecol 1988; 159:309-11.
258. James MFM, Cork RC, Dennett JE. Succinylcholine pretreatment with magnesium sulfate. Anesth Analg 1986; 65:373-6.
259. Thompson SW, Moscicki JC, DiFazio CA. The anesthetic contribution of magnesium sulfate and ritodrine hydrochloride in rats. Anesth Analg 1988; 67:31-4.
260. Koinig H, Wallner T, Marhofer P, et al. Magnesium sulfate reduces intra- and postoperative analgesic requirements. Anesth Analg 1998; 87:206-10.
261. Fuentes A, Rajas A, Porter K, et al. The effects of magnesium sulfate on bleeding time in pregnancy. Am J Obstet Gynecol 1995; 173:1246-9.
262. Zuckerman H, Shalev E, Gilad G, Katzuni E. Further study of the inhibition of premature labor by indomethacin. Part I. J Perinat Med 1984; 12:19-23.
263. Spearing G. Alcohol, indomethacin, and salbutamol: A comparative trial of their use in preterm labor. Obstet Gynecol 1979; 53:171-4.
264. Schorr SJ, Ascarelli MH, Rust OA, et al. A comparative study of ketorolac (Toradol) and magnesium sulfate for arrest of preterm labor. South Med J 1998; 91:1028-32.
265. Kramer WB, Saade GR, Belfort M, et al. A randomized double-blind study comparing fetal effects of sulindac to terbutaline during management of preterm labor. Am J Obstet Gynecol 1999; 180:390-401.
266. Carlan SJ, O'Brien WF, O'Leary TD, et al. Randomized comparative trial of indomethacin and sulindac for the treatment of refractory preterm labor. Obstet Gynecol 1992; 79:223-8.
267. Kramer WB, Saade G, Ou CN, et al. Placental transfer of sulindac and its active metabolite in humans. Am J Obstet Gynecol 1995; 172: 886-90.
268. Karim SMM, Devlin J. Prostaglandin content of amniotic fluid during pregnancy and labor. J Obstet Gynaecol Br Commonw 1967; 74:230-4.
269. Karim SMM. Appearance of prostaglandin F2 in human blood during labour. Br Med J 1968; 4:618-21.
270. Weitz CM, Ghodgaonkar RB, Dubin NH, Niebyl JR. Prostaglandin F metabolite concentration as a prognostic factor in preterm labor. Obstet Gynecol 1986; 67:496-9.
271. Repke JR, Niebyl JR. Role of prostaglandin synthetase inhibitors in the treatment of preterm labor. Semin Reprod Endocrinol 1985; 3:259-72.
272. Kocsis JJ, Hernandovich J, Silver MJ, et al. Duration of inhibition of platelet prostaglandin formation and aggregation by ingested aspirin or indomethacin. Prostaglandins 1973; 3:141-4.
273. Moise KJ, Huhta JC, Sharif DS, et al. Indomethacin in the treatment of premature labor: Effects on the fetal ductus arteriosus. N Eng J Med 1988; 319:327-31.
274. Rudolph AM, Heymann MA. Hemodynamic changes induced by blockers of prostaglandin synthesis in the fetal lamb in utero. Adv Prostaglandin Thromboxane Res 1978; 4:231-7.
275. Dudley DKL, Hardie MJ. Fetal and neonatal effects of indomethacin used as a tocolytic agent. Am J Obstet Gynecol 1985; 151:181-4.
276. Niebyl JR, Witter FR. Neonatal outcome after indomethacin treatment for preterm labor. Am J Obstet Gynecol 1986; 155:747-9.
277. Moise KJ. Effect of advancing gestational age on the frequency of fetal ductal constriction in association with maternal indomethacin use. Am J Obstet Gynecol 1993; 168:1350-3.
278. Vermillion ST, Scardo JA, Lashus AG, Wiles HB. The effect of indomethacin tocolysis on fetal ductus arteriosus constriction with advancing gestational age. Am J Obstet Gynecol 1997; 177:256-61.
279. Novy MJ. Effects of indomethacin on labor, fetal oxygenation and fetal development in Rhesus monkeys. Adv Prostaglandin Thromboxane Res 1978; 4:285-300.
280. Kirshon B, Moise KJ, Wasserstrum N, et al. Influence of short-term indomethacin therapy on fetal urine output. Obstet Gynecol 1988; 72:51-3.
281. Kirshon B, Moise KJ, Mari G, Willis R. Long-term indomethacin therapy decreases fetal urine output and results in oligohydramnios. Am J Perinat 1991; 8:86-8.
282. Anderson R, Berl T, McDonald D, et al. Prostaglandins: Effects on blood pressure, renal blood flow, sodium and water excretion. Kidney Int 1976; 10:205-15.
283. Wurtzel D. Prenatal administration of indomethacin as a tocolytic agent: Effect on neonatal renal function. Obstet Gynecol 1990; 76: 689-92.
284. Norton ME, Merrill J, Cooper BA, et al. Neonatal complications after administration of indomethacin for preterm labor. N Engl J Med 1993; 329:1602-7.
285. Mayer CA, Lewis DF, Harding JA, et al. Tocolysis with indomethacin increases the incidence of necrotizing enterocolitis in the low birth weight neonate. Am J Obstet Gynecol 1994; 170:102-6.

286. Pietrantoni M, Weeks J, Bridges S, et al. Adverse neonatal outcomes following antenatal indomethacin use (abstract). Am J Obstet Gynecol 1995; 172:A565.

287. Ment LR, Oh W, Ehrenkranz RA, et al. Low dose indomethacin and prevention of intraventricular hemorrhage: A multicenter randomized trial. Pediatrics 1994; 93:543-50.

288. Fausett MB, Esplin MS, Yoder B, et al. Indomethacin for preterm labor prolongs gestation and is not associated with increased neonatal complicationin infants delivered prior to 32 weeks. Am J Obstet Gynecol 2000; 182:S48.

289. Parilla B, Grobman W, Holtzman R et al. Indocin tocolysis is not associated with increased risk of necrotizing enterocolitis. Am J Obstet Gynecol 2000; 182:S62.

290. Lunt CC, Sain AS, Barth WH, Hankins GD. The effect of indomethacin tocolysis in maternal coagulation states. Obstet Gynecol 1994; 84:820-2.

291. Rodgers RPC, Levin J. A critical reappraisal of the bleeding time. Semin Thromb Hemost 1990; 16:1-20.

292. deSwiet M, Redman CWG. Aspirin, extradural anesthesia and the MRC collaborative low-dose aspirin study in pregnancy (CLASP) (letter). Br J Anaesth 1992; 69:109.

293. Horlocker TT, Wedel DJ, Offord KP. Does preoperative antiplatelet therapy increase the risk of hemorrhagic complications associated with regional anesthesia? Anesth Analg 1990; 70:631-4.

294. Horlocker TT, Wedel DJ, Schroder DR, et al. Preoperative antiplatelet does not increase the risk of spinal hematoma associated with regional anesthesia. Anesth Analg 1995; 80:303-9.

295. Williams KN, Jackowski A, Evans PJD. Epidural haematoma requiring surgical decompression following repeated cervical epidural steroid injections for chronic pain. Pain 1990; 42:197-9.

296. Ulmsten U, Andersson K-E, Wingerup L. Treatment of premature labor with the calcium antagonist nifedipine. Arch Gynecol 1980; 229:1-5.

297. Papatsonis DNM, VanGeijn HP, Ader HJ, et al. Nifedipine and ritodrine in the management of preterm labor: A randomized multicentre trial. Obstet Gynecol 1997; 90:230-4.

298. Kupferminc M, Lessing JB, Yarm Y, Peyser MR. Nifedipine versus ritodrine for suppression of preterm labor. Br J Obstet Gynaecol 1993; 100:1090-4.

299. Tsatsaris V, Papatsonis D, Goffinett F, et al. Tocolysis with nifedipine or beta-adrenergic agonists: A meta-analysis. Obstet Gynecol 2001; 97: 840-7.

300. Ducsay CA, Thompson JS, Wu AT, Novy MJ. Effects of calcium entry blocker (nicardipine) tocolysis in rhesus macaques: Fetal plasma concentrations and cardiorespiratory changes. Am J Obstet Gynecol 1987; 157:1482-6.

301. Harake B, Gilbert RD, Ashwal S, Power GG. Nifedipine: Effects on fetal and maternal hemodynamics in pregnant sheep. Am J Obstet Gynecol 1987; 157:1003-8.

302. Blea CW, Barnard JM, Magness RR, et al. Effect of nifedipine on fetal and maternal hemodynamics and blood gases in the pregnant ewe. Am J Obstet Gynecol 1997; 176:922-30.

303. Mari G, Kirshon B, Moise KJ, et al. Doppler assessment of the fetal and uteroplacental circulation during nifedipine therapy for preterm labor. Am J Obstet Gynecol 1989; 161:1514-8.

304. Pirhonen JP, Erkkola RU, Ekblad UU, Nyman L. Single dose of nifedipine in normotensive pregnancy: Nifedipine concentrations, hemodynamic responses, and uterine and fetal flow velocity waveforms. Obstet Gynecol 1990; 76:807-11.

305. Ray D, Dyson D, Crites Y. Nifedipine tocolysis and neonatal acid-base status at delivery (abstract). Am J Obstet Gynecol 1994; 170:405A.

306. Economy KE, Abuhamad AZ. Calcium channel blockers as tocolytics. Sem Perinatol 2001; 25:264-71.

307. Papastonis DNM, Lok CAR, Bos JM, et al. Calcium channel blockers in the management of preterm labor and hypertension in pregnancy. Eur J Obstet Gynecol Reprod Biol 2001; 97:122-40.

308. Forman A, Andersson KE, Ulmsten U. Inhibition of myometrial activity by calcium antagonists. Semin Perinatol 1981; 5:288-94.

309. Struyker-Boudier HAJ, Smits JFM, DeMey JGR. The pharmacology of calcium antagonists: A review. J Cardiovasc Pharmacol 1990; 15 (suppl 4): S1-10.

310. Tosone SR, Reves JG, Kissin I, et al. Hemodynamic responses to nifedipine in dogs anesthetized with halothane. Anesth Analg 1983; 62:903-8.

311. Ben-Ami M, Giladi Y, Shalev E. The combination of magnesium sulfate and nifedipine: A cause of neuromuscular blockade. Br J Obstet Gynaecol 1994; 101:262-3.

312. Csapo AI, Puri CP, Tarro S, Henzl MR. Deactivation of the uterus during normal and premature labor by the calcium antagonist nicardipine. Am J Obstet Gynecol 1982; 142:483-91.

313. Goodwin TM, Valenzuela GJ, Silver H, Creasy G. Dose ranging study of the oxytocin antagonist atosiban in the treatment of preterm labor. Obstet Gynecol 1996; 88:331-6.

314. Goodwin TM, Millar L, North L, et al. The pharmacokinetics of the oxytocin antagonist atosiban in pregnant women with preterm uterine contractions. Am J Obstet Gynecol 1995; 173:913-7.

315. Valenzuela GJ, Craig J, Bernhardt MD, Holland ML. Placental passage of the oxytocin antagonist atosiban. Am J Obstet Gynecol 1995; 172:1304-6.

316. Romero R, Sibai BM, Sanchez-Ramos L, et al. An oxytocin receptor antagonist (atosiban) in the treatment of preterm labor: A randomized, double-blind, placebo-controlled trial with tocolytic rescue. Am J Obstet Gynecol 2000; 182:1191-9.

317. The Canadian and Israeli Atosiban Study Group. Double blind, randomized, controlled trial of atosiban and ritodrine in the treatment of preterm labor: A multicenter effectiveness and safety study. Am J Obstet Gynecol 2000; 182:1184-90.

318. The European Atosiban Study Group. The oxytocin antagonist atosiban versus the beta-agonist terbutaline in the treatment of preterm labor. A randomized double-blind controlled study. Acta Obstet Gynecol Scand 2001; 80:413-2.

319. The Worldwide Atosiban versus Beta-agonists Study Group. Effectiveness and safety of the oxytocin antagonist atosiban versus beta-adrenergic agonists in the treatment of preterm labour. Br J Obstet Gynaecol 2001; 108:133-42.

320. Phaneuf S, Asboth G, Mackenzie LZ, et al. Effect of oxytocin antagonists on the activation of human myometrium in vitro: Atosiban prevents oxytocin-induced desensitization. Am J Obstet Gynecol 1994; 171:1627-34.

321. Riley ET, Flanagan B, Cohen SE, Chitkara U. Intravenous nitroglycerin: A potent uterine relaxant for emergency obstetric procedures. Review of literature and report of three cases. Internat J Obstet Anesth 1996; 5:264-8.

322. Bukowski R, Saade GR. New developments in the management of preterm labor. Sem Perinatol 2001; 25:272-4.

323. Bradley KK, Buxton ILO, Barber JE, et al. Nitric oxide relaxes human myometrium by a cGMP-independent mechanism. Am J Physiol (Cell Physiol) 1998; 275:C1668-73.

324. Caponas G. Glyceryl trinitrate and acute uterine relaxation: A literature review. Anaesth Intensive Care 2001; 29:163-77.

325. Heymann MA, Bootstaylor B, Roman C, et al. Glyceryl trinitrate stops active labour in sheep. In Moncada S, Feelisch M, Busse R, Higgs EA, editors. The Biology of Nitric Oxide. London, Portland Press, 1994; 3:201-3.

326. Bootstaylor BS, Roman C, Parer JT, Heymann MA. Fetal and maternal hemodynamic and metabolic effects of maternal nitroglycerin infusion in sheep. Am J Obstet Gynecol 1997; 176:644-50.

327. Buhimschi CS, Buhimschi IA, Malinow AM, Weiner CP. Effects of sublingual nitroglycerin on human uterine contractility during the active phase of labor. Am J Obstet Gynecol 2002; 187:235-8.

328. El-Sayed YY, Riley ET, Holbrook H, et al. Randomized comparison of intravenous nitroglycerin and magnesium sulfate for treatment of preterm labor. Obstet Gynecol 1999; 93:79-83.

329. Lees CC, Lojacona A, Thompson C, et al. Glyceryl trinitrate and ritodrine in tocolysis: An international multicenter randomized study. Obstet Gynecol 1999; 94:403-8.

330. Bukowski R, Mackay L, Fittkow C, et al. Inhibition of cervical ripening by local application of cyclooxygenase-2 inhibitor. Am J Obstet Gynecol 2001; 184:1374-9.

331. Cole S, Smith R, Bisits A. Pharmacotherapy for Preterm Labor. Front Horm Res 2001; 27:279-307.

Chapter 35
Abnormal Presentation and Multiple Gestation

BettyLou Koffel, M.D.

The labor and delivery of a patient with a multiple gestation and/or fetal breech presentation represents a major challenge for the obstetrician and the anesthesiologist. Anesthetic requirements may change from moment to moment, and an obstetric emergency may require immediate intervention. All members of the perinatal care team must communicate directly and clearly with each other as well as with the parturient and her family.

The **presentation** denotes that portion of the fetus that overlies the pelvic inlet. In most cases, the fetal presenting part can be palpated through the cervix during a vaginal examination. The presentation may be **cephalic, breech,** or **shoulder.** Breech and shoulder presentations occur with increased frequency in patients with multiple gestation. Cephalic presentations are further subdivided into **vertex, brow,** and **face** presentations according to the degree of flexion of the neck.

The **lie** refers to the alignment of the fetal spine with the maternal spine. The fetal lie can be either longitudinal or transverse. A fetus with a vertex or breech presentation has a longitudinal lie. A persistent oblique or transverse lie typically requires abdominal delivery.

The **position** of the fetus denotes the relationship of a specific fetal bony point to the maternal pelvis. The position of the **occiput** defines the position for vertex presentations. Other markers for position include the **sacrum** for breech presentations, the **mentum** for face presentations, and the **acromion** for shoulder presentations. The **attitude** of the fetus describes the relationship of the fetal parts to each other. This typically refers to the position of the head with regard to the trunk, as in flexed, military, or hyperextended.

ABNORMAL POSITION

During normal labor the fetal occiput rotates from a transverse or oblique position to a direct **occiput anterior** position. In a minority of patients with an oblique posterior position, the occiput rotates directly posteriorly and results in a **persistent occiput posterior** position. Most cases of persistent occiput posterior position develop through malrotation from an initially occiput anterior position.[1] The occiput posterior position may lead to a prolonged labor that is associated with

increased maternal discomfort. Less often, the vertex remains in the **occiput transverse** position; this condition is known as **deep transverse arrest.**

In the past, obstetricians performed manual or forceps rotation to hasten delivery and lessen perineal trauma in women with an abnormal position of the vertex. Today, many obstetricians are reluctant to perform rotational forceps delivery for fear of causing excessive maternal and/or fetal trauma. In cases of persistent occiput posterior position, the contemporary obstetrician is more likely to allow the head to remain in the occiput posterior position at vaginal delivery. Some cases of persistent occiput posterior position and many cases of deep transverse arrest require cesarean delivery for dystocia.

During administration of epidural analgesia in a patient with an abnormal position, it is helpful to add a lipid-soluble opioid to a dilute solution of local anesthetic. This provides analgesia while preserving pelvic muscle tone. Relaxation of the pelvic floor and perineum may deter the spontaneous rotation of the vertex during labor. In contrast, profound pelvic floor relaxation is needed to facilitate instrumental vaginal delivery.

BREECH PRESENTATION

Breech presentation describes a longitudinal lie in which the fetal buttocks and/or lower extremities overlie the pelvic inlet. Figure 35-1 shows three varieties of breech presentation:
1. **Frank breech**—Lower extremities flexed at the hips and extended at the knees
2. **Complete breech**—Lower extremities flexed at both the hips and the knees
3. **Incomplete breech**—One or both of the lower extremities extended at the hips

Ultrasound or radiographic examination typically allows the obstetrician to confirm the type of breech presentation and to exclude the presence of severe congenital anomalies (e.g., anencephaly). The type of breech presentation affects the obstetrician's decision regarding the mode of delivery. The fetus with a frank breech presentation tends to remain in that presentation throughout labor. In contrast, a complete breech presentation may change to an incomplete breech presentation at any time before or during labor.

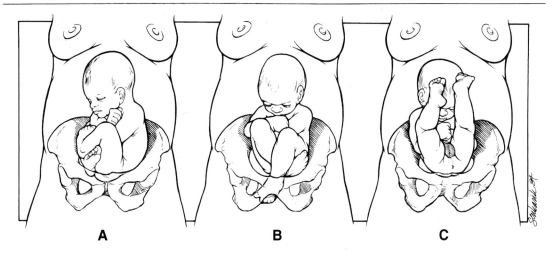

FIGURE 35-1. Three possible breech presentations. **A,** The **complete breech** demonstrates flexion of the hips and flexion of the knees. **B,** The **incomplete breech** demonstrates intermediate deflexion of one or both hips and knees. **C,** The **frank breech** shows flexion of the hips and extension of both knees. (From Lanni SM, Seeds JW. Malpresentations. In Gabbe SG, Niebyl JR, Simpson JL, editors. Obstetrics: Normal and Problem Pregnancies, 4th ed. New York, Churchill Livingstone, 2002:482.)

Epidemiology

The breech presentation is the most common of the abnormal presentations. Both the incidence and the type of breech presentation vary with gestational age (Table 35-1). Before 28 weeks' gestation, as many as 40% of fetuses are in a breech presentation. Most of these convert to a vertex presentation by 34 weeks' gestation, but 2% to 3% of fetuses remain in a breech presentation at term.

Many factors predispose to breech presentation, but the exact etiology is unknown (Box 35-1). Abnormalities of the fetus or the maternal pelvis or uterus may play a role. Among patients with pelvic or uterine abnormalities, a breech presentation may allow more room for fetal growth and movement. Likewise, hydrocephalic fetuses are more likely to assume a breech presentation. Multiparity, multiple gestation, polyhydramnios, and anencephaly also predispose to breech presentation. These conditions may interfere with the normal process of accommodation between the fetal head and the uterine cavity and maternal pelvis.[2]

Obstetric Complications

Obstetric complications are more likely with a breech presentation (Table 35-2). Cesarean delivery decreases the risk of some of these complications. Vaginal breech delivery entails a higher risk of neonatal trauma than does delivery of an infant with a vertex presentation, but cesarean delivery does not eliminate the risk of trauma to the infant. Rather, cesarean delivery of a breech presentation can be difficult and traumatic, especially if the skin and uterine incisions are inadequate or if inadequate muscle relaxation occurs.

The risk of umbilical cord prolapse varies with the type of breech presentation (Table 35-3). In the patient with an incomplete breech presentation, the presenting part does not fill the cervix as well as the vertex or buttocks, which allows the umbilical cord to slip into the vagina before delivery. Umbilical cord prolapse typically necessitates prompt cesarean delivery.

MORBIDITY AND MORTALITY

There is an increased risk of **perinatal morbidity** and **mortality** with breech presentation, even when the risk is adjusted for preterm gestation. The factors that cause breech presentation

---

TABLE 35-1   TYPES OF BREECH PRESENTATION

Type of breech	% of all breech presentations	Proportion with preterm gestation
Frank	48-73	38
Complete	5-12	12
Incomplete	12-38	50

Modified from Lanni SM, Seeds JW. Malpresentations. In Gabbe SG, Niebyl JR, Simpson JL, editors. Obstetrics: Normal and Problem Pregnancies, 4th ed. New York, Churchill Livingstone, 2002:482.

Box 35-1 FACTORS ASSOCIATED WITH BREECH PRESENTATION

- Uterine distention or relaxation
  Multiparity
  Multiple gestation
  Polyhydramnios
  Macrosomia
- Abnormalities of the uterus or pelvis
  Pelvic tumors
  Uterine anomalies
  Pelvic contracture
- Abnormalities of the fetus
  Hydrocephalus
  Anencephaly
- Obstetric conditions
  Previous breech delivery
  Preterm gestation
  Oligohydramnios
  Cornual-fundal placenta
  Placenta previa

Modified from Cunningham FG, MacDonald PC, Gant NF, et al. Williams Obstetrics, 21st ed. New York, McGraw-Hill, 2001; 509-35; and Lanni SM, Seeds JW. Malpresentations. In Gabbe SG, Niebyl JR, Simpson JL, editors. Obstetrics: Normal and Problem Pregnancies. New York, Churchill Livingstone, 2002:473-501.

often are more important than the presentation itself. For example, the severe congenital anomalies that predispose to breech presentation (e.g., hydrocephalus, anencephaly) significantly contribute to neonatal morbidity and mortality. Morgan and Kane[3] reviewed 16,327 breech deliveries that occurred at 147 hospitals during 1961 and 1962. Breech presentation was associated with an increased incidence of perinatal mortality, even after correction for preterm gestation, cord prolapse, placenta previa, and placental abruption. Relative perinatal mortality rates (calculated from data for linked siblings from the Norway Medical Birth Registry) confirm that breech presentation is a marker of perinatal risk, regardless of the mode of delivery.[4] Both fetal distress and dystocia occur more frequently in these patients, even in those parturients who have undergone successful external cephalic version.[5] After an analysis of outcome for 57,819 pregnancies, Schutte et al.[6] concluded, "It is possible that breech presentation is not coincidental but a consequence of poor fetal quality, in which case medical intervention is unlikely to reduce the perinatal mortality associated with breech presentation to the level associated with vertex presentation."

Breech presentation is also associated with an increased risk of **maternal morbidity** and **mortality**. Vaginal breech delivery entails an increased risk of maternal perineal trauma and hemorrhage.[2] Cesarean delivery is associated with an increased risk of maternal morbidity and mortality,[2,7] especially febrile morbidity.[8] These risks may be even higher for patients who require emergency abdominal delivery.[9] However, in a study of outcome following breech delivery, Schiff et al.[8] did not demonstrate an increased risk of maternal morbidity in women who underwent cesarean section during labor, when compared with women who underwent elective cesarean section.

Obstetric Management

EXTERNAL CEPHALIC VERSION

The process of external cephalic version converts a breech or shoulder presentation to a vertex presentation. This procedure is successful in 35% to 86% of nonlaboring patients at term.[10-12] External cephalic version is most likely to be successful if (1) the presenting part has not entered the pelvis, (2) amniotic fluid volume is normal, (3) the fetal back is not positioned posteriorly, (4) the patient is not obese, (5) the patient is parous, and (6) the presentation is frank breech or transverse.[10,12] Early labor does not preclude successful external cephalic version.[10] External cephalic version rarely is successful when the cervix is fully dilated or when the membranes have ruptured,[11] although anecdotal cases of success have been reported.[13]

Obstetricians often administer a tocolytic agent (e.g., terbutaline) before performing external cephalic version. The optimal timing of external cephalic version is unclear. The procedure is more likely to be successful if it is performed before term, but in these cases, the fetus may spontaneously return to a breech presentation before the onset of labor. For this reason, many obstetricians prefer to delay version until 38 to 39 weeks' gestation. If external cephalic version is successful, the obstetrician may then proceed with amniotomy induction of labor.

Successful external cephalic version helps reduce the perinatal morbidity and mortality associated with breech delivery. After a successful external cephalic version, labor and vaginal delivery occur in 66% to 89% of patients,[11,14] albeit with an increased risk of fetal distress and dystocia, when compared with patients with a spontaneous cephalic presentation.

External cephalic version is associated with a low rate of morbidity in contemporary obstetric practice. Safe external cephalic version requires continuous fetal heart rate (FHR) monitoring because placental separation or umbilical cord compression may occur. Fetomaternal hemorrhage is another potential complication of external cephalic version.[11] In one study, 16 (18%) of 89 patients undergoing external cephalic version had Kleihauer-Betke stains that signaled the occurrence of a fetomaternal hemorrhage.[15]

Several studies have described the use of epidural or spinal anesthesia for external cephalic version.[12,14,16-19] Some obstetricians argue that the absence of anesthesia limits the force that the obstetrician can apply during the procedure. They contend that administration of anesthesia may encourage the obstetrician to use excessive force, which may increase the risk of perinatal morbidity and mortality. Schorr et al.[14] randomized 69 women to receive epidural anesthesia or no epidural anesthesia for external cephalic version. The success rate was better in the epidural group than in the no-epidural group (67% versus 32%), and there was no evidence of adverse outcome as a result of administration of epidural anesthesia. Neiger et al.[16] reported outcome for 16 patients in whom the first attempt at external cephalic version had been unsuccessful *without* epidural anesthesia. These patients elected to undergo another attempt *with* epidural anesthesia. Nine (56%) of these 16 procedures were successful, and 7 of those 9 women delivered vaginally. In a prospective but nonrandomized study of external cephalic version, Birnbach et al.[17]

TABLE 35-2	INCIDENCE OF COMPLICATIONS ASSOCIATED WITH BREECH PRESENTATION

Complication	Incidence
Intrapartum fetal death	Increased sixteenfold
Intrapartum asphyxia	Increased 3.8-fold
Umbilical cord prolapse	Increased fivefold to twentyfold
Birth trauma	Increased thirteenfold
Arrest of aftercoming head	8.8%
Spinal cord injuries with deflexion	21%
Major congenital anomalies	6%-18%
Preterm delivery	16%-33%
Hyperextension of head	5%

Modified from Lanni SM, Seeds JW. Malpresentations. In Gabbe SG, Niebyl JR, Simpson JL, editors. Obstetrics: Normal and Problem Pregnancies, 4th ed. New York, Churchill Livingstone, 2002:487.

TABLE 35-3	RISK OF UMBILICAL CORD PROLAPSE

Type of breech	Risk of cord prolapse (%)
Frank	0.5
Complete	4-6
Incomplete	15-18

Modified from Lanni SM, Seeds JW. Malpresentations. In Gabbe SG, Niebyl JR, Simpson JL, editors. Obstetrics: Normal and Problem Pregnancies, 4th ed. New York, Churchill Livingstone, 2002:482.

observed a higher rate of success in patients who received spinal analgesia (sufentanil 10 μg) than in patients who received no spinal analgesia (80% versus 30%, respectively). In contrast, Dugoff et al.[18] observed no difference in the rate of success of external cephalic version in patients randomized to receive spinal anesthesia (bupivacaine 2.5 mg and sufentanil 10 μg) or no spinal anesthesia. In some of the studies in which regional analgesia/anesthesia seemed to result in a greater likelihood of successful external cephalic version, the success rates in the non-intervention groups seem lower than expected. One retrospective report described the practice of an experienced obstetrician who has obtained success rates of 83% and 89% using spinal or epidural lidocaine anesthesia in patients who had an earlier, same-day, failed attempt at external cephalic version at 37 weeks' gestation. Intravenous nitroglycerin was also used to facilitate the version in these patients.[19]

The American College of Obstetricians and Gynecologists (ACOG)[12] has concluded that "there is not enough consistent evidence to make a recommendation favoring spinal or epidural anesthesia" during external cephalic version. In the Kaiser Permanente Northwest and Providence Health Systems, we do not routinely give spinal or epidural anesthesia during external cephalic version.

MODE OF DELIVERY

A substantial number of obstetricians recommend the routine performance of cesarean section in patients with a breech presentation. Approximately 85% of pregnancies with a breech presentation are delivered abdominally in contemporary obstetric practice in the United States.

Advocates of elective cesarean delivery of fetuses with a breech presentation cite the increased maternal morbidity and mortality associated with emergency cesarean section, as well as an increased risk of perinatal morbidity and mortality associated with labor and traumatic vaginal delivery.[9] Earlier analysis of both retrospective and prospective studies[20,21] resulted in the development of various protocols that allowed selected patients with a breech presentation to labor and deliver vaginally (Box 35-2).

Cheng and Hannah[7] performed a meta-analysis of studies of singleton term pregnancies with a breech presentation, published between 1966 and 1992. Short-term neonatal morbidity was higher in the planned vaginal delivery groups, as

---

Box 35-2 CRITERIA FOR A TRIAL OF LABOR AND VAGINAL DELIVERY FOR PATIENTS WITH A FETAL BREECH PRESENTATION

1. Frank breech presentation
2. Adequate pelvis by imaging pelvimetry
3. Estimated fetal weight between 2500 and 3500 g by ultrasonography or by two experienced examiners
4. Flexion of the fetal head (The neutral position—the so-called military position—also is acceptable.)
5. Continuous electronic FHR monitoring
6. Spontaneous progression of labor, with timely effacement and dilation of the cervix and timely descent of the breech
7. Availability of an individual skilled in vaginal breech delivery
8. Availability of an individual skilled in the administration of obstetric anesthesia
9. Spontaneous delivery to the level of the umbilicus
10. Ability to perform an abdominal delivery promptly
11. Availability of an individual with skills in neonatal resuscitation

---

was long-term infant morbidity. Overall maternal morbidity and mortality were lower among the women in the planned vaginal delivery groups compared with the planned cesarean delivery groups. However, the maternal benefit from a planned vaginal delivery depends on the occurrence of successful vaginal delivery. As Bingham and Lilford[9] demonstrated with their decision theory analysis, "the greater dangers of emergency compared with nonelective surgery may abolish the advantages of attempting a vaginal delivery." These authors suggested that "a policy of elective cesarean section for all cases would not necessarily increase maternal mortality and morbidity." Another meta-analysis,[22] which used a "random effects model" (which accounts for both within-study and between-study variations in outcome) also supports this view.

The Term Breech Trial Collaborative Group[23] enrolled 2088 women from 26 countries with a singleton fetus in a frank or complete breech presentation. These women were randomly assigned to undergo planned cesarean section or planned vaginal delivery. Using an intention-to-treat analysis, the investigators noted that perinatal mortality, neonatal mortality, and serious neonatal morbidity were significantly lower for the planned cesarean section group. This difference was greatest in those countries with a low perinatal mortality rate (e.g., Canada, United Kingdom, United States). Maternal morbidity and mortality did not differ between the two groups for the first 6 weeks postpartum.[23] Women who underwent planned cesarean delivery were less likely to report urinary incontinence at 3 months postpartum.[24]

Despite these results, controversy continues within the obstetric community. Some obstetricians from Canada, the United Kingdom, and the United States contend that there is no longer "any room . . . for disagreement," and that "vaginal breech delivery is no longer justified."[25-27] Meanwhile, other obstetricians continue to argue that, when strict criteria are used, a trial of vaginal breech delivery is not only safe but advisable.[28,29] However, the ACOG Committee on Obstetric Practice[30] has stated:

> Planned vaginal delivery of a singleton term breech may no longer be appropriate . . . . Patients with a persistent breech presentation at term in a singleton gestation should undergo a planned cesarean delivery . . . . A planned cesarean delivery does not apply to patients presenting with advanced labor and likely to have an imminent delivery of a fetus in a breech presentation or to patients whose second twin is in a nonvertex presentation.

There is less controversy regarding the mode of delivery for the preterm fetus with a breech presentation. Retrospective studies suggest that if the estimated fetal weight is less than 1500 g, vaginal breech delivery may increase the risk of trauma and cerebral hemorrhage. These studies suggested an advantage associated with abdominal delivery of the preterm fetus with a breech presentation.[2,31] Cibils et al.[32] noted that the route of delivery did not significantly affect outcome for 262 very low birth weight (VLBW, less than 1500 g) infants with a frank or complete breech presentation, who were delivered between 1980 and 1987. However, their data suggested that abdominal delivery may offer some advantage for infants with a *footling* breech presentation. Overall, they noted a high perinatal mortality rate for these VLBW infants, which they attributed to factors other than presentation and route of delivery.

To my knowledge, there is only one published, randomized study of vaginal breech delivery of preterm fetuses.

Zlatnik[33] randomized 38 women (with a breech presentation between 28 and 36 weeks' gestation) to undergo either a trial of labor or an immediate cesarean section. Unfortunately, the sample size was too small to permit definite conclusions.

Trial of labor and vaginal breech delivery occur infrequently in most hospitals in North America and the United Kingdom. The availability of personnel experienced in obstetric anesthesia and neonatal resuscitation are prerequisites to a trial of labor (Box 35-2). Most patients undergoing a trial of labor for breech presentation receive epidural analgesia.[8] Finally, hyperextension of the fetal head remains an absolute contraindication to a trial of labor in the patient with a breech presentation.

VAGINAL BREECH DELIVERY

During a trial of labor, the cervix must be fully dilated before the patient begins to push. Some obstetricians delay maternal expulsive efforts until 30 minutes after the diagnosis of full cervical dilation. Others delay expulsive efforts until the breech is at the perineum.

There are three varieties of vaginal breech delivery. **Spontaneous breech delivery** is delivery without any traction or manipulation other than support of the infant's body. With **assisted breech delivery** (also known as partial breech extraction), the infant deliveries spontaneously as far as the umbilicus; at that time, the obstetrician assists delivery of the chest and the aftercoming head. With **total breech extraction,** the obstetrician applies traction on the feet and ankles to deliver the entire body of the infant. Except for vaginal delivery of a second twin, obstetricians almost never perform total breech extraction. Total breech extraction increases the likelihood of difficult, traumatic delivery, including fetal head entrapment.[34]

During assisted breech delivery or total breech extraction, the obstetrician attempts to maintain flexion of the cervical spine during delivery of the aftercoming head. This may be accomplished manually or by the application of Piper forceps (Figures 35-2 through 35-4). In most cases the obstetrician performs a generous episiotomy to prevent perineal obstruction of the aftercoming head.

CESAREAN SECTION

Cesarean section does not guarantee an atraumatic delivery, especially if the skin and uterine incisions are inadequate. Before 32 weeks' gestation, the lower uterine segment may be inadequate to allow an atraumatic delivery through a low transverse uterine incision. In such cases, the obstetrician should perform a low vertical incision that can be extended to facilitate an atraumatic delivery. Unfortunately, such incisions often extend to the body of the uterus, which does not heal as well as the lower uterine segment. It is unclear whether this increases the risk of uterine rupture during a trial of labor in a subsequent pregnancy (see Chapter 23).

Anesthetic Management

Benefits of epidural anesthesia during labor include the following: (1) pain relief, (2) inhibition of early pushing, (3) a relaxed pelvic floor and perineum at delivery, and (4) the option to extend anesthesia for emergency cesarean section if needed. The patient must not push before the cervix is fully dilated; otherwise, the patient might push a lower extremity through a partially dilated cervix, which may result in fetal head entrapment. Early pushing also may increase the risk of a prolapsed umbilical cord. At delivery, a relaxed pelvic floor and perineum facilitates an atraumatic delivery of the aftercoming fetal head.

Provision of analgesia for a trial of labor in patients with a breech presentation presents a challenge for the anesthesiologist:

1. The anesthesiologist must provide sacral analgesia to inhibit early pushing during the first stage of labor.
2. The anesthesiologist must tailor epidural analgesia to ensure that the patient is able to push adequately during the second stage. If the patient is unable to achieve a spontaneous delivery of a vertex presentation, the obstetrician may perform instrumental vaginal delivery. In contrast, total breech extraction of a singleton fetus is unacceptable in modern obstetric practice. Most obstetricians insist on spontaneous delivery of the infant to the level of the umbilicus.

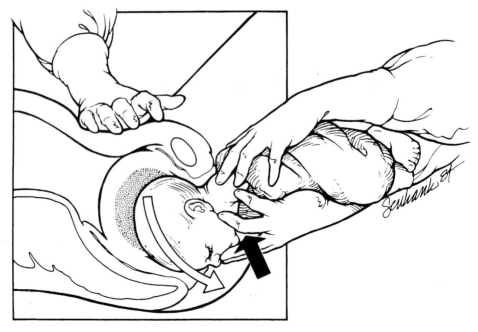

FIGURE 35-2. Vaginal breech delivery. The heavy arrow indicates the direction of pressure from two fingers of the operator's right hand on the fetal maxilla (not the mandible). This maneuver assists in maintaining appropriate flexion of the fetal vertex, as does moderate suprapubic pressure from an assistant. Delivery of the head may be accomplished with continued maternal expulsive forces and gentle downward traction. (From Lanni SM, Seeds JW. Malpresentations. In Gabbe SG, Niebyl JR, Simpson JL, editors. Obstetrics: Normal and Problem Pregnancies, 4th ed. New York, Churchill Livingstone, 2002:486.)

3. At delivery, the anesthesiologist is challenged to quickly provide profound perineal anesthesia to facilitate delivery of the aftercoming head. Many obstetricians routinely apply Piper forceps to the aftercoming head. This maneuver requires adequate anesthesia and muscle relaxation.

Older studies of the use of epidural analgesia for vaginal breech delivery either did not specify the local anesthetic regimen[35,36] or used concentrated solutions of bupivacaine (0.25%).[37] These studies found a small[35,37] or no[36] increase in the length of the second stage of labor but no effect on the type

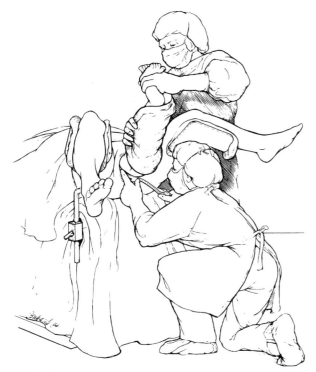

FIGURE 35-3. Vaginal breech delivery. Demonstration of INCORRECT assistance during the application of Piper forceps; the assistant hyperextends the fetal neck. Positioning as such increases the risk for neurologic injury. (From Lanni SM, Seeds JW. Malpresentations. In Gabbe SG, Niebyl JR, Simpson JL, editors. Obstetrics: Normal and Problem Pregnancies, 4th ed. New York, Churchill Livingstone, 2002:486.)

of delivery.[35-37] Neonatal condition was not affected[37] or was slightly better[35,36] when mothers received epidural analgesia.

Van Zundert et al.[38] have argued that the expulsion time (i.e., the interval between the first expulsive effort by the mother and the delivery of the baby) is a more important indicator of fetal risk than the total duration of the second stage. They retrospectively evaluated the use of epidural analgesia during a trial of labor in 281 women with a breech presentation. They excluded 62 women who underwent cesarean section for failure to progress, and they excluded another 54 women for miscellaneous reasons. They subsequently evaluated obstetric outcome for the remaining 165 women. Their anesthetic technique included the intermittent epidural bolus injection of 0.125% bupivacaine with 1:800,000 epinephrine. The mean ± SEM expulsion time was only 8.7 ± 0.4 minutes. This retrospective analysis represents one of the few studies that includes a description of the anesthetic technique. The expulsion times noted in this report are remarkably short.

Chadha et al.[39] retrospectively evaluated obstetric outcome in 643 women with a singleton breech presentation and a spontaneous onset of labor at term. Epidural analgesia was associated with an increased need for oxytocin augmentation of labor as well as a prolongation of the first (approximately 3 hours) and second (approximately 18 to 30 minutes) stages of labor. The administration of epidural analgesia also was associated with an increased likelihood of cesarean section during the second stage of labor. The authors did not discuss why some patients received epidural analgesia and others did not. They also did not describe their epidural analgesic technique. In a subsequent letter to the editor, the authors[40] acknowledged that they had injected 0.25% to 0.5% bupivacaine to establish analgesia and had maintained analgesia with a continuous epidural infusion of 0.08% bupivacaine at a rate of 15 to 20 mL/hr. They also acknowledged that their objective was to provide "complete pain relief," which suggests that some patients may have had excessive anesthesia (see Chapter 21).

The results of retrospective studies are clouded by the potential for selection bias. Higher levels of pain during early labor are associated with an increased incidence of prolonged labor and other obstetric complications (e.g., abnormal FHR

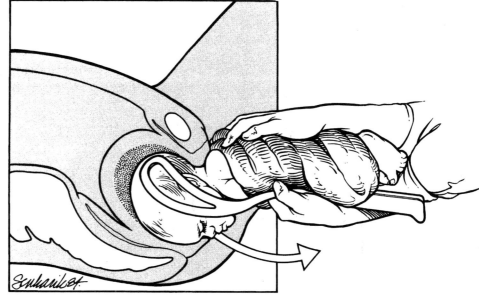

FIGURE 35-4. Vaginal breech delivery. Once the Piper forceps are applied, the fetal trunk is supported by one hand, and gentle traction on the forceps *(arrow)* in the direction of the pelvic axis results in a controlled delivery, as illustrated here. (From Lanni SM, Seeds JW, Malpresentations. In Gabbe SG, Niebyl JR, Simpson JL, editors. Obstetrics: Normal and Problem Pregnancies, 4th ed. New York, Churchill Livingstone, 2002:486.)

patterns, instrumental delivery, requirement for neonatal resuscitation). Women who experience severe pain and have a prolonged labor are more likely to request and receive epidural analgesia.[41] Moreover, obstetricians may be more likely to suggest or request the administration of epidural analgesia when they believe that operative delivery will be required.

ANALGESIA FOR LABOR

Emergency cesarean section may be required at any time during a trial of labor. Epidural analgesia is an excellent choice during a trial of labor in patients with a breech presentation. The anesthesiologist should tailor the epidural analgesic technique to the needs of the individual patient. These patients often have earlier complaints of rectal pressure than patients with a vertex presentation. It is important to provide sufficient sacral analgesia to inhibit pushing during the first stage of labor. I prefer to add a lipid-soluble opioid (e.g., fentanyl, sufentanil) to a dilute solution of local anesthetic, and I administer that solution by continuous epidural infusion. Use of a local anesthetic alone to eliminate low back and perineal discomfort results in extensive motor block, which may decrease the effectiveness of maternal expulsive efforts during the second stage. The advantages of the epidural administration of both a local anesthetic and a lipid-soluble opioid were recently confirmed by Benhamou et al.,[42] who observed that a continuous epidural infusion of bupivacaine 0.0625% with sufentanil 0.25 μg/mL produced better maternal analgesia and less motor block than administration of bupivacaine 0.125% in parturients with a breech presentation.

ANESTHESIA FOR VAGINAL BREECH DELIVERY

Patients with a breech presentation should deliver in a room where an emergency abdominal delivery can be performed immediately. I administer a nonparticulate antacid at the time of transfer to the delivery room. The anesthesiologist should be prepared for emergency administration of general anesthesia at any time. Umbilical cord compression is common during the second stage of labor in patients with a breech presentation. For that reason, the mother should receive supplemental oxygen during all cases of vaginal breech delivery.

Provision of effective anesthesia for vaginal breech delivery represents a true challenge for the anesthesiologist. During the second stage of labor, the anesthesiologist is asked to provide analgesia while maintaining adequate maternal expulsive efforts. At any time, the anesthesiologist may be asked to quickly provide dense anesthesia for vaginal or cesarean delivery. Because I typically administer a dilute solution of local anesthetic during the first stage of labor, it often is necessary to administer a more concentrated solution of local anesthetic at the time of delivery. I prefer to maintain analgesia with bupivacaine, but I always have a syringe of 3% 2-chloroprocaine immediately available. I begin to inject 3% 2-chloroprocaine at the first evidence of difficulty to ensure the presence of adequate anesthesia for operative delivery.

In the past some anesthesiologists favored the **double-catheter technique** for administration of epidural analgesia. With this method, one epidural catheter is placed through a high lumbar interspace and a second catheter is placed through the caudal canal. A small volume of a dilute solution of local anesthetic is injected through the lumbar epidural catheter for relief of pain during the first stage of labor. When the mother has the urge to push, a larger volume of a concentrated solution of local anesthetic (e.g., 10 mL of 1.5% lidocaine or 2% 2-chloroprocaine) is injected through the caudal epidural catheter. This technique allows the anesthesiologist to provide a rapid onset of profound sacral analgesia and a relaxed pelvic floor and perineum while maintaining rectus muscle tone.

Alternatively, **combined spinal-epidural (CSE) analgesia** may be a useful technique for patients with a breech presentation. This technique offers advantages for patients who request analgesia in either very early or advanced labor. One disadvantage of CSE analgesia is that it delays confirmation of correct placement of the epidural catheter. It is preferable that the epidural catheter be placed "perfectly" in patients with a breech presentation.

Perhaps the obstetrician's greatest fear is the risk of **fetal head entrapment.** Most of these cases result from entrapment of the fetal head behind a partially dilated cervix. Fetal head entrapment is more likely to occur in patients who are less than 32 weeks' gestation. Before 32 weeks' gestation, the fetal head is larger than the wedge formed by the fetal buttocks and thighs. The lower extremities, buttocks, and abdomen may deliver before the cervix is fully dilated, and the cervix may then entrap the head. If this occurs, the obstetrician may choose one of three options: (1) performance of Dührssen incisions in the cervix, (2) request for relaxation of skeletal and cervical smooth muscle, or (3) cesarean section.

The performance of **Dührssen incisions** may be difficult technically. The obstetrician makes two or three radial incisions in the cervix at the 2, 6, and 10 o'clock positions.[2] This procedure is associated with an increased risk of maternal morbidity (e.g., genitourinary trauma, hemorrhage). The blood loss may be substantial and concealed. Bleeding within the peritoneal cavity may not be visible externally.

More often, the obstetrician chooses the second option and requests that the anesthesiologist provide relaxation of skeletal and cervical smooth muscle. Smooth muscle represents only 15% of total cervical tissue,[43] and some physicians argue that it is not possible to provide profound relaxation of the cervix through relaxation of smooth muscle. Nonetheless, the provision of both skeletal and smooth muscle relaxation often facilitates vaginal delivery of the aftercoming head. In the past, the technique of choice included a rapid sequence induction of general anesthesia, followed by administration of a high concentration (2 to 3 MAC) of a volatile halogenated agent. It is unnecessary to administer nitrous oxide because such a large dose of the volatile halogenated agent is being given. Moreover, the distressed fetus should benefit from a high inspired concentration of oxygen. This technique results in uterine and cervical relaxation in 2 to 3 minutes. When fetal head entrapment results from *perineal* obstruction, delivery may soon follow the administration of succinylcholine.

Immediately after delivery, the anesthesiologist should discontinue administration of the volatile halogenated agent and substitute nitrous oxide, with or without an opioid. Administration of a high concentration of a volatile halogenated agent increases the risk of uterine atony after delivery. Prompt discontinuation of the volatile halogenated agent, along with intravenous administration of oxytocin, should provide adequate uterine tone in most patients. Anesthesia should be maintained until the placenta is delivered, the episiotomy and lacerations are repaired, and hemostasis is secured.

Intravenous or sublingual **nitroglycerin** has nearly replaced the use of volatile halogenated agents as agents for uterine relaxation. This common, widespread practice has been based on case reports and small series of cases. However, a review of 32 publications did not provide unequivocal support for the use of nitroglycerin to provide uterine relaxation in obstetric emergencies.[44] Administration of nitroglycerin results in the release of nitric oxide, which helps mediate the relaxation of smooth muscle. Other factors (e.g., pregnancy, labor) may affect the human myometrial response to nitroglycerin and nitric oxide. Administration of nitroglycerin seems safe, but there is a paucity of evidence that confirms the efficacy of nitroglycerin for providing uterine relaxation for treatment of obstetric emergencies in laboring women.[44]

Buhimschi et al.[45] attempted to provide an objective assessment of the effect of nitroglycerin on human uterine tone and contractility in laboring women. In a double-blind fashion, 12 parturients were randomized to receive either placebo or sublingual nitroglycerin (three doses, 800 µg each) 10 minutes apart. Intrauterine pressure was measured with a sensor-tip catheter. Sublingual nitroglycerin did not reduce either uterine activity or tone, despite a significant (20%) reduction in maternal mean arterial pressure. In emergency cases, the lack of maternal hypotension after nitroglycerin administration may reflect intravenous fluid administration, position changes, and maternal anxiety associated with emergency situations.

I continue to use one or two sublingual sprays of nitroglycerin (400 to 800 µg) rather than intravenous nitroglycerin, because the metered dose spray is stable and convenient and does not require dilution with crystalloid, with the attendant chance of preparation error. Published reports have described intravenous doses ranging from 50 to 500 µg or more. In my experience, both the sublingual and intravenous routes of administration provide a rapid onset of uterine relaxation, and the effect typically is very brief. I simultaneously prepare for the induction of general anesthesia should nitroglycerin not provide enough relaxation.

The use of epidural analgesia most likely has decreased the incidence of fetal head entrapment during vaginal breech delivery for at least two reasons. First, epidural analgesia inhibits early pushing during the first stage of labor. Second, although epidural analgesia does not relax the cervix at delivery, it provides effective pain relief and skeletal muscle relaxation. A relaxed pelvic floor and perineum facilitates delivery of the aftercoming head. Moreover, effective analgesia and skeletal muscle relaxation allow an assistant to provide maternal suprapubic pressure, which helps maintain flexion of the fetal cervical spine during delivery.

ANESTHESIA FOR CESAREAN SECTION

Spinal, epidural, or general anesthesia can be given for cesarean section. At cesarean section, the obstetrician should perform a uterine incision that allows an atraumatic delivery of the infant. Rarely, the obstetrician may request provision of uterine relaxation, even when a vertical uterine incision has been performed. Uterine relaxation may be necessary in cases of fetal malformations (e.g., sacral teratoma, hydrocephalus). When general anesthesia is used, the anesthesiologist may increase the concentration of the volatile halogenated agent. When regional anesthesia is used, a small dose of nitroglycerin or a beta-adrenergic tocolytic agent such as terbutaline typically provides adequate relaxation. Rarely, it may be necessary to perform intraoperative induction of general anesthesia followed by administration of a high concentration of a volatile halogenated agent.

Regardless of the route of delivery, all members of the obstetric care team should remember that infants with a breech presentation tend to be more depressed than infants with a vertex presentation. An individual skilled in neonatal resuscitation should be immediately available.

OTHER ABNORMAL PRESENTATIONS

Face Presentation

A face presentation occurs in 1 in 500 live births. Approximately 70% to 80% of infants with a face presentation can be delivered vaginally.[34] In general, the infant can be delivered vaginally only if the mentum rotates to an anterior position. Manual efforts to flex the fetal cervical spine or convert an unfavorable mentum posterior position to a more favorable mentum anterior position rarely are successful.[34]

Brow Presentation

In patients with a brow presentation, the cervical spine is intermediate between the full flexion of a normal vertex presentation and the full extension of a face presentation. A brow presentation occurs in approximately 1 in 1500 deliveries. Persistent brow presentation typically requires cesarean section for dystocia. Spontaneous flexion or extension of the neck may occur during labor, which may allow vaginal delivery.[34]

Compound Presentation

A compound presentation occurs in 1 in 400 to 1 in 1200 deliveries. Most often, an upper extremity presents with the vertex. Umbilical cord prolapse is common (10% to 20%), as is neurologic or musculoskeletal damage to the involved extremity.[34] Labor and delivery may occur safely, but abdominal delivery is necessary for cord prolapse or failure to progress. Vaginal manipulation should be avoided.[34]

Shoulder Presentation

A shoulder presentation (also known as a **transverse lie**) mandates performance of cesarean section except in two circumstances. First, successful external cephalic version may allow vaginal delivery. Second, the obstetrician may perform internal podalic version and total breech extraction of a second twin with a shoulder presentation.

Cesarean delivery of a fetus with a **back-down transverse lie** can be especially difficult. This presentation represents one of the few indications for a classic uterine incision in contemporary obstetric practice.

MULTIPLE GESTATION

Epidemiology

Monozygotic twins (those that occur when a single fertilized ovum divides into two distinct individuals after a variable number of divisions) exhibit a constant incidence of approximately 4 per 1000 births. The incidence of **dizygotic twins** (those that occur when two separate ova are fertilized) varies among races and by maternal age. Dizygotic twins occur most frequently among blacks, least frequently among Asians, and with an intermediate frequency among Caucasians. The incidence increases from 3 per 1000 among women less than 20 years of age to 14 per 1000 among women 35 to 40 years of age. The incidence also increases with parity, independent of maternal age.[46] In the United States the rate of multiple births has increased more than 50% since 1980. Twin births represented 3% of all births in 2001. Nearly 0.2% of all births were triplets, quadruplets, quintuplets, or other higher-order multiples. The increased rate of multiple births reflects delayed childbearing and increased use of assisted reproductive techniques.[47]

Placentation

Placenta classification includes (1) **dichorionic diamniotic,** (2) **monochorionic diamniotic,** and (3) **monochorionic monoamniotic** (Figure 35-5). All dizygotic twins develop a dichorionic diamniotic placenta. A dichorionic diamniotic placenta also is present if monozygotic twinning occurs during the first 2 to 3 days after fertilization. Twinning between 3 and 8 days commonly results in a monochorionic diamniotic placenta. Monochorionic monoamniotic placentas are found when twinning occurs at 8 to 13 days. Embryonic cleavage between 13 and 15 days results in **conjoined twins** with a monochorionic monoamniotic placenta. Twinning cannot occur beyond 15 days.[48]

The type of placentation determines the likelihood of vascular communications. Vascular communications occur in nearly all monochorionic placentas and are rare in dichorionic placentas.[48] Vascular communications may result in **twin-twin transfusion syndrome** and **intrauterine fetal death (IUFD)**. Monochorionic placentation also increases the risk of IUFD from other causes (e.g., cord accident).[48-50] Some obstetricians favor early cesarean section in patients with a monochorionic monoamniotic placenta. However, this may be unnecessary. Among these patients, most cases of IUFD occur before 32 weeks' gestation. In a retrospective study, labor and vaginal delivery were not associated with an increased risk of IUFD in patients with monoamniotic twins.[49]

Physiologic Changes

Multiple gestation accelerates and exaggerates the physiologic and anatomic changes of pregnancy. Of interest to the anesthesiologist, multiple gestation exaggerates the cardiovascular and pulmonary changes of pregnancy. In contrast, the renal, hepatic, and central nervous system (CNS) changes resemble those that occur in women with a singleton fetus.

Increased uterine size, especially near term, results in decreased total lung capacity and functional residual capacity (FRC). During periods of hypoventilation or apnea, hypoxemia develops more rapidly because of the decreased FRC and an increased maternal metabolic rate. A recent cross-sectional study demonstrated no significant difference in respiratory function between 68 women with a twin pregnancy and 140 women with a singleton pregnancy.[51] Maternal weight increases at a greater rate after 30 weeks' gestation in women

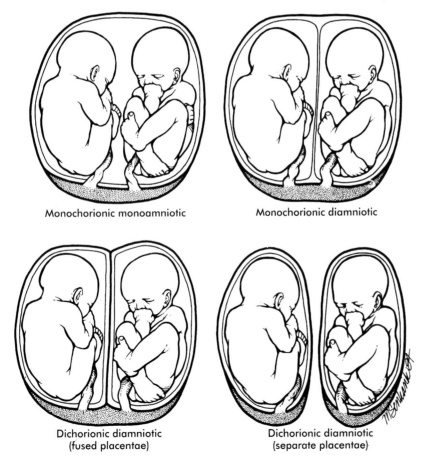

Monochorionic monoamniotic

Monochorionic diamniotic

Dichorionic diamniotic
(fused placentae)

Dichorionic diamniotic
(separate placentae)

FIGURE 35-5. Placentation in twin pregnancies. (From Chitkara U, Berkowitz RL. Multiple gestations. In Gabbe SG, Niebyl JR, Simpson JL, editors. Obstetrics: Normal and Problem Pregnancies, 4th ed. New York, Churchill Livingstone, 2002:828.)

with multiple gestation,[52] which may increase the risk of difficult intubation and ventilation. Increased uterine size displaces the stomach cephalad, which decreases the competence of the lower esophageal sphincter and increases the risk of pulmonary aspiration of gastric contents.

Maternal blood volume increases an additional 500 mL with twin gestation.[50] Relative or actual anemia often occurs. Likewise, multiple gestation results in a greater increase in cardiac output than that which occurs in women with a singleton fetus.[53] The greater fetal weight and larger volume of amniotic fluid predispose the mother to aortocaval compression and the supine hypotension syndrome.

Obstetric Complications

FETAL COMPLICATIONS

Fetal complications include those related solely to multiple gestation (e.g., twin-twin transfusion) and complications related to abnormal presentation (e.g., prolapsed cord) (Box 35-3).

Twin-Twin Transfusion

Deep arteriovenous vascular communications in a monochorionic placenta may result in twin-twin transfusion,[54] in which one twin becomes the donor and the other twin becomes the recipient. The donor twin is smaller and is at risk for intrauterine growth restriction (IUGR) and anemia. The recipient twin is plethoric and is at risk for volume overload and cardiac failure. Twin-twin transfusion may result in a perinatal mortality rate as high as 100%,[55] although aggressive therapy may decrease this rate to 20%.[56] The therapeutic options that are most often considered currently include decompression amniocentesis, interruption of the placental vessel communications, amniotic septostomy, and selective feticide.[57] Only vessel occlusion addresses the etiology of the problem; other interventions attempt to lessen the fetal/neonatal effects of twin-twin transfusion. Decompression amniocentesis or serial amnioreduction may improve circulation to a "stuck" donor twin, which allows restoration of normal amniotic fluid volume and "catch-up" fetal growth. Early experience with percutaneous endoscopic laser coagulation suggests that this technique results in death of the donor twin in approximately half of the cases.[58] This is considered unacceptable by some, despite the decreased risk of cerebral palsy in the surviving twin.[59,60] Comorbidity/mortality is also common in the surviving twin after fetal death associated with twin-twin transfusion.[61,62] No clear evidence supports one therapy over another.[57]

Intrauterine Growth Restriction

Twin-twin transfusion represents only one of the potential etiologies of IUGR in patients with multiple gestation. The

---

Box 35-3 FETAL COMPLICATIONS ASSOCIATED WITH MULTIPLE GESTATION

- Preterm delivery
- Congenital anomalies
- Polyhydramnios
- Cord entanglement
- Umbilical cord prolapse
- Intrauterine growth restriction
- Twin-twin transfusion
- Malpresentation

---

polyhydramnios within one fetal sac may limit the growth of the other fetus. In patients with three or more fetuses, limited intrauterine size may restrict fetal growth. Of course, factors that cause IUGR in singleton pregnancies also may cause IUGR in patients with multiple gestation (e.g., uteroplacental insufficiency, chromosomal abnormalities).

Preterm Labor

Patients with multiple gestation are at high risk for preterm labor and delivery. Preterm labor occurs in 40% to 50% of pregnant women with multiple gestation, and 30% to 40% deliver before 37 weeks' gestation.[63] Some obstetricians favor prophylactic oral administration of a tocolytic drug and/or bedrest. The role of prophylactic cerclage in high-order multiple gestations has not been determined.[64]

When preterm labor occurs, the patient may receive parenteral tocolytic therapy. Often the anesthesiologist is asked to administer anesthesia after tocolytic therapy has failed. The side effects of these tocolytic agents may affect the response to anesthesia (see Chapter 34). Multiple gestation most likely increases the risk of pulmonary edema associated with tocolytic therapy.

Abnormal Presentation

Multiple gestation is associated with an increased incidence of abnormal presentation, which results in part from the need to accommodate two or more fetuses within the uterine cavity. Malpresentation increases the risk of umbilical cord prolapse, which may occur either before or after delivery of the first fetus.

Morbidity and Mortality

Approximately 10% of all cases of **perinatal mortality** result from multiple gestation. The perinatal mortality rate in twin pregnancies is four times greater than that associated with singleton pregnancies (i.e., 43 deaths per 1000 births compared with 10 per 1000 births).[50] Preterm delivery accounts for most of this increase, although twins and triplets also have a higher weight-specific mortality, which may be related to twin-twin transfusion, congenital malformations, preeclampsia, malpresentation, and/or a prolapsed umbilical cord.[65] Improved obstetric and neonatal care have reduced the overall perinatal mortality rate for monoamniotic twins and triplets.[66] Some maternal-fetal medicine specialists advocate selective multifetal reduction to reduce the maternal morbidity and the perinatal morbidity and mortality associated with three or more fetuses. This is a matter of great controversy, both ethically and medically.[48,50]

A recent study evaluated outcome for 150,386 sets of twins and 5240 sets of triplets born between 1995 and 1997; fetal death at 20 weeks' gestation or later occurred in 2.6% of twin gestations and 4.3% of triplet gestations.[67] The authors noted that "survival of the remaining fetuses was inversely related to the time of the first fetal demise." Opposite gender twins were more likely to survive; this may reflect the absence of monochorionic placentation.[67] In monochorionic twin gestations complicated by twin-twin transfusion and fetal death, approximately half of the surviving twins experience mortality or serious morbidity.[61] Death of one fetus may occur well before term. Despite concerns about the development of consumptive coagulopathy in either the mother or the surviving fetus(es), conservative management with weekly assessment is considered the wisest choice.[50] A possible exception may be the management of cases of fetal death related to twin-twin transfusion; in these cases the risk of comorbidity/mortality may warrant early delivery, despite the risks of prematurty.[61,62]

Multiple gestation also is associated with an increased risk of **neonatal morbidity and mortality.** Despite a 95% neonatal survival rate, triplets have a significantly greater risk for intraventricular hemorrhage and retinopathy of prematurity.[68]

Order of Delivery
Given current obstetric practice, birth order does not seem to influence perinatal outcome.[68,69] The choice of anesthetic technique may affect outcome for the second twin. For example, Crawford[70] observed that among women who received epidural anesthesia, the first and second twins had similar umbilical cord blood pH measurements. In contrast, among women who received general anesthesia, the second twin tended to be more acidotic than the first. Likewise, Jarvis and Whitfield[71] observed no difference in the outcome for twins A and B when the mother received epidural analgesia. Administration of general anesthesia is increasingly rare for cesarean delivery in women with multiple gestation.[72] The interval between deliveries does not affect the outcome for twin B.[73]

MATERNAL COMPLICATIONS
Multiple gestation increases the incidence of maternal morbidity and mortality (Box 35-4), even with adjustment for confounding factors.[74] The incidence of maternal complications increases in proportion to the number of fetuses. Nearly all triplet gestations are associated with antenatal and/or postnatal maternal complications.[75] Maternal consumptive coagulopathy may occur after the IUFD of one or more fetuses.[76]

Abdominal distention and diaphragmatic elevation can cause respiratory distress and may necessitate early delivery in some patients with three or more fetuses. The increased incidence of cesarean section contributes to the increased risk of maternal morbidity and mortality associated with multiple gestation.

Multiple gestation (and the use of assisted reproductive techniques[77]) increases both the incidence and severity of preeclampsia.[50,75] Preeclampsia prompts delivery by 34 weeks' gestation in as many as 70% of patients with quadruplet pregnancies.[78]

Blood loss with delivery is increased by approximately 500 mL.[50] Uterine distention increases the risk of uterine atony and postpartum hemorrhage. Most cases of atony respond to standard pharmacologic therapy (e.g., oxytocin, methylergonovine, 15-methylprostaglandin $F_{2\text{-alpha}}$ [carboprost, Hemabate]). Persistent uterine atony requires the performance of emergency hysterectomy.

Box 35-4 MATERNAL COMPLICATIONS ASSOCIATED WITH MULTIPLE GESTATION

- Preterm premature rupture of membranes
- Preterm labor
- Prolonged labor
- Preeclampsia/eclampsia
- Placental abruption
- Disseminated intravascular coagulation
- Operative delivery (forceps and abdominal)
- Uterine atony
- Obstetric trauma
- Antepartum and/or postpartum hemorrhage

Obstetric Management
Twin gestation itself does not contraindicate labor and vaginal delivery. However, multiple gestation is associated with an increased incidence of cesarean section. Most obstetricians favor cesarean section for all patients with three or more fetuses.[48,50] A meta-analysis of 1932 infants does not support planned cesarean section for twins unless Twin A is breech.[79]

Both fetuses have a vertex presentation in 30% to 50% of cases of twin gestation. Approximately 25% to 40% have a vertex/breech combination. The remaining patients have various combinations of vertex, breech, and transverse lie. Most obstetricians allow a trial of labor if both twins have a vertex presentation. Similarly, a majority of obstetricians opt for cesarean section if the first twin has a breech or shoulder presentation. Controversy remains regarding the ideal management in those cases in which twin A has a vertex presentation and twin B has a nonvertex presentation.

TWIN A
Decisions regarding the method of delivery typically revolve around the gestational age and presentation of twin A. An obstetrician who is unwilling to allow a trial of labor in a patient with a *singleton* breech presentation is highly unlikely to allow a trial of labor in a patient with a breech presentation for twin A. Moreover, if twin A has a breech presentation and twin B has a vertex presentation, interlocking chins may occur during labor and delivery. This complication occurs infrequently (approximately 1 in 1000 cases of twin delivery), but the consequences can be devastating.[48] Other indications for cesarean delivery of twin A include (1) evidence of discordant growth (especially if twin B is larger than twin A), (2) twin-twin transfusion, (3) selected congenital anomalies, and (4) evidence of uteroplacental insufficiency.[48,50] A trial of labor mandates continuous FHR monitoring of both fetuses. After amniotomy, an electrocardiographic (ECG) lead may be placed on the scalp of twin A, and Doppler ultrasonography may be used to monitor twin B.

The unanticipated case of head entrapment, a deflexed head, or locked twins may necessitate emergency abdominal delivery of both twins A and B. The obstetrician proceeds with cesarean section while an assistant supports the exteriorized body of twin A. The obstetrician applies gentle traction on the head while the infant's body is guided back into the vagina. This can be accomplished without major injury to the infant or the mother.[80]

TWIN B
If twin A is delivered vaginally, the obstetrician must make a decision regarding the method of delivery for twin B. If twin B has a vertex presentation and if the head is well applied to the cervix, the obstetrician may allow the patient to resume labor and may await spontaneous vaginal delivery. Rarely, if twin B has a vertex presentation but the head is not well applied to the cervix, the obstetrician may perform internal podalic version and total breech extraction.

If twin B has a nonvertex presentation, options include (1) external cephalic version, followed by a resumption of labor; (2) internal podalic version and total breech extraction; and (3) performance of cesarean section. Real-time ultrasonography facilitates the performance of external cephalic version. This procedure is successful in approximately 70% of cases. The likelihood of success is not associated with parity, gestational age, or birth weight.[81] One study noted that patients who received epidural anesthesia were more relaxed and tolerated the procedure better than those who did not receive epidural anesthesia.[81]

Delivery of twin B is the one situation in which internal podalic version and total breech extraction are considered appropriate in contemporary obstetric practice. At least two studies have noted that second twins delivered by total breech extraction have obstetric outcomes similar to second twins with a vertex presentation.[82,83] Other studies have observed similar perinatal outcomes after the performance of either total breech extraction or cesarean delivery of twin B. These studies noted no difference between groups in birth weight, Apgar scores, perinatal mortality, incidence of neonatal complications (e.g., RDS, necrotizing enterocolitis, severe intracranial hemorrhage), or the duration of mechanical ventilation, oxygen therapy, or hospitalization.[84,85] Based on their analysis of published studies, Houlihan and Knuppel[86] concluded that assisted breech extraction is appropriate for a nonvertex second twin ≥ 1700 g.

The obstetrician will opt for total breech extraction of twin B only if there is evidence that twin B is not larger than twin A. Antepartum sonographic examination allows the obstetrician to assess the head size and weight of both fetuses. If twin B is not larger than twin A, the pelvis and cervical dilation are probably adequate for vaginal delivery of twin B, provided that the cervix has not begun to contract.

In the past, obstetricians favored the delivery of twin B within 15 to 30 minutes of delivery of twin A. However, most data supporting that management plan were obtained before the use of intrapartum FHR monitoring.[48] Using continuous FHR and uterine monitoring, Rayburn et al.[87] noted that the interval between deliveries averaged 21 minutes (with a range of 1 to 134 minutes) in 115 patients with live-born twins. A total of 28 infants delivered between 16 and 30 minutes after the delivery of twin A, and 17 delivered more than 30 minutes after the delivery of twin A. All 45 infants who delivered more than 15 minutes after the delivery of twin A did well. In fact, all 17 neonates who delivered after 30 minutes had a 5-minute Apgar score of at least 8. In a review of 118 twin deliveries, Leung et al.[88] demonstrated an association but not a causal relationship between the twin-twin delivery interval and the umbilical cord blood gas and pH measurements for the second twin. The authors noted that continuous FHR monitoring is essential; 73% of the second twins not delivered by 30 minutes required operative delivery for evidence of fetal distress.[88] Successful delays of 41 to 143 days have occurred when the first twin delivered before the age of viability.[89] Porreco et al.[90] described outcome for nine cases of multiple gestation in which one fetus was delivered preterm and the obstetrician attempted to delay delivery of the remaining fetuses. The latency interval ranged from 3 to 76 days. The incidence of neonatal mortality was 70% among the firstborn infants, but was only 18% among the infants whose delivery was delayed. Antibiotics, tocolytic agents, and cerclage are used by some obstetricians when attempting to delay delivery in such patients.[90]

Anesthetic Management

LABOR AND VAGINAL DELIVERY

Epidural anesthesia provides optimal analgesia and flexibility for subsequent anesthetic needs. The anesthesiologist must be vigilant because obstetric conditions and anesthetic requirements may change rapidly. Given the increased risk for cesarean section in these patients, the anesthesiologist should demand a perfect epidural anesthetic. If there is any question regarding the location of the catheter or the efficacy of the block, the catheter should be removed and another one should be placed within the epidural space.

Patients with multiple gestation are at increased risk for aortocaval compression and hypotension during the administration of regional anesthesia. Use of the full lateral position, both during and after induction of epidural anesthesia, decreases the risk of aortocaval compression. Because these patients are at increased risk for uterine atony and postpartum hemorrhage, I establish large-bore intravenous access before delivery.

Patients with multiple gestation should deliver in a room where an emergency abdominal delivery can be performed immediately. I administer supplemental oxygen to all women with multiple gestation, because it may improve fetal condition, and it provides an added margin of maternal safety if emergency induction of general anesthesia should become necessary.

As the patient nears the time of delivery for twin A, I augment the intensity of the block. I extend the sensory level to approximately T8 to T6 using a solution of local anesthetic that is more concentrated than that used earlier during labor. Effective anesthesia facilitates the performance of internal podalic version and total breech extraction of twin B; it also facilitates the extension of anesthesia for cesarean section if necessary. I prepare a syringe of 3% 2-chloroprocaine to be used if emergency extension of epidural anesthesia is required.

I prefer not to administer spinal anesthesia for vaginal delivery because of its lack of flexibility in cases of rapidly changing conditions. However, spinal or CSE anesthesia may be appropriate when delivery appears imminent in a patient without preexisting epidural anesthesia.

VAGINAL DELIVERY OF TWIN A/ABDOMINAL DELIVERY OF TWIN B

The flexibility associated with epidural anesthesia is especially advantageous if the obstetrician delivers twin A vaginally and twin B abdominally. I administer a nonparticulate antacid at the first sign of obstetrician distress (not to be confused with fetal distress), and I inject additional local anesthetic to extend the sensory level to approximately T4. In cases of dire fetal distress, it may be necessary to administer general anesthesia if adequate anesthesia cannot be achieved rapidly. Typically this can be avoided if both the level and intensity of anesthesia are augmented at the time of delivery for twin A and if the anesthesiologist gives attention to both the FHR tracing and the obstetrician.

If the obstetrician opts for internal podalic version and total breech extraction of twin B, it is better to perform the procedure shortly after the delivery of twin A, before the uterus and the cervix begin to contract. Pain relief and skeletal muscle relaxation (both provided by epidural anesthesia) facilitate internal version and total breech extraction of twin B in most patients. In some cases, pharmacologic uterine relaxation may be required to facilitate internal version and breech extraction of twin B. Sublingual or intravenous nitroglycerin may provide adequate relaxation for internal podalic version.[91,92] If this is unsuccessful, it may be necessary to perform rapid-sequence induction of general anesthesia, followed by administration of a high concentration of a volatile halogenated agent (vide supra).

CESAREAN SECTION

Epidural, spinal, or general anesthesia can be safely given for scheduled abdominal delivery. I prefer epidural anesthesia over spinal anesthesia because of the increased risk of hypotension during administration of spinal anesthesia in patients with multiple gestation. Epidural anesthesia results in a gradual onset of sympathetic blockade, which reduces the incidence of severe hypotension. The use of spinal anesthesia is associated with a greater requirement for ephedrine, but objective evidence does not suggest that this adversely affects neonatal outcome.[72] Comparison of brachial artery and popliteal artery blood pressures allows the detection of occult supine hypotension, which results in decreased uteroplacental perfusion in the presence of a normal brachial artery pressure. If either hypotension or occult supine hypotension is detected, additional left uterine displacement or displacement to the opposite side may resolve the problem. Jawan et al.[93] observed that spinal anesthesia in patients with multiple gestation has a more rapid onset and higher cephalad spread (T3 versus T5) than in patients with a singleton pregnancy. In contrast, in a retrospective study, Behforouz et al.[94] noted that the dose of *epidural* lidocaine required to achieve a T4 sensory level was similar in women with singleton versus high-order (i.e., triplets, quadruplets) pregnancies. In a recent study, mean umbilical venous (UV) and umbilical arterial (UA) lidocaine concentrations were 35% to 53% higher in twin newborn infants than in singleton infants exposed to epidural anesthesia for cesarean section. Mean fetal:maternal lidocaine ratios were at least 18% higher in the twin newborns than in the singleton newborns. The authors speculated that this may be a result of the increased maternal cardiac output and plasma volume associated with twin gestation, as well as the decreased total plasma protein concentration, which results in an increase in the free lidocaine concentration.[95]

When general anesthesia is used, the increased oxygen consumption and decreased FRC associated with multiple gestation increase the risk of hypoxemia during periods of apnea. Adequate denitrogenation (preoxygenation) is essential.

The presence of two or more fetuses results in prolonged uterine incision-to-delivery intervals because of the increased time required to deliver multiple infants. A prolonged interval increases the risk of umbilical cord blood acidemia and neonatal depression. Neonatal depression is less likely if regional anesthesia is administered.[70]

KEY POINTS

- An increased incidence of breech presentation occurs among patients who present with preterm labor.
- Both breech presentation and multiple gestation are associated with an increased incidence of perinatal morbidity and mortality, regardless of the method of delivery.
- Epidural anesthesia offers several advantages during a trial of labor in the patient with a breech presentation. Specifically, epidural anesthesia (1) provides effective pain relief; (2) inhibits early pushing; (3) provides a relaxed pelvic floor and perineum, which facilitates atraumatic delivery of the aftercoming head; and (4) facilitates provision of anesthesia for emergency cesarean section.
- Multiple gestation exaggerates the physiologic and anatomic changes of pregnancy.
- Multiple gestation increases the risk of aortocaval compression and hypotension during administration of regional anesthesia.
- Epidural analgesia is the analgesic technique of choice during labor in the patient with multiple gestation. Provision of pain relief and skeletal muscle relaxation facilitates the vaginal delivery of twin B. Provision of epidural analgesia also facilitates the administration of anesthesia for emergency cesarean section if it is needed.
- The obstetrician may request pharmacologic provision of uterine and/or cervical relaxation to facilitate vaginal delivery of twin B or to facilitate the delivery of the aftercoming fetal head in cases of breech presentation. Intravenous or sublingual nitroglycerin may provide rapid-onset uterine relaxation of short duration. Rapid-sequence induction of general anesthesia followed by administration of a high concentration of a volatile halogenated agent also represents a reliable method of providing uterine and cervical relaxation.

REFERENCES

1. Gardberg M, Laakkonen E, Sälevaara M. Intrapartum sonography and persistent occiput posterior position: A study of 408 deliveries. Obstet Gynecol 1998; 91:746-9.
2. Cunningham FG, Gant NF, Leveno KJ, et al. Williams Obstetrics, 21st ed. New York, McGraw-Hill, 2002; 451-67, 509-35.
3. Morgan HS, Kane SH. An analysis of 16,327 breech births. JAMA 1964; 187:262-4.
4. Albrechtsen S, Rasmussen S, Dalaker K, et al. Perinatal mortality in breech presentation. Obstet Gynecol 1998; 92:775-80.
5. Lau TK, Lo KWK, Rogers M. Pregnancy outcome after successful external cephalic version for breech presentation at term. Am J Obstet Gynecol 1997; 176:218-23.
6. Schutte MF, Van Hemel OJS, van de Berg C, van de Pol A. Perinatal mortality in breech presentations as compared to vertex presentations in singleton pregnancies: An analysis based upon 57,819 computer-registered pregnancies in the Netherlands. Eur J Obstet Gynecol Reprod Biol 1985; 19:391-400.
7. Cheng M, Hannah M. Breech delivery at term: A critical review of the literature. Obstet Gynecol 1993; 82:605-18.
8. Schiff E, Friedman SA, Mashiach S, et al. Maternal and neonatal outcome of 846 term singleton breech deliveries: Seven-year experience at a single center. Am J Obstet Gynecol 1996; 175:18-23.
9. Bingham P, Lilford RJ. Management of the selected term breech presentation: Assessment of the risks of selected vaginal delivery versus cesarean section for all cases. Obstet Gynecol 1987; 69:965-78.
10. Fortunato SJ, Mercer LJ, Guzick DS. External cephalic version with tocolysis: Factors associated with success. Obstet Gynecol 1988; 72:59-62.
11. Zhang J, Bowes WA, Fortney JA. Efficacy of external cephalic version: A review. Obstet Gynecol 1993; 82:306-12
12. American College of Obstetricians and Gynecologists. External Cephalic Version. ACOG Practice Bulletin No. 13, February 2000.
13. Brost BC, Adams JD, Hester M. External cephalic version after rupture of membranes. Obstet Gynecol 2000;95:1041.
14. Schorr SJ, Speights SE, Ross EL, et al. A randomized trial of epidural anesthesia to improve external cephalic version success. Am J Obstet Gynecol 1997; 177:1133-7.
15. Fernandez CO, Bloom SL, Smulian JC, et al. A randomized placebo-controlled evaluation of terbutaline for external cephalic version. Obstet Gynecol 1997; 90:775-9.

16. Neiger R, Hennessy MD, Patel M. Reattempting failed external cephalic version under epidural anesthesia. Am J Obstet Gynecol 1998; 179: 1136-9.
17. Birnbach DJ, Matut J, Stein DJ, et al. The effect of intrathecal analgesia on the success of external cephalic version. Anesth Analg 2001; 93:410-3.
18. Dugoff L, Stamm CA, Jones OW 3rd, et al. The effect of spinal anesthesia on the success rate of external cephalic version: A randomized trial. Obstet Gynecol 1999; 93:345-9.
19. Cherayil G, Feinberg B, Robinson J, et al. Central neuraxial blockade promotes external cephalic version success after a failed attempt. Anesth Analg 2002;94:1589-92.
20. Collea JV, Chein C, Quilligan EJ. The randomized management of term frank breech presentation: A study of 208 cases. Am J Obstet Gynecol 1980; 137:235-44.
21. Gimovsky ML, Wallace RL, Schifrin BS, Paul RH. Randomized management of the nonfrank breech presentation at term: A preliminary report. Am J Obstet Gynecol 1983; 146:34-40.
22. Gifford DS, Morton SC, Fiske M, Kahn K. A meta-analysis of infant outcomes after breech delivery. Obstet Gynecol 1995; 85:1047-54.
23. Hannah ME, Hannah WJ, Hewson SA, et al. Planned caesarean section versus planned vaginal birth for breech presentation at term: A randomized multicentre trial. Lancet 2000; 356:1375-83.
24. Hannah ME, Hannah WJ, Hodnett ED, et al. Outcomes at 3 months after planned cesarean vs planned vaginal delivery for breech presentation at term. JAMA 2002; 287:1822-31.
25. Greene MF. Vaginal breech delivery is no longer justified. Obstet Gynecol 2002; 99:113-4.
26. Lumley J. Any room left for disagreement about assisting breech births at term? The Lancet 2000;356:1368-9.
27. McNiven P, Kaufman K, McDonald H. Prevention: planned cesarean delivery reduces early perinatal and neonatal complications for term breech presentations. Can J Anesth 2001;48:1114-6.
28. Hauth JC, Cunningham FG. Vaginal breech is still justified. Obstet Gynecol 2002;99:1115-6.
29. van Roosmalen J. There is still room for disagreement about vaginal delivery of breech infants at term. BJOG 2002;109:967-9.
30. American College of Obstetricians and Gynecologists. Mode of term singleton breech delivery. ACOG Committee Opinion No. 265 (Obstet Gynecol 2001;98:1189-90).
31. Confino E, Ismajovich B, Sherzer A, et al. Vaginal versus cesarean section oriented approaches in the management of breech delivery. Int J Gynaecol Obstet 1985; 23:1-6.
32. Cibils LA, Karrison T, Brown L. Factors influencing neonatal outcomes in the very-low-birth weight fetus (<1500 grams) with a breech presentation. Am J Obstet Gynecol 1994; 171:35-42.
33. Zlatnik FJ. The Iowa premature breech trial. Am J Perinatol 1993; 10:60-3.
34. Lanni SM, Seeds JW. Malpresentations. In Gabbe SG, Niebyl JR, Simpson JL, editors. Obstetrics: Normal and Problem Pregnancies, 4th ed. New York, Churchill Livingstone, 2002:473-501.
35. Crawford JS. An appraisal of lumbar epidural blockade in patients with a singleton fetus presenting by the breech. J Obstet Gynaecol Br Commonw 1974; 81:867-72.
36. Breeson AJ, Kovacs GT, Pickles BG, Hill JG. Extradural analgesia: The preferred method of analgesia for vaginal breech delivery. Br J Anaesth 1978; 50:1227-30.
37. Confino E, Ismajovich B, Rudick V, David MP. Extradural analgesia in the management of singleton breech delivery. Br J Anaesth 1985; 57:892-5.
38. Van Zundert A, Vaes L, Soetens M, et al. Are breech deliveries an indication for lumbar epidural analgesia? Anesth Analg 1991; 72:399-403.
39. Chadha YC, Mahmood TA, Dick MJ, et al. Breech delivery and epidural analgesia. Br J Obstet Gynaecol 1992; 99:96-100.
40. Chadha YC, Mahmood TA, Dick MJ, et al. Author's reply (letter). Br J Obstet Gynaecol 1992; 99:782-3.
41. Wuitchik M, Bakal D, Lipshitz J. The clinical significance of pain and cognitive activity in latent labor. Obstet Gynecol 1989; 73:35-42.
42. Benhamou D, Mercier FJ, Ayed MB, et al. Continuous epidural analgesia with bupivacaine 0.125% or bupivacaine 0.0625% plus sufentanil 0.25 μg mL⁻¹: A study in singleton breech presentation. Internat J Obstet Anesth 2002;11:13-8.
43. Danforth DN. The distribution and functional activity of the cervical musculature. Am J Obstet Gynecol 1954; 68:1261-71.
44. Caponas G. Glyceryl trinitrate and acute uterine relaxation: A literature review. Anaesth Intensive Care 2001;29:163-77.
45. Buhimschi CS, Buhimschi IA, Malinow AM, et al. Effects of sublingual nitroglycerin on human uterine contractility during the active phase of labor. Am J Obstet Gynecol 2002;187:235-8.
46. Hrubec Z, Robinette CD. The study of human twins in medical research. N Engl J Med 1984; 310:435-41.
47. Martin JA, Hamilton BE, Ventura SJ, et al. Births: Final data for 2000. National Vital Statistics Reports 50 (5), February 12, 2002.
48. Chitkara U, Berkowitz RL. Multiple gestations. In Gabbe SG, Niebyl JR, Simpson JL, editors. Obstetrics: Normal and Problem Pregnancies, 4th ed. New York, Churchill Livingstone, 2002: 827-67.
49. Tessen JA, Zlatnik FJ. Monoamniotic twins: A retrospective controlled study. Obstet Gynecol 1991; 77:832-4.
50. Cunningham FG, Gant NF, Leveno KJ, et al. Williams Obstetrics, 21st ed. New York, McGraw-Hill, 2002;765-810.
51. McAuliffe F, Kametas N, Costello J, et al. Respiratory function in singleton and twin pregnancy. BJOG 2002;109:765-9.
52. Pederson AL, Worthington-Roberts BM, Hickok DE. Weight gain patterns during twin gestation. J Am Diet Assoc 1989; 89:642-6.
53. Veille JC, Morton MJ, Burry KJ. Maternal cardiovascular adaptations to twin pregnancy. Am J Obstet Gynecol 1985; 153:261-3.
54. Bermudez C, Becerra CH, Bornick PW, et al. Placental types and twin-twin transfusion syndrome. Am J Obstet Gynecol 2002;187:489-94.
55. Gonsoulin W, Moise KJ Jr, Kirshon B, et al. Outcome of twin-twin transfusion diagnosed before 28 weeks of gestation. Obstet Gynecol 1990; 75:214-6.
56. Elliott JP, Urig MA, Clewell WH. Aggressive therapeutic amniocentesis for treatment of twin-twin transfusion syndrome. Obstet Gynecol 1991; 77:537-40.
57. Roberts D, Neilson JP, Weindling AM. Interventions for the treatment of twin-twin transfusion syndrome. The Cochrane Library 2002;4.
58. Ville Y, Hyett J, Hecher K, Nicolaides K. Preliminary experience with endoscopic laser surgery for severe twin-twin transfusion syndrome. N Engl J Med 1995; 332:224-7.
59. Elliott JP. Twin-twin transfusion (letter). N Engl J Med 1995; 333:387-8.
60. Fisk NM, Bajoria R, Wigglesworth J. Twin-twin transfusion (letter). N Engl J Med 1995; 333:388.
61. Van Heteren CF, Nijhuis JG, Semmekrot BA, et al. Risk for surviving twin after fetal death of co-twin in twin-twin transfusion syndrome. Obstet Gynecol 1998;92:215-9.
62. Denbow ML, Battin MR, Cowan F, et al. Neonatal cranial ultrasonographic findings in preterm twins complicated by severe fetofetal transfusion syndrome. Am J Obstet Gynecol 1998;178:479-83.
63. Roberts WE, Morrison JC, Hamer C, Wiser WL. The incidence of preterm labor and specific risk factors. Obstet Gynecol 1990; 76:85S-9S.
64. Elimian A, Figueroa R, Nigam S, et al. Perinatal outcome of triplet gestation: Does prophylactic cerclage make a difference? J Matern Fetal Med 1999; 8:119-22.
65. Buekens P, Wilcox A. Why do small twins have a lower mortality rate than small singletons? Am J Obstet Gynecol 1993; 168:937-41.
66. Rodis JF, McIlveen PF, Egan JFX, et al. Monoamniotic twins: improved perinatal survival with accurate prenatal diagnosis and antenatal fetal surveillance. Am J Obstet Gynecol 1997;177:1046-9.
67. Johnson CD, Zhang J. Survival of other fetuses after a fetal death in twin or triplet pregnancies. Obstet Gynecol 2002;99:698-703.
68. Kaufman GE, Malone FD, Harvey-Wilkes KB, et al. Neonatal morbidity and mortality associated with triplet pregnancy. Obstet Gynecol 1998;91:342-8.
69. Antoine C, Kirshenbaum NW, Young BK. Biochemical differences related to birth order in triplets. J Reprod Med 1996;31:330-2.
70. Crawford JS. A prospective study of 200 consecutive twin deliveries. Anaesthesia 1987; 42:33-43.
71. Jarvis GJ, Whitfield MF. Epidural analgesia and the delivery of twins. J Obstet Gynaecol 1981; 2:90-2.
72. Marino T, Goudas LC, Steinbok V, et al. The anesthetic management of triplet cesarean delivery: A retrospective case series of maternal outcomes. Anesth Analg 2001;93:991-5.
73. American College of Obstetricians and Gynecologists. Special problems of multiple gestation. ACOG Education Bulletin No. 253, 1998.
74. Conde-Agudelo A, Belizan JM, Lindmark G. Maternal morbidity and mortality associated with multiple gestations. Obstet Gynecol 2000;95:899-904.
75. Malone FD, Kaufman GE, Chelmow D, et al. Maternal morbidity associated with triplet pregnancy. Am J Perinatol 1998; 15:73-7.
76. Skelly H, Marivate M, Norman R, et al. Consumptive coagulopathy following fetal death in a triplet pregnancy. Am J Obstet Gynecol 1982; 142:595-6.
77. Lynch A, McDuffie R, Jr., Murphy J, et al. Preeclampsia in multiple gestation: The role of assisted reproductive technologies. Obstet Gynecol 2002;99:445-51.
78. Elliott JP, Radin TG. Quadruplet pregnancy: Contemporary management and outcome. Obstet Gynecol 1992; 80:421-4.
79. Hogle, KL, Hutton EK, McBrien KA, et al. Cesarean delivery for twins: a systematic review and meta-analysis. Obstet Gynecol 2003;188:220-7.

80. Swartjes JM, Bleker OP, Schutte MF. The Zavanelli maneuver applied to locked twins. Am J Obstet Gynecol 1992; 166:532-3.

81. Tchabo J, Tomai T. Selected intrapartum external cephalic version of the second twin. Obstet Gynecol 1992; 79:421-3.

82. Blickstein I, Schwartz-Shoham Z, Lancet M, Borenstein R. Vaginal delivery of the second twin in breech presentation. Obstet Gynecol 1987; 69:774-6.

83. Fishman A, Grubb DK, Kovacs BW. Vaginal delivery of the nonvertex second twin. Am J Obstet Gynecol 1993; 168:861-4.

84. Davison L, Easterling TR, Jackson JC, Benedetti TJ. Breech extraction of low-birth weight second twins: Can cesarean section be justified? Am J Obstet Gynecol 1992; 166:497-502.

85. Greig PC, Veille J, Morgan T, Henderson L. The effect of presentation and mode of delivery on neonatal outcome in the second twin. Am J Obstet Gynecol 1992; 167:901-6.

86. Houlihan C, Knuppel RA. Intrapartum management of multiple gestations. Clin Perinatol 1996;23:91-116.

87. Rayburn WF, Lavin JP, Miodovnik M, Vainer MW. Multiple gestation: Time interval between delivery of the first and second twins. Obstet Gynecol 1984; 63:502-6.

88. Leung R, Tam W, Leung T, et al. Effect of twin-to-twin delivery interval on umbilical cord blood gas in the second twins. BJOG 2002;109:63-7.

89. Wittmann BK, Farquharson D, Wong GP, et al. Delayed delivery of second twin: Report of four cases and review of the literature. Obstet Gynecol 1992; 79:260-3.

90. Porreco RP, Diss Sabin E, Heyborne KD, Lindsay LG. Delayed-interval delivery in multifetal pregnancy. Am J Obstet Gynecol 1998; 178:20-3.

91. Vinatier D, Dufour P, Bérard J. Utilization of intravenous nitroglycerin for obstetrical emergencies. Int J Gynecol Obstet 1996; 55:129-34.

92. Dufour P, Vinatier D, Vanderstichele S, et al. Intravenous nitroglycerin for internal podalic version of the second twin in transverse lie. Obstet Gynecol 1998; 92:416-9.

93. Jawan B, Lee JH, Chong ZK, Chang CS. Spread of spinal anesthesia for caesarean section in singleton and twin pregnancies. Br J Anaesth 1993; 70:639-41.

94. Behforouz N, Dounas M, Benhamou D. Epidural anaesthesia for caesarean delivery in triple and quadruple pregnancies. Acta Anaesthesiol Scand 1998; 42:1088-91.

95. Vallejo MC, Ramanathan S. Plasma lidocaine concentrations are higher in twin compared to singleton newborns following epidural anesthesia for cesarean delivery. Can J Anesth 2002;49:701-5.

Chapter 36
Fever and Infection
Scott Segal, M.D. · Harvey Carp, M.D., Ph.D. · David H. Chestnut, M.D.

Infection and fever are common clinical problems in obstetric patients. The purpose of this chapter is to review the obstetric and anesthetic management of pregnant women with fever and/or infection.

FEVER

Definition and Pathophysiology

In 1868, Carl Wunderlich[1] analyzed more than 1 million axillary temperature measurements from 25,000 patients. He concluded that the average normal temperature of healthy adults was 37.0° C. However, he found a range of temperatures, with a nadir of 36.2° C between 2:00 and 8:00 AM and a zenith of 37.5° C between 4:00 and 9:00 PM. He also observed that women had slightly higher mean temperatures than men. A more recent study using modern oral thermometers largely confirmed Wunderlich's original data.[2]

Well-regulated temperature results from hypothalamic integration of afferent thermal information from the skin, spinal cord, and other sites within the central nervous system (CNS). When this integrated temperature deviates from normal, thermoregulatory responses are triggered.[3] In humans, the first (and least metabolically "expensive") response to temperature perturbations is behavioral (e.g., moving to a different environment, putting on appropriate clothing, adjusting room temperature). Such responses obviously are unavailable to an anesthetized patient, although some may be implemented by those caring for the patient. Further responses to temperature perturbations are mediated by the autonomic nervous system. Hypothermia prompts vasoconstriction in peripheral tissues to decrease skin blood flow, decrease heat loss, and retain heat in the core compartment. If vasoconstriction is not adequate to prevent hypothermia, thermoregulatory shivering is triggered to increase heat production. The CNS controls the metabolic activity of skeletal muscle, which converts chemical energy into heat by shivering.

Increased body temperature initially prompts vasodilation. This vasodilation is passive. It results from the release of sympathetic tone, and it is seen in unanesthetized adults exposed to a hot environment before any significant change in central temperature occurs. If vasodilation is not adequate to prevent hyperthermia, thermoregulatory sweating occurs, which increases evaporative heat loss.

An abnormal body temperature can result from drugs or diseases that either change thermoregulatory thresholds or impair thermoregulatory responses. Hypothalamic activity and fever may be triggered by endogenous pyrogens released from immune effector cells in response to invasion by microorganisms (Figure 36-1). Although no single endogenous pyrogen has been identified conclusively as the mediator of the febrile response, tumor necrosis factor seems capable of reproducing many components of the febrile response.[3] Endogenous pyrogen activity appears to depend largely on increased endothelial cell production of prostaglandins. Of interest, many of these products help mediate uterine activity and parturition.[4]

Clinically, temperature measurements greater than 38° C represent fever. During episodes of fever, the thermoregulatory setpoint is elevated, and the normal thermoregulatory mechanisms are used to maintain the elevated temperature. However, there are circumstances in which an abnormally high temperature is measured in the absence of a change in thermoregulatory setpoint. This may occur when thermoregulatory responses to hyperthermia are prevented (e.g., block of sympathetically mediated sweating) or overwhelmed (e.g., immersion in hot water, malignant hyperthermia).

The fetus, by virtue of its intraabdominal location, has a unique problem with heat elimination. The only anatomic routes for egress of heat are the fetal skin surface (through the amniotic fluid) or the uteroplacental circulation. Current evidence suggests that the fetus relies on heat exchange across the uteroplacental circulation to dissipate most of its metabolic heat. The normal fetus maintains a temperature that is approximately 0.5° to 0.75° C higher than the maternal temperature.[5]

Interaction with Pregnancy

Maternal-fetal infection is associated with increased perinatal morbidity.[6] The increased morbidity is the result of many factors, including preterm delivery (perhaps related to an increased release of prostaglandins) and direct effects of the infection. In addition, experimental evidence suggests that extreme levels of fever, independent of the infection itself, also may have a deleterious effect on the fetus. Morishima et al.[7] reported increased uterine activity and fetal deterioration during maternal hyperthermia produced by radiant heat in

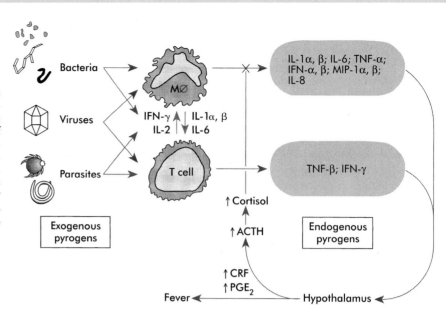

FIGURE 36-1. Production of endogenous pyrogens by macrophages and T lymphocytes. A variety of microbial pathogens produce molecules that function as exogenous pyrogens, which trigger the release of endogenous pyrogens from mononuclear cells. *ACTH,* Adrenocorticotropic hormone; *CRF,* corticotropin-releasing factor; *IFN,* interferon; *IL,* interleukin; *MIP,* macrophage inflammatory protein; PGE_2, prostaglandin E_2; *TNF,* tumor necrosis factor. (From Beutler B, Beutler AM. The pathogenesis of fever. In Wyngaarden JB, Smith LH, Bennett JC, editors. Textbook of Medicine, 19th ed. Philadelphia, WB Saunders, 1992:1570.)

anesthetized baboons. However, the extreme degree of hyperthermia (approximately 107° F [41.7° C]) employed in this study produced maternal as well as fetal deaths. Such extreme hyperthermia exceeds the modest fever that often occurs clinically, and the clinical relevance of this study is unclear.

Similarly, Cefalo and Hellegers[8] observed fetal deterioration at levels of hyperthermia that produced maternal cardiovascular collapse in anesthetized gravid ewes. However, these investigators reported increased umbilical blood flow with lesser (more clinically relevant) degrees of hyperthermia (approximately 0.5° to 1.5° C above baseline). They suggested that increased umbilical blood flow (in response to moderate degrees of hyperthermia) might be beneficial to the fetus by increasing oxygen delivery and heat removal.

Harris et al.[9] demonstrated the preservation of fetal oxygenation and acid-base status during moderate degrees of fever (approximately 1° C above baseline) produced by the injection of bacterial pyrogen in awake pregnant ewes. However, they also observed an increase in fetal heart rate (FHR) and a greater incidence of fetal arrhythmias during fever.

Recent epidemiologic evidence has suggested that mild maternal fever may not be as benign as has been assumed on the basis of animal studies. Lieberman et al.[10] retrospectively reviewed the records of 1218 nulliparous women with singleton pregnancies with a vertex presentation, and who were afebrile on admission for spontaneous labor at term gestation. The authors noted the occurrence of fever >100.4° F (38° C) in 10% of the patients, nearly all of whom had received epidural analgesia. One-minute Apgar scores < 7 and hypotonia were more common in the babies of febrile mothers. Maternal fever >101° F was associated with a more frequent requirement for bag-and-mask ventilation of the newborn infant in the delivery room and a greater need for supplemental oxygen in the nursery.[10] In a case-control study, the same group also found a strong association between intrapartum fever and neonatal seizures (odds ratio = 3.4) in infants born at term.[11] Likewise, Perlman[12] found a high incidence of maternal fever among a cohort of infants who had a 5-minute Apgar score of 5 or less and/or who required chest compressions in the delivery room.

Even more ominous is the suggestion that maternal fever may correlate with neonatal brain injury. In a large epidemiologic study, otherwise unexplained cerebral palsy was over nine times more common in babies whose mothers had intrapartum fever >38° C than in babies whose mothers were afebrile.[13] An equally strong association has been observed between maternal fever and neonatal encephalopathy.[14] Dammann et al.[15] recently reported an increased risk of cognitive deficits at age 9 among children whose mothers were febrile in labor. The mechanism linking neurologic injuries to maternal fever remains unknown but may involve the liberation of inflammatory cytokines during fever.[16] It remains unclear whether temperature elevation itself can cause neurologic injury, as distinct from the underlying infection or other inflammatory processes that cause both fever and liberation of inflammatory cytokines.

Fever also produces significant maternal effects. Elevated temperature is associated with increased maternal heart rate, cardiac output, oxygen consumption, and catecholamine production. Recent evidence has linked postcesarean fever to an increased risk of uterine rupture during a subsequent trial of labor.[17] Even low-grade fever may prompt obstetricians to perform instrumental vaginal delivery or cesarean section rather than continue expectant management of labor. In a retrospective analysis, Lieberman et al.[18] found a twofold increase in the incidence of both operative vaginal and cesarean delivery among nulliparous women who were afebrile on admission but subsequently developed fever > 99.5° F (37.5° C) during labor, when compared with parturients who remained afebrile, even after controlling for birth weight, length of labor, and choice of analgesia.

Together, these studies suggest that the fetus typically tolerates modest levels of maternal fever. Transient neonatal depression and possibly neonatal seizures and other neurologic disorders may be associated with processes that produce maternal fever, but it is not clear that these adverse outcomes are associated with fever *per se.* However, it is clear that an extremely high fever adversely affects both the mother and fetus.

Infections in Pregnant Women

Fever most often is the result of an infectious process. The most common sites of infection in pregnant women are the fetal membranes, the urinary tract, the respiratory tract, and the postpartum uterine cavity.

CHORIOAMNIONITIS

Chorioamnionitis is one of the most common infections in pregnant women. It occurs in approximately 1% of all pregnancies.[6,19-23] The diagnosis of chorioamnionitis is based on clinical signs, which include a temperature of greater than 38.0° C and maternal or fetal tachycardia, uterine tenderness, and/or foul-smelling amniotic fluid. Unfortunately, the laboratory diagnosis of chorioamnionitis is neither sensitive nor specific and may not correlate with the clinical presentation.[6,19-23] Moreover, the classical clinical signs of chorioamnionitis often are absent. Goodman et al.[24] reviewed the records of 531 women with pathologically proven chorioamnionitis. They found that only 10% of the patients had abdominal tenderness and only 1% had foul-smelling amniotic fluid.

In most cases, bacteria gain access to the amniotic cavity and the fetus by ascending through the cervix after rupture of the membranes. Chorioamnionitis develops in a significant number of parturients with premature rupture of the membranes (PROM). Alternatively, infectious agents present in the maternal circulation may undergo transplacental transport and gain access to the amniotic cavity.[6] Similar to other pelvic infections, chorioamnionitis often is polymicrobial in origin, and bacteria normally present in the genital tract most likely are responsible for most cases of infection. *Bacteroides* species, group B streptococci, and *Escherichia coli* are organisms commonly isolated from the amniotic fluid of parturients with chorioamnionitis.[6] In addition, maternal bacteremia occurs in approximately 10% of women with the clinical diagnosis of chorioamnionitis.[6,19-24] Candida species occasionally cause chorioamnionitis, especially in women with preterm labor, and have been associated with severe sequelae, including maternal sepsis and fetal demise.[25]

Maternal complications include preterm labor,[26] postpartum infection,[27] postpartum hemorrhage,[8] sepsis, and sometimes death. In addition, several studies have noted an increased incidence of cesarean section for dystocia in women with chorioamnionitis.[6,19-21,23,28] Some investigators have suggested that infection adversely affects uterine contractility and contributes to an increased risk of cesarean section.[20] However, in some cases, chorioamnionitis may represent an ascending infection developing late in a labor that is already prolonged and dysfunctional.[23] Satin et al.[23] observed no increase in the incidence of cesarean section when chorioamnionitis was diagnosed before the administration of oxytocin. However, they observed a 44% incidence of cesarean delivery when the diagnosis was made after the administration of oxytocin.

Neonatal complications of chorioamnionitis include pneumonia, meningitis, sepsis, and death.[19,21] Recently a strong association between chorioamnionitis and **cerebral palsy** has been identified.[13,16,29,30] Meta-analyses of over 20 published studies have demonstrated relative risks of cerebral palsy of 1.9 to 4.7 in preterm and term infants whose mothers had clinical evidence of chorioamnionitis.[30,31] The link between maternal infection and neonatal neurologic injury appears to be related to intraamniotic infection or inflammation, especially when there is evidence of fetal systemic inflammation (funisitis).[16,29] Chorioamnionitis has also been linked epidemiologically to **cystic periventricular leukomalacia**, which often produces devastating neurologic impairment in the child.[30,32] The effect of intraamniotic inflammation on the fetal lung is complex. Elevated amniotic fluid cytokines may reduce the incidence of acute respiratory distress syndrome in preterm neonates by stimulating surfactant production.[33]

However, the incidence of **chronic lung disease** is increased in infants exposed to chorioamnionitis, apparently as a result of inflammatory mediators.[34,35]

Historically, prompt delivery has been the cornerstone of obstetric management of patients with chorioamnionitis. However, Gibbs et al.[19] obtained excellent maternal and neonatal outcome without the use of arbitrary time limits for delivery. They performed cesarean section only for standard obstetric indications and not for the diagnosis of chorioamnionitis alone.[19] However, no recent studies have reevaluated this practice and its relationship to the risk of neonatal neurologic injury.

For many years pediatricians requested that obstetricians delay antibiotic therapy until after delivery. They cited the theoretical concern that intrapartum therapy might "obscure the results of neonatal blood cultures."[36] However, studies suggest that early, antepartum treatment results in decreased maternal and neonatal morbidity when compared with delayed, postpartum treatment.[37,38] Gibbs et al.[37] randomized 45 women with intraamniotic infection to receive either intrapartum or postpartum antibiotic therapy with ampicillin and gentamicin. Intrapartum antibiotic therapy resulted in a decreased incidence of neonatal sepsis and a shorter neonatal hospital stay. Mothers who received intrapartum antibiotics also had a shorter hospitalization, fewer days with fever, and a lower peak postpartum temperature than did mothers whose antibiotic therapy was delayed until after delivery. Most obstetricians currently give antibiotics before delivery in women with chorioamnionitis. The early use of antibiotics also may affect the anesthesiologist's decision regarding the administration of regional anesthesia (*vide infra*).

UROLOGIC INFECTIONS

Urinary tract infections are common during pregnancy. Increased concentrations of progesterone cause the relaxation of ureteral smooth muscle. In addition, the gravid uterus causes partial ureteral obstruction. Both factors cause urinary stasis, which increases the risk of urinary tract infection.[6,39,40] Further, these physiologic changes make it more likely that asymptomatic bladder infection will ascend into the kidneys and produce pyelonephritis.

Acute pyelonephritis is a serious threat to maternal and fetal well-being. Symptoms of acute pyelonephritis include fever, chills, flank pain, and other symptoms of lower urinary tract infection. Laboratory tests reveal pyuria and leukocytosis with a left shift. Pregnant women with pyelonephritis may appear severely ill. Approximately 10% of pregnant women with pyelonephritis will develop transient bacteremia during the course of this infection.[6,38,39] The most common organisms found in such patients are *E. coli*, *Klebsiella*, and *Proteus* species.

Hospitalization is generally required to initiate aggressive parenteral antibiotic treatment of this serious maternal infection, although limited data support outpatient treatment during the first and second trimesters.[41] Pyelonephritis is associated with an increased risk of preterm labor and delivery.[42] Thus obstetricians should observe for evidence of preterm labor.

Obstetricians also should monitor renal and respiratory function. Nearly 20% of affected women have transient renal dysfunction.[39] Cunningham et al.[43] suggested that acute pyelonephritis during pregnancy may be associated with pulmonary injury and respiratory failure. They suggested that "this syndrome was probably caused by permeability pulmonary edema, likely mediated by endotoxin-induced alveolar-capillary membrane injury."[43] Towers et al.[44] compared 11 pregnant women who had pyelonephritis and pulmonary injury with 119 women who had pyelonephritis only. They noted that "the presence of a maternal heart rate >110 beats/min and a fever to 103° F (39.4° C) 12 to 24 hours before the occurrence of respiratory symptoms was highly predictive of pulmonary injury."[44] Further, they observed that fluid overload and the use of tocolytic therapy were the most significant predictive factors associated with pulmonary injury. Finally, there was a trend toward a greater risk of pulmonary injury with the use of ampicillin alone for the treatment of pyelonephritis. The authors concluded the following:

> Tocolytic agents should be used only to treat the contractions of those pregnant patients with pyelonephritis who have documented and significant cervical change. The perceived benefit of tocolytic therapy must be weighed against the significant risk of pulmonary injury. Furthermore, strict management of fluids should occur so that patients do not have fluid overload.[44]

Hemodynamic alterations may be present even in infected women who do not demonstrate overt signs of sepsis. Twickler et al.[45] used ultrasonographic techniques to evaluate the central hemodynamic measurements in 37 pregnant women with uncomplicated pyelonephritis. They found decreased mean arterial pressure and systemic vascular resistance (SVR), and increased heart rate and cardiac output, compared with measurements obtained from the same patients after they had recovered from their infections.[45]

Recent reviews also strongly support the practice of screening and treating pregnant women for asymptomatic bacteruria, up to 30% of whom will eventually develop pyelonephritis. Treatment is associated with a reduced incidence of pyelonephritis (odds ratio = 0.25) and preterm labor (odds ratio = 0.6).[46]

RESPIRATORY TRACT INFECTION

Most respiratory tract infections during pregnancy are upper respiratory tract viral infections that do not pose a serious threat to the mother or fetus. However, upper respiratory tract infection precedes approximately 50% of the cases of pneumonia that occur during pregnancy.[47] Pregnancy results in a number of changes that may predispose the pregnant woman to the development of serious respiratory tract infection. Hyperemia and hypersecretion are characteristic of the respiratory tract mucosa during pregnancy, and these changes may intensify the effect of the initial infection. In the case of a viral infection, the excess secretions may predispose the patient to bacterial superinfection. Further, the increased oxygen consumption and decreased functional residual capacity characteristic of pregnancy may increase the likelihood that infection will result in maternal hypoxemia.

Benedetti et al.[48] emphasized the importance of early diagnosis and treatment as well as the direct measurement of maternal oxygenation in cases of pneumonia during pregnancy. Most community-acquired pneumonias in healthy young women are bacterial in origin. *Streptococcus pneumoniae* is the most common pathogen.[47,48] *Mycoplasma pneumoniae* and influenza are other common pathogens. *Legionella pneumophila,* chlamydia, and varicella are less common pathogens in this population. Varicella pneumonia has been associated with maternal and fetal morbidity. Acyclovir has been used successfully to treat varicella pneumonia during pregnancy.[49] *Pneumocystis carinii* pneumonia represents the most common cause of AIDS-related death in pregnancy and is associated with 50% mortality.[50]

POSTPARTUM INFECTION

The most common source of postpartum infection is the genital tract. However, the urinary tract and less often the breasts and the lungs may be infected.[6] Postpartum uterine infection typically results in fever, malaise, abdominal pain, and purulent lochia. Bacteremia may occur in as many as 20% of patients with uterine infection after cesarean section.[6,22] Although obstetricians typically refer to postpartum uterine infection as *endometritis,* this infection involves the decidua, myometrium, and parametrial tissues. Bacteria that colonize the cervix and vagina gain access to the amniotic fluid during labor, and they may invade devitalized uterine tissue postpartum.

Patients who undergo cesarean section are at increased risk for postpartum endometritis when compared with similar patients who deliver vaginally.[6,22] Prolonged rupture of membranes and/or prolonged duration of labor increase the incidence of postpartum uterine infection. Prophylactic administration of antibiotics decreases the incidence of postpartum uterine infection and wound infection after cesarean section in all women, whether performed electively or emergently.[51] Endometritis typically responds to appropriate antibiotic therapy. However, serious complications (e.g., peritonitis, abscess, septic thrombophlebitis) may occur.[6,22] In future pregnancies, women who have experienced endometritis are at increased risk for uterine rupture, and obstetricians and anesthesiologists should demonstrate extra vigilance for this serious complication.[17]

Epidural Analgesia and Noninfectious Fever

Epidural anesthesia administered for surgery—including cesarean section—typically results in hypothermia. This occurs because vasodilation produced by the block causes a redistribution of body heat from the core to the periphery, where it is lost to the environment.[52] Conversely, laboring women who receive regional analgesia may experience a rise in temperature.

In 1989, Fusi et al.[53] first observed that epidural analgesia was associated with progressive intrapartum maternal pyrexia. They reported that the vaginal temperatures of 18 parturients who received epidural analgesia increased approximately 1° C over 7 hours, whereas the temperatures of 15 women who received intramuscular meperidine and metoclopramide remained constant. There was no evidence of infection in any of the women. The authors suggested that epidural analgesia may cause an "imbalance between the heat-producing and heat-dissipating mechanisms."[53]

Fusi et al.[53] measured vaginal temperature; this measurement may be affected by the sympathectomy and vaginal mucosal vasodilation associated with epidural analgesia. Tympanic membrane temperature should not be affected by the local vasodilation associated with epidural analgesia, and it may provide a more accurate assessment of core temperature. Camann et al.[54] studied the effect of epidural analgesia on maternal oral and tympanic membrane temperature measurements in 53 laboring women. They studied three groups of patients; one group received intravenous nalbuphine, one group received epidural bupivacaine only, and one group received epidural bupivacaine with fentanyl. The patients were not randomized to receive either nalbuphine or epidural analgesia; however, those women who requested epidural analgesia were randomized to receive either epidural bupivacaine only or epidural bupivacaine with fentanyl. The authors maintained ambient room temperature at 20° to 22° C. They found that epidural analgesia did not affect maternal temperature during the first 4 hours of the study. At 5 hours and thereafter, the mean tympanic membrane temperatures were significantly higher in both of the epidural groups when compared with the intravenous nalbuphine group (Figure 36-2). Among women in the bupivacaine-only group, mean tympanic temperature increased from approximately 36.6° C at 1 hour to 37.1° C at 9 hours, a rate of rise of less than 0.07° C per hour. There was no difference between the epidural bupivacaine-only and the epidural bupivacaine-fentanyl groups in maternal tympanic membrane temperature measurements.

Several other investigators have documented similar patterns of temperature elevation and an increased incidence of clinical fever (>38.0° C) in laboring women receiving epidural analgesia.[55-59] These studies typically have found the rate of temperature increase to be approximately 0.1° C per hour of epidural analgesia, usually after a lag of 4 to 5 hours. However, the incidence of clinical fever has varied strikingly, from 1% to 36%.[55-60]

The mechanisms by which epidural analgesia produces maternal hyperthermia during labor remain unclear. Fusi et al.[53] attributed the maternal pyrexia to the high ambient temperature (24° to 26° C) found in most British delivery rooms. However, other investigators have failed to find an association between ambient temperature and maternal[55] or fetal[61] temperature. A second possible explanation for epidural analgesia-associated fever in laboring women is that the decreased sweating and the lack of hyperventilation that follow the provision of effective pain relief may predispose these women to pyrexia.[53,54,62] In volunteers, epidural anesthesia raised the sweating threshold by 0.55° C.[63] Moreover, epidural analgesia attenuates but does not eliminate a significant increase in $\dot{V}O_2$ that occurs during labor.[64] This increased energy expenditure may manifest as increased heat production in the laboring patient. Third, opioids given to women without epidural analgesia might suppress fever that otherwise would have been apparent. However, differences in opioid use did

not explain the difference in the occurrence of fever in one large retrospective study,[65] and Camann et al.[54] did not find a difference in temperature curves between women randomized to receive epidural bupivacaine with or without fentanyl. Fourth, the high incidence of shivering among laboring women who receive epidural analgesia may predispose them to the development of fever. Gleeson et al.[66] found that laboring patients who shivered after the administration of epidural analgesia developed pyrexia as early as 1 hour after initiation of the block, compared with more than 4 hours after initiation of the block in patients who did not shiver. Moreover, the maximum temperature reached was higher, and the incidence of clinical fever was three times more common, in the women who shivered.[66] Some shivering and sweating in labor is nonthermoregulatory, in that it is not accompanied by changes in core temperature or vasomotor tone.[67]

Finally, it is important to note that nearly all clinical studies of epidural analgesia-associated fever have been nonrandomized. Women who are more likely to request epidural analgesia during labor also are more likely to have other risk factors for fever during labor. These may include nulliparity,[59] prolonged rupture of membranes,[55,59] prolonged labor,[54,55,59,61] higher temperature on admission,[59] early chorioamnionitis,[59] and more frequent cervical examinations.[68] In a case-control study, Vallejo et al.[60] compared women without epidural analgesia and with clinical chorioamnionitis to two groups of women who received epidural analgesia, one with and the other without chorioamnionitis. The clinical diagnosis of chorioamnionitis was confirmed histologically. Not surprisingly, fever was far more common in the infected women. However, the incidence of fever in uninfected women with epidural analgesia was only 1%.[60] Similarly, Dashe et al.[69] reviewed the records and placental pathology reports for 149 women who delivered >6 hours after membrane rupture. The authors found an increased incidence of fever in those patients who had received epidural analgesia. However, histologic evidence of placental inflammation was also more common among the women who received epidural analgesia. In the absence of placental inflammation, the incidence of maternal fever was similar in patients who did and did not receive epidural analgesia (11% versus 9%).[69] Goetzl et al.[70]

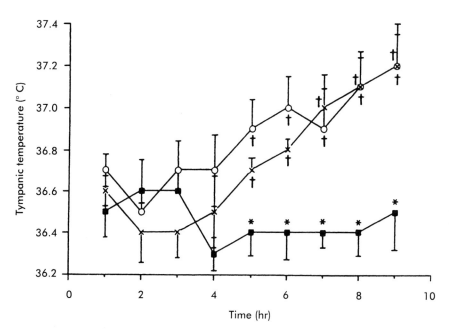

FIGURE 36-2. Mean tympanic temperatures during labor in three groups of patients: Epidural bupivacaine-fentanyl (O), epidural bupivacaine–only (X), and parenteral opioid (●) groups.
*P <0.01 compared with the epidural group.
†P <0.01 compared with the preepidural temperature.
(From Camann WR, Hortvet LA, Hughes N, et al. Maternal temperature regulation during extradural analgesia for labour. Br J Anaesth 1991; 657:565-8.)

recently randomized women with epidural analgesia to receive either acetaminophen or placebo in labor. The incidence of fever >100.4° F (38° C) was identical in the two groups. The authors demonstrated elevated maternal and umbilical cord blood markers of inflammation (e.g., interleukin 6) in febrile women.

Among the published studies of women randomized to receive epidural or intravenous opioid analgesia during labor, the only trial that specifically evaluated the influence of analgesic technique on maternal fever confirmed an increased incidence of fever in the women randomized to receive epidural analgesia.[71] However, the association was confined to nulliparous women. Further, febrile patients had a longer duration of labor, greater use of internal fetal monitoring, and increased use of oxytocin for augmentation of labor.[71] Meta-analysis of other randomized trials of epidural versus intravenous opioid analgesia has confirmed the association between epidural analgesia and maternal fever.[72]

Epidural analgesia-associated maternal hyperthermia has become a subject of significant controversy. In theory, the fetus is at risk for hyperthermia when the mother is febrile because the fetus dissipates heat by means of its transmission to the amniotic fluid and the maternal blood. In the study by Fusi et al.,[53] although the maximum mean maternal temperature in the epidural group was approximately 37.7° C, the authors applied their results to those of the study by Morishima et al.,[7] in which detrimental maternal and fetal effects were produced by warming pregnant baboons to a temperature of approximately 42° C (107° F). Fusi et al.[53] did not report Apgar scores or umbilical cord blood gas or acid-base measurements.

In contrast, Camann et al.[54] argued that the small temperature rise seen with epidural analgesia is unlikely to affect the fetus. They concluded the following:

> The clinical significance of these findings remains unclear. Although statistically significant differences between extradural and non-extradural groups were noted in the mean temperature readings during labor, this difference did not exceed 1° C. The extradural patients, despite greater temperatures, were not clinically febrile, and there was only a weak correlation between maternal temperature and fetal heart rate. Thus, it is unlikely that this degree of temperature increase was sufficient to result in an adverse intrauterine environment with subsequent fetal compromise.[54]

Subsequently, Macaulay et al.[61] evaluated the effect of epidural analgesia on maternal oral, intrauterine, and fetal skin temperature during labor. The authors studied 57 women, 33 of whom received epidural analgesia and 24 of whom received either no analgesia, nitrous oxide, or intramuscular meperidine. The authors noted that the ambient temperatures ranged from 23.3° to 29° C. They reported a maximum fetal skin temperature greater than 38.0° C in 10 of 33 patients in the epidural group but in none of 24 in the no-epidural group. Three fetuses (all in the epidural group) developed estimated core temperatures of greater than 40.0° C. Conversely, only two women had an oral temperature greater than 37.5° C during the study. Administration of epidural analgesia did not affect Apgar scores or umbilical cord blood gas and acid-base measurements. The authors did not report neonatal temperature measurements. Nonetheless, they concluded that "the fetus whose mother has a long labor using epidural analgesia in a hot environment may reach a temperature at which heat-induced neurologic injury can occur."[61] They also cited the study of Morishima et al.,[7] in which detrimental maternal and

fetal effects were produced by warming pregnant baboons to near-lethal temperatures. They did not acknowledge other evidence that suggests that modest increases in temperature do not cause fetal injury and actually may increase fetal blood flow.[8,9] Nonetheless, the epidemiologic association between maternal fever and neonatal neurologic injuries suggests that efforts to avoid maternal fever—and to reduce fever when it occurs—may be warranted.

The neonate may also be placed at risk *indirectly* as a result of the interventions triggered by the occurrence of maternal fever.[57,58] Mayer et al.[58] retrospectively reviewed the records of 300 low-risk nulliparous women who received systemic opioids, epidural analgesia, or both (n = 100 per group). They found a 2% incidence of maternal fever in the opioid group, compared with an incidence of 16% and 24% in the two epidural groups. The incidence of intrapartum maternal antibiotic administration was 6% in those women who received systemic opioids only, versus 19% and 22% in the two groups of women who received epidural analgesia. Among the 10 patients with culture- or pathology-proven chorioamnionitis, none had fever as the *only* presenting sign or symptom. They concluded: "Rather than treating all women with temperature elevations and epidural [analgesia] for presumed chorioamnionitis, it is reasonable to target treatment to those with fetal tachycardia, meconium-stained fluid, or abnormal amniotic fluid studies."[58] Further, these authors suggested that "by seeking further evidence that the source of the fever is infectious prior to committing both the mother and her neonate to antibiotic therapy, one can limit. . . the use of antibiotics by about 50% without undertreating amnionitis."[58]

In another retrospective study, Lieberman et al.[57] reevaluated the records of 1657 low-risk nulliparous women originally enrolled in a trial of active management of labor. They too found a higher incidence of maternal temperature >38.0° C in parturients who received epidural analgesia compared with those who did not (15% versus 1%). Neonates in the epidural group had a higher incidence of sepsis evaluation (34% versus 10%) and antibiotic treatment (15% versus 4%) compared with neonates in the no-epidural group. The incidence of actual neonatal sepsis was exceedingly low in both groups (0.3% versus 0.2%). As in all studies in which women self-select their analgesia, the women receiving epidural analgesia were already at risk for intrapartum fever. (For example, they had larger infants, longer labors, and a twofold increase in the rate of induction.[57]) Moreover, the active labor management protocol mandated frequent cervical examinations and early amniotomy, which may have increased the risk of fever.[73] In contrast to most prospective studies of epidural analgesia-associated hyperthermia, the authors found fever even in women with labor of less than 6 hours' duration, which suggests the possibility that an increase in maternal temperature may have already begun at the time epidural analgesia was initiated.[68] Of interest, 63% of the sepsis evaluations occurred in infants of mothers who did *not* have intrapartum fever.[73] Because the authors did not provide data on the indications for sepsis evaluations, it is not possible to explain the association between these evaluations and the presence of epidural analgesia.

In a subsequent study, the same group of investigators analyzed a cohort in which intrapartum temperature remained below 100.4° F (38° C) throughout labor.[74] Neonatal sepsis evaluations were more common in women with epidural analgesia than those without (20% versus 9%) after controlling for gestational age, birth weight, maternal smoking history, active labor management, PROM, and admission cervical dilation. Epidural analgesia was associated with both major (rupture of membranes >24 hours, FHR >160 bpm) and minor criteria (maternal temperature >99.5° F [37.5° C] rupture of membranes for 12 to 24 hours) for sepsis evaluation. As with this group's earlier study, women were not randomized to receive epidural or intravenous opioid analgesia, and it is likely that many of the features of labor that led to sepsis evaluations also predisposed women to choose epidural analgesia.

Subsequent work by other investigators has suggested the paramount influence of maternal temperature elevation on the likelihood of neonatal sepsis evaluations. In the study of Philip et al.,[71] women randomized to receive epidural analgesia had more fever (>38° C [100.4° F]) than those randomized to receive intravenous opioid analgesia (15% versus 4%). Neonatal sepsis evaluations were also far more common in women with fever than in those without (96% versus 13%). However, within both the febrile and the afebrile cohorts, the incidence of neonatal sepsis evaluation was independent of the type of analgesia. The authors concluded:

> Our results indicate that in the absence of maternal fever, epidural analgesia during labor has no bearing on the need for such neonatal management and therefore should not be considered a predictor *per se* for neonatal sepsis evaluations. We attribute this finding to the minimization of ascertainment bias as a result of randomization of analgesia.[71]

Other investigators have highlighted the importance of neonatology practice style in determining the rate of sepsis evaluations. Yancey et al.[75] studied the rates of maternal fever and neonatal sepsis evaluation during a period in which the use of epidural analgesia rapidly increased from 1% to 83% following the introduction of a round-the-clock, on-demand epidural analgesia service. Fever >99.5° F (37.5° C) increased threefold and fever >100.4° F (38° C) increased 18-fold following the increased use of epidural analgesia, although numerous indices of the patients' admission status and intrapartum obstetric management did not change. There was a modest increase (relative risk = 1.5 to 1.7) in the incidence of neonatal laboratory testing (e.g., blood counts, blood cultures), but there was no change in the incidence of neonatal antibiotic treatment. The authors contrasted their results to those of Lieberman et al.,[57] and attributed the difference to neonatal practice patterns that did not require antibiotic therapy solely on the basis of maternal fever or antibiotic exposure.[75] Kaul et al.[76] also emphasized the importance of neonatology practice style. These authors reviewed the records of 1177 nulliparous women and their newborn babies. Women with epidural analgesia had more fever, longer duration of ruptured membranes, more instrumental and cesarean deliveries, and larger babies. However, the incidence of neonatal sepsis evaluation was not different between babies whose mothers did and did not receive epidural analgesia (7.5% versus 9.4%). The authors attributed the lower rate of neonatal sepsis evaluation and the lack of effect of epidural analgesia to the use of more stringent guidelines for neonatal sepsis evaluation, which specifically did not include maternal fever in the absence of clinical chorioamnionitis.[76]

In our judgment, published data do not support a conclusion that mild maternal hyperthermia *per se* adversely affects the fetus during labor. Inflammatory conditions associated with maternal fever and/or the decision to request epidural analgesia may have direct effects on the neonatal CNS as well as indirect effects on the practice of neonatologists. Further study of the effect of epidural analgesia on maternal and fetal temperature regulation is warranted. Perhaps pediatricians and neonatologists should attempt to develop practice guidelines that limit neonatal sepsis evaluations to infants who are at increased risk for infection. Efforts to understand the etiology of—and to prevent—noninfectious maternal temperature elevation associated with epidural analgesia are warranted. Meanwhile, we conclude that epidural analgesia is unlikely to cause hyperthermia of sufficient severity to adversely affect the fetus. When maternal pyrexia occurs, good clinical practice dictates that efforts be made to lower maternal temperature and identify and treat a presumed maternal infection.

SEPTIC SHOCK

Septic shock is a rare, life-threatening complication of maternal infection. This clinical syndrome is characterized by hypotension and multiorgan hypoperfusion and failure.[6] Septic shock largely is an effect of the mediators released from immune effector cells, including endotoxin, tumor necrosis factor, interleukins, and cyclooxygenase metabolites of arachidonic acid.[77] Antibodies directed against tumor necrosis factor, interleukin-1 antagonists, and nonsteroidal antiinflammatory agents are being tested to determine their efficacy in the treatment of septic shock.[77] Current evidence suggests that nitric oxide may be responsible for the vasodilation characteristic of septic shock. A preliminary study has suggested that inhibition of nitric oxide synthesis may increase blood pressure in patients with septic shock.[78]

In pregnant women, septic shock typically is associated with gram-negative bacteremia, although it can occur in association with gram-positive aerobic and anaerobic infections. Untreated chorioamnionitis, pyelonephritis, endometritis, wound infection, incomplete abortion, and self-induced abortion may result in maternal sepsis and septic shock. The mainstay of therapy is elimination and/or aggressive treatment of the source of infection. Antibiotic therapy should include broad-spectrum coverage for bacteria such as *E. coli*, enterococcus, and anaerobic organisms. A combination of ampicillin, gentamicin, and clindamycin represents an effective regimen, as does a combination of imipenem, cilastatin, and vancomycin.[77]

Laboratory studies have suggested that pregnancy makes laboratory animals more susceptible to infection or products of infection. Beller et al.[79] infused *E. coli* B6 lipopolysaccharide into both nonpregnant and pregnant minipigs. The average length of survival for the nonpregnant animals was 16 hours, whereas the average length of survival for the pregnant animals was only 3.5 hours. The pregnant animals suffered more pronounced cardiovascular abnormalities and metabolic acidosis. The authors concluded that pregnant minipigs are more susceptible to the harmful effects of lipopolysaccharide than nonpregnant minipigs. They acknowledged that it is unclear whether pregnant women are more susceptible to endotoxin than nonpregnant women. However, clinical studies have noted that once septic shock develops in pregnant patients, maternal mortality is as high as 30% to 66%.[80-82]

Only a few reports have described the management of these seriously ill patients. All reports have included single cases or a small number of patients. Lee et al.[81] reviewed 10 cases of septic shock in obstetric patients. Of the 10 women, 8 developed septic shock during the postpartum period. Risk factors included prolonged rupture of membranes (n = 2), retained products of conception (n = 3), and previous instrumentation of the genitourinary tract (n = 2); 2 of the 10 women died. Other maternal complications included adult respiratory distress syndrome (ARDS) (n = 3), disseminated intravascular coagulation (DIC) (n = 2), pulmonary edema (n = 1), and septic pulmonary embolus (n = 1). The primary hemodynamic abnormalities were decreased SVR and depressed myocardial function; three patients, including one who died, had markedly depressed myocardial function.

Mabie et al.[82] reported 18 cases of pregnancy-associated septic shock that occurred during 11 years in a single institution, with an incidence of 1 per 8338 deliveries. The most common etiologies were pyelonephritis (n = 6), chorioamnionitis (n = 3), endometritis (n = 2), and toxic shock syndrome (n = 2). Five (28%) patients died with infected products of conception or toxic shock syndrome. The hemodynamic profiles of the patients in this series were similar to those described by Lee et al.[61]; four of the five patients who died had mildly or severely depressed myocardial function.[82]

Complications of amniocentesis have recently been implicated in the etiology of septic shock.[83-86] In some cases, perfo-

ration of the bowel with the amniocentesis needle has been implicated, while in one case overwhelming Candida sepsis occurred in an immunocompetent woman.[84]

In most cases, concomitant supportive therapy is required to decrease maternal and fetal morbidity. Physicians must give attention to the maintenance of maternal oxygenation, circulation, and coagulation. These patients are at risk for respiratory, renal, and/or hepatic failure. Both Lee et al.[81] and Mabie et al.,[82] as well as the American College of Obstetricians and Gynecologists (ACOG),[77] agree that the mainstay of therapy is eradication of the infectious source. Hemodynamic management should begin with rapid infusion of crystalloid (1 to 2 L), with subsequent fluid and pharmacologic therapy guided by hemodynamic data obtained from a pulmonary artery catheter. A management scheme based on these authors' recommendations is shown in Figure 36-3, and inotropic and vasoactive drugs useful in the treatment of these patients are shown in Table 36-1.

Although the effects of maternal therapy on the fetus should be considered, treatment of the mother has first priority. Often what is best for the mother will be best for the fetus. However, in some cases, maternal sepsis may require preterm

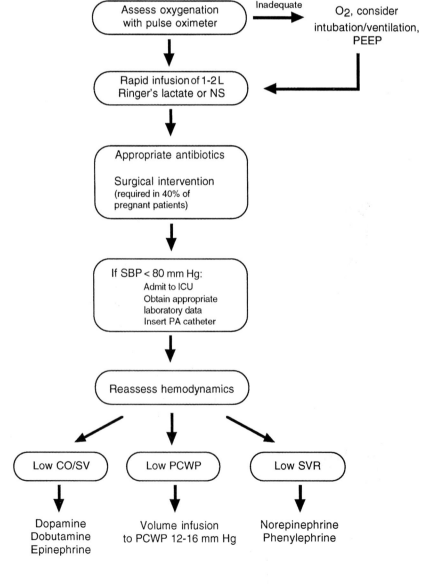

FIGURE 36-3. Management algorithm for obstetric septic shock. *CO,* cardiac output; *ICU,* intensive care unit; *NS,* Normal saline; *PA,* pulmonary artery; *PCWP,* pulmonary capillary wedge pressure; *PEEP,* positive end-expiratory pressure; *SBP,* Systolic blood pressure; *SV,* stroke volume; *SVR,* systemic vascular resistance. (Adapted from Lee W, Clark SL, Cotton DB, et al. Septic shock during pregnancy. Am J Obstet Gynecol 1988; 159:410-6; Mabie WC, Baron JR, Sibai BM. Septic shock in pregnancy. Obstet Gynecol 1997; 90:553-61; and American College of Obstetricians and Gynecologists. Septic Shock. ACOG Technical Bulletin No. 204, April 1995.)

TABLE 36-1	SYMPATHOMIMETIC AND VASOPRESSOR DRUGS USEFUL FOR TREATMENT OF OBSTETRIC SEPTIC SHOCK	
Agent	**Maintenance dose range**	
Dopamine	1-10 μg/kg/min	
Dobutamine	2-10 μg/kg/min	
Epinephrine	1-8 μg/min	
Norepinephrine	2-8 μg/min	
Phenylephrine	20-200 μg/min	

Modified from Lee W, Clark SL, Cotton DB, et al. Septic shock during pregnancy. Am J Obstet Gynecol 1988; 159:410-6, and American College of Obstetricians and Gynecologists. Septic Shock. ACOG Technical Bulletin No. 204, April 1995.

delivery before the age of viability. The ACOG recommends delivery only in cases in which the pregnancy itself is the source of the infection.[77]

REGIONAL ANESTHESIA IN THE FEBRILE PATIENT

Clinical Studies

Clinicians have long suspected an association between the performance of dural puncture during a period of bacteremia and the subsequent development of meningitis. Some clinicians have feared that diagnostic lumbar puncture may cause meningitis rather than aid in its diagnosis. They reasoned that lumbar puncture may disrupt the rich venous plexus surrounding the spinal cord and allow the direct introduction of infected blood into the CNS by the spinal needle. Alternatively, some have speculated that disruption of the dural barrier may permit hematogenous spread of infection into the CNS without direct vessel trauma. Similar concerns apply to the performance of epidural anesthesia and the development of epidural abscess (see Chapter 33). Administration of continuous epidural analgesia often results in blood vessel trauma, and it almost always includes the introduction of a foreign body. Theoretically, this technique could produce a nidus for subsequent infection.

At least six retrospective clinical studies have evaluated the risk of diagnostic lumbar puncture.[87-92] (These studies did not evaluate the administration of regional anesthesia.) These reports provided conflicting conclusions regarding the risk of meningitis after the performance of dural puncture in bacteremic patients. Two studies suggested an association between dural puncture and meningitis.[87,90] However, both studies had serious methodologic flaws. One study was performed during an epidemic of meningitis.[87] Although the authors observed a high rate of meningitis after lumbar puncture, they did not evaluate a comparable control group who did not undergo lumbar puncture. Teele et al.[90] reported an association between lumbar puncture and meningitis only in bacteremic children less than 1 year of age. However, they acknowledged the possibility that clinical judgment might have prompted their pediatricians to perform diagnostic lumbar puncture in children with incipient meningitis before the cerebrospinal fluid (CSF) provided diagnostic evidence of infection.

The remaining four studies clearly did not support an association between dural puncture and meningitis.[88,89,91,92] Shapiro et al.[92] concluded the following:

The development of bacterial meningitis in children with occult bacteremia is strongly associated with the species of bacteria that causes the infection, but not with a lumbar puncture. . . . Children with high-density bacteremia may appear to be more severely ill than children who have bacteremia with lower concentrations of bacteria, and therefore may be more likely to undergo a lumbar puncture.

Chestnut[93] stated, "Physicians often perform diagnostic lumbar puncture in patients with fever and/or bacteremia of unknown origin. If dural puncture during bacteremia results in meningitis, one would expect that unequivocal clinical data should exist." However, no epidemiologic study has clearly established a causal relationship between the performance of dural puncture during bacteremia and the subsequent development of meningitis or epidural abscess. Part of the uncertainty regarding the risk of dural puncture results from awareness that processes other than meningeal integrity may help protect against the occurrence of CNS infection. For example, as many as 35% of epidural catheters used postoperatively are colonized by bacteria, but epidural abscess is a *very rare* complication.[94]

Some anesthesiologists have cited anecdotal reports of meningitis after spinal anesthesia during presumed bacteremia as evidence that dural puncture may cause meningitis.[95-98] In one of these reports, the physicians used reusable equipment, and the source of infection was traced to inadequately sterilized supplies.[95] The use of sterile, disposable equipment and strict attention to aseptic technique have largely eliminated these factors as a source of infection.

However, most evidence points to external contamination, not blood-borne pathogens, as the source of meningitis after spinal anesthesia. Kilpatrick and Girgis[97] reported 17 cases of meningitis after spinal anesthesia in nonpregnant patients. In 10 cases CSF cultures were positive, and all grew unusual or nosocomial organisms. Ready and Helfer[99] reported two cases of meningitis after the administration of epidural anesthesia in obstetric patients. Both patients were afebrile and without clinical signs of infection at the time of epidural catheter placement. The epidural catheter was in place for less than 1 hour in one of the two patients. Davis et al.[100] reported a case of postpartum meningitis after administration of epidural analgesia during labor. The meningitis apparently was caused by a group B beta-hemolytic streptococcus that was cultured from the patient's blood and vagina. Videira et al.[101] reported three cases of meningitis following 38,128 spinal anesthetics (i.e., an incidence of 1:12,709). In two cases, streptococci presumed to be skin flora were cultured. The authors concluded that lapses in sterile technique may have been responsible for the meningitis. Likewise, in another report, poor attention to asepsis was apparently responsible for three cases of meningitis occurring in a 3-year period in a single hospital.[102] In one case, the offending organism was cultured from the nose of the anesthesiologist performing the block.

Several reports have recently described the occurrence of meningitis after the administration of combined spinal-epidural (CSE) analgesia in obstetric patients.[103-105] None of these patients was febrile during administration of CSE analgesia. Further, in the cases with positive CSF cultures, the authors concluded that contamination by skin flora was the most likely mechanism of infection. There is no evidence that supports a conclusion that use of the CSE technique is associated with an increased risk of meningitis. Rather, these anecdotal cases likely reflect a reporting bias that resulted in the publication of complications associated with the use of a relatively new technique.[106]

Large epidemiologic studies have found a very low incidence of CNS infection after the administration of regional anesthesia. Dripps and Vandam[107] prospectively studied 8460 patients who received 10,098 spinal anesthetics between 1948 and 1951. Similarly, Phillips et al.[108] reported the administration of spinal anesthesia to 10,440 patients between 1964 and 1966. A large number of the patients in both studies underwent obstetric or urologic procedures. Undoubtedly some patients had bacteremia during or after the performance of spinal anesthesia. However, neither study reported a single case of CNS infection.[107,108] Similarly, four reviews of more than 500,000 obstetric patients who received epidural anesthesia reported no cases of meningitis and only two cases of epidural space infection.[109-112] Undoubtedly some of these parturients were bacteremic during the administration of epidural anesthesia, given the frequency with which parturients develop fever and infection during labor. For example, Blanco et al.[22] found a 1% incidence of bacteremia in a random sample of patients on the labor ward. Other studies have noted an 8% to 10% incidence of bacteremia in parturients with chorioamnionitis.[19-21,24]

Unfortunately, there are no good predictive factors for identifying the subgroup of febrile patients with chorioamnionitis who are bacteremic at the time of anesthesia. The severity of fever does not reliably predict the likelihood of bacteremia in these patients. For example, Blanco et al.[22] reported that 86 (49%) of 176 patients with documented bacteremia had a temperature below 38.8° C. Furthermore, Bader et al.[113] reported no significant difference between the mean temperatures of bacteremic and nonbacteremic patients with chorioamnionitis. Similarly, in a study of 146 women with chorioamnionitis, Goodman et al.[24] found no differences in temperature, leukocytosis, or maternal symptoms between patients with positive or negative blood cultures.

Bader et al.[113] retrospectively observed no cases of CNS infection after the administration of epidural or spinal anesthesia for labor and/or cesarean section in 279 patients with chorioamnionitis. Only 43 of these 279 women received antibiotic therapy before the administration of regional anesthesia. At least three women had positive blood cultures consistent with bacteremia, and none of these three women received antibiotics before the administration of anesthesia. Similarly, Ramanathan et al.[114] reviewed their experience with administration of epidural anesthesia in 113 parturients with chorioamnionitis. The diagnosis of chorioamnionitis was made before the placement of the epidural catheter in 39 of these 113 women. Antibiotic therapy was begun soon after the diagnosis of chorioamnionitis in most patients; in 16 women, antibiotic therapy was delayed until after delivery. None of these 113 patients developed any signs or symptoms of bacterial meningitis or epidural abscess. More recently, Goodman et al.[24] found no cases of meningitis or epidural abscess among 531 patients with chorioamnionitis (proven by culture or pathologic examination) who received epidural (n = 517) or spinal (n = 14) anesthesia. Eleven of 45 patients with fever before initiation of the block and 174 of 229 patients with pre-existing leukocytosis received no antibiotics before instrumentation of the epidural or subarachnoid space.

Together, clinical studies suggest that meningitis or epidural abscess is a very rare complication of epidural or spinal anesthesia. Further, bacteremia itself does not appear to increase the risk of CNS infection after the administration of

regional anesthesia. However, published studies of regional anesthesia in patients with chorioamnionitis were small and retrospective. Given the infrequent occurrence of CNS infection among noninfected patients undergoing regional anesthesia, none of these studies was sufficiently large to exclude the possibility that chorioamnionitis increases the risk of meningitis or epidural abscess. Moreover, the retrospective study design introduces the possibility of selection bias. That is, the anesthesiologists may have avoided regional anesthesia in the sickest patients with chorioamnionitis.

Laboratory Studies

Carp and Bailey[115] performed a study to assess the risk of meningitis after the performance of dural puncture in bacteremic animals. In this study, rats were made bacteremic by producing a flank abscess using *E. coli* bacteria. The bacteremia was similar in magnitude to that which occurs during the early phase of sepsis in humans. Cisternal dural puncture was performed after the onset of bacteremia. After 24 hours, the cisterna magna was drained surgically, and the CSF was cultured for evidence of meningitis. Of the 40 animals that underwent dural puncture during *E. coli* bacteremia, 12 developed meningitis (Table 36-2). None of the 40 bacteremic animals not subjected to dural puncture developed meningitis. Further, dural puncture did not result in infection in the 30 animals without bacteremia. Importantly, *none* of the 30 bacteremic animals given a dose of gentamicin 15 minutes before dural puncture developed meningitis.

This study augments earlier laboratory studies that observed the development of meningitis after the performance of dural puncture in bacteremic laboratory animals.[116-118] Although animal models of disease permit careful control of experimental conditions, these studies do not duplicate clinical conditions. Thus there are limitations in the application of this study to clinical practice.[115] First, the level of bacteremia produced in the rats exceeded the transient, low-grade bacteremia that often occurs clinically. Also, these animals most likely had hemodynamic and metabolic changes characteristic of early sepsis. Second, although *E. coli* is a common cause of bacteremia in surgical and obstetric patients, it is an uncommon cause of meningitis. Third, the relative size of the dural

TABLE 36-2	THE ASSOCIATION BETWEEN BACTEREMIA AND THE RECOVERY OF *E. COLI* FROM CSF AFTER DURAL PUNCTURE			
n	**Bacteremia (CFU/ml)***	**Gentamicin†**	**Dural puncture**	**CSF *E. coli*‡**
40	40 ± 22 (5-100)	No	Yes	12/40§
40	48 ± 25¶ (2-100)	No	No	0/40
30	0 (0)	No	Yes	0/30
30	49 ± 35 (5-110)	Yes	Yes	0/30

n, Number of rats in each group.
*Data expressed as mean ± SD (range in parentheses).
†Gentamicin administered before dural puncture.
‡Data expressed as the number of animals with *E. coli* cultured from spinal fluid per total number of animals in that group.
§*P* < 0.05 compared with other groups.
¶Not significantly different compared with the bacteremic groups undergoing cisternal puncture.
Modified from Carp H, Bailey S. The association between meningitis and dural puncture in bacteremic rats. Anesthesiology 1992; 76:739-42.

tear produced by the 26-gauge needle used in this study is greater in rats compared with that in humans. Fourth, the cisternal site of dural puncture is not used clinically. Fifth, spinal and epidural anesthesia involves the injection of local anesthetics, and these drugs appear to be bacteriostatic.[119] Finally, the investigators knew the identity of the organism (e.g., *E. coli*) and also knew that it was susceptible to gentamicin.

In summary, this study suggests that high-grade bacteremia may increase the risk of meningitis after dural puncture. However, antibiotic therapy before dural puncture appears to reduce if not eliminate this risk.

Recommendations

In our judgment, the anesthesiologist may safely give spinal or epidural anesthesia to healthy patients at risk for bacteremia. The anesthesiologist need not avoid administration of regional anesthesia in patients at risk for transient, low-grade bacteremia after the administration of anesthesia. Moreover, appropriate antibiotic therapy may lessen the risk of meningitis or epidural abscess in patients with established infection. In our practice, we administer spinal or epidural anesthesia to patients with evidence of systemic infection, provided that appropriate antibiotic therapy has begun. Thus it often is appropriate for the anesthesiologist to request the institution of antibiotic therapy before administration of anesthesia. Finally, although the choice of anesthesia must be individualized, it seems prudent to avoid spinal or epidural anesthesia in untreated patients with overt clinical signs of sepsis.

Chestnut[93] reviewed this subject and concluded the following:

> We do not give regional anesthesia in the absence of other relevant information. Rather, we provide care for febrile patients who require anesthesia for labor, delivery, or emergency surgery. When one considers the risks of infection with regional anesthesia, one should ask: What are the alternatives? What are the consequences of withholding regional anesthesia in a febrile patient? For example, what is the greater risk in a febrile parturient: meningitis or epidural abscess after spinal or epidural anesthesia, or failed intubation and aspiration during general anesthesia?

Finally, both physicians and patients should recognize that most cases of meningitis and epidural abscess occur spontaneously. Eng and Seligman[89] concluded, "Even if an appropriate temporal sequence . . . is documented . . . one cannot differentiate spontaneous meningitis from lumbar puncture-induced meningitis in the individual patient."

GENITAL HERPES INFECTION

The herpes simplex virus type 2 (HSV-2) causes a locally recurring disease that is characterized by asymptomatic periods interrupted by episodes of viral reactivation from sites in the sensory ganglia.[6] Genital herpes infection typically presents as painful vesicular or papular lesions on the skin or mucous membranes of the genital tract, including the labia, vulva, perineum, cervix, and urethra. Primary maternal HSV-2 infection is associated with transient viremia.[120] Patients with primary infection often have systemic symptoms, including fever, headache, and lymphadenopathy. Hepatitis, aseptic meningitis, encephalitis, and cauda equina syndrome are uncommon complications of primary genital herpes infection. During recurrent (i.e., secondary) infection, maternal antibodies prevent the recurrence of viremia. Thus systemic symptoms are less severe—or do not occur at all—during episodes of recurrent infection. However, recurrent infection may result in severe symptoms localized to the site of the lesions on the external genitalia. Unfortunately, asymptomatic shedding of the virus also may occur in the genital tract.

Interaction with Pregnancy

During the first 20 weeks of pregnancy, primary genital herpes infection may be associated with an increase in the frequency of pregnancy loss and congenital malformations,[121] although recent cohort studies have disputed the risk of fetal death.[122] However, the major obstetric concern is the potential for transmission of the virus to the infant at the time of birth. The infant may become infected in one of two ways. First, infection can occur as the fetus comes in direct contact with the virus during vaginal delivery. Second, intrauterine infection can occur by ascent of the organism after rupture of membranes. Neonatal HSV infection is a life-threatening infection with the potential for permanent CNS sequelae.[6,120,121] The severity of the neonatal infection may be modified by the early institution of antiviral therapy.[123] Retrospective studies suggest that the risk of neonatal HSV infection associated with a primary maternal infection is much greater than that associated with recurrent maternal infection or asymptomatic shedding of the virus.[121,124-126] Most likely there is a greater risk that the infant will be exposed to the virus during episodes of primary maternal infection.

Obstetric Management

The ACOG has reviewed the obstetric management of parturients with HSV infections and has concluded the following[125]:

> It is now well established that abdominal delivery in women with active infection, especially primary infection, will significantly reduce the risk and incidence of neonatal HSV infection. Cesarean delivery, however, will not prevent all cases of neonatal infection. Currently it is recommended that term patients who have visible lesions and are in labor or who have ruptured membranes should undergo cesarean delivery. Although it has been classically taught that cesarean delivery of women with visible lesions should be performed if membranes have been ruptured for less than 4-6 hours, not all neonates born to mothers with HSV infections become infected even with membranes ruptured for more than 24 hours. In contrast, neonates born within 2 hours of ruptured membranes have developed HSV infection. For patients with active HSV infections and premature rupture of membranes remote from term, there are not enough data to recommend a management protocol that would apply in all clinical situations. The risk of extreme immaturity must be weighed against the risk of neonatal HSV infection.

A large epidemiologic study of 58,362 women recently provided the first direct evidence that cesarean section dramatically reduces the overall risk of HSV transmission to the neonate when HSV cultures of the cervix and external genitalia taken at the time of labor are positive (odds ratio = 0.14).[127] Other risk factors for neonatal infection include maternal HSV seronegativity, positive cervical culture for HSV, use of invasive fetal monitoring, and HSV-1 (versus HSV-2) isolation at the time of labor.[127]

Of interest, the mothers of most infants infected with HSV have no history of HSV infection and no obvious lesions at the time of delivery.[125,126] Previously, it was thought that antenatal viral cultures could predict asymptomatic viral shedding at the time of delivery and reduce the incidence of neonatal infection. Unfortunately, there is little correlation between antepartum HSV culture results and viral shedding at the time of delivery, even in women with a history of previous HSV infection.[126] However, recent studies support the value of prophylactic acyclovir in reducing the occurrence of viral lesions during late pregnancy in women with a history of HSV infection.[128,129]

Apparently, asymptomatic shedding is both infrequent and transient, and antenatal cultures may not reflect the situation at the time of delivery. Current clinical recommendations suggest that the route of delivery should be guided by a careful pelvic examination after the onset of labor rather than by antepartum viral cultures. The ACOG has stated, "If there are no visible lesions at the onset of labor, vaginal delivery is acceptable."[125]

Anesthetic Management

There are at least four published retrospective studies of the use of regional anesthesia in patients with genital herpes infection. These studies reported no serious neurologic sequelae related to the use of regional anesthesia.[114,130-132] However, most of the patients in these studies had recurrent (secondary) infection. Two studies[114,131] were limited to patients with recurrent infection, and a third study[130] did not indicate whether the patients had primary or recurrent infection. Bader et al.[132] reported outcome for 169 women with genital herpes infection who underwent cesarean section:

> None of the 164 patients with secondary infections had septic or neurologic complications related to the type of anesthetic administered. Therefore, it is our practice to use either spinal or epidural anesthesia when possible for cesarean delivery in these patients.

Only 5 of the 169 women in this study had primary infections, and 3 of those women received spinal anesthesia. Of those 3 women, 1 had transient, postoperative weakness of the left leg. The authors[132] stated the following:

> None of the cases of primary infection had associated systemic symptoms; it is therefore possible that some of these cases were actually misdiagnosed recurrent infections. The safety of regional anesthesia in patients with primary HSV infection remains unclear.

Viremia may accompany primary episodes of genital herpes infection. However, viremia rarely complicates recurrent episodes of genital herpes infection. It is unlikely that a spinal or epidural needle could introduce virus into the CNS in patients with recurrent genital herpes infection. Thus there is consensus that it is safe to give spinal or epidural anesthesia in women with recurrent genital herpes infection and no systemic symptoms. There are insufficient data to allow a definitive recommendation regarding the safety of regional anesthesia in patients with primary infection who may be viremic. When the anesthesiologist confronts a patient with primary infection, the theoretical risk of CNS infection should be weighed against the risks of alternative methods of analgesia and anesthesia.

Finally, several studies have suggested that postcesarean spinal or epidural administration of morphine increases the incidence of recurrence of oral HSV infection (e.g., HSV-1).

This phenomenon was confirmed in a prospective randomized trial.[133] The exact etiology is unknown, but some investigators have speculated that pruritus and scratching play a role. Boyle[134] concluded that facial pruritus is a marker of the migration of morphine to the trigeminal nucleus but not the cause of HSV-1 recrudescence. Boyle[134] suggested that immunologic modulation by the opioid within this ganglion is the primary cause of the viral reactivation. To our knowledge, there are no reports suggesting that epidural or intrathecal administration of opioids increases the risk of recurrent *genital* herpes infection.

KEY POINTS

- Fever may be produced by endogenous pyrogens released from immune effector cells in response to infection.
- Fetal temperature typically is slightly greater than maternal temperature.
- Modest maternal fever does not seem to adversely affect the fetus, but maternal infection and other inflammatory states may cause fetal neurologic injury.
- Pyelonephritis and chorioamnionitis are the antepartum infections most likely to result in maternal and perinatal morbidity and mortality.
- Septic shock is an uncommon but devastating complication of maternal infection that demands aggressive hemodynamic support, broad-spectrum antibiotic therapy, and in some cases, surgical intervention.
- Epidural analgesia may produce a modest increase in maternal temperature. No study has shown that the modest increase in maternal temperature associated with epidural analgesia adversely affects the fetus. However, maternal fever during labor may prompt the neonatologist to evaluate the neonate for possible sepsis.
- The anesthesiologist may safely administer epidural or spinal anesthesia to patients at risk for transient bacteremia.
- The anesthesiologist may safely administer epidural or spinal anesthesia to patients with established infection, provided there is no evidence of frank sepsis. However, it seems prudent to begin antibiotic therapy before the administration of anesthesia.
- Recurrent genital herpes infection does not contraindicate the administration of regional anesthesia.

REFERENCES

1. Wunderlich C. Das Verhalten der Eiaenwarme in Krankenheiten. Leipzig, Germany: Ott Wigard, 1868.
2. Mackowiak PA, Wasserman SS, Levine MM. A critical appraisal of 98.6 degrees F, the upper limit of the normal body temperature, and other legacies of Carl Reinhold August Wunderlich. Jama 1992; 268:1578-80.
3. Beutler B, Beutler AM. The pathogenesis of fever. In: Wyngaarden JB, Smith LH, Bennett JC, eds. Textbook of Medicine. Philadelphia: WB Saunders, 1992:1568-71.

4. Novy MJ, Liggins GC. Role of prostaglandins, prostacyclin, and thromboxanes in the physiologic control of the uterus and in parturition. Semin Perinatol 1980; 4:45-66.

5. Walker DW, Wood C. Temperature relationship of the mother and fetus during labor. Am J Obstet Gynecol 1970; 107:83-7.

6. Gibbs RS, Sweet RL. Maternal and fetal infections. In: Creasy RK, Resnik R, eds. Maternal-Fetal medicine: Principles and Practice. Philadelphia: WB Saunders, 1989:656-725.

7. Morishima HO, Glaser B, Niemann WH, James LS. Increased uterine activity and fetal deterioration during maternal hyperthermia. Am J Obstet Gynecol 1975; 121:531-8.

8. Cefalo RC, Hellegers AE. The effects of maternal hyperthermia on maternal and fetal cardiovascular and respiratory function. Am J Obstet Gynecol 1978; 131:687-94.

9. Harris WH, Pittman QJ, Veale WL, et al. Cardiovascular effects of fever in the ewe and fetal lamb. Am J Obstet Gynecol 1977; 128:262-5.

10. Lieberman E, Lang J, Richardson DK, et al. Intrapartum maternal fever and neonatal outcome. Pediatrics 2000; 105:8-13.

11. Lieberman E, Eichenwald E, Mathur G, et al. Intrapartum fever and unexplained seizures in term infants. Pediatrics 2000; 106:983-8.

12. Perlman JM. Maternal fever and neonatal depression: Preliminary observations. Clin Pediatr 1999; 38:287-91.

13. Grether JK, Nelson KB. Maternal infection and cerebral palsy in infants of normal birth weight. JAMA 1997; 278:207-11.

14. Impey L, Greenwood C, MacQuillan K, et al. Fever in labour and neonatal encephalopathy: A prospective cohort study. BJOG 2001; 108:594-7.

15. Dammann O, Drescher J, Veelken N. Maternal fever at birth and nonverbal intelligence at age 9 years in preterm infants. Dev Med Child Neurol 2003; 45:148-51.

16. Yoon BH, Romero R, Park JS, et al. Fetal exposure to an intra-amniotic inflammation and the development of cerebral palsy at the age of three years. Am J Obstet Gynecol 2000; 182:675-81.

17. Shipp TD, Zelop C, Cohen A, et al. Post-cesarean delivery fever and uterine rupture in a subsequent trial of labor. Obstet Gynecol 2003; 101:136-9.

18. Lieberman E, Cohen A, Lang J, et al. Maternal intrapartum temperature elevation as a risk factor for cesarean delivery and assisted vaginal delivery. Am J Pub Health 1999; 89:506-10.

19. Gibbs RS, Castillo MS, Rodgers PJ. Management of acute chorioamnionitis. Am J Obstet Gynecol 1980; 136:709-13.

20. Duff P, Sanders R, Gibbs RS. The course of labor in term patients with chorioamnionitis. Am J Obstet Gynecol 1983; 147:391-5.

21. Yoder PR, Gibbs RS, Blanco JD, et al. A prospective, controlled study of maternal and perinatal outcome after intra-amniotic infection at term. Am J Obstet Gynecol 1983; 145:695-701.

22. Blanco JD, Gibbs RS, Castaneda YS. Bacteremia in obstetrics: clinical course. Obstet Gynecol 1981; 58:621-5.

23. Satin AJ, Maberry MC, Leveno KJ, et al. Chorioamnionitis: a harbinger of dystocia. Obstet Gynecol 1992; 79:913-5.

24. Goodman EJ, DeHorta E, Taguiam JM. Safety of spinal and epidural anesthesia in parturients with chorioamnionitis. Reg Anesth 1996; 21:436-41.

25. Qureshi F, Jacques SM, Bendon RW, et al. Candida funisitis: A clinicopathologic study of 32 cases. Pediatr Dev Pathol 1998; 1:118-24.

26. Ustun C, Kocak I, Baris S, et al. Subclinical chorioamnionitis as an etiologic factor in preterm deliveries. Internat J Gynaecol Obstet 2001; 72:109-15.

27. Tran TS, Jamulitrat S, Chongsuvivatwong V, Geater A. Risk factors for postcesarean surgical site infection. Obstet Gynecol 2000; 95:367-71.

28. Mark SP, Croughan-Minihane MS, Kilpatrick SJ. Chorioamnionitis and uterine function. Obstet Gynecol 2000; 95:909-12.

29. Gaudet LM, Smith GN. Cerebral palsy and chorioamnionitis: The inflammatory cytokine link. Obstet Gynecol Surv 2001; 56:433-6.

30. Wu YW. Systematic review of chorioamnionitis and cerebral palsy. Ment Retard Dev Disabil Res Rev 2002; 8:25-9.

31. Wu YW, Colford JM, Jr. Chorioamnionitis as a risk factor for cerebral palsy: A meta-analysis. Jama 2000; 284:1417-24.

32. Resch B, Vollaard E, Maurer U, et al. Risk factors and determinants of neurodevelopmental outcome in cystic periventricular leucomalacia. Eur J Pediatr 2000; 159:663-70.

33. Shimoya K, Taniguchi T, Matsuzaki N, et al. Chorioamnionitis decreased incidence of respiratory distress syndrome by elevating fetal interleukin-6 serum concentration. Hum Reprod 2000; 15:2234-40.

34. Schmidt B, Cao L, Mackensen-Haen S, et al. Chorioamnionitis and inflammation of the fetal lung. Am J Obstet Gynecol 2001; 185:173-7.

35. Van Marter LJ, Dammann O, Allred EN, et al. Chorioamnionitis, mechanical ventilation, and postnatal sepsis as modulators of chronic lung disease in preterm infants. J Pediatr 2002; 140:171-6.

36. Mead PB. When to treat intra-amniotic infection. Obstet Gynecol 1988; 72:935-6.

37. Gibbs RS, Dinsmoor MJ, Newton ER, Ramamurthy RS. A randomized trial of intrapartum versus immediate postpartum treatment of women with intra-amniotic infection. Obstet Gynecol 1988; 72:823-8.

38. Gilstrap LC, Leveno KJ, Cox SM, et al. Intrapartum treatment of acute chorioamnionitis: impact on neonatal sepsis. Am J Obstet Gynecol 1988; 159:579-83.

39. Gilstrap LC, Cunningham FG, Whalley PJ. Acute pyelonephritis in pregnancy: An anteorspective study. Obstet Gynecol 1974; 57:409-13.

40. Kass EH. Bacteriuria and pyelonephritis of pregnancy. Arch Intern Med 1960; 205:194-205.

41. Wing DA. Pyelonephritis in pregnancy: Treatment options for optimal outcomes. Drugs 2001; 61:2087-96.

42. Schaeffer AJ. Experimental gestational pyelonephritis induces preterm births and low birth weights in C3H/HeJ mice. J Urol 2000; 164:260-1.

43. Cunningham FG, Lucas MJ, Hankins GD. Pulmonary injury complicating antepartum pyelonephritis. Am J Obstet Gynecol 1987; 156:797-807.

44. Towers CV, Kaminskas CM, Garite TJ, et al. Pulmonary injury associated with antepartum pyelonephritis: can patients at risk be identified? Am J Obstet Gynecol 1991; 164:974-8; discussion 978-80.

45. Twickler DM, Lucas MJ, Bowe L, et al. Ultrasonographic evaluation of central and end-organ hemodynamics in antepartum pyelonephritis. Am J Obstet Gynecol 1994; 170:814-8.

46. Smaill F. Antibiotics for asymptomatic bacteriuria in pregnancy. Cochrane Database Syst Rev 2000:CD000490.

47. Leontic EA. Respiratory disease in pregnancy. Med Clin North Am 1977; 61:111-28.

48. Benedetti TJ, Valle R, Ledger WJ. Antepartum pneumonia in pregnancy. Am J Obstet Gynecol 1982; 144:413-7.

49. Landsberger EJ, Hager WD, Grossman JH. Successful management of varicella pneumonia complicating pregnancy. A report of three cases. J Reprod Med 1986; 31:311-4.

50. Ahmad H, Mehta NJ, Manikal VM, et al. *Pneumocystis carinii* pneumonia in pregnancy. Chest 2001; 120:666-71.

51. Smaill F, Hofmeyr GJ. Antibiotic prophylaxis for cesarean section. Cochrane Database Syst Rev 2002:CD000933.

52. Matsukawa T, Sessler DI, Christensen R, et al. Heat flow and distribution during epidural anesthesia. Anesthesiology 1995; 83:961-7.

53. Fusi L, Steer PJ, Maresh MJ, Beard RW. Maternal pyrexia associated with the use of epidural analgesia in labour. Lancet 1989; 1:1250-2.

54. Camann WR, Hortvet LA, Hughes N, Bader AM, Datta S. Maternal temperature regulation during extradural analgesia for labour. Br J Anaesth 1991; 67:565-8.

55. Vinson DC, Thomas R, Kiser T. Association between epidural analgesia during labor and fever. J Fam Pract 1993; 36:617-22.

56. Ploeckinger B, Ulm MR, Chalubinski K, Gruber W. Epidural anaesthesia in labour: influence on surgical delivery rates, intrapartum fever and blood loss. Gynecol Obstet Invest 1995; 39:24-7.

57. Lieberman E, Lang JM, Frigoletto F, et al. Epidural analgesia, intrapartum fever, and neonatal sepsis evaluation. Pediatrics 1997; 99:415-9.

58. Mayer DC, Chescheir NC, Spielman FJ. Increased intrapartum antibiotic administration associated with epidural analgesia in labor. Am J Perinatol 1997; 14:83-6.

59. Herbst A, Wolner-Hanssen P, Ingemarsson I. Risk factors for fever in labor. Obstet Gynecol 1995; 86:790-4.

60. Vallejo MC, Kaul B, Adler LJ, et al. Chorioamnionitis, not epidural analgesia, is associated with maternal fever during labour. Can J Anaesth 2001; 48:1122-6.

61. Macaulay JH, Bond K, Steer PJ. Epidural analgesia in labor and fetal hyperthermia. Obstet Gynecol 1992; 80:665-9.

62. Goodlin RC, Chapin JW. Determinants of maternal temperature during labor. Am J Obstet Gynecol 1982; 143:97-103.

63. Glosten B, Savage M, Rooke GA, Brengelmann GL. Epidural anesthesia and the thermoregulatory responses to hyperthermia—preliminary observations in volunteer subjects. Acta Anaesthesiol Scand 1998; 42:442-6.

64. Hagerdal M, Morgan CW, Sumner AE, Gutsche BB. Minute ventilation and oxygen consumption during labor with epidural analgesia. Anesthesiology 1983; 59:425-7.

65. Gross JB, Cohen AP, Lang JM, et al. Differences in systemic opioid use do not explain increased fever incidence in parturients receiving epidural analgesia. Anesthesiology 2002; 97:157-61.

66. Gleeson NC, Nolan KM, Ford MR. Temperature, labour, and epidural analgesia. Lancet 1989; 2:861-2.

67. Panzer O, Ghazanfari N, Sessler DI, et al. Shivering and shivering-like tremor during labor with and without epidural analgesia. Anesthesiology 1999; 90:1609-16.

68. Dolak JA, Brown RE. Epidural analgesia and neonatal fever. Pediatrics 1998; 101:492; author reply 493-4.

69. Dashe JS, Rogers BB, McIntire DD, Leveno KJ. Epidural analgesia and intrapartum fever: placental findings. Obstet Gynecol 1999; 93:341-4.

70. Goetzl L, Evans T, Rivers J, et al. Elevated maternal and fetal serum interleukin-6 levels are associated with epidural fever. Am J Obstet Gynecol 2002; 187:834-8.

71. Philip J, Alexander JM, Sharma SK, et al. Epidural analgesia during labor and maternal fever. Anesthesiology 1999; 90:1271-5.

72. Leighton BL, Halpern SH. The effects of epidural analgesia on labor, maternal, and neonatal outcomes: A systematic review. Am J Obstet Gynecol 2002; 186:S69-77.

73. Tarshis J, Camann WR, Datta S. Epidural analgesia and neonatal fever (letter). Pediatrics 1998; 101:490-1.

74. Goetzl L, Cohen A, Frigoletto F, et al. Maternal epidural use and neonatal sepsis evaluation in afebrile mothers. Pediatrics 2001; 108:1099-102.

75. Yancey MK, Zhang J, Schwarz J, et al. Labor epidural analgesia and intrapartum maternal hyperthermia. Obstet Gynecol 2001; 98:763-70.

76. Kaul B, Vallejo M, Ramanathan S, Mandell G. Epidural labor analgesia and neonatal sepsis evaluation rate: A quality improvement study. Anesth Analg 2001; 93:986-90.

77. American College of Obstetricians and Gynecologists. Septic Shock. ACOG Technical Bulletin No. 204, April 1995.

78. Petros A, Bennett D, Vallance P. Effect of nitric oxide synthase inhibitors on hypotension in patients with septic shock. Lancet 1991; 338:1557-8.

79. Beller FK, Schmidt EH, Holzgreve W, Hauss J. Septicemia during pregnancy: a study in different species of experimental animals. Am J Obstet Gynecol 1985; 151:967-75.

80. Ledger WJ, Norman M, Gee C, Lewis W. Bacteremia on an obstetric-gynecologic service. Am J Obstet Gynecol 1975; 121:205-12.

81. Lee W, Clark SL, Cotton DB, et al. Septic shock during pregnancy. Am J Obstet Gynecol 1988; 159:410-6.

82. Mabie WC, Barton JR, Sibai B. Septic shock in pregnancy. Obstet Gynecol 1997; 90:553-61.

83. Ayadi S, Carbillon L, Varlet C, et al. Fatal sepsis due to Escherichia coli after second-trimester amniocentesis. Fetal Diagn Ther 1998; 13:98-9.

84. Rode ME, Morgan MA, Ruchelli E, Forouzan I. Candida chorioamnionitis after serial therapeutic amniocenteses: A possible association. J Perinatol 2000; 20:335-7.

85. Winer N, David A, Leconte P, et al. Amniocentesis and amnioinfusion during pregnancy. Report of four complicated cases. Eur J Obstet Gynecol Reprod Biol 2001; 100:108-11.

86. Hamanishi J, Itoh H, Sagawa N, et al. A case of successful management of maternal septic shock with multiple organ failure following amniocentesis at midgestation. J Obstet Gynaecol Res 2002; 28:258-61.

87. Wegefroth P, Lastham JR. Lumbar puncture as a factor in the causation of meningitis. Am J Med Sci 1919; 158:183-5.

88. Pray L. Lumbar puncture as a factor in the pathogenesis of meningitis. Am J Dis Child 1941; 295:62-8.

89. Eng RH, Seligman SJ. Lumbar puncture-induced meningitis. Jama 1981; 245:1456-9.

90. Teele DW, Dashefsky B, Rakusan T, Klein JO. Meningitis after lumbar puncture in children with bacteremia. N Engl J Med 1981; 305:1079-81.

91. Smith KM, Deddish RB, Ogata ES. Meningitis associated with serial lumbar punctures and post-hemorrhagic hydrocephalus. J Pediatr 1986; 109:1057-60.

92. Shapiro ED, Aaron NH, Wald ER, Chiponis D. Risk factors for development of bacterial meningitis among children with occult bacteremia. J Pediatr 1986; 109:15-9.

93. Chestnut DH. Spinal anesthesia in the febrile patient. Anesthesiology 1992; 76:667-9.

94. Kost-Byerly S, Tobin JR, Greenberg RS, et al. Bacterial colonization and infection rate of continuous epidural catheters in children. Anesth Analg 1998; 86:712-6.

95. Barrie H. Meningitis following spinal anesthesia. Lancet 1941; i:242-3.

96. Lee JJ, Parry H. Bacterial meningitis following spinal anaesthesia for caesarean section. Br J Anaesth 1991; 66:383-6.

97. Kilpatrick ME, Girgis NI. Meningitis: A complication of spinal anesthesia. Anesth Analg 1983; 62:513-5.

98. Roberts SP, Petts HV. Meningitis after obstetric spinal anaesthesia. Anaesthesia 1990; 45:376-7.

99. Ready LB, Helfer D. Bacterial meningitis in parturients after epidural anesthesia. Anesthesiology 1989; 71:988-90.

100. Davis L, Hargreaves C, Robinson PN. Postpartum meningitis. Anaesthesia 1993; 48:788-9.

101. Videira RL, Ruiz-Neto PP, Brandao Neto M. Post spinal meningitis and asepsis. Acta Anaesthesiol Scand 2002; 46:639-46.

102. Trautmann M, Lepper PM, Schmitz FJ. Three cases of bacterial meningitis after spinal and epidural anesthesia. Eur J Clin Microbiol Infect Dis 2002; 21:43-5.

103. Harding SA, Collis RE, Morgan BM. Meningitis after combined spinal-extradural anaesthesia in obstetrics. Br J Anaesth 1994; 73:545-7.

104. Cascio M, Heath G. Meningitis following a combined spinal-epidural technique in a labouring term parturient. Can J Anaesth 1996; 43: 399-402.

105. Bouhemad B, Dounas M, Mercier FJ, Benhamou D. Bacterial meningitis following combined spinal-epidural analgesia for labour. Anaesthesia 1998; 53:292-5.

106. Rawal N, Holmstrom B, Crowhurst JA, Van Zundert A. The combined spinal-epidural technique. Anesthesiol Clin North America 2000; 18:267-95.

107. Dripps RD, Vandam LD. Long-term follow-up of patients who received 10,098 spinal anesthetics. JAMA 1954; 156:1486-91.

108. Phillips OC, Ebner H, Nelson AT, Black MH. Neurologic complications following spinal anesthesia with lidocaine: a prospective review of 10,440 cases. Anesthesiology 1969; 30:284-9.

109. Hellmann K. Epidural anaesthesia in obstetrics: a second look at 26,127 cases. Can Anaesth Soc J 1965; 12:398-404.

110. Crawford JS. Some maternal complications of epidural analgesia for labour. Anaesthesia 1985; 40:1219-25.

111. Scott DB, Hibbard BM. Serious non-fatal complications associated with extradural block in obstetric practice. Br J Anaesth 1990; 64:537-41.

112. Paech MJ, Godkin R, Webster GS. Complications of obstetric epidural analgesia and anaesthesia: A prospective analysis of 10,995 cases. Internat J Obstet Anesth 1998; 7:5-11.

113. Bader AM, Gilbertson L, Kirz L, Datta S. Regional anesthesia in women with chorioamnionitis. Reg Anesth 1992; 17:84-6.

114. Ramanathan S, Sheth R, Turndorf H. Anesthesia for cesarean section in patients with genital herpes infections: a retrospective study. Anesthesiology 1986; 64:807-9.

115. Carp H, Bailey S. The association between meningitis and dural puncture in bacteremic rats. Anesthesiology 1992; 76:739-42.

116. Weed LH, Wegeforth P, Ayer JB, Felton LD. The production of meningitis by release of cerebrospinal fluid during an experimental septicemia: Preliminary note. JAMA 1919; 72:190-3.

117. Idzumi G. Experimental pneumococcus meningitis in rabbits and dogs. J Infect Dis 1920; 26:373-87.

118. Petersdorf RG, Swarner DR, Garcia M. Studies on the pathogenesis of meningitis. II.Development of meningitis during pneumococcal bacteremia. J Clin Invest 1962; 41:320-27.

119. James FM, George RH, Naiem H, White GJ. Bacteriologic aspects of epidural analgesia. Anesth Analg 1976; 55:187-90.

120. Corey L, Adams HG, Brown ZA, Holmes KK. Genital herpes simplex virus infections: clinical manifestations, course, and complications. Ann Intern Med 1983; 98:958-72.

121. Brown ZA, Vontver LA, Benedetti J, et al. Effects on infants of a first episode of genital herpes during pregnancy. N Engl J Med 1987; 317:1246-51.

122. Eskild A, Jeansson S, Stray-Pedersen B, Jenum PA. Herpes simplex virus type-2 infection in pregnancy: no risk of fetal death: results from a nested case-control study within 35,940 women. Bjog 2002; 109:1030-5.

123. Whitley RJ, Corey L, Arvin A, et al. Changing presentation of herpes simplex virus infection in neonates. J Infect Dis 1988; 158:109-16.

124. Prober CG, Sullender WM, Yasukawa LL, et al. Low risk of herpes simplex virus infections in neonates exposed to the virus at the time of vaginal delivery to mothers with recurrent genital herpes simplex virus infections. N Engl J Med 1987; 316:240-4.

125. American College of Obstetricians and Gynecologists. Perinatal Herpes Simplex Virus Infections. ACOG Technical Bulletin No. 122, 1988.

126. Arvin AM, Hensleigh PA, Prober CG, et al. Failure of antepartum maternal cultures to predict the infant's risk of exposure to herpes simplex virus at delivery. N Engl J Med 1986; 315:796-800.

127. Brown ZA, Wald A, Morrow RA, et al. Effect of serologic status and cesarean delivery on transmission rates of herpes simplex virus from mother to infant. JAMA 2003; 289:203-9.

128. Scott LL, Hollier LM, McIntire D, et al. Acyclovir suppression to prevent recurrent genital herpes at delivery. Infect Dis Obstet Gynecol 2002; 10:71-7.

129. Watts DH, Brown ZA, Money D, et al. A double-blind, randomized, placebo-controlled trial of acyclovir in late pregnancy for the reduction of herpes simplex virus shedding and cesarean delivery. Am J Obstet Gynecol 2003; 188:836-43.

130. Ravindran RS, Gupta CD, Stoops CA. Epidural analgesia in the presence of herpes simplex virus (type 2) infection. Anesth Analg 1982; 61:714-5.

131. Crosby ET, Halpern SH, Rolbin SH. Epidural anaesthesia for caesarean section in patients with active recurrent genital herpes simplex infections: a retrospective review. Can J Anaesth 1989; 36:701-4.

132. Bader AM, Camann WR, Datta S. Anesthesia for cesarean delivery in patients with herpes simplex virus type-2 infections. Reg Anesth 1990; 15:261-3.

133. Boyle RK. Herpes simplex labialis after epidural or parenteral morphine: a randomized prospective trial in an Australian obstetric population. Anaesth Intensive Care 1995; 23:433-7.

134. Boyle RK. A review of anatomical and immunological links between epidural morphine and herpes simplex labialis in obstetric patients. Anaesth Intensive Care 1995; 23:425-32.

Chapter 37

Antepartum and Postpartum Hemorrhage

David C. Mayer, M.D. · Fred J. Spielman, M.D. ·
Elizabeth A. Bell, M.D., M.P.H.

The increased blood volume associated with normal pregnancy typically accommodates the obligatory blood loss that occurs during vaginal or cesarean delivery. In some parturients, blood loss overwhelms compensatory mechanisms and results in hypovolemia and shock that threaten both the mother and the fetus. Although maternal mortality associated with hemorrhage has steadily declined in Western nations, peripartum hemorrhage remains a leading cause of maternal and fetal morbidity and mortality. Hemorrhage accounted for 17% of maternal deaths in the United States from 1991 to 1999.[1] A survey of maternal morbidity in the United Kingdom suggests that severe hemorrhage occurs in approximately 6.7 per 1000 deliveries.[2] *Why Mothers Die 1997-1999,* the most recent *Report on Confidential Enquiries into Maternal Deaths in the United Kingdom,* suggests that older parturients (age > 35) are at greatest risk.[3] In addition to age differences, significant disparity exists in the rates of death in white and African-American subpopulations in the United States.[1,4] In underdeveloped countries, postpartum hemorrhage is the leading cause of maternal death.[5] Many of these deaths are preventable; common problems include failure to recognize risk factors, failure to estimate the degree of blood loss correctly, and failure to initiate treatment for severe hemorrhage quickly. Anesthesiologists should become involved early in the care of bleeding parturients.

Peripartum hemorrhage includes a wide range of pathophysiologic events. An individual patient may have more than one etiology for hemorrhage. Further, patients with antepartum hemorrhage are at risk for postpartum bleeding.

MECHANISMS OF HEMOSTASIS

After disruption of vascular integrity, mechanisms of hemostasis include (1) platelet aggregation and plug formation, (2) local vasoconstriction, (3) clot polymerization, and (4) fibrous tissue fortification of the clot. Platelet activation and aggregation occur rapidly after endothelial damage. Activated platelets release adenosine diphosphate (ADP), serotonin, catecholamines, and other factors that promote local vasoconstriction and hemostasis. These factors also activate the coagulation cascade. The end result of the cascade is conversion of fibrinogen into fibrin (see Chapter 42).

Contraction of the uterus represents the primary mechanism for controlling blood loss at parturition. Endogenous oxytocics effect myometrial contraction after delivery.

Underestimation of peripartum hemorrhage is a frequent problem. Visual assessments typically underestimate the true amount of blood loss. The larger the blood loss, the greater the discrepancy.[6] Inadequate fluid administration is common. The aforementioned report from the United Kingdom noted that substandard care was a contributing factor in 79% of direct maternal deaths that resulted from hemorrhage.[3] The primary problems were delayed recognition of hypovolemia and inadequate volume resuscitation. Various schemes have been developed to help determine the severity of hypovolemia secondary to pathologic blood loss (Table 37-1). The clinical utility of these classification schemes is unclear.

ANTEPARTUM HEMORRHAGE

Antepartum vaginal bleeding occurs in nearly 6% of pregnant women.[7] Most cases of bleeding do not result from serious pathology; for example, some patients experience modest bleeding from cervicitis. However, a significant proportion of patients who experience antepartum hemorrhage have abnormalities in placentation—either placenta previa or placental abruption.

The greatest threat of antepartum hemorrhage is not to the mother but to her fetus. Two decades ago, vaginal bleeding during the second and third trimester was associated with perinatal mortality rates as high as 80%.[8] More recent data suggest that antepartum bleeding secondary to placenta previa or abruption is responsible for perinatal mortality rates as high as 22% and 37%, respectively.[9]

Placenta Previa

A placenta previa is present when the placenta implants in advance of the fetal presenting part. Further classification can be made depending on the relationship between the cervical os and the placenta. A total placenta previa completely covers the cervical os. A partial placenta previa covers part, but not all of the cervical os. A marginal placenta previa lies close to, but does not cover the cervical os (Figure 37-1).

EPIDEMIOLOGY

The incidence of placenta previa is approximately 1 in 200 pregnancies.[10] The exact etiology is unclear, but prior uterine trauma is a common element among the associated conditions. The placenta implants in the scarred area, which typically includes the lower uterine segment. Conditions associated with placenta previa include multiparity, advanced maternal age, previous cesarean section or other uterine surgery, and previous placenta previa.[11] The presence of placenta previa increases the likelihood that the patient will require a peripartum hysterectomy.[12]

DIAGNOSIS

The classic sign of placenta previa is painless vaginal bleeding during the second or third trimester. The first episode of bleeding typically occurs preterm. (A minority of patients

TABLE 37-1	STAGING SCHEME FOR ASSESSMENT OF OBSTETRIC HEMORRHAGE	
Severity of shock	**Findings**	**% Blood loss**
None	None	< 15% to 20%
Mild	Tachycardia (< 100 bpm) Mild hypotension Peripheral vasoconstriction	20% to 25%
Moderate	Tachycardia (100 to 120 bpm) Hypotension (SBP 80 to 100 mm Hg) Restlessness Oliguria	25% to 35%
Severe	Tachycardia (>120 bpm) Hypotension (SBP < 60 mm Hg) Altered consciousness Anuria	> 35%

SBP, Systolic blood pressure.
From Gonik B. Intensive care monitoring of the critically ill pregnant patient. In Creasy RK, Resnik R, editors. Maternal-Fetal Medicine, 3rd ed. Philadelphia, WB Saunders, 1994:865-90.

with placenta previa have no vaginal bleeding before term.) With the first episode of bleeding, contractions typically are absent, and the onset of bleeding is not related to any particular event. The lack of abdominal pain and abnormal uterine tone help distinguish this event from placental abruption, but their absence may be misleading and does not exclude abruption. As many as 10% of patients with placenta previa have a coexisting placental abruption.[13] The first episode of bleeding rarely causes shock, and it typically stops spontaneously. Fetal distress or demise is uncommon with the first episode of hemorrhage.

OBSTETRIC MANAGEMENT

Ultrasonography is the mainstay for confirming the presence of placenta previa. With current equipment, ultrasonographic examination is accurate in confirming or excluding the diagnosis of placenta previa. It also helps the obstetrician assess gestational age. Magnetic resonance imaging (MRI) may be used to determine the etiology of third-trimester bleeding, but it is not practical in most clinical situations.[14]

Vaginal examinations are best avoided. If they are needed to rule out lacerations as a cause of bleeding, vaginal examinations typically are performed using a "double set-up" (*vide infra*).

Obstetric management is based on the severity of vaginal bleeding and the maturity of the fetus. Active labor, persistent bleeding, or a mature fetus should prompt abdominal delivery, provided the diagnosis of placenta previa is confirmed by ultrasonography or double set-up examination.

The fetus is at risk from two distinct pathophysiologic processes: (1) progressive or sudden placental separation that causes uteroplacental insufficiency and (2) preterm delivery and its sequelae.[15] In the past, delivery frequently was performed after the second episode of bleeding that required transfusion. Currently, most obstetricians favor expectant management within the hospital. A few obstetricians manage selected patients without recent bleeding or anemia who live within 20 to 30 minutes of the hospital on an outpatient basis. Discharge to home occurs only after evaluation in the hospital for 24 to 48 hours and cessation of bleeding for 1 day. The goal is to delay delivery until the fetus is mature. Maternal vital signs are assessed frequently, and the hemoglobin concentration is checked at regular intervals. Fetal evaluation includes frequent performance of a nonstress test or biophys-

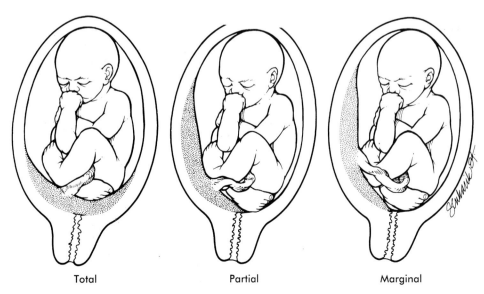

FIGURE 37-1. Three variations of placenta previa. (From Benedetti TJ. Obstetric hemorrhage. In Gabbe SG, Niebyl JR, Simpson JL, editors. Obstetrics: Normal and Problem Pregnancies, 4th ed. New York, Churchill Livingstone, 2001: 516.)

Total   Partial   Marginal

ical profile, ultrasonographic assessment of fetal growth, and fetal lung maturity studies as indicated. Hemorrhage is prevented by the enforcement of strict bed rest and avoidance of vaginal examinations and coitus.

Expectant management requires immediate access to a medical center with 24-hour obstetric and anesthesia coverage and a neonatal intensive care unit. Expectant management is terminated when the patient begins active labor, the fetus has documented lung maturity, the gestational age reaches 37 weeks, excessive bleeding occurs, or another obstetric complication (e.g., preeclampsia) develops.[16] The obstetrician may administer a glucocorticoid (e.g., betamethasone) to accelerate fetal lung maturity if delivery is anticipated between 28 and 32 weeks' gestation.

A significant number of patients with placenta previa have preterm labor. Because vaginal examinations to confirm cervical dilation are contraindicated, it is difficult to document the diagnosis of preterm labor.[17] Decisions regarding tocolytic therapy also are problematic. Obstetricians must balance the potential cardiovascular consequences of tocolytic therapy in the presence of maternal hemorrhage versus the consequences of preterm delivery.[18] In a retrospective study of patients with symptomatic placenta previa, Besinger et al[19] observed that tocolytic therapy was associated with a clinically significant delay in delivery and an increase in birth weight, but such therapy did not reduce the frequency or severity of recurrent vaginal bleeding. Tocolytic therapy is not recommended for patients with uncontrolled hemorrhage or those suspected of having placental abruption.

The choice of tocolytic drug is controversial. Some maternal-fetal medicine specialists favor magnesium sulfate because they believe it is less likely to cause maternal hypotension during hemorrhage than the beta-adrenergic agents. In addition, the beta-adrenergic agents produce maternal tachycardia, which makes it more difficult to assess maternal intravascular volume.[17] Chestnut et al.[20] evaluated the hemodynamic response to maternal hemorrhage during infusion of either magnesium sulfate or ritodrine in gravid ewes. Magnesium sulfate but not ritodrine worsened maternal hypotension during hemorrhage. The fetal pH decreased significantly only in the magnesium sulfate group. The authors speculated that hypermagnesemia attenuated the maternal compensatory response to hemorrhage. Vincent et al.[21] hypothesized that administration of calcium chloride might help restore cardiovascular stability during hemorrhage in hypermagnesemic gravid ewes. Although administration of calcium chloride 10 mg/kg slightly increased maternal cardiac output, it did not substantially improve maternal mean arterial pressure (MAP), uterine blood flow, or fetal oxygenation.

Expectant management has reduced the incidence of neonatal morbidity and mortality. Ultrasonography allows the obstetrician to perform serial assessment of placental location and fetal growth. Tocolysis and blood transfusion allow the obstetrician to delay delivery, and assessment of fetal lung maturity helps determine the appropriate timing of delivery. Nevertheless, prematurity remains the most common cause of neonatal mortality and morbidity, especially if bleeding begins before 20 weeks' gestation. McShane et al.[22] observed that the onset of bleeding before 20 weeks' gestation was associated with a very poor fetal outcome. The authors found a significant correlation between antepartum maternal hemorrhage and the need for neonatal transfusion.

Fetuses of women with placenta previa may be at risk for other problems. Naeye[23] noted an increased incidence of asymmetric intrauterine growth restriction (IUGR) in fetuses of women with placenta previa. Several factors may account for the association between placenta previa and IUGR. First, the lower uterine segment may be less vascular than normal sites of placental implantation. Second, the placenta often is adherent to an area of fibrosis. Third, patients with placenta previa have an increased incidence of first-trimester bleeding, which may promote a partial placental separation, decreasing the placental exchange surface area. Fourth, although the blood loss from placenta previa is almost entirely maternal, trauma to the placenta with vaginal examination or coitus may result in some fetal blood loss, which could retard fetal growth.[24] Some studies have reported an increased incidence of congenital anomalies in the fetuses of women with placenta previa.

ANESTHETIC MANAGEMENT

All patients admitted with antepartum vaginal bleeding should be evaluated by anesthesia personnel on arrival. Special consideration should be given to the airway, and intravascular volume should be assessed carefully. At least one large-gauge intravenous catheter should be placed, the patient's hematocrit should be determined, and a blood type and cross-match should be performed. Volume resuscitation should be initiated using non-dextrose-containing balanced salt solution (Ringer's lactate or normal saline).

Double Set-Up

The accuracy of ultrasonography for the identification of placenta previa has almost eliminated the need for the double set-up examination. Nonetheless, there remain some cases for which a double set-up examination is required. The examination is performed in the operating room. All members of the obstetric care team (including the anesthesiologist, obstetrician, and pediatrician) make full preparation for cesarean section. Full preparation includes application of maternal monitors, insertion of two large-gauge intravenous cannulae, administration of a nonparticulate antacid, and a sterile prep and draping of the abdomen. Two units of packed red blood cells (PRBCs) should be in the operating room. The obstetrician subsequently performs a careful vaginal examination. A cesarean section is performed if significant bleeding occurs or if the obstetrician confirms the presence of placenta previa in a woman with a mature fetus.

Cesarean Section

The choice of anesthetic technique depends on the indication and urgency for cesarean section and the degree of maternal hypovolemia. No consensus exists among anesthesiologists regarding the appropriate use of regional anesthesia in patients with a placenta previa *without* active bleeding. Surveys of obstetric anesthesiologists have revealed that epidural and spinal anesthesia are commonly employed in patients who are not actively bleeding or hypotensive before the induction of anesthesia.[25,26] However, such patients remain at risk for increased intraoperative blood loss for at least three reasons. First, the obstetrician may cut into the placenta during uterine incision. Second, after delivery, the lower uterine segment implantation site does not contract as well as the normal fundal implantation site. Third, a patient with placenta previa is at increased risk for placenta accreta, especially if there is a history of previous cesarean section.[11] For these reasons, we place two large-gauge intravenous cannulae before the start of *either* elective or emergency cesarean section. Further, it seems unwise to perform only a type and screen, even among those patients undergoing an elective cesarean section for placenta previa. Rather, we insist that two units of PRBCs are present before the start of surgery. A prospective trial comparing epidural versus general anesthesia for cesarean section in patients with placenta previa demonstrated that general anesthesia was associated with a lower postoperative hematocrit. Operative times, estimated blood loss, urine output, and neonatal Apgar scores were similar between the two groups.[27] A reasonable conclusion would be that single-shot spinal anesthesia is also acceptable for this group of patients, provided there is a low risk of placenta accreta.

Bleeding patients represent a significant challenge for the anesthesia care team. Frequently such a patient has just presented to the hospital, and minimal time exists for evaluation. In these cases, patient evaluation, resuscitation, and preparation for operative delivery all proceed simultaneously. Because the placental site is the source of hemorrhage, the bleeding may continue unabated until the placenta is removed and the uterus contracts. Preoperative evaluation requires careful assessment of the parturient's airway and intravascular volume. Two large-gauge intravenous catheters should be placed, and four units of PRBCs should be ordered. Blood administration sets, fluid warmers, and equipment for invasive monitoring should be available. Initially, non-dextrose-containing crystalloid and/or colloid are infused rapidly. In some cases, there is not enough time for the cross-match to be completed, and type-specific blood must be given.

Rapid-sequence induction of general anesthesia is the preferred technique for bleeding patients. The choice of intravenous induction agent depends on the degree of cardiovascular instability. In patients with severe hypovolemic shock, intubation may require only a muscle relaxant, but this is rare. It is best to avoid sodium thiopental in patients with ongoing, severe hemorrhage. (If sodium thiopental is selected, a reduced dose should be given.) Likewise, propofol should not be used in hypovolemic patients.

Ketamine and etomidate are the best induction agents for bleeding patients. **Ketamine** (0.5 to 1.0 mg/kg) has an excellent record of safety and efficacy in obstetric anesthesia practice. Postoperative hallucinations and nightmares are uncommon when the dose does not exceed 1 mg/kg. Ketamine may cause myocardial depression in patients with severe hypovolemia. **Etomidate** is an acceptable alternative to ketamine and also is safe for use in obstetric patients.[28] When it is used for induction of anesthesia, etomidate (0.3 mg/kg) causes minimal cardiac depression. A reduced dose is appropriate in patients with severe hemorrhage. Disadvantages of etomidate include venous irritation, myoclonus, and possible adrenal suppression.

For the maintenance of anesthesia, the choice of agents depends on maternal cardiovascular stability. In patients with modest bleeding and no preexisting fetal distress, 50% nitrous oxide and 50% oxygen can be given with a low concentration of a volatile halogenated agent to prevent maternal awareness. The concentration of nitrous oxide can be reduced (or omitted) in cases of fetal distress. Oxytocin (20 U/L) should be infused immediately after delivery. The lower uterine segment implantation site does not contract as well as the fundus. All uterine relaxants should be eliminated if bleeding continues. Thus it may be best to eliminate the volatile halogenated agent after delivery and substitute nitrous oxide (70%) and an intravenous opioid. Small doses of opioid (e.g., fentanyl, alfentanil, remifentanil) can be given without causing significant cardiovascular depression.

If the placenta does not separate easily, a placenta accreta may exist. In such cases, massive blood loss and the need for cesarean hysterectomy should be expected (*vide infra*). The need for invasive hemodynamic monitoring varies among patients. A central venous catheter can guide intravenous fluid therapy in cases of persistent oliguria. Likewise, an indwelling arterial catheter is useful for patients with labile blood pressure or those who require frequent determination of hematocrit and blood gas measurements. Coagulopathy rarely occurs with placenta previa; the most common deficit is a dilutional thrombocytopenia.

Placental Abruption

Placental abruption is defined as separation of the placenta from the decidua basalis before delivery of the fetus. Acute bleeding results from exposed decidual vessels. Fetal distress occurs because of loss of area for maternal-fetal gas exchange. Acute and chronic varieties exist, and further grading schemes have been described.[17]

EPIDEMIOLOGY

The etiology is not known, but several conditions are associated with placental abruption. Known risk factors include hypertension, advanced age and parity, tobacco use, cocaine use, trauma, premature rupture of membranes, and a history of previous abruption. A review of maternal deaths from 1979 to 1992 reported to the National Pregnancy Mortality Surveillance System of the Centers for Disease Control suggested that the risk of mortality increased with age and was three times greater in nonwhite than in white populations.[29] Placental abruption occurs in approximately 1% of pregnancies, and the incidence may be increasing.[30] An increase in the number of women using cocaine may be partly responsible for the increased incidence. Placental abruption also is associated with IUGR and fetal malformations, which may signal "a long-standing pathologic process involving both mother and fetus."[31]

DIAGNOSIS

The classic presentation includes vaginal bleeding, uterine tenderness, and increased uterine activity. An atypical presentation does not exclude the diagnosis. In addition, the amount of vaginal bleeding can lead to an underestimation of the true intravascular volume deficit, especially when a large retroplacental hematoma is present. In this situation, the uterus may contain more than 2500 mL of blood.[32] Ultrasonographic examination often can determine the presence of a retroplacental hematoma, but a normal sonographic examination does not exclude the diagnosis. Sonographic examination does help estimate gestational age and determine placental location.

PATHOPHYSIOLOGY

The major complications of placental abruption are hemorrhagic shock, acute renal failure (ARF), coagulopathy, and fetal distress or demise. Abruption is the most common cause of disseminated intravascular coagulation (DIC) in pregnancy. Coagulopathy occurs in 10% of all cases of placenta abruption. The incidence of coagulopathy increases when fetal distress or demise exists.[30]

The major fetal risk is hypoxia. Fetal distress and intrauterine fetal death occur more frequently with abruption than with placenta previa.[30] Approximately 15% to 25% of all perinatal deaths occur secondary to abruption. As many as 20% of these fetuses die in utero before maternal hospitalization.[16]

Fetal oxygenation depends on adequate maternal oxygen-carrying capacity, uteroplacental blood flow, and transplacental exchange. Large maternal blood loss causes maternal hypotension, decreased uterine blood flow, and decreased maternal oxygen-carrying capacity. Abruption also causes a decrease in the placental surface available for exchange of oxygen. Fetal anemia may occur with blood loss from the fetal side of the uteroplacental circulation.

Prematurity also is responsible for perinatal morbidity and mortality. A vicious cycle may be established in which a small placental abruption stimulates uterine contractions, causing further separation of the placenta. It may be possible to inhibit uterine contractions in selected cases with no signs of fetal distress. In cases of known or suspected abruption, the risks of tocolytic therapy and intrauterine fetal death must be weighed against the risks of perinatal morbidity and mortality from preterm delivery. Respiratory distress syndrome is the most common neonatal complication; it occurs in as many as 50% of deliveries complicated by abruption.[16]

Ylä-Outinen et al.[33] studied 85,177 deliveries. Perinatal mortality among deliveries complicated by abruption was 34%. Gestational age at the time of diagnosis was an important prognostic factor. The location and extent of the placental abruption seen sonographically have clinical significance. A retroplacental hematoma has a less favorable prognosis for fetal survival than subchorionic hemorrhage. Large retroplacental bleeding is associated with a mortality rate of 50% or greater, whereas a similar-sized subchorionic abruption may lead to a 10% rate of mortality.[16,34]

The incidence of infants who are small for gestational age (SGA) also increases with abruption. This suggests a long-standing pathologic process. Naeye et al.[35] prospectively studied more than 53,000 deliveries. They found that decidual necrosis at the placental margin and large placental infarcts were the most common placental abnormalities. Infants who died had 14% less placental weight, 8% less body weight, and 3% shorter body length than surviving control infants of the same gestational age.

OBSTETRIC MANAGEMENT

Once the diagnosis of abruption is suspected, the fetal heart rate (FHR) should be monitored, and if feasible, an internal scalp electrode and internal pressure catheter should be placed. A large-gauge intravenous catheter should be placed, and blood should be obtained for cross-match and assessment of hematocrit and coagulation. Supplemental oxygen should be administered and left uterine displacement should be maintained.

The apparent blood loss may not reflect the true degree of intravascular volume deficit, which often is caused by a retroplacental hematoma. Placement of a urethral catheter helps the physician determine the adequacy of renal perfusion.

The definitive treatment is delivery of the fetus and placenta, but the degree of maternal and fetal compromise determines the timing and route of delivery. If the patient is preterm, the degree of abruption is minimal, and the fetus shows no signs of distress, the patient is hospitalized, and the pregnancy is allowed to continue for fetal lung maturation. In the majority of cases, however, prompt delivery is desired. The route of delivery depends on several factors. Some studies have noted an increased survival rate among babies delivered by cesarean section versus those delivered vaginally, but these studies may be flawed by selection bias. Tragically, some patients present with a live fetus only to have the fetus die

while waiting for delivery. Therefore no unnecessary delay in delivery should occur once the diagnosis of abruption is confirmed; further placental separation may cause fetal death.

Induction of labor is preferred when there is no evidence of fetal distress and a favorable cervix is present. Vaginal delivery also is desirable for the delivery of a dead fetus. In most other cases, cesarean section is performed without delay.

The obstetrician should exclude major congenital malformations before performing cesarean delivery. Moreover, a rapid but complete evaluation of the parturient must be performed. Cesarean section is hazardous in the unstable mother with severe hypovolemia or coagulopathy.

ANESTHETIC MANAGEMENT

The anesthesiologist should consider the severity of the abruption and the urgency of delivery.

Labor and Vaginal Delivery

The patient undergoing induction of labor may receive epidural analgesia if she has normal coagulation studies and no intravascular volume deficit. The appropriateness of epidural anesthesia for patients at risk for extension of abruption and further hemorrhage has been questioned. Vincent et al.[36] observed that epidural anesthesia significantly worsened maternal hypotension, uterine blood flow, and fetal PaO_2 and pH during untreated hemorrhage (20 mL/kg) in gravid ewes. Curiously, maternal heart rate decreased during hemorrhage in the epidural group but not in the control group (Figure 37-2). However, intravascular volume replacement promptly eliminated the difference between groups in maternal MAP, cardiac output, and fetal PaO_2. The authors concluded that epidural anesthesia may adversely affect the compensatory response to untreated hemorrhage in pregnant women. At the University of North Carolina, we do not deny epidural anesthesia to a patient with a partial abruption, provided she has no coagulopathy and is not hypovolemic. We continually look for evidence of further bleeding and maintain normal intravascular volume.

Cesarean Section

More problematic is the patient who requires anesthesia for cesarean section because of acute fetal distress. General anesthesia is preferred for most of these cases. Sodium thiopental may precipitate severe hypotension in patients with unrecognized hypovolemia. Ketamine and etomidate are better options for the patient with unknown or decreased intravascular volume. Large doses of ketamine may increase uterine tone during early gestation, which is deleterious to a stressed fetus.[37] This is an unlikely problem with administration of a single dose (1 mg/kg) for induction of anesthesia. Severe hypotension after the administration of sodium thiopental is more likely to be harmful than the possibility of increased uterine tone after administration of a single dose of ketamine.

Aggressive volume resuscitation is critical. Both crystalloid and colloid may be used; the choice is less important than adequate restoration of intravascular volume. In cases of severe hemorrhage, management is aided by the insertion of central venous and arterial catheters. An antecubital vein can be used for central line placement when a coagulopathy is suspected or present.

These patients are at risk for persistent hemorrhage resulting from uterine atony or a coagulopathy. After delivery, oxytocin (20 U/L) should be infused promptly to stimulate uterine tone. Persistent uterine atony requires the administration of

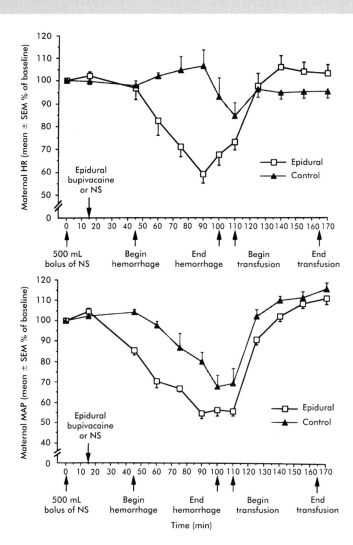

FIGURE 37-2. Maternal heart rate *(HR)* and mean arterial pressure *(MAP)* responses over time. Maternal HR was lower during hemorrhage ($P < 0.05$) in the epidural group than in the control group. During transfusion, maternal HR was slightly higher ($P < 0.05$) in the epidural group than in the control group. Maternal MAP was lower during hemorrhage ($P < 0.05$) in the epidural group than in the control group. (From Vincent RD, Chestnut DH, Sipes SL, et al. Epidural anesthesia worsens uterine blood flow and fetal oxygenation during hemorrhage in gravid ewes. Anesthesiology 1992; 76:799-806.)

Box 37-1 CONDITIONS ASSOCIATED WITH UTERINE RUPTURE
Previous uterine surgery
Trauma
• Indirect
Blunt (e.g., seat belt injury)
Excessive manual fundal pressure
Extension of cervical laceration
• Direct
Penetrating wound
Intrauterine manipulation
Forceps application and rotation
Postpartum curettage
Manual placental extraction
Version and extraction
External version
Inappropriate use of oxytocin
Grand multiparity
Uterine anomaly
Placenta percreta
Tumors (trophoblastic disease, cervical carcinoma)
Fetal problems (macrosomia, malposition, anomaly)

From Plauché WC. Surgical problems involving the pregnant uterus: Uterine inversion, uterine rupture, and leiomyomas. In Plauché WC, Morrison JC, O'Sullivan MJ, editors. Surgical Obstetrics. Philadelphia, WB Saunders, 1989:224.

Because of the variation in nomenclature and severity, accurate determination of the maternal and fetal morbidity secondary to uterine rupture is difficult. The most frequent variety of disruption is uterine scar separation or dehiscence. Some cases of uterine scar dehiscence are asymptomatic. Uterine scar dehiscence is more common and less likely to cause maternal or fetal morbidity than uterine rupture. **Uterine scar dehiscence** is a uterine wall defect that does not result in fetal distress or excessive hemorrhage and does not require emergency cesarean section or postpartum laparotomy. In contrast, **uterine rupture** is a uterine wall defect that results in fetal distress and/or maternal hemorrhage sufficient to require cesarean section or postpartum laparotomy.[38,41]

The rupture of a classic uterine scar increases morbidity and mortality because the anterior uterine wall is highly vascular and also may include the area of placental implantation. Lateral extension of the rupture can involve the major uterine vessels and typically is associated with massive bleeding. Plauché et al.[41] reviewed 23 cases of catastrophic uterine rupture; they noted no maternal deaths but a fetal mortality rate of 35%. The aforementioned report from the United Kingdom included only one maternal death from uterine rupture.[3]

DIAGNOSIS

The variable presentation of uterine rupture makes the diagnosis difficult. True uterine rupture should be suspected when vaginal bleeding, hypotension, cessation of labor, and fetal distress are noted. Historically, obstetricians have considered abdominal pain to be a consistent, sensitive sign of uterine rupture. One retrospective study reported the occurrence of pain in less than 10% of patients with either scar dehiscence or true rupture.[38] Fetal distress is the most reliable sign of uterine scar dehiscence or rupture (see Chapter 23).

In patients with an unscarred uterus, uterine rupture is rare. Risk factors include grand multiparity, malpresentation, and administration of oxytocin and/or prostaglandin. Postpartum hemorrhage, maternal tachycardia, and FHR decelerations

other ecbolic drugs *(vide infra)*. In cases of coagulopathy, coagulation factors should be replaced.

Most parturients recover quickly and completely after delivery. A minority of patients, notably those with prolonged hypotension, coagulopathy, and massive blood volume/product replacement, are best monitored and followed in a multidisciplinary intensive care unit.

Uterine Rupture

EPIDEMIOLOGY

Rupture of the gravid uterus can be disastrous to both the mother and fetus. Fortunately, it does not occur often. Previous uterine trauma increases the risk, but the incidence of true uterine rupture is less than 1% among parturients who have a scarred uterus.[38,39] Uterine rupture is rare in primigravid women or in women with an unscarred uterus.[40] Trauma during attempted forceps delivery may cause uterine rupture in a patient with an unscarred uterus. Box 37-1 lists other conditions associated with uterine rupture.

may signal uterine rupture. The diagnosis is confirmed by manual exploration of the uterus or during laparotomy.

OBSTETRIC MANAGEMENT

Treatment options include repair, arterial ligation, and hysterectomy. **Uterine repair** is appropriate for most cases of separation of an old transverse uterine scar and for some cases of rupture of an old classic incision. However, there remains the risk of rupture in a future pregnancy. A disadvantage of **arterial ligation** is that it may not control the bleeding and may delay the performance of definitive treatment. **Hysterectomy** is the preferred, definitive procedure for most cases of uterine rupture.[38,41] Patients with rupture of an unscarred uterus are more likely to require blood transfusion than patients with rupture of a scarred uterus. The fibrous edges of a scar bleed less readily than the rough edges of a newly ruptured uterus.[42]

ANESTHETIC MANAGEMENT

Patient evaluation and resuscitation are begun while the patient is prepared for emergency laparotomy. If rupture has occurred antepartum, fetal distress is likely. General anesthesia often is necessary, except in some stable patients with preexisting epidural anesthesia. Aggressive volume replacement and maintenance of urine output are essential. Invasive hemodynamic monitoring is appropriate when there is uncertainty regarding the intravascular volume.

Vasa Previa

Vasa previa is associated with a velamentous insertion of the cord where fetal vessels traverse the fetal membranes ahead of the fetal presenting part. Rupture of the membranes may be accompanied by a tear of a fetal vessel, leading to exsanguination of the fetus.

EPIDEMIOLOGY

Vasa previa occurs rarely (1 in 2000 to 3000 deliveries). It poses no threat to the mother, but because it involves the loss of fetal blood, vasa previa is associated with one of the highest fetal mortality rates (50% to 75%) of any of the complications of pregnancy. The term fetus has approximately 250 mL of blood. The amount of blood that can be lost without fetal death is relatively small compared with the volume of maternal blood lost with placenta previa or abruption.[43] Thus the combination of modest vaginal bleeding and fetal distress suggest vasa previa. In many cases in which infants have survived, an emergency cesarean delivery was performed for the mistaken diagnosis of placenta previa or abruption.

DIAGNOSIS

Early diagnosis and treatment are essential to reduce the chance of fetal death. Unfortunately, the diagnosis is most often made by examination of the placenta after delivery. A high index of suspicion is mandatory, and this requires a familiarity with the various features associated with vasa previa: (1) vasa previa is more common with multiple gestation, particularly with triplets; (2) the umbilical vessels do not always traverse the cervical opening; (3) bleeding may not be present, but the umbilical vessels may be compressed against the maternal pelvis by the fetal head, resulting in hypoxia; (4) hemorrhage may occur with intact membranes and may be concealed; (5) bleeding can begin long after the membranes have ruptured; and (6) the fetal vessels can be observed or palpated through the dilated cervix. In some cases the fetal vessels can be seen on ultrasonographic examination or at amnioscopy.[44]

It often is difficult to distinguish vasa previa from placental abruption. The presence of fetal bleeding can be confirmed by examining the shed blood for evidence of fetal hemoglobin (the Kleihauer-Betke test) or nucleated red blood cells.

OBSTETRIC MANAGEMENT

The treatment of vasa previa is directed solely toward ensuring fetal survival. Ruptured vasa previa is a true obstetric emergency that requires immediate delivery, almost always by cesarean section. Neonatal resuscitation requires immediate attention to neonatal volume replacement. Initially, the physician may transfuse some of the baby's own blood drawn from umbilical-placental vessels into a heparinized syringe. However, adequate volume replacement also requires administration of colloid or balanced salt solution.

ANESTHETIC MANAGEMENT

The choice of anesthetic technique depends on the urgency of cesarean section (see Chapter 26).

POSTPARTUM HEMORRHAGE

Postpartum hemorrhage is a major cause of maternal morbidity and mortality. It occurs in as many as 10% of deliveries. In many underdeveloped countries, postpartum hemorrhage is the leading cause of maternal mortality.[5] Table 37-2 lists some predisposing factors for postpartum hemorrhage.

Postpartum hemorrhage is defined as blood loss of greater than 500 mL after delivery.[45] This is an arbitrary and confusing definition. Some studies have suggested that the average blood loss at vaginal delivery is 500 to 600 mL, and that the average blood loss at cesarean section is approximately 1000 mL.[46] Duthie et al.[47] reported that the average measured blood loss at vaginal delivery is 320 to 400 mL, and is just under 500 mL for a cesarean section. Regardless, most studies agree that physicians and nurses often underestimate the severity of obstetric hemorrhage.[6,46,47] Postpartum hemorrhage may be identified clinically (albeit retrospectively) by a 10% decrease in hematocrit from admission to the postpartum period or by the need to administer PRBCs.[48]

Primary postpartum hemorrhage occurs during the first 24 hours after delivery, and **secondary** postpartum hemorrhage occurs between 24 hours and 6 weeks postpartum. Primary postpartum hemorrhage is more likely to result in maternal morbidity or mortality. A recent study noted evidence of myocardial ischemia in 28 (51%) of 55 patients with hemorrhagic shock resulting from severe postpartum hemorrhage.[49] The authors concluded that "clinical objectives for the management of hemorrhagic shock in this patient subpopulation should focus on the early simultaneous restoration of blood pressure and hemoglobin levels and the reduction of tachycardia if prevention fails."[49] Figure 37-3 provides an overview of the obstetric management of postpartum hemorrhage.

Uterine Atony

EPIDEMIOLOGY

Uterine atony is the most common cause of postpartum hemorrhage. Atony is one of the most common reasons to perform a peripartum hysterectomy, and it is the most common

TABLE 37-2   FACTORS PREDISPOSING TO POSTPARTUM HEMORRHAGE

	Atony	Lacerations, disruptions	Placental abnormalities	Coagulation disorders
Precipitous labor	X	X		
Instrumental delivery		X		
General anesthesia	X			
Prolonged labor	X			
Uterine leiomyomas	X	X	X	
Macrosomia	X	X		
Twins	X	X		
Chorioamnionitis	X			
Multiparity	X		X	
Prior cesarean section		X	X	
Prior hysterotomy or curettage		X	X	
Stimulated labor	X	X		
History of postpartum hemorrhage	X		X	X
Fetal demise	X			X
Amniotic fluid embolism	X			X
Tocolytic therapy	X			

PPH, Postpartum hemorrhage.
From Herbert WNJ, Cefalo R. Management of postpartum hemorrhage. Clin Obstet Gynecol 1984; 27:139-47.

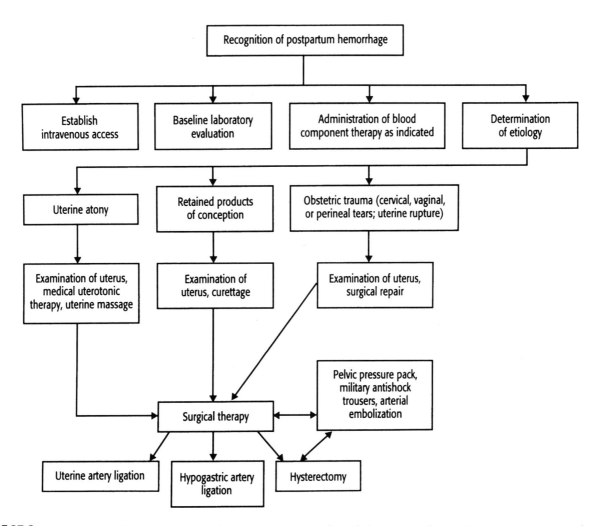

FIGURE 37-3. Management plan for postpartum hemorrhage. (From American College of Obstetricians and Gynecologists. Postpartum Hemorrhage. ACOG Educational Bulletin No. 243, Washington, D.C., January 1998.)

indication for peripartum blood transfusion.[50,51] Postpartum hemostasis involves the release of endogenous uterotonic agents in addition to normal hemostatic mechanisms. Although the role of oxytocin and prostaglandins in the initiation of parturition is not well understood, these substances are responsible for uterine contraction and involution during the third stage of labor. Contraction of the uterus represents the primary mechanism for controlling blood loss at parturition. Uterine atony represents a failure of this process. Parturients with obstetric hemorrhage also have uterine arteries that are relatively unresponsive to vasoconstrictor substances.[52]

Many cases of atony result from overdistention of the uterus. Box 37-2 lists conditions associated with uterine atony.

DIAGNOSIS

The diagnosis of atony often is complicated by the presence of other problems. A soft postpartum uterus and vaginal bleeding are the most common physical findings. The absence of vaginal bleeding does not exclude this disorder because the atonic, engorged uterus may contain more than 1000 mL of blood.

OBSTETRIC MANAGEMENT

Uterine atony often occurs immediately after delivery, but it may occur several hours later. Initial treatment includes bimanual compression, uterine massage, and intravenous infusion of oxytocin. These measures are successful in most patients. Only a small percentage of these patients require transfusion and/or hysterectomy. However, each patient with atony should be evaluated by an anesthesiologist. The physician should administer supplemental oxygen, ensure the presence of adequate intravenous access, and make certain that appropriate crystalloid resuscitation has been initiated.

Oxytocin is the first-line drug for the prophylaxis or treatment of uterine atony. The number of uterine high-affinity receptors for oxytocin increases greatly near term. Endogenous oxytocin is a 9-amino acid polypeptide produced in the posterior pituitary. The exogenous form of the drug (Pitocin, Syntocinon) is a synthetic preparation. Older preparations were derived from animal extracts that were contaminated with antidiuretic hormone (ADH). This was problematic during the administration of large doses. Because ADH is only two amino acids different from oxytocin, even the synthetic form may produce a small ADH effect. This rarely is a problem, especially when the drug is administered with normal saline (NS) or Ringer's lactate (RL). Oxytocin should not be given with a hypotonic solution.

Bolus administration of oxytocin causes peripheral vasodilation, which may result in hypotension. Weis et al.[53] administered oxytocin 0.1 U/kg intravenously to pregnant women in the first trimester. They noted that heart rate increased, MAP

decreased by 30%, and total peripheral resistance decreased by 50%. Secher et al.[54] noted that bolus intravenous administration of 5 or 10 U of oxytocin increased pulmonary artery pressures in pregnant women. An oxytocin infusion at a rate of 80 mU/min for 10 minutes resulted in no cardiovascular changes.[54] Various electrocardiographic (ECG) changes also may occur during the administration of oxytocin, but their significance is unclear. Fortunately, cardiovascular changes are short lived (less than 10 minutes). The liver, the kidneys, and the enzyme oxytocinase are responsible for the short plasma half-life of oxytocin.

At the University of North Carolina, we avoid bolus intravenous administration of oxytocin. Rather, we add 20 U of oxytocin to a liter of NS or RL and start an intravenous infusion. The onset is almost immediate.[55] Some physicians advocate giving a more concentrated solution of oxytocin (e.g., 40 U/L) before giving other uterotonic agents in patients with mild uterine atony. Munn el al.[56] compared two oxytocin regimens (333 mU/min versus 2667 mU/min, infused intravenously over 30 minutes) after cord clamping in women who underwent cesarean delivery during labor. The authors observed a significant decrease in the number of requests for additional uterotonic medications in the high-dose oxytocin group. The incidence of hypotension was similar in the two groups. A recent study suggests that there is no clinical advantage associated with administration of oxytocin by the *intramyometrial* route.[57]

Prostaglandins of the E and F families represent the most recent additions to the pharmacologic treatment of uterine atony and have received wide acceptance as effective uterotonic agents. Concentrations of endogenous prostaglandins increase during labor, but their peak concentrations do not occur until placental separation. In some women, uterine atony may be caused by failure of prostaglandins to increase during the third stage of labor.[58,59] Prostaglandins increase myometrial intracellular free calcium concentrations, which ultimately lead to increases in myosin light-chain kinase activity.[60] Common side effects noted after administration of any of the prostaglandins are fever, diarrhea, nausea, and vomiting.

Prostaglandin E$_2$ is one option for the treatment of uterine atony. It causes bronchodilation, decreased systemic vascular resistance (SVR) and blood pressure, and increased heart rate and cardiac output in normovolemic patients. Pulmonary vascular resistance does not change.[61,62] In one study,[61] intravenous administration of prostaglandin E$_2$ caused an increase in PaO$_2$, with no change in PaCO$_2$. In the United States, the only available formulation of prostaglandin E$_2$ is a 20-mg vaginal suppository, which limits the usefulness of this drug during significant vaginal bleeding. (Some obstetricians give the suppositories rectally rather than vaginally.) There is limited experience with an intravenous formulation of the drug.[63] None of the prostaglandins currently available in the United States are approved for intravenous administration.

Administration of **prostaglandin F$_{2\text{-alpha}}$** increases cardiac output, systemic and pulmonary artery pressures, and pulmonary vascular resistance in anesthetized pregnant women.[61] Increased PaCO$_2$ and decreased PaO$_2$ suggest alterations of ventilation/perfusion ratios after prostaglandin F$_{2\text{-alpha}}$ administration.[61,64] Overt bronchospasm may occur. One patient received an overdose (40 mg) of the drug and developed pulmonary edema and cardiovascular collapse.[65] The starting dose is 1 mg given intramuscularly or intramyometrially. Prostaglandin F$_{2\text{-alpha}}$ is not approved for the treatment of uterine atony in the United States.

Box 37-2 CONDITIONS ASSOCIATED WITH UTERINE ATONY

Multiple gestation	Precipitous labor
Macrosomia	Augmented labor
Polyhydramnios	Tocolytic agents
High parity	High concentration of a volatile
Prolonged labor	halogenated agent
Chorioamnionitis	

15-Methyl prostaglandin F$_{2\text{-alpha}}$ (carboprost, Hemabate) is the preferred prostaglandin for the treatment of refractory uterine atony, and its use may succeed in controlling hemorrhage when all other pharmacologic treatments have failed. The use of 15-methyl prostaglandin F$_{2\text{-alpha}}$ most likely has decreased the need to perform obstetric hysterectomy for uterine atony. Unfortunately, this valuable obstetric drug compound also may result in bronchospasm, disturbed ventilation/perfusion ratios, increased intrapulmonary shunt fraction, and hypoxemia.[66,67] The dose of 15-methyl prostaglandin F$_{2\text{-alpha}}$ is 250 μg administered intramuscularly or intramyometrially. The dose may be repeated every 15 to 30 minutes. The total dose should not exceed 2 mg. One small series[68] reported success using this drug as an intravenous infusion, but more data are needed. It is not approved for intravenous administration.

Misoprostol is a prostaglandin E$_1$ analogue developed for the treatment of peptic ulcer disease. This drug has been successfully administered for cervical priming and/or induction of labor at term, and also as an alternative to oxytocin in the management of the third stage of labor. O'Brien et al.[69] concluded that rectally administered misoprostol appears to be an effective treatment for postpartum hemorrhage unresponsive to oxytocin and ergometrine. High-dose intravaginal misoprostol does not alter maternal cardiac function as measured by transthoracic electrical bioimpedance during midpregnancy.[70]

The **ergot alkaloids** represent a third class of drugs for the treatment of uterine atony. The natural ergot alkaloids are produced by a fungus that commonly infests rye and other grains. **Ergonovine** and **methylergonovine** (a semisynthetic preparation) are the two ergot alkaloids currently used for treatment of uterine atony. Ergots are restricted to postpartum use. Some obstetricians routinely administer an ergot alkaloid after vaginal delivery, but most obstetricians restrict their use to patients with uterine atony.

Ergonovine and methylergonovine are identical in their pharmacologic profiles and activity. Both drugs rapidly produce tetanic uterine contraction. The uterotonic effect is most likely mediated by means of alpha-adrenergic receptors.

Parenteral administration of an ergot alkaloid is associated with a high incidence of nausea and vomiting, which is problematic for the awake patient. Ergonovine and methylergonovine have been reported to be less cardiotoxic than other ergot alkaloids, but they may cause serious cardiovascular system derangements (e.g., vasoconstriction, hypertension). Pulmonary artery pressure increases after intravenous administration of an ergot alkaloid, and the duration is longer than that noted after bolus administration of oxytocin.[71] Pulmonary edema may occur. Ergot alkaloids also cause coronary artery vasoconstriction and have been used to induce coronary vasospasm during cardiac catheterization. Tsui el al.[72] reported one case of cardiac arrest and myocardial infarction after administration of intravenous ergonovine. Hypertension, severe enough to cause a cerebrovascular accident and seizures, may occur.[73] Patients at greatest risk are those with preexisting hypertension; however, sudden and marked hypertension also may occur in nonhypertensive patients. The combination of an ergot alkaloid followed by a vasopressor may lead to exaggerated hypertension and morbidity.[74] Concurrent use of these drugs should be avoided. Other relative contraindications for ergot alkaloids are chronic hypertension, preeclampsia, peripheral vascular disease, and ischemic heart disease. Treatment of ergot-induced vasoconstriction and hypertension may require administration of a potent vasodilator (e.g., hydralazine, nitroglycerin, sodium nitroprusside).

Ergot alkaloids have an almost immediate onset when they are given intravenously. When given intramuscularly, the onset also is rapid (a few minutes). Both ergonovine and methylergonovine are dispensed in ampules containing 0.2 mg. Obstetricians typically ask the anesthesiologist to administer 0.2 mg intramuscularly. This large dose should *not* be given as an intravenous bolus. Another approach is to dilute 0.2 mg in 10 mL, give intravenous boluses of 1 mL (i.e., 0.02 mg), and check the maternal blood pressure before giving another dose 2 to 3 minutes later. The effect is rapid, and frequently a response occurs after the administration of a small dose. Typically, the uterotonic effect lasts for 2 to 3 hours. Regardless of the route of administration, blood pressure and the ECG should be monitored closely. At the University of North Carolina—for patients *without* reactive airway disease—we prefer to administer 15-methyl prostaglandin F$_{2\text{-alpha}}$ before resorting to ergot alkaloids in cases of uterine atony that has not responded to an oxytocin infusion.

If these uterotonic drugs do not result in successful hemostasis, invasive techniques must be considered. Invasive techniques include embolization of arteries supplying the uterus, surgical ligation of arteries, and hysterectomy *(vide infra)*.

Genital Trauma

The most common injuries incurred at childbirth are lacerations and hematomas of the perineum, vagina, and cervix. Most injuries have minimal consequence, but some puerperal lacerations and hematomas are associated with significant hemorrhage, either immediate or delayed. Prompt recognition and treatment can minimize morbidity and mortality.[75] Genital tract lacerations should be suspected in all patients who have vaginal bleeding despite a firm, contracted uterus. The cervix and vagina must be inspected carefully in these patients.

Pelvic hematomas may be divided into three types: vaginal, vulvar, and retroperitoneal.[17] **Vaginal hematomas** result from soft tissue injury during delivery. The use of forceps or vacuum extraction increases the risk. Other risk factors include a prolonged second stage of labor, multiple gestation, preeclampsia, and vulvovaginal varicosities. Bleeding often is occult and gradual. Injury may be detected only after significant blood loss has occurred. The patient may complain of severe rectal pressure, and examination discloses a large hematoma extending into the vagina. Treatment consists of incision, drainage, and packing of the wound. Often a discreet source of bleeding is not found.

Vulvar hematomas commonly involve branches of the pudendal artery. Approximately 80% of these cases appear soon after delivery; the remainder do not become apparent until 1 to 3 days later. Extreme vulvar pain and signs of hypovolemia may follow. Small hematomas that are not enlarging may be observed and treated conservatively with ice packs and oral analgesics. Large hematomas must be incised and evacuated.

Retroperitoneal hematomas are the least common and most dangerous. A retroperitoneal hemorrhage occurs after laceration of one of the branches of the hypogastric artery. Injury typically occurs during cesarean section or, infrequently, after rupture of a low transverse uterine scar during labor. These hematomas may be large and may extend as far as the kidneys.

The symptoms of concealed bleeding depend on the size of the hematoma and the rate at which it forms. In some instances, abrupt hypotension may be the first sign of bleeding. The diagnosis of a retroperitoneal hematoma must be considered whenever a postpartum patient has an unexpected fall in hematocrit or unexplained tachycardia and hypotension. Other signs and symptoms are restlessness, lower abdominal pain, a tender mass above the inguinal ligament that displaces a firm uterus to the contralateral side, and vaginal bleeding with hypotension out of proportion to the external blood loss. Ileus, unilateral leg edema, urinary retention, and hematuria also may occur. Computed tomography is a useful technique for determining the location and size of the hematoma. It is especially useful for detecting collections of blood in inaccessible areas such as the presacral space.[76]

Occasionally a retroperitoneal hematoma may be self-limiting and require no surgical intervention. Often these life-threatening hematomas require exploratory laparotomy and ligation of the hypogastric vessels. Fliegner[77] reported that 38 of 39 patients with a broad ligament hematoma received a blood transfusion. (The average amount given was 4000 mL.) Of the total, 8 (21%) of the patients required an abdominal hysterectomy.

ANESTHETIC MANAGEMENT

Choice of anesthetic technique for the repair of genital lacerations and evacuation of pelvic hematomas depends on the affected area, surgical requirements, physical status of the patient, and urgency of the procedure. Local infiltration and a small dose of intravenous opioid suffice for most vulvar hematomas. Repair of extensive lacerations and drainage of vaginal hematomas require significant levels of analgesia or anesthesia. Previously administered spinal or epidural anesthesia may have regressed. It may be inappropriate to initiate a regional block again because it may cause hypotension in a hypovolemic patient. Pudendal nerve block may not be technically feasible because of anatomic distortion and/or severe pain from the hematoma. For a brief examination, nitrous oxide (40% to 50%) analgesia can be administered safely and effectively. The analgesia has a rapid onset and is easily reversible. The patient should remain awake and alert, with spontaneous ventilation. The major risk of inhalation analgesia is that the anesthetic depth may change insidiously, especially if opioids or sedatives were administered before the nitrous oxide. Laryngeal reflexes may become lost, in which case the airway is unprotected. The anesthesiologist must maintain continual verbal contact with the patient. An alternative to nitrous oxide analgesia is ketamine. Low doses of ketamine (10-mg boluses, up to a total dose of 0.5 mg/kg) sufficient to produce sedation and analgesia do not alter laryngeal reflexes. A nonparticulate antacid should be administered before administration of either nitrous oxide or ketamine.

Exploratory laparotomy for a retroperitoneal hematoma typically requires the administration of general anesthesia. A rapid-sequence induction is mandatory unless a difficult intubation is expected.

Retained Placenta

Not all cases of retained placenta result in postpartum hemorrhage. In some patients, the uterus contracts, the placenta does not separate, and little or no hemorrhage occurs. (One possible cause of this problem is the early administration of oxytocin at vaginal delivery.) In other cases, the placenta appears to separate, but fragments of the placenta remain within the uterus. Retained placental fragments are a leading cause of both early and delayed postpartum hemorrhage.[78] The degree of hemorrhage often is not severe, but it may be insidious, and visual estimates are inaccurate.

OBSTETRIC MANAGEMENT

Treatment of retained placenta during the early postpartum period involves manual removal and inspection of the placenta. After removal of the placenta, uterine tone should be enhanced with oxytocin, and the patient should be observed for evidence of recurrent hemorrhage.

ANESTHETIC MANAGEMENT

Choice of anesthetic technique depends on the presence or absence of hemorrhage and the use of regional anesthesia for delivery. Epidural anesthesia previously administered for labor and delivery often is adequate. If not, analgesia can be provided by giving additional local anesthetic agent through the epidural catheter. Spinal anesthesia is a good choice for patients who are not bleeding and who did not have epidural anesthesia for delivery. In some cases, the administration of 40% to 50% nitrous oxide is effective. An alternative is the administration of small doses of ketamine (10-mg boluses, up to a total dose of 0.5 mg/kg) or fentanyl (50 to 100 µg). Often this is adequate to allow examination and manual placental extraction by a skilled obstetrician. Maintenance of protective airway reflexes is imperative, and a nonparticulate antacid should be administered first.

In some cases, the obstetrician requests uterine relaxation to facilitate manual removal. Historically, anesthesiologists have performed rapid-sequence induction of general anesthesia, followed by the administration of a high dose of a volatile halogenated agent to relax the uterus. (Equipotent doses of all the volatile halogenated agents depress uterine contractility equally.[79,80]) This technique provides both anesthesia and uterine relaxation, but it entails all of the risks (e.g., failed intubation, aspiration) associated with general anesthesia in obstetric patients. Many anesthesiologists currently advocate the administration of **nitroglycerin** for this purpose. Two small studies[81,82] evaluated the intravenous administration of nitroglycerin to postpartum women in a nonrandomized, nonblinded manner. The dose used in one study[82] was 50 µg, whereas 500 µg was administered to each patient in the other study.[81] Both studies claimed good results and no major side effects, but an intravenous bolus dose of 500 µg may be excessive. Others have administered nitroglycerin by different routes and in varying doses (e.g., sublingual spray, 800 µg) and have reported that it is an effective uterine relaxant.[83-85] Ley et al.[85] observed that intravenous nitroglycerin 500 µg decreased intrauterine pressure from 38 to 23 mm Hg in one patient with a retained placenta. Buhimschi et al.[86] studied 12 parturients in active labor with epidural analgesia. Each patient received either placebo or three 800-µg doses of sublingual nitroglycerin, given 10 minutes apart. The nitroglycerin failed to reduce uterine activity or tone, despite the fact that it reduced maternal blood pressure. The authors suggested that higher doses of nitroglycerin might be effective in reducing uterine tone, but "at the cost of increasing maternal and fetal risk." (Of course, fetal safety is not an issue in the setting of retained placenta.) Nitroglycerin most likely results in uterine relaxation by releasing nitric oxide, and it may require the presence of placental tissue to be effective.[87] To date, no randomized, controlled trials have documented the efficacy of nitroglycerin for the provision of uterine relaxation. However, anecdotal case reports consistently suggest that nitroglycerin is an effective uterine relaxant clinically. Further, it seems safe to administer modest doses of nitroglycerin in most situations in which uterine relaxation is required.

Placenta Accreta

Placenta accreta is defined as an abnormally adherent placenta. There are three types of placenta accreta (Figure 37-4). **Placenta accreta vera** is defined as adherence to the myometrium without invasion of or passage through uterine muscle. **Placenta increta** represents invasion of the myometrium. **Placenta percreta** includes invasion of the uterine serosa or other pelvic structures.

EPIDEMIOLOGY

The incidence of this devastating problem may be increasing because of the increased incidence of cesarean section.[88] Prior uterine trauma is a risk factor for the development of placenta accreta. The combination of one or more prior cesarean sections and a current placenta previa or low-lying placenta should prompt suspicion regarding the presence of a placenta accreta. In a prospective study, Chattopadhyay et al.[89] noted a 5% incidence of placenta accreta when placenta previa occurred in patients with an unscarred uterus. In patients with one previous cesarean section, the incidence of placenta accreta was 10%, but the incidence increased to 59% in patients with a history of two or more cesarean sections. Two thirds of the patients with placenta previa, placenta accreta, and a preexisting uterine scar required cesarean hysterectomy.[89] Clark et al.[11] made similar observations (Table 37-3). However, the number of patients studied with more than two cesarean deliveries was small. Placenta accreta may be present even when no antepartum hemorrhage occurs in association with the placenta previa.

DIAGNOSIS

Antepartum diagnosis is unusual. In some cases the condition is first suspected at vaginal delivery when the obstetrician notes difficulty in separating the placenta. The definitive diagnosis often is made at laparotomy. The use of ultrasonography may help identify those patients with placenta previa and previous cesarean section who have placenta accreta.[90] If the placenta appears to extend anteriorly in the region of the old uterine scar, a high likelihood of placenta accreta is expected. Transvaginal color Doppler ultrasonography and MRI have correctly identified placenta accreta and placenta percreta, respectively.[91,92] In contrast, Lam et al.[93] retrospectively reviewed imaging studies of patients who had pathologic diagnoses of placenta accreta, percreta, or increta. The authors concluded that both MRI and ultrasonography had poor predictive capability for the diagnosis of placenta accreta.

OBSTETRIC MANAGEMENT

In selected cases, the obstetrician may opt for uterine curettage, followed by over-sewing of the bleeding placental bed. This rarely is successful. Conservative nonsurgical treatment options have been attempted, with varying success. Most cases require cesarean or postpartum hysterectomy, which should proceed without delay. The obstetrician must recognize the problem and make a prompt decision to proceed with definitive therapy (i.e., hysterectomy). However, nonsurgical techniques may aid the management of patients with placenta percreta and extensive extrauterine involvement. O'Brien et al.[94] reported 109 cases of placenta percreta; 101 of these 109 cases were managed surgically. Forty percent of the patients required more than 10 units of PRBCs, and 7% of the patients died. Balloon occlusion and/or embolization techniques may reduce the severity of intraoperative blood loss in patients with placenta percreta.[95,96]

Placenta accreta currently is the most common indication for obstetric hysterectomy in many hospitals. Unfortunately, many obstetricians have little or no experience with the performance of obstetric hysterectomy. When we prepare to anesthetize a patient at high risk for placenta accreta, we ask the obstetrician whether the diagnosis of placenta accreta has been considered and whether preparations for hysterectomy are complete. It is desirable that two obstetricians be scrubbed for cesarean section when a patient is at high risk for placenta accreta. Blood loss in these cases can be substantial. Of greatest importance is the ability to get large amounts of blood products to the operating room quickly.

ANESTHETIC MANAGEMENT

Preoperative diagnosis of placentation abnormalities—especially those that are associated with substantial intraoper-

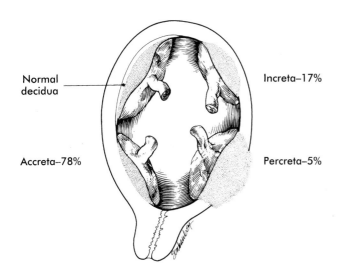

FIGURE 37-4. Uteroplacental relationships found in abnormal placentation. (From Bendetti TJ. Obstetric hemorrhage. In Gabbe SG, Niebyl JR, Simpson JL, editors. Obstetrics: Normal and Problem Pregnancies, 4th ed. New York, Churchill Livingstone, 2001:519.)

TABLE 37-3	PLACENTA PREVIA WITH PRIOR UTERINE INCISION: EFFECT ON INCIDENCE OF PLACENTA ACCRETA		
No. of prior cesarean sections	Patients with placenta previa (n = 286)	Placenta previa/accreta (n = 29)	%
0	238	12	5
1	25	6	24
2	15	7	47
3	5	2	40
4	3	2	67

From Clark SL, Koonings PP, Phelan JP. Placental previa/accreta and prior cesarean section. Obstet Gynecol 1985; 89:92.

ative blood loss—may help the anesthesiologist choose the most appropriate anesthetic technique. Such knowledge is especially important with regard to patients with placenta percreta (*vide supra*).

Uterine Inversion

EPIDEMIOLOGY

Uterine inversion—or the turning inside out of all or part of the uterus—is a rare but potentially disastrous event during the peripartum period. Inversions may be acute or chronic, but only acute peripartum inversions are of interest to the obstetric anesthesiologist. The reported incidence of this disorder varies widely, but acute peripartum inversions most likely occur in 1 in 5000 to 1 in 10,000 pregnancies. Maternal mortality secondary to uterine inversion is very low in the Western world. The most recent report of maternal mortality in the United Kingdom included no maternal deaths secondary to hemorrhage from uterine inversion.[3]

Risk factors for uterine inversion include uterine atony, inappropriate fundal pressure, umbilical cord traction, and uterine anomalies. An abnormally implanted placenta (i.e., placenta accreta) may be first recognized when uterine inversion occurs.

DIAGNOSIS

Many cases of uterine inversion are obvious because of hemorrhage and a mass in the vagina, but others may not be readily apparent. Inversion should be suspected in all cases of postpartum hemorrhage and hypotension. Historically, obstetricians have stated that the shock is out of proportion to the blood loss, but an underestimation of obstetric hemorrhage is more likely. The atonic uterus frequently seen with uterine inversion contributes to the ongoing blood loss.

OBSTETRIC MANAGEMENT

Early replacement of the uterus is the best treatment. Once the uterus has been replaced, a firm, well-contracted uterus is desired. Oxytocin (20 U/L) should be infused initially, but additional drugs (e.g., 15-methyl prostaglandin $F_{2-alpha}$) may be needed.

ANESTHETIC MANAGEMENT

In some cases, uterine tone precludes immediate replacement, and uterine relaxation is needed before successful replacement can be performed. The ideal technique should produce rapid uterine relaxation with no side effects and should have a short duration to facilitate restoration of uterine tone after replacement of the uterus. Administration of general anesthesia with a volatile halogenated agent is the most proven method for producing uterine relaxation. *Endotracheal intubation is mandatory.* Equipotent doses of all volatile halogenated agents produce a similar degree of uterine relaxation.[79,80] There are anecdotal reports of the use of terbutaline, magnesium sulfate, and organic nitrates to facilitate relaxation and reduction of the inverted uterus. Altabef et al.[97] reported the intravenous administration of two 50-μg doses of nitroglycerin to relax and facilitate replacement of the uterus in one patient. Bayhi et al.[98] reported the successful intravenous administration of nitroglycerin 200 μg for this purpose. (Others have reported the use of nitroglycerin to relax the uterus in cases of a retained placenta[81,85] [*vide supra*].) These anecdotal reports suggest that administration of nitroglycerin may obviate the need for general anesthesia.

Invasive Treatment Options

Regardless of the cause of obstetric hemorrhage, conservative measures sometimes fail to stop the bleeding. In these cases, invasive procedures must be used promptly to avoid severe morbidity and mortality. Options include angiographic arterial embolization, balloon occlusion, surgical arterial ligation, and hysterectomy.

The uterine arteries, which are branches of the anterior trunk of the internal iliac arteries, provide the primary blood supply to the uterus. However, the ovarian arteries also make a sizable contribution to uterine blood flow during pregnancy. During **angiography** the radiologist can identify the vessels responsible for bleeding and embolize these vessels safely and effectively with gelatin sponge and pledgets (Gelfoam).[99,100] **Embolization** is attractive because only local anesthesia is needed, complications are few, preservation of fertility is likely, and this procedure has been performed safely in the presence of a coagulopathy. This procedure requires rapid access to an angiography facility and a skilled radiologist. The patient must be observed and monitored properly while in the angiography suite. Unfortunately, logistic problems prevent physicians from using this very effective technique to full advantage. Options such as arterial ligation and hysterectomy may be performed subsequently if needed. However, if arterial ligation is attempted first, embolization techniques are more difficult to perform and may not be successful.

Bilateral surgical ligation of the uterine, ovarian, and internal iliac arteries may be useful when other measures have failed. The decrease in pulse pressure distal to the ligature may allow normal hemostatic mechanisms to function. This technique, when successful, also permits the preservation of fertility. Arterial ligation may result in damage to other pelvic structures (e.g., ureter). The vascular anatomy is variable, and lower extremity ischemia is another potential complication of the procedure. Although high failure rates have been published, early bilateral hypogastric artery ligation after delivery, but before hemodynamic instability occurs, has been associated with a 90% success rate.[101] Another study noted that arterial ligation eliminated the need for hysterectomy in 65% of the patients.[102] There were fewer complications in the ligation group, and the estimated blood loss and amount of blood transfused also were less in this group (Table 37-4). Ligation was less effective if the cause of hemorrhage was uterine atony. This study was flawed because the authors included patients with failed hypogastric artery ligation in the hysterectomy group. Failure to arrest hemorrhage by this technique may result from the presence of a rich collateral circulation.[103]

Cesarean or **postpartum hysterectomy** often represents the definitive treatment for postpartum hemorrhage. Obstetric hysterectomy is more difficult than hysterectomy in a nonpregnant patient. The uterus is enlarged, the vessels are engorged, and exposure may be difficult. Tissues are edematous, and suture ligatures often slip. The amount of blood loss depends in part on whether the hysterectomy is elective or emergent. A multicenter review showed that the average blood loss for emergent cases was 2526 mL, with an average transfusion requirement of 6.6 units of blood.[104] In elective cases, the mean blood loss was 1319 mL, and the average replacement was 1.6 units of blood (Table 37-5). Wenhem and Matijevic[105] evaluated data from 28 postpartum hysterectomies and found that emergency operations, as compared to elective procedures, were associated with a significantly greater blood loss, requirement for transfusion of blood products, and utilization of intensive care.

ANESTHETIC MANAGEMENT

Anesthetic considerations for arterial ligation and obstetric hysterectomy are similar. The obstetrician requires good skeletal muscle relaxation and a quiet operative field. Patients without preexisting regional anesthesia almost always require general anesthesia for emergency obstetric hysterectomy. In these cases, all the considerations noted for patients with antepartum hemorrhage should be applied. Massive blood loss can be expected, and large amounts of crystalloid and blood products are required. In a report of 117 emergency peripartum hysterectomies, Zelop et al.[106] noted that respiratory complications occurred in 21% of the patients, and DIC occurred in 27%.

If hemorrhage complicates cesarean section in a patient with spinal or epidural anesthesia, the anesthesiologist may need to give general anesthesia to protect the patient's airway. However, an early decision by the obstetrician to proceed with a controlled hysterectomy may allow the anesthesiologist to avoid administration of general anesthesia, provided that severe hypotension does not occur and that the patient remains alert and comfortable. An experienced, skilled obstetric team is invaluable during this difficult operation.

Controversy exists regarding the type of anesthesia that should be administered to the patient who is scheduled for elective cesarean hysterectomy or who is at high risk for emergency hysterectomy during elective cesarean section (e.g., the patient with a present placenta previa and a history of cesarean section). Chestnut and Redick[107] reviewed their experience with administration of epidural anesthesia for elective cesarean hysterectomy in 25 patients between 1972 and 1984. Of these patients, 7 (28%) required intraoperative induction of general anesthesia because of patient discomfort and/or inadequate operating conditions. The authors stated that epidural anesthesia may not be adequate for elective cesarean hysterectomy for three reasons. First, the operative time for cesarean hysterectomy is twice that required for cesarean section alone, predisposing the patient to fatigue and restlessness. Second, intraperitoneal manipulation, dissection, and traction typically exceed that required with cesarean section alone and may result in pain, nausea, and vomiting. Third, "hyperemic pelvic viscera with engorged, edematous

TABLE 37-4 COMPARISON OF COMPLICATIONS BETWEEN HYPOGASTRIC ARTERY LIGATION (HAL) AND HYSTERECTOMY OR HAL REQUIRING HYSTERECTOMY

	HAL successful (n = 19)	Hysterectomy or HAL with hysterectomy (n = 45)
Estimated blood loss (mL) mean (range)	2230 (1000-3000)	3500 (1500-5500)
Blood transfusion (mL) mean (range)	2000 (1000-5000)	3500 (2000-8000)
Hospital stay (days) mean (range)	7 (5-12)	9 (6-24)
Intraoperative hypotension	9 (47%)	33 (73%)
Reexploration	0	6 (13%)
Injury to bladder	0	4 (9%)
Febrile morbidity	2 (11%)	16 (36%)
Pelvic hematoma	0	2 (4%)
Wound infection	1 (5%)	7 (16%)
Deep vein thrombosis	0	1 (2%)
Maternal mortality	0	3 (7%)

From Chattopadhyay SK, Deb Roy B, Edrees YB. Surgical control of obstetric hemorrhage: Hypogastric artery ligation or hysterectomy? Int J Gynecol Obstet 1990; 32:345-51.

TABLE 37-5 OPERATIVE MANAGEMENT AND COMPLICATIONS OF ELECTIVE VERSUS EMERGENT OBSTETRIC HYSTERECTOMIES

	Elective (n = 21)	Emergent (n = 21)	P
Anesthesia			
Epidural	8	4	
Spinal	0	1	
General	13	16	
Operative time (min)*	137 ± 55	148 ± 62	NS
Hysterectomy			
Total	21	19	NS
Subtotal	0	2	
Estimated blood loss (mL)*	1319 ± 396	2526 ± 1240	< 0.001
Intraoperative hypotension	6 (29%)	13 (62%)	< 0.05
Intraoperative crystalloid (mL)*	4062 ± 1512	5374 ± 2340	< 0.05
Intraoperative transfusion	7 (33%)	17 (81%)	< 0.01
Intraoperative or postoperative transfusion	10 (48%)	18 (86%)	< 0.01
Total units transfused*	1.6 ± 1.9	6.6 ± 5.4	< 0.001
Discharge hematocrit (%)*	30 ± 4	30 ± 4	NS
Intraoperative injury			
Ureteral	1 (5%)	0	NS
Cystotomy	1 (5%)	0	NS
Reoperation required	0	1 (5%)	NS
Days in hospital*	5.5 ± 1.3	7.3 ± 4.3	< 0.05
Mortality	0	0	NS

*Mean ± SD.
NS, not significant.
Modified from Chestnut DH, Dewan DM, Redick LF, et al. Anesthetic management for obstetric hysterectomy: A multi-institutional study. Anesthesiology 1989; 70:607-10.

vasculature require careful dissection facilitated by a quiet operative field."[107] Subsequently, in a multi-institutional study of obstetric hysterectomy, none of the 12 patients who received continuous epidural anesthesia for elective or emergency hysterectomy required intraoperative induction of general anesthesia. Chestnut et al.[104] noted the following:

> Many parturients want to be awake and alert during cesarean delivery. Maintenance of a T-4 sensory level, prophylaxis against nausea and vomiting, and judicious sedation should reduce the need for intraoperative induction of general anesthesia.

At the University of North Carolina, we do not withhold administration of regional anesthesia from normovolemic women undergoing elective, repeat cesarean section for placenta previa, despite the risk for placenta accreta and emergency hysterectomy in those women. It seems prudent to choose a continuous anesthetic technique for these patients. We inform patients that intraoperative induction of general anesthesia may be required if significant hemorrhage should occur. The anesthesiologist should spend time maintaining intravascular volume rather than holding an emesis basin. Further, the hypotensive patient may not be able to protect her airway.

The presence of a known placenta *percreta* may greatly increase the risk for significant bleeding, even when compared to placenta accreta. For these cases, general anesthesia may be preferable. In cases of known abnormal placentation, preoperative prophylactic bilateral hypogastric artery balloons can be placed via angiography. At surgery, the balloons are inflated after cesarean delivery of the fetus, which allows the surgeons to perform cesarean hysterectomy with good tissue exposure and minimal blood loss.[108]

Regardless of the anesthetic technique used, two large-gauge intravenous catheters should be inserted, and at least two units of packed PRBCs should be immediately available. Additional units should be available without delay. Vasoactive drugs (e.g., phenylephrine, dopamine, epinephrine) should be immediately available. It is useful to have a skilled assistant who can help establish invasive monitoring if it is needed. A fluid warmer, a forced air warmer, and equipment for rapid infusion of fluids must be available when anticipating and managing significant blood loss.

TRANSFUSION THERAPY

As early as 1818, James Blundell, the obstetrician credited with performing the first transfusion and advancing the concept of blood compatibility, recognized the efficacy of transfusion in women with postpartum hemorrhage.[109] Despite advances in the prevention, diagnosis, and treatment of the hemorrhagic complications of pregnancy, the potential for massive blood loss remains a threat during pregnancy. All physicians who provide care for pregnant women should understand the indications, requirements, risks, and benefits of transfusion.

Concerns regarding bloodborne infectious disease have led to a reevaluation of indications for red blood cell transfusion, particularly during the perioperative period. Combs et al.[110] studied 14,267 consecutive term deliveries without placenta previa and found that red blood cell transfusion was used in only 150 (1.1%) deliveries. Camann and Datta[111] reviewed records for 9596 women who had a cesarean delivery between 1984 and 1987. They noted that 336 (3.5%) parturients received blood products during or after cesarean section.

Placenta previa was the most frequent indication for transfusion. The incidence of transfusion declined from 6.2% to 3.2% during the study period.[111] The authors attributed the decline in transfusion to an increasing awareness by physicians and patients about infectious risks from blood products, as well as physicians' acceptance of a lower perioperative hemoglobin concentration. During the study period, the American Association of Blood Banks (AABB) mandated a confidential donor history as well as laboratory testing to screen for human immunodeficiency virus (HIV).[112]

Although long-standing tradition states that patients undergoing elective surgery should have a hemoglobin concentration of at least 10 g/dL, current guidelines have been individualized. The Consensus Development Conference on Perioperative Red Cell Transfusion concluded that healthy patients tolerate a hemoglobin concentration as low as 7 g/dL.[113] Oxygen delivery is maintained with a low hemoglobin concentration as long as the patient is normovolemic. As the red blood cell mass decreases, both blood viscosity and resistance to blood flow markedly decrease, which results in an increase in cardiac output and tissue blood flow without a concomitant increase in cardiovascular work. Tissue oxygen delivery is maintained despite the decreased red blood cell mass. Although anecdotal evidence and case reports suggest that maternal well-being and perinatal outcome are not altered by mild anemia, the increased metabolic rate during pregnancy suggests that the pregnant patient may have less tolerance for the additional cardiovascular stress of severe anemia. The minimum hemoglobin concentration required to sustain a normal pregnancy has not been clearly defined. However, it seems intuitive that transfusion should be performed in *all* obstetric patients with clinical evidence of inadequate oxygen-carrying capacity, and in *most* obstetric patients with a hemoglobin concentration of less than 7 g/dL. Likewise, it seems intuitive that *ongoing* blood loss should prompt the anesthesiologist to begin transfusion in some patients with a hemoglobin concentration *greater* than 7 g/dL.

In our judgment, the potential for transfusion and the occasional patient who develops an antibody from fetal antigen exposure during pregnancy warrant the performance of an admission type and screen in all parturients. (The necessity of an admission type and screen for *all* parturients is currently a matter of some dispute.[114] See Appendix B on page 953.) Only those patients with risk factors (e.g., placenta previa, a positive antibody screen, preoperative bleeding, coagulopathy) require a prophylactic cross-match. The need to obtain a type and screen for patients before elective cesarean section has also been questioned. One recent study noted that in patients without admission risk factors, the overall urgent blood transfusion rate was 0.8 per 1000 cesarean sections.[115] Risk factors associated with the need for transfusion in patients undergoing cesarean section include preoperative anemia, previous cesarean section, placenta previa, abnormal presentation, multiple gestation, chorioamnionitis, and placental abruption.[115] Nonetheless, in our judgment, a type and screen *should* be performed in all patients undergoing cesarean section.

With the type and screen, the blood bank identifies the ABO and Rh status of the patient's blood. The antibody screen is conducted using patient serum mixed with commercially processed O-positive red blood cells that contain most of the antigens that react with the common, clinically significant antibodies. Excluding the Rh-negative patient, approximately 1 in 1000 women develop an antibody to a fetal red blood cell antigen (transferred across the placenta) during pregnancy. In these women, the blood bank requires additional time to identify the antibody, especially if the antibody is uncommon. For patients in whom the antibody cannot be identified rapidly, the final in vitro cross-match of donor and recipient blood is of critical importance in determining whether donor blood is compatible.

In the patient who has a negative screen for antibodies to the antigens present on the processed red blood cells, the cross-match rarely, if ever, contributes further to the care of the patient. A transfusion reaction would be extremely uncommon in the presence of a negative antibody screen, and for this reason, some blood banks abbreviate or even dispense with the final cross-match for patients who have a negative screen. (The abbreviated cross-match is conducted using a rapid-spin cross-match technique that can quickly provide a final check to ensure compatible blood products. This 10-minute technique requires less time than the three-stage cross-match, which requires 45 minutes.) The benefits of not performing a cross-match on all obstetric patients include the ability to maintain a limited blood-bank inventory, decreased wastage of banked blood, and monetary savings derived from avoiding unnecessary cross-matches.

If blood is required quickly and the results of an antibody screen are not available, the safest option is administration of ABO Rh type-specific blood. (Antibody formation from previous sensitization is unusual.) If the blood type is unknown and blood is required immediately, type O, Rh-negative blood can be given.

Autologous Transfusion

The advantages of autologous blood transfusion include avoiding the risks of alloimmunization and hemolytic reactions, reducing the demands on the blood supply, and the psychological benefits of patients participating in their own treatment. Three methods of autologous transfusion exist: preoperative (antepartum) donation, intraoperative blood salvage, and normovolemic hemodilution. Preoperative donation and normovolemic hemodilution are blood conservation techniques that are used when blood loss can be predicted before surgery.

ANTEPARTUM DONATION

Although the concept of preoperative autologous donation is not new, the risks of bloodborne infection from donor blood have made the procedure more popular during the last decade. In 1992, approximately 1,117,000 autologous units of blood were donated before elective surgery.[116] Women with placenta previa who are stable and who do not require immediate delivery are potential candidates for antepartum donation. Patients with a rare blood type (for whom there may be great difficulty in locating suitable blood for transfusion) also may benefit from antepartum donation. The standards of the American Association of Blood Banks state that the patient's hemoglobin and hematocrit should be at least 11 g/dL and 33%, respectively, which would exclude some pregnant patients with physiologic and/or iron-deficiency anemia. Some physicians have suggested that a *pre-donation* hemoglobin and hematocrit of 10 g/dL and 30%, respectively, are acceptable for pregnant women. However, most published studies of pregnant patients have required a pre-donation hematocrit of at least 34%.[117-119]

In the past, antepartum donation has been discouraged for pregnant women because of concern over their ability to tolerate an acute volume change and the possibility of causing preterm labor or fetal distress. Droste et al.[117] measured maternal cardiac output, total peripheral vascular resistance, and fetal umbilical artery systolic/diastolic ratios before and after donation of 450 mL of whole blood by 16 women during the third trimester of pregnancy. Except for a small increase in maternal heart rate, the donation of a unit of blood had no significant maternal or fetal effect. Likewise, Kruskall[118] demonstrated that autologous blood donation during pregnancy was safe for both mother and fetus.

Andres et al.[119] cautioned that antepartum donation by obstetric patients may not be justified. They stated that the commonly accepted risk factors for postpartum hemorrhage and transfusion do not permit physicians to correctly identify those patients who will require blood transfusion and that many patients who donate blood will not require a transfusion. They identified 251 patients with traditionally accepted risk factors for postpartum bleeding: repeat cesarean section, multiple gestation, and placenta previa. Only four (1.6%) of these patients required blood transfusion (0.7% of those with a prior cesarean section, 3.7% with multiple gestation, and 25% with a placenta previa). They suggested that preoperative donation may not be beneficial or cost effective when the low frequency of blood transfusion in high-risk patients and the difficulty in correctly predicting those patients likely to require transfusion are considered. In addition, their data showed that the transfusion of a single unit of PRBCs is uncommon. Among *all* patients who required transfusion, 12 of 13 (92%) required more than one unit of red cells. Many obstetric patients are unable to donate more than one unit of blood. Thus it is likely that homologous blood would be required in addition to autologous transfusion.

Combs et al.[110] suggested that the small decrease in infection risk does not justify the expense of antepartum autologous blood donation in patients without placenta previa. They concluded that a hypothetical antepartum blood donation program restricted to patients with known risk factors would cost $32,800 to $130,700 to prevent one case of transfusion-related hepatitis and $26,000,000 to $78,000,000 to prevent one case of HIV infection. They concluded: "In obstetric patients without placenta previa, the need for peripartum red-cell transfusion cannot be predicted with sufficient accuracy to justify the costs of antepartum autologous blood donation."[110]

INTRAOPERATIVE BLOOD SALVAGE

Intraoperative blood salvage or autotransfusion is a technique of scavenging blood lost during operation, processing it by centrifugation, and washing and transfusing the scavenged, autologous red blood cells.[120] Red blood cells that are salvaged, processed, and transfused have an excellent survival rate. This technique, which can rapidly provide large quantities of autologous blood, is widely used in cardiovascular and general surgery and is acceptable to many Jehovah's Witness patients.

Malignancy, infection, the presence of old hemolyzed blood, and the use of collagen or hemostatic material are relative contraindications to the use of intraoperative blood salvage. A concern in the peripartum period is that blood processing and washing may not adequately remove amniotic fluid and fetal debris and that transfusion may precipitate the anaphylactoid syndrome of pregnancy (amniotic fluid embolism). Recent studies of in vitro washing of scavenged maternal blood mixed with amniotic fluid showed elimination (or greatly reduced concentrations) of alpha-fetoprotein, phospholipids, tissue factor, fetal squamous cells, and other cellular debris.[121,122] The best washed product for transfusion results from the addition of a leukocyte depletion filter to the system. Even with this added filter, the washed blood is likely to contain fetal red blood cells.[121,122] Therefore, isoimmunization of the mother is possible, and anti-D immune globulin should be administered when appropriate.

In a randomized study, Rainaldi et al.[123] observed that 34 patients who underwent intraoperative salvage and reinfusion of autologous blood (mean ± SD volume = 363 ± 153 mL) required fewer transfusions of homologous blood and had a shorter hospital stay than a control group. Rebarber et al.[124] performed a retrospective, multicenter study of 139 patients in whom autologous blood transfusion was performed during cesarean section between 1988 and 1997. The range of auto-transfused volumes was 200 to 11,250 mL. The authors identified no cases of acute respiratory distress syndrome or amniotic fluid embolism, and they identified no increase in the incidence of other complications (e.g., DIC) when compared with 87 control patients who underwent similar surgical procedures *without* autotransfusion at the same hospitals.

Intraoperative blood salvage may be appropriate in cases of massive obstetric hemorrhage when blood bank resources might not be sufficient to provide timely restoration of maternal oxygen-carrying capacity. In cases of suspected placenta accreta, the American College of Obstetricians and Gynecologists has stated that "cell saver technology should be considered if available."[125] Although there may be a small increase in the risk of the anaphylactoid syndrome of pregnancy (amniotic fluid embolism), it is outweighed by the potential benefits in cases of life-threatening hemorrhage. Suction of blood into the cell-washing system should be initiated only after delivery of the fetoplacental unit.

At the University of North Carolina, our experience with peripartum blood salvage has been limited to cases of massive bleeding during peripartum hysterectomy. Cell salvage techniques may also be indicated in less extreme situations in Jehovah's Witness patients. (Editor's note: In most published reports of the use of intraoperative blood salvage in obstetric patients, the average volume of salvaged blood returned to the patient was equivalent to one unit of blood or less. Rarely does transfusion of such a small amount of blood make the difference in outcome. Given the ongoing uncertainty regarding maternal safety, a decision to use intraoperative cell salvage in obstetric patients should be made with great care. In an editorial, Weiskopf[126] suggested that "the use of this technique during cesarean section should be limited to those times when it is the only way to augment the patient's oxygen-carrying capacity, when it is necessary to preserve function or life.")

NORMOVOLEMIC HEMODILUTION
The potential advantages of this technique include (1) no wastage of collected blood, (2) the ability to transfuse fresh blood with active clotting factors and platelets, and (3) little risk of storage or clerical errors. Limited experience with normovolemic hemodilution exists in obstetrics.[127,128] Grange et al.[128] employed normovolemic hemodilution before cesarean section in 38 women at increased risk for significant blood loss (e.g., placenta previa). The authors collected 500 to 1000 mL of blood from each patient, and the collected blood was reinfused at the end of surgery or earlier, if required. They observed no

maternal or fetal complications during or after phlebotomy. One patient also received homologous blood, and 14 received previously donated autologous blood. The authors concluded that acute hemodilution is well tolerated in parturients undergoing cesarean section and may be used with or without preoperative autologous blood donation. This technique may be acceptable to Jehovah's Witnesses who are at increased risk for significant blood loss during cesarean section.

Treatment of Massive Blood Loss
Peripartum hemorrhage can lead to massive blood loss. *Why Mothers Die 1997–1999: Confidential Enquiries into Maternal Deaths in the United Kingdom*[3] emphasizes the importance of clinical guidelines in the management of massive hemorrhage in obstetric patients, and stresses the importance of a functioning blood bank, accurate estimation of blood loss, prompt treatment of clotting disorders, and the early involvement of a hematologist.

In previously healthy parturients, blood pressure may remain near normal until blood loss exceeds 1500 mL. Blood is shifted from venous capacitance vessels to the central circulation by peripheral and splanchnic vasoconstriction. In the initial resuscitation from hemorrhage, warmed non-dextrose-containing crystalloid (e.g., RL, NS) and colloid solution (e.g., hydroxyethyl starch) are acceptable choices for volume replacement. When blood is required for replacement, whole blood would appear to be an ideal choice for maintaining intravascular volume. Few if any donor units are maintained as whole blood in the modern blood bank. The high demand for blood components such as platelets, fresh frozen plasma, and cryoprecipitate is one reason more than 90% of donor blood is fractionated into blood components. Blood component therapy provides the patient with only those products that are required and helps extend the shelf life of each component. Components and derivatives from one unit of blood can be used to treat several patients.[129] Products such as Rh-immune globulin currently are available only from donor blood.

Red blood cells are prepared from citrate phosphate dextrose adenine (CPDA) whole blood by centrifuging the blood and removing 200 to 250 mL of plasma. Each unit of CPDA PRBCs contains 250 mL and has a hematocrit of 70%, thus providing the same increase in hemoglobin as one unit of whole blood but with approximately half the volume. (Transfusion of one unit of PRBCs increases the hemoglobin by approximately 1.5 g/dL and the hematocrit by 4% to 5% in a 70-kg woman.) The shelf life of the preserved cells is 35 days. A solution of adenine, dextrose, mannitol, and saline may be added to the CPDA PRBCs after plasma has been removed. This solution extends the red cell shelf life to 42 days, and has a hematocrit of 60%.

Fresh frozen plasma maintains the viability of all clotting factors. Even though most coagulation factors are stable during storage at 4° C, factors V and VIII gradually decline to 15% to 30% of normal during storage as whole blood or plasma. The only clear indication for fresh frozen plasma is the replacement of coagulation factors in clotting disorders.[129] Fresh frozen plasma should not be used to treat hypovolemia or used as a protein supplement. The prophylactic use of fresh frozen plasma has not proved to be effective in decreasing blood loss in massive blood loss situations.[130,131] Administration of fresh frozen plasma should be considered when urgent reversal of warfarin is desired and for correction of microvascular bleeding in the presence of an elevated prothrombin time (PT) and activated partial thromboplastin time (aPTT). Cryoprecipitate (which contains factor VIII, fibrinogen, fibronectin, von Willebrand factor, and factor XIII) is useful when there is evidence of consumptive coagulopathy with depleted fibrinogen and elevated D-dimer measurements.

Platelets are difficult to store, and inventories in most blood banks are very low. The average platelet storage period is 72 hours. One unit of donor platelets increases the platelet count by 5000 to 10,000/mm³ in the average adult woman. Each platelet concentrate contains a small amount of red blood cells; thus the potential for sensitization exists. The blood bank typically provides platelets from a blood group and Rh-compatible donor. Platelets should be transfused only to prevent or correct bleeding associated with a decrease in platelet count or abnormality of platelet function.[132] Prophylactic platelet transfusion does not benefit patients with immune idiopathic thrombocytopenic purpura. (Such patients often do not have clinical bleeding, even with a low platelet count.) A patient undergoing surgery, including vaginal delivery, is unlikely to benefit from a platelet transfusion unless the platelet count is less than 50,000/mm³.[132]

A coagulopathy can develop rapidly in an obstetric patient. Although confirmatory laboratory tests (e.g., platelet count, fibrinogen concentration, PT, aPTT) are required to diagnose coagulopathy, one of the best guides to the need for coagulation factor replacement is observation of the surgical field for the presence of microvascular bleeding.[130,131] The absence of clot formation and the failure of bleeding to respond to attempts at surgical hemostasis suggest a coagulopathy. Hemostasis typically is adequate when clotting factors are greater than 30% of normal.[130,131,133,134] Surgical bleeding in the presence of clotting factor levels of 30% or greater (i.e., in those patients with a PT or aPTT measurement of less than 1.5 times the control) suggests an etiology other than low levels of coagulation factors.[130,131]

It often is difficult to separate a dilutional coagulopathy from a disseminated coagulopathy. A **dilutional coagulopathy** results from the replacement of blood loss with crystalloid and PRBCs, which dilute concentrations of coagulation factors and/or platelets. Increased bleeding as a result of decreased coagulation factors and platelets develops gradually and typically does not occur until more than one blood volume of loss (i.e., approximately 8 to 10 units of PRBC or whole blood replacement) occurs.[130,131] A dilutional coagulopathy responds rapidly to small aliquots of fresh frozen plasma and platelets.

Disseminated coagulopathy leads to a dramatic decline in coagulation factors and platelets because of clotting factor and platelet consumption.[130,131] Disseminated coagulopathy often develops early and rapidly in obstetric patients, particularly in women with amniotic fluid embolism or placental abruption. Multiple coagulation components (fresh frozen plasma, platelets, cryoprecipitate) may be required. In these catastrophic settings, the clinician must be prepared to titrate blood component therapy to hemostasis, obtain frequent coagulation testing, and obtain early consultation from a hematologist and the director of the blood bank and/or clinical laboratory.

Complications of Transfusion of Blood Products

Transfusion-related complications can be broadly divided into infectious, immunologic, storage, and infusion. The risk of parenteral transfusion of known viruses, including HIV,

hepatitis B, hepatitis C, and cytomegalovirus, continues to decrease with good donor screening and newer donor blood assays that decrease the window period. Current mathematical models for transfusion-related HIV transmittal suggest a risk of 1 in 200,000 to 1 in 2,000,000 transfusions.[135] Emerging viruses (e.g., hepatitis G), as yet unknown viruses, and bacterial infection will continue to be challenges in transfusion medicine.

Viral hepatitis is the most frequent infection associated with transfusion but has decreased dramatically with screening of donor blood for hepatitis C.[136] Currently the incidence is approximately 1 per 103,000 units of blood transfused.[135] Unfortunately, the major sequelae of hepatitis C may not be clinically evident for several months after the transfusion. Approximately 20% to 30% of those infected develop chronic active hepatitis, 20% to 50% of these people later develop cirrhosis, and 1% to 5% develop hepatocellular carcinoma.[137]

Cytomegalovirus (CMV) infection may occur frequently as a result of blood transfusion.[138] The virus is carried in asymptomatic donors in the neutrophil. Most of these infections are asymptomatic or mild, but infection in the immunocompromised patient and fetal transmission can produce serious sequelae. The virus is very prevalent; approximately 40% of Americans have experienced infection. Most are asymptomatic, but a congenitally acquired infection can produce severe infection in some infants. CMV infection can be prevented effectively by using CMV-negative blood or by eliminating neutrophils from donor blood by filtration or washing the donor unit.[139]

The most common cause of an acute transfusion-related death is **hemolytic transfusion reaction.**[140] Most of these reactions are preventable because blood group incompatibility typically occurs as the result of errors in blood-product labeling or patient identification. Acute intravascular hemolysis is manifested as fever, chills, nausea, chest and flank pain, hypotension, DIC, hemoglobinemia, hemoglobinuria, and ARF. These symptoms are masked by general anesthesia. Immediate supportive care should include stopping the transfusion, treating hypotension and hyperkalemia, administering a diuretic, and alkalinizing the urine. Assays for urine and plasma hemoglobin concentration and an antibody screen confirm the diagnosis. A repeat cross-match must be performed. Coagulation studies and blood counts to guide component therapy are helpful.

The biochemical and additional changes that occur during blood storage can lead to problems in the recipient, particularly when blood is infused rapidly. Plasma potassium concentration increases in stored blood. Transfused potassium rapidly moves intracellularly in a recipient who has adequate perfusion and oxygenation. However, rapid infusion of multiple units can lead to **hyperkalemia,** particularly in the hypothermic, acidotic patient. Blood maintained at 4° C also can contribute to **hypothermia,** especially if the patient is anesthetized in a cold operating room. If the temperature of the patient's blood is less than 30° C, ventricular irritability and cardiac arrest may occur.[141]

The decreased pH of stored blood is caused by the addition of citrate phosphate dextrose and the accumulation of lactic and pyruvic acids as a result of red blood cell metabolism and glycolysis. Despite the lower pH, transfusion of large amounts of stored blood rarely causes an acidosis.

The anticoagulant used for blood collection and storage contains a large amount of citrate, which binds ionized calcium. Citrate is rapidly metabolized in the liver and typically does not lead to significant hypocalcemia. In patients who are cold, who have liver disease, or who require rapid infusion of multiple units of blood, citrate may accumulate and cause a decrease in ionized calcium. The hypocalcemia results in decreased cardiac contractility, hypotension, and elevated central venous pressure.

KEY POINTS

- The visual estimate of vaginal bleeding often does not reflect the extent of intravascular volume deficit.
- Two hemorrhagic disorders often coexist in the same patient.
- Approximately 15% to 25% of all perinatal deaths occur as a result of placental abruption, and as many as 20% of these deaths occur before hospitalization of the mother.
- Fetal heart rate abnormalities represent the most reliable sign of uterine rupture.
- Uterine atony is the most common cause of postpartum hemorrhage.
- The use of 15-methyl prostaglandin $F_{2\text{-alpha}}$ (carboprost, Hemabate) most likely has decreased the need to perform obstetric hysterectomy for uterine atony.
- A history of cesarean section and current placenta previa increase the risk of placenta accreta. Placenta accreta may result in massive hemorrhage, which often requires the performance of obstetric hysterectomy.
- Nonsurgical invasive techniques, such as embolization of uterine and other pelvic vessels, may aid the management of severe postpartum hemorrhage.
- Fresh frozen plasma should not be given to correct hypovolemia or as prophylaxis against coagulopathy during blood transfusion.

REFERENCES

1. Chang J, Elam-Evans LD, Berg CJ, et al. Pregnancy-related mortality surveillance-United States, 1991-1999. In: Surveillance Summaries, February 21, 2003. MMWR 2003;52(No.SS-2):1-8.
2. Waterstone M, Bewley S, Wolfe C. Incidence and predictors of severe obstetric morbidity: case control study. BMJ 2001; 322:1089-93.
3. Why Mothers Die 1997-1999: Confidential Enquiries into Maternal Deaths in the United Kingdom. Department of Health, London, HMSO, 2001; 36-7.
4. NCCDPHP, CDC. State-specific maternal mortality among black and white women—United States 1987-1996. MMWR 1999; 48:492-6.
5. Li XF, Fortney JA, Kotelchuck M, Glover LH. The postpartum period: The key to maternal mortality. Int J Gynecol Obstet 1996; 54:1-10.
6. Duthie SJ, Ven D, Yung GLK, et al. Discrepancy between laboratory determination and visual estimation of blood loss during normal delivery. Eur J Obstet Gynecol Reprod Biol 1990; 38:119-24.
7. Clark SL. Placenta previa and abruptio placentae. In Creasy RK, Resnik R, editors. Maternal-Fetal Medicine, 4th ed. Philadelphia, WB Saunders, 1999:616-31.
8. Scott JR. Vaginal bleeding in the midtrimester of pregnancy. Am J Obstet Gynecol 1972; 113:329-34.
9. Nielson EC, Varner MW, Scott JR. The outcome of pregnancies complicated by bleeding during the second trimester. Surg Gynecol Obstet 1991; 173:371-4.
10. Hayashi RH. Hemorrhagic shock in obstetrics. Clin Perinatol 1986; 13:755-63.
11. Clark SL, Koonings PP, Phelan JP. Placenta previa/accreta and prior cesarean section. Obstet Gynecol 1985; 66:89-92.
12. Stanco LM, Schrimmer DB, Paul RH, Mishell DR. Emergency peripartum hysterectomy and associated risk factors. Am J Obstet Gynecol 1993; 168:879-83.
13. Ramin SM, Gilstrap LC. Placental abnormalities: Previa, abruption, and accreta. In Plauché WC, Morrison JC, O'Sullivan MJ, editors. Surgical Obstetrics. Philadelphia, WB Saunders, 1992:203-15.
14. Kay HH, Spritzer CE. Preliminary experience with magnetic resonance imaging in patients with third-trimester bleeding. Obstet Gynecol 1991; 78:424-9.
15. Gatt SP. Anaesthetic management of the obstetric patient with antepartum or intrapartum haemorrhage. Clin Anaesthesiol 1986; 4:373-88.
16. Pozaic S. Hemorrhagic complications in pregnancy. In Harvey CJ, editor. Critical Care Obstetrical Nursing. Gaithersburg, Md, Aspen Publications, 1991:115-46.
17. Benedetti TJ. Obstetric hemorrhage. In Gabbe SG, Niebyl JR, Simpson JL, editors. Obstetrics: Normal and Problem Pregnancies, 4th ed. New York, Churchill Livingstone, 2001:503-38.
18. Silver R, Depp R, Sabbagha RE, et al. Placenta previa: Aggressive expectant management. Am J Obstet Gynecol 1984; 150:15-22.
19. Besinger RE, Moniak CW, Paskiewicz LS, et al. The effect of tocolytic use in the management of symptomatic placenta previa. Am J Obstet Gynecol 1995; 172:1770-8.
20. Chestnut DH, Thompson CS, McLaughlin GL, Weiner CP. Does the intravenous infusion of ritodrine or magnesium sulfate alter the hemodynamic response to hemorrhage in gravid ewes? Am J Obstet Gynecol 1988; 159:1467-73.
21. Vincent RD, Chestnut DH, Sipes SL, et al. Does calcium chloride help restore maternal blood pressure and uterine blood flow during hemorrhagic hypotension in hypermagnesemic gravid ewes? Anesth Analg 1992; 74:670-6.
22. McShane PM, Heyl PS, Epstein MF. Maternal and perinatal morbidity resulting from placenta previa. Obstet Gynecol 1985; 65:176-82.
23. Naeye RL. Placenta praevia: Predisposing factors and effects on the fetus and surviving infants. Obstet Gynecol 1978; 52:521-5.
24. Dommisse J. Placenta praevia and intra-uterine growth retardation. S Afr Med J 1985; 67:291-2.
25. Society for Obstetric Anesthesia and Perinatology Newsletter. Winter, 1998:9.
26. Bonner SM, Haynes SR, Ryall D. The anaesthetic management of Caesarean section for placenta previa: A questionnaire survey. Anasthesia 1995; 50:992-4.
27. Hong J-Y, Jee Y-S, Hoon H-J, Kim SM. Comparison of general and epidural anesthesia in elective cesarean section for placenta previa totalis: Maternal hemodynamics, blood loss and neonatal outcome. Internat J Obstet Anesth 2003; 12:12-6.
28. Downing JW, Buley RJR, Brock-Utne JG, Houlton PC. Etomidate for induction of anaesthesia at caesarean section: Comparison with thiopentone. Br J Anaesth 1979; 51:135-9.
29. Chichakli LO, Atrash HK MacKay AP, et al. Pregnancy-related mortality in the United States due to hemorrhage: 1979-1992. Obstet Gynecol 1999; 94:721-5.
30. Saftlas AF, Olson DR, Atrash HK, et al. National trends in the incidence of abruptio placentae. Obstet Gynecol 1991; 78:1081-6.
31. Raymond EG, Mills JL. Placental abruption. Maternal risk factors and associated fetal conditions. Acta Obstet Gynecol Scand 1993; 12:440-3.
32. Pritchard JA, Brekken AL. Clinical and laboratory studies on severe abruptio placentae. Am J Obstet Gynecol 1967; 97:681-95.
33. Ylä-Outinen A, Palander M, Heinonen PK. Abruptio-placentae: Risk factors and outcome of the newborn. Eur J Obstet Gynaecol Reprod Biol 1987; 25:23-8.
34. Nyberg DA, Mack LA, Benedetti TJ, et al. Placental abruption and placental hemorrhage: Correlation of sonographic findings with fetal outcome. Radiology 1987; 164:357-61.
35. Naeye RL, Harkness WL, Utts J. Abruptio placentae and perinatal death: A prospective study. Am J Obstet Gynecol 1977; 128:740-6.
36. Vincent RD, Chestnut DH, Sipes SL, et al. Epidural anesthesia worsens uterine blood flow and fetal oxygenation during hemorrhage in gravid ewes. Anesthesiology 1992; 76:799-806.
37. Oats JN, Vasey DP, Waldron BA. Effects of ketamine on the pregnant uterus. Br J Anaesth 1979; 51:1163-5.

38. Farmer RM, Kirschbaum T, Potter D, et al. Uterine rupture during trial of labor after previous cesarean section. Am J Obstet Gynecol 1991; 165:996-1001.

39. Plauché WC. Surgical problems involving the pregnant uterus: Uterine inversion, uterine rupture, and leiomyomas. In Plauché WC, Morrison JC, O'Sullivan MJ, editors. Surgical Obstetrics. Philadelphia, WB Saunders, 1989.

40. Miller DA, Goodwin TM, Gherman RB, Paul RH. Intrapartum rupture of the unscarred uterus. Obstet Gynecol 1997; 89:671-3.

41. Plauché WC, Von Almen W, Muller R. Catastrophic uterine rupture. Obstet Gynecol 1984; 64:792-7.

42. Flannelly GM, Turner MJ, Rassmussen MJ, Stronge JM. Rupture of the uterus in Dublin: An update. J Obstet Gynecol, 1993; 12:440-3.

43. Ramin SM, Gilstrap LC. Placental abnormalities: Previa, abruption, and accreta. In Plauché WC, Morrison JC, O'Sullivan MJ, editors. Surgical Obstetrics. Philadelphia, WB Saunders, 1992:193-216.

44. Cunningham FG, Gant NF, Leveno KJ, Gilstrap III LC, Hauth JC, Wenstrom KD. Williams Obstetrics, 21st ed. New York, McGraw-Hill, 2001:827-52.

45. World Health Organization. The prevention and management of postpartum hemorrhage. Report of a Technical Working Group, Geneva, July 3-6, 1989. Document WHO/MCM/90.7, Geneva.

46. Ueland K. Maternal cardiovascular dynamics. VII. Intrapartum blood volume changes. Am J Obstet Gynecol 1976; 126:671-7.

47. Duthie SJ, Ghosh A, Ng A, Ho PC. Intra-operative blood loss during elective lower segment caesarean section. Br J Obstet Gynaecol 1992; 99:364-7.

48. Combs CA, Murphy EL, Laros RK Jr. Factors associated with hemorrhage with vaginal birth. Obstet Gynecol 1991; 77:69-76.

49. Karpati PCJ, Rossignol M, Pirot M, et al. High incidence of myocardial ischemia during postpartum hemorrhage. Anesthesiology 2004; 100:30-6.

50. Clark Sl, Yeh S, Phelan JP, et al. Emergency hysterectomy for obstetric hemorrhage. Obstet Gynecol 1984; 64:376-80.

51. Kamani AA, McMorland GH, Wadsworth LD. Utilization of red blood cell transfusion in an obstetric setting. Am J Obstet Gynecol 1988; 159:1177-81.

52. Nelson SH, Suresh MS. Lack of reactivity of uterine arteries from patients with obstetric hemorrhage. Am J Obstet Gynecol 1992; 166:1436-43.

53. Weis FR, Markello R, Mo B, Bochiechio P. Cardiovascular effects of oxytocin. Obstet Gynecol 1975; 46:711-4.

54. Secher NJ, Arnsbro P, Wallin L. Haemodynamic effects of oxytocin (Syntocinon) and methyl ergometrine (Methergine) on the systemic and pulmonary circulations of pregnant anaesthetized women. Acta Obstet Gynecol Scand 1978; 57:97-103.

55. Spielman FJ, Herbert WNP. Maternal cardiovascular effects of drugs that alter uterine activity. Obstet Gynecol Surv 1988; 43:516-22.

56. Munn MB, Owen J, Vincent R, et al. Comparison of two oxytocin regimens to prevent uterine atony at cesarean delivery: a randomized controlled trial. Obstet Gynecol 2001; 98:386-90.

57. Dennehy KC, Rosaeg OP, Cicutti NJ, et al. Oxytocin injection after caesarean delivery: Intravenous or intramyometrial? Can J Anaesth 1998; 45:635-9.

58. Fuchs A-R, Husslein P, Sumulong L, Fuchs F. The origin of circulating 13,14-dihydro-15-keto-prostaglandin $F_{2-alpha}$ during delivery. Prostaglandins 1982; 24:715-22.

59. Noort WA, Van Bulck B, Vereecken A, et al. Changes in plasma levels of $PGF_{2-alpha}$ and PGI_2 metabolites at and after delivery at term. Prostaglandins 1989; 37:3-12.

60. Challis JRG, Lye SJ. Physiology and endocrinology of term and preterm labor. In Gabbe SG, Niebyl JR, Simpson JL, editors. Obstetrics: Normal and Problem Pregnancies, 4th ed. New York, Churchill Livingstone, 2002:93-104.

61. Secher NJ, Thayssen P, Arnsbro P, Olsen J. Effect of prostaglandin E_2 and $F_{2-alpha}$ on the systemic and pulmonary circulation in pregnant anesthetized women. Acta Obstet Gynecol Scand 1982; 61:213-8.

62. Hughes WA, Hughes SC. Hemodynamic effects of prostaglandin E_2. Anesthesiology 1989; 70:713-5.

63. Sarkar PK, Mamo J. Successful control of atonic primary postpartum haemorrhage and prevention of hysterectomy, using IV prostaglandin E_2. Br J Clin Pract 1990; 44:756-7.

64. Thayssen P, Secher NJ, Arnsbro P. Systolic time intervals and haemodynamic changes during intravenous infusions of prostaglandins $F_{2-alpha}$ and E_2. Br Heart J 1981; 45:447-56.

65. Douglas MJ, Farquharson DF, Ross PLE, Renwick JE. Cardiovascular collapse following an overdose of prostaglandin $F_{2-alpha}$: A case report. Can J Anaesth 1989; 36:466-9.

66. Andersen LH, Secher NJ. Pattern of total and regional lung function in subjects with bronchoconstriction induced by 15-me $PGF_{2\alpha}$. Thorax 1976; 31:685-92.

67. O'Leary AM. Severe bronchospasm and hypotension after 15-methyl prostaglandin $F_{2-alpha}$ in atonic postpartum haemorrhage. Internat J Obstet Anesth 1994; 3:42-4.

68. Granstrom L, Ekman G, Ulmsten U. Intravenous infusion of 15-methyl-prostaglandin $F_{2-alpha}$ (Prostinfenem) in women with heavy post-partum hemorrhage. Acta Obstet Gynecol Scand 1989; 68:365-7.

69. O'Brien P, El-Refaey H, Gordon A, et al. Rectally administered misoprostol for the treatment of postpartum hemorrhage unresponsive to oxytocin and ergometrine: A descriptive study. Obstet Gynecol 1998; 92:212-4.

70. Ramsey PS, Hogg BB, Savage KG, et al. Cardiovascular effects of intravaginal misoprostol in the mid trimester of pregnancy. Am J Obstet Gynecol 2000; 183:1100-2.

71. Sanders-Bush E, Mayer SE. 5-Hydroxytryptamine (serotonin): Receptor agonists and antagonists. In Hardman JG, Limbird LE, editors. Goodman & Gilman's The Pharmacological Basis of Therapeutics, 10th ed. New York, McGraw-Hill, 2001:269-90.

72. Tsui BC, Stewart B, Fitzmaurice A, Williams R. Cardiac arrest and myocardial infarction induced by postpartum intravenous ergonovine administration. Anesthesiology 2001; 94:363-4.

73. Abouleish E. Postpartum hypertension and convulsion after oxytocic drugs. Anesth Analg 1976; 55:813-5.

74. Casady GN, Moore DC, Bridenbaugh LD. Postpartum hypertension after use of vasoconstrictor and oxytocic drugs. JAMA 1960; 172:1011-5.

75. Zahn CM, Yeomans ER. Postpartum hemorrhage: Placenta accreta, uterine inversion, and puerperal hematomas. Clin Obstet Gynecol 1990; 33:422-31.

76. Plauché WC. Obstetric genital trauma. In Plauché WC, Morrison JC, O'Sullivan MJ, editors. Surgical Obstetrics. Philadelphia, WB Saunders, 1992:383-404.

77. Fliegner JRH. Postpartum broad ligament haematomas. J Obstet Gynaecol Brit Commonw 1971; 78:184-9.

78. King PA, Duthie SJ, Dong ZG, Ma HK. Secondary postpartum haemorrhage. Aust N Z J Obstet Gynaecol 1989; 29:394-8.

79. Munson ES, Embro WJ. Enflurane, isoflurane, and halothane and isolated human uterine muscle. Anesthesiology 1977; 46:11-4.

80. Turner RJ, Lambros M, Keyway L, Gatt SP. The in-vitro effects of sevoflurane and desflurane on the contractility of pregnant human uterine muscle. Internat J Obstet Anesth 2002; 11:246-51.

81. Peng ATC, Gorman RS, Shulman SM, et al. Intravenous nitroglycerin for uterine relaxation in the postpartum patient with retained placenta (letter). Anesthesiology 1989; 71:172-3.

82. DeSimone CA, Norris MC, Leighton BL. Intravenous nitroglycerin aids manual extraction of a retained placenta (letter). Anesthesiology 1990; 73:787.

83. Greenspoon JS, Kovacic A. Breech extraction facilitated by glyceryl trinitrate sublingual spray (letter). Lancet 1991; 338:124-5.

84. Mayer DC, Weeks SK. Antepartum uterine relaxation with nitroglycerin at caesarean delivery. Can J Anaesth 1992; 39:166-9.

85. Ley SJ, Scheller J, Jones BR, Slotnick N. Intrauterine pressure during administration of nitroglycerin for extraction of retained placenta. Anesthesiol Rev 1993; 20:95-7.

86. Buhimschi CS, Buhimschi IA, Malinow AM, Weinder CP. Effects of sublingual nitroglycerin on human uterine contractility during the active phase of labor. Am J Obstet Gynecol 2002; 187:235-8.

87. Segal S, Csavoy AN, Datta S. Placental tissue enhances uterine relaxation by nitroglycerin. Anesth Analg 1998; 86:304-9.

88. Weckstein LN, Masserman JSH, Garite TJ. Placenta accreta: A problem of increasing clinical significance. Obstet Gynecol 1986; 69:480-2.

89. Chattopadhyay SK, Kharif H, Sherbeeni MM. Placenta praevia and accreta after previous caesarean section. Eur J Obstet Gynecol Reprod Biol 1993; 52:151-6.

90. Finberg HJ, Williams JW. Placenta accreta: Prospective sonographic diagnosis in patients with placenta previa and prior cesarean section. J Ultrasound Med 1992; 11:333-43.

91. Rosemund RL, Kepple DM. Transvaginal color Doppler sonography in the prenatal diagnosis of placenta accreta. Obstet Gynecol 1992; 80:508-10.

92. Thorp JM Jr, Councell RB, Sandridge DA, Wiest HH. Antepartum diagnosis of placenta previa percreta by magnetic resonance imaging. Obstet Gynecol 1992; 80:506-8.

93. Lam G, Kuller J, McMahon M. Use of magnetic resonance imaging and ultrasound in the antenatal diagnosis of placenta accreta. J Soc Gynecol Investig 2002; 9:37-40.

94. O'Brien JM, Barton JR, Donaldson ES. The management of placenta percreta: Conservative and operative strategies. Am J Obstet Gynecol 1996; 175:1632-8.

95. Paull JD, Smith J, Williams L, et al. Balloon occlusion of the abdominal aorta during caesarean hysterectomy for placenta percreta. Anaesth Intens Care 1995; 23:731-34.

96. Dubois J, Gabel L, Grignon A, et al. Placenta percreta: Balloon occlusion and embolization of the internal iliac arteries to reduce intraoperative blood losses. Am J Obstet Gynecol 1997; 176:723-6.

97. Altabef KM, Spencer JT, Zinberg S. Intravenous nitroglycerin for uterine relaxation of an inverted uterus. Am J Obstet Gynecol 1992; 166:1237-8.

98. Bayhi DA, Sherwood CDA, Campbell CE. Intravenous nitroglycerin for uterine inversion. J Clin Anesth 1992; 4:487-8.

99. Pelage JP, Le Dref O, Jacob D, et al. Selective arterial embolization of the uterine arteries in the management of intractable post-partum hemorrhage. Acta Obstet Gynecol Scand 1999; 78:698-703.

100. Hansch, E., Chitkara U, McAlpine J, et al. Pelvic arterial embolization for control of obstetric hemorrhage: a five-year experience. Am J Obstet Gynecol 1999; 180:1454-60.

101. Ledee N, Ville Y, Musset D, et al. Management in intractable obstetric haemorrhage: an audit study on 61 cases. Eur J Obstet Gynecol Reprod Biol 2001; 94:189-96.

102. Chattopadhyay SK, Deb Roy B, Edrees YB. Surgical control of obstetric hemorrhage: Hypogastric artery ligation or hysterectomy? Internat J Gynecol Obstet 1990; 32:345-51.

103. O'Leary JA. Uterine artery ligation in the control of postcesarean hemorrhage. J Reprod Med 1995; 40:189-93.

104. Chestnut DH, Dewan DM, Redick LF, et al. Anesthetic management for obstetric hysterectomy: A multi-institutional study. Anesthesiology 1989; 70:607-10.

105. Wenham J, Matijevic R. Postpartum hysterectomies: Revisited. J Perinat Med 2001; 29:260-5.

106. Zelop CM, Harlow BL, Frigoletto FD, et al. Emergency peripartum hysterectomy. Obstet Gynecol 1993; 168:1443-8.

107. Chestnut DH, Redick LF. Continuous epidural anesthesia for elective cesarean hysterectomy. South Med J 1985; 78:1168-9.

108. Kidney DD, Nguyen AM, Ahdoot D, et al. Prophylactic perioperative hypogastric artery balloon occlusion in abnormal placentation. Am J Roentgenol 2001; 176:1521-4.

109. Young JH. James Blundell (1790-1878): Experimental physiologist and obstetrician. Med Hist 1964; 8:159-69.

110. Combs CA, Murphy EL, Laros RK. Cost-benefit analysis of autologous blood donation in obstetrics. Obstet Gynecol 1992; 80:621-5.

111. Camann WR, Datta S. Red cell use during cesarean delivery. Transfusion 1991; 31:12-5.

112. Consensus Conference. The impact of routine HLTV-III antibody testing of blood and plasma donors on public health. JAMA 1986; 256:1178-80.

113. Consensus Conference. Perioperative red blood cell transfusion. JAMA 1988; 260:2700-3.

114. Ransom SB, Fundaro G, Dombrowski MP. The cost-effectiveness of routine type and screen admission testing for expected vaginal delivery. Obstet Gynecol 1998; 92:493-5. (In reply: Eisenbrey AB. Letter to the Editor. Obstet Gynecol 1999; 93:321-2.)

115. Ransom SB, Fundaro G, Dombrowski MP. Cost-effectiveness of routine blood type and screen testing for cesarean section. J Reprod Med 1999; 44:592-4.

116. McCullough J. Transfusion Medicine. New York, McGraw-Hill, 1998: 99-118.

117. Droste S, Sorensen T, Price T, et al. Maternal and fetal hemodynamic effects of autologous blood donation during pregnancy. Am J Obstet Gynecol 1992; 167:89-93.

118. Kruskall MS, Leonard S, Klapholz H. Autologous blood donation during pregnancy: Analysis of safety and blood use. Obstet Gynecol 1987; 70:938-40.

119. Andres RL, Piacquadio KM, Resnick R. A reappraisal of the need for autologous blood donation in the obstetric patient. Am J Obstet Gynecol 1990; 163:1551-3.

120. Williamson KR, Taswell HF. Intraoperative blood salvage: A review. Transfusion 1991; 31:662-75.

121. Catling SJ, Williams S, Fielding AM. Cell salvage in obstetrics: an evaluation of the ability of cell salvage combined with leucocyte depletion filtration to remove amniotic fluid from operative blood loss at caesarean section. Internat J Obstet Anesth 1999; 8:79-84.

122. Waters JH, Biscotti C, Potter ES, Phillipson E. Amniotic fluid removal during cell salvage in the cesarean section patient. Anesthesiology 2000; 92:1531-6.

123. Rainaldi MP, Tazzari PL, Scagliarini G, et al. Blood salvage during caesarean section. Br J Anaesth 1998; 80:195-8.

124. Rebarber A, Lonser R, Jackson S, et al. The safety of intraoperative autologous blood collection and autotransfusion during cesarean section. Am J Obstet Gynecol 1998; 179:715-20.

125. American College of Obstetricians and Gynecologists Committee on Obstetrics. Placenta accreta. Obstet Gynecol 2002; 99:169-70.

126. Weiskopf RB. Erythrocyte salvage during cesarean section (editorial). Anesthesiology 2000; 92:1519-22.

127. Estella NM, Berry DL, Baker BW, et al. Normovolemic hemodilution before cesarean hysterectomy for placenta percreta. Obstet Gynecol 1997; 90:669-70.

128. Grange CS, Douglas MJ, Adams TJ, Wadsworth LD. The use of acute hemodilution in parturients undergoing cesarean section. Am J Obstet Gynecol 1998; 178:156-60.

129. Transfusion alert: Indications for the use of red blood cells, platelets, and fresh frozen plasma. US Department of Health and Human Services, Public Health Service, National Institutes of Health, 1989.

130. Ciavarella D, Reed RL, Counts RB, et al. Clotting factor levels and the risk of diffuse microvascular bleeding in the massively transfused patient. Br J Haematol 1987; 67:365-8.

131. Murray DJ, Olson J, Strauss R, et al. Coagulation changes during packed red cell replacement of major blood loss. Anesthesiology 1988; 69: 839-45.

132. Consensus Conference. Platelet transfusion therapy. JAMA 1987; 257:1777-80.

133. Consensus Conference. Fresh-frozen plasma: Indications and risks. JAMA 1985; 253:551-3.

134. Aggeler PM. Physiological basis for transfusion therapy in hemorrhagic disorders: A critical review. Transfusion 1961; 1:71-85.

135. Goodnough LT, Brecher ME, Kanter MH, AuBuchon JP. Transfusion medicine. First of two parts–blood transfusion. N Engl J Med 1999; 340:438-47.

136. Alter HJ. To C or not to C: These are the questions. Blood 1995; 85:1681-95.

137. Tong MJ, el-Farra NS, Reikes AR, Co RL. Clinical outcomes after transfusion-associated hepatitis C. N Engl J Med 1995; 332:1463-6.

138. Rader DL. Cytomegalovirus infection in patients undergoing noncardiac surgical procedures. Surg Gynecol Obstet 1985; 160:13-5.

139. Pamphilon DH, Rider JH, Barbara JA, Williamson LM. Prevention of transfusion-transmitted cytomegalovirus infection. Transfus Med 1999; 9:115-23.

140. Honig CL, Bove JR. Transfusion associated fatalities: Review of Bureau of Biologics report. Transfusion 1980; 20:653-6.

141. Miller RD. Transfusion therapy. In Miller RD, editor. Anesthesia, 5th ed. New York, Churchill Livingstone, 2000:1613-44.

Chapter 38
Embolic Disorders

Andrew M. Malinow, M.D.

Embolic disease during pregnancy includes pulmonary thromboembolism, amniotic fluid embolism, and venous air embolism. The presentation of each of these entities varies in incidence and clinical course. For example, venous air embolism frequently occurs during cesarean section.[1-6] Symptoms, if present, are transient, and the diagnosis often is missed (or dismissed if detected) by the anesthesiologist.[1] In contrast, amniotic fluid embolism is rare, but its clinical presentation is cataclysmic.[7]

In obstetric patients, many embolic events occur intrapartum or postpartum. Together, these disorders make up the most common cause of direct maternal mortality in the Western world.[8] The anesthesiologist is most often involved in resuscitation of the patient. Early recognition, diagnosis, and treatment are necessary to reduce associated morbidity and mortality.

THROMBOEMBOLISM

Incidence
Pulmonary thromboembolism (PTE) occurs in approximately 0.05% of all pregnancies.[9] It most often occurs secondary to deep vein thrombosis, but it also can occur after superficial vein, puerperal septic pelvic vein, and puerperal ovarian vein thrombosis.

Superficial vein thrombosis occurs during the antepartum period in as many as 0.15% of all pregnancies.[9] However, the incidence increases as much as eightfold during the postpartum period. **Deep vein thrombosis** occurs in 0.02% to 0.36% of all pregnancies.[9-12] In the past, the incidence increased fivefold to eightfold during the postpartum period.[9,11] Published evidence suggests that the incidence of postpartum deep vein thrombosis has decreased in recent years, most likely because of more aggressive efforts toward early ambulation and the use of other means of prophylaxis after delivery.[13,14] As many as half of pregnancy-related episodes of deep vein thrombosis occur by 15 weeks' gestation, and two thirds occur by 20 weeks' gestation.[13,14] **Puerperal ovarian vein thrombosis** and **septic pelvic vein thrombosis** present during the early postpartum period with an incidence of 0.025% and 0.1%, respectively.[9,15]

Approximately 33% of patients with untreated septic pelvic vein thrombosis experience a pulmonary embolus. However, most cases of PTE during pregnancy occur as a result of deep vein thrombosis.[9] Although most cases of deep vein thrombosis occur antepartum, almost two thirds of all pregnancy-associated cases of PTE occur postpartum.[13] Approximately 13% to 24% of pregnant patients with untreated deep vein thrombosis experience a pulmonary embolus, and the mortality rate is 12% to 15%.[9,16,17] Appropriate treatment of deep vein thrombosis reduces the incidence of PTE to 0.7% to 4.5%,[11,17] and it reduces the mortality rate to 0.7%.[17,18] Although the incidence of maternal mortality from PTE has declined by more than 50% during the last two decades, PTE still accounts for approximately 12% to 25% of direct maternal mortality.[19-23]

Etiology
Half of the cases of thromboembolism in women of childbearing years occur during pregnancy or the puerperium.[24] In fact, pregnancy results in a fivefold to sixfold increase in the relative risk of thromboembolism.[16] The increased frequency of thromboembolic disease during pregnancy is a result of at least three factors: (1) an increase in venous stasis, (2) the hypercoagulable state of pregnancy, and (3) the vascular injury associated with vaginal or cesarean delivery.

VENOUS STASIS
Pregnancy results in an enormous increase in uterine size and blood flow. Maternal blood volume and cardiac output increase approximately 50% during pregnancy. Uterine blood flow increases to 700 to 900 mL/min at term, which represents approximately 10% to 12% of maternal cardiac output.[25] The uterus—normally a pelvic organ—becomes an abdominal organ by term. The gravid uterus compresses the inferior vena cava as well as other anatomic structures (e.g., the ureter). Vena caval compression results in venous stasis distal to the compression, in the pelvis and lower extremities.

CHANGES IN COAGULATION
Pregnancy is associated with enhanced platelet turnover, coagulation, and fibrinolysis. It also is associated with an

increase in the concentration of clotting factors, including I (fibrinogen), V, VII, VIII, IX, X, and XII. Thrombin generation also increases. Platelet count typically remains unchanged (or is decreased by hemodilution) during pregnancy. In summary, pregnancy represents a state of accelerated but compensated intravascular coagulation.

Parturition accelerates platelet activation, coagulation, and fibrinolysis.[26,27] Unlike coagulation activity, fibrinolytic activity decreases during the 48 hours after delivery.[27] Therefore coagulation activity is increased relative to fibrinolytic activity.

VASCULAR DAMAGE

Both vaginal delivery and separation of the placenta result in vascular trauma. Vascular trauma may initiate a series of physiologic events leading to an acceleration of coagulation activity. This increased coagulation activity most likely is responsible for the increased incidence of PTE during the puerperium. Surgery (e.g., cesarean section) results in a further increase in the risk of thromboembolism. The risks of both deep vein thrombosis and PTE are five to eight times higher after cesarean delivery than after vaginal delivery.[24,28] Even tubal ligation after vaginal delivery seems to increase the risk of thromboembolism when compared with vaginal delivery alone.[24]

OBSTETRIC CONDITIONS

A recent population-based study of more than a million deliveries noted an increased risk of PTE in women whose pregnancies were complicated by preeclampsia and multiple gestation (i.e., an increased relative risk of sevenfold to eightfold, and twofold to threefold, respectively).[28] Both of these obstetric conditions—or the management of these conditions—are associated with risk factors for thromboembolic disease (e.g., bed rest, increased venous stasis, increased risk of operative delivery and vascular injury).

COINCIDENTAL DISEASE

A history of previous thromboembolism increases the risk of PTE during pregnancy. Early in pregnancy there is an increase in the level of D-dimers and thrombin/antithrombin complexes in patients with prior thromboembolic events, when compared with normal controls.[29] In addition, coincidental diseases further increase the risk of thromboembolism in obstetric patients. These diseases include smoking, obesity, antiphospholipid antibody syndrome, protein S and C deficiencies, antithrombin III deficiency, hyperhomocysteinemia, and prothrombin gene or factor V Leiden mutation.[18,24,30,31]

Pathophysiology

The manifestations and prognosis of PTE depend on several factors: (1) the size and number of emboli, (2) concurrent cardiopulmonary function, (3) the rate of clot fragmentation and lysis, and (4) the presence or absence of a source for recurrent emboli.[32] After a pulmonary embolus occurs, respiratory failure results from either extensive occlusion of the pulmonary vasculature (which results in cardiorespiratory decompensation) or pulmonary edema.[33] Pulmonary hypertension may result from direct vascular obstruction by a large embolus (e.g., a saddle embolus). However, a small embolus also may be associated with severe pulmonary hypertension, especially if there is underlying cardiac or pulmonary disease or recurrent pulmonary embolization.[32,33] In any case, right

ventricular overload can occur. In addition, disruption of normal capillary integrity may occur.[33] Simultaneous cardiorespiratory compromise may prompt aggressive intravenous volume replacement. The increase in hydrostatic forces and the disruption of normal capillary integrity can lead to pulmonary edema.[33]

Diagnosis

CLINICAL

The diagnosis of a pulmonary embolus requires a high index of suspicion and prompt evaluation (Table 38-1). The patient may complain of dyspnea, palpitations, anxiety, and chest pain, which may be pleuritic. The patient may appear cyanotic and diaphoretic. The patient may have a cough, with or without hemoptysis. Physical examination often reveals tachycardia. Signs of right ventricular failure, including an accentuated or split second heart sound, jugular venous distention, a parasternal heave, and hepatic enlargement, may be seen. The electrocardiogram (ECG) may show signs of right ventricular strain, including a right-axis shift, P pulmonale, ST-T segment abnormalities, T-wave inversion, and supraventricular arrhythmias.[18,33]

Embolism leads to a redistribution in pulmonary blood flow. This redistribution of perfusion can lead to "hyperperfusion" of otherwise low ventilation-perfusion zones in unaffected areas of the lung.[34] In cases of right ventricular failure, a decrease in cardiac output leads to decreased mixed-venous oxygen content, which enhances the effects of ventilation-perfusion mismatch.[34] Arterial hypoxemia often results. However, as many as 30% of all patients with a pulmonary embolus have a PaO_2 greater than 85 mm Hg.[35]

Invasive hemodynamic monitoring typically reveals (1) normal to low (less than 15 mm Hg) pulmonary artery occlusion pressure, (2) increased mean pulmonary artery pressure (but typically less than 35 mm Hg), and (3) increased (greater than 8 mm Hg) central venous pressure (CVP).[32,33] Calculated pulmonary vascular resistance typically is more than 2.5 times normal.[33] Right ventricular failure occurs when the mean pulmonary artery pressure exceeds 35 to 45 mm Hg.[33] In severe cases, left ventricular failure results because of poor left ventricular filling and arterial hypoxemia.

DIAGNOSTIC EVALUATION

A negative D-dimer assay can be a reassuring diagnostic test in cases of PTE that are of "low" clinical suspicion.[36] However, a positive D-dimer assay is not specific for PTE in pregnant women.

TABLE 38-1	PHYSICAL FINDINGS OF PULMONARY EMBOLISM
Finding	**Percent of patients**
Tachypnea	85%
Tachycardia	40%
Fever	45%
Accentuated second heart sound	50%
Localized rales	60%
Thrombophlebitis	40%
Supraventricular dysrhythmia	15%

From Spence TH. Pulmonary embolization syndrome. In Civetta JM, Taylor RW, Kirby RR, editors. Critical Care. Philadelphia, JB Lippincott, 1988: 1091-102.

Chest radiographs may show atelectasis, pleural effusion, an elevated hemidiaphragm, and a peripheral segmental or subsegmental infiltrate.[9,33] However, the chest radiograph is neither specific nor sensitive in the diagnosis of PTE. In fact, 25% to 40% of patients with a pulmonary embolus have a normal chest radiograph.[9,32]

Some clinicians use spiral (helical) computed tomography (CT) for the initial radiographic evaluation. In nonpregnant patients, spiral CT is very sensitive and specific for a central pulmonary artery embolus. The sensitivity of spiral CT for isolated subsegmental PTE is approximately 30%, and such emboli account for approximately 20% of cases of symptomatic thromboembolism.[36]

Chest radiography facilitates the interpretation of a subsequent nuclear scan because not all perfusion defects on lung scan are a result of PTE. In addition, it aids in the diagnosis of other conditions (e.g., pleurisy, pneumothorax, and fractured rib) that may mimic PTE.

If the perfusion scan is normal, the diagnosis of PTE can be excluded. Multiple perfusion defects and ventilation-perfusion mismatch on lung scan suggest a high probability of PTE.[33] A high clinical suspicion of PTE and a high-probability lung scan (e.g., segmental perfusion defect with normal ventilation) obviate the need for further diagnostic imaging.[32,37] In such cases, the diagnosis of PTE most likely is correct, and heparin therapy should begin. If the lung scan reveals subsegmental defects with normal ventilation or matched perfusion and ventilation defects, the probability of PTE is between 10% and 40%.[32,37] Pulmonary angiography (preferably performed by means of the brachial route) should be considered if clinical suspicion is high.[37]

Although the physician should limit unnecessary fetal radiation exposure, small amounts of radiation exposure most likely increase fetal risk to a very limited degree.[33,37-40] The absolute risk of childhood cancer in the general population is approximately 0.1%. The increased relative risk of childhood cancer after radiation exposure (e.g., radiographic pelvimetry) in utero is 2.4.[37] Most studies suggest that fetal radiation exposure to less than 5 rads does not result in an increased incidence of teratogenesis.[33,37-39]

Fetal radiation exposure during maternal diagnostic radiologic testing has been estimated (Table 38-2).[33,37,38] It is possible to use a chest radiograph, a ventilation-perfusion scan, and pulmonary angiography to make the diagnosis of PTE, with a total fetal radiation exposure of less than 60 mrads.[39] Even when pulmonary angiography must be performed by means of the femoral route, total fetal radiation exposure is less than 400 mrads.[39]

There are published case reports of echocardiographic diagnosis of both an intracardiac embolus and a pulmonary artery embolus after cesarean section.[41] Although it is not as sensitive as pulmonary angiography in the detection of a pulmonary artery embolus, echocardiographic confirmation of a clot may obviate the need for the more invasive procedure (especially if there is a delay in beginning the angiography procedure) and may hasten the time to anticoagulation.

Left-sided proximal iliac or femoral vein occlusion occurs in approximately 70% of all cases of deep vein thrombosis during pregnancy.[10,14,42] It has been suggested that an increased incidence of left-sided stasis occurs (compared with the right side) because the left iliac vein crosses beneath a low bifurcation of the aorta or the right iliac artery.[10] Compression ultrasonography (e.g., comparison of flow before and after compression of a venous segment) is especially effective in diagnosing proximal deep vein thromboses (iliac or femoral).[10,43] Compression ultrasonography and color flow Doppler imaging may substitute for contrast venography in the diagnosis of symptomatic deep vein thrombosis during pregnancy.[10,43] ^{125}I-fibrinogen leg scanning is not used during pregnancy. Free ^{125}I crosses the placenta and accumulates in the fetal thyroid gland.

Puerperal ovarian vein and septic pelvic vein thromboses appear to represent different manifestations of the same clinical process. These disorders may occur after vaginal or cesarean delivery. Physicians should suspect these entities when a postpartum patient has a prolonged (i.e., greater than 72 hours) fever that is unresponsive to antibiotic therapy. The patient may not complain of pelvic pain or have a pelvic mass.[15,18] Some patients also may have deep vein thrombosis.[18] Therefore complaints of leg pain, tenderness, and edema also may accompany puerperal ovarian vein or septic pelvic vein thrombosis. In the past, the diagnosis of ovarian vein or septic pelvic vein thrombosis was often made after an empiric trial of heparin resulted in the amelioration of signs and symptoms. Rarely, the diagnosis was made at surgery.[15,18] In recent years, computed axial tomography (with contrast) and magnetic resonance imaging have helped confirm the diagnosis of these disorders.[15,44] In fact, the physician can perform sequential imaging studies to follow the clinical resolution of ovarian vein and septic pelvic vein thromboses.[15,44]

Therapy

DEEP VEIN THROMBOSIS

The anesthesiologist must understand whether and how the obstetrician will anticoagulate the patient. Controversy exists regarding the dose and even the use of anticoagulant therapy in patients with a history of deep vein thrombosis and PTE in a previous pregnancy or in those gravidae who have other risk factors for thromboembolism. Thus the American College of Obstetricians and Gynecologists (ACOG) has published an educational bulletin that presents the scientific rationale for the use of anticoagulant therapy in various scenarios (Table 38-3).[45] It is clear that prevention of PTE represents the primary focus of therapy for deep vein thrombosis. **Heparin**

TABLE 38-2	ESTIMATED DOSES OF ABSORBED FETAL RADIATION FROM PROCEDURES USED TO DIAGNOSE MATERNAL VENOUS THROMBOEMBOLISM
Procedure	**Estimated fetal radiation exposure (mrads)**
Chest radiograph (with shielding)	< 1
Ventilation lung scan (using ^{99m}Tc sulfur colloid submicronic aerosol)	1-5
Perfusion lung scan (using 1-2 mCI ^{99m}Tc microaggregates of human albumin)	6-12
Pulmonary angiography	
Via brachial route	< 50
Via femoral route	< 375
Limited contrast venography (with shielding)	< 50

Note: 1 mRad = 0.01 mGy.
From Ginsberg JS, Hirsh J, Rainbow AJ, Cuates G. Risks to the fetus of radiologic procedures used in the diagnosis of maternal venous thromboembolic disease. Thromb Haemost 1992; 61:189-96.

TABLE 38-3   AN ACCEPTABLE REGIMEN FOR ANTICOAGULANT THERAPY IN OBSTETRIC PATIENTS

Clinical situation	Anticoagulation regimen
Varicosities	None
Superficial thrombophlebitis	None
Hypercoagulable states	Therapeutic
Previous deep vein thrombosis/ pulmonary embolism	
Post trauma	None
Oral contraceptives	Prophylactic
Antiphospholipid antibody syndrome	Prophylactic or therapeutic
Unexplained	Prophylactic
Recurrent	Prophylactic or therapeutic
Deep vein thrombosis/ pulmonary embolism (current pregnancy)	Therapeutic until 6 to 12 weeks postpartum *or* therapeutic for 4 to 6 months and then prophylactic until 6 to 12 weeks postpartum
Deep vein thrombosis (prior pregnancy)	Prophylactic beginning in early pregnancy
Pulmonary embolism (prior pregnancy)	Prophylactic or therapeutic

Prophylactic, Subcutaneous administration of 5000 U heparin bid without prolongation of aPTT; *Therapeutic*, parenteral administration of heparin to achieve a prolongation of aPTT to 1.5 to 2.5 times control or a circulating blood heparin level of 0.3 U/mL, or LMWH (to achieve a trough antifactor Xa level of approximately 0.4 to 0.7 U/mL).
Modified from American College of Obstetricians and Gynecologists. Thromboembolism in Pregnancy. ACOG Practice Bulletin No. 19, Washington, D.C., August 2000.

therapy should be started immediately after the diagnosis of deep vein thrombosis. During pregnancy, dose requirements may be increased because of increased levels of clotting factors. The adequacy of heparin therapy should be monitored by performing serial activated partial thromboplastin time (aPTT) measurements. The loading dose of heparin is 5000 U (i.e., 80 U/kg) intravenously, followed by an initial intravenous infusion rate of 15 to 20 U/kg/hr (i.e., at least 30,000 U/day).[18,45] The aPTT should be kept 1.5 to 2.5 times normal (corresponding to a circulating blood heparin level of approximately 0.3 U/mL or an antifactor Xa trough level of approximately 0.7 U/mL) for 7 to 10 days.[18,45] Intravenous anticoagulation in typically maintained for at least 5 to 7 days. Subsequently, subcutaneous administration can be substituted for intravenous administration. Specifically, the daily heparin dose is given subcutaneously in divided doses every 8 hours to prolong the aPTT at least 1.5 to 2.5 times control. The subcutaneous route of administration appears to decrease the incidence of bleeding complications.[9] The aPTT is evaluated 6 hours after a subcutaneous dose. The dose of heparin may need to be increased, even by as much as 50%, in the second and third trimesters of pregnancy.[45]

A continuous infusion pump has been used in an effort to increase patient compliance with subcutaneous heparin therapy. Although early reports are conflicting, it appears that infusion pump delivery of subcutaneous heparin (by means of a soft indwelling catheter) helps maintain therapeutic levels of anticoagulation in the ambulatory (and perhaps noncompliant) patient.[46]

Heparin therapy is continued until labor begins; heparin is discontinued when the patient begins active labor.[18] Contraction of the uterus represents the primary mechanism for control-ling blood loss at parturition. However, operative vaginal or abdominal delivery entails the risk of traumatic hemorrhage. The timing of the last dose of heparin is important, and it may be reassuring to assess anticoagulant activity by determining the aPTT or by directly measuring the blood concentration of heparin. Routine use of protamine is not suggested. However, if necessary, incremental doses of protamine can be given up to a calculated dose of 1 mg protamine/100 U of heparin. The dose should be titrated to surgical hemostasis.[9]

Once the postpartum patient is stable and hemostasis is ensured, heparin therapy can be reinstituted. **Warfarin** can be administered concurrently. Once warfarin-induced anticoagulation (as monitored by an international normalized ratio [INR] of 2.0 to 3.0) is achieved, heparin can be discontinued.[45] Anticoagulation is continued for 3 months postpartum.[9] Most evidence suggests that maternal administration of warfarin is compatible with breast-feeding[47] (see Chapter 13).

Over the last decade the use of **low molecular weight heparin (LMWH)**, both for *prophylactic* and *therapeutic* anticoagulation, has become commonplace during pregnancy.[45] Because LMWH has greater antithrombotic activity (antifactor Xa) than anticoagulant activity (antifactor IIa), it does not affect the aPTT. However, it is not clear that the antifactor Xa level predicts the risk of bleeding, and monitoring of antifactor Xa activity is not routinely available in many hospitals.

In the United States, **enoxaparin** (Lovenox, Rhone-Poulenc Rohrer) injected once or twice daily at a dose of 40 mg (1 mg = 100 U), is often used for thromboprophylaxis during pregnancy.[45] (This is a larger dose than that typically given to nonpregnant patients who have undergone orthopedic surgery.[48]) Peak antifactor Xa activity occurs within 3 to 5 hours of administration, and 50% of the total antifactor Xa activity disappears within 6 hours.[48] Enoxaparin is also used for *therapeutic* anticoagulation in doses of 30 to 80 mg twice daily.[45] **Dalteparin** (Fragmin, Pharmacia and Upjohn) is another LMWH also used in pregnancy. In a dose that is greater than that given to nonpregnant patients, dalteparin is injected twice daily (i.e., 2500 to 5000 U once or twice daily for thrombo*prophylaxis* and 100 U/kg twice daily for *therapeutic* anticoagulation).[45]

Purported advantages of LMWH therapy include a decreased risk of heparin-induced thrombocytopenia, osteoporosis, and bleeding. However, these advantages have not been clearly established in pregnant patients. As with unfractionated heparin, the pharmacokinetics of LMWH are altered during pregnancy.[49] Therefore, if the drug is being used for therapeutic anticoagulation, antifactor Xa activity levels must be monitored, with a desired trough level of 0.4 U/mL to 0.7 U/mL.[50] The other major disadvantage is that the cost of LMWH is as high as ten times the cost of standard unfractionated heparin.

PULMONARY EMBOLISM

Approximately 10% of all afflicted patients die within the first hour after a pulmonary embolus.[51] Of those who survive this acute phase, long-term survival depends on rapid diagnosis and institution of therapy. Therapy focuses on providing (1) adequate maternal and fetal oxygenation; (2) support of maternal circulation, including uteroplacental perfusion; and (3) immediate anticoagulation or venous interruption to prevent recurrence of a (perhaps lethal) pulmonary embolus.[32] Acute decompensation from a pulmonary embolus warrants fibrinolytic therapy or, in severe cases, surgical embolectomy.[9,32,33]

Standard heparin is the anticoagulant of choice. Heparin therapy should be started immediately. A bolus intravenous dose of 150 U/kg is followed by a continuous infusion of 15 to 25 U/kg/hr to maintain the aPTT at twice-normal values.[9,32,33,45]

Inferior vena caval interruption should be considered in any patient who cannot be anticoagulated or who suffers from recurrent emboli while on anticoagulant therapy.[52,53] Caval ligation has an operative mortality of 10% to 15%. However, in nonpregnant patients, insertion of an inferior vena caval filter has a mortality rate of less than 1% and a recurrence rate of lethal emboli of less than 1%. Transvenous placement of a Greenfield filter has a long-term patency rate of 97%.[52]

Thrombolytic therapy should be considered in patients with a massive pulmonary embolus.[32,33,54-57] Both urokinase and streptokinase have been used during pregnancy.[24,33,54-57] Urokinase is less antigenic and, in theory, should have fewer side effects.[54,57] A suggested course of urokinase therapy is an initial dose of 4400 IU/kg followed by 4400 IU/kg/hr.[57] Although an increase in the aPTT and fibrin degradation products can be used to follow thrombolytic therapy, the most sensitive measure is the thrombin time.[57] The thrombin time should be no greater than five times normal. Nonetheless, the risk of bleeding is always present.[57] Antepartum and intrapartum complications include maternal hemorrhage and placental abruption.[18,54,55]

Recombinant tissue plasminogen activator (rt-PA) has a theoretical advantage over streptokinase and urokinase in that it does not induce systemic fibrinolysis. Instead, rt-PA is active when bound to thrombin and is therefore clot specific.[58] Recombinant tissue plasminogen factor has been used successfully in pregnant women who have experienced massive pulmonary embolism.[59-62] Bleeding is a risk of rt-PA therapy.[63]

Surgical embolectomy is an extreme measure that is reserved for the rapidly deteriorating patient.[16,61,62] It is associated with a high mortality rate.[16]

Anesthetic Management

Cardiopulmonary sequelae of PTE often dictate the anesthetic management for labor and vaginal or cesarean delivery. More often, **asymptomatic women** with a history of deep vein thrombosis present for labor and vaginal or cesarean delivery. In such cases the anesthesiologist must consider the risks versus the benefits of regional anesthesia.

The medical literature is peppered with reports of patients who suffered epidural hematoma after epidural anesthesia,[64] after epidural anesthesia and anticoagulation,[65,66] and after anticoagulation alone.[57,67] Vandermeulen et al.[65] reviewed 61 cases of a spinal epidural and/or subdural hematoma following spinal or epidural anesthesia, published between 1906 and 1994. (Approximately 53 of these cases were published during the last 30 years.) Likewise, Wulf[66] reviewed 51 cases of spinal hematoma associated with epidural anesthesia, published between 1966 and 1995. In contrast, there have been at least 326 published cases of spontaneous epidural or subdural hematoma—not associated with epidural or spinal anesthesia—during the last 30 years.[65]

Insertion of an epidural needle causes some amount of bleeding into the epidural space in 5% to 40% of healthy patients.[68,69] However, studies have reported the safe use of epidural or spinal anesthesia in more than 30,000 patients receiving thromboprophylaxis with *standard* heparin during the last 15 years.

In December 1997, the U.S. Food and Drug Administration (FDA) issued a warning calling attention to the risk of epidural or spinal hematoma with concurrent use of LMWH and epidural or spinal anesthesia.[70] There are at least 30 spontaneous safety reports of patients in the United States who suffered epidural or subdural hematoma after regional anesthesia or spinal puncture while receiving thromboprophylaxis with enoxaparin. Most of these patients were elderly female patients undergoing orthopedic surgery.[70,71] The risk of hematoma seems to be increased by "traumatic or repeated spinal or epidural punctures."[70] The apparent increase in the risk of an epidural hematoma following concurrent administration of regional anesthesia and prophylactic LMWH may be related to the relatively greater bioavailability and longer biologic half-life of LMWH after subcutaneous injection, when compared with standard heparin.[65]

The risk of epidural hematoma associated with each specific therapy is unknown. Obviously, both the anesthesiologist and the patient would like reassurance that there is little or no increase in risk when compared with that for the patient who is not receiving anticoagulation therapy. The following guidelines represent those used by anesthesiologists at the University of Maryland:

1. Patients who require full anticoagulation receive anticoagulant doses of subcutaneous heparin (approximately 8000 to 10,000 U every 8 to 12 hours) in an effort to keep the aPTT at twice-normal values.

2. Heparin is discontinued with the onset of active labor. In these patients, we withhold regional anesthesia until the aPTT is normal or the blood heparin concentration is near zero. If these conditions are not met, the patient is offered intravenous opioid analgesia for labor until the aPTT is near normal or the blood heparin concentration is near zero. Many of our pregnant patients currently receive thromboprophylaxis with LMWH, but not many patients are therapeutically anticoagulated with LMWH, because of the cost and need for monitoring of therapeutic antifactor Xa activity levels. Patients and their obstetricians are counseled during early pregnancy that the use of LMWH thromboprophylaxis precludes the use of regional anesthesia until at least 12 hours have elapsed since the time of the last dose. Therapeutic anticoagulation with high-dose LMWH precludes the use of regional anesthesia for 24 hours from the time of the last dose. Our obstetricians typically substitute standard unfractionated heparin for LMWH near term so that they can use the aPTT to monitor anticoagulation activity.

3. Protamine may be administered in selected patients who require emergency cesarean section. Regional anesthesia is administered only if a coagulation profile is normal. We do not routinely reverse heparin therapy with protamine to allow administration of regional anesthesia. Further, protamine is unpredictable in reversing the antifactor Xa activity caused by LMWH.[71] Therefore, we do not give protamine to patients who have received LMWH.[72]

4. If cesarean section is needed in a patient with abnormal coagulation, general anesthesia is administered.

5. We discuss with the obstetrician the reinstitution of anticoagulation therapy after delivery. (There is some published sentiment for routine thromboprophylaxis after elective and/or uncomplicated cesarean delivery in healthy patients.[73]) For patients scheduled to receive postpartum thromboprophylaxis with single-daily doses of LMWH, at least 6 to 8 hours should elapse after spinal or epidural nee-

dle placement *before* the first dose of LMWH is given; the second postoperative dose should be given no sooner than 24 hours after the first dose.[74] For patients receiving higher (i.e., twice-daily) doses of LMWH, at least 24 hours should elapse after spinal or epidural needle placement before the first postpartum dose of LMWH is given. Likewise, in patients in whom blood is detected during needle and/or catheter placement, initiation of LMWH therapy should be delayed for at least 24 hours.

6. Removal of the epidural catheter may cause venous disruption and bleeding into the epidural space. Therefore we prefer to remove the epidural catheter before the reinstitution of heparin therapy. The 2002 Consensus Statement of the American Society of Regional Anesthesia and Pain Medicine[74] states that neuraxial catheters may be "safely maintained" in patients receiving single-daily dosing of LMWH postoperatively. The Consensus Statement also states that the catheter should be removed at least 10 to 12 hours after the last dose of LMWH, and that subsequent doses of LMWH should occur a minimum of 2 hours after catheter removal.[74] For patients receiving twice-daily doses of LMWH, the Consensus Statement recommends that indwelling catheters should be removed *before* initiation of LMWH thromboprophylaxis.[74] In these patients, the first dose of LMWH should not be administered until at least 2 hours after catheter removal.[74]

Concomitant fibrinolytic therapy places the patient at high risk for hemorrhage and contraindicates the administration of epidural anesthesia if delivery has not occurred. There is one published case of a nonpregnant patient who developed an epidural hematoma after administration of epidural anesthesia for a vascular surgical procedure that included administration of urokinase.[75] Fibrinolytic agents are associated with a significant risk of placental abruption and maternal hemorrhage. Therefore labor and delivery represent relative contraindications to the use of fibrinolytic therapy, and the question regarding epidural anesthesia is moot.

Peripartum anticoagulation or fibrinolytic therapy (administered before, during, or after the administration of regional anesthesia) requires that the anesthesiologist, obstetrician, and nursing staff remain vigilant for any of the signs and symptoms that herald epidural hematoma. These include (1) severe, unremitting backache; (2) neurologic deficit, including bowel or bladder dysfunction or radiculopathy; (3) tenderness over the spinous or paraspinous area; and (4) unexplained fever.[71,75] Suspicion of epidural hematoma should lead to immediate diagnostic imaging of the spinal cord and neurosurgical consultation for possible spinal cord decompression.[75]

Risks of general anesthesia in the anticoagulated patient include the risk of airway bleeding. Laryngoscopy and tracheal intubation should be atraumatic if possible. The anesthesiologist should be aware that placement of nasopharyngeal and oropharyngeal airways, gastric tubes, and other devices (e.g., temperature probes, stethoscopes) carries the tangible risk of traumatic hemorrhage. Emergency surgery may necessitate the administration of protamine to reverse anticoagulation and decrease the risk of hemorrhage during and after surgery.

AMNIOTIC FLUID EMBOLISM

Amniotic fluid embolism is a devastating condition that is unique to pregnancy. First reported in 1926,[76] it was not until 1941 that Steiner and Lushbaugh[77] reviewed a series of autopsies and described the syndrome of sudden peripartum shock characterized by pulmonary edema.

Incidence

Reports of incidence vary greatly, in part because amniotic fluid embolism is a diagnosis of exclusion that often is correctly assigned only after autopsy. In the United States, the incidence of amniotic fluid embolism is approximately 4 to 5 per 100,000 live births.[78] However, amniotic fluid embolism accounts for as many as 12% of maternal deaths.[8] The overall mortality rate for afflicted parturients is reported to be between 25% and 80%.[78-80] Two thirds of these deaths occur within the first 5 hours.[79,80] Among survivors, the incidence of severe and permanent neurologic dysfunction is disappointingly high for a group of young, previously healthy patients. In a review of 46 cases of amniotic fluid embolism reported to a national registry, only 3 (25%) of 12 patients who had *survived* a cardiac arrest were judged neurologically intact.[80]

Pathophysiology

The etiology of the amniotic fluid embolism syndrome is unclear. In primate models, the injection of autologous amniotic fluid does not produce amniotic fluid embolism.[79] The amount of particulate matter found in the lungs does not correlate with the severity of the clinical presentation.[79] Experimental injection of filtered amniotic fluid has produced the picture of amniotic fluid embolism in some animals. Some investigators have suggested that arachidonic acid metabolites, especially leukotrienes, are responsible for the clinical and pathophysiologic features of amniotic fluid embolism.[81,82] One study suggested the presence of a heat-stable pressor agent in meconium, which enhances the cardiopulmonary response to the infusion of autologous amniotic fluid in goats.[83] In the review of cases reported to the national registry for amniotic fluid embolism, the presence of meconium in the amniotic fluid was associated with a uniformly dismal prognosis, with no neurologically intact survivors.[80]

Experience with hemodynamic monitoring during the resuscitation of parturients with amniotic fluid embolism has challenged traditional beliefs garnered from earlier work in nonprimate (and in some cases nonpregnant) models. Clark[79] has described a **biphasic** response to amniotic fluid embolism. The **early phase** consists of transient (but perhaps intense) pulmonary vasospasm, which most likely results from the release of vasoactive substances. This may account for the right heart dysfunction that often is fatal. Low cardiac output leads to increased ventilation-perfusion mismatch, hypoxemia, and hypotension. This phase most likely has a duration of less than 30 minutes.[79] Right heart function and pulmonary artery pressures are typically reported close to "normal" by the time invasive hemodynamic monitoring is begun in humans resuscitated from amniotic fluid embolism.[79,84] However, a recent report of transesophageal echocardiography initiated within 15 minutes of the onset of symptoms of a fatal amniotic fluid embolism confirmed the occurrence of acute, massive right heart failure and severe pulmonary artery hypertension.[85] A **second phase** of left ventricular failure and pulmonary edema occurs in those women who survive the initial insult.[79,84,86] Case reports that include invasive hemodynamic monitoring have consistently noted the occurrence of left ventricular dysfunction in women afflicted with amniotic fluid embolism. The etiology of the left ventricular dysfunction is unclear.[79]

Disruption of the normal clotting cascade occurs in as many as 66% of women with amniotic fluid embolism.[78,79] The etiology of the coagulopathy is unclear. Although amniotic fluid contains procoagulant, it is doubtful that this amount of factor-X activator is sufficient to cause the clotting abnormalities seen with amniotic fluid embolism. It has been suggested that circulating trophoblast may be responsible for the disruption of the normal clotting cascade.[79] In addition, uterine atony (perhaps a result of a circulating myometrial depressant factor[79] or uterine hypoperfusion) occurs in some women. Massive hemorrhage also may contribute to a consumptive coagulopathy.

Clinical Presentation

Amniotic fluid embolism has occurred during first-trimester abortion,[87] in the second trimester,[88,89] after abdominal trauma,[90] and even in the postpartum period.[78,91,92] In an analysis of the 46 cases reported to the national registry, Clark et al.[80] found that three cases occurred during second-trimester termination of pregnancy. Of the remaining 43 cases, 30 (70%) occurred during labor, and 13 (30%) occurred after cesarean ($n = 8$) or vaginal ($n = 5$) delivery. Of the latter 13, the mean ± SD time from delivery to initial clinical presentation was 8 ± 8 minutes. Nine of the 13 patients who demonstrated amniotic fluid embolism after delivery did so within 5 minutes of delivery.

Overall, labor was not tumultuous, and analysis of the data suggested "no causative link between hypertonic contractions and the occurrence of amniotic fluid embolism."[80] Among the 30 patients who had amniotic fluid embolism during labor, only 15 (50%) had received oxytocin, and only one demonstrated uterine hyperstimulation at the time of the acute event. The authors concluded that uterine hyperstimulation is a result rather than a cause of amniotic fluid embolism (Figure 38-1).

Thirty-eight (88%) of 43 patients experienced amniotic fluid embolism at some time after spontaneous ($n = 12$) or artificial ($n = 26$) rupture of membranes. In six of these patients, signs and symptoms of amniotic fluid embolism occurred within 3 minutes of artificial rupture of membranes and/or placement of an intrauterine pressure catheter. Meconium-stained amniotic fluid was noted in a minority of cases.[80]

The diagnosis of amniotic fluid embolism is one of exclusion. The clinical presentation often is compatible with other malignant events (Table 38-4). Obviously, the differential diagnosis should include (1) other **obstetric complications** (e.g., placental abruption, eclampsia), (2) **nonobstetric complications** (e.g., PTE, venous air embolism, septic shock, myocardial infarction, anaphylaxis), and (3) **anesthetic complications** (e.g., total spinal anesthesia, systemic local anesthetic toxicity).[42]

In the past, physicians thought that the detection of fetal squamous cells in the pulmonary circulation was pathognomonic of amniotic fluid embolism.[93,94] However, in the cases reported to the national registry, cells of fetal origin were found in the pulmonary circulation in only 73% of those patients who expired and underwent autopsy.[80] Further, cells of fetal origin were found in only 50% of patients diagnosed with amniotic fluid embolism who had aspirates of pulmonary arterial blood.[80] Conversely, obstetricians have detected fetal squamous cells in the pulmonary circulation of both antepartum and postpartum patients with no clinical evidence of amniotic fluid embolism.[95,96]

Kobayashi et al.[97] described the use of a monoclonal antibody for detection of an amniotic fluid-specific antigen (fetal mucin) in the maternal circulation of patients with signs and symptoms of amniotic fluid embolism. Measurement of the maternal plasma concentration of zinc coproporphyrin, a component of meconium, also has been proposed as a sensitive test for the diagnosis of amniotic fluid embolism.[98]

In summary, Clark et al.[80] have concluded that the syndrome of amniotic fluid embolism is "not consistent with an embolic event, as it is commonly understood." Thus they suggested that the term *amniotic fluid embolism* is a misnomer that should be discarded. They acknowledged that this syndrome seems to occur after maternal intravascular exposure to fetal tissue during normal labor, vaginal delivery, or cesarean section. They suggested that "the syndrome of acute peripartum hypoxia, hemodynamic collapse, and coagulopathy should be designated in a more descriptive manner as *anaphylactoid syndrome of pregnancy*"[80] Further, they called attention to the "striking similarities between clinical and hemodynamic findings in amniotic fluid embolism and both anaphylaxis and septic shock, [which] suggests a common pathophysiologic mechanism for all these conditions" (Figure 38-2).[80]

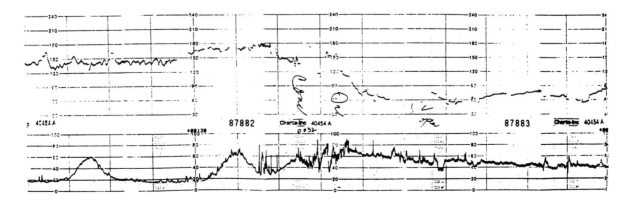

FIGURE 38-1. Fetal heart rate tracing in a patient with amniotic fluid embolism. Maternal symptoms began just *before* the onset of spontaneous uterine hypertonus and fetal bradycardia. (From Clark SL, Hankins GDV, Dudley DA, et al. Amniotic fluid embolism: Analysis of the national registry. Am J Obstet Gynecol 1995; 172:1158-69.)

Management

Prompt recognition and institution of resuscitative measures may influence maternal and fetal outcome (Box 38-1). Most patients require endotracheal intubation, mechanical ventilation, and administration of supplemental oxygen. Prompt support of oxygenation and circulation may decrease the severity of neurologic sequelae. Early recognition and communication with the blood bank often are necessary to facilitate the provision of the large quantities of blood and blood products required during resuscitation.

These patients are young and typically healthy before the onset of amniotic fluid embolism. Resuscitative measures should be aggressive. Esposito et al.[99] reported the successful use of cardiopulmonary bypass and pulmonary artery thromboembolectomy for the treatment of postpartum shock caused by amniotic fluid embolism. Large-volume, rapid intravenous infusion devices may be invaluable during resus-

citation. In recent years there have been several published cases of patients who survived amniotic fluid embolism.[100-105]

During resuscitation, the obstetrician should make an early decision regarding delivery of the fetus. Among the cases reported to the national registry, at least 28 patients had amniotic fluid embolism while the fetus was alive in utero.[80] Twenty-two (79%) infants survived, but of those, only 11 were neurologically intact. Among those patients who experienced cardiac arrest while the fetus was in utero, a cardiac arrest-to-delivery interval greater than 15 minutes was associated with a decreased likelihood of intact survival. However, the authors noted some cases of fetal neurologic injury even when delivery occurred within 5 minutes of maternal cardiac arrest. The authors concluded:

> Intact maternal survival after cardiac arrest is rare, and delivery may, on theoretical grounds, actually be of benefit to the mother undergoing cardiopulmonary resuscitation. For these reasons we recommend that perimortem cesarean section be initiated as soon as possible after maternal cardiac arrest in patients with clinical amniotic fluid embolism.[80]

If the patient received regional anesthesia before the onset of amniotic fluid embolism, the subsequent coagulopathy should alert physicians and nurses to the potential for bleeding within the epidural space. Neurologic function should be assessed frequently, as allowed by the physical condition of the patient. It has been suggested that an indwelling epidural catheter should be removed as soon as possible, preferably after the transfusion of blood and replacement of coagulation factors has temporarily created a state of normal coagulation.[106-108]

Finally, Clark[105] reported two cases of successful pregnancy outcomes in women who survived amniotic fluid embolism during earlier pregnancies. He concluded the following[105]:

> This report supports the role of a qualitatively abnormal amniotic fluid, which may be different in a subsequent pregnancy, as opposed to any unusual maternal sensitivity to amniotic fluid per se in the genesis of this condition. Although any conclusions based on two cases must be regarded as tenu-

TABLE 38-4	SIGNS AND SYMPTOMS NOTED IN PATIENTS WITH AMNIOTIC FLUID EMBOLISM		
Sign or symptom		**No. of patients**	**%**
Hypotension		43	100
Fetal distress*		30	100
Pulmonary edema or adult respiratory distress syndrome†		28	93
Cardiopulmonary arrest		40	87
Cyanosis		38	83
Coagulopathy‡		38	83
Dyspnea§		22	49
Seizure		22	48
Atony		11	23
Bronchospasm‖		7	15
Transient hypertension		5	11
Cough		3	7
Headache		3	7
Chest pain		1	2

*n = 30. Includes all live fetuses in utero at time of event.
†n = 30. Sixteen patients did not survive long enough for these diagnoses to be confirmed.
‡n = 38. Eight patients did not survive long enough for this diagnosis to be confirmed.
§n = 45. One patient was intubated at the time of the event and could not be assessed.
‖Difficult ventilation was noted during cardiac arrest in six patients, and wheezes were auscultated in one patient.
From Clark SL, Hankins GDV, Dudley DA, et al. Amniotic fluid embolism: Analysis of the national registry. Am J Obstet Gynecol 1995; 172:1158-69.

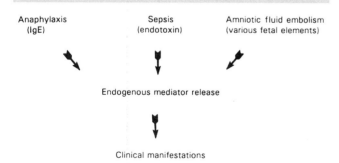

FIGURE 38-2. Proposed pathophysiologic relation between amniotic fluid embolism, septic shock, and anaphylactic shock. Each syndrome also may have specific direct physiologic effects (e.g., fever in endotoxin-mediated sepsis). (From Clark SL, Hankins GDV, Dudley DA, et al. Amniotic fluid embolism: Analysis of the national registry. Am J Obstet Gynecol 1995; 172:1158-69.)

Box 38-1 RESUSCITATION OF THE PATIENT WITH AMNIOTIC FLUID EMBOLISM

1. Initiate cardiopulmonary resuscitation if necessary.
2. Support maternal circulation.
3. Perform intravenous volume resuscitation.
   - Establish intravenous access with several large-gauge catheters.
   - Insert an intraarterial catheter and a pulmonary artery catheter.
   - Begin inotropic support if needed (e.g., dopamine, norepinephrine).
4. Perform fetal monitoring.
   - Make a decision regarding delivery—either before impending maternal demise or to improve chances of maternal resuscitation.
5. Treat the coagulopathy.
   - Decide between component therapy versus fresh whole blood.
   - Obtain early consultation from a hematologist and a blood bank pathologist.
6. Manage sequelae of shock (e.g., cardiac failure, pulmonary edema, adult respiratory distress syndrome, renal failure, hepatic failure, neurologic sequelae).
7. Anticipate a prolonged intensive care unit stay.

ous, it appears that on a theoretic basis. . . repeat amniotic fluid embolism syndrome is probably unlikely.

VENOUS AIR EMBOLISM

Venous air embolism is a recognized complication of many surgical procedures. Numerous case reports of venous air embolism in obstetric patients have appeared in the medical literature since the early nineteenth century.[109] Even recently, published reports have documented the occurrence of maternal morbidity as a result of venous air embolism during cesarean section.[110-112] In 1987, we published the first study of venous air embolism during cesarean section.[1] Subsequently, others have confirmed our observation that venous air embolism is a common occurrence during cesarean section[2-5] and vaginal delivery.[113] Venous air embolism may account for symptoms (e.g., dyspnea, chest pain) and signs (e.g., sudden decrease in SaO_2, hypotension, arrhythmias) commonly encountered during cesarean delivery.[1-4]

Incidence

One study determined that subclinical venous air embolism (as determined by analysis of end-tidal nitrogen) occurred in 97% of patients receiving *general* anesthesia for cesarean section.[6] Other studies have noted that venous air embolism occurs in as many as 67% of patients receiving *regional* anesthesia for cesarean section.[1-5] Precordial Doppler monitoring is able to detect a volume of intracardiac air as small as 0.1 mL. In one study, concurrent transthoracic echocardiography confirmed all episodes of Doppler-detected venous air embolism during cesarean section.[2] Together, these studies suggest that either one third of the episodes of venous air embolism during cesarean section are missed by listening to the Doppler signal, or that general anesthesia is associated with an increased risk of venous air embolism during cesarean section.[2,6] In either case, venous air embolism is a common occurrence and can occur at any time during delivery.[1-6,114]

Pathophysiology

A gradient as small as −5 cm H_2O between the surgical field and the heart allows a significant amount of air to be entrained into the venous circulation. Routine left uterine displacement and use of the Trendelenburg position (which often is requested during cesarean delivery) increases this gradient. In theory, any cause of decreased CVP (e.g., hemorrhage) also may increase the chance for venous air embolism.

Three studies have provided conflicting data regarding the influence of maternal position on the occurrence of venous air embolism during cesarean section.[3,6,115] The steep Trendelenburg position is probably best avoided. Placement of the patient in the reverse Trendelenburg position most likely does not significantly decrease the incidence of venous air embolism. However, at least two studies have observed that uterine exteriorization is associated with an increased incidence of Doppler changes suggestive of venous air embolism during cesarean section.[5,116]

Morbidity and mortality from venous air embolism are related to the volume and rate of the infusion of air into the central circulation as well as the site of embolization. Large volumes (more than 3 mL/kg) of air are fatal, most likely because of right ventricular outflow tract obstruction (i.e., "air lock"). Smaller amounts of air can result in ventilation-perfusion mismatch, hypoxemia, right heart failure, arrhythmias, and hypotension. A paradoxical air embolus into the arterial circulation (by means of a patent foramen ovale) can lead to cardiovascular and neurologic sequelae and morbidity.

Clinical Presentation

Massive venous air embolism can present as a sudden, dramatic, and devastating event with hypotension, hypoxemia, and even cardiac arrest.[110,111,117] However, venous air embolism causes significant hemodynamic compromise (i.e., a more than 20% decrease in blood pressure) in only 0.7% to 2% of parturients at delivery.[2,4] Typically, the clinical picture is much less dramatic. Venous air embolism has been associated with chest pain (less than 50% of cases),[1,3-5,114] decreased SaO_2 (25% of cases),[4,5] and dyspnea (20% to 50% of cases).[1,4]

ECG changes, including ST-segment depression, are seen in 25% to 50% of all patients undergoing cesarean delivery.[114,118,119] It is unclear whether venous air embolism is responsible for these ECG changes. The clinical significance of these ECG changes also is unclear. One study used precordial Doppler monitoring, transthoracic echocardiography, and ST-segment analysis to supplement ECG monitoring during elective cesarean section. Although decreased ejection fraction as measured by echocardiography was sometimes associated with episodes of ST-segment depression, regional wall motion abnormalities were not detected.[114] Doppler evidence of venous air embolism was not associated with ST-segment depression in this study, but both modalities were used concurrently in only one fourth of the subjects.[114]

Recommendations

Kaunitz et al.[8] reported that venous air embolism is responsible for 1% of maternal deaths in the United States. However, it is likely that some of these deaths resulted from episodes of venous air embolism during orogenital sex.[120,121] Although there is evidence that venous air embolism is a common occurrence during cesarean section, maternal morbidity and mortality are rare. I do not recommend the routine use of precordial Doppler monitoring during cesarean section. However, high-risk patients (those who are hypovolemic or those with known intracardiac shunts) may benefit from the use of precordial Doppler monitoring. A high index of suspicion should accompany any complaints of chest pain or dyspnea, decreased SaO_2, hypotension, or arrhythmia. Early recognition of the signs and symptoms associated with venous air embolism should prompt the appropriate response (Box 38-2).

Box 38-2 RESUSCITATION OF THE PATIENT WITH MASSIVE VENOUS AIR EMBOLISM

1. Prevent further air entrainment (e.g., flood surgical field, change position).
2. Discontinue nitrous oxide and give 100% oxygen.
3. Support ventilation as needed.
4. Support circulation.
5. If hemodynamic instability persists, consider placement of a multi-orifice central venous catheter to attempt aspiration of air.
6. Expedite delivery.
7. If there is delayed emergence from general anesthesia, consider neurodiagnostic imaging to rule out intracerebral air. Patients with evidence of parodoxical cerebral arterial gas embolism may benefit from hyperbaric oxygen therapy.

REFERENCES

1. Malinow AM, Naulty JS, Hunt CO, et al. Precordial ultrasonic Doppler monitoring during cesarean delivery. Anesthesiology 1987; 66:816-9.
2. Fong J, Gadalla F, Piorri MK, Druzin M. Are Doppler detected venous emboli during cesarean section air emboli? Anesth Analg 1990; 71:254-7.
3. Karapurthy VK, Downing JW, Husain FJ, et al. Incidence of venous air embolism during cesarean section is unchanged by 5 to 10 degree head up tilt. Anesth Analg 1989; 69:620-3.
4. Vartikar JV, Johnson MD, Datta S. Precordial Doppler monitoring and pulse oximetry during cesarean delivery and detection of venous air embolism. Reg Anesth 1989; 14:145-8.
5. Handler JS, Bromage PR. Venous air embolism during cesarean delivery. Reg Anesth 1990; 15:170-3.
6. Lew TWK, Tay DHB, Tomas E. Venous air embolism during cesarean section: More common than previously thought. Anesth Analg 1993; 77:448-52.
7. Resnik R, Swartz WH, Plumer MH, et al. Amniotic fluid embolism and survival. Obstet Gynecol 1976; 47:295-8.
8. Kaunitz AM, Hughes JW, Grimes DA, et al. Causes of maternal death in the United States. Obstet Gynecol 1985; 65:605-12.
9. Weiner CP. Diagnosis and management of thromboembolic disease during pregnancy. Clin Obstet Gynecol 1985; 28:107-18.
10. Polak JF, Wilkinson DL. Ultrasonographic diagnosis of symptomatic deep venous thrombosis in pregnancy. Am J Obstet Gynecol 1991; 165:625-9.
11. Rothbard MJ, Gluck D, Stone ML. Anticoagulation therapy in antepartum pulmonary embolism. N Y State J Med 1976; 76:582-4.
12. Friend JR, Kakkar VV. The diagnosis of deep vein thrombosis in the puerperium. J Obstet Gynecol Br Commonw 1970; 77:820-33.
13. Barbour LA, Pickard J. Controversies in thromboembolic disease during pregnancy: A critical review. Obstet Gynecol 1995; 86:621-33.
14. Gherman RB, Goodwin TM, Leung B, et al. Incidence, clinical characteristics and timing of objectively diagnosed venous thromboembolism during pregnancy (abstract). Pri Care Update Obstet Gynecol 1998; 5:155-6.
15. Brown CEL, Lowe TW, Cunningham FG, Weinreb JC. Puerperal pelvic thrombophlebitis: Impact on diagnosis and treatment using x-ray computed tomography and magnetic resonance imaging. Obstet Gynecol 1986; 68:789-94.
16. Bolan JC. Thromboembolic complications of pregnancy. Clin Obstet Gynecol 1981; 26:913-22.
17. Villasanta U. Thromboembolic disease in pregnancy. Am J Obstet Gynecol 1965; 93:142-60.
18. Sipes SL, Weiner CP. Venous thromboembolic disease in pregnancy. Semin Perinatol 1990; 14:103-18.
19. Rochat RW, Koonin LM, Atrash HK, Jewitt JF. Maternal Mortality Collaborative. Maternal mortality in the United States: 1980-1985. Obstet Gynecol 1988; 72:91-7.
20. Lewis G, Drife J, Botting B, et al., editors. Why Mothers Die 1997-1999: The Confidential Enquiries into Maternal Deaths in the United Kingdom. London, RCOG Press, 2001.
21. Högberg U, Innala E, Sandstrom A. Maternal mortality in Sweden, 1980-1988. Obstet Gynecol 1994; 84:240-4.
22. Jacob S, Bloebaum L, Shah G, Varner MW. Maternal mortality in Utah. Obstet Gynecol 1998; 91:187-91.
23. Franks AL, Atrash HK, Lawson HW, Colberg KS. Obstetrical pulmonary embolism mortality: United States 1970-1985. Am J Pub Health 1990; 80:720-1.
24. Bonnar J. Venous thromboembolism and pregnancy. Clin Obstet Gynecol 1981; 8:455-73.
25. Palmer SK, Zamudio S, Coffin C, et al. Quantitative estimation of human uterine artery blood flow and pelvic blood flow redistribution in pregnancy. Obstet Gynecol 1992; 80:1000-6.
26. Gerbasi FR, Bottoms S, Farag A, Mammen EF. Increased intravascular coagulation associated with pregnancy. Obstet Gynecol 1990; 75:385-9.
27. Gerbasi FR, Bottoms S, Farag A, Mammen EF. Changes in hemostatic activity during delivery and the immediate postpartum period. Am J Obstet Gynecol 1990; 162:1158-63.
28. Ros HR, Lichtenstein P, Bellocco R, et al. Pulmonary embolism and stroke in relation to pregnancy: How can high-risk women be identified? Am J Obstet Gynecol 2002; 186:198-203.
29. Bremme K, Lind H, Blomback M. The effect of prophylactic heparin treatment in enhanced thrombin generation in pregnancy. Obstet Gynecol 1993; 78:78-83.
30. Gerhardt A, Scharf RE, Beckman MW, et al. Prothrombin and factor V Leiden mutation in women with a history of thrombosis during pregnancy and the puerperium. N Engl J Med 2000; 342:374-80.
31. Danilenko-Dixon DR, Heit JA, Silverstein MD, et al. Risk factors for deep venous thrombosis and pulmonary embolism during pregnancy or post partum: A population based, case control study. Am J Obstet Gynecol 2001; 184:104-10.
32. Spence TH. Pulmonary embolization syndrome. In Civetta JM, Taylor RM, Kirby RR, editors. Critical Care. ; Philadelphia, JB Lippincott, 1988:1091-102.
33. Hollingsworth HM, Pratter MR, Irwin RS. Acute respiratory failure in pregnancy. J Intensive Care Med 1989; 4:11-34.
34. Gal TJ. Causes and consequences of impaired gas exchange. In Benumof J, Saidman L, editors. Anesthesia and Perioperative Complications. St Louis, Mosby, 1992:203-27.
35. Powrie RD, Larson L, Rosene-Montella K, et al. Alveolar-arterial oxygen gradient in acute pulmonary embolism in pregnancy. Am J Obstet Gynecol 1998; 178:394-6.
36. Kearon C. Diagnosis of pulmonary embolism. CMAJ 2003; 168:183-94.
37. Ginsberg JS, Hirsh J, Rainbow AJ, Coates G. Risks to the fetus of radiologic procedures used in the diagnosis of maternal venous thromboembolic disease. Thromb Haemost 1992; 61:189-96.
38. Barron WM. The pregnant surgical patient: Medical evaluation and management. Ann Int Med 1984; 101:683-91.
39. Mossman KL, Hill LT. Radiation risks in pregnancy. Obstet Gynecol 1982; 60:237-42.
40. American College of Obstetricians and Gynecologists. Guidelines for Diagnostic Imaging During Pregnancy. ACOG Committee Opinion No. 158, Washington, D.C., September 1995.
41. Rosenberg JM, Lefor AT, Kenien G, et al. Echocardiographic diagnosis and surgical treatment of postpartum pulmonary embolism. Ann Thoracic Surg 1990; 49:667-9.
42. Bergqvist A, Bergqvist D, Lindhagen A, Matzsch T. Late symptoms after pulmonary-related deep vein thrombosis. Br J Obstet Gynaecol 1990; 97:338-41.

43. Greer IA, Barry J, Mackon N, Allan PW. Diagnosis of deep venous thrombosis in pregnancy: A new role for diagnostic ultrasound. Br J Obstet Gynaecol 1990; 97:53-7.

44. Mintz MC, Levy DW, Axel L, et al. Puerperal ovarian vein thrombosis: MR diagnosis. Am J Radiol 1987; 149:1273-4.

45. American College of Obstetricians and Gynecologists Committee on Practice Bulletin. Thromboembolism in Pregnancy. ACOG Practice Bulletin No. 19, Washington, D.C., August 2000.

46. Floyd RC, Gookin KS, Hess LW, et al. Administration of heparin by subcutaneous infusion with a programmable pump. Am J Obstet Gynecol 1991; 165:931-3.

47. American Academy of Pediatrics, Committee on Drugs. The transfer of drugs and other chemicals into human milk. Pediatrics 1994; 93:137-50.

48. Eisenach JC. Safety issues concerning the use of spinal/epidural anesthesia in patients receiving low molecular weight heparin prophylaxis. ASRA News. American Society of Regional Anesthesia Nov 1995:5-6.

49. Sephton V, Farquharson RG, Topping J, et al. A longitudinal study of maternal dose response to low molecular weight heparin in pregnancy. Obstet Gynecol 2003; 101:1307-11.

50. Katz V. Thrombophilias in Ob/Gyn, part II: Treatment strategies. Contemp Ob/Gyn 2002; 11:59-70.

51. Dalen JE, Alpert JS. Natural history of pulmonary embolism. Prog Cardiovasc Dis 1975; 17:259-70.

52. Jones TK, Barnes RW, Greenfield J. Greenfield vena caval filter: Rationale and current indications. Ann Thorac Surg 1986; 42:S48-55.

53. Arbogast JD, Blessed WB, Lacoste H, et al. Use of two Greenfield caval filters to prevent recurrent pulmonary embolism in a heparin allergic gravida. Obstet Gynecol 1994; 84:652-4.

54. Declos GL, Davies F. Thrombolytic therapy for pulmonary embolism in pregnancy: A case report. Am J Obstet Gynecol 1986; 155:375-6.

55. Fagher B, Ahlgren M, Astedt B. Acute massive pulmonary embolism treated with streptokinase during labor and the early puerperium. Acta Obstet Gynecol Scand 1990; 69:659-62.

56. Hall RJC, Young C, Sutton GC, Cambell S. Treatment of acute massive pulmonary embolism by streptokinase during labor and delivery. Br Med J 1972; 4:647-9.

57. Kramer WB, Belfort M, Saade GR et al. Successful urokinase therapy of massive pulmonary embolism in pregnancy. Obstet Gynecol 1995; 86:660-2.

58. Skerman JH, Huckaby T, Otterson WN. Emboli in pregnancy. In Datta S, editor. Anesthetic and Obstetric Management of High-Risk Pregnancy. St Louis, Mosby, 1991:495-521.

59. Baudo F, Caimi TM, Redaelli R, et al. Emergency treatment with recombinant tissue plasminogen activator of pulmonary embolism in a pregnant woman with antithrombin III deficiency. Am J Obstet Gynecol 1990; 163:1274-5.

60. Blegvad S, Lund O, Nielsen TT, Guldholt I. Emergency embolectomy in a patient with massive pulmonary embolism during second trimester pregnancy. Acta Obstet Gynecol Scand 1989; 68:267-70.

61. Ilsaas C, Husby P, Koller ME, et al. Cardiac arrest due to massive pulmonary embolism following caesarean section. Successful resuscitation and pulmonary embolectomy. Acta Anesth Scand 1998; 42:264-6.

62. Splinter WM, Dwane PD, Wigle RD, McGrath MJ. Anaesthetic management of emergency cesarean section followed by pulmonary embolectomy. Can J Anaesth 1989; 36:689-92.

63. Nishimura K, Kawaguchi M, Shimokawa M, et al. Treatment of pulmonary embolism during cesarean section with recombinant tissue plasminogen activator. Anesthesiology 1998; 89:1027-8.

64. Stephanov S, dePreux J. Lumbar epidural hematoma following epidural anesthesia. Surg Neurol 1982; 18:351-3.

65. Vandermeulen EP, Van Aken H, Vermylen J. Anticoagulants and spinal-epidural anesthesia. Anesth Analg 1994; 79:1165-77.

66. Wulf H. Epidural anaesthesia and spinal haematoma. Can J Anaesth 1996; 43:1260-71.

67. Harik SI, Raichle ME, Reis DJ. Spontaneously remitting spinal epidural hematoma in a patient on anticoagulants. New Engl J Med 1971; 284:1355-7.

68. Crawford JS. Principles and Practice of Obstetric Anaesthesia, 5th ed. Oxford, Blackwell Scientific Publications, 1984:181-283.

69. Naulty JS, Ostheimer GW, Datta S, et al. Incidence of venous air embolism during epidural catheter insertion. Anesthesiology 1982; 57:410-2.

70. Lumpkin M. FDA Public Health Advisory: Reports of epidural or spinal hematomas with the concurrent use of low-molecular weight heparin and spinal/epidural anesthesia or spinal puncture. U.S. Department of Health and Human Services, Public Health Service, Food and Drug Administration, Rockville, MD, December 15, 1997.

71. Horlocker TT, Wedel DJ. Spinal and epidural blockade and perioperative low molecular weight heparin: Smooth sailing on the Titanic (editorial). Anesth Analg 1998; 86:1153-6.

72. Wakefield TW, Andrews PC, Wrobleski SK, et al. A [+RGD] protamine variant for non-toxic and effective reversal of conventional heparin and low molecular weight heparin anticoagulation. J Surg Research 1996; 63:280-6.

73. Black WA. Thromboembolism prophylaxis and cesarean section (editorial). S Med J 2003; 96:121.

74. Horlocker TT, Wedel DJ, Benzon H, et al. Regional anesthesia in the anticoagulated patient: Defining the risks. (The second ASRA Consensus Conference on Neuraxial Anesthesia and Anticoagulation.) Reg Anesth Pain Med 2003; 28:172-97.

75. Dickman CA, Shedd SA, Spetzler RF, et al. Spinal epidural hematoma associated with epidural anesthesia: Complications of systemic heparinization in patients receiving peripheral vascular thrombolytic therapy. Anesthesiology 1990; 72:947-50.

76. Meyer JR. Embolia pulmonar amnio-caseo. Brasil Med 1926; 2:301-3.

77. Steiner PE, Lushbaugh CC. Maternal pulmonary embolism by amniotic fluid. JAMA 1941; 117:1245-54.

78. Gilbert WM, Danielson B. Amniotic fluid embolism: decreased mortality in a population-based study. Obstet Gynecol 1999; 93973-7.

79. Clark SL. New concepts of amniotic fluid embolism: A review. Obstet Gynecol Surv 1990; 45:360-8.

80. Clark SL, Hankins GDV, Dudley DA, et al. Amniotic fluid embolism: Analysis of the national registry. Am J Obstet Gynecol 1995; 172:1158-69.

81. Clark SL. Arachidonic acid metabolites and the pathophysiology of amniotic fluid embolism. Semin Reprod Endocrinol 1985; 3:253-7.

82. Azegami M, Mori N. Amniotic fluid embolism and leukotrienes. Am J Obstet Gynecol 1986; 155:1119-24.

83. Hankins GDV, Snyder RR, Clark SL, et al. Acute hemodynamic and respiratory effects of amniotic fluid embolism in the pregnant goat model. Am J Obstet Gynecol 1993; 168:1113-30.

84. Clark SC, Cotton DB, Gonik B, et al. Central hemodynamic alterations in amniotic fluid embolism. Am J Obstet Gynecol 1988; 158:1124-6.

85. Schechtman M, Ziser A, Markovits R, Rozenberg B. Amniotic fluid embolism: Early findings of tranesophageal echocardiography. Anesth Analg 1999;89: 1456-8.

86. Clark SL, Montz FJ, Phelan JP. Hemodynamic alterations associated with amniotic fluid embolism: A reappraisal. Am J Obstet Gynecol 1985; 151:617-21.

87. Cromley MG, Taslov PJ, Cummings DC. Probable amniotic fluid embolism after first trimester abortion. J Reprod Med 1983; 18:209-11.

88. Kelly MC, Bailie K, McCourt KC. A case of amniotic fluid embolism in a twin pregnancy in the second trimester. Internat J Obstet Anesth 1995; 4:175-7.

89. Weksler N, Ovadia L, Stav A, et al. Continuous arteriovenous hemofiltration in the treatment of amniotic fluid embolism. Internat J Obstet Anesth 1994; 3:92-6.

90. Olcott CO, Robinson AJ, Maxwell TM, et al. Amniotic fluid embolism and disseminated intravascular coagulation after maternal trauma. J Trauma 1973; 13:737-40.

91. Quinn A, Barrett T. Delayed onset of coagulopathy following amniotic fluid embolism: Two case reports. Internat J Obstet Anesth 1993; 2: 177-80.

92. Margarson MP. Delayed amniotic fluid embolism following cesarean section under spinal anaesthesia. Anaesthesia 1995; 50:804-6.

93. Schaerf RHM, DeCampo T, Civetta JM. Hemodynamic alterations and rapid diagnosis in a case of amniotic-fluid embolus. Anesthesiology 1977; 46:155-7.

94. Dolyniuk M, Orfei E, Vania H, et al. Rapid diagnosis of amniotic fluid embolism. Obstet Gynecol 1983; 61:28-30S.

95. Lee W, Ginsburg KA, Cotton DB, Kaufman RH. Squamous and trophoblastic cells in the maternal pulmonary circulation identified by hemodynamic monitoring during the peripartum period. Am J Obstet Gynecol 1986; 155:999-1001.

96. Clark S, Pavlova Z, Greenspoon J, et al. Squamous cells in the maternal circulation. Am J Obstet Gynecol 1986; 154:104-6.

97. Kobayashi H, Ohi H, Terao T. A simple, noninvasive, sensitive method for diagnosis of amniotic fluid embolism by monoclonal antibody TKH-2 that recognizes NeuAcα2-6GalNAc. Am J Obstet Gynecol 1993; 168:848-53.

98. Kanayama N, Yamazaki T, Naruse H, et al. Determining zinc coproporphyrin in maternal plasma: A new method for diagnosing amniotic fluid embolism. Clin Chem 1992; 38:526-9.

99. Esposito RA, Grossi EA, Coppia G, et al. Successful treatment of postpartum shock caused by amniotic fluid embolism with cardiopul-

monary bypass and pulmonary artery thromboembolectomy. Am J Obstet Gynecol 1990; 163:571-4.

100. Girard P, Mal H, Laine J-F, et al. Left heart failure in amniotic fluid embolism. Anesthesiology 1986; 64:262-5.

101. Shah K, Karlman R, Heller J. Ventricular tachycardia and hypotension with amniotic fluid embolism during cesarean section. Anesth Analg 1986; 65:533-5.

102. Mainprize TC, Maltby JR. Amniotic fluid embolism: A report of four probable cases. Can Anaesth Soc J 1986; 33:382-7.

103. Dashow EE, Cotterill R, Benedetti TJ, et al. Amniotic fluid embolus: A report of two cases resulting in maternal survival. J Reproduct Med 1989; 34:660-6.

104. Alon E, Atanassoff PG. Successful cardiopulmonary resuscitation of a parturient with amniotic fluid embolism. Internat J Obstet Anesth 1992; 1:205-7.

105. Clark SL. Successful pregnancy outcomes after amniotic fluid embolism. Am J Obstet 1992; 167:511-2.

106. Sprung J, Cheng SY, Patel S. When to remove an epidural catheter in a parturient with disseminated intravascular coagulation. Reg Anesth 1992; 17:351-4.

107. Sprung J, Cheng EY, Patel S, Kampine JP. Understanding and management of amniotic fluid embolism. J Clin Anesth 1992; 4:235-40.

108. Sprung J, Rakic M, Patel S. Amniotic fluid embolism during epidural anesthesia for cesarean section. Acta Anaesth Belg 1991; 42:225-31.

109. Amussat JZ. Recherces sur l'introduction accidentelle de l'air dans les veins. Paris Germer Bailliere, 1839:255.

110. Kostash MA, Mensink F. Lethal air embolism during cesarean delivery for placenta previa. Anesthesiology 2002; 96: 753-4.

111. Fong J, Gadalla F, Gimbel AA. Precordial Doppler diagnosis of haemodynamically compromising air embolism during cesarean section. Can J Anaesth 1990; 37:262-4.

112. Davis FM, Clover PW, Maycock E. Hyperbaric oxygen for cerebral air arterial embolism occurring during cesarean section. Anesth Intensive Care 1990; 18:403-5.

113. Flanagan J, Slimack J, Black D, et al. The incidence of venous air embolism in the parturient (abstract). Reg Anesth 1990; 15:A10.

114. Mathew JP, Fleisher LA, Rinehouse JA, et al. ST segment depression during labor and delivery. Anesthesiology 1992; 77:635-41.

115. Fong J, Gadalla F, Druzin M. Venous emboli occurring during caesarean section: The effect of patient position. Can J Anaesth 1991; 38:191-5.

116. Bromage PR, Hohman WA. Uterine posture and incidence of venous air embolism (VAE) during cesarean section (CS) (abstract). Reg Anesth 1991; 15:S29.

117. Epps SN, Robbins AJ, Marx GF. Complete recovery after near-fatal venous air embolism during cesarean section. Int J Obstet Anesth 1998; 7:131-3.

118. Palmer CM, Norris MC, Giudici MC, et al. Incidence of electrocardiographic changes during cesarean delivery under regional anesthesia. Anesth Analg 1990; 70:36-43.

119. McLintic AJ, Pringle SD, Lilley S, et al. Electrocardiographic changes during cesarean section under regional anesthesia. Anesth Analg 1992; 74:51-6.

120. Aronson ME, Nelson PK. Fatal air embolism in pregnancy resulting from an unusual sexual act. Obstet Gynecol 1967; 30:127-30.

121. Fyke FE, Kazmier FJ, Harms RW. Venous air embolism: Life-threatening complication of orogenital sex during pregnancy. Am J Med 1985; 78:333-6.

Part X

The Parturient with Systemic Disease

John Snow, the London physician who twice anesthetized Queen Victoria for childbirth, made the first notes of an anesthetic administered to a parturient with systemic disease. On February 12, 1852, he was called to anesthetize a 23-year-old pregnant woman with osteosarcoma of the left shoulder. Her labor had begun 6 hours earlier. As Snow describes it, "the chloroform was not given to the extent of causing unconsciousness but it removed the suffering and caused fits of laughter in the patient after each time of inhaling it for the first half hour." The child was stillborn, "ill-nourished and small." From the child's condition, Snow believed that it had been dead for some time. He noted that the woman died a few weeks later.[1]

Snow wrote extensively about anesthesia. He was acutely aware that systemic disease affected the patient's response to anesthesia. In his last book, published posthumously, he described in detail various physical conditions that influenced a patient's response. Snow stated: "The comparative strength of debility of the patient has considerable influence on the way in which chloroform acts. Usually the more feeble the patient is, whether from illness, or from any other cause, the more quietly does he become insensible."[2] Snow's approach to patients with systemic disease was the same as that used today. The management of the parturient with severe diseases did not become a significant clinical problem until the twentieth century, when medical care had improved to the point that such a patient could survive into adulthood, and become pregnant with a reasonable chance of carrying a child into the third trimester. Snow's experience with this seriously ill patient was probably unique for his day.

Donald Caton, M.D.

REFERENCES

1. The Case Books of Dr. John Snow. Ellis RH, editor. Wellcome Institute for the History of Medicine, Medical History, Supplement No. 14, 1994:218.

2. Snow J. On Chloroform and Other Anaesthetics: Their Action and Administration. John Churchill 1858:53.

Chapter 39
Autoimmune Disorders

Robert W. Reid, M.D.

In the late nineteenth century, Ehrlich proposed the dictum of *horror autotoxicus*, the belief that immunity is directed against foreign material and never against one's own body.[1] We now know that autoimmune disorders represent a violation of this dictum—a failure of self-tolerance. The induction of autoimmunity is multifactorial, involving both genetic and environmental factors. More than 40 diseases result from autoimmunity, and many lead to chronic illness and severe disability. Genes within the major histocompatibility complex govern these disorders. Women of childbearing age have the highest incidence of several autoimmune disorders. Occasionally the initial diagnosis is made during pregnancy.

During normal pregnancy, altered immune function allows maternal tolerance of the fetal allograft. Both the mother and fetus produce immunologic factors that inhibit maternal cell-mediated immunity.[2,3] This helps prevent rejection of the fetus and limit the expression of autoimmunity. However, the high estrogen environment of pregnancy may enhance immune function.[4] Teleologically, this enhancement may be required to protect the mother and fetus from the risks of peripartum infection.

Systemic lupus erythematosus, lupus anticoagulant, scleroderma and polymyositis/dermatomyositis are discussed in this chapter. Other autoimmune disorders—insulin-dependent diabetes mellitus (see Chapter 41), autoimmune thrombocytopenic purpura and autoimmune hemolytic anemia (see Chapter 42), rheumatoid arthritis and ankylosing spondylitis (see Chapter 47), and myasthenia gravis (see Chapter 48)—are discussed elsewhere in this text.

SYSTEMIC LUPUS ERYTHEMATOSUS

Definition and Epidemiology
Systemic lupus erythematosus (SLE) is a multisystem inflammatory disease of unknown etiology that is characterized by the production of autoantibodies against nuclear, cytoplasmic, and cell membrane antigens. Although SLE may occur at any age, it is recognized most commonly between the ages of 13 and 40, with a female-to-male ratio of 10:1. The prevalence among childbearing women is 1 in 700. African-Americans, Asians, and Native Americans are affected more often than Caucasians.[5]

Pathophysiology
The etiology of SLE remains unclear. Affected individuals have both hyperactivity of the antibody-producing B cells and defects of the helper and suppressor T cells. Genetic defects in immune regulation and environmental triggers (e.g., food, drugs, ultraviolet light, microorganisms) lead to a proliferation of B cells capable of producing autoantibodies. More than 30 classes of antigens have been identified as targets of these antibodies. Diverse antigen-antibody immune complexes are formed, followed by secondary inflammatory responses. Deposition of immune complexes and continued inflammation within the glomerulus may lead to irreversible renal injury. Deposits also occur within the skin, choroid plexus, and other endothelial surfaces, with or without an inflammatory response. The view of SLE as an immune complex disorder is an oversimplification. For example, some of the autoantibodies actively bind to erythrocytes, granulocytes,

lymphocytes, and macrophages, which lead to the removal of these cells from the circulation.[5]

Diagnosis

Because of the widespread antigenic targets of SLE, clinical manifestations of this disorder are diverse. Box 39-1 outlines objective criteria for the diagnosis of SLE.[6] Although epidemiologic studies require the presence of four or more of these criteria, the clinical diagnosis may be suspected if fewer features are present without another explanation. Typically the diagnosis of SLE is made before conception; however, the initial diagnosis is made during pregnancy in 20% of cases.[7]

Effect of Pregnancy

Pregnancy does not worsen the long-term course of SLE.[8,9] However, controversy exists regarding whether pregnancy is associated with an increased risk of acute exacerbation of the disease. Lack of objective indicators of disease severity, the highly variable disease course, and lack of adequate controls complicate efforts to determine the effect of pregnancy on SLE. Ruiz-Irastorza et al.[10] prospectively assessed disease activity with the Lupus Activity Index during 78 pregnancies in 68 parturients with previously diagnosed SLE. Sixty-five percent of these patients exhibited worsened disease activity, most often during the second and third trimester and the puerperium. These flares of SLE activity were not more severe than in nonpregnant patients, and most responded to conservative management. Similar findings were reported in a prospective study of 40 pregnancies in 37 women with SLE.[11] In a case-control study, Urowitz et al.[12] noted that quiescent SLE at the onset of pregnancy was associated with a decreased risk of exacerbation during pregnancy.

Box 39-1 DIAGNOSTIC CRITERIA FOR SYSTEMIC LUPUS ERYTHEMATOSUS

Malar rash
- Butterfly rash over malar region
Discoid rash
- Erythematous, raised patches with scaling
Photosensitivity
Oral ulceration
Arthritis
- Nonerosive arthritis, generally of two or more peripheral joints
Serositis
- Pleuritis
- Pericarditis
Renal disorder
- Persistent proteinuria or cellular casts
Neurologic disorder
- Seizures
- Psychosis
Hematologic disorder
- Hemolytic anemia, leukopenia, lymphopenia, or thrombocytopenia
Immunologic disorder
- Positive LE preparation
- Anti-DNA
- Anti-Sm
- False-positive syphilis test
Antinuclear antibody

Modified from Tan EM, Cohen AS, Fries JF, et al. The 1982 revised criteria for the classification of systemic lupus erythematosus. Arthritis Rheum 1982; 25:1271-7.

Effect on the Mother

Most women with SLE do not have renal impairment at conception, probably because renal insufficiency impairs fertility. However, pregnancy may worsen preexisting renal dysfunction. There is a 30% incidence of transient renal dysfunction and a 7% incidence of permanent renal dysfunction during pregnancy in women with SLE.[13] It is not clear whether preeclampsia occurs more often in patients with SLE. It often is difficult to distinguish between lupus nephritis and preeclampsia; both may present with hypertension, edema, and proteinuria. The difference is a critical one, however, because the corresponding treatments are quite different (i.e., immunosuppressive therapy for lupus nephritis versus delivery for preeclampsia). An increased serum uric acid concentration and a decline in creatinine clearance, in the absence of an active urinary sediment, suggest preeclampsia rather than SLE.[14]

SLE may cause thrombocytopenia. When thrombocytopenia occurs in a pregnant woman, preeclampsia, HELLP syndrome (i.e., **H**emolysis, **E**levated **L**iver enzymes, and **L**ow **P**latelets), and disseminated intravascular coagulation (DIC) also must be considered. Although anemia is a common manifestation of SLE, it must be differentiated from nutritional anemia and the physiologic anemia of late pregnancy.

The loosening of ligaments, which often occurs during late pregnancy, worsens the pain of lupus arthritis. Patients with SLE occasionally require joint replacement because of osteonecrosis, most commonly of the femoral head. These prostheses may become painful, dislocated, or infected during pregnancy.[15] Finally, neurologic complications of SLE are rare during pregnancy but may include seizures, chorea gravidarum, and stroke.

Effect on the Fetus

Maternal SLE impairs fetal survival. The incidence of spontaneous abortion ranges from 5% to 28%, intrauterine fetal demise from 1% to 18%, and preterm delivery from 6% to 47%.[4,16,17] Markers that predict poor pregnancy outcome include disease severity, the presence of lupus nephritis, and the presence of lupus anticoagulant and anticardiolipin antibodies.

Neonatal lupus erythematosus is a syndrome characterized by lupus dermatitis and/or congenital heart block. Although this disorder has been associated with maternal SLE, in most instances the mother is asymptomatic. Rather, the presence of maternal anti-Ro (SS-A) or anti-La (SS-B) antibody is linked with the disorder. These autoantibodies are found in as many as 87% of patients with SLE[18] and 60% of mothers of children with complete congenital heart block.[19] Among children of mothers with anti-Ro antibody, the incidence of lupus dermatitis is 25%, and the incidence of congenital heart block is 3%.[20] Fetal echocardiography reveals atrioventricular dissociation, cardiac dilation, and pericardial effusion in those infants with congenital heart block. Treatment includes antepartum administration of corticosteroids and digitalis, prompt delivery, and newborn cardiac pacing.[15]

Medical Management

Because of the wide clinical spectrum of SLE, medical management is directed toward specific manifestations of the disease process. Women who begin pregnancy with active disease should continue their preconception medications.

Low-dose prednisolone, azathioprine, and hydroxychloroquine modulate the immune and inflammatory processes and are used to treat SLE flares during pregnancy.[21] Immunosuppressive therapy is associated with an increased rate of abortion, preterm delivery, intrauterine growth restriction (IUGR), and low birth weight, but evidence of teratogenicity does not exist.[22] Maternal use of azathioprine has been associated with reversible neonatal lymphopenia, depressed serum immunoglobin levels, and decreased thymic size in the newborn.[23]

Antenatal exposure to prednisone appears to be safe, and most children develop normally. However, there is growing concern that prolonged fetal exposure to other glucocorticoids such as dexamethasone or betamethasone may lead to decreased intrauterine growth and abnormal neuronal development.[24] Corticosteroid therapy may precipitate gestational diabetes, and patients are monitored for evidence of glucose intolerance. Striae, gastrointestinal ulceration, and bone demineralization may complicate chronic corticosteroid therapy. These patients should receive postprandial and bedtime antacids.[25] The pediatrician should be alerted to the possibility of fetal adrenal suppression.

Aspirin and other nonsteroidal antiinflammatory drugs (NSAIDs) have been used to manage lupus arthritis. These drugs have shown no evidence of teratogenicity.[26] However, they may cause premature closure of the ductus arteriosus in the fetus,[27] and they may impair maternal and neonatal hemostasis.[28]

Obstetric Management

The obstetrician should be aware of the increased risk of spontaneous abortion, preterm delivery, and IUGR. Accurate dating of the fetus is obtained with ultrasonography at the first prenatal visit and again at 20 weeks' gestation. Because the coexistence of antiphospholipid antibodies predicts a much higher fetal risk, maternal serum is obtained to check for these serologic markers. Kaaja et al.[29] suggested that the presence of antiphospholipid antibodies in SLE may lead to thromboxane dominance and contribute to adverse gestational outcome. Low-dose aspirin therapy (e.g., 50 to 80 mg daily) eliminates this dominance and may improve outcome.

The platelet count, creatinine clearance, 24-hour urine protein, and presence or absence of anti-Ro/La should be determined. Platelet count determination is repeated monthly. If anti-Ro/La is detected or the fetal heart rate (FHR) is 60 beats per minute with no beat-to-beat variability in the second trimester, fetal echocardiography and FHR testing are performed to evaluate for early signs of congenital heart block or failure. In normal pregnancy, serial complement levels gradually rise. However, hypocomplementemia and an elevation of complement split products should be attributed to disease activity in the parturient with SLE.[14] Hypocomplementemia and high anticardiolipin antibody activity at initial evaluation are associated with pregnancy loss and preterm birth.[30]

The obstetrician monitors for the onset of preeclampsia with the regular assessment of blood pressure, weight gain, and proteinuria. Samuels and Pfeifer[25] have recommended weekly nonstress or contraction-stress testing from 28 to 34 weeks' gestation and then twice weekly until delivery. Amniotic fluid volume is assessed weekly after 34 weeks' gestation. The timing and route of delivery are individualized. Although vaginal delivery is preferred, the cesarean delivery rate is 38% to 51%.[15]

Anesthetic Management

The obstetrician, anesthesiologist, and rheumatologist should discuss the condition of both the mother and fetus and formulate a plan for delivery. Maternal organ system involvement and the current severity of the disease should be evaluated systematically.

Pericarditis is common in patients with SLE; although it typically is asymptomatic, cardiac tamponade has been reported.[31] Prolongation of the P-R interval or nonspecific T-wave changes may be noted on the electrocardiogram (ECG). A history of dyspnea on exertion or unexplained tachycardia may suggest significant pericarditis or myocarditis. Rarely, coronary artery vasculitis or accelerated atherosclerosis lead to myocardial ischemia and infarction, even in young women.[32] Ozaki et al.[33] reported an episode of myocardial ischemia during emergency anesthesia in an elderly patient with SLE and undiagnosed antiphospholipid syndrome.

Roldan et al.[34] performed echocardiographic studies on 69 patients with SLE and discovered a high incidence of valvular abnormalities. These findings included valvular thickening in 52%, vegetations in 43%, regurgitation in 25%, and stenosis in 4% of the study subjects. These valvular abnormalities were associated with substantial morbidity and mortality during the follow-up period. Parturients with known valvular involvement should receive prophylactic antibiotic coverage (see Chapter 40).

Winslow et al.[35] studied the prevalence and progression of pulmonary hypertension in 28 patients with SLE. The prevalence of pulmonary hypertension was 14% at initial evaluation and 43% 5 years later. Epidural anesthesia for cesarean delivery in parturients with pulmonary hypertension has been reported (see Chapter 40). However, an abrupt onset of sympathetic blockade and subsequent decreased venous return to the right atrium may cause precipitous systemic hypotension and hypoxemia in the parturient with pulmonary hypertension. A recent report described the administration of general anesthesia in a parturient with SLE and pulmonary hypertension, with co-existing SLE-related restrictive lung disease, pulmonary edema, and orthopnea.[36]

Subclinical pleuritis is common, but significant pleural effusions rarely occur. Patients may suffer from infectious pneumonia or lupus pneumonitis. The latter condition is characterized by fleeting, hemorrhagic infiltrates that may become consolidated. Pulmonary embolism and diaphragmatic dysfunction have been reported.[32]

Peripheral neuropathies are observed in 15% of patients with SLE. These include mononeuritis multiplex (e.g., foot drop) and sensory neuropathies.[5] Mild autonomic nerve dysfunction also has been noted in some of these patients.[37] These deficits should be documented before the administration of either regional or general anesthesia. Migraine headache and sterile meningitis resulting from SLE must be considered in the differential diagnosis of a postpartum headache. Psychological disorders and frank psychosis may occur during disease exacerbation. Seizures may occur, especially if chronic anticonvulsant medications are discontinued inadvertently.

The anesthesiologist should evaluate the parturient for hematologic abnormalities, including anemia, thrombocytopenia, and coagulopathy. An abnormality of the activated partial thromboplastin time (aPTT), which is not corrected with a 1:1 control plasma mix, suggests the presence of either lupus anticoagulant (a coexistent but separate disease entity) or, more rarely, true autoantibodies against specific coagulation factors (e.g., VIII, IX, XII). Lupus anticoagulant is a laboratory artifact, which does *not* cause clinical coagulopathy. True coagulation factor autoantibodies (or inhibitors) may result in a significant bleeding diathesis, which would contraindicate the administration of regional anesthesia.

Chronic use of an NSAID leads to qualitative platelet defects and rarely has been associated with epidural hematoma.[38-40] However, NSAIDs are widely used, and their potential role in causing spinal epidural hematoma remains conjectural. Horlocker et al.[41] prospectively studied 924 patients undergoing orthopedic procedures with spinal or epidural anesthesia. Preoperative antiplatelet medications were taken by 39% of these patients; however no cases of spinal epidural hematoma were observed. In a large, multicenter randomized trial,[42] 9364 parturients received either low-dose aspirin (60 mg daily) or placebo for prevention and treatment of preeclampsia. A preliminary analysis of outcome for more than 5000 enrollees noted that at least 1069 patients had received epidural analgesia, and no cases of epidural hematoma were observed.[43] In the past some anesthesiologists have determined the bleeding time in patients taking aspirin or another NSAID. However, the predictive value of the bleeding time measurement is unclear in these patients, and the bleeding time test is not recommended in patients whose only risk factor is ingestion of an NSAID.

Occasionally, atypical blood antibodies complicate efforts to type and cross-match blood for a patient with SLE. Additional time should be allowed for this possibility.

Prosthetic orthopedic joints should be positioned carefully during vaginal or cesarean delivery. Lupus arthritis rarely involves the cervical spine. Women who have received chronic corticosteroid therapy should receive a peripartum stress dose of a corticosteroid.

ANTIPHOSPHOLIPID SYNDROME

Definition and Epidemiology

The antiphospholipid syndrome has generated great interest in recent years. Harris[44] stated that it "likely occurs less frequently than the number of papers published on the subject." This syndrome is characterized by the presence of two autoantibodies, **lupus anticoagulant** and **anticardiolipin antibody**. These antibodies do not bind directly to phospholipids. Instead, antiphospholipid antibodies bind to phospholipid-binding plasma proteins.[5] The prevalence of lupus anticoagulant and anticardiolipin antibody among patients with SLE is 34% and 44%, respectively. However, only 35% of patients with lupus anticoagulant have SLE.[45] The antiphospholipid antibody syndrome is considered an entity that is distinct from SLE.

Pathophysiology

The term *lupus anticoagulant* is a misnomer, because it has no true anticoagulant activity in vivo. Instead, the anticoagulant activity of lupus anticoagulant is a laboratory artifact that affects the phospholipid-dependent coagulation assays—the aPTT, the kaolin clotting time (KCT), the tissue thromboplastin inhibition (TTI) test, and the dilute Russell viper venom time (dRVVT). These tests remain prolonged even when repeated with a 1:1 mixture of the patient's plasma and control plasma. The prothrombin time (PT) typically is normal. Lupus anticoagulant appears to block in vitro assembly

of prothrombinase (a phospholipid complex), thus preventing the conversion of prothrombin to thrombin.[45]

True bleeding caused by lupus anticoagulant is extremely rare and, in most cases, is explained by an underlying factor deficiency or inhibitor.[45,46] Paradoxically, lupus anticoagulant and anticardiolipin antibody are associated with thrombotic events, both arterial and venous. The mechanism by which this thrombotic tendency occurs remains unknown. Possibilities include decreased plasminogen activity, enhanced platelet aggregation, decreased release and inhibition of prostacyclin, inhibition of protein C,[47] and elevated factor VIII activity.[46]

Diagnosis

The diagnosis of antiphospholipid syndrome depends on a positive IgG or IgM anticardiolipin antibody test or unequivocal evidence of lupus anticoagulant. The latter is demonstrated by (1) evidence of abnormal phospholipid-dependent coagulation (elevated aPTT), (2) evidence that this abnormality is caused by an inhibitor rather than factor deficiency (elevated aPTT with 1:1 mix), and (3) proof that the inhibitor is directed against phospholipid rather than specific coagulation factors.[48] High titers of IgG antibodies to cardiolipin are more likely to be associated with thrombotic complications than IgM antibodies.[5] Because tests for syphilis are designed to detect the antiphospholipid antibodies present in syphilis, the VDRL and Wasserman tests often are falsely positive.

Effect on the Mother

The parturient with antiphospholipid antibodies may suffer from venous and arterial thrombosis, including deep vein thrombosis, pulmonary embolism, myocardial infarction, and cerebral infarction. Silver et al.[49] published a historic cohort study of 130 women with antiphospholipid syndrome. During the observation interval (median = 3.2 years), 48% of these women developed at least one of the following disorders: transient ischemic attack, peripheral thrombosis, stroke, amaurosis fugax, autoimmune thrombocytopenia, and SLE. Twenty-three percent of the thrombotic events occurred during pregnancy. Cuadrado et al.[50] reported a 23% prevalence of thrombocytopenia among 171 patients with antiphospholipid syndrome.

Effect on the Fetus

Antiphospholipid antibodies place the fetus at high risk for death in utero. In one study of women with lupus anticoagulant, only 13 (7.5%) of 173 pregnancies resulted in the delivery of a live newborn.[51] In another study of 105 pregnancies complicated by fetal death, 31% fulfilled criteria for antiphospholipid syndrome.[52]

Most fetal deaths occur during midpregnancy and late pregnancy. Placental infarction is the apparent mechanism of mortality. Rand et al.[53] described a mechanism by which antiphospholipid antibodies could cause placental thrombosis and infarction. They demonstrated that these antibodies decrease levels of annexin V, an anticoagulant present on the surface of vascular endothelium and trophoblast cells, and subsequently accelerate coagulation on these surfaces. After delivery, infants of women with antiphospholipid syndrome do not have an increased rate of neonatal or childhood complications.[54]

Medical and Obstetric Management

Some studies have suggested that fetal survival is improved when affected pregnant women are treated with low-dose aspirin, high-dose corticosteroids, heparin, or a combination of these.[55,56] Heparin, usually combined with low-dose aspirin, is typically used in patients at risk for thrombosis.[57] Pattison et al.[58] performed a double-blind, randomized trial of 50 women with a history of recurrent miscarriages (three or more) and antiphospholipid antibodies, who received either aspirin (75 mg daily) or placebo during pregnancy. This study suggested that low-dose aspirin has no additional benefit when added to supportive obstetric management. However, Branch and Khamashta[57] noted that the majority of subjects in this study were otherwise healthy with low titers of antiphospholipid antibodies.

Anesthetic Management

Management of the patient with antiphospholipid antibodies is similar to that of the patient with SLE. Coexisting autoimmune disorders, secondary organ involvement, and thrombotic phenomena should be evaluated. The anesthesiologist must remain aware that the term *lupus anticoagulant* is a misnomer and does *not* warrant denial of regional anesthesia. Infrequently, antiphospholipid antibodies may cause coagulation factor deficiencies. In such patients, regional anesthesia is relatively contraindicated. However, in the absence of an underlying coagulation deficit or anticoagulant therapy, the elevated aPTT does not suggest a bleeding tendency, and regional anesthesia may be administered safely.

Ralph[59] reviewed the anesthetic management of 27 pregnancies complicated by antiphospholipid syndrome. In this series, all parturients received aspirin (100 to 150 mg daily) throughout pregnancy. Uninterrupted aspirin therapy alone was not considered a contraindication to regional anesthesia. In those parturients who had also received thromboprophylaxis with standard unfractionated heparin, the author waited at least 4 hours after the last dose of heparin before administration of spinal or epidural anesthesia. Documentation of a normal aPTT was obtained when the heparin dose was greater than 10,000 IU twice daily by subcutaneous injection or when heparin had been administered intravenously. The author affirmed that the administration of low molecular weight heparin (LMWH) for thromboprophylaxis precludes the administration of regional anesthesia until at least 12 hours have elapsed since the time of the last dose. Further, therapeutic anticoagulation with high-dose LMWH precludes the administration of regional anesthesia until at least 24 hours have elapsed since the time of the last dose[59] (see Chapter 38).

If there is evidence of fetal distress secondary to multiinfarct placental insufficiency, hypotension from sympathetic blockade should be prevented. The gradual onset of epidural anesthesia seems preferable to the abrupt onset of single-shot spinal anesthesia. Parturients with antiphospholipid syndrome who undergo general anesthesia are at risk for venous thrombosis. To lessen this risk, Ralph[59] recommends the use of compression stockings and warmed fluids to prevent hypothermia and dehydration.

SYSTEMIC SCLEROSIS (SCLERODERMA)

Definition and Epidemiology

Systemic sclerosis or scleroderma is a chronic progressive disease of unknown etiology characterized by deposition of fibrous connective tissue in the skin and other tissues. It is a heterogeneous disorder that is separated into **limited cutaneous** and **diffuse cutaneous scleroderma.** A subset of patients may have systemic sclerosis without cutaneous involvement.

The annual incidence of scleroderma is between 2 and 10 per million, with a prevalence of 240 per million in the United States—four to nine times greater than the global prevalence.[60] Limited cutaneous scleroderma is three times more common among women than among men and primarily occurs between 30 and 50 years of age. Diffuse cutaneous scleroderma occurs equally among women and men, most often in the fourth decade but occasionally earlier in life.[61] As more women delay childbearing until later in life, scleroderma will become more common among the population of pregnant women.

Pathophysiology

In systemic sclerosis, fibroblasts produce excess collagen and other matrix constituents through an unknown process or regulatory defect. This excess collagen leads to microvascular obliteration and fibrosis within the skin and other target organs. Endothelial cells undergo vasomotor and permeability changes, which manifest as cyclic vasoconstriction-vasodilation and edema. Patients with scleroderma produce autoantibodies against nuclear and centromere structures, but the significance of these antibodies is unknown.

Scleroderma exhibits a strong female predilection, a steep increase in incidence after the childbearing years, and some clinical similarities to the chronic graft-versus-host disease (GVHD) that may occur after bone marrow transplantation. Because of these observations, some investigators have hypothesized that microchimerism may be involved in the pathogenesis of scleroderma. Fetal cells and DNA have been detected in maternal blood for decades after normal pregnancy and delivery. In a fascinating investigation, Nelson et al.[62] sought to determine whether human leukocyte antigen (HLA) compatibility of a child was associated with later development of scleroderma in the mother. These investigators found that HLA-class II compatibility between the child and mother (a condition favorable for microchimerism) was more common among those women who developed scleroderma. Artlett et al.[63] confirmed this finding and suggested that the fetal cells remain unrecognized by the host because of this HLA compatibility and that later activation of the fetal cells, by an unknown stimulus, results in development of the disease. However, this theory of pathogenesis does not explain why scleroderma patients have the Raynaud phenomenon and renal disease, whereas patients with chronic graft-versus-host disease do not.[60]

Diagnosis

The triad of Raynaud's phenomenon, nonpitting edema, and hidebound skin establishes the diagnosis of scleroderma. Raynaud's phenomenon is characterized by cyclic pallor and cyanosis of the digits in response to cold or emotion. This phenomenon is a frequent prodrome to scleroderma, but only 1 in 100 patients with Raynaud's phenomenon progress to scleroderma. Limited cutaneous scleroderma, also termed **CREST syndrome**, involves calcinosis, Raynaud's phenomenon, esophageal dysfunction, sclerodactyly, and telangiectasia. Skin involvement is limited to the hands, face, and feet in this form of the disease. Clinical manifestations of diffuse cutaneous scleroderma are summarized in Box 39-2.

Effect of Pregnancy

Most patients with scleroderma have slow but progressive skin and organ involvement. More than 70% of those patients with diffuse cutaneous scleroderma and more than 95% of those with limited cutaneous scleroderma are still alive 15 years after diagnosis. When death occurs, it most often

---

Box 39-2 MANIFESTATIONS OF DIFFUSE CUTANEOUS SYSTEMIC SCLEROSIS

SKIN

Raynaud's phenomenon
Nonpitting edema
Hidebound skin (involves all but back and buttocks)

GASTROINTESTINAL

Hypomotility
Dysphagia
Reflux esophagitis
Postprandial fullness
Constipation
Abdominal pain
Intermittent diarrhea
Malnutrition
Ileus

PULMONARY

Interstitial fibrosis
Pleuritis
Pleural effusion
Chest wall restriction
Pulmonary hypertension

RENAL

Proteinuria
Renal insufficiency and failure
Malignant hypertension

CARDIAC

Chronic pericardial effusion
Myocardial ischemia and infarction
Conduction disturbances
Heart failure

MUSCULOSKELETAL

Arthritis (symmetric, small joints)
Myopathy
Muscle wasting

OTHER

Peripheral or cranial neuropathy
Facial pain
Trigeminal neuralgia
Keratoconjunctivitis sicca
Xerostomia
Absence of anticentromere antibodies (ANA)
Coagulopathy secondary to vitamin K deficiency

From LeRoy EC. Systemic sclerosis (scleroderma). In Wyngaarden JB, Smith LH, Bennett JC, editors. Cecil Textbook of Medicine. 19th ed. Philadelphia. WB Saunders, 1992:1530-5.

---

results from renal failure and malignant hypertension. Steen et al.[64] reviewed the clinical course for 231 women with a history of scleroderma—69 with and 162 without concomitant pregnancy. These authors observed no difference in survival between these two groups. They reported only one pregnancy-related death. Steen[65] also reported a prospective study of 91 pregnancies among 59 women with systemic sclerosis. In this study, parturients indicated that their scleroderma symptoms were unchanged in 57 (62%) of the pregnancies. Eighteen pregnancies (20%) were accompanied with some improvement, usually in the symptoms of Raynaud's phenomenon. In 16 (18%) of the pregnancies, esophageal reflux, cardiac arrhythmias, arthritis, skin thickening, and renal crisis occurred or worsened.

Effect on Pregnancy and the Fetus

The prospective study by Steen[65] revealed no increased frequency of miscarriage, except in those women with diffuse scleroderma of greater than 4 years' duration. Preterm birth occurred in 29% of these pregnancies, but only one perinatal death occurred.

Medical Management

No proven treatment exists for the arrest of scleroderma. At best, therapy is directed toward improving existing symptoms and slowing end-organ damage. D-penicillamine is no longer recommended because of toxicity and minimal evidence of efficacy.[66] Glucocorticoids only ameliorate inflammatory myositis and have no effect on disease progression. The immunosuppressive agents chlorambucil and azathioprine have no beneficial effect.[67,68] Unproved and potentially teratogenic drugs should be discontinued during pregnancy. Plasmapheresis may improve severe localized scleroderma.[69] Stanozolol and prostacyclin analogs help ameliorate the vasospastic component of Raynaud's phenomenon.[70] Captopril and enalapril are the agents of choice for treating the hypertensive crisis of scleroderma in *non*pregnant patients.[71] However, the use of angiotensin-converting enzyme (ACE) inhibitors during pregnancy is associated with teratogenicity, IUGR, preterm delivery, and neonatal renal dysfunction. Thus ACE inhibitors should be avoided during pregnancy in the absence of renal crisis.[72] NSAIDs are used to relieve the pain of joint and skin involvement.

Obstetric Management

Parturients with scleroderma should be evaluated for evidence of renal, pulmonary, and cardiac dysfunction. Some physicians recommend the termination of pregnancy if advanced disease is present.[73] However, intensive antenatal observation for onset of renal disease, systemic hypertension, pulmonary hypertension, cardiac dysfunction, and fetal distress allows most mothers to deliver healthy infants. Renal crisis is difficult to diagnose and treat in parturients with scleroderma. Despite the aforementioned risks of ACE inhibitors,[72] these drugs should be used urgently in cases of renal crisis, because they provide the only effective control of hypertension during renal crisis.[65] Obstructive uropathy may result from an enlarging uterus, which is trapped within a noncompliant abdomen.[74] Uterine and cervical wall thickening may lead to ineffective uterine contractions or cervical dystocia at delivery.[64]

Anesthetic Management

The pregnant woman with scleroderma presents several challenges to the anesthesiologist.[75-85] As with SLE, management is based on a multidisciplinary approach. When possible, an anesthesiologist should evaluate the pregnant woman before labor and delivery.

History and physical examination should be directed toward disclosure of underlying systemic dysfunction. Laboratory testing includes a complete blood count, coagulation screen, determination of electrolytes and creatinine clearance, arterial blood gas analysis, urinalysis, and urine protein determination. An ECG and pulmonary function testing should be obtained in all of these patients. Echocardiography is a useful adjuvant to evaluate ventricular dysfunction, pericardial and pleural effusions, and pulmonary hypertension. In addition, arterial pulses, noninvasive blood pressure measurement, peripheral venous access, extent of Raynaud's involvement, and special positioning requirements should be assessed.

A thorough evaluation of the patient's upper airway is necessary. Severe limitation of the oral opening may result from perioral hidebound skin, making direct laryngoscopy impossible. The anesthesiologist should determine the maximal mouth opening, ability to sublux the mandible, visualization of oropharyngeal structures, degree of atlantooccipital joint extension, and presence of oral or nasal telangiectasias. From this evaluation, the anesthesiologist can determine whether direct laryngoscopy will be difficult if general anesthesia is required.[86] The patient should be prepared for the possibility of an awake intubation. Equipment for fiberoptic intubation and emergency cricothyrotomy must be immediately available in the labor and delivery suite.

Epidural anesthesia has been used successfully in parturients with scleroderma.[78] If otherwise appropriate, the anesthesiologist should encourage the early administration of epidural anesthesia in laboring women at risk for difficult intubation. Even when severe, diffuse cutaneous involvement is present, the skin of the lumbar back is spared. Spinal anesthesia for cesarean delivery in a parturient with scleroderma has recently been reported,[84] although this case was complicated by precipitous hypotension. Full sensation returned 3.5 hours after administration of spinal anesthesia in this parturient.

A prolonged duration of regional anesthesia has been observed in some patients with scleroderma. Eisele and Reitan[75] reported a case of an axillary block (performed with 1% lidocaine with epinephrine) that persisted for 24 hours. Lewis[77] reported a case of a digital nerve block (performed with 1% lidocaine without epinephrine) that persisted for 10 hours. Neill[81] reported a case of a sciatic nerve block that lasted 16 hours. Thompson and Conklin[78] used 2% 2-chloroprocaine to establish epidural anesthesia from T6 to S5, which persisted for nearly 6 hours in a laboring woman. Prolonged anesthesia may result from microvasculature changes and diminished uptake of the local anesthetic agent. This does not represent a contraindication to regional anesthesia; rather, it should prompt the anesthesiologist to give small incremental boluses of the local anesthetic agent and to prepare the patient for the possibility of a prolonged block. Incremental bolus injection also seems preferable to the continuous infusion of local anesthetic agent; continuous infusion may result in the administration of an excessive dose with a prolonged block. Epidural anesthesia seems preferable to spinal anesthesia because of the ability to titrate the dose response to the desired level of anesthesia.

If cesarean delivery is required, the decision to use epidural or general anesthesia depends on the urgency of delivery, anticipated airway difficulty, and the anesthesiologist's skills. The anesthesiologist should be aware that gastric hypomotility results in a risk of esophageal reflux and aspiration greater than that associated with pregnancy alone. Central venous catheterization may be required for venous access in those patients with diffuse cutaneous involvement. Extensive skin involvement may lead to inaccurate noninvasive blood pressure cuff measurement and may necessitate invasive arterial monitoring. Radial artery catheterization is contraindicated in those patients with Raynaud's phenomenon because of the risk of hand ischemia. Brachial artery catheterization may be necessary. Pulmonary artery catheterization may be indicated in the presence of cardiac dysfunction or pulmonary hypertension.[87] The patient—and especially those extremities affected by Raynaud's phenomenon—should be kept warm. Scleroderma decreases tear production; therefore eyes should be protected against corneal abrasions.

POLYMYOSITIS AND DERMATOMYOSITIS

Definition and Epidemiology

Polymyositis and dermatomyositis represent two members of a larger disease group, the idiopathic inflammatory myopathic diseases. **Polymyositis** is characterized by nonsuppurative inflammation of muscle, primarily those skeletal muscles of the proximal limbs, neck, and pharynx. This inflammation leads to symmetric weakness, atrophy, and fibrosis of affected muscle groups. **Dermatomyositis** represents the same disorder, with the addition of a characteristic heliotrope eruption (blue-purple discoloration of the upper eyelid) and Gottron's papules (raised, scaly, violet eruptions over the knuckles). These disorders are quite rare, with a prevalence of 10 per million and an annual incidence of 5.5 per million. Women are affected twice as often as men. The age of onset is bimodal, with peaks before puberty and during the fifth decade.[88,89]

Pathophysiology

Both polymyositis and dermatomyositis are associated with other autoimmune disorders, notably scleroderma. The etiology of inflammatory muscle disease is unknown and likely multifactorial. An initial insult mediated by viral infection or another infectious agent, or exposure to environmental substances, may lead to initial muscle damage in genetically susceptible individuals. This initial process may then trigger an autoimmune response involving chronic muscle inflammation. A viral etiology is suggested by seasonal and geographic clustering of new cases. However, viral genomic material has not been identified in affected muscle tissue. Many drugs, including lipid-lowering drugs in the statin group and anti-retroviral drugs, are associated with the development of myopathy. The presence of cellular infiltrates within affected muscle tissue and complement-mediated capillary damage are features of inflammatory muscle diseases. More than 12 autoantibodies have been identified within affected individuals. Underlying malignancy has been associated with polymyositis and dermatomyositis, although the cause-and-effect relationship is unclear.[88,89]

Diagnosis

Bohan and Peter[90] proposed the diagnostic criteria for polymyositis and dermatomyositis (Box 39-3). The level of serum creatine kinase correlates with disease activity. Electromyography and muscle biopsy provide confirmation of the diagnosis.

As with other autoimmune disorders, variable systemic involvement is present. Pharyngeal muscle involvement leads to dysphagia and reflux. Most patients exhibit impaired gastric and esophageal motility.[91] Chronic aspiration pneumonitis is the most common pulmonary manifestation of polymyositis and dermatomyositis.[92] Myositis of the respiratory muscles may cause respiratory insufficiency. Interstitial lung disease is seen in 5% to 10% of patients. Cardiac involvement includes nonspecific repolarization abnormalities, conduction disturbances, arrhythmias, coronary artery vasculitis, and rarely heart failure.[93] Arthritis generally involves the small hand and finger joints. Renal or hematologic involvement is rare.

Effect of Pregnancy

Reports of polymyositis or dermatomyositis during pregnancy are rare. Ishii et al.[94] reviewed 12 reports of 29 pregnancies during a 30-year period. In 11 patients (40%), the initial diagnosis was made during gestation or during the immediate postpartum period. Among the 18 patients with previously diagnosed disease, the disease remained inactive in 11 patients (61%), and only 2 (11%) had an exacerbation of disease activity. Kanoh et al.[95] described a patient who was diagnosed with dermatomyositis after the delivery of a healthy infant. Additional similar reports suggest that pregnancy may be a trigger for the induction of dermatomyositis in some women.

Effect on the Fetus

Fetal survival is affected by concurrent polymyositis/dermatomyositis. Ishii et al.[94] noted that 10 (32%) of 29 pregnancies (with 31 fetuses) ended with fetal death or abortion, and that 8 infants (26%) were delivered preterm. Fetal outcome was strongly influenced by disease activity. Of the women who had minimal disease activity, nearly 60% delivered healthy babies at term. Kofteridis et al.[96] described a parturient with an acute onset of dermatomyositis with rhabdomyolysis and myoglobinuria, which presented at 14 weeks' gestation and resulted in spontaneous abortion of the fetus. Subsequently the patient's condition improved with corticosteroid therapy.

Box 39-3 DIAGNOSTIC CRITERIA FOR POLYMYOSITIS AND DERMATOMYOSITIS

POLYMYOSITIS

Symmetric weakness of proximal muscles
Histologic evidence of muscle inflammation and necrosis
Elevation of serum skeletal-muscle enzymes
Electromyographic evidence of myopathy

DERMATOMYOSITIS

Three or four of the above, plus heliotrope eruption or Gottron's papules

---

From Bohan A, Peter JB. Polymyositis and dermatomyositis. N Engl J Med 1975; 292:344-7, 403-7.

Medical and Obstetric Management

Pregnancy should be planned during periods of disease inactivity. Serum creatine kinase, glutamic oxaloacetic transaminase, and aldolase determinations can guide this decision. Glucocorticoid treatment is the mainstay of medical management of the active disease. Although no controlled studies have demonstrated the efficacy of steroids, most clinicians note improvement in muscle strength and decreased creatine kinase levels after 1 to 2 months of steroid therapy. Although methotrexate and azathioprine have been used in nonpregnant patients, they have unproven value. Obstetric management involves frequent monitoring of disease activity and fetal well-being.

Anesthetic Management

Anesthetic management of the parturient with polymyositis or dermatomyositis begins with the evaluation of disease activity and underlying cardiopulmonary involvement. If muscle weakness is present, spirometry should be obtained to determine whether respiratory muscles are affected. Maximum breathing capacity and peak expiratory flow rate are the most helpful measurements. Pharyngeal weakness may cause chronic aspiration, which may lead to pulmonary diffusion defects. Arterial blood gas analysis and a chest radiograph should be obtained in those patients with a history of aspiration. An ECG should be obtained to exclude conduction abnormalities and arrhythmias.

The anesthesiologist must exercise care when performing regional anesthesia in the patient with muscle weakness. Excessive cephalad spread may further impair intercostal muscle function and lead to ventilatory insufficiency. Abdominal muscle paralysis may slow progress of the second stage of labor. Careful epidural administration of a dilute solution of local anesthetic agent should provide effective pain relief without adverse effect on the progress of labor. Intrathecal opioid administration is an attractive, alternative method of pain relief during labor in these patients.

Patients with polymyositis or dermatomyositis may exhibit an atypical response to succinylcholine. Johns et al.[97] reported a short-lived thumb contracture response after succinylcholine administration in a child with dermatomyositis. Direct laryngoscopy was not impaired, the contracture resolved in 3 minutes, and normal neuromuscular recovery occurred. In this patient, a 20% rise in potassium concentration was observed—a response similar to that seen in normal subjects after succinylcholine administration. Eielsen and Stovner[98] reported a prolonged duration (50 minutes) of paralysis after succinylcholine administration in a patient with dermatomyositis who had homozygous atypical pseudocholinesterase. They obtained dibucaine determinations for four other patients with dermatomyositis and discovered one with heterozygous atypical pseudocholinesterase. Neither the occurrence of benign contractures nor the possibility of atypical pseudocholinesterase precludes the use of succinylcholine if it is required for cesarean delivery. Neuromuscular recovery should be documented before extubation. Some authors have advocated the avoidance of agents known to trigger malignant hyperthermia in those patients with polymyositis/dermatomyositis and elevated creatine kinase levels.[99,100] This is speculative and is not supported by published clinical experience.

An atypical response to nondepolarizing muscle relaxants has been reported. Flusche et al.[101] reported a case of prolonged paralysis (9.5 hours) after the administration of vecuronium in a patient with polymyositis. Underlying malignancy with associated myasthenic syndrome may prolong neuromuscular blockade. Other reports of nondepolarizing neuromuscular blockade in patients with polymyositis/dermatomyositis have indicated a normal response and recovery.[99,102] Parturients who have received chronic corticosteroid therapy should receive a peripartum stress dose of a corticosteroid.

KEY POINTS

- Pregnancy does not worsen the long-term course of autoimmune disorders.
- Autoimmune disorders lead to renal, cardiac, and pulmonary dysfunction.
- The term *lupus anticoagulant* is a misnomer because it has no true anticoagulant activity in vivo.
- Patients with scleroderma are at increased risk for difficult airway management.

REFERENCES

1. Himmelweit F, Marguardt M, Dale H. The collected papers of Paul Ehrlich. London: Pergamon, 1900:205-12.
2. Rocklin RE, Kitzmiller JL, Carpenter CB, et al. Maternal-fetal relation. Absence of an immunologic blocking factor from the serum of women with chronic abortions. N Engl J Med 1976; 295:1209-13.
3. Olding LB, Murgita RA, Wigzell H. Mitogen-stimulated lymphoid cells from human newborns suppress the proliferation of maternal lymphocytes across a cell-impermeable membrane. J Immunol 1977; 119:1109-14.
4. Dombroski RA. Autoimmune disease in pregnancy. Med Clin North Am 1989; 73:605-21.
5. Robinson DR. Systemic Lupus Erythematosus. In: Dale DC, Federman DD, Antman K, et al., eds. Scientific American Medicine. Vol. 2. New York City: WebMD Professional Publishing, 1999:15-IV.
6. Tan EM, Cohen AS, Fries JF, et al. The 1982 revised criteria for the classification of systemic lupus erythematosus. Arthritis Rheum 1982; 25:1271-7.
7. Gimovsky ML, Montoro M, Paul RH. Pregnancy outcome in women with systemic lupus erythematosus. Obstet Gynecol 1984; 63:686-92.
8. Tincani A, Balestrieri G, Faden D, DiMario C. Systemic lupus erythematosus in pregnancy. Lancet 1991; 338:756-7.
9. Meehan RT, Dorsey JK. Pregnancy among patients with systemic lupus erythematosus receiving immunosuppressive therapy. J Rheumatol 1987; 14:252-8.
10. Ruiz-Irastorza G, Lima F, Alves J, et al. Increased rate of lupus flare during pregnancy and the puerperium: A prospective study of 78 pregnancies. Br J Rheumatol 1996; 35:133-8.
11. Petri M, Howard D, Repke J. Frequency of lupus flare in pregnancy: The Hopkins Lupus Pregnancy Center experience. Arthritis Rheum 1991; 34:1538-45.
12. Urowitz MB, Gladman DD, Farewell VT, et al. Lupus and pregnancy studies. Arthritis Rheum 1993; 36:1392-7.
13. Ramsey-Goldman R. Pregnancy in systemic lupus erythematosus. Rheum Dis Clin North Am 1988; 14:169-85.
14. Buyon JP, Kalunian KC, Ramsey-Goldman R, et al. Assessing disease activity in SLE patients during pregnancy. Lupus 1999; 8:677-84.
15. Lockshin MD. Pregnancy associated with systemic lupus erythematosus. Semin Perinatol 1990; 14:130-8.
16. Le Huong D, Wechsler B, Vauthier-Brouzes D, et al. Outcome of planned pregnancies in systemic lupus erythematosus: a prospective study on 62 pregnancies. Br J Rheumatol 1997; 36:772-7.
17. Carmona F, Font J, Cervera R, et al. Obstetrical outcome of pregnancy in patients with systemic Lupus erythematosus. A study of 60 cases. Eur J Obstet Gynecol Reprod Biol 1999; 83:137-42.
18. Petri M, Watson R, Hochberg MC. Anti-Ro antibodies and neonatal lupus. Rheum Dis Clin North Am 1989; 15:335-60.
19. Press J, Uziel Y, Laxer RM, et al. Long-term outcome of mothers of children with complete congenital heart block. Am J Med 1996; 100:328-32.
20. McCune AB, Weston WL, Lee LA. Maternal and fetal outcome in neonatal lupus erythematosus. Ann Intern Med 1987; 106:518-23.
21. Lima F, Buchanan NM, Khamashta MA, et al. Obstetric outcome in systemic lupus erythematosus. Semin Arthritis Rheum 1995; 25:184-92.
22. Tendron A, Gouyon JB, Decramer S. In utero exposure to immunosuppressive drugs: experimental and clinical studies. Pediatr Nephrol 2002; 17:121-30.
23. Cote CJ, Meuwissen HJ, Pickering RJ. Effects on the neonate of prednisone and azathioprine administered to the mother during pregnancy. J Pediatr 1974; 85:324-8.
24. Scott JR. Risks to the children born to mothers with autoimmune diseases. Lupus 2002; 11:655-60.
25. Samuels P, Pfeifer SM. Autoimmune diseases in pregnancy. The obstetrician's view. Rheum Dis Clin North Am 1989; 15:307-22.
26. Ostensen M, Ostensen H. Safety of nonsteroidal antiinflammatory drugs in pregnant patients with rheumatic disease. J Rheumatol 1996; 23:1045-9.
27. Moise KJ, Huhta JC, Sharif DS, et al. Indomethacin in the treatment of premature labor. Effects on the fetal ductus arteriosus. N Engl J Med 1988; 319:327-31.
28. Stuart MJ, Gross SJ, Elrad H, Graeber JE. Effects of acetylsalicylic-acid ingestion on maternal and neonatal hemostasis. N Engl J Med 1982; 307:909-12.
29. Kaaja R, Julkunen H, Viinikka L, Ylikorkala O. Production of prostacyclin and thromboxane in lupus pregnancies: effect of small dose of aspirin. Obstet Gynecol 1993; 81:327-31.
30. Petri M, Howard D, Repke J, Goldman DW. The Hopkins Lupus Pregnancy Center: 1987-1991 update. Am J Reprod Immunol 1993; 28:188-91.
31. Averbuch M, Bojko A, Levo Y. Cardiac tamponade in the early postpartum period as the presenting and predominant manifestation of systemic lupus erythematosus. J Rheumatol 1986; 13:444-5.
32. Carette S. Cardiopulmonary manifestations of systemic lupus erythematous. Rheum Dis Clin North Am 1988; 14:135-47.
33. Ozaki M, Minami K, Shigematsu A. Myocardial ischemia during emergency anesthesia in a patient with systemic lupus erythematosus resulting from undiagnosed antiphospholipid syndrome. Anesth Analg 2002; 95:255.
34. Roldan CA, Shively BK, Crawford MH. An echocardiographic study of valvular heart disease associated with systemic lupus erythematosus. N Engl J Med 1996; 335:1424-30.
35. Winslow TM, Ossipov MA, Fazio GP, et al. Five-year follow-up study of the prevalence and progression of pulmonary hypertension in systemic lupus erythematosus. Am Heart J 1995; 129:510-5.
36. Cuenco J, Tzeng G, Wittels B. Anesthetic management of the parturient with systemic lupus erythematosus, pulmonary hypertension, and pulmonary edema. Anesthesiology 1999; 91:568-70.
37. Altomonte L, Mirone L, Zoli A, Magaro M. Autonomic nerve dysfunction in systemic lupus erythematosus: evidence for a mild involvement. Lupus 1997; 6:441-4.
38. Onishchuk JL, Carlsson C. Epidural hematoma associated with epidural anesthesia: complications of anticoagulant therapy. Anesthesiology 1992; 77:1221-3.
39. Locke GE, Giorgio AJ, Biggers SL, et al. Acute spinal epidural hematoma secondary to aspirin-induced prolonged bleeding. Surg Neurol 1976; 5:293-6.
40. Greensite FS, Katz J. Spinal subdural hematoma associated with attempted epidural anesthesia and subsequent continuous spinal anesthesia. Anesth Analg 1980; 59:72-3.
41. Horlocker TT, Wedel DJ, Schroeder DR, et al. Preoperative antiplatelet therapy does not increase the risk of spinal hematoma associated with regional anesthesia. Anesth Analg 1995; 80:303-9.
42. CLASP (Collaborative Low-dose Aspirin Study in Pregnancy) Collaborative Group. CLASP: A randomised trial of low-dose aspirin for the prevention and treatment of pre-eclampsia among 9364 pregnant women. Lancet 1994; 343:619-29.
43. de Swiet M, Redman CW. Aspirin, extradural anaesthesia and the MRC Collaborative Low-dose Aspirin Study in Pregnancy (CLASP) (letter). Br J Anaesth 1992; 69:109-10.
44. Harris EN. A reassessment of the antiphospholipid syndrome. J Rheumatol 1990; 17:733-5.
45. Love PE, Santoro SA. Antiphospholipid antibodies: anticardiolipin and the lupus anticoagulant in systemic lupus erythematosus (SLE) and in non-SLE disorders. Prevalence and clinical significance. Ann Intern Med 1990; 112:682-98.

46. Espinoza LR, Hartmann RC. Significance of the lupus anticoagulant. Am J Hematol 1986; 22:331-7.
47. Derksen RH, Hasselaar P, Oosting JD, De Groot PG. The antiphospholipid antibody dilemma. Clin Rheumatol 1990; 9:39-44.
48. Triplett DA. Clinical significance of antiphospholipid antibodies. ASCP Thrombosis and Hemostasis, Check Sample (No TH 88-1), vol 10. Chicago: American Society of Clinical Pathologists, 1985.
49. Silver RM, Draper ML, Scott JR, et al. Clinical consequences of antiphospholipid antibodies: an historic cohort study. Obstet Gynecol 1994; 83:372-7.
50. Cuadrado MJ, Mujic F, Munoz E, et al. Thrombocytopenia in the antiphospholipid syndrome. Ann Rheum Dis 1997; 56:194-6.
51. Lubbe WF, Liggins GC. Lupus anticoagulant and pregnancy. Am J Obstet Gynecol 1985; 153:322-7.
52. Carbone J, Orera M, Rodriguez Mahou M, et al. Immunological abnormalities in primary APS evolving into SLE: 6 years follow-up in women with repeated pregnancy loss. Lupus 1999; 8:274-8.
53. Rand JH, Wu XX, Andree HA, et al. Pregnancy loss in the antiphospholipid-antibody syndrome: A possible thrombogenic mechanism. N Engl J Med 1997; 337:154-60.
54. Pollard JK, Scott JR, Branch DW. Outcome of children born to women treated during pregnancy for the antiphospholipid syndrome. Obstet Gynecol 1992; 80:365-8.
55. Lubbe WF, Butler WS, Palmer SJ, Liggins GC. Fetal survival after prednisone suppression of maternal lupus-anticoagulant. Lancet 1983; 1:1361-3.
56. Rai R, Cohen H, Dave M, Regan L. Randomised controlled trial of aspirin and aspirin plus heparin in pregnant women with recurrent miscarriage associated with phospholipid antibodies (or antiphospholipid antibodies). BMJ 1997; 314:253-7.
57. Branch DW, Khamashta A. Antiphospholipid syndrome: Obstetric diagnosis, management, and controversies. Obstet Gynecol 2003; 101:1333-44.
58. Pattison NS, Chamley LW, Birdsall M, et al. Does aspirin have a role in improving pregnancy outcome for women with the antiphospholipid syndrome? A randomized controlled trial. Am J Obstet Gynecol 2000; 183:1008-12.
59. Ralph CJ. Anaesthetic management of parturients with the antiphospholipid syndrome: A review of 27 cases. Internat J Obstet Anesth 1999; 8:249-52.
60. Moxley G. Scleroderma and Related Diseases. In: Dale DC, Federman DD, Antman K, et al., eds. Scientific American Medicine. Vol. 2. New York City: WebMD Professional Publishing, 2001:15-V.
61. LeRoy EC. Systemic sclerosis (scleroderma). In: Wyngaarden JB, Smith LH, Bennett JC, eds. Cecil Textbook of Medicine. Philadelphia: WB Saunders, 1992:1530-5.
62. Nelson JL, Furst DE, Maloney S, et al. Microchimerism and HLA-compatible relationships of pregnancy in scleroderma. Lancet 1998; 351:559-62.
63. Artlett CM, Welsh KI, Black CM, Jimenez SA. Fetal-maternal HLA compatibility confers susceptibility to systemic sclerosis. Immunogenetics 1997; 47:17-22.
64. Steen VD, Conte C, Day N, et al. Pregnancy in women with systemic sclerosis. Arthritis Rheum 1989; 32:151-7.
65. Steen VD. Pregnancy in women with systemic sclerosis. Obstet Gynecol 1999; 94:15-20.
66. Furst DE, Clements PJ. D-penicillamine is not an effective treatment in systemic sclerosis. Scand J Rheumatol 2001; 30:189-91.
67. Seibold JR. Scleroderma. In: Kelley WN, Harris ED, Ruddy S, Sledge CB, eds. Textbook of Rheumatology. Philadelphia: WB Saunders, 1989: 1215-44.
68. Tuffanelli DL. Systemic scleroderma. Med Clin North Am 1989; 73: 1167-80.
69. Wach F, Ullrich H, Schmitz G, et al. Treatment of severe localized scleroderma by plasmapheresis–report of three cases. Br J Dermatol 1995; 133:605-9.
70. Muller-Ladner U, Benning K, Lang B. Current therapy of systemic sclerosis (scleroderma). Clin Investig 1993; 71:257-63.
71. Lopez-Ovejero JA, Saal SD, D'Angelo WA, et al. Reversal of vascular and renal crises of scleroderma by oral angiotensin-converting-enzyme blockade. N Engl J Med 1979; 300:1417-9.
72. Mastrobattista JM. Angiotensin converting enzyme inhibitors in pregnancy. Semin Perinatol 1997; 21:124-34.
73. Black CM. Systemic sclerosis and pregnancy. Baillieres Clin Rheumatol 1990; 4:105-24.
74. Moore M, Saffran JE, Baraf HS, Jacobs RP. Systemic sclerosis and pregnancy complicated by obstructive uropathy. Am J Obstet Gynecol 1985; 153:893-4.
75. Eisele JH, Reitan JA. Scleroderma, Raynaud's phenomenon, and local anesthetics. Anesthesiology 1971; 34:386-7.
76. Birkhan J, Heifetz M, Haim S. Diffuse cutaneous scleroderma: an anaesthetic problem. Anaesthesia 1972; 27:89-90.
77. Lewis GB. Prolonged regional analgesia in scleroderma. Can Anaesth Soc J 1974; 21:495-7.
78. Thompson J, Conklin KA. Anesthetic management of a pregnant patient with scleroderma. Anesthesiology 1983; 59:69-71.
79. Smith GB, Shribman AJ. Anaesthesia and severe skin disease. Anaesthesia 1984; 39:443-55.
80. Younker D, Harrison B. Scleroderma and pregnancy. Anaesthetic considerations. Br J Anaesth 1985; 57:1136-9.
81. Neill RS. Progressive systemic sclerosis. Prolonged sensory blockade following regional anaesthesia in association with a reduced response to systemic analgesics. Br J Anaesth 1980; 52:623-5.
82. D'Angelo R, Miller R. Pregnancy complicated by severe preeclampsia and thrombocytopenia in a patient with scleroderma. Anesth Analg 1997; 85:839-41.
83. Hseu SS, Sung CS, Mao CC, et al. Anesthetic management in a parturient with progressive systemic sclerosis during cesarean section–a case report. Acta Anaesthesiol Sin 1997; 35:161-6.
84. Bailey AR, Wolmarans M, Rhodes S. Spinal anaesthesia for caesarean section in a patient with systemic sclerosis. Anaesthesia 1999; 54:355-8.
85. Wilkes NJ, Peachey T, Beard C. Spinal anaesthesia for Caesarean section in a patient with systemic sclerosis. Anaesthesia 1999; 54:1020-1.
86. Benumof JL. Management of the difficult adult airway. With special emphasis on awake tracheal intubation. Anesthesiology 1991; 75:1087-110.
87. Anonymous. Case records of the Massachusetts General Hospital. Weekly clinicopathological exercises. Case 4-1999. A 38-year-old woman with increasing pulmonary hypertension after delivery. N Engl J Med 1999; 340:455-64.
88. Plotz PH, Dalakas M, Leff RL, et al. Current concepts in the idiopathic inflammatory myopathies: polymyositis, dermatomyositis, and related disorders. Ann Intern Med 1989; 111:143-57.
89. Olsen NJ. Idiopathic Inflammatory Myopathies. In: Dale DC, Federman DD, Antman K, et al., eds. Scientific American Medicine. Vol. 2. New York City: WebMD Professional Publishing, 2000:15-VI.
90. Bohan A, Peter JB. Polymyositis and dermatomyositis (second of two parts). N Engl J Med 1975; 292:403-7.
91. Horowitz M, McNeil JD, Maddern GJ, et al. Abnormalities of gastric and esophageal emptying in polymyositis and dermatomyositis. Gastroenterology 1986; 90:434-9.
92. Dickey BF, Myers AR. Pulmonary disease in polymyositis/dermatomyositis. Semin Arthritis Rheum 1984; 14:60-76.
93. Caro I. Dermatomyositis as a systemic disease. Med Clin North Am 1989; 73:1181-92.
94. Ishii N, Ono H, Kawaguchi T, Nakajima H. Dermatomyositis and pregnancy. Case report and review of the literature. Dermatologica 1991; 183:146-9.
95. Kanoh H, Izumi T, Seishima M, et al. A case of dermatomyositis that developed after delivery: the involvement of pregnancy in the induction of dermatomyositis. Br J Dermatol 1999; 141:897-900.
96. Kofteridis DP, Malliotakis PI, Sotsiou F, et al. Acute onset of dermatomyositis presenting in pregnancy with rhabdomyolysis and fetal loss. Scand J Rheumatol 1999; 28:192-4.
97. Johns RA, Finholt DA, Stirt JA. Anaesthetic management of a child with dermatomyositis. Can Anaesth Soc J 1986; 33:71-4.
98. Eielsen O, Stovner J. Dermatomyositis, suxamethonium action and atypical plasmacholinesterase. Can Anaesth Soc J 1978; 25:63-4.
99. Saarnivaara LH. Anesthesia for a patient with polymyositis undergoing myectomy of the cricopharyngeal muscle. Anesth Analg 1988; 67:701-2.
100. Farag HM, Naguib M, Gyasi H, Ibrahim AW. Anesthesia for a patient with eosinophilic myositis. Anesth Analg 1986; 65:903-4.
101. Flusche G, Unger-Sargon J, Lambert DH. Prolonged neuromuscular paralysis with vecuronium in a patient with polymyositis. Anesth Analg 1987; 66:188-90.
102. Ganta R, Campbell IT, Mostafa SM. Anaesthesia and acute dermatomyositis/polymyositis. Br J Anaesth 1988; 60:854-8.

Chapter 40
Cardiovascular Disease

Miriam Harnett, M.B., FFARCSI ·
Philip S. Mushlin, M.D. · William R. Camann, M.D.

The prevalence of cardiac disease in pregnancy has remained relatively constant over the last several decades, ranging between 0.4% and 4.1%.[1-3] In the developed world, congenital heart disease has supplanted rheumatic heart disease as the major cause of cardiac disease in pregnancy.

Maternal outcome seems to correlate best with the functional classification of the patient according to the criteria of the New York Heart Association (NYHA) (Box 40-1).[4] Exceptions include patients with pulmonary hypertension, significant left ventricular dysfunction, and severe cases of Marfan syndrome (especially those women with significant enlargement of the aortic root). These lesions pose a very high risk and may contraindicate pregnancy, regardless of functional class. Otherwise, class I or II patients have a maternal mortality rate of less than 1%, whereas class III or IV patients have a mortality rate between 5% and 15%. Perinatal loss also is associated with maternal functional class; patients who are class III or IV have a perinatal mortality rate between 20% and 30%.[4,5]

The optimal management of women with cardiovascular disease begins before conception, for several reasons. First, if the woman is not examined until she becomes pregnant, the physician may underestimate the severity of the lesion. For example, the murmurs of aortic insufficiency and mitral regurgitation decrease in intensity during pregnancy, presumably because of a decrease in systemic vascular resistance (SVR). Second, some patients (e.g., women with a prosthetic valve) may require a change in medication before conception. Third, in some cases it may be best for the patient to avoid pregnancy altogether.

CONGENITAL HEART DISEASE

Congenital heart disease is now the major cause of cardiac disease in pregnant women in the United States, accounting for 60% to 80% of all cases.[6] Improvements in the early diagnosis and treatment of complex congenital cardiac anomalies have led to an increase in the number of women with congenital heart disease who survive to childbearing age. In some cases, successful surgery during infancy and childhood results in complete repair and normal cardiovascular function. These women may be asymptomatic and may have relatively normal intracardiac pressures and blood flow patterns. Such patients often require no special treatment, with two exceptions. First, antibiotic prophylaxis may be warranted. Second, the presence of a neonatologist at delivery is desirable as there is a 0.7% to 1.0% incidence of congenital cardiac lesions in the offspring of these women.[6] Some of the more common lesions that may be repaired successfully in childhood include atrial and ventricular septal defects, patent ductus arteriosus, tetralogy of Fallot, transposition of the great vessels, and tricuspid atresia.

In contrast, some women may present during pregnancy with an uncorrected lesion or a lesion that has undergone partial correction. Obstetric and anesthetic management of these patients is more challenging and complex.

Left-to-Right Shunts

Lesions such as a *small* atrial septal defect (ASD), ventricular septal defect (VSD), or patent ductus arteriosus (PDA) may produce a modest degree of left-to-right intracardiac shunting, which often is well tolerated during pregnancy. Anesthetic management of patients with these defects should include attention to the following details. First, care should be taken to avoid the accidental intravenous infusion of air bubbles. Second, if epidural anesthesia is used, the anesthesiologist should use a loss-of-resistance to saline rather than air to identify the epidural space. Epidural injection of even small amounts of air can result in systemic embolization. Transient reversals of atrial pressure gradients during the cardiac cycle may allow paradoxical air emboli to occur, even when mean right atrial pressure is lower than mean left atrial pressure.[7] Third, early administration of epidural anesthesia is desirable. Pain causes increased maternal concentrations of catecholamines and increased maternal SVR and may increase the severity of left-to-right shunt resulting in pulmonary hypertension and right ventricular failure. Early administration of epidural anesthesia allows a pain-free labor and prevents the increased maternal concentrations of catecholamines and increased maternal SVR. Fourth, a slow onset of epidural anesthesia is preferred. A rapid decrease in SVR could result in a reversal of shunt flow, and an asymptomatic left-to-right shunt may become a right-to-left shunt with maternal hypox-

emia. Finally, the patient should receive supplemental oxygen, and it seems prudent to monitor hemoglobin oxygen saturation. Even mild hypoxemia can result in increased pulmonary vascular resistance and reversal of shunt flow. It also is important to avoid hypercarbia and acidosis, which may increase pulmonary vascular resistance.

Coarctation of the Aorta

Coarctation of the aorta is a congenital lesion that is more common in males than in females. Patients who have undergone successful corrective surgery and who have normal arm and leg blood pressures do not require special precautions or monitoring. An arm-to-leg gradient of less than 20 mm Hg is associated with a good outcome of pregnancy.[8] Pregnant women with uncorrected coarctation or a residual decrease in aortic diameter are at high risk for left ventricular failure, aortic rupture or dissection, and endocarditis. In such pregnancies the fetal mortality rate may approach 20% because of decreased uterine perfusion distal to the aortic lesion.[9] The incidence of congenital heart disease is approximately 3% in the offspring of mothers with aortic coarctation.[8] Compared with the general population, patients with aortic coarctation are more likely to have a bicuspid aortic valve (hence the increased risk of endocarditis) or an aneurysm in the circle of Willis. Thus these patients may be at increased risk for a cerebrovascular accident.[10]

Physical examination should be directed toward the comparison of the right-sided versus left-sided blood pressures and upper versus lower extremity pressures. The electrocardiogram (ECG) may show left ventricular hypertrophy. Magnetic resonance imaging may be a useful means of confirming the diagnosis in a pregnant patient.

The pathophysiologic manifestations include a fixed obstruction to aortic outflow and distal hypoperfusion. The cardiovascular demands of pregnancy tend to exacerbate both the risk and consequences of this lesion. Attention should be directed toward maintaining normal to slightly elevated SVR, a normal to slightly increased heart rate, and adequate intravascular volume. In patients with uncorrected coarctation, neuraxial anesthesia should be administered with great caution, if at all. For cesarean section, general anesthesia is preferred. Remifentanil has been used and facilitates maintenance of hemodynamic stability.[11] Invasive hemodynamic monitoring can help guide the administration of intravenous fluids. Uterine perfusion pressure is usually reflected more accurately by using a postductal intraarterial catheter instead of a preductal catheter. Ephedrine and dopamine are the vasopressors of choice because of their mild positive chronotropic effects.

Tetralogy of Fallot

Tetralogy of Fallot accounts for 5% of cases of congenital heart disease in pregnant women. This lesion includes four components: (1) a VSD, (2) right ventricular hypertrophy, (3) pulmonic stenosis with right ventricular outflow tract obstruction, and (4) an overriding aorta (i.e., the aortic outflow tract receives blood from both the right and left ventricles). Tetralogy of Fallot is the most common congenital heart lesion associated with a right-to-left shunt. Patients typically present with cyanosis.

INTERACTION WITH PREGNANCY

In the absence of corrective surgery, the number of women who reach childbearing age and become pregnant is quite small. Most pregnant women with tetralogy of Fallot have had corrective surgery. The surgical treatment, typically performed in childhood, involves closure of the VSD and widening of the pulmonary outflow tract. This surgery generally is successful and results in an asymptomatic patient. In some cases, a small VSD may recur, or progressive hypertrophy of the pulmonary outflow tract may occur slowly over the first several decades of life. The cardiovascular changes of pregnancy (e.g., increased blood volume, increased cardiac output, decreased SVR) may unmask these previously asymptomatic residua of corrected tetralogy of Fallot. The severity of symptoms depends on the size of the VSD, the magnitude of the pulmonic stenosis, and the contractile performance of the right ventricle. Patients with corrected tetralogy of Fallot, even if they have been asymptomatic for many years, should undergo echocardiography before and during early pregnancy.

ANESTHETIC MANAGEMENT

Anesthetic management for patients with successful correction of tetralogy of Fallot often does not differ from that for a woman without this lesion. Patients with corrected tetralogy of Fallot may manifest various atrial and ventricular arrhythmias, owing to surgical injury to the cardiac conduction channels. Thus a 12-lead ECG and ECG monitoring during labor are desirable.

Greater attention should be given to the parturient with uncorrected tetralogy of Fallot or corrected tetralogy of Fallot with residua. The anesthesiologist should avoid causing a decrease in SVR, which increases the severity of right-to-left shunt. It also is important to maintain adequate intravascular volume and venous return. In the presence of right ventricular compromise, high filling pressures are needed to enhance right ventricular performance and ensure adequate pulmonary blood flow. Administration of a neuraxial block during early labor is advisable and helps prevent an increase in pulmonary vascular resistance and consequent right-to-left shunting. For cesarean delivery, regional anesthesia should be administered slowly; single-shot spinal anesthesia is a poor choice because the abrupt reduction in SVR may cause shunt reversal and hypoxemia.

Eisenmenger Syndrome

A chronic, uncorrected left-to-right shunt may produce right ventricular hypertrophy, elevated pulmonary artery pressures, right ventricular dysfunction, and ultimately, the syndrome first described by Eisenmenger in 1897.[12] The primary lesion may be either an ASD or VSD, or an aortopulmonary communication, such as PDA or truncus arteriosus. The pulmonary and right ventricular musculature undergoes remodeling in response to chronic pulmonary volume overload. High, fixed pulmonary arterial pressure gradually limits flow through the pulmonary vessels. A reversal of shunt flow occurs when pulmonary artery pressure exceeds the level of systemic pressure. The primary left-to-right shunt becomes a right-to-left shunt. Initially the shunt may be bidirectional; acute changes in pulmonary vascular resistance or SVR may influence the primary direction of intracardiac blood flow. However, the pulmonary vascular occlusive disease ultimately leads to irreversible pulmonary hypertension. Therefore correction of the primary intracardiac lesion is not helpful at this stage.

The clinical manifestations of Eisenmenger syndrome include the sequelae of arterial hypoxemia and right ventricular failure (e.g. dyspnea, clubbing of the nails, polycythemia, engorged neck veins, peripheral edema).

INTERACTION WITH PREGNANCY

These women often are unable to respond to the increased demands for oxygen during pregnancy. Maintenance of satisfactory oxygenation requires adequate pulmonary blood flow. The decrease in pulmonary vascular resistance seen in normal pregnancy does not occur in these women because pulmonary vascular resistance is fixed. The decrease in SVR associated with pregnancy tends to exacerbate the severity of the right-to-left shunt. The pregnancy-associated decrease in functional residual capacity also may predispose the patient to maternal hypoxemia. Maternal hypoxemia results in decreased oxygen delivery to the fetus, which results in a high incidence of intrauterine growth restriction (IUGR) and fetal demise.[13] Maternal mortality is as high as 30% to 50% among these patients.[5,14] Thromboembolic phenomena are responsible for as many as 43% of all maternal deaths in patients with Eisenmenger syndrome. Many of these deaths occur postpartum—as late as 4 to 6 weeks after delivery.[5]

OBSTETRIC MANAGEMENT

Patients with Eisenmenger syndrome who become pregnant should be counseled to terminate the pregnancy.[15] If the patient desires to remain pregnant, a multidisciplinary approach with close communication among the obstetrician, cardiologist, and anesthesiologist is essential. The obstetrician most likely will want to perform an early instrumental vaginal delivery to minimize maternal expulsive efforts. Some obstetricians favor prophylactic anticoagulation during the intrapartum period, but it is unclear whether this improves maternal outcome.[5]

ANESTHETIC MANAGEMENT

The primary goals of anesthetic management are as follows[16-18]:
1. Maintain adequate SVR.
2. Maintain intravascular volume and venous return. Avoid aortocaval compression.
3. Prevent pain, hypoxemia, hypercarbia, and acidosis, which may cause an increase in pulmonary vascular resistance.
4. Avoid myocardial depression during general anesthesia.

Treatment of Pulmonary Hypertension

Inhaled nitric oxide (iNO) selectively dilates the pulmonary vascular bed without producing systemic hemodynamic effects. Thus, iNO can improve right ventricular function and may consequently enhance left ventricular function by improving oxygenation. Experience with iNO in parturients is limited. Goodwin et al.[19] reported its use during the second stage of labor and postpartum in a parturient with Eisenmenger syndrome. The administration of iNO was associated with an improvement in the patient's hypoxemia and a reduction in her pulmonary artery pressure. It was discontinued after 48 hours and vasodilator therapy was maintained with an infusion of prostacyclin; however, the patient died 2 days later.[19] In a similar case the woman died 3 weeks postpartum.[20] However, use of iNO has been associated with good outcome in women with severe primary pulmonary hypertension.[21]

Labor

Supplemental oxygen should be provided at all times. The pulse oximeter is the most useful monitor for detecting acute changes in shunt flow.[22] Pollack et al.[17] described the simultaneous use of pulse oximeters on the right hand and left foot of a parturient whose severe Eisenmenger syndrome resulted from an uncorrected PDA. The right hand receives preductal blood flow, whereas the flow to the lower extremities is postductal. Thus the authors could rapidly estimate relative changes in shunt fraction.

An intraarterial catheter facilitates the rapid detection of sudden changes in blood pressure, and a central venous pressure (CVP) catheter can help reveal clinically significant changes in cardiac filling pressures. However, the insertion of a CVP catheter occasionally produces complications (e.g., air emboli, infection, hematoma, pneumothorax), which can be disastrous in these patients. Although some physicians have stated that a pulmonary artery catheter is "essential" for the intrapartum management of pregnant women with Eisenmenger syndrome,[18] we and others[17,23] disagree and believe that a pulmonary artery catheter may be relatively contraindicated for several reasons. First, it is difficult, if not impossible, to properly position the balloon-tipped, flow-directed catheter within the pulmonary artery. Second, if the catheter does go into the pulmonary artery, the risks of pulmonary artery rupture and hemorrhage are great. Third, these patients may not tolerate catheter-induced arrhythmias. Fourth, measurements of cardiac output by thermodilution are uninterpretable in the presence of a large intracardiac shunt. Fifth, pulmonary artery pressure monitoring rarely yields clinically useful information in the presence of severe, fixed pulmonary hypertension. Sixth, the pulmonary artery catheter may predispose to pulmonary thromboembolism.[24] Finally, the risks of placing/using a pulmonary artery catheter include the entire spectrum of complications associated with placement of a CVP catheter.

Effective analgesia is necessary to prevent labor-induced increases in plasma catecholamines, which may further increase pulmonary vascular resistance. During the first stage of labor, intrathecal administration of an opioid is ideal, because it produces profound analgesia with minimal sympathetic blockade. For the second stage of labor, epidural or intrathecal doses of a local anesthetic and an opioid will provide satisfactory analgesia; alternatively, a pudendal block can be placed early in the second stage of labor. In some instances, maternal anticoagulation may complicate or contraindicate the use of regional anesthetic techniques. In such cases an intravenous infusion of remifentanil, with or without patient-controlled analgesia (PCA), may be the next best option.[25] However, the quality and reliability of intravenous opioid analgesia is not as good as that provided by a regional anesthetic technique.[26]

Cesarean Section

Historically, anesthesiologists have avoided regional anesthesia because the vasodilation that accompanies sympathectomy can worsen a right-to-left shunt. However, favorable outcomes have been achieved with epidural anesthesia, which has become the technique of choice for parturients with Eisenmenger syndrome.[18,27] The key to the safe use of spinal or epidural anesthesia is incremental injection of local anesthetic while carefully correcting any adverse hemodynamic sequelae.[28] It is critical that the anesthesiologist avoid aortocaval compression and maintain adequate venous return. Intravenous crystalloid and small doses of phenylephrine are administered as needed to maintain maternal preload, SVR, and oxygen saturation.

Several disadvantages are associated with the use of general anesthesia. Positive-pressure ventilation results in decreased venous return, which compromises cardiac output. The volatile halogenated agents can cause myocardial depression and decreased SVR. Rapid-sequence induction with agents such as thiopental or propofol characteristically decreases both contractility and SVR, which may exacerbate a right-to-left shunt. On the other hand, a slow induction of general anesthesia predisposes to maternal aspiration. This risk notwithstanding, a rapid-sequence induction of general anesthesia is usually avoided in patients with Eisenmenger syndrome. Measures to decrease the risk of anesthesia-related aspiration include (1) maintaining the patient NPO for solids for at least 8 hours before the induction of anesthesia, (2) preoperative pharmacologic therapy (e.g., H_2-receptor antagonist, metoclopramide, sodium citrate), and (3) the use of cricoid pressure. Although opioids are not routinely used when giving general anesthesia in healthy women undergoing cesarean section, it seems appropriate to include a systemic opioid during administration of general anesthesia to help maintain hemodynamic stability in women with severe cardiovascular disease.

Regardless of the anesthetic technique used, these women are at high risk for hemodynamic compromise immediately after delivery. Large losses of blood should be replaced promptly with crystalloid, colloid, and/or appropriate blood products. Cautious fluid therapy is important when the blood loss is minimal, because the postpartum autotransfusion may cause intravascular volume overload in women with myocardial dysfunction.

PRIMARY PULMONARY HYPERTENSION

The syndrome of primary pulmonary hypertension is characterized by markedly elevated pulmonary artery pressures in the absence of an intracardiac or aortopulmonary shunt.[29] Unlike those with Eisenmenger syndrome, patients with primary pulmonary hypertension often have a reactive pulmonary vasculature that can respond to vasodilator therapy. The maternal mortality rate may be as high as 30% to 40%. These patients also have a high incidence of IUGR, fetal loss, and preterm delivery.[30]

The hemodynamic goals of obstetric and anesthetic management are similar to those for the patient with Eisenmenger syndrome[16,31,32]:

1. Prevent pain, hypoxemia, acidosis, and hypercarbia, which cause an increase in pulmonary vascular resistance.
2. Maintain intravascular volume and venous return. Avoid aortocaval compression and replace blood loss at delivery.
3. Maintain adequate SVR, as women with fixed pulmonary hypertension cannot increase their cardiac output to compensate for a decrease in blood pressure that results from a decrease in SVR.
4. Avoid myocardial depression during general anesthesia, especially in women with fixed pulmonary hypertension.

Supplemental oxygen is a superb pulmonary vasodilator and should be administered routinely in these patients. Monitoring typically includes placement of both an arterial and a CVP catheter. A pulmonary artery catheter can guide treatment when the pulmonary vascular resistance (PVR) is responsive to vasodilator therapy; however, the physician should weigh carefully the risks versus benefits of pulmonary artery catheterization (*vide supra*).[33] Transesophageal echocardiography has been used intraoperatively during cesarean delivery.[34]

Agents that have been used to treat primary pulmonary hypertension include iNO, nitroglycerin, calcium-entry blocking agents, prostaglandins, and endothelin antagonists.[21,35-39] A successful maternal and fetal outcome was recently reported in a woman with primary pulmonary hypertension who had received epoprostenol throughout pregnancy.[40]

Continuous neuraxial block is preferred for labor and delivery.[41,42] Epidural anesthesia allows for a pain-free first and second stage of labor and facilitates elective forceps delivery. Several reports have noted the successful use of epidural anesthesia for cesarean section.[31,43] Slow induction of epidural anesthesia is of critical importance. If hypotension occurs it should be treated initially with intravenous fluid. Vasopressors such as ephedrine should be used with caution because these agents can further increase the pulmonary artery pressures. Single-shot spinal anesthesia may cause severe hemodynamic instability and should be avoided except in those rare instances when it is used in preference to general anesthesia. Continuous spinal anesthesia[44] and general anesthesia have also been successfully used in patients with primary pulmonary hypertension.

Weeks and Smith[32] reviewed all published cases of intrapartum anesthetic management for women with primary pulmonary hypertension. They concluded the following:

> Epidural anesthesia has been used with success, but in the presence of pre-existing right ventricular failure, any large decrease in systemic vascular resistance may lead to a further decrease in cardiac output. Refractory hypotension may also cause right ventricular ischemia, leading to a further deterioration in right ventricular function. The potential hazards of general anesthesia include increased pulmonary artery pressure during laryngoscopy and intubation, the adverse effects of positive pressure ventilation on venous return and the negative inotropic effects of certain anesthetic agents. However, these adverse effects can be minimized by the use of a narcotic-based induction and maintenance technique. Any resulting narcotic-induced neonatal depression should be easily treated. Intensive postoperative management is of critical importance and should probably continue for one week because of the high incidence of sudden death during this period.[32]

HYPERTROPHIC OBSTRUCTIVE CARDIOMYOPATHY

Hypertrophic obstructive cardiomyopathy (HOCM) is an uncommon form of cardiomyopathy that affects the interventricular septum in the area of the left ventricular outflow tract. This disorder is characterized by left ventricular hypertrophy, decreased left ventricular chamber size, and left ventricular dysfunction. Patients with HOCM require a **slow heart rate** and a **modest expansion of intravascular volume** to ensure adequate ventricular filling. It is important to avoid increases in myocardial contractility and decreases in SVR, which tend to exacerbate the degree of outflow tract obstruction. Sudden death, usually from ventricular arrhythmias, is a major cause of mortality in patients with HOCM.

Interaction with Pregnancy

Women with HOCM have an increased risk of maternal mortality.[45] Some patients with HOCM tolerate pregnancy well. The increased blood volume of pregnancy helps maintain adequate ventricular filling, which helps decrease the severity of outflow tract obstruction. However, pregnancy also results in increased heart rate and myocardial contractility and decreased SVR. All three of these physiologic changes may worsen the outflow tract obstruction. Aortocaval compression results in decreased venous return, which decreases left ventricular chamber size and results in increased obstruction. Thus pregnancy may exacerbate HOCM in some parturients.

Medical Management

Good outcome depends on careful attention to control of heart rate, maintenance of adequate vascular volume, and prevention of arrhythmias. Medical management includes treatment with a beta-adrenergic receptor antagonist, which should be continued during pregnancy.[46] Women of childbearing age who are symptomatic or have a history of syncope or presyncope should be considered candidates for insertion of a pacemaker or an automatic implantable cardioverter defibrillator (AICD) before conception.[47]

Obstetric Management

Most obstetricians reserve cesarean section for obstetric indications. These patients typically tolerate the second stage of labor well, given the fact that increased SVR helps maintain ventricular function. If oxytocin is needed after delivery, it should be given slowly; bolus administration may cause systemic vasodilation and an increase in outflow tract obstruction. Methylergonovine may be acceptable as an alternative uterotonic agent.

Anesthetic Management

The goals of anesthetic management are as follows[16,48,49,50]:
1. Maintain intravascular volume and venous return. Avoid aortocaval compression.
2. Maintain adequate SVR.
3. Maintain a slow heart rate and sinus rhythm. Aggressively treat atrial fibrillation and other tachyarrhythmias.
4. Prevent an increase in myocardial contractility.

Beta-adrenergic receptor blockade should be maintained during labor and delivery. Regional analgesic/anesthetic techniques, including combined spinal-epidural (CSE) analgesia using intrathecal opioids, may be administered during labor. Phenylephrine is the preferred vasopressor for treatment of hypotension in these patients.

An elective cesarean delivery may be performed safely with epidural anesthesia.[48] HOCM represents a relative contraindication to the use of single-shot spinal anesthesia for cesarean section. The rapid onset of sympathectomy is hazardous in these patients. Patients with HOCM tolerate general anesthesia well.[50] The volatile halogenated agents cause decreased myocardial contractility, which is advantageous in patients with HOCM. Whether one volatile agent offers any advantage over the others in patients with HOCM has not been demonstrated. The most common adverse occurrence following general anesthesia in patients with HOCM is reversible congestive heart failure.[50] Remifentanil has been successfully used during cesarean delivery in a woman with severe heart dysfunction secondary to HOCM.[51]

ISCHEMIC HEART DISEASE

Myocardial infarction accounts for nearly 2000 deaths yearly in women under the age of 45.[52] Fortunately, myocardial infarction is a rare event during pregnancy. In 1952, Ginz[53] estimated that the incidence was less than 1 in 10,000 pregnancies. However, the incidence of myocardial ischemia during pregnancy may be increasing for several reasons. First, there is a greater prevalence of delayed childbearing. Indeed, assisted reproductive techniques have resulted in pregnancies in postmenopausal women older than 50 years of age. Second, many young women continue to abuse tobacco. Third, there is an increased incidence of cocaine abuse by women of childbearing age. Fourth, the use of oral contraceptives after age 35 may increase the risk of ischemic heart disease.

Badui and Enciso[54] reviewed reports of 136 parturients with peripartum myocardial infarction. The average maternal age was 32; some 43% of affected women had no obvious risk factors, and 47% had no evidence of atherosclerosis. The maternal mortality rate was 19%, and the perinatal mortality rate was 17%.[54]

Pathophysiology

The etiology of myocardial infarction during pregnancy is multifactorial. Coronary artery morphology has been studied in 125 patients who had a myocardial infarction during pregnancy. Coronary atherosclerosis (with or without intracoronary thrombus) was found in 43% of patients, coronary thrombus without atherosclerotic disease was found in 21%, coronary dissection was noted in 16%, and normal coronary arteries were found in 29% of patients.[55] An intrapartum myocardial infarction in a woman with normal coronary arteries may be caused by disorders such as pheochromocytoma, collagen vascular disease, sickle cell anemia, or protracted coronary artery spasm (secondary to cocaine abuse, pregnancy-induced hypertension, or administration of an ergot alkaloid).

Interaction with Pregnancy

Pregnancy results in increased heart rate, myocardial wall tension and contractility, basal metabolic rate, and oxygen consumption. Labor causes a further, progressive increase in oxygen consumption. Pain results in increased maternal concentrations of catecholamines, which increase myocardial oxygen demand. Each uterine contraction results in an autotransfusion of 300 to 500 mL of blood to the central circulation. Autotransfusion increases preload and may further compromise the balance between myocardial oxygen supply and demand. Oxygen consumption peaks at delivery. Maternal expulsive efforts at delivery may result in a 150% increase in oxygen consumption. Oxygen consumption remains 25% higher than nonpregnant levels in the immediate postpartum period. Elective cesarean section does not eliminate the cardiovascular stress of delivery; cardiac output increases as much as 50% during and after elective cesarean section.

The cardiovascular changes of pregnancy, labor, and delivery may precipitate myocardial ischemia or infarction in women with coronary artery disease or other cardiac lesions (Table 40-1 and Box 40-2). Cocaine abuse can cause myocardial ischemia as a result of tachycardia, hypertension, arrhythmias, coronary artery spasm, coronary thrombosis, and the acceleration of atherosclerotic disease.[56] Thus the possibility of cocaine abuse should be considered when a pregnant woman develops myocardial ischemia or infarction.

TABLE 40-1   BALANCE BETWEEN MYOCARDIAL OXYGEN SUPPLY AND DEMAND

Parameter	Effect of pregnancy
Supply	
Diastolic time	Decreased
Coronary perfusion pressure	May be decreased
Arterial oxygen content	
Arterial oxygen tension	Increased
Hemoglobin concentration	Decreased
Coronary vessel diameter	Unchanged
Demand	
Basal oxygen requirements	Increased
Heart rate	Increased
Wall tension	
Preload (ventricular radius)	May be increased
Afterload	Decreased
Contractility	Increased

Box 40-2 CAUSES OF MYOCARDIAL ISCHEMIA IN PREGNANT WOMEN

Cocaine abuse
Atherosclerosis
Coronary artery vasospasm
Coronary artery aneurysm
Coronary artery dissection
Coronary artery hematoma
Severe hypertension
Tachycardia (in association with left ventricular hypertrophy)
Severe hypotension
Hypoxemia
Anemia
Severe aortic stenosis or regurgitation

Diagnosis

The diagnosis of myocardial ischemia is made by history, physical examination, and ECG. Among nonpregnant patients, the most significant symptoms include chest pain, dyspnea, diaphoresis, poor exercise tolerance, and syncope. However, all of these symptoms may occur in normal pregnant women. Chest pain that radiates to the left arm or syncope not explained by supine hypotension should prompt further evaluation. The diagnosis of myocardial infarction may be confirmed by serum cardiac enzyme determinations. The serum creatine kinase MB fraction may increase twofold 30 minutes after delivery in the absence of myocardial ischemia. Plasma troponin-1 is a useful test in patients with suspected peripartum myocardial infarction because it remains within the normal range unless myocardial injury has occurred.

The ECG may be misleading; during pregnancy the normal ECG may show sinus tachycardia, a leftward axis shift, ST-segment depression, flattened or inverted T waves, and a Q wave in lead III.[57] Holter monitoring and echocardiography are noninvasive tests that remain useful during pregnancy. During early pregnancy, cardiac catheterization is used with caution because of the teratogenic effects of ionizing radiation.[58] However, the risk-benefit analysis may favor intrapartum cardiac catheterization with appropriate lead shielding.[59] The simultaneous use of echocardiography may decrease the need for cineangiography, thereby reducing fetal radiation exposure.

Medical Management

Optimal management of the pregnant woman with coronary artery disease requires attention to the needs of both mother and fetus. Physicians should treat disease states (e.g., anemia, thyrotoxicosis, hypertension, infection, substance abuse) that may adversely affect myocardial oxygen supply and demand.[60]

The pharmacologic agents (e.g., nitrates, beta-adrenergic receptor antagonists, calcium-entry antagonists) used in the treatment of myocardial ischemia in nonpregnant patients are also used during pregnancy. Treatment of myocardial ischemia improves cardiac function, which should increase uteroplacental perfusion. Conversely, overly aggressive therapy may adversely affect the fetus. For example, if nitroglycerin is given intravenously, the physician must beware of a sudden reduction in preload, which may decrease cardiac output and uterine blood flow and result in undesired uterine atony. It is useful to monitor the fetal heart rate (FHR) in such cases.

Ischemia that is unresponsive to medical management may require percutaneous transluminal coronary angioplasty,[61,62] stent placement,[63] or cardiopulmonary bypass surgery.[64]

Schumacher et al.[65] reported a case of myocardial infarction that was treated with tissue plasminogen activator (TPA) at 21 weeks' gestation. Maternal outcome was good, and cesarean section for preterm labor was performed at 33 weeks. The safety of thrombolytic agent use during pregnancy has not yet been established. TPA has a short half-life, and because of its large molecular weight (65,000 d) it does not cross the placenta. Nevertheless, TPA increases the risk of placental abruption, intrauterine hemorrhage, and resultant fetal demise. The administration of TPA close to delivery may increase blood loss during operative procedures.

Obstetric Management

The risk of recurrent myocardial infarction in pregnant women with a history of previous infarction is unknown. Frenkel et al.[66] reviewed 24 published cases of patients who conceived after myocardial infarction. They noted that "each woman had an uneventful pregnancy with no cardiac or obstetric complications related to the myocardial infarction."[66] They concluded that previous myocardial infarction does not contraindicate labor, and they recommended that cesarean section be reserved "for obstetric situations and . . . situations that are life-threatening to the mother and cannot be corrected immediately."[66]

It has been suggested that acute myocardial infarction complicated by refractory congestive heart failure should prompt early cesarean section. Listo and Bjorkenheim[67] described a patient with an acute anterior wall myocardial infarction during labor who developed cardiogenic shock, which led to intrapartum fetal death. Cesarean section resulted in a rapid resolution of pulmonary edema. Mabie et al.[68] reported a 42-year-old woman with no known cardiac risk factors who had an acute myocardial infarction at 32 weeks' gestation and developed preterm labor. Symptoms of congestive heart failure improved promptly after cesarean section. The initial left ventricular dysfunction ultimately resolved. These authors suggested that early cesarean section may help protect stunned but viable myocardium.

The risk of recurrent perioperative myocardial infarction is increased in patients who undergo major surgery within 6 months of a prior myocardial infarction. Invasive hemodynamic monitoring, maintenance of normal intravascular volume, and aggressive prophylaxis and therapy of ischemia may reduce this risk.[69]

Cohen et al.[70] reviewed the advantages and disadvantages of cesarean section versus vaginal delivery in patients with a history of recent myocardial infarction. An elective cesarean section allows the obstetrician to control the timing of delivery. The performance of an elective cesarean section averts the prolonged maternal stress of labor and the hyperdynamic circulatory changes associated with maternal expulsive efforts during the second stage of labor. Disadvantages of cesarean section are related to (1) an increased risk of blood loss, (2) an increased risk of infection, (3) greater postpartum pain, (4) delayed ambulation, and (5) an increased risk of pulmonary morbidity after delivery. The use of epidural anesthesia throughout labor minimizes hyperdynamic circulatory changes associated with vaginal delivery.

Early studies suggested that oxytocin decreases coronary artery blood flow; however, these studies used pituitary extracts that contained arginine vasopressin, a potent coronary artery vasoconstrictor. Intravenous infusion of synthetic oxytocin is considered safe for the induction of labor and treatment of postpartum uterine atony in women with coronary artery disease. However, a bolus injection of oxytocin may cause hypotension, and a prolonged infusion of large doses of oxytocin may result in hyponatremia and congestive heart failure.

In summary, no consensus exists regarding the optimal method of delivery in these patients. Some obstetricians recommend the liberal use of cesarean section; but others argue that cesarean section is major surgery, which does not eliminate maternal hemodynamic stress and predisposes to hemorrhagic and infectious complications. It seems reasonable to reserve cesarean section for obstetric indications unless maternal hemodynamic instability mandates immediate delivery.

Anesthetic Management

Optimal management requires a multidisciplinary approach. The therapeutic options for parturients with coronary artery disease or active ischemia are similar to those for nonpregnant patients. The ECG and SpO_2 should be monitored continuously during labor and vaginal or cesarean delivery. An arterial catheter and occasionally a pulmonary artery catheter may facilitate management of women who have had a recent myocardial infarction or who have left ventricular and/or valvular dysfunction.

LABOR

Supplemental oxygen should be administered during labor and delivery. Epidural anesthesia provides excellent pain relief, prevents hyperventilation, and reduces maternal concentrations of catecholamines. (Hypocapnia and catecholamines both cause coronary artery vasoconstriction.) Amniotomy should be delayed until satisfactory epidural analgesia is established. A dense epidural block ensures total relief of pain during labor, minimizes maternal expulsive efforts during the second stage of labor, and facilitates the rapid achievement of satisfactory anesthesia if urgent cesarean delivery is required.

We usually do not include epinephrine in the local anesthetic solution because an unintentional intravascular injection of epinephrine can produce maternal tachycardia, and the systemic absorption of epidural epinephrine increases the likelihood of maternal hypotension. Treatment with ephedrine increases maternal heart rate, which increases myocardial oxygen demand and may aggravate myocardial ischemia. For this reason, phenylephrine is the preferred vasopressor for treatment of hypotension in patients with ischemic heart disease.

A continuous epidural infusion technique facilitates hemodynamic stability during labor. Continuous spinal anesthesia may be used safely, but the placement of a large-gauge catheter is associated with a high incidence of postdural puncture headache (PDPH).

CESAREAN SECTION
Single-shot spinal anesthesia results in a rapid onset of sympathectomy and an increased risk of severe hypotension. Continuous epidural anesthesia is the preferred technique for cesarean section.[71,72] It is reasonable to use local anesthetic solutions without epinephrine such as 0.75% ropivacaine or 0.5% levobupivacaine. When general anesthesia is required, a modified rapid-sequence induction (e.g., using etomidate, remifentanil, and succinylcholine) can be performed over 1 to 2 minutes without compromising hemodynamic stability.

These women remain at increased risk for cardiovascular instability (myocardial infarction, pulmonary edema) after vaginal or cesarean delivery. Thus we often maintain an epidural infusion of a dilute solution of local anesthetic during the immediate postpartum period to achieve a partial sympathectomy, which decreases the effective intravascular volume and therefore decreases the risk of postpartum pulmonary edema. We monitor the patient in an obstetric intensive care setting for at least 24 hours after delivery. Cardiology consultation is helpful for postpartum management.

VALVULAR DISORDERS
Published guidelines address diagnostic testing, physical activity, thromboprophylaxis, and treatment during pregnancy in patients with valvular heart disease.[73-75]

Aortic Stenosis
Aortic stenosis is classified as valvular, subvalvular, or supravalvular. In women of childbearing age, valvular aortic stenosis is usually rheumatic in origin. Subvalvular and supravalvular aortic stenosis are typically congenital. A bicuspid aortic valve is perhaps the most common congenital anomaly of the heart.[76]

PATHOPHYSIOLOGY
Patients with rheumatic aortic stenosis may remain asymptomatic for years. This lesion does not become hemodynamically significant until the valve diameter is one third of its normal size.[5] (The normal aortic valve area is 2.6 to 3.5 cm^2.) A valvular gradient of 50 mm Hg signals the presence of severe stenosis. Patients with a gradient that exceeds 100 mm Hg are at high risk for myocardial ischemia. Patients with moderate-to-severe disease have a relatively fixed stroke volume; they may be unable to maintain adequate coronary or cerebral perfusion during exertion. The onset of angina, dyspnea, or syncope is ominous and signals a life expectancy of less than 5 years.[77]

DIAGNOSIS
A coarse systolic murmur, which reaches its maximal intensity at midsystole and radiates to the apex and the neck, is characteristic of aortic stenosis. The ECG may show evidence of left ventricular hypertrophy, conduction disturbances, and ischemia. In patients with severe aortic stenosis, the chest radiographic examination may reveal left ventricular enlargement, aortic valve calcification, and poststenotic dilation of the ascending aorta. Echocardiography is an accurate, noninvasive method for monitoring the cardiac status of parturients with aortic stenosis throughout pregnancy.[78]

INTERACTION WITH PREGNANCY
The increased blood volume of pregnancy allows women with mild aortic stenosis to tolerate pregnancy well,[5] although they are at risk for infective endocarditis after delivery. Women with severe aortic stenosis have a limited ability to compensate for increased demands during pregnancy. They may develop dyspnea, angina, or syncope. In one review of pregnant women with aortic stenosis, the maternal mortality rate was 17%.[79] The rate of perinatal fetal loss may approach 20%.[77] Women with severe aortic stenosis are advised to have corrective surgery before conception. Symptoms early in gestation may warrant the termination of pregnancy; nonsurgical[80] or surgical intervention (valve replacement) should be considered if a woman's clinical condition worsens or is refractory to medical treatment.

OBSTETRIC MANAGEMENT
No consensus exists regarding the ideal method of delivery. These patients are at high risk during early termination of pregnancy, vaginal delivery, or cesarean section. Regardless of the method of delivery, it is critical to maintain intravascular volume, venous return, and sinus rhythm. Aortocaval compression, peripartum hemorrhage, and sympathectomy may cause decreased cardiac output. Many obstetricians favor instrumental vaginal delivery early during the second stage of labor.

ANESTHETIC MANAGEMENT
The goals of anesthetic management are as follows[16,81,82]:
1. Maintain a normal heart rate and sinus rhythm.
2. Maintain adequate SVR.
3. Maintain intravascular volume and venous return. Avoid aortocaval compression.
4. Avoid myocardial depression during general anesthesia.

It is important to maintain a normal heart rate and sinus rhythm. Because these patients have a fixed stroke volume, a slow heart rate decreases cardiac output. Severe tachycardia increases myocardial oxygen demand and decreases time for diastolic perfusion of the hypertrophic left ventricle. Patients with aortic stenosis do not tolerate arrhythmias well. Atrial systole is critical for the maintenance of adequate ventricular filling and cardiac output. Prompt treatment of arrhythmias is essential.

Patients with aortic stenosis do not tolerate a significant decrease in SVR, which results in hypotension and decreased perfusion of the hypertrophic left ventricle. Normal patients compensate for decreased SVR by increasing stroke volume and heart rate. Patients with aortic stenosis have a fixed stroke volume, and they must increase their heart rate to increase cardiac output. However, severe tachycardia is undesirable and hazardous.

Patients with aortic stenosis do not tolerate decreased venous return and left ventricular filling pressure. Adequate end-diastolic volume is necessary to maintain left ventricular stroke volume.

It is helpful to place an intraarterial catheter early in labor or before cesarean section. Many anesthesiologists prefer to place a pulmonary artery catheter in patients with aortic stenosis. Others contend that placement of a pulmonary artery catheter entails a high risk of ventricular arrhythmias and cardiovascular collapse and that often it is adequate to monitor CVP in these patients. The left ventricle is relatively noncompliant, and the anesthesiologist may observe an increased pulmonary capillary wedge pressure (PCWP) in a patient with a normal left ventricular end-diastolic volume (LVEDV). During labor, hypovolemia is a greater threat than pulmonary edema. Thus, CVP or PCWP should be maintained at high-normal levels (e.g., PCWP of 18 mm Hg) to protect cardiac output during unexpected peripartum hemorrhage.[5]

Historically, anesthesiologists have avoided spinal and epidural anesthesia in pregnant women with aortic stenosis. Moderate-to-severe aortic stenosis remains a relative contraindication for single-shot spinal anesthesia. However, numerous reports have described the safe use of continuous epidural or continuous spinal anesthesia for vaginal or cesarean delivery in women with aortic stenosis.[82,83] Slow epidural administration of small bolus doses of local anesthetic with fentanyl allows the anesthesiologist to titrate appropriate volumes of crystalloid and allows the patient to achieve compensatory vasoconstriction above the level of the block. Typically we do not use local anesthetic solutions that contain epinephrine for patients with moderate-to-severe aortic stenosis. An unintentional intravascular injection of epinephrine can precipitate tachycardia, whereas systemic absorption of epinephrine from the epidural space can decrease SVR and lower venous return.

It is essential to maintain left uterine displacement during the induction and maintenance of anesthesia. Maintenance of venous return and LVEDV are critical. Invasive hemodynamic monitoring is invaluable during the use of regional anesthesia in parturients with severe aortic stenosis.

When general anesthesia is needed, a combination of etomidate and a modest dose of opioid is a good choice for the induction of anesthesia and is generally preferable to agents such as sodium thiopental (which causes myocardial depression) and ketamine (which causes tachycardia). Redfern et al.[84] reported the use of alfentanil 1.75 mg (35 µg/kg), etomidate 12 mg, and succinylcholine for the administration of general anesthesia in a pregnant woman with severe aortic stenosis. After induction, the mother had transient hypotension. At delivery, the infant showed evidence of severe depression but responded to controlled ventilation and administration of naloxone. Alternatively, a combination of low-dose thiopental and ketamine may be a suitable induction regimen if etomidate is unavailable. Recent reports have described the successful use of remifentanil-based general anesthesia in women with severe cardiac disease.[85-87]

Aortic Insufficiency

Aortic insufficiency occurs more often than aortic stenosis in women of childbearing age.[88] Rheumatic heart disease is the etiology in almost 75% of affected patients. Women with rheumatic aortic insufficiency typically have mitral valve disease. When aortic insufficiency occurs as an isolated lesion, it is less likely to have a rheumatic etiology.

Fifteen percent of patients with VSD develop prolapse of an aortic cusp and **chronic, progressive aortic insufficiency**. Congenital fenestrations of the aortic valve occasionally produce mild aortic insufficiency. Syphilis or ankylosing spondylitis may be associated with cellular infiltration and scarring of the media of the thoracic aorta, which may lead to aortic dilation, aneurysm formation, and severe regurgitation. Syphilitic involvement of the aorta also may narrow the coronary ostia, which may result in coronary insufficiency. Cystic medial necrosis of the ascending aorta, idiopathic dilation of the aorta, and severe hypertension may widen the aortic annulus and lead to progressive aortic insufficiency.

Acute aortic insufficiency may result from infective endocarditis, which may involve a valve previously affected by rheumatic disease, a congenitally deformed valve, or rarely a normal aortic valve. Traumatic rupture of the aortic valve is an uncommon cause of acute aortic insufficiency. Occasionally, retrograde dissection of the aorta involves the aortic annulus and produces aortic insufficiency. Acute aortic insufficiency is a life-threatening condition.[88,89] However, in one case, acute dissection was managed medically with nifedipine and labetalol, and successful cesarean delivery was accomplished several weeks later, using epidural anesthesia.[88]

PATHOPHYSIOLOGY

Regurgitation of blood from the aorta to the left ventricle occurs when the aortic valve fails to close normally. Aortic insufficiency results in left ventricular volume overload, which over time leads to left ventricular dilation and hypertrophy. Initially, the enlarging left ventricle tolerates the increased work. Eventually left ventricular contractility decreases, the ejection fraction and forward stroke volume progressively decline, and LVEDV continues to rise. Deterioration of left ventricular function often precedes the development of symptoms. A competent mitral valve can protect the pulmonary circulation from the initial increases in LVEDV and LVEDP. However, as the ventricle begins to fail, further increases in LVEDV and LVEDP occur, which leads to pulmonary edema.

Equilibration between aortic and left ventricular pressures may occur toward the end of diastole, particularly when the heart rate is slow. The LVEDP may increase to extremely high levels (greater than 40 mm Hg). Rarely the left ventricular pressure exceeds the left atrial pressure toward the end of diastole. This may cause premature closure of the mitral valve or diastolic mitral regurgitation.

Myocardial ischemia occurs in patients with aortic insufficiency because left ventricular dilation and increased left ventricular systolic pressure result in increased myocardial oxygen demand. In addition, decreased coronary flow during diastole results in decreased myocardial perfusion.

CLINICAL PRESENTATION

The average interval between the first episode of acute rheumatic fever and the development of hemodynamically significant aortic insufficiency is 7 years. The disease typically remains asymptomatic for another 10 to 20 years, but during this time, aortic insufficiency typically worsens.

With **chronic aortic insufficiency,** the first complaint often is a pounding sensation in the chest, especially when the patient is lying down. Exertional dyspnea typically is the first symptom of diminished cardiac reserve. This is followed by orthopnea, paroxysmal nocturnal dyspnea, and diaphoresis. Symptoms of left ventricular failure are more common than symptoms of myocardial ischemia. However, chest pain may result from coronary insufficiency or excessive pounding of the heart on the chest wall. Late in the course of the disease, peripheral edema, congestive hepatomegaly, and ascites may develop.

Acute aortic insufficiency (secondary to trauma or infective endocarditis) is associated with abrupt increases in LVEDV that result in markedly elevated LVEDP. Left atrial and pulmonary artery pressures increase rapidly, and hemodynamic deterioration ensues; emergent surgery is often necessary as a life-saving measure.[88,89]

DIAGNOSIS

The arterial pulse pressure is widened. However, the severity of aortic insufficiency does not correlate directly with pulse pressure; some patients with severe aortic insufficiency have a normal blood pressure. Patients characteristically have a rapidly rising "water hammer" pulse, which collapses suddenly as arterial pressure plummets during late systole and diastole. A diastolic thrill often is palpable along the left sternal border, and a third heart sound is common. The murmur of aortic insufficiency typically is a high-pitched, blowing decrescendo diastolic murmur that is heard best along the left sternal border in the third intercostal space. The ECG may be totally normal in patients with mild aortic insufficiency, whereas the ECG may show left ventricular hypertrophy and myocardial ischemia in women with severe disease. The presence of atrial fibrillation is suggestive of coexisting mitral valvular disease.

MEDICAL MANAGEMENT

The left ventricular failure of chronic aortic insufficiency initially responds to treatment with digoxin, salt restriction, and diuretics. Cardiac arrhythmias and infections are poorly tolerated and require prompt therapy.

OBSTETRIC MANAGEMENT

Aortic insufficiency often is tolerated well during pregnancy for at least three reasons. First, pregnancy typically results in a modest increase in maternal heart rate, and this decreases the time for regurgitant blood flow during diastole. Second, pregnancy results in decreased SVR, which favors the forward flow of blood and decreases the amount of regurgitant blood flow. Third, the increased blood volume of pregnancy helps maintain adequate filling pressures.

ANESTHETIC MANAGEMENT

The goals of anesthetic management are as follows[16]:
1. Maintain a heart rate that is normal or slightly increased.
2. Prevent an increase in SVR.
3. Avoid aortocaval compression.
4. Avoid myocardial depression during general anesthesia.

Epidural anesthesia may result in decreased afterload and is preferred for either vaginal or cesarean delivery. During labor, early administration of epidural anesthesia prevents the pain-associated increase in SVR, which can precipitate acute left ventricular volume overload in women with aortic insufficiency. These patients do not tolerate bradycardia, which

should be treated promptly. Wadsworth et al.[51] described the use of remifentanil for general anesthesia for cesarean delivery in a woman with aortic insufficiency.

Mitral Stenosis

Mitral stenosis is the most common lesion associated with rheumatic heart disease.[90] The incidence of rheumatic heart disease has declined in most developed countries, presumably as a result of improved socioeconomic conditions and perhaps as a result of a change in the prevalence or virulence of the hemolytic streptococcal pathogen.[91] Rheumatic heart disease remains a common problem in many parts of Africa and Asia.

PATHOPHYSIOLOGY

The rheumatic mitral valve is fused along the edges of the cusps or the chordae tendineae. Commissural band stenosis (defined as thickening and rigidity of the commissures) appears to be more common than cuspal stenosis with calcification in pregnant women with mitral stenosis (Figure 40-1). The valve thickens and becomes funnel-shaped or fish-mouthed. Calcium can accumulate on the cusps, leaflets, and annulus.

The normal mitral valve orifice has a surface area of 4 to 6 cm². Symptoms typically develop when the size of the orifice is 2 cm² or less. A reduction to 1 cm² or less is considered severe and often requires surgical intervention.

Mitral stenosis prevents filling of the left ventricle, which results in decreased stroke volume and decreased cardiac

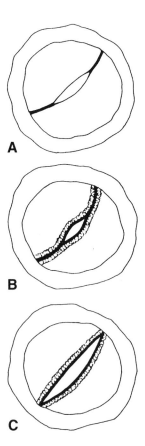

FIGURE 40-1. Types of mitral valve stenosis. **A,** Commissural band stenosis. **B,** Commissural cuspal stenosis. **C,** Commissural stenosis after splitting of the valve. (From Stephen SJ. Changing patterns of mitral stenosis. J Am Coll Cardiol 1992; 19:1277.)

output. By definition, mitral stenosis prevents emptying of the left atrium. This results in left atrial dilation and increased left atrial and pulmonary arterial pressures. Atrial fibrillation may occur and mural thrombi may develop. Increased pulmonary arterial pressure results in dyspnea, hemoptysis, and pulmonary edema.

Progressive pulmonary hypertension results in compensatory right ventricular hypertrophy. Increased pulmonary vascular resistance worsens with exercise and may lead to right heart failure. Severe, fixed pulmonary hypertension limits the compensatory changes in pulmonary vascular resistance that normally accompany changes in cardiac output and SVR.

DIAGNOSIS

After an acute episode of rheumatic fever, mitral stenosis progresses slowly for 20 to 30 years. Approximately 25% of women with mitral stenosis first experience symptoms during pregnancy. Symptoms and signs associated with mitral stenosis include dyspnea, hemoptysis, chest pain, right heart failure, and thromboembolism. Auscultation may reveal a diastolic murmur, an accentuated S1, an audible S4, and an opening snap. The ECG may show left atrial enlargement, atrial fibrillation, and right ventricular hypertrophy. Echocardiography helps confirm the diagnosis, although careful measurements are critical because mitral valve-area calculation by Doppler may be inaccurate during pregnancy.[92]

INTERACTION WITH PREGNANCY

Women with severe mitral stenosis often do not tolerate the cardiovascular demands of pregnancy. Mitral stenosis limits the patient's ability to increase cardiac output during pregnancy. The increased heart rate of pregnancy limits the time available for filling of the left ventricle and results in increased left atrial and pulmonary arterial pressures and an increased likelihood of pulmonary edema.[93] Atrial fibrillation is associated with an increased risk of maternal morbidity and mortality in women with mitral stenosis. Both the loss of atrial systole and the increased ventricular rate result in decreased cardiac output and an increased risk of pulmonary edema. Approximately 80% of cases of systemic emboli occur in patients with atrial fibrillation.[93]

Women with mitral stenosis who are asymptomatic before pregnancy usually tolerate pregnancy well. Women with previous pulmonary congestion have an increased incidence of pulmonary edema and a higher risk of mortality during or after pregnancy. The risk of maternal death is greatest during labor and during the postpartum period. The sudden increase in preload immediately after delivery may flood the central circulation and result in the development of severe pulmonary edema. However, hypovolemia and a sudden decrease in venous return, which can occur with hemorrhage or assumption of the supine position, should be avoided.

MEDICAL MANAGEMENT

Beta-adrenergic receptor blockade is useful to prevent tachycardia during pregnancy. Al Kasab et al.[94] found that maternal administration of propranolol or atenolol decreased the incidence of maternal pulmonary edema without adverse effect on the fetus or neonate.

Atrial fibrillation requires aggressive treatment with digoxin and beta-adrenergic receptor blockade. If pharmacologic therapy fails to control the ventricular response, cardioversion should be performed. After cardioversion,

pulmonary edema typically responds well to bed rest in the left lateral decubitus position and to administration of a diuretic.

SURGICAL MANAGEMENT

If significant mitral stenosis is recognized before pregnancy, surgery is recommended. Mitral commissurotomy is preferred. If valve replacement is required, a bioprosthetic valve is preferred.

Some women require mitral valvotomy during pregnancy. This palliative procedure results in a temporary delay in the progression of mitral stenosis, but it may be life saving and may enable a woman to complete her pregnancy successfully. The second trimester most likely is the best time for this palliative procedure. However, severe maternal symptoms may prompt the performance of mitral commissurotomy at any stage of gestation.[95] Mitral balloon valvuloplasty is usually a relatively safe and highly effective intervention for women with a pliable valve and no signs of regurgitation; this procedure circumvents open heart surgery and the risks of anesthesia and surgery for the mother and fetus.[96-100]

OBSTETRIC MANAGEMENT

Pregnancy usually is well tolerated by women with mild mitral stenosis. However, for women with moderate to severe stenosis (valve area <1.5 cm^2), pregnancy worsens the functional NYHA status by an average of 1 or 2 classes.[101-103] Parturients with symptomatic mitral stenosis require invasive hemodynamic monitoring during labor and vaginal or cesarean delivery. Mitral stenosis does not affect management of the first stage of labor except that adequate analgesia is essential. During the second stage, the Valsalva maneuver may result in a sudden, undesirable increase in venous return. Thus it is best to prevent maternal expulsive efforts during the second stage. The obstetrician should allow the force of uterine contractions rather than maternal pushing to facilitate fetal descent to a level where low forceps or vacuum extraction delivery can be accomplished.

Clark et al.[104] used invasive hemodynamic monitoring to study eight pregnant women with severe mitral stenosis. All eight women delivered vaginally. Five of the eight women received furosemide for preload reduction during the intrapartum period. The authors observed no significant hemodynamic changes in the three patients who received epidural anesthesia. Two of the eight patients had clinical evidence of pulmonary edema on admission. No patient developed a new onset of pulmonary edema during the immediate postpartum period. However, the authors observed a mean increase in PCWP of 10 mm Hg in the immediate postpartum period. One patient, who had an uncomplicated labor and delivery, was hospitalized on postpartum day 31 with severe congestive heart failure, and she died 5 days later. The authors made the following recommendations for intrapartum management of patients with severe mitral stenosis:

1. Give supplemental oxygen during labor and delivery, and maintain left uterine displacement.
2. Place a pulmonary artery catheter before induction of labor or during early labor.
3. Restrict fluids and maintain a PCWP of approximately 14 mm Hg.
4. Prevent tachycardia. Treat severe tachycardia with intravenous administration of a beta-adrenergic receptor antagonist.

5. Give epidural anesthesia during active labor, and maintain epidural anesthesia during the immediate postpartum period to reduce preload and prevent postpartum pulmonary edema.

6. Reserve cesarean section for obstetric indications.

We concur with these recommendations, except that intravenous hydration often is necessary during the administration of epidural anesthesia. Moreover, we object to the somewhat arbitrary recommendation that physicians maintain PCWP at 14 mm Hg. Rather, it is more appropriate to determine the best PCWP for an individual patient and maintain it at that level during labor and the puerperium.

ANESTHETIC MANAGEMENT

The goals of anesthetic management are as follows[16,93]:

1. Maintain a slow heart rate.
2. Maintain a sinus rhythm, if present. Aggressively treat acute atrial fibrillation.
3. Avoid aortocaval compression. Maintain venous return and PCWP to maximize LVEDV without causing pulmonary edema.
4. Maintain adequate SVR.
5. Prevent pain, hypoxemia, hypercarbia, and acidosis, which may increase pulmonary vascular resistance.

A slow heart rate allows increased diastolic filling time through the fixed, obstructed mitral valve. It is important to prevent a significant decrease in SVR, given the patient's limited ability to increase cardiac output to maintain perfusion pressure. We give supplemental oxygen to all parturients with mitral stenosis, and we monitor hemoglobin oxygen saturation with a pulse oximeter.

It is important to provide adequate analgesia with the onset of painful contractions. In some cases, we have administered fentanyl intravenously to help control maternal heart rate. Intrathecal administration of an opioid provides excellent analgesia during the first stage of labor without causing sympathetic blockade. An intrathecal opioid and modest doses of a local anesthetic agent may provide satisfactory anesthesia during the second stage. Clark et al.[104] and Hemmings et al.[105] have reported the successful administration of epidural anesthesia in parturients with severe mitral stenosis. Epidural anesthesia is the most reliable method for providing perineal anesthesia during the second stage of labor.

An alternative approach is to use a CSE technique. The anesthesiologist may give an intrathecal dose of opioid, with or without a small dose of a local anesthetic agent, followed by slow epidural administration of a dilute solution of local anesthetic, with or without an opioid (e.g., 0.125% bupivacaine with fentanyl 2 μg/mL). Prior intrathecal administration of an opioid often allows the anesthesiologist to give smaller doses of local anesthetic epidurally. The presence of an epidural catheter facilitates the provision of perineal anesthesia during the second stage of labor. Phenylephrine rather than ephedrine is the preferred vasopressor in patients with mitral stenosis. Small bolus doses of phenylephrine help maintain SVR and do not cause maternal tachycardia.

Epidural anesthesia is preferred for cesarean section. Invasive hemodynamic monitoring, judicious intravenous administration of crystalloid, slow induction of anesthesia, and administration of small bolus doses of phenylephrine help ensure maternal hemodynamic stability.

If general anesthesia is required, caution is indicated when using drugs that can produce tachycardia (e.g., atropine, ketamine, pancuronium, meperidine). A beta-adrenergic receptor antagonist and a modest dose of opioid should be administered before or during the induction of general anesthesia. Esmolol is a good choice in these patients; it has both a rapid onset and a brief duration of action. However, esmolol may cause adverse fetal effects.[106-110] The FHR should be monitored until delivery when possible.

After delivery, the anesthesiologist and obstetrician should be aware that bolus administration of either oxytocin, methylergonovine, or 15-methyl prostaglandin $F_{2-alpha}$ may result in increased pulmonary vascular resistance. Regardless of the method of delivery or anesthetic technique, the patient is at risk for hemodynamic compromise and pulmonary edema during the postpartum period. Cesarean section does not eliminate the hemodynamic stress of the puerperium, except that the greater loss of blood during cesarean section may be beneficial for women with mitral stenosis. These patients require intensive care during the immediate postpartum period.

Mitral Regurgitation

The most common causes of noncongenital mitral regurgitation are myxomatous degeneration, ischemic papillary muscle disease, rheumatic fever, and endocarditis.[111] These processes can cause a variety of anatomic abnormalities that involve the valve annulus, leaflets, and subvalvular apparatus. The result is a backflow of blood into the left atrium during systole.

PATHOPHYSIOLOGY

The variable features that influence atrial and ventricular enlargement include the severity of the systolic regurgitant flow and whether the mitral regurgitation is acute or chronic. **Acute mitral regurgitation** may follow rheumatic fever, bacterial endocarditis, blunt chest trauma, myocardial ischemia, and prosthetic valve dysfunction. Acute mitral regurgitation also may occur in patients with Marfan syndrome and left atrial myxoma. Acute mitral regurgitation imposes a large volume overload on the left atrium. Blood is pumped across the incompetent valve into a noncompliant left atrium. Forward cardiac output decreases, and compensatory peripheral vasoconstriction aggravates the lesion. Pulmonary congestion ensues and results in pulmonary edema. If the patient survives the acute episode, pulmonary arterial pressures continue to increase and right heart failure may develop. In some cases emergency surgery may be necessary.

Common causes of **chronic mitral regurgitation** include rheumatic heart disease, myxomatous degeneration of valve leaflets, Marfan syndrome, hypertrophic cardiomyopathy, and prosthetic valve dysfunction. Chronic mitral regurgitation causes less hemodynamic stress on the left ventricle. The left atrium accommodates the regurgitant blood flow by gradual dilation and increased compliance. Left atrial dilation predisposes to atrial fibrillation. The onset of atrial fibrillation may produce palpitations. However, patients with mitral regurgitation withstand atrial fibrillation better than patients with mitral stenosis because there is no obstruction to diastolic blood flow. Pulmonary hypertension also is less common in those with chronic mitral regurgitation than in patients with mitral stenosis. Typically, there is only a modest increase in left atrial pressure. Severe, long-standing mitral regurgitation results in increased left atrial pressure and pulmonary congestion.

DIAGNOSIS

Patients with acute mitral regurgitation complain of dyspnea. Physical examination reveals a pansystolic murmur, an accentuated pulmonary component of the second heart sound, and in severe cases, an S3. ECG findings include left ventricular hypertrophy and atrial arrhythmias. With severe, acute mitral regurgitation, the pulmonary artery catheter tracing includes a V wave with a wide pulse pressure.

Symptoms of chronic mitral regurgitation include chronic weakness and fatigue secondary to a low cardiac output. The ECG may demonstrate atrial fibrillation. Left ventricular dilation and hypertrophy are more common in those with chronic mitral regurgitation than in patients with acute mitral regurgitation. Prominent atrial waves reflect atrial hypertrophy. Chest radiographs may show a moderately enlarged heart and marked left atrial enlargement.

INTERACTION WITH PREGNANCY

Mitral regurgitation typically is well tolerated during pregnancy. Pregnant women with rheumatic mitral regurgitation typically tolerate the increased blood volume and heart rate of pregnancy, especially if sinus rhythm is maintained. In one series of 28 maternal deaths associated with rheumatic valvular disease, no patient died of complications of mitral regurgitation unless coexisting mitral stenosis was present. Valve repair is usually feasible for nonrheumatic causes of mitral regurgitation, and women with severe regurgitation should have the repair before conception.[112]

There is an increased risk of atrial fibrillation during pregnancy in women with mitral regurgitation. Some physicians recommend prophylactic digoxin therapy to decrease the risk of a rapid ventricular response, if atrial fibrillation should occur.[5]

The hypercoagulability of pregnancy increases the risk of systemic embolization. Systemic embolization may occur in as many as 20% of pregnant women with mitral regurgitation. Anticoagulation may be indicated if (1) cardioversion is planned, (2) there is a history of embolic phenomena, or (3) a new onset of atrial fibrillation occurs.

During labor, SVR is increased by pain, expulsive efforts (e.g., Valsalva maneuver), and aortic compression by the uterus. Increased SVR is poorly tolerated by parturients with regurgitant valvular lesions.

These women are at increased risk for infective endocarditis, and antibiotic prophylaxis is indicated.[113]

ANESTHETIC MANAGEMENT

The goals of anesthetic management for patients with mitral regurgitation are as follows[16]:
1. Prevent an increase in SVR.
2. Maintain a heart rate that is normal or slightly increased.
3. Maintain sinus rhythm, if present. Aggressively treat acute atrial fibrillation.
4. Avoid aortocaval compression and maintain venous return, but prevent an increase in central vascular volume.
5. Avoid myocardial depression during general anesthesia.
6. Prevent pain, hypoxemia, hypercarbia, and acidosis, which may increase pulmonary vascular resistance.

Maternal monitoring during labor should include continuous ECG monitoring. Invasive monitoring is rarely warranted except in cases of severe mitral regurgitation. If pulmonary edema or refractory hypotension develops, the information obtained from a pulmonary artery catheter will help guide treatment.

Continuous epidural anesthesia is preferred for labor and vaginal or cesarean delivery. Epidural anesthesia prevents the increase in SVR that is associated with pain. Epidural anesthesia may result in some decrease in SVR, which promotes the forward flow of blood and helps prevent pulmonary congestion. However, epidural anesthesia also may result in decreased venous return. Careful administration of intravenous crystalloid and left uterine displacement are necessary to maintain venous return and left ventricular filling. In contrast to patients with mitral stenosis, patients with mitral regurgitation may benefit from the chronotropic effect of ephedrine if a vasopressor is required.

If general anesthesia is required, the anesthesiologist should give attention to the maintenance of adequate heart rate and decreased afterload. The increased heart rate associated with ketamine and pancuronium may be desirable in these patients. Myocardial depression should be avoided. Hypoxemia, hypercarbia, acidosis, and hypothermia produce an undesirable increase in pulmonary vascular resistance, and these perturbations should be avoided.

Acute atrial fibrillation must be treated promptly and aggressively. Hemodynamic instability warrants the immediate performance of cardioversion.

Mitral Valve Prolapse

Mitral valve prolapse (MVP) occurs in approximately 2% to 6% of the general population and 12% to 17% of women of childbearing age.[114] Women with MVP generally tolerate pregnancy very well.[115]

PATHOPHYSIOLOGY

Myxomatous degeneration of the mitral valve affects the cusps, chordae tendineae, and annulus and may cause the valve to billow into the left atrium during systole. Involvement of the chordae tendineae can lead to chordal rupture and subsequent mitral regurgitation.

MVP with or without mitral regurgitation can result from papillary muscle ischemia or endocarditis. MVP also is associated with many medical conditions, including von Willebrand disease, Ehlers-Danlos syndrome, kyphoscoliosis, pectus excavatum, osteogenesis imperfecta, myotonic dystrophy, and most notably, Marfan syndrome.

DIAGNOSIS

Most patients with MVP are asymptomatic. However, some women develop palpitations, chest pain, anxiety, fatigue, and lightheadedness.

The auscultatory hallmarks are the midsystolic click and late systolic murmur. The intensity of these auscultatory findings may decrease during pregnancy because of the expansion of the maternal intravascular volume and decreased SVR. These conditions increase ventricular volume, enhance forward blood flow, and lessen the prolapse of the mitral valve.

The diagnosis often is made by echocardiography. The most common echocardiographic finding is abrupt posterior movement of both valve leaflets (or only the posterior leaflet) in midsystole. These patients frequently have exaggerated motion of the anterior leaflet; however, actual prolapse into the left atrium appears to be more common with the posterior leaflet.

The ECG typically is within normal limits in asymptomatic patients. However, nonspecific changes in the inferior and anterolateral leads and a variety of arrhythmias may occur. Paroxysmal supraventricular tachycardia is the most common tachyarrhythmia. Ventricular arrhythmias have been implicated in rare cases of sudden death. There also is a high incidence of MVP among patients with Wolff-Parkinson-White syndrome.

Neurologic complications include acute hemiplegia, transient ischemic attacks, cerebellar infarcts, amaurosis fugax, and retinal arteriolar occlusions. These complications likely result from an embolic etiology. Cardiac arrhythmias may contribute to the likelihood of embolic events.

MEDICAL MANAGEMENT

The prognosis with MVP is dependent on the presence or absence of coexisting cardiovascular disease such as HOCM, Marfan syndrome, ASD, and coronary artery disease. A beta-adrenergic receptor antagonist may be necessary to treat arrhythmias, chest pain, and palpitations. Because progressive mitral regurgitation occurs in approximately 15% of patients with MVP, treatment of left ventricular failure with digoxin and a diuretic may become necessary.

OBSTETRIC MANAGEMENT

Most patients with MVP tolerate pregnancy very well. There appears to be no increased risk of obstetric complications or fetal stress in patients with MVP. The American Heart Association (AHA) recommends that patients with MVP associated with mitral regurgitation receive antibiotic prophylaxis for all genitourinary procedures, especially complicated vaginal delivery.[116] Patients with only a mid-systolic click, no murmur, and no echocardiographic evidence of regurgitation need not receive prophylactic antibiotics. However, an isolated click may be an indication for more thorough evaluation of valve morphology and function, including Doppler-echocardiographic imaging.[116]

ANESTHETIC MANAGEMENT

The severity of coexisting disease often dictates whether invasive hemodynamic monitoring is required. Regional anesthesia is an excellent choice for labor and vaginal or cesarean delivery. The sympathectomy and decreased concentrations of catecholamines are beneficial for these patients. In some circumstances, sedation with small parenteral doses of an opioid or a benzodiazepine may be warranted. Because cardiac arrhythmias occur with increased frequency in patients with MVP, the differential diagnosis of hypotension and neurologic events during regional anesthesia must include cardiac arrhythmias.

When general anesthesia is required, sympathomimetic agents (e.g., ketamine, pancuronium) most likely should be avoided because of the high incidence of arrhythmias. It also seems prudent to avoid agents that sensitize the myocardium to catecholamines. Ephedrine may precipitate or exacerbate tachyarrhythmias. Hypotension can be treated with small bolus doses of a dilute solution of phenylephrine. Management of the rare patient with MVP and evidence of decreased cardiac reserve is similar to that for the patient with mitral regurgitation.

Prior Prosthetic Valve Surgery

The pregnant woman with a prosthetic valve is at high risk for maternal and fetal complications. Maternal complications include thromboembolic phenomena, valve failure, and bacterial endocarditis. Endocarditis is a serious threat to any parturient with a prosthetic heart valve. The AHA has recommended that all patients with prosthetic valves receive antibiotic prophylaxis when undergoing genitourinary procedures.[116]

Complications of maternal anticoagulation therapy include fetal teratogenicity and maternal and fetal hemorrhage.[117] Selecting a prosthetic valve for women of childbearing age is not an easy matter.[112] The advantage of a bioprosthetic valve is that anticoagulation therapy is avoided unless the woman requires therapy for another condition (e.g., atrial fibrillation, thromboembolism).[5] A major disadvantage of porcine tissue valves is their greater likelihood of failure during the course of a lifetime when compared with mechanical valves. Newer-generation mechanical valves have an excellent hemodynamic profile and seldom require replacement[118]; however, anticoagulation therapy is still required.

Pregnant women are hypercoagulable and at increased risk for the development of thromboemboli. Discontinuation of anticoagulation therapy results in a very high risk of thromboembolic complications in pregnant women with mechanical heart valves. Thus it is essential to maintain anticoagulation therapy during pregnancy (Box 40-3). When the risk of valve thrombosis is very high, heparin can be administered intravenously or subcutaneously to achieve an aPTT measurement of 2.5 to 3.0 times control. Some women choose to take warfarin from weeks 13 to 35 to avoid self-administration of heparin. Warfarin (Coumadin) crosses the placenta, is teratogenic, and has other adverse fetal effects (see Chapter 13). The teratogenic effects of warfarin are limited to the first trimester, and warfarin can be used safely during the second and third trimesters. In such cases, the obstetrician or cardiologist typically substitutes subcutaneous heparin for warfarin several weeks before the anticipated date of delivery to avoid the onset of labor during warfarin treatment.[119,120] Heparin does not cross the placenta, and it has no adverse fetal effects. The use of heparin also facilitates the reversal of anticoagulation before delivery.

Low molecular weight heparin (LMWH) does not seem to provide adequate anticoagulation efficacy for women with a mechanical heart valve. The package labeling for enoxaparin specifically warns that it is "not recommended for thromboprophylaxis in pregnant women with prosthetic heart valves"

Box 40-3 GENERAL CONSIDERATIONS IN A PATIENT WITH A PROSTHETIC VALVE

1. Bioprosthetic valves are the valves of choice for women of childbearing age.
2. Anticoagulation should be monitored closely. All pregnant women with a mechanical valve require anticoagulation. The presence of atrial fibrillation or thromboemboli should prompt use of anticoagulation therapy in women with a porcine valve.
3. Warfarin derivatives cross the placenta and have been associated with fetal malformations and hemorrhage.
4. Heparin does not cross the placenta, but it can cause maternal hemorrhage.
5. All women who have undergone valve replacement surgery should receive prophylactic antibiotic therapy during the peripartum period.
6. The obstetrician and anesthesiologist should anticipate some degree of residual myocardial, valvular, and pulmonary dysfunction.

and that "cases of prosthetic heart valve thrombosis have been reported in patients with prosthetic valves who have received enoxaparin for thromboprophylaxis."

OBSTETRIC MANAGEMENT

Cesarean section is reserved for obstetric indications.[117] Some obstetricians may perform elective forceps or vacuum extraction delivery to shorten the duration of the second stage of labor. The cardiologist may recommend maintenance of anticoagulation during labor and delivery, which may predispose to increased hemorrhage during and after delivery.

ANESTHETIC MANAGEMENT

The maintenance of anticoagulation therapy may contraindicate the administration of regional anesthesia. Normal or near-normal coagulation should be documented before administration of epidural or spinal anesthesia to these patients. Also, the chronic use of heparin may result in thrombocytopenia. Systemic opioid administration is an alternative form of analgesia for anticoagulated patients; however the quality of analgesia is not as good as that provided by regional techniques.

If cesarean section is required, the anticoagulated patient will require general anesthesia. Residual valvular and myocardial dysfunction will affect decisions regarding the use of invasive hemodynamic monitoring and the choice of anesthetic agents.

Cardiac Surgery During Pregnancy

Closed mitral valve procedures during pregnancy were reported as early as 1952.[121] The first reported case of cardiopulmonary bypass (CPB) during pregnancy occurred in 1958 and consisted of an aortic valvuloplasty at 4 months of gestation.[122] Although the outcome for the mother was good, the infant died at 4 months of age as a result of multiple congenital anomalies. Published reports have noted a moderate maternal mortality rate of 5% to 6%, which exceeds the rate for similar surgery in nonpregnant patients.[123] The fetal mortality rate remains high (30% to 50%)[123,124]; the reasons are multifactorial. Women who undergo cardiac surgery during pregnancy often have chronic hypoxemia and chronic compromise of uteroplacental perfusion. Additionally, CPB adds additional insults, including nonpulsatile blood flow and hypothermia.

CPB may induce regional alterations in flow to selected vascular beds.[124] Therefore measurement of maternal arterial blood pressure may not reliably reflect uteroplacental perfusion. Relatively high pump flows (e.g., greater than 2 L/min/m^2) should ensure adequate uteroplacental perfusion. Several authors have noted that both the baseline FHR and beat-to-beat FHR variability decrease during CPB.[123-129] In some cases a sinusoidal FHR pattern is noted.[129] These changes occur in addition to the decreased FHR variability that occurs during general anesthesia. An increase in pump flow results in an increased FHR in some but not all cases.[125]

Nonpulsatile flow results in a greater reduction in peripheral muscle blood flow than pulsatile flow, but the implications for uteroplacental perfusion are unclear. One report examined uterine-umbilical artery velocimetry during CPB with nonpulsatile pump flow.[126] Surprisingly, the uterine artery blood flow remained pulsatile during CPB. Nonetheless, it seems logical to use pulsatile flow if it is available.

Systemic hypothermia is used during CPB to help preserve the myocardium and to decrease total-body oxygen demands. It is not clear whether the hypothermia itself is the cause of adverse fetal outcomes. If possible, it seems prudent to maintain normothermia or only moderate hypothermia (e.g., not less than 32° C).

Adequate anticoagulation often is difficult to achieve in pregnant women; this increases the risks of valve thrombosis during pregnancy.[119] In some cases, it may be necessary to perform emergency cesarean section immediately before or during CPB.[130,131] After delivery, the placental implantation site and uterine surface may bleed profusely in the setting of profound anticoagulation during CPB. Lamarra et al.[132] described the adjunctive use of aprotinin, a potent inhibitor of fibrinolysis, to control bleeding after emergency surgery for mitral valve thrombosis immediately after cesarean section. The authors claimed that the use of aprotinin was the single most important factor in affording an uncomplicated outcome.

The second trimester is probably the optimal time for cardiac surgery during pregnancy. Management should focus on the optimization of maternal conditions before, during, and after surgery. Fortunately, women who have had successful repair of cardiac lesions can expect good reproductive outcome in subsequent pregnancies.[133]

PERIPARTUM CARDIOMYOPATHY

Peripartum cardiomyopathy (PPCM) is a rare but devastating form of heart failure, which by definition has its onset during the last month of pregnancy or during the first 5 months postpartum.[134] The incidence is 1 in 3000 to 4000 live births.[135,136] The presentation is often insidious. Initially, the clinical presentation may be limited to symptoms of a mild upper respiratory infection, chest congestion, and fatigue. These symptoms can rapidly progress to florid cardiac failure with biventricular hypokinesis, low cardiac output, elevated filling pressures, and ventricular ectopy.

The etiology of PPCM is unknown. Viral, autoimmune, and toxic factors have been implicated.[137] Some investigators have speculated that nutritional deficiencies, small-vessel coronary artery disease, myocarditis, excessive salt intake, and peripartum fluid shifts may have a role in the etiology.[138-140] PPCM seems to be more common in women with multiple gestation, preeclampsia, obesity, or advanced maternal age, and also in women who breast-feed. It remains unclear whether PPCM represents a unique syndrome or a pregnancy-related exacerbation of some other form of cardiomyopathy.

Diagnosis

The diagnosis of PPCM is one of exclusion. The cardiologist should investigate and exclude the more common causes of cardiomyopathy.

Management

The management of PPCM is largely supportive. Patients who are symptomatic should receive the usual treatment for heart failure and be managed by a multidisciplinary team. If PPCM occurs in the antepartum period, the patient may benefit from prompt vaginal or cesarean delivery.

Early studies suggested that the maternal mortality was as high as 30% to 60%; more recently a 5-year survival of 94% has been quoted.[141] Approximately 50% of women will have complete or near-complete recovery of ventricular function.

The remaining women will undergo progressive clinical deterioration resulting in cardiac transplantation or early death.[142] Women with a history of PPCM and normal ventricular function have a relapse rate of 20% and a mortality rate of 0% to 2% with a subsequent pregnancy. If residual ventricular dysfunction exists before conception, the relapse rate is as high as 50%, with a mortality rate of 8% to 17%.[143]

It is unclear whether recurrent PPCM represents true recurrence of a distinct syndrome or pregnancy-induced exacerbation of ongoing, subclinical ventricular dysfunction. To our knowledge there are no published reports of women with PPCM who received cardiac transplantation and developed recurrent disease in a subsequent pregnancy. However, the numbers of such patients are small; thus the effect of transplantation on the recurrence rate of PPCM is unknown.

Obstetric management involves expedient delivery of the fetus by cesarean or instrumental vaginal delivery. Anticoagulation is indicated, given that PPCM increases the risk of thromboembolic events.[144,145] A small retrospective study suggested that intravenous immune globulin may improve cardiac function.[146]

Anesthetic management for vaginal or cesarean delivery for women with PPCM should reflect principles that are the same as those for any patient with severe cardiomyopathy. General anesthesia may result in profound myocardial depression or cardiac arrest.[147] A combination of remifentanil and propofol has been used for cesarean delivery in a woman with congestive cardiac failure secondary to PPCM.[148] The use of regional anesthesia (i.e., slow induction of epidural anesthesia guided by pulmonary artery pressure measurements) has also been reported.[149]

THE PREGNANT PATIENT WITH A TRANSPLANTED HEART

Current survival rates after cardiac transplantation average approximately 90% at 1 year and 80% at 5 years.[150] A growing number of women have undergone cardiac transplantation for the treatment of end-stage cardiomyopathy and subsequently have undergone successful pregnancy and uncomplicated vaginal or cesarean delivery.[151,152] Morini et al.[153] reviewed the outcome of 23 pregnancies in women with a transplanted heart; they noted that many of these women delivered healthy babies at term, either vaginally or by cesarean section. Successful pregnancies following heart-lung transplantation have also been reported.[154]

The two most common indications for cardiac transplantation in the adult population are viral cardiomyopathy and ischemic cardiomyopathy. Viral cardiomyopathy is by far the most common indication in women of childbearing age.[150] Other conditions such as congenital heart disease and PPCM represent less frequent indications for transplantation.

Pathophysiology

The transplanted heart has no afferent or efferent autonomic or somatic innervation,[155,156] which results in the following consequences. First, the lack of vagal innervation causes the baseline heart rate to be fast (100 to 120 bpm), and reflex slowing of the heart rate (e.g., oculocardiac reflex, carotid massage) does not occur. In addition, the normal heart rate variation with respiration (sinus arrhythmia) is absent. Drugs that act by means of the vagus nerve (e.g., atropine, neostigmine) have no cardiac effects, although these agents stimulate peripheral cholinergic receptors. Second, only direct-acting sympathomimetic agents (e.g., isoproterenol) reliably produce chronotropic or inotropic effects. Third, chronic denervation results in the "up-regulation" of cardiac beta-adrenergic receptors. This results in increased sensitivity to beta-adrenergic receptor stimulation.[157] Camann et al.[158] observed profound tachycardia after epidural administration of 12 mL of 2% lidocaine with 1:200,000 epinephrine in a pregnant patient with a transplanted heart. Fourth, the chronotropic response to stress is delayed. Adequate cardiac output depends on maintenance of adequate preload (the Starling mechanism).

Interaction with Pregnancy

Many women with a renal transplant subsequently have undergone successful pregnancy after renal transplantation. Maternal immunosuppressive therapy does not appear to have an adverse effect on fetal and neonatal outcome.[152] Similar observations have been made in women who became pregnant after cardiac transplantation, but the numbers are small. Patients receiving cyclosporine and prednisone often develop hypertension, which typically requires antihypertensive therapy.[152] The physiologic changes of normal pregnancy (e.g., increased blood volume, increased renal blood flow, altered drug clearance) may require a change in the dose of cyclosporine. Complications related to pregnancy (e.g., preeclampsia, premature rupture of membranes, infection) occur more commonly in women with a transplanted heart.[159]

Anesthetic Management

Preanesthetic assessment should include special attention to exercise tolerance after transplantation and during pregnancy. Recent reports of cardiac catheterization and echocardiography should be sought. Most cardiac transplant recipients undergo routine yearly cardiac catheterization for at least three reasons: (1) coronary atherosclerosis is accelerated in transplanted hearts, (2) complete afferent denervation prevents the occurrence of angina during myocardial ischemia, (3) endomyocardial biopsies may provide early evidence of allograft rejection.

These women will require a "stress" dose of corticosteroid during or after delivery if corticosteroids are part of their immunosuppressive regimen. Regardless of the method of delivery or anesthetic technique, strict antiseptic techniques must be employed in these immunosuppressed patients.

It is essential to avoid aortocaval compression and to maintain adequate intravascular volume and venous return. Some physicians favor the measurement of CVP. However, women with good ventricular function and no evidence of rejection should tolerate volume changes during labor quite well.[150] Infection is a major cause of morbidity in these immunosuppressed patients, and in most cases, the risk of catheter-induced sepsis likely outweighs the benefit of CVP monitoring during labor and vaginal delivery.

Women with a heart transplant have delivered vaginally with[153] and without[160] epidural anesthesia. Slow induction of epidural analgesia with a dilute solution of local anesthetic with opioid may decrease the extent of sympathectomy and the incidence and severity of hypotension. If hypotension should occur, small doses of phenylephrine may be administered safely. Ephedrine has both a direct and indirect mechanism of action, and it may be less effective than expected. If a chronotropic agent is required, isoproterenol (not atropine) should be administered.

Epidural anesthesia is the preferred anesthetic technique for cesarean section. With slow induction of epidural anesthesia, compensatory mechanisms (e.g., vasoconstriction above the level of sympathetic blockade) decrease the likelihood of severe hypotension. Additional crystalloid can be given to maintain adequate intravascular volume and venous return. Spinal anesthesia has been administered successfully for cesarean delivery in women who have undergone heart-lung transplantation.[161] Both spinal and general anesthesia have been used successfully for a wide variety of surgical procedures in nonpregnant patients with a transplanted heart.[150] If general anesthesia is required, it seems reasonable to use ketamine rather than thiopental to preserve sympathetic tone during the induction of anesthesia.

CARDIOPULMONARY RESUSCITATION DURING PREGNANCY

Cardiac arrest during late pregnancy occurs in approximately 1 in 30,000 pregnancies.[162] The incidence is higher among women with cardiovascular disease. The duration of the interval between cardiac arrest and the start of resuscitation and the expertise of the resuscitation team affect the likelihood of survival. The potential etiologies for cardiac arrest in pregnant women include amniotic fluid embolism, pulmonary embolism, arrhythmia, hemorrhage, myocardial infarction, congestive heart failure, and intracranial hemorrhage. Iatrogenic causes include local anesthetic toxicity, high spinal anesthesia, hypermagnesemia, and hypoxemia resulting from failed intubation.

The pregnant woman should be intubated soon after the initiation of cardiopulmonary resuscitation (CPR), not only to facilitate oxygenation and ventilation, but also to protect the airway from the aspiration of gastric contents. If maternal cardiac arrest occurs before 24 weeks' gestation (i.e., before the onset of fetal viability), the rescuers' only concern should be directed toward saving the mother.[162]

Beyond 24 weeks' gestation, the resuscitation team must consider the lives of both the mother and fetus. It is essential that the resuscitation team maintain left uterine displacement during CPR. A folded pillow, wedge, or similar device should be placed beneath the mother's right hip and flank. Alternatively, the uterus can be displaced leftward manually, but this is a less reliable means of avoiding aortocaval compression. Cardiac compressions are most efficiently accomplished with the patient on a hard surface. Rees and Willis[162] described the Cardiff wedge, which provides both relief of aortocaval compression and a firm surface for chest compressions. In the absence of a Cardiff wedge, a hard surface and a "human wedge" may be used.[163] A person designated as a human wedge kneels on the floor, sitting on the heels. This person, who need not be medically trained, subsequently uses one arm to stabilize the patient's shoulders and the other arm to stabilize the pelvis (Figure 40-2).

Optimal care of the mother is the best therapy for the fetus. Regarding the use of vasoactive agents to support or restore the circulation, the AHA[164] has stated the following:

When cardiac arrest occurs in a pregnant woman, standard resuscitative measures and procedures can and should be taken without modification. If ventricular fibrillation (VF) is present, it should be treated with defibrillation according to the VF algorithm. Closed-chest compressions and support-

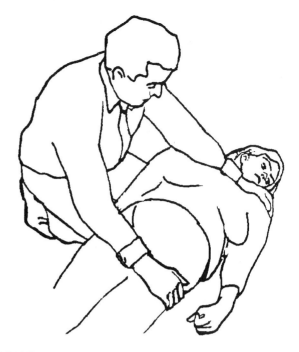

FIGURE 40-2. The human wedge position for cardiopulmonary resuscitation of a pregnant woman.

ive ventilation should be done in accord with usual protocols. To minimize the effects of the gravid uterus on venous return and cardiac output, a wedge, such as a pillow, should be placed under the right abdominal flank and hip to displace the uterus to the left side of the abdomen.... Standard pharmacologic therapy should also be used without modification. Specifically, vasopressors such as epinephrine, norepinephrine, and dopamine should not be withheld when clinically indicated.

If initial efforts to restore oxygenation, ventilation, and circulation are unsuccessful in a pregnant woman beyond 24 weeks' gestation, the physician should consider immediate delivery of the fetus. Immediate delivery may save the life of the fetus and also may facilitate resuscitation of the mother.[164-166] Evacuation of the uterus allows relief of aortocaval compression and restoration of venous return to the heart. Marx[167] reviewed five cases wherein resuscitation was required for more than 10 minutes after unintentional intravenous injection of bupivacaine. The three patients who underwent immediate cesarean section survived with no neurologic deficit, whereas those in whom delivery was delayed suffered irreversible brain damage. Even if the fetus is nonviable, a cesarean delivery may facilitate resuscitation of the mother by (1) relieving aortocaval compression and restoring venous return, (2) decreasing metabolic demands, and (3) allowing more effective chest compressions.[168,169] One report described dramatic improvement in maternal hemodynamics after cesarean delivery in a woman who 12 hours earlier had undergone mitral valve repair.[170]

If delivery does not facilitate successful maternal resuscitation, physicians should consider other measures, including thoracotomy, open-chest cardiac massage, and CPB.[171,172] Maternal complications that can occur when CPR is performed during pregnancy include laceration of the liver, uterine rupture, hemothorax, and hemopericardium.[173]

Early delivery (within 4 to 5 minutes of maternal cardiac arrest) "maximize(s) the chances of both maternal and infant survival."[164] The AHA noted that "while the optimum interval from arrest to delivery is within 5 minutes, there are case reports of intact infant survival after more than 20 minutes of complete maternal arrest."[164]

The infant is likely to be hypoxic and acidotic, and it also may be preterm. Fetal complications include cardiac arrhythmias or asystole from maternal defibrillation and drug therapy, central nervous system (CNS) toxicity from antiarrhythmic drugs, and decreased oxygenation as a result of decreased maternal cardiac output, uteroplacental vasoconstriction, and maternal hypoxemia and acidosis.[174]

There are no specific AHA guidelines for CPR in the immediate postpartum period. Right hip displacement should be maintained because the postpartum uterus may still cause significant aortocaval compression. The patient should lie on a firm surface to facilitate chest compressions. Open-chest cardiac massage is used when standard closed-chest algorithms fail.

Cardiopulmonary bypass (CPB) has been used as part of maternal resuscitation in the following situations:

1. As a method of rewarming patients who have become hypothermic as a result of rapid, massive volume infusion.[175]
2. In the management of bupivacaine-induced cardiac toxicity (CPB provides circulatory support while bupivacaine is slowly dissociated from the myocardial sodium channels).[176]
3. During performance of pulmonary embolectomy in patients with a massive pulmonary embolus.[177]

ARRHYTHMIAS

Arrhythmias occur with increased frequency during pregnancy.[178,179] The majority of these arrhythmias are atrial in origin and have no adverse hemodynamic sequelae. Nonetheless, they may be of great concern to the patient and

her obstetrician. Occasionally arrhythmias may adversely affect maternal and fetal homeostasis. In some cases these arrhythmias represent the first manifestation of underlying organic heart disease. Ideally, the patient's cardiologist will have performed the appropriate assessment and instituted pharmacologic therapy before the patient presents to the labor and delivery unit (Figure 40-3). Unfortunately, some women have hemodynamically significant rhythm disturbances during labor and delivery. Rarely, electrical cardioversion or catheter ablation is required during gestation.[180]

Antiarrhythmic Medications

DIGITALIS

Digoxin is widely used for the treatment of a variety of maternal atrial tachyarrhythmias and has been used extensively in pregnancy for decades. Enhanced renal function during pregnancy facilitates the excretion of digoxin. Nonetheless, transplacental fetal and neonatal digitalis intoxication may occur.[181] The maternal digoxin concentration should be monitored at regular intervals. In the past, some women received digoxin for treatment of a fetal tachyarrhythmia. However, now some maternal-fetal medicine specialists give digoxin directly to the fetus. There are no published reports of fetal malformations associated with maternal use of digoxin.

QUINIDINE

This drug is used to treat a variety of atrial tachyarrhythmias. Quinidine has been used safely during pregnancy for decades, and no evidence suggests that it is teratogenic. This drug has mild oxytocic properties and may be associated with preterm labor.[182] Quinidine has a high affinity for plasma protein, and it may be necessary to adjust the dose during pregnancy.

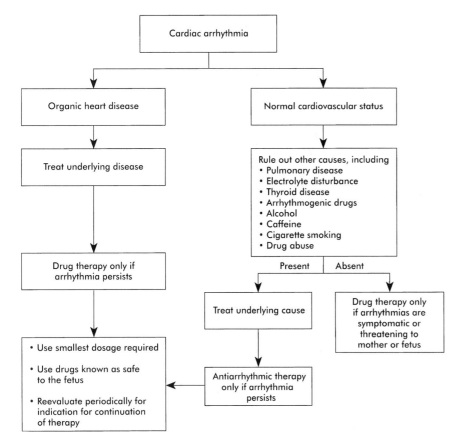

FIGURE 40-3. Management of cardiac arrhythmias during pregnancy. (From Rotmensch HH, Rotmensch S. Elkayam U, et al. Management of cardiac arrhythmias during pregnancy. Drugs 1987; 33:628.)

parallel decrease in TRAb, but the responsible mechanism is unknown.

Surgical therapy (e.g., subtotal thyroidectomy) generally is reserved for pregnant patients for whom medical therapy has failed.[239,240] The pregnant patient should receive preoperative preparation with a glucocorticoid, a beta-adrenergic receptor antagonist, and iodine to minimize the risk of thyroid storm. Clinical data suggest that the treatment of maternal Graves' disease with iodine does not result in fetal hypothyroidism.[296] These data imply that short-term, preoperative maternal treatment with iodine should be safe for the fetus.

There are no published data on the safety of thyroid surgery at various times during pregnancy. It seems prudent to delay surgery during pregnancy until the end of the first trimester, when organogenesis is complete.[240,297] The relative risks and benefits for the mother and fetus should be compared, with an emphasis on the severity of the maternal hyperthyroidism and its resistance to medical therapy.

Thyroid storm occurs in 2% to 4% of pregnant patients with hyperthyroidism.[298,299] Most contemporary cases of thyroid storm during pregnancy occur in patients who have received either incomplete or no treatment of the preexisting hyperthyroidism.[298-306] Precipitating events for thyroid storm during pregnancy include infection, thyroid cancer, normal labor, hemorrhage, cesarean section, and eclampsia.[298-301,305-307]

The treatment of thyroid storm in pregnant patients is identical to that in nonpregnant patients (Box 41-7). The use of beta-adrenergic receptor antagonists during pregnancy may be associated with intrauterine growth restriction (IUGR) or preterm labor,[308] but these medications are commonly prescribed for pregnant patients. **Propranolol** is the most widely used beta-adrenergic receptor antagonist for treatment of thyroid storm. Several case reports have described the use of the beta-adrenergic receptor antagonist **esmolol** for treatment of hyperthyroidism in nonpregnant and pregnant patients.[269-272] However, laboratory and clinical observations suggest that maternal administration of esmolol may result in fetal bradycardia and acidosis.[309-312] I recommend the use of esmolol for the treatment of hyperthyroidism during pregnancy only when propranolol is contraindicated or when the patient's hemodynamic status necessitates the use of a short-acting beta-adrenergic receptor antagonist. For example, hyperthyroid cardiomyopathy during pregnancy or the puerperium may require invasive monitoring and the use of multiple medications that can be titrated to effect.[299,313-315]

In general, maternal and fetal interests are best served by the use of optimal maternal therapy. In some cases, the physician may opt for maternal therapy that, in theory, may have an adverse effect on fetal well-being. In these cases, the physician should document the rationale for the choice of therapy in the medical record.

OBSTETRIC MANAGEMENT

Hyperthyroidism during pregnancy is associated with increased rates of spontaneous abortion (8% to 14%), preterm delivery (9% to 22%), and congenital goiter (3% to 7%).[299,304,316,317] Poorly controlled hyperthyroidism is associated with a higher incidence of preeclampsia.[318] The presence of hyperthyroidism does not affect the obstetric management of these problems. In a retrospective study, Davis et al.[299] suggested that early diagnosis and treatment of hyperthyroidism during pregnancy is associated with better maternal and fetal outcome.

The use of a nonselective beta-adrenergic receptor antagonist may precipitate or aggravate preterm labor. In women with Graves' disease, fetal goiter may develop as a result of the placental transfer of antithyroid medications or thyroid-stimulating antibodies.[319] Fetal goiter can interfere with vaginal delivery, or it may lead to airway obstruction in the neonate. Fetal goiter can be diagnosed by ultrasonography. Fetal hypothyroidism can be diagnosed by percutaneous umbilical cord blood sampling, and it can be treated with intraamniotic injections of thyroxine.[320] In pregnant patients with Graves' disease, maternal serum concentrations of TRAbs during the third trimester may be predictive of neonatal thyroid function.[321]

Normal somatic and intellectual development have been reported in the children of hyperthyroid mothers who were treated with antithyroid medications.[322] Breast-feeding is not contraindicated for mothers receiving antithyroid medications[238] (see Chapter 13).

ANESTHETIC MANAGEMENT

No prospective, randomized studies have evaluated the efficacy or safety of various anesthetic techniques in pregnant or nonpregnant patients with hyperthyroidism. Several features of hyperthyroidism may affect anesthetic management: (1) the hyperdynamic cardiovascular system and the possibility of cardiomyopathy, (2) partial airway obstruction secondary to an enlarged thyroid gland, (3) respiratory muscle weakness, and (4) electrolyte abnormalities.[234,323]

Halpern[324] described two patients with uncontrolled hyperthyroidism who required anesthesia for cesarean section. He suggested that either regional or general anesthesia can be safely administered in hyperthyroid patients. Based on theoretical concerns, he suggested the omission of epinephrine from the epidural solution of local anesthetic agent and the use of an alpha-adrenergic receptor agonist (e.g., phenylephrine) for the treatment of hypotension. However, earlier clinical studies in nonpregnant subjects with spontaneous hyperthyroidism have shown normal hemodynamic responses to exogenous epinephrine, norepinephrine, phenylephrine or clonidine.[325-327] Thus it appears safe to give epinephrine to minimize local anesthetic uptake and toxicity during the administration of epidural anesthesia in euthyroid and hyperthyroid patients.

Hyperthyroid patients should receive glucocorticoid supplementation because they may have a relative deficiency of glucocorticoid reserves.[264,265] It seems prudent to avoid medications associated with tachycardia (e.g., ketamine, atropine).[234,324] Thiopental may be the induction agent of choice because it has an antithyroid effect in male rats that persists for several days.[328] Patients with Graves' disease may have exophthalmos, which necessitates additional care to prevent corneal abrasions during general anesthesia.[324] Clinical data suggest that postoperative hepatic dysfunction is unlikely after halothane or enflurane anesthesia in hyperthyroid patients.[329] Other authors have emphasized the efficacy of deep preoperative sedation in nonpregnant hyperthyroid patients.[234,263] I do not recommend this technique in pregnant patients because of the risks of maternal aspiration and neonatal depression.

Adequate preoperative preparation of the patient minimizes the risk of perioperative thyroid storm. When time permits, the goal of preoperative preparation is to make the patient euthyroid. In an emergency, a hyperthyroid patient can be prepared for surgery with oral propylthiouracil and intravenous glucocorticoid, sodium iodide, and propranolol. The anesthesiologist should be prepared to treat perioperative thyroid storm (Box 41-7).

Hypothyroidism

DEFINITION AND EPIDEMIOLOGY

Hypothyroidism is defined as an abnormal decrease in the serum concentration of unbound or free thyroid hormones. The prevalence of hypothyroidism in the general population is 0.4% to 1.7%, which is similar to that for hyperthyroidism.[227,228,330,331] Hypothyroidism is more common in women and among the elderly. The American College of Physicians has published guidelines suggesting that women older than 50 years of age undergo laboratory screening for unsuspected but symptomatic thyroid disease.[332] The preferred screening test is a sensitive assay for serum TSH.

PATHOPHYSIOLOGY

The etiologies of hypothyroidism can be divided into two categories: primary and secondary (Box 41-8). Primary hypothyroidism is more common than secondary hypothyroidism. The clinical manifestations of hypothyroidism represent the effects of withdrawal of thyroid hormone from its many target organs and tissues.

CLINICAL PRESENTATION AND DIAGNOSIS

The clinical presentation of hypothyroidism is dominated by constitutional signs and symptoms: hoarseness, paresthesias, cold intolerance, delayed relaxation of deep tendon reflexes, slow movements, coarse skin and hair, periorbital puffiness, and bradycardia.[333] During the preanesthetic history and physical examination, the following clues may suggest the diagnosis of hypothyroidism: (1) a history of neck irradiation or radioiodine therapy; (2) the use of lithium, iodine, amiodarone, antithyroid medications, or thyroid replacement medications; and (3) a history of thyroid surgery or the presence of a surgical scar overlying the site of the thyroid gland.

By definition, hypothyroidism is diagnosed by measuring a decreased serum concentration of unbound or free T_4. In the presence of an intact feedback loop, the serum concentration of TSH should be increased in patients with primary hypothyroidism. The serum TSH concentration is a more sensitive indicator of primary hypothyroidism than the serum T_4 concentration. Therefore a serum TSH determination is the best initial laboratory test in a patient with suspected hypothyroidism.[334]

INTERACTION WITH PREGNANCY

The prevalence of hypothyroidism during pregnancy is approximately 0.3%.[335] This estimate is based on laboratory screening of all obstetric patients in a given geographic area. Pregnant women most likely exhibit overt or symptomatic hypothyroidism at a much lower rate. Hypothyroid women have a lower fertility rate than euthyroid women, which reflects neuroendocrine and ovarian dysfunction.[230,336] The immunosuppressive effects of pregnancy may lead to a temporary improvement of Hashimoto's thyroiditis during pregnancy.[240]

MEDICAL MANAGEMENT

Hypothyroidism is treated by replacement therapy with oral thyroid hormones. The medication most commonly used in replacement therapy is **levothyroxine,** which has a half-life of 7 days.[333] Prior studies have shown that the required dose of thyroid hormone replacement often increases during pregnancy in hypothyroid women.[337] Recent data suggest that this phenomenon results from an inhibition of thyroid hormone gastrointestinal uptake by prenatal vitamins and supplements.[338] The effect can be minimized by administering thyroid hormone and the vitamins/supplements at least 4 hours apart. Serial measurements of the serum TSH concentration allow titration of the appropriate dose.

OBSTETRIC MANAGEMENT

Hypothyroidism is associated with an increased incidence of the following obstetric complications: anemia, preeclampsia, IUGR, placental abruption, postpartum hemorrhage, and fetal distress during labor.[339-344] However, several reports have emphasized the successful pregnancy outcomes observed in some hypothyroid patients.[345,346] Early diagnosis and treatment of hypothyroidism appears to be associated with improved maternal and fetal well-being.[339,341] In one series, low birth weight resulted from early delivery for PIH rather than hypothyroidism itself.[341]

In most instances of maternal hypothyroidism, neonatal thyroid function is normal because fetal thyroid development typically is independent of maternal thyroid function. However, the fetus depends on maternal thyroxine until the fetal thyroid system is fully functional at approximately 20 weeks' gestation. Therefore, maternal hypothyroidism in the first half of pregnancy may affect fetal brain development. The appropriate maternal screening procedures and therapeutic interventions currently are controversial, pending additional data.[238,239,347,348] In addition, fetal hypothyroidism

---

Box 41-8 CAUSES OF HYPOTHYROIDISM

PRIMARY

AUTOIMMUNE
- Hashimoto's thyroiditis
- Atropic hypothyroidism

IATROGENIC
- Radioiodine therapy for hyperthyroidism
- Subtotal thyroidectomy

DRUGS
- Iodine deficiency or excess
- Lithium
- Amiodarone
- Antithyroid drugs

CONGENITAL
- Dyshormonogenesis
- Thyroid gland dysgenesis or agenesis

SECONDARY

PITUITARY DYSFUNCTION
- Irradiation
- Surgery
- Neoplasm
- Sheehan's syndrome
- Idiopathic

HYPOTHALAMIC DYSFUNCTION
- Irradiation
- Granulomatous disease
- Neoplasm

From Gavin LA. The diagnostic dilemmas of hyperthyroxinemia and hypothyroxinemia. Adv Intern Med 1988; 33:185-203.

during the second half of pregnancy (i.e., iodine deficiency) may also affect normal maturation of the fetal CNS.[349] With universal newborn screening for hypothyroidism, these neonates should be readily identified. Published data suggest that cognitive development is relatively normal in hypothyroid infants who receive appropriate thyroid hormone replacement, with an initial dose of 10 to 15 µg/kg/day.[350]

A syndrome of proteinuria and hypothyroidism has been described in patients with pregestational type 1 DM.[351] The overall clinical implications of this disease entity are unclear, but untreated hypothyroidism is associated with decreased insulin requirements in these patients.

ANESTHETIC MANAGEMENT

Hypothyroidism has several clinical manifestations that may affect anesthetic management: (1) reversible myocardial dysfunction, (2) coronary artery disease, (3) reversible defects in hypoxic and hypercapnic ventilatory drives, (4) obstructive sleep apnea, (5) paresthesias, (6) prolonged somatosensory evoked potential central conduction time, (7) increased CSF protein concentrations, (8) increased peripheral nociceptive thresholds, (9) hyponatremia, (10) decreased glucocorticoid reserves, (11) anemia, and (12) abnormal coagulation factors and platelets.[334,352-364] Hypothyroid patients may have an abnormal response to peripheral nerve stimulation, which decreases the clinical utility of a nerve stimulator during neuromuscular blockade.[365] Clinical studies of vasopressors in nonpregnant hypothyroid patients show normal responses to exogenous epinephrine and decreased responses to phenylephrine.[366,367]

Whether elective surgery should be delayed to adequately treat hypothyroidism is controversial.[368-375] In my judgment, a number of patient safety issues remain unresolved, which justifies a delay of elective surgery. For emergency procedures, anesthesia care should include glucocorticoid supplementation. Myxedema (hypothyroid) coma most likely is the only clinical setting in which acute intravenous thyroid hormone replacement is indicated. In most hypothyroid patients, acute intravenous replacement therapy entails a significant risk of myocardial ischemia.[354]

No prospective, randomized studies have compared the safety or efficacy of various anesthetic techniques in pregnant or nonpregnant hypothyroid patients. Hypothyroidism is associated with qualitative platelet dysfunction and is a rare cause of acquired von Willebrand disease.[364,376,377] The anesthesiologist should use results from the history, physical examination, and laboratory testing to verify the presence of normal coagulation before regional anesthesia is administered. Epidural hematoma represents a theoretical risk in these patients. To my knowledge, there are no published reports of this complication in this patient population.

PHEOCHROMOCYTOMA

Definition and Epidemiology

Pheochromocytoma is a tumor of chromaffin cells of neurectodermal origin. Ninety percent of these tumors are located in the medulla of one or both adrenal glands. Most of the remaining tumors arise from paraaortic chromaffin cells within the abdominal cavity (e.g., the organ of Zuckerkandl). Rarely, pheochromocytomas have been found in extraabdominal sites.[378] Pheochromocytomas occur bilaterally (e.g., in the medulla of both adrenal glands) in 5% to 10% of cases.[379,380] Approximately 10% of pheochromocytomas are malignant.[378-381]

Approximately 0.04% to 1.0% of hypertensive patients have a pheochromocytoma.[378-380,382] Males and females are affected relatively equally, and the peak incidence varies between the third and seventh decades of life.

Pheochromocytoma is one of the tumors in two of the multiple endocrine neoplasia (MEN) syndromes: **type IIa** or **Sipple syndrome** (e.g., medullary thyroid carcinoma, hyperparathyroidism, pheochromocytoma); and **type IIb** (e.g., medullary thyroid carcinoma, mucocutaneous neuromas, pheochromocytoma).[382] Other disease processes associated with pheochromocytoma include von Recklinghausen disease, von Hippel-Lindau disease, Sturge-Weber syndrome, and tuberous sclerosis.[381] Approximately 10% of pheochromocytomas represent a familial form of the disease, and these tumors are more likely to be bilateral.[382]

Pathophysiology

The pathophysiology of pheochromocytoma is related almost entirely to the systemic effects of its endocrine secretory products. In most cases, these are norepinephrine and epinephrine. However, some pheochromocytomas may secrete other catecholamines (e.g., dopamine, dihydroxyphenylalanine [DOPA]) or peptide hormones (e.g., vasoactive intestinal peptide [VIP], endorphins, calcitonin, adrenocorticotropic hormone [ACTH]).[379,383] In an individual patient, the clinical manifestations of pheochromocytoma represent the net systemic effects of the tumor's secretory products.

Clinical Presentation and Diagnosis

Pheochromocytoma can present with a variety of common or uncommon symptoms.[378-381] Patients typically have **paroxysmal symptoms** because of the episodic nature of hormone secretion by the tumor (Table 41-4). The attacks may remain

TABLE 41-4	SYMPTOMS OF PHEOCHROMOCYTOMA DURING PAROXYSMAL ATTACKS (% OF PATIENTS)		
	Previous series		**Ross and Griffith series**
Symptom	**Mean**	**Range**	
Headache	59.9	43-80	57
Sweating	52.2	37-71	61
Palpitations	49.2	44-71	63
Pallor	42.9	42-44	43
Nausea	34.5	10-42	33
Tremor	33.5	30-38	13
Anxiety	28.9	15-72	30
Abdominal pain	25.8	15-62	14
Chest pain	25.0	19-50	0
Weakness	19.4	8-58	25
Dyspnea	17.0	15-39	23
Weight loss	16.5	14-23	7
Flushing	14.8	10-19	4
Visual disturbances	12.4	11-22	19

From Ross EJ, Griffith DNW. The clinical presentation of phaeochromocytoma. Q J Med 1989; 71:485-96.

the same, or the symptoms may evolve over time.[381] Pallor is common, but flushing is uncommon in patients with pheochromocytoma. Paroxysmal symptoms may be triggered by a wide variety of physical activities that patients learn to avoid.[381] Typically, these activities directly or indirectly increase the pressure around the tumor. One study suggested that the diagnosis of pheochromocytoma can be excluded with 99.9% certainty if a patient does not have attacks of sweating, tachycardia, or headaches.[384] As the tumor grows, the attacks may last longer and may occur more frequently.[381]

Pheochromocytomas have frustrated and confused several generations of physicians because of their ability to mimic other diseases. In one series of patients with pheochromocytoma, 76% of the tumors were not diagnosed before autopsy.[380] Newer technology does not hold the key because recent publications include a number of examples of pheochromocytomas that were initially confused with other medical or psychiatric disorders.[385-388] In addition to their systemic endocrine effects, pheochromocytomas occasionally may cause local abdominal symptoms.[389]

Hypertension is a frequent but not universal finding; it occurs in 77% to 98% of patients with a pheochromocytoma.[381,383] Most patients have paroxysmal episodes of hypertension, but 50% also may have sustained hypertension.[381] **Orthostatic hypotension** occurs in 70% of patients with a pheochromocytoma.[381,383] The presumed mechanisms for orthostatic hypotension include chronic vasoconstriction with intravascular volume depletion and impaired reflex responses secondary to receptor down-regulation or synaptic effects of circulating catecholamines.[381,383] Ambulatory blood pressure monitoring for 24 hours may be useful in documenting paroxysmal hypertension in patients with suspected pheochromocytoma.[379]

The first step in the laboratory diagnosis of pheochromocytoma is to look for increased catecholamine secretion. This is accomplished by measuring concentrations of norepinephrine and epinephrine or their metabolites (metanephrine, normetanephrine, or vanillylmandelic acid) in plasma or urine samples.[379,383,390] Unfortunately, controversy exists regarding the best laboratory test or combination of tests for evaluating a suspected pheochromocytoma.[390-397] A recent retrospective series showed that urinary total metanephrines and plasma total catecholamines were the most sensitive laboratory tests.[398] Spot urine samples are much easier to collect than 24-hour urine samples. When corrected for creatinine, spot urine samples have comparable accuracy in the diagnosis of pheochromocytoma.[399] Another option is to substitute an overnight urine sample for the 24-hour collection.[400] It is best to consult with a clinical pathologist before ordering diagnostic tests for a patient with suspected pheochromocytoma.

For patients in whom the initial laboratory tests are equivocal, several pharmacologic tests can be performed. In patients with a pheochromocytoma, clonidine fails to suppress catecholamine secretion, and glucagon stimulates catecholamine secretion.[383,384,392] The baseline plasma catecholamine concentrations dictate which of these pharmacologic tests should be used.[401,402] A stimulatory test carries some risk of provoking a symptomatic attack and hemodynamic instability.[383]

After the diagnosis is confirmed, the site of the tumor should be identified. Computed tomography (CT) and magnetic resonance imaging (MRI) are the preferred initial studies.[379,383] A nuclear medicine scan with ^{131}I-labeled metaiodobenzylguanidine (MIBG) may be useful in nonpregnant patients.[403] This agent is an analog of guanethidine that is concentrated by adrenergic neurons or tumor cells. Recent retrospective data suggest that MRI and MIBG-scintigraphy are the most sensitive imaging studies for localization of a pheochromocytoma.[398] An additional localization technique involves the analysis of catecholamine concentrations in venous blood samples from the inferior vena cava and adrenal veins.[379,383,404]

Interaction with Pregnancy

Pheochromocytoma is a rare medical problem during pregnancy. The overall incidence of pheochromocytoma in pregnancy is estimated to be less than 0.2 per 10,000 pregnancies.[405,406] Although pregnancy may accelerate the growth of some tumors, there are no data to suggest that this is true for pheochromocytoma.[407] There are approximately 350 reported cases of pheochromocytoma during pregnancy. Both sporadic and familial types of pheochromocytoma may occur during pregnancy.[408-412] Malignant and benign pheochromocytomas have been described during pregnancy.[413-415]

The clinical signs and symptoms of pheochromocytoma are similar in pregnant and nonpregnant patients.[405,416-419] Noninvasive hemodynamic measurements demonstrated intense vasoconstriction and decreased cardiac output during episodes of hypertension in two pregnant patients with pheochromocytoma.[420,421] The clinical recognition of pheochromocytoma during pregnancy is especially difficult because of its rarity and its similarity to preeclampsia, a common obstetric disease.[416,420] The diagnosis of pheochromocytoma before labor and delivery may reduce maternal mortality from 35% to near zero.[405] Easterling et al.[421] demonstrated that either an inverse relationship between blood pressure and heart rate or an increasing hematocrit during treatment with a beta-adrenergic receptor antagonist in a patient with suspected preeclampsia suggests the presence of pheochromocytoma.

Plasma concentrations of epinephrine, norepinephrine, and dopamine in normal pregnant women are not significantly different from those in nonpregnant controls.[422] Treadway et al.[423] noted that the concentration of norepinephrine was decreased and the concentration of normetanephrine was increased in urine from normal pregnant women when compared with nonpregnant controls (although the magnitudes of these differences were not stated). Pregnant and nonpregnant women have similar urine concentrations of metanephrine and vanillylmandelic acid.[423,424] These data suggest that the same cut-off values can be used to interpret most laboratory tests (except urinary norepinephrine and normetanephrine) for the diagnosis of pheochromocytoma in pregnant and nonpregnant patients. During pregnancy, intraabdominal pheochromocytomas can be localized with ultrasound, CT, or MRI.[405,417-419,425,426]

Medical and Surgical Management

The definitive therapy of pheochromocytoma is surgical resection of the tumor.* The greatest challenge in the perioperative management of these patients is to prevent or effectively treat wide swings in hemodynamic measurements. Typically, these patients may experience severe hypertension during the induction of anesthesia and surgical manipulation of the tumor. Severe hypotension frequently occurs after excision of the tumor because of an abrupt decline in circulating concentrations of catecholamines. The perioperative management of a patient with pheochromocytoma can be divided into two phases: preoperative and intraoperative.

---

* References 378,379,382-384,427-429.

PREOPERATIVE PREPARATION

The preoperative preparation of a patient with pheochromocytoma relies on pharmacologic therapy to return the patient to a near-normal physiologic state. Patients with a norepinephrine-dominant pheochromocytoma have intense peripheral vasoconstriction and severe intravascular volume depletion. In these patients, preoperative preparation includes alpha-adrenergic receptor blockade and intravascular volume repletion.[382-384,427-429] The most commonly used alpha-adrenergic receptor antagonist is **phenoxybenzamine.** The initial dose is 10 mg orally twice a day and this dose is titrated upward to 40 to 50 mg twice a day. **Doxazosin, prazosin,** and **phentolamine** are other alpha-adrenergic receptor antagonists that have been used successfully in this setting.[428-430] Beta-adrenergic receptor antagonists may be added to treat arrhythmias, but their use must be preceded by effective alpha-adrenergic receptor blockade to avoid a paradoxical hypertensive response.[378,382-384] Beta-adrenergic receptor blockade must be individualized because patients with pheochromocytoma are at risk for a catecholamine-induced cardiomyopathy.[431-434]

The administration of **nicardipine,** a calcium-entry blocking agent, is an alternative approach in the preoperative preparation of these patients.[429,435] **Metyrosine** is another therapeutic option for preoperative preparation. It interferes with catecholamine synthesis and has been used as an adjunct to preoperative alpha-adrenergic receptor blockade at doses of 250 to 1000 mg orally twice a day.[436] Patients whose symptoms or early responses to alpha-adrenergic receptor blockade are suggestive of an epinephrine-dominant pheochromocytoma may need beta-adrenergic receptor blockade as their primary preoperative therapy.[427]

Alpha-adrenergic receptor blockade with phenoxybenzamine is the most commonly used technique for preoperative preparation of the patient with pheochromocytoma.[437] Administration of a long-acting alpha-adrenergic receptor antagonist (such as phenoxybenzamine) may be desirable before tumor excision, but it may contribute to hypotension after removal.[384] Prospective randomized clinical studies comparing different methods of patient preparation have not been performed. A retrospective review of pheochromocytoma patients preoperatively treated with phenoxybenzamine, prazosin, or doxazosin suggests that each of these agents is effective and safe.[438] Regardless of the method chosen, the patient must be prepared adequately. Careful patient preparation undoubtedly is a major reason for the recent decline in operative mortality in patients with pheochromocytoma.[382,427] Hull[427] stated, "Emergency surgery to remove a phaeochromocytoma from an unprepared patient should never be contemplated." Roizen[439] has established four widely accepted criteria for adequate preoperative alpha-adrenergic receptor blockade in patients with pheochromocytoma[439] (Box 41-9). In his experience, most patients require 10 to 14 days of treatment to meet these criteria.[439]

INTRAOPERATIVE MANAGEMENT

Intraoperative management includes the treatment of episodic **hypertension** and **tachycardia** *before* excision and profound **hypotension** *after* excision. Many medications have been used successfully to manage intraoperative hypertension and tachycardia in these patients, including calcium-entry blocking agents, nitroprusside, nitroglycerin, esmolol, magnesium sulfate, and adenosine.[428,429,435,440-445] Because of the episodic nature of catecholamine secretion and the change in cardiovascular status that occurs after tumor excision, agents

---

Box 41-9 CRITERIA FOR ADEQUATE PREOPERATIVE ALPHA-ADRENERGIC BLOCKADE IN PATIENTS WITH PHEOCHROMOCYTOMA

1. No in-hospital blood pressure reading higher than 165/90 mm Hg should be evident for 48 hours before surgery. We often measure arterial blood pressure every minute for 1 hour in a stressful environment (our PostAnesthesia Care Unit). If no blood pressure reading is greater than 165/90, this criterion is considered satisfied.
2. Orthostatic hypotension should be present, but blood pressure on standing should not be lower than 80/45 mm Hg.
3. The electrocardiogram (ECG) should be free of ST-T changes that are not permanent.
4. No more than one premature ventricular contraction should occur every 5 minutes.

From Roizen MF. Anesthetic implications of concurrent diseases. In Miller RD, editor. Anesthesia, 5th ed. New York. Churchill Livingstone, 2000:903-1015.

---

with a short duration of action may be advantageous.[446] The successful use of various regimens implies that the intraoperative treatment of hypertension and tachycardia depends more on the vigilance and skill of the anesthesiologist than on the specific medication used.

The intraoperative monitoring of a patient with pheochromocytoma should include the standard monitors, an intraarterial catheter, and a Foley catheter. Ongoing assessments of cardiac filling pressures and volumes and cardiac contractility facilitate the successful treatment of catecholamine-induced cardiomyopathy or postexcision hypotension. This information may be acquired with a pulmonary artery catheter or transesophageal echocardiography.[447] Surgery for resection of pheochromocytoma may be by the open or laparoscopic approaches.[448] The perioperative courses are similar for either surgical approach, but the laparoscopic approach results in a shorter postoperative hospital stay.[449] A retrospective review of 143 patients who underwent resection of a pheochromocytoma or paraganglioma at the Mayo Clinic from 1983-1996 showed a 25% incidence of sustained intraoperative hypertension but very few serious perioperative complications.[450]

Hypoglycemia also may be a serious problem after the resection of a pheochromocytoma.[451,452] Insulin secretion is inhibited by alpha-adrenergic receptor stimulation, and removal of the tumor may result in a rebound of insulin release. The blood glucose concentration should be measured frequently after excision of a pheochromocytoma.

Medical therapy of pheochromocytoma is used only as a temporizing measure during pregnancy or in patients with inoperable or metastatic disease. Pheochromocytoma recurs in 6.5% of patients who have had a complete surgical resection.[453] With advanced disease, therapeutic options include chemotherapy, ^{131}I-MIBG, tumor embolization, and palliative external radiation therapy.[382,383,403,415,454] Symptomatic relief can be achieved by means of adrenergic receptor blockade or administration of metyrosine.

MANAGEMENT DURING PREGNANCY

When pheochromocytoma presents during pregnancy, surgical resection of the tumor is the desired therapy.[405,416,420,455] Before 24 weeks' gestation, surgery should proceed as soon as the patient is adequately prepared with adrenergic blockade.[456,457] Anecdotal reports suggest that laparoscopy can be safely used for pheochromocytoma resection during pregnancy.[448] After 24 weeks' gestation, the gravid uterus represents a mechanical obstruction to surgery for most abdominal

pheochromocytomas. These patients should receive adrenergic blockade for the remainder of the pregnancy.[456] The tumor can be removed at the time of cesarean section, once fetal maturation has occurred.[415,416]

Phenoxybenzamine is the most widely used medication for preoperative preparation of the pregnant patient with pheochromocytoma. Although phenoxybenzamine easily crosses the placenta,[458] it does not have long-term adverse fetal effects.* Other alpha-adrenergic receptor antagonists have been used successfully in pregnant patients with pheochromocytoma, including phentolamine, prazosin, and labetalol.† Beta-adrenergic blockade may be added if needed to control tachycardia or arrhythmias or to treat an epinephrine-dominant pheochromocytoma. The following beta-adrenergic receptor antagonists have been used successfully in pregnant patients with a pheochromocytoma: propranolol, atenolol, timolol, metoprolol, and labetalol.‡ Clinical experience with metyrosine during pregnancy is very limited.[405] The current package insert lists metyrosine in "pregnancy category C." The use of metyrosine in pregnant patients with pheochromocytoma should be restricted to those who are resistant to adrenergic blockade, pending additional clinical data on the safety of metyrosine during pregnancy.

The following medications have been successfully used to control intraoperative hypertension and tachycardia in pregnant patients with a pheochromocytoma: phentolamine, nitroprusside, nitroglycerin, magnesium sulfate, trimethaphan, and propranolol.§ Safety of maternal administration of nitroprusside has been questioned on the basis of possible fetal cyanide toxicity.[466] Adverse effects were noted in fetal lambs when high doses of nitroprusside were administered in pregnant ewes who had developed tachyphylaxis.[466] Clinical case reports suggest that a low-dose maternal infusion of nitroprusside (approximately 1 μg/kg/min) should be safe during the peripartum period.[467,468] If maternal tachyphylaxis develops, nitroprusside should be discontinued and a different vasodilator should be used. Nitroprusside decreases uteroplacental vascular resistance in hypertensive sheep, and it antagonizes norepinephrine-induced uterine artery vasoconstriction in humans and guinea pigs.[469-471] These data suggest theoretical advantages for the perioperative use of nitroprusside in pregnant patients with pheochromocytoma. Some reports suggest that esmolol may not be an ideal medication during pregnancy.[309,312]

Early diagnosis and adequate adrenergic blockade are essential to optimize maternal and fetal safety.[405,416,456] I recommend the administration of phenoxybenzamine for preoperative preparation of the pregnant patient. If beta-adrenergic receptor blockade is necessary, I recommend the use of propranolol unless there is a specific contraindication to nonselective beta-adrenergic blockade. During surgery, I recommend the use of short-acting cardiovascular medications with which the anesthesiologist is very familiar. Monitoring and therapy should be directed toward optimization of preload, afterload, and cardiac contractility in the face of rapid changes in circulating concentrations of catecholamines. Attention to detail most likely is more important than the choice of specific medications.

Obstetric Management

Pheochromocytoma during pregnancy is associated with an increased incidence of fetal death and IUGR.[405] The presumed mechanism is decreased uterine blood flow secondary to catecholamines secreted by the tumor because the metabolic activity of the placenta is an effective barrier to the transplacental passage of maternal catecholamines.[472] When pheochromocytoma is diagnosed and effective maternal alpha-adrenergic receptor blockade is instituted before delivery, the fetal death rate declines from 50% to near zero.[456]

Several cases of placental abruption have been reported in patients with pheochromocytoma.[473,474] From a hemodynamic standpoint, this may be analogous to the occurrence of placental abruption in patients with acute cocaine intoxication.[475] The association between pheochromocytoma and preeclampsia is unclear because of the overlap in clinical presentation. For example, proteinuria occasionally occurs in patients with pheochromocytoma.[476]

The preferred method of delivery is cesarean section to minimize the increased pressure on the tumor that can occur during active labor.[405,416,474]

Anesthetic Management

Preoperative preparation and intraoperative monitoring and management were discussed earlier in this chapter. A variety of general anesthetic agents and spinal and epidural anesthesia have been used successfully in nonpregnant patients with pheochromocytoma.[427,429,477-481] A small, prospective randomized comparison of three general anesthetic techniques and one regional anesthetic technique for pheochromocytoma resection in nonpregnant patients did not demonstrate any intraoperative or postoperative differences between groups.[482] Box 41-10 lists perioperative medications that should be avoided to minimize hormone secretion by a pheochromocytoma. There are two published cases of nonpregnant patients with a pheochromocytoma who received an incorrect intraoperative diagnosis of malignant hyperthermia.[484,485]

In pregnant patients with pheochromocytoma, analgesia during labor is not an issue because cesarean section is the preferred method of delivery. Cesarean section, with or without concurrent tumor resection, has been accomplished safely with **general**,* **epidural**,[457,459,461] and **combined epidural-general anesthetic techniques**.[417,419,421] There are no prospective, randomized studies of anesthetic management of pregnant patients with pheochromocytoma. It seems reasonable to avoid the abrupt hemodynamic changes that may occur during spinal anesthesia and to avoid the medications listed in Box 41-10. Either epidural or general anesthesia for cesarean section should be selected based on factors other than the presence or absence of a pheochromocytoma. The care with which anesthesia is administered is more important than the technique that is selected.

Box 41-10 PEROPERATIVE MEDICATIONS TO AVOID IN PATIENTS WITH PHEOCHROMOCYTOMA[161,378,382,427,483]	
Atracurium	Pancuronium
Droperidol	Pentazocine
Halothane	Succinylcholine
Metoclopramide	Tubocurarine
Metocurine	Vancomycin
Morphine	

These medications may increase either directly or indirectly the release of catecholamines by the tumor. Also, halothane potentiates cardiac arrhythmias in the presence of increased plasma concentrations of catecholamines.

---

*References 405,413,416-421,455-463.
†References 405,415-417,455,456,463,464.
‡References 405,413,415,417,419,421,457,459,461-464.
§References 416,418,443,455,457,462,463,465.

*References 418,419,455,460,462,464,465.

- Pregnancy is characterized by a progressive increase in peripheral resistance to insulin.
- Diabetes mellitus is associated with an increased incidence of polyhydramnios, preterm labor, preeclampsia, fetal macrosomia, and cesarean section.
- Insulin requirements decrease during the first stage of labor, increase during the second stage, and decrease again after delivery.
- Fetal structural malformations are the leading cause of perinatal mortality in patients with diabetes mellitus. Strict glycemic control before conception results in a decreased risk of fetal structural malformations in diabetic patients.
- Maternal diabetes mellitus results in an increased risk of neonatal hypoglycemia.
- Adequate maternal glycemic control and aggressive treatment of maternal hypotension with non-dextrose-containing crystalloid and ephedrine are factors associated with normal neonatal acid-base status during the administration of regional anesthesia in patients with diabetes mellitus.
- Normal pregnancy is a euthyroid state because the serum concentrations of unbound or free thyroid hormones are within the normal nonpregnant range.
- Radioactive iodine therapy is contraindicated during pregnancy.
- Thyroid storm is a rare but life-threatening disorder during pregnancy. It is best prevented by the effective treatment of preexisting hyperthyroidism and adequate preparation of the patient before surgery.
- Hypothyroidism is unusual during pregnancy, most likely because hypothyroid patients have decreased fertility.
- The required dose of a thyroid hormone replacement medication increases during pregnancy.
- Neonatal thyroid function is normal in most cases of maternal hypothyroidism.
- Pheochromocytoma during pregnancy is difficult to distinguish clinically from preeclampsia.
- Maternal and fetal safety are enhanced by the early diagnosis of pheochromocytoma and effective adrenergic receptor blockade, pending definitive surgical therapy. Adequate adrenergic receptor blockade is mandatory before the resection of pheochromocytoma.
- Cesarean section is the preferred method of delivery in the patient with pheochromocytoma.
- At the time of pheochromocytoma resection, the anesthesiologist should anticipate the potential for episodic hypertension and tachycardia *during* manipulation of the tumor, followed by severe hypotension *after* tumor resection.
- Hypoglycemia may occur after the excision of a pheochromocytoma.
- The relative merits of general and regional anesthesia have not been studied adequately in pregnant patients with the following endocrine disorders: diabetes mellitus, hyperthyroidism, hypothyroidism, and pheochromocytoma.

REFERENCES

1. Geiss LS, Herman WH, Goldschmid MG, et al. Surveillance for diabetes mellitus: United States, 1980-1989. MMWR CDC Surveill Summ 1993; 42(ss-2):1-20.
2. Rubin RJ, Altman WM, Mendelson DN. Health care expenditures for people with diabetes mellitus, 1992. J Clin Endocrinol Metab 1994; 78:809A-F.
3. American Diabetes Association Expert Committee on the Diagnosis and Classification of Diabetes Mellitus. Report of the Expert Committee on the Diagnosis and Classification of Diabetes Mellitus. Diabetes Care 1997; 20:1183-97.
4. Gerich JE, Charles MA, Grodsky GM. Regulation of pancreatic insulin and glucagon secretion. Ann Rev Physiol 1976; 38:353-88.
5. Steiner DF, James DE. Cellular and molecular biology of the beta cell. Diabetologia 1992; 35(suppl 2):S41-8.
6. Blackshear PJ. Early protein kinase and biosynthetic responses to insulin. Biochem Soc Trans 1992; 20:682-5.
7. Denton RM, Tavare JM, Borthwick A, et al. Insulin-activated protein kinases in fat and other cells. Biochem Soc Trans 1992; 20:659-64.
8. Cohen P. Signal integration at the level of protein kinases, protein phosphatases and their substrates. Trends Biochem Sci 1992; 17:408-13.
9. Kitabachi AE, Murphy MB. Diabetic ketoacidosis and hyperosmolar hyperglycemic nonketotic coma. Med Clin North Am 1988; 72:1545-63.
10. Shafir E, Bergman M, Felig P. The endocrine pancreas: Diabetes mellitus. In Felig P, Baxter JD, Broadus AE, et al, editors. Endocrinology and Metabolism, 2nd ed. New York, McGraw-Hill, 1987:1043-178.
11. Laffel L. Ketone bodies: A review of physiology, pathophysiology and application of monitoring to diabetes. Diabetes Metab Res Rev 1999; 15:412-26.
12. Turpin BP, Duckworth WC, Solomon SS. Simulated hyperglycemic hyperosmolar syndrome: Impaired insulin and epinephrine effects upon lipolysis in the isolated rat fat cell. J Clin Invest 1979; 63:403-9.
13. Zierler, KL, Rabinowitz D. Roles of insulin and growth hormone, based on studies of forearm metabolism in man. Medicine 1963; 42:385-402.
14. Hoeldtke RD, Boden G, Shuman CR, et al. Reduced epinephrine secretion and hypoglycemia unawareness in diabetic autonomic neuropathy. Ann Intern Med 1982; 96:459-62.
15. Popp DA, Tse TF, Shah SD, et al. Oral propranolol and metoprolol both impair glucose recovery from insulin-induced hypoglycemia in insulin-dependent diabetes mellitus. Diabetes Care 1984; 7:243-7.
16. Fisher K, Lees JA, Newman JH. Hypoglycemia in hospitalized patients: Causes and outcomes. N Engl J Med 1986; 315:1245-50.
17. Sheehy TW. Case report: Factitious hypoglycemia in diabetic patients. Am J Med Sci 1992; 304:298-302.
18. Santiago JV. Overview of the complications of diabetes. Clin Chem 1986; 32:B48-53.
19. The Diabetes Control and Complications Trial Research Group. The effect of intensive treatment of diabetes on the development and progression of long-term complications in insulin-dependent diabetes mellitus. N Engl J Med 1993; 329:977-86.
20. King P, Peacock I, Donnelly R. The UK Prospective Diabetes Study (UKPDS): Clinical and therapeutic implications for type 2 diabetes. J Clin Pharmacol 1999; 48:643-8.
21. Rodriques B, McNeill JH. The diabetic heart: Metabolic causes for the development of a cardiomyopathy. Cardiovasc Res 1992; 26:913-22.
22. Coustan DR. Screening and diagnosis of gestational diabetes. Baillieres Clin Obstet Gynaecol 1991; 5:293-313.
23. Cousins L, Baxi L, Chez R, et al. Screening recommendations for gestational diabetes mellitus. Am J Obstet Gynecol 1991; 165:493-6.
24. Jovanovic L, Petitit DJ. Gestational diabetes mellitus. JAMA 2001; 286:2516-8
25. American College of Obstetricians and Gynecologists. Gestational Diabetes. ACOG Practice Bulletin No. 30. September, 2001 (Obstet Gynecol 2001; 98:525-38).

26. Homko CJ, Reece EA. To screen or not to screen for gestational diabetes: The clinical quagmire. Clin Perinatol 2001; 28:407-14.

27. U.S. Preventive Services Task Force. Screening for gestational diabetes mellitus: Recommendations and rationale. Obstet Gynecol 2003; 101:393-4.

28. Magee MS, Walden CE, Benedetti TJ, Knopp RH. Influence of diagnostic criteria on the incidence of gestational diabetes and perinatal morbidity. JAMA 1993; 269:609-15.

29. Kaufmann RC, Schleyhahn FT, Huffman DG, et al. Gestational diabetes diagnostic criteria: Long-term maternal follow-up. Am J Obstet Gynecol 1995; 172:621-5.

30. Ferrara A, Hedderson MM, Queseenberry CP, et al. Prevalence of gestational diabetes mellitus detected by the National Diabetes Data Group or the Carpenter and Coustan plasma glucose thresholds. Diabetes Care 2002; 25:1625-30.

31. O'Kane MJ, Lynch PLM, Moles KW, et al. Determination of a Diabetes Control and Complications Trial: Aligned HbA$_{1C}$ reference range in pregnancy. Clin Chim Acta 2001; 311:157-9.

32. Ciaraldi TP, Kettel M, El-Roeiy A, et al. Mechanisms of cellular insulin resistance in human pregnancy. Am J Obstet Gynecol 1994; 170:635-41.

33. Buchanan TA. Glucose metabolism during pregnancy: Normal physiology and implications for diabetes mellitus. Isr J Med Sci 1991; 27:432-41.

34. Crombach G, Siebolds M, Mies R. Insulin use in pregnancy; clinical pharmacokinetic considerations. Clin Pharmcaokinet 1993; 24:89-100.

35. Boden G. Fuel metabolism in pregnancy and in gestational diabetes mellitus. Obstet Gynecol Clin NA 1996; 23:1-10.

36. Coustan DR, Carpenter MW, O'Sullivan PS, et al. Gestational diabetes: Predictors of subsequent disordered glucose metabolism. Am J Obstet Gynecol 1993; 168:1139-45.

37. Kim C, Newton KM, Knopp RH. Gestational diabetes and the incidence of type 2 diabetes. Diabetes Care 2002; 25:1862-8.

38. Gaudier FL, Hauth JC, Poist M, et al. Recurrence of gestational diabetes mellitus. Obstet Gynecol 1992; 80:755-8.

39. Spong CY, Guitlermo L, Kuboshige J, et al. Recurrence of gestational diabetes mellitus: Identification of risk factors. Am J Perinatol 1998; 15:29-33.

40. Jovanovic-Peterson L, Peterson CM. Pregnancy in the diabetic woman: Guidelines for a successful outcome. Endocrinol Metab Clin North Am 1992; 21:433-56.

41. Hubinot CJ, Balasse H, Dufrane SP, et al. Changes in pancreatic B cell function during late pregnancy, early lactation, and postlactation. Gynecol Obstet Invest 1988; 25:89-95.

42. Sorenson RL, Brelje TC. Adaptation of islets of Langerhans to pregnancy: Beta-cell growth, enhanced insulin secretion and the role of lactogenic hormones. Horm Metab Res 1997; 29:301-7.

43. Picard F, Wanatabe M, Schoonjans K, et al. Progesterone receptor knockout mice have an improved glucose homeostasis secondary to beta-cell proliferation. Proc Natl Acad Sci USA 2002; 99:15644-8.

44. Felig P, Lynch V. Starvation in human pregnancy: Hypoglycemia, hypoinsulinemia, and hyperketonemia. Science 1970; 170:990-2.

45. Hare JW. Insulin management of type I and type II diabetes in pregnancy. Clin Obstet Gynecol 1991; 34:494-504.

46. Maheux PC, Bonin B, Dizazo A, et al. Glucose homeostasis during spontaneous labor in normal human pregnancy. J Clin Endo Metab 1996; 81:209-15.

47. Holst N, Jenssen TG, Burhol PG, et al. Plasma vasoactive intestinal peptide, insulin, gastric inhibitory polypeptide, and blood glucose in late pregnancy and during and after delivery. Am J Obstet Gynecol 1986; 155:126-31.

48. Jovanovic L, Peterson CM. Insulin and glucose requirements during the first stage of labor in insulin-dependent diabetic women. Am J Med 1983; 75:607-12.

49. Caplan RH, Pagliara AS, Beguin EA, et al. Constant intravenous insulin infusion during labor and delivery in diabetes mellitus. Diabetes Care 1982; 5:6-10.

50. Nattrass M, Alberti KGMM, Dennis KJ, et al. A glucose-controlled insulin infusion system for diabetic women during labour. Br Med J 1978; 2:599-601.

51. Davies HA, Clark JDA, Dalton KJ, Edwards OM. Insulin requirements of diabetic women who breast-feed. Br Med J 1989; 298:1357-8.

52. Lev-Ran A. Sharp temporary drop in insulin requirement after cesarean section in diabetic patients. Am J Obstet Gynecol 1974; 120:905-8.

53. Yen SSC, Vela P, Tsai CC. Impairment of growth hormone secretion in response to hypoglycemia during early and late pregnancy. J Clin Endocr 1970; 31:29-32.

54. Singer F, Horlick M, Poretsky L. Recovery of beta-cell function postpartum in a patient with insulin-dependent diabetes mellitus. NY State J Med 1988; 88:496-8.

55. Garner PR, Tsang R. Insulinoma complicating pregnancy presenting with hypoglycemic coma after delivery: A case report and review of the literature. Obstet Gynecol 1989; 73:847-9.

56. Feudtner C, Gabbe SG. Diabetes and pregnancy: Four motifs of modern medical history. Clin Obstet Gynecol 2000; 43:4-16.

57. Cousins L. Pregnancy complications among diabetic women: Review 1965-1985. Obstet Gynecol Surv 1987; 42:140-9.

58. White P. Pregnancy complicating diabetes. Am J Med 1949; 7:609-16.

59. White P. Classification of obstetric diabetes. Am J Obstet Gynecol 1978; 130:228-30.

60. Lufkin EG, Nelson RL, Hill LM, et al. An analysis of diabetic pregnancies at Mayo Clinic, 1950-79. Diabetes Care 1984; 7:539-47.

61. Maislos M, Harman-Bohem I, Weitzman S. Diabetic ketoacidosis, a rare complication of gestational diabetes. Diabetes Care 1992; 15:968-70.

62. Montoro MN, Myers VP, Mestman JH, et al. Outcome of pregnancy in diabetic ketoacidosis. Am J Perinatol 1993; 10: 17-20.

63. Gabbe SG, Mestman JH, Hibbard LT. Maternal mortality in diabetes mellitus: An 18-year survey. Obstet Gynecol 1976; 48:549-51.

64. Rodgers BD, Rodgers DE. Clinical variables associated with diabetic ketoacidosis during pregnancy. J Reprod Med 1991; 36:797-800.

65. Cullen MT, Reece EA, Homko CJ, et al. The changing presentations of diabetic ketoacidosis during pregnancy. Am J Perinatol 1996; 13:449-32.

66. Stamler EF, Cruz ML, Mimouni F, et al. High infectious morbidity in pregnant women with insulin-dependent diabetes: An understated complication. Am J Obstet Gynecol 1990; 163:1217-21.

67. Robertson G, Wheatley T, Robinson RE. Ketoacidosis in pregnancy: An unusual presentation of diabetes mellitus, case reports. Br J Obstet Gynecol 1986; 93:1088-90.

68. Richards SR, Klingelberger CE. Intravenous ritodrine as a possibly provocative predictive test in gestational diabetes: A case report. J Reprod Med 1987; 32:798-800.

69. Bernstein IM, Catalano PM. Ketoacidosis in pregnancy associated with the parenteral administration of terbutaline and betamethasone: A case report. J Reprod Med 1990; 35:818-20.

70. Tibaldi JM, Lorber DL, Nerenberg A. Diabetic ketoacidosis and insulin resistance with subcutaneous terbutaline infusion: A case report. Am J Obstet Gynecol 1990; 163:509-10.

71. Foley MR, Lanon MB, Gabbe SG, et al. Effect of prolonged oral terbutaline therapy on glucose tolerance in pregnancy. Am J Obset Gynecol 1993; 168:100-5.

72. Steel JM, Parboosingh J. Insulin requirements in pregnant diabetics with premature labor controlled by ritodrine. Br Med J 1977; 1:880.

73. LoBue C, Goodlin RC. Treatment of fetal distress during diabetic ketoacidosis. J Reprod Med 1978; 20:101-4.

74. Rhodes RW, Ogburn PL. Treatment of severe diabetic ketoacidosis in the early third trimester in a patient with fetal distress: A case report. J Reprod Med 1984; 29:621-4.

75. Hughes AB. Fetal heart rate changes during diabetic ketosis: Case report. Acta Obstet Gynecol Scand 1987; 66:71-3.

76. Blechner JN, Stenger VG, Prystowsky H. Blood flow to the human uterus during maternal metabolic acidosis. Am J Obstet Gynecol 1975; 121:789-94.

77. Miodovnik M, Lavin JP, Harrington DJ, et al. Effect of maternal ketoacidemia on the pregnant ewe and the fetus. Am J Obstet Gynecol 1982; 144:585-93.

78. Takahashi Y, Kawabata I, Shinohara A, et al. Transient fetal blood flow redistribution induced by maternal diabetic ketoacidosis diagnosed by Doppler ultrasonography. Prenat Diagn 2000; 20:524-5.

79. Raziel A, Schreyer P, Zabow P, et al. Hyperglycemic hyperosmolar syndrome complicating severe pregnancy-induced hypertension: Case report. Br J Obstet Gynaecol 1989; 96:1385-6.

80. ter Braak EWM, Evers IM, Erkelens DW, et al. Maternal hypoglycemia during pregnancy in type 1 diabetes: Maternal and fetal consequences. Diabetes Metab Res Rev 2002; 18:96-105.

81. Lankford HV, Bartholomew SP. Severe hypoglycemia in diabetic pregnancy. VA Med Q 1992; 119:172-4.

82. Kimmerle R, Heinemann L, Delecki A, Berger M. Severe hypoglycemia incidence and predisposing factors in 85 pregnancies of type I diabetic women. Diabetes Care 1992; 15:1034-7.

83. Rosenn BM, Miodovnik M, Holcberg G, et al. Hypoglycemia: The price of intensive insulin therapy for pregnant women with insulin-dependent diabetes mellitus. Obstet Gynecol 1995; 85:417-22.

84. Diabetes Control and Complications Trial Research Group. Epidemiology of severe hypoglycemia in the Diabetes Control and Complications Trial. Am J Med 1991; 90:450-9.

85. Diamond MP, Reece EA, Caprio S, et al. Impairment of counterregulatory hormone responses to hypoglycemia in pregnant women with

insulin-dependent diabetes mellitus. Am J Obstet Gynecol 1992; 166: 70-7.

86. Simonson DC, Tamborlane WV, DeFronzo RA, Sherwin RS. Intensive insulin therapy reduces counter regulatory hormone responses to hypoglycemia in patients with type I diabetes. Ann Int Med 1985; 103:184-90.

87. Amiel SA, Sherwin RS, Simonson DC, Tamborlane WV. Effect of intensive insulin therapy on glycemic thresholds for counter regulatory hormone release. Diabetes 1988; 37:901-7.

88. Reece EA, Hagay Z, Roberts AB, et al. Fetal doppler and behavioral responses during hypoglycemia induced with the insulin clamp technique in pregnant diabetic women. Am J Obstet Gynecol 1995; 172:151-5.

89. Airaksinen KEJ, Anttila LM, Linnaluoto MK, et al. Autonomic influence on pregnancy outcome in IDDM. Diabetes Care 1990; 13:756-61.

90. Peterson CM, Jovanovic-Peterson L, Mills JL, et al. The Diabetes in Early Pregnancy Study: Changes in cholesterol, triglycerides, body weight, and blood pressure. Am J Obstet Gynecol 1992; 166:513-8.

91. Siddiqi T, Rosenn B, Mimouni F, et al. Hypertension during pregnancy in insulin-dependent diabetic women. Obstet Gynecol 1991; 77:514-9.

92. Sibai BM, Caritis S, Hauth J, et al. Risks of preeclampsia and adverse neonatal outcomes among women with pregastational diabetes mellitus. Am J Obstet Gynecol 2000; 182:364-9.

93. Reece EA, Eagan JFX, Coustan DR, et al. Coronary artery disease in diabetic pregnancies. Am J Obstet Gynecol 1986; 154:150-1.

94. Rosenn B, Miodovnik M, Kranias G, et al. Progression of diabetic retinopathy in pregnancy: Association with hypertension in pregnancy. Am J Obstet Gynecol 1992; 166:1214-8.

95. Klein BEK, Moss SE, Klein R. Effect of pregnancy on progression of diabetic retinopathy. Diabetes Care 1990; 13:34-40.

96. Buchbinder A, Miodovnik M, McElvy S, et al. Is insulin lispro associated with the development or progression of diabetic retinopathy during pregnancy? Am J Obstet Gynecol 2000; 183:1162-5.

97. Kitzmiller JL. Insulin lispro and the development of proliferative diabetic retinopathy during pregnancy. Am J Obstet Gynecol 2001; 185:774-5.

98. Reece EA, Winn HN, Hayslett JP, et al. Does pregnancy alter the rate of progression of diabetic nephropathy? Am J Perinatol 1990; 7:193-7.

99. Rossing K, Jacobsen P, Hommel E, et al. Pregnancy and progression of diabetic nephropathy. Diabetologia 2002; 45:36-41.

100. Coleman TL, Randall H, Graves W, et al. Vaginal birth after cesarean among women with gestational diabetes. Am J Obstet Gynecol 2001; 184:1104-7.

101. Roberts AB, Pattison NS. Pregnancy in women with diabetes mellitus, twenty years experience: 1968-1987. NZ Med J 1990; 103:211-3.

102. Goldman M, Kitzmiller JL, Abrams B, et al. Obstetric complications with GDM: Effects of maternal weight. Diabetes 1991; 40(suppl 2): 79-82.

103. Jacobson JD, Cousins L. A population-based study of maternal and perinatal outcome in patients with gestational diabetes. Am J Obstet Gynecol 1989; 161:981-6.

104. Keller JD, Lopez-Zeno JA, Dooley SL, Socol ML. Shoulder dystocia and birth trauma in gestational diabetes: A five-year experience. Am J Obstet Gynecol 1991; 165:928-30.

105. Kjaer K, Hagen C, Sando SH, Eshoj O. Infertility and pregnancy outcome in an unselected group of women with insulin-dependent diabetes mellitus. Am J Obstet Gynecol 1992; 166:1412-8.

106. Greene MF, Hare JW, Krache M, et al. Prematurity among insulin-requiring diabetic gravid women. Am J Obstet Gynecol 1989; 161: 106-11.

107. Peck RW, Price DE, Lang GD, et al. Birth weight of babies born to mothers with type I diabetes: Is it related to blood glucose control in the first trimester? Diabetic Med 1990; 8:258-62.

108. Schaefer-Graf UM, Heuer R, Kilavuz O, et al. Maternal obesity not maternal glucose values correlates best with high rates of fetal macrosomia in pregnancies complicated by gestational diabetes. J Perinat Med 2002; 30:313-21.

109. Hod M, Merlob P, Freidman S, et al. Gestational diabetes mellitus: A survey of perinatal complication in the 1980s. Diabetes 1991; 40(suppl 2): 74-8.

110. Spellacy WN, Miller S, Winegar A, Peterson PQ. Macrosomia: Maternal characteristics and infant complications. Obstet Gynecol 1985; 66: 158-61.

111. Mimouni F, Miodovnik M, Rosenn B, et al. Birth trauma in insulin-dependent diabetic pregnancies. Am J Perinatol 1992; 9:205-8.

112. Johnstone FD, Nasrat AA, Prescott RJ. The effect of established and gestational diabetes on pregnancy outcome. Br J Obstet Gynaecol 1990; 97:1009-15.

113. Pederson J. Weight and length at birth of infants of diabetic mothers. Acta Endocrinol 1954; 16:330-42.

114. Menon RK, Cohen RM, Sperling MA, et al. Transplacental passage of insulin in pregnant women with insulin-dependent diabetes mellitus: Its role in fetal macrosomia. N Engl J Med 1990; 323:309-15.

115. Modanlou HD, Komatsu G, Dorchester W, et al. Large-for-gestational-age neonates: Anthropometric reasons for shoulder dystocia. Obstet Gynecol 1982; 60:417-23.

116. Cousins L. Etiology and prevention of congenital anomalies among infants of overt diabetic women. Clin Obstet Gynecol 1991; 34:481-93.

117. Becerra JE, Khoury MJ, Cordero JF, Erickson JD. Diabetes mellitus during pregnancy and the risks for specific birth defects: A population-based case-control study. Pediatrics 1990; 85:1-9.

118. Tamura RK, Dooley SL. The role of ultrasonography in the management of diabetic pregnancy. Clin Obstet Gynecol 1991; 34:526-34.

119. Sheffield JS, Butler-Koster EL, Casey BM, et al. Maternal diabetes mellitus and infant malformations. Obstet Gynecol 2002; 100:925-30.

120. Reece EA, Homko CJ, Wu Y-K. Multifactorial basis of the syndrome of diabetic embryopathy. Teratology 1996; 54:171-82.

121. Steel JM, Johnstone FD, Hepburn DA, Smith AF. Can prepregnancy care of diabetic women reduce the risk of abnormal babies? Br Med J 1990; 301:1070-4.

122. Kitzmiller JL, Gavin LA, Gin GD, et al. Preconception care of diabetes: Glycemic control prevents congenital anomalies. JAMA 1991; 265:731-6.

123. The Diabetes Control and Complications Trial Research Group. Pregnancy outcomes in the Diabetes Control and Complications Trial. Am J Obstet Gynecol 1996; 174:1343-53.

124. Ray JG, O'Brien TE, Chan WS. Preconception care and the risk of congenital anomalies in the offspring of women with diabetes mellitus: A meta-analysis. QJ Med 2001; 94:435-44.

125. Rosenn B, Miodovnik M, Combs CA, et al. Pre-conception management of insulin-dependent diabetes: Improvement of pregnancy outcome. Obstet Gynecol 1991; 77:846-9.

126. Dicker D, Ben-Rafael Z, Ashkenazi J, Feldberg D. In vitro fertilization and embryo transfer in well-controlled, insulin-dependent diabetics. Fertil Steril 1992; 58:430-2.

127. Landon MB, Gabbe SG. Diabetes mellitus and pregnancy. Obstet Gynecol Clin North Am 1992; 19:633-54.

128. Robert MF, Neff RK, Hubbell JP, et al. Association between maternal diabetes and the respiratory-distress syndrome in the newborn. N Engl J Med 1976; 294:357-60.

129. Mimouni F, Miodovnik M, Whitsett JA, et al. Respiratory distress syndrome in infants of diabetic mothers in the 1980s: No direct adverse effect of maternal diabetes with modern management. Obstet Gynecol 1987; 69:191-5.

130. Piper JM, Langer O. Does maternal diabetes delay fetal pulmonary maturity? Am J Obstet Gynecol 1993; 168:783-6.

131. Piper JM. Lung maturation in pregnancy: If and when to test. Sem Perinatol 2002; 26:206-9.

132. Obenshain SS, Adam PAJ, King KC, et al. Human fetal insulin response to sustained maternal hyperglycemia. N Engl J Med 1970; 283:566-70.

133. Oakley NW, Beard RW, Turner RC. Effect of sustained maternal hyperglycaemia on the fetus in normal and diabetic pregnancies. Br Med J 1972; 1:466-9.

134. Kenepp NB, Shelley WC, Kumar S, et al. Effects on newborn of hydration with glucose in patients undergoing caesarean section with regional anaesthesia. Lancet 1980; 1:645.

135. Hagay Z, Reece EA. Diabetes mellitus in pregnancy and periconceptual genetic counseling. Am J Perinatol 1992; 9:87-93.

136. Hod M, Diamant YZ. The offspring of a diabetic mother: Short and long-range implications. Isr J Med Sci 1992; 28:81-6.

137. Aerts L, Holemans K, Van Assche FA. Maternal diabetes during pregnancy: Consequences for the offspring. Diabetic Metab Rev 1990; 6:147-67.

138. Gauguier D, Bihoreau M-T, Picon L, Ktorza A. Insulin secretion in adult rats after intrauterine exposure to mild hyperglycemia during late gestation. Diabetes 1991; 40(suppl 2):109-14.

139. Greene MF, Benacerraf BR. Prenatal diagnosis in diabetic gravidas: Utility of ultrasound and maternal serum alpha-fetoprotein screening. Obstet Gynecol 1991; 77:520-4.

140. Mazze RS. Measuring and managing hyperglycemia in pregnancy: from glycosuria to continuous blood glucose monitoring. Sem Perinatol 2002; 26:171-80.

141. Zinman B. The physiologic replacement of insulin: an elusive goal. N Engl J Med 1989; 321:363-70.

142. Owens DR, Zinman B, Bolli GB. Insulins today and beyond. Lancet 2001; 358:739-46.

143. Hoffman A, Ziv E. Pharmacokinetic considerations of new insulin formulations and routes of administration. Clin Pharmacokinet 1997; 33:285-301.

144. Lorenz RA. Modern insulin therapy for type I diabetes mellitus. Primary Care 1999; 26:917-29.

145. Bolli GB, DiMarchi, RD, Park GD, et al. Insulin analogues and their potential in the management of diabetes mellitus. Diabetologia 1999; 42:1151-67.

146. Vajo Z, Fawcett J, Duckworth WC. Recombinant DNA technology in the treatment of diabetes: Insulin analogs. Endocrine Reviews 2001; 22:706-17.

147. Gerich JE. Novel insulins: Expanding options in diabetes management. Am J Med 2002; 113:308-16.

148. Levien TL, Baker DE, White JR, et al. Insulin glargine: A new basal insulin. Ann Pharmacother 2002; 36:1019-27.

149. Binder C, Lauritzen T, Faber O, et al. Insulin pharmacokinetics. Diabetes Care 1984; 7:188-89.

150. Chauhan SP, Perry Jr KG. Management of diabetic ketoacidosis in the obstetric patient. Obstet Gyneocl Clin NA 1995; 22:143-55.

151. Prihoda JS, Davis LE. Metabolic emergencies in obstetrics. Obstet Gynecol Clin North Am 1991; 18:301-18.

152. Landon MB, Gabbe SG. Fetal surveillance in the pregnancy complicated by diabetes mellitus. Clin Obstet Gynecol 1991; 34:535-43.

153. Jovanovic-Peterson L, Peterson CM. New strategies for the treatment of gestational diabetes. Isr J Med Sci 1991; 27:510-5.

154. Hare JW. Gestational diabetes mellitus: Levels of glycemia as management goals. Diabetes 1991; 40 (suppl 2):193-6.

155. Coustan DR. Management of gestational diabetes. Clin Obstet Gynecol 1991; 34:558-64.

156. Langer O, Conway DL, Berkus MD, et al. A comparison of glyburide and insulin in women with gestational diabetes mellitus. N Engl J Med 2000; 343:1134-8.

157. Landon MB, Gabbe SG, Sachs L. Management of diabetes mellitus and pregnancy: A survey of obstetricians and maternal-fetal specialists. Obstet Gynecol 1990; 75:635-40.

158. Johnstone FD, Steel JM, Haddad NG, et al. Doppler umbilical artery flow velocity waveforms in diabetic pregnancy. Br J Obstet Gynaecol 1992; 99:135-40.

159. Landon MB, Langer O, Gabbe SG, et al. Fetal surveillance in pregnancies complicated by insulin-dependent diabetes mellitus. Am J Obstet Gynecol 1992; 167:617-21.

160. Rosenn BM. Antenatal fatal testing in pregnancies complicated by gestational diabetes mellitus. Sem Perinatol 2002; 26:210-4.

161. Wissler RN. The patient with endocrine disease. Prob Anesth 1992; 6:61-89.

162. Burgos LG, Ebert TJ, Asiddao C, et al. Increased intraoperative cardiovascular morbidity in diabetics with autonomic neuropathy. Anesthesiology 1989; 70:591-7.

163. Tentolouris N, Katsilambros N, Papazachos G, et al. Corrected QT interval in relation to the severity of diabetic autonomic neuropathy. Eur J Clin Invest 1997; 27:1049-54.

164. Ishihara H, Singh H, Giesecke AH. Relationship between diabetic autonomic neuropathy and gastric contents. Anesth Analg 1994; 78:943-7.

165. Behera D, Das S, Dash RJ, et al. Cough reflex threshold in diabetes mellitus with and without autonomic neuropathy. Respiration 1995; 62;263-8.

166. Ficker JH, Dertinger SH, Siegfried W, et al. Obstructive sleep apnea and diabetes mellitus: The role of cardiovascular autonomic neuropathy. Eur Respir J 1998; 11:14-9.

167. Datta S, Brown WU. Acid-base status in diabetic mothers and their infants following general or spinal anesthesia for cesarean section. Anesthesiology 1977; 47:272-6.

168. Datta S, Brown WU, Ostheimer GW, et al. Epidural anesthesia for cesarean section in diabetic parturients: Maternal and neonatal acid-base status and bupivacaine concentration. Anesth Analg 1981; 60: 574-8.

169. Datta S, Kitzmiller JL, Naulty S, et al. Acid-base status of diabetic mothers and their infants following spinal anesthesia for cesarean section. Anesth Analg 1982; 61:662-5.

170. Ramanathan S, Khoo P, Arismendy J. Perioperative maternal and neonatal acid-base status and glucose metabolism in patients with insulin-dependent diabetes mellitus. Anesth Analg 1991; 73:105-11.

171. Jouppila P, Jouppila R, Barinoff T, Koivula A. Placental blood flow during caesarean section performed under subarachnoid blockade. Br J Anaesth 1984; 56:1379-83.

172. Thalme B, Engstrom L. Acid-base and electrolyte balance in newborn infants of diabetic mothers. Acta Paediatr Scand 1969; 58:133-40.

173. Gabbe SG, Mestman JH, Freeman RK, et al. Management and outcome of class A diabetes mellitus. Am J Obstet Gynecol 1977; 127:465-9.

174. Hirsch IB, McGill JB, Cryer PE, White PF. Perioperative management of surgical patients with diabetes mellitus. Anesthesiology 1991; 74:346-59.

175. Gavin LA. Perioperative management of the diabetic patient. Endocrinol Metab Clin North Am 1992; 21:457-75.

176. McAnulty GR, Robertshaw HJ, Hall GM. Anaesthetic management of patients with diabetes mellitus. Br J Anaesth 2000; 85:80-90.

177. Abboud TK, Artal R, Henriksen EH, et al. Effects of spinal anesthesia on maternal circulating catecholamines. Am J Obstet Gynecol 1982; 142:252-4.

178. Shnider SM, Abbound TK, Artal R, et al. Maternal catecholamines decrease during labor after lumbar epidural anesthesia. Am J Obstet Gynecol 1983; 147:13-5.

179. Crites J, Ramanathan J. Acute hypoglycemia following combined spinal-epidural anesthesia (CSE) in a parturient with diabetes mellitus. Anesthesiology 2000; 93:591-2.

180. Verma SR, Plaat F. CSE in labor and hypoglycemia (letter). Anesthesiology 2001; 94:1150-1.

181. Attallah MM, Daif AA, Saied MMA, Sonbul ZM. Neuromuscular blocking activity of tubocurarine in patients with diabetes mellitus. Br J Anaesth 1992; 68:567-9.

182. Bromage PR. Epidural Analgesia. Philadelphia, WB Saunders, 1978:658-9.

183. Peeyush M, Ravishankar M, Adithan C, Shashindran CH. Altered pharmacokinetics of lignocaine after epidural injection in type II diabetics. Eur J Clin Pharmacol 1992; 43:269-71.

184. Jones HD. Ulnar nerve damage following general anaesthetic: A case possibly related to diabetes mellitus. Anaesthesia 1967; 22:471-5.

185. Navalgund AA, Jahr JS, Gieraerts R, et al. Multiple nerve palsies after anaesthesia and surgery. Anesth Analg 1988; 67:1002-4.

186. Kalichman MW, Calcutt NA. Local anesthetic-induced conduction block and nerve fiber injury in streptozotocin-diabetic rats. Anesthesiology 1992; 77:941-7.

187. Salzarulo HH, Taylor LA. Diabetic "stiff-joint syndrome" as a cause of difficult endotracheal intubation. Anesthesiology 1986; 64:366-8.

188. Hogan K, Rusy D, Springman SR. Difficult laryngoscopy and diabetes mellitus. Anesth Analg 1988; 67:1162-5.

189. Rosenbloom AL. Skeletal and joint manifestations of childhood diabetes. Pediatr Clin North Am 1984; 31:569-89.

190. Nadal JLY, Fernandez BG, Escobar IC, et al. The palm print as a sensitive predictor of difficult laryngoscopy in diabetics. Acta Anaesthesiol Scand 1998; 42:199-203.

191. Meyer RM. Difficult intubation in severe diabetics (letter). Anesth Analg 1989; 69:419.

192. Warner ME, Contreras MG, Warner MA, et al. Diabetes mellitus and difficult laryngoscopy in renal and pancreatic transplant patients. Anesth Analg 1998; 86:516-9.

193. Eastwood DW. Anterior spinal artery syndrome after epidural anesthesia in a pregnant diabetic patient with scleredema. Anesth Analg 1991; 73:90-1.

194. Goucke CR, Graziotti P. Extradural abscess following local anaesthetic and steroid injection for chronic low back pain. Br J Anaesth 1990; 65:427-9.

195. Van Herle AJ, Vassart G, Dumont JE. Control of thyroglobulin synthesis and secretion. N Engl J Med 1979; 301:239-49.

196. Lemansky P, Herzog V. Endocytosis of thyroglobulin is not mediated by mannose-6-phosphate receptors in thyrocytes: Evidence for low-affinity-binding sites operating in the uptake of thyroglobulin. Eur J Biochem 1992; 209:111-9.

197. Chopra IJ. Biologic effects of iodothyronines. Monogr Endocrinol 1981; 18:118-42.

198. Weintraub BD, Wondisford FE, Farr EA, et al. Pre-translational and post-translational regulation of TSH synthesis in normal and neoplastic thyrotrophs. Horm Res 1989; 32:22-4.

199. Taylor T, Wondisford FE, Blaine T, Weintraub BD. The paraventricular nucleus of the hypothalamus has a major role in thyroid hormone feedback regulation of thyrotropin synthesis and secretion. Endocrinology 1990; 126:317-24.

200. Schimmel M, Utiger RD. Thyroid and peripheral production of thyroid hormones: Review of recent findings and their clinical implications. Ann Int Med 1977; 87:760-8.

201. Westgren U, Melander A, Ingemansson S, et al. Secretion of thyroxine, 3,5,3'-triiodothyronine, and 3,3',5'-triiodothyronine in euthyroid man. Acta Endocrinol 1977; 84:281-9.

202. Tegler L, Gillquist J, Lindvall R, Almqvist S. Secretion rates of thyroxine, triiodothyronine, and reverse triiodothyronine in man during surgery. Acta Endocrinol 1982; 101:193-8.

203. Laurberg P. Mechanisms governing the relative proportions of thyroxine and 3,5,3'-triiodothyronine in thyroid secretion. Metabolism 1984; 33:379-92.

204. Glinoer D, DeNayer P, Bourboux P, et al. Regulation of maternal thyroid during pregnancy. J Clin Endocrinol Metab 1990; 71:276-87.

205. Hohtari H, Pakarinen A, Kauppila A. Serum concentrations of thyrotropin, thyroxine, triiodothyronine and thyroxine binding globulin in female endurance runners and joggers. Acta Endocrinol 1987; 114:41-6.

206. Juan-Pereira L, Navarro MA, Roca M, Fuentes-Arderiu X. Within-subject variation of thyroxin and triiodothyronine concentrations in serum. Clin Chem 1991; 37:772-3.

207. Bartalena L, Robbins J. Variations in thyroid hormone transport proteins and their clinical implications. Thyroid 1992; 2:237-45.

208. Davies PH, Franklyn JA. The effects of drugs on tests of thyroid function. Eur J Clin Pharmacol 1991; 40:439-51.

209. Bartalena L. Recent achievements in studies on thyroid hormone-binding proteins. Endocr Rev 1990; 11:47-64.

210. Mendel CM, Cavalieri RR. Transport of thyroid hormone in health and disease: Recent controversy surrounding the free hormone hypothesis. Thyroid Today 1988; 11(3):1-9.

211. Sakurai A, Nakai A, DeGroot LJ. Expression of three forms of thyroid hormone receptor in human tissues. Mol Endocrinol 1989; 3:392-9.

212. Glass CK, Holloway JM. Regulation of gene expression by the thyroid hormone receptor. Biochim Biophys Acta 1990; 1032:157-76.

213. Safran M, Leonard JL. Comparison of the physicochemical properties of type I and type II iodothyronine 5′-deiodinase. J Biol Chem 1991; 266:3233-8.

214. Arthur JR, Nicol F, Beckett GJ. Selenium deficiency, thyroid hormone metabolism, and thyroid hormone deiodinases. Am J Clin Nutr Suppl 1993; 57:236S-9S.

215. DeGroot LJ. Mechanism of thyroid hormone action. Adv Exp Med Biol 1991; 299:1-10.

216. Evans RM. The steroid and thyroid hormone receptor superfamily. Science 1988; 240:889-95.

217. Weiss RE, Refetoff S. Thyroid hormone resistance. Ann Rev Med 1992; 43:363-75.

218. Capen CC. Pathophysiology of chemical injury of the thyroid gland. Toxicol Lett 1992; 64/65:381-8.

219. Krieg AF, Gambino R, Galen RS. Why are clinical laboratory tests performed? When are they valid? JAMA 1975; 233:76-8.

220. Silva de Sa MF, Maranhao TMO, Iasigi N, et al. Measurement of T4, T3 and reverse T3 levels, resin T3 uptake, and free thyroxin index in blood from the intervillous space of the placenta, in maternal peripheral blood, and in the umbilical artery and vein of normal parturients and their conceptuses. Gynecol Obstet Invest 1988; 25:223-9.

221. Yoshikawa N, Nishikawa M, Horimoto M, et al. Thyroid-stimulating activity in sera of normal pregnant women. J Clin Endocrinol Metab 1989; 69:891-5.

222. Yoshimura M, Nishikawa M, Yoshikawa N, et al. Mechanism of thyroid stimulation by human chorionic gonadotropin in sera of normal pregnant women. Acta Endocrinol 1991; 124:173-8.

223. Beckmann MW, Wuerfel W, Austin RJ, et al. Suppression of human chorionic gonadotropin in the human placenta at term by human thyroid-stimulating hormone in vitro. Gynecol Obstet Invest 1992; 34: 164-70.

224. Burrow GN. Thyroid status in normal pregnancy (editorial). J Clin Endocrinol Metab 1990; 71:274-5.

225. Glinoer D. Regulation of thyroid function in pregnancy: Maternal and neonatal repercussions. Adv Exp Med Biol 1991; 299:197-201.

226. Romano R, Jannini EA, Pepe M, et al. The effects of iodoprophylaxis on thyroid size during pregnancy. Am J Obstet Gynecol 1991; 164:482-5.

227. Tunbridge WMG, Evered DC, Hall R, et al. The spectrum of thyroid disease in a community: The Whickham survey. Clin Endocrinol 1977; 7:481-93.

228. Remedios LV, Weber PM, Feldman R, et al. Detecting unsuspected thyroid dysfunction by the free thyroxine index. Arch Int Med 1980; 140:1045-9.

229. Sakiyama R. Common thyroid disorders. Am Fam Physician 1988; 38:227-38.

230. Adlersberg MS, Burrow GN. Focus on primary care: Thyroid function and dysfunction in women. Obstet Gynecol Surv 2002; 57(Suppl):51-7.

231. Weetman AP. Grave's disease. N Engl J Med 2000; 343:1236-48.

232. Klein I, Trzepacz PT, Roberts M, Levey GS. Symptom rating scale for assessing hyperthyroidism. Arch Int Med 1988; 148:387-90.

233. Char DH. The ophthalmopathy of Graves' disease. Med Clin North Am 1991; 75:97-119.

234. Stehling LC. Anesthetic management of the patient with hyperthyroidism. Anesthesiology 1974; 41:585-95.

235. Spaulding SW, Lippes H. Hyperthyroidism: Causes, clinical features, and diagnosis. Med Clin North Am 1985; 69:937-51.

236. Forfar JC, Muir AL, Sawers SA, Toft AD. Abnormal left ventricular function in hyperthyroidism: Evidence for a possible reversible cardiomyopathy. N Engl J Med 1982; 307:1165-70.

237. Fisher JN. Management of thyrotoxicosis. Southern Med J 2002; 95: 493-505.

238. American College of Obstetricians and Gynecologists. Thyroid Disease in Pregnancy. ACOG Practice Bulletin No. 37. August 2002. (Reprinted in Obstet Gynecol 2002; 100:387-96.)

239. Lazarus JH, Kokandi A. Thyroid disease in relation to pregnancy: A decade of change. Clin Endocrinol 2000; 53:265-78.

240. Ecker JL, Musci TJ. Treatment of thyroid disease in pregnancy. Obstet Gynecol Clin N Am 1997; 24:575-89.

241. Kung AWC, Lau KS, Kohn LD. Epitope mapping of TSH receptor-blocking antibodies in Grave's disease that appear during pregnancy. J Clin Endocrinol Metab 2001; 86:3647-53.

242. Kuscu NK, Koyuncu F. Hyperemesis gravidarum: current concepts and management. Postgrad Med J 2002; 78:76-9.

243. Kung AWC, Ma JTC, Wang C, Young RTT. Hyperthyroidism during pregnancy due to coexistence of struma ovarii and Graves' disease. Postgrad Med J 1990; 66:132-3.

244. Kung AWC, Chau MT, Lao TT, et al. The effect of pregnancy on thyroid nodule formation. J Clin Endocrine Metab 2002; 87:1010-4.

245. Vini L, Hyer S, Pratt B, et al. Management of differentiated thyroid cancer diagnosed during pregnancy. Eur J Endocrinol 1999; 140:404-6.

246. Driggers RW, Kopelman JN, Satin AJ. Delaying surgery for thyroid cancer in pregnancy: A case report. J Reprod Med 1998; 43:909-12.

247. Klein I, Becker DV, Levey GS. Treatment of hyperthyroid disease. Ann Int Med 1994; 121:281-8.

248. Kaplan MM, Meier DA, Dworkin HJ. Treatment of hyperthyroidism with radioactive iodine. Endo Metab Clin NA 1998; 27:205-23.

249. Feliciano DV. Everything you wanted to know about Graves' disease. Am J Surg 1992; 164:404-11.

250. Netterville JL, Aly A, Ossoff RH. Evaluation and treatment of complications of thyroid and parathyroid surgery. Otolaryngol Clin North Am 1990; 23:529-52.

251. McArthur JW, Rawson RW, Means JH, Cope O. Thyrotoxic crisis: An analysis of the thirty-six cases seen at the Massachusetts General Hospital during the past twenty-five years. JAMA 1947; 134: 868-74.

252. Waldstein SS, Slodki SJ, Kaganiec GI, Bronsky D. A clinical study of thyroid storm. Ann Int Med 1960; 52:626-42.

253. Mazzaferri EL, Skillman TG. Thyroid storm: A review of 22 episodes with special emphasis on the use of guanethidine. Arch Int Med 1969; 124:684-90.

254. Tietgens ST, Leinung MC. Thyroid storm. Med Clin NA 1995; 79: 169-84.

255. Nicoloff JT. Thyroid storm and myxedema coma. Med Clin North Am 1985; 69:1005-17.

256. Roth RN, McAuliffe MJ. Hyperthyroidism and thyroid storm. Emerg Med Clin N Am 1989; 7:873-83.

257. Brooks MH, Waldstein SS, Bronsky D, Sterling K. Serum triiodothyronine concentration in thyroid storm. J Clin Endocrinol Metab 1975; 40:339-41.

258. Jacobs HS, Eastman CJ, Ekins RP, et al. Total and free triiodothyronine and thyroxine levels in thyroid storm and recurrent hyperthyroidism. Lancet 1973; 2:236-8.

259. Brooks MH, Waldstein SS. Free thyroxine concentrations in thyroid storm. Ann Int Med 1980; 93:694-7.

260. Coulombe P, Dussault JH, Letarte J, Simard SJ. Catecholamine metabolism in thyroid diseases. I. Epinephrine secretion rate in hyperthyroidism and hypothyroidism. J Clin Endocrinol Metab 1976; 42:125-31.

261. Coulombe P, Dussault JH, Walker P. Catecholamine metabolism in thyroid disease. II. Norepinephrine secretion rate in hyperthyroidism and hypothyroidism. J Clin Endocrinol Metab 1977; 44:1185-9.

262. Wilson WR, Theilen EO, Hege JH, Valenca MR. Effects of beta-adrenergic receptor blockade in normal subjects before, during, and after triiodothyronine-induced hypermetabolism. J Clin Invest 1966; 45:1159-69.

263. Knight RT. The use of spinal anesthesia to control sympathetic overactivity in hyperthyroidism. Anesthesiology 1945; 6: 225-30.

264. Levin ME, Daughaday WH. The influence of the thyroid on adrenocortical function. J Clin Endocrinol Metab 1955; 15:1499-511.

265. Mikulaj L, Nemeth S. Contribution to the study of adrenocortical secretory function in thyrotoxicosis. J Clin Endocrinol Metab 1958; 18:539-42.

266. Saunders J, Hall SEH, Crowther A, Soenksen PH. The effect of propranolol on thyroid hormones and oxygen consumption in thyrotoxicosis. Clin Endocrinol 1978; 9:67-72.

267. Heyma P, Larkins RG, Higginbotham L, Ng KW. D-propranolol and L-propranolol both decrease conversion of L-thyroxine to L-triiodothyronine. Br Med J 1980; 281:24-5.

268. Aanderud S, Aarbakke J, Sundsfjord J. Effect of different beta-blocking drugs and adrenaline on the conversion of thyroxine to triiodothyronine in isolated rat hepatocytes. Horm Metab Res 1986; 18:110-3.

269. Thorne AC, Bedford RF. Esmolol for perioperative management of thyrotoxic goiter. Anesthesiology 1989; 71:291-4.

270. Vijayakumar HR, Thomas WO, Ferrara JJ. Perioperative management of severe thyrotoxicosis with esmolol. Anaesthesia 1989; 44:406-8.

271. Isley WL, Dahl S, Gibbs H. Use of esmolol in managing a thyrotoxic patient needing emergency surgery. Am J Med 1990; 89:122-3.

272. Brunette DD, Rothong C. Emergency department management of thyrotoxic crisis with esmolol. Am J Emerg Med 1991; 9:232-4.

273. Ikram H. The nature and prognosis of thyrotoxic heart disease. Q J Med 1985; 54:19-28.

274. Ashikaga H, Abreu R, Schneider RF. Propranolol administration in a patient with thyroid storm. Ann Int Med 2000; 132:681-2.

275. Redahan C, Karski JM. Thyrotoxicosis factitia in a post-aortocoronary bypass patient. Can J Anaesth 1994; 41:969-72.

276. Gronert GA. Malignant hyperthermia. Anesthesiology 1980; 53: 395-423.

277. Stevens JJ. A case of thyrotoxic crisis that mimicked malignant hyperthermia. Anesthesiology 1983; 59:263.

278. Christensen PA, Nissen LR. Treatment of thyroid storm in a child with dantrolene. Br J Anaesth 1987; 59:523.

279. Bennett MH, Wainwright AP. Acute thyroid crisis on induction of anaesthesia. Anaesthesia 1989; 44:28-30.

280. Nishiyama K, Kitahara A, Natsume H, et al. Malignant hyperthermia in a patient with Grave's disease during subtotal thyroidectomy. Endocrine J 2001; 48:227-32.

281. Tajiri J, Katsuya H, Kiyokawa T, et al. Successful treatment of thyrotoxic crisis with plasma exchange. Crit Care Med 1984; 12:536-7.

282. Heimann P. Choice of preoperative treatment in hyperthyroidism. World J Surg 1978; 2:289-92.

283. Hamilton WFD, Forrest AL, Gunn A, et al. Beta-adrenoceptor blockade and anaesthesia for thyroidectomy. Anaesthesia 1984; 39:335-42.

284. Tan TT, Morat P, Ng ML, Khalid BAK. Effects of Lugol's solution on thyroid function in normals and patients with untreated thyrotoxicosis. Clin Endocrinol 1989; 30:645-9.

285. Caswell HT, Marks AD, Channick BJ. Propranolol for the preoperative preparation of patients with thyrotoxicosis. Surg Gynecol Obstet 1978; 146:908-10.

286. Eriksson M, Rubenfeld S, Garber AJ, Kohler PO. Propranolol does not prevent thyroid storm. N Engl J Med 1977; 296:263-4.

287. Jamison MH, Done HJ. Post-operative thyrotoxic crisis in a patient prepared for thyroidectomy with propranolol. Br J Clin Prac 1979; 33:82-3.

288. Strube PJ. Thyroid storm during beta blockade. Anaesthesia 1984; 39:343-6.

289. Peden NR, Gunn A, Browning MCK, et al. Nadolol and potassium iodide in combination in the surgical treatment of thyrotoxicosis. Br J Surg 1982; 69:638-40.

290. Feek CM, Sawers JSA, Irvine WJ, et al. Combination of potassium iodide and propranolol in preparation of patients with Graves' disease for thyroid surgery. N Engl J Med 1980; 302:883-5.

291. Baeza A, Aguayo J, Barria M, Pineda G. Rapid preoperative preparation in hyperthyroidism. Clin Endocrinol 1991; 35:439-42.

292. Kleinmann RE, Vagenakis AG, Braverman LE. The effect of iopanoic acid on the regulation of thyrotropin secretion in euthyroid subjects. J Clin Endocrinol Metab 1980; 51:399-403.

293. Wing DA, Miller LK, Koonings PP, et al. A comparison of propylthiouracil versus methimazole in the treatment of hyperthyroidism in pregnancy. Am J Obstet Gynecol 1994; 170:90-5.

294. Diav-Citrin O, Ornoy A. Teratogen update: Antithyroid drugs-methimazole, carbimazole, and propylthiouracil. Teratology 2002; 65:38-44.

295. Hashizume K, Ichikawa K, Nishii Y, et al. Effect of administration of thyroxine on the risk of postpartum recurrence of hyperthyroid Graves' disease. J Clin Endocrinol Metab 1992; 75:6-10.

296. Momotani N, Hisaoka T, Noh J, et al. Effects of iodine on thyroid status of fetus versus mother in treatment of Graves' disease complicated by pregnancy. J Clin Endocrinol Metab 1992; 75:738-44.

297. Steinberg ES, Santos AC. Surgical anesthesia during pregnancy. Int Anesth Clin 1990; 28:58-66.

298. Hawe P, Francis HH. Pregnancy and thyrotoxicosis. Br Med J 1962; 2:817-22.

299. Davis LE, Lucas MJ, Hankins GDV, et al. Thyrotoxicosis complicating pregnancy. Am J Obstet Gynecol 1989; 160:63-70.

300. Kamm ML, Weaver JC, Page EP, Chappell CC. Acute thyroid storm precipitated by labor: Report of a case. Obstet Gynecol 1963; 21:460-3.

301. Guenter KE, Friedland GA. Thyroid storm and placenta previa in a primigravida. Obstet Gynecol 1965; 26:403-7.

302. Horrocks P, Leonard JC. Thyrotoxic crisis and transient myasthenia gravis in pregnancy. Postgrad Med J 1966; 42:46-9.

303. Langer A, Hung CT, McAnulty JA, et al. Adrenergic blockade: A new approach to hyperthyroidism during pregnancy. Obstet Gynecol 1974; 44:181-6.

304. Pekonen F, Lamberg BA, Ikonen E. Thyrotoxicosis and pregnancy: An analysis of 43 pregnancies in 42 thyrotoxic mothers. Ann Chir Gynaecol 1978; 67:1-7.

305. Menon V, McDougall WW, Leatherdale BA. Thyrotoxic crisis following eclampsia and induction of labour. Postgrad Med J 1982; 58:286-7.

306. Pugh S, Lalwani K, Awal A. Thyroid storm as a cause of loss of consciousness following anaesthesia for emergency caesarean section. Anaesthesia 1994; 49:35-7.

307. Tewari K, Balderston KD, Carpenter SE, et al. Papillary thyroid carcinoma manifesting as thyroid storm of pregnancy: case report. Am J Obstet Gynecol 1998; 179:818-9.

308. Frishman WH, Chesner M. Beta-adrenergic blockers in pregnancy. Am Heart J 1988; 115:147-52.

309. Eisenach JC, Castro MI. Maternally administered esmolol produces fetal beta-adrenergic blockade and hypoxemia in sheep. Anesthesiology 1989; 71:718-22.

310. Losasso TJ, Muzzi DA, Cucchiara RF. Response of fetal heart rate to maternal administration of esmolol. Anesthesiology 1991; 74:782-4.

311. Gilson GJ, Knieriem KJ, Smith JF, et al. Short-acting beta-adrenergic blockade and the fetus: A case report. J Reprod Med 1992; 37:277-9.

312. Ducey JP, Knape KG. Maternal esmolol administration resulting in fetal distress and cesarean section in a term pregnancy. Anesthesiology 1992; 77:829-32.

313. Hankins GDV, Lowe TW, Cunningham FG. Dilated cardiomyopathy and thyrotoxicosis complicated by septic abortion. Am J Obstet Gynecol 1984; 149:85-6.

314. Clark SL, Phelan JP, Montoro M, Mestman J. Transient ventricular dysfunction associated with cesarean section in a patient with hyperthyroidism. Am J Obstet Gynecol 1985; 151:384-6.

315. Valko PC, McCarty DL. Peripartum cardiac failure in a woman with Graves' disease. Am J Emerg Med 1992; 10:46-9.

316. Ayromlooi J, Zervoudakis IA, Sadaghat A. Thyrotoxicosis in pregnancy. Am J Obstet Gynecol 1973; 117:818-23.

317. Sugrue D, Drury MI. Hyperthyroidism complicating pregnancy: Results of treatment by antithyroid drugs in 77 pregnancies. Br J Obstet Gynaecol 1980; 87:970-5.

318. Millar LK, Wing DA, Leung AS, et al. Low birth weight and preeclampsia in pregnancies complicated by hyperthyroidism. Obstet Gynecol 1994; 84:946-9.

319. Anonymous. Thyroid dysfunction in utero (editorial). Lancet 1992; 339:155.

320. Davidson KM, Richards DS, Schatz DA, Fisher DA. Successful in utero treatment of fetal goiter and hypothyroidism. N Engl J Med 1991; 324:543-6.

321. Mortimer RH, Tyack SA, Galligan JP, et al. Graves' disease in pregnancy: TSH receptor binding inhibiting immunoglobulins and maternal and neonatal thyroid function. Clin Endocrinol 1990; 32:141-52.

322. Messer PM, Hauffa BP, Olbricht T, et al. Antithyroid drug treatment of Graves' disease in pregnancy: Long-term effects on somatic growth, intellectual development and thyroid function of the offspring. Acta Endocrinol 1990; 123:311-6.

323. Nandwani N, Tidmarsh M, May AE. Retrosternal goiter: A cause of dyspnoea in pregnancy. Int J Obstet Anesth 1998; 7:46-9.

324. Halpern SH. Anaesthesia for caesarean section in patients with uncontrolled hyperthyroidism. Can J Anaesth 1989; 36:454-9.

325. Aoki VS, Wilson WR, Theilen EO. Studies on the reputed augmentation of the cardiovascular effects of catecholamines in patients with spontaneous hyperthyroidism. J Pharmacol Exp Therapent 1972; 181: 362-8.

326. Theilen EO, Wilson WR. Hemodynamic effects of peripheral vasoconstriction in normal and thyrotoxic subjects. J Appl Physiol 1967; 22:207-210.

327. Del Rio G, Zizzo G, Marrama P, et al. Alpha-2 adrenergic activity is normal in patients with thyroid disease. Clin Endocrinol (Oxf). 1994; 40:235-9.

328. Wase AW, Foster WC. Thiopental and thyroid metabolism. Proc Soc Exp Biol Med 1956; 91:89-91.

329. Seino H, Dohi S, Aiyoshi Y, et al. Postoperative hepatic dysfunction after halothane or enflurane anesthesia in patients with hyperthyroidism. Anesthesiology 1986; 64:122-5.

330. Riniker M, Tieche M, Lupi GA, et al. Prevalence of various degrees of hypothyroidism among patients of a general medical department. Clin Endocrinol 1981; 14:69-74.

331. Sawin CT, Castelli WP, Hershman JM, et al. The aging thyroid: Thyroid deficiency in the Framingham study. Arch Intern Med 1985; 145:1386-8.

332. American College of Physicians. Screening for thyroid disease. Ann Int Med 1998; 129:141-3.

333. Utiger RD. The thyroid: Physiology, hyperthyroidism, hypothyroidism, and the painful thyroid. In Felig P, Baxter JD, Broadus AE, editors. Endocrinology and Metabolism, 2nd ed. New York, McGraw-Hill, 1987:389-472.

334. Nordyke RA, Gilbert FI. Management of primary hypothyroidism. Comp Ther 1990; 16:28-32.

335. Klein RZ, Haddow JE, Faix JD, et al. Prevalence of thyroid deficiency in pregnant women. Clin Endocrinol 1991; 35:41-6.

336. Maruo T, Katayama K, Barnea ER, Mochizuki M. A role for thyroid hormone in the induction of ovulation and corpus luteum function. Horm Res 1992; 37(suppl 1):12-8.

337. Mandel SJ, Larsen PR, Seely EW, Brent GA. Increased need for thyroxine during pregnancy in women with primary hypothyroidism. N Engl J Med 1990; 323:91-6.

338. Chopra IJ, Baber K. Treatment of primary hypothyroidism during pregnancy: Is there an increase in thyroxine dose requirement in pregnancy? Metabolism 2003; 52:122-8.

339. Davis LE, Leveno KJ, Cunningham FG. Hypothyroidism complicating pregnancy. Obstet Gynecol 1988; 72:108-12.

340. Buckshee K, Kriplani A, Kapil A, et al. Hypothyroidism complicating pregnancy. Aust NZ J Obstet Gynaecol 1992; 32:240-2.

341. Leung, AS, Millar LK, Koonings PP, et al. Perinatal outcome in hypothyroid pregnancies. Obstet Gynecol 1993; 81:349-53.

342. Mizgala L, Lao TT, Hannah ME. Hypothyroidism presenting as hypothermia following pre-eclampsia at 23 weeks gestation: Case report and review of the literature. Br J Obstet Gynaecol 1991; 98:221-4.

343. Patel S, Robinson S, Bidgood RJ, Edmonds CJ. A pre-eclamptic-like syndrome associated with hypothyroidism during pregnancy. Q J Med 1991; 79:435-41.

344. Wasserstrum N, Anania CA. Perinatal consequences of maternal hypothyroidism in early pregnancy and inadequate replacement. Clin Endocrinal 1995; 42:353-8.

345. Montoro M, Collea JV, Frasier SD, Mestman JH. Successful outcome of pregnancy in women with hypothyroidism. Ann Int Med 1981; 94:31-4.

346. Balen AH, Kurtz AB. Successful outcome of pregnancy with severe hypothyroidism: Case report and literature review. Br J Obstet Gynaecol 1990; 97:536-9.

347. American College of Obstetricians and Gynecologists. Screening for hypothyroidism. Committee on Obstetric Practice, Committee Opinion No. 241. September 2000 (Int J Gynaecol Obstet 2001; 75:342-3).

348. Smallridge RC, Ladenson PW. Hypothyroidism in pregnancy: consequences to neonatal health. J Clin Endocrinol Metab 2001; 86: 2349-53.

349. Thilly CH, Delange F, Lagasse R, et al. Fetal hypothyroidism and maternal thyroid status in severe endemic goiter. J Clin Endocrinol Metab 1978; 47:354-60.

350. Fisher DA, Foley BL. Early treatment of congenital hypothyroidism. Pediatrics 1989; 83:785-9.

351. Jovanovic-Peterson L, Peterson CM. De novo clinical hypothyroidism in pregnancies complicated by type I diabetes, subclinical hypothyroidism, and proteinuria: A new syndrome. Am J Obstet Gynecol 1988; 159:442-6.

352. Bough EW, Crowley WF, Ridgway EC, et al. Myocardial function in hypothyroidism: Relation to disease severity and response to treatment. Arch Intern Med 1978; 138:1476-80.

353. Becker C. Hypothyroidism and atherosclerotic heart disease: Pathogenesis, medical management, and the role of coronary artery bypass surgery. Endocr Rev 1985; 6:432-40.

354. Ellyin FM, Kumar Y, Somberg JC. Hypothyroidism complicated by angina pectoris: Therapeutic approaches. J Clin Pharmacol 1992; 32:843-7.

355. Zwillich CW, Pierson DJ, Hofeldt FD, et al. Ventilatory control in myxedema and hypothyroidism. N Engl J Med 1975; 292:662-5.

356. Duranti R, Gheri RG, Gorini M, et al. Control of breathing in patients with severe hypothyroidism. Am J Med 1993; 95: 29-37.

357. Rajagopal KR, Abbrecht PH, Derderian SS, et al. Obstructive sleep apnea in hypothyroidism. Ann Intern Med 1984; 101:491-4.

358. Ozkardes A, Ozata M, Beyhan Z, et al. Acute hypothyroidism leads to reversible alterations in central nervous system as revealed by somatosensory evoked potentials. Electroenceph Clin Neurophysiol 1996; 100:500-4.

359. Nystroem E, Hamberger A, Lindstedt G, et al. Cerebrospinal fluid proteins in subclinical and overt hypothyroidism. Acta Neurol Scand 1997; 95:311-4.

360. Guieu R, Harley JR, Blin O, et al. Nociceptive threshold in hypothyroid patients. Acta Neurol 1993; 15:183-8.

361. Skowsky WR, Kikuchi TA. The role of vasopressin in the impaired water excretion of myxedema. Am J Med 1978; 64:613-21.

362. Ridgway EC, McCammon JA, Benotti J, et al. Acute metabolic responses in myxedema to large doses of intravenous L-thyroxine. Ann Intern Med 1972; 77:549-55.

363. Tudhope GR, Wilson GM. Anaemia in hypothyroidism: Incidence, pathogenesis, and response to treatment. Q J Med 1960; 29:513-37.

364. Hofbauer LC, Heufelder AE. Coagulation disorders in thyroid diseases. Eur J Endocrinol 1997; 136:1-7.

365. Miller LR, Benumof JL, Alexander L, et al. Completely absent response to peripheral nerve stimulation in an acutely hypothyroid patient. Anesthesiology 1989; 71:779-81.

366. Johnson AB, Webber J, Mansell P, et al. Cardiovascular and metabolic responses to adrenaline infusion in patients with short-term hypothyroidism. Clin Endocrinol 1995; 43:747-51.

367. Polikar R, Kennedy B, Ziegler M, et al. Decreased sensitivity to alpha-adrenergic stimulation in hypothyroid patients. J Clin Endocrinol Metab 1990; 70:1761-4.

368. Hay ID, Duick DS, Vlietstra RE, et al. Thyroxine therapy in hypothyroid patients undergoing coronary revascularization: A retrospective analysis. Ann Intern Med 1981; 95:456-7.

369. Finlayson DC, Kaplan JA. Myxoedema and open heart surgery: Anaesthesia and intensive care unit experience. Can Anaesth Soc J 1982; 29:543-9.

370. Weinberg AD, Brennan MD, Gorman CA, et al. Outcome of anesthesia and surgery in hypothyroid patients. Arch Intern Med 1983; 143:893-7.

371. Ladenson PW, Levin AA, Ridgway EC, et al. Complications of surgery in hypothyroid patients. Am J Med 1984; 77:261-6.

372. Litt L, Roizen MF. Anesthetic and surgical risk in hypothyroidism. Arch Intern Med 1984; 144:657-8.

373. Sherry KM, Hutchinson IL. Postoperative myxoedema: A report of coma and upper airway obstruction. Anaesthesia 1984; 39:1112-4.

374. Levelle JP, Jopling MW, Sklar GS. Perioperative hypothyroidism: An unusual postanesthetic diagnosis. Anesthesiology 1985; 63:195-7.

375. Bennett-Guerrero E, Kramer DC, Schwinn DA. Effect of chronic and acute thyroid hormone reduction on perioperative outcome. Anesth Analg 1997; 85:30-6.

376. Myrup B, Bregengard C, Faber J. Primary haemostasis in thyroid disease. J Int Med 1995; 238:59-63.

377. Aylesworth CA, Smallridge RC, Rick ME, et al. Acquired von Willebrand's Disease: A rare manifestation of postpartum thyroiditis. Am J Hematol 1995; 50:217-9.

378. Samaan NA, Hickey RC, Shutts PE. Diagnosis, localization, and management of pheochromocytoma: Pitfalls and follow-up in 41 patients. Cancer 1988; 62:2451-60.

379. Sheps SG, Jiang N-S, Klee GG. Diagnostic evaluation of pheochromocytoma. Endocrinol Metab Clin North Am 1988; 17: 397-414.

380. Sutton MGSJ, Sheps SG, Lie JT. Prevalence of clinically unsuspected pheochromocytoma: Review of a 50-year autopsy series. Mayo Clin Proc 1981; 56:354-60.

381. Ross EJ, Griffith DNW. The clinical presentation of phaeochromocytoma. Q J Med 1989; 71:485-96.

382. Shapiro B, Fig LM. Management of pheochromocytoma. Endocrinol Metab Clin North Am 1989; 18:443-81.

383. Benowitz NL. Pheochromocytoma. Adv Intern Med 1990; 35:195-220.

384. Bravo EL, Gifford RW. Pheochromocytoma: Diagnosis, localization and management. N Engl J Med 1984; 311:1298-303.

385. Greaves DJ, Barrow PM. Emergency resection of phaeochromocytoma presenting with hyperamylasaemia and pulmonary oedema after abdominal trauma. Anaesthesia 1989; 44:841-2.

386. Murai K, Hirota K, Niskikimi T, et al. Pheochromocytoma with electrocardiographic change mimicking angina pectoris, and cyclic change in direct arterial pressure: A case report. Angiology 1991; 42:157-61.

387. Evans TC, Van Hare RS. Abrupt onset of weakness and seizure in a 39-year-old woman. Ann Emerg Med 1992; 21:1145-52.

388. Lambert MT. Pheochromocytoma presenting as exacerbation of post-traumatic stress disorder symptomology. Int J Psych Med 1992; 22:265-8.

389. Counselman FL, Brenner CJ, Brenner DW. Adrenal pheochromocytoma presenting with persistent abdominal and flank pain. J Emerg Med 1991; 9:241-6.

390. Mornex R, Peyrin L, Pagliari R, Cottet-Emard J-M. Measurement of plasma methoxyamines for the diagnosis of pheochromocytoma. Horm Res 1991; 36:220-6.

391. Plouin PF, Duclos JM, Menard J, et al. Biochemical tests for diagnosis of phaeochromocytoma: Urinary versus plasma determinations. Br Med J 1981; 282:853-4.

392. Bravo EL. Diagnosis of pheochromocytoma, reflections on a controversy. Hypertension 1991; 17:742-4.

393. Stewart MF, Reed P, Weinkove C, et al. Biochemical diagnosis of phaeochromocytoma: Two instructive case reports. J Clin Pathol 1993; 46:280-2.

394. Eisenhofer G, Lenders JWM. Clues to the diagnosis of pheochromocytoma from differential tissue metabolism of catecholamines. Adv Pharmacol 1998; 42:374-7.

395. Heron E, Chattelier G, Billaud E, et al. The urinary metanephrine-to-creatinine ratio for the diagnosis of pheochromocytoma. Ann Int Med 1996; 125:300-3.

396. Gerlo EAM, Sevens C. Urinary and plasma catecholamines and urinary catecholamine metabolites in pheochromocytoma: Diagnostic value in 19 cases. Clin Chem 1994; 40:250-6.

397. Peaston RT, Lai LC. Biochemical detection of phaeochromocytoma. Should we still be running HMMA? J Clin Pathol 1993; 46:734-7.

398. Witteles RM, Kaplan EL, Roizen MF. Sensitivity of diagnostic and localization tests for pheochromocytoma in clinical practice. Arch Int Med 2000; 160:2521-4.

399. Kaplan NM, Kramer NJ, Holland OB, et al. Single-voided urine metanephrine assays in screening for pheochromocytoma. Arch Intern Med 1977; 137:190-3.

400. Peaston RT, Lennard TWJ, Lai LC. Overnight excretion of urinary catecholamines and metabolites in the detection of pheochromocytoma. J Clin Endo Metab 1996; 81:1378-84.

401. Sjoberg RJ, Simcic KJ, Kidd GS. The clonidine suppression test for pheochromocytoma: A review of its utility and pitfalls. Arch Int Med 1992; 152:1193-7.

402. Elliott WJ, Murphy MB. Reduced specificity of the clonidine suppression test in patients with normal plasma catecholamine levels. Am J Med 1988; 84:419-24.

403. Troncone L, Rufini V, Montemaggi P, et al. The diagnostic and therapeutic utility of radioiodinated metaiodobenzylguanidine (MIBG): 5 years experience. Eur J Nuc Med 1990; 16:325-35.

404. Newbould EC, Ross GA, Dacie JE, et al. The use of venous catheterization in the diagnosis and localization of bilateral phaeochromocytomas. Clin Endocrinol 1991; 35:55-9.

405. Harper MA, Murnaghan GA, Kennedy L, et al. Phaeochromocytoma in pregnancy: Five cases and a review of the literature. Br J Obstet Gynaecol 1989; 96:594-606.

406. Osler M. Pregnancy and endocrine disorders: Incidence and obstetrical considerations. Acta Obstet Gynecol Scand 1967; 46(suppl 9): 49-57.

407. Doll DC. Cancer and pregnancy: Introduction. Semin Oncol 1989; 16:335-6.

408. Ringenberg QS, Doll DC. Endocrine tumors and miscellaneous cancers in pregnancy. Semin Oncol 1989; 16:445-55.

409. Chodankar CM, Abhyankar SC, Deodhar KP, Shanbhag AM. Sipple's syndrome (multiple endocrine neoplasia) in pregnancy: Case report. Aust NZ J Obstet Gynaecol 1982; 22:243-4.

410. Nishikawa K, Yukioka H, Tatekawa S, Fujimori M. Phaeochromocytoma crisis in Sipple's syndrome with intrauterine death and disseminated intravascular coagulation. Int J Obstet Anesth 1993; 2:45-8.

411. Epstein H, Morehouse M, Cowles T, King CR. MEA III presenting as pheochromocytoma and complicating pregnancy and the puerperium: A case report. J Reprod Med 1985; 30:501-4.

412. Strauss S, Pansky M, Lewinsohn G. Hemorrhagic pheochromocytoma in a pregnant patient with neurofibromatosis: Sonographic appearance. J Ultrasound Med 1990; 9:165-7.

413. Simanis J, Amerson JR, Hendee AE, Anton AH. Unresectable pheochromocytoma in pregnancy: Pharmacology and biochemistry. Am J Med 1972; 53:381-5.

414. Devoe LD, O'Dell BE, Castillo RA, et al. Metastatic pheochromocytoma in pregnancy and fetal biophysical assessment after maternal administration of alpha-adrenergic, beta-adrenergic, and dopamine antagonists. Obstet Gynecol 1986; 68(suppl):15S-8S.

415. Ellison GT, Mansberger JA, Mansberger AR. Malignant recurrent pheochromocytoma during pregnancy: Case report and review of the literature. Surgery 1988; 103:484-9.

416. Brunt LM. Phaechromocytoma in pregnancy. Br J Surg 2001; 88:481-3.

417. Hopkins PM, MacDonald R, Lyons G. Caesarean section at 27 weeks gestation with removal of phaeochromocytoma. Br J Anaesth 1989; 63:121-4.

418. Pattison J, Harrop-Griffiths AW, Whitlock JE, Roberts JC. Caesarean section in a patient with haemoglobin SC disease and a phaeochromocytoma. Anaesthesia 1990; 45:958-9.

419. Bakri YN, Ingemansson SE, Ali A, Parikh S. Pheochromocytoma and pregnancy: Report of three cases. Acta Obstet Gynecol Scand 1992; 71:301-4.

420. Combs CA, Easterling TR, Schmucker BC, Benedetti TJ. Hemodynamic observations during paroxysmal hypertension in a pregnancy with pheochromocytoma. Obstet Gynecol 1989; 74:439-41.

421. Easterling TR, Carlson K, Benedetti TJ, Mancuso JJ. Hemodynamics associated with the diagnosis and treatment of pheochromocytoma in pregnancy. Am J Perinatol 1992; 9:464-6.

422. Ratge D, Knoll E, Wisser H. Plasma free and conjugated catecholamines in clinical disorders. Life Sci 1986; 39:557-64.

423. Treadway CR, Kane FJ, Jarrahi-Zadeh A, Lipton MA. A psychoendocrine study of pregnancy and puerperium. Am J Psychiatr 1969; 125:1380-6.

424. Pekkarinen A, Castren O. Excretion of vanillylmandelic acid (VMA) in the third trimester of normal and toxaemic pregnancy and other clinical conditions. Ann Chir Gynaecol 1968; 57:373-81.

425. Stanley JH, Sanchez F, Frey GD, Schabel SI. Computed tomography evaluation of pheochromocytoma in pregnancy. J Comput Tomogr 1985; 9:369-72.

426. Greenberg M, Moawad AH, Wieties BM, et al. Extraadrenal pheochromocytoma: Detection during pregnancy using MR imaging. Radiology 1986; 161:475-6.

427. Hull CJ. Phaeochromocytoma: Diagnosis, preoperative preparation and anesthetic management. Br J Anaesth 1986; 58:1453-68.

428. Prys-Roberts C. Phaechromocytoma-recent progress in its management. Br J Anaesth 2000; 85:44-57.

429. Kinney MAO, Narr BJ, Warner MA. Perioperative management of pheochromocytoma. J Cardiothor Vasc Anesth 2002; 16:359-69.

430. Prys-Roberts C, Farndon JR. Efficacy and safety of doxazosin for perioperative management of patients with pheochromocytoma. World J Surg 2002; 26:1037-42.

431. Scott I, Parkes R, Cameron DP. Phaeochromocytoma and cardiomyopathy. Med J Aust 1988; 148:94-6.

432. Sadowski D, Cujec B, McMeekin JD, Wilson TW. Reversibility of catecholamine-induced cardiomyopathy in a woman with pheochromocytoma. Can Med Assoc J 1989; 141:923-4.

433. Sardesai SH, Mourant AJ, Sivathandon Y, et al. Phaeochromocytoma and catecholamine induced cardiomyopathy presenting as heart failure. Br Heart J 1990; 63:234-7.

434. Hicks RJ, Wood B, Kalff V, et al. Normalization of left ventricular ejection fraction following resection of pheochromocytoma in a patient with dilated cardiomyopathy. Clin Nucl Med 1991; 16:413-6.

435. Proye C, Thevenin D, Cecat P, et al. Exclusive use of calcium channel blockers in preoperative and intraoperative control of pheochromocytomas: Hemodynamics and free catecholamine assays in ten consecutive patients. Surgery 1989; 106:1149-54.

436. Perry RR, Keiser HR, Norton JA, et al. Surgical management of pheochromocytoma with the use of metyrosine. Ann Surg 1990; 212:621-8.

437. Stenstrom G, Haljamae H, Tisell LE. Influence of pre-operative treatment with phenoxybenzamine on the incidence of adverse cardiovascular reactions during anaesthesia and surgery for phaeochromocytoma. Acta Anaesthesiol Scand 1985; 29:797-803.

438. Kocak S, Aydintug S, Canakci N. Alpha blockade in preoperative preparation of patients with pheochromocytomas. Int Surg 2002; 87:191-4.

439. Roizen MF. Anesthetic implications of concurrent diseases. In Miller RD, editor. Anesthesia, 4th ed. New York, Churchill Livingstone, 1994:903-1014.

440. Arai T, Hatano Y, Ishida H, Mori K. Use of nicardipine in the anesthetic management of pheochromocytoma. Anesth Analg 1986; 65:706-8.

441. Lipson A, Hsu T-H, Sherwin B, Geelhoed GW. Nitroprusside therapy for a patient with a pheochromocytoma. JAMA 1978; 239:427-8.

442. Zakowski M, Kaufman B, Berguson P, et al. Esmolol use during resection of pheochromocytoma: Report of three cases. Anesthesiology 1989; 70:875-7.

443. James MFM. Use of magnesium sulphate in the anaesthetic management of phaeochromocytoma: A review of 17 anaesthetics. Br J Anaesth 1989; 62:616-23.

444. Groedal S, Bindslev L, Sollevi A, Hambergr B. Adenosine: A new antihypertensive agent during pheochromocytoma removal. World J Surg 1988; 12:581-5.

445. Doi M, Ikeda K. Sevoflurane anesthesia with adenosine triphosphate for resection of pheochromocytoma. Anesthesiology 1989; 70:360-3.

446. Baraka A, Usta N, Yamut F, Haroun S. Verapamil may not be the drug of choice for control of hemodynamic changes during surgical excision of pheochromocytoma. Anesthesiology 1987; 66:705-6.

447. Ryan T, Timoney A, Cunningham AJ. Use of transesophageal echocardiography to manage beta-adrenoceptor block and assess left ventricular function in a patient with phaeochromocytoma. Br J Anaesth 1993; 70:101-3.

448. Janetschek G, Neumann HPH. Laparoscopic surgery for pheochromocytoma. Urol Clin NA 2001; 28:97-105.

449. Sprung J, O'Hara JF, Gill IS, et al. Anesthetic aspects of laparoscopic and open adrenalectomy for pheochromocytoma. Urology 2000; 55:339-43.

450. Kinney MAO, Warner MF, van Heerden JA, et al. Perianesthetic risks and outcomes of pheochromocytoma and paraganglioma resection. Anesth Analg 2000; 91:1118-23.

451. Akiba M, Kodama T, Ito Y, et al. Hypoglycemia induced by excessive rebound secretion of insulin after removal of pheochromocytoma. World J Surg 1990; 14:317-24.

452. Levin H, Heifetz M. Phaeochromocytoma and severe protracted postoperative hypoglycaemia. Can J Anaesth 1990; 37:477-8.

453. van Heerden JA, Roland CF, Carney JA, et al. Long-term evaluation following resection of apparently benign pheochromocytoma(s)/paraganglioma(s). World J Surg 1990; 14:325-9.

454. Krempf M, Lumbroso J, Mornex R, et al. Use of I-131-metaiodobenzylguanidine in the treatment of malignant pheochromocytoma. J Clin Endocrinol Metab 1991; 72:455-61.

455. Fudge TL, McKinnon WMP, Geary WL. Current surgical management of pheochromocytoma during pregnancy. Arch Surg 1980; 115:1224-5.

456. Burgess GE. Alpha blockade and surgical intervention of pheochromocytoma in pregnancy. Obstet Gynecol 1979; 53:266-70.

457. Mitchell SZ, Freilich JD, Brant D, Flynn M. Anesthetic management of pheochromocytoma resection during pregnancy. Anesth Analg 1987; 66:478-80.

458. Santiero ML, Stromquist C, Wyble L. Phenoxybenzamine placental transfer during the third trimester. Ann Pharmacotherapy 1996; 30:1249-51.

459. Stonham J, Wakefield C. Phaeochromocytoma in pregnancy: Caesarean section under epidural analgesia. Anaesthesia 1983; 38:654-8.

460. Stenstrom G, Swolin K. Pheochromocytoma in pregnancy: Experience of treatment with phenoxybenzamine in three patients. Acta Obstet Gynecol Scand 1985; 64:357-61.

461. Lyons CW, Colmorgen GHC. Medical management of pheochromocytoma in pregnancy. Obstet Gynecol 1988; 72:450-1.

462. James MFM, Huddle KRL, vander Veen BW. Use of magnesium sulphate in the anaesthetic management of phaeochromocytoma in pregnancy. Can J Anaesth 1988; 35:178-82.

463. Hamilton A, Sirrs S, Schmidt N, et al. Anaesthesia for phaeochromocytoma in pregnancy. Can J Anaesth 1997; 44:654-7.

464. Venuto R, Burstein P, Schneider R. Pheochromocytoma: Antepartum diagnosis and management with tumor resection in the puerperium. Am J Obstet Gynecol 1984; 150:431-2.

465. Burgess GE, Cooper JR, Marino RJ, Peuler MJ. Anesthetic management of combined cesarean section and excision of pheochromocytoma. Anesth Analg 1978; 57:276-9.

466. Naulty J, Cefalo RC, Lewis PE. Fetal toxicity of nitroprusside in the pregnant ewe. Am J Obstet Gynecol 1981; 139: 708-11.

467. Shoemaker CT, Meyers M. Sodium nitroprusside for control of severe hypertensive disease of pregnancy: A case report and discussion of potential toxicity. Am J Obstet Gynecol 1984; 149:171-3.

468. Stempel JE, O'Grady JP, Morton MJ, Johnson KA. Use of sodium nitroprusside in complications of gestational hypertension. Obstet Gynecol 1982; 60:533-8.

469. Lieb SM, Zugaib M, Nuwayhid B, et al. Nitroprusside-induced hemodynamic alterations in normotensive and hypertensive pregnant sheep. Am J Obstet Gynecol 1981; 139:925-31.

470. Nelson SH, Suresh MS. Comparison of nitroprusside and hydralazine in isolated uterine arteries from pregnant and nonpregnant patients. Anesthesiology 1988; 68:541-7.

471. Weiner C, Liu KZ, Thompson L, et al. Effect of pregnancy on endothelium and smooth muscle: Their role in reduced adrenergic sensitivity. Am J Physiol 1991; 261:H1275-83.

472. Dahia PLM, Hayashida CY, Strunz C, et al. Low cord blood levels of catecholamine from a newborn of a pheochromocytoma patient. Eur J Endocrinol 1994; 130:217-9.

473. Pestelek B, Kapor M. Pheochromocytoma and abruptio placentae. Am J Obstet Gynecol 1963; 85:538-40.

474. Davies AE, Navaratnarajah M. Vaginal delivery in a patient with phaeochromocytoma: A case report. Br J Anaesth 1984; 56:913-6.

475. Flowers D, Clark JFJ, Westney LS. Cocaine intoxication associated with abruptio placentae. J Natl Med Assoc 1991; 83:230-2.

476. Hendee AE, Martin RD, Waters WC. Hypertension in pregnancy: Toxemia or pheochromocytoma. Am J Obstet Gynecol 1969; 105:64-72.

477. Braude BM, Leiman BC, Moyes DG. Etomidate infusion for resection of phaeochromocytoma: A report of 2 cases. S Afr Med J 1986; 69:60-2.

478. Strebel S, Scheidegger D. Propofol-fentanyl anesthesia for pheochromocytoma resection. Acta Anaesthesiol Scand 1991; 35:275-7.

479. Bromage PR, Millar RA. Epidural blockade and circulating catecholamine levels in a child with phaeochromocytoma. Can Anaesth Soc J 1958; 5:282-7.

480. Cousins MJ, Rubin RB. The intraoperative management of phaeochromocytoma with total epidural sympathetic blockade. Br J Anaesth 1974; 46:78-81.

481. Miller D, Robblee JA. Perioperative management of a patient with a malignant pheochromocytoma. Can Anaesth Soc J 1985; 32:278-82.

482. Roizen MF, Horrigan RW, Koike M, et al. A prospective randomized trial of four anesthetic techniques for resection of pheochromocytoma (abstract). Anesthesiology 1982; 57:A43.

483. Takai Y, Seki H, Kinoshita K. Pheochromocytoma in pregnancy manifesting hypertensive crisis induced by metoclopramide. Int J Gynecol Obstet 1997; 59:133-7.

484. Allen GC, Rosenberg H. Phaeochromocytoma presenting as acute malignant hyperthermia: A diagnostic challenge. Can J Anaesth 1990; 37:593-5.

485. Crowley KJ, Cunningham AJ, Conroy B, et al. Phaeochromocytoma: A presentation mimicking malignant hyperthermia. Anaesthesia 1988; 43:1031-2.

Chapter 42
Hematologic and Coagulation Disorders
Shiv K. Sharma, M.D., FRCA · Robert B. Lechner, M.D., Ph.D.

ANEMIA

Normal Hemoglobin Morphology

Normal adult hemoglobin consists of four polypeptides (two alpha and two beta chains) and the iron-containing prosthetic group (heme or ferroprotoporphyrin IX). In the early embryo, theta (θ) and zeta (ζ) chains are present instead of the alpha (α) chains, and epsilon (ε) chains are present instead of the beta (β) chains. After early embryogenesis, pairs of alpha chains are linked with pairs of either beta, gamma (γ), or delta (δ) chains to form adult hemoglobin (Hgb A = $\alpha_2\beta_2$), fetal hemoglobin (Hgb F = $\alpha_2\gamma_2$), or hemoglobin A_2 (Hgb A_2 = $\alpha_2\delta_2$). By term gestation, the ratio of hemoglobin F to hemoglobin A is approximately 1:1. By 1 year of age, hemoglobin F typically constitutes less than 1% of total hemoglobin. Although hemoglobin A_2 is present, it constitutes less than 2.5% of total adult hemoglobin.

The sequence of amino acids (141 amino acids for alpha chains and 146 for beta chains) defines the **primary structure**. The three-dimensional shape of each chain defines the **secondary structure**, and the relationship between the four chains and the heme prosthetic group defines the **tertiary structure**. The binding of the ligands 2,3-diphosphoglycerate (2,3-DPG) and oxygen defines the **quaternary structure**.

The affinity of hemoglobin for oxygen is expressed as the P_{50} (i.e., the oxygen tension at which half of hemoglobin's oxygen-carrying capacity is used). Increased temperature and increased hydrogen ion and 2,3-DPG concentrations reduce the affinity of hemoglobin for oxygen, which results in an increase in the P_{50}. This facilitates the unloading of oxygen at peripheral tissues. When compared with purified hemoglobin A, purified hemoglobin F has a lower oxygen affinity and a greater response to changes in pH but only a minimal response to changes in 2,3-DPG concentration. The decreased interaction between hemoglobin F and intraerythrocyte 2,3-DPG accounts for the increased affinity of fetal blood for oxygen in vivo.

Dilutional Anemia of Pregnancy

During normal pregnancy, plasma volume increases by approximately 50%, but red blood cell (RBC) mass increases by only 30%. This results in a dilutional anemia. RBC mass increases linearly after the first trimester until delivery, and plasma volume plateaus or falls slightly near term. Therefore hemoglobin concentrations are lowest between 28 and 34 weeks' gestation. If the hemoglobin concentration falls below 10.5 g/dL, the physician should consider etiologies other than the dilutional anemia of pregnancy.

Thalassemia

The thalassemias are a diverse group of microcytic, hemolytic anemias that result from the reduced synthesis of one or more of the polypeptide globin chains. This reduced synthesis leads to (1) an imbalance in globin chain synthesis, (2) defective hemoglobin synthesis, and (3) erythrocyte damage resulting from excess globin subunits. In α-thalassemia, alpha-chain production is reduced, and in β-thalassemia, beta-chain production is reduced.

α-THALASSEMIA

There are two alpha-chain loci on each chromosome 16; therefore there are four genes that can produce alpha chains. Because mutations can affect any or all of these genes, four types of α-thalassemia exist: **silent carrier** (three functioning genes), α-**thalassemia trait** (two functioning genes), **hemoglobin H disease** (one functioning gene), and α^0-**thalassemia** or **Barts hydrops** (no functioning genes). As the number of functioning genes decreases from four to zero, the ratio of alpha to beta chains decreases from 0.8:1 to 0.6:1

to 0.3:1 to 0:1. The mRNA production from the second alpha gene exceeds that of the first alpha gene by a factor of 1.5 to 3.[1,2] Therefore deletions of the second alpha gene may produce a greater clinical effect. As beta (or beta-like) chains accumulate, they can form tetramers in utero (e.g., hemoglobin Barts = γ_4) or after delivery (e.g., hemoglobin H = β_4).

In the United States, 30% of black women are **silent carriers** and have only slightly decreased (78 to 80 fL) mean corpuscular volume (MCV); other indices for these women are normal.[3] A chromosome lacking one alpha gene is common in the Mediterranean basin, the Middle East, India, Southeast Asia, Indonesia, and the South Pacific Islands. These patients are *not* at increased risk during pregnancy or surgery.

The **α-thalassemia trait** affects 3% of black women in the United States. These women have an MCV of 70 to 75 fL and mild anemia. They typically are asymptomatic. The diagnosis of α-thalassemia trait should be considered if a black patient with microcytic anemia does not respond to oral iron therapy. The diagnosis is confirmed by alpha-gene analysis. These patients are *not* at increased risk during pregnancy or surgery.

Patients with **hemoglobin H disease** have moderately severe anemia, splenomegaly, fatigue, and generalized discomfort. Hemoglobin H (β_4) constitutes 2% to 15% of total hemoglobin in these patients. These patients do not have a decreased life span, and hospitalization for the treatment of their anemia rarely is required.

α⁰-Thalassemia generally is incompatible with life. This disease is relatively common in Southeast Asia, China, and the Philippines. Affected individuals die either in utero or shortly after birth of hydrops fetalis, or they die in early childhood if transfusions are administered in utero.

Molecular genetic testing can identify couples at increased risk for offspring with a hemoglobinopathy and provides guidance as to whether to perform prenatal testing. If patients at increased risk for thalassemia have a low MCV, and their hemoglobin electrophoresis results are inconsistent with β-thalassemia trait, they should undergo DNA-based testing to detect α-globin gene deletion characteristic of α-thalassemia. Counseling for prenatal genetic testing should be offered if both parents have α-thalassemia trait or if one parent has hemoglobin H disease and the other either is a silent carrier or has α-thalassemia trait.[4]

β-THALASSEMIA

In β-thalassemia, the production of beta chains is reduced. There are more than 50 genetic causes for ineffective beta-chain production, including gene deletion, transcription mutations, and RNA-processing mutations.[5] Unlike the alpha chains, which have four genes (two on each chromosome 16), beta chains have only one gene on each chromosome 11. mRNA production from the second beta-like gene (i.e., delta) is almost completely suppressed. Therefore there are only two primary forms of β-thalassemia: **β⁰-thalassemia,** in which there is no beta-chain formation, and **β⁺-thalassemia,** in which some beta-chain production exists. β⁰-Thalassemia also is called β-*thalassemia major* or *Cooley's anemia.* Patients who receive β-thalassemia genes from both parents but with mutations of different types often develop a milder form of the disease and require fewer or no transfusions. This condition is known as **thalassemia intermedia.** Finally, **β-thalassemia minor** refers to the heterozygous carrier of β-thalassemia.

β-Thalassemia is found most often in persons from the Mediterranean basin, the Middle East, India, and Southeast Asia. It occurs less frequently among persons from southern Russia, China, and Africa.

Individuals with β-thalassemia have inadequate beta-chain production; thus they have a relative excess of alpha chains. Excess alpha chains precipitate and form inclusion bodies in RBC precursors, which results in anemia secondary to ineffective erythropoiesis and splenic hemolysis. In the fetus, the gamma chain is unaffected; therefore anemia only develops as gamma-chain production ceases during the first year of life. In some patients, gamma-chain production continues to a variable degree. Thus the ongoing production of hemoglobin F (even in adults) may minimize the effects of decreased beta-chain production.

β-Thalassemia major

In patients with β-thalassemia major, severe anemia develops in the first few months of extrauterine life. The anemia results in tissue hypoxia, increased intestinal absorption of iron, and increased erythropoietin production. The resulting expansion of marrow cavities causes skeletal abnormalities and pathologic fractures. Splenomegaly leads to thrombocytopenia and leukopenia. Transfusions are required to maintain life, and the resulting iron load leads to iron accumulation, first in Kupffer's cells (noncirculating macrophages found in the liver), then in liver parenchymal cells, and finally in endocrine and myocardial cells. Deposition of iron in endocrine tissues may result in diabetes mellitus, adrenal insufficiency, and infertility.[6,7] Myocardial accumulation of iron can lead to conduction abnormalities and intractable heart failure, which is exacerbated by anemia-induced tachycardia. Heart failure and infection are the most common causes of death.

Patients with β-thalassemia major who present at less than 2 years of age often have hepatomegaly and a hemoglobin concentration as low as 2 g/dL. Patients who present later in life (2 to 12 years of age) typically have a hemoglobin concentration between 4 and 10 g/dL, with marked anisopoikilocytosis and numerous target cells, nucleated RBCs, and inclusion bodies. Levels of hemoglobin F range from 10% to 90% of the total hemoglobin, and hemoglobin A_2 constitutes the remainder of the hemoglobin that is present. Prenatal diagnosis is possible using fetal cells obtained by means of chorionic villus sampling or amniocentesis and subjected to DNA analysis.[8]

Treatment includes (1) transfusion of leukocyte-poor RBCs every 2 to 3 weeks to maintain a hemoglobin concentration greater than 10 g/dL, thus preventing endogenous erythropoiesis; (2) splenectomy; and (3) iron chelation therapy to prevent hemosiderosis.[9] Deferoxamine is the most effective chelation agent currently available. It is given by continuous subcutaneous administration or by intermittent intramuscular injection. Oral chelation drugs and bone marrow transplantation are possible future treatment options.

It is unusual for patients with β-thalassemia major to become pregnant. If patients do conceive, the metabolic demands of pregnancy result in increased transfusion requirements, which may worsen hemosiderosis and cardiac failure. These patients have an increased incidence of spontaneous abortion, intrauterine fetal death, and intrauterine growth restriction (IUGR).[10]

During pregnancy, the transfusion of 600 to 8400 mL of blood typically is required to maintain the hemoglobin concentration above 10 g/dL. It is unclear whether chelation therapy should be continued because the fetal effects of deferoxamine are unknown. A trial of labor is appropriate, and operative delivery should be reserved for obstetric indications.

Extramedullary hematopoiesis can result in vertebral cortical weakening, pathologic fractures, and rarely paraplegia.[11] In our judgment, these skeletal abnormalities do not contraindicate the administration of regional anesthesia. Patients with splenomegaly may have thrombocytopenia. The anesthesiologist should exclude a history of spontaneous hemorrhage and determine the platelet count before administration of regional anesthesia.

β-Thalassemia minor

In patients with β-thalassemia minor, the clinical course typically is benign. The anemia typically is mild (e.g., hemoglobin concentration of 9 to 11 g/dL) and is characterized by microcytosis and hypochromatosis. Levels of hemoglobin F range from 1% to 3%, and levels of hemoglobin A$_2$ range from 3.5% to 7%.

Moderate anemia develops only during periods of stress, such as pregnancy and severe infection. Nonetheless, most patients with β-thalassemia minor tolerate pregnancy well. Folate supplementation is recommended. Supplemental iron is administered only to patients with laboratory evidence of iron deficiency. Transfusions are reserved for patients with hemorrhage or a hemoglobin concentration below 8 g/dL. Infection, which can cause bone marrow suppression, must be treated promptly and vigorously. β-Thalassemia minor typically does not affect anesthetic management during labor or cesarean section.

Sickle Cell Disease

More than 380 abnormal alpha, beta, gamma, and delta chains have been identified.[12] Structural hemoglobinopathies result when these abnormal chains are used to form hemoglobin molecules. The most common abnormal hemoglobins are hemoglobin S, hemoglobin C, hemoglobin D, and hemoglobin E. Patients can be homozygous for an abnormal hemoglobin (e.g., **hemoglobin SS** or **sickle cell anemia**), heterozygous for an abnormal hemoglobin (e.g., **hemoglobin SA** or **sickle cell trait**), or doubly heterozygous for an abnormal hemoglobin (e.g., **hemoglobin SC** or **sickle cell hemoglobin C disease**). Both the heterozygous state for the thalassemias and the structural hemoglobinopathies appear to afford a degree of protection against malaria, which may explain their geographic distribution and continued presence in the gene pool.

A **sickle cell disorder** refers to a state in which erythrocytes undergo sickling when they are deoxygenated. Normal erythrocytes have a biconcaval shape. Sickle cells are elongated and crescent shaped, with two pointed ends. *Sickle cell disease* refers to disorders in which sickling results in clinical signs and symptoms and includes hemoglobin SS disease, hemoglobin SC disease, hemoglobin SD disease, and sickle cell β-thalassemia.

SICKLE CELL ANEMIA

Epidemiology

Table 42-1 lists the prevalence of sickle cell anemia and the other most common hemoglobinopathies in the United States adult black population.[13] In Africa, the prevalence of the sickle cell trait is as high as 20% to 40%.

Pathophysiology

In hemoglobin S molecules, valine is substituted for glutamic acid as the sixth amino acid in the beta chains. This results in a propensity for hemoglobin molecules to aggregate when the hemoglobin is in the deoxygenated state. The hemoglobin molecules stack on top of one another and form microtubules. The primary cause of sickling is the abnormal hemoglobin; however, erythrocyte metabolic and membrane abnormalities may contribute to sickling, which may explain the variable clinical presentation of patients with hemoglobin SS.

Oxygen tension is the most important determinant in sickling. Hemoglobin S begins to aggregate at a PO_2 of less than 50 mm Hg, and all of the hemoglobin S is aggregated at a PO_2 of approximately 23 mm Hg. The formation of hemoglobin S aggregates is time dependent. Therefore even though 85% of hemoglobin S would eventually sickle after prolonged exposure to the oxygen tension in venous blood, less than 5% does because the hemoglobin typically reaches the lungs and becomes oxygenated before aggregates form. If an erythrocyte sickles, it can return to its normal shape once the hemoglobin S becomes oxygenated. However, the cellular membrane remains altered, and after it has undergone repeated sickling cycles, it remains sickled regardless of oxygen tension. As a result, the erythrocyte life span is reduced to approximately 12 days.[14]

Other factors that affect sickling are listed in Box 42-1. The sickled cells can form aggregates and lead to vasoocclusive disease. Sickled cells also are cleared more rapidly from the circulation by the reticuloendothelial system, which results in a reduced erythrocyte life span.

The incidence of pneumonia and pyelonephritis is increased in pregnant patients with sickle cell disease when compared with other pregnant patients. Marked ventricular hypertrophy can occur in pregnant women with sickle cell disease secondary to increased cardiac output. This may lead

TABLE 42-1	PREVALENCE OF HEMOGLOBINOPATHIES IN THE UNITED STATES IN PERSONS OF AFRICAN DESCENT	
Type	**Estimated prevalence**
Traits	
Hemoglobin AS	1:12.5
Hemoglobin AC	1:33
β-Thalassemia minor	1:67
Persistent hemoglobin F	1:1000
Sickling Disorders	
Hemoglobin SS	1:625
Hemoglobin SC	1:833
Hemoglobin S–β-thalassemia	1:1667
Hemoglobin S–persistent hemoglobin F	1:25,000
Hemoglobin CC	1:4444
β-Thalassemia major	1:17,778
Hemoglobin C–β-thalassemia	1:4444

From Motulsky AG. Frequency of sickling disorders in U.S. Blacks. N Engl J Med 1973; 288:31-3.

Box 42-1 FACTORS THAT INCREASE SICKLING IN WOMEN WITH SICKLE CELL ANEMIA

Hemoglobin S more than 50% of the total hemoglobin
Dehydration leading to increased blood viscosity
Hypotension causing vascular stasis
Hypothermia
Acidosis

to a decrease in ventricular compliance and a deterioration in ventricular diastolic function.[15] The reduced erythrocyte life span results in anemia, jaundice, cholecystitis, and a hyperdynamic cardiac state. Anemia results in erythroblastic hyperplasia, expansion of medullary spaces, and a loss of cortex in long bones, vertebral bodies, and the skull. Vasoocclusive events can lead to **infarctive crises** (which most often occur in the chest, abdomen, back, and long bones), **cerebrovascular accidents,** and rarely **peripheral neuropathy**.[16] Aggregate formation in the spleen can result in microinfarcts. **Aplastic crises** can result from depression of erythropoiesis secondary to infection (especially parvovirus) or from marrow failure secondary to folate deficiency during pregnancy. During an aplastic crisis, the hemoglobin concentration can drop 2 g/dL per day and result in high-output cardiac failure and death. **Sequestration crises** can result from the massive pooling of erythrocytes, especially in the spleen. This occurs more frequently in patients with hemoglobin SC disease or sickle cell β-thalassemia than in patients with other forms of sickle cell disease. In general, a major sequestration crisis is one in which the hemoglobin concentration is less than 6 g/dL and has fallen more than 3 g/dL from the baseline measurement.

Diagnosis

In the adult, sickle cell anemia is characterized by (1) a hemoglobin concentration of approximately 6 to 8 g/dL, (2) macrocytosis, (3) elevated reticulocyte count, and (4) the presence of sickle cells on a peripheral blood smear. The diagnosis is confirmed by electrophoresis. Because most hemoglobinopathies are inherited as autosomal recessive conditions, prenatal screening for abnormal hemoglobin by electrophoresis is recommended in couples at high risk for sickle cell disease.[4] In utero, the diagnosis can be made by using restriction endonucleases specific for the sickle mutation and cells obtained during amniocentesis[17] or chorionic villus sampling.[18]

Interaction with Pregnancy

Pregnancy typically exacerbates the complications of sickle cell anemia. Maternal mortality is as high as 1%.[19] Pulmonary embolism and infection are the leading causes of death. Fetal mortality is as high as 20%.[19] Patients with sickle cell anemia have an increased incidence of preterm labor, placental abruption, placenta previa, and pregnancy-induced hypertension (PIH).[20]

Medical Management

Sickle cell anemia is a chronic anemia, and blood transfusions are given only when they are specifically indicated (e.g., aplastic crisis, pneumonia with hypoxemia, before or during surgery). The goals of transfusion are to achieve a hemoglobin concentration greater than 8 g/dL and to ensure that hemoglobin A represents more than 40% of the total hemoglobin present. Maintaining a hemoglobin concentration above 10 g/dL during pregnancy decreases the incidence of painful crises but does not appear to alter fetal or maternal mortality.[20] If the patient's baseline hemoglobin concentration is less than 6 g/dL, simple transfusions with buffy coat poor, hemoglobin S-free, washed RBCs should be adequate to meet treatment goals. Otherwise, partial exchange transfusions may be necessary.

Hemoglobin F does not form aggregates with hemoglobin S. Administration of hydroxyurea[21] (or another chemotherapeutic drug) may enhance the production of hemoglobin F, which may decrease the morbidity and mortality of sickle cell anemia. Bone marrow transplantation is another experimental treatment that shows promise.[22]

Obsteric Management

During prenatal visits, the obstetrician should monitor maternal weight gain and blood pressure as well as intrauterine fetal growth. Cervical examinations are performed regularly to detect impending preterm labor. Antepartum fetal surveillance is begun at the time of extrauterine viability (i.e., approximately 25 to 26 weeks' gestation). If obstetric complications develop, immediate and aggressive treatment is required. Blood transfusions are reserved for specific indications (e.g., severe anemia, hypoxemia, preeclampsia, septicemia, renal failure, acute chest pain syndrome, anticipated surgery). A hemoglobin concentration of 8 g/dL is adequate for vaginal delivery. It is common practice to increase the hemoglobin concentration to 10 g/dL in patients scheduled for cesarean section, but no study has shown that this increased hemoglobin concentration decreases morbidity or mortality.

Anesthetic Management

The anesthetic management of the patient with severe sickle cell anemia resembles that for the patient with high-output heart failure. Pain control during labor is essential, and continuous lumbar epidural analgesia is recommended. For operative delivery, either regional or general anesthesia is acceptable. The choice depends on the patient's preference and physical status and the anesthesiologist's preference. Principles of anesthetic management include (1) use of crystalloid to maintain intravascular volume, (2) transfusion of RBCs to maintain oxygen-carrying capacity, (3) administration of supplemental oxygen and the use of a pulse oximeter to monitor oxygen saturation, (4) maintenance of normothermia, and (5) prevention of peripheral venous stasis.

SICKLE CELL DISEASE VARIANTS

If a patient carries one sickle cell gene and another gene for a hemoglobin that has a propensity to sickle, that patient is considered to have sickle cell disease. The resulting diseases form a spectrum between the asymptomatic sickle cell trait (hemoglobin SA) and sickle cell anemia (SS disease). Patients with hemoglobin SD disease tend to have the mildest form, and patients with SC disease or sickle cell β-thalassemia tend to have a more severe disease.

As with the hemoglobin S gene, hemoglobin C is most prevalent among persons of West African descent, whereas hemoglobin D is most prevalent among persons of Northwest Indian descent, and hemoglobin E is most prevalent among persons of Southeast Asian descent. Patients with hemoglobin SC and hemoglobin SD disease tend to be asymptomatic during childhood, with only mild anemia. A hemoglobin concentration of 11 to 13 g/dL, with the presence of target cells, is consistent with sickle cell disease in nonpregnant patients. The diagnosis is confirmed by electrophoresis. Typically these individuals do not develop symptoms until the second half of pregnancy. During late pregnancy, these patients may develop severe anemia (secondary to splenic sequestration) and splenomegaly. Patients with hemoglobin SC disease also have a tendency to develop marrow necrosis, which predisposes to fat emboli. The other clinical manifestations are similar to those for patients with sickle cell anemia.

In the past, vigorous transfusion therapy was recommended for patients with sickle cell disease. However, current recommendations are to transfuse patients only when the hemoglobin concentration is less than 8 g/dL. Obstetric and anesthetic management are similar to that for patients with sickle cell anemia.

Patients who are homozygous for hemoglobin C, D, or E typically have mild anemia. Target cells often are seen, and splenomegaly is common. Patients who are heterozygous (i.e., one gene for hemoglobin C, D, or E and one gene for normal hemoglobin) are asymptomatic. The diagnosis is confirmed with electrophoresis. Pregnancy typically is well tolerated, and no specific change in obstetric or anesthetic management is required.

SICKLE CELL TRAIT

Sickle cell trait is the most benign form of the sickle cell disorders. It occurs in approximately 8% of black women in the United States. The RBCs of patients with sickle cell trait do not sickle until the Po_2 falls below 15 mm Hg; therefore RBC life span is normal.[23] A study of 65,000 patients with sickle cell trait found only a slight increase in the incidence of renal (hematuria) and pulmonary (emboli) complications when compared with patients without sickle cell trait.[24] Pregnant women with sickle cell trait are at increased risk for **asymptomatic bacteriuria**, which predisposes them to **pyelonephritis**. Similar to women with sickle cell disease, women with sickle cell trait also are at increased risk for preeclampsia.[25] Otherwise, patients with sickle cell trait are not at increased risk during surgery.

Autoimmune Hemolytic Anemia

Patients with autoimmune hemolytic anemia produce antibodies to their own RBCs; this results in hemolysis and varying degrees of anemia. Table 42-2 lists the characteristics of the four main types of autoimmune hemolytic anemia.[26,27] In patients with warm antibodies, the antibodies react with RBCs at a temperature of 35° to 40° C, whereas cold antibodies react optimally at a temperature of less than 30° C. The annual incidence of new cases of autoimmune hemolytic anemia is approximately 1 per 80,000 persons. Table 42-3 lists the various etiologies of autoimmune hemolytic anemia.[28]

Patients with warm-reacting antibodies typically respond to treatment with glucocorticoids; splenectomy is reserved for those patients who are refractory to steroid therapy. After splenectomy, steroid requirements typically decrease, but relapses (which require steroid therapy) are common. Cytotoxic drugs (e.g., cyclophosphamide, 6-mercaptopurine) have not proven to be beneficial in these patients.

In patients with cold-reacting antibodies, the anemia typically is mild, and maintenance of normal body and ambient temperatures typically is all that is required.

COAGULATION

Thrombotic and Thrombolytic Pathways

Hemostasis depends on the normal function of vascular tissue, platelets, and coagulation factors. During the initial response to a loss of vessel integrity, **primary hemostasis** results as platelets adhere to exposed collagen. (This response is facilitated by the von Willebrand factor.) Platelet activation results in the release of substances that constrict the injured vessels and cause other platelets to adhere and form a hemostatic plug. These platelet-released mediators include (1) arachidonic acid, which is converted to thromboxane A_2 (TXA_2); (2) 12-hydroxyeicosatetraenoic acid (12-HETE); (3) serotonin (5-HT); and (4) adenosine diphosphate.

The platelet plug is not stable, and initiation of the coagulation cascade, followed by deposition and stabilization of fibrin, is required for **secondary hemostasis**. Most coagulation factors circulate in the blood as zymogens, which are converted to active enzymes that in turn convert other zymogens to active enzymes. For example, Factor X (a zymogen) is converted to factor Xa (an enzyme), which converts prothrombin to thrombin. A simplified diagram of the coagulation cascade appears in Figure 42-1. In the **intrinsic system**, factor XII binds to negatively charged substrate (e.g., collagen) and may undergo autolysis to form factor XIIa, or it may be converted to XIIa by trace amounts of XIIa. In addition to activating its own zymogen, factor XIIa converts prekallikrein to kallikrein and factor XI to XIa. High-molecular-weight kininogen can bind factor XI and facilitate its conversion to XIa by XIIa.

TABLE 42-2   CHARACTERISTICS OF AUTOIMMUNE HEMOLYTIC ANEMIAS

Disease	Immunoglobulin	Complement involved	Site of RBC destruction	Treatment	Transfusion requirements
Incomplete warm autoantibodies	Typically IgG	No	Spleen	Corticosteroids, splenectomy, gamma-globulin	Rarely needed; if given, combined with corticosteroids
	Rarely IgA	No	Spleen		
	Rarely IgM	C4b and C3b	Liver		
Complete warm autoantibodies					
Type 1	IgM	C4b and C3b	Liver	Corticosteroids, splenectomy	Rarely needed
Type 2	IgM	C1-9	Intracellular	Plasma exchange, corticosteroids	Frequently needed
Cold autoagglutinins and hemolysins	IgM	No	Intracellular	Corticosteroids, keeping patient warm	Very rarely needed
Biphasic hemolysins					
Acute	IgG	Yes	Intracellular agglutination	Treatment of underlying infection	Occasionally needed
Chronic	IgG	Yes	Intracellular hemolysis	Plasmapheresis, chlorambucil	Frequently needed

IgA, Immunoglobulin A; *IgG*, immunoglobulin G; *IgM*, immunoglobulin M.
From Gibson J. Autoimmune hemolytic anemia: Current concepts. Aust NZ J Med 1988: 18:625-37; and Engelfriet CD, Overbeeke MAM, Kr von dem Borne AEG. Autoimmune hemolytic anemia. Semin Hematol 1992; 29:3-12.

Kallikrein and high molecular weight kininogen also can convert factor XII to XIIa. Factor XIa converts factor IX to IXa, which, with factor VIIIa, converts factor X to Xa.

In the **extrinsic system**, tissue damage causes the release of thromboplastin (also known as *factor III* or *tissue factor*). This binds with either factor VII or VIIa and converts factor X to Xa. The thromboplastin factor VII complex has only 3% of the activity of the thromboplastin factor VIIa complex, but the former may be important in the initiation of coagulation in response to tissue damage. Once factor Xa is formed, it converts factor VII to VIIa, thus increasing the proportion of factor VIIa present, which increases the conversion of factor X to Xa. The thromboplastin factor VII complex also can convert factor IX to IXa, which indicates an interrelation between the intrinsic and extrinsic systems[29]; however, the physiologic significance of this reaction is unclear because it proceeds at a much slower rate than does the conversion of factor X to Xa.

Factor Xa promotes platelet aggregation, and it converts factors V and VIII to factors Va and VIIIa, respectively. Factor Xa, combined with factor Va, converts factor II (prothrombin) to factor IIa (thrombin). According to cell-based coagulation theory,[30] activated platelets provide the primary surface for conversion of factor X to Xa and prothrombin to thrombin. Thrombin converts factors I (fibrinogen), V, VIII, and XIII to factors Ia (fibrin), Va, VIIIa, and XIIIa, respectively. Thrombin also causes platelet activation. Factor XIIIa is required to cross-link fibrin strands, which helps form a stable clot.

Clot formation is limited by antithrombin III and proteins C and S. Antithrombin III, whose activity is enhanced by heparin, inhibits factors IXa and Xa and thrombin. Protein C is activated by a thrombin-thrombomodulin complex. With protein S as a cofactor, protein C breaks down factors Va and VIIIa.

The final component of the hemostatic system is the fibrinolytic system, in which plasmin breaks down fibrin. Tissue-type plasminogen activator (t-PA) circulates as an active

TABLE 42-3	ETIOLOGIES OF AUTOIMMUNE HEMOLYTIC ANEMIAS

Etiology	Approximate percent
Primary or idiopathic	43
Secondary	
Neoplasms	22
Drug-related	15
Infections	8
Connective tissue diseases	5
Other diseases	5
Pregnancy	2

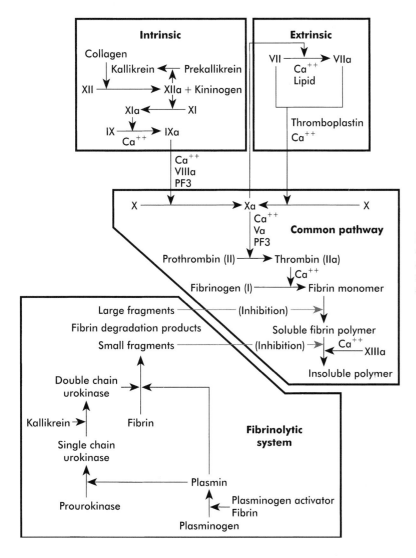

FIGURE 42-1. Components of the extrinsic, intrinsic, and common pathways and the fibrinolytic system. The term *cascade* is a misnomer that stems from the presence of positive and negative feedback loops in both the coagulation and fibrinolytic systems.

protease; however, its activity increases dramatically when it binds to fibrin, at which time it converts plasminogen to plasmin. Urokinase-like plasminogen activator (u-PA) is secreted as the relatively inactive pro-urokinase; it is converted to the active form (single-chain urokinase) by plasmin. Single chain urokinase is converted to its most active form (double-chain urokinase) by kallikrein, which is released during activation of the coagulation cascade. Plasmin activity is localized to the clot by the local availability of fibrin and by plasminogen activator inhibitors, which are secreted by many cells. The drug epsilon-aminocaproic acid (EACA) inhibits fibrinolysis by binding to plasminogen and plasmin and preventing their binding to fibrin.

Box 2-1 outlines the changes in the concentrations of coagulation factors during pregnancy. The levels of most procoagulants increase during pregnancy, and this is accompanied by a similar change in the levels of plasminogen and plasminogen activator inhibitors.[31] Deficiencies in these procoagulant factors or an increase in fibrinolytic factors cause **hemorrhagic disorders**. Deficiencies in antithrombin III, protein C or S, or the fibrinolytic system cause **thromboembolic disorders**.

Assessment of Coagulation

ROUTINE HEMATOLOGY

The increase in the concentration of most coagulation factors is associated with a shortening of the prothrombin time (PT) and the activated partial thromboplastin time (aPTT) during *normal* pregnancy (see Chapter 2). In contrast, in severely preeclamptic women with a platelet count of less than 100,000/mm[3], the concentration of coagulation factors may decrease because of their excessive consumption. Therefore, assessment of coagulation in these patients should include the determination of PT, aPTT, and the fibrinogen level.[32]

BLEEDING TIME

The cutaneous bleeding time measurement is used by some physicians to (1) diagnose platelet-related bleeding disorders, (2) predict abnormal bleeding, and (3) monitor therapy for bleeding disorders. Most investigators agree on the validity of the bleeding time measurement when it is applied to a population of patients. (For example, the mean bleeding time of a group of patients with von Willebrand disease will exceed that of a population of normal persons.) However, it is unclear whether the bleeding time correctly predicts the risk of bleeding in an individual patient.

Rodgers and Levin[33] identified and reviewed 862 printed documents that discussed the bleeding time measurement. They constructed receiver operating characteristic (ROC) curves (which characterize the sensitivity and specificity of a test) in every study in which published data were adequate. They concluded the following[33]:
1. No evidence confirms that the utility of the bleeding time measurement has been enhanced by recent advances in the standardization of the method.
2. The bleeding time is not a specific in vivo indicator of platelet function.
3. No evidence confirms that the bleeding time predicts the risk of hemorrhage.
4. No evidence confirms that bleeding from a standardized cut in the skin reflects the risk of bleeding elsewhere in the body.
5. No evidence suggests that abnormalities in the test occur sufficiently in advance of other indicators of bleeding to allow actions to be taken that could favorably alter outcome.
6. No evidence confirms that the bleeding time is a useful indicator of the efficacy of therapy.

Others disagree with these conclusions. Burns and Lawrence[34] concluded that "patients with known disorders of primary hemostasis, as a result of either hereditary functional platelet disorders or von Willebrand disease, should be assessed preoperatively with a bleeding time and treated on the basis of the test results."

There is no evidence to suggest that the bleeding time correctly predicts the risk of epidural hematoma following administration of regional anesthesia in a woman with preeclampsia or in a patient who has been taking a nonsteroidal antiinflammatory drug (NSAID) (e.g., indomethacin, low-dose aspirin). As a result, many anesthesiologists have abandoned the use of the bleeding time measurement before administration of regional anesthesia in these patients.

THROMBOELASTOGRAPHY

Thromboelastography (TEG) is a simple test that measures whole blood coagulation and can rapidly provide information about the adequacy of platelet function and other coagulation factors.[35] Thromboelastographic parameters are interrelated and reflect activities of coagulation proteins, platelets, and their interaction. A simplified diagram of TEG parameters related to intrinsic and extrinsic coagulation appears in Figure 42-2. TEG has been used to determine the coagulation status in normal and high-risk pregnant women,[36] to manage peripartum coagulopathy,[37] and to assess hemostasis before the administration of epidural anesthesia in pregnant patients with thrombocytopenia.[38] Some investigators found a correlation between TEG measurements and low-molecular-weight heparin (LMWH) anticoagulation activity, as measured by serum anti-Xa concentrations. They concluded that TEG might be a useful test to monitor LMWH activity.[39] TEG has been criticized for its inability to diagnose a specific coagulation defect.[40] A recent study suggests that the modified TEG using the monoclonal antibody fragment c7E3 Fab, which inhibits platelet interaction with fibrinogen by binding to glycoprotein IIb/IIIa platelet surface receptors, may provide information about the independent contribution of fibrinogen and platelets to the blood clot strength.[41] Further studies are required to determine the ability of TEG to predict the risk for epidural hematoma after the administration of epidural or spinal anesthesia in pregnant patients.

PFA-100™ (PLATELET FUNCTION ANALYZER)

The PFA-100™ has been designed to measure platelet function in vitro, especially platelet activation and aggregation. This simple test evaluates the capacity of a sodium-citrated whole blood sample to form a platelet plug at the aperture situated on a collagen/ADP or collagen/epinephrine surface under high-shear conditions. The time required for full occlusion of the aperture by the platelet plug is designated as the *closure time*. Some investigators have found this test equally sensitive to platelet aggregometry and more sensitive than the bleeding time in detecting both congenital and acetylsalicylic acid-induced platelet defects.[42] In a study involving pregnant women, the PFA-100 measurements were increased in preeclamptic women with or without thrombocytopenia.[43] More studies are

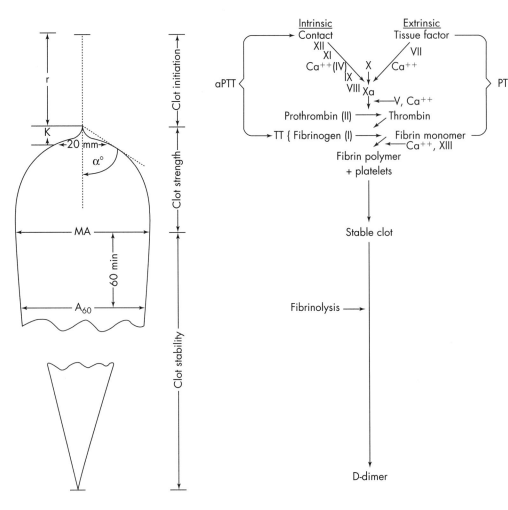

FIGURE 42-2. Simplified side-by-side presentation of thromboelastographic parameters and the routine coagulation profile. *r,* reaction time; *K,* clot formation time; α *angle,* clot formation rate; *MA,* maximum amplitude; *A60,* amplitude 60 minutes after MA; *aPTT,* activated partial thromboplastin time; *PT,* prothrombin time; *TT,* thrombin time. (From Sharma SK, Vera RL, Stegall WC, Whitten CW. Management of a postpartum coagulopathy using thromboelastography. J Clin Anesth 1997; 9:243-7.)

warranted to determine the clinical value of PFA-100 measurements in pregnant women.

THROMBOCYTOPENIC COAGULOPATHIES

Autoimmune Thrombocytopenic Purpura

Several terms have been used to describe this disease. *Idiopathic thrombocytopenic purpura* was used first, but the name was changed to *immune thrombocytopenic purpura* when it was discovered that immunoglobulin G (IgG) antibodies were responsible for the increased platelet destruction.[44] Currently the preferred term is **autoimmune thrombocytopenic purpura (ATP)**. This disease should not be confused with neonatal alloimmune thrombocytopenia, in which maternal antibodies to a fetal platelet antigen cause fetal and neonatal thrombocytopenia.

The incidence of mild thrombocytopenia during pregnancy is between 4.6% and 8.3%,[45,46] but the incidence of ATP most likely is much closer to 0.01%.[47] Antibodies directed against platelet antigens are produced primarily in the spleen, where phagocytosis by macrophages also occurs. Antibody production and phagocytosis also can occur in the liver and bone marrow. The binding of complement to platelets can facilitate their clearance,[48] and antibody binding to megakaryocytes can result in the ineffective production of platelets.[49]

DIAGNOSIS

The diagnosis of ATP must be considered if the platelet count is less than 100,000/mm³ and normal or increased numbers of megakaryocytes are present in the bone marrow. Moreover, the blood smear often reveals the presence of increased platelet volume and diameter.[50] Other **nonimmunologic conditions** that must be considered include (1) **gestational or essential thrombocytopenia,** (2) **preeclampsia,** (3) **disseminated intravascular coagulation (DIC)**, and (4) **thrombotic thrombocytopenic purpura.** Other **immunologic** conditions that must be considered include (1) **drug-induced thrombocytopenia,**[51] (2) **posttransfusion purpura** (in this case, a blood transfusion in the previous 2 weeks is likely),[52] and (3) **pseudothrombocytopenia.** Pseudothrombocytopenia is a laboratory artifact. In cases of pseudothrombocytopenia, chelation of Ca++ by ethylenediamine-tetraacetate (EDTA) exposes antigenic sites that react with antibodies, which causes clumping and artificially lowers the platelet count.[53] In these cases, the automated platelet count is normal if citrate anticoagulant is used.

INTERACTION WITH PREGNANCY

If ATP is diagnosed during pregnancy, conservative management typically is sufficient. Corticosteroids are administered if the platelet count is less than 20,000/mm³ before the onset of labor or less than 50,000/mm³ at the time of delivery.[54] High-dose intravenous immunoglobulin produces a rapid but transient increase in the platelet count and is administered if the patient fails to respond to corticosteroid therapy. In some women with preexisting ATP who become pregnant, thrombocytopenia becomes sufficiently severe that administration of high-dose corticosteroids and immunoglobulin is inadequate, and splenectomy eventually may be necessary.[55]

Some obstetricians have observed significant hemorrhage during the immediate postpartum period in as many as 33% of women with a platelet count of less than 100,000/mm³.[56] In contrast, others have noted no increase in peripartum blood loss in women with a platelet count of between 60,000/mm³ and 100,000/mm³.[57] Because episiotomies and perineal lacerations pose the greatest potential for intrapartum bleeding, it is preferable to avoid performing an episiotomy in thrombocytopenic women, if possible. Bleeding occurs less often from the placental implantation site.[58] (Contraction of the uterus represents the primary mechanism for postpartum hemostasis.) After delivery, platelet count often returns to normal in these patients.[59]

OBSTETRIC MANAGEMENT

Maternal IgG can cross the placenta and cause fetal thrombocytopenia, which increases the risk of neonatal hemorrhage. Although there is a correlation between maternal platelet-associated IgG and fetal thrombocytopenia,[58] it is not possible to predict the degree of fetal thrombocytopenia based on maternal platelet count[60] or serology.[61] No study has demonstrated a correlation between the fetal platelet count and intrapartum fetal risk. To our knowledge, there are no definitive reports of fetal intracranial hemorrhage secondary to ATP. Neonatal intracranial hemorrhage is rare and is not related to the method of delivery.[62] Thus some obstetricians have concluded that cesarean section should be reserved for obstetric indications.[62] Others contend that a fetal platelet count of less than 50,000/mm³ mandates the performance of cesarean section.[63] Fetal scalp blood sampling during labor represents a conservative management approach. Percutaneous umbilical cord blood sampling at 38 weeks' gestation has been suggested. However, it is likely that the risk of the procedure is greater than the risk of intrapartum fetal hemorrhage.

Thrombotic Thrombocytopenic Purpura

The classic pentad that defines the syndrome of thrombotic thrombocytopenic purpura (TTP) includes (1) fever; (2) thrombocytopenia (platelet count as low as 20,000/mm³); (3) microangiopathic hemolytic anemia; (4) neurologic signs such as photophobia, headache, and seizures; and (5) renal failure.[64] These five characteristics need not be present simultaneously. The neurologic and renal changes result from the deposition of platelet emboli and may be of variable intensity in the acute presentation and during recurrences. Diseases that share some of the clinical findings of TTP include DIC, preeclampsia, and hemolytic uremia syndrome.

Disseminated platelet aggregation is a hallmark of TTP.[64,65] Decreased levels of the large multimeric forms of von Willebrand factor are seen in the acute phase of TTP,[66] and these levels return to normal during remission. This is in contrast to hemolytic uremic syndrome, in which the large multimeric forms of von Willebrand factor are present in normal amounts. The affinity of von Willebrand factor for platelet membrane glycoprotein IIb/IIIa also is increased in TTP.[65] The presence of von Willebrand factor (but not fibrinogen) in platelet aggregates helps to differentiate TTP from DIC.[67] (In patients with DIC, fibrinogen but not von Willebrand factor is found in the platelet aggregates.)

Approximately 70% of patients who achieve remission develop at least one recurrence.[68] Whether pregnancy affects the incidence of primary or recurrent episodes of TTP is controversial.[69,70] Fetal death typically occurs if TTP devel-

TABLE 42-4	DRUGS THAT AFFECT PLATELET FUNCTION
Category	**Drugs**
Inhibitors of cyclooxygenase	Aspirin, NSAIDs
Stimulators of adenylcyclase	Prostaglandin E₁, prostacyclin
Inhibitors of phosphodiesterase	Caffeine, theophylline
Antibiotics	Penicillins, cephalosporins
Anticoagulants	Heparin
Volume expanders	Dextran, hydroxyethyl starch

ops during the first trimester.[69] Effective treatments include (1) infusion of 30 to 50 mL/kg of plasma, combined with plasmapheresis (approximately 75% plasma exchange); (2) intravenous IgG (400 mg/kg/day); (3) prednisone (1 to 2 mg/kg/day); and (4) infusion of prostacyclin (4 to 9 ng/kg/min).[71-73] Platelet transfusions should be avoided. Termination of pregnancy may be beneficial if the treatment is ineffective[74]; however, evacuation of uterine contents does not always result in clinical improvement.[69,70] Because of the coagulopathy present in these patients, regional anesthesia is not recommended.

Drug-Induced Platelet Disorders

Drugs can **accelerate platelet destruction** by an immunologic mechanism[75]; however, the drugs that are most likely to result in this complication are not used often in obstetric patients (e.g., quinidine, quinine, gold salts, heparin).

In contrast, drugs that **decrease platelet function** often are used in obstetric patients (Table 42-4). Aspirin irreversibly inactivates cyclooxygenase and increases the bleeding time 1.5 to 2 times.[76] The bleeding time is prolonged for 1 to 4 days after the ingestion of aspirin,[77] and in vitro platelet function tests can remain abnormal for as long as 1 week.[78] It has been suggested that the maternal ingestion of aspirin may increase the risk of both maternal and neonatal hemorrhage.[79] However, one controlled study demonstrated that doses of aspirin that prolonged the bleeding time did not result in prolonged bleeding after gastric punch biopsy.[80] Therefore in the *absence* of a preexisting hemostatic defect (e.g., von Willebrand disease, hemophilia A, uremia) in which aspirin's effect is more pronounced,[81,82] recent ingestion of aspirin does *not* contraindicate the administration of epidural or spinal anesthesia.[83]

Other NSAIDs (e.g., ibuprofen, indomethacin, naproxen) reversibly inhibit cyclooxygenase. These drugs have only a transient effect on the bleeding time[76,77] and have been given to patients with hemostatic diseases (e.g., hemophilia A) without deleterious effect.[84] Maternal ingestion of these drugs should not affect anesthetic management.

Drugs that increase platelet cyclic adenosine monophosphate (cAMP) levels decrease platelet responsiveness. This increase in cAMP levels can occur after the administration of prostaglandin E₁ or prostacyclin (which stimulates adenyl cyclase)[85] or after the administration of drugs that decrease the destruction of cAMP (e.g., caffeine, theophylline).

Most penicillins and some cephalosporins decrease platelet activity.[86] In addition to heparin's effect on the coagulation system, heparin decreases platelet function by decreasing the production of thrombin, which is a potent platelet activator. Dextran, which is absorbed onto platelet membranes, can

reduce platelet aggregation. Because platelet membranes are a substrate for steps in the coagulation system, clot formation also may be impaired by dextran. Hydroxyethyl starch also appears to decrease platelet function.[87]

CONGENITAL COAGULOPATHIES

von Willebrand Disease

This hemostatic disorder was first described in 1926 by Erich von Willebrand.[88] von Willebrand factor is synthesized by endothelial cells and megakaryocytes. The von Willebrand factor subunit is approximately 260 to 275 kilodaltons (kDa) in size. A dimer is formed by a combination of two subunits, and variable numbers of the dimers are combined to form multimers that range in size from 500 to 200,000 kDa. von Willebrand factor plays two primary roles in coagulation: (1) it forms a complex with factor VIII, which decreases the excretion of factor VIII, and (2) it mediates platelet adhesion by binding to platelets (a reaction enhanced by ristocetin) and collagen. von Willebrand disease typically is inherited as an autosomal dominant trait, and it has an incidence that ranges from 1:100 to 1:2500 for the mild form[89,90] and from 1:200,000 to 1:2,000,000 for the severe homozygous form.[91,92]

Multiple factors control the synthesis of von Willebrand factor. Patients with von Willebrand disease have variable levels of both von Willebrand factor and factor VIII. Thus some patients with von Willebrand disease are asymptomatic. Because von Willebrand factor aids in platelet binding to sites of vascular damage, symptoms of von Willebrand disease (e.g., bleeding from skin and mucosae) can mimic those of platelet disorders. Because von Willebrand factor slows clearance of factor VIII, a deficiency can result in decreased factor VIII levels, and patients with severe disease can present with hemorrhages into muscles and joints similar to those seen in patients with classic hemophilia.

Patients with von Willebrand disease differ from those with hemophilia in several respects. In von Willebrand disease, platelet function is affected, and the bleeding time typically is prolonged. In contrast, the bleeding time typically is normal in patients with hemophilia. Patients with von Willebrand disease typically have decreased platelet aggregation in response to ristocetin. In patients with hemophilia, the infusion of small amounts of normal serum or serum from patients with hemophilia have minimal effect on factor VIII levels. Patients with von Willebrand disease have a prolonged increase in factor VIII levels after the infusion of small amounts of serum from normal patients or patients with hemophilia.

von Willebrand disease can be divided into several subtypes based on quantitative and qualitative defects in von Willebrand factor.[93] If patients lack the larger multimers, they can have normal factor VIII activity, but they have decreased platelet adhesion and a prolonged bleeding time.

During pregnancy, prophylactic treatment is reserved for those patients with a factor VIII level below 25%. For patients with von Willebrand disease type I or IIa, 0.3 μg/kg of l-deamino-8-D-arginine vasopressin (DDAVP) is administered as labor begins, and the dose is repeated every 12 hours. For patients who are not responsive to DDAVP, fresh frozen plasma or cryoprecipitate (500 to 1500 units of factor VIII activity) should be administered. Most commercial preparations of factor VIII lose von Willebrand factor in the manufacturing process; however, this factor is retained in the processing of Humate-P, a pasteurized factor VIII concentrate, which may control hemorrhage in patients with von Willebrand disease who are unresponsive to cryoprecipitate.[94]

During labor, factor VIII levels should be maintained at 50% of normal. If cesarean section is required, treatment should be instituted to increase the factor VIII level to 80% of normal. The factor VIII level should be checked daily during the postpartum period, and treatment should be initiated if the factor VIII level falls below 25% or if significant bleeding occurs.[95]

Other Coagulation Factor Deficiencies

In males, the two most common coagulation factor deficiencies are factor VIII (hemophilia A) and factor IX (hemophilia B). Both occur as X-linked traits. A female can have hemophilia if her father is a hemophiliac and her mother is a carrier for hemophilia and passes the abnormal X chromosome to her daughter. A female also can have hemophilia if she is a carrier (i.e., she received one abnormal gene from a carrier mother or an affected father) and there is either a new mutation of the other gene for factor VIII or IX or there is another X-chromosome abnormality.[96]

In early embryogenesis, half of the X chromosomes are inactivated. As a population, half of the abnormal genes and half of the normal genes are inactivated in females who are heterozygous for hemophilia A or B. On average, these women will have half of the normal concentration of factor VIII or IX, which typically is adequate for coagulation. Because the chromosome inactivation is random, more abnormal genes are inactivated in a certain percentage of carriers, and these women will have a normal concentration of factor VIII or IX. However, if most of the normal genes are inactivated, the individual can have severely depressed levels of factor VIII or IX. If such a patient becomes pregnant, factor supplementation or plasma exchange (with fresh frozen plasma) may be necessary before or during delivery.[97]

Half of the male children of heterozygous carriers for hemophilia A or B will have hemophilia. These infants have an increased incidence of excessive bleeding after circumcision, but the incidence of cephalohematoma does not appear to be increased.[98] It is not clear whether the mode of delivery affects the incidence of cephalohematoma. Heterozygous carriers may undergo a trial of labor and vaginal delivery, but the following procedures should be avoided: (1) placement of a fetal scalp electrode, (2) fetal scalp blood pH determination, (3) vacuum extraction, and (4) difficult forceps delivery.[99] Maternal considerations should affect the decision to administer (or not administer) regional anesthesia.

Other congenital factor deficiencies occur as autosomal recessive traits and manifest symptoms only in the homozygous state. Detailed descriptions of these rare disorders can be found elsewhere.[100,101]

Table 42-5 lists the plasma concentrations of coagulation factors that are required for hemostasis. If liver disease or a vitamin K deficiency is responsible for the coagulopathy, the patient may benefit from intramuscular administration of vitamin K. A deficiency can be corrected more rapidly by the administration of 10 to 20 mL/kg of fresh frozen plasma.

ACQUIRED COAGULOPATHIES

Disseminated Intravascular Coagulation

DIC results from an abnormal activation of the coagulation system, which results in (1) formation of large amounts of

TABLE 42-5	MINIMUM COAGULATION FACTOR LEVELS

Coagulation factor	Plasma concentration required for hemostasis (U or IU/dL)
I	10-25
II	40
V	10-15
VII	5-10
VIII	10-40
IX	10-40
X	10-15
XI	20-30
XIII	1-5

thrombin, (2) depletion of coagulation factors, (3) activation of the fibrinolytic system, and (4) hemorrhage. In the obstetric population, the most frequent causes of DIC are preeclampsia, placental abruption, sepsis, retained dead fetus syndrome, and amniotic fluid embolism.[102]

Laboratory findings consistent with DIC include a decreased platelet count; decreased fibrinogen and antithrombin III concentrations; variable increases in prothrombin, partial thromboplastin, thrombin, and reptilase times; and increased concentrations of *D*-dimer, fibrin monomer, and fibrin degradation products.

Therapeutic goals for these patients are as follows: (1) treat or remove the precipitating cause, (2) stop ongoing proteolytic activity (i.e., both the coagulation and fibrinolytic pathways), (3) replace depleted coagulation factors, and (4) provide multisystem support as required. In obstetric patients, evacuation of the uterine contents often results in removal of the precipitating cause. A vaginal delivery can be attempted if the mother is stable and delivery can be achieved in a timely manner. If delivery cannot be achieved quickly, cesarean section may be required. Rarely, it may be necessary to perform cesarean section to deliver a dead fetus.

Considerable controversy exists regarding the medical management of these patients. Management may vary according to the etiology of DIC. If the patient has placental abruption, the physician should give cryoprecipitate or fresh frozen plasma to maintain a fibrinogen concentration above 150 mg/dL and platelets to maintain a platelet count above 100,000/mm³.

The use of heparin is controversial. Some physicians have advocated the use of heparin in patients with retained dead fetus syndrome and hypofibrinogenemia,[103] in patients with amniotic fluid embolism who do not have severe hemorrhage,[102] in patients who are septic,[104] and in patients with evidence of peripheral deposition of fibrin.[105] Standard heparin can be administered either intravenously or subcutaneously at a dose of 300 to 700 U/hr.[102] LMWH can be given subcutaneously at a rate of 75 U/kg/day.[106] Heparin can cause thrombocytopenia by a nonimmunologic or an immunologic mechanism,[107] but the risk of this problem may be reduced by administration of LMWH.[106,108] Both standard heparin and LMWH are effective only in the presence of an adequate concentration of antithrombin III. Patients with DIC may have a depleted concentration of antithrombin III, and administration of fresh frozen plasma may be necessary. In addition to fresh frozen plasma, infusion of cryoprecipitate and platelets may be necessary to restore adequate levels of coagulation factors. The use of epsilon-aminocaproic acid, aprotinin, and

antithrombin III concentrates as treatment for DIC is controversial. Recent evidence suggests that administration of antithrombin III is beneficial in the treatment of DIC and sometimes improves organ function.[109]

These patients often have multiorgan system failure and require mechanical ventilatory support. DIC almost always mandates the administration of general anesthesia for those patients who require cesarean section.

Therapeutic Anticoagulation

Most pregnant women who require chronic anticoagulation receive heparin throughout pregnancy. If warfarin is administered during pregnancy, it typically is discontinued in favor of heparin before the onset of labor. If a patient begins labor while she is still taking warfarin, the effects can be reversed by intramuscular administration of vitamin K. Because reversal of anticoagulation requires time for the synthesis of new procoagulants, acute reversal can be accomplished by the administration of 10 to 20 mL/kg of fresh frozen plasma.

If the patient is receiving standard heparin, the drug can be stopped, and the normalization of coagulation can be monitored by following the aPTT or the activated coagulation time (ACT). If conditions require immediate reversal, 50 mg of protamine can be administered intravenously, with additional doses given as determined by the aPTT or the ACT.

If coagulation is deemed adequate for cesarean section, a regional anesthetic technique can be considered. The anesthesiologist should weigh the risks and benefits of regional and general anesthesia for the individual patient. Ideally, we would prefer not to administer regional anesthesia to a patient with a persistent laboratory abnormality of coagulation. However, in selected circumstances, we may offer regional anesthesia to a patient with an isolated laboratory abnormality and no clinical evidence of coagulopathy. In such patients, frequent neurologic examinations are performed to facilitate the early detection of an epidural hematoma during the postpartum period.

Other Acquired Coagulopathies

Coagulopathies associated with pregnancy-induced hypertension and volume resuscitation after hemorrhage are discussed in Chapters 44 and 37, respectively.

REGIONAL ANESTHESIA IN THE PATIENT WITH ONGOING COAGULOPATHY

Concern exists that an epidural hematoma may develop after the administration of regional anesthesia in patients with coagulopathy. There are only eight published cases of epidural or spinal subdural hematoma after the administration of epidural anesthesia in pregnant patients.[110,111] This suggests that epidural hematoma after regional anesthesia either is very rare (and the risk has been overstated) or is underreported. However, in view of the serious consequences of an epidural hematoma, the anesthesiologist should carefully assess the risks and benefits of performing regional anesthesia in a patient with either clinical or laboratory evidence of coagulopathy.

Frank coagulopathy represents an absolute contraindication to the administration of epidural or spinal anesthesia. The anesthesiologist can use PT/INR, aPTT, and ACT measurements or TEG to assess the extent of anticoagulation

and the effectiveness of reversal in patients receiving standard heparin or oral anticoagulation therapy. If a regional anesthetic technique is considered in a patient with a congenital coagulopathy, the factor assays (e.g., factor VIII activity and factor VIII ristocetin cofactor activity in patients with von Willebrand disease; factor VIII and factor IX levels in patients with hemophilia A and B, respectively) should be within the normal range before needle placement.[93]

Through the years, a large number of patients have received regional anesthesia while receiving subcutaneous thromboprophylaxis with standard, unfractionated heparin, without neurologic complications. Safe practice typically includes the following precautions: (1) proper dosing of heparin, (2) atraumatic placement of the needle and/or catheter, and (3) measurement of a platelet count in patients on prolonged heparin therapy. Some anesthesiologists prefer to avoid needle/catheter placement or removal within 4 hours of the last dose of standard heparin.

The American Society of Regional Anesthesia and Pain Medicine (ASRA) convened its second Consensus Conference on Neuraxial Anesthesia and Anticoagulation in April, 2002, to provide guidelines to improve the safety of regional anesthesia/analgesia in anticoagulated patients.[112] The Consensus Conference concluded that subcutaneous (mini-dose) thromboprophylaxis with standard, unfractionated heparin does *not* contraindicate the use of neuraxial anesthetic techniques. However, the platelet count should be assessed before the administration of neuraxial anesthesia and/or catheter removal in patients who have received standard heparin for more than 4 days. In patients receiving chronic *oral* anticoagulation therapy, the anticoagulation therapy should be stopped at least 4 to 5 days before the planned procedure, and the PT/INR should be measured before needle placement.

LMWH (e.g., exoxaparin) is considered to be more efficacious for thromboprophylaxis compared with standard, unfractionated heparin, and has been used safely in pregnant women.[108] At least 53 cases of epidural/spinal hematoma after spinal or epidural anesthesia in nonobstetric patients receiving LMWH have been reported.[112,113] The Food and Drug Administration issued a warning in December, 1997, calling attention to the risk of epidural or spinal hematoma with the concurrent use of LMWH and epidural or spinal anesthesia. The apparent increase in the risk of an epidural hematoma after concurrent administration of regional anesthesia and prophylactic LMWH may be related to the use of higher doses of LMWH, and the relatively greater bioavailability and longer biologic half-life of LMWH after subcutaneous injection, when compared with standard heparin.

The ASRA Consensus Conference concluded that in patients receiving preoperative LMWH for thromboprophylaxis, needle placement should occur at least 10 to 12 hours after the last LMWH dose.[112] In patients receiving higher doses of LMWH (e.g., enoxaparin 1 mg/kg every 12 hours, enoxaparin 1.5 mg/kg daily, dalteparin 120 U/kg every 12 hours, dalteparin 200 U/kg daily, or tinzaparin 175 U/kg daily), needle placement should not occur until at least 24 hours after the last dose of LMWH.[112]

In patients receiving a single daily dose of LMWH thromboprophylaxis, the first postoperative LMWH dose should be administered 6 to 8 hours after surgery. An indwelling epidural catheter may be safely maintained in these patients; however, it should be removed at least 10 to 12 hours after the last dose of LMWH, and the next dose of LMWH should be administered at least 2 hours *after* catheter removal. In patients receiving higher (e.g., twice-daily) doses of LMWH, the first dose of LMWH should be delayed for 24 hours postoperatively, and an indwelling catheter should be removed at least 2 hours *before* initiation of LMWH therapy.[112]

The anti-Xa level is not predictive of the risk of bleeding during/following administration of regional anesthesia. Concomitant administration of medications affecting hemostasis (e.g., administration of both LMWH and an antiplatelet drug) further increases the risk of hemorrhagic complications.[112]

The assessment of risk is more problematic in the patient with isolated laboratory evidence of coagulopathy. Thrombocytopenia (with variable degrees of decreased platelet function) is common in women with severe preeclampsia (see Chapter 44). Asymptomatic thrombocytopenia also may occur in healthy obstetric patients. Some anesthesiologists have reported the safe administration of epidural anesthesia—without any neurologic complications—in thrombocytopenic (i.e., platelet count less than 100,000/mm^3) healthy pregnant women, preeclamptic women, and women with ATP.[114] These anesthesiologists state that in the absence of clinical evidence of bleeding, regional anesthesia should not necessarily be withheld in pregnant women with a platelet count of less than 100,000/mm^3. These studies of regional anesthesia in thrombocytopenic patients are small and retrospective and do not exclude the possibility that modest thrombocytopenia increases the risk for epidural hematoma. However, no published evidence suggests that a specific platelet count predicts the risk of epidural hematoma in obstetric patients.

When determining whether regional anesthesia is safe in a thrombocytopenic patient, multiple factors should be considered. These include (1) clinical evidence of bleeding, (2) recent platelet count, (3) a recent change in the platelet count, (4) quality of platelets, (5) adequacy of coagulation factors, and most important, (6) the risk versus the benefit of performing regional anesthesia. In our judgment, the bleeding time measurement is *not* helpful in determining the risk of epidural hematoma. TEG provides a qualitative assessment of circulating platelets and coagulation factor activity. Although TEG shows some promise, its usefulness in predicting the risk for epidural hematoma is unproved.

Clinical judgment represents the most important means of assessing the risk for epidural hematoma in an individual patient. Clearly, the anesthesiologist would not want to perform regional anesthesia in a patient with clinical evidence of coagulopathy (e.g., bleeding from nasal or oral mucosae or venipuncture sites, presence of petechiae and/or ecchymoses). In contrast, consider the example of a patient with severe preeclampsia, severe upper airway edema, a stable platelet count of 100,000/mm^3, and no clinical evidence of coagulopathy. In our judgment, the risk of a failed intubation is greater than the risk of an epidural hematoma in such a patient. We would offer epidural analgesia to such a patient after a thorough discussion of the risks and benefits. In contrast, some anesthesiologists advocate a more conservative approach in such cases, and recommend alternative methods of analgesia during labor, followed by awake laryngoscopy and intubation if cesarean section should become necessary.

We do not obtain a bleeding time measurement in patients who have received low-dose aspirin during pregnancy for the prevention of preeclampsia and who have no other risk factors for bleeding. Low-dose aspirin (i.e., 60 to 75 mg) does not significantly prolong the bleeding time in pregnant women.[115] Moreover, a large number of women receiving low-dose

aspirin therapy for the prevention or treatment of preeclampsia have received uncomplicated epidural analgesia for labor and delivery.[116]

There are several modifications of technique that may decrease the risk of venous injury during the administration of epidural analgesia. These include (1) administration of epidural analgesia during early labor before the platelet count or platelet function declines, (2) use of a midline technique, (3) use of a small needle and catheter, and (4) administration of saline through the needle to distend the epidural space before insertion of the catheter. In addition, the epidural catheter may be placed several hours before the patient requires analgesia. This interval allows the anesthesiologist to observe for symptoms and signs of epidural hematoma formation (e.g., back pain, radicular pain, leg weakness) before the administration of an analgesic/anesthetic solution. This last recommendation is impractical in most circumstances. Further, it is unclear that any of these recommendations decrease the likelihood of epidural hematoma in patients with platelet dysfunction or coagulopathy.

During the administration of epidural analgesia, the anesthesiologist can minimize motor blockade by administering a dilute solution of local anesthetic with an opioid (e.g., 0.0625% bupivacaine with 2 μg/mL of fentanyl). The anesthesiologist should subsequently perform a neurologic examination at 1- to 2-hour intervals to detect evidence of neurologic compromise secondary to an epidural hematoma. If unexplained neurologic deficits occur, immediate steps should be taken to exclude the occurrence of an epidural hematoma (see Chapter 33).

Similar precautions should be taken during the administration of postoperative analgesia. Bromage[117] made the following observations:

Severe back pain and, later, root pain emanating from the site of compression are the earliest signs calling for urgent neurologic assessment. This implies that postoperative pain management interventions must not distort normal neurologic function. Therefore, intraspinal local anesthetic and opioids should be short acting so that any analgesic intraspinal infusion can be shut off periodically and at least 6 and 12 hours after surgery, so that a valid neurologic examination can be carried out and documented at those times. If signs of hematoma arise, the patient is then committed to the serious and costly course of early and appropriate imaging—magnetic resonance imaging and/or myelography—followed by urgent laminectomy if cord compression is confirmed. This is a formidable contingency plan, costly and risky at best, but with the prospect of catastrophic paralysis if spinal-cord compression is delayed beyond the short period of 6 to 12 hours when full recovery may be expected.

In some cases, severe thrombocytopenia and coagulopathy may develop *after* the placement of an epidural catheter. In such cases, many anesthesiologists contend that the catheter should *not* be removed until the patient has normal coagulation.[118,119] They argue that movement or removal of the catheter may dislodge a clot, resulting in fresh bleeding and an epidural hematoma. This is a matter of dispute. Others recommend leaving the catheter in situ until delivery and removing it promptly after delivery.[120]

HYPERCOAGULABLE STATES

Effective hemostasis is maintained by an appropriate balance of procoagulant and anticoagulant activity. A congenital deficiency in anticoagulant activity occurs in approximately 0.02% of the population and in 2% to 5% of persons with a history of venous thrombosis.[121] Protein C, protein S, and antithrombin III deficiencies are the most common causes of hypercoagulability, with plasminogen deficiency and dysfibrinogenemia less common.[122] Venous thromboses are more common than arterial thromboses, and their incidence increases with surgery, pregnancy, oral contraceptive use, and immobilization.[121] These patients have an increased incidence of IUGR and intrauterine fetal death, perhaps as a result of placental thrombosis and insufficiency.

Protein C Deficiency

Protein C is produced in the liver, and it requires vitamin K for its synthesis. It acts by inhibiting *activated* factors V and VIII. The incidence of protein C deficiency is approximately 1 in 15,000.

Protein C levels normally increase by 35% during pregnancy, but this increase is attenuated in patients with protein C deficiency.[123] In patients with protein C deficiency, thrombosis occurs in 25% of pregnancies unless anticoagulation therapy is administered.[124] Two thirds of these episodes occur during the postpartum period. Heparin should be administered during the first and third trimesters, and either heparin or warfarin is administered during the second trimester and postpartum period.

Protein C is a vitamin K-dependent protein with a short half-life (8 hours). If warfarin is administered without prior heparin anticoagulation, protein C levels fall before the levels of factors II, VII, IX, and X fall. Thrombosis with skin necrosis can result.[121]

Protein S Deficiency

In contrast to protein C, the plasma levels of protein S normally *decrease* during pregnancy.[123] Protein S also is produced in the liver and depends on vitamin K for its synthesis. Protein S acts as a cofactor for protein C. Circulating protein S binds to C4b-binding protein (a protein of the complement system), but it is the free fraction that acts as a cofactor for protein C. Immunologic assays measure total protein S concentrations; therefore a diagnosis of protein S deficiency is made either by using a functional assay or by calculating the percent of protein S bound to C4b-binding protein. The treatment for protein S deficiency is identical to that for protein C deficiency.

Antithrombin III Deficiency

Antithrombin III is synthesized in the liver and endothelial cells. It inactivates thrombin and factors IXa, Xa, XIa, and XIIa. Its activity is potentiated by heparin. Deficiency of antithrombin III occurs in 1 in 5000 persons.[125] Quantitative (type I) and qualitative (type II) deficiencies can exist; thus both immunologic and functional assays are required to detect abnormalities.

The risk of thrombosis during pregnancy increases from 0.1% in normal persons[126] to 55% to 68% in untreated patients with antithrombin III deficiency.[124,127] Anticoagulation or antithrombin III replacement is indicated during pregnancy.[128] Heparin is administered during the first and third trimesters, and heparin or warfarin is administered during the second trimester and postpartum period. Heparin acts by

potentiating the activity of antithrombin III. Therefore if antithrombin III levels are decreased, heparin's activity also is decreased. This may necessitate the administration of more heparin to patients with antithrombin III deficiency[128] or administration of antithrombin III concentrate (20 to 40 mg/kg) along with the heparin.[121] Alternatively, some experts recommend the administration of antithrombin III only during labor and the postpartum period.[129]

Lupus Anticoagulant

The term *lupus anticoagulant* is a misnomer. These patients do not have a coagulopathy; rather, they are at risk for thromboembolic events. The hypercoagulable state associated with lupus anticoagulant is discussed in Chapter 39.

KEY POINTS

- Regional anesthetic techniques can be used safely during labor and delivery in patients with hemoglobinopathies.
- The first goal in the treatment of disseminated intravascular coagulation is to treat or remove the precipitating cause. In pregnant patients, evacuation of the uterine contents often results in removal of the precipitating cause.
- No evidence suggests that the bleeding time correctly predicts the risk of bleeding within the epidural space in an individual patient.
- Uncorrected, frank coagulopathy represents an absolute contraindication to the administration of epidural or spinal anesthesia.
- In a patient with an isolated laboratory abnormality and no clinical evidence of coagulopathy, the anesthesiologist should assess the risks and benefits of performing regional anesthesia.

REFERENCES

1. Liebhaber SA, Kan YW. Differentiation of the mRNA transcripts originating from the α_1- and α_2-globin loci in normals and α-thalassemics. J Clin Invest 1981; 68:439-46.
2. Orkin SH, Goff SC. The duplicated human α-globin genes: Their relative expression as measured by RNA analysis. Cell 1981; 24:345-51.
3. Dozy AM, Kan YW, Embury SH, et al. α-Globin gene organization in blacks precludes the severe form of α-thalassaemia. Nature 1979; 280:605-7.
4. American College of Obstetricians and Gynecologists. Genetic Screening for Hemoglobinopathies. ACOG Committee Opinion No. 168. Washington, DC, 1996.
5. Weatherall DJ. The thalassemias. In Williams WJ, Beutler E, Erslev AJ, Lichtman MA, editors. Hematology. New York, McGraw-Hill, 1990:510-39.
6. Lassman MN, O'Brien RT, Pearson HA, et al. Endocrine evaluation in thalassemia major. Ann NY Acad Sci 1974; 232:226-37.
7. Canale VC, Steinherz P, New M, Erlandson M. Endocrine function in thalassemia major. Ann NY Acad Sci 1974; 232:333-45.
8. Kazazian HH Jr, Boehm CD. Molecular basis and prenatal diagnosis of β-thalassemia. Blood 1988; 72:1107-16.
9. Piomelli S, Loew T. Management of thalassemia major (Cooley's anemia). Hematol Oncol Clin North Am 1991; 5:557-69.
10. Mordel N, Birkenfeld A, Goldfarb AN, Rachmilewitz EA. Successful full-term pregnancy in homozygous β-thalassemia major: Case report and review of the literature. Obstet Gynecol 1989; 73:837-40.
11. Singounas EG, Sakas DE, Hadley DM, et al. Paraplegia in a pregnant thalassemic woman due to extramedullary hematopoiesis: Successful management with transfusions. Surg Neurol 1991; 36:210-5.
12. Beutler E. The sickle cell diseases and related disorders. In Williams WJ, Beutler E, Erslev AJ, Lichtman MA, editors. Hematology. New York, McGraw-Hill, 1990:613-44.
13. Motulsky AG. Frequency of sickling disorders in U.S. Blacks. N Engl J Med 1973; 288:31-3.
14. Solanki DL, McCurdy PR, Cuttitta FF, Schechter GP. Hemolysis in sickle cell disease as measured by endogenous carbon monoxide production. Am J Clin Path 1988; 89:221-5.
15. Veille JC, Hanson R. Left ventricular systolic and diastolic function in pregnant patients with sickle cell disease. Am J Obstet Gynecol 1994; 170:107-10.
16. Tsen LC, Cherayil G: Sickle cell-induced peripheral neuropathy following spinal anesthesia for cesarean delivery. Anesthesiology 2001; 95:1298-9.
17. Chang JC, Kan YW. A sensitive new prenatal test for sickle-cell anemia. N Engl J Med 1982; 307:30-2.
18. Goossens M, Dumez Y, Kaplan L, et al. Prenatal diagnosis of sickle-cell anemia in the first trimester of pregnancy. N Engl J Med 1983; 309:831-3.
19. Poddar D, Maude GH, Plant MJ, et al. Pregnancy in Jamaican women with homozygous sickle cell disease: Fetal and maternal outcome. Br J Obstet Gynaecol 1986; 93:727-32.
20. Koshy M, Burd L, Wallace D, et al. Prophylactic red-cell transfusions in pregnant patients with sickle cell disease. N Engl J Med 1988; 319:1447-52.
21. Platt OS, Orkin SH, Dover G, et al. Hydroxyurea enhances fetal hemoglobin production in sickle cell anemia. J Clin Invest 1984; 74:652-6.
22. Vermylen C, Fernandez-Robles E, Ninane J, Cornu G. Bone marrow transplantation in five children with sickle cell anaemia. Lancet 1988; 1:1427-8.
23. Barbedo MMR, McCurdy PR. Red cell life span in sickle cell trait. Acta Haematol 1974; 51:339-43.
24. Heller P, Best WR, Nelson RB, Becktel J. Clinical implications of sickle-cell trait and glucose-6-phosphate dehydrogenase deficiency in hospitalized black male patients. N Engl J Med 1979; 300:1001-5.
25. Larrabee KD, Monga M. Women with sickle cell trait are at increased risk for preeclampsia. Am J Obstet Gynecol 1997; 177:425-8.
26. Gibson J. Autoimmune hemolytic anemia: Current concepts. Aust NZ J Med 1988; 18:625-37.
27. Engelfriet CP, Overbeeke MAM, Kr von dem Borne AEG. Autoimmune hemolytic anemia. Semin Hematol 1992; 29:3-12.
28. Sokol RJ, Hewitt S. Autoimmune hemolysis: A critical review. Crit Rev Oncol Hematol 1985; 4:125-54.
29. Osterud B, Rapaport SI. Activation of factor IX by the reaction product of tissue factor and factor VII: Additional pathway for initiating blood coagulation. Proc Natl Acad Sci USA 1977; 74:5260-4.
30. Roberts HR, Monroe DM III, Hoffman M. Molecular biology and biochemistry of the coagulation factors and pathways of hemostasis. In Buetler E, Lichtman MA, Coller BS, et al., editors. Williams Hematology, 6th edition. New York, McGraw-Hill, 2001: 1409-34.
31. Bonnar J, Daly L, Sheppard BL. Changes in the fibrinolytic system during pregnancy. Semin Thromb Hemostas 1990; 16:221-9.
32. Leduc L, Wheeler JM, Kirshon B, et al. Coagulation profile in severe preeclampsia. Obstet Gynecol 1992; 79:14-8.
33. Rodgers RPC, Levin J. A critical reappraisal of the bleeding time. Semin Thromb Hemostas 1990; 16:1-20.
34. Burns ER, Lawrence C. Bleeding time: A guide to its diagnostic and clinical utility. Arch Pathol Lab Med 1989; 113:1219-24.
35. Mallett SV, Cox DJA. Thrombelastography. Br J Anaesth 1992; 69:307-13.
36. Sharma SK, Philip J, Whitten CW, et al. Assessment of changes in coagulation in parturients with preeclampsia using thromboelastography. Anesthesiology 1999; 90:385-90.
37. Sharma SK, Vera RL, Stegall WC, Whitten CW. Management of postpartum coagulopathy using thromboelastography. J Clin Anesth 1997; 9:243-7.
38. Campos CJ, Pivalizza EG, Abouleish EI. Thromboelastography in a parturient with immune thrombocytopenic purpura (letter). Anesth Analg 1998; 86:675.
39. Klein SM, Slaughter TF, Vail PT, et al. Thromboelastography as a perioperative measure of anticoagulation resulting from low molecular

weight heparin: A comparison with anti-xa concentrations. Anesth Analg 2000; 9l:1091-5.

40. Whitten CW, Greilich PE: Thromboelastography: Past, present, and future. Anesthesiology 2000; 92:1223-5.

41. Gottumukkala VNR, Sharma SK, Philip J. Assessing platelet and fibrinogen contribution to clot strength using modified thromboelastography in pregnant women. Anesth Analg 1999; 89:1453-5.

42. Mammen EF, Comp PC, Gosselin R, et al. PFA-100™ system: A new method for assessment of platelet dysfunction. Semin Thromb Hemost 1998; 24:195-202.

43. Vincelot A, Nathan N, Collet D, et al. Platelet function during pregnancy: An evaluation using the PFA-100 analyser. Br J Anaesth 2001; 87:890-3.

44. Shulman NR, Marder VJ, Weinrach RS. Similarities between known antiplatelet antibodies and the factor responsible for thrombocytopenia in idiopathic purpura: Physiologic, serologic and isotopic studies. Ann NY Acad Sci 1965; 124:499-542.

45. Freedman J, Musclow E, Garvey B, Abbott D. Unexplained periparturient thrombocytopenia. Am J Hematol 1986; 21:397-407.

46. Burrows RF, Kelton JG. Incidentally detected thrombocytopenia in healthy mothers and their infants. N Engl J Med 1988; 319:142-5.

47. Kessler I, Lancet M, Borenstein R, et al. The obstetrical management of patients with immunologic thrombocytopenic purpura. Int J Gynaecol Obstet 1982; 20:23-8.

48. McMillan R. Chronic idiopathic thrombocytopenic purpura. N Engl J Med 1981; 304:1135-47.

49. Gernsheimer T, Stratton J, Ballem PJ, Slichter SJ. Mechanisms of response to treatment in autoimmune thrombocytopenic purpura. N Engl J Med 1989; 320:974-80.

50. Greinacher A, Mueller-Eckhardt C. Hereditary types of thrombocytopenia with giant platelets and inclusion bodies in the leukocytes. Blut 1990; 60:53-60.

51. Mueller-Eckhardt C, Salama A. Drug-induced immune cytopenias: A unifying pathogenetic concept with special emphasis on the role of drug metabolites. Transfusion Med Rev 1990; 4:69-77.

52. Waters AH. Post-transfusion purpura. Blood Rev 1989; 3:83-7.

53. Pegels JG, Bruynes ECE, Engelfriet CP, Kr von dem Borne AEG. Pseudothrombocytopenia: An immunologic study on platelet antibodies dependent on ethylene diamine tetra-acetate. Blood 1982; 59:157-61.

54. Pillai M. Platelets and pregnancy. Br J Obstet Gynaecol 1993; 100:201-4.

55. Laros RK, Sweet RL. Management of idiopathic thrombocytopenic purpura during pregnancy. Am J Obstet Gynecol 1975; 122:182-90.

56. O'Reilly RA, Taber B-Z. Immunologic thrombocytopenic purpura and pregnancy. Obstet Gynecol 1978; 51:590-7.

57. Druzin ML, Stier E. Maternal platelet count at delivery in patients with idiopathic thrombocytopenic purpura, not related to perioperative complications. J Am Coll Surg 1994; 179:264-6.

58. Heys RF. Child bearing and idiopathic thrombocytopenic purpura. J Obstet Gynaecol Br Common 1966; 73:205-14.

59. Kelton JG, Inwood MJ, Barr RM, et al. The prenatal prediction of thrombocytopenia in infants of mothers with clinically diagnosed immune thrombocytopenia. Am J Obstet Gynecol 1982; 144:449-54.

60. Cines DB, Dusak B, Tomaski A, et al. Immune thrombocytopenic purpura and pregnancy. N Engl J Med 1982; 306:826-31.

61. Aster RH. "Gestational" thrombocytopenia: A plea for conservative management. N Engl J Med 1990; 323:264-6.

62. Payne SD, Resnik R, Moore TR, et al. Maternal characteristics and risk of severe neonatal thrombocytopenia and intracranial hemorrhage in pregnancies complicated by autoimmune thrombocytopenia. Am J Obstet Gynecol 1997; 177:149-55.

63. Scott JR, Cruikshank DP, Kochenour NK, et al. Fetal platelet counts in the obstetric management of immunologic thrombocytopenic purpura. Am J Obstet Gynecol 1980; 136:495-9.

64. Murphy WG, Moore JC, Warkentin TE, et al. Thrombotic thrombocytopenic purpura. Blood Coagul Fibrinolysis 1992; 3:655-9.

65. Moore JC, Murphy WG, Kelton JG. Calpain proteolysis of von Willebrand factor enhances its binding to platelet membrane glycoprotein IIb/IIIa: An explanation for platelet aggregation in thrombotic thrombocytopenic purpura. Br J Haematol 1990; 74:457-64.

66. Murphy WG, Moore JC, Baar RD, et al. Relationship between platelet aggregating factor and von Willebrand factor in thrombotic thrombocytopenic purpura. Br J Haematol 1987; 66:509-13.

67. Asada Y, Sumiyoshi A, Hayashi T, et al. Immunohistochemistry of vascular lesions in thrombotic thrombocytopenic purpura with special reference to factor VIII–related antigen. Thromb Res 1985; 38:469-79.

68. Bell WR, Braine HG, Ness PM, Kickler TS. Improved survival in thrombotic thrombocytopenic purpura-hemolytic uremic syndrome. N Engl J Med 1991; 325:398-403.

69. Pinette MG, Vintzileos AM, Ingardia CJ. Thrombotic thrombocytopenic purpura as a cause of thrombocytopenia in pregnancy: Literature review. Am J Perinatol 1989; 6:55-7.

70. Miller JM, Pastorek JG. Thrombotic thrombocytopenic purpura and hemolytic uremic syndrome in pregnancy. Clin Obstet Gynecol 1991; 34:64-71.

71. Rock GA, Shumak KH, Buskard NA, et al. Comparison of plasma exchange with plasma infusion in the treatment of thrombotic thrombocytopenic purpura. N Engl J Med 1991; 325:393-7.

72. Finn NG, Wang JC, Hong KJ. High dose intravenous gamma immunoglobulin infusion in the treatment of thrombotic thrombocytopenic purpura. Arch Intern Med 1987; 147:2165-7.

73. Tardy B, Page Y, Comtet C, et al. Intravenous prostacyclin in thrombotic thrombocytopenia purpura: Case report and review of the literature. J Int Med 1991; 230: 279-82.

74. Natelson EA, White D. Recurrent thrombotic thrombocytopenic purpura in early pregnancy: Effect of uterine evacuation. Obstet Gynecol 1985; 66(suppl 3):54S-6S.

75. Aster RH, George JN. Thrombocytopenia due to enhanced platelet destruction by immunologic mechanisms. In Williams WJ, Beutler E, Erslev AJ, Lichtman MA, editors. Hematology. New York, McGraw-Hill, 1990:1370-98.

76. Buchanan GR, Martin V, Levine PH, et al. The effects of "anti-platelet" drugs on bleeding time and platelet aggregation in normal human subjects. Am J Clin Path 1977; 68:355-9.

77. Nadell J, Bruno J, Varady J, Segre EJ. Effect of naproxen and of aspirin on bleeding time and platelet aggregation. J Clin Pharmacol 1974; 14:176-82.

78. Weiss HJ, Aledort LM, Kochwa S. The effect of salicylates on the hemostatic properties of platelets in man. J Clin Invest 1968; 47:2169-80.

79. Stuart MJ, Gross SJ, Elrad H, Graeber JE. Effects of acetylsalicylic-acid ingestion on maternal neonatal hemostasis. N Engl J Med 1982; 307:909-12.

80. O'Laughlin JC, Hoftiezer JW, Mahoney JP, Ivey KJ. Does aspirin prolong bleeding from gastric biopsies in man? Gastrointest Endosc 1981; 27:1-5.

81. Gaspari F, Vigano G, Orisio S, et al. Aspirin prolongs bleeding time in uremia by a mechanism distinct from platelet cyclooxygenase inhibition. J Clin Invest 1987; 79:1788-97.

82. Kaneshiro MM, Mielke CH, Kasper CK, Rapaport SI. Bleeding time after aspirin in disorders of intrinsic clotting. N Engl J Med 1969; 281:1039-42.

83. Orlikowski CEP, Payne AJ, Moodley J, Rocke DA. Thromboelastography after aspirin ingestion in pregnant and non-pregnant subjects. Br J Anaesth 1992; 69:159-61.

84. Thomas P, Hepburn B, Kim HC, Saidi P. Nonsteroidal anti-inflammatory drugs in the treatment of hemophilic arthropathy. Am J Hematol 1982; 12:131-7.

85. Fisher CA, Kappa JR, Sinha AK, et al. Comparison of equimolar concentrations of iloprost, prostacyclin, and prostaglandin E1 on human platelet function. J Lab Clin Med 1987; 109:184-90.

86. Fass RJ, Copeland EA, Brandt JT, et al. Platelet-mediated bleeding caused by broad-spectrum penicillins. J Infect Dis 1987; 155:1242-8.

87. Boldt J, Knothe C, Zickmann B, et al. Influence of different intravascular volume therapies on platelet function in patients undergoing cardiopulmonary bypass. Anesth Analg 1993; 76:1185-90.

88. von Willebrand EA. Hereditors pseudohamofile. Finska Laeksaellsk 1926; 68: 87-122.

89. Bloom AL. The von Willebrand syndrome. Semin Hematol 1980; 17:215-27.

90. Rodeghiero F, Castaman G, Dini E. Epidemiological investigation of the prevalence of von Willebrand's disease. Blood 1987; 69:454-9.

91. Mannucci PM, Bloom AL, Larrieu MJ, et al. Atherosclerosis and von Willebrand factor. Br J Haematol 1984; 57:163-9.

92. Berliner SA, Seligsohn U, Zivelin A, et al. A relatively high frequency of severe (type III) von Willebrand's disease in Israel. Br J Haematol 1986; 62:535-43.

93. Roqué H, Funai E, Lockwood CJ. von Willebrand disease and pregnancy. J Mater Fetal Med 2000; 9:257-66.

94. Rose E, Forster A, Aledort LM. Correction of prolonged bleeding time in von Willebrand's disease with Humate-P (letter). Transfusion 1990; 30:381.

95. Lipton RA, Ayromlooi J, Coller BS. Severe von Willebrand's disease during labor and delivery. JAMA 1982; 248:1355-7.

96. Mori PG, Pasino M, Rosanda Vadala C, et al. Haemophilia 'A' in a 46,X, i(X_q) female. Br J Haematol 1979; 43:143-7.

97. Seeds JW, Cefalo RC, Miller DT, Blatt PM. Obstetric care of the affected carrier of hemophilia B. Obstet Gynecol 1983; 62:23S-5S.

98. Baehner RL, Strauss HS. Hemophilia in the first year of life. N Engl J Med 1966; 275:524-8.

99. Nagey DA, editor. Management of pregnancy in hemophiliac patient. Collected Letters of the International Correspondence Society of Obstetricians and Gynecologists 1982; 23:38-40.

100. Roberts HR, Jones MR. Hemophilia and related conditions: Congenital deficiencies of prothrombin (factor II), factor V, and factors VII to XII. In Williams WJ, Beutler E, Erslev AJ, Lichtman MA, editors. Hematology. New York, McGraw-Hill, 1990:1453-73.

101. Gralnick HR. Congenital abnormalities of fibrinogen. In Williams WJ, Beutler E, Erslev AJ, Lichtman MA, editors. Hematology. New York, McGraw-Hill, 1990:1474-90.

102. Brandjes DPM, Schenk BE, Buller HR, ten Cate JW. Management of disseminated intravascular coagulation in obstetrics. Eur J Obstet Gynaecol Reprod Biol 1991; 42:S87-9.

103. Thiagarajah S, Wheby MS, Jain R, et al. Disseminated intravascular coagulation in pregnancy: The role of heparin therapy. J Repro Med 1981; 26:17-20.

104. Risberg B, Andreasson S, Eriksson E. Disseminated intravascular coagulation. Acta Anaesthesiol Scand 1991; 35(suppl 95):60-71.

105. Feinstein DI. Diagnosis and management of disseminated intravascular coagulation: The role of heparin therapy. Blood 1982; 60:284-7.

106. Oguma Y, Sakuragawa N, Maki M, et al. Treatment of disseminated intravascular coagulation with low molecular weight heparin. Semin Thromb Hemostas 1990; 16:34-40.

107. Cines DB, Kaywin P, Bina M, et al. Heparin-associated thrombocytopenia. N Engl J Med 1980; 303:788-95.

108. American College of Obstetricians and Gynecologists. Anticoagulation with low-molecular-weight heparin during pregnancy. ACOG Committee Opinion No. 211. Washington, DC, 1998.

109. Eisele B, Lamy M, Thijs LG, et al. Antithrombin III in patients with severe sepsis: A randomized placebo-controlled, double-blind multicenter trial plus meta-analysis on all randomized, placebo-controlled, double-blind trials with antithrombin III in severe sepsis. Intensive Care Med 1998; 24:663-72.

110. Vandermeulen EP, Van Aken HV, Vermylen J. Anticoagulants and spinal-epidural anesthesia. Anesth Analg 1994; 79:1165-77.

111. Loo CC, Dahlgren G, Irestedt L. Neurological complications in obstetric regional anaesthesia. Internat J Obstet Anesth 2000; 9:99-124.

112. Horlocker TT, Wedel DJ, Benzon H, et al. Regional anesthesia in the anticoagulated patient: Defining the risks. (The second ASRA Consensus Conference on Neuraxial Anesthesia and Anticoagulation.) Reg Anesth Pain Med 2003; 28:172-97.

113. Horlocker TT, Wedel DJ. Neuraxial block and low molecular weight heparin: Balancing perioperative analgesia and thromboprophylaxis. Reg Anesth Pain Med 1998; 23(Supplement):164-77.

114. Beilin Y, Zahn J, Comerford M. Safe epidural analgesia in thirty parturients with platelet counts between 69,000 and 98,000 mm^{-3}. Anesth Analg 1997;85:385-8.

115. Williams HD, Howard R, O'Donnell N, Findley I. The effect of low dose aspirin on bleeding times. Anaesthesia 1993; 48:331-3.

116. CLASP (Collaborative Low-dose Aspirin Study in Pregnancy) Collaborative Group. CLASP: A randomized trial of low-dose aspirin for the prevention and treatment of pre-eclampsia among 9364 pregnant women. Lancet 1994; 343:619-29.

117. Bromage PR. Epidural anesthesia in the anticoagulated patient. Anesthesiol Rev 1992; 19:22-4.

118. Ruskin KJ, Kaufman BS. Epidural anesthesia in the anticoagulated patient. Anesthesiol Rev 1992; 19:25-6.

119. Rosinia FA. Epidural anesthesia and anticoagulation (letter). Anesthesiology 1993; 79:203.

120. Sprung J, Cheng EY, Patel S. When to remove an epidural catheter in a parturient with disseminated intravascular coagulation. Reg Anesth 1992; 17:351-4.

121. Conard J, Horellou MH, Samama M. Incidence of thromboembolism in association with congenital disorders in coagulation and fibrinolysis. Acta Chir Scand Suppl 1988; 543:15-25.

122. Comp PC. Overview of the hypercoagulable states. Semin Thromb Hemostas 1990; 16:158-61.

123. Malm J, Laurell M, Dahlback B. Changes in the plasma levels of vitamin K dependent proteins C and S and of C4b-binding protein during pregnancy and oral contraception. Br J Haematol 1988; 68:437-43.

124. Conard J, Horellou MH, Van Dreden P, Samama M. Pregnancy and congenital deficiency in antithrombin III or protein C (abstract). Thromb Haemostas 1987; 58:39.

125. Odegard OR, Abildgaard U. Antithrombin III: Critical review of assay methods. Significance of variations in health and disease. Haemostas 1978; 7:127-34.

126. Letsky EA, de Swiet M. Thromboembolism in pregnancy and its management. Br J Haematol 1984; 57:543-52.

127. Hellgren M, Tengborn L, Abildgaard U. Pregnancy in women with congenital antithrombin III deficiency: Experience of treatment with heparin and antithrombin. Gynecol Obstet Invest 1982; 14:127-41.

128. Owen J. Antithrombin III replacement therapy in pregnancy. Semin Hematol 1991; 28:46-52.

129. Menache D, O'Malley JP, Schorr JB, et al. Evaluation of the safety, recovery, half-life, and clinical efficacy of antithrombin III (human) in patients with hereditary antithrombin III deficiency. Blood 1990; 75:33-9.

Chapter 43
Human Immunodeficiency Virus

David J. Wlody, M.D.

In 1981, a cluster of cases of an unusual disorder, *Pneumocystis carinii* pneumonia, initiated the search that culminated in the characterization of a new disease, the acquired immunodeficiency syndrome (AIDS), and the identification of its causative agent, the human immunodeficiency virus (HIV). Subsequently we have witnessed an explosion of this disease in the United States. Geographically, a disease that once was limited to two or three urban areas is now found in every area of the country. Further, the number of cases of HIV infection has reached epidemic levels. As of December 2002, more than 886,000 cases of AIDS have been reported to the Centers for Disease Control and Prevention (CDC). Approximately 384,000 people were reported living with AIDS at that time. Some 501,000 people have been reported to have died from AIDS and its complications.[1] The number of asymptomatic individuals who are infected with HIV is undoubtedly greater than 1 million. HIV infection has exploded demographically from its initial isolation within the homosexual community to its current endemic status among intravenous drug users, their sexual partners, and children born to women infected with HIV.

In the United States, women represent the fastest growing population of persons with AIDS.[2] In 1994, AIDS was the third leading cause of death among women between the ages of 25 and 44 nationally, and it was the leading cause of death among black women in that age group.[3] Clearly, anyone providing anesthesia to pregnant women in the United States in the early years of the twenty-first century will care for patients who are infected with HIV. Neither medicolegal concerns nor fear of contracting HIV should prevent anesthesiologists from providing effective intrapartum analgesia and anesthesia to HIV-infected women.

PATHOPHYSIOLOGY

HIV, previously known as *lymphadenopathy-associated virus (LAV)* and *human T-cell lymphotropic virus type III (HTLV-III)*, is a member of the lentivirus subfamily of human retroviruses. The lentiviruses typically cause indolent infections in their hosts. These infections are notable for central nervous system (CNS) involvement, long periods of clinical latency, and persistent viremia caused by an impaired humoral immune response.[4] As a retrovirus, HIV carries the enzyme reverse transcriptase. This enzyme converts the single-stranded viral RNA into double-stranded DNA, which subsequently can be integrated into the DNA of the infected cell. HIV displays similarity to HIV-2, a virus that is endemic in western Africa and that produces a similar syndrome. HIV-2 is even more closely related to the simian immunodeficiency virus (SIV). This has led to the unproven theory that transmission of SIV to humans in the form of HIV-2 was followed by rapid evolution into HIV and its subsequent escape from an isolated human population.[5]

For infection of the host cell to occur, HIV must bind to a cell-surface receptor, the CD4 antigen complex. This protein molecule was first detected on helper T cells, and it subsequently was identified on B cells, macrophages, and monocytes.[6] It also is found on placental cells[7] and may provide a route of vertical transmission to the fetus during early pregnancy. The interaction between HIV and host cells requires an interaction with an additional cell-surface protein; binding with either the CCR5 or CXCR4 co-receptor is required for infection to occur.[8] A number of potential therapeutic agents target this interaction.[9]

Infection of helper T cells is the key to immune suppression in HIV disease. These cells play a major role in cell-mediated immunity, and they also are essential to the activation of B cells and subsequent antibody production.[10] Macrophage activation also depends on adequate numbers of helper T cells. In addition to these T cell–mediated effects, both neutropenia and disturbances of neutrophil function are common in the later stages of HIV infection.[11] Abnormalities of these elements of the immune system render the HIV patient vulnerable to bacterial, viral, fungal,

parasitic, and mycobacterial infection. In addition, for reasons that are not entirely clear, patients infected with HIV are susceptible to several malignancies (e.g., Kaposi's sarcoma, B-cell lymphoma, invasive cervical carcinoma). AIDS-associated Kaposi's sarcoma is almost exclusively limited to homosexual males with HIV, or to women whose sexual partner is a bisexual male; this suggests that the malignancy is related to another sexually transmitted disease. In fact, DNA sequences from human herpes virus 8 (HHV8) have been identified in AIDS-associated Kaposi's sarcoma.[12,13]

DIAGNOSIS

There are several techniques for diagnosing HIV infection, including viral culture, p24 antigen detection tests, viral polymerase chain reaction (PCR), and immune function tests. Most often, the diagnosis is made on the basis of one of two antibody detection tests: either enzyme immunoassay (EIA) or the Western blot test. EIA measures the binding of anti-HIV antibody from the patient's serum to a mixture of antigens that typically have been obtained through recombinant DNA techniques (third generation test). The use of third generation tests has improved the reliability of EIA, but false positives (caused by autoimmune disorders, vaccination against influenza and hepatitis B, and/or high parity) and false negatives (caused by immunosuppressive therapy and various malignancies) can occur.[14] For these reasons, a Western blot test typically is performed after a positive EIA. False-positive Western blot tests can occur, but they are less common than false-positive EIA tests. The Western blot test allows the identification of antibodies to nine specific HIV antigens. Different organizations have different criteria for a positive Western blot test, but a positive test generally requires the presence of antibody to at least three different antigens. If there is no detectable antibody to any of these antigens, the test is negative.[14] Any combination of antibodies that does not meet the criteria for a positive test is considered indeterminate and is an indication for retesting in 4 to 8 weeks.

Quantitative PCR techniques, through the amplification of viral RNA, can detect extremely low levels of infection. This technique can detect viremia as early as 2 weeks after exposure, during the period of primary symptomatic infection.[15] Although this technique can be used to diagnose acute HIV infection, it is used almost exclusively to monitor the response to ongoing antiretroviral therapy.

Both the EIA and Western blot tests rely on the detection of antibody to HIV antigens. Unfortunately, there may be an interval of several weeks to months after the initial infection before detectable levels of antibody are present. A patient infected with HIV who is tested during this "window period" will have a negative test result but will be fully capable of infecting others. This is a strong argument for instituting universal precautions. If barrier precautions are instituted only for patients with a positive test result, health care workers will be exposed unnecessarily to seronegative but infectious patients.

Patients may be chronically infected with HIV for many years yet appear clinically well or have only minor evidence of immune suppression, such as oral candidiasis or recurrent herpes zoster. The diagnosis of AIDS is made when any one of a number of AIDS-indicator conditions develops (Box 43-1).

Box 43-1 AIDS-INDICATOR CONDITIONS

Candidiasis of bronchi, trachea, or lungs
Candidiasis, esophageal
Cervical cancer, invasive
Coccidioidomycosis, disseminated or extrapulmonary
Cryptococcosis, extrapulmonary
Cryptosporidiosis, chronic intestinal (greater than 1 month's duration)
Cytomegalovirus disease (other than liver, spleen, or nodes)
Cytomegalovirus retinitis (with loss of vision)
Encephalopathy, HIV-related
Herpes simplex: chronic ulcer(s) (greater than 1 month's duration); or bronchitis, pneumonitis, or esophagitis
Histoplasmosis, disseminated or extrapulmonary
Isosporiasis, chronic intestinal (greater than 1 month's duration)
Kaposi's sarcoma
Lymphoma, Burkitt's (or equivalent term)
Lymphoma, immunoblastic (or equivalent term)
Lymphoma, primary, of brain
Mycobacterium avium complex or *M. kansasii*, disseminated or extrapulmonary
Mycobacterium tuberculosis, any site (pulmonary or extrapulmonary)
Mycobacterium, other species or unidentified species, disseminated or extrapulmonary
Pneumocystis carinii pneumonia
Pneumonia, recurrent
Progressive multifocal leukoencephalopathy
Salmonella septicemia, recurrent
Toxoplasmosis of brain
Wasting syndrome due to HIV
CD4+ T-lymphocyte count < 200 cells/µL

From MMWR 41(RR-17), December 18, 1992.

CLINICAL MANIFESTATIONS

In the early stages of the AIDS epidemic, the predominant symptoms were those of immune suppression (e.g., opportunistic infections, unusual malignancies). Disturbances of gastrointestinal function were also prominent. As improvements in prophylaxis and treatment of opportunistic infections have increased longevity, it has become apparent that HIV eventually affects multiple organ systems. The aggressive use of highly active antiretroviral therapy (HAART) can significantly prolong the symptom-free interval, and it is highly unusual for a pregnant patient to present with significant organ system involvement.

Neurologic Abnormalities

Neurologic involvement can occur at any time during HIV infection (Box 43-2). Viral particles can be isolated from the cerebrospinal fluid (CSF) at the time of primary infection.[16] The manifestations of nervous system involvement vary with the stage of the disease.

During **initial systemic HIV infection,** a variety of CNS disorders may occur. Headache, photophobia, and retroorbital pain are common.[15] Aseptic meningoencephalitis has been reported. Cognitive and affective changes (e.g., depression, irritability) may be noted. Finally, cranial and peripheral neuropathies often are seen. Most of these disorders are self-limited, but persistent neurologic dysfunction may occur.[17]

A demyelinating neuropathy similar to the Guillain-Barré syndrome is the most common neurologic disorder seen during the **asymptomatic or latent phase of HIV infection**. It is

presumably autoimmune in nature, and it typically responds to intravenous immunoglobulin (IVIG) or plasmapheresis.[17]

A subset of patients remains neurologically asymptomatic during the latent phase of HIV infection. Nevertheless, these patients typically have CSF abnormalities, including the local synthesis of HIV antibody and the presence of HIV particles or viral nucleic acid.[17] This is an important consideration when determining the risk of introducing virus into the CNS during the performance of regional anesthesia in an asymptomatic patient. It is almost certain that CNS infection has already occurred.

Finally, the **late stages of HIV infection** are marked by significant neurologic deterioration in almost all patients. **Meningitis** is common; etiologies include tuberculosis, cryptococcus, metastatic lymphoma, and direct infection of the meninges by HIV. **Diffuse encephalopathy** can occur; cytomegalovirus (CMV), herpes simplex virus (HSV), and toxoplasma typically produce a simultaneous impairment of both cognition and alertness. Diffuse encephalopathy also may be seen as a consequence of systemic disease, such as sepsis or hypoxemia secondary to respiratory disease. Patients with the **AIDS dementia complex** also present with a diffuse encephalitic picture; however, unlike other forms of encephalitis in which cognitive function is diminished, the level of alertness remains unimpaired. In addition, the complex is associated with impairment of motor function and behavioral changes (apathy, agitation). **Focal brain disorders** can occur, secondary to toxoplasmosis, primary CNS lymphoma, and progressive multifocal leukoencephalopathy (PML), an opportunistic viral infection that causes selective destruction of white matter tracts. **Myelopathy** is common; it can present in an acute, segmental form, as in the transverse myelitis produced by varicella infection, or as a more progressive and diffuse disorder—vacuolar myelopathy—which is marked by a progressive, painless gait disturbance and spasticity. A distal, predominantly sensory **peripheral neuropathy** is quite common in late HIV infection. The etiology is unknown; it has been suggested that it is secondary to cytokine-mediated neurotoxicity.[17] Sensory and motor dysfunction typically are minimal, but pain can be severe enough to prevent walking. CMV infection can also lead to a polyradiculopathy that usually

responds to anti-CMV therapy. **Autonomic neuropathy** can present with mild postural hypotension or severe cardiovascular instability during invasive procedures. Autonomic dysfunction also can contribute to the chronic diarrhea that occurs in some patients with AIDS. An **inflammatory myopathy** resembling dermatomyositis has been reported, although this disorder is less common than the neuropathies.[17] Finally, neurologic side effects of antiretroviral and other therapies also may occur (*vide infra*).

Pulmonary Abnormalities

The pulmonary manifestations of HIV disease are not caused by a direct effect of the virus but rather by the opportunistic infections associated with the disease. The most prominent of these is *P. carinii,* a fungal organism to which most humans develop an antibody response by 4 years of age.[18] Despite this evidence of widespread exposure to the organism, symptomatic ***Pneumocystis carinii* pneumonia (PCP)** typically is seen only in patients with severe immune suppression. The clinical picture is similar to the adult respiratory distress syndrome (ARDS), with severe hypoxemia and a pattern of diffuse interstitial infiltrates on chest radiograph. The mortality rate of patients with PCP who require intubation may be as high as 75%.[19] Early initiation of steroid therapy decreases the likelihood of progression to respiratory failure.[20] Patients who survive the disease are at risk for the development of pneumatoceles; subsequent rupture leading to pneumothorax is common. Survivors of PCP also are at risk for developing chronic airway disease, including chronic bronchitis and bronchiectasis.[18]

Reactivation of latent **tuberculosis** is common in patients with HIV infection because of the impairment of cellular immunity that ordinarily maintains the disease in a quiescent state; HIV-infected individuals also may be more susceptible to acquiring tuberculosis when they are exposed to an infectious individual.[21] The impairment of humoral immunity is responsible for an increased incidence of bacterial pneumonia caused by encapsulated organisms (e.g., *Streptococcus pneumoniae, Haemophilus influenzae*).[22] Finally, although less frequent than PCP, pneumonia secondary to other fungal organisms (e.g., aspergillus, cryptococcus, coccidioides) is much more common in patients infected with HIV than in the general population.[22]

Gastrointestinal Abnormalities

The presence of large quantities of lymphoid tissue in the gastrointestinal tract implies a major role for the gut in HIV replication,[23] and gastrointestinal disturbances occur at some time in almost all patients with HIV infection (Box 43-3). Painful or difficult swallowing is common and typically is caused by herpetic, CMV, or candida **esophagitis**; the contribution of these disorders to gastroesophageal reflux is unclear.[24]

Severe diarrhea resulting from infection with CMV, HSV, candida, cryptosporidia, *Mycobacterium avium* complex (MAC), or HIV itself can lead to significant cachexia and electrolyte abnormalities. Finally, **hepatobiliary disease** is common. Causes of parenchymal liver disease include hepatitis B and C, CMV, mycobacterial infection (both *Mycobacterium tuberculosis* and *M. avium* complex), and cryptococcus. Kaposi's sarcoma and non-Hodgkin's lymphoma may involve the liver. Cryptosporidiosis and CMV can cause cholangitis in patients with severe immune dysfunction.[23]

Hematologic Abnormalities

HIV infection is associated with hematologic abnormalities that affect each of the peripheral cell lines.[25] **Leukopenia** is a hallmark of the disease, especially the depletion of CD4 lymphocytes; qualitative alterations in the function of neutrophils and macrophages also occur. **Anemia** is quite common. Causes include direct HIV infection of erythroid precursors, suppression of erythropoiesis caused by inappropriate release of tumor necrosis factor, infiltration of bone marrow with MAC, and occult GI blood loss.

Coagulation disturbances are common in patients with HIV. **Immune thrombocytopenia (ITP)** is common and typically is only mildly symptomatic. Platelet production may be impaired because of direct infection of megakaryocytes with HIV. Thrombocytopenia frequently responds to the initiation of antiretroviral therapy. The response to corticosteroid therapy is variable. Intravenous immune globulin produces a rapid but transient effect, and it may be indicated in patients with life-threatening hemorrhage. The activated partial thromboplastin time (aPTT) may be prolonged because of the presence of the lupus anticoagulant; this appears to be an in vitro abnormality with no clinical significance (see Chapter 39). Finally, many of the antiretroviral agents and other drugs used in these patients have hematologic toxicity.

Cardiovascular Abnormalities

When echocardiography and autopsy evidence of lymphocytic infiltration of the myocardium are used as evidence of cardiovascular involvement in patients with HIV, the prevalence of such involvement is as high as 50%.[25] Nevertheless, clinically significant cardiovascular disease is rare in patients with HIV. **Pericarditis** has been reported to be the most prevalent cardiovascular disorder seen in these patients. The most common etiology appears to be mycobacterial infection; CMV, HSV, Kaposi's sarcoma, malignant lymphoma, and HIV itself have also been implicated.[27] **Pulmonary hypertension** can develop secondary to repeated episodes of PCP and may also be a consequence of cytokine-mediated endothelial injury.[26] Direct **myocardial involvement**—typically focal myocarditis—is identified in 15% to 50% of autopsy studies, but clinical myocarditis or cardiomyopathy is rare.[26] **Infective endocarditis** among patients with HIV occurs almost exclusively in intravenous drug users. Finally, the elevations in serum cholesterol and triglycerides produced by the protease inhibitors appear to increase the risk of coronary artery disease in patients receiving these drugs.

Endocrine Abnormalities

Endocrine dysfunction can result from HIV infection, opportunistic infections, or drug therapy.[28] There is a relatively high incidence of pathologic findings in the pituitary gland at autopsy, yet clinical evidence of pituitary dysfunction is rare. Similarly, whereas adrenal involvement with CMV is a common autopsy finding, glucocorticoid insufficiency is uncommon, although clearly more prevalent in HIV-positive patients than in the general population. Patients with AIDS frequently have abnormal thyroid function tests, similar to the findings seen in patients with other chronic illnesses, yet clinical hypothyroidism is unusual. Hyperglycemia, presumably secondary to insulin resistance, has been reported in patients receiving protease inhibitors. Finally, intravenous pentamidine therapy for CMV infection may cause islet cell injury, which may lead to hypoglycemia caused by the release of insulin from damaged islet cells. If sufficient islet cells are destroyed, diabetes mellitus can develop.

Renal Abnormalities

Patients with HIV are at risk for acute renal failure secondary to sepsis, dehydration, and drug toxicity.[29] A common cause of chronic renal insufficiency is proliferative glomerulonephritis secondary to deposition of immune complexes containing HIV antigen within the glomeruli. Renal failure may also occur because of a specific disorder, **HIV-associated nephropathy (HIVAN)**.[31] This entity, seen almost exclusively in black patients, is characterized by a focal segmental glomerulosclerosis. Hypertension is uncommon, deterioration of renal function is extremely rapid, and the long-term prognosis is worse than that seen in renal failure due to other causes. The underlying cause appears to be direct infection of renal cells by HIV. Antiretroviral therapy appears to modify the course of the disease.[30]

INTERACTION WITH PREGNANCY

The rapidly increasing incidence of HIV infection among heterosexual women limits the credibility of any estimate of the seroprevalence of HIV among pregnant women. In 1991, the CDC reported a nationwide seroprevalence rate of 1.5 per 1000 pregnant women. There is a considerable geographic variation in these figures; the highest rates of seroprevalence were found in New York (5.8 per 1000), the District of Columbia (5.5 per 1000), and New Jersey (4.9 per 1000). Seropositive women were identified in all but 2 of the 39 reporting areas.[31] More recently, the nationwide seroprevalence of HIV during pregnancy has been reported to be 1.7 per 1000.[32]

The diagnosis of HIV infection in the offspring of HIV-infected mothers has been hampered by the persistence of passively acquired maternal antibody in the newborn for as long as 18 months. Until 18 months of age, an infant's HIV status must be confirmed by viral culture or DNA PCR. Measurement of circulating p24 antigen has been used for rapid diagnosis of neonatal HIV infection,[33] but this is no longer recommended because it is less sensitive than PCR and is associated with false positives.[34]

There is intense interest in the identification of those factors that promote perinatal transmission of HIV from mother to infant (i.e., vertical transmission) (Box 43-4). Clinical severity of maternal disease is associated with an increased risk of transmission, as reflected by an increased rate of infection in infants born to women with symptomatic AIDS.[35] Maternal viral burden correlates with transmission. In one study, 13 of 13 women with more than 80,000 viral RNA

Box 43-4   RISK FACTORS FOR VERTICAL TRANSMISSION OF HIV

Severity of maternal disease
Maternal viral burden
Prolonged ruptured membranes
Sexually transmitted disease
Chorioamnionitis
Lack of maternal antiviral therapy
Invasive procedures (?)
Vaginal delivery
Breast-feeding

---

copies/mL transmitted the disease, but none of the 63 women with less than 20,000 copies/mL transmitted HIV.[36] Other factors that have been implicated in vertical transmission include the presence of ruptured membranes for more than 4 hours,[37] coexisting sexually transmitted diseases,[38] chorioamnionitis,[39] and invasive procedures such as amniocentesis and cerclage.[38] At least one study has demonstrated that fetal scalp blood pH sampling and the use of fetal scalp electrodes do not increase vertical transmission[40]; however, the documented presence of HIV in maternal cervical secretions has caused some clinicians to be reluctant to use this monitoring technique.[41] Finally, there is considerable evidence that breast-feeding may double the rate of perinatal transmission in women with established HIV infection.[42] Thus breast-feeding should be discouraged unless bottle feeding is not a safe alternative, as is true in many underdeveloped countries.

In addition to identifying risk factors for vertical transmission, there is a significant effort to determine which active interventions might decrease the transmission of HIV. The first such intervention that was identified is the administration of zidovudine (ZDV, formerly AZT). In a study known as the AIDS Clinical Trial Group (ACTG) protocol 076, administration of ZDV orally during pregnancy, intravenously during labor, and orally to the infant for the first 6 weeks of life decreased the transmission rate from 25.5% to 8.3%. No significant adverse effects were noted in these infants.[43] Because transmission is highly correlated with maternal viral load, it has been recommended that HAART (i.e., triple drug therapy) be initiated whenever maternal viral load exceeds 1000 RNA copies/mL.[44]

The demonstration that low rates of newborn infection occur when the interval between rupture of membranes and delivery was shortened suggested that cesarean delivery might decrease vertical transmission. In fact, at least four studies suggest that elective cesarean section may decrease the rate of transmission by as much as 80%.[44] The American College of Obstetricians and Gynecologists (ACOG) has recommended that HIV-infected women be offered the option of elective cesarean delivery to decrease the rate of transmission below that which would be expected with ZDV therapy alone.[45] Although the ACOG acknowledged that the data were insufficient to demonstrate a benefit for women with viral loads less than 1000 viral copies/mL of plasma, there is some evidence that abdominal delivery may be beneficial even in the setting of viral loads below that threshold[46]; thus it has been suggested that elective cesarean section be offered to patients in this group as well.[44]

A number of studies have assessed the effect of HIV infection on pregnancy outcome. Alger et al.[47] followed 97 seronegative and 101 seropositive but asymptomatic women throughout pregnancy. There was no difference between groups in the incidence of low birth weight (LBW) (less than 2500 g), small for gestational age (SGA) infants, or low 5-minute Apgar scores.[47] However, in a study of 315 seropositive and 311 seronegative women in Kenya, HIV seropositivity was associated with an increased risk of preterm delivery and LBW but not with an increased incidence of SGA infants.[48] These different results may reflect the higher incidence of symptomatic HIV disease in the Kenyan patients. Another study noted that the incidence of serious infectious complications (e.g., PCP, CNS toxoplasmosis) is greater than 30% in pregnant women with advanced HIV infection (CD4 counts of less than 300 cells/mm^3).[49] The fetal implications of such infections are obvious. There is no evidence that drug therapy *per se* affects pregnancy outcome; neither preterm delivery, LBW, low Apgar scores, nor stillbirth increased in women receiving therapy compared with controls.[50]

There also is concern that pregnancy itself may have an adverse effect on the progression of HIV infection. However, no evidence suggests that pregnancy accelerates clinical deterioration in the HIV-infected patient, or that viral RNA load changes significantly during pregnancy.[47,51,52]

DRUG THERAPY

Patients who are infected with HIV are treated with an ever-increasing number of antiretroviral medications, singly but more commonly in combination, as well as agents used for the prevention or treatment of opportunistic infections (Box 43-5). The following represents only a partial list of these drugs.

Maternal Side Effects

NUCLEOSIDE REVERSE TRANSCRIPTASE INHIBITORS (NRTI)

Zidovudine (ZDV, AZT, Retrovir®)

ZDV is a thymidine analog that interferes with the replication of HIV within host cells by interfering with viral transcriptase and elongation of the viral DNA chain. No longer used as monotherapy (except during pregnancy in women with less than 1000 viral RNA copies/mL), it is usually part of the initial treatment regimen in patients with newly diagnosed HIV, because it acts synergistically or additively with the other nucleoside analogues, non-nucleoside reverse transcriptase inhibitors, and protease inhibitors.[53]

Common side effects include headache, nausea, insomnia, and malaise. These symptoms typically are self-limited and seldom require termination of therapy. The major toxicity associated with ZDV is hematologic; anemia and neutropenia can occur. In general, hematologic toxicity is more severe in patients with more advanced disease. **Bone marrow suppression** may require the substitution of a less toxic agent or the addition of recombinant erythropoietin and granulocyte colony stimulating factor (G-CSF). Long-term therapy with ZDV may be associated with a myopathy that is characterized by myalgias, elevated creatine-phosphokinase (CPK) levels, and proximal muscle weakness that predominantly affects the lower extremities. This myopathy has been suggested as resulting from inhibition of mitochondrial DNA synthesis.

Didanosine (ddI, dideoxyinosine, Videx®)

Didanosine, once used as a single-agent substitute for ZDV in patients who could not tolerate that drug, is now used as a

Box 43-5 SIDE EFFECTS OF MATERNAL DRUG THERAPY

ZIDOVUDINE (ZDV)

Anemia
Neutropenia
Thrombocytopenia
Myopathy

DIDANOSINE (ddI)

Peripheral neuropathy
Pancreatitis

ZALCITABINE (ddC)

Peripheral neuropathy
Pancreatitis

STAVUDINE (d4T)

Peripheral neuropathy

LAMIVUDINE (3TC)

Pancreatitis (more common in children than in adults)

ABACAVIR

Hypersensitivity reaction

NEVIRAPINE

Skin rash
Induction of cytochrome P-450 system

DELAVIRDINE

Skin rash
Increased levels of drugs with hepatic metabolism

EFAVIRENZ

CNS symptoms
Increased levels of drugs with hepatic metabolism

PROTEASE INHIBITORS

Abdominal discomfort, nausea, diarrhea
Hyperglycemia
Elevated cholesterol and triglycerides
Lipodystrophy
Increased levels of drugs with hepatic metabolism
Nephrolithiasis (with indinavir only)

GANCICLOVIR

Neutropenia
Anemia
Peripheral neuropathy

FOSCARNET

Renal toxicity
Disturbances of calcium metabolism
Hypomagnesemia

TRIMETHOPRIM-SULFAMETHOXAZOLE

Elevation of liver enzymes
Neutropenia
Rash
Fever

DAPSONE

Methemoglobinemia
Hyperkalemia

AEROSOLIZED PENTAMIDINE

Bronchospasm

INTRAVENOUS PENTAMIDINE

Hypoglycemia
Hyperglycemia
Ventricular arrhythmias
Renal toxicity

---

component of combination drug therapy.[54] The major toxicity of didanosine is **peripheral neuropathy**. Predominantly sensory, it is usually symmetrical and distal, typically limited to the lower extremities. It initially presents with dysesthesias, described as burning, aching, or tingling. It can progress to pain on walking or at rest that can be severe enough to interfere with ambulation. Risk factors include low CD4+ counts and preexisting neuropathy. Peripheral neuropathy usually resolves when administration of the drug is stopped, and although some patients can resume treatment without recurrence of symptoms, it is more common for a different agent to be substituted.[54] The mechanism of neuropathy is not completely understood, but it has been ascribed to inhibition of mitochondrial DNA synthesis.

Pancreatitis has been associated with didanosine therapy; this may manifest as an asymptomatic elevation of plasma amylase or mild abdominal pain, but a fulminant course and death rarely may occur. Risk factors for the development of pancreatitis include history of drug or alcohol abuse, preexisting pancreatitis, and the coadministration of other drugs (e.g., pentamidine) that are associated with pancreatic injury. Life-threatening lactic acidosis has also been described, in common with the other nucleoside analogues. Hematologic toxicity is absent.

Zalcitabine (ddC, dideoxycytidine, HIVID®)

Because of the availability of equally effective but less toxic agents, zalcitabine is used relatively infrequently in current treatment regimens.[55] Its primary toxicities are peripheral neuropathy, a self-limited maculopapular skin eruption, and pancreatitis, although the incidence of this is lower than with didanosine.

Stavudine (d4T, Zerit®)

This thymidine analogue is often used as a substitute for ZDV as part of an initial treatment regimen. Because of similar placental transfer and lack of reported fetal side effects, it has also been used as an alternative to ZDV monotherapy in pregnant women who cannot tolerate the older drug.[56] It is associated with peripheral neuropathy to a greater extent than ZDV, but less commonly than with didanosine or zalcitabine. Pancreatitis is rare. Stavudine appears to be associated with a higher risk of lactic acidosis than the other NRTIs.

Lamivudine (3TC, Epivir®)

Because of its low affinity for human DNA polymerases, lamivudine is one of the least toxic NRTIs.[57] Pancreatitis has been reported in pediatric patients, although the contribution of other medications cannot be discounted.

Abacavir (Ziagen®)

This purine analogue is commonly administered as a component of Trizivir®, a fixed dose combination of abacavir, zidovudine, and lamivudine. Neurologic and hematologic toxicity are rare. The most significant adverse effect is an acute hypersensitivity reaction, typically seen soon after initiation of the drug.[58]

NON-NUCLEOSIDE REVERSE TRANSCRIPTASE INHIBITORS (NNRTI)

The NNRTIs bind directly to a site on the reverse transcriptase enzyme and thereby inhibit the enzyme's ability to function. Resistance to the NNRTIs develops rapidly when they are administered as single agents. Thus these agents are used only in combination with an NRTI.

Nevirapine (Viramune®)

The major toxicity of nevirapine is skin rash, including Stevens-Johnson syndrome and toxic epidermal necrolysis, which can be life-threatening.[59] Fatal hepatitis has been reported. Nevirapine causes induction of the cytochrome P-450 system and may decrease levels of other drugs metabolized by that mechanism.

Delavirdine (Rescriptor®)

Delavirdine is associated with a maculopapular skin rash that often resolves with continued drug administration.[60] Because it inhibits the P-450 system, delavirdine may increase plasma levels of CNS depressants, particularly the benzodiazepines, which should be used with caution in patients receiving this drug.[60]

Efavirenz (Sustiva®)

The newest of the NNRTIs has been used both as a component of initial treatment regimens as well as in patients with progression of disease during first-line treatment.[61] Resistance is less likely to develop with this drug than with the other drugs of its class. The most common side effects are rash and CNS symptoms, including dizziness, insomnia, somnolence, and confusion. Benzodiazepines should be used cautiously because of the potential for impaired metabolism.

PROTEASE INHIBITORS

Amprenavir (Agenerase®), Saquinavir (Invirase®), Indinavir (Crixivan®), Nelfinavir (Viracept®), Lopinavir (Kaletra®) and Ritonavir (Norvir®)

Used as a component of a multiple drug regimen, the protease inhibitors have revolutionized the treatment of HIV and have contributed significantly to long-term survival of patients with HIV.[62] Abdominal discomfort, nausea, vomiting, and diarrhea have been reported with each of these agents. Indinavir appears to have the unique side effect of crystalluria and nephrolithiasis. As the administration of these agents has become increasingly widespread, metabolic complications secondary to their prolonged use currently are becoming quite common; these include hyperglycemia, significant elevations of cholesterol and triglycerides, and an unusual redistribution of body fat from the extremities to the thorax and abdomen (lipodystrophy).[63]

The protease inhibitors are metabolized by the CYP3A isoenzyme of the cytochrome P-450 system, and they competitively inhibit this enzyme. Because many CNS depressants, particularly the benzodiazepines, are metabolized by this mechanism, the protease inhibitors can be expected to increase the sedative effects of these drugs. In fact, the package insert for several of these agents states that simultaneous use of these CNS depressants is contraindicated.[64,65] However, clinical experience suggests that these drugs (e.g., benzodiazepines) can be used safely if they are titrated carefully. The effects of the ergot alkaloids may also be increased by the simultaneous use of the protease inhibitors.[64]

CYTOMEGALOVIRUS (CMV) PROPHYLAXIS

Ganciclovir

Ganciclovir is indicated for the treatment of established CMV infection, particularly retinitis, as well as CMV prophylaxis in patients with advanced HIV disease. Associated leukopenia and anemia are common and are seen in approximately 40% and 25% of patients, respectively, receiving intravenous therapy; oral prophylactic therapy can lead to similar disturbances of hematopoesis, but this is less common.[66] Thrombocytopenia occurs in 6% of treated patients. Ganciclovir's hematologic toxicity is enhanced by concurrent ZDV therapy. The drug also has been associated with peripheral neuropathy in approximately 20% of patients.[66]

Foscarnet

This drug is used to treat CMV retinitis. It can produce renal toxicity, especially when used concurrently with other nephrotoxic drugs. Foscarnet also may produce electrolyte abnormalities, including hypocalcemia, hypophosphatemia, and hypomagnesemia.[67]

PCP PROPHYLAXIS

Trimethoprim-sulfamethoxazole (TMP-SMX)

This drug is used for the treatment and prophylaxis of PCP. In one study, 57% of patients receiving the drug developed toxicity severe enough to require cessation of therapy.[68] The most common reason for terminating therapy was elevation of the liver enzymes aspartate transaminase (AST) and alanine transaminase (ALT). Neutropenia, rash, and fever also are common.[18]

Dapsone

This agent is used in patients who cannot tolerate TMP-SMX. It can produce rash, fever, hyperkalemia and methemoglobinemia.[69]

Pentamidine

Aerosolized pentamidine is useful in the prophylaxis of PCP, although it is less effective than TMP-SMX.[70] It has the advantage of producing minimal systemic toxicity, but it can cause significant bronchospasm.[69] **Intravenous pentamidine** is indicated for the treatment of PCP. It has a direct toxic effect on pancreatic islet cells; initial **hypoglycemia** (from the release of insulin from damaged cells) is followed by **hyperglycemia**. Ventricular arrhythmias (*torsade de pointes*) and nephrotoxicity (including acute tubular necrosis) also have been reported.[69]

Fetal Side Effects

There are few published data regarding the use of these agents in pregnant women. Fortunately, clinical experience suggests that fetal risk is minimal. This is best demonstrated by ACTG

protocol 076, which demonstrated a significant reduction of vertical transmission of HIV with maternal ZDV therapy.[43] There was no difference between the ZDV and the placebo groups in the number and type of birth defects. The only apparent difference in neonatal outcome was a mild transient anemia (which required no treatment) in the treatment group. Ongoing observation of these infants is planned, but no difference in growth or neurodevelopmental status has been identified in the ZDV group.

Historically, physicians have worried that the use of TMP-SMX during the third trimester may increase the risk of neonatal kernicterus. This complication has not been reported, and TMP-SMX should be continued until delivery in women who can tolerate the drug.[71]

Of the other antiretroviral agents or drugs used to treat opportunistic infections during pregnancy, there are none that are listed in FDA pregnancy category A, which signifies a lack of fetal effect in controlled human trials.[72] The use of such drugs may require a careful evaluation and extrapolation from animal studies, as well as a full discussion of the risks and benefits with the mother.[73] Minkoff and DeHovitz[71] concluded the following:

> The guiding principle in the use of medications by HIV-infected women who become pregnant is to adhere strictly to standards promulgated for nonpregnant women, unless there are documented and compelling fetal concerns that would justify a modification of those standards.

ANESTHETIC MANAGEMENT

Coexisting Diseases

Many parturients infected with HIV have health problems that are related to those behaviors that led to their infection with HIV. The most significant of these is substance abuse. Approximately 44% of women with AIDS contracted the virus through intravenous drug use. An additional 18% of women with AIDS contracted the virus from a sexual partner who used intravenous drugs.[1] It can be expected that many of these patients also abuse alcohol and crack cocaine.

The HIV-positive parturient is at high risk for harboring other sexually transmitted diseases. From the anesthesiologist's perspective, the most significant of these diseases is syphilis because of the neurologic effects of this disease in its later stages. If regional anesthesia is performed, a careful neurologic examination should be completed and documented. Hepatitis B also is a sexually transmitted disease, and it should be investigated in HIV-positive parturients. Severe hepatic impairment affects anesthetic management. Of equal importance are the infectivity of hepatitis B and the high likelihood of transmission after needlestick injury. For this reason, it is unacceptable for health care workers to remain unvaccinated against hepatitis B.

Regional Anesthesia

Whether HIV-infected patients are more prone to the infectious complications of regional anesthesia is an important concern. This question was addressed in a study of 30 HIV-positive pregnant women, of whom 18 received regional anesthesia and 12 did not. There was no evidence of accelerated disease progression or increased infectious or neurologic complications in the regional anesthesia group.[74] A more recent study demonstrated no postoperative changes in viral load or CD4+/CD8+ ratio and no increased hemodynamic instability or blood loss in HIV-infected patients undergoing elective cesarean section under spinal anesthesia.[75] The lack of infectious complications of regional anesthesia is of course predicated on the maintenance of strict aseptic technique. The American Society of Anesthesiologists (ASA) Subcommittee on Infection Control Policy has recommended that a gown be worn during invasive procedures performed on an HIV-infected patient.[76]

Some physicians may question whether it is prudent to administer regional anesthesia to a patient who almost certainly will develop neurologic deficits at some time in the future. Some worry that these deficits might be ascribed to the regional anesthetic technique. Because such deficits are unlikely to be temporally related to the anesthetic, this does not seem to be a significant concern. Further, it seems cruel to deny the most effective intrapartum analgesic techniques to HIV-positive women simply because of fear of future litigation.

Another question is whether an anesthesiologist can ethically or legally refuse to provide care to an HIV-positive patient. Specifically, can an anesthesiologist refuse to provide epidural analgesia during labor? The American Medical Association has taken the position that physicians have an ethical duty to treat HIV-positive patients. Refusing to treat patients with HIV also places the physician at legal risk because numerous federal, state, and local statutes prohibit discrimination against patients with HIV disease. Any physician who refuses to provide care for patients with HIV must participate in a referral system that ensures that such patients receive prompt medical care.[77]

Despite the use of small conical (i.e., pencil-point) spinal needles and despite careful technique during administration of epidural anesthesia, postdural puncture headache (PDPH) remains a problem in pregnant patients. Clearly, the onset of headache and photophobia in an immunosuppressed patient who has recently undergone a major regional anesthetic can be worrisome, but the typical postural nature of a PDPH should allay fears of bacterial meningitis.

Once the diagnosis of PDPH is made, an initial course of conservative therapy is indicated. This typically consists of bed rest, analgesics, and oral hydration. Although dehydration can worsen PDPH, there is no evidence that forced oral or intravenous overhydration has any beneficial effect.

Should conservative therapy fail, a number of additional pharmacologic interventions have been proposed, including intravenous or oral caffeine and the 5-HT receptor agonist sumatriptan, with varying degrees of success. However, the gold standard for treatment of PDPH is the performance of an autologous epidural blood patch. Such treatment can be expected to produce permanent and complete pain relief in the great majority of patients; a second epidural blood patch typically produces relief in most patients who fail to respond to the initial procedure.

Some physicians have expressed concern that the introduction of HIV-infected blood into the neuraxis might lead to the introduction of HIV into a previously uninfected CNS.[78] The magnetic resonance imaging (MRI) demonstration of subarachnoid extension of an epidural blood patch heightens these concerns.[79] However, it is likely that CNS infection occurs quite early in the course of the disease, even in asymptomatic patients. Nevertheless, it seems prudent to at least acknowledge the possibility that epidural blood patch can accelerate the CNS manifestations of the disease. This question was addressed in a study of six seropositive patients who

developed PDPH after diagnostic lumbar puncture and who subsequently received an epidural blood patch.[80] These patients subsequently underwent serial neuropsychologic testing for as long as 2 years. The authors stated that "none of these six subjects had a decline in neurocognitive performance or other adverse neurologic or infectious sequelae" during the period of the study. Admittedly these numbers are small, but this study provides the best evidence to date of the safety of epidural blood patch in the HIV-infected patient.

An alternative to autologous epidural blood patch is the epidural infusion of normal saline or colloidal solutions such as hetastarch. Unfortunately, the relief obtained from this technique often is transient, lasting only as long as the infusion continues. It may provide palliation until the dural puncture site heals spontaneously. Another proposed alternative is epidural blood patch with fresh homologous blood. However, there are no published data on this technique.

General Anesthesia

As with regional anesthesia, it is appropriate to ask whether patients with HIV might be more susceptible to the infectious (e.g., pulmonary) complications of general anesthesia. To my knowledge, there is no published study that addresses this question. However, it seems appropriate to handle the endotracheal tube in as sterile a manner as possible and to minimize the duration of postoperative ventilation.

Another question involves the effect of general anesthesia on immune function. Several published studies suggest that general anesthesia can transiently depress immune function, but this appears to be clinically insignificant in normal patients.[10] It is appropriate to ask whether this effect might be exaggerated to the point of clinical significance in patients with HIV disease. Unfortunately, studies regarding this issue are lacking. At present, it would be inappropriate to recommend one anesthetic technique over another on the basis of their effects on immune function.[81]

Evron et al.[82] recently reviewed anesthetic considerations for patients with HIV.

STRATEGIES TO MINIMIZE HIV TRANSMISSION
To The Uninfected Patient

Any survey of HIV and anesthesia must include a discussion of those measures that can decrease the risk of HIV transmission to the uninfected patient. By far the greatest cause of such transmission is the transfusion of infected blood. Thus the most significant impact anesthesiologists can have on disease transmission is to minimize the transfusion of homologous blood.

In healthy patients, oxygen delivery is satisfactorily maintained at hemoglobin levels much lower than the traditional transfusion threshold of 10 g/dL. The Consensus Development Conference on perioperative red blood cell transfusion concluded that healthy patients tolerate a hemoglobin concentration as low as 7 g/dL.[83] Patients with chronic anemia have an increased concentration of 2,3-diphosphoglycerate, which allows effective oxygen delivery at even lower hemoglobin concentrations. Of course, patients with significant cardiopulmonary disease require a higher hemoglobin concentration.

It is not clear whether these guidelines can be applied to the antepartum patient. An association between preterm delivery and hemoglobin concentrations of less than 10 g/dL

has been reported,[84] as has a similar association between LBW and hemoglobin concentrations of less than 9 g/dL.[85] However, it is unknown whether this is a causal relationship or whether anemia serves as a marker of poor nutrition and/or lower socioeconomic status, which may independently lead to perinatal morbidity. Although it is impossible to designate a minimum acceptable hemoglobin level during pregnancy, anemia clearly is undesirable. Once a cause is determined, appropriate therapy should be initiated; this may include transfusion if the anemia is life threatening for the mother or fetus.

Patients often want to use blood specifically donated by friends or relatives for their use (**directed donation**). There are disadvantages of directed donation. First, a directed unit is unavailable to another patient who may need it more emergently. Second, directed donation may discourage the routine voluntary donation of blood. Third, the directed donor sacrifices anonymity and legal protection.[86] More pertinent to the issue of HIV transmission, there is no evidence that blood from designated donors is safer than anonymously donated bank blood[87]; this may be related to the slightly higher rate of HIV-seropositivity among first-time donors.[88] Further, fatal graft-versus-host disease has been reported in patients receiving blood from first-degree relatives.[89]

Another approach is the use of **autologous blood donation** during pregnancy in those patients at high risk of peripartum hemorrhage, such as those with placenta previa or suspected placenta accreta. Several studies have demonstrated the safety of autologous donation in pregnant women with a hematocrit of at least 34%.[90,91] However, it may be impossible to identify those patients who are more likely to require transfusion. In one study, only 4 (1.6%) of 251 high-risk patients eventually required transfusion. Further, only 2 of 13 patients who did receive blood during the peripartum period had identifiable risk factors. This casts doubt on the benefits and cost effectiveness of autologous donation during pregnancy.[92]

In patients at risk for hemorrhage during cesarean section, the use of **acute normovolemic hemodilution** may decrease the need for transfusion. This involves the collection of blood immediately before surgery with the simultaneous infusion of an appropriate volume of crystalloid or colloid to maintain normovolemia. In one study of 38 patients at risk for hemorrhage, 750 to 1000 mL of blood was removed with the simultaneous infusion of an equal volume of pentastarch. The hemoglobin concentration decreased from 10.9 to 8.3 g/dL; fetal monitoring revealed no change in the fetal heart rate pattern. The blood was reinfused during surgery. Neonatal outcome was normal, and only one patient required homologous blood.[93] It may be unrealistic to expect that this technique will totally eliminate the need for homologous blood in all patients, but it may play a valuable role in the reducing the need for transfusion.

A final option for minimizing heterologous transfusion is **intraoperative blood salvage**. Unfortunately, it is as difficult to determine those patients who might benefit from the use of the cell saver as it is to identify patients who might benefit from autologous donation. Further, the cell saver eliminates functionally active tissue factor but does not completely remove *all* tissue factor from blood heavily contaminated with amniotic fluid.[94]

There are few published data regarding the use of intraoperative blood salvage in obstetric patients.[95-98] Jackson and Lonser[96] reported the safe use of intraoperative blood salvage in 64 parturients between 1980 and 1991. They observed no evidence of amniotic fluid embolism or other adverse

response to the transfusion of salvaged red blood cells. In a randomized study, Rainaldi et al.[97] observed that 34 patients who underwent intraoperative salvage and reinfusion of autologous blood (mean ± SD volume = 363 ± 153 mL) required fewer transfusions of homologous blood and had a shorter hospital stay than a control group. Rebarber et al.[98] performed a retrospective, multicenter study of 139 patients in whom autologous blood transfusion was performed during cesarean section between 1988 and 1997. (This study likely included some of the cases previously reported by Jackson and Lonser.[96]) The authors identified no cases of acute respiratory distress syndrome or amniotic fluid embolism, and they identified no increase in the incidence of other perioperative complications when outcome was compared with that of 87 control patients who underwent similar surgical procedures *without* autotransfusion at the same hospitals.

Together, these results are reassuring. However, additional studies are needed to confirm the safety of intraoperative blood salvage in pregnant women. Uncertainty remains regarding the etiology of the syndrome of amniotic fluid embolism (including uncertainty as to which agent[s] trigger the syndrome and which patients are at risk). Thus I believe that intraoperative blood salvage should be reserved for those situations in which sufficient banked blood is unavailable, or for situations in which homologous blood is unacceptable to the patient, and only after the surgical field has been irrigated and gross contamination with amniotic fluid has been eliminated. Use of a leukocyte depletion filter may provide a further margin of safety.[99]

STANDARDS FOR EQUIPMENT DISINFECTION

The ASA Subcommittee on Infection Control Policy has made specific recommendations regarding the disinfection of reusable anesthesia equipment that comes in contact with mucous membranes. In practice, this includes laryngoscope blades, endoscopes, and face masks. The ASA Subcommittee recommends that such items be washed as soon as possible to remove gross contamination, followed by either high-level disinfection or sterilization. Functionally, each of these procedures kills fungi, viruses, and vegetative bacteria (including mycobacteria). In addition, sterilization kills larger numbers of endospores.[76]

In many institutions, disposable carbon dioxide absorbers and unidirectional valves are used when anesthetizing HIV-infected patients. However, no evidence suggests that HIV is transmitted in respiratory aerosols.[100] This practice is unnecessary and is not recommended by the ASA Subcommittee. An exception involves the HIV patient with active pulmonary tuberculosis; if a disposable absorber is not used, the entire assembly distal to the fresh gas source must be disassembled and sterilized.

The rate of nosocomial transmission of HIV is negligible, and the only documented cases of such transmission apparently occurred in a setting in which disinfection procedures were notably lax.[100] Common sense measures should effectively reduce the rate of transmission to zero.

To The Health Care Worker

The primary means of preventing the transmission of HIV to health care workers is the mandatory use of universal blood and body fluid barrier precautions. This policy has three crucial components. First, it must be universal. Establishing a higher level of concern when dealing with known HIV-positive patients implies a lower level of concern when caring for patients not known to be HIV positive. Unfortunately, even a patient who is infected with HIV may be living within the window between the acquisition of infection and seroconversion. Further, we should be equally concerned with the transmission of other blood-borne infections of higher infectivity and sometimes equal deadliness, such as hepatitis B and C.

Second, this policy must be followed whenever contact with infectious material is anticipated. Blood obviously is the primary source of exposure, but other body fluids that are considered to be potentially infectious include amniotic fluid, CSF, synovial fluid, pleural fluid, and pericardial fluid. Saliva is not thought to be infectious, but manipulations of the oral mucosa (e.g., laryngoscopy, endotracheal intubation) likely lead to the contamination of saliva with blood.

Third, the barrier precautions must be effective. These barriers should include gloves, mask, and eye shields. The use of gloves prevents 98% of an anesthesiologist's contact with patient blood.[101] When gross contamination is likely (e.g., during neonatal resuscitation), full-length gowns are indicated.

An additional component of universal precautions is the avoidance of needlestick injuries. The recapping of needles is the most common cause of needlestick injuries. Contaminated needles, including needles that have been injected into intravenous tubing, should *not* be recapped by hand. If recapping is necessary, a mechanical protective device should be used. The use of needleless systems can be expected to significantly decrease the risk of injury, and the use of such systems should be encouraged.[102]

A problem that is unique to obstetric anesthesia practice is the appropriate means of removing meconium from the neonate's trachea. The traditional practice of applying direct suction by mouth to an endotracheal tube, even with the interposition of a face mask, is clearly unacceptable. The use of an in-line trap can reduce the risk of contamination when oral suction is applied, but unless the trap is maintained in the vertical position, it is possible for meconium to be aspirated by the operator. The ideal way of removing meconium includes the use of a mechanical device that allows direct application of wall suction to the endotracheal tube. The use of extreme negative pressure may cause tracheal invagination.[103] The preferred range of negative pressure is −80 to −120 mm Hg.

POSTEXPOSURE PROPHYLAXIS FOR HEALTH CARE WORKERS

Occupational exposure to HIV is perhaps the most frightening work-related injury that an anesthesiologist can sustain. The risk of seroconversion after percutaneous exposure to HIV-infected blood is approximately 0.3%,[104] but this provides little reassurance to the exposed health care worker in view of the presumed 100% fatality rate of HIV infection. As of June 2000, the CDC had received voluntary reports of 56 United States health care providers with documented HIV seroconversion temporally related to occupational exposure, and an additional 138 reports of seroconversion that were considered possibly a result of occupational exposure.[104]

Certain measures should be taken after any parenteral exposure to potentially infectious body fluids, even those of the HIV-negative patient (Box 43-6). Although it is of uncertain efficacy in preventing HIV seroconversion, local wound care with an antiseptic solution is indicated.[105] In view of the exceedingly high transmission rate of hepatitis B infection, it

is mandatory to determine the health care worker's antibody status after parenteral exposure to body fluids from a patient with known hepatitis B or a patient at high risk for infection with hepatitis B. A previously vaccinated health care worker with an absent or insufficient antibody titer should receive a booster dose of vaccine and hepatitis B immune globulin (HBIG) to provide protection until an adequate antibody response develops. A health care worker with no history of vaccination and an absent antibody titer should undergo primary immunization and should receive HBIG.[104]

Several primate studies have demonstrated that the administration of antiretroviral drugs shortly after inoculation with SIV or HIV-2 can prevent seroconversion.[106,107] Further, although prospective data are lacking, a retrospective case-control study demonstrated an 81% reduction in transmission of HIV to exposed health care workers who received ZDV prophylaxis.[108] Finally, the reduction of vertical transmission by ZDV therapy demonstrated by ACTG 076 was only partly a result of the reduction of maternal viral load; inhibition of viral replication clearly played some role.[104] Altogether, these results suggest that postexposure prophylaxis may play a significant role in preventing seroconversion.

The U.S. Public Health Service has issued postexposure prophylaxis guidelines for health care workers exposed to HIV via percutaneous injury (Table 43-1).[104] These recommendations attempt to determine the relative risk of transmission based on the nature of the material to which the worker was exposed, the size of the inoculum, the route of exposure, and the presumed viral titer in the inoculum. Although encouraging results have been obtained, the primary strategy for the prevention of occupational transmission should focus on the prevention of exposure, especially the prevention of needlestick injuries.

Box 43-6 TREATMENT OF OCCUPATIONAL EXPOSURE TO HIV

- Local wound care
- Administration of tetanus toxoid
- Determination of worker's hepatitis B antibody titers
- Risk stratification
- Chemoprophylaxis as indicated (see Table 43-1)

TABLE 43-1   U.S. PUBLIC HEALTH SERVICE GUIDELINES FOR POSTEXPOSURE HIV PROPHYLAXIS FOR PERCUTANEOUS INJURIES

	HIV positive Class 1*	HIV positive Class 2†	Source of unknown HIV status‡	Unknown source§	HIV negative
Less severe exposure‖	Basic two-drug PEP¶	Expanded three-drug PEP#	No PEP warranted; consider basic two-drug PEP for source with HIV risk factors	No PEP warranted; consider basic two-drug PEP in settings where exposure to HIV-infected patients is likely	No PEP warranted
More severe exposure**	Expanded three-drug PEP	Expanded three-drug PEP	No PEP warranted; consider basic two-drug PEP for source with HIV risk factors	No PEP warranted; consider basic two-drug PEP in settings where exposure to HIV-infected patients is likely	No PEP warranted

PEP, Postexposure prophylaxis.
*Asymptomatic HIV infection or known low viral load (<1500 RNA copies/mL).
†Symptomatic HIV infection, AIDS, acute seroconversion, known high viral load.
‡If PEP is initiated and source is later found to be HIV negative, PEP can be discontinued.
§For example, needle from sharps disposal container.
‖Solid needle, superficial injury.
¶ZDV 600 mg/day in two to three divided doses and 3TC 150 mg bid; alternative basic two-drug regimen: 3TC 150 mg bid and d4T 40 mg bid, *or* ddI 400 mg qd and d4T 40 mg bid.
#Basic regimen plus indinavir 800 mg q8h.
**Large-bore hollow needle, deep puncture, visible blood on device, needle used in patient's artery or vein.
From Centers for Disease Control and Prevention. Updated Public Health Service Guidelines for the Management of Occupational Exposures to HBV, HCV, and HIV and Recommendations for Postexposure Prophylaxis. MMWR 2001; 50(RR-11):24-5.

9. DeClercq E. New developments in anti-HIV chemotherapy. Biochim Biophys Acta 2002; 1587:258-75.
10. Layon AJ, Peck AB. Anesthetic effects on immune function: Where do we stand? In Stoelting RK, Barash PG, Gallagher TJ, editors. Advances in Anesthesia, vol 10. St Louis, Mosby, 1993:69-93.
11. Noel, GJ. Host defense abnormalities associated with HIV infection. Pediatr Clin North Am 1991; 38:37-43.
12. Chang Y, Cesarman E, Pessin MS, et al. Identification of herpesvirus-like DNA sequences in AIDS-associated Kaposi's sarcoma. Science 1994; 266:1865-9.
13. Moore PS, Chang Y. Detection of herpesvirus-like DNA sequences in Kaposi's sarcoma in patients with and those without HIV infection. N Engl J Med 1995; 332:1181-5.
14. Holodniy M, Busch MP. Establishing the diagnosis of HIV infection. In Dolin R, Masur H, Saag MS, editors. AIDS Therapy, 2nd ed. New York, Churchill-Livingstone, 2003:3-20.
15. Carr A, Cooper DA. Primary HIV infection. In Sande MA, Volberding PA, editors. The Medical Management of AIDS, 6th ed. Philadelphia, WB Saunders, 1999:67-78.
16. Denning DW, Anderson J, Rudge P, Smith H. Acute myelopathy associated with primary infection with human immunodeficiency virus. Br Med J 1987; 294:143-4.
17. Price RW. Management of the neurologic complications of HIV-1 infection and AIDS. In Sande MA, Volberding PA, editors. The Medical Management of AIDS, 6th ed. Philadelphia, WB Saunders, 1999:217-40.
18. Huang L, Stansell JD. Pneumocystis carinii pneumonia. In Sande MA, Volberding PA, editors. The Medical Management of AIDS, 6th ed. Philadelphia, WB Saunders, 1999:305-30.
19. Wachter RM, Luce JM, Safrin S, et al. Cost and outcome of intensive care for patients with AIDS, Pneumocystis carinii pneumonia, and severe respiratory failure. JAMA 1995;273:230-5.
20. Bozette SA, Sattler FR, Chiu J, et al. A controlled trial of early adjunctive treatment with corticosteroids for Pneumocystis carinii pneumonia in the acquired immunodeficiency syndrome. N Engl J Med 1990; 323:1451-7.
21. Chambers HF. Tuberculosis in the HIV-infected patient. In Sande MA, Volberding PA, editors. The Medical Management of AIDS, 6th ed. Philadelphia, WB Saunders, 1999:353-60.
22. Bartlett JG Other HIV-related pneumonias. In Sande MA, Volberding PA, editors. The Medical Management of AIDS, 6th ed. Philadelphia, WB Saunders, 1999:331-42.
23. Talal AH, Dieterich DT. Gastrointestinal and hepatic manifestations of HIV infection. In Sande MA, Volberding PA, editors. The Medical Management of AIDS, 6th ed. Philadelphia, WB Saunders, 1999: 195-216.
24. Connolly GM, Hawkins D, Harcourt-Webster JN et al. Oesophageal symptoms, their causes, treatment and prognosis in patients with the acquired immunodeficiency syndrome. Gut 1989;30:1033-9.
25. Hambleton J. Hematologic complications of HIV infection. In Sande MA, Volberding PA, editors. The Medical Management of AIDS, 6th ed. Philadelphia, WB Saunders, 1999:265-74.
26. Cheitlin MD. Cardiovascular complications of HIV infection. In Sande MA, Volberding PA, editors. The Medical Management of AIDS, 6th ed. Philadelphia, WB Saunders, 1999:275-84.
27. Barbaro G. Cardiovascular manifestations of HIV infection. Circulation 2002;106:1420-5.
28. Schambelan M, Sellmeyer DE, Grunfeld C. Endocrinologic manifestations of HIV infection. In Sande MA, Volberding PA, editors. The Medical Management of AIDS, 6th ed. Philadelphia, WB Saunders, 1999:285-96.
29. Rodriguez RA, Humphreys MH. Renal complications of HIV infection. In Sande MA, Volberding PA, editors. The Medical Management of AIDS, 6th ed. Philadelphia, WB Saunders, 1999:297-302.
30. Herman ES, Klotman PE. HIV-associated nephropathy: epidemiology, pathogenesis, and treatment. Semin Nephrol 2003;23:200-8.
31. Gwinn M, Pappaioanou M, George JR, et al. Prevalence of HIV infection in childbearing women in the United States: Surveillance using newborn blood samples. JAMA 1991; 265:1704-8.
32. Centers for Disease Control and Prevention. US Public Health Service recommendations for human immunodeficiency virus counseling and voluntary testing for pregnant women. MMWR 1995; 44 (RR-7):1-15.
33. Miles SA, Balden E, Magpantay L, et al. Rapid serologic testing with immune-complex-dissociated HIV p24 antigen for early detection of HIV infection in neonates. N Engl J Med 1993; 328:297-302.
34. Pavia AT, Christenson JC. Pediatric AIDS. In Sande MA, Volberding PA, editors. The Medical Management of AIDS, 6th ed. Philadelphia, WB Saunders, 1999:525-35.

KEY POINTS

- HIV is the third most common cause of death among women of reproductive age in the United States.
- The prevalence of HIV seropositivity among pregnant women in the United States has been estimated to be as high as 1.7 per 1000.
- HIV infection eventually can be expected to involve every organ system. CNS involvement occurs as early as the period of initial infection and seroconversion.
- ZDV therapy during pregnancy results in a 67% reduction in the rate of vertical transmission of HIV to the infant. Elective cesarean section reduces the rate of vertical transmission of HIV by almost 50%. The *combination* of ZDV therapy during pregnancy *and* elective cesarean section reduces vertical transmission of HIV to a rate of 2% or less.
- HIV-infected patients often are treated with multiple medications, each of which has side effects that are relevant to anesthetic management.
- Regional anesthesia is safe in the HIV-infected parturient.
- Autologous epidural blood patch is safe in the HIV-infected patient.
- Our greatest contribution to minimizing the spread of HIV to uninfected patients is the minimization of homologous blood transfusion.
- The most effective method of minimizing HIV transmission to health care workers is strict adherence to universal blood and body fluid barrier precautions.
- Postexposure prophylaxis has the potential to decrease transmission of HIV by as much as 81%. It is indicated for all health care workers who experience high-risk exposures to potentially infectious materials.

REFERENCES

1. Centers for Disease Control and Prevention. HIV/AIDS Surveillance Report, 2002; 14:1-48. URL http://www.cdc.gov/hiv/stats/hasrlink.htm. (Accessed Dec. 18, 2003.)
2. Ahdieh L. Pregnancy and infection with human immunodeficiency virus. Clin Obstet Gynecol 2001; 44:154-66.
3. Centers for Disease Control. Update: Mortality attributable to HIV infection among persons aged 25-44 years, United States 1994. MMWR 1996; 45(6):121-5.
4. Geleziunas R, Greene WC. Molecular insights into HIV-1 infection and pathogenesis. In Sande MA, Volberding PA, editors. The Medical Management of AIDS, 6th ed. Philadelphia, WB Saunders, 1999:23-39.
5. Bryant ML, Ratner L. Biology and molecular biology of human immunodeficiency virus. Pediatr Infect Dis J 1992; 11:390-400.
6. Staprans SI, Feinberg MB. Natural history and immunopathogenesis of HIV-1 disease. In Sande MA, Volberding PA, editors. The Medical Management of AIDS, 5th ed. Philadelphia, WB Saunders, 1997:29-56.
7. Maury W, Potts BJ, Rabson AB. HIV-1 infection of first-trimester and term human placental tissue: A possible mode of maternal-fetal transmission. J Infect Dis 1989; 160:583-8.
8. Kilby JM. Inhibitors of HIV attachment and fusion. In Dolin R, Masur H, Saag MS, editors. AIDS Therapy, 2nd ed. New York, Churchill-Livingstone, 2003:252-62.

35. Ryder RW, Nsa W, Hassig SE, et al. Perinatal transmission of the human immunodeficiency virus type 1 to infants of seropositive women in Zaire. N Engl J Med 1989; 320:1637-42.

36. Dickover RE, Garratty EM, Herman SA, et al. Identification of levels of maternal HIV-1 RNA associated with risk of perinatal transmission. JAMA 1996; 275:599-605.

37. Landesman SH, Kalish LA, Burns DN, et al. Obstetrical factors and the transmission of human immunodeficiency virus type I from mother to child. N Engl J Med 1996; 334:1617-23.

38. Mandelbrot L, Mayaux M-J, Bongain A, et al. Obstetric factors and mother-to-child transmission of human immunodeficiency virus type 1: The French perinatal cohorts. Am J Obstet Gynecol 1996; 175:661-7.

39. St. Louis ME, Kamenga M, Brown C, et al. Risk for perinatal HIV-1 transmission according to maternal immunologic, virologic, and placental factors. JAMA 1993; 269:2853-9.

40. Viscarello RR, Copperman AB, DeGennaro NJ. Is the risk of perinatal transmission of human immunodeficiency virus increased by the intrapartum use of spiral electrodes or fetal pH sampling? Am J Obstet Gynecol 1994; 170:740-3.

41. Beckerman KP. Conception, pregnancy, and parenthood: maternal health care and the HIV epidemic. In Sande MA, Volberding PA, editors. The Medical Management of AIDS, 6th ed. Philadelphia, WB Saunders, 1999:555-73.

42. Dunn DT, Newell ML, Ades AE, Peckham CS. Risk of human immunodeficiency virus type 1 transmission through breast-feeding. Lancet 1992; 340:585-8.

43. Connor EM, Sperling RS, Gelber R, et al. Reduction of maternal-infant transmission of human immunodeficiency virus type 1 with zidovudine treatment. N Engl J Med 1994; 331:1173-80.

44. Minkoff H. Human immunodeficiency virus infection in pregnancy. Obstet Gynecol 2003;101:797-810.

45. American College of Obstetricians and Gynecologists. Scheduled cesarean delivery and prevention of vertical transmission of HIV infection. ACOG Committee Opinion No. 219, 1999.

46. Ioannidis JPA, Abrams EJ, Ammann A, et al. Perinatal transmission of human immunodeficiency virus type 1 by pregnant women with RNA viral loads <1000 copies/ml. J Infect Dis 2001;183:539-45.

47. Alger LS, Farley JJ, Robinson BA, et al. Interactions of human immunodeficiency virus infection and pregnancy. Obstet Gynecol 1993; 82:787-96.

48. Temmerman M, Chomba EN, Ndinya-Achola J, et al. Maternal human immunodeficiency virus-1 infection and pregnancy outcome. Obstet Gynecol 1994; 83:495-501.

49. Minkoff H, Willoughby A, Mendez H, et al. Serious infections during pregnancy among women with advanced human immunodeficiency virus infection. Am J Obstet Gynecol 1990; 162:30-4.

50. Tuomala RE, Shapiro DE, Mofenson LM, et al. Antiretroviral therapy during pregnancy and the risk of an adverse outcome. N Engl J Med 2002; 346:1863-70.

51. Burns DN, Landesman S, Minkoff H, et al. The influence of pregnancy on human immunodeficiency virus type 1 infection: Antepartum and postpartum changes in human immunodeficiency virus type 1 viral load. Am J Obstet Gynecol 1998; 178:355-9.

52. Bessinger R, Clark R, Kissinger P et al. Pregnancy is not associated with the progression of HIV disease in women attending an HIV outpatient program. Am J Epidemiol 1998; 147:434-40.

53. Fischl MA. Zidovudine. In Dolin R, Masur H, Saag MS, editors. AIDS Therapy, 2nd ed. New York, Churchill-Livingstone, 2003:23-38.

54. Dolin R. Didanosine. In Dolin R, Masur H, Saag MS, editors. AIDS Therapy, 2nd ed. New York, Churchill-Livingstone, 2003:39-56.

55. Bartlett JA. Zalcitabine. In Dolin R, Masur H, Saag MS, editors. AIDS Therapy, 2nd ed. New York, Churchill-Livingstone, 2003:57-65.

56. Pavia AT. Stavudine. In Dolin R, Masur H, Saag MS, editors. AIDS Therapy, 2nd ed. New York, Churchill-Livingstone, 2003:66-83.

57. Eron JJ. Lamivudine. In Dolin R, Masur H, Saag MS, editors. AIDS Therapy, 2nd ed. New York, Churchill-Livingstone, 2003:84-101.

58. Johnson VA. Abacavir. In Dolin R, Masur H, Saag MS, editors. AIDS Therapy, 2nd ed. New York, Churchill-Livingstone, 2003:110-21.

59. Montaner JSG, Lange JMA. Nevirapine. In Dolin R, Masur H, Saag MS, editors. AIDS Therapy, 2nd ed. New York, Churchill-Livingstone, 2003:134-44.

60. Demeter LM, Reichman RC. Delavirdine. In Dolin R, Masur H, Saag MS, editors. AIDS Therapy, 2nd ed. New York, Churchill-Livingstone, 2003:122-33.

61. Mayers DL. Efavirenz. In Dolin R, Masur H, Saag MS, editors. AIDS Therapy, 2nd ed. New York, Churchill-Livingstone, 2003:145-56.

62. Deeks SG, Volberding PA. Antiretroviral therapy. In Sande MA, Volberding PA, editors. The Medical Management of AIDS, 6th ed. Philadelphia, WB Saunders, 1999:97-115.

63. Hadigan C, Grinspoon S. Diabetes, insulin resistance, lipid disorders, and fat redistribution syndromes. In Dolin R, Masur H, Saag MS, editors. AIDS Therapy, 2nd ed. New York, Churchill-Livingstone, 2003:862-73.

64. Norvir (Ritonavir). In Physicians' Desk Reference, 57th ed. Montvale, NJ, Medical Economics, 2003:484.

65. Agenerase (Amprenavir). In Physicians' Desk Reference, 57th ed. Montvale, NJ, Medical Economics, 2003:1440.

66. Drew WL, Stempien MJ, Kheraj M, Erlich KS. Management of herpesvirus infections (cytomegalovirus, herpes simplex virus, and varicella zoster virus). In Sande MA, Volberding PA, editors. The Medical Management of AIDS, 6th ed. Philadelphia, WB Saunders, 1999: 429-52.

67. Polis MA. Cytomegalovirus disease. In Dolin R, Masur H, Saag MS, editors. AIDS Therapy, 2nd ed. New York, Churchill-Livingstone, 2003:582-603.

68. Medina I, Mills J, Leoung G, et al. Oral therapy for *Pneumocystis carinii* pneumonia in the acquired immunodeficiency syndrome: A controlled trial of trimethoprim-sulfamethoxazole versus trimethoprim-dapsone. N Engl J Med 1990; 323:776-82.

69. Masur H. Pneumocystis. In Dolin R, Masur H, Saag MS, editors. AIDS Therapy, 2nd ed. New York, Churchill-Livingstone, 2003:403-18.

70. Schneider MME, Hoepelman AIM, Schattenkerk JKME, et al. A controlled trial of aerosolized pentamidine or trimethoprim-sulfamethoxazole as primary prophylaxis against *Pneumocystis carinii* pneumonia in patients with human immunodeficiency virus infection. N Engl J Med 1992; 327:1836-41.

71. Minkoff HL, DeHovitz JA. Care of women infected with the human immunodeficiency virus. JAMA 1991; 266:2253-8.

72. Piscitelli SC, Pau AK. AIDS-related medications. In Dolin R, Masur H, Saag MS, editors. AIDS Therapy, 2nd ed. New York, Churchill-Livingstone, 2003:940-70.

73. Minkoff HL, Moreno JD. Drug prophylaxis for human immunodeficiency virus-infected pregnant women: Ethical considerations. Am J Obstet Gynecol 1990; 163:1111-4.

74. Hughes SC, Dailey PA, Landers D, et al. Parturients infected with human immunodeficiency virus and regional anesthesia: Clinical and immunologic response. Anesthesiology 1995; 82:32-7.

75. Avidan MS, Groves P, Blott M, et al. Low complication rate associated with cesarean section under spinal anesthesia for HIV-1 infected women on antiretroviral therapy. Anesthesiology 2002; 97:320-4.

76. American Society of Anesthesiologists Subcommittee on Infection Control Policy. Recommendations for Infection Control for the Practice of Anesthesiology. Park Ridge, Ill, 1994.

77. Kern JMD, Croy BB. AIDS litigation for the primary care physician. In Sande MA, Volberding PA, editors. The Medical Management of AIDS, 3rd ed. Philadelphia, WB Saunders, 1992:477-83.

78. Gibbons JJ. Post-dural puncture headache in the HIV-positive patient (letter). Anesthesiology 1991; 74:953.

79. Griffiths AG, Beards SC, Jackson A, Horsman EL. Visualization of extradural blood patch for post lumbar puncture headache by magnetic resonance imaging. Br J Anaesth 1993; 70:223-5.

80. Tom DJ, Gulevich SJ, Shapiro HM, et al. Epidural blood patch in the HIV-positive patient: Review of clinical experience. Anesthesiology 1992; 76:943-7.

81. Gershon RY, Manning-Williams D. Anesthesia and the HIV-infected parturient: A retrospective study. Int J Obstet Anesth 1997; 6:76-81.

82. Evron S, Glezerman M, Harow E, et al. Human immunodeficiency virus: Anesthetic and obstetric considerations. Anesth Analg 2004; 98:503-11.

83. Consensus Conference. Perioperative red blood cell transfusion. JAMA 1988; 260:2700-3.

84. Klein L. Premature birth and maternal prenatal anemia. Am J Obstet Gynecol 1962; 83:588-90.

85. Kaltreider DF, Johnson JWC. Patients at high risk for low-birth weight delivery. Am J Obstet Gynecol 1976; 124:251-6.

86. American Society of Anesthesiologists Committee on Transfusion Medicine. Questions and Answers About Transfusion Practices, 3rd ed. Park Ridge, Ill, 1998.

87. Cordell RR, Yalon VA, Cigahn-Haskell C, et al. Experience with 11,916 designated donors. Transfusion 1986; 26:484-6.

88. Cumming PD, Wallace EL, Schorr JB, Dodd RY. Exposure of patients to human immunodeficiency virus through the transfusion of blood components that test antibody-negative. N Engl J Med 1989; 321:941-6.

89. Thaler M, Shamiss A, Orgad S, et al. The role of blood from HLA-homozygous donors in fatal transfusion-associated graft-versus-host disease after open-heart surgery. N Engl J Med 1989; 321:25-8.

90. Herbert WP, Owen HG, Collins ML. Autologous blood storage in obstetrics. Obstet Gynecol 1988; 72:166-70.

91. McVay PA, Hoag RW, Hoag MS, Toy PTCY. Safety and use of autologous blood donation during the third trimester of pregnancy. Am J Obstet Gynecol 1989; 160:1479-88.

92. Andres RL, Piacquadio KM, Resnik R. A reappraisal of the need for autologous blood donation in the obstetric patient. Am J Obstet Gynecol 1990; 163:1551-3.

93. Grange CS Douglas MJ, Adams TJ, Wadsworth.LD. The use of acute hemodilution in parturients undergoing cesarean section. Am J Obstet Gynecol 1998; 178:156-60.

94. Bernstein HH, Rosenblatt MA, Gettes M, Lockwood C. The ability of the Haemonetics 4 cell saver to remove tissue factor from blood contaminated with amniotic fluid. Anesth Analg 1997; 85:831-3.

95. Grimes DA. A simplified device for intraoperative autotransfusion. Obstet Gynecol 1988; 72:947-50.

96. Jackson SH, Lonser RE. Safety and effectiveness of intracesarean blood salvage (letter). Transfusion 1993; 33:181.

97. Rainaldi MP, Tazzari PL, Scagliarini G, et al. Blood salvage during cesarean section. Br J Anaesth 1998; 80:195-8.

98. Rebarber A, Lonser R, Jackson S, et al. The safety of intraoperative autologous blood collection and autotransfusion during cesarean section. Am J Obstet Gynecol 1998; 179:715-20.

99. Waters JH, Biscotti C, Potter PS, Phillipson E. Amniotic fluid removal during cell salvage in the cesarean section patient. Anesthesiology 2000; 92:1519-22.

100. Gerberding JL. Limiting the risks to health care workers. In Sande MA, Volberding PA, editors. The Medical Management of AIDS, 5th ed. Philadelphia, WB Saunders, 1997:75-85.

101. Kristensen MS, Sloth E, Jensen TK. Relationship between anesthetic procedure and contact of anesthesia personnel with patient body fluids. Anesthesiology 1990; 73:619-24.

102. Greene ES, Berry AJ, Arnold WP, Jagger J. Percutaneous injuries in anesthesia personnel. Anesth Analg 1996; 83:273-8.

103. Bent RC, Wiswell TE, Chang A. Removing meconium from infant tracheae: What works best? Am J Dis Child 1992; 146:1085-9.

104. Centers for Disease Control and Prevention. Updated Public Health Service guidelines for the management of occupational exposures to HBV, HCV, and HIV and recommendations for postexposure prophylaxis. MMWR 2001; 50(RR-11):1-52.

105. Henderson DK, Fahey BJ, Willy M, et al. Risk for occupational transmission of human immunodeficiency virus type 1 (HIV-1) associated with clinical exposures: A prospective evaluation. Ann Intern Med 1990; 113:740-6.

106. Böttiger D, Johansson N-G, Samuelsson B, et al. Prevention of simian immunodeficiency virus, SIV_{sm}, or HIV-2 infection in cynomolgus monkeys by pre- and postexposure administration of BEA-005. AIDS 1997; 11:157-62.

107. Otten RA, Smith DK, Adams DR, et al. Efficacy of postexposure prophylaxis after intravaginal exposure of pig-tailed macaques to a human-derived retrovirus (HIV-2). J Virol 2000; 74:9771-5.

108. Cardo DM, Culver DH, Ciesielski CA, et al. A case-control study of HIV seroconversion in health care workers after percutaneous exposure. N Engl J Med 1997; 337:1485-90.

Chapter 44
Hypertensive Disorders

David R. Gambling, M.B., B.S., FRCPC

The hypertensive disorders of pregnancy are a leading cause of maternal death, with an estimated 50,000 women dying from preeclampsia each year, worldwide.[1] Hypertensive disease is the third highest cause of direct maternal death in the United States, after thromboembolism (number 1) and hemorrhage (number 2), accounting for 15% of direct maternal deaths.[2] In the United Kingdom, hypertensive disease of pregnancy remains the second leading cause of direct maternal death, after thromboembolism.[3]

In the past, the terminology used to define hypertension during pregnancy has been confusing. The National High Blood Pressure Education Program Working Group has recommended that the term *gestational hypertension* replace the term *pregnancy-induced hypertension* to describe cases in which high blood pressure without proteinuria develops after 20 weeks' gestation and subsequently resolves postpartum (Box 44-1).[2] As many as 25% of women with gestational hypertension will develop proteinuria and the syndrome of preeclampsia.[4]

Preeclampsia is a syndrome defined by hypertension and proteinuria, and can be associated with other signs and symptoms such as edema, visual disturbances, headache, and epigastric pain. The term *eclampsia* is used when central nervous system (CNS) involvement results in seizures in a woman with preeclampsia. The term *HELLP syndrome* is applied to preeclamptic women with *H*emolysis, *E*levated *L*iver enzymes, and *L*ow *P*latelets, although the exact relationship between preeclampsia and HELLP syndrome is unclear. Proteinuria may not always be present in patients with HELLP syndrome.[1]

Chronic hypertension exists in 5% of pregnant women and is defined as hypertension present before 20 weeks' gestation or present before pregnancy.[5] If it develops in late pregnancy, chronic hypertension may be difficult to distinguish from gestational hypertension and preeclampsia, but if the hypertension persists beyond 12 weeks postpartum it is classified as chronic. Chronic hypertension is commonly complicated by superimposed preeclampsia, which is often difficult to diagnose.

PREECLAMPSIA

The term *preeclampsia* describes the development of hypertension with proteinuria after 20 weeks' gestation. (Patients with gestational trophoblastic disease, such as hydatidiform mole, can develop preeclampsia before 20 weeks' gestation [Box 44-2].) Preeclampsia is defined as mild unless one or more co-existing conditions make it severe (Box 44-3).

Epidemiology

A disorder of unknown etiology, preeclampsia affects 5% to 9% of all pregnancies, although the incidence may vary considerably from one institution to another.[6] Between 1979 and 1986, the incidence of preeclampsia increased from 2.4 per 1000 deliveries to 5.2 per 1000 deliveries in the United States[7]; this may reflect both a true increase in the incidence of the disease, as well as improved record keeping. The increasing rate of preeclampsia is in part a result of an increase in the birth rates among older women, as well as the large increase in the number of high-order multiple gestations associated with assisted reproductive techniques.

Approximately 85% of cases of preeclampsia affect women during their first pregnancy.[6] Box 44-4 lists other risk factors for the development of preeclampsia. In the past, low socioeconomic status and young maternal age were considered risk factors, but their independent contribution to the risk for preeclampsia is not clear. In a study of 4024 pregnancy-related deaths after 20 weeks' gestation in the United States between 1979 and 1992, MacKay et al.[8] reported a maternal death rate from preeclampsia or eclampsia of 1.5 deaths/100,000 live

---

Box 44-1 CLASSIFICATION OF HYPERTENSIVE DISORDERS IN PREGNANCY[2]

- **GESTATIONAL HYPERTENSION**
  - Transient hypertension of pregnancy, if preeclampsia is not present at time of delivery, and blood pressure returns to normal by 12 weeks postpartum (a retrospective diagnosis)
- **PREECLAMPSIA**
  - Mild
  - Severe
- **HELLP SYNDROME (HEMOLYSIS, ELEVATED LIVER ENZYMES, LOW PLATELETS)**
- **CHRONIC HYPERTENSION**
- **CHRONIC HYPERTENSION WITH SUPERIMPOSED PREECLAMPSIA**

Box 44-2 CRITERIA FOR THE DIAGNOSIS OF PREECLAMPSIA[1]

HYPERTENSION*

A sustained systolic blood pressure of at least 140 mm Hg, or a sustained diastolic blood pressure of at least 90 mm Hg, that occurs after 20 weeks' gestation in a woman with previously normal blood pressure.

PROTEINURIA

≥ 300 mg protein in a 24-hour urine collection

---

*Preeclampsia is a pregnancy-specific syndrome that usually occurs after 20 weeks' gestation.

Box 44-3 FEATURES OF SEVERE PREECLAMPSIA[1]

Blood pressure: ≥ 160 mm Hg systolic or ≥ 110 mm Hg diastolic on two occasions at least 6 hours apart while the patient is on bed rest; diagnosis not delayed if the diastolic blood pressure exceeds 110 mm Hg

Proteinuria: ≥ 5 g in a 24-hour urine specimen (or ≥ 3+ on two random urine samples at least 4 hours apart.)

Oliguria: Urine output < 500 mL in 24 hours

Cerebral or visual disturbances: Headache, blurred vision, or altered consciousness

Pulmonary edema or cyanosis

Epigastric or right upper quadrant pain: Believed to be caused by stretching of Glisson's capsule by hepatic edema

Hepatic rupture: Fortunately a rare complication

Impaired liver function

Thrombocytopenia

Fetal growth restriction

---

births. The highest risk of death was at 20 to 28 weeks' gestation. Black women were at greater risk for maternal death than white women. Other risk factors include no antenatal care and advanced maternal age.[9]

Pathogenesis

Preeclampsia is a systemic disorder that occurs only in the presence of placental tissue. However, the exact pathogenic mechanisms responsible for the initiation and progression of preeclampsia are not well defined. Preeclampsia is most likely

---

Box 44-4 RISK FACTORS FOR PREECLAMPSIA[11]

I. PRECONCEPTIONAL AND/OR CHRONIC RISK FACTORS

PARTNER-RELATED RISK FACTORS

- Nulliparity/primipaternity/teenage pregnancy
- Limited sperm exposure, donor insemination, oocyte donation
- Oral sex (risk reduction)
- Partner who fathered a preeclamptic pregnancy in another woman

NON-PARTNER-RELATED RISK FACTORS

- History of previous preeclampsia
- Age, interval between pregnancies
- Family history

PRESENCE OF SPECIFIC UNDERLYING DISORDERS

- Chronic hypertension and renal disease
- Obesity, insulin resistance, low birth weight
- Gestational diabetes, type I diabetes mellitus
- Activated protein C resistance (factor V mutation), protein S deficiency
- Antiphospholipid antibodies
- Hyperhomocysteinemia
- Sickle cell disease, sickle cell trait (?)

EXOGENOUS FACTORS

- Smoking (risk reduction)
- Stress, work-related psychosocial strain
- In utero diethylstilbestrol exposure

II. PREGNANCY-ASSOCIATED RISK FACTORS

- Multiple pregnancy
- Structural congenital anomalies
- Hydrops fetalis
- Chromosomal anomalies (trisomy 13, triploidy)
- Hydatidiform mole
- Urinary tract infection

---

a disease with heterogeneous causes linked to maternal, paternal, fetal, and placental factors.[10,11]

IMMUNOLOGIC FACTORS

The fetus acquires 50% of its genes from the father; thus it represents, in part, a paternal allograft that interacts with maternal tissue as fetal trophoblast migrates into the maternal decidua after implantation. True intervillous flow is established by 12 weeks' gestation, and in normal pregnancy, a second wave of trophoblastic invasion occurs at 14 to 16 weeks' gestation. This invasion results in the disruption of the muscular integrity of the maternal spiral arteries, which leads to their adrenergic denervation and converts them from high-resistance to low-resistance vessels.[11] At the same time, biochemical adaptations occur in the maternal vasculature, with an increased dominance of the endothelium-dependent vasodilators **prostacyclin (PGI$_2$)** and **nitric oxide**.

In women with preeclampsia, a failure of this secondary trophoblastic invasion at the deciduo-myometrial junction occurs.[12] This failure can result in a high-resistance, low-flow uteroplacental circulation and consequent placental ischemia and hypoxia. These changes antedate the full clinical development of preeclampsia and may represent an aberrant immunologic mechanism.[11] In some women, these changes lead to

preeclampsia; other women do not develop hypertension but have babies with intrauterine growth restriction (IUGR).

Zuspan[13] considered preeclampsia "a birth defect, acquired at the time of implantation." Other factors consistent with an immunologic etiology include the occurrence of the disease in a subsequent pregnancy when a woman changes her partner[14] and occurrence after a woman has discontinued birth-control methods that prevent exposure to sperm.[15] Further, the risk of developing preeclampsia decreases with an increased duration of unprotected, preconception sexual activity with the father of the child.[16] However, the hypothesis that the risk of preeclampsia may be reduced with repeated maternal exposure and adaptation to specific foreign antigens of the partner was challenged in a study from Norway, which suggested that the interval between births was more important.[17] The authors concluded that "the protective effect of previous pregnancy against preeclampsia is transient" and that "a change of partner is not associated with an increased risk of preeclampsia." A major difficulty in identifying an immunologic origin for preeclampsia is that the immunologic changes associated with normal early pregnancy are not yet fully explained.[18]

GENETIC FACTORS

The genetic inheritance of preeclampsia is complex, and genetic studies of preeclampsia are difficult to perform. A familial tendency toward preeclampsia exists in some populations[19] and may result from a recessive fetal inheritance or maternal-fetal sharing of a recessive gene.[20] A number of genes are presently being studied by the Genetics of Preeclampsia Collaborative Study in the United Kingdom. These include the following:

Angiotensinogen

A molecular variant of angiotensinogen (angiotensinogen gene T235) has been described in association with preeclampsia[21]; in homozygous carriers, it increases the risk for developing preeclampsia by a factor of 20.

Angiotensin II Type I Receptor

Preeclamptic women are very sensitive to the vasopressor effects of angiotensin II. Preliminary evidence suggests that maternal-to-fetal transmission of an angiotensin II receptor dinucleotide repeat allele is increased in preeclampsia.[22]

Factor V Leiden

Recent evidence suggests that an increased resistance to activated protein C, caused by a mutation of the gene encoding coagulation factor V (factor V Leiden mutation), predisposes affected women to severe preeclampsia.[23,24] The Leiden mutation consists of an amino-acid substitution of glutamine for arginine at position 506 in the factor V molecule. This renders the protein resistant to proteolytic inactivation by activated protein C and predisposes carriers to thrombosis. Dizon-Townson et al.[23] postulated that the association between severe preeclampsia and factor V Leiden mutation results from an increased occurrence of thrombosis and infarction in the placenta. This thrombophilic mutation may also interact with a factor II mutation (G20210A), which is also more prevalent in women with preeclampsia and HELLP syndrome than in normotensive pregnant controls.[25]

Tumor Necrosis Factor-Alpha

It is unclear whether polymorphism of the tumor necrosis factor-alpha gene increases the risk or protects against the development of preeclampsia.[26]

Redman et al.[27] have suggested that preeclampsia represents an excessive maternal inflammatory response to pregnancy, and they have predicted that a single preeclampsia gene will not be found.

ENDOTHELIAL FACTORS

The vascular endothelium is a highly specialized, metabolically active interface between blood and underlying tissues.[10] Vascular endothelial damage and dysfunction is the common pathologic feature of preeclampsia and occurs in the placental decidual vessels and renal microvasculature.[28] Figure 44-1 shows a possible cascade of pathogenic factors that may lead to endothelial dysfunction in preeclampsia.[10] Endothelial injury also may cause (or result from) arteriolar vasospasm in the hepatic, myocardial, and cerebral circulations of patients with severe preeclampsia. Endothelial cell dysfunction in response to these postulated (but unknown) factor(s) may cause a hormonal imbalance in women with preeclampsia (Figure 44-2).

The metabolic end-products of normal vascular endothelium include the endothelium-derived relaxing factors (EDRF), nitric oxide, endothelium-derived hyperpolarizing factor (EDHF), and prostaglandins, including PGI_2. Both PGI_2 and nitric oxide are potent vasodilators. In preeclamptic women, the failure of trophoblast to invade the uteroplacental vascular bed may encourage an increased production of free radicals and lipid peroxides by the decidual lymphoid tissue.[29] Free radicals are a highly reactive and damaging species that augment endothelial damage and exacerbate the disease process by means of oxidative stress.[30] Lipid peroxides activate cyclooxygenase and impair PGI_2 synthetase. As a result, an imbalance occurs between the production of the vasoconstrictor **thromboxane (TXA_2)**, which is derived from platelets, and the production of endothelium-derived PGI_2.

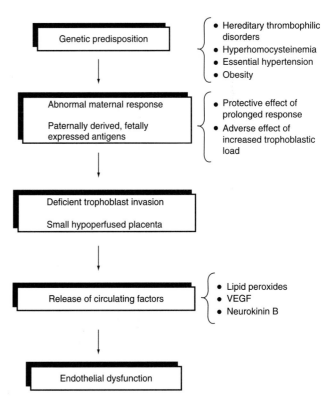

FIGURE 44-1. The proposed pathogenesis of preeclampsia. *VEGF,* Vascular endothelial growth factors. (From Kenny LC, Baker PN. The etiology of preeclampsia. In Belfort MA, Thornton S, Saade G [eds]. Hypertension in Pregnancy. New York, Marcel Dekker, 2003:17-36.)

This imbalance results in a reduced perfusion of the intervillous space. Lipid peroxide activity also may result in decreased release of nitric oxide from the endothelium in patients with preeclampsia.[31] Using a low-dose endotoxin infusion as a model for preeclampsia in rats, Sakawi et al.[32] showed that nitric oxide, either directly or via secondary species, plays a significant role in the biochemical and physiologic changes seen in preeclampsia.

Free radicals also may increase the plasma levels of the potent vasoconstrictor **endothelin,** which has the potential to contribute to the generalized vasoconstriction that occurs in patients with preeclampsia. Although there is evidence for the activation of the endothelin system in preeclampsia, the exact role of endothelin in the pathogenesis of preeclampsia is unclear.[33]

Healthy, normotensive pregnant women demonstrate a marked increase in the concentrations of plasma renin, angiotensin II, and aldosterone, which is accompanied by a blunted pressor response to exogenous angiotensin II.[34] They also show evidence of reduced adrenergic sensitivity.[35] In women with preeclampsia, the normal stimulation of the **renin-angiotensin-aldosterone system (RAAS)** does not occur. This lack of stimulation and an associated increase in vascular sensitivity to angiotensin II and norepinephrine (which antedates the development of clinical disease) may be explained by endothelial cell injury and reduced nitric oxide production.[35] **Endothelium-derived hyperpolarizing factor (EDHF)** is another potent vasodilator that has yet to be identified but could be an arachidonic acid product, an endogenous canniboid, or an increase in extracellular potassium.[36] In the absence of nitric oxide, EDHF can mediate vasodilator responses to bradykinin during normal pregnancy but not in preeclampsia. The up-regulation of EDHF activity may represent a vascular adaptation to normal pregnancy that is absent in preeclampsia and thus contributes to clinical features of the disease.[37]

PLATELET FACTORS

Redman[38] described preeclampsia as a "trophoblast-dependent process, mediated by platelet dysfunction and prevented at least in part by anti-platelet agents." Platelet dysfunction may be mediated by vascular endothelial damage. In the absence of adequate PGI₂ and nitric oxide,[39] surface-mediated platelet activation occurs, which favors platelet adhesion to the damaged surface lining of the spiral arteries. Platelet adhesion subsequently releases the constituents of the dense granules, including TXA₂ and serotonin (5-hydroxytryptamine, or 5-HT), which promote further platelet aggregation.

In patients with mild preeclampsia, some intact endovascular trophoblast and endothelium may persist in the spiral arteries.[34] The serotonin released from aggregating platelets interacts with endothelial 5-HT₁ receptors, resulting in a partial recovery of vascular PGI₂ and nitric oxide release. The PGI₂ stimulates the uteroplacental RAAS, inducing the release of uteroplacental angiotensin II and improving uteroplacental perfusion by increased pressure. The needs of the fetus are ensured but at the cost of increased maternal blood pressure (Figure 44-3).

In patients with early-onset severe preeclampsia, a greater degree of injury occurs in the walls of the uteroplacental vessels. They cannot respond with an endothelium-dependent 5-HT₁ effect, and the released serotonin interacts instead with 5-HT₂ receptors on the vascular smooth muscle cells. Platelet-derived serotonin also activates 5-HT₂ platelet receptors, which amplifies the platelet aggregation process and establishes a positive feedback loop.[34] Ketanserin (a 5-HT₂ serotonergic-receptor blocker) effectively reduces preeclamptic hypertension and platelet aggregation, which supports the hypothesis that platelet-derived serotonin plays a major role in the pathophysiology of preeclampsia.[40]

Determining platelet aggregability in early pregnancy may allow for early detection of the disease. One study demonstrated that aggregation responses to collagen were universally

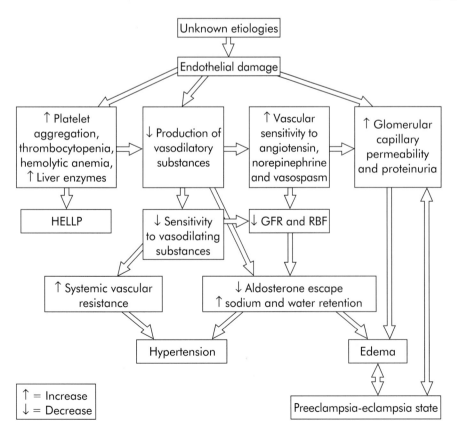

FIGURE 44-2. Hypothesis of the mechanisms by which endothelial damage leads to preeclampsia and eclampsia. *HELLP, Hemolysis, Elevated Liver enzymes, and Low Platelets; SVR,* systemic vascular resistance. (Modified from Boxer LM, Malinow AM Preeclampsia and eclampsia. Curr Opin Anesth 1997; 10:188-98.)

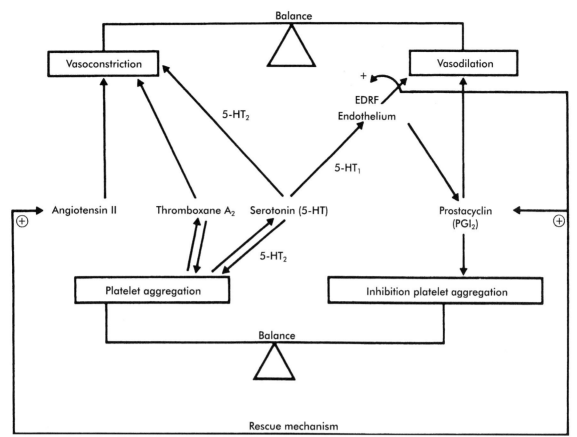

FIGURE 44-3. Control of uteroplacental perfusion in mild and early-onset severe preeclampsia. In mild preeclampsia, serotonin (5-HT) released from aggregating platelets interacts with endothelial 5-HT$_1$ receptors, resulting in the release of prostacyclin and nitric oxide *(EDRF)*. The released prostacyclin induces angiotensin II release, improving uteroplacental perfusion. In early-onset severe preeclampsia, damaged uteroplacental vessels cannot respond to a 5-HT$_1$ effect. Instead, serotonin interacts with 5-HT$_2$ receptors on vascular smooth muscle cells, inducing vasoconstriction. Platelet-derived serotonin also activates 5-HT$_2$ platelet receptors, establishing a positive feedback loop, and intensifying platelet aggregation. The loss of 5-HT$_1$ receptors prevents stimulation of the uteroplacental renin-angiotensin-aldosterone system and the rescue mechanism of angiotensin II release. (From deJong CL, Dekker GA, Sibai BM. The renin-angiotensin-aldosterone system in preeclampsia: A review. Clin Perinatol 1991; 18:683-711.)

higher in early pregnancy in women who developed preeclampsia than in normotensive controls.[41]

CALCIUM
Intracellular free calcium is an important determinant of vascular tone and contractility. In normal pregnancy, the intracellular free calcium concentration increases slowly, but this increase is significantly greater in the third trimester in women with preeclampsia.[42] Increased lipid peroxidation of cell membranes (which occurs in women with preeclampsia) increases cell permeability to calcium by partially inhibiting cell membrane calcium adenosine triphosphatase (ATPase) activity, which leads to an increase in cytoplasmic calcium levels.[43] This increase is enhanced by angiotensin II, and the enhancement is greater in women with preeclampsia than in normotensive women.[44] This response to angiotensin II occurs long before signs of preeclampsia become evident and is a sensitive predictor of its subsequent development.

COAGULATION FACTORS
The coagulation abnormalities seen in preeclampsia are likely the result of endothelial activation by one of a number of circulating factors.[45] One of these is **vascular endothelial growth factor (VEGF)**, a family of glycoproteins that causes endothelial cell PGI$_2$ production and promotes endothelial expression of procoagulant activity. VEGF levels are increased in women

with preeclampsia, and VEGF has a vasodilator effect on resistance vessels via production of nitric oxide.[45]

Platelet activation in preeclampsia is surface-mediated. Thrombocytopenia commonly occurs, although the platelet count rarely falls below 100,000/mm^3.[6] This compensated thrombolytic state resembles that which occurs in thrombotic thrombocytopenic purpura (TTP) and in the hemolytic uremic syndrome. Women with preeclampsia have an increased tendency toward thromboembolism *(vide infra)*, which may result in part from an alteration in the plasma ratio between von Willebrand factor (vWF) and factor VIII coagulant (F VIII C) activity. Endothelial cell damage releases von Willebrand factor into the circulation, and thrombin inactivates factor VIII coagulant activity, thus increasing the vWF/F VIII C ratio.[46]

FATTY ACID METABOLISM
A growing body of evidence suggests that altered handling of fatty acids by the liver is a key factor in the pathogenesis of preeclampsia.[47] Both increased hepatic uptake of free fatty acids and hypertriglyceridemia are seen more frequently in women who develop preeclampsia. These observations are compelling, given that various degrees of liver dysfunction occur in preeclampsia and endothelial cell accumulation of triglyceride can inhibit the release of PGI$_2$ (Figure 44-4). In addition, changes in lipoprotein metabolism seen in preeclampsia and HELLP syndrome may contribute to the coagulopathy occasionally associated with these conditions.[48]

In summary, the pathogenesis of preeclampsia is incompletely understood. It is possible that there are different subsets of preeclampsia that have yet to be defined. For example, the pathogenesis of preeclampsia may differ between nulliparous and parous women, and between women with early-onset disease and late-onset disease. In a recent editorial, Roberts[49] concluded that "it is unlikely that what we call preeclampsia is one disease."

Pathophysiology

Preeclampsia is a multisystem disorder that primarily affects the maternal cardiovascular, central nervous, and genitourinary systems. However, all systems become involved to some degree.

CARDIOVASCULAR CHANGES

Blood Pressure

Preeclamptic women often have a flattening or reversal of the normal diurnal blood pressure pattern.[50] Their characteristically labile blood pressure may reflect their increased sensitivity to endogenous pressor hormones and autocoids, which antedates the appearance of clinical signs.[6] Power spectral analysis confirms that heart rate and blood pressure variability is increased in women with preeclampsia.[51] This variability appears to result from an increase in the sympathetic and parasympathetic control of the cardiovascular system.[51] Moutquin et al.[52] noted significantly higher systolic and diastolic blood pressures during early pregnancy in nulliparous

women who later developed preeclampsia. Other investigators have not observed higher pressures until the second trimester (Figure 44-5).[53]

Some investigators believe that the increase in blood pressure results from an increase in peripheral vascular resistance secondary to a state of sympathetic overactivity. In a study that used a microneurographic technique to obtain recordings of postganglionic sympathetic nerve activity, both blood pressure and sympathetic activity were greater in preeclamptic patients than in normotensive pregnant controls.[54] The increase in sympathetic nerve activity in preeclamptic women was three times that of normotensive pregnant women and twice that of nonpregnant women with hypertension. Both blood pressure and the increase in postganglionic sympathetic nerve activity normalized shortly after delivery.[54]

Blood Volume

The preponderance of evidence suggests that blood volume is reduced in women with preeclampsia.[55] At least one study found no difference in mean plasma volumes between normotensive gravidae and women with mild preeclampsia (Figure 44-6).

Mabie et al.[56] observed normal central venous pressure (CVP) and pulmonary capillary wedge pressure (PCWP) in antepartum patients with severe preeclampsia and without pulmonary edema. They suggested that if preeclamptic women have decreased plasma volume, normal filling pressures may result from a redistribution of intravascular volume to the central circulation. The authors noted that many preeclamptic patients behave as if they are venoconstricted

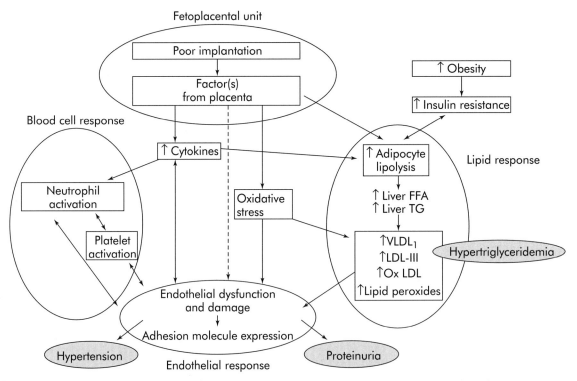

FIGURE 44-4. Summary of the potential role of a disturbance in fatty acid and lipoprotein metabolism in the pathogenesis of preeclampsia. Increased plasma cytokine (IL-1, TNF-a) concentrations resulting from the activation of macrophages/neutrophils either directly or indirectly through endothelial activation, or by the placenta itself, may enhance peripheral lipolysis, which already is stimulated in normal pregnancy by HPL. This results in an increased flux of free fatty acids (FFA) to the liver. These are channeled predominantly into hepatic triglyceride synthesis; thus there is an increased secretion (greater than that of normal pregnancy) of large, triglyceride-rich VLDL particles, which also are removed less efficiently than in normal pregnancy. Accumulation of triglyceride occurs in the hepatocyte when this pathway is saturated, and this response is a possible explanation for the fatty changes in liver that occur with preeclampsia and acute fatty liver of pregnancy (AFLP). Increased concentrations of triglyceride-rich lipoproteins in the circulation may contribute both directly and, through the generation of small, dense LDL, indirectly to endothelial dysfunction and therefore expression of preeclampsia in the mother. (From Sattar N, Gaw A, Packard CJ, Greer IA. Potential pathogenic roles of aberrant lipoprotein and fatty acid metabolism in preeclampsia. Br J Obstet Gynaecol 1996; 103:614-20.)

and are at risk for pulmonary congestion and edema after excessive fluid administration. Pouta et al.[57] demonstrated that an intravenous fluid bolus resulted in a greater increase in CVP in preeclamptic women than in normotensive controls undergoing spinal anesthesia. The authors suggested that this resulted from hypovolemia and decreased capacitance vessel compliance in the preeclamptic patients. Of interest, the same study demonstrated that basal levels of **atrial natriuretic peptide (ANP)** were higher in preeclamptic women; further, the fluid bolus resulted in a greater

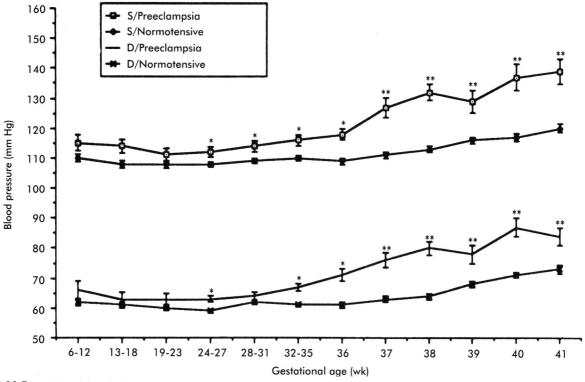

FIGURE 44-5. Systolic and diastolic blood pressures in normotensive pregnant women and in women destined to develop preeclampsia. *S/Preeclampsia,* Systolic blood pressure in the preeclamptic group; *S/Normotensive,* systolic blood pressure in the normotensive group; *D/Preeclampsia,* diastolic blood pressure in the preeclamptic group; *D/Normotensive,* diastolic blood pressure in the normotensive group. Values are expressed as ± SEM. *P < 0.01; **P < 0.001. (From Villar MA, Sibai BM. Clinical significance of elevated mean arterial blood pressure in second trimester and threshold increase in systolic or diastolic blood pressure during third trimester. Am J Obstet Gynecol 1989; 160:419-23.)

FIGURE 44-6. Plasma volume measurements (Evans blue dye-dilution technique) in the early and late third trimester in normotensive pregnant women and women with mild pregnancy-induced hypertension *(PIH)* with singleton pregnancies. *BSA,* Body surface area; *NS,* not significant. (From Sibai BM, Anderson GD, Spinnato JA, et al. Plasma volume findings in patients with mild pregnancy-induced hypertension. Am J Obstet Gynecol 1983; 147:16-9.)

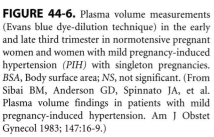
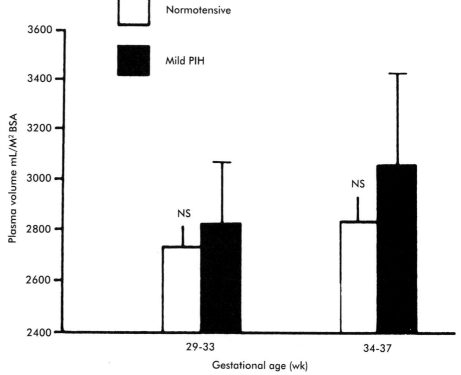

increase in ANP levels in preeclamptic patients than in control patients *(vide infra)*.[57]

Hemodynamic Changes

Early studies suggested that cardiac output is increased in preeclamptic women. Since the introduction of the pulmonary artery catheter and Doppler echocardiography, many investigators have measured cardiac output in preeclamptic women, with heterogenous findings.[58] Unfortunately, these studies often included patients with complicating factors, such as chronic hypertension, renal disease, oliguria, pulmonary edema, and prior treatment with intravenous fluids or antihypertensive drugs. Some investigators have studied parous women, despite the fact that "the purest form" of preeclampsia occurs in nulliparous women.[58]

Easterling et al.[59] used a noninvasive Doppler technique to measure cardiac output in preeclamptic women. The hemodynamic findings varied. However, as the severity of preeclampsia increased, the findings in individual patients changed from a hyperdynamic state (i.e., high cardiac output) to one characterized predominantly by high systemic vascular resistance (SVR). These same investigators also conducted a longitudinal study of uncomplicated nulliparous women who were enrolled before 22 weeks' gestation.[60] Women who subsequently developed preeclampsia had higher cardiac output than normotensive controls, but the authors found no evidence of increased SVR. Furthermore, no subjects crossed over to high-resistance hypertension as in their previous study, despite evidence of preeclampsia. More recent work has demonstrated a hyperdynamic state in preeclampsia, with elevated cardiac output before the onset of symptoms and a crossover to low cardiac output and high SVR with the onset of the clinical syndrome.[61] Cotton et al.[62] studied women with severe preeclampsia who had not received therapy. They suggested that three hemodynamic subsets exist. The majority of the subjects were hyperdynamic, with evidence of increased cardiac output, normal or slightly increased SVR, and normal or slightly decreased blood volume and filling pressures. A second subset had normal cardiac output and lower filling pressures but higher SVR. The third group demonstrated markedly increased SVR but significantly reduced blood volume and depressed left ventricular function (Figures 44-7 and 44-8).

In summary, the hemodynamic findings in preeclampsia are varied and complex. Hemodynamic measurements change during the course of the disease, with the stage of pregnancy, and in response to therapy.

Cardiac Function

Preeclamptic women typically have a normal heart rate, although significant tachycardia may occur after hydralazine administration. CVP measurements can be misleading; they vary significantly, and there is a poor correlation between CVP and PCWP in both treated[63] and untreated[64] women with severe preeclampsia (Figure 44-9). It is hazardous to give preeclamptic women a large bolus of fluid to achieve an arbitrary, predetermined CVP. Such management entails a definite risk of pulmonary edema.

Colloid Oncotic Pressure

The plasma colloid oncotic pressure (COP), which already is reduced in normal pregnancy because of the decreased albumin concentration, often is decreased further in preeclamptic women (Figure 44-10).[65] Mean COP measurements are approximately 18 mm Hg antepartum and 14 mm Hg postpartum in preeclamptic women. (This latter figure may reflect aggressive fluid administration.) In contrast, normal pregnant women have measurements of 22 and 17 mm Hg, respectively. The low COP, coupled with increased vascular perme-

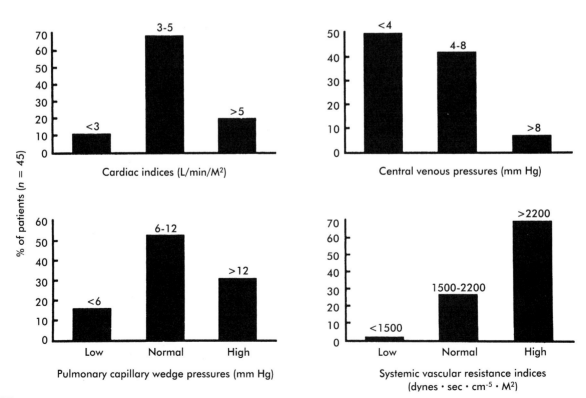

FIGURE 44-7. Hemodynamic subsets in 45 untreated subjects with severe preeclampsia. (From Cotton DB, Lee W, Huhta JC, Dorman KF. Hemodynamic profile of severe pregnancy-induced hypertension. Am J Obstet Gynecol 1988; 158:523-9.)

ability and the loss of intravascular fluid and protein into interstitial tissues, increases the risk of pulmonary edema.[66]

HEMATOLOGIC CHANGES

Well-documented coagulation abnormalities occur, typically in patients with severe disease. These include (1) hypercoagulability (i.e., accentuation of the normal pregnancy-associated hypercoagulability), (2) activation of the fibrinolytic system, and (3) platelet activation (Box 44-5).[67] Virtually all preeclamptic women have at least some evidence of abnormal activation of the clotting cascade.

Hypercoagulability

Evidence of hypercoagulability in the common pathway includes an accelerated prothrombin time (PT), increased activation of the common pathway factors (i.e., II, V, X), and decreased fibrinogen.[67]

Preeclamptic women may have a red blood cell membrane anomaly that may enhance and accelerate the occurrence of a

hypercoagulable state. This anomaly includes an altered configuration of phospholipids within the cell membrane, which results in a procoagulant cell surface that may trigger thrombin formation.[68]

Fibrin represents the end-point of the coagulation cascade. The subsequent degradation of fibrin polymer by plasmin produces non-cross-linked fragments and more stable dimeric fragments (e.g., D-dimer).[69] Hematologists historically have

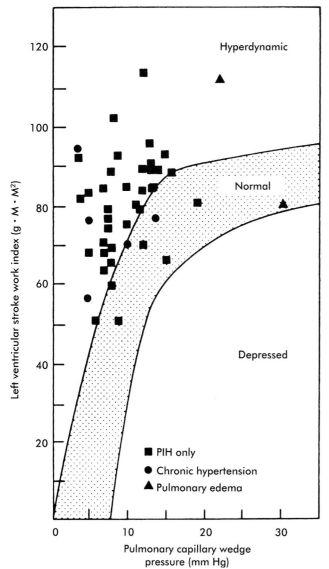

FIGURE 44-8. Left ventricular function curve in 45 untreated women with severe preeclampsia. Patients with the same values are represented by a single point. (From Cotton DB, Lee W, Huhta JC, Dorman KF. Hemodynamic profile of severe pregnancy-induced hypertension. Am J Obstet Gynecol 1988; 158:523-9.)

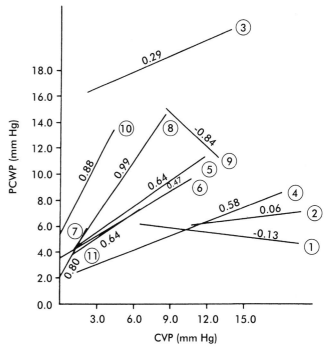

FIGURE 44-9. Pulmonary capillary wedge pressure *(PCWP)* and central venous pressure *(CVP)* in 11 untreated patients with severe preeclampsia. Regression lines and correlation coefficients are shown. PCWP and CVP correlated poorly in several patients, and the dispersion of data around individual regression lines was large. (From Newsome LR, Bramwell RS, Curling PE. Severe preeclampsia: Hemodynamic effects of lumbar epidural anesthesia. Anesth Analg 1986; 65:31-6.)

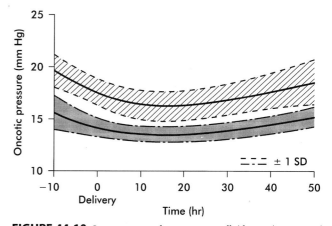

FIGURE 44-10. Intrapartum and postpartum colloid oncotic pressure in nine normotensive women *(hatched curve)* and nine women with severe preeclampsia *(stippled curve)*. Oncotic pressure, already reduced in normal pregnancy because of the decreased albumin concentration, is lowered further in preeclampsia. Values decline even further during labor and delivery and during the first postpartum day. The dashed lines indicate the standard deviation. (From Zinaman M, Rubin J, Lindheimer MD. Serial plasma oncotic pressure levels and echoencephalography during and after delivery in severe pre-eclampsia. Lancet 1985; 1:1245-50.)

measured fibrin/fibrinogen degradation products (FDPs) to detect intravascular coagulation, but most assays cannot distinguish between FDPs originating from fibrinogen and those originating from fibrin. In contrast, the presence of fibrin D-dimer specifically reflects the formation and breakdown of fibrin and indicates intravascular coagulation and fibrinolysis. Trofatter et al.[69] used a monoclonal antibody to detect fibrin D-dimer in preeclamptic women. The presence of D-dimer correlated with increased FDPs, detectable fibrin monomer, and a platelet count of 100,000/mm^3 or less. D-dimer–positive women had significantly higher blood pressure measurements, greater proteinuria, more abnormal liver function tests, and higher serum creatinine and blood urea nitrogen (BUN) measurements. Some authors consider increased fibrinopeptide A levels to be a better indicator of hypercoagulability; preeclamptic women have significantly higher concentrations than normal pregnant women.

The increased factor VIII antigen/activity ratio indicates increased thrombin formation. Some studies have suggested that higher ratios indicate proportionately more severe disease.[70]

Antithrombin III (AT III), a circulating protease inhibitor, inhibits the active forms of coagulation factors IX, X, XI, and XII. In preeclampsia, AT-III levels are low and correlate with the severity of maternal morbidity. Increased thrombin AT-III (TAT) complexes reflect increased thrombin production.[71,72] Purified human AT-III concentrate has been given intravenously to women with severe preeclampsia.[73]

Fibrinolysis

Studies of fibrinolytic activity have provided conflicting results. Most investigators have reported an altered relationship between plasminogen activators and inhibitors, with a resultant decrease in fibrinolytic activity, which probably contributes to the persistence of fibrin in the renal and placental microvasculature.[67] Preeclamptic women have higher concentrations of **lipoprotein(a),** which may be a marker for the severity of disease.[74] Lipoprotein(a) enhances blood coagulation by competing with plasminogen for its binding sites on fibrin clots and endothelial cells.

Platelet Activation

Thrombocytopenia. Most cases of thrombocytopenia in pregnancy are benign gestational states,[75] but thrombocytopenia occurs in 15% to 30% of women with preeclampsia or eclampsia. However, the platelet count is less than 100,000/mm^3 in fewer than 10% of all preeclamptic women,

and it shows marked daily variation. Women with severe preeclampsia are at increased risk for having a platelet count of less than 100,000/mm^3.[76]

McDonagh et al.[77] identified a relationship between a prolonged bleeding time (BT) and a platelet count of less than 75,000/mm^3 in women with severe preeclampsia. This indicates that preeclampsia may be associated with a significant defect in both platelet function and number. In an accompanying editorial, Samama and Simon[78] noted that the BT is a nonpredictive test[79] and, to date, there is no laboratory test that can reliably predict whether it is safe to perform regional anesthesia in these patients. They recommended use of the platelet count alone as a first-line test of hemostasis in preeclamptic women. Thrombocytopenia without other coagulation abnormalities, but with evidence of hemolysis and increased liver enzymes, characterizes **HELLP syndrome,** an uncommon variant of severe preeclampsia.

Burrows et al.[80] found elevated platelet-associated immunoglobulin G (IgG) in 35% of preeclamptic patients, which suggests that an immune mechanism is partly responsible for the thrombocytopenia. Samuels et al.[81] also observed abnormal platelet antiglobulin in a substantial number of preeclamptic women and their neonates.

Additional evidence of platelet activation in women with preeclampsia includes the following: (1) a significant increase in the release of beta-thromboglobulin by platelets, (2) a shorter production time, consistent with a reduced platelet half-life, and (3) the appearance of megathrombocytes (giant platelets) in peripheral blood, which indicates a younger platelet population.[82]

Platelet Sensitivity to PGI$_2$. PGI$_2$ normally inhibits platelet aggregation. Although PGI$_2$ production increases in normal pregnancy, platelets in pregnant women are less responsive to PGI$_2$-induced inhibition than platelets in nonpregnant controls. In preeclamptic women, platelets demonstrate a 50% reduction in sensitivity to a PGI$_2$ analog.[67]

Neonatal Coagulation Disturbances

Several investigators have described clotting abnormalities in neonates whose mothers had preeclampsia. However, it is likely that these disturbances reflect the condition of the newborn rather than the passage of a placental factor.[67]

RENAL FUNCTION

The characteristic renal lesion is glomerular enlargement with resultant ischemia—primarily as a result of swollen intracapillary cells. These changes result in a glomerular filtration rate (GFR) that is on average 25% below that in normal pregnancy. (GFR is 122 mL/min in nonpregnant patients, and it increases to 170 mL/min by the beginning of the second trimester in normal pregnancy.) The glomerulopathy causes proteinuria, which occurs as a result of an increased permeability to most large molecular weight proteins.[6] The amount of proteinuria may correlate positively with the extent of histologic change and the degree of hypertension.[83] In addition to albumin, other proteins (e.g., globulins, hemoglobin, transferrin) appear in the urine, which underlines the severity of glomerulopathy.

Serum creatinine levels seldom increase above normal nonpregnant measurements, and a level greater than 1 mg/dL may indicate substantial renal involvement.[6] Urate clearance decreases, and serum uric acid concentrations increase. Hyperuricemia may provide an early indication of preeclampsia. A uric acid concentration greater than 5.5 mg/dL has been associated with an increase in perinatal morbidity and

---

Box 44-5 CHANGES THAT IMPLY HYPERCOAGULATION IN PREECLAMPSIA

↑ Common pathway activity
↓ Fibrinogen
↑ Fibrin degradation products
D-dimer positive
↑ Fibrinopeptide A
↑ Factor VIII antigen: factor VIII activity
↓ Antithrombin III
↑ Thrombin-antithrombin III complexes
↓ Platelets
↑ Beta-thromboglobulin
↑ Platelet aggregability
↓ Sensitivity to prostacyclin

Modified from Perry KG, Martin JN. Abnormal hemostasis and coagulopathy in preeclampsia and eclampsia. Clin Obstet Gynecol 1992; 35:338-50.

mortality.[84] A normal uric acid concentration (i.e., less than 5 mg/dL) is inconsistent with significant disease; however, the uric acid level is not a good prognostic indicator for the severity of maternal or fetal complications associated with preeclampsia.[85] Sodium excretion also diminishes, although the extent of impairment varies. Rarely, some oliguric preeclamptic women have a high urinary sodium concentration during labor or in the early puerperium, possibly as a result of severe intrarenal arteriolar spasm. In these patients, serum creatinine levels may increase[70] two to three times the normal nonpregnant level.[6,83]

Oliguria parallels the severity of preeclampsia, and persistent oliguria (less than 400 mL in 24 hours) calls for immediate assessment of intravascular volume. Renal failure occurs only rarely, and complete recovery of renal function can be anticipated in almost all cases *(vide infra).*

ENDOCRINE AND METABOLIC CHANGES

The RAAS constitutes one arm of an integrated control system, which includes other vasoactive hormones (e.g., prostaglandins, vasopressin, ANP), the sympathetic nervous system, the heart, blood vessels, and circulating blood volume. The purpose of this control system is to maintain a constant blood pressure. This system undergoes complex changes during both normal and preeclamptic pregnancies.[86] During **normal pregnancy,** high concentrations of pro-renin and active renin appear in the circulation, and the levels of angiotensinogen, angiotensin I, angiotensin II, and aldosterone increase markedly. Intuitively, the increased RAAS activity seems paradoxical because the high renin secretion coincides with extracellular volume expansion, increased renal blood flow, and increased GFR—factors that normally should lead to a feedback reduction in RAAS activity. However, studies have shown that increased PGI_2 synthesis and vasodilation together play a role in this paradoxical stimulation. Moreover, angiotensin II is less effective in its feedback suppression of renin release.[86]

In women with **preeclampsia,** a breakdown of the normal balance between vasodilators (e.g., PGI_2, nitric oxide) and vasoconstrictors (e.g., angiotensin II, TXA_2, serotonin, endothelin) occurs. The RAAS becomes suppressed, and most studies indicate decreased plasma renin concentration (PRC) and activity (PRA). Possible reasons include (1) the "normalization" of vascular response to angiotensin II, with increased effectiveness of the negative feedback mechanism; (2) deficient production of PGI_2; and (3) lower blood ionized calcium levels. However, PRC and PRA increase significantly in the uterine venous blood of preeclamptic women. Broughton-Pipkin[87] postulated that the resultant increase in angiotensin II concentration would increase systemic pressure, which would increase blood flow to the uterus and its contents. In patients with severe preeclampsia, a deficiency in PGI_2 (and perhaps nitric oxide) allows angiotensin II to exert its unopposed uteroplacental vasoconstrictor effect.

RESPIRATORY FUNCTION

Women with preeclampsia have an increased risk of upper airway narrowing from **pharyngolaryngeal edema.**[88] In addition, **pulmonary edema** is a severe, sometimes frightening complication of severe preeclampsia and eclampsia. It occurs in approximately 3% of cases. Sibai et al.[89] reviewed 37 consecutive cases of pulmonary edema associated with severe preeclampsia and eclampsia. The onset occurred antepartum in 30% of cases. (Approximately 90% of these women had evidence of preexisting chronic hypertension.) The remaining 70% of patients developed pulmonary edema *after* delivery. Many postpartum cases resulted from excessive infusion of crystalloid or colloid before delivery. Sciscione et al.[90] recently reviewed 51 cases of acute pulmonary edema during pregnancy or postpartum at their hospital. Preeclampsia was the cause of 9 (18%) of the cases of pulmonary edema. In this study, the majority of cases of pulmonary edema associated with preeclampsia occurred *before* delivery. Further, five of the nine preeclamptic women had preexisting essential hypertension.

HEPATIC FUNCTION

Serum transaminase levels frequently increase in patients with mild preeclampsia.[83] Epigastric or subcostal pain is an ominous symptom that typically is caused by distention of the liver capsule by edema or subcapsular or parenchymal bleeding. Manas et al.[91] used computed tomography (CT) scans to demonstrate hepatic hemorrhage in five of seven preeclamptic women with upper abdominal pain. Ultrasonography also may be used to confirm the diagnosis. Rarely, severe subcapsular hemorrhage disrupts the liver capsule and causes intraperitoneal bleeding—a major surgical emergency.

Liver biopsy in preeclampsia may show mild periportal fibrin deposition, periportal hemorrhage, ischemic lesions, or no apparent change.[2] Subendothelial deposits of fibrin, similar to those seen in the kidney, suggest endothelial damage.

NEUROLOGIC CHANGES

The classic manifestations of preeclampsia include severe headache, visual disturbances, CNS hyperexcitability, and hyperreflexia. The occurrence of seizures indicates eclampsia until proved otherwise. The etiology of eclamptic seizures remains unclear. Some investigators attribute them to hypertensive encephalopathy and loss of cerebral blood flow autoregulation when the mean arterial pressure (MAP) exceeds a critical threshold.[92] However, gross retinal signs occur rarely, and approximately 20% of women with eclampsia have a systolic blood pressure of 140 mm Hg or less and a diastolic pressure of 90 mm Hg or less. Other proposed etiologies for eclamptic seizures include vasospasm, microinfarctions and punctate hemorrhages, thrombosis, and cerebral edema.[93]

UTEROPLACENTAL PERFUSION

Preeclamptic women have decreased uteroplacental perfusion.[94] During normal pregnancy, the uteroplacental bed constitutes a low-resistance circuit, and Doppler waveforms demonstrate continuous diastolic flow (i.e., a low systolic/diastolic ratio). In women with preeclampsia, downstream resistance increases, diastolic velocity decreases, and the systolic/diastolic ratio increases.[95] This is most common in fetuses with IUGR. Preeclampsia can be categorized as severe if there is evidence of IUGR and/or oligohydramnios. In these cases the fetus often does not tolerate severe or protracted hypotension during the induction of regional anesthesia. Continuous fetal heart rate (FHR) monitoring is recommended during the induction of anesthesia in these patients.

Prophylaxis

ASPIRIN PROPHYLAXIS

In low doses (i.e., 60 to 100 mg daily), aspirin alters the imbalance in TXA_2 and PGI_2 production that occurs in preeclamptic

women. Specifically, low-dose aspirin increases PGI_2 production, and it also inhibits platelet synthesis of TXA_2 for the duration of the platelets' lifespan.[95]

Initial studies suggested that low-dose aspirin has a beneficial effect in preventing preeclampsia. Dekker and Sibai[96] reviewed the results of randomized trials conducted between 1985 and 1991 and concluded that low-dose aspirin was effective in the prevention of gestational hypertension, preeclampsia, and IUGR in women at risk for these complications. These results were confirmed by Hauth et al.,[97] who found that daily ingestion of 60 mg of aspirin beginning at 24 weeks' gestation significantly reduced the incidence of preeclampsia. These authors confirmed patient compliance by measuring serum levels of thromboxane B_2 (TXB_2), a metabolite of TXA_2. They noted a significant reduction in TXB_2 levels at 29 to 31 weeks' gestation, 34 to 36 weeks' gestation, and at delivery. In contrast, they observed increased TXB_2 levels in the placebo group.[97]

Unfortunately, these encouraging results were not confirmed in subsequent large, multicenter, randomized, placebo-controlled trials. (It has been suggested that the encouraging findings of the early studies may reflect publication bias, given that small studies with positive findings are more likely to be published than those with negative results.[98]) Data from these studies suggest that low-dose aspirin provides no benefit in the prevention of preeclampsia in either low-risk[8] or high-risk[99] patients. Sibai et al.[100] reported the results of a trial involving 3135 healthy women from 10 medical centers, who were randomly assigned to receive aspirin 60 mg/day or placebo beginning at 13 to 26 weeks' gestation. This study found a small difference (of borderline significance) between groups in the incidence of preeclampsia. There was no difference between groups in the incidence of gestational hypertension alone. Of interest, more women in the low-dose aspirin group developed placental abruption. In view of this increased risk for placental abruption, these investigators concluded that routine use of low-dose aspirin prophylaxis in healthy nulliparous women is unwarranted.

Another study evaluated the impact of daily treatment with aspirin 60 mg compared with placebo, beginning at 13 to 26 weeks' gestation, in 2539 women at high risk for developing preeclampsia.[99] The study subjects included women with pregestational insulin-dependent diabetes mellitus ($n = 471$), chronic hypertension ($n = 774$), multifetal gestation ($n = 688$), and a history of preeclampsia during a previous pregnancy ($n = 606$). The incidence of preeclampsia was similar in the low-dose aspirin and placebo groups, whether analyzed as a whole or according to individual risk factors.

Despite these discouraging results, some investigators believe that low-dose aspirin may benefit certain groups of women at high risk for developing severe, early-onset preeclampsia.[101,102] Recent studies may be criticized because patient compliance was not confirmed by measurement of serum TXB_2 levels. Future studies may define new criteria for determining which patients are at high risk for developing preeclampsia. Further, the timing of aspirin administration may prove to be an important factor.[101] Perhaps new criteria for low-dose aspirin prophylaxis will emerge. Indeed, a recent meta-analysis of randomized trials that evaluated the efficacy of prophylactic aspirin showed that uterine artery Doppler assessment identifies high-risk women in whom aspirin results in a significant reduction in preeclampsia.[103]

CALCIUM PROPHYLAXIS

Epidemiologic studies have suggested an inverse relationship between calcium intake and the incidence of eclampsia. This prompted investigators to conduct randomized clinical trials of calcium supplementation for the prevention of preeclampsia. A meta-analysis of 14 randomized trials, involving 2459 women, confirmed that prenatal administration of supplemental calcium reduced blood pressure and the incidence of preeclampsia; the authors did not have sufficient data to evaluate the impact of supplemental calcium on maternal and fetal morbidity.[104] However, a large, multicenter, randomized trial of daily 2-g calcium supplements (beginning at 13 to 21 weeks' gestation) showed that calcium did *not* lessen the risk of preeclampsia in healthy nulliparous women.[105] This is the most definitive study to date. However, some investigators argue that the pathophysiologic events that occur in patients with preeclampsia are well established by 13 weeks' gestation, and that calcium prophylaxis should begin *before* conception. A study that addresses this hypothesis has not been performed.

ANTIOXIDANT PROPHYLAXIS

Oxidative stress may play a role in the pathogenesis of preeclampsia.[106] Recent evidence suggests that antioxidant therapy with 1000 mg/day of vitamin C and 400 mg/day of vitamin E may help prevent preeclampsia.[107] Large randomized studies are needed to confirm these preliminary results.

Diagnosis

Preeclampsia occurs more frequently in nulliparous women than in parous women. It typically becomes apparent during the third trimester—often near term. Its principal features include hypertension and proteinuria, with or without edema (which may manifest clinically as significant weight gain). Women who develop the disorder during the second trimester fare worse than those who manifest it after 34 weeks' gestation.[108] Women with early-onset severe disease have a higher incidence of chronic hypertension,[109] unrecognized renal disease, and rarely, other underlying disease (e.g., systemic lupus erythematosus, pheochromocytoma).

Typically, preeclampsia regresses rapidly after delivery, and signs and symptoms resolve within 48 hours. Occasionally, late postpartum eclampsia occurs and is manifest by increased blood pressure, proteinuria, and the occurrence of seizures within 10 days of delivery.

BLOOD PRESSURE

The use of phase IV Korotkoff sounds (i.e., muffling) may lead to an overestimation of the diastolic blood pressure by 7 to 15 mm Hg. Muffling also can prove difficult to detect. Although European and Australian physicians typically assess muffling, United States obstetricians typically use phase V (i.e., diastolic pressure at which the sound disappears).[2] In hyperkinetic pregnancies, phase V also may be difficult to detect because sounds continue to an abnormally low level. Sibai,[108] therefore, has recommended the use of both phase IV and V sounds (e.g., 120/80/70 mm Hg).

Automatic noninvasive blood pressure (NIBP) devices correlate well with intraarterial measurements in pregnancy. They eliminate observer bias and generally give reproducible results and are often used in practice. However, NIBP devices vary in the way that they determine blood pressure. Those

that use oscillometry overestimate systolic pressures and underestimate diastolic pressures in healthy pregnant women when compared with their nonpregnant counterparts.[110] The Dinamap (Critikon) may provide a misleadingly low measurement of diastolic blood pressure, which may adversely affect management decisions in women with preeclampsia. Hasan et al.[110] recommended that 10 mm Hg be added to the Dinamap diastolic measurement. Blood pressure should be measured by mercury sphygmomanometer, at least in the first instance and until measurements stabilize.[2] An appropriate sized cuff should be used (length 1.5 times the upper arm circumference or cuff bladder that encircles at least 80% of the arm).[2]

PROTEINURIA

Several factors affect the diagnosis of proteinuria by urinalysis (e.g., contamination, exercise, specific gravity, pH greater than 8.0). Sibai[108] recommended that diagnostic measures be quantitative (e.g., more than 300 mg protein/24 hr for the diagnosis of mild preeclampsia or more than 5 g protein/24 hr for the diagnosis of severe preeclampsia).

EDEMA AND WEIGHT GAIN

It often is difficult to distinguish between physiologic and pathologic edema. Thus, most obstetricians consider edema an unreliable sign that should not be used in the diagnosis of preeclampsia. However, significant weight gain typically points to pathologic fluid retention, and a gain of more than 2 lb per week, especially in the third trimester, is associated with an increased risk of preeclampsia.[111]

OMINOUS SIGNS AND SYMPTOMS

Headache, visual disturbances, and epigastric pain indicate severe preeclampsia or incipient eclampsia (see Box 44-3). Premonitory symptoms of eclampsia typically occur, but seizures may develop without warning in an asymptomatic woman with no evidence of severe hypertension.

Interaction with Pregnancy

HOW DOES PREGNANCY AFFECT PREECLAMPSIA?

This may seem to be an odd question, given that preeclampsia occurs only in pregnant women. Nonetheless, it should be emphasized that preeclampsia requires the presence of trophoblastic tissue, and the only definitive "cure" is to end the pregnancy. Preeclampsia continues as long as trophoblast remains in situ, although treatment may lessen its severity. The severity also appears related to the amount of trophoblast that is present. Thus, multiple pregnancies and other situations of hyperplacentation (e.g., molar pregnancy, diabetes mellitus) increase the risk of developing the disorder and may increase its severity.[1]

Ananth et al.[112] observed that women with placenta previa are at decreased risk of developing preeclampsia, which may be a result of altered placental perfusion. However, patients with placenta previa often deliver preterm, and thus may not reach a gestational age at which preeclampsia would otherwise have developed. With this criticism in mind, the authors stratified the patients by gestational age and found that the inverse relationship between placenta previa and preeclampsia persisted at each gestational age (Figure 44-11). However, it should be emphasized that preeclampsia/eclampsia and placenta previa are not mutually exclusive.[113]

HOW DOES PREECLAMPSIA AFFECT PREGNANCY?

In women with mild preeclampsia and an immature fetus, expectant management involves retarding the hypertensive process without endangering maternal or fetal welfare. This allows time for the fetus to mature, and it allows the cervix to ripen, which increases the probability of vaginal delivery. Recent recommendations for women with mild preeclampsia who are remote from term include initial hospitalization for maternal and fetal evaluation. This is followed by regular outpatient assessments—either at home or in the clinic—in selected reliable individuals who demonstrate an understanding of the nonreassuring symptoms of the disease.[114]

Indications for induction of labor include (1) gestational age of 37 weeks or more, (2) fetal lung maturity, (3) a favorable cervix, and (4) increasing blood pressure despite conservative measures. Only rarely does an obstetrician allow a patient with mild preeclampsia to continue beyond 37 weeks' gestation (e.g., if the biophysical profile remains normal and the cervix remains unfavorable). Evidence of maternal or fetal deterioration should prompt delivery, regardless of the gestational age.[1]

Both controlled and uncontrolled trials have evaluated the use of antihypertensive drugs to lower maternal blood pressure in preeclamptic women in an attempt to prolong gestation and improve perinatal outcome.[108] No study has demonstrated that antihypertensive therapy improves perinatal outcome when compared with hospitalization alone.[115] Likewise, no trial has suggested that antihypertensive therapy masks the progress of the disease.

Sibai et al.[116] prospectively evaluated outcome for 95 women who developed severe preeclampsia between 28 and 32 weeks' gestation. The authors either delayed delivery with bed rest, oral antihypertensive agents, and intensive antenatal fetal assessments, or they treated patients "aggressively" with induction of labor or cesarean section 48 hours after the administration of a glucocorticoid to accelerate fetal lung maturity. The authors found that expectant management

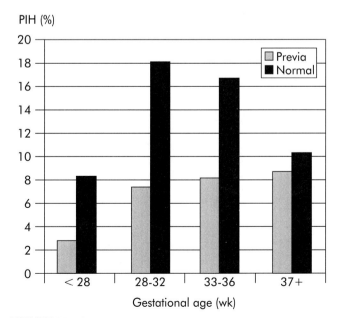

FIGURE 44-11. Risk of pregnancy-induced hypertension *(PIH)* in relation to placenta previa, stratified according to gestational age at delivery. (From Ananth CV, Bowes WA, Savitz DA, Luther ER. Relationship between pregnancy-induced hypertension and placenta previa: A population-based study. Am J Obstet Gynecol 1997; 177:997-1002.)

(which included careful monitoring of both the mother and fetus at a perinatal center) increased the gestational age at delivery by 2 weeks and reduced neonatal complications. There were no cases of eclampsia or perinatal death in either group, and the incidence of placental abruption was similar in the two groups (approximately 4%).[116] Schiff et al.[117] also recommended conservative management of severe preeclampsia remote from term, provided that maternal blood pressure is well controlled, laboratory measurements remain stable, and the fetal biophysical profile remains reassuring (Table 44-1).

Obstetric Management

Regardless of gestational age, any of the following complications mandates immediate delivery: (1) severe hypertension that persists after 24 to 48 hours, (2) progressive thrombocytopenia, (3) liver dysfunction, (4) progressive renal dysfunction (including severe oliguria), (5) premonitory signs of eclampsia, and (6) evidence of fetal jeopardy.

INITIAL LABORATORY INVESTIGATIONS

The laboratory tests required for women who develop hypertension after midpregnancy are listed in Box 44-6.[2] The platelet count represents the most important feature of the complete blood count. The admission platelet count is an excellent predictor of subsequent thrombocytopenia.[76] If the platelet count exceeds 100,000/mm^3 in patients with mild preeclampsia, "routine" coagulation assessment is unnecessary.

Liver function tests should be obtained from all preeclamptic women because approximately 20% have elevated transaminase levels.[118,119] If levels are elevated, delivery is encouraged. If the patient is not delivered, she should be observed for signs and symptoms of liver hematoma.

A clean-catch specimen of urine should be evaluated for evidence of proteinuria. Serum BUN and creatinine concentrations allow assessment of renal function. A normal serum uric acid concentration argues against the presence of significant disease.

CLINICAL EVALUATION

The initial neurologic examination should determine the extent of hyperexcitability (e.g., hyperreflexia, clonus). The presence and severity of headache should be determined. A severe, retroorbital headache suggests incipient eclampsia. Seizure prophylaxis includes the administration of magnesium sulfate to prevent progression to eclampsia.

The initial fetal evaluation includes the performance of a biophysical profile (see Chapter 6). The patient should have continuous FHR monitoring with the onset of labor, or earlier if there is evidence of fetal compromise. The absence of FHR accelerations may be an ominous sign. Persistent late FHR decelerations, whether subtle or obvious, indicate uteroplacental dysfunction and herald the possible need for early cesarean section.

FURTHER MANAGEMENT

Urine output should be followed closely, and maintenance crystalloid administration generally should not exceed 2 mL/kg/hr (and should be less in patients with severe preeclampsia) to avoid the possibility of fluid overload. Other sources of fluid intake (e.g., magnesium sulfate, oxytocin) frequently complicate management, and it may prove necessary to double (or triple) the concentrations of magnesium sulfate and oxytocin to avoid the infusion of excessive amounts of fluid. Unfortunately this precaution increases the risk of unintentional administration of an excessive dose of magnesium sulfate or oxytocin. Hourly urine output must be monitored closely, and oliguria should be treated appropriately.

Intravenous crystalloid administration decreases COP.[65] Jones et al.[120] observed that intravenous colloid decreased

TABLE 44-1	GUIDELINES FOR SELECTION OF PATIENTS FOR CONSERVATIVE MANAGEMENT OF SEVERE PREECLAMPSIA REMOTE FROM TERM	

Expedited delivery	Conservative management
Maternal	
Uncontrolled severe hypertension[a]	Controlled hypertension
Eclampsia	Urinary protein < 5 g/day
Thrombocytopenia (platelet count < 100,000/μL)	Oliguria < 0.5 mL/kg/hr that resolves with fluid intake or bed rest
AST, ALT[b] > 2 × upper limit of normal, with epigastric or right upper quadrant pain	Elevated AST or ALT[b], without abdominal tenderness
Pulmonary edema	
Renal compromise[c]	
Persistent neurologic symptoms[d]	
Fetal	
Fetal distress, diagnosed with NST[e] or BPP[f]	BPP[f] ≥ 6
Amniotic fluid index ≤ 2	Amniotic fluid index > 2
Ultrasonographically estimated fetal weight < 5th percentile	Ultrasonographically estimated fetal weight > 5th percentile
Reverse umbilical artery end-diastolic flow	

[a]Systolic blood pressure > 160 mm Hg or diastolic blood pressure > 110 mm Hg despite maximum recommended doses of two antihypertensive medications.
[b]AST, aspartate aminotransferase; ALT, alanine aminotransferase.
[c]Persistent oliguria (< 0.5 mL/kg/hr) or elevation in serum creatinine ≥ 1 mg/dL over baseline.
[d]Persistent headache or visual changes.
[e]NST, nonstress test.
[f]BPP, biophysical profile.
From Lewis R, Sibai B. Recent advances in the management of preeclampsia. J Matern-Fetal Med 1997; 6:6-15.

Box 44-6 INITIAL LABORATORY INVESTIGATIONS FOR WOMEN WHO DEVELOP HYPERTENSION AFTER 20 WEEKS' GESTATION[2]

HEMOGLOBIN AND HEMATOCRIT

- Hemoconcentration supports diagnosis of preeclampsia and is an indicator of severity.
- Values are reduced if there is hemolysis.

PLATELET COUNT

- Thrombocytopenia suggests severe preeclampsia.

QUANTIFICATION OF PROTEIN EXCRETION

- Pregnancy-associated hypertension with proteinuria should be considered preeclampsia (pure or superimposed).

SERUM CREATININE

- Abnormal or rising creatinine suggests severe preeclampsia, especially in presence of oliguria.

SERUM URIC ACID

- Increased serum uric levels suggest the diagnosis of preeclampsia.

SERUM TRANSAMINASE LEVELS

- Rising serum transaminase measurements suggest severe preeclampsia with hepatic involvement.

SERUM ALBUMIN, LACTIC ACID DEHYDROGENASE (LDH), BLOOD SMEAR, COAGULATION PROFILE*

- For women with severe disease, hypoalbuminemia indicates the extent of endothelial leak. An increase in LDH and evidence of schizocytosis and spherocytosis indicates hemolysis.

*aPTT, PT, fibrinogen, D-dimer: Reserve for patients with right upper quadrant pain, possible HELLP syndrome, or clinical evidence of coagulopathy.

COP less than crystalloid. However, there appears to be no benefit to the administration of colloid, except in selected patients with renal or cardiopulmonary compromise. Kirshon et al.[121] recommended colloid administration when the COP becomes markedly decreased (less than 12 mm Hg) or when a negative COP-PCWP gradient exists. I do not routinely measure COP, and because few subjects require invasive hemodynamic monitoring, PCWP measurements typically are unavailable. In practice, I typically reserve colloid administration for the management of selected patients with oliguria (vide infra).

Women with severe preeclampsia are more likely to proceed to cesarean section. Factors that contribute to this outcome include an increased incidence of placental abruption and fetal distress. Further, many preterm parturients with preeclampsia have an unfavorable cervix, which diminishes the possibility of vaginal delivery despite the infusion of oxytocin.

Drug Therapy

ANTICONVULSANTS

Magnesium sulfate remains the treatment of choice for seizure prophylaxis in North America and has gained popularity throughout the world as a result of the recently published Magpie Trial.[122] The primary results from this multicenter trial were first announced by Lelia Duley from the United Kingdom

at the 13th World Congress of the International Society for the Study of Hypertension in Pregnancy in Toronto, Canada, in June 2002. She explained that the Magpie Trial started in 1998, and that 10,110 women from around the globe were studied. Women with a blood pressure of at least 140/90 mm Hg and proteinuria, either antepartum or within 24 hours of delivery, were randomly assigned to receive magnesium sulfate 4 g or placebo intravenously, followed by a maintenance dose (1 g/hr intravenously or 5 g intramuscularly every 4 hours) or placebo for 24 hours. Monitoring was done clinically and, if eclampsia occurred, magnesium sulfate 2 or 4 g was given intravenously to women who had received magnesium or placebo, respectively. Those women who received magnesium sulfate had a 58% lower risk of having a seizure (95% confidence interval [CI] = 40% to 71%). There was also a 55% lower risk of maternal death (95% CI = 26% to 114%), although this was not statistically significant, ($P = 0.11$). Side effects of magnesium sulfate were common (e.g., flushing, nausea, vomiting, pain at the intramuscular injection site, muscle weakness), but there was no difference between groups in serious side effects (e.g., cardiac arrest, stroke, pulmonary edema). Somewhat disappointing to anesthesiologists was the fact that the investigators did not evaluate the impact of epidural analgesia on outcome. Other unanswered questions relate to the optimal dose, timing, and duration of magnesium sulfate therapy.[123]

Other studies have supported the claim that magnesium sulfate is the preferred agent for seizure prophylaxis in preeclamptic women. Lucas et al.[124] randomized 2138 women with preeclampsia to receive either intramuscular magnesium sulfate or intravenous and oral phenytoin. None of the 1049 women in the magnesium sulfate group, versus 10 (0.9%) of 1089 women in the phenytoin group, had a seizure. The Eclampsia Trial Collaborative Group[125] compared magnesium sulfate, phenytoin, and diazepam administration for the prevention of recurrent seizures in women with eclampsia. They found that magnesium sulfate therapy was more effective in preventing recurrent seizures than either phenytoin (5.7% versus 17.1%; relative risk = 0.33; 95% CI = 0.21 to 0.53) or diazepam (13.2% versus 27.9%; relative risk = 0.48; 95% CI = 0.36 to 0.63).

In a recently published randomized trial of magnesium sulfate versus placebo in 222 women with mild preeclampsia (blood pressure of at least 140/90 mm Hg and 1+ proteinuria), there was no difference between groups in the percentage of women who progressed to severe preeclampsia or in maternal and infant outcomes.[126] The study was underpowered, so that valid conclusions cannot be made. Over 2500 women with mild preeclampsia would need to be studied in an appropriately powered study. However, this small, well-designed study was published for inclusion in any future meta-analysis.[127]

In the United States, most obstetricians give an intravenous bolus of magnesium sulfate 4 to 6 g over 20 minutes and follow with an intravenous infusion of 1 to 2 g/hr. During maintenance therapy, patients are monitored clinically (e.g., patellar reflexes, respiratory rate, urine output). If oliguria or the suspicion of magnesium toxicity develops, the serum magnesium concentration should be measured, and the maintenance dose adjusted accordingly. Interpretation of the serum magnesium concentration is confounded by the fact that three sets of units can be used. In this chapter, I express magnesium concentrations in mg/dL (2.4 mg/dL = 2 mEq/L = 1 mmol/L). Obviously it is important to know the units that are used by your laboratory because these differences could contribute to clinical errors in dosing. In untreated patients,

the normal range for serum magnesium concentrations is 1.7 to 2.4 mg/dL. The therapeutic range for serum magnesium concentrations lies between 5 and 9 mg/dL.[126] Loss of patellar reflexes occurs at approximately 12 mg/dL, respiratory arrest at 15 to 20 mg/dL, and asystole at more than 25 mg/dL (although magnesium's potential to cause cardiac arrest when ventilation is maintained is unclear).[128]

In the event of suspected magnesium toxicity, magnesium sulfate must be discontinued immediately and the patient should be treated with intravenous calcium gluconate (1 g) or calcium chloride (300 mg). Sodium bicarbonate should be administered if metabolic acidemia is suspected. In the rare event of respiratory impairment, the patient may require endotracheal intubation and mechanical ventilation until spontaneous respiration resumes. Magnesium toxicity is more likely in patients with renal dysfunction, and serial measurements of serum magnesium levels are of increased importance in this subgroup of women.

Magnesium sulfate exerts a peripheral effect at the neuromuscular junction, and it may have a central anticonvulsant effect that is mediated by means of cerebral N-methyl-D-aspartate (NMDA) receptors.[129] Other potentially beneficial effects of magnesium sulfate include (1) vasodilation in vascular beds (including small-diameter cerebral vessels) by a direct or indirect (Ca^{2+} competing) effect, (2) increased cyclic guanosine monophosphate (GMP) production, (3) attenuation of the vascular responses to pressor substances, (4) decreased PRA and angiotensin-converting enzyme (ACE) levels, and (5) increased production of PGI_2 by endothelial cells.[128]

Magnesium sulfate may prevent eclampsia by reducing cerebral vasoconstriction and ischemia. In order to test whether nimodipine, a calcium-entry blocking agent with specific cerebral vasodilator activity, is more effective than magnesium sulfate for seizure prophylaxis in women with severe preeclampsia, Belfort et al.[130] conducted an unblinded, multicenter trial in which 1650 women with severe preeclampsia were randomly assigned to receive either nimodipine (60 mg orally every 4 hours) or intravenous magnesium sulfate from enrollment until 24 hours postpartum. High blood pressure was controlled with intravenous hydralazine as needed. The primary outcome measure was the development of eclampsia, as defined by a witnessed tonic–clonic seizure. The women who received nimodipine were more likely to have a seizure than those who received magnesium sulfate (21 of 819 [2.6%] versus 7 of 831 [0.8%], P = 0.01). The adjusted risk ratio for eclampsia associated with nimodipine, as compared with magnesium sulfate, was 3.2 (95% CI = 1.1 to 9.1). The antepartum seizure rates did not differ significantly between groups, but the nimodipine group had a higher rate of postpartum seizures (9 of 819 [1.1%] versus 0 of 831, P = 0.01). The fact that magnesium sulfate is more effective than nimodipine for seizure prophylaxis in women with severe preeclampsia suggests that the mechanism for magnesium's anticonvulsant activity remains unknown.

Magnesium sulfate has an enviable safety record in pregnant patients. With therapeutic doses, mothers remain awake and alert, and their protective laryngeal reflexes remain intact. Earlier reports noted possible adverse effects, such as decreased FHR variability, decreased uterine activity, prolonged labor, excessive blood loss, and neonatal depression (e.g., low Apgar scores, respiratory depression, hyporeflexia).[131] Indeed, Donaldson[132] (a neurologist) has argued against the use of magnesium sulfate because of the poten-tial for acute hypermagnesemia, neuromuscular block, hyporeflexia, respiratory impairment, and electrocardiogram (ECG) changes. However, most obstetricians currently believe that the benefits of magnesium sulfate therapy outweigh its potential risks in preeclamptic patients.[133] (In contrast, there is some controversy regarding the risk:benefit ratio for magnesium sulfate when it is used for tocolysis [see Chapters 10 and 34].)

Magnesium sulfate can produce favorable hemodynamic effects in the maternal circulation, especially at the level of the placenta. Using a bioimpedance monitor, Scardo et al.[134] demonstrated a rapid, sustained fall in SVR and an increase in the cardiac index in preeclamptic women who received a bolus—followed by a continuous intravenous infusion—of magnesium sulfate. Magnesium attenuates peroxide-induced vasoconstriction in the human placenta by two mechanisms: (1) inhibition of TXA_2 synthesis, and (2) calcium-channel blockade.[135] Uterine blood flow is either unaffected or increased after magnesium sulfate therapy.[136] Hypermagnesemia does not significantly reduce systemic blood pressure at the serum concentrations used to treat preeclampsia.[137]

Magnesium sulfate therapy does not prolong the duration of normal or induced labor,[138] and it does not increase the rate of cesarean section.[139]

ANTIHYPERTENSIVE DRUGS

Obstetricians use **methyldopa** for the treatment of chronic hypertension and for expectant management of preeclampsia. There is no clear benefit to drug treatment in women with mild preeclampsia who are remote from term.[115] Most obstetricians and anesthesiologists reserve parenteral antihypertensive therapy for short-term blood pressure control in severely preeclamptic women. No evidence suggests that antihypertensive drugs delay or prevent the development of preeclampsia or its associated problems, such as IUGR or perinatal death.[1] However, short-term use of methyldopa during the third trimester has no adverse impact on the uteroplacental or fetal circulation.[140] The principal rationale for the use of antihypertensive drugs in this setting is to prevent maternal morbidity associated with encephalopathy, cerebrovascular accidents, or other end-organ damage. The threshold for treatment is a diastolic blood pressure of 105 to 110 mm Hg or a MAP of 125 mm Hg. The aim of therapy is to maintain a diastolic blood pressure of 90 to 105 mm Hg or a MAP of 105 to 125 mm Hg.[115]

Hydralazine

Hydralazine is the antihypertensive agent most commonly used for acute blood pressure control during pregnancy. Hydralazine preferentially relaxes arterioles, which results in decreased SVR.[119] Hydralazine increases cyclic GMP concentrations in severely preeclamptic women, which helps explain its antihypertensive effect.[141] The dose is 5 mg administered intravenously every 20 minutes, as needed, up to a cumulative dose of 20 mg. If this dose does not produce the desired response or if side effects such as tachycardia, headache, or nausea occur, labetalol 10 to 20 mg intravenously, or nifedipine 10 mg orally, may be added.[115] Heart rate, stroke volume, and cardiac output increase after the administration of hydralazine—a result of a compensatory response that is mediated by baroceptors and the sympathetic nervous system.

In a study of 70 women who received intravenous hydralazine 5 mg for the treatment of severe hypertension, the dose was repeated every 15 minutes to reduce the MAP to

less than 125 mm Hg. Mean arterial pressure decreased by 12 mm Hg (95% CI = 10 to 14 mm Hg) after the first bolus, 9 mm Hg (95% CI = 6.5 to 12 mm Hg) after the second bolus, and 5 mm Hg (95% CI = 1 to 10 mm Hg) after the third bolus. There was no significant difference in the incidence of FHR abnormalities or umbilical cord acidemia between women treated before delivery and those treated after delivery. The authors concluded that hydralazine administered in 5-mg boluses is a safe and effective drug for the treatment of severe hypertension in women with preeclampsia.[142] However, this study did not include a control group, and its conclusions have attracted criticism.[143]

Gudmundsson et al.[144] used Doppler ultrasonography to evaluate the effects of oral hydralazine (50 mg twice daily for 3 days) on the placental and renal circulations in 12 women whose pregnancies were complicated by preeclampsia. Hydralazine administration resulted in increased maternal heart rate and decreased blood pressure, but it did not affect uteroplacental, renal, or umbilical blood flow velocity, suggesting that at recommended doses oral hydralazine has no effect on uteroplacental, fetoplacental, or maternal renal vascular resistance.[144]

Labetalol

Labetalol is a combined alpha- and beta-adrenergic receptor antagonist (ratio 1:3 when given orally and 1:7 when given intravenously). Its affinity for $alpha_1$ receptors is less than that of phentolamine, and its beta-blocking potency is somewhat lower than that of propranalol.[145]

Labetalol is typically used as a second-line drug to treat hypertension in preeclamptic women. Labetalol decreases maternal SVR without increasing maternal heart rate or decreasing cardiac index, uterine blood flow, or FHR, when it is given in a total dose of less than 1 mg/kg.[146,147] When given intravenously, typically in an initial dose of 10 to 20 mg, it has a faster onset of action than hydralazine. If necessary, the dose is doubled every 10 minutes to a maximum dose of 220 to 300 mg or administered as an infusion at 2 mg/min.[2] Labetalol should be avoided in women with asthma or congestive heart failure.

Mabie et al.[148] compared labetalol and hydralazine for the acute management of severe preeclampsia and concluded that hydralazine lowered MAP more effectively, although labetalol had a more rapid effect. There was considerable variability in the dose of labetalol that was required to produce the desired reduction of blood pressure. As would be expected, maternal heart rate decreased with labetalol and increased with hydralazine. Thus some obstetricians recommend combination therapy with both labetalol and hydralazine.[115]

The accumulated experience with labetalol testifies to its efficacy and safety, but it has not supplanted hydralazine as the drug of choice in patients with severe preeclampsia. Some reports have described transplacental transfer of labetalol causing neonatal beta-adrenergic receptor blockade with concomitant adverse sequelae such as bradycardia, hypotension, and hypoglycemia.[149] One study that compared labetalol with hydralazine for the treatment of hypertension in patients with preeclampsia found no signs of either adrenergic blockade or depressed neurobehavioral scores at 24 hours of age in neonates whose mothers had received labetalol.[150] However, the authors acknowledged the potential for a type-2 statistical error because of the small sample size.

Nitroglycerin

Nitroglycerin (NTG) has a rapid onset of action, and it may cause abrupt hypotension. Hence, it is mostly used for short-term treat-

ment (e.g., to control the pressor response to tracheal intubation). Small (50 to 100 µg) boluses may be given intravenously, or NTG may be given sublingually in a 400-µg metered spray.

NTG causes vascular smooth muscle relaxation by means of its intracellular degradation to nitric oxide, which stimulates guanylate cyclase and thus results in increased cGMP production. It relaxes all segments of the vascular system, but it has a more pronounced effect on the venous circulation; thus it decreases preload more effectively than it decreases afterload. NTG readily crosses the placenta. One study noted that maternal administration of NTG decreased both maternal blood pressure and umbilical artery vascular resistance without affecting uterine vascular resistance (suggesting that NTG causes fetoplacental vasodilation while protecting uteroplacental perfusion).[151]

Volume expansion is essential before NTG administration in women with severe preeclampsia.[152] NTG should be diluted to a concentration of 100 µg/mL (50 mg/500 mL) and administered by infusion pump. Many physicians prefer to give NTG by means of nonabsorbent tubing because of its absorption by polyvinyl chloride. An initial dose of 0.5 to 1 µg/kg/min may be increased by 0.5 µg/kg/min until a satisfactory response occurs.

Sodium Nitroprusside

Also a powerful smooth muscle vasodilator, sodium nitroprusside (SNP) interacts with the sulfhydryl groups on endothelial cells to release nitric oxide. It predominantly relaxes the arterial vessels, thus reducing afterload. However, to some extent SNP also reduces venous return. SNP acts rapidly, and its potency demands careful titration. Typically administered at an initial dose of 0.5 µg/kg/min, the dose is increased gradually to control blood pressure. Because SNP metabolism results in the production of cyanide, some physicians have expressed concern about the safety of SNP during pregnancy. Transplacental transfer of SNP does occur, and fetal cyanide toxicity could occur with high doses of SNP.[153] However, short-term use of SNP, in typical clinical doses up to 2 µg/kg/min, is unlikely to cause fetal injury. Cyanide toxicity is more likely with prolonged infusion rates that exceed 4 µg/kg/min over several hours to days. Some investigators have suggested the coinfusion of sodium thiosulfate with SNP to prevent cyanide toxicity.[154]

Nifedipine

Nifedipine, a calcium-entry blocking agent, inhibits the influx of extracellular Ca^{2+} into smooth muscle cells through slow channels. Its effects predominate in arterial and arteriolar smooth muscle. Of the calcium-entry blockers, nifedipine has the most selective vasodilator properties and the least cardiodepressant effects. Common maternal side effects include facial flushing, headache, and tachycardia. Currently available only in capsules, nifedipine rapidly lowers blood pressure after either oral or sublingual administration, although the FDA has not approved the use of sublingual nifedipine for the treatment of hypertensive emergencies. After an initial dose of 10 mg orally, it may be repeated in 30 minutes and subsequently given in a maintenance dose of 10 to 20 mg every 3 to 6 hours. In randomized trials comparing oral nifedipine to intravenous labetalol for treatment of hypertensive emergencies in preeclamptic women, nifedipine had a more rapid onset (25 versus 43 minutes) and was associated with improved urine output and an increase in cardiac index.[155,156] Physicians should be aware of the potential for an exaggerated hypotensive response in patients receiving magnesium sulfate.[157] One report[158] described severe hypotension and fetal distress 20 minutes after a 10-mg dose of sublingual

nifedipine alone; hence the sublingual route should be avoided in preeclamptic women. Nifedipine has been used to attenuate the hypertensive response to tracheal intubation in women with preeclampsia.[159]

Esmolol

Esmolol is a ultrashort-acting cardioselective beta-adrenergic receptor antagonist with a rapid onset that can be given intravenously in a dose of 1mg/kg, with or without lidocaine 1.5 mg/kg, to effectively attenuate the hemodynamic responses to laryngoscopy and tracheal intubation in preeclampsia.[160]

Complications

SEVERE REFRACTORY HYPERTENSION

Most patients with severe preeclampsia respond well to intermittent boluses of hydralazine, but some require other agents for the management of refractory hypertension. Cotton et al.[152] studied the effects of NTG administration, with and without plasma volume expansion. They achieved a more controlled reduction in blood pressure in the volume-expanded group. Volume expansion may attenuate the hypotensive effect, but it helps maintain cardiac index and oxygen delivery.

SNP has been used to treat refractory hypertension in patients with severe preeclampsia. Many authorities recommend volume expansion *before* the administration of SNP. Wasserstrum[161] administered SNP to 10 invasively monitored women with preeclampsia. The subjects were divided into two groups, according to whether tachycardia or bradycardia accompanied the hypotensive effect. Wasserstrum[161] concluded that bradycardia and an associated extreme hypotensive response indicated severe circulatory compromise, similar to the cardiac and vasomotor depression that characterizes severe hemorrhage. I use SNP rarely and cautiously in women with severe preeclampsia, and only after consideration (and appropriate correction) of the patient's blood volume. Further, SNP administration mandates the placement of an arterial catheter to facilitate continuous assessment of maternal blood pressure.

Intravenous labetalol is a useful drug in the management of refractory hypertension. Ramanathan et al.[162] reported that labetalol effectively treated severe hypertension and blunted the pressor response to tracheal intubation in preeclamptic women. Large bolus doses (e.g., 50 mg intravenously) are potentially dangerous, especially in hypovolemic patients, and have caused maternal cardiovascular collapse[163] and fetal death.[164]

Fenakel et al.[165] evaluated nifedipine as a first-line agent in women who developed severe preeclampsia between 26 and 36 weeks' gestation. Patients received nifedipine or hydralazine to stabilize blood pressure, and then labetalol 20 mg every 6 hours until delivery, plus methyldopa if necessary. The authors observed that 20 of 24 women who received nifedipine, versus 17 of 25 who received hydralazine, obtained adequate control of blood pressure. Neonatal intensive care unit stay was significantly shorter in the nifedipine group (15 versus 32 days). Scardo et al.[166] noted no adverse maternal or neonatal effects from oral nifedipine administration in women with severe preeclampsia, despite the fact that each patient received a concurrent infusion of magnesium sulfate. The authors found that one dose of nifedipine was adequate for blood pressure control in 60% of subjects, two doses were needed in 20% of subjects, and the remainder needed three or more doses. No episodes of "overshoot" hypotension or fetal

distress occurred, and a gradual decrease in MAP and SVR index was accompanied by an increase in cardiac index.[166] Blea et al.[167] demonstrated a transient decrease in uteroplacental blood flow after infusion of nifedipine in pregnant ewes. However, they also noted that "the deterioration of fetal blood gases is out of proportion to the transient decreases in uteroplacental blood flow and demonstrates that another mechanism for this fetal acidosis and hypoxia exists during nifedipine infusion." The relevance of these observations to clinical practice is unclear.

ACE inhibitors are *contraindicated* before delivery because of potentially lethal fetal and neonatal sequelae, which include IUGR, oligohydramnios, congenital malformations, and neonatal renal failure (see Chapter 13). However, ACE inhibitors may prove useful during the postpartum period, when blood pressure control is otherwise difficult to achieve, provided the mother does not breast-feed.

In summary, physicians have a choice of drugs for the treatment of refractory hypertension. Although it is not primarily an antihypertensive agent, magnesium sulfate has a transient vasodilator effect, and it should be administered before the administration of an antihypertensive agent. Hydralazine and labetalol alone, or in combination, are first-line antihypertensive drugs. Some investigators have questioned the preferential choice of hydralazine for treatment of severe hypertension in pregnant women. A recent meta-analysis[168] did not provide support for the use of hydralazine as first-line treatment of severe hypertension in pregnant women. The authors called for the performance of adequately powered clinical trials and suggested that studies should compare the use of labetalol versus nifedipine.[168] Nifedipine can be administered orally, but concern regarding its interaction with magnesium sulfate may limit its use. NTG and SNP may help attenuate the pressor response to tracheal intubation, but they rarely are required in the management of refractory hypertension.

OLIGURIA

Oliguria implies a persistent reduction in urine output, which is best diagnosed after serial measurements over time. The etiology of oliguria may be *prerenal* (resulting from systemic vasoconstriction and decreased intravascular volume), or less commonly, *renal*. Renal causes of oliguria include tubular damage from hemolysis and hemoglobinuria, and acute tubular necrosis that is precipitated by severe hypotension in a kidney already ischemic from vasospasm.[169] However, it should be noted that acute renal failure (ARF) is *uncommon* in oliguric patients with severe preeclampsia and generally does not result in chronic renal dysfunction.[170]

Clark et al.[171] defined refractory oliguria as a urine output of less than 30 mL/hr for 3 consecutive hours, which does not improve with a 300- to 500-mL bolus of intravenous crystalloid. Three mechanisms of oliguria have been described, based on the patient's hemodynamic status.[171] Category I patients are oliguric on the basis of intravascular volume depletion, with a low or low-normal PCWP, a moderately increased SVR, and a hyperdynamic left ventricle. These patients have improved urine output after an intravenous fluid challenge. Category II patients have selective renal artery spasm with normal or increased PCWP and cardiac output and a normal SVR. These patients respond to preload reduction with NTG and furosemide and afterload reduction with hydralazine. One study has shown that low-dose dopamine is useful as a selective renal vasodilator in this class of patients,[172] although it is unclear whether this practice is

beneficial.[169] Category III patients have intense, generalized vasospasm with a decreased cardiac output, markedly elevated PCWP and SVR, and a decreased left ventricular stroke work index (LVSWI). This group responds to afterload reduction.

When confronted with the problem of oliguria in a preeclamptic patient, the placement and patency of the urinary catheter should be confirmed. In the absence of macroscopic hematuria, a modest fluid challenge (e.g., 300 to 500 mL of Ringer's lactate) may be administered without invasive monitoring, but rarely should this volume be exceeded without first obtaining additional information regarding intravascular volume. In this setting, some physicians administer 250 to 500 mL of colloid (e.g., 5% albumin) in an attempt to increase intravascular volume and decrease SVR; this increases the low COP that accompanies preeclampsia, but it places the patient at risk for pulmonary edema. In cases of refractory oliguria, placement of a CVP catheter allows assessment of right-sided filling pressures, but it should be remembered that CVP measurements do not consistently predict PCWP and left ventricular function in patients with severe preeclampsia.[63] Alternatively, the physician may place a pulmonary artery catheter in patients with severe oliguria that persists despite intravenous hydration.[173] Intravascular volume may be expanded until the PCWP is 12 to 14 mm Hg. If the SVR is high, an afterload-reducing agent is used to achieve an SVR of 1000 to 1200 dyne · sec · cm^{-5}. Other indications for a pulmonary artery catheter in patients with severe preeclampsia include refractory hypertension and pulmonary edema (Box 44-7).

Administration of a diuretic (e.g., furosemide) may be indicated if the aforementioned therapy fails, but only after consultation with a nephrologist.[169] Conversion of oliguric to non-oliguric ARF with the use of high-dose diuretics has not been shown to improve mortality or reduce the need for dialysis.[169]

HELLP SYNDROME

The term *HELLP syndrome* describes a clinical state that may represent a severe form of preeclampsia, and is characterized by *H*emolysis, *E*levated *L*iver enzymes, and *L*ow *P*latelets. HELLP syndrome may be confused with hepatitis, gallbladder disease, acute fatty liver of pregnancy, and TTP (Box 44-8). Three classes of HELLP syndrome have been described based on the nadir in perinatal platelet count.[174] Class 1 patients have a platelet count of less than 50,000/mm^3. Class 2 is defined by a platelet count nadir of 50,000 to 100,000/mm^3, and class 3 is defined by a platelet count nadir of 100,000 to 150,000/mm^3.

The etiology of HELLP syndrome remains poorly understood. Its clinical and pathologic manifestations result from an unknown insult that leads to intravascular platelet activation and microvascular endothelial damage. *Hemolysis*, which is defined as the presence of microangiopathic hemolytic anemia, represents the hallmark of the disorder.

Sibai[175] reviewed published reports and noted a lack of consensus regarding the diagnostic features of HELLP syndrome. He recommended the following diagnostic criteria: (1) hemolysis, defined by an abnormal peripheral blood smear and an increased bilirubin level (1.2 mg/dL or greater); (2) elevated liver enzymes, defined as an increased SGOT (AST) of at least 70 U/L and an LDH greater than 600 U/L; and (3) a low platelet count (less than 100,000/mm^3). Audibert et al.[176] subsequently evaluated the clinical utility of these criteria. A diagnosis of HELLP syndrome was made only if all three abnormalities were present. A diagnosis of *partial* HELLP syndrome was made if only one or two of the three criteria were present, and a diagnosis of severe preeclampsia was made if none of these laboratory findings was present. Patients with full HELLP syndrome had a higher incidence of serious maternal complications, including stroke, cardiac arrest, disseminated intravascular coagulation (DIC), placental abruption, need for blood transfusion, pleural effusion, acute renal failure, and wound infection.[176] Prior to the routine use of high-dose corticosteroid treatment *(vide infra)*, maternal mortality associated with HELLP syndrome occurred mostly in women with class 1 disease and was often associated with a delay in diagnosis.[177] Increased risk for mortality may result from hepatic or CNS hemorrhage or vascular insult to the cardiopulmonary or renal systems.[177]

Most cases of HELLP syndrome present preterm, although 20% may present postpartum. The majority of patients initially complain of malaise and epigastric or right upper quadrant pain. Nausea and vomiting occur in 50% of patients.

Box 44-7 INDICATIONS FOR INVASIVE HEMODYNAMIC MONITORING IN OBSTETRIC PATIENTS*

Sepsis with refractory hypotension or oliguria
Unexplained or refractory pulmonary edema, heart failure, or oliguria
Severe pregnancy-induced hypertension with pulmonary edema or persistent oliguria
Intraoperative or intrapartum cardiovascular decompensation
Massive blood and volume loss or replacement
Adult respiratory distress syndrome
Shock of undefined etiology
Some chronic conditions, particularly when associated with labor or major surgery:
• New York Heart Association class III (symptoms with normal activity) or IV (symptoms at bed rest) cardiac disease (structural or physiologic)
• Peripartum or perioperative coronary artery disease (ischemia, myocardial infarction)

*Invasive monitoring will not be necessary in every patient with one of these conditions, nor is this an all-inclusive list of indications for monitoring. In most instances, the conditions and indications for invasive monitoring are identical to those found in other areas of medicine or surgery.
From the American College of Obstetricians and Gynecologists. Invasive Hemodynamic Monitoring in Obstetrics and Gynecology. ACOG Technical Bulletin No. 175, Washington, D.C., December 1992.

Box 44-8 CONDITIONS SOMETIMES CONFUSED WITH PREECLAMPSIA OR ECLAMPSIA

Viral hepatitis
Acute fatty liver of pregnancy
Acute pancreatitis
Gallbladder disease
Appendicitis
Kidney stones
Glomerulonephritis
Hemolytic-uremic syndrome
Exacerbation of systemic lupus erythematosus
Autoimmune thrombocytopenia
Thrombotic thrombocytopenic purpura
Cerebral venous thrombosis
Encephalitis of various causes
Cerebral hemorrhage

From Sibai BM. Treatment of hypertension in pregnant women. N Engl J Med 1996; 335:257-65.

Nonspecific viral-like symptoms also affect many patients.[175] Approximately 80% of affected women have evidence of preeclampsia before delivery. However, hypertension and proteinuria may be slight or absent, and a lack of these signs may cause physicians to overlook the possibility of HELLP syndrome.

Although most patients develop HELLP syndrome before delivery, it reaches its peak intensity 24 to 48 hours postpartum. The LDH levels typically peak on the first postpartum day. Hemolysis typically ceases within 48 hours of delivery. The platelet count typically returns to greater than 100,000/mm^3 within 72 hours of its lowest level, but thrombocytopenia may persist for as many as 11 days. Maternal morbidity increases significantly as the platelet count falls below 50,000/mm^3, and perinatal morbidity also increases with increasing severity of the disease. Provided that there is no DIC, hemostasis often is normal until the platelet count is less than 40,000/mm^3.[178] However, the platelet count may fall quickly, leading to a risk of clinical bleeding. The time course of thrombocytopenia is important. For example, if the platelet count has been stable at 80,000/mm^3 and there is no evidence of bleeding, regional anesthesia can be considered. However, if the platelet count drops from 120,000/mm^3 to 80,000/mm^3 within 2 hours, regional anesthesia most likely is contraindicated[179] (vide infra).

When HELLP syndrome develops postpartum, the onset ranges from a few hours to 6 days after delivery. Patients who develop the syndrome postpartum have a higher incidence of pulmonary edema and renal failure.[180] A number of studies have demonstrated better maternal outcome with administration of dexamethasone 10 mg intravenously at 12-hour intervals until disease remission is noted.[181] Dexamethasone therapy is continued until the following occur: (1) the blood pressure is 150/100 or less, (2) urine output is at least 100 mL/hr for 2 consecutive hours without a fluid bolus or the use of diuretics, (3) the platelet count is greater than 100,000/mm^3, (4) the LDH level begins to decline, and (5) the patient appears stable clinically. At that point, two doses of dexamethasone 5 mg are given intravenously 12 hours apart.[181]

DeBoer et al.[182] investigated the incidence of DIC in patients with HELLP syndrome. All patients had evidence of compensated DIC (i.e., stimulation of the coagulation cascade, leading to the formation of thrombin AT-III complexes, with decreased plasma AT-III and protein C concentrations but normal coagulation). Decompensated DIC (i.e., a full-blown activation of the coagulation cascade, with consumption of all clotting factors) was not observed. In another study of adverse outcomes associated with HELLP syndrome, the incidence of DIC was 8% and was more common in women with placental abruption and/or with acute renal failure.[183]

Patients with HELLP syndrome who experience right upper quadrant pain and neck pain, shoulder pain, or relapsing hypotension should undergo imaging of the liver. Barton and Sibai[184] noted that CT examination was abnormal in 45% of HELLP-syndrome patients with these clinical presentations. The most common abnormal hepatic imaging findings were subcapsular hematoma and intraparenchymal hemorrhage. Abnormalities in liver function tests did not accurately reflect the presence of abnormal hepatic imaging findings, but the severity of thrombocytopenia did correlate with the hepatic imaging findings. An abnormal hepatic imaging finding was noted in 77% of patients with a platelet count of 20,000/mm^3 or less.[184]

Delivery represents the only definitive treatment of HELLP syndrome and should be undertaken immediately, with few exceptions. Conservative treatment (e.g., bed rest, antithrombotic agents, plasma volume expansion) typically is unsuccessful and often results in early maternal or fetal deterioration. In cases of profound prematurity, if the patient's clinical condition allows, glucocorticoid therapy may be administered to accelerate lung maturity, followed by delivery 48 hours later. However, this course of management should only be undertaken in tertiary care centers. Administration of high-dose steroids to women with HELLP syndrome may facilitate the subsequent administration of regional anesthesia, especially if a latency of 24 hours is achieved before delivery. This is a result of the substantial increase in the platelet count after steroid therapy.[185]

PULMONARY EDEMA

Pulmonary edema occurs in approximately 3% of patients with severe preeclampsia.[89,186] Pulmonary edema often occurs as a result of low COP, increased intravascular hydrostatic pressure, and/or increased pulmonary capillary permeability.[66] Echocardiography may be required to exclude cardiogenic causes of pulmonary edema.[187,188] Many cases develop 2 to 3 days postpartum, and resolution requires management of the underlying cause (e.g., overhydration, sepsis, cardiac failure).[119] The initial treatment measures include (1) administration of supplemental oxygen, (2) fluid restriction, and (3) administration of a diuretic (e.g., furosemide). Placement of a pulmonary artery catheter facilitates management in patients with severe pulmonary edema. Further management may include vasodilator therapy to reduce preload or afterload, and dopamine or dobutamine in women with evidence of left ventricular failure. Colloid administration may prove beneficial if the COP-PCWP gradient is lowered. Rarely, tracheal intubation and ventilation may be required if respiratory failure complicates refractory pulmonary edema.[119] Adult respiratory distress syndrome (ARDS) can complicate severe preeclampsia,[189] especially if an increase in pulmonary capillary permeability exists.

PLACENTAL ABRUPTION

Placental abruption occurs in approximately 2% of women with preeclampsia and contributes to the increase in perinatal morbidity and mortality that occurs with this disease. The incidence of abruption is higher in those with preexisting chronic hypertension.[119] The obstetric management depends on its severity and the presence of complications such as hypotension, coagulopathy, and fetal distress (see Chapter 37). An abruption sufficient to kill the fetus indicates major blood loss—as much as 50% of maternal blood volume.

DIC may complicate severe abruption. The definitive management is immediate delivery. Administration of packed red blood cells, fresh frozen plasma, and rarely, platelets may be necessary.[119]

FETAL DISTRESS

Fetal distress frequently complicates preeclampsia, either chronically (because of uteroplacental insufficiency) or acutely (because of a deterioration in maternal status). FHR decelerations are more common in term hypertensive pregnancies than in term normotensive pregnancies.[190] IUGR is not uncommon and results from marginal placental function and limited fetal reserve.[190]

LONG-TERM EFFECTS

A recent retrospective cohort study suggests that preeclamptic women may be at increased risk for diseases related to hypertension later in life.[191]

Preanesthetic Assessment

FLUID BALANCE

Evaluation of the patient's fluid balance must include a strict intake/output chart, placement of an indwelling urinary catheter, and assessment of the patient's current weight. The aim of fluid therapy is to (1) provide an adequate volume to meet daily maintenance requirements and compensate for insensible losses, (2) maintain a satisfactory urine output, (3) act as a conduit for the administration of therapeutic agents (e.g., magnesium sulfate, hydralazine), and (4) compensate for any reduction in preload and afterload during the administration of epidural anesthesia.

Excessive administration of crystalloid or colloid may result in pulmonary or cerebral edema (vide supra).[6,192] It would seem reasonable to recommend converting a negative CVP to a positive CVP (e.g., 2 to 3 cm H_2O) to avoid postepidural hypotension, and additional crystalloid (e.g., 250 to 500 mL) can be infused if hypotension ensues. One study demonstrated a beneficial effect of volume expansion with colloid in patients with severe preeclampsia.[193] These investigators found that moderate volumes of colloid infused over 20 minutes caused a desired increase in oxygen delivery and consumption ($\dot{V}O_2$) secondary to an increase in cardiac output. However, there was no change in the arteriovenous oxygen content difference or in the oxygen extraction ratio. The SVR index was reduced and there was improved regional perfusion, as reflected by an increase in total body $\dot{V}O_2$.[193]

Two studies have investigated the effects of intravenous volume loading with crystalloid on atrial natriuretic peptide (ANP) secretion in preeclamptic women.[57,194] ANP is a vasodilator secreted from the cardiac atria in response to an acute volume load, and this response is more pronounced in preeclamptic women. ANP has properties that counteract vasospasm and improve renal elimination of excess extracellular fluid. These studies support the use of volume expansion before administration of regional anesthesia in preeclamptic women. Pouta et al.[57] confirmed that rapid intravenous infusion of crystalloid results in exaggerated ANP release in women with preeclampsia. They concluded that ANP release is not sufficient to decrease maternal blood pressure but may help counter regional vasospasm in the uteroplacental circulation. Grunewald et al.[194] also found an augmented ANP response to volume expansion in preeclamptic women. In addition, they noted that volume expansion did not affect the uterine artery pulsatility index (PI). These observations suggest that volume expansion per se (with the accompanying increased release of ANP) neither improves nor reduces uteroplacental perfusion in preeclamptic women.[194]

HEMODYNAMIC STATUS

Blood pressure must be measured accurately by meticulous examination. The cuff width must be appropriate (20% to 25% greater than the diameter of the upper arm) to avoid overestimation of systolic pressure, and readings should be standardized (e.g., lower arm, left lateral position).[108] Automated NIBP monitors determine mean pressure as well as systolic and diastolic pressures and provide consistent measurements, which help avoid interobserver unreliability.

The NIBP measurements should be compared intermittently with direct auscultatory findings. Quinn[195] demonstrated that automated devices underestimate systolic and diastolic blood pressures in preeclamptic women. In some cases the difference between auscultatory findings and NIBP measurements exceeds 30 mm Hg.[195] Thus, the same method of BP measurement should be used consistently in order to guide therapy. However, it should be remembered that current management guidelines are based on auscultatory measurements and not on automated NIBP measurements.[1]

A radial artery catheter may be indicated when NIBP measurement proves difficult (e.g., from obesity) or when other conditions (e.g., diabetes mellitus, pulmonary edema) necessitate frequent blood sampling. When contemplating general anesthesia for cesarean section, I will often insert an arterial catheter to assess the effects of antihypertensive agents and the impact of endotracheal intubation.

It rarely is necessary to measure CVP before delivery, and the benefits of careful clinical assessment (e.g., examination of the jugular veins to exclude venous engorgement and increased jugular venous pressure) should not be overlooked. Clues to increased SVR also may be apparent during careful examination (e.g., cold, poorly perfused extremities and a low pulse pressure).

If a central venous catheter is placed, it should allow passage of a pulmonary artery catheter because serial monitoring of PCWP, cardiac output, biventricular function, and mixed venous blood gases enables superior definition of the patient's hemodynamic status.[173] Some physicians argue that administration of regional anesthesia in preeclamptic patients with severe volume depletion requires the placement of a pulmonary artery catheter, but I am unaware of data that support this argument. No study has demonstrated improved outcome with the use of a pulmonary artery catheter in preeclamptic women. A pulmonary artery catheter may be useful in selected patients with severe preeclampsia (e.g., with hypertension unresponsive to hydralazine, oliguria unresponsive to an initial fluid challenge, or pulmonary edema).[196] Some physicians have called attention to the complications associated with the use of a pulmonary artery catheter.[173] However, aggressive volume resuscitation can prove hazardous without invasive hemodynamic monitoring. Management must be individualized. The patient's status, the facilities available, and the risks of invasive hemodynamic monitoring must be considered. In view of the potential for serious—and even fatal—complications, the anesthesiologist should perform a careful assessment of the risks and benefits associated with the management of an individual patient in that institution. I rarely use a pulmonary artery catheter in the management of preeclamptic women, but have done so in selected parturients with refractory hypertension, persistent oliguria, pulmonary edema, or other coexisting cardiopulmonary disorders. Box 44-7 outlines the indications for invasive hemodynamic monitoring in obstetric patients, as proposed by the American College of Obstetricians and Gynecologists (ACOG).

COAGULATION

Bleeding Time

Channing-Rodgers and Levin[79] have questioned the usefulness of the BT as an indicator of platelet function and a predictor of the risk of hemorrhage. They analyzed 862 publications that discussed the BT measurement (664 of which contained

original data). They called attention to several major assumptions that could not be supported by the available data.

The BT does not specifically measure platelet function, and it can be abnormal in a number of coagulation disorders, such as factor deficiencies. Other variables (e.g., red blood cell mass, low hematocrit) also affect the test. No evidence suggests that the skin BT predicts the potential for bleeding from a traumatized epidural vein in a woman with severe preeclampsia.

Anesthesiologists have long presumed a connection between a prolonged BT and the putative risk of epidural hematoma in a patient with severe preeclampsia. Because there are few published reports of this complication after administration of epidural anesthesia in pregnant patients,[197,198] such presumption seems unwarranted. I do not determine the BT before performing epidural or spinal anesthesia in preeclamptic women. In view of the test's unpredictability and unreliability, I cannot justify or recommend its use. Some anesthesiologists suggest measurement of the BT in women with a platelet count of less than 100,000/mm³. In my view, this represents an illogical approach. Either the BT is unreliable (which currently seems beyond question) or it is not. Its use in specific situations cannot be justified. One possible exception to this statement may include situations involving inherited disorders of platelet function (e.g., von Willebrand syndrome)[79]; however a PFA-100™ test would be less traumatic to the patient and provide just as much information (*vide infra*).

Platelet Count

Platelets play a major role in the arrest of bleeding. The widespread belief that a platelet count of less than 100,000/mm³ indicates an increased risk of bleeding stems from earlier studies in which the platelet count and BT were measured concurrently. Channing-Rodgers and Levin[79] noted the broad scatter of published data and emphasized that one of these variables could not be used to make a precise prediction of the other. A specific platelet count that predicts the risk of complications from regional anesthesia has *not* been determined. Indeed, it seems illogical to place an arbitrary limit on a platelet count below which epidural anesthesia should not be performed. Women have received uncomplicated epidural anesthesia with platelet counts as low as 2000 to 4000/mm³.[179] The platelet count is *one* indicator of the woman's hematologic status, but it remains the most commonly performed test of coagulation status in preeclamptic women. If obvious evidence of clinical bleeding (e.g., ecchymoses, petechiae) accompanies the thrombocytopenia, I consider this significant and avoid regional block.

More problematic is the patient who has a significant drop in the platelet count during a short interval (e.g., from 150,000/mm³ to 100,000/mm³ over 2 to 3 hours). Many anesthesiologists are reluctant to administer regional anesthesia in such cases. I believe that this becomes a matter of clinical judgment. The anesthesiologist must balance the very remote risk of epidural hematoma against the established benefits of epidural anesthesia in preeclamptic women.

There is little science to guide one's decision as to what level of thrombocytopenia requires platelet transfusion. In the absence of clinical bleeding, many physicians would not transfuse unless the platelet count was less than 30,000 to 40,000/mm³. However, a spinal epidural hematoma has been described in an eclamptic woman who received epidural anesthesia after receiving six units of platelets. Her pre-transfusion platelet count was 71,000/mm³.[199]

Prothrombin Time (PT) and Activated Partial Thromboplastin Time (aPTT)

Disseminated intravascular coagulation is a rare occurrence in preeclamptic patients, in the absence of placental abruption, amniotic fluid embolism, or sepsis.[200] Low-grade DIC is associated with preeclampsia and can be monitored by serial platelet counts and serum fibrin degradation products.[200] If there are no signs of placental abruption, hemorrhage, sepsis, or a consumptive coagulopathy, routine PT and aPTT measurements in preeclamptic patients are of limited value, even in the presence of thrombocytopenia.[201] Further, a preeclamptic patient with a platelet count greater than 100,000/mm³ is unlikely to have a prolonged PT or aPTT, in the absence of other evidence of a coagulopathy. In patients with evidence of a clinical coagulopathy or significant liver dysfunction, a prolonged PT and aPTT represent a legitimate risk for the occurrence of bleeding in a confined area (e.g., the epidural space), and it would be wise to avoid regional anesthetic techniques.

Thromboelastography

Thromboelastography (TEG) can be used as a bedside measure of the viscoelastic changes that occur during coagulation. Using a single sample of whole blood, the TEG measures all phases of coagulation and resultant clot stability. The original technique involves the use of a rotating cuvette in which a piston is suspended. Blood in the cuvette slowly coagulates, and as coagulation advances, fibrin strands form between the cuvette wall and the piston. In the past, the apparatus measured shear elasticity as the fibrin transferred motion from the cuvette to the piston, a torsion wire, and a moving pen and paper trace. Today the TEG parameters are derived in a similar way, but the equipment is more sophisticated and computerized.[202] The following parameters are recorded:

1. The *r (reaction) time* (in minutes) is the interval between the start and a 1-mm width trace deflection (Figure 44-12). It represents the reaction time, which indicates clotting factor activity.
2. The *k (clot formation) time* (in minutes) is the interval between the end of the r time and a 20-mm width trace deflection. This interval reflects the period of rapid fibrin build-up and cross-linking.
3. The *maximum amplitude (MA) of the trace* (in mm) and the *r + k time* (in minutes) depend on the fibrinogen concentration, platelet count, and platelet function. In addition, these measurements reflect clot strength.

During pregnancy, "normal" measurements demonstrate the presence of a hypercoagulable state. Table 44-2 shows the reduction in r time and k time that occurs during pregnancy and as late as 24 hours postpartum. The MA, alpha angle (which indicates clot formation rate), and G force (which

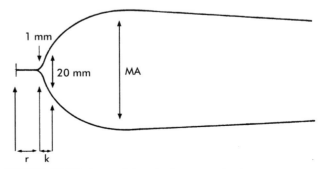

FIGURE 44-12. A normal thromboelastogram, showing measurement of r, k, and MA. (See text for explanation.)

indicates clot strength or "elastic shear modulus") also increase significantly during pregnancy.[202]

It remains to be seen whether TEG will prove useful in preeclamptic women (Table 44-3). A number of studies have compared TEG measurements in preeclamptic women with those in normotensive pregnant women.[203-205] Wong et al.[203] compared TEG measurements with the platelet count and PT, aPTT, and BT measurements in both preeclamptic women and healthy parturients. They concluded that TEG did not predict abnormal coagulation. Orlikowski et al.[204] attempted to correlate platelet count, BT, and TEG measurements in 49 pregnant women with preeclampsia or eclampsia. There was no significant correlation between the TEG and the PT, aPTT, or BT measurements. However, there was a strong correlation between the platelet count and the TEG k time and MA of the trace. None of these studies had a sufficiently large sample size

to demonstrate that TEG is a superior method for predicting clinically significant hemorrhage. At best, TEG may provide an estimate of the risk for surgical bleeding, but it is unlikely that TEG will improve our ability to reduce the already low incidence of epidural hematoma following epidural or spinal anesthesia.

PFA-100™ Analysis

The PFA-100™ system is a bench-top test of platelet function that uses whole citrated blood. The blood is aspirated through a capillary to the central aperture of a membrane coated with collagen and a platelet agonist (either epinephrine or adenosine diphosphate). The time to obtain occlusion of the aperture by a platelet plug is called the *closure time*. In one study the closure time was significantly longer in hypertensive pregnant women than in normotensive controls.[206] In another study of PFA-100™,[207] normal pregnant controls were

TABLE 44-2	THROMBOELASTOGRAPHIC VARIABLES		
	Nonpregnant **Native (*n* = 17)** **Celite (*n* = 15)**	**Pregnant** **(*n* = 134)** **(*n* = 38)**	**Postpartum** **(*n* = 69)** **(*n* = 34)**
r (mm)			
Native	30.8 ± 5.3 (24-43)	26.3 ± 6.7 (13-41)*	27.9 ± 4.7 (18-38)*
Celite	14.3 ± 2.4 (11-17)	7.2 ± 1.9 (4-11)*	6.3 ± 2 (4-10)*
k (mm)			
Native	11.6 ± 2.5 (9-17)	9.3 ± 3.2 (5-17)*	8.6 ± 2.1 (5-14)*
Celite	4.4 ± 1.2 (3-7)	2.5 ± 0.5 (1.5-3)*	2.3 ± 0.4 (2-3)*
MA (mm)			
Native	56.8 ± 5.1 (46-63)	66.4 ± 7.1 (54-80)*	67.7 ± 7.8 (52-80)*
Celite	61.5 ± 4.5 (55-68)	71.7 ± 4.5 (58-76)*	72.4 ± 2.8 (67-78)*
α angle (°)			
Native	33.4 ± 6.1 (24-42)	42.5 ± 9 (27-65)*	47.1 ± 8.1 (37-67)*†
Celite	64 ± 6.1 (54-74)	73.4 ± 4.2 (65-81)*	74.2 ± 5.3 (61-80)*
G force (1000 × dyn/cm²)			
Native	6.7 ± 1.3	10.6 ± 3.8*	11.4 ± 3.9*
Celite	8.2 ± 1.6	13.0 ± 2.4*	13.3 ± 2.0*
LY60 (%)			
Native	4.8 ± 1.5 (2-7)	4.8 ± 2.5 (0.5-10)	5.1 ± 2 (2-10)
Celite	4.8 ± 2.4 (1-8)	4.4 ± 1.9 (1-9)	5 ± 1.5 (3-9)

Values are mean ± SD (range).
Native = native whole blood, Celite = celite-activated whole blood.
r = reaction time, k = clot formation time, α angle = clot formation rate, MA = maximum amplitude (clot strength), G = shear elastic modulus, LY60 = % reduction in MA at 60 min.
*P < 0.05 versus nonpregnant, †P < 0.05 versus pregnant.
From Sharma SK, Philip J, Wiley J. Thromboelastic changes in healthy parturients and postpartum women. Anesth Analg 1997; 85:94-8.

TABLE 44-3	TEG MEASUREMENTS IN NORMAL PREGNANT AND PREECLAMPTIC WOMEN			
TEG	**Normal pregnancy** **(*n* = 25)**	**Mild preeclampsia** **(*n* = 28)**	**Severe preeclampsia** **(PC > 150)** **(*n* = 16)**	**Severe** **preeclampsia** **(PC < 150) (*n* = 24)**
r (mm)	7.1 ± 2	7.9 ± 2.9	7.2 ± 1.3	10.2 ± 3.1*
k (mm)	2.7 ± 0.4	2.9 ± 0.7	3 ± 0.5	3.1 ± 1
MA (mm)	75 ± 3.8	75.5 ± 3.0	71.4 ± 6.4**	67.9 ± 5.9**
α angle (°)	73.5 ± 4	72.3 ± 3.4	70.1 ± 3.1	70.9 ± 6.7
LY 60	4.2 ± 2.5	3.8 ± 1.5	3.9 ± 1.1	3.7 ± 1.1
Hct (%)	35 ± 3	36 ± 3	36 ± 3	35 ± 1
PC	224 ± 45	219 ± 63	215 ± 54	80 ± 31†

Values are mean ± SD. *P < 0.05, **P < 0.01, †P < 0.001 compared to normal group and other subgroups of preeclampsia. PC = platelet count × 1000/mm³; Hct = hematocrit.
r = reaction time; k = clot parmation time; α angle = clot formation rate; MA = maximum amplitude (clot strength); LY 60 = MA after 60 minutes (clot lysis). All measurements were made using celite-activated whole blood. Measurements made with native whole blood were obtained in a separate study.[205]
From Sharma SK, Philip J, Wiley J, Cross S. Activated thromboelastography: Assessment of coagulation abnormalities in preeclamptic patients (abstract). Anesth Analg 1998; 86:S387.

compared with women with gestational thrombocytopenia, preeclampsia without thrombocytopenia, and preeclampsia with thrombocytopenia. The authors concluded that platelet function may be decreased in thrombocytopenic preeclamptic women, when compared to controls.[207] The ability of the PFA-100™ to quantify or predict the risk of surgical bleeding or epidural hematoma formation has not been demonstrated.

RENAL FUNCTION
BUN and creatinine concentrations, as well as the serial urine output during the previous several hours, should be noted. In patients with severe preeclampsia and HELLP syndrome, a reduced GFR may compromise urea and creatinine clearance, and the plasma levels may approximate those in healthy non-pregnant subjects. A creatinine level exceeding 1 mg/dL may indicate substantial renal involvement. Likewise, a uric acid concentration of 7.5 mg/dL or more signals severe renal compromise.

RESPIRATORY FUNCTION
From the anesthesiologist's perspective, the possibility of severe upper airway edema constitutes a major concern.[88,208,209] Any suggestion of stridor or dyspnea should alert the anesthesiologist to the possible hazards of general anesthesia and should prompt the use of a regional anesthetic technique. Although airway edema may increase the difficulty of tracheal intubation, it should not compromise alveolar ventilation and gas exchange. A low Pao_2 (or Sao_2) is more likely to indicate pulmonary edema.

HEPATIC FUNCTION
The occurrence of epigastric pain suggests hepatic involvement and impending clinical deterioration. When liver function tests suggest impaired hepatic function, the diagnosis of HELLP syndrome should be considered, and coagulation deficits secondary to the hepatic damage should be excluded. Liver hematomas can be associated with severe preeclampsia, and if they rupture are associated with life-threatening hemorrhage. Our center has successfully managed cases of preeclampsia-associated hepatic hemorrhage with selective embolization of branches of the hepatic artery by an interventional radiologist.[210]

FETAL STATUS
Although fetal condition infrequently affects the anesthesiologist's choice of anesthetic technique, an informed preanesthetic assessment requires knowledge of the estimated gestational age, the presence or absence of IUGR, and the obstetrician's most recent assessment of fetal well-being.

ANESTHETIC IMPLICATIONS OF MAGNESIUM SULFATE
Magnesium Sulfate and Regional Anesthesia
Past studies have assessed the effects of hypermagnesemia on maternal hemodynamic responses during epidural anesthesia and hemorrhage.[211-214] In gravid ewes receiving either magnesium sulfate or normal saline, the establishment of epidural anesthesia (with a T10 sensory level) resulted in a greater decrease in maternal MAP in animals who received magnesium sulfate than in those who received saline-control.[211] The authors suggested that administration of magnesium sulfate may increase the likelihood of modest hypotension during epidural anesthesia in normotensive pregnant women. However, they speculated that this modest hypotension may not increase fetal risk because magnesium sulfate did not worsen maternal cardiac output or uterine blood flow (UBF) in this study.

Administration of magnesium sulfate also worsens the maternal compensatory hemodynamic response to hemorrhage in gravid ewes.[212] Sipes et al.[213] speculated that this attenuation may represent a decreased response to endogenous vasopressors. They investigated the cardiovascular response of gravid ewes to exogenous vasopressors, with and without concurrent magnesium sulfate infusion. Hypermagnesemia antagonized the effects of alpha$_1$- and alpha$_2$-adrenergic agonists and angiotensin II on the uterine vasculature. The authors speculated that this antagonism might help protect UBF and the fetus during periods of stress. Sipes et al.[214] subsequently determined that ephedrine was superior to phenylephrine in restoring UBF during the treatment of hypotension induced by a high thoracic level of epidural anesthesia in hypermagnesemic gravid ewes. If applicable to humans, these studies collectively suggest that hypermagnesemia worsens the hypotensive response to a low thoracic level of epidural anesthesia, without an adverse effect on UBF and the fetus. This situation is comparable to the institution of epidural analgesia during labor, and it suggests that the epidural block should be titrated carefully during magnesium sulfate infusion. With more extensive blockade (e.g., for cesarean section), concurrent magnesium sulfate infusion and epidural block may significantly impair MAP and UBF. If hypotension occurs, ephedrine is the preferred vasopressor to restore blood pressure and UBF.

Reynolds et al.[215] investigated the effect of fetal hypermagnesemia on the compensatory response to hypoxia resulting from maternal hemorrhage and hypotension in fetal lambs. In this study, fetal hypermagnesemia inhibited the compensatory increase in fetal cerebral blood flow that typically occurs in response to hypoxia. Further, hypermagnesemia resulted in increased fetal mortality. Other investigators have expressed concern regarding the possible adverse effects of hypermagnesemia (when used for tocolysis) on the fetus and neonate.[216] However, recent evidence suggests that prenatal exposure to magnesium sulfate is not associated with increased neonatal morbidity or mortality.[217] Hence, the collective effects of magnesium on the fetus and neonate remain a matter of dispute (see Chapter 10.) However, it should be emphasized that questions regarding the safety of magnesium sulfate are primarily confined to the use of magnesium sulfate as a tocolytic agent (see Chapter 34.) The beneficial effects (e.g., seizure prophylaxis) of magnesium sulfate in preeclamptic patients are well established (*vide supra*).[122]

Prolonged magnesium sulfate administration is associated with a decreased baseline FHR and decreased FHR variability, although these changes are of small magnitude and questionable clinical significance.[218] Magnesium also blocks the positive correlation between gestational age and the number of accelerations observed in control subjects, which may be more important clinically.[218]

Magnesium Sulfate and Neuromuscular Function
At the motor end plate, magnesium inhibits calcium-facilitated presynaptic transmitter release, which produces evidence of neuromuscular blockade at serum magnesium concentrations greater than 12 mg/dL.[128] Hypermagnesemia enhances sensitivity to all nondepolarizing muscle relaxants.[219,220] Small, incremental doses of the muscle relaxant should be used only if a relaxant is required, and the response should be monitored closely with a peripheral nerve stimulator.

The interaction between magnesium and succinylcholine is less clear. Studies in vitro have suggested that hypermagnesemia prolongs the duration of action of succinylcholine, but

this has not been demonstrated in clinical studies.[128] Kambam et al.[221] found significantly lower plasma cholinesterase levels in women with preeclampsia when compared with healthy pregnant controls (179 ± 26 U/mL versus 264 ± 24 U/mL). However, they noted that administration of magnesium sulfate had no effect on plasma cholinesterase activity. They concluded that the low level of plasma cholinesterase activity is responsible for the prolonged action of succinylcholine in preeclamptic patients receiving magnesium sulfate.[221] I use a normal dose of succinylcholine in preeclamptic women who are receiving magnesium sulfate, and I have never had a problem with a prolonged effect in these patients. It is unnecessary to administer a defasciculating dose of a nondepolarizing muscle relaxant before administration of succinylcholine in patients receiving magnesium sulfate. Indeed, even a small dose of a nondepolarizing muscle relaxant can result in profound neuromuscular blockade in patients receiving magnesium sulfate.

Other Drug Interactions with Magnesium Sulfate

Magnesium blunts the contractile response to vasoconstrictors (e.g., norepinephrine) and inhibits catecholamine release after sympathetic stimulation. Because of these properties, magnesium sulfate may facilitate the action of other drugs used to control the pressor response to tracheal intubation. For this reason it may be beneficial to continue the magnesium sulfate infusion during the induction of general anesthesia.

Because calcium plays a major role in the coagulation cascade, the use of magnesium sulfate in preeclampsia raises the troubling possibility that coagulation abnormalities may be exacerbated by magnesium sulfate. One study demonstrated an increase in the BT in preeclamptic patients receiving magnesium sulfate (i.e., from 4.7 ± 1.8 minutes before therapy to 11.5 ± 4.1 minutes after therapy).[222] Serum magnesium concentrations were not determined in this study. Another study of healthy volunteers noted a more modest increase in BT (from 8.0 to 11.8 minutes) during infusion of magnesium sulfate. In this study, the mean serum magnesium concentration was 1.5 mmol/L (3.6 mg/dL).[223] The recognized unreliability of the BT renders these findings of little significance. However, a more recent study (using TEG) showed that the coagulation index is unchanged by a bolus of magnesium sulfate.[224] The authors concluded that magnesium therapy should not influence the use of regional anesthesia.[224]

Clinically, magnesium sulfate does not increase the risk of perioperative blood loss, and an epidural hematoma is a rare event. Thousands of parturients have received epidural or spinal anesthesia while receiving magnesium sulfate, yet there are few published cases of epidural hematoma in these patients. I do not measure the BT before deciding whether to administer regional anesthesia in preeclamptic patients receiving magnesium sulfate.

Since magnesium acts as an antagonist at the NMDA receptor, it can prevent central sensitization caused by peripheral nociceptive stimulation. Although animal studies and some clinical studies suggest an antinociceptive effect for magnesium sulfate, a recent randomized study showed that perioperative administration of magnesium sulfate does not increase CSF magnesium concentration and has no effect on postoperative pain.[225]

Epidural Analgesia/Anesthesia for Labor and Delivery

Most anesthesiologists and obstetricians consider epidural analgesia the preferred form of pain relief for labor and deliv-

ery in preeclamptic women for several reasons. First, epidural block affords the best pain relief—it is superior to all other analgesic methods. Second, preeclamptic women have an exaggerated hypertensive response to pain, which is attenuated by epidural analgesia. Third, epidural analgesia reduces the circulating levels of catecholamines and stress-related hormones, which facilitates blood pressure control.[226] Fourth, epidural analgesia may result in improved intervillous blood flow in preeclamptic women.[227] Fifth, epidural analgesia results in stable cardiac output.[64] Finally, preeclamptic women are at increased risk for cesarean section compared with normotensive parturients, and early administration of epidural analgesia for labor facilitates the subsequent administration of epidural anesthesia for emergency cesarean section. It is especially important to obtain early confirmation of satisfactory placement of the epidural catheter in preeclamptic patients, so that epidural anesthesia can be provided if emergency cesarean section is needed.

Administration of epidural analgesia during labor does not increase the cesarean section rate in preeclamptic women, when compared with intravenous opioid analgesia. Lucas et al.[228] randomly assigned 738 preeclamptic women to receive either epidural analgesia ($n = 372$) or patient-controlled analgesia (PCA) with intravenous meperidine ($n = 366$) during labor. Pain relief was superior in the epidural group, but the overall cesarean section rate was the same (17%) in both groups, and neonatal outcomes were similar.[228] In a secondary retrospective analysis of a subset of enrollees from a multicenter evaluation of aspirin therapy for prevention of preeclampsia, Hogg et al.[229] found that epidural analgesia for laboring women with severe preeclampsia was not associated with an increase in the cesarean delivery rate. The frequency of pulmonary edema and renal failure was also not affected by the use of epidural analgesia. Head et al.[230] randomly assigned 116 laboring women with severe preeclampsia to receive either epidural analgesia or intravenous PCA opioid analgesia during labor. There was no significant difference between groups in the rate of cesarean delivery. Ephedrine administration for hypotension was more frequent in the epidural group (9% versus 0%), and neonatal naloxone administration was more common in the intravenous opioid group (54% versus 9%).[230]

Combined spinal-epidural (CSE) analgesia has been used for patients with severe preeclampsia. A preliminary study noted modest maternal hemodynamic changes with satisfactory neonatal outcomes.[231] My own experience with CSE analgesia for patients with preeclampsia has been very satisfactory.

Long-term epidural analgesia recently has been used to treat women with severe preeclampsia. In a prospective but nonrandomized study,[232] 10 women received prolonged epidural analgesia and 10 controls were treated with bedrest and antihypertensive therapy. The mean ± SD admission-to-delivery interval was 36 ± 10 days in the epidural group and 10 ± 6 days in the control group. Neonatal birth weight was greater in the epidural group than in the control group (2240 ± 310 g versus 1590 ± 380 g).[232]

INTRAVENOUS HYDRATION

I typically give a bolus of crystalloid that does not exceed 10 mL/kg current body weight. I adjust this figure downward when there is evidence of recent excessive weight gain or if the fluid balance chart suggests overhydration (e.g., input exceeds output by 2 L or more). When initiating epidural analgesia, I use 0.125% bupivacaine with 2 µg/mL fentanyl, augment the block slowly, and observe the patient's blood pressure at frequent (1 to 3 minute) intervals for 20 to 30 minutes. An addi-

tional fluid bolus (e.g., 200 to 300 mL) can be given to treat hypotension if necessary.

CHOICE OF LOCAL ANESTHETIC

Bupivacaine is a commonly used local anesthetic. It provides potent analgesia with less motor block than an equipotent concentration of lidocaine. Moreover, dilute solutions cause less hypotension than more concentrated solutions. Initially, I inject 3 mL of a 0.125% solution through the epidural catheter, and I give additional 3- to 5-mL bolus injections until the patient is comfortable and has a T10 sensory level bilaterally. I also give fentanyl 50 to 100 μg through the epidural catheter before starting an epidural infusion.

TREATMENT OF HYPOTENSION

Prevention of hypotension—by appropriate hydration and careful titration of the block—is preferable to treatment. However, hypotension does occur in some patients. If the blood pressure falls, I give an additional bolus of crystalloid and place the parturient in a full lateral position, preferably on her left side. Supplemental oxygen is administered until the hypotension resolves. If these measures fail, I give ephedrine 5 to 10 mg, taking into account the increased sensitivity to vasopressors that characterize preeclampsia, although clinically this is rarely a problem.

MAINTENANCE OF ANALGESIA

Continuous infusion epidural analgesia (CIEA) and patient-controlled epidural analgesia (PCEA) are both reasonable options, although the latter is associated with less total dose of drug. We use a PCEA program exclusively at our hospital. We give 0.125% bupivacaine with fentanyl 2 μg/mL. The PCEA parameters are as follows: bolus dose of 5 mL, a lockout interval of 5 minutes, a background infusion of 6 mL/hr, and an hourly maximum dose of 26 mL. For continuous epidural infusion, analgesia can be maintained using 0.0625% bupivacaine plus fentanyl 2 μg/mL at a rate of approximately 15 mL/hr. Administration of 0.0625% to 0.125% bupivacaine with fentanyl or sufentanil results in better pain relief than administration of bupivacaine alone. Although no randomized studies have confirmed that the addition of opioid to the local anesthetic benefits preeclamptic women, the advantages seem self-evident. Maintenance of satisfactory epidural analgesia facilitates the subsequent extension of epidural anesthesia for emergency cesarean section.

EPINEPHRINE

In common with many obstetric anesthesiologists, I do not believe that epidural epinephrine is contraindicated in women with preeclampsia, although I rarely use it during labor. Epinephrine improves epidural analgesia, but it has the disadvantage of increasing motor block.[233] I prefer to supplement the local anesthetic with an opioid.

Marx et al.[234] demonstrated that epidural administration of an epinephrine-containing local anesthetic in patients with high umbilical vascular resistance resulted in a further increase in vascular resistance. Other investigators[235] have found an increase in vascular resistance of the uteroplacental circulation when epinephrine is added to bupivacaine for cesarean delivery under epidural anesthesia. This was associated with decreased flow in fetal renal and middle cerebral arteries, but there was no difference between groups in neonatal Apgar scores or umbilical cord blood pH.[235] Whereas some reports support the safety of epidural administration of an epinephrine-containing local anesthetic in preeclamptic women,[236,237] others suggest caution.[238]

ANESTHESIA FOR VAGINAL DELIVERY

When a parturient has an epidural catheter in place, I augment the block for vaginal delivery, if necessary, and choose a local anesthetic concentration appropriate to the circumstance (i.e., spontaneous or instrumental vaginal delivery). In the few women who come to vaginal delivery without epidural anesthesia, a low subarachnoid block is a reasonable choice. However, if time allows, I administer epidural anesthesia. Even a low subarachnoid (saddle) block has the potential to produce significant hypotension in a patient with severe preeclampsia. Whenever possible, anesthesiologists should avoid administration of general anesthesia for vaginal delivery in *all women,* but especially in those with preeclampsia *(vide infra).*

POSSIBLE CONTRAINDICATIONS TO REGIONAL ANESTHESIA

Few absolute contraindications to regional anesthesia exist. If the patient refuses an epidural or subarachnoid block, I do not proceed to general anesthesia without first trying to counter her views by persuasive argument. The anesthesiologist should discuss the inherent risks and benefits of all techniques, including the legitimate concerns about general anesthesia. A woman's refusal to accept a regional anesthetic technique may result from misinformation and an unrealistic fear of remote risks. Sympathetic explanation may assuage her fears and allow her to reconsider regional anesthesia.

Coagulation Disturbances

Evidence of a consumptive process—with a rapidly declining platelet count and a prolonged PT and aPTT—should deter the anesthesiologist from proceeding to regional anesthesia. However, audits of "coagulation screens" have revealed only a small percentage of such abnormalities in high-risk preeclamptic women. Prieto et al.[239] assessed coagulation studies in 48 women with severe preeclampsia and a platelet count of less than 100,000/mm^3 but with no clinical evidence of bleeding. None of these patients had an abnormal PT or aPTT. Some anesthesiologists prefer to establish early epidural anesthesia in patients with severe preeclampsia in anticipation of a subsequent decline in the platelet count.

Despite their sometimes benign clinical manifestations, patients with HELLP syndrome have severe disease and often require cesarean delivery. Regional anesthesia is contraindicated if thrombocytopenia is severe, if the platelet count has fallen rapidly during a short period (because of microvascular platelet consumption) or if there is clear evidence of a consumptive coagulopathy characterized by an increased PT, aPTT, and D-dimer concentration. In one report of 31 women with HELLP syndrome who required cesarean delivery, 23 patients received general anesthesia and 8 had epidural anesthesia, but the epidural catheter was placed before the development of thrombocytopenia.[240]

Difficult Airway

Upper airway edema rarely precludes the administration of regional anesthesia. If the woman has stridor, her SaO$_2$ and arterial blood gas tensions must be assessed. In the event of respiratory compromise, awake intubation and general anesthesia is the more prudent choice for cesarean section.

If anatomic airway problems exist, the choice of anesthetic technique calls for careful risk-benefit analysis. What repre-

sents the greater risk—total spinal anesthesia in the presence of a difficult airway *or* difficult/failed tracheal intubation during general anesthesia? I believe the potential combination of total spinal anesthesia and an inability to ventilate the patient has been greatly overemphasized. I give continuous epidural anesthesia to patients with evidence of a difficult airway. Of course, the block requires careful and slow titration, and if there is any possibility of its inadequacy, it must be repeated.

Anesthesia for Cesarean Section

PREANESTHETIC ASSESSMENT

Even when the anesthesiologist plans regional anesthesia, judicious preoperative assessment requires meticulous airway examination (see Chapter 31). I assess airway patency by listening for hoarseness or stridor. This assessment includes asking the patient to take a quick, deep breath while listening over the trachea. This maneuver may detect inspiratory stridor caused by edematous vocal cords.

INTRAOPERATIVE MONITORING

NIBP measurement suffices for patients with mild preeclampsia. Many anesthesiologists consider an arterial catheter desirable in patients with severe preeclampsia because it permits continuous measurement of blood pressure. I typically reserve an arterial catheter for those patients with severe preeclampsia who require general anesthesia. In patients with severe disease (especially those with oliguria), measurement of CVP or PCWP helps guide fluid replacement. Urine output must be continuously monitored intraoperatively and after delivery for at least 24 hours.

EPIDURAL VERSUS GENERAL ANESTHESIA

In a landmark study, Hodgkinson et al.[241] studied systemic and pulmonary artery pressures during administration of either epidural or general anesthesia for cesarean section in 20 severely preeclamptic women. In the general anesthesia group, systemic and pulmonary artery pressures increased significantly during tracheal intubation and during suction and extubation at the end of surgery. In the epidural group, MAP fell slightly with the induction of anesthesia, whereas pulmonary artery pressures remained essentially unchanged (Figure 44-13).

Ramanathan et al.[226] compared the hemodynamic and neuroendocrine stress responses during administration of either epidural or general anesthesia for cesarean section in 21 women with severe preeclampsia. As in Hodgkinson's study, all patients received magnesium sulfate for variable periods before surgery. In addition, the majority of women had received antihypertensive therapy. The authors obtained a T4 sensory level in the epidural group, and they gave ephedrine and additional crystalloid if maternal systolic pressure fell below 100 mm Hg or if MAP decreased by 20% below baseline. Patients in the general anesthesia group received either labetalol or NTG to reduce diastolic pressure to less than 100 mm Hg (or to reduce MAP by 20% below baseline) before the induction of anesthesia. In the epidural group, baseline MAP decreased from 133 to 115 mm Hg when the block reached the T4 level. A further drop occurred at the time of delivery. In the general anesthesia group, pretreatment with labetalol or NTG decreased the MAP from 131 to 112 mm Hg before induction of anesthesia. A transient but significant increase in MAP occurred with the skin incision immediately after tracheal intubation[226] (Figure 44-14).

Ramanathan et al.[226] also examined the levels of stress hormones during anesthesia. In the general anesthesia group, adrenocorticotrophic hormone (ACTH) and beta-endorphin levels increased significantly at the time of skin incision. No such change occurred in the epidural group (Figure 44-15). Plasma epinephrine and norepinephrine levels also increased significantly with skin incision in the general anesthesia group, whereas dopamine levels increased steadily throughout surgery and into the postpartum period. In the epidural group, no significant change in levels of epinephrine and dopamine occurred during the study period. Norepinephrine concentrations decreased significantly at skin incision and continued to decline thereafter (Figure 44-16). Babies whose mothers received general anesthesia were more likely to have an Apgar score of less than 7 at 1 minute but not at 5 minutes. Umbilical artery blood gas measurements and umbilical cord plasma concentrations of ACTH, catecholamines, and cortisol did not differ between the two groups.[226]

In summary, epidural anesthesia (with a T4 sensory level) blunts the maternal hemodynamic and neuroendocrine stress responses during elective cesarean section in women with severe preeclampsia. Epidural anesthesia also avoids the transient neonatal depression associated with general anesthesia.

The presence of coagulopathy, placental abruption, severe fetal distress, or unanticipated technical difficulties with regional anesthesia may mandate the administration of general anesthesia. Wallace et al.[242] randomized 80 women with severe preeclampsia to receive general, epidural, or CSE anesthesia for cesarean delivery. The authors noted that no serious maternal or fetal complications resulted from any of the anesthetic techniques, and that each has a role in clinical practice, provided that a careful approach is taken. However, general anesthesia for cesarean section entails definite risks in preeclamptic women, including (1) the potential for aspiration of gastric contents, (2) difficult endotracheal intubation (accentuated by the risk of pharyngolaryngeal edema), (3) severe hypertension with endotracheal intubation, and (4) impairment of intervillous blood flow.[243]

EPIDURAL ANESTHESIA FOR ELECTIVE OR NONURGENT CESAREAN SECTION

After appropriate intravenous hydration, I establish anesthesia with small increments of 2% lidocaine with epinephrine (or 0.5% ropivacaine or bupivacaine) and fentanyl 100 μg. I allow at least 30 minutes for the induction of adequate anesthesia. I aim to achieve a sensory level of at least T4 to T6, and confirm a good sacral block by testing sensation on the posterior thigh or in the popliteal fossa.

Blood pressure should be monitored at frequent intervals during the onset of the block. A modest fall (e.g., 20 to 30 mm Hg systolic or 10 to 15 mm Hg diastolic) often occurs and requires no treatment other than observation and perhaps an additional fluid bolus (e.g., Ringer's lactate 200 to 500 mL), unless the patient has symptoms. Persistent hypotension should be treated with small (5- to 10-mg) increments of ephedrine intravenously.

I begin an intravenous infusion of oxytocin (20 U/1000 mL of Ringer's lactate) after delivery of the infant. I prefer to avoid administration of methylergonovine or 15-methyl prostaglandin $F_{2\text{-alpha}}$ because of their pressor effects. However, it may be necessary to give one of these potent drugs if the patient suffers from persistent uterine atony.

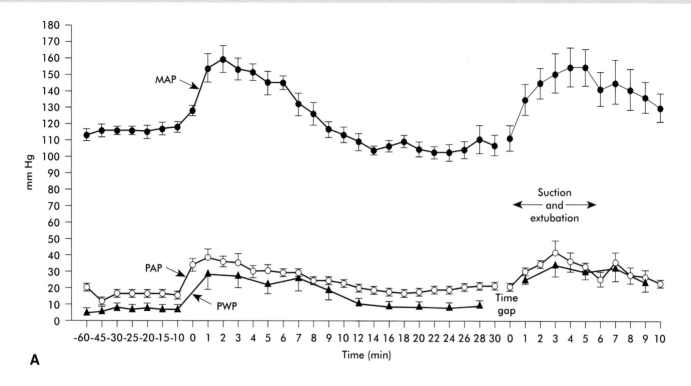

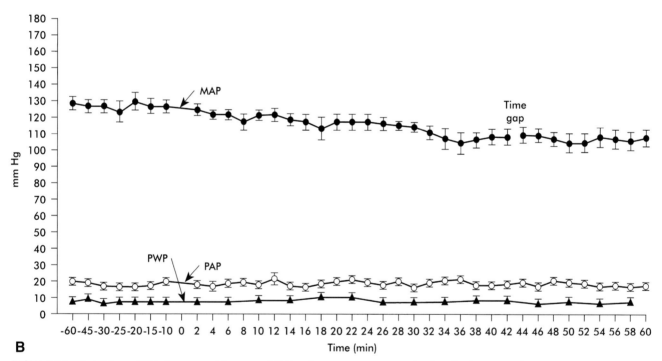

FIGURE 44-13. A, Mean ± SEM of mean arterial pressure *(MAP)*, pulmonary artery pressure *(PAP)*, and pulmonary wedge pressure *(PWP)* in 10 preeclamptic patients who underwent cesarean section under thiopental, nitrous oxide (40%), and halothane (0.5%) anesthesia. Measurements before the induction of anesthesia are indicated at −60 to −10 minutes. The start of induction is indicated by the first 0. The second 0 refers to the start of suction and extubation. The *time gap* refers to the time elapsed between the completion of the first 30 minutes of anesthesia and the start of suction and extubation. **B,** Mean ± SEM of MAP, PAP, and PWP in 10 preeclamptic patients who underwent cesarean section under epidural bupivacaine anesthesia. Measurements before epidural injection of bupivacaine (at 0 minutes) are indicated at −60 to −10 minutes, and measurements during epidural anesthesia are indicated at 2 to 60 minutes. (From Hodgkinson R, Husain FJ, Hayashi RH. Systemic and pulmonary blood pressure during caesarean section in parturients with gestational hypertension. Can Anaesth Soc J 1980; 27:389-94.)

SPINAL ANESTHESIA FOR ELECTIVE OR NONURGENT CESAREAN SECTION

Most anesthesiologists would agree that either epidural or spinal anesthesia may be administered safely in women with *mild* preeclampsia. I often administer spinal anesthesia in patients with well-defined mild disease. To offset the possibility of brisk hypotension, I typically infuse 10 to 15 mL/kg of crystalloid or 500 mL of 5% albumin or other colloid. Hyperbaric bupivacaine 0.75% is the local anesthetic of choice, in a dose of 1.2 to 1.6 mL (9 to 12 mg). I typically add fentanyl (10 μg) and morphine (0.1 to 0.15 mg) to the bupivacaine solution. In women with incipient coagulopathy (e.g.,

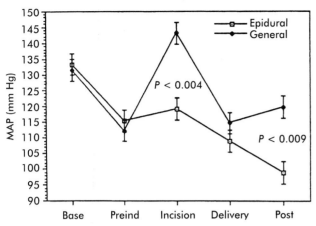

FIGURE 44-14. Changes in mean arterial pressure *(MAP)* in 21 severely preeclamptic women who underwent cesarean section. *Base,* Baseline measurements; *preind* in the general group, the MAP obtained after pretreatment with labetalol or nitroglycerin; *preind* in the epidural group, the MAP obtained with a T4 sensory block; *incision,* at skin incision; *delivery,* at delivery of infant; *post,* postpartum. (From Ramanathan J, Coleman P, Sibai B. Anesthetic modification of hemodynamic and neuroendocrine stress responses to cesarean delivery in women with severe preeclampsia. Anesth Analg 1991; 73:772-9.)

thrombocytopenia), I consider spinal anesthesia preferable to epidural block because the technique does not involve the use of a catheter (which has the potential to lacerate epidural veins) and a smaller-bore needle is used.

However, the situation is different in the woman with severe preeclampsia, especially if there is evidence of fetal compromise. The risks and benefits of spinal anesthesia for cesarean section in women with severe preeclampsia have been debated at length.[244-246] The advantages of spinal anesthesia include: (1) avoidance of general anesthesia and the risks of airway misadventure and hypertension associated with laryngoscopy and endotracheal intubation, (2) a rapid onset, which allows timely cesarean delivery in cases of fetal distress, (3) more reliable anesthesia than that provided with an epidural technique, and (4) less risk of trauma in the epidural space (and thus a decreased risk of epidural hematoma). Some anesthesiologists also contend that epidural anesthesia eventually produces a complete sympathectomy, which causes the same degree of hypotension as spinal anesthesia (albeit with a slower onset).[247]

The arguments against spinal anesthesia in this setting are as follows: (1) spinal anesthesia may produce abrupt and profound hypotension secondary to sympathetic blockade of rapid onset; this is more likely to occur in a patient with a constricted intravascular volume, which is common in women with severe preeclampsia; (2) this degree of hypotension may not be tolerated by a fetus with evidence of chronic compromise (e.g., decreased uteroplacental perfusion, IUGR, oligohydramnios); and (3) studies and reports that spinal anesthesia is less likely to cause hypotension in women with severe preeclampsia are either poorly designed or too small to exclude the potential for catastrophic hypotension.[246]

Can hypotension be prevented consistently in *any* group of patients receiving spinal anesthesia for cesarean section? The answer is no. Neither volume expansion nor prophylactic ephedrine consistently prevents the occurrence of hypotension during spinal anesthesia for cesarean section. Some anesthesiologists argue that patients with severe preeclampsia suffer less severe hypotension during administration of spinal anesthesia than other pregnant patients. Indeed, a recent

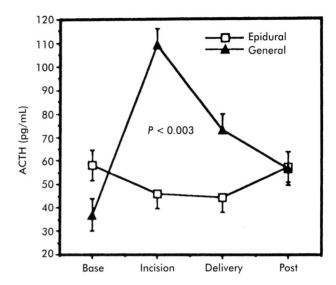

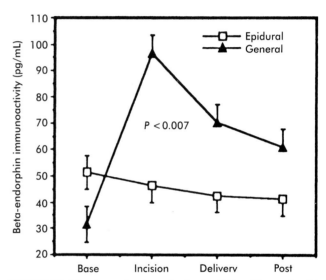

FIGURE 44-15. Changes in plasma levels of ACTH and beta-endorphin like immunoactivity in 21 severely preeclamptic women who received either general or epidural anesthesia for cesarean section. *Base,* Before induction of anesthesia; *incision,* at skin incision, *delivery,* at delivery of the infant; *post,* postpartum. (From Ramanathan J, Coleman P, Sibai B. Anesthetic modification of hemodynamic and neuroendocrine stress responses to cesarean delivery in women with severe preeclampsia. Anesth Analg 1991; 73:772-9.)

prospective cohort study noted that the risk of hypotension was almost six times *less* in severely preeclamptic women than in healthy pregnant women receiving spinal anesthesia for elective cesarean section.[248]

Pouta et al.[57] compared the response to spinal anesthesia in six preeclamptic women (with unknown severity of disease) versus seven normotensive pregnant women. After receiving a 1000-mL bolus of crystalloid, each patient received 13 mg of hyperbaric spinal bupivacaine and another 1000 mL of intravenous crystalloid. Administration of the first 1000 mL of crystalloid resulted in an increase in CVP in all patients. No patient in either group required ephedrine. Karinen et al.[249] administered spinal bupivacaine to 12 preeclamptic patients undergoing cesarean section; 6 of the 12 patients had severe preeclampsia. There were no control subjects. Each patient received a 1000-mL bolus of crystalloid before the administration of spinal anesthesia. Only 2 (17%) of the 12 patients had a decrease in blood pressure of at least 20%, which

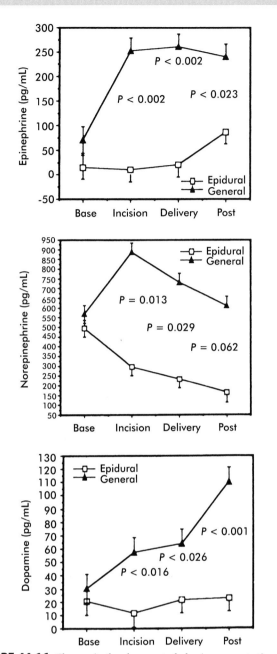

FIGURE 44-16. Changes in the plasma catecholamine concentrations in 21 severely preeclamptic women who received either general or epidural anesthesia for cesarean section. *Base,* Before induction of anesthesia; *incision,* at skin incision; *delivery,* at delivery of the infant; *post,* postpartum. (From Ramanathan J, Coleman P, Sibai B. Anesthetic modification of hemodynamic and neuroendocrine stress responses to cesarean delivery in women with severe preeclampsia. Anesth Analg 1991; 73:772-9.)

required treatment with ephedrine. One of those two patients experienced profound hypotension associated with a C-5 sensory block. Overall there was no change in mean uterine artery vascular resistance, as determined by measurement of the uterine artery pulsatility index (PI). However, the authors noted an increase in the uterine artery PI in both patients who experienced hypotension. All Apgar scores were acceptable, but the authors did not determine umbilical cord blood gas and pH measurements in all of the patients. In summary, the incidence of significant hypotension was 17%, but the hypotension was easily treated.[249]

Wallace et al.[242] performed a prospective study in which 80 women with severe preeclampsia were randomized to receive either general, epidural, or CSE anesthesia for cesarean sec-

tion. (Designation of one group as a CSE group is somewhat misleading, given that each patient in the CSE group received 1.5 mL [11.25 mg] of hyperbaric 0.75% bupivacaine intrathecally. This dose is essentially a full dose of spinal bupivacaine.) The authors excluded patients with a platelet count of less than 100,000/mm[3] and/or a nonreassuring FHR pattern. The authors observed a similar reduction in blood pressure in the epidural and CSE groups. Hypotension was easily treated in both groups, and no patient required an excessive volume of intravenous fluid. Likewise, these two groups had similar requirements for ephedrine, and the authors observed no evidence of rebound hypertension when ephedrine was given in 5-mg doses.[242]

Hood and Curry[247] performed a retrospective review of their experience with regional anesthesia for cesarean section in patients with severe preeclampsia. They reviewed the records of 103 severely preeclamptic women who underwent cesarean section during a 2-year period; 35 women received epidural anesthesia, and 103 received spinal anesthesia. The blood pressure nadir was similar between groups, as was the use of ephedrine, but patients in the spinal group received more intravenous crystalloid solution. Maternal and neonatal outcomes were similar between groups.[247] Another retrospective report from Malaysia found no difference in maternal or neonatal outcomes between epidural and spinal anesthesia for cesarean delivery in women with mild or severe preeclampsia.[250]

A small prospective randomized trial of spinal anesthesia for cesarean section in severe preeclampsia confirmed that spinal anesthesia can be used without significant hypotension when compared to an epidural technique.[251] Sharwood-Smith et al.[251] even suggested that spinal anesthesia is *preferred* for patients with severe preeclampsia because it is associated with better quality of anesthesia and more efficient use of the operating room. Another preliminary study from Sharwood-Smith et al.[252] evaluated the changes in pulse transit time associated with induction of spinal anesthesia in women with preeclampsia. Pulse transit time was determined by measuring the time between the ECG R-wave and the maximum rate of change of the optical plethysmograph at the second toe. Compared with normotensive controls, the increase in pulse transit time resulting from spinal anesthesia occurred more slowly in preeclamptic women, suggesting that their arteries relaxed more slowly. Despite this finding, there was no significant difference between the two groups in the occurrence of hypotension.[252]

One published case report described the successful use of continuous spinal anesthesia in a morbidly obese parturient with severe preeclampsia.[253]

When considering these reports a number of points must be remembered: (1) severe preeclampsia is a heterogenous disease; (2) the hemodynamic profile, the level of hydration, and the degree of renal impairment for each patient vary, and the use of various pharmacotherapeutic agents differs from one hospital to another; (3) patients may present to the anesthesiologist in various stages of the "therapy spectrum"; (4) obstetricians remain concerned about the risk of pulmonary edema resulting from overzealous hydration, and pulmonary edema is a leading cause of maternal mortality among preeclamptic women; and (5) fetal well-being varies from one patient to another, and published studies of spinal anesthesia in preeclamptic women have largely excluded women with nonreassuring FHR tracings.[246] (In a recent prospective, randomized trial of spinal versus general anesthesia for cesarean section in preeclamptic women with a nonreassuring FHR

tracing, spinal anesthesia was associated with a greater mean umbilical arterial blood base deficit and a lower median umbilical arterial blood pH.[254]) It seems reasonable to suggest that until large, randomized studies determine otherwise, epidural anesthesia remains preferable to spinal anesthesia for women with severe preeclampsia. Of course, in some cases (e.g., urgent cesarean section in a patient with a difficult airway), the perceived benefits of spinal anesthesia may outweigh the risks. When possible, I prefer incremental administration of epidural anesthesia in women with severe preeclampsia who require cesarean section. Further, I encourage early administration of epidural analgesia in preeclamptic women who are in spontaneous labor or who undergo induction of labor.

URGENT CESAREAN SECTION

Many parturients already have an epidural catheter in situ for labor analgesia, unless they require surgery shortly after admission. There is little excuse for not having a functioning epidural block in a preeclamptic woman who requires emergency cesarean section after several hours in the labor and delivery area. To augment a preexisting block rapidly, I typically administer either 3% 2-chloroprocaine or pH adjusted 2% lidocaine with epinephrine 1:200,000. The FHR should be monitored in the operating room until the last possible moment.

In women *without* an epidural catheter in situ, I consider spinal anesthesia to be the preferred technique, even in the presence of fetal distress. Satisfactory anesthesia can be achieved rapidly—without delaying surgery—while the nursing team prepares the operating room. Although it may not be possible to avoid hypotension in all patients, the risks represent a lesser hazard than the emergency administration of general anesthesia. I recommend the administration of a 5-mg dose of prophylactic intravenous ephedrine immediately after the intrathecal injection of bupivacaine. In patients with severe preeclampsia, hypotension responds rapidly to additional boluses of ephedrine, and a transient "overshoot" rarely proves to be deleterious. I have used spinal anesthesia for women with severe preeclampsia and have never had a serious unwanted outcome, but my patients usually arrive in the operating room after receiving intravenous hydration and magnesium sulfate therapy. In this situation, it is important to have the obstetrician scrubbed and ready to proceed with surgery shortly after induction of spinal anesthesia in order to reduce the induction-to-delivery interval.

General Anesthesia

The possibility of difficult intubation should be minimized by meticulous preoperative airway assessment and preparation. Unfortunately, airway edema may not become apparent until laryngoscopy.[208] I try to avoid emergency general anesthesia if there is any prospect of difficult intubation secondary to anatomic factors.

The transient but severe hypertension that accompanies tracheal intubation in preeclamptic women can significantly increase maternal intracranial pressure (ICP), with the attendant risks of cerebrovascular accident. Fortunately, the incidence of hemorrhagic stroke is low in both normal pregnant and preeclamptic women,[255] but intracranial hemorrhage remains the largest single cause of death in women with preeclampsia.[256] Other reasons to attenuate the pressor response include the maternal risks of increased myocardial oxygen consumption, cardiac arrhythmias, and pulmonary edema, as well as the sig-

nificant reduction in UBF, which may harm the fetus.[243] Many regimens have been proposed to attenuate the pressor response during laryngoscopy and intubation. Hood et al.[257] documented the successful use of intravenous NTG, titrated to reduce MAP by approximately 20% before the induction of general anesthesia in women with severe preeclampsia. All patients received magnesium sulfate before anesthesia, but none underwent preoperative volume expansion.

I use SNP rarely. If I use SNP, I start the infusion at 0.5 µg/kg/min, and then titrate it to blood pressure response. I aim for a systolic blood pressure of approximately 140 mm Hg, and rarely have found it necessary to exceed a dose of 1.5 µg/kg/min.

Sosis and Leighton[258] recommended trimethaphan (Arfonad) for acute blood pressure control during induction and emergence from general anesthesia. In contrast to NTG and SNP, trimethaphan does not significantly change cerebral blood flow or ICP. Administered in a 0.1% solution and titrated to response, it effectively attenuates the pressor response to intubation. The potential problems of histamine release and prolonged neuromuscular blockade after succinylcholine administration have little significance during short-term administration. I have no experience with this drug.

Ramanathan et al.[162] used labetalol to attenuate the pressor response in a prospective, randomized study of preeclamptic women who subsequently received general anesthesia for cesarean section. The labetalol group received 20 mg intravenously, followed by 10-mg increments (up to a maximum total dose of 1 mg/kg over a 10-minute period), and patients in the control group received no antihypertensive therapy before the induction of anesthesia. Maternal MAP increased with tracheal intubation in both groups, but a significantly greater rise occurred in the control group. Control subjects but not patients in the labetalol group developed significant tachycardia. I consider labetalol the drug of choice in this setting and administer it by bolus injection or continuous infusion, according to the severity of hypertension and the urgency of the situation.

Lawes et al.[259] administered both intravenous fentanyl 100 µg and droperidol 5 mg to obtund the pressor response to intubation in 26 women with severe preeclampsia. After a 5-minute waiting period, they gave additional fentanyl 100 µg, plus bolus doses of trimethaphan 2.5 mg, if required. This regimen satisfactorily reduced arterial pressure in approximately 80% of cases. However, I suspect that administration of these doses of fentanyl and droperidol results in heavy sedation. Furthermore, few pharmacies stock droperidol these days because of the concern that droperidol administration is associated with cardiac arrhythmias. A better approach is to give 1 to 3 µg/kg of intravenous fentanyl—*without* droperidol—to reduce the hemodynamic sequelae of laryngoscopy and intubation. The neonatal resuscitation team should be informed that the fetus has been exposed to this modest dose of fentanyl.

Technique of General Anesthesia

I give 30 mL of 0.3 M sodium citrate orally and metoclopramide 10 mg intravenously immediately before the induction of anesthesia. After denitrogenation, induction of anesthesia proceeds in a rapid-sequence manner, with application of cricoid pressure until the endotracheal tube is in place and the cuff is inflated. In the past, I gave 4 to 5 mg/kg of sodium thiopental (a slightly higher dose than usual) to induce anesthesia; however, propofol 2 mg/kg has replaced sodium

thiopental for this purpose in our hospital. Succinylcholine 1.5 mg/kg is given to achieve effective intubation conditions. I use a 6- or 6.5-mm endotracheal tube in case there is undetected airway edema. Rocuronium, vecuronium, or atracurium are reasonable choices for the maintenance of neuromuscular blockade (if necessary), once the patient has demonstrated recovery from succinylcholine. To ensure an adequate depth of anesthesia, I give isoflurane 0.7% to 1% or sevoflurane 1% to 2% in 50% nitrous oxide and 50% oxygen before delivery, to control hypertension and prevent awareness.

After delivery of the infant, I give fentanyl (approximately 3 to 5 μg/kg) intravenously while increasing the concentration of nitrous oxide to approximately 66%. Hypertension rarely requires treatment after delivery. In fact, immediately after delivery, hypotension is more common than hypertension, regardless of the anesthetic technique. I typically continue administration of magnesium sulfate throughout anesthesia unless hypotension becomes an issue. Prior to awakening I give ondansetron 4 mg and dexamethasone 4 mg intravenously for nausea prophylaxis. Morphine 5 to 10 mg intravenously is given for early postoperative analgesia.

Postpartum Management

Women receiving magnesium sulfate initially return to the Postanesthesia Care Unit (PACU) for 1 to 2 hours. Subsequently, in our hospital we closely observe all women with severe preeclampsia in a monitored-care environment for at least 24 hours after delivery. Patients with coagulation abnormalities, fluid balance problems, sepsis, or other complications may remain for a longer period. The principles of postpartum care include the following:

1. **Analgesia:** Women who undergo cesarean section receive epidural or intrathecal opioids unless contraindications exist. I give morphine 2.5 to 3.0 mg epidurally or 0.1 to 0.15 mg intrathecally, regardless of the woman's concurrent therapy, because she will remain under close observation for at least 24 hours. Concurrent administration of a nonsteroidal antiinflammatory drug both improves and prolongs intraspinal opioid analgesia after cesarean section (see Chapter 28).
2. **Fluid balance:** A strict intake/output chart should be maintained for at least 24 hours or until a diuresis develops. A total intake of 75 mL/hr should not be exceeded until the patient begins to mobilize her excess extracellular water.[6]
3. **Magnesium sulfate:** Magnesium sulfate is continued for at least 24 hours postpartum or until there is evidence of maternal diuresis. The duration of therapy varies from one institution to another and seems to be somewhat empirical but typically is related to the rate of recovery from hypertension, oliguria, and/or coagulopathy, as well as the patient's general well-being.[260] Late postpartum seizures have been described. In some institutions, postpartum seizures are more common than antepartum seizures.
4. **Hemodynamic control:** It may be necessary to reinstitute antihypertensive therapy to avoid rebound hypertension as the patient begins to experience postoperative pain.

Infrequently, severe preeclampsia-eclampsia, with or without HELLP syndrome, persists more than 24 to 48 hours postpartum. Parturients with persistent hypertension, oliguria, and thrombocytopenia are at increased risk for morbidity and mortality, especially if these abnormalities do not resolve within 72 to 96 hours postpartum. Ultrasound-directed uterine curettage appears to be effective in promoting resolution of the thrombocytopenia associated with severe preeclampsia,[261] but this therapy has not gained widespread acceptance in clinical practice.

ECLAMPSIA

Eclampsia is defined as convulsions and/or coma not caused by coincidental neurologic disease (e.g., epilepsy), which occur(s) during pregnancy or the puerperium in a woman whose condition also meets the criteria for preeclampsia. The relationship between preeclampsia and eclampsia remains controversial.[262]

Epidemiology

The reported incidence of eclampsia varies greatly among countries and communities and ranges from 1 in 110 to 1 in 3448 pregnancies. (The lower incidence was reported in Sweden, where appropriate prenatal care and early hospitalization of preeclamptic women effectively prevents most cases of eclampsia.) Sibai[263] reported an incidence of 1 in 320 pregnancies in a tertiary care hospital in Tennessee. Most centers have a much lower incidence.

In the United Kingdom, the incidence of eclampsia is approximately 1 in 2000 pregnancies.[264] Leitch et al.[265] described a significant reduction in both the incidence of eclampsia and its associated morbidity in the United Kingdom. The overall incidence of eclampsia has declined by more than 90% since 1931, but the incidence of antepartum and intrapartum eclampsia has declined more than the incidence of postpartum eclampsia (i.e., a relatively greater proportion of cases of eclampsia occurs postpartum than in previous years). Leitch et al.[265] noted that between 1931 and 1940, 15% of cases of eclampsia resulted in maternal death. However, they identified no maternal deaths resulting from eclampsia after 1964. The perinatal mortality rate declined from 433 perinatal deaths per 1000 cases of eclampsia between 1931 and 1940 to 169 per 1000 cases between 1961 and 1970. The most recent *Confidential Enquiries into Maternal Deaths in the United Kingdom: 1997-1999*, noted five maternal deaths associated with eclampsia.[3]

In the United States, eclampsia remains a significant complication of pregnancy, with high mortality and morbidity rates. In a study of 399 consecutive women with eclampsia, the mortality rate was 1%, and antepartum onset carried the greatest risk, especially before 32 weeks' gestation. However, postpartum eclampsia was more likely to be associated with neurologic deficits.[266] Eclampsia remains a common condition and a leading cause of maternal and perinatal mortality in developing countries.[267]

Eclampsia is a life-threatening emergency that occurs suddenly, most commonly in the third trimester near term. Approximately 60% of seizures precede delivery. (In some populations with good prenatal care, the majority of cases of eclampsia occur postpartum.) Most postpartum cases occur during the first 24 hours, but seizures attributed to eclampsia have been reported as late as 22 days after delivery. Approximately 50% of all patients have evidence of severe preeclampsia, but the classic triad of hypertension, proteinuria, and edema may be absent or only mildly abnormal in 30% of eclamptic women.[262] Risk factors for eclampsia include nulliparity, multiple gestation, molar pregnancy, triploidy, preexisting hypertension or renal disease, previous severe preeclampsia or eclampsia, nonimmune hydrops

fetalis, and systemic lupus erythematosus.[263] Major maternal complications include placental abruption, HELLP syndrome, DIC, neurologic deficits, pulmonary aspiration, pulmonary edema, cardiopulmonary arrest, and acute renal failure.[266]

Pathophysiology

Any of the pathophysiologic changes of preeclampsia may be present. Headache, visual disturbances, and epigastric or right upper quadrant pain are consistent with severe preeclampsia and may portend eclampsia. Seizures have an abrupt onset, typically beginning as facial twitching and followed by a tonic phase that persists for 15 to 20 seconds. This progresses to a generalized clonic phase characterized by apnea, which lasts approximately 1 minute. Breathing typically resumes with a long stertorous inspiration, and the patient enters a postictal state, with a variable period of coma. Cardiorespiratory arrest and pulmonary aspiration of gastric contents may complicate a seizure. The number of seizures varies from 1 to 2 to as many as 100 in severe, untreated cases.

Cerebral vasospasm, ischemia, edema, hemorrhage, hypertensive encephalopathy, and DIC have been implicated in the pathogenesis of seizures.[268] However, the causes are poorly understood, and no single process accounts for the clinical features of eclampsia.[269]

Diagnosis

Until proven otherwise, the occurrence of seizures during pregnancy should be considered eclampsia. All delivery room personnel must be alert to premonitory symptoms (e.g., transient visual disturbances, headache, epigastric pain). Conditions simulating eclampsia include epilepsy, encephalitis, meningitis, cerebral tumor, and cerebrovascular accidents (e.g., ruptured berry aneurysm, arteriovenous malformation), but none should be considered until eclampsia has been ruled out (Table 44-4).[270] The CT scan may be normal, or it may show evidence of cerebral edema, infarction, or hemorrhage. The last complication occurs more frequently in elderly gravidae with preexisting hypertension and may result in death or permanent disability (e.g., hemiplegia).[270] Other neurologic abnormalities include transient neurologic deficits, temporary cortical blindness,[271] retinal detachment, and postpartum psychosis.[263] Electroencephalography typically is abnormal

and shows focal or diffuse slowing as well as focal or generalized epileptiform activity.[269]

Obstetric Management

The immediate goals are to stop the convulsions, establish a clear airway, and prevent major complications (e.g., hypoxemia, aspiration). Further management includes antihypertensive therapy, induction or augmentation of labor, and expeditious (preferably vaginal) delivery. Fetal bradycardia typically occurs during and immediately after a seizure but does not mandate immediate delivery unless it persists.

Resuscitation and Seizure Control

During the seizure, oxygenation may prove impossible, but supplemental oxygen should be delivered by means of an Ambu bag and face mask (Box 44-9). Attempts to insert an oral airway should be withheld until the seizure abates, but a soft nasopharyngeal airway may facilitate oxygenation. As soon as breathing resumes, ventilation may be gently augmented by bag and face-mask oxygen. A pulse oximeter probe should be applied to assess maternal oxygenation. Blood pressure and the ECG should be monitored to identify hypertension, arrhythmia, or cardiac arrest. While initial resuscitation is underway, an assistant should establish intravenous access, which is occasionally difficult to do in a combative post-ictal woman. Midazolam (i.e., as much as 10 to 20 mg intravenously, in divided doses) may be required to sedate the combative individual in order to allow further treatment. However, an expert in airway management must be present if a potent benzodiazepine is used.

Magnesium sulfate is the preferred drug for the definitive treatment of seizures. After an immediate loading dose of 4 to 6 g is infused intravenously over 20 minutes, a maintenance dose of 1 to 2 g/hr is given, assuming the patient has adequate urine output. Recurrent convulsions should prompt administration of an additional bolus dose of 2 to 4 g, infused over 5 to 10 minutes. Observations for evidence of magnesium toxicity include (1) hourly monitoring of urine output, (2) regular evaluation of deep tendon reflexes, and (3) observation of respiratory rate (vide supra).

Unless other contraindications exist, eclamptic patients should undergo expeditious delivery. The most frequent indications for cesarean section include fetal distress, placental

TABLE 44-4	DIFFERENTIAL DIAGNOSIS OF PERIPARTUM SEIZURES
Cerebrovascular compromise	Cerebral infarction
	Cerebral hemorrhage
	Subarachnoid hemorrhage
	Cerebral venous thrombosis
	Cerebral edema and malignant hypertension
Mass lesions	Vascular malformations
	Benign and malignant tumors
	Cerebral abscess
Infectious diseases	Viral
	Bacterial
	Parasitic infestations
	HIV
Epilepsy	Central stimulants (e.g., cocaine, theophylline)
Toxic/metabolic disorders	Hyponatremia, hypocalcemia, hypoglycemia, hyperglycemia

Adapted from Sibai BM. Eclampsia. In Goldstein PJ, Stern BJ, editors. Neurologic Disorders of Pregnancy, 2nd ed. Mount Kisco, New York, Futura Publishing Company, 1992:1-24; and Kaplan PW, Repke JT. Eclampsia. Neurologic Clinics. 1994; 12:565-82.

abruption, extreme prematurity with an unfavorable cervix, and failed induction of labor. Other indications might include recurrent seizures and persistent postictal agitation.

CT scans are of limited clinical value in eclampsia and should be performed on affected women with focal neurologic signs, atypical seizures, and/or delayed recovery.[272]

Anesthetic Management

The preanesthetic assessment of an eclamptic parturient parallels that for a patient with severe preeclampsia. Key points include the following:

1. **Assessment of seizure control and neurologic function.** The possibility of increased ICP need not concern the anesthesiologist if the patient remains conscious, alert, and seizure free. Persistent coma and localizing signs may indicate major intracranial pathology, which would affect anesthetic management.
2. **Maintenance of fluid balance.** Intake should be restricted to 75 to 100 mL/hr.
3. **Blood pressure control.** Appropriate treatment must be instituted if the diastolic pressure exceeds 110 mm Hg.
4. Monitoring of **maternal oxygenation** by continuous pulse oximetry.
5. **Continuous FHR monitoring.**
6. **Laboratory investigations** follow the routine for preeclamptic patients, but in eclamptic patients, coagulation studies should be undertaken, regardless of the platelet count.

In conscious eclamptic women with no evidence of increased ICP or coagulopathy and whose seizures have been well controlled, I consider epidural analgesia the technique of choice for labor pain. Concern about unintentional dural puncture in a patient with unsuspected increased ICP is largely theoretical in conscious patients. However, epidural analgesia should be withheld in a woman with a possible neurologic deficit until the diagnosis becomes clear. Opioids, in

large doses, should be avoided because of the possible exacerbation of increased ICP from respiratory depression.

I recommend epidural anesthesia for cesarean section in selected cases, provided that the patient remains seizure free, has stable vital signs, and is conscious and rational. This approach is supported by a study from South Africa, where Moodley et al.[273] found no difference in maternal and neonatal outcomes when comparing epidural versus general anesthesia for cesarean section in conscious women with eclampsia. Contraindications to epidural anesthesia include patient refusal, DIC, and placental abruption. In a study of eclamptic patients in Bangladesh, spinal anesthesia was associated with a lower mortality rate than general anesthesia for cesarean delivery.[274]

Unconscious or obtunded patients or those with evidence of increased ICP should have a "neurosurgical" anesthetic, with an opioid/relaxant technique and deliberate hyperventilation. To avoid the possibility of awareness, the anesthesiologist can administer a small dose of a volatile halogenated agent after hyperventilation is established. The patient should be extubated while in the left lateral position and only when fully conscious. I routinely leave these patients intubated and transfer them to an intensive care unit for blood pressure control, assessment of neurologic recovery, and a controlled wean from assisted ventilation. Magnesium sulfate administration should continue until blood pressure stabilizes and CNS hyperexcitability disappears. In the event of prolonged unconsciousness, the patient should undergo CT scan.

Maternal Outcome after Eclampsia

The reported incidence of recurrent eclampsia ranges from zero to 20%.[275] Sibai et al.[276] estimated the risk of eclampsia in a second pregnancy to be 1.4%. The risk of stroke is greatest during the postpartum period.[277]

CHRONIC HYPERTENSION

Definition

Hypertension that precedes pregnancy or occurs before 20 weeks' gestation represents **chronic hypertension.** Other criteria that aid in the diagnosis of chronic hypertension include use of antihypertensive drugs before pregnancy and persistence of hypertension beyond 12 weeks postpartum.[5]

Hypertension is defined as **mild** with a systolic blood pressure of ≥ 140 mm Hg or diastolic blood pressure of ≥ 90 mm Hg on at least two occasions and at least 4 hours apart. A blood pressure of ≥ 180 mm Hg systolic and/or ≥ 110 mm Hg diastolic constitutes **severe** hypertension. The patient is considered to be **low risk** if she has mild hypertension without organ involvement.[278] A patient with chronic hypertension in pregnancy is deemed to be **high risk** in the presence of one or more of the following: (1) secondary hypertension, (2) target organ damage, (3) previous perinatal loss, and (4) severe hypertension.

Superimposed preeclampsia refers to a patient with preexisting hypertension whose pregnancy is complicated by preeclampsia.[6] Women with chronic hypertension have a fivefold increase in the incidence of preeclampsia, compared with normotensive women.[115]

Gestational hypertension is the development of hypertension after 20 weeks' gestation in a previously normotensive woman. Drug therapy typically is not required, and the out-

---

Box 44-9 ECLAMPSIA: THE ABCs OF SEIZURE CONTROL

AIRWAY

Turn patient to left side; apply jaw thrust.
Attempt bag and mask ventilation ($FiO_2 = 1.0$).
Insert soft nasopharyngeal airway if necessary.

BREATHING

Continue bag and mask ventilation ($FiO_2 = 1.0$).
Apply pulse oximeter and monitor SaO_2.

CIRCULATION

Secure intravenous access.
Check blood pressure at frequent intervals.
Monitor ECG.

DRUGS

Magnesium sulfate
• 4 to 6 g intravenously over 20 minutes
• 1-2 g/hr for maintenance therapy
• 2 g intravenously, over 10 minutes, for recurrent seizures

HYDRALAZINE

• 5 to 10 mg intravenously or labetalol 10 to 20 mg intravenously as needed to treat hypertension

come of pregnancy typically is good. However, gestational hypertension may progress to preeclampsia and/or chronic hypertension (Table 44-5).[115]

Epidemiology

Approximately 5% of pregnant women have chronic hypertension. Hypertensive vascular disease occurs more frequently in pregnant women who are older, obese, and/or African-American.[115] Most women (90%) with chronic hypertension have **essential** or **primary hypertension,** and the remainder have **secondary hypertension** with an underlying cause (e.g., renal disease, renal artery stenosis, endocrine disorder).[5] Because an increasing number of women now delay childbearing until an older age, it is likely that the incidence of chronic hypertension in pregnancy will continue to rise.

Pathophysiology and Interaction with Pregnancy

Blood pressure normally declines during early pregnancy, which makes it difficult to diagnose chronic hypertension before 24 weeks' gestation. During late pregnancy, the normal blood pressure rise may be exaggerated, leading to confusion with preeclampsia.[5] However, the pattern of hypertension is different in women with chronic hypertension when compared with that in preeclamptic women. For example, women with chronic hypertension are more likely to maintain a diurnal variation in blood pressure than preeclamptic women. Most women with mild chronic hypertension fare well during pregnancy and have a normal outcome. However, some develop superimposed preeclampsia, and they are at increased risk for perinatal morbidity and mortality. Progressive hyperuricemia, abnormal activation of coagulation, and proteinuria typically indicate superimposed preeclampsia.[115]

Sibai et al.[279] assessed risk factors for adverse pregnancy outcomes in 763 pregnant women with chronic hypertension. Risk factors for the occurrence of superimposed preeclampsia included (1) a history of preeclampsia in a previous pregnancy, (2) chronic hypertension of at least 4 years' duration, and (3) a diastolic blood pressure of at least 100 mm Hg during early pregnancy. The presence of proteinuria early in pregnancy was associated with adverse neonatal outcome, independent of the development of preeclampsia. Administration of low-dose aspirin did not reduce the incidence of superimposed preeclampsia.[279]

In 10% of cases, chronic hypertension is secondary to one or more underlying disorders such as renal disease, collagen vascular disorders, or endocrine disease. Many of these patients do not tolerate pregnancy well; significant deterioration may occur in patients with Cushing syndrome, and fetal prognosis is poor with this condition. Pheochromocytoma, if undetected, is also associated with a significant risk of maternal and fetal morbidity and mortality (see Chapter 41).

In contrast, hyperaldosteronism improves with pregnancy, and pregnant patients sustain less potassium loss than nonpregnant patients. Similarly, the resistance to the pressor effects of angiotensin II—which characterizes normal pregnancy—may ameliorate hypertension in pregnant women with renal artery stenosis.[6]

Medical Management

It is unclear whether effective control of mild chronic hypertension brings long-term benefits with respect to end-organ function. Further, antihypertensive therapy does not reduce the incidence of superimposed preeclampsia, and good outcomes occur in most women, regardless of whether they receive antihypertensive medications.[5] In one randomized clinical trial, perinatal outcome was not improved in women with mild-to-moderate hypertension who received methyldopa or labetalol when compared with similar patients who received no treatment.[280] Sibai[278] recommends antihypertensive treatment for women with *high-risk* chronic hypertension. The aim of treatment is to keep the blood pressure below 140/90 mm Hg. Initial blood pressure control with intravenous agents, such as hydralazine and labetalol, may be needed. Methyldopa is commonly used for the long-term treatment of hypertension, especially if the patient was taking it before conception. However, there are contraindications (e.g., liver dysfunction) to its use, and the drug causes side effects, including dry mouth and drowsiness. Occasionally methyldopa is ineffective. Some physicians recommend oral labetalol as the first-line treatment of chronic hypertension, in an initial dose of 100 mg twice daily up to a maximum of 2400 mg per day.[278] A thiazide diuretic or nifedipine can be added if labetalol alone is ineffective. Nifedipine is useful in women with diabetes and vascular disease and, when used in combination with a diuretic, is effective in young black women with a low-renin type or salt-sensitive hypertension.[278] The use of diuretics during pregnancy is controversial because of the associated reduction in plasma volume. However, this reduction in plasma

TABLE 44-5	HYPERTENSIVE DISORDERS OF PREGNANCY		
Clinical finding	**Chronic hypertension**	**Gestational hypertension**	**Preeclampsia**
Time of onset of hypertension	< 20 Weeks' gestation	Typically in third trimester	≥ 20 Weeks' gestation
Degree of hypertension	Mild or severe	Mild	Mild or severe
Proteinuria*	Absent	Absent	Typically present
Serum urate > 5.5 mg/dL (0.33 mmol/L)	Rare	Absent	Present in almost all cases
Hemoconcentration	Absent	Absent	Present in severe disease
Thrombocytopenia	Absent	Absent	Present in severe disease
Hepatic dysfunction	Absent	Absent	Present in severe disease

*Defined as ≥ 1+ by dipstick testing on two occasions or ≥ 300 mg in a 24-hour urine collection.
From Sibai BM. Treatment of hypertension in pregnant women. N Engl J Med 1996; 335:257-65.

volume is not usually associated with adverse fetal outcome. Sibai[278] recommends the use of a diuretic alone or in combination, unless preeclampsia and/or IUGR develops. ACE inhibitors must be avoided during pregnancy because their use is associated with fetal hypocalvaria, renal failure, oligohydramnios, and fetal or neonatal death. Atenolol is not recommended during pregnancy because of its association with decreased fetal weight.[281]

Obstetric Management

Because of the typically favorable outcome in more than 85% of pregnancies, the obstetric management of women with *low-risk* chronic hypertension differs little from that of normal pregnancy. These patients require more intensive surveillance of blood pressure, but the majority are candidates for home monitoring. The patient measures her blood pressure as often as twice daily but at least two to three times per week. If blood pressure remains stable and within acceptable limits, the patient attends the antenatal clinic every 2 weeks until 30 weeks' gestation. Thereafter, she should have weekly clinic visits and regular antenatal testing (e.g., nonstress test, biophysical profile). Although a single elevated blood pressure has little significance, persistent elevation typically requires hospitalization. If superimposed preeclampsia develops, early delivery becomes a priority.

High-risk women will require aggressive antihypertensive treatment and frequent evaluations of maternal and fetal well-being. These women are at increased risk for postpartum pulmonary edema, renal failure, and hypertensive encephalopathy.[278]

Anesthetic Management

The anesthetic management of patients with chronic hypertension differs little from that previously outlined for women with preeclampsia. Although hypertension is the only demonstrable finding in approximately 85% of patients, the presence of more severe complications (e.g., myocardial disease, renal insufficiency) must be excluded in those with long-standing disease or severe hypertension. Because of the concurrent pregnancy, estimation of exercise tolerance becomes more difficult, but the anesthesiologist should ask about the patient's cardiovascular status before and during pregnancy. The assessment also should elicit the presence of other complicating diseases (e.g., obesity, diabetes).

Important points to note during the physical examination include heart size, the presence or absence of significant bruits, evidence of impaired left ventricular function (e.g., basal pulmonary rales), and ophthalmoscopic findings (if reported). In addition to routine laboratory tests, patients with long-standing disease or severe hypertension require a 12-lead ECG to discern evidence of left ventricular hypertrophy or ischemic heart disease. Special attention should be given to the serum creatinine level. A concentration greater than 1 mg/dL suggests significant renal involvement.

ANALGESIA FOR LABOR
The previously recommended technique of epidural analgesia applies equally well to these parturients. In women with severe hypertension from superimposed disease, efforts should be made to control the blood pressure with hydralazine or labetalol before the administration of epidural analgesia. Persistent hypertension does not contraindicate epidural analgesia, but brisk hypotension must be avoided during establishment of the block.

Women with chronic hypertension often are parous, and painful labor may progress rapidly. In these patients I typically institute epidural analgesia with 0.125% bupivacaine plus fentanyl 100 μg and maintain analgesia with a patient-controlled epidural infusion of bupivacaine and fentanyl. This helps ensure cardiovascular stability and often eliminates the need for further top-up injections.

The CSE technique offers an excellent alternative for inducing labor analgesia in parous women who are experiencing strong contractions with rapid descent of the fetus. I inject 1 mL of 0.25% bupivacaine, with or without 10 μg of fentanyl. Intrathecal injection provides a rapid onset of analgesia, which often remains satisfactory during the second stage of labor if PCEA is started immediately after CSE is induced. Maternal hypotension can occur in the first 5 to 20 minutes after the intrathecal dose and needs immediate treatment with small intravenous increments of ephedrine and fluid boluses. By avoiding intrathecal fentanyl my patients do not complain of pruritus and yet still have satisfactory analgesia with minimal motor block.

ANESTHESIA FOR CESAREAN SECTION
When women with chronic hypertension or superimposed preeclampsia require elective or emergency cesarean section, the previously discussed anesthetic guidelines and techniques for preeclampsia apply. I administer either epidural or spinal anesthesia in patients with moderate elevation of blood pressure. I prefer to avoid spinal anesthesia if the woman has severe uncontrolled hypertension, but in urgent situations, spinal anesthesia is preferable to general anesthesia.

However, general anesthesia may be required if a coagulopathy exists. Women with chronic hypertension more frequently develop placental abruption, with the associated risks of profound fetal distress and maternal DIC. In such situations, general anesthesia is the technique of choice. It is especially important to secure adequate intravenous access before surgery because the risk of perioperative hemorrhage is high. Care is taken to obtund the hypertensive response to tracheal intubation with intravenous agents such as lidocaine, labetalol, and fentanyl.

POSTPARTUM CARE
The risk of postpartum pulmonary edema, encephalopathy, and renal failure is increased in women with target organ involvement, superimposed preeclampsia, and placental abruption. Blood pressure should be closely controlled for at least 48 hours after delivery. In patients with superimposed preeclampsia, postpartum treatment should include administration of magnesium sulfate. After the discontinuation of magnesium sulfate, women with chronic hypertension typically revert to their previous antihypertensive regimens. Patients with pregestational diabetes mellitus and those with cardiomyopathy may need to receive an ACE inhibitor, but these drugs should be avoided if mother is breast-feeding. Mothers who breast-feed are most safely managed with methyldopa or labetalol.[278]

KEY POINTS

- Preeclampsia/eclampsia is a multisystem disorder of unknown etiology that primarily affects nulliparous women. It remains a leading cause of maternal and perinatal morbidity and mortality.
- The pathogenesis of preeclampsia is multifactorial. Multiple clinical subsets of preeclampsia probably exist.
- The vacular endothelial cell appears to be the target of the disease process in preeclampsia, although the exact nature of endothelial cell activation has not been elucidated completely.
- The principal features of preeclampsia include (1) hypertension, associated with a hyperdynamic circulation and/or increased systemic vascular resistance; (2) glomerulopathy, evidenced by proteinuria; and (3) edema, which may manifest as excessive weight gain. Although preeclampsia typically includes edema, most experts agree that it is no longer a diagnostic criterion for the disease.
- Important hematologic changes may occur in patients with preeclampsia, including thrombocytopenia, a hypercoagulable state, and compensated disseminated intravascular coagulation (DIC).
- Efforts to prevent preeclampsia have been unsuccessful. *Neither* low-dose aspirin *nor* supplemental calcium is effective in preventing preeclampsia in patients with either low or high risk for developing the disease. The use of antioxidants to prevent preeclampsia is now undergoing evaluation.
- The cornerstone of obstetric management of preeclampsia is to "stabilize and deliver." This includes intravenous magnesium sulfate for seizure prophylaxis, judicious fluid administration to avoid pulmonary edema, selective use of antihypertensive agents, and timely delivery. Cesarean section should be reserved for obstetric indications.
- Expectant management of early-onset severe preeclampsia is possible but should be undertaken only in tertiary care centers because of the risk of significant maternal and fetal morbidity and the need for close monitoring of both maternal and fetal condition.
- Major complications of severe preeclampsia include severe refractory hypertension, oliguria, HELLP syndrome, placental abruption, cerebral hemorrhage, and pulmonary edema.
- Important elements of preanesthetic consultation and care for patients with severe preeclampsia include (1) seizure prophylaxis, (2) consideration of the patient's hemodynamic status and need for invasive monitoring, (3) restoration of the volume deficit, (4) review of the platelet count (and coagulation studies in selected patients), and (5) exclusion of upper airway or pulmonary edema.

- Epidural analgesia confers significant maternal and fetal benefits during labor in preeclamptic women. The block requires careful titration in those receiving a concurrent infusion of magnesium sulfate.
- Either epidural or spinal anesthesia may be safely administered for elective or emergency cesarean section in most women with mild preeclampsia. However, the safety of spinal anesthesia for women with severe preeclampsia is controversial. The risk of fetal compromise secondary to severe hypotension is the principal concern with spinal anesthesia. General anesthesia carries significant risks in women with severe preeclampsia, but studies have shown that general and regional anesthesia result in similar maternal and neonatal outcomes when careful attention is paid to the technique. Significant coagulation abnormalities occur rarely, even in patients with severe preeclampsia; when present, these abnormalities preclude the administration of regional anesthesia.
- Women with preeclampsia require observation and care in a high-density nursing environment for the first 24 hours postpartum or until there is evidence of diuresis.
- Until proven otherwise, the occurrence of seizures during pregnancy should be considered eclampsia.
- The anesthetic management of patients with eclampsia parallels that of patients with severe preeclampsia, but the possibility of increased intracranial pressure should be excluded, especially in obtunded patients.
- Chronic hypertension more frequently complicates pregnancy in older women. The majority do well during pregnancy, but some experience dangerous exacerbations of their disease. Women with chronic hypertension are at increased risk for superimposed preeclampsia or eclampsia.

REFERENCES

1. American College of Obstetricians and Gynecologists. Diagnosis and Management of Preeclampsia and Eclampsia. ACOG Practice Bulletin No. 33, January 2002 (Obstet Gynecol 2002; 99:159-67).
2. Report on the National High Blood Pressure Education Program Working Group on High Blood Pressure in Pregnancy. Am J Obstet Gynecol 2000; 183: S1-22.
3. Why Mothers Die: Report on Confidential Enquiries into Maternal Deaths in the United Kingdom, 1997-1999. London, RCOG Press, 2001.
4. Saudan P, Brown MA, Buddle ML, Jones M. Does gestational hypertension become preeclampsia? Br J Obstet Gynaecol 1998; 105: 1177-84.
5. American College of Obstetricians and Gynecologists. Chronic Hypertension in Pregnancy. ACOG Practice Bulletin No. 29, July, 2001 (Obstet Gynecol 2001; 98:177-85).
6. Cunningham FG, Gant NF, Leveno KJ, et al. Hypertensive disorders in pregnancy. In: Williams Obstetrics, 21st ed. New York: McGraw-Hill, 2001: 567-618.
7. Saftlas AF, Olson DR, Franks AL, et al. Epidemiology of preeclampsia and eclampsia in the United States, 1979-1986. Am J Obstet Gynecol 1990; 163:460-5.
8. MacKay AP, Berg CJ, Atrash HK. Pregnancy-related mortality from preeclampsia and eclampsia. Obstet Gynecol 2001; 97:533-8.
9. Sibai BM, Gordon T, Thom E, et al. Risk factors for preeclampsia in healthy nulliparous women: A prospective multicenter study. Am J Obstet Gynecol 1995; 172:642-8.

10. Kenny LC, Baker PN. The etiology of preeclampsia. In Belfort MA, Thornton S, Saade G, editors. Hypertension in Pregnancy. New York, Marcel Dekker, 2003: 17-36.

11. Dekker GA. The immunological aspects of preeclampsia: Links with current concepts on etiology and pathogenesis. In Belfort MA, Thornton S, Saade G, editors. Hypertension in Pregnancy. New York, Marcel Dekker, 2003: 37-56.

12. Zhou Y, Damsky CH, Fisher SJ. Preeclampsia is associated with failure of human cytotrophoblasts to mimic vascular adhesion phenotype. J Clin Invest 1997; 99:2152-64.

13. Zuspan FP. New concepts in the understanding of hypertensive diseases during pregnancy: An overview. Clin Perinatol 1991; 18:653-9.

14. Feeney JG, Scott JS. Preeclampsia and changed paternity. Eur J Obstet Gynaecol Reprod Biol 1980; 11:35-8.

15. Klonoff-Cohen HS, Savitz DA, Cefalo RC, McCann MF. An epidemiologic study of contraception and preeclampsia. JAMA 1989; 262:3143-7.

16. Robillard P-Y, Hulsey TC, Perianin J, et al. Association of pregnancy-induced hypertension with duration of sexual cohabitation before conception. Lancet 1994; 344:973-5.

17. Skjaerven R, Wilcox AJ, Lie RT. The interval between pregnancies and the risk of preeclampsia. N Engl J Med 2002; 346: 33-8.

18. Broughton-Pipkin F, Rubin PC. Pre-eclampsia: The 'disease of theories'. Brit Med Bull 1994; 50:381-96.

19. Arngrimsson R, Björnsson S, Geirsson RT, et al. Genetics and familial predisposition to eclampsia and preeclampsia in a defined population. Br J Obstet Gynaecol 1990; 97:762-9.

20. Hayward C, Livingstone J, Holloway S, et al. An exclusion map for preeclampsia: Assuming autosomal recessive inheritance. Am J Hum Genet 1992; 50:749-57.

21. Ward K, Hata A, Jeunemaitre X, et al. A molecular variant of angiotensinogen associated with pre-eclampsia. Nature Genetics 1993; 4:59-61.

22. Morgan L, Crawshaw S, Baker PN, et al. Distortion of maternal-fetal angiotensin II type I receptor allele transmission in preeclampsia. J Med Genet 1998; 35:632-6.

23. Dizon-Townson DS, Nelson LM, Easton K, Ward K. The factor V Leiden mutation may predispose women to severe preeclampsia. Am J Obstet Gynecol 1996; 175:902-5.

24. Lindoff C, Ingemarsson I, Martinsson G, et al. Preeclampsia is associated with a reduced response to activated protein C. Am J Obstet Gynecol 1997; 176:457-60.

25. Benedetto C, Marozio L, Salton L, et al. Factor V Leiden and factor II G20210A in preeclampsia and HELLP syndrome. Acta Obstet Gynecol Scand 2002; 81:1095-100.

26. Heiskanen J, Romppanen EL, Hiltunen M, et al. Polymorphism in the tumor-necrosis factor-α gene in women with preeclampsia. J Assist Reprod Genet 2002; 19:220-3.

27. Redman CWG, Sacks GP, Sargent IL. Preeclampsia: An excessive maternal inflammatory response to pregnancy. Am J Obstet Gynecol 1999; 180:499-506.

28. Dekker GA, Sibai BM. Etiology and pathogenesis of preeclampsia: Current concepts. Am J Obstet Gynecol 1998; 179:1359-75.

29. Wang Y, Walsh SW, Kay HH. Placental lipid peroxides and thromboxane are increased and prostacyclin is decreased in women with preeclampsia. Am J Obstet Gynecol 1992; 167:946-9.

30. Vaughan JE, Walsh SW. Oxidative stress reproduces placental abnormalities of preeclampsia. Hypertens Pregnancy 2002; 21:205-23.

31. Seligman SP, Buyon JP, Clancy RM, et al. The role of nitric oxide in the pathogenesis of preeclampsia. Am J Obstet Gynecol 1994; 171:944-8.

32. Sakawi Y, Tarpey M, Chen YF, et al. Evaluation of low-dose endotoxin administration during pregnancy as a model of preeclampsia. Anesthesiology 2000; 93:1446-55.

33. Slowinski T, Neumayer HH, Stoize T, et al. Endothelin system in normal and hypertensive pregnancy. Clin Sci (London) 2002; 103 Suppl 48: 446S-9S.

34. deJong CL, Dekker GA, Sibai BM. The renin-angiotensin-aldosterone system in preeclampsia: A review. Clin Perinatol 1991; 18:683-711.

35. Weiner C, Liu KZ, Thompson L, et al. Effect of pregnancy on endothelium and smooth muscle: Their role in reduced adrenergic sensitivity. Am J Physiol 1991; 261:H1275-83.

36. Triggle CR, Ding H. Endothelium-derived hyperpolarizing factor: Is there a novel chemical mediator? Clin Exp Pharmacol Physiol 2002; 29:153-60.

37. Kenny LC, Baker PN, Kendall DA, et al. Differential mechanisms of endothelium-dependent vasodilator responses in human myometrial small arteries in normal pregnancy and preeclampsia. Clin Sci (London) 2002; 103:67-73.

38. Redman CW. Platelets and the beginnings of preeclampsia (editorial). N Engl J Med 1990; 323:478-80.

39. Yoneyama Y, Suzuki S, Sawa R, et al. Plasma nitric oxide levels and the expression of P-selectin on platelets in preeclampsia. Am J Obstet Gynecol 2002; 187:676-80.

40. Bolte AC, van Geijn HP, Dekker GA. Pathophysiology of preeclampsia and the role of serotonin. Eur J Obstet Gynecol Biol 2001; 95:12-21.

41. Felfernig-Boehm D, Salat A, Vogl SE, et al. Early detection of preeclampsia by determination of platelet aggregability. Thromb Res 2000; 98:136-46.

42. Kilby MD, Broughton-Pipkin F, Symonds EM. Changes in platelet intracellular free calcium in normal pregnancy. Br J Obstet Gynaecol 1993; 100:375-9.

43. Matteo R, Proverbio T, Córdova K, et al. Preeclampsia, lipid peroxidation, and calcium adenosine triphosphatase activity of red blood cell ghosts. Am J Obstet Gynecol 1998; 178:402-8.

44. Baker PN, Kilby MD, Broughton Pipkin F. The effect of angiotensin II on platelet intracellular free calcium concentrations in human pregnancy. J Hypertens 1992; 10:55-60.

45. Hayman R, Brockelsby J, Kenny L, Baper P. Preeclampsia: The endothelium, circulating factor(s) and vascular endothelial growth factor. J Soc Gynecol Invest 1999; 6:3-10.

46. Scholtes MC, Gerretsen G, Haak HL. The factor VIII ratio in normal and pathological pregnancies. Eur J Obstet Gynecol Reprod Biol 1983; 16:89-95.

47. Sattar N, Gaw A, Packard CJ, Greer IA. Potential pathogenic roles of aberrant lipoprotein and fatty acid metabolism in preeclampsia. Br J Obstet Gynaecol 1996; 103:614-20.

48. Wetzka B, Winkler K, Kinner M, et al. Altered lipid metabolism in preeclampsia and HELLP syndrome: Links to enhanced platelet reactivity and fetal growth. Semin Thromb Hemost 1999; 25:455-62.

49. Roberts JM. Preeclampsia: Is there value in assessing before clinically evident disease? Obstet Gynecol 2001; 98:596-9.

50. Benedetto C, Zonca M, Marozio L, et al. Blood pressure patterns in normal pregnancy and in pregnancy-induced hypertension, preeclampsia, and chronic hypertension. Obstet Gynecol 1996; 88:503-10.

51. Ekholm EMK, Tahvanainen KUO, Metsälä T. Heart rate and blood pressure variabilities are increased in pregnancy-induced hypertension. Am J Obstet Gynecol 1997; 177:1208-12.

52. Moutquin JM, Rainville C, Giroux L, et al. A prospective study of blood pressure in pregnancy: Prediction of preeclampsia. Am J Obstet Gynecol 1985; 151:191-6.

53. Villar MA, Sibai BM. Clinical significance of elevated mean arterial blood pressure in second trimester and threshold increase in systolic or diastolic blood pressure during third trimester. Am J Obstet Gynecol 1989; 160:419-23.

54. Schobel HP, Fischer T, Heuszer K, et al. Preeclampsia: A state of sympathetic overactivity. N Engl J Med 1996; 335:1480-5.

55. Silver HM, Seebeck M, Carlson R. Comparison of total blood volume in normal, preeclamptic, and nonproteinuric gestational hypertensive pregnancy by simultaneous measurement of red blood cell and plasma volumes. Am J Obstet Gynecol 1998; 179:87-93.

56. Mabie WC, Ratts TE, Sibai BM. The central hemodynamics of severe preeclampsia. Am J Obstet Gynecol 1989; 161:1443-8.

57. Pouta A, Karinen J, Vuolteenaho O, Laatikainen T. Preeclampsia: The effect of intravenous fluid preload on atrial natriuretic peptide secretion during caesarean section under spinal anaesthesia. Acta Anaesthesiol Scand 1996; 40:1203-9.

58. Easterling TR. The maternal hemodynamics of preeclampsia. Clin Obstet Gynecol 1992; 35:375-86.

59. Easterling TR, Watts DH, Schmucker BC, Benedetti TJ. Measurement of cardiac output during pregnancy: Validation of doppler technique and clinical observations in preeclampsia. Obstet Gynecol 1987; 69:845-50.

60. Easterling TR, Benedetti TJ, Schmucker BC, Millard SP. Maternal hemodynamics in normal and preeclamptic pregnancies: A longitudinal study. Obstet Gynecol 1990; 76:1061-9.

61. Bosio PM, McKenna PJ, Conroy R, O'Herlihy C. Maternal central hemodynamics in hypertensive disorders of pregnancy. Obstet Gynecol 1999; 94:978-84.

62. Cotton DB, Lee W, Huhta JC, Dorman KF. Hemodynamic profile of severe pregnancy-induced hypertension. Am J Obstet Gynecol 1988; 158:523-9.

63. Bolte AC, Dekker GA, van Eyck J, van Schijndel RS, van Geijn HP. Lack of agreement between central venous pressure and pulmonary capillary wedge pressure in preeclampsia. Hypertens Pregnancy 2000; 19:261-71.

64. Newsome LR, Bramwell RS, Curling PE. Severe preeclampsia: Hemodynamic effects of lumbar epidural anesthesia. Anesth Analg 1986; 65:31-6.

65. Zinaman M, Rubin J, Lindheimer MD. Serial plasma oncotic pressure levels and echoencephalography during and after delivery in severe preeclampsia. Lancet 1985; 1:1245-50.

66. Benedetti TJ, Kates R, Williams V. Hemodynamic observations in severe preeclampsia complicated by pulmonary edema. Am J Obstet Gynecol 1985; 152:330-4.

67. Perry KG, Martin JN. Abnormal hemostasis and coagulopathy in preeclampsia and eclampsia. Clin Obstet Gynecol 1992; 35:338-50.

68. Grisaru D, Zwang E, Peyser MR, et al. The procoagulant activity of red blood cells from patients with severe preeclampsia. Am J Obstet Gynecol 1997; 177:1513-6.

69. Trofatter KF, Howell ML, Greenberg CS, Hage ML. Use of the fibrin D-dimer in screening for coagulation abnormalities in preeclampsia. Obstet Gynecol 1989; 73:435-40.

70. Thornton CA, Bonnar J. Factor VIII-related antigen and factor VIII coagulant activity in normal and preeclamptic pregnancy. Br J Obstet Gynaecol 1977; 84: 919-23.

71. Weiner CP, Brandt J. Plasma antithrombin III activity: An aid in the diagnosis of preeclampsia-eclampsia. Am J Obstet Gynecol 1982; 142:275-81.

72. deBoer K, ten Cate JW, Sturk A, et al. Enhanced thrombin generation in normal and hypertensive pregnancy. Am J Obstet Gynecol 1989; 160: 95-100.

73. Jackson UC, Fox HE, Owen J, Friedman KD. The administration of antithrombin III in the management of severe preeclampsia: A pilot study. J Mat Fetal Med 1992; 1:308-12.

74. Wang J, Mimuro S, Lahoud R, et al. Elevated levels of lipoprotein(a) in women with preeclampsia. Am J Obstet Gynecol 1998; 178:146-9.

75. Saino S, Kekomaki R. Riikonen S, Trramo K. Maternal thrombocytopenia at term: A population-based study. Acta Obstet Gynecol Scand 2000; 79:744-9.

76. Leduc L, Wheeler JM, Kirshon B, et al. Coagulation profile in severe preeclampsia. Obstet Gynecol 1992; 79:14-8.

77. McDonagh RJ, Ray JG, Burrows RF, et al. Platelet count may predict abnormal bleeding time among pregnant women with hypertension and preeclampsia. Can J Anesth 2001; 48:563-9.

78. Samama CM, Simon L. Detecting coagulation disorders of pregnancy: Bleeding time or platelet count? Can J Anesth 2001; 48:515-8.

79. Channing-Rodgers RP, Levin J. A critical reappraisal of the bleeding time. Semin Thromb Hemost 1990; 16:1-30.

80. Burrows RF, Hunter DJ, Andrew M, Kelton JG. A prospective study investigating the mechanism of thrombocytopenia in preeclampsia. Obstet Gynecol 1987; 70:334-8.

81. Samuels P, Main EK, Tomaski A, et al. Abnormalities in platelet antiglobulin tests in preeclamptic mothers and their neonates. Am J Obstet Gynecol 1987; 157:109-13.

82. Inglis TC, Stuart J, George AJ, Davies AJ. Haemostatic and rheological changes in normal pregnancy and preeclampsia. Br J Haematol 1982; 50:461-5.

83. Weiner CP. The clinical spectrum of preeclampsia. Am J Kidney Dis 1987; 9:312-6.

84. Many A, Hubel CA, Roberts JM. Hyperuricemia and xanthine oxidase in preeclampsia, revisited. Am J Obstet Gynecol 1996; 174:288-91.

85. Williams KP, Galerneau F. The role of serum uric acid as a prognostic indicator of the severity of maternal and fetal complications in hypertensive pregnancies. J Obstet Gynecol Can 2002; 24:628-32.

86. Hubel CA, Roberts JM, Taylor RN, et al. Lipid peroxidation in pregnancy: New perspectives on preeclampsia. Am J Obstet Gynecol 1989; 161:1025.34

87. Broughton-Pipkin F. Hypertension in pregnancy: Physiology or pathology? In Jones CT, Nathanielsz PW, editors. The Physiological Development of the Fetus and the Newborn. London, Academic Press, 1985:699-709.

88. Heller PJ, Scheider EP, Marx GF. Pharyngolaryngeal edema as a presenting symptom in preeclampsia. Obstet Gynecol 1983; 62:523-5.

89. Sibai BM, Mabie BC, Harvey CJ, Gonzalez AR. Pulmonary edema in severe preeclampsia-eclampsia: Analysis of 37 consecutive cases. Am J Obstet Gynecol 1987; 156:1174-9.

90. Sciscione AC, Ivester T, Largoza M, et al. Acute pulmonary edema in pregnancy. Obstet Gynecol 2003; 101:511-5.

91. Manas KG, Welsh JD, Rankin RA, Miller DD. Hepatic hemorrhage without rupture in preeclampsia. N Engl J Med 1985; 312:424-6.

92. Richards A, Graham D, Bullock R. Clinicopathological study of neurological complications due to hypertensive disorders of pregnancy. J Neurol Neurosurg Psychiatr 1988; 51:416-21.

93. Lewis LK, Hinshaw DB, Will AD, et al. CT and angiographic correlation of severe neurological disease in toxemia of pregnancy. Neuroradiol 1988; 30:59-64.

94. Kaar K, Jouppila P, Kuikka J, et al. Intervillous blood flow in normal and complicated late pregnancy by means of an intravenous ^{133}Xe method. Acta Obstet Gynecol Scand 1980; 59:7-10.

95. Trudinger BJ, Cook CM. Doppler umbilical and uterine flow waveforms in severe pregnancy hypertension. Br J Obstet Gynaecol 1990; 97:142-8.

96. Dekker GA, Sibai BM. Low-dose aspirin in the prevention of preeclampsia and fetal growth retardation: Rationale, mechanisms, and clinical trials. Am J Obstet Gynecol 1993; 168:214-27.

97. Hauth JC, Goldenberg RL, Parker R, et al. Low-dose aspirin therapy to prevent preeclampsia. Am J Obstet Gynecol 1993; 168:1083-93.

98. Broughton-Pipkin F, Crowther C, DeSwiet M, et al. Where next for prophylaxis against preeclampsia? Report of a workshop. Br J Obstet Gynaecol 1996; 103:603-7.

99. Caritis S, Sibai B, Hauth J, et al. Low-dose aspirin to prevent preeclampsia in women at high risk. N Engl J Med 1998; 338:701-5.

100. Sibai BM, Caritis SN, Thom E, et al. Prevention of preeclampsia with low-dose aspirin in healthy nulliparous pregnant women. N Engl J Med 1993; 329:1213-8.

101. Heybourne KD. Preeclampsia prevention: Lessons from the low-dose aspirin therapy trials. Am J Obstet Gynecol 2000; 183:523-8.

102. Coomarasamy A, Honest H, Papaioannou S, et al. Aspirin for prevention of preeclampsia in women with historical risk factors: A systematic review. Obstet Gynecol 2003; 101:1319-32.

103. Coomarasamy A, Papaioannou S, Gee H, Khan KS. Aspirin for the prevention of preeclampsia in women with abnormal uterine artery Doppler: A meta-analysis. Obstet Gynecol 2001; 98:861-6.

104. Bucher HC, Guyatt GH, Cook RJ, et al. Effect of calcium supplementation on pregnancy-induced hypertension and preeclampsia: A meta-analysis of randomized controlled trials. JAMA 1996; 275:1113-7.

105. Levine RJ, Hauth JC, Curet LB, et al. Trial of calcium to prevent preeclampsia. N Engl J Med 1997; 337:69-76.

106. Vaughan JE, Walsh SW. Oxidative stress reproduces placental abnormalities of preeclampsia. Hypertens Pregnancy 2002; 21:205-23.

107. Chappell LC, Seed PT, Briley AL, et al. Effect of antioxidants on the occurrence of preeclampsia in women at increased risk: A randomized trial. Lancet 1999; 354:810-6.

108. Sibai BM. Pitfalls in diagnosis and management of preeclampsia. Am J Obstet Gynecol 1988; 159:1-5.

109. Dekker GA, de Vries JIP, Doelitzsch PM, et al. Underlying disorders associated with severe early-onset preeclampsia. Am J Obstet Gynecol 1995; 173:1042-8.

110. Hasan MA, Thomas TA, Prys-Roberts C. Comparison of automatic oscillometric arterial pressure measurement with conventional auscultatory measurement in the labour ward. Br J Anaesth 1993; 70:141-4.

111. Sibai BM, Ewell M, Levine RJ, et al. Risk factors associated with preeclampsia in healthy nulliparous women. Am J Obstet Gynecol 1997; 177:1003-10.

112. Ananth CV, Bowes WA, Savitz DA, Luther ER. Relationship between pregnancy-induced hypertension and placenta previa: A population-based study. Am J Obstet Gynecol 1997; 177:997-1002.

113. Cobo E, Canaval H, Fonseca J. Severe preeclampsia and postpartum eclampsia associated with placenta previa and cesarean hysterectomy: A case report. Am J Perinatol 1994; 11:288-9.

114. Lewis R, Sibai B. Recent advances in the management of preeclampsia. J Mat Fetal Med 1997; 6:6-15.

115. Sibai BM. Treatment of hypertension in pregnant women. N Engl J Med 1996; 335:257-65.

116. Sibai BM, Mercer BM, Schiff E, Friedman SA. Aggressive versus expectant management of severe preeclampsia at 28-32 weeks' gestation: A randomized controlled trial. Am J Obstet Gynecol 1994; 171: 818-22.

117. Schiff E, Friedman SA, Sibai BM. Conservative management of severe preeclampsia remote from term. Obstet Gynecol 1994; 84:626-30.

118. Romero R, Vizoso J, Emamian M, et al. Clinical significance of liver dysfunction in pregnancy-induced hypertension. Am J Perinatol 1988; 5:146-51.

119. Dildy GA, Cotton DB. Management of severe preeclampsia and eclampsia. Crit Care Clin 1991; 7:829-50.

120. Jones MM, Longmire S, Cotton DB, et al. Influence of crystalloid versus colloid infusion on peripartum colloid osmotic pressure changes. Obstet Gynecol 1986; 68:659-61.

121. Kirshon B, Moise KJ, Cotton DB, et al. Role of volume expansion in severe preeclampsia. Surg Gynecol Obstet 1988; 167:367-71.

122. The Magpie Trial Collaborative Group. Do women with preeclampsia, and their babies, benefit from magnesium sulphate? The Magpie Trial: A randomized placebo-controlled trial. Lancet 2002; 359:1877-91.

123. Yentis SM. The Magpie has landed: Preeclampsia, magnesium sulphate and rational decisions (editorial). Internat J Obstet Anesth 2002; 11: 238-41.

124. Lucas MJ, Leveno KJ, Cunningham FG. A comparison of magnesium sulfate with phenytoin for the prevention of eclampsia. N Engl J Med 1995; 333:201-5.

125. Eclampsia Trial Collaborative Group. Which anticonvulsant for women with eclampsia? Evidence from the collaborative eclampsia trial. Lancet 1995; 345:1455-63.

126. Livingstone JC, Livingstone LW, Ramsey R, et al. Magnesium sulfate in women with mild preeclampsia: A randomized controlled trial. Obstet Gynecol 2003; 101:217-20.

127. Scott JR. Magnesium sulfate for mild preeclampsia (editorial). Obstet Gynecol 2003; 101-213.

128. James MFM. Magnesium in obstetric anesthesia. Internat J Obstet Anesth 1998; 7:115-23.

129. Cotton DB, Hallak M, Janusz C, et al. Central anticonvulsant effects of magnesium sulfate on N-methyl-D-aspartate-induced seizures. Am J Obstet Gynecol 1993; 168:974-8.

130. Belfort MA, Anthony J, Saade GA, Allen JC. A comparison of magnesium sulfate and nimodipine for the prevention of eclampsia. N Engl J Med 2003; 348:304-11.

131. Sibai BM, Ramanathan J. The case for magnesium sulfate in preeclampsia-eclampsia. Internat J Obstet Anesth 1992; 1:167-75.

132. Donaldson JO. The case against magnesium sulfate for eclamptic convulsions. Internat J Obstet Anesth 1992; 1:159-66.

133. Witlin AG, Sibai BM. Magnesium sulfate therapy in preeclampsia and eclampsia. Obstet Gynecol 1998; 92:883-9.

134. Scardo JA, Hogg BB, Newman RB. Favorable hemodynamic effects of magnesium sulfate in preeclampsia. Am J Obstet Gynecol 1995; 173:1249-53.

135. Walsh SW, Romney AD, Wang Y, Walsh MD. Magnesium sulfate attenuates peroxide-induced vasoconstriction in the human placenta. Am J Obstet Gynecol 1998; 178:7-12.

136. Belfort MA, Saade GR, Moise KJ. The effect of magnesium sulfate on maternal and fetal blood flow in pregnancy-induced hypertension. Acta Obstet Gynecol Scand 1993; 72:526-30.

137. Greene MF. Magnesium sulfate for preeclampsia. N Engl J Med 2003; 348:275-6.

138. Atkinson MW, Guinn D, Owen J, Hauth JC. Does magnesium sulfate affect the length of labor induction in women with pregnancy-associated hypertension? Am J Obstet Gynecol 1995; 173:1219-22.

139. Witlin AG, Friedman SA, Sibai BM. The effect of magnesium sulfate therapy on the duration of labor in women with mild preeclampsia at term: A randomized, double-blind, placebo-controlled trial. Am J Obstet Gynecol 1997; 176:623-7.

140. Montan S, Anandakumar C, Arulkumaran S, et al. Effects of methyldopa on uteroplacental and fetal hemodynamics in pregnancy-induced hypertension. Am J Obstet Gynecol 1993; 168:152-6.

141. Lopez-Jaramillo P, Narvaez M, Calle A, et al. Cyclic guanosine 3`,5` monophosphate concentrations in preeclampsia: Effects of hydralazine. Br J Obstet Gynaecol 1996; 103:33-8.

142. Paterson-Brown S, Robson SC, Redfern N, et al. Hydralazine boluses for the treatment of severe hypertension in preeclampsia. Br J Obstet Gynaecol 1994; 101:409-13.

143. Duley L. Hydralazine boluses (letter). Br J Obstet Gynaecol 1995; 102:83.

144. Gudmundsson S, Gennser G, Marsal K. Effects of hydralazine on placental and renal circulation in preeclampsia. Acta Obstet Gynecol Scand 1995; 74:415-8.

145. Hoffman BB. Adrenoceptor-blocking drugs. In Katzung BG, editor. Basic and Clinical Pharmacology, 6th ed. Norwalk, Conn, Appleton & Lange, 1995:132-46.

146. Morgan MA, Silavin SL, Dormer KJ, et al. Effects of labetalol on uterine blood flow and cardiovascular hemodynamics in hypertensive gravid baboon. Am J Obstet Gynecol 1993; 168:1574-9.

147. Rodgers RC, Sibai BM, Whybrew WD. Labetalol pharmacokinetics in pregnancy-induced hypertension. Am J Obstet Gynecol 1990; 162:362-6.

148. Mabie WC, Gonzalez AR, Sibai BM, Amon E. A comparative trial of labetalol and hydralazine in the acute management of severe hypertension complicating pregnancy. Obstet Gynecol 1987; 70:328-33.

149. Klarr JM, Bhatt-Mehta V, Donn SM. Neonatal adrenergic blockade following single dose maternal labetalol administration. Am J Perinatol 1994; 11:91-3.

150. Hjertberg R, Faxelius G, Lagercrantz H. Neonatal adaptation in hypertensive pregnancy: A study of labetalol versus hydralazine treatment. J Perinat Med 1993; 21:69-75.

151. Grunewald C, Kublickas M, Carlstrom K, et al. Effects of nitroglycerin on the uterine and umbilical circulation in severe preeclampsia. Obstet Gynecol 1995; 86:600-4.

152. Cotton DB, Longmire S, Jones MM, et al. Cardiovascular alterations in severe pregnancy-induced hypertension: Effects of intravenous nitroglycerin coupled with blood volume expansion. Am J Obstet Gynecol 1986; 154:1053-9.

153. Naulty J, Cefalo RC, Lewis PE. Fetal toxicity of nitroprusside in the pregnant ewe. Am J Obstet Gynecol 1981; 139:708-11.

154. Curry SC, Carlton MW, Raschke RA. Prevention of fetal and maternal cyanide toxicity from nitroprusside with coinfusion of sodium thiosulfate in gravid ewes. Anesth Analg 1997; 84:1121-6.

155. Vermillion ST, Scardo JA, Newman RB, Chauhan SP. A randomized, double-blind trial of oral nifedipine and intravenous labetalol in hypertensive emergncies of pregnancy. Am J Obstet Gynecol 1999; 181: 858-61.

156. Scardo JA, Vermillion ST, Newman RB, et al. A randomized, double-blind hemodynamic evaluation of nifedipine and labetalol in preeclamptic hypertensive emergencies. Am J Obstet Gynecol 1999; 181:862-6.

157. Waisman GD, Mayorga LM, Camera MI, et al. Magnesium plus nifedipine: Potentiation of hypotensive effect in preeclampsia? Am J Obstet Gynecol 1988; 159:308-9.

158. Impey L. Severe hypotension and fetal distress following sublingual administration of nifedipine to a patient with severe pregnancy induced hypertension at 33 weeks. Br J Obstet Gynaecol 1993; 100:959-61.

159. Kumar N, Batra YK, Bala I, Gopalan S. Nifedipine attenuates the hypertensive response to tracheal intubation in pregnancy-induced hypertension. Can J Anaesth 1993; 40:329-33.

160. Bansal S, Pawar M. Hemodynamic responses to laryngoscopy and intubation in patients with pregnancy-induced hypertension: Effect of intravenous esmolol with or without lidocaine. Internat J Obstet Anesth 2002; 11:4-8.

161. Wasserstrum N. Nitroprusside in preeclampsia: Circulatory distress and paradoxical bradycardia. Hypertension 1991; 18:79-84.

162. Ramanathan J, Sibai BM, Mabie WC, et al. The use of labetalol for attenuation of the hypertensive response to endotracheal intubation in preeclampsia. Am J Obstet Gynecol 1988; 159:650-4.

163. Skovgaard Olsen K, Beier-Holgersen R. Hemodynamic collapse following labetalol administration in preeclampsia. Acta Obstet Gynecol Scand 1992; 71:151-2.

164. Skovgaard Olsen K, Beier-Holgersen R. Fetal death following labetalol administration in preeclampsia. Acta Obstet Gynecol Scand 1992; 71:145-7.

165. Fenakel K, Fenakel G, Appleman Z, et al. Nifedipine in the treatment of severe preeclampsia. Obstet Gynecol 1991; 77:331-7.

166. Scardo JA, Vermillion ST, Hogg BB, Newman RB. Hemodynamic effects of oral nifedipine in preeclamptic hypertensive emergencies. Am J Obstet Gynecol 1996; 175:336-40.

167. Blea CW, Barnard JM, Magness RR, et al. Effect of nifedipine on fetal and maternal hemodynamics and blood gases in the pregnant ewe. Am J Obstet Gynecol 1997; 176:922-30.

168. Magee LA, Cham C, Waterman EJ, et al. Hydralazine for treatment of severe hypertension in pregnancy: Meta-analysis. Br Med J 2003; 327: 955-60.

169. Singri N, Ahya SN, Levin ML. Acute renal failure. JAMA 2003; 289: 747-51.

170. Drakeley AJ, LeRoux PA, Anthony J, Penny J. Acute renal failure complicating severe preeclampsia requiring admission to an obstetric intensive care unit. Am J Obstet Gynecol 2002; 186:253-6.

171. Clark S, Greenspoon J, Aldahl D, et al. Severe preeclampsia with persistent oliguria: Management of hemodynamic states. Am J Obstet Gynecol 1986; 154:490-4.

172. Kirshon B, Lee W, Mauer M, et al. Effects of low-dose dopamine therapy in the oliguric patient with preeclampsia. Am J Obstet Gynecol 1988; 159:604-7.

173. Gilbert WM, Towner DR, Field NT, Anthony J. The safety and utility of pulmonary artery catheterization in severe preeclampsia and eclampsia. Am J Obstet Gynecol 2000; 182:1379-403.

174. Martin JN, Rinehart BK, May WL, et al. The spectrum of severe preeclampsia: Comparative analysis by HELLP (hemolysis, elevated liver enzymes, and low platelets) syndrome classification. Am J Obstet Gynecol 1999; 180:1373-84.

175. Sibai BM. The HELLP syndrome (hemolysis, elevated liver enzymes, and low platelets): Much ado about nothing? Am J Obstet Gynecol 1990; 162:311-6.

176. Audibert F, Friedman SA, Frangieh AY, Sibai BM. Clinical utility of strict diagnostic criteria for the HELLP (hemolysis, elevated liver enzymes, and low platelets) syndrome. Am J Obstet Gynecol 1996; 175:460-4.

177. Isler CM, Rinehart BK, Terrone DA, et al. Maternal mortality associated with HELLP (hemolysis, elevated liver enzymes, and low platelets) syndrome. Am J Obstet Gynecol 1999; 181:924-8.

178. Roberts WE, Perry KG, Woods JB, et al. The intrapartum platelet count in patients with HELLP (hemolysis, elevated liver enzymes, and low platelets) syndrome: Is it predictive of later hemorrhagic complications? Am J Obstet Gynecol 1994; 171:799-804.

179. Douglas MJ. Platelets, the parturient and regional anesthesia. Internat J Obstet Anesth 2001; 10:113-20.

180. Sibai BM, Ramadan MK, Chari RS, et al. Pregnancies complicated by HELLP syndrome (hemolysis, elevated liver enzymes, and low platelets): Subsequent pregnancy outcome and long-term prognosis. Am J Obstet Gynecol 1995; 172:125-9.

181. Magann EF, Martin JN. Critical care of HELLP syndrome with corticosteroids. Am J Perinatol 2000; 17:417-22.

182. deBoer K, Buller HR, ten Cate JW, Treffers PE. Coagulation studies in the syndrome of hemolysis, elevated liver enzymes and low platelets. Br J Obstet Gynaecol 1991; 98:42-7.

183. Haddad B, Barton JC, Livingstone R, et al. Risk factors for adverse maternal outcomes among women with HELLP (hemolysis, elevated liver enzymes, and low platelet count) syndrome. Am J Obstet Gynecol 2000; 183:444-8.

184. Barton JR, Sibai BM. Hepatic imaging in HELLP syndrome (hemolysis, elevated liver enzymes, and low platelet count). Am J Obstet Gynecol 1996; 174:1820-5.

185. O'Brien JM, Shumate SA, Satchwell SL, et al. Maternal benefit of corticosteroid therapy in patients with HELLP (hemolysis, elevated liver enzymes, and low platelet count) syndrome: Impact on the rate of regional anesthesia. Am J Obstet Gynecol 2002;186:475-9.

186. Fox DB, Troiano NH, Graves CR. Use of the pulmonary artery catheter in severe preeclampsia: A review. Obstet Gynecol Surv 1996; 51:684-95.

187. Mabie WC, Hackmann BB, Sibai BM. Pulmonary edema associated with pregnancy: Echocardiographic insights and implications for treatment. Obstet Gynecol 1993; 81:227-34.

188. Desai DK, Moodley J, Naidoo DP, Bhorat I. Cardiac abnormalities in pulmonary oedema associated with hypertensive crisis in pregnancy. Br J Obstet Gynaecol 1996; 103:523-8.

189. Catanzarite VA, Willms D. Adult respiratory distress syndrome in pregnancy and the puerperium: Causes, courses and outcomes. Obstet Gynecol 2001; 97:760-4.

190. Andrews WW, Cox SM, Sherman ML, Leveno KJ. Maternal and perinatal effects of hypertension at term. J Reprod Med 1992:37:73-6.

191. Wilson BJ, Watson MS, Prescott GJ, et al. Hypertensive diseases of pregnancy and risk of hypertension and stroke in later life: Results from cohort study. BMJ 2003; 326:845.

192. Benedetti TJ, Quilligan EJ. Cerebral edema in severe pregnancy-induced hypertension. Am J Obstet Gynecol 1980; 137:860-2.

193. Belfort MA, Saade GR, Wasserstrum N, et al. Acute volume expansion with colloid increases oxygen delivery and consumption but does not improve oxygen extraction in severe preeclampsia. J Mat Fetal Med 1995; 4:57-64.

194. Grunewald C, Nisell H, Carlstrom K, et al. Acute volume expansion in normal pregnancy and preeclampsia. Effects on plasma atrial natriuretic (ANP) and cyclic guanosine monophosphate (cGMP) concentrations and feto-maternal circulation. Acta Obstet Gynecol Scand 1994; 73:294-9.

195. Quinn M. Automated blood pressure measurement devices: A potential source of morbidity in preeclampsia? Am J Obstet Gynecol 1994; 170:1303-7.

196. Leibowitz AB, Beilin Y. Pulmonary artery catheters and outcome in the perioperative period. New Horizons, 1997; 5:214-21.

197. Wulf H. Epidural anaesthesia and spinal haematoma. Can J Anaesth 1996; 43: 1260-71.

198. Loo CC, Dahlgren G, Irestedt L. Neurological complications in obstetric regional anaesthesia. Internat J Obstet Gynecol 2000; 9:99-124.

199. Yuen TST, Kua JSW, Tan IKS. Spinal hematoma following epidural anaesthesia in a patient with eclampsia. Anaesthesia 1999; 54:350-4.

200. Letsky EA. Disseminated intravascular coagulation. Best Pract Res Clin Obstet Gynecol 2001; 15:623-44.

201. Prieto JA, Mastrobattista JM, Blanco JD. Coagulation studies in patients with marked thrombocytopenia due to severe preeclampsia. Am J Perinatol 1995; 12:220-2.

202. Sharma SK, Philip J, Wiley J. Thromboelastic changes in healthy parturients and postpartum women. Anesth Analg 1997; 85:94-8.

203. Wong CA, Liu S, Glassenberg R. Comparison of thromboelastography with common coagulation tests in preeclamptic and healthy parturients. Reg Anesth 1995; 20:521-7.

204. Orlikowski CEP, Rocke DA, Murray WB, et al. Thromboelastography changes in preeclampsia and eclampsia. Br J Anaesth 1996; 77:157-61.

205. Sharma SK, Philip J, Whitten CW, et al. Assessment of changes in coagulation in parturients with preeclampsia using thromboelastography. Anesthesiology 1999; 90:385-90.

206. Marietta M, Castelli I, Piccinini F, et al. The PFA-100 system for the assessment of platelet function in normotensive and hypertensive pregnancies. Clin Lab Haematol 2001; 23:131-4.

207. Vincelot A, Nathan N, Collet D, et al. Platelet function during pregnancy: An evaluation using the PFA100 analyser. Br J Anaesth 2001; 87:890-3.

208. Brimacombe J. Acute pharyngolaryngeal oedema and preeclamptic toxaemia. Anaesth Intens Care 1992; 20:97-8.

209. Rocke DA, Scoones GP. Rapidly progressive laryngeal oedema associated with pregnancy-aggravated hypertension. Anaesthesia 1992; 47: 141-3.

210. Rinehart BK, Terron DA, Magann EF, et al. Preeclampsia-associated hepatic haemorrhage and rupture: Mode of management related to maternal and perinatal outcome. Obstet Gynecol Surv 1999; 54: 196-202.

211. Vincent RD, Chestnut DH, Sipes SL, et al. Magnesium sulfate decreases maternal blood pressure but not uterine blood flow during epidural anesthesia in gravid ewes. Anesthesiology 1991; 74:77-82.

212. Chestnut DH, Thompson CS, McLaughlin GL, Weiner CP. Does the intravenous infusion of ritodrine or magnesium sulfate alter the hemodynamic response to hemorrhage in gravid ewes? Am J Obstet Gynecol 1988; 159:1467-73.

213. Sipes SL, Chestnut DH, Vincent RD, et al. Does magnesium sulfate alter the maternal cardiovascular response to vasopressor agents in gravid ewes? Anesthesiology 1991; 75:1010-8.

214. Sipes SL, Chestnut DH, Vincent RD, et al. Which vasopressor should be used to treat hypotension during magnesium sulfate infusion and epidural anesthesia? Anesthesiology 1992; 77:101-8.

215. Reynolds JD, Chestnut DH, Dexter F, et al. Magnesium sulfate adversely affects fetal lamb survival and blocks fetal cerebral blood flow response during maternal hemorrhage. Anesth Analg 1996; 83:493-9.

216. Scudiero R, Khoshnood B, Pryde PG, et al. Perinatal death and tocolytic magnesium sulfate. Obstet Gynecol 2000; 96:178-82.

217. Elimian A, Verma R, Ogburn P, et al. Magnesium sulfate and neonatal outcomes in preterm neonates. J Matern Fetal Neonatal Med 2002; 12:118-22.

218. Hallak M, Martinez-Poyer J, Kruger ML, et al. The effect of magnesium sulfate on fetal heart rate parameters: A randomized, placebo-controlled trial. Am J Obstet Gynecol 1999; 181:1122-7.

219. Kussmann B, Shorten G, Uppington J, Comunale ME. Administration of magnesium sulphate before rocuronium: Effects on speed of onset and duration of neuromuscular block. Br J Anaesth 1997; 79:122-4.

220. Hodgson RE, Rout CC, Rocke DA, Louw NJ. Mivacurium for caesarean section in hypertensive parturients receiving magnesium sulphate therapy. Internat J Obstet Anesth 1998; 7:12-7.

221. Kambam JR, Perry SM, Entman S, Smith BE. Effect of magnesium on plasma cholinesterase activity. Am J Obstet Gynecol 1988; 159:309-11.

222. Kynczl-Leisure M, Cibils LA. Increased bleeding time after magnesium sulfate infusion. Am J Obstet Gynecol 1996; 175:1293-4.

223. Ravn HB, Vissinger H, Kristensen SD, et al. Magnesium inhibits platelet activity: An infusion study in healthy volunteers. Thromb Haemost 1996; 75:939-44.

224. Harnett MJP, Datta S, Bhavani-Shankar K. The effect of magnesium on coagulation in parturients with preeclampsia. Internat J Obstet Anesth 2001; 92:1257-60.

225. Seong-Hoon K, Lim H-R, Kim D-C, et al. Magnesium sulfate does not reduce postoperative analgesic requirements. Anesthesiology 2001; 95:640-6.

226. Ramanathan J, Coleman P, Sibai B. Anesthetic modification of hemodynamic and neuroendocrine stress responses to cesarean delivery in women with severe preeclampsia. Anesth Analg 1991; 73:772-9.

227. Jouppila P, Jouppila R, Hollmen A, Koivula A. Lumbar epidural analgesia to improve intervillous blood flow during labor in severe preeclampsia. Obstet Gynecol 1982; 59:158-61.

228. Lucas MJ, Sharma SK, McIntire DD, et al. A randomized trial of labor analgesia in women with pregnancy-induced hypertension. Am J Obstet Gynecol 2001; 185:970-5.

229. Hogg B, Haugh JC, Caritis SN, et al. Safety of labor epidural anesthesia for women with severe hypertensive disease. Am J Obstet Gynecol 1999; 181:1096-1101.

230. Head BB, Owen J, Vincent RD, et al. A randomized trial of intrapartum analgesia in women with severe preeclampsia. Obstet Gynecol 2002; 99:452-7.

231. Ramanathan J, Vaddadi AK, Arheart KL. Combined spinal and epidural anesthesia with low doses of intrathecal bupivacaine in women with

severe preeclampsia: A preliminary report. Reg Anesth Pain Med 2001; 26:46-51.

232. Kanayama N, Belayet HM, Khatun S, et al. A new treatment of severe preeclampsia by long-term epidural anesthesia. J Human Hypertens 1999; 13:167-71.

233. Lysak SZ, Eisenach JC, Dobson CE. Patient-controlled epidural analgesia during labor: A comparison of three solutions with a continuous infusion control. Anesthesiology 1990; 72:44-9.

234. Marx GF, Elstein ID, Schuss M, et al. Effects of epidural block with lignocaine and lignocaine-adrenaline on umbilical artery velocity wave ratios. Br J Obstet Gynaecol 1990; 97:517-20.

235. Alahuta S, Rasanen J, Jouppila P, Jouppila R, Hollmen AI. Uteroplacental and fetal circulation during extradural bupivacaine-adrenaline and bupivacaine for caesarean section in hypertensive pregnancies with chronic fetal asphyxia. Br J Anaesth 1993; 71:348-53.

236. Heller PJ, Goodman C. Use of local anesthetics with epinephrine for epidural anesthesia in preeclampsia. Anesthesiology 1986; 65:224-6.

237. Dror A, Abboud TK, Moore J, et al. Maternal hemodynamic responses to epinephrine-containing local anesthetics in mild preeclampsia. Reg Anesth 1988; 13:107-11.

238. Hadzic A, Vloka J, Patel N, Birnbach D. Hypertensive crisis after a successful placement of an epidural anesthetic in a hypertensive parturient. Case report. Reg Anesth 1995; 20:156-8.

239. Prieto JA, Mastrobattista JM, Blanco JD. Coagulation studies in patients with marked thrombocytopenia due to severe preeclampsia. Am J Perinatol 1995; 12:220-2.

240. Crosby ET. Obstetrical anaesthesia for patients with the syndrome of haemolysis, elevated liver enzymes and low platelets. Can J Anaesth 1991; 38:227-33.

241. Hodgkinson R, Husain FJ, Hayashi RH. Systemic and pulmonary blood pressure during caesarean section in parturients with gestational hypertension. Can Anaesth Soc J 1980; 27:389-94.

242. Wallace DH, Leveno KJ, Cunningham FG, et al. Randomized comparison of general and regional anesthesia for cesarean delivery in pregnancies complicated by severe preeclampsia. Obstet Gynecol 1995; 86:193-9.

243. Jouppila P, Kuikka J, Jouppila R, Hollmen A. Effect of induction of general anesthesia for cesarean section on intervillous blood flow. Acta Obstet Gynecol Scand 1979; 58:249-53.

244. Santos AC. Spinal anesthesia in severely preeclamptic women. When is it safe? (editorial) Anesthesiology 1999; 90:1252-4.

245. Malinow AM. Spinal anesthesia in preeclamptic patients: Supportive evidence (letter). Anesthesiology 2000; 92:622.

246. Howell P. Spinal anesthesia in severe preeclampsia: Time for reappraisal, or time for caution? (editorial) Internat J Obstet Anesth 1998; 7:217-9.

247. Hood DD, Curry R. Spinal versus epidural anesthesia for cesarean section in severely preeclamptic patients: A retrospective survey. Anesthesiology 1999; 90:1276-82.

248. Aya AGM, Mangin R, Vialles N, et al. Patients with severe preeclampsia experience less hypotension during spinal anesthesia for elective cesarean delivery than healthy parturients: A prospective cohort comparison. Anesth Analg 2003; 97:867-72.

249. Karinen J, Räsänen J, Alahuhta S, et al. Maternal and uteroplacental haemodynamic state in preeclamptic patients during spinal anaesthesia for Caesarean section. Br J Anaesth 1996; 76:616-20.

250. Chiu CL, Mansor M, Ng KP, Chan YK. Retrospective review of spinal versus epidural anestheisia for cesarean section in preeclamptic patients. Internat J Obstet Anesth 2003; 12:23-7.

251. Sharwood-Smith G, Watson CE. Regional anesthesia for cesarean section in severe preeclampsia: Spinal anesthesia is the preferred choice. Internat J Obstet Anesth 1999; 8:85-9.

252. Sharwood-Smith G, Drummond G, Bruce J. Pulse transit time confirms altered hemodynamic response to spinal anesthesia in pregnancy induced hypertension. Hypertens Pregnancy 2002;21:P016 (abstracts from the 13th World Congress of the International Society for the Study of Hypertension in Pregnancy, June 2-5, 2002, Toronto, Canada).

253. Overdyk FJ, Harvey SC. Continuous spinal anesthesia for cesarean section in a parturient with severe preeclampsia. J Clin Anesth 1998; 10:510-3.

254. Dyer RA, Els L, Ped FC, et al. Prospective, randomized trial comparing general with spinal anesthesia for cesarean delivery in preeclamptic patients with a nonreassuring fetal heart trace. Anesthesiology 2003; 99:561-69.

255. Simolke GA, Cox SM, Cunningham FG. Cerebrovascular accidents complicating pregnancy and the puerperium. Obstet Gynecol 1991; 78:37-42.

256. Cooper GM, Lewis G, Neilson J. Confidential enquiries into maternal deaths, 1997-1999 (editorial). Br J Anaesth 2002; 89:369-72.

257. Hood DD, Dewan DM, James FM, et al. The use of nitroglycerin in preventing the hypertensive response to tracheal intubation in severe preeclampsia. Anesthesiology 1985; 63:329-32.

258. Sosis M, Leighton B. In defense of trimethaphan for use in preeclampsia. Anesthesiology 1986; 64:657-8.

259. Lawes EG, Downing JW, Duncan PW, et al. Fentanyl-droperidol supplementation of rapid sequence induction in the presence of severe pregnancy-induced and pregnancy-aggravated hypertension. Br J Anaesth 1987; 59:1381-91.

260. Isler CM, Barrilleaux PS, Rinehart BK, Magann EF, Martin JN. Postpartum seizure prophylaxis: Using maternal clinical parameters to guide therapy. Obstet Gynecol 2003; 101:66-9.

261. Magann EF, Bass JD, Chauhan SP, et al. Accelerated recovery from severe preeclampsia: Uterine curettage versus nifedipine. J Soc Gynecol Invest 1994; 1:210-4.

262. Broughton-Pipkin F. The hypertensive disorders of pregnancy. Br Med J 1995; 311:609-13.

263. Sibai BM. Eclampsia. VI. Maternal-perinatal outcome in 254 consecutive cases. Am J Obstet Gynecol 1990; 163:1049-55.

264. Douglas KA, Redman CWG. Eclampsia in the United Kingdom. Br Med J 1994; 309:1395-400.

265. Leitch CR, Cameron AD, Walker JJ. The changing pattern of eclampsia over a 60-year period. Br J Obstet Gynaecol 1997; 104:917-22.

266. Mattar F, Sibai BM. Eclampsia VIII. Risk factors for maternal morbidity. Am J Obstet Gynecol 2000; 182:307-12.

267. Usta IM, Sibai BM. Emergent management of puerperal eclampsia. Obstet Gynecol Clin N Am 1995; 22:315-35.

268. Barton JR, Sibai BM. Cerebral pathology in eclampsia. Clin Perinatol 1991; 18:891-910.

269. Kaplan PW, Repke JT. Eclampsia. Neurol Clin 1994; 12:565-82.

270. Witlin AG, Friedman SA, Egerman RS, et al. Cerebrovascular disorders complicating pregnancy-beyond eclampsia. Am J Obstet Gynecol 1997; 176:1139-48.

271. Cunningham FG, Fernadez CO, Hernadez C. Blindness associated with preeclampsia and eclampsia. Am J Obstet Gynecol 1995; 172:1291-8.

272. Moodley J, Bobat SM, Hoffman M, Bill PLA. Electroencephalogram and computerised cerebral tomography findings in eclampsia. Br J Obstet Gynaecol 1993; 100:984-8.

273. Moodley J, Jjuuko G, Rout C. Epidural compared with general anaesthesia for caesarean delivery in conscious women with eclampsia. Br J Obstet Gynaecol 2001; 108:378-82.

274. Razzaque M, Rahman K, Sashidharan R. Spinal is safer than GA for LSCS in eclamptics (abstract). Anesthesiology 2001; 94:A34.

275. Barton JR, Bronstein SJ, Sibai BM. Management of the eclamptic patient. J Matern Fetal Med 1992; 1:313-9.

276. Sibai BM, El-Nazer A, Gonzalez-Ruiz AR. Severe preeclampsia-eclampsia in young primigravidas: Subsequent pregnancy outcome and remote prognosis. Am J Obstet Gynecol 1986; 155:1011-6.

277. Kittner SJ, Stern BJ, Feeser BR, et al. Pregnancy and the risk of stroke. N Engl J Med 1996; 335:768-74.

278. Sibai BM. Chronic hypertension in pregnancy. Obstet Gynecol 2002; 100:369-77.

279. Sibai BM, Lindheimer M, Hauth J, et al. Risk factors for preeclampsia, placental abruption, and adverse neonatal outcomes among women with chronic hypertension. N Engl J Med 1998; 339:667-71.

280. Sibai BM, Mabie WC, Shamsa F, et al. A comparison of no medication versus methyldopa or labetalol in chronic hypertension during pregnancy. Am J Obstet Gynecol 1990; 162:960-7.

281. Sibai BM. Chronic hypertension in pregnancy (letter). Obstet Gynecol 2002; 100:1358-9.

Chapter 45
Liver Disease

Robert W. Reid, M.D.

VIRAL HEPATITIS

Definition

Acute viral hepatitis is the most common cause of jaundice during pregnancy. It represents one of the most serious infections of pregnant women. Epstein-Barr virus, cytomegalovirus, herpes simplex, yellow fever, and rubella viruses are infrequent causes of acute viral hepatitis. More than 80% of cases of viral hepatitis are caused by hepatitis viruses A, B, or C; these agents have a specific affinity for the hepatocyte. Hepatitis viruses D, E, and G also have been identified. Infection may cause mild nonclinical illness or fulminant hepatic necrosis. In some cases, chronic infection may lead to cirrhosis, hepatic failure, hepatocellular carcinoma, or death. Vertical transmission to the infant during the perinatal period may lead to neonatal hepatitis.

Pathophysiology and Epidemiology

Table 45-1 summarizes the clinical and epidemiologic properties of the seven major causative agents.[1-4] **Hepatitis A virus (HAV)** is responsible for nearly half of known cases of viral hepatitis. This virus replicates in the liver, is secreted in the bile, and is then shed through feces. Transmission between individuals occurs almost exclusively through fecal-oral contamination. Occasionally, the virus is spread through intravenous drug use or sexual contact.[5] Rare cases of vertical transmission have been reported.[6,7] Although it is very contagious, the duration of viremia is short. Clinical illness typically is mild, is limited to 2 or 3 weeks, and is never associated with a chronic carrier state. Fulminant hepatic necrosis is a rare but devastating complication of HAV infection.

Hepatitis B virus (HBV) is transmitted through parenteral or sexual exposure. Women at risk include those with a history of intravenous drug use, multiple sexual partners, sexually transmitted diseases, or exposure to cryoprecipitate; those who work or are treated in a hemodialysis unit; those who work in a health or public safety field; those with a recent tattoo; and those who have resided in a prison or an institution for the developmentally disabled. However, these risk factors identify only half of all HBV-positive pregnant women.[8] In the United States, 0.2% of persons are seropositive for HBV.[9] In contrast to HAV infection, 5% to 10% of those infected with HBV progress to a chronic carrier state; 30% of those individuals continue to experience active hepatocellular destruction and are at risk for cirrhosis, hepatocellular carcinoma, and death. Vertical transmission of active HBV infection to the newborn is common in the absence of neonatal immunoprophylaxis.[4,10]

Hepatitis C virus (HCV) poses a serious public health problem. In the United States, over 4 million persons are infected with HCV. The prevalence of HCV is approximately 1.8%. This virus is responsible for most cases of non-A, non-B viral hepatitis and is predominantly transmitted through parenteral, sexual, nasal, and intrauterine routes. Before the advent of blood-bank screening for HCV in July 1992, most cases of posttransfusion hepatitis were caused by HCV. Intravenous drug users exhibit seropositive rates of 60% to 90%. The virus is also transmitted via intranasal use of cocaine. Sexual transmission of HCV occurs less readily than occurs with HBV. Most infections with HCV are asymptomatic, and many people are unaware of their infection. Nevertheless, up to 90% of infected individuals slowly develop cirrhosis,

TABLE 45-1	SOME AGENTS THAT CAUSE ACUTE VIRAL HEPATITIS[1-37]					
	Hepatitis A	**Hepatitis B**	**Hepatitis C**	**Hepatitis D**	**Hepatitis E**	**Hepatitis G**
Viral family	Picronaviridae	Hepadnaviridae	Flaviviridae	Satellite virus or subviral particle	Caliciviridae	Flaviviridae variant
Genomic type	27 nm RNA	42 nm DNA	9.4 kb RNA	36 nm hybrid	7.5 kb RNA	9.4 kb RNA
Typical transmission	Fecal-oral	P/S	P/S	P/S	Fecal-oral	P/S
Proportion of cases	25%	32%	20%	–	–	9%
Incidence in pregnancy	1:1000	1:500	Unknown	Unknown	Unknown	Unknown
Incubation period	15-50 days	60-110 days	37-70 days	Comparable to HBV	10-56 days	Unknown
Progression to chronic liver disease	No	1%-5% in adults; 80%-90% in children	85%	Chronic liver disease common if HDV superinfection is present in HBV-infected individuals	No	Unknown
Vertical transmission	Rarely	10%-20%	2%-10%	Comparable to HBV	Commonly	40%-60%
Immunoglobulin available	Yes	Yes	No	No	No	No
Vaccine	Yes	Yes	No	HBV vaccine	No	No

P/S, Parenteral or sexual transmission; *nm*, nanometer; *kb*, kilobase.

hepatocellular carcinoma, hepatic failure, and death over two decades or longer. Women of reproductive age are at particular risk for unrecognized, asymptomatic HCV infection.[1,3] The risk of perinatal transmission is approximately 1% to 5%.[1,11]

Hepatitis D virus (HDV or **delta agent)** is an incomplete RNA virus that is dependent on coinfection with HBV. Chronic HDV infection carries an increased risk of fulminant hepatic failure. Although vertical transmission of HDV does occur, measures that protect against HBV infection also protect the neonate against HDV infection.

The **hepatitis E virus (HEV)** was identified and cloned in 1990.[12,13] This RNA virus is transmitted by the fecal-oral route and is responsible for major epidemics of viral hepatitis in developing countries. In 1997, Kwo et al.[14] reported the first case of an HEV isolate acquired in the United States. Among nonpregnant patients, HEV infection typically is self-limited and does not lead to a chronic carrier state. However, HEV infection during pregnancy is associated with a high risk of maternal and fetal morbidity and mortality.[15] Vertical transmission of this virus has been reported.[16]

A virus was isolated in fecal extracts from several patients in France with viral hepatitis not caused by HAV, HBV, HCV, or HEV. This virus was tentatively called the **Hepatitis F virus (HFV)**.[17] However, the existence of this virus has not been confirmed and is now considered doubtful.[1]

Hepatitis G virus (HGV; also called **hepatitis GB virus C** or **HGBV-C)** was characterized in 1996.[18] This RNA virus is closely related to the HCV virus. Alter et al.[19] reported that HGV is common among volunteer blood donors; they demonstrated that HGV may be transmitted by means of blood transfusion. Vertical transmission of HGV from mother to infant has been reported.[20,21] However, the clinical significance of HGV infection is unknown, and no causal relation between HGV and hepatitis has been established. In fact, the liver/serum concentration ratio of HGV RNA is less than one, suggesting that HGV may not even be hepatotropic.[22]

Diagnosis

Clinical symptoms of acute viral hepatitis range from vague constitutional symptoms (e.g., malaise, nausea, anorexia)

to overt jaundice. Physical examination often reveals tender hepatomegaly. Bilirubinuria and acholic stool are noted. Hepatic transaminase enzymes rise to the 1000 IU range during acute infection. Serologic testing confirms the diagnosis. Acute HAV infection is marked by the presence of immunoglobulin M (IgM)–class anti-HAV antibody. Hepatitis B surface antigen (HBsAg) or anti-HBc antibody indicates either an acute HBV infection or the presence of a chronic active infection. The presence of hepatitis B virus core component e-antigen (HBeAg) suggests a high degree of infectivity and neonatal risk.[1,10] The current generation of enzyme immunoassay detects anti-HCV antibody with 95% sensitivity. Positive or indeterminate results should be confirmed with recombinant immunoblot assay. Anti-HCV antibodies are not detectable until 15 weeks after acute infection. Qualitative testing for HCV virus RNA by polymerase chain reaction (PCR) may detect infection as early as 2 weeks after acute infection.[3] Hepatitis D viral infection is indicated by serology for IgM anti-HDV or HDV RNA. Laboratory techniques for the diagnosis of HEV infection include PCR and serologic antibody detection. At this time, HGV infection can be identified only through PCR assay, which is not readily available or standardized.

Effect on the Fetus

Preterm labor and delivery is more common among mothers with viral hepatitis.[23] A single report[24] suggested that Down syndrome is more common after HAV infection, but there has been no further suggestion of hepatitis-induced teratogenicity.

Vertical transmission of HBV from mother to fetus remains a significant public health concern. Without proper neonatal immunoprophylaxis, 10% to 20% of infants born to HBsAg seropositive mothers will have clinical infection. If the mother also is HBeAg seropositive, the risk of infection is greater than 85%.[25] Because infants do not show evidence of HBV infection until the second or third month postpartum, most investigators believe that transmission occurs during the immediate peripartum period—when the infant is exposed to vaginal blood and secretions—rather than by transplacental exposure.

Jabeen et al.[11] studied a large cohort of women in Ireland who were inadvertently infected with HCV after exposure to contaminated anti-D immunoglobulin between 1977 and 1978; the infection was discovered in 1994. In the 20 years following infection, all of these women experienced at least one pregnancy (mean parity = 3.5). Of the 100 total pregnancies, 85 went to term. Of the children born to HCV RNA-positive mothers, only one (2.3%) tested positive for the virus. This vertical transmission rate is significantly less than the vertical transmission rate for HBV infection. Comparison with a control group showed no difference in the rate of spontaneous abortion, birth weight, or other obstetric complications.[11] Agha et al.[26] reported transplacental transmission in 85 (11%) of 767 HCV-infected parturients. In this study, HCV-infected women who exhibited positive PCR, high aspartate aminotransferase, and positive anti-HCV IgM were most likely to transmit HCV to their babies.

Hepatitis E viral infection is associated with a very high risk of maternal and fetal morbidity and mortality. Tsega et al.[15] reported that HEV infection caused death in 8 (42%) of 19 pregnant Ethiopian women (mostly during the third trimester), as well as 10 fetal complications.

Medical and Obstetric Management

Management of the pregnant woman with acute viral hepatitis involves supportive care and prevention of newborn transmission. Although most women may be managed at home, hospitalization is indicated for severe nausea and vomiting, encephalopathy, coagulopathy, or debilitation. These women should avoid strenuous activity or trauma to the upper abdomen. Family contacts should receive immunoprophylaxis.[22,27]

Two new inactivated HAV vaccines are available and safe for use in pregnancy.[5] The Advisory Committee on Immunization Practices (ACIP)[28] recently recommended that these vaccines should replace HAV immune globulin for preexposure prophylaxis. HAV vaccination should be considered for parturients at risk for HAV exposure. This includes women who travel to developing countries; use illicit intravenous drugs; or work in neonatal intensive care units, day care centers, institutions for persons having developmental disabilities, public food preparation facilities, medical laboratories, and non-human primate research facilities.

Because of the risk of newborn infection, the Centers for Disease Control and Prevention (CDC)[29] and the American College of Obstetricians and Gynecologists (ACOG)[30] currently recommend HBV screening for all pregnant women. The CDC also recommends HBV vaccination for all newborns, regardless of maternal serology. If the mother is HBsAg negative, the newborn is vaccinated with either Recombivax HB or Engerix-B (1) before hospital discharge, (2) at 1 to 2 months of age, and (3) at 6 to 18 months of age. If the mother is HBsAg positive or has unknown serology, initial vaccination should be performed within 12 hours of delivery and hepatitis B immune globulin (HBIG) should be administered.

Lin et al.[31] prospectively demonstrated that mother-to-fetus microtransfusion occurred least among women who delivered by elective cesarean section. In a retrospective analysis, Lee et al.[32] suggested that cesarean section significantly reduced the risk of neonatal HBV infection when it was combined with vaccination and administration of immune globulin. In a population of infants who were born to HBeAg- and HBsAg-seropositive mothers, the rate of newborn HBV infection was

20% after vaginal delivery, compared with 6% after cesarean delivery, when a 50-IU dose of HBIG was administered to both groups of infants within 9 hours of delivery. Schalm and Pit-Grosheide[33] have argued that increasing the dose of HBIG to 200 IU, administered within 2 hours of birth, reduces the infection rate to 5% and may negate the need for cesarean delivery.

Although routine prenatal testing for HCV infection is not yet recommended, women who present with known risk factors should be tested for HCV.[3] Alpha-interferon-2b effectively reduces HCV RNA titers and improves the clinical outcome of patients with chronic HCV infection.[34] At least two reports have described normal pregnancy outcome during inadvertent interferon therapy[35,36]; however, interferon currently is not considered safe during gestation. No published data support the administration of immune globulin as HCV immunoprophylaxis during labor.[37]

INTRAHEPATIC CHOLESTASIS OF PREGNANCY

Definition and Epidemiology

Intrahepatic cholestasis of pregnancy is the second most common cause of jaundice during pregnancy. It is a syndrome that is characterized by pruritus followed by jaundice. It occurs most often in the third trimester, but it may occur anytime during pregnancy. In most areas, the incidence is less than 1 in 500 pregnancies; however, in Scandinavian and South American countries, intrahepatic cholestasis occurs during as many as 10% of all pregnancies. Nulliparous women with multiple gestation are at highest risk. In a report from Chile, the prevalence of intrahepatic cholestasis of pregnancy was 21% among women with twin pregnancies versus 4.7% among women with single pregnancies.[38] Although the disorder resolves promptly after delivery, it commonly recurs in subsequent pregnancies or with the administration of estrogenic oral contraceptives. The specific etiology of intrahepatic cholestasis of pregnancy is unknown; however, it seems to represent an enhanced sensitivity to the cholestatic effects of estrogenic steroids. Sulphation is an important step in reducing the cholestatic potential of estrogens and bile acids. Davies et al.[39] demonstrated decreased sulphotransferase activity during pregnancy.

Diagnosis

The diagnosis of intrahepatic cholestasis of pregnancy is considered in the pregnant woman who develops pruritus followed by jaundice 2 to 4 weeks later. Pruritus is the most distressing symptom and may lead to irritability, insomnia, and depression. Although physical examination reveals mild hepatomegaly, the presence of abdominal pain or hepatic tenderness should exclude the diagnosis of intrahepatic cholestasis of pregnancy. Biochemical abnormalities include markedly elevated serum bile acids and moderate conjugated hyperbilirubinemia. Serum transaminase enzymes may be normal or elevated. Although liver biopsy rarely is indicated, histopathology reveals acinar cholestasis and canalicular bile plugs. Inflammation and necrosis are not observed.[40] Impaired bile salt excretion causes steatorrhea, fat malabsorption, and mild malnutrition.[41]

Effect on the Mother and Fetus

Intrahepatic cholestasis of pregnancy has minimal impact on maternal health during gestation. Although pruritus is

distressing, the mother should be assured that the disorder will resolve within 2 weeks after delivery. There is no risk of developing chronic liver disease. Vitamin K malabsorption, if uncorrected, may lead to clinical coagulopathy. Fisk et al.[42] reported an 11% incidence of postpartum hemorrhage among women with intrahepatic cholestasis of pregnancy.

Although maternal outcome is good, the fetus is at increased risk.[43,44] Fisk and Storey[45] reported the outcome of 86 infants born to women with intrahepatic cholestasis of pregnancy. Spontaneous preterm labor occurred in 44%, meconium-stained amniotic fluid in 45%, and intrapartum fetal distress in 22% of these cases. The perinatal mortality rate was 3.5%. In a retrospective review of 320 consecutive parturients with intrahepatic cholestasis of pregnancy, Rioseco et al.[46] reported a similar incidence of meconium-stained amniotic fluid and spontaneous preterm delivery. Israel et al.[47] demonstrated that myometrial strips from patients with intrahepatic cholestasis of pregnancy exhibit an enhanced contractile response to oxytocin, which correlates with the clinical observation of uterine hypertonus. Neonatal hypoprothrombinemia places the infant at increased risk for intracranial hemorrhage.

Medical and Obstetric Management

Medical management is directed toward improving bile secretion and reducing intestinal reabsorption of bile salts to provide symptomatic relief. Cholestyramine resin relieves the pruritus in many women but may aggravate fat malabsorption and has been associated with severe fetal intracranial hemorrhage.[48] Marpeau et al.[49] demonstrated that ursodeoxycholic acid modifies the pool of biliary acids and provides marked regression of clinical and biologic markers of intrahepatic cholestasis of pregnancy. Subsequent clinical trials[50-52] demonstrated improved maternal and fetal outcome after the administration of ursodeoxycholic acid. Vitamin K should be administered subcutaneously if prolongation of the prothrombin time (PT) is noted during gestation. Mullally and Hansen[44] recommend induction of labor and delivery near term (after confirmation of fetal lung maturity) or earlier if fetal compromise is identified.

ACUTE FATTY LIVER OF PREGNANCY (REVERSIBLE PERIPARTUM LIVER FAILURE)

Definition and Epidemiology

Idiopathic acute fatty liver of pregnancy (AFLP) or reversible peripartum liver failure is an uncommon disorder of late pregnancy that is characterized by impaired hepatic metabolic activity, which may progress to liver failure, disseminated intravascular coagulation (DIC), profoundly depressed antithrombin III level, hypoglycemia, and renal insufficiency. The liver failure resolves shortly after delivery in all but rare cases. Histologic examination of the liver reveals microvesicular fatty infiltration of the liver. In 1856, Tarnier[53] likened the affected liver of a parturient with probable AFLP to greasy, fat-laden goose livers and paint-splattered canvases. In 1934, Stander and Cadden[54] described this disorder in a pregnant woman who developed third-trimester jaundice and drowsiness. Less than 100 cases of AFLP were reported before 1980, and the incidence was estimated at 1 per 1 million pregnancies.[55,56] In recent years, however, heightened awareness and early recognition suggest that the disorder may occur in 1 per 6700 gestations.[57]

Pathophysiology

The pathogenesis of AFLP remains unknown. However, similarities in the clinical presentation and hepatic histology of children with long-chain-3-hydroxyacyl-CoA dehydrogenase (LCHAD) deficiency, an inborn error causing impairment of mitochondrial beta-oxidation, have suggested a role for fatty acid accumulation in the etiology of AFLP. Rinaldo et al.[58] have hypothesized that abnormal fatty-acid metabolites produced by a fetus with LCHAD deficiency may enter the maternal circulation and overwhelm the mitochondrial-oxidation pathways of the heterozygous mother. Indeed, this would occur at a time when the maternal liver is already responding to the increased demands of fatty acid oxidation during late pregnancy. AFLP is more common in twin than in singleton pregnancies. Davidson et al.[59] reported three cases of AFLP in parturients with triplet gestation. Multiple gestation may further stress the fatty acid oxidation capacity in susceptible parturients.

Similarities between AFLP and preeclampsia or eclampsia are intriguing. Both disorders primarily occur near term and are associated with nulliparity and multiple gestation. Hepatic involvement occurs with preeclampsia in the form of the HELLP syndrome (i.e., *Hemolysis, Elevated Liver* enzymes, and *Low Platelets*). Riely[60] reported that 64 of 140 cases of AFLP occurred along with preeclampsia or eclampsia. Minakami et al.[61] reviewed 41 liver biopsy specimens from preeclamptic women with and without hepatic dysfunction. They documented microvesicular fat in all 41 of these specimens. Thus AFLP may represent a severe variant on the pathologic continuum of preeclampsia/eclampsia. Tyni et al.[62] reviewed records for 18 mothers of 28 infants with LCHAD deficiency. Preeclampsia, HELLP syndrome, and AFLP occurred in 31% of these pregnancies. These fascinating results further support the role of fatty acid accumulation in the pathogenesis of the preeclampsia-AFLP continuum.

Diagnosis

The diagnosis of AFLP must be considered in any woman who presents with hepatic dysfunction during late pregnancy. Castro et al.[57] described 28 consecutive cases of AFLP over a 15-year period. Affected parturients recounted a prodromal period of 1 to 21 days (average = 9 days) with symptoms including nausea and vomiting (reported by 71%), malaise (64%), abdominal pain (50%), fever (32%), jaundice or dark urine (29%), headache (21%), pruritus (11%), and sore throat (11%). Pruritus is uncommon and typically suggests the more common diagnosis of intrahepatic cholestasis of pregnancy. Hepatic encephalopathy is a late and ominous finding. In this study, the diagnosis of AFLP was established before delivery in only 36% of cases.[57] Physical examination reveals an afebrile patient with mild hypertension and modest peripheral edema and jaundice.

The hallmark laboratory findings are those of prolonged PT, profoundly depressed antithrombin III levels, and elevated liver enzyme levels. All patients exhibit evidence of persistent DIC.[57] Leukocytosis and elevated total bilirubin, creatinine, and alkaline phosphatase concentrations are observed in nearly all cases. Profound hypoglycemia (secondary to impaired hepatic glycogenolysis) is common. Thrombocytopenia develops only in those patients with clinical bleeding. Similarly, oliguria is observed only in those parturients with hypovolemia caused by hemorrhage.

Liver biopsy is rarely required for the diagnosis because clinical findings exclude all other possibilities except preeclampsia. In the latter case, biopsy findings are identical to AFLP and do not alter treatment (i.e., delivery of the infant). Further, biopsy may be precluded by coagulopathy. However, if performed, characteristic histology includes microvesicular fatty infiltration of the pericentral hepatocytes with oil red-O stain on frozen section. Hepatocellular necrosis, portal inflammation, and cholestasis are noted in most cases. Rolfes and Ishak[63] have cautioned that the histology of AFLP often is variable and may be misinterpreted as viral hepatitis. Liver biopsy is recommended only for those parturients with an atypical presentation of AFLP.[60]

Diagnostic imaging rarely contributes to the diagnosis. Fatty infiltration of the liver may be documented by ultrasonography and computed tomography (CT) in approximately half the cases.[57]

Effect on the Mother and Fetus

With improved clinical recognition, prompt delivery of the infant, and aggressive medical management of the parturient, maternal and fetal mortality rates have decreased over the last half century. The maternal mortality rate was 70%, 10%, and 0%, in series reported in 1965, 1985, and 1999, respectively.[57,64,65] Maternal complications may include DIC, profound hypoglycemia, hepatic encephalopathy, pancreatitis, acute renal failure, and hepatic rupture. Fetal distress and death may occur secondary to uteroplacental insufficiency. Moise and Shah[66] have cautioned that replacement of maternal coagulation factors may lead to the deposition of fibrin at the choriodecidual interface and subsequent uteroplacental insufficiency.

Of the 30 fetuses (two sets of twins) reported by Castro et al.[57], there was one stillbirth and one neonatal death resulting from perinatal asphyxia. Despite aggressive maternal support, fetal compromise occurred frequently. Meconium-stained amniotic fluid was noted in 60% of cases.[57]

Before 1990, it was thought that AFLP did not recur during subsequent gestation. Watson and Seeds[67] reviewed the records of 21 women with a history of AFLP during a previous pregnancy. There was no recurrence among the 25 subsequent gestations. However, four cases of recurrent AFLP subsequently have been reported.[68-70]

Medical and Obstetric Management

AFLP is a medical emergency that demands rapid evaluation and treatment. Hepatic failure and fetal death may develop within a few days. There are no reported cases of maternal recovery before delivery. As soon as the diagnosis is established and the mother is stabilized, plans must be made for delivery of the infant. There is no clear advantage for cesarean section over expeditious vaginal delivery. Immediate maternal supportive care includes fluid and electrolyte support, treatment of hypoglycemia, and attention to coagulopathy and anemia. The maternal glucose level should be checked every 1 to 2 hours. All patients will require infusion of at least 5% dextrose solution, and many will require 10% dextrose solution with multiple supplemental doses. Hepatic encephalopathy may improve with a low-protein, high-carbohydrate diet and enteral lactulose.

Postpartum hemorrhage should be anticipated; adequate intravenous access should be established, and cross-matched blood should be immediately available. In most cases, the maternal condition improves within 24 to 48 hours after delivery, with continued recovery during the subsequent week. Survivors experience no hepatic residua, and follow-up liver biopsies show no evidence of fibrosis.[57,60]

Orthotopic liver transplantation is an option for the rare parturient who shows no evidence of recovery by 3 days postpartum.[71-73] However, AFLP is a reversible form of acute hepatic failure in nearly all patients, and this option must be considered with great caution. Doepel et al.[74] described a young, previously healthy parturient who was diagnosed with AFLP at delivery. Fulminant hepatic failure with severe encephalopathy and hepatorenal syndrome rapidly ensued. Hepatic imaging showed 90% parenchymal damage, and liver biopsy revealed necrosis. She was placed on the Scandinavian liver transplant waiting list with high urgent status. However, no suitable liver was found. After 8 days, her clinical condition improved, and she was removed from the transplant waiting list. Four weeks after delivery, the patient was discharged in good condition. Six months later, the patient was feeling well, and clinical tests were normal.

SPONTANEOUS HEPATIC RUPTURE OF PREGNANCY

Spontaneous hepatic rupture is a rare complication of late pregnancy or the early puerperium. Approximately 140 published cases have been reported; more than 90% of these occurred in women with preeclampsia. The typical presentation is a triad of preeclampsia, right upper quadrant pain, and acute hypotension. Historically, few cases have been diagnosed correctly before laparotomy or autopsy. When cases have been diagnosed at surgery, the preoperative diagnosis typically was placental abruption, uterine rupture, or perforated gastrointestinal ulcer.[75]

By definition, spontaneous hepatic rupture of pregnancy occurs in the absence of antecedent trauma. Instead, rupture is preceded by an intraparenchymal hepatic hematoma. The strong association with preeclampsia suggests that periportal hemorrhagic necrosis, hypertension, and coagulopathy may lead to hematoma formation. With expansion of the hematoma, the hepatic capsule is progressively distended and dissected from the parenchyma, which leads to rupture.[75,76]

The mortality rate is greater than 60%; however, increased awareness and improved diagnostic modalities may improve survival.[77] Ultrasonography, CT, and technetium scanning may reveal the expanding hematoma before rupture. Paracentesis with lavage is highly sensitive for the detection of intraabdominal hemorrhage. Although contained hepatic hematoma may be managed with blood products and close observation, rupture almost always demands immediate laparotomy and prompt control of hemorrhage.[77,78] Transcatheter hepatic arterial embolization has been reported as an alternative to surgical intervention.[79,80] Hunter et al.[81] reported a case of massive, spontaneous hepatic rupture at 36 weeks' gestation in a woman with severe preeclampsia. The patient underwent life-saving total hepatectomy with the creation of an end-to-side portocaval shunt. The patient subsequently underwent orthotopic liver transplantation after being maintained in an anhepatic state for almost 13 hours.

PORTAL HYPERTENSION

Portal hypertension is a disorder that commonly follows cirrhosis of the liver but also may occur secondary to noncirrhotic portal fibrosis or extrahepatic portal venous

obstruction. It is uncommon during pregnancy because it rarely afflicts women of reproductive age and chronic liver disease impairs fertility.[82] Clinical manifestations of portal hypertension include the development of portal-systemic collaterals, splenomegaly, and ascites. The portal-systemic collaterals of greatest significance are those within the gastric and esophageal mucosae. Hemorrhage from these varices is the most significant complication of portal hypertension and is associated with a 30% to 60% mortality rate per bleeding episode.[83]

Risk of Variceal Hemorrhage during Pregnancy

During normal pregnancy, uterine compression of the inferior vena cava causes diversion of venous return through the azygos and vertebral venous systems.[84] This has led some physicians to believe that pregnancy may result in an increased rate of variceal hemorrhage. In addition, some physicians have advocated delivery by cesarean section to avoid straining and variceal rupture during vaginal delivery.

Schreyer et al.[85] reviewed 99 pregnancies in women with cirrhosis. A total of 69 of these pregnancies occurred in women without a portosystemic shunt, and 30 occurred in women with a shunt. The incidence of severe variceal hemorrhage was eight times greater in the nonshunted patients (24%) than in the shunted patients (3%). The maternal mortality rate was 13% in the nonshunted group. The authors recommended consideration of prophylactic portosystemic shunting for cirrhotic women who might become pregnant.

Britton[86] reviewed 83 pregnancies among 53 women with cirrhotic portal hypertension and 77 pregnancies among 38 women with noncirrhotic portal hypertension. When women with prior shunting were excluded, the incidence of variceal hemorrhage was 30%. An 18% mortality rate followed these hemorrhagic events. The majority of bleeding episodes occurred during the second trimester. Only 1 of the 61 patients who underwent vaginal delivery suffered intrapartum variceal bleeding, suggesting that the mode of delivery had little influence on the risk of bleeding.

A recent study by Kochhar et al.[87] described 116 pregnancies among 44 women with noncirrhotic portal hypertension. The incidence of fetal loss was 8%, which did not differ from the incidence (10%) in an age-matched control group. The incidence of variceal bleeding was 14%, and all events were successfully managed with sclerotherapy.

Medical and Obstetric Management

Endoscopic sclerotherapy is the preferred management of variceal hemorrhage during pregnancy.[88] It currently is recommended that all women with portal hypertension who wish to conceive should undergo endoscopy and prophylactic sclerotherapy before conception.[89] Endoscopic evaluation should be repeated at least once each trimester. If uncontrolled hemorrhage occurs despite sclerotherapy, portosystemic shunting may be considered.[88,89] Zeeman and Moise[90] recently reported the use of prophylactic banding in a parturient with severe esophageal varices not deemed manageable with endoscopic sclerotherapy alone.

The transjugular intrahepatic portosystemic stent-shunt (TIPS) procedure has been introduced for the management of portal hypertension in nonpregnant patients.[91] The outcome of this procedure has not been proven to be better than that provided by traditional endoscopic sclerotherapy.[92]

Nevertheless, Wildberger et al.[93] recently reported the use of TIPS at mid-gestation in a parturient with recurrent variceal bleeding due to cirrhosis. Fetal radiation exposure during this procedure was less than 1 rem—a level not considered prohibitive by the authors of this report.

Frequent antenatal assessment of hepatic function, hematologic status, and fetal well-being are performed. Sodium restriction or diuresis should be approached cautiously during pregnancy. Prophylactic H_2-receptor antagonist therapy may prevent reflux esophagitis. Cesarean section should be reserved for obstetric indications. Facilities and personnel to manage massive gastrointestinal hemorrhage must be immediately available.[94]

LIVER TRANSPLANTATION

Since 1967, orthotopic liver transplantation has become a lifesaving treatment for patients with end-stage hepatic failure. Approximately 11% of those who have received transplants have been young women of reproductive age.[95] Although chronic liver disease is associated with a high rate of infertility, transplantation consistently returns reproductive function to normal.[96] To date, over 100 pregnancies have been reported after liver transplantation. In addition, there have been at least 12 reports of liver transplantation during pregnancy.[97]

Effect of Pregnancy on the Hepatic Allograft

Two of the largest series of pregnancy after liver transplantation are from the Universities of Pittsburgh and Colorado.[95,98] These two studies describe the outcome of 34 deliveries in 30 patients. Most of these patients experienced stable hepatic function throughout pregnancy and the postpartum period. Although 26% experienced hepatic enzyme abnormalities during pregnancy, only two women suffered acute rejection and two women developed chronic rejection. One patient with chronic rejection required re-transplantation 2 months postpartum. Thrombosis of the graft hepatic artery was noted at surgery. All patients except one continued prepregnancy immunosuppression, including prednisone, cyclosporine, azathioprine, and/or tacrolimus. In a series of 19 pregnancies in 19 orthotopic liver recipients in France,[99] 3 women experienced graft dysfunction—2 during early pregnancy (which prompted elective abortion) and 1 at 37 weeks' gestation. A 2001 report from the National Transplantation Pregnancy Registry[100] confirmed that pregnancy does not adversely affect graft function when the graft function is stable before pregnancy. Female recipients of liver transplantation should be advised to wait 2 years before conception to ensure stable graft function.[101]

Obstetric Course and Perinatal Outcome

In the Pittsburgh-Colorado series,[95,98] major gestational complications included renal insufficiency (50%), hypertension (30%), preeclampsia (20%), and anemia (30%). A total of 31 live births occurred—two thirds by cesarean section and one third by vaginal delivery. Half of the infants were delivered preterm. Three neonatal deaths occurred. These neonatal deaths were associated with cytomegalovirus (CMV) infection, preterm delivery, and a time interval between transplantation and pregnancy of less than 6 months. Despite intrauterine exposure to immunosuppressive agents, no congenital

abnormalities were observed. Perinatal renal dysfunction was the primary determinant of adverse pregnancy outcome. Immunosuppression with cyclosporine during pregnancy was more often associated with antenatal complications than was the use of tacrolimus. Within the series of patients from France,[99] complications included spontaneous abortion (21%) and hypertension (27%). Among the 11 pregnancies that progressed beyond the first trimester, no cases of perinatal death or congenital abnormalities were observed.

ANESTHETIC MANAGEMENT OF THE PARTURIENT WITH LIVER DISEASE

Anesthetic management is determined by the extent of hepatic impairment. The woman with inactive viral hepatitis, mild intrahepatic cholestasis of pregnancy, or uncomplicated liver transplantation may be managed in the same manner as a healthy parturient, assuming that hepatic synthetic and metabolic function are intact. Coagulopathy should be excluded or corrected before the administration of regional anesthesia. In contrast, the parturient with acute viral hepatitis, advanced cirrhosis, portal hypertension, or AFLP presents many challenges to the anesthesiologist (Box 45-1).

Systemic Abnormalities Associated with Hepatic Disease

Acute and chronic parenchymal liver disease results in impaired synthesis of clotting factors I, II, V, VII, and X. Cholestasis leads to malabsorption of vitamin K, an important cofactor required for the synthesis of factors II, VII, IX, and X. The plasma half-life of factor VII is 5 hours; thus coagulopathy may develop rapidly. Vitamin K administration rapidly corrects coagulopathy if malabsorption is the primary defect. However, impaired hepatic synthesis does not respond to vitamin K administration. Fresh frozen plasma or cryoprecipitate may be needed if clinical bleeding develops.

Cardiovascular manifestations of hepatic insufficiency include increased cardiac output and low systemic vascular resistance (SVR). The latter is caused by extensive arteriovenous shunting. Hepatic insufficiency results in an increase in blood volume that is greater than that of normal pregnancy. Cardiomyopathy may develop. Although cardiac filling pressures typically are normal, tense ascites may impair venous return. Central venous or pulmonary artery pressure monitoring should be considered in those patients with ascites or cardiomyopathy who require cesarean delivery.

Box 45-1 ANESTHETIC GUIDELINES FOR THE PARTURIENT WITH LIVER DISEASE

- Evaluate the extent of hepatic impairment.
- Recognize and evaluate underlying systemic abnormalities.
- Assist the obstetric team with stabilization of maternal condition before delivery.
- Exclude or correct coagulopathy before administration of regional anesthesia.
- Prevent further hepatic injury by optimizing hepatic blood flow and oxygenation.
- Recognize altered pharmacokinetics and pharmacodynamics.
- Prevent transmission of viral hepatitis to the health care team.
- Monitor the patient for evidence of postoperative hepatic dysfunction.

Impaired hypoxic pulmonary vasoconstriction and portopulmonary venous communication lead to significant hypoxemia. Ascites and the gravid uterus cause diaphragmatic elevation, decrease functional residual capacity, and lead to further intrapulmonary shunting. Patients with liver disease have increased 2,3-diphosphoglycerate levels within red blood cells and a right shift of the oxyhemoglobin dissociation curve.[102]

Hepatic encephalopathy is a reversible neuropsychiatric disorder that occurs in patients with advanced hepatic failure. Inadequate hepatic clearance of ammonia and mercaptan toxins, altered gamma-aminobutyric acid levels, and increased brain influx of false neurotransmitters are proposed mechanisms of this syndrome.[103] Impairments may range from mild confusion to coma. These patients are at risk for pulmonary aspiration of gastric contents. The integrity of the blood-brain barrier is altered, and anesthetic agents should be titrated carefully.[102]

Metabolic abnormalities associated with hepatic disease include hypoglycemia, hyponatremia, hypokalemia, and acid-base disturbances. Hypoglycemia, which results from impaired hepatic gluconeogenesis and glycogenolysis, is especially common in patients with AFLP. Glucose concentrations should be determined frequently in these patients.

Albumin is synthesized exclusively by the liver. However, the half-life of albumin is approximately 15 days. Therefore, a change in the serum albumin concentration is not a sensitive marker of hepatic function. Acute hepatic failure is associated with increased plasma triglyceride and abnormal lipoprotein concentrations. These metabolic changes may be sensitive markers for hepatic function.

Abnormal renal sodium retention often accompanies hepatic disease and contributes to ascites formation. The pathogenesis is unclear but seems to involve increased plasma aldosterone, increased sympathetic activity, altered renal prostaglandins and kinins, and reduced renal blood flow. Overt oliguric renal failure may occur, which heralds the onset of the hepatorenal syndrome. Renal vasoconstriction and central hypovolemia may be involved in the pathogenesis of this syndrome. The prognosis for these patients is poor.[83]

Effect of Anesthesia on Hepatic Blood Flow and Oxygenation

Failure to maintain hepatic blood flow or oxygenation may lead to further hepatic necrosis and hepatic failure in a parturient with compromised hepatic function. Gelman[104] has shown that halothane anesthesia decreases hepatic blood flow to 84% of baseline and that upper abdominal surgery further decreases hepatic blood flow to 42% of baseline. Frink et al.[105] examined the effects of four volatile halogenated agents on hepatic blood flow and oxygenation in dogs. Hepatic oxygen delivery was reduced to 86% (sevoflurane), 81% (isoflurane), 57% (enflurane), and 57% (halothane) of control at 1.0 minimum alveolar concentration (MAC). Kanaya et al.[106] confirmed that isoflurane has a more favorable effect on liver perfusion than does halothane. Adequate hepatic oxygenation is especially important in the presence of halothane because hypoxia forces halothane metabolism into a reductive rather than an oxidative pathway. Subsequent reductive metabolites are more reactive and hepatotoxic.[107,108] Admittedly, there is no indisputable proof that general anesthesia of any type causes postoperative hepatic

dysfunction. Nonetheless, it seems prudent to avoid halothane in patients with hepatic disease, if only for medicolegal reasons.

Regional anesthesia also may reduce hepatic blood flow.[109,110] This largely reflects the effects of systemic arterial hypotension secondary to sympathetic blockade. However, Tanaka et al.[111] recently demonstrated a reduction in hepatic blood flow during epidural anesthesia, despite normotension maintained by continuous infusion of colloid. This decrease in hepatic blood flow was reversed by the addition of a dopamine infusion, which suggests that decreased cardiac output, secondary to sympathetic blockade, was responsible for the observed decrease in hepatic blood flow. Nevertheless, most anesthesiologists believe that judicious hydration, slow induction of epidural anesthesia, and avoidance of systemic hypotension should prevent a clinically significant reduction in hepatic blood flow.

Regional Anesthesia

In the absence of coagulopathy, regional anesthesia may be administered to the parturient with hepatic disease. Local anesthetic agents of the amide type undergo hepatic biotransformation. In patients with cirrhosis, the half-life of lidocaine is increased almost threefold (from 108 to 296 minutes), and the volume of distribution is increased from 1.3 to 2.3 L/kg.[112] An expanded volume of distribution offers some protection against toxicity despite impaired clearance. 2-Chloroprocaine undergoes hydrolysis with pseudocholinesterase. Although hepatic pseudocholinesterase production may be decreased in patients with liver disease, the effect this may have on the overall clearance of 2-chloroprocaine is uncertain. Some anesthesiologists have recommended avoiding epidural anesthesia because of the high volume of local anesthetic agent required, although there are no published studies of drug disposition after administration of epidural anesthesia in patients with liver disease.[108] Ascites and portal hypertension lead to engorged epidural veins; thus the use of a test dose to exclude intravascular injection is essential. Heriot et al.[113] reported the successful administration of epidural anesthesia to a parturient with portal hypertension and esophageal varices. On a theoretic basis, spinal anesthesia may be safer than epidural anesthesia because less total drug is used. However, spinal anesthesia has the disadvantage of a rapid onset of sympathetic blockade.

General Anesthesia

Coagulopathy, obstetric hemorrhage, dire fetal distress, or altered mental status may necessitate the use of general anesthesia for cesarean section. Intravascular volume should be evaluated before the induction of anesthesia. In the presence of ascites or cardiovascular compromise, arterial and central venous pressure monitoring may be helpful. Large-gauge intravenous access should be established. Patients with bleeding esophageal varices should be intubated awake. Nasogastric suction is contraindicated. Rapid-sequence induction may be facilitated with thiopental, propofol, ketamine, or etomidate, depending on the patient's hemodynamic status. Liver disease and reduced pseudocholinesterase concentrations may delay the patient's metabolism of succinylcholine, but this is of minimal clinical importance. Thus succinylcholine remains the muscle relaxant of choice for rapid-sequence induction and should be given in the same bolus dose as that used for

healthy parturients. Airway trauma must be avoided in the patient with coagulopathy; profound neuromuscular blockade facilitates atraumatic tracheal intubation. After documentation of neuromuscular recovery, paralysis may be maintained with atracurium or cisatracurium. Inhalation anesthesia may be maintained with isoflurane and nitrous oxide. Reversal of neuromuscular blockade must be documented before extubation. Although the clearance of opioids is delayed in patients with severe liver disease, they may be administered cautiously to provide postoperative analgesia.

KEY POINTS

- All pregnant women should be screened for hepatitis B virus (HBV), and all newborns should be vaccinated against HBV.
- Acute fatty liver of pregnancy may represent a severe variant on the pathologic continuum of preeclampsia/eclampsia.
- Acute fatty liver of pregnancy is a rare but life-threatening complication of pregnancy that demands rapid evaluation and prompt delivery.
- Women with portal hypertension should undergo endoscopy and prophylactic sclerotherapy before conception.
- Pregnancy does not affect the long-term survival of hepatic allografts.
- Posttransplantation immunosuppression is well tolerated during pregnancy.
- Coagulopathy must be excluded or corrected before the administration of regional anesthesia in parturients with liver disease.

REFERENCES

1. Keeffe EB. Acute Viral Hepatitis. In: Dale DC, Federman DD, Antman K, et al., eds. Scientific American Medicine. Vol. 1. New York City: WebMD Professional Publishing, 2001:4-VII.
2. Duff P. Hepatitis in pregnancy. Semin Perinatol 1998; 22:277-83.
3. Burns DN, Minkoff H. Hepatitis C: screening in pregnancy. Obstet Gynecol 1999; 94:1044-8.
4. American College of Obstetricians and Gynecologists Committee on Obstetric Practice. Hepatitis Virus Infections in Obstetrician-Gynecologists. ACOG Committee Opinion Number 203, July 1998. (Int J Gynecol Obstet 1998; 63:203-4).
5. Duff B, Duff P. Hepatitis A vaccine: ready for prime time. Obstet Gynecol 1998; 91:468-71.
6. Watson JC, Fleming DW, Borella AJ, et al. Vertical transmission of hepatitis A resulting in an outbreak in a neonatal intensive care unit. J Infect Dis 1993; 167:567-71.
7. Leikin E, Lysikiewicz A, Garry D, Tejani N. Intrauterine transmission of hepatitis A virus. Obstet Gynecol 1996; 88:690-1.
8. Jonas MM, Schiff ER, O'Sullivan MJ, et al. Failure of Centers for Disease Control criteria to identify hepatitis B infection in a large municipal obstetrical population. Ann Intern Med 1987; 107:335-7.
9. Arevalo JA, Washington AE. Cost-effectiveness of prenatal screening and immunization for hepatitis B virus. JAMA 1988; 259:365-9.
10. Lok AS, McMahon BJ. Chronic hepatitis B. Hepatology 2001; 34:1225-41.
11. Jabeen T, Cannon B, Hogan J, et al. Pregnancy and pregnancy outcome in hepatitis C type 1b. QJM 2000; 93:597-601.
12. Reyes GR, Purdy MA, Kim JP, et al. Isolation of a cDNA from the virus responsible for enterically transmitted non-A, non-B hepatitis. Science 1990; 247:1335-9.

13. Velazquez O, Stetler HC, Avila C, et al. Epidemic transmission of enterically transmitted non-A, non-B hepatitis in Mexico, 1986-1987. JAMA 1990; 263:3281-5.
14. Kwo PY, Schlauder GG, Carpenter HA, et al. Acute hepatitis E by a new isolate acquired in the United States. Mayo Clin Proc 1997; 72: 1133-6.
15. Tsega E, Hansson BG, Krawczynski K, Nordenfelt E. Acute sporadic viral hepatitis in Ethiopia: Causes, risk factors, and effects on pregnancy. Clin Infect Dis 1992; 14:961-5.
16. Khuroo MS, Kamili S, Jameel S. Vertical transmission of hepatitis E virus. Lancet 1995; 345:1025-6.
17. Deka N, Sharma MD, Mukerjee R. Isolation of the novel agent from human stool samples that is associated with sporadic non-A, non-B hepatitis. J Virol 1994; 68:7810-5.
18. Linnen J, Wages J, Zhang Keck ZY, et al. Molecular cloning and disease association of hepatitis G virus: a transfusion-transmissible agent. Science 1996; 271:505-8.
19. Alter HJ, Nakatsuji Y, Melpolder J, et al. The incidence of transfusion-associated hepatitis G virus infection and its relation to liver disease. N Engl J Med 1997; 336:747-54.
20. Zanetti AR, Tanzi E, Romano L, et al. Multicenter trial on mother-to-infant transmission of GBV-C virus. The Lombardy Study Group on Vertical/Perinatal Hepatitis Viruses Transmission. J Med Virol 1998; 54:107-12.
21. Inaba N, Okajima Y, Kang XS, et al. Maternal-infant transmission of hepatitis G virus. Am J Obstet Gynecol 1997; 177:1537-8.
22. Pessoa MG, Terrault NA, Detmer J, et al. Quantitation of hepatitis G and C viruses in the liver: evidence that hepatitis G virus is not hepatotropic. Hepatology 1998; 27:877-80.
23. Smithwick EM, Pascual E, Go SC. Hepatitis-associated antigen: A possible relationship to premature delivery. J Pediatr 1972; 81:537-40.
24. Stoller A, Collmann RD. Incidence of infective hepatitis followed by Down's syndrome nine months later. Lancet 1965; 2:1221-3.
25. Beasley RP, Trepo C, Stevens CE, Szmuness W. The e antigen and vertical transmission of hepatitis B surface antigen. Am J Epidemiol 1977; 105:94-8.
26. Agha S, Sherif LS, Allam MA, Fawzy M. Transplacental transmission of hepatitis C virus in HIV-negative mothers. Res Virol 1998; 149: 229-34.
27. American College of Obstetricians and Gynecologists. Hepatitis in Pregnancy. ACOG Technical Bulletin Number 174, November 1992. (Int J Gynecol Obstet 1993; 42:189-98).
28. Advisory Committee on Immunization Practices (ACIP). Prevention of hepatitis A through active or passive immunization. MMWR Recomm Rep 1999; 48(RR-12):1-37.
29. Centers for Disease Control and Prevention. 1998 Guidelines for Treatment of Sexually Transmitted Diseases. MMWR Recomm Rep 1998; 47(RR-1):1-111.
30. American College of Obstetricians and Gynecologists (ACOG). Viral Hepatitis in Pregnancy. ACOG Educational Bulletin Number 248, July 1998. (Int J Gynecol Obstet 1998; 63:195-202).
31. Lin HH, Kao JH, Hsu HY, et al. Least microtransfusion from mother to fetus in elective cesarean delivery. Obstet Gynecol 1996; 87:244-8.
32. Lee SD, Lo KJ, Tsai YT, et al. Role of caesarean section in prevention of mother-infant transmission of hepatitis B virus. Lancet 1988; 2:833-4.
33. Schalm SW, Pit-Grosheide P. Prevention of hepatitis B transmission at birth (letter). Lancet 1989; 1:44.
34. Keeffe EB, Hollinger FB. Therapy of hepatitis C: consensus interferon trials. Consensus Interferon Study Group. Hepatology 1997; 26:101S-7S.
35. Ruggiero G, Andreana A, Zampino R. Normal pregnancy under inadvertent alpha-interferon therapy for chronic hepatitis C. J Hepatol 1996; 24:646.
36. Ozaslan E, Yilmaz R, Simsek H, Tatar G. Interferon therapy for acute hepatitis C during pregnancy. Ann Pharmacother 2002; 36:1715-8.
37. Hunt CM, Carson KL, Sharara AI. Hepatitis C in pregnancy. Obstet Gynecol 1997; 89:883-90.
38. Gonzalez MC, Reyes H, Arrese M, et al. Intrahepatic cholestasis of pregnancy in twin pregnancies. J Hepatol 1989; 9:84-90.
39. Davies MH, Ngong JM, Yucesoy M, et al. The adverse influence of pregnancy upon sulphation: a clue to the pathogenesis of intrahepatic cholestasis of pregnancy? J Hepatol 1994; 21:1127-34.
40. Rolfes DB, Ishak KG. Liver disease in pregnancy. Histopathology 1986; 10:555-70.
41. Reyes H, Radrigan ME, Gonzalez MC, et al. Steatorrhea in patients with intrahepatic cholestasis of pregnancy. Gastroenterology 1987; 93:584-90.
42. Fisk NM, Bye WB, Storey GN. Maternal features of obstetric cholestasis: 20 years experience at King George V Hospital. Aust N Z J Obstet Gynaecol 1988; 28:172-6.
43. Germain AM, Carvajal JA, Glasinovic JC, et al. Intrahepatic cholestasis of pregnancy: an intriguing pregnancy-specific disorder. J Soc Gynecol Investig 2002; 9:10-4.
44. Mullally BA, Hansen WF. Intrahepatic cholestasis of pregnancy: Review of the literature. Obstet Gynecol Surv 2002; 57:47-52.
45. Fisk NM, Storey GN. Fetal outcome in obstetric cholestasis. Br J Obstet Gynaecol 1988; 95:1137-43.
46. Rioseco AJ, Ivankovic MB, Manzur A, et al. Intrahepatic cholestasis of pregnancy: a retrospective case-control study of perinatal outcome. Am J Obstet Gynecol 1994; 170:890-5.
47. Israel EJ, Guzman ML, Campos GA. Maximal response to oxytocin of the isolated myometrium from pregnant patients with intrahepatic cholestasis. Acta Obstet Gynecol Scand 1986; 65:581-2.
48. Sadler LC, Lane M, North R. Severe fetal intracranial haemorrhage during treatment with cholestyramine for intrahepatic cholestasis of pregnancy. Br J Obstet Gynaecol 1995; 102:169-70.
49. Marpeau L, Chazouilliere O, Rhimi Z, et al. Pregnancy-associated idiopathic intrahepatic cholestasis. Hypotheses of physiopathology: a therapeutic case report. Fetal Diagn Ther 1991; 6:120-5.
50. Floreani A, Paternoster D, Melis A, Grella PV. S-adenosylmethionine versus ursodeoxycholic acid in the treatment of intrahepatic cholestasis of pregnancy: preliminary results of a controlled trial. Eur J Obstet Gynecol Reprod Biol 1996; 67:109-13.
51. Diaferia A, Nicastri PL, Tartagni M, et al. Ursodeoxycholic acid therapy in pregnant women with cholestasis. Int J Gynaecol Obstet 1996; 52:133-40.
52. Berkane N, Cocheton JJ, Brehier D, et al. Ursodeoxycholic acid in intrahepatic cholestasis of pregnancy. A retrospective study of 19 cases. Acta Obstet Gynecol Scand 2000; 79:941-6.
53. Tarnier M. Note sur l'état graisseux du foie dans la fièvre puérperale. C R Mem Soc Biol (Paris) 1856; 3:209-14.
54. Stander HJ, Cadden JF. Acute yellow atrophy of the liver in pregnancy. Am J Obstet Gynecol 1934; 28:61-9.
55. Haemmerli UP. Jaundice during pregnancy: With special emphasis on recurrent jaundice during pregnancy and its differential diagnosis. Acta Med Scand 1966; 4444:1-111.
56. Kaplan MM. Acute fatty liver of pregnancy. N Engl J Med 1985; 313:367-70.
57. Castro MA, Fassett MJ, Reynolds TB, et al. Reversible peripartum liver failure: A new perspective on the diagnosis, treatment, and cause of acute fatty liver of pregnancy, based on 28 consecutive cases. Am J Obstet Gynecol 1999; 181:389-95.
58. Rinaldo P, Treem WR, Riely CA. Liver disease in pregnancy. N Engl J Med 1997; 336:377-8.
59. Davidson KM, Simpson LL, Knox TA, D'Alton ME. Acute fatty liver of pregnancy in triplet gestation. Obstet Gynecol 1998; 91:806-8.
60. Riely CA. Acute fatty liver of pregnancy. Semin Liver Dis 1987; 7:47-54.
61. Minakami H, Oka N, Sato T, et al. Preeclampsia: a microvesicular fat disease of the liver? Am J Obstet Gynecol 1988; 159:1043-7.
62. Tyni T, Ekholm E, Pihko H. Pregnancy complications are frequent in long-chain 3-hydroxyacyl-coenzyme A dehydrogenase deficiency. Am J Obstet Gynecol 1998; 178:603-8.
63. Rolfes DB, Ishak KG. Acute fatty liver of pregnancy: a clinicopathologic study of 35 cases. Hepatology 1985; 5:1149-58.
64. Kunelis CT, Peters JL, Edmondson HA. Fatty liver of pregnancy and its relationship to tetracycline therapy. Am J Med 1965; 33:427-40.
65. Pockros PJ, Reynolds TB. Acute fatty liver of pregnancy. Dig Dis Sci 1985; 30:601-2.
66. Moise KJ, Shah DM. Acute fatty liver of pregnancy: Etiology of fetal distress and fetal wastage. Obstet Gynecol 1987; 69:482-5.
67. Watson WJ, Seeds JW. Acute fatty liver of pregnancy. Obstet Gynecol Surv 1990; 45:585-91.
68. Visconti M, Manes G, Giannattasio F, Uomo G. Recurrence of acute fatty liver of pregnancy. J Clin Gastroenterol 1995; 21:243-5.
69. MacLean MA, Cameron AD, Cumming GP, et al. Recurrence of acute fatty liver of pregnancy. Br J Obstet Gynaecol 1994; 101:453-4.
70. Barton JR, Sibai BM, Mabie WC, Shanklin DR. Recurrent acute fatty liver of pregnancy. Am J Obstet Gynecol 1990; 163:534-8.
71. Ockner SA, Brunt EM, Cohn SM, et al. Fulminant hepatic failure caused by acute fatty liver of pregnancy treated by orthotopic liver transplantation. Hepatology 1990; 11:59-64.
72. Amon E, Allen SR, Petrie RH, Belew JE. Acute fatty liver of pregnancy associated with preeclampsia: management of hepatic failure with postpartum liver transplantation. Am J Perinatol 1991; 8:278-9.
73. Franco J, Newcomer J, Adams M, Saeian K. Auxiliary liver transplant in acute fatty liver of pregnancy. Obstet Gynecol 2000; 95:1042.
74. Doepel M, Backas HN, Taskinen EI, et al. Spontaneous recovery of postpartum liver necrosis in a patient listed for transplantation. Hepatogastroenterology 1996; 43:1084-7.

75. Bis KA, Waxman B. Rupture of the liver associated with pregnancy: a review of the literature and report of 2 cases. Obstet Gynecol Surv 1976; 31:763-73.

76. Minuk GY, Lui RC, Kelly JK. Rupture of the liver associated with acute fatty liver of pregnancy. Am J Gastroenterol 1987; 82:457-60.

77. Herbert WN, Brenner WE. Improving survival with liver rupture complicating pregnancy. Am J Obstet Gynecol 1982; 142:530-4.

78. Manas KJ, Welsh JD, Rankin RA, Miller DD. Hepatic hemorrhage without rupture in preeclampsia. N Engl J Med 1985; 312:424-6.

79. Loevinger EH, Vujic I, Lee WM, Anderson MC. Hepatic rupture associated with pregnancy: Treatment with transcatheter embolotherapy. Obstet Gynecol 1985; 65:281-4.

80. Terasaki KK, Quinn MF, Lundell CJ, et al. Spontaneous hepatic hemorrhage in preeclampsia: Treatment with hepatic arterial embolization. Radiology 1990; 174:1039-41.

81. Hunter SK, Martin M, Benda JA, Zlatnik FJ. Liver transplant after massive spontaneous hepatic rupture in pregnancy complicated by preeclampsia. Obstet Gynecol 1995; 85:819-22.

82. Cundy TF, O Grady JG, Williams R. Recovery of menstruation and pregnancy after liver transplantation. Gut 1990; 31:337-8.

83. Boyer TD. Cirrhosis of the liver and its major sequelae. In: Wyngaarden JB, Smith LH, Bennett JC, eds. Cecil Textbook of Medicine. Philadelphia: WB Saunders, 1992:786-96.

84. Kerr MG, Scott DB, Samuel E. Studies of the inferior vena cava in late pregnancy. Br Med J 1964; 1:532-3.

85. Schreyer P, Caspi E, El Hindi JM, Eshchar J. Cirrhosis. Pregnancy and delivery: A review. Obstet Gynecol Surv 1982; 37:304-12.

86. Britton RC. Pregnancy and esophageal varices. Am J Surg 1982; 143:421-5.

87. Kochhar R, Kumar S, Goel RC, et al. Pregnancy and its outcome in patients with noncirrhotic portal hypertension. Dig Dis Sci 1999; 44:1356-61.

88. Kochhar R, Goenka MK, Mehta SK. Endoscopic sclerotherapy during pregnancy. Am J Gastroenterol 1990; 85:1132-5.

89. Pauzner D, Wolman I, Niv D, et al. Endoscopic sclerotherapy in extrahepatic portal hypertension in pregnancy. Am J Obstet Gynecol 1991; 164:152-3.

90. Zeeman GG, Moise KJ. Prophylactic banding of severe esophageal varices associated with liver cirrhosis in pregnancy. Obstet Gynecol 1999; 94:842.

91. Rossle M, Haag K, Ochs A, et al. The transjugular intrahepatic portosystemic stent-shunt procedure for variceal bleeding. N Engl J Med 1994; 330:165-71.

92. Conn HO. Transjugular intrahepatic portosystemic shunts versus sclerotherapy: A discussion of discordant results. Ann Intern Med 1997; 126:907-10.

93. Wildberger JE, Vorwerk D, Winograd R, et al. New TIPS placement in pregnancy in recurrent esophageal varices hemorrhage: Assessment of fetal radiation exposure. Rofo Fortschr Geb Rontgenstr Neuen Bildgeb Verfahr 1998; 169:429-31.

94. Pajor A, Lehoczky D. Pregnancy and extrahepatic portal hypertension. Review and report on the management. Gynecol Obstet Invest 1990; 30:193-7.

95. Scantlebury V, Gordon R, Tzakis A, et al. Childbearing after liver transplantation. Transplantation 1990; 49:317-21.

96. Riely CA. Contraception and pregnancy after liver transplantation. Liver Transpl 2001; 7:S74-6.

97. Eguchi S, Yanaga K, Fujita F, et al. Living-related right lobe liver transplantation for a patient with fulminant hepatic failure during the second trimester of pregnancy: Report of a case. Transplantation 2002; 73:1970-1.

98. Casele HL, Laifer SA. Association of pregnancy complications and choice of immunosuppressant in liver transplant patients. Transplantation 1998; 65:581-3.

99. Ville Y, Fernandez H, Samuel D, et al. Pregnancy in liver transplant recipients: course and outcome in 19 cases. Am J Obstet Gynecol 1993; 168:896-902.

100. Armenti VT, Radomski JS, Moritz MJ, et al. Report from the National Transplantation Pregnancy Registry (NTPR): Outcomes of pregnancy after transplantation. Clin Transpl 2001:97-105.

101. Nagy S, Bush MC, Berkowitz R, et al. Pregnancy outcome in liver transplant recipients. Obstet Gynecol 2003; 102:121-8.

102. Gelman S. Anesthesia and the liver. In: Barash PG, Cullen BF, Stoelting RK, eds. Clinical Anesthesia. Philadelphia: JB Lippincott, 1992:1185-214.

103. Scharschmidt BF. Acute and chronic hepatic failure. In: Wyngaarden JB, Smith LH, Bennett JC, eds. Cecil Textbook of Medicine. Philadelphia: WB Saunders, 1992:796-9.

104. Gelman SI. Disturbances in hepatic blood flow during anesthesia and surgery. Arch Surg 1976; 111:881-3.

105. Frink EJ, Morgan SE, Coetzee A, et al. The effects of sevoflurane, halothane, enflurane, and isoflurane on hepatic blood flow and oxygenation in chronically instrumented greyhound dogs. Anesthesiology 1992; 76:85-90.

106. Kanaya N, Iwasaki H, Namiki A. Noninvasive ICG clearance test for estimating hepatic blood flow during halothane and isoflurane anaesthesia. Can J Anaesth 1995; 42:209-12.

107. McLain GE, Sipes IG, Brown BR. An animal model of halothane hepatotoxicity: roles of enzyme induction and hypoxia. Anesthesiology 1979; 51:321-6.

108. Ross WT, Daggy BP, Cardell RR. Hepatic necrosis caused by halothane and hypoxia in phenobarbital-treated rats. Anesthesiology 1979; 51:327-33.

109. Greene NM. Anesthesia risk factors in patients with liver disease. Contemp Anesth Pract 1981; 4:87-109.

110. Kennedy WF, Everett GB, Cobb LA, Allen GD. Simultaneous systemic and hepatic hemodynamic measurements during high peridural anesthesia in normal man. Anesth Analg 1971; 50:1069-77.

111. Kennedy WF, Everett GB, Cobb LA, Allen GD. Simultaneous systemic and hepatic hemodynamic measurements during high spinal anesthesia in normal man. Anesth Analg 1970; 49:1016-24.

112. Tanaka N, Nagata N, Hamakawa T, Takasaki M. The effect of dopamine on hepatic blood flow in patients undergoing epidural anesthesia. Anesth Analg 1997; 85:286-90.

113. Thomson PD, Melmon KL, Richardson JA, et al. Lidocaine pharmacokinetics in advanced heart failure, liver disease, and renal failure in humans. Ann Intern Med 1973; 78:499-508.

114. Heriot JA, Steven CM, Sattin RS. Elective forceps delivery and extradural anaesthesia in a primigravida with portal hypertension and oesophageal varices. Br J Anaesth 1996; 76:325-7.

Chapter 46
Malignant Hyperthermia

M. Joanne Douglas, M.D., FRCPC

Malignant hyperthermia (MH) is an inherited disorder of skeletal muscle. On exposure to triggering agents (e.g., succinylcholine, volatile halogenated anesthetic agents), affected individuals develop a hypermetabolic syndrome characterized by muscle rigidity, hypercapnia, acidosis, arrhythmias, and hyperthermia. MH was first described in 1960 by Denborough and Lovell[1] but may have been responsible for some of the earlier deaths attributed to ether and chloroform anesthesia.[2]

EPIDEMIOLOGY

Ording[3] reviewed the incidence of MH in Denmark and noted that the incidence of the fulminant syndrome (e.g., muscle rigidity, acidosis, hyperkalemia, arrhythmias, hyperthermia, increased creatine kinase [CK] levels, myoglobinuria) was 1 in 220,000 patients who received general anesthesia, and 1 in 62,000 when succinylcholine was combined with a volatile halogenated agent. MH (either mild or fulminant) was suspected in 1 in 16,000 patients who received anesthesia of any type. The male to female ratio was 1.4:1.[3] There is some geographic variation in the incidence of MH.

There are few reports of MH developing during pregnancy and parturition.[4-10] The infrequent occurrence during pregnancy probably reflects both the low frequency of this disorder in the general population and the widespread use of local and regional anesthetic techniques in obstetric patients.

PATHOPHYSIOLOGY

MH is the result of a disorder in the regulation of calcium in skeletal muscle. In MH-susceptible pigs the ryanodine receptor is the calcium-release channel of the sarcoplasmic reticulum.[11] The ryanodine receptor is a protein that spans the gap between the terminal cisternae of the sarcoplasmic reticulum and the transverse tubule.[12,13] When an electrical impulse sets off a wave of depolarization down the T tubule, it causes the ryanodine receptor to open up channels, allowing calcium to escape into the myoplasm.[14] This binds troponin, allowing actin and myosin filaments to interact, resulting in contraction.

In the muscle of MH-susceptible patients, the activation threshold for the release of sarcoplasmic calcium is reduced. In the presence of volatile halogenated agents an increased release of calcium from the sarcoplasmic reticulum[15,16] and activation of the actin-myosin contraction system occur, causing an augmentation of contraction. This process is accompanied by the use of energy (adenosine triphosphate [ATP]), increased oxygen consumption, and increased production of carbon dioxide, lactate, and heat. When the heat within the muscle cannot be dispersed, irreversible contracture results. Ultimately, breakdown of the muscle cell and the release of CK, potassium, and myoglobin occur. Increased hormone-sensitive lipase activity in the mitochondria may augment calcium release, leading to calcium-induced calcium release, which further increases contraction.[17,18] Dantrolene inhibits excitation-contraction coupling, and succinylcholine, caffeine, and volatile halogenated agents increase it.

Wappler et al.[19] recently suggested that the 5-hydroxytryptamine (5-HT) system might be involved in the development of MH. In vivo and in vitro experiments using 5-HT agonists and antagonists demonstrated that 5-HT agonists may initiate MH in MH-susceptible pigs and humans. The precise mechanism is unknown.[19]

GENETICS

MH is a heterogeneous disorder with more than one gene defect responsible for production of the clinical syndrome.[20,21] It is inherited in an autosomal dominant fashion with variable penetrance, although this has been questioned in some families.[22] Porcine MH is transmitted as a recessive gene. The defective gene in MH-susceptible pigs has been localized to the glucose phosphate isomerase locus,[23] close to the site of

the ryanodine receptor gene responsible for the calcium-release channel.[24]

Investigators have demonstrated a defect in a similar region in some families with MH (chromosome 19q12.1-13.2, MHS-1), and several mutations have been linked to MH susceptibility.[25] Central core disease, a myopathy associated with MH, has been mapped to a similar region,[26] but this is being questioned.[25] Mutations responsible for MH in some families are located on chromosomes 5p, 17, 7q, 3q and 1q.[25] Other myopathies may be characterized by a hyperthermic state with muscle damage and metabolic derangements similar to MH, but their chromosomal abnormality has not been mapped to the same area.[27-31]

TRIGGERS

Known triggers of MH include the depolarizing muscle relaxants (e.g., succinylcholine) and all the volatile halogenated anesthetic agents (i.e., halothane, enflurane, isoflurane, desflurane, sevoflurane) (Box 46-1). The dose and duration of exposure to the triggering agent may influence the onset and severity of a reaction. Previous uneventful general anesthesia with triggering anesthetic agents does not rule out the diagnosis of MH.[32,33]

In contrast to the porcine model, reports of stress-induced MH in humans are rare.[34-36] The sympathetic nervous system is active during an episode of acute MH, but there is insufficient evidence to implicate increased sympathetic activity as a cause in humans. Muscle biopsy testing helps distinguish MH from exercise-induced myolysis, exertional heat stroke, and other myopathies.[36-39] However, evidence is accumulating that some cases of heat stroke and exercise-induced rhabdomyolysis are linked to MH susceptibility.[40-42]

Investigators have explored other possible triggers of MH both in the porcine model and in humans. No evidence suggests that exogenous calcium,[43] digoxin,[43] hypercarbia,[43] potassium,[43] or norepinephrine[44] triggers MH. Exercise[45] and environmental temperature[46-48] may intensify an existing reaction or modify a developing reaction. Sodium thiopental[49] and pancuronium[50] delay the onset in pigs and may modify the reaction in humans.

There are case reports of MH occurring during regional anesthesia and non-triggering general anesthesia.[37,51-54] The cases that occurred during regional anesthesia appeared mild and responded readily to treatment. In some cases, however, the diagnosis was not confirmed with muscle biopsy or appropriate laboratory investigation at the time of the event.

CLINICAL PRESENTATION

Individuals who are MH-susceptible may develop the fulminant syndrome when anesthetized with a triggering agent. During an acute episode, the diagnosis is based on the finding of an elevated end-tidal CO_2 concentration, muscle rigidity (generalized and/or masseter), respiratory and metabolic acidosis, and rhabdomyolysis, which causes an elevated concentration of CK, hyperkalemia, and myoglobinuria. Hypoxemia, unstable blood pressure, and evidence of sympathetic hyperactivity (e.g., tachycardia, arrhythmias) are other signs. Hyperthermia may occur early, but often it is a late sign (Box 46-2). Perioperative rhabdomyolysis, without any of the previously mentioned clinical signs, also may indicate MH susceptibility.[55,56]

With the advent of routine end-tidal CO_2 monitoring, MH may be detected early, often before the development of rhabdomyolysis and hyperthermia.[57] This may lead to uncertainty about the clinical diagnosis of MH, given that many of the confirmatory signs and laboratory abnormalities may be absent during the early phase of MH. Thus, this could present a dilemma as to whether these patients should undergo diagnostic muscle biopsy.

Masseter Muscle Rigidity

Masseter muscle rigidity is one of the early signs of MH.[58] The masseter muscles are sensitive to the action of succinylcholine and respond with increased tension in normal individuals.[59,60] Often this increased tension is imperceptible, but in some patients it is impossible to open the mouth for laryngoscopy and intubation. The duration of rigidity parallels the duration of action of succinylcholine. Typically there is no difficulty with mask ventilation. Masseter muscle rigidity rarely occurs after the use of nondepolarizing muscle relaxants such as vecuronium, atracurium, and mivacurium.[61] Patients with myopathies and other neuromuscular disorders also may present with masseter muscle rigidity after the administration of succinylcholine.[29,62]

If masseter muscle rigidity is accompanied by generalized rigidity, anesthesia should be discontinued, dantrolene should be administered, and the patient should be monitored closely.[63] However, there is controversy regarding the management of isolated masseter muscle rigidity.[64] Options include (1) discontinuation of the anesthetic agents and administration of dantrolene; (2) continuation of anesthesia with non-

---

Box 46-1 TRIGGERS FOR MH

FACTORS KNOWN TO TRIGGER MH

- Volatile anesthetic agents
  - Halothane
  - Enflurane
  - Isoflurane
  - Desflurane
  - Sevoflurane
- Succinylcholine

FACTORS THAT DO NOT TRIGGER MH IN SWINE

- Exogenous calcium
- Digoxin
- Hypercarbia
- Potassium
- Norepinephrine

Box 46-2 SIGNS AND SYMPTOMS OF MH

- Tachycardia
- Tachypnea
- Masseter spasm
- Generalized rigidity
- Elevated end-tidal CO_2 concentration
- Cyanosis
- Arrhythmia
- Acidosis
- Hyperkalemia
- Hyperpyrexia
- Myoglobinuria
- Increased CK level

triggering, "safe" agents and close attention to the end-tidal CO_2 concentration; and (3) continuation of anesthesia with triggering agents and careful monitoring. In my judgment, the anesthesiologist should either discontinue anesthesia altogether or continue anesthesia with nontriggering agents. If the anesthesiologist continues anesthesia, the end-tidal CO_2 concentration, electrocardiogram (ECG), temperature, and arterial blood gases should be monitored. The anesthesiologist also should look for evidence of rhabdomyolysis by monitoring CK levels and looking for myoglobinuria and should recommend that the patient undergo muscle biopsy.[65]

DIAGNOSIS

Several authors[66-68] have correlated clinical presentation (i.e., evidence of metabolic and muscle derangements) with muscle biopsy results. The greater the number of clinical signs or abnormal laboratory findings, the greater the risk of MH (Table 46-1).[66] An early assessment of the risk of MH allows the anesthesiologist to initiate appropriate treatment. The mortality rate for MH is as high as 80% without dantrolene therapy.[69] Early administration of dantrolene lowers the mortality rate to 4%.[69]

An international group of experts has developed a clinical grading scale to predict MH susceptibility.[70] This scale consists of six processes (rigidity, muscle breakdown, respiratory acidosis, temperature increase, cardiac involvement, family history) and their clinical indicators. Points are assigned for each indicator and the total represents a raw score. A rank subsequently is assigned to this score, which indicates the likelihood of the patient developing MH.

TABLE 46-1	RISK OF MH WITH ASSOCIATED SIGNS AND SYMPTOMS	
Type	**Symptoms/signs**	**Risk**
Fulminant/classic	Metabolic acidosis Muscle rigidity Hyperthermia (> 38.5° C) Arrhythmias Hyperkalemia Myoglobinuria Increased CK level	0.96
Moderate	Inconclusive signs of MH involving metabolic and muscle abnormalities, with MH the probable diagnosis	0.88
Mild	Signs of metabolic derangement (pH > 7.3, body core temperature ≤ 38.5° C)	0.14
Masseter spasm with rhabdomyolysis	CK level > 1500, myoglobinuria	0.76
Masseter spasm with signs of metabolic disturbance	Arrhythmias, rising core temperature	0.57
Masseter spasm only		0.28
Unexplained perioperative death or cardiac arrest		0.66
Other	Postoperative pyrexia or rhabdomyolysis	0.07

Data from Ellis FR, Halsall PJ, Christian AS. Clinical presentation of suspected malignant hyperthermia during anaesthesia in 402 probands. Anaesthesia 1990; 45:838-41.

TESTING

Susceptibility to MH is determined by a positive caffeine-halothane contracture test. During this test, fresh muscle is exposed to halothane and caffeine, and the degree of contraction is measured. The caffeine-halothane contracture test has been standardized in MH units throughout North America (the North American protocol)[71] and Europe (the European protocol).[72] This test is the "gold standard" for the diagnosis of MH. The sensitivity and specificity of the North American protocol are 97% and 78%, respectively.[73] Some false-positive results may occur.[74] Patients with a negative caffeine-halothane contracture test subsequently have received anesthesia with triggering agents without incident.[75-77] Some centers now add ryanodine or 4-chloro-m-cresol to the test to increase its accuracy.[78]

Other centers are investigating the use of nuclear magnetic resonance spectroscopy as a noninvasive screening test for MH. Early acidosis and decreased phosphocreatine content occur during graded exercise in MH-susceptible patients.[79] Some of these changes occur with myopathies other than MH, and the investigators have emphasized that further studies are needed to determine whether this technology is suitable for screening for MH susceptibility.

In the absence of muscle biopsy results, a parturient with a positive family history should be treated as if she were MH susceptible.

PREGNANCY AND MH

In 1972, Crawford[80] wondered "whether or not there was a record of a pregnant or newly born patient or animal having developed hyperpyrexia and . . . whether hyperpyrexia has been encountered in a patient undergoing an operation under regional block anesthesia." Subsequently there have been few reports of MH during parturition and fewer reports of maternal mortality attributable to MH. Wadhwa[4] reported a fatality in a woman with a known family history of MH, who developed muscle rigidity during twilight sleep for parturition. Douglas et al.[5] subsequently reported one fatal case of MH in a parturient undergoing general anesthesia for cesarean section.

There are three published reports of nonfatal MH during cesarean section. The triggering agents were succinylcholine and halothane,[6] cyclopropane,[7] and succinylcholine alone (without a volatile halogenated agent).[8] There are several reports of the successful administration of epidural anesthesia during labor and cesarean section in MH-susceptible parturients.[4,81-89]

The rarity of these events suggests that pregnancy protects against the occurrence of MH. However, it also may reflect the widespread use of regional anesthesia for labor, vaginal delivery, and cesarean section.

Maternal Physiology

Basal metabolic rate, oxygen consumption, and minute ventilation increase during pregnancy.[90] Serum bicarbonate, buffer base, and base excess decrease to maintain normal pH. Thus the pregnant patient typically has a compensated respiratory alkalosis. The decreased buffering capacity could adversely affect the pregnant woman during an episode of MH.

Oxygen consumption and minute ventilation increase further during labor.[91] Maternal lactate and pyruvate concentrations increase steadily during labor, indicating an increase in

both aerobic and anaerobic metabolism.[92] Hyperventilation during contractions may result in periods of hypoventilation between contractions, which may adversely affect the PaO_2 of both the mother and fetus. These metabolic and physiologic responses to pain are similar to those that occur during MH. Effective epidural analgesia decreases oxygen consumption and minute ventilation.[91] If tachycardia and hyperventilation occur despite effective analgesia, they are more likely to signal an episode of MH.

Aortocaval compression from the pregnant uterus results in decreased cardiac output, hypotension, and decreased uteroplacental perfusion. Thus aortocaval compression may accelerate the occurrence of acidosis during an episode of MH. Aortocaval compression hinders resuscitative efforts during cardiac arrest,[93,94] and evacuation of the uterus (i.e., delivery of the fetus) facilitates maternal resuscitation. The same may be true during an episode of MH. The obstetrician may need to deliver the fetus to facilitate maternal resuscitation during a fulminant case of MH.

CK concentrations are not diagnostic of MH. During pregnancy, there is a slight decrease in CK levels during the first trimester. CK levels remain stable until term, when they increase by approximately 50%. At delivery, there is an abrupt increase in the CK concentration, followed by a return to normal by 6 weeks postpartum (Figure 46-1 and Table 46-2).[95] The increased CK concentration results from increases in both the CK-M fraction (skeletal muscle) and the CK-B fractions (myometrium, placenta, and fetal blood). Postpartum CK levels are higher in nulliparous patients, regardless of differences in length of labor.[96] Mean plasma CK activity is approximately 50% higher in African-Americans than in Caucasians or Asians.[95]

Acute cocaine toxicity may mimic MH. Although cocaine does not induce contractures in MH-susceptible muscle,[97] elevated CK levels and myoglobinemia can occur secondary to rhabdomyolysis and renal failure from cocaine intoxication.[98] Umbilical cord blood CK and myoglobin levels are elevated when cocaine metabolites are present in maternal urine.[99]

Effects on the Fetus and Newborn

MH often is inherited as an autosomal dominant gene. In these cases, there is a 50% chance that the infant of an MH-susceptible parent also will be MH susceptible. All anesthetic agents cross the placenta. Small quantities of succinylcholine also cross the placenta. This knowledge should prompt the anesthesiologist to question the choice of anesthetic agents for an MH-negative mother whose fetus has an MH-susceptible father. In this situation, the anesthesiologist should avoid the use of triggering agents until after delivery.

There is only one published report of suspected MH in a newborn.[100] The condition is rare in infancy, and some reports of infant MH may represent an undiagnosed myopathy.[62,101,102]

MANAGEMENT OF THE MH-SUSCEPTIBLE PARTURIENT

Ideally, an anesthesiologist evaluates every MH-susceptible patient before hospitalization for labor and delivery. Clearly, the obstetrician should consult an anesthesiologist immediately after the admission of each MH-susceptible patient. All hospitals and birthing facilities should be prepared to provide care for MH-susceptible patients. Adequate supplies of dantrolene (at least 36 vials), sterile water, and sodium bicarbonate should be immediately available.

Analgesia for Labor

Soon after admission, a large-gauge intravenous catheter should be placed in each MH-susceptible patient. Maternal temperature, heart rate, and blood pressure should be monitored throughout labor. During early labor, it may be acceptable to monitor temperature and heart rate intermittently to facilitate maternal ambulation, if desired. Once active labor is established, frequent monitoring of the maternal heart rate and temperature should be initiated. Continuous ECG and axillary temperature monitoring are ideal once the parturient is confined to bed. (Measurement of axillary temperature allows placement of a temperature probe in close proximity to large muscle groups.) Of course, aortocaval compression should be avoided throughout labor and delivery.

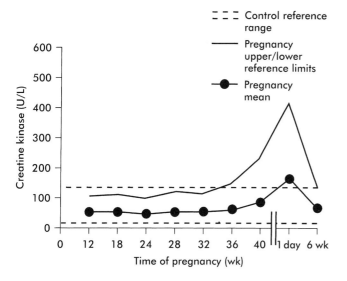

FIGURE 46-1. Changes in CK activity during and after pregnancy. (Modified from Lockitch G, editor. Handbook of Diagnostic Biochemistry and Hematology in Normal Pregnancy. Boca Raton, Fla, CRC Press, 1993:59.)

TABLE 46-2	GESTATIONAL CHANGES IN CK ACTIVITY		
	CK (U/L)		
Time of gestation	**Range**	**Mean (SD)**	**% of control**
Nonpregnant control	20-137	63 (31)	—
12 weeks	0-111	55 (28)	87
18 weeks	0-113	55 (29)	87
24 weeks	0-100	50 (25)	79
28 weeks	0-122	54 (34)	86
32 weeks	0-114	54 (30)	86
36 weeks	0-145	57 (44)	90
Term	0-227	85 (71)	135
1 day postpartum	0-410	162 (124)	257
6 weeks postpartum	0-139	63 (37)	100

SD, Standard deviation
From Lockitch G, editor. Handbook of Diagnostic Biochemistry and Hematology in Normal Pregnancy. Boca Raton, Fla, CRC Press, 1993:59.

Most agents that are used to provide intrapartum analgesia are considered safe for the MH-susceptible parturient (Table 46-3). Both the obstetrician and anesthesiologist should encourage the early administration of epidural analgesia. Relief of pain causes decreased maternal stress (as reflected by decreased catecholamine,[103] cortisol,[104] and adrenocorticotrophic hormone [ACTH] concentrations) and decreased maternal metabolism and oxygen consumption.[105] Although experts continue to debate the role of stress in human MH,[17] it is best to decrease stress when possible. Further, the anesthesiologist may extend epidural anesthesia for vaginal delivery or cesarean section if necessary. Extension of epidural anesthesia allows the anesthesiologist to avoid administration of general anesthesia.

All local anesthetic agents appear safe for MH-susceptible patients. Epinephrine can be safely added to the local anesthetic agent to improve the quality and duration of analgesia, if appropriate clinically.

Anesthesia for Cesarean Section

General anesthesia should be avoided for operative delivery. Spinal or epidural anesthesia can be safely given using either amide or ester local anesthetic agents. Spinal anesthesia entails a greater risk of hypotension, which requires treatment with adrenergic agents such as ephedrine. Ephedrine should be used as required, but it should be avoided during an acute episode of MH. In doses greater than those used clinically, ephedrine increases halothane-induced muscle contractures in vitro.[106] Epidural anesthesia may be preferred because slow induction of anesthesia and administration of an adequate volume of intravenous fluid decrease the risk of hypotension.

Rarely, the mother may refuse regional anesthesia. In other cases, regional anesthesia may be contraindicated (e.g., maternal hemorrhage, coagulopathy, dire fetal distress). When the anesthesiologist encounters an MH-susceptible parturient, a "clean" anesthesia machine and delivery circuit should be obtained or prepared. These can be prepared by replacing the carbon dioxide absorbent and the delivery tubing and purging the machine of residual anesthetic agent with a 10 L/min flow of oxygen through the circuit for 10 minutes.[107,108]

In cases of general anesthesia, the anesthesiologist should administer a nonparticulate antacid and perform adequate denitrogenation. Unless a difficult intubation is expected, the anesthesiologist should plan a rapid-sequence induction, with application of cricoid pressure. The anesthesiologist should administer nontriggering agents (Table 46-3 and Box 46-3). All commonly used induction agents (e.g., thiopental, ketamine, etomidate, propofol, midazolam) are safe in MH-susceptible patients. Succinylcholine and the volatile halogenated agents (e.g., halothane, enflurane, isoflurane, sevoflurane, and desflurane) are contraindicated. For intubation, a rapid onset (approximately 60 to 90 seconds) of

TABLE 46-3	COMMON ANESTHETIC DRUGS AND THEIR SAFETY IN MH-SUSCEPTIBLE WOMEN		
Drug	**Route**	**Use**	**Safe MH**
Local Anesthetic Agents			
Bupivacaine	Regional	Analgesia/anesthesia	Yes
Lidocaine	Regional	Analgesia/anesthesia	Yes
	Intravenous	Intubation/arrhythmia	Yes*
Ropivacaine	Regional	Analgesia/anesthesia	Yes
2-Chloroprocaine	Regional	Analgesia/anesthesia	Yes
Opioids			
Fentanyl	Regional, intravenous	Analgesia	Yes
Meperidine	Regional, intravenous	Analgesia	Yes
Morphine	Regional, intravenous	Analgesia	Yes
Induction Agents			
Sodium thiopental	Intravenous	Induction	Yes
Propofol	Intravenous	Induction	Yes
Etomidate	Intravenous	Induction	Yes
Ketamine	Intravenous	Analgesia/induction	Yes
Benzodiazepines	Intravenous	Amnesia/anxiolysis	Yes
Neuromuscular Blocking Agents			
Succinylcholine	Intravenous	Muscle relaxation	No
Rocuronium	Intravenous	Muscle relaxation	Yes
Atracurium	Intravenous	Muscle relaxation	Yes
Vecuronium	Intravenous	Muscle relaxation	Yes
Pancuronium	Intravenous	Muscle relaxation	Yes
General Anesthetic Agents			
Halothane, enflurane, isoflurane, sevoflurane, desflurane	Inhalation	Anesthesia, uterine relaxation	No
Nitrous oxide	Inhalation	Analgesia/anesthesia	Yes

*Do not use during a crisis (see text).

muscle relaxation can be achieved with rocuronium (0.6 to 0.9 mg/kg, which is 2 to 3 times ED_{95}).[109] Other options are vecuronium (0.25 mg/kg)[110] or pancuronium (0.15 mg/kg). Nitrous oxide (delivered with a vapor-free machine), opioids, and propofol are safe agents for the maintenance of anesthesia. Midazolam administered after delivery provides amnesia. It is safe to reverse neuromuscular blockade with glycopyrrolate and neostigmine or edrophonium. Atropine may cause an increase in temperature, which could cause a diagnostic dilemma.

At delivery, maternal and umbilical cord blood gas and pH measurements should be determined. This may provide information regarding an impending reaction in either the mother or neonate. If uterine relaxation (tocolysis) is required to assist with delivery of the baby or to facilitate the removal of a retained placenta, I prefer to give 100-μg bolus doses of nitroglycerin intravenously[111]; its action is brief and easily reversed with oxytocin. Clearly, a volatile halogenated agent should *never* be given to effect uterine relaxation in an MH-susceptible patient.

Box 46-3 GENERAL ANESTHESIA FOR CESAREAN SECTION IN THE MH-SUSCEPTIBLE PATIENT

Monitors: end-tidal CO_2, pulse oximeter, ECG, automatic blood pressure, peripheral nerve stimulator, temperature (axillary and rectal or esophageal)

Induction: denitrogenation, rapid-sequence induction (thiopental 4 mg/kg, ketamine 1 mg/kg, propofol 2.0 to 2.5 mg/kg), intubation

Muscle relaxant: intubation: rocuronium 0.6 to 0.9 mg/kg; maintenance: rocuronium

Maintenance of anesthesia: nitrous oxide/oxygen, propofol, opioid

Amnesia: midazolam

Reversal of neuromuscular blockade: glycopyrrolate and neostigmine

---

Obstetric Drugs in MH-Susceptible Patients

Information on obstetric drugs is scant (Table 46-4). The beta-sympathomimetic tocolytic agents (e.g., ritodrine, terbutaline) produce anxiety and tachycardia in normal parturients. These side effects may be confused with MH, but these agents most likely are safe in the MH-susceptible parturient.

Magnesium sulfate attenuates but does not prevent MH in MH-susceptible swine.[112] There is one report of a fatal adverse interaction between dantrolene and the calcium entry-blocker diltiazem.[113] Administration of calcium entry-blockers most likely should be avoided during an episode of MH. These agents also do not prevent the development of MH.[114]

Oxytocin is safe. Some of the commercial preparations of oxytocin contain a preservative (chlorbutol) that has been shown to reverse the development of MH in susceptible pigs in vitro.[115] The ergot alkaloids cause vasoconstriction, which may cause decreased muscle perfusion and an increased tendency toward lactic acidosis. The prostaglandins may be associated with changes in blood pressure and maternal oxygen desaturation.[116] Prostaglandin E_2 also may cause pyrexia.[117] The routine postpartum administration of ergot alkaloids or prostaglandins most likely should not be performed in MH-susceptible patients. However, persistent uterine atony and postpartum hemorrhage may warrant the administration of either or both of these agents.

ASSESSMENT OF HYPERTHERMIA AND TACHYCARDIA

The hallmark signs of MH may be present during normal labor (Boxes 46-4 and 46-5). Other causes of fever and tachycardia in the MH-susceptible parturient should be excluded. Tachycardia and tachypnea are normal responses to pain, anxiety, and fever. Fever may be a sign of dehydration and infection. Pain and infection (e.g., chorioamnionitis, urinary tract infection) are much more common during parturition than MH. Normal par-

---

TABLE 46-4	DRUGS COMMONLY USED FOR LABOR AND DELIVERY AND THEIR SAFETY IN MH-SUSCEPTIBLE WOMEN		
Drug	**Route**	**Use**	**Safe**
Tocolytics			
Ritodrine	Intravenous	Tocolysis	Yes
Magnesium sulfate	Intravenous	Tocolysis, seizure prophylaxis	Yes
Nitroglycerin	Intravenous	Tocolysis, antihypertensive	Yes
Calcium entry-blockers	Intravenous	Tocolysis, antihypertensive	Yes*
Oxytocics			
Oxytocin	Intravenous	Uterine atony	Yes
Prostaglandin $F_{2-alpha}$	Intramuscular, intramyometrial	Uterine atony	†
Ergot alkaloids	Intramuscular	Uterine atony	†
Cardiovascular Drugs			
Ephedrine	Intravenous	Vasopressor	Yes*
Epinephrine	Intravenous, regional	Prolongation of regional block	Yes*
Beta-blockers	Oral, intravenous	Beta blockade	Yes
Antiemetics			
Droperidol	Intravenous	Prophylaxis, therapeutic	Yes
Metoclopramide	Intravenous	Prophylaxis, therapeutic	Yes

*Do not use during a crisis (see text).
†Inadequate information available.

Box 46-4 DIFFERENTIAL DIAGNOSIS OF FEVER DURING PARTURITION

- Infection: chorioamnionitis, urinary tract infection, other infections (e.g., influenza, viral illness)
- Environmental temperature
- Epidural anesthesia
- Dehydration/labor
- MH
- Drug reactions: cocaine, atropine, tricyclic antidepressants, monoamine oxidase (MAO) inhibitors, neuroleptic malignant syndrome, prostaglandins

---

Box 46-5 DIFFERENTIAL DIAGNOSIS OF TACHYCARDIA DURING PARTURITION

- Pain
- Fever
- Anxiety
- Blood loss
- Hypotension
- Drug reactions: cocaine, atropine, beta-adrenergic tocolytic agents
- MH

Box 46-6 MANAGEMENT OF MH CRISIS

1. Discontinue all triggering agents.
2. Hyperventilate with 100% oxygen. Disconnect vaporizers if possible. Change carbon dioxide absorbent and tubing when possible. (The machine does not have to be changed immediately.)
3. Administer dantrolene 2.5 mg/kg intravenously (up to 10 mg/kg).
4. Continue dantrolene until temperature, heart rate, and end-tidal CO_2 return to normal.
5. Perform serial blood gas measurements. Treat acidosis with sodium bicarbonate 1 to 2 mEq/kg.
6. Treat hyperkalemia with glucose and insulin.
7. Treat arrhythmias with procainamide. (Arrhythmias may not develop if dantrolene is administered early.)
8. Cool the patient (e.g., cold intravenous solutions, cooling blanket, lavage of body cavities with cold solutions).
9. Maintain urine output with fluids, mannitol, and/or furosemide.
10. Postoperatively, counsel the patient and refer her for muscle biopsy.

Modified from Malignant Hyperthermia Association of the United States and the North American Malignant Hyperthermia Registry. Updated technical bulletin for malignant hyperthermia. American Society of Anesthesiologists Newsletter, 1992; 56:30-1.

---

turients may have a gradual increase in temperature during epidural analgesia.[118] This may be accompanied by a corresponding increase in maternal and fetal heart rate.

The butyrophenones, phenothiazines, thioxanthenes, and other miscellaneous antipsychotic agents may produce tachycardia, fever, and rigidity (i.e., neuroleptic malignant syndrome [NMS]).[119] There is one published report of NMS in a pregnant woman.[120] Drugs capable of increasing serotonin in the central nervous system (serotonin reuptake inhibitors [SSRIs]) also can produce a hypermetabolic reaction. Cocaine intoxication produces severe vasoconstriction, fever, and rhabdomyolysis.[121]

TREATMENT

Box 46-6 summarizes the treatment of MH. All triggering agents must be stopped immediately, and the patient should be hyperventilated with 100% oxygen. The anesthetic tubing and carbon dioxide absorbent should be changed as soon as possible. The level of volatile agent decreases rapidly with flushing of the machine with 100% oxygen.[106,107] Therefore substitution with a vapor-free machine is not an immediate priority.

The anesthesiologist should give dantrolene intravenously in a dose of 2.5 mg/kg, up to a total dose of 10 mg/kg, until the signs (e.g., tachycardia, rigidity, fever) have subsided.[122] (There are case reports in which higher doses of dantrolene were required.) Oxygen saturation, end-tidal CO_2, ECG, blood pressure, arterial and venous blood gas measurements, core temperature, potassium levels, lactate concentration, CK levels, coagulation profile, urine output, and urine myoglobin should be monitored.

The anesthesiologist must initiate treatment of acidosis, hyperkalemia, arrhythmias, and hyperthermia. Metabolic acidosis is treated by giving sodium bicarbonate in 1- to 2-mEq/kg increments as guided by blood gas and pH measurements. The anesthesiologist should treat hyperkalemia by administration of bicarbonate, glucose, and insulin.

Early administration of dantrolene often prevents or successfully treats arrhythmias. If arrhythmias persist, pro-

cainamide is the treatment of choice. Calcium entry-blockers should be avoided because simultaneous administration of dantrolene and a calcium entry-blocker may precipitate cardiovascular collapse.

The anesthesiologist and obstetrician should actively cool the patient. Options include: (1) intravenous administration of iced saline (15 mL/kg three times, 15 minutes apart); (2) lavage of stomach, bladder, rectal, peritoneal, and thoracic cavities with iced saline; and (3) surface cooling with ice and/or a hypothermia blanket.

Myoglobin is excreted in the urine. Thus diuresis should be maintained by giving adequate volumes of crystalloid and furosemide 1 mg/kg and/or mannitol 0.25 g/kg (up to four doses of each drug intravenously). Mannitol is present in dantrolene, and separate administration of a diuretic agent may not be necessary.

After an acute episode of MH, postoperative administration of dantrolene (1 mg/kg or more intravenously every 4 to 6 hours for 24 to 48 hours) is recommended.[123] In addition, the patient should be monitored closely in an intensive care unit for at least 24 to 48 hours). Counseling and diagnostic muscle biopsy should be performed after recovery from the acute episode. The Malignant Hyperthermia Association of the United States (MHAUS) provides a registry and an informative newsletter for MH-susceptible patients. An MH hotline (800-MH-HYPER [800-644-9737] or, outside the United States, 315-464-7079) is available 24 hours a day to assist physicians with questions on treatment, diagnosis, and follow-up.

DANTROLENE IN PREGNANCY

Dantrolene is the drug of choice for the treatment of an MH crisis. It crosses the placenta and can be detected in the fetus after maternal administration.[124] Clinical doses do not adversely affect maternal or fetal cardiovascular and acid-base measurements in gravid ewes. After an infusion of 2.2 mg/kg/hr in an MH-susceptible parturient, Glassenberg and Cohen[87] reported a fetal-to-maternal ratio of 0.48. This is

similar to the fetal-to-maternal ratio reported by Morison[86] after prophylactic oral administration of dantrolene.

There is one published report of postpartum uterine atony after the administration of dantrolene.[9] Laboratory testing of the effects of dantrolene sodium on pregnant uterine muscle suggests that the relaxant effect is secondary to the mannitol.[125]

The anesthesiologist need not give prophylactic dantrolene to an MH-susceptible patient, especially when all triggering agents are avoided. The anesthesiologist should give dantrolene promptly when an MH crisis is suspected. Dantrolene crosses the placenta and may result in neonatal hypotonia if it is administered before delivery. A new preparation may allow easier mixing of dantrolene for injection.[126]

Fricker et al.[127] reported serial measurements of dantrolene concentrations in breast milk after administration of dantrolene in a patient with suspected MH during cesarean section (Figure 46-2). They estimated that the half-life of dantrolene in breast milk is approximately 9 hours. They concluded that "breast-feeding can be expected to be safe for the newborn 2 days after discontinuation of intravenous dantrolene administration in the mother."[127]

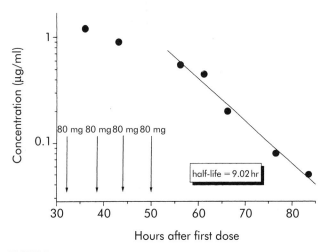

FIGURE 46-2. Estimation of half-life of dantrolene in breast milk by log-linear fitting of the terminal elimination phase (dantrolene measured in breast milk by HPLC, reverse-phase high-pressure liquid chromatographic column, by in-line ultraviolet absorption spectrometer; detection limit, 0.02 μg/ml). (From Fricker RM, Hoerauf KH, Drewe J, Kress HG. Secretion of dantrolene into breast milk after acute therapy of a suspected malignant hyperthermia crisis during cesarean section. Anesthesiology 1998; 89:1023-5.)

KEY POINTS

- The anesthesiologist may extend epidural anesthesia and thus avoid administration of general anesthesia for emergency cesarean section.
- All local anesthetic agents are safe in MH-susceptible patients.
- Intravenous administration of dantrolene is the treatment of choice for an MH crisis.
- Dantrolene crosses the placenta and may result in neonatal hypotonia.
- Dantrolene may cause uterine atony.
- The anesthesiologist need not administer dantrolene prophylactically to MH-susceptible parturients.

KEY POINTS

- MH is a heterogeneous disorder of skeletal muscle with variable clinical expressivity.
- Affected individuals develop a hypermetabolic syndrome on exposure to triggering agents (e.g., succinylcholine, volatile halogenated agents).
- The current diagnostic test is the caffeine-halothane contracture test.
- It is unclear whether pregnancy alters susceptibility to MH.
- Both the obstetrician and anesthesiologist should encourage early administration of epidural anesthesia during labor in MH-susceptible patients.

REFERENCES

1. Denborough MA, Lovell RRH. Anaesthetic deaths in a family (letter). Lancet 1960; 2:45.
2. Harrison GG, Isaacs H. Malignant hyperthermia: A historical vignette. Anaesthesia 1992; 47:54-6.
3. Ording H. Incidence of malignant hyperthermia in Denmark. Anesth Analg 1985; 64:700-4.
4. Wadhwa RK. Obstetric anesthesia for a patient with malignant hyperthermia susceptibility. Anesthesiology 1977; 46:63-4.
5. Douglas MJ, O'Connor GA, Allanson JE. Malignant hyperthermia in British Columbia. BC Med J 1983; 25:299-300.
6. Liebenschütz F, Mai C, Pickerodt VWA. Increased carbon dioxide production in two patients with malignant hyperpyrexia and its control by dantrolene. Br J Anaesth 1979; 51:899-903.
7. Lips FJ, Newland M, Dutton G. Malignant hyperthermia triggered by cyclopropane during cesarean section. Anesthesiology 1982; 56:144-6.
8. Cupryn JP, Kennedy A, Byrick RJ. Malignant hyperthermia in pregnancy. Am J Obstet Gynecol 1984; 150:327-8.
9. Weingarten AE, Korsh JI, Neuman GG, Stern SB. Postpartum uterine atony after intravenous dantrolene. Anesth Analg 1987; 66:269-70.
10. Tettambel M. Malignant hyperthermia in an obstetric patient. J Am Osteopathic Assoc 1980; 79:773-5.
11. Imagawa T, Smith JS, Coronado R, Campbell KP. Purified ryanodine receptor from skeletal muscle sarcoplasmic reticulum is the Ca^{2+}-permeable pore of the calcium release channel. J Biol Chem 1987; 262:16636-43.
12. Inui M, Saito A, Fleischer S. Purification of the ryanodine receptor and identity with feet structures of junctional terminal cisternae of sarcoplasmic reticulum from fast skeletal muscle. J Biol Chem 1987; 262:1740-7.
13. Lai FA, Erickson HP, Rousseau E, et al. Purification and reconstitution of the calcium release channel from skeletal muscle. Nature 1988; 331:315-9.
14. Fill M, Coronado R. Ryanodine receptor channel of sarcoplasmic reticulum. Trends Neurol 1988; 11:453-7.
15. Nelson TE. Abnormality in calcium release from skeletal sarcoplasmic reticulum of pigs susceptible to malignant hyperthermia. J Clin Invest 1983; 72:862-70.
16. Lopez JR, Allen PD, Alamo L, et al. Myoplasmic free [CA^{2+}] during a malignant hyperthermia episode in swine. Muscle Nerve 1988; 11:82-8.
17. Sessler DI. Malignant hyperthermia. Acta Anaesthesiol Scand (suppl) 1996; 109: 25-30.
18. Zucchi R, Ronca-Testoni S. The sarcoplasmic reticulum Ca^{2+} channel/ryanodine receptor: Modulation by endogenous effectors, drugs and disease states. Pharmacol Rev 1997; 49:1-51.
19. Wappler F, Fiege M, Schulte am Esch J. Pathophysiological role of the serotonin system in malignant hyperthermia. Br J Anaesth 2001; 87:794-8.
20. Levitt RC. Prospects for the diagnosis of malignant hyperthermia susceptibility using molecular genetic approaches. Anesthesiology 1992; 76:1039-48.
21. Levitt RC, Nouri N, Jedlicka AE, et al. Evidence for genetic heterogeneity in malignant hyperthermia susceptibility. Genomics 1991; 11:543-7.
22. Fagerlund TH, Islander G, Twetman ER, Berg K. Malignant hyperthermia susceptibility, an autosomal dominant disorder? Clin Genet 1997; 51:365-9.

23. Davies W, Harbitz I, Fries R, et al. Porcine malignant hyperthermia carrier detection and chromosomal assignment using a linked probe. Anim Genet 1988; 19: 203-12.

24. Fujii J, Ostu K, Zorzato F, et al. Identification of a mutation in porcine ryanodine receptor associated with malignant hyperthermia. Science 1991; 253:448-51.

25. Hopkins PM. Malignant hyperthermia: Advances in clinical management and diagnosis. Br J Anaesth 2000; 85:118-28

26. Kausch K, Lehmann-Horn F, Janka M, et al. Evidence for linkage of the central core disease locus to the proximal long arm of human chromosome 19. Genomics 1991; 10:765-9.

27. Wang JM, Stanley TH. Duchenne muscular dystrophy and malignant hyperthermia: Two case reports. Can Anaesth Soc J 1986; 33:492-7.

28. Heytens L, Martin JJ, Van de Kelft E, Bossaert LL. In vitro contracture tests in patients with various neuromuscular diseases. Br J Anaesth 1992; 68:72-5.

29. Lehmann-Horn F, Iaizzo PA. Are myotonias and periodic paralyses associated with susceptibility to malignant hyperthermia? Br J Anaesth 1990; 65:692-7.

30. Moslehi R, Langlois S, Yam I, Friedman JM. Linkage of malignant hyperthermia and hyperkalemic periodic paralysis to the adult skeletal muscle sodium channel (SCN4A) gene in a large pedigree. Am J Med Genet 1998; 76:21-7.

31. Lambert C, Blanloeil Y, Krivosic Horber R, et al. Malignant hyperthermia in a patient with hypokalemic periodic paralysis. Anesth Analg 1994; 79:1012-4.

32. Prather Strazis K, Fox AW. Malignant hyperthermia: A review of published cases. Anesth Analg 1993; 77:297-304.

33. Bendixen D, Skovgaard LT, Ørding H. Analysis of anaesthesia in patients suspected to be susceptible to malignant hyperthermia before diagnostic in vitro contracture test. Acta Anaesthesiol Scand 1997; 41:480-4.

34. Britt BA. Combined anesthetic- and stress-induced malignant hyperthermia in two offspring of malignant hyperthermic-susceptible parents. Anesth Analg 1988; 67:393-9.

35. Feuerman T, Gade GF, Reynolds R. Stress-induced malignant hyperthermia in a head-injured patient. J Neurosurg 1988; 68:297-9.

36. Hackl W, Winkler M, Mauritz W, et al. Muscle biopsy for diagnosis of malignant hyperthermia susceptibility in two patients with severe exercise-induced myolysis. Br J Anaesth 1991; 66:138-40.

37. Gronert GA, Thompson RL, Onofrio BM. Human malignant hyperthermia: Awake episodes and correction by dantrolene. Anesth Analg 1980; 59:377-8.

38. Hopkins PM, Ellis FR, Halsall PJ. Evidence for related myopathies in exertional heat stroke and malignant hyperthermia. Lancet 1991; 338:1491-2.

39. Iaizzo PA, Lehmann-Horn F. Anesthetic complications in muscle disorders (editorial). Anesthesiology 1995; 82:1093-6.

40. Wappler F, Fiege M, Steinfath M, et al. Evidence for susceptibility to malignant hyperthermia in patients with exercise-induced rhabdomyolysis. Anesthesiology 2001; 94:95-100.

41. Davis M, Brown R, Dickson A, et al. Malignant hyperthermia associated with exercise-induced rhabdomyolysis or congenital abnormalities and a novel RYR1 mutation in New Zealand and Australian pedigrees. Br J Anaesth 2002; 88:508-15.

42. Tobin JR, Jason DR, Challa VR, et al. Malignant hyperthermia and apparent heat stroke, (letter). JAMA 2001; 286:168-9.

43. Gronert GA, Ahern CP, Milde JH, White RD. Effect of CO_2, calcium, digoxin and potassium on cardiac and skeletal muscle metabolism in malignant hyperthermia susceptible swine. Anesthesiology 1986; 64:24-8.

44. Maccani RM, Wedel DJ, Hofer RE. Norepinephrine does not potentiate porcine malignant hyperthermia. Anesth Analg 1996; 82:790-5.

45. Allsop P, Jorfeldt L, Rutberg H, et al. Delayed recovery of muscle pH after short duration, high intensity exercise in malignant hyperthermia susceptible subjects. Br J Anaesth 1991; 66:541-5.

46. Nelson TE. Porcine malignant hyperthermia: Critical temperatures for in vivo and in vitro responses. Anesthesiology 1990; 73:449-54.

47. Denborough M, Hopkinson KC, O'Brien RO, Foster PS. Overheating alone can trigger malignant hyperthermia in piglets. Anaesth Intensive Care 1996; 24:348-54.

48. Iaizzo PA, Kehler CH, Carr RJ, et al. Prior hypothermia attenuates malignant hyperthermia in susceptible swine. Anesth Analg 1996; 82:803-9.

49. Gronert GA, Milde JH. Variations in onset of malignant hyperthermia. Anesth Analg 1981; 60:499-503.

50. Jones DE, Ryan JF, Taylor B, et al. Pancuronium in large doses protects susceptible swine from halothane induced malignant hyperthermia (abstract). Anesthesiology 1985; 63:A344.

51. Katz JD, Krich LB. Acute febrile reaction complicating spinal anaesthesia in a survivor of malignant hyperthermia. Can Anaesth Soc J 1976; 23:285-9.

52. Kemp DR, Choong LS. Malignant hyperthermia and the conscious patient. Aust NZJ Surg 1988; 58:423-7.

53. Motegi Y, Shirai M, Arai M, et al. Malignant hyperthermia during epidural anesthesia. J Clin Anesth 1996; 8:157-60.

54. Pollock N, Hodges M, Sendall J. Prolonged malignant hyperthermia in the absence of triggering agents. Anaesth Intensive Care 1992; 20:520-3.

55. Fierobe L, Nivoche Y, Mantz J, et al. Perioperative severe rhabdomyolysis revealing susceptibility to malignant hyperthermia. Anesthesiology 1998; 88:263-5.

56. Harwood TN, Nelson TE. Massive postoperative rhabdomyolysis after uneventful surgery: A case report of subclinical malignant hyperthermia. Anesthesiology 1998; 88:265-8.

57. Karan SM, Crowl F, Muldoon SM. Malignant hyperthermia masked by capnographic monitoring. Anesth Analg 1994; 78:590-2.

58. Flewellen EH, Nelson TE. Halothane-succinylcholine induced masseter spasm: Indication of malignant hyperthermia susceptibility? Anesth Analg 1984; 63:693-7.

59. Van Der Spek AFL, Fang WB, Ashton-Miller JA, et al. Increased masticatory muscle stiffness during limb muscle flaccidity with succinylcholine administration. Anesthesiology 1988; 69:11-6.

60. Smith CE, Donati F, Bevan DR. Effects of succinylcholine at the masseter and adductor pollicis muscles in adults. Anesth Analg 1989; 69:158-62.

61. Albrecht A, Wedel DJ, Gronert GA. Masseter muscle rigidity and nondepolarizing neuromuscular blocking agents. Mayo Clin Proc 1997; 72:329-32.

62. Hinkle AJ, Dorsch JA. Maternal masseter muscle rigidity and neonatal fasciculations after induction for emergency cesarean section. Anesthesiology 1993; 79:175-7.

63. O'Flynn RP, Shutack JG, Rosenberg H, Fletcher JE. Masseter muscle rigidity and malignant hyperthermia susceptibility in pediatric patients. An update on management and diagnosis. Anesthesiology 1994; 80:1228-33.

64. Kaplan RF. Clinical controversies in malignant hyperthermia susceptibility. Anesthesiol Clin North Am 1994; 12:537-51.

65. Allen GC, Rosenberg H. Malignant hyperthermia susceptibility in adult patients with masseter muscle rigidity. Can J Anaesth 1990; 37:31-5.

66. Ellis FR, Halsall PJ, Christian AS. Clinical presentation of suspected malignant hyperthermia during anaesthesia in 402 probands. Anaesthesia 1990; 45:838-41.

67. Hackl W, Mauritz W, Schemper M, et al. Prediction of malignant hyperthermia susceptibility: Statistical evaluation of clinical signs. Br J Anaesth 1990; 64:425-9.

68. Larach MG, Rosenberg H, Larach DR, Broennle AM. Prediction of malignant hyperthermia susceptibility by clinical signs. Anesthesiology 1987; 66:547-50.

69. Allen GC. Malignant hyperthermia susceptibility. Anesth Clin North Am 1994; 12:513-35.

70. Larach MG, Localio AR, Allen GC, et al. A clinical grading scale to predict malignant hyperthermia susceptibility. Anesthesiology 1994; 80:771-9.

71. Larach MG. Standardization of the caffeine halothane muscle contracture test. Anesth Analg 1989; 69:511-5.

72. The European Malignant Hyperpyrexia Group. A protocol for the investigation of malignant hyperpyrexia (MH) susceptibility. Br J Anaesth 1984; 56:1267-9.

73. Allen GC, Larach MG, Kunselman AR. The sensitivity and specificity of the caffeine-halothane contracture test. A report from the North American malignant hyperthermia registry. Anesthesiology 1998; 88:579-88.

74. Serfas KD, Bose D, Patel L, et al. Comparison of the segregation of the RYR1 C1840T mutation with segregation of the caffeine/halothane contracture test results for malignant hyperthermia susceptibility in a large Manitoba Mennonite family. Anesthesiology 1996; 84:322-9.

75. Allen GC, Rosenberg H, Fletcher JE. Safety of general anesthesia in patients previously tested negative for malignant hyperthermia susceptibility. Anesthesiology 1990; 72:619-22.

76. Ørding H, Hedengran AM, Skovgaard LT. Evaluation of 119 anaesthetics received after investigation for susceptibility to malignant hyperthermia. Acta Anaesthesiol Scand 1991; 35:711-6.

77. Islander G, Ranklev-Twetman E. Evaluation of anaesthesias in malignant hyperthermia negative patients. Acta Anaesthesiol Scand 1995; 39:819-21.

78. Rosenberg H, Antognini JF, Muldoon S. Testing for malignant hyperthermia. Anesthesiology 2002; 96:232-7.

79. Bendahan D, Kozak-Ribbens G, Rodet L, et al.[31] Phosphorus magnetic resonance spectroscopy characterization of muscular metabolic anomalies in patients with malignant hyperthermia: Application to diagnosis. Anesthesiology 1998; 88:96-107.

80. Crawford JS. Hyperpyrexia during pregnancy (letter). Lancet 1972; i:1244.

81. Willatts SM. Malignant hyperthermia susceptibility: Management during pregnancy and labour. Anaesthesia 1979; 34:41-6.

82. Isherwood DM, Ridley J, Wilson J. Creatine phosphokinase (CPK) levels in pregnancy: A case report and a discussion of the value of CPK levels in the prediction of possible malignant hyperpyrexia. Br J Obstet Gynaecol 1975; 82:346-9.

83. Douglas MJ, McMorland GH. The anaesthetic management of the malignant hyperthermia susceptible parturient. Can Anaesth Soc J 1986; 33:371-8.

84. Khalil SN, Williams JP, Bourke DL. Management of a malignant hyperthermia susceptible patient in labor with 2-chloroprocaine epidural anesthesia. Anesth Analg 1983; 62:119-21.

85. Sorosky JJ, Ingardia CJ, Botti JJ. Diagnosis and management of susceptibility to malignant hyperthermia in pregnancy. Am J Perinatol 1989; 6:46-8.

86. Morison DH. Placental transfer of dantrolene (letter). Anesthesiology 1983; 59:265.

87. Glassenberg R, Cohen H. Intravenous dantrolene in a pregnant malignant hyperthermia susceptible (MHS) patient (abstract). Anesthesiology 1984; 61:A404.

88. Lucy SJ. Anaesthesia for caesarean delivery of a malignant hyperthermia susceptible parturient. Can J Anaesth 1994; 41:1220-6.

89. Pollock NA, Langton EE. Management of malignant hyperthermia susceptible parturients. Anaesth Intensive Care 1997; 25:398-407.

90. Cohen SE. Physiological alterations of pregnancy. In Clinics in Anaesthesiology. London, WB Saunders, 1986:33-46.

91. Bonica JJ. Pain of parturition. In Clinics in Anaesthesiology. London, WB Saunders, 1986:1-31.

92. Marx GF, Greene NM. Maternal lactate, pyruvate and excess lactate production during labor and delivery. Am J Obstet Gynecol 1964; 90:786-93.

93. Kasten GW, Martin ST. Resuscitation from bupivacaine-induced cardiovascular toxicity during partial inferior vena cava occlusion. Anesth Analg 1986; 65:341-4.

94. Marx GF. Cardiopulmonary resuscitation of late-pregnant women (letter). Anesthesiology 1982; 56:156.

95. Lockitch G, editor. Handbook of Diagnostic Biochemistry and Hematology in Normal Pregnancy. Boca Raton, Fla, CRC Press, 1993:48,59.

96. Abramov Y, Abramov D, Abrahamov A, et al. Elevation of serum creatine phosphokinase and its MB isoenzyme during normal labor and early puerperium. Acta Obstet Gynecol Scand 1996; 75:255-60.

97. Sato N, Brum JM, Mitsumoto H, DeBoer GE. Effect of cocaine on the contracture response to 1% halothane in patients undergoing diagnostic muscle biopsy for malignant hyperthermia. Can J Anaesth 1995; 42:158-62.

98. Lampley EC, Williams S, Myers SA. Cocaine-associated rhabdomyolysis causing renal failure in pregnancy. Obstet Gynecol 1996; 87:804-6.

99. Roby PV, Glenn CM, Watkins SL, et al. Association of elevated umbilical cord blood creatine kinase and myoglobin levels with the presence of cocaine metabolites in maternal urine. Am J Perinatol 1996; 13:453-5.

100. Sewall K, Flowerdew RMM, Bromberger P. Severe muscular rigidity at birth: Malignant hyperthermia syndrome? Can Anaesth Soc J 1980; 27:279-82.

101. Wilhoit RD, Brown RE, Bauman LA. Possible malignant hyperthermia in a 7-week-old infant. Anesth Analg 1989; 68:688-91.

102. Allen G, Rosenberg H. Diagnosis of malignant hyperthermia in infants (letter). Anesth Analg 1990; 70:115.

103. Lederman RP, McCann DS, Work Jr B, Huber MJ. Endogenous plasma epinephrine and norepinephrine in last-trimester pregnancy and labor. Am J Obstet Gynecol 1977; 129:5-8.

104. Thornton CA, Carrie LES, Sayers L, et al. A comparison of the effect of extradural and parenteral analgesia on maternal plasma cortisol concentrations during labour and the puerperium. Br J Obstet Gynaecol 1976; 83:631-5.

105. Pearson JF, Davies P. The effect of continuous lumbar epidural analgesia on the acid-base status of maternal arterial blood during the first stage of labour. J Obstet Gynaecol Br Commonw 1973; 80:218-24.

106. Urwyler A, Censier K, Seeberger MD, et al. In vitro effect of ephedrine, adrenaline, noradrenaline and isoprenaline on halothane-induced contractures in skeletal muscle from patients potentially susceptible to malignant hyperthermia. Br J Anaesth 1993; 70:76-9.

107. Beebe JJ, Sessler DI. Preparation of anesthesia machines for patients susceptible to malignant hyperthermia. Anesthesiology 1988; 69:395-400.

108. McGraw TT, Keon TP. Malignant hyperthermia and the clean machine. Can J Anaesth 1989; 36:530-2.

109. Abouleish E, Abboud T, Lechevalier T, et al. Rocuronium (Org 9426) for caesarean section. Br J Anaesth 1994; 73:336-41.

110. Lennon RL, Olson RA, Gronert GA. Atracurium or vecuronium for rapid sequence endotracheal intubation. Anesthesiology 1986; 64:510-3.

111. Mayer DC, Weeks SK. Antepartum uterine relaxation with nitroglycerin at caesarean delivery. Can J Anaesth 1992; 39:166-9.

112. Lopez JR, Sanchez V, Lopez I, et al. The effects of extracellular magnesium on myoplasmic [CA^{2+}] in malignant hyperthermia susceptible swine. Anesthesiology 1990; 73:109-17.

113. Yoganathan T, Casthely PA, Lamprou M. Dantrolene-induced hyperkalemia in a patient with diltiazem and metoprolol. J Cardiothorac Anesth 1988; 2:363-4.

114. Harrison GG, Wright IG, Morrell DF. The effects of calcium channel blocking drugs on halothane initiation of malignant hyperthermia in MHS swine and on the established syndrome. Anaesth Intensive Care 1988; 16:197-201.

115. Sim ATR, White MD, Denborough MA. The effect of oxytocin on porcine malignant hyperpyrexia susceptible skeletal muscle. Clin Exper Pharmacol Physiol 1987; 14:605-10.

116. Hankins GDV, Berryman GK, Scott RT, Hood D. Maternal arterial desaturation with 15-methyl prostaglandin F_2 alpha for uterine atony. Obstet Gynecol 1988; 72:367-9.

117. Hughes WA, Hughes SC. Hemodynamic effects of prostaglandin E_2. Anesthesiology 1989; 70:713-6.

118. Mercier FJ, Benhamou D. Hyperthermia related to epidural analgesia during labor. Int J Obstet Anesth 1997; 6:19-24.

119. Heiman-Patterson TD. Neuroleptic malignant syndrome and malignant hyperthermia. Important issues for the medical consultant. Med Clin North Am 1993; 77:477-92.

120. Russell CS, Lang C, McCambridge M, Calhoun B. Neuroleptic malignant syndrome in pregnancy. Obstet Gynecol 2001; 98:906-8.

121. Chan TC, Evans SD, Clark RF. Drug-induced hyperthermia. Crit Care Clin 1997; 13:785-807.

122. Flewellen EH, Nelson TE, Jones WP, et al. Dantrolene dose response in awake man: Implications for management of malignant hyperthermia. Anesthesiology 1983; 59:275-80.

123. Wedel DJ. Malignant hyperthermia: Prevention and treatment. American Society of Anesthesiologists Newsletter 1997; 61:13-5.

124. Craft JB, Goldberg NH, Lim M, et al. Cardiovascular effects and placental passage of dantrolene in the maternal-fetal sheep model. Anesthesiology 1988; 68:68-72.

125. Shin YK, Kim YD, Collea JV, Belcher MD. Effect of dantrolene sodium on contractility of isolated human uterine muscle. Int J Obstet Anesth 1995; 4:197-200.

126. Karan SM, Lojeski EW, Haynes DH, et al. Intravenous lecithin-coated microcrystals of dantrolene are effective in the treatment of malignant hyperthermia: An investigation in rats, dogs, and swine. Anesth Analg 1996; 82:796-802.

127. Fricker RM, Hoerauf KH, Drewe J, Kress HG. Secretion of dantrolene into breast milk after acute therapy of a suspected malignant hyperthermia crisis during cesarean section. Anesthesiology 1998; 89:1023-5.

Chapter 47
Musculoskeletal Disorders

Edward T. Crosby, M.D., FRCPC

Pregnancy commonly results in musculoskeletal complaints. Although they typically are benign and self-limited, symptoms may be disabling in some women. In addition, preexisting musculoskeletal disorders interact with pregnancy to a variable degree. These interactions range from an ameliorating effect of pregnancy on the course of the disease (e.g., rheumatoid arthritis) to the potential for a significant and possibly life-threatening deterioration in maternal condition (e.g., uncorrected severe thoracic scoliosis). The purpose of this chapter is to discuss the most common musculoskeletal disorders encountered in pregnant women and their implications for obstetricians and anesthesiologists.

GESTATIONAL BACK PAIN

Low back pain is the most common musculoskeletal complaint during pregnancy.[1-3] It occurs at some time during gestation in more than 50% of pregnant women. After the first trimester the point prevalence ranges from 22% to 28%.[3] Risk factors include an antecedent history of low back pain, young age, low socioeconomic class, multiparity, spondylolisthesis, and excessive weight gain during pregnancy.[1-5]

The etiology includes hormonal and mechanical factors. The corpus luteum synthesizes and releases relaxin, and maternal blood concentrations of this peptide hormone increase tenfold during gestation. Relaxin induces ligamentous softening and peripheral and pelvic joint laxity, which cause instability of the symphysis pubis and sacroiliac joints. These ligamentous changes may cause low back pain as early as the first trimester. The degree of instability and disability may be related to the maternal concentration of relaxin. There is a correlation between mean serum levels of relaxin and the occurrence of back pain during pregnancy, and women with incapacitating symptoms have the highest serum concentrations of relaxin.[6,7]

Mechanical changes have a later onset than hormonal changes. Uterine enlargement results in a forward rotation of the sacrum and an increase in the lumbar lordotic curve, which tends to close the lumbar interlaminar space (Figure 47-1). This exaggerates the mechanical load borne by both the facet joints and the posterior aspect of the intervertebral discs. These mechanical changes also may compromise nerve root foramina. Sciatica occurs in 1% of pregnant women, and most cases occur late in pregnancy.[3] Sciatica may be confused with the more common *posterior pelvic pain,* located in the posterior pelvis distal to the lumbosacral junction. Although posterior pelvic pain may radiate to the posterior thighs and extend to below the knees, it does not extend to the ankle or involve the foot and is not associated with neurologic changes, which distinguishes it from sciatica.[8] Disc herniation is rare in pregnancy but does occur.[9] Incapacitating pain that radiates below the knee—typically accompanied by progressive neurologic deficits or bowel and bladder dysfunction—distinguishes disc herniation from the more common and benign gestational back pains.[3,9]

In summary, hormonal changes cause sacroiliac joint dysfunction, which is responsible for the back pain that occurs early in pregnancy. Mechanical changes are primarily responsible for the back pain that presents during late gestation, although symphysis pubis and sacroiliac joint instability also

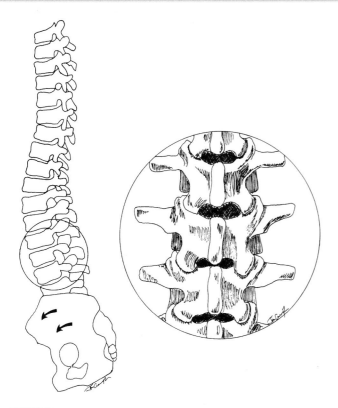

FIGURE 47-1. Musculoskeletal changes of pregnancy. Forward rotation of the pelvis and increased lumbar lordosis increase the load borne by the posterior vertebral elements and tend to close the lumbar interlaminar spaces. Lumbar vertebrae L2 to L4 are shown in the insert.

may continue to cause pain. Disc herniation is uncommon and is characterized by the presence of neurologic findings.

Obstetric Management

Treatment is conservative in the absence of neurologic compromise.[8] Exercise therapy may increase abdominal muscle strength and reduce the lumbar lordosis in women with benign complaints. However, exercise therapy may worsen symptoms in parturients with posterior pelvic pain and should be individually prescribed.[8] Bed rest is reserved for patients with neurologic symptoms or disability secondary to pelvic instability. Patients with severe neurologic signs or symptoms of disc herniation should be assessed by a consultant neurologist or surgeon who can provide recommendations for intrapartum and postpartum care. Surgical intervention may be required in parturients with incapacitating pain or progressive neurologic deficits.[9] The obstetrician may choose to perform elective instrumental vaginal delivery to decrease maternal work and back stress during the second stage of labor in women with severe symptoms.

Anesthetic Management

No evidence suggests that epidural or spinal anesthesia is contraindicated in patients with gestational back pain. The anesthesiologist may provide regional anesthesia, even to those patients with sciatica. However, neurologic signs and symptoms should be first identified and delineated. It seems prudent to administer a dilute solution of local anesthetic, with or without an opioid, to minimize motor block associated with epidural analgesia during labor.

All members of the obstetric care team must pay careful attention to the positioning of the patient with back complaints. The patient must not be placed in a position that she could not tolerate before the administration of regional anesthesia. The lithotomy position places significant stress on the lower back and should be avoided whenever possible. If it is used, care must be taken to raise and lower both legs simultaneously to prevent injury to the lumbar spine and to avoid extremes when positioning the legs. Finally, caregivers should avoid rotational movements of the spine during transfer of the patient between the bed and the operating table.

CHRONIC LOW BACK PAIN

Most instances of acute low back pain do not involve neural structures and represent minor, self-limited injuries. Prolapse of an intervertebral disc occurs in approximately 1% of acute low back injuries, and the resultant compression of neural elements results in sciatica. This injury most commonly occurs in the L4 to L5 or L5 to S1 motion segments in patients 20 to 50 years of age.[10] Most instances of acute low back injury resolve spontaneously after a short period of time, but symptoms persist in some patients. About 5% of patients have persistent symptoms and chronic low back pain 3 months after an episode of acute low back pain. Approximately 50% of pregnant women with a previous history of back pain and/or those with chronic low back pain experience a recurrence or exacerbation of their symptoms during pregnancy.[4,5]

Regional anesthesia is more likely to fail in patients with chronic low back pain and in those who have had back surgery.[11-14] Benzon et al.[11] reported a delayed onset of epidural anesthesia in patients with back pain or sciatica; the affected roots were blocked 10 to 70 minutes later than the contralateral roots at the same level. The delay in block onset most likely results from the inability of the local anesthetic agent to diffuse into the area of the injured root. Central disc herniations also result in a delayed onset of the block beyond the level of the lesion. Luyendijk and van Voorthuisen[15] evaluated 600 epidurograms and confirmed that contrast material failed to reach the nerve root in 33% of patients with uncomplicated disc prolapse and did not move beyond the affected disc space in 5% of cases. Schachner and Abram[13] suggested that this is caused by epidural scarring and adhesions that may develop during healing after disc injury. During epidurography, they noted that contrast material did not diffuse past the level of an injured disc and exited through the foramina below the abnormal disc. Thus prolapse of an intervertebral disc may result in relative or total obstruction to the flow of local anesthetic agent within the epidural space. The unblocked area includes the affected segment but also may include all segments (either ipsilateral or bilateral) distal to the affected level.

Sharrock et al.[12] reported a high rate (91%) of successful epidural anesthesia in patients with a history of limited spinal surgery. However, the success rate was lower than that achieved by the same group of anesthetists in a population with no history of back surgery (98.7%). They attributed the increased rate of failure to the distortion of surface anatomy and the tethering of the dura to the ligamentum flavum by scar formation. The latter renders the epidural space discontinuous. Support for this hypothesis is provided by LaRocca and MacNab's description of the postlaminectomy membrane.[16] They noted the postlaminectomy formation of organized fibrous tissue surrounding the dura and, at times,

binding the nerves to the posterior aspect of the disc and adjacent vertebral body. The fibrous response was proportional to the extent of surgical trauma and was more marked with greater operative exposure. The peridural fibrosis extended beyond the laminectomy defect in the more extensive exposures and obliterated the epidural space at that level. Consequently, a local anesthetic agent injected into the epidural space may not diffuse beyond the area of scarring, and an inadequate block may result.[14] Postlaminectomy spinal stenosis also may result in attenuation or obliteration of the epidural space, and the most common site of obstructive stenosis is immediately above the fusion mass.[17]

Obstetric Management

It is not uncommon for obstetricians to offer pregnant women who have had persistent back pain the option of cesarean delivery to decrease the potential for further back injury during labor. There are no data to either encourage or discourage this option.

Anesthetic Management

The anesthesiologist may offer epidural or spinal anesthesia to patients with previous lumbar spine pathology or surgery. A decreased incidence of successful epidural anesthesia may be expected, especially in patients who have had extensive surgery. Nonetheless, the experienced anesthesiologist will administer epidural anesthesia successfully in the majority of patients. Sharrock et al.[12] recommended administration of epidural anesthesia one to two interspaces above the operated segment to improve the likelihood of a successful block. Rarely, a high block may result if there is a total obstruction to flow of the local anesthetic agent at lower spinal levels.[14] Subarachnoid anesthesia most likely is more reliable than epidural anesthesia in this patient population.

POSTPARTUM BACKACHE

Postpartum backache (PPB) is a common complaint. MacArthur et al.,[18,19] citing data obtained from a postal survey of 11,701 women who had delivered 1 to 9 years previously, reported that PPB—starting within 3 months of delivery and persisting for 6 weeks or longer—occurred in 23% of women. Approximately 25% of these women had experienced backache before delivery, but 14% reported new PPB. In many women, the pain was persistent; 70% had had it for more than 2 years and 65% had it at the time of questioning 1 to 9 years later. Back pain was more common in women who delivered vaginally with epidural analgesia than in those who did not have epidural analgesia (18.9% versus 10.5%, respectively). Women who had epidural analgesia also were more likely to have had induced labor, an abnormal fetal position, a multiple pregnancy, a prolonged first and/or second stage of labor, forceps delivery, episiotomy, cesarean section, postpartum hemorrhage, and/or a large baby. MacLeod et al.[20] also performed a postal survey of 2065 patients 1 year postpartum and reported a 26.2% incidence of PPB in parturients who had epidural analgesia compared with a 1.7% incidence in those who did not; the latter incidence of PPB (1.7%) is the lowest, by far, of any reported by any author in a postpartum population in the first year after delivery.

A number of authors have carried out prospective evaluations to eliminate the potential for reporting bias that confounds these retrospective surveys. Breen et al.[21] performed a 6-month prospective assessment of 1042 parturients. Although 44% of women experienced PPB, there was no difference between those who had epidural analgesia compared with those who did not. The most significant predictor of PPB was antenatal back pain. Weight gain was greater in patients with postpartum and new-onset back pain. Groves et al.[22] assessed the incidence of late (12 to 18 months) PPB in this same cohort of patients. The incidence of late PPB was 49%, and there was no difference in the incidence among patients who had epidural analgesia (49%) compared with those who did not (50%). The incidence was significantly greater among women who had reported early PPB (66%) than among those who did not (33%). The incidence of late-onset PPB, not present in the first 2 months postpartum, was 21%. MacArthur et al.[23] also prospectively studied the association between epidural analgesia and early, new-onset PPB in 329 parturients. In patients who labored without epidural analgesia, the incidence of PPB was 43% at 1 day, 23% at 7 days, and 7% at 6 weeks. The incidence of PPB in patients who had epidural analgesia was higher on the first postpartum day (53%), but this increase was not persistent. At 1 year postpartum, 12% had back pain (9.9% in the epidural group and 13.8% in the no-epidural group). The numeric rating score for the intensity of back pain was the same in both groups. Howell et al.[24] performed a randomized controlled trial of epidural *versus* non-epidural analgesia during labor in 369 nulliparous women. There was no difference in the incidence of PPB at 3 and 12 months postpartum, and there was no difference in the characteristics of the pain.[24] In a follow-up study, there was no difference between the two groups in the incidence of long-term low back pain, disability, or movement restriction more than 2 years after delivery.[25]

The type of epidural analgesia provided also has been reviewed to determine whether manipulation of the technique alters the outcome related to PPB. Patel et al.[26] studied 340 nulliparous women and compared parturients who had received a combined spinal-epidural (CSE) technique for labor analgesia with those who had not received regional analgesia. Pre-pregnancy backache was present in 23% of the patients studied, and 41% had new-onset gestational backache before the onset of labor. The incidence of backache at 6 to 8 months postpartum was 33% overall and was not different between the groups. There was a 7% incidence of new backache in the CSE group and a 6% incidence in the no-CSE group. Russell et al.[27] studied 616 women who requested epidural analgesia for labor and randomized them to one of two study groups; one group received a local anesthetic (0.125% bupivacaine) infusion, and the other received a more dilute solution of local anesthetic with an opioid (0.0625% bupivacaine with either fentanyl 2.5 μg/mL or sufentanil 0.25 μg/mL). A third group who did not wish to have epidural analgesia served as the control group. There was a higher incidence of induced and augmented labor as well as a higher incidence of instrumental delivery and cesarean section in both epidural groups. Thirty-three women reported new-onset PPB after delivery; there was no difference among the three groups. The only factor linked with backache or new PPB developing within the first 3 months postpartum was antenatal backache. Finally, MacArthur and Lewis[28] observed no association between the management of epidural analgesia (e.g., local anesthetic used, infusion type, duration of analgesia, extent of motor and sensory blockade) and the occurrence of PPB.

Both transient and more persistent postpartum backaches are common, but there is little evidence that they are related to the provision of epidural analgesia during labor. Similarly, no evidence suggests that denying a parturient epidural analgesia results in a lower incidence of back problems during the postpartum period. Factors that are associated with more persistent PPB include the presence of back pain before pregnancy, the presence of gestational backache, performance of physically heavy work, and multiparity.[29]

SCOLIOSIS

Scoliosis is a lateral deviation in the vertical axis of the spine. The severity of scoliosis is determined by measurement of the angle of the spinal curve—the Cobb angle, which is expressed in degrees (Figure 47-2). The incidence of minor curves is 4 per 1000 in the North American population. Larger curves occur less frequently and predominantly in females. Severe scoliosis is relatively rare in parturients; it is present in 0.03% of pregnancies.[30] Most cases of scoliosis are idiopathic although some are associated with other conditions (Box 47-1).

Scoliotic curves can be divided into structural and nonstructural varieties. *Nonstructural* curves are those seen with postural scoliosis, sciatica, and leg-length discrepancies. They do not affect the mobility of the spine and are nonprogressive.

Structural curves are seen in patients with idiopathic scoliosis and with scoliosis resulting from the conditions listed in Box 47-1. Structural curves result in reduced spinal mobility, and these patients typically have a fixed prominence (rib hump) on the convex side of the curve. There is also a rotatory component associated with the scoliotic curve. The axial rotation of the vertebral body is such that the spinous processes rotate away from the convexity of the curve and back toward the midline of the patient (Figures 47-3 and 47-4).[31] Deformation of the vertebral bodies results in shorter, thinner pedicles and laminae and a more narrow vertebral canal on the concave side. Vertebral deformation does not occur in patients with a Cobb angle of less than 40 degrees.

Scoliosis interferes with the formation, growth, and development of the lungs. The number of alveoli normally increases tenfold between birth and age 8. The occurrence of scoliosis before lung maturity may reduce the number of alveoli that form. The pulmonary vasculature develops in parallel with the alveoli. Early-onset scoliosis may result in increased pulmonary vascular resistance, leading to pulmonary hypertension and eventually right heart failure.

Vertebral and rib cage deformities also affect the mechanical function of the lungs. The most common pulmonary function abnormality is a restrictive pattern with decreased vital capacity, total lung capacity, and lung compliance. This pattern occurs in all patients with a thoracic curve greater than 65 degrees. The functional residual capacity (FRC) is reduced, and airways may close during normal tidal breathing. If the FRC is reduced to such an extent that it falls below the closing capacity, basal alveoli and small airways remain open during only part of the respiratory cycle, whereas others may remain closed throughout the entire cycle. The most common blood gas abnormality is an increased alveolar-to-arterial oxygen gradient, with reduced Pa_{O_2} and a normal Pa_{CO_2}. This results from both venoarterial shunting and altered regional perfusion. Venous admixture may result in arterial hypoxemia. The natural history of severe, progressive scoliosis includes early death from cardiopulmonary failure.[32]

Scoliosis and cardiac anomalies may have a common embryogenic etiology. The incidence of mitral valve prolapse exceeds 25% in patients with adolescent scoliosis. Children with congenital heart disease also have an increased incidence of scoliosis.[33]

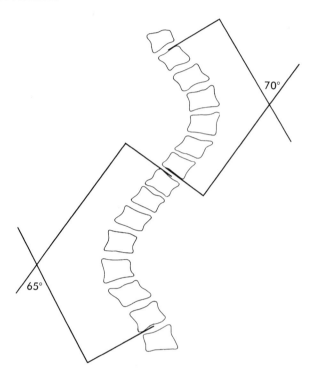

FIGURE 47-2. Schematic representation of the Cobb angle. A line is drawn parallel to the superior cortical plate of the proximal end vertebrae and parallel to the inferior cortical plate of the distal end vertebrae. A perpendicular line is erected to each of these lines. The angle of intersection is the Cobb angle of the curve.

Box 47-1 CONDITIONS ASSOCIATED WITH SCOLIOSIS

CONGENITAL (VERTEBRAL) ANOMALIES

- Hemivertebra
- Spina bifida

NEUROLOGIC DISORDERS

- Cerebral palsy
- Polio
- Neurofibromatosis

MYOPATHIC DISORDERS

- Myotonic dystrophy
- Muscular dystrophy

CONNECTIVE TISSUE DISORDERS

- Marfan syndrome
- Rheumatoid disease

OSTEOCHONDRODYSTROPHIES

- Achondroplasia/hypochondroplasia
- Osteogenesis imperfecta

INFECTION

- Tuberculosis

PREVIOUS TRAUMA

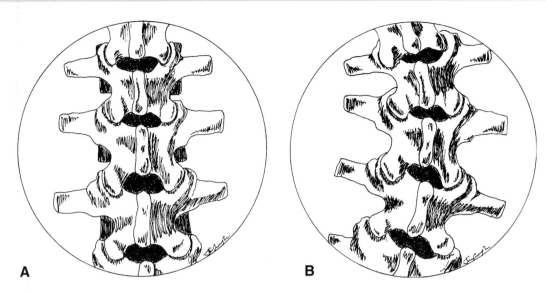

FIGURE 47-3. Spinal rotation with scoliosis. **A,** Posterior anatomy of the midlumbar spine (L2 to L4) in a patient with a normal back. **B,** Anatomy at the same level in a patient with a 30-degree lumbar scoliosis. There is a reduction in the dimensions of the interlaminar space on the concave side and an expansion on the convex side of the curve. These changes are enhanced with increased severity of the curve. As the curve increases, the spinous processes will rotate into the concavity of the curve, further altering the local anatomy.

Scoliosis Associated with Neuromuscular Disease

When scoliosis develops secondary to a primary neurologic or myopathic disorder, abnormal respiratory function results not only from the skeletal deformity of scoliosis but also from abnormalities in both the central control of respiration and the supraspinal innervation of the respiratory muscles, as well as from the loss of muscle function caused by the myopathy or lesions of the motor neurons and peripheral nerves. Respiratory function may be further compromised by the following: (1) impairment of the defense mechanisms of the airways caused by loss of control of the pharynx and the larynx, (2) an ineffective cough mechanism, and (3) infrequent or reduced large breaths. Recurrent aspiration pneumonitis may result from compromised protective airway reflexes. In general, the prognosis of scoliosis caused by neuromuscular disease is worse than that of idiopathic scoliosis and is determined predominantly by progression of the primary disorder. These patients typically develop irreversible respiratory failure at a younger age, and pregnancy is uncommon in this population.

Interaction with Pregnancy

Pregnancy may exacerbate both the severity of spinal curvature and cardiopulmonary abnormalities in women with uncorrected scoliosis. Progression of a curve is defined as an increase in the Cobb angle of 5 degrees or more over subsequent assessments. Curves that are less than 25 degrees or curves that have been stable before pregnancy typically do not progress during pregnancy.[34,35] In contrast, more severe curves and those that have not stabilized may progress during pregnancy. Some investigators have described a correlation between the severity of the curve and maternal morbidity and mortality. However, it is likely that the severity of functional cardiopulmonary impairment before pregnancy is a better predictor of maternal outcome than the severity of the curve.[29,36-38] Patients with a severe curve (i.e., Cobb angle of more than 60 degrees)

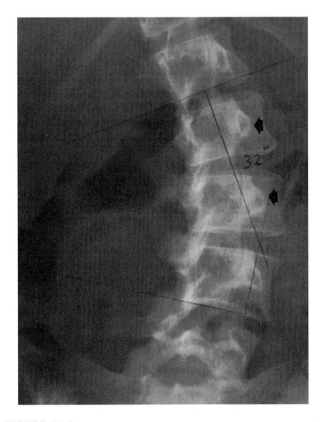

FIGURE 47-4. Radiographic study of the lumbar spine in a 26-year-old woman with idiopathic scoliosis. The spinous processes and pedicles *(arrows)* are rotated away from the convexity and into the concavity of the curve. (The epidural space was entered easily by directing the needle approximately 15 degrees off the perpendicular at the skin level toward the convexity of the curve.)

but good cardiopulmonary function tolerate pregnancy well.[38]

The physiologic changes of pregnancy include a decrease in the FRC and the closing capacity and an increase in minute ventilation and oxygen demand. The patient with scoliosis has

a noncompliant thoracic cage. As the enlarging uterus causes elevation of the diaphragm, further decreases in FRC and closing capacity may occur, which may lead to greater ventilation-perfusion mismatch and decreased arterial oxygen content. The antepartum onset of significant respiratory symptoms or the exacerbation of preexistent symptomatology is associated with increased maternal morbidity and an increased risk for assisted ventilation after operative delivery.[37]

The thoracic cage normally increases in circumference during pregnancy as a result of increases in both anteroposterior and transverse diameters. If the chest cage is relatively fixed by scoliosis, the diaphragm is responsible for all increments in minute ventilation. As the enlarging uterus enters the abdominal cavity during mid-gestation, diaphragmatic activity is restricted. Minute ventilation typically increases by 45% during pregnancy. In the normal parturient, the increase is primarily a result of increased tidal volume. In the scoliotic patient with restrictive lung disease, such increases in tidal volume may not be possible, and the increased minute ventilation is achieved by means of increased respiratory rate and increased work of breathing. The peak increases in pulmonary activity are reached by the middle of the third trimester. However, because the uterus continues to grow, it may further encroach on the noncompliant thorax and cause deterioration despite the fact that respiratory demand has stabilized.

Dyspnea on exertion is uncommon in patients with scoliosis who have curves of less than 70 degrees, but it becomes more common as the deformity exceeds 100 degrees. In younger patients with a curve of less than 70 degrees, exercise capacity may be impaired because of the lack of regular aerobic exercise and deconditioning rather than intrinsic ventilatory impairment.[39] Dyspnea occurs in most pregnant women by the middle of the third trimester. It typically begins in the first or second trimester and is most prevalent at term. Two features help distinguish physiologic from pathologic dyspnea.[40] Physiologic dyspnea tends to occur earlier in pregnancy and often plateaus or even improves as term approaches. The dyspnea of cardiopulmonary decompensation more often begins in the second half of pregnancy and is progressive, often becoming most severe as gestation advances, when the physiologic loading is maximal. Second, physiologic dyspnea is rarely extreme, and patients typically can maintain daily activities. Dyspnea that is extreme or has a limiting impact on normal activity may signal maternal cardiorespiratory decompensation. Dyspnea at rest also is rare in the absence of cardiopulmonary dysfunction. Dyspnea that is acute in onset or progressive and intractable, especially if it is coupled with other signs and symptoms, is more likely to represent cardiopulmonary decompensation.

Minute ventilation of the unmedicated parturient increases by a further 75% to 150% and 150% to 300% in the first and second stages of labor, respectively. Oxygen consumption increases above prelabor values by 40% in the first stage and 75% in the second stage. These levels may be unattainable by the scoliotic parturient with restrictive lung disease, and respiratory failure and hypoxemia may result during labor.

Parturients with pulmonary hypertension have a limited ability to increase cardiac output. During normal pregnancy, cardiac output increases 40% to 50% above nonpregnant measurements; during labor and delivery, even greater increases are observed. These increases are achieved with both increased stroke volume and an increased heart rate. These demands may result in an excessive burden on the cardiovascular system in parturients who had marginal cardiac reserve before pregnancy. If the right ventricle fails in the presence of pulmonary hypertension, left ventricular filling will decrease and low output failure and sudden death may occur.

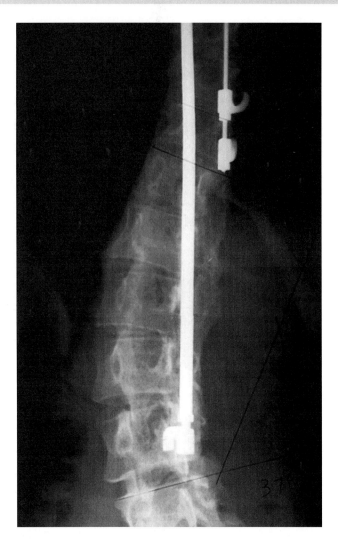

FIGURE 47-5. Harrington rod instrumentation. Radiographic study of the lumbar spine in a 31-year-old woman with thoracolumbar scoliosis corrected with spinal instrumentation. There is rotation of the vertebrae into the curve (toward the rod), and extensive bone grafting is evident adjacent to the rod. Two lumbar interspaces (L4 to L5 and L5 to S1) are not involved in the fusion.

Surgical Management

During spinal fusion and instrumentation, the spinal musculature is reflected off the vertebrae over the course of the curve and the spinous processes and interspinous ligaments are removed. The spine subsequently is extended, correcting the curve. The vertebrae are decorticated throughout the extent of the planned fusion, and the instrumentation is placed. Bone graft material is obtained from the ilium and is placed over the decorticated vertebrae. A number of techniques for fusion have been described; all of these involve spinal instrumentation and extensive bone grafting in the axial spine (Figure 47-5).

During the last three decades, scoliosis screening programs and early intervention (e.g., orthotic braces for curves of 25 to 40 degrees and spinal fusion for curves greater than 40 degrees) have been used to prevent the natural progression of

the disease. Early diagnosis and intervention have resulted in a reduced incidence of uncorrected major curves in adults. Patients who undergo early fusion and instrumentation have a lower incidence of the cardiopulmonary complications that afflict patients with severe uncorrected disease.[41,42]

Obstetric Management

Patients with corrected scoliosis tolerate pregnancy, labor, and delivery well. In patients without major lumbosacral deformity, there is little alteration of the pelvic cavity, and malpresentation is not more common than in normal pregnancy. Uterine function is normal, and labor is not prolonged. Spontaneous vaginal delivery is anticipated, and cesarean section should be reserved for obstetric indications.

Patients with severe disease (especially those with gestational decompensation) may require elective cesarean section because of maternal compromise. One uncontrolled study suggested a higher incidence of operative delivery among patients with previous Harrington rod instrumentation for correction of idiopathic scoliosis.[43]

Pelvic abnormalities are more common when scoliosis is associated with neuromuscular disorders[44] (Figure 47-6). In addition, abdominal and pelvic muscle weakness predisposes parturients to problems with expulsion of the infant during the second stage and may necessitate instrumental vaginal delivery.

Anesthetic Management

Parturients who have thoracolumbar scoliosis with a Cobb angle of greater than 30 degrees or who have undergone spinal instrumentation and fusion for scoliosis should be referred

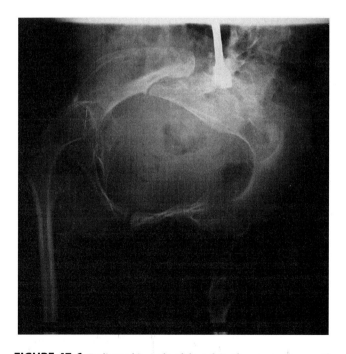

FIGURE 47-6. Radiographic study of the pelvis of a young woman with progressive spinal muscular atrophy (Kugelberg-Welander syndrome) and severe kyphoscoliosis, demonstrating an inadequate pelvic outlet. She delivered two children by cesarean section under general anesthesia after failed attempts to perform epidural anesthesia. (Reprinted with permission from Crosby ET. Scoliosis and major spinal surgery. In Gambling D, Douglas MJ, editors. Obstetric Anesthesia and Uncommon Disorders. Philadelphia, WB Saunders, 1998:205.)

for antepartum anesthetic consultation. The anesthesiologist needs to determine the underlying etiology of the scoliosis as well as the severity and stability of the curve. The anesthesiologist should seek a history of maternal cardiopulmonary symptoms and back pain and should review prior obstetric and anesthetic experiences. In patients with scoliosis secondary to neuromuscular disorders, the anesthesiologist should review anesthetic considerations specific to those disorders.

Women with evident pulmonary compromise should undergo evaluation by a pulmonologist. Pulmonary function studies and arterial blood gas measurements on room air should be obtained. These patients must be reevaluated periodically to ensure that they are tolerating the increasing physiologic demands of pregnancy. Echocardiography is useful to assess right heart function in patients with a curve of 60 degrees or more, in those with pulmonary symptoms or arterial hypoxemia, and in patients with lung volumes or flows that are less than 50% of predicted measurements.

Radiographic studies performed before pregnancy and operative notes describing spinal surgical procedures need to be reviewed. When possible, the anesthesiologist should also review the radiographs of the lumbar spine before giving regional anesthesia to any patient with significant scoliosis or previous spinal surgery. The anesthesiologist also should examine the spine and note the surface landmarks and interspaces that are least affected by the deformity. Modes of analgesia and anesthesia for labor and delivery can be discussed during antepartum consultation.

Invasive hemodynamic monitoring rarely is indicated during labor and delivery. Evidence of significant respiratory compromise on pulmonary function studies and evidence of impending respiratory failure warrant placement of an arterial catheter and serial measurement of blood gases. Echocardiographic demonstration of significant right heart dysfunction may warrant placement of a pulmonary artery catheter.

The anesthesiologist may offer epidural anesthesia for labor and delivery to patients with severe thoracolumbar scoliosis. Identification of the epidural space is more difficult in such patients, and the anesthesiologist should anticipate an increased incidence of complications. It is useful to remember the presence of the vertebral rotation during the performance of regional anesthesia in a patient with a significant lumbar curve. The midline of the epidural space is deviated toward the convexity of the curve relative to the spinous process palpable at the skin level (see Figures 47-3 and 47-4). The degree of lateral deviation is largely determined by the severity of the deformity. The needle should enter the selected interspace and be directed toward the convexity of the curve. The experienced anesthesiologist can track the resistance of both the interspinous ligament and the ligamentum flavum to maintain the correct course into the epidural space. The extent of the local anatomic distortion is the limiting factor, and the selection of spaces that are least involved in the curve is advised (Figure 47-7). Patients with scoliosis resulting from myopathic or neurologic disease may have a distortion of spinal anatomy significant enough to prohibit the administration of regional anesthesia.

Structural curves of 20 degrees or less and minor functional curves, such as those commonly seen in pregnant women at term, rarely result in any significant rotatory deviation of the vertebrae. Little if any accommodation in technique is required for successful needle placement in these patients.

Local anesthetic dose requirements for epidural and spinal anesthesia are variable. Moreover, during administration of spinal anesthesia in a patient with a severe curve, hyperbaric local anesthetic solution may pool in dependent portions of the spine and result in an inadequate block.[45] Thus it is preferable to use a continuous technique so that the dose of local anesthetic agent can be titrated to the desired segmental level of anesthesia.

Some physicians believe that corrective spinal surgery represents a relative contraindication to the subsequent use of regional anaesthesia. I disagree, and I offer regional anesthesia to selected patients with a history of corrective surgery. However, the following potential problems must be considered. First, persistent back pain occurs in almost half of patients with corrected scoliosis and correlates with both increased duration since surgery and increased extent of fusion.[46,47] Second, degenerative changes occur in the spine below the area of fusion at a greater than usual rate. There is an increased incidence of both retrolisthesis and spondylolisthesis.[47] Third, 20% of patients undergo fusion to the L4 or L5 level. Thus few lumbar interspaces remain uninvolved.[43,48] Fourth, either midline or paramedian insertion of an epidural needle in the fused area may not be possible

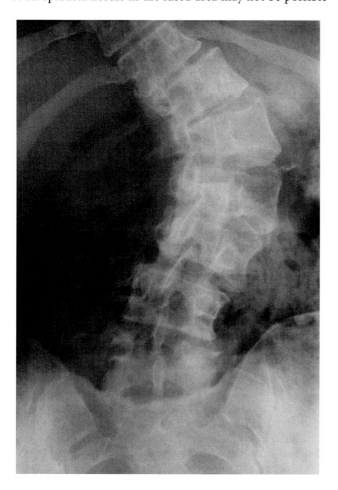

FIGURE 47-7. Radiograph of the lower thoracolumbar spine in a young woman with scoliosis predominantly affecting the lumbar spine and markedly distorting her local anatomy. She received lumbar epidural analgesia for labor during her first pregnancy, after a catheter was placed with some difficulty. She received patient-controlled intravenous nalbuphine for labor analgesia during her second pregnancy after persistent, unsuccessful attempts to insert an epidural catheter. The radiograph directed the practitioner toward the lower lumbar spaces, where anatomic distortion is less pronounced.

because of the presence of instrumentation, scar tissue, and bone graft material. Fifth, intraoperative trauma to the ligamentum flavum may result in adhesions in the epidural space or obliteration of the epidural space, and this may interfere with spread of the local anesthetic agent injected into the epidural space.[16] Sixth, obliteration of the epidural space may increase the incidence of unintentional dural puncture, and it may not be possible to provide an epidural blood patch if postdural puncture headache (PDPH) should result. Finally, these patients often manifest a high degree of anxiety about their backs and may be reluctant to have regional anesthesia.

Several reports have described the use of epidural anesthesia in obstetric patients with spinal instrumentation and fusion.[43,49] These reports have detailed a high incidence of difficulties encountered during the administration of epidural anesthesia in these patients. Complications included (1) unsuccessful identification of the epidural space, (2) multiple attempts before successful identification of the space and insertion of the catheter, (3) false loss of resistance, (4) unintentional dural puncture, and (5) failed block or inadequate analgesia. Complications seem to occur more frequently in patients with fusion that extends to the lower lumbar and lumbosacral interspaces than in those with fusion that ends in the upper lumbar spine.

Both the anesthesiologist and patient should anticipate the possibility that blind attempts to identify the epidural space may fail. Yeo and French[50] reported the use of ultrasonography to facilitate the administration of regional anesthesia in a patient with Harrington rod instrumentation. Although the technique resulted in successful subarachnoid block, the epidural catheter functioned poorly and the resulting block was inadequate. Alternative modes of intrapartum analgesia include administration of intraspinal opioids, caudal anesthesia,[51] patient-controlled intravenous opioid analgesia, and inhalation analgesia. Spinal (subarachnoid) analgesia or anesthesia is a reasonable alternative to epidural anesthesia for labor or cesarean section in parturients who have undergone major spinal surgery with instrumentation. It is possible to make an intentional dural puncture with a small-gauge needle either through or adjacent to a fusion mass in some patients in whom it had not been possible to identify the epidural space (Figure 47-8). A catheter subsequently may be passed, or alternatively, repeat injections through the same site can be made. Finally, Gerancher et al.[52] reported the successful performance of caudal epidural blood patch for the treatment of PDPH in a patient with Harrington rod instrumentation.

RHEUMATOID ARTHRITIS

Rheumatoid arthritis is a chronic systemic disorder characterized by synovial proliferation that leads to joint destruction and subsequent deformity. The population prevalence is 0.35%, but it occurs more frequently in women.[53]

The lumbosacral spine is affected in only 5% of patients with rheumatoid arthritis. In contrast, the cervical spine is commonly involved, and atlantoaxial subluxation occurs in 25% of patients with rheumatoid arthritis.[54] Although atlantoaxial subluxation may occur early in the course of the disease, it most often occurs only in patients with highly active and erosive disease and a history of 10 years or more of mutilating peripheral joint lesions.[55,56] Atlantoaxial subluxation occurs as a result of an attenuation or disruption of the trans-

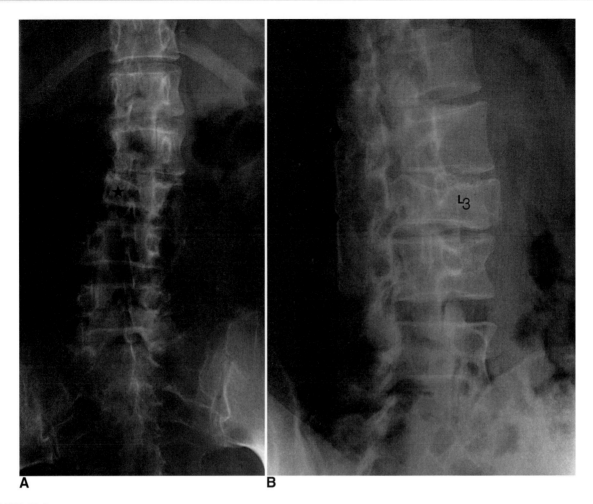

FIGURE 47-8. Radiographs of the lumbar spine in a young woman who had spine fusion after a back injury. **A,** Detailed anteroposterior view, demonstrating vertebral compression at L3 *(star)* and a mild local scoliosis. **B,** Detailed lateral view, demonstrating the considerable bone graft *(arrows)* used to create the fusion. After attempts to insert an epidural catheter failed, she was provided labor analgesia with two small-gauge needle (24-gauge Sprotte) dural punctures and injection of bupivacaine 2.5 mg and fentanyl 10 μg.

verse ligament, which allows anterior movement of C1 on C2 during neck flexion. Radiographically, atlantoaxial subluxation is marked by an increase in the atlas-dens interval, which is best demonstrated on the lateral cervical spine radiograph with the neck flexed (Figure 47-9).

Vertical subluxation of the odontoid process occurs primarily in elderly patients with severe and longstanding disease. A scoliotic deformity of the trachea and larynx has been reported in patients with vertical subluxation.[57] The deformity is complex, involving both rotation and deviation of the larynx from the midline. This deformity may make endotracheal intubation difficult. However, vertical subluxations occur primarily in older patients with severe, longstanding disease, and are unlikely to be seen in pregnant women.

Extraarticular features are common in patients with rheumatoid arthritis. Anesthesiologists have a special interest in abnormalities that affect the airway and the cardiovascular and respiratory systems (Box 47-2).[58] These abnormalities occur primarily in patients with longstanding disease and rarely are a problem in young patients.[58]

Interaction with Pregnancy

Rheumatoid arthritis typically does not complicate pregnancy. In the absence of vasculitis, fetal outcome is good. Pregnancy has a beneficial, ameliorating effect on the activity

of rheumatoid arthritis.[58] Approximately 75% of women note improved symptoms during pregnancy, and this typically is evident by the end of the first trimester. A gradual resolution of pain, swelling, and stiffness occurs. The clinical improvement typically continues throughout pregnancy and recurs in future pregnancies. This remission often occurs despite the elimination of second-line antirheumatic drugs and a substantial reduction in the dosage of first-line drugs. Relapse occurs postpartum, beginning as early as the second week after delivery. It appears that most patients return to a disease status comparable to their prepregnant state.

Medical Management

Acetylsalicylic acid (aspirin) is the mainstay of treatment for rheumatoid arthritis.[59] No evidence suggests that it is teratogenic, and it most likely is the safest antirheumatic agent for administration during pregnancy. Potential complications (especially when high doses are continued until delivery) include anemia, postterm delivery, prolonged labor, antepartum and postpartum hemorrhage, neonatal cephalohematoma, and intracranial hemorrhage in preterm infants.[59,60] Most of these complications occur at delivery; therefore aspirin should be discontinued near term. There is little evidence that most nonsteroidal antiinflammatory agents (NSAIDs) are a major problem during pregnancy, although dystocia has been

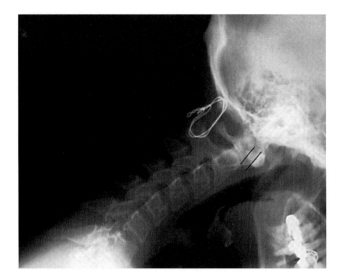

FIGURE 47-9. Lateral radiographic study of the cervical spine (in flexion) in a 32-year-old woman with rheumatoid arthritis. There is isolated atlantoaxial subluxation (6 mm) in the absence of other radiologic changes of rheumatoid arthritis. She presented with neck pain, and a wire was placed between the occiput and the spinous process of C2 to limit the subluxation.

attributed to their use. Because there is less clinical experience with these agents, some physicians recommend that they be stopped during pregnancy.[60] Indomethacin may suppress labor and has been implicated in premature closure of the ductus arteriosus and the occurrence of persistent fetal circulation and pulmonary hypertension. It should be avoided for the treatment of rheumatoid arthritis during pregnancy.[60]

Corticosteroids appear safe; placental inactivation results in low fetal levels of pharmacologically active drug.[59,60] Prednisone is an appropriate second-line antirheumatic agent during pregnancy. Gold, antimalarial agents, and *D*-penicillamine typically are discontinued, although few problems have been attributed to their use during pregnancy.[58] Azathioprine may be used safely during pregnancy at doses less than 2 mg/kg/day, but other immunosuppressive agents (e.g., methotrexate, cyclophosphamide, chlorambucil) are highly teratogenic and should be discontinued before conception.[60] An attempt often is made to reduce the dose of all antirheumatic agents during pregnancy and, if possible, to discontinue them in the final weeks of gestation.

Obstetric Management

Vaginal delivery is preferred, and cesarean section should be reserved for obstetric indications. A major concern is maternal positioning during labor. Rheumatoid joints are unstable because of ligament loosening associated with chronic swelling and because of the destruction of ligaments and cartilage. It is important to determine the permissible range of motion and activity for affected joints. Special emphasis should be given to the hips, knees, and neck. Physicians and nurses should be aware of the potential risks of forcing motion beyond the disease-imposed limits.

Anesthetic Management

The preanesthetic evaluation should include a careful evaluation of the airway. Patients with rheumatoid arthritis may have a small mandible, temporomandibular joint (TMJ) dysfunction, cricoarytenoid arthritis, and laryngeal deviation.

Box 47-2 EXTRAARTICULAR FEATURES OF RHEUMATOID ARTHRITIS

CARDIOVASCULAR

- Pericarditis
- Pericardial effusions
- Endocardial vegetations
- Myocardial nodules—conduction disturbance
- Arteritis/vasculitis

AIRWAY

- Mandibular hypoplasia
- Cricoarytenoid arthritis
- Temporomandibular joint dysfunction
- Laryngeal deviation and rotation

PULMONARY

- Pleural effusion
- Pulmonary fibrosis
- Pulmonary nodules

CHEST WALL

- Costochondritis

NEUROLOGIC

- Peripheral nerve compression
- Cervical nerve root compression

HEMATOLOGIC

- Anemia
- Felty syndrome

OPHTHALMIC

- Keratoconjunctivitis

These findings are unusual in young patients, but both mandibular hypoplasia and TMJ dysfunction may be present in young women with juvenile rheumatoid arthritis (JRA) and may complicate direct laryngoscopy. Cervical spine involvement is not common in young patients but may occur in patients with disease of long duration and in those with severe, deforming disease, typically parturients with JRA. Cervical spine radiographs should be evaluated in parturients who have severe erosive disease, neck symptoms, or a history of disease of 10 years' duration or longer. The cardiac and pulmonary features of rheumatoid arthritis are not common in young patients, but signs and symptoms of pleural and pericardial effusions and pulmonary parenchymal involvement should be sought.

No evidence contraindicates the administration of spinal or epidural anesthesia to patients with rheumatoid arthritis. Moreover, no evidence suggests that the bleeding time correctly predicts the risk of bleeding into the epidural space.[61] I do not determine the bleeding time in patients who have taken aspirin or NSAIDs. Care should be taken to avoid excessive manipulation of the neck during administration of general anesthesia. Finally, joints should be padded and protected appropriately during anesthesia.

ANKYLOSING SPONDYLITIS

Ankylosing spondylitis is a chronic inflammatory arthropathy characterized by infiltration of granulation tissue into the

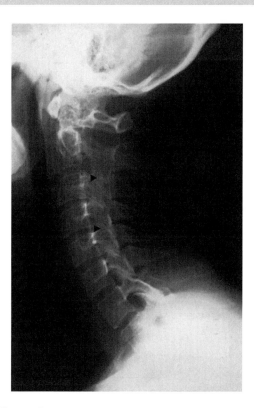

FIGURE 47-10. Lateral radiographic study of the cervical spine in a 31-year-old woman with ankylosing spondylitis. There is evidence of facet joint ankylosis *(arrowheads),* although the lordotic curve remains well preserved. The ligaments of the thoracic spine are undergoing calcification with the spine in flexion, and there is a compensatory increase in the lumbar lordosis to maintain erect posture. (Flexion of the lumbar spine proved difficult, and a paramedian approach was used to enter the epidural space.)

> **Box 47-3   EXTRAARTICULAR FEATURES OF ANKYLOSING SPONDYLITIS**
>
> **SYSTEMIC**
> - Fever
> - Weight loss
> - Fatigue
>
> **CARDIOVASCULAR**
> - Aortitis
> - Aortic insufficiency
> - Conduction disorders—heart block
>
> **PULMONARY**
> - Restrictive lung disease
> - Pulmonary fibrosis
>
> **NEUROLOGIC**
> - Cauda equina syndrome
> - Vertebrobasilar insufficiency
> - Peripheral nerve lesions
>
> **HEMATOLOGIC**
> - Anemia
>
> **UROLOGIC**
> - Prostatitis
>
> **OPHTHALMIC**
> - Uveitis

---

bony insertions of ligaments and joint capsules. Subsequent fibrosis, ossification, and ankylosis occur.[62] The sacroiliac, facet, and costovertebral joints are primarily affected. There is progressive flexion and fusion of the spine and fixation of the rib cage. The clinical spectrum is wide, and only a small proportion of patients progress to total spinal ankylosis.[63]

Ankylosing spondylitis occurs in 0.3% to 0.6% of women. The onset commonly occurs during the second and third decades, a period of peak childbearing potential.[63] The disease is milder in women than in men, but women are more likely to have peripheral arthritis and involvement of the cervical spine and symphysis pubis.[63] Although clinically significant lesions of the cervical spine may occur early in the course of the disease, they are far more common in patients with long-standing ankylosing spondylitis (Figure 47-10).[64] A slower development of radiologic changes of the dorsolumbar spine occurs in women, and spinal rigidity or deformity occurs rarely in young patients.[65] Extraarticular manifestations of ankylosing spondylitis also are rare in young patients (Box 47-3).[62]

Interaction with Pregnancy

Unlike rheumatoid arthritis, there is no evidence that pregnancy ameliorates the symptoms or progression of spinal abnormalities in patients with ankylosing spondylitis, and a significant number of patients experience an aggravation of morning stiffness and back pain.[63,66] However, pregnancy may ameliorate the extraarticular features of this disease (e.g., psoriasis, inflammatory bowel disease, small joint arthritis).

Ankylosing spondylitis does not adversely affect pregnancy, labor, or delivery, and, in the absence of pelvic joint ankylosis and/or hip joint involvement, an uncomplicated vaginal delivery at term should be anticipated in most patients.

Acetaminophen and antiinflammatory medications (i.e., aspirin and other NSAIDs) represent the mainstay of medical treatment. Most patients require treatment at some point during gestation.[63] The aim of treatment during pregnancy is to provide the lowest effective dose for the shortest time during gestation. An attempt is made to withdraw the analgesic medications in the late stages of pregnancy to prevent complications during and after delivery.

Anesthetic Management

The anesthesiologist should review the patient's history with respect to the duration of the disease, the presence of extraarticular features, and the recent use of analgesics. TMJ dysfunction, cervical spine involvement, and cardiopulmonary complications are rare early in the disease course and uncommon in parturients. Back symptoms often are out of proportion to the radiographic appearance of the spine, and calcification of the spinal ligaments typically is not advanced in young patients. The anesthesiologist may administer spinal or epidural anesthesia to patients with ankylosing spondylitis. It is unusual to experience complications during the provision of regional anesthesia to young patients with ankylosing spondylitis. However, calcification of the interspinous ligaments and osteophyte formation may make it difficult for the parturient to flex forward, making midline needle placement

difficult. A paramedian approach can be considered in this instance.

SPINA BIFIDA

Spina bifida is a condition that results from the failure of the bony vertebrae to completely enclose the neural elements in a bony canal. There is a wide spectrum with respect to the severity of the deformity and its implications. *Spina bifida occulta* is defined as failed fusion of the neural arch without herniation of the meninges or neural elements. A defect limited to a single vertebra, typically L5 or S1, is so common (occurring in 5% to 36% of the population) that it can be considered a normal variant.[67] Superficial signs of this lesion may include a tuft of hair, cutaneous angioma, lipoma, or a skin dimple, but such signs are not common in patients with isolated vertebral arch anomalies and an underlying normal cord. Patients with spina bifida occulta rarely have symptoms related to this anomaly, although they may have a higher incidence of posterior disc herniation.[67]

Spina bifida cystica is defined as failed closure of the neural arch with herniation of the meninges (i.e., meningocele) or the meninges and neural elements (i.e., myelomeningocele) through the vertebral defect. These conditions are relatively uncommon and occur in 1 to 3 per 1000 births.[68-70] Neurologic deficits involving the lower extremities and sphincters occur in almost all patients. These deficits vary only in degree of severity. Hydrocephalus is present in most patients, and shunting of the ventricular system often is required. By puberty as many as 50% of shunted patients have little or no requirement for the shunt.[71] Early and aggressive surgical treatment of the lesion has increased survival from 45% in the early 1970s to 70% to 90% by the mid-1980s. Obstetricians and anesthesiologists can expect to encounter an increasing number of pregnant women with symptomatic spina bifida.[72] Unfortunately, many surviving patients have significant residual neurologic impairment.[73,74] Myelomeningocele is a progressive neurologic disease that eventually produces orthopedic, neurologic, and genitourinary complications. Kyphoscoliosis is common in patients with a thoracic lesion, and it occurs in 20% of patients with a lumbosacral defect.[75] Paralytic scoliosis is the most common type and results from an imbalance of paravertebral muscle tone; it also undergoes rapid progression with growth.

There is an intermediate group of conditions wherein the bony defect is associated with one or more anomalies of the spinal cord, including intraspinal lipomas, dermal sinus tracts, dermoid cysts, fibrous bands, and diastematomyelia (split cord). These lesions are called *occult spinal dysraphism* to differentiate them from the more benign occulta lesions described previously.[76] These patients may have no neurologic symptoms or may have minor motor and sensory deficits of the lower limbs and bowel and bladder. Patients with cord abnormalities have cutaneous stigmata in 50% to 70% of cases.

Tethered Cord

The spinal cord may be attached to a congenitally abnormal structure in the lumbar spine, resulting in a tethered spinal cord.[76-78] This condition is marked by a low-lying (L2 to L3) conus medullaris anchored by a thick filum terminale. Magnetic resonance imaging (MRI) studies suggest that teth-

ering is present in virtually all patients with spina bifida cystica and myelomeningocele.[77] Tethered cord also is common in patients with occult spinal dysraphism.[78] It is not clear what proportion of patients with spina bifida occulta have a tethered cord, but the incidence is low. The presence of a low-lying tethered cord may be associated with a more caudal termination of the subarachnoid space.[79]

Obstetric Management

Pregnancy is not complicated by the presence of an occulta lesion. Recurrent urinary tract infection is the most common antenatal complication in patients with spina bifida cystica and is associated with preterm labor.[75] Uterine enlargement may compromise pulmonary function, especially in patients with kyphoscoliosis. The obstetrician should evaluate the adequacy of the pelvis to determine whether a trial of labor is appropriate. Cesarean section is reserved for obstetric indications, but there is an increased likelihood of dystocia in these patients.[75]

Anesthetic Management

The epidural space may be incomplete or discontinuous across the level of occulta lesions because of the absent lamina and variable formation of the ligamentum flavum at this site. An attempt to identify the epidural space at the site of this lesion will likely result in unintentional dural puncture.[68] However, successful epidural analgesia has been reported with the catheter placed within the zone of the lesion.[69] Flow of local anesthetic solution through the lateral and anterolateral epidural space may result in extension of the block beyond the level of the lesion, but the block may be incomplete and inadequate.

Despite its common occurrence in the population and the inevitability of dural puncture if epidural analgesia is attempted at affected spinal levels, spina bifida occulta rarely complicates the administration of regional anesthesia for two reasons. First, the lesion typically occurs at the L5 to S1 segments, below the level at which most epidural and spinal anesthetics are administered.[69,70] Second, the most common anomaly is a simple midline split in the lamina; this defect rarely interferes with either the performance or development of spinal or epidural anesthesia. More extensive lesions involving multiple vertebral segments are less common.

In patients with cystica lesions, the anesthesiologist should determine the level of the lesion and whether the patient has residual spinal cord function below the level of the lesion. Patients with a complete lesion at or above T11 are likely to experience painless labor. However, the risk of autonomic hyperreflexia in patients with thoracic lesions should be evaluated, and prophylaxis must be provided if the patient is deemed to be at risk. This is especially important if the lesion is between T5 and T8, but such lesions are rare in parturients.[80]

If the patient has had a ventricular shunt placed in the past, the current status of the shunt should be determined. Neurosurgical consultation should be obtained if questions remain about the requirement for or function of the shunt. Pulmonary function should be assessed, especially in patients with scoliosis. Baseline renal function also should be assessed.

There are published reports of the use of epidural and spinal anesthesia in patients with spina bifida cystica.[69-71,81-84] Unfortunately, the experience is limited, and most published series of pregnant women with spina bifida cystica report neither the type of anesthesia provided nor the complications

experienced. Tidmarsch and May[84] recently reported management of intrapartum analgesia in 16 patients with spina bifida, of whom 8 had spina bifida cystica. Of those 8, 5 received epidural anesthesia for labor and/or delivery. Three patients had a "normal" block, one patient had a somewhat high block (sensory level of T3 following 10 mL of 0.25% bupivacaine), and one patient had poor sacral analgesia.

It seems appropriate to administer epidural or spinal anesthesia in patients with well-preserved neurologic function. The anesthesiologist should be aware that the terminal portion of the spinal cord typically lies at a vertebral level that is lower than normal in these patients. These patients typically have had imaging studies performed in the past, which may facilitate the anesthesiologist's assessment of the anatomy. Subarachnoid injection should be performed in the lower lumbar spine (below the conus) or avoided in favor of epidural anesthesia. Unfortunately, inadequate epidural anesthesia is more likely because of the abnormal, discontinuous epidural space. In the majority of patients with negligible function of the extremities and sphincters, the presence of a low-lying tethered cord is clinically irrelevant, and it need not alter the level of subarachnoid injection. In these patients, spinal anesthesia may be easier technically, and it may provide anesthesia more reliably.[81,82] A subarachnoid hematoma after spinal anesthesia in an elderly woman with occult spinal dysraphism and a tethered cord (L4) has been reported.[83] Dural puncture was made at the L3 to L4 level and was complicated initially by blood in the CSF, which cleared. During laminectomy, a bleeding vessel was identified on the surface of the cord.

ACHONDROPLASIA

Achondroplasia is an inherited disorder of bone metabolism. The incidence is 1 in 26,000.[85] Although it is inherited in an autosomal dominant mode, most cases arise from spontaneous mutation.[86,87]

Achondroplasia is the most common cause of disproportionate dwarfism.[85] There is normal periosteal bone formation but a quantitative decrease in endochondral bone formation. This results in short tubular bones, frontal bossing, a short maxilla, a large mandible, and abnormalities at the base of the spine. The range of cervical motion may be decreased.[88,89] Lumbar lordosis and thoracic kyphosis are increased, and thoracic kyphoscoliosis occurs.[90,91] The vertebral pedicles are short, and there is a decreased length of the neural arch, which leads to shortened anteroposterior and transverse diameters of the vertebral canal, resulting in foramen magnum and spinal stenosis.[92,93] Symptomatic spinal stenosis often does not present until the fourth or fifth decade, when kyphosis, scoliosis, osteophytes, and herniated discs cause further narrowing of the spinal canal. There is considerable interindividual variation in the clinical and radiographic characteristics. Skeletal abnormalities often show more variation than consistency.[92,94]

Hypochondroplasia is a variant disorder of achondroplasia. The clinical and radiographic findings tend to be less marked in hypochondroplasia than in achondroplasia, but there is interindividual variation.[92] Spinal stenosis is less severe and less often results in symptoms in patients with hypochondroplasia.

Obstetric Management

The uterus is an abdominal organ in the achondroplastic patient.[95] With advancing pregnancy it may encroach on the small thoracic cage and result in further decreases in the FRC and closing capacity. Severe dyspnea may occur during the third trimester. On a theoretic basis, the abdominal location of the uterus increases the risk of supine hypotension syndrome from aortocaval compression.

Back discomfort is common during pregnancy, and the reported incidence of sciatica is higher than in normal parturients.[96] This most likely is related to the underlying spinal abnormalities.

Typically, an inadequate maternal pelvis combined with a normal-sized fetus results in cephalopelvic disproportion. Pelvimetry may be used to confirm this, and the obstetrician should anticipate the need to deliver most patients by cesarean section.[88,91,94]

Anesthetic Management

The presence of short, obese limbs may make it difficult to obtain measurements of blood pressure with a noninvasive cuff and an intra-arterial catheter may be necessary. Prominent paraspinal muscles and the marked lumbar lordosis may complicate attempts to palpate landmarks during the administration of spinal or epidural anesthesia.[91,95] Scoliosis of the spine also may cause technical difficulties. The small stature of the patient and the spinal stenosis reduce the dose of local anesthetic required for major regional anesthesia.[88,91,94,95] It is difficult to estimate the appropriate dose of local anesthetic for single-shot spinal anesthesia. Continuous epidural anesthesia is preferable because it allows the anesthesiologist to titrate the dose of local anesthetic to the desired level of anesthesia. Although local anesthetic dose requirements are typically less than doses required by parturients of normal stature, this is variable and supports the use of a regional anesthetic technique that may be titrated to the desired effect.[90,97-99]

Difficult intubation has been reported in achondroplastic patients and should be anticipated.[89,90] It is not invariable, and most reports that comment on the subject note no difficulties in airway management.[85,87,100,101]

OSTEOGENESIS IMPERFECTA

Osteogenesis imperfecta (OI) is an inherited condition that occurs with an incidence of between 1 in 21,000 and 1 in 60,000.[102,103] The genetic defect is within the genome that encodes for type I collagen, the major collagen in tissues that require structural strength. The disease is a generalized connective tissue disorder, and expression ranges from mild osteoporosis to the classical clinical stigmata characterized by multiple bone fractures and skeletal deformities, blue sclera, and middle ear deafness (otosclerosis). Four types may be distinguished clinically, and a system of classification (types I through IV) has been proposed.[104] Type I is the prototype disease. It is inherited as an autosomal dominant trait and is the most common and mildest form of this disease. It typically presents in childhood with multiple fractures after minor trauma.[104] Types II and III are inherited as autosomal recessive traits and are characterized by extreme bone fragility. Type II is uniformly lethal, and stillbirth or early neonatal death is common; death in utero is caused by skeletal collapse, and early neonatal death typically results from chest wall failure and respiratory insufficiency. Infants affected with type III may have fractures at birth and may develop progressive skeletal deformities during the first two decades of life.

Type IV, also autosomal dominant, is much less common and is variable in its expressivity.

The majority of parturients with OI have type I disease, although pregnancy has been reported in more severe forms of the disease.[105] There is considerable variability among affected patients as to the age of onset and frequency of fractures. Dwarfism is typical, and kyphoscoliosis is common, as are other chest wall abnormalities. These chest and spinal abnormalities result in restrictive lung disorders (Figure 47-11). Other abnormalities include a decrease in the range of motion of the shortened cervical spine, micrognathia, and malformed brittle teeth.[103,105,106] Poor platelet adhesion may cause platelet dysfunction and a modest bleeding tendency. Hyperthyroidism occurs in 40% of patients; an elevated concentration of thyroxine leads to both increased oxygen consumption and heat production.[105,106] Hyperthermia may occur, and there is a case report of the occurrence of malignant hyperthermia (MH) in a patient with OI. However, most patients—when tested with the halothane-caffeine contracture test—are not MH susceptible.[107]

Obstetric Management

Platelet dysfunction results in an increased incidence of intrapartum and postpartum hemorrhage, although this is uncommon. Labor and vaginal delivery are associated with an increased risk of uterine rupture and pelvic fracture. These complications are also uncommon and most likely are influenced primarily by the severity of the disease. Cephalopelvic disproportion typically mandates delivery by cesarean section in severely affected parturients.

Anesthetic Management

The anesthesiologist must be aware of the fragility of the bones, the potential for difficult intubation, and the presence and severity of restrictive lung disease. Transfers, positioning, and any invasive intervention must be accomplished with extreme care. Blood pressure cuffs and tourniquets to facilitate placement of intravenous catheters should be applied gently to prevent fractures. Difficult intubation may occur because of a short neck with limited range of motion.[105] The anesthesiologist should take care not to hyperextend the neck, and laryngoscopy should be gentle to avoid fractures. Alternatives to direct laryngoscopy may be considered to reduce the applied forces necessary. If succinylcholine is used, a defasciculating dose of a nondepolarizing muscle relaxant should be employed to prevent fasciculations.[106] An alternative to succinylcholine (e.g., rocuronium) also may be administered to prevent fasciculations. Hyperthermia should be anticipated, and there should be provisions to cool the patient if a significant rise in body temperature should occur. Although there is a case report of probable MH in a patient with osteogenesis imperfecta, most patients are not MH susceptible.[107]

Before giving regional anesthesia, the anesthesiologist should consider the technical difficulties inherent in performing regional anesthesia in a patient with spinal deformities. The anesthesiologist also should be aware of the platelet function defect in these patients. In my judgment, this risk is best evaluated by obtaining a thorough history *rather* than by laboratory evaluation (e.g., bleeding time) before the administration of regional anesthesia. In the setting of a reassuring history, regional anesthesia need not be withheld. Small stature and spinal abnormalities decrease the local anesthetic dose requirements and increase the risk of both misplaced injection and local anesthetic toxicity. It may be difficult to estimate the appropriate dose for single-shot spinal anesthesia in these patients. Thus continuous epidural or subarachnoid anesthesia are the regional anesthetic techniques of choice, barring a contraindication. Yeo and Paech[108] reported the successful use of both epidural and subarachnoid block for cesarean section on five occasions over 9 years in a single patient with type I OI.

SPONDYLOLISTHESIS

Isthmic spondylolisthesis is a condition in which a defect in the pars interarticularis of a vertebra allows anterior slippage of the subjacent portion of the spine. As the body slips forward, it does not carry the neural arch with it; thus there is little tendency toward spinal canal stenosis. Isthmic spondylolisthesis typically occurs at the lumbosacral junction, although it is not uncommon in the lumbar spine. Approximately 38% of cases occur in women.[109] The onset is common in the second to fourth decades, a period of peak childbearing potential.

Back pain is the presenting feature. Strenuous physical activity often precipitates the onset of pain. Pregnancy increases back symptoms in approximately half of these patients, but obstetric complications are unusual.[109,110]

There is no published case of regional anesthesia during labor in a parturient with severe spondylolisthesis (e.g., lumbosacral subluxation). Ideally, an anesthesiologist will see the patient during pregnancy to assess her symptoms and lumbar spinal anatomy. In the absence of evidence of a neurologic deficit, it seems appropriate to administer either epidural or spinal anesthesia.

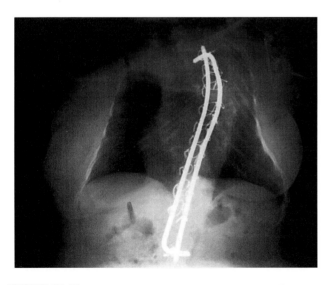

FIGURE 47-11. A chest radiograph of a 30-year-old woman with osteogenesis imperfecta, type I. Generalized osteoporosis, corrected thoracic kyphoscoliosis, a restricted thoracic cage, and multiple old fractures are demonstrated. (General anesthesia was provided for cesarean section and tubal ligation.)

KEY POINTS

- Low back pain is the most common musculoskeletal complaint during pregnancy. It results from both hormonal and mechanical factors.
- Low back pain does not contraindicate the administration of spinal or epidural anesthesia.
- Corrected idiopathic thoracolumbar scoliosis is the most common major musculoskeletal disorder seen in pregnant women. Prepregnancy pulmonary function is a better predictor of maternal outcome than the severity of the curve.
- Regional anesthesia is more challenging technically in patients with scoliosis, and the anesthesiologist should anticipate an increased incidence of complications and inadequate anesthesia.
- Maternal rheumatoid arthritis and ankylosing spondylitis do not adversely affect the outcome of pregnancy.
- Pregnancy often ameliorates the symptoms of rheumatoid arthritis.
- Spina bifida occulta is a common incidental finding in normal patients; it does not contraindicate the administration of spinal or epidural anesthesia.
- Spina bifida cystica and occult spinal dysraphism are associated with a high incidence of tethered cord; this may complicate the administration of subarachnoid (spinal) anesthesia.
- Cephalopelvic disproportion often mandates the performance of cesarean section in patients with achondroplasia or osteogenesis imperfecta.

REFERENCES

1. Orvieto R, Achiron A, Ben-Rafael Z, et al. Low back pain of pregnancy. Acta Obstet Gynecol Scand 1994; 73:209-14.
2. Kristiansson P, Svärdsudd K, von Schoultz B. Back pain during pregnancy: A prospective study. Spine 1996; 21:702-9.
3. Ostgaard HC, Anderson GBJ, Karlsson K. Prevalence of back pain in pregnancy. Spine 1991; 16:549-52.
4. MacEvilly M, Buggy D. Back pain and pregnancy: A review. Pain 1996; 64:405-14.
5. Brynhildsen J, Hansson A, Persson A, et al. Follow-up of patients with low back pain during pregnancy. Obstet Gynecol 1998; 91:182-6.
6. Kristiansson P, Svärdsudd K, von Schoultz B. Serum relaxin, symphyseal pain, and back pain during pregnancy. Am J Obstet Gynecol 1996; 175:1342-7.
7. MacLennan AH, Nicolson R, Green RC. Serum relaxin and pelvic pain of pregnancy. Lancet 1986; 2:241-3.
8. Ostgaard HC, Zutherström G, Roos-Hansson E, et al. Reduction of back and posterior pelvic pain in pregnancy. Spine 1994; 19:894-900.
9. Garmel SH, Guzelian GA, D'Alton JG, et al. Lumbar disk disease in pregnancy. Obstet Gynecol 1997; 89:821-2.
10. Frymoyer JW. Back pain and sciatica. N Engl J Med 1988; 318:291-300.
11. Benzon HT, Braunschweig R, Molloy RE. Delayed onset of epidural anesthesia in patients with back pain. Anesth Analg 1981; 60:874-7.
12. Sharrock ME, Urqhart B, Mineo R. Extradural anaesthesia in patients with previous lumbar spine surgery. Br J Anaesth 1990; 65:237-9.
13. Schachner SM, Abram SE. Use of two epidural catheters to provide analgesia of unblocked segments in a patient with lumbar disc disease. Anesthesiology 1982; 56:150-1.
14. Calleja MA. Extradural analgesia and previous spinal surgery: A radiological appraisal. Anaesthesia 1991; 40:946-7.
15. Luyendijk W, van Voorthuisen AE. Contrast examination of the spinal epidural space. Acta Radiol 1966; 5:1051-66.
16. LaRocca H, MacNab I. The laminectomy membrane: Studies in its evolution, effects and prophylaxis in dogs. J Bone Joint Surg 1974; 56:545-50.
17. Brodsky AE. Post-laminectomy and post-fusion stenosis of the lumbar spine. Clin Orthop 1976; 115:130-9.
18. MacArthur C, Lewis M, Crawford S. Epidural anaesthesia and longterm backache after childbirth. Br Med J 1990; 301:9-12.
19. MacArthur C, Lewis M, Crawford S. Investigation of longterm problems after obstetric epidural anaesthesia. Br Med J 1992; 304:1279-82.
20. MacLeod J, MacIntyre C, McClure JH, et al. Backache and epidural analgesia. A retrospective survey of mothers 1 year after childbirth. Int J Obstet Anesth 1995; 4:21-5.
21. Breen TW, Ransil BJ, Groves PA, et al. Factors associated with back pain after childbirth. Anesthesiology 1994; 81:29-34.
22. Groves PA, Breen TW, Ransil BJ, et al. The natural history of postpartum back pain and its relationship with epidural anaesthesia. Anesthesiology 1994; 81:A1167.
23. Macarthur A, Macarthur C, Weeks S. Epidural anaesthesia and low back pain after delivery: A prospective cohort study. Br Med J 1995; 311:1336-9.
24. Howell CJ, Kidd C, Roberts P, et al. A randomized controlled trial of epidural compared with non-epidural analgesia in labour. Br J Obstet Gynaecol 2001; 108:27-33.
25. Howell CJ, Dean T, Lucking L, et al. Randomised study of long term outcome after epidural versus non-epidural analgesia during labour. BMJ 2002; 325:357-9.
26. Patel M, Fernando P, Gill P, et al. A prospective study of long-term backache after childbirth in primigravidae: The effect of ambulatory epidural analgesia during labour. Int J Obstet Anesth 1995; 4:187.
27. Russell R, Dundas R, Reynolds R. Long term backache after childbirth: Prospective search for causative factors. Brit Med J 1996; 312:1384-8.
28. MacArthur C, Lewis M. Anaesthetic characteristics and long-term backache after obstetric epidural anaesthesia. Internat J Obstet Anesth 1996; 5:8-13.
29. Ostgaard HC, Andersson GBJ. Postpartum low-back pain. Spine 1992; 17:53-5.
30. To WWK, Wong MWN. Kyphoscoliosis complicating pregnancy. Int J Gynecol Obstet 1996; 55:123-8.
31. White AA III, Panjabi MM. Practical biomechanics of scoliosis and kyphosis. In White AA III, Panjabi MM, editors. Clinical Biomechanics of the Spine, 2nd ed. Philadelphia, JB Lippincott, 1990:127-68.
32. Pehrsson K, Larsson S, Oden A, et al. Long-term follow-up of patients with untreated scoliosis: A study of mortality, causes of death, and symptoms. Spine 1992; 17:1091-6.
33. Hirschfeld SS, Ruder C, Nasch CL, et al. The incidence of mitral valve prolapse in adolescent scoliosis and thoracic hypokyphosis. Pediatrics 1982; 70:451-4.
34. Berman AT, Cohen DL, Schwentker EP. The effects of pregnancy on idiopathic scoliosis: A preliminary report on eight cases and a review of the literature. Spine 1982; 7:76-7.
35. Blount WP, Mellencamp DD. The effect of pregnancy on idiopathic scoliosis. J Bone Joint Surg 1980; 62A:1083-7.
36. Kopenhager T. A review of 50 pregnant patients with kyphoscoliosis. Br J Obstet Gynecol 1977; 84:585-7.
37. Sawicka EH, Spencer GT, Branthwaite MA. Management of respiratory failure complicating pregnancy in severe kyphoscoliosis: A new use for an old technique? Br J Dis Chest 1986; 80:191-6.
38. Siegler D, Zorab PA. Pregnancy in thoracic scoliosis. Br J Dis Chest 1981; 75:367-70.
39. Kesten S, Garfinkel SK, Wright T, et al. Impaired exercise capacity in adults with moderate scoliosis. Chest 1991; 99:663-6.
40. Zeldis SM. Dyspnea during pregnancy: Distinguishing cardiac from pulmonary causes. Clin Chest Med 1992; 13:567-85.
41. Torell G, Nordwall A, Nachemson A. The changing pattern of scoliosis treatment due to screening. J Bone Joint Surg 1981; 63A:337-41.
42. Moskowitz A, Moe JH, Winter RB, et al. Long-term follow-up of scoliosis fusion. J Bone Joint Surg 1980; 62A:364-76.
43. Crosby ET, Halpern SH. Obstetric epidural anaesthesia in patients with Harrington instrumentation. Can J Anaesth 1989; 36:693-6.
44. Schneerson JM. Pregnancy in neuromuscular and skeletal disorders. Monaldi Arch Chest Dis 1994; 49:227-30.
45. Moran DH, Johnson MD. Continuous spinal anesthesia with combined hyperbaric and isobaric bupivacaine in a patient with scoliosis. Anesth Analg 1990; 70:445-7.
46. Cochran T, Irstam L, Nachemson A. Long term anatomic and functional changes in patients with adolescent idiopathic scoliosis treated by Harrington rod fusion. Spine 1983; 8:576-84.

47. Sponseller PD, Cohen MS, Nachemson AL, et al. Results of surgical treatment of adults with idiopathic scoliosis. J Bone Joint Surg 1987; 69A:667-75.

48. Aaro S, Ohlen G. The effect of Harrington instrumentation on the sagittal mobility of the spine in scoliosis. Spine 1983; 8:570-5.

49. Daley MD, Morningstar BA, Rolbin SH, et al. Epidural anesthesia for obstetrics after spinal surgery. Reg Anesth 1990; 15:280-4.

50. Yeo ST, French R. Combined spinal-epidural in the obstetric patient with Harrington rods assisted by ultrasonography. Br J Anaesth 1999; 83:670-2.

51. Sudunagunta S, Eckersall SJ, Gowrie-Mohan S. Continuous caudal analgesia in labour for a patient with Harrington rods. Int J Obstet Anesth 1998; 7:128-30.

52. Gerancher JC, D'Angelo R, Carpenter R. Caudal epidural blood patch for the treatment of postdural puncture headache. Anesth Analg 1998; 87:394-5.

53. O'Sullivan JB, Cathcart ES. The prevalence of rheumatoid arthritis: Follow-up evaluation of the effect of criteria on rates in Sudbury, Massachusetts. Ann Intern Med 1972; 76:573-7.

54. Grantham SA, Lipson SJ. Rheumatoid arthritis and other noninfectious inflammatory diseases: Rheumatoid arthritis of the cervical spine. In The Cervical Spine Research Society Editorial Committee. The Cervical Spine, 2nd ed. Philadelphia, JB Lippincott, 1989:564-98.

55. Wolfe BK, O'Keeffe D, Mitchell DM, et al. Rheumatoid arthritis of the cervical spine: Early and progressive radiographic features. Radiology 1987; 165:145-8.

56. Santavirta S, Kankaanpaa U, Sandelin J, et al. Evaluation of patients with rheumatoid cervical spine. Scan J Rheum 1987; 16:9-16.

57. Keenan MA, Stiles CM, Kaufman RL. Acquired laryngeal deviation associated with cervical spine disease in erosive polyarticular arthritis: Use of the fiberoptic bronchoscope in rheumatoid arthritis. Anesthesiology 1983; 58:441-9.

58. Klipple GL, Cecere FA. Rheumatoid arthritis and pregnancy. Rheum Clin North Am 1989; 15:213-39.

59. Bulmash JM. Rheumatoid arthritis and pregnancy. Obstet Gynecol Clin North Am 1985; 8:223-76.

60. Lockshin MD, Druzin ML. Rheumatic disease. In Barron WM, Lindheimer MD, Davison JM, editors. Medical Disorders in Pregnancy, 2nd ed. Mosby, St. Louis, 1995:307-37.

61. Channing Rodgers RP, Levin J. A critical reappraisal of the bleeding time. Semin Thromb Hem 1990; 16:1-20.

62. Sinclair JR, Mason RA. Ankylosing spondylitis: The case for awake intubation. Anaesthesia 1984; 39:3-11.

63. Ostensen M, Husby G. Ankylosing spondylitis and pregnancy. Rheum Dis Clin North Am 1989; 15:241-54.

64. Sorin S, Askari A, Moskowitz RW. Atlantoaxial subluxation as complication of early ankylosing spondylitis: Two case reports and a review of the literature. Arthrit Rheum 1979; 22:273-6.

65. Hunter T. The spinal complications of ankylosing spondylitis. Semin Arthrit Rheum 1989; 19:172-82.

66. Ostensen M, Husby G. A prospective clinical study of the effect of pregnancy on rheumatoid arthritis and ankylosing spondylitis. Arthrit Rheum 1983; 26:1155-9.

67. Aavrahami E, Frishman E, Fridman Z, et al. Spina bifida occulta of S1 is not an innocent finding. Spine 1994; 19:12-5.

68. McGrady EM, Davis AG. Spina bifida occulta and epidural anaesthesia. Anaesthesia 1988; 43:867-9.

69. Cooper MG, Sethna NF. Epidural analgesia in patients with congenital lumbosacral spinal anomalies. Anesthesiology 1991; 75:370-4.

70. Vaagenes P, Fjaerestad I. Epidural block during labour in a patient with spina bifida cystica. Anaesthesia 1981; 36:299-301.

71. Farine D, Jackson U, Portale A. Pregnancy complicated by maternal spina bifida. J Reprod Med 1988; 33:323-6.

72. Richmond D, Zaharievski I, Bond A. Management of pregnancy in mothers with spina bifida. Eur J Obstet Gynecol Reprod Biol 1987; 25:341-5.

73. Evans RC, Tew B, Thomas MD, et al. Selective surgical management of neural tube malformations. Arch Dis Child 1985; 60:415-9.

74. Charney EB, Weller SC, Sutton LN, et al. Management of the newborn with myelomeningocele: Time for the decision making process. Pediatrics 1985; 75:58-64.

75. Muller EB, Nordwall A. Prevalence of scoliosis in children with myelomeningocele. Spine 1992; 17:1097-102.

76. Page LK. Occult spinal dysraphism and related disorders. In Wilkins RH, Rengachary SS, editors. Neurosurgery. New York, McGraw-Hill, 1985:2053-7.

77. Rekate HL. Neurosurgical management of the child with spina bifida. In Rekate HL, editor. Comprehensive Management of Spina Bifida. Boca Raton, Fla, CRC Press, 1991:93-111.

78. James CCM, Lassman LP. Tight filum terminale and tethered cord syndromes. In James CCM, Lassman LP, editors. Spina Bifida Occulta. London, Academic Press, 1981:202-9.

79. Brooks SB, El Gammal T, Hartlage P, et al. Myelography of sacral agenesis. AJNR 1981; 2:319.

80. Crosby E, St-Jean B, Reid D, et al. Obstetrical anaesthesia and analgesia in chronic spinal cord-injured women. Can J Anaesth 1992; 39:487-94.

81. Broome IJ. Spinal anaesthesia for caesarean section in a patient with spina bifida cystica. Anaesth Intensive Care 1989; 17:377-9.

82. Nuyten F, Gielen M. Spinal catheter anaesthesia in a patient with spina bifida. Anaesthesia 1990; 45:846-7.

83. Wood GG, Jacka MJ. Spinal hematoma following spinal anesthesia in a patient with spina bifida occulta. Anesthesiology 1997; 87:983-4.

84. Tidmarsh MD, May AE. Epidural anaesthesia and neural tube defects. Int J Obstet Anesth 1998; 7:111-14.

85. Mayhew JF, Katz J, Miner M, et al. Anaesthesia for the achondroplastic dwarf. Can Anaesth Soc J 1986; 33:216-21.

86. Berkowitz ID, Raja SN, Bender KS, et al. Dwarfs: Pathophysiology and anesthetic implications. Anesthesiology 1990; 73:739-59.

87. Kalla GN, Fening E, Obiaya MO. Anaesthetic management of achondroplasia. Br J Anaesth 1986; 58:117-9.

88. Cohen SA. Anesthesia for cesarean section in achondroplastic dwarfs. Anesthesiology 1980; 52:264-6.

89. Mather JS. Impossible direct laryngoscopy in achondroplasia: A case report. Anaesthesia 1966; 21:244-8.

90. Walts LF, Finerman G, Wyatt GM. Anaesthesia for dwarfs and other patients of pathological small stature. Can Anaesth Soc J 1975; 22:703-9.

91. Carstoniu J, Yee I, Halpern S. Epidural anaesthesia for caesarean section in an achondroplastic dwarf. Can J Anaesth 1992; 39:708-11.

92. Wynne-Davies R, Walsh WK, Gormley J. Achondroplasia and hypochondroplasia. J Bone Joint Surg 1981; 63B:508-15.

93. Lutter LD, Lonstein JE, Winter RB, et al. Anatomy of the achondroplastic lumbar canal. Clin Orthop 1977; 126:139-42.

94. Wardall GJ, Frame WT. Extradural anaesthesia for caesarean section in achondroplasia. Br J Anaesth 1990; 64:367-70.

95. Brimacombe JR, Caunt JA. Anaesthesia in a gravid achondroplastic dwarf. Anaesthesia 1990; 45:132-4.

96. Allanson JE, Hall JG. Obstetric and gynecologic problems in women with chondrodystrophies. Obstet Gynecol 1986; 67:74-8.

97. Beilin Y, Leibowitz AB. Anesthesia for an achondroplastic dwarf presenting for urgent cesarean section. Int J Obstet Anesth 1993; 2:96-7.

98. Ratner EF, Hamilton CL. Anesthesia for cesarean section in a pituitary dwarf. Anesthesiology 1998; 89:253-4.

99. Morrow MJ, Black IH. Epidural anaesthesia for caesarean section in an achondroplastic dwarf. Br J Anaesth 1998; 81:619-21.

100. Bancroft GH, Lauria JI. Ketamine induction for cesarean section in a patient with acute intermittent porphyria and achondroplastic dwarfism. Anesthesiology 1983; 59:143-4.

101. McArthur RDA. Obstetrical anaesthesia in an achondroplastic dwarf at a regional hospital. Anaesth Intensive Care 1992; 20:376-8.

102. Cunningham AJ, Donnelly M, Comerford J. Osteogenesis imperfecta. Anesthetic management of a patient for cesarean section: A case report. Anesthesiology 1984; 61:91-3.

103. Carlson JW, Harlass FE. Management of osteogenesis imperfecta in pregnancy. J Reprod Med 1093; 38:228-32.

104. Sillence D. Osteogenesis imperfecta: An expanding panorama of variants. Clin Orthop 1981; 159:11-25.

105. Vogel TM, Ratner EF, Thomas RC Jr, Chitkara U. Pregnancy complicated by severe osteogenesis imperfecta: report of two cases. Anesth Analg 2002; 94:1315-7.

106. Cho E, Dayan SS, Marx GF. Anaesthesia in a parturient with osteogenesis imperfecta. Br J Anaesth 1992; 68:422-3.

107. Rampton AJ, Kelly DA, Shanahan EC, et al. Occurrence of malignant hyperpyrexia in a patient with osteogenesis imperfecta. Br J Anaesth 1984; 56:1443-6.

108. Yeo ST, Paech MJ. Regional anaesthesia for multiple cesarean sections in a parturient with osteogenesis imperfecta. Int J Obstet Anesth 1999; 8:284-7.

109. Vebostad A. Spondylolisthesis. Acta Orthop Scand 1974; 45:711-23.

110. Dandy DJ, Shannon MJ. Lumbo-sacral subluxation. J Bone Joint Surg 1971; 53B:578-95.

Chapter 48
Neurologic and Neuromuscular Disease

Angela M. Bader, M.D.

The choice of anesthetic technique for pregnant women with neurologic disease requires knowledge of the pathophysiology of the disorder and the controversies involved. If a patient's neurologic condition deteriorates postpartum, the cause may be unclear and the anesthetic technique may be blamed. There are limited published data on specific neurologic and neuromuscular disorders in pregnant women. However, few of these disorders contraindicate the use of regional anesthesia. In most cases, the obstetrician should obtain early antepartum consultation from an anesthesiologist. Early consultation allows accurate antepartum documentation of the extent and pattern of the neurologic deficit and discussion and formulation of the anesthetic plan.

MULTIPLE SCLEROSIS

Multiple sclerosis is a major cause of neurologic disability in young adults. The prevalence of the disorder varies with the population. A geographic gradient appears to exist. The prevalence is less than 1 per 100,000 near the equator, but it increases to 3 to 8 per 1000 in the northern United States and Canada.[1]

The disease is characterized by its variability and consists of altered patterns of neurologic disability over years. Two general patterns have been identified: (1) **exacerbating remitting,** in which attacks appear abruptly and resolve over several months, and (2) **chronic progressive.**[2] Most relapses reproduce previous neurologic deficits and cause pyramidal, cerebellar, or brainstem symptoms.

The etiology remains unclear. Exposure to a viral agent early in life may trigger an autoimmune response in patients with certain histocompatibility antigens.[3] Pathologic findings include inflammation and loss of myelin in the central nervous system (CNS).

The more common symptoms include motor weakness, impaired vision, ataxia, bladder and bowel dysfunction, and emotional lability. Cerebrospinal fluid (CSF) immunoglobulin and lymphocyte concentrations are increased, and magnetic resonance imaging (MRI) studies demonstrate white matter plaques. Lesions may be documented by demonstration of prolonged evoked potentials in the involved areas.

There is no curative treatment. Immunosuppressive therapies may hasten recovery from a relapse, but no evidence suggests that these agents influence the progressive course of the disease. Recent work suggests that beta-interferon may be the first therapeutic agent to significantly reduce the relapse rate and retard disability.[4] Postpartum administration of high-dose intravenous immunoglobulin may also reduce the risk of relapse.[5] The relapse rate is approximately 0.3 to 0.4 attacks per year, and the deficits tend to become more progressive and debilitating over time. Environmental factors such as stress, infection, and increased body temperature may provoke relapse.[6]

Interaction with Pregnancy

Multiple sclerosis does not affect fertility, pregnancy, or the management of labor and delivery. The length of the three stages of labor is normal, and there is no increase in the incidence of preterm labor, difficult delivery, or stillbirth.[7] Infants of women with multiple sclerosis may be at increased risk for meconium aspiration.[7] Immunologically active substances such as beta- interferon are increased during pregnancy and may influence T-cell function and hence the course of the disease.[8]

Patients with exacerbating-remitting multiple sclerosis have a slightly decreased relapse rate during pregnancy and an increase in exacerbation during the first 3 to 6 months postpartum.[8-10] Stress, exhaustion, infection, and hyperpyrexia exacerbate multiple sclerosis, and all of these factors may contribute to the increased relapse rate after delivery. The loss of antenatal immunosuppression and the postpartum decline in maternal concentrations of reproductive hormones also may be responsible.

Pregnancy does not negatively affect the long-term outcome of multiple sclerosis. Rather, at least one study suggests that parturition may have a slightly favorable effect on long-term disease activity.[11]

Anesthetic Management

The anesthesiologist should assess the patient's degree of compromise, document the pattern of deficits, and give special attention to respiratory involvement. Historically, there has been great controversy regarding the administration of anesthesia in patients with multiple sclerosis. Most anesthesiologists have considered general anesthesia to be safe, although published data are limited.[12,13] Many anesthesiologists have been reluctant to administer spinal or epidural anesthesia because the effect of local anesthetic drugs on the course of the disease is unclear. Some anesthesiologists have worried that spinal or epidural anesthesia may expose demyelinated areas of the spinal cord to the potential neurotoxic effects of local anesthetic agents. Several animal studies have investigated the possible neurotoxic effects of local anesthetic agents on the normal spinal cord. In one study, subarachnoid injection of small doses of a local anesthetic agent produced no histologic changes in the cord or meninges. Injection of very large doses caused reversible inflammatory and degenerative changes; all changes were absent by 14 days after injection.[14]

Diagnostic lumbar puncture is not associated with an increased rate of relapse.[15] Two reports have implicated spinal anesthesia in the exacerbation of multiple sclerosis.[13,16] However, these two series included only a small number of relapses. Bamford et al.[13] described only one relapse after nine spinal anesthetics, and Stenuit and Marchand[16] identified only two relapses after the administration of spinal anesthesia in 19 patients. The relationship of these relapses to spinal anesthesia or other postoperative conditions (e.g., stress, infection, hyperpyrexia) known to exacerbate multiple sclerosis is unclear.

There are few published data regarding the use of epidural anesthesia in patients with multiple sclerosis. Warren et al.[17] reported minor exacerbations after the administration of epidural anesthesia for two separate vaginal deliveries in one patient. Crawford et al.[18] reported only one postoperative relapse in 50 nonobstetric and seven obstetric patients who received epidural anesthesia. Confavreux et al.[9] reported a study of 269 pregnancies in 254 women with multiple sclerosis, of whom 42 received epidural analgesia. They noted that epidural analgesia did not have an adverse effect on the rate of relapse or on the progression of disability in these patients. We retrospectively evaluated 32 pregnancies in women with multiple sclerosis and observed that women who received epidural anesthesia for vaginal delivery did not have a higher incidence of relapse than those who received only local infiltration. Among the five patients who underwent cesarean delivery, one had a postpartum relapse. The data suggested that the concentration of local anesthetic used for epidural anesthesia may influence the relapse rate because all patients in the relapse group had received higher concentrations of bupivacaine or lidocaine.[19] The concentration of local anesthetic in the CSF progressively increases during prolonged administration of epidural anesthesia. The increased concentration may overwhelm the protective effect of dilution within the CSF. These observations suggest that anesthesiologists should use dilute solutions of local anesthetic for epidural anesthesia during labor.

The addition of an opioid reduces the total dose of local anesthetic required for epidural analgesia during labor. Leigh et al.[20] described the successful use of intrathecal diamorphine in a patient with multiple sclerosis.

The administration of anesthesia for cesarean section is more problematic. However, given the limited duration of surgery, multiple doses of local anesthetic are not needed, and the CSF concentrations should not increase over time. At the Brigham and Women's Hospital, either spinal or epidural anesthesia may be administered for cesarean delivery in patients with multiple sclerosis.

In summary, published data do not contraindicate the use of regional anesthesia for labor, delivery, or cesarean section. The patient should be aware that there is a high incidence of relapse during the postpartum period, regardless of the type of anesthesia used. However, pregnancy does not have a negative influence on the long-term course of the disease. In an editorial, Whitaker[10] stated, "Women with multiple sclerosis can be informed that conception, gestation, and epidural

anesthesia will not alter the natural history of their disease. However, the increased frequency of relapses during the postpartum period can reduce the ability of the mother to provide care for her newborn when relapses occur."

HEADACHE DURING PREGNANCY

Headache is one of the most common neurologic symptoms during pregnancy (Table 48-1). The most common kinds of headache during pregnancy include tension headache, migraine headache, and headache associated with pregnancy-induced hypertension (PIH).

Tension Headache

Tension or muscle contraction headache is the most common headache that occurs during pregnancy.[21] The symptoms typically include dull, persistent pain that extends over the entire head. The onset typically is gradual, and the symptoms may persist for long periods of time. The etiology is unknown. These headaches are more common in women, are frequently associated with anxiety, and may be a symptom of postpartum depression.[22]

TREATMENT

In the nonpregnant patient, treatment may include acetaminophen, aspirin, opioids, tricyclic antidepressants, and benzodiazepines. Most experts avoid the administration of benzodiazepines during pregnancy because of conflicting evidence regarding the incidence of orofacial clefts after fetal exposure during the first trimester.[23] Opioids have a long record of safe use during pregnancy. Tricyclic antidepressants also have been used safely during pregnancy; recent work suggests that these agents do not have a detrimental effect on the neurodevelopment of children exposed in utero.[24]

OBSTETRIC AND ANESTHETIC MANAGEMENT

Tension headache may signal an increased risk of postpartum depression.[22] The presence and treatment of tension headache rarely affect obstetric and anesthetic management.

Migraine Headache

Migraine headaches are classically described as unilateral, throbbing headaches sometimes accompanied by nausea and vomiting. The duration varies from hours to days. Visual disturbances (e.g., scotomata) typically precede the onset of these headaches. Focal neurologic symptoms (e.g., aphasia, hemiplegia) also may occur. Most investigators favor neurovascular vasospasm, followed by cerebral vasodilation, as the etiology. This results from either a primary vascular disorder or a disturbance in the noradrenergic nervous system.[25]

Migraine occurs in 4% to 6% of men and 13% to 17% of women.[26] Symptoms generally occur early in adult life. Headache occurs less frequently with advancing age. Hormonal influences are well known; estrogen withdrawal is associated with an exacerbation of symptoms.[27] Approximately 79% of women improve during pregnancy, and 21% remain unchanged or worsen.[28] After delivery, the decrease in hormonal concentrations coincides with an increase in migraine symptoms.[29]

TREATMENT

In nonpregnant patients, therapy often includes ergotamine tartrate, typically in combination with caffeine (Cafergot). However, ergot alkaloids are contraindicated during pregnancy because of associated oxytocic effects and uncertain teratogenic effects.[28,30] Promethazine relieves nausea and vomiting. Beta-adrenergic receptor antagonists (e.g., propranolol) are used for prophylaxis. These agents cross the placenta, and they are used for prophylaxis during pregnancy only when a patient's symptoms are severe. Occasionally calcium entry-blocking agents are used. The use of sumatriptan, a selective serotonin agonist, is controversial. An increased incidence of congenital anomalies has been observed after administration of high doses of sumatriptan in animals.[28] However, a recent review of human studies found no evidence that sumatriptan has any specific effect on pregnancy outcome.[31]

OBSTETRIC MANAGEMENT

There are conflicting data regarding the relationship between migraine and preeclampsia. Recent evidence suggests that women who have a history of migraine may have a higher

TABLE 48-1	HEADACHE DURING PREGNANCY		
Etiology	**Symptoms**	**Pattern**	**Treatment**
Tension headache	Dull, widespread headache	Increased incidence during peripartum period	Analgesics Tricyclic antidepressants
Migraine headache	Frontotemporal throbbing Prodrome of scotomata	Improvement in 79% of patients during pregnancy	Ergotamine contraindicated during pregnancy Promethazine Beta-blockers for prophylaxis
Preeclampsia	Generalized headache Occasional scotomata and/or blurred vision	Occurrence during pregnancy and occasionally postpartum	Blood pressure control Delivery
Meningeal irritation (subarachnoid hemorrhage, meningitis)	Generalized headache	Increased risk of subarachnoid hemorrhage during pregnancy	Based on etiology
Brain tumor	Variable	No increase in incidence during pregnancy, possible increased growth rate	Based on etiology
Pseudotumor cerebri	Generalized headache Visual symptoms	Increased incidence and worsened symptoms during pregnancy	Typically remits within 1 to 3 months or after childbirth

risk of PIH; however, other studies report no increase in the incidence of miscarriage, preeclampsia, congenital anomalies, or stillbirth despite the treatment of migraine during pregnancy.[28,32]

Cerebral ischemia has been reported after the administration of terbutaline in pregnant patients with migraine. Rosene et al.[33] recommended that physicians avoid the administration of terbutaline in pregnant women with a history of vascular headache.

ANESTHETIC MANAGEMENT

There are no published data regarding the relationship between intrapartum anesthesia and postpartum migraine headache.

SPINAL CORD INJURY

Spinal cord injuries occur with an incidence of approximately 30 per million population.[34] Improved handling and stabilization of victims at the site of an accident and the availability of extensive rehabilitative services have resulted in an increased number of women who present for obstetric care after spinal cord injury.

Patient disability and residual function depend on the anatomic location of the injury.[35] Cord injuries below S2 involve only bladder, bowel, and sexual functions. These patients have relaxed perineal muscles, and women with such injuries experience pain during labor. Women with a lesion above T10 do not experience labor pain. Patients with a lesion above T6 have varying degrees of respiratory compromise and are at risk for autonomic hyperreflexia.

Immediately after the injury, the patient suffers a loss of reflex function within the isolated spinal cord.[36] This stage is called *spinal shock* and is characterized by flaccid paralysis with loss of tendon and autonomic reflexes for a period of weeks to months. These patients lose vasomotor tone, temperature regulation, sweating, and piloerection in the parts of the body below the lesion. Pulmonary edema, hemodynamic instability, and circulatory collapse can develop in the absence of brainstem regulation of vasomotor tone. The patient is at risk for aspiration, infection, and other pulmonary complications.

After a variable period, the patient progresses to a chronic stage in which reflex activity is regained. In most cases, this occurs within 1 to 6 weeks after the injury; rarely it may take several months to regain reflex activity.[37] This stage is characterized by disuse atrophy, flexor spasms, and an exaggeration of reflexes. The *mass motor reflex* results from the absence of central inhibitory mechanisms. A stimulus that normally would result in the contraction of a few muscle units results in the widespread spasm of entire muscle groups. The mass motor reflex can occur with any level of spinal cord injury. It may occur with autonomic hyperreflexia in a patient with a lesion above T6.[38]

Approximately 85% of patients with chronic spinal cord injuries at T6 or above experience the syndrome of **autonomic hyperreflexia.**[39] This is a life-threatening complication that results from the absence of central inhibition on the sympathetic neurons in the cord below the injury. Noxious stimuli, bladder or bowel distention, and uterine contractions result in afferent transmission by means of the dorsal spinal root (Figure 48-1).[40] These afferent neurons synapse with sympathetic neurons, and the impulse is propagated both cephalad and caudad in the sympathetic chain, without central inhibition. This results in extreme sympathetic hyperactivity and

severe systemic hypertension secondary to vasoconstriction below the level of the lesion. In response, the reflex arcs involving the baroreceptors of the aortic and carotid bodies lead to bradycardia and vasodilation above the level of the lesion. In patients with lesions of T6 and above, these compensatory mechanisms are insufficient to compensate for the severe hypertension. Intracranial hemorrhage occurs in some cases. A variety of agents have been used for control of the hypertension of autonomic hyperreflexia (Figure 48-2).[41]

Obstetric Management

Pregnancy may aggravate many of the medical complications of spinal cord injury (Box 48-1).[40] The loss of both functional residual capacity and expiratory reserve volume during pregnancy may increase the likelihood of respiratory compromise associated with spinal cord injury. Pregnancy increases the risk of deep vein thrombosis, thromboembolic phenomena, and urinary tract infection. Uterine contractions can stimulate autonomic hyperreflexia.

Women with a lesion above T11 have an increased risk of preterm labor.[42] Because these women do not experience labor pain, obstetric management includes weekly cervical examinations during the third trimester. Vaginal delivery is preferred. The use of forceps may be necessary because of the parturient's inability to push.[43] In a study of 52 pregnancies in spinal cord-injured women, 9 of 12 patients with a lesion above T5 had symptoms of autonomic hyperreflexia. The

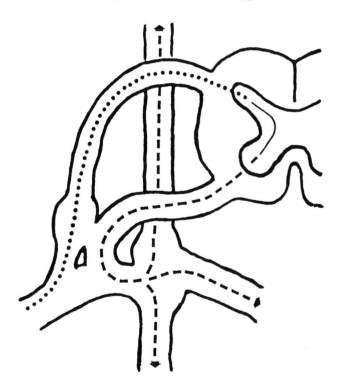

FIGURE 48-1. Noxious stimuli enter the dorsal horn of the spinal cord through the dorsal spinal root *(dotted line)*. These afferent neurons synapse either directly or by means of interneurons *(solid line)* with sympathetic neurons in the intermediolateral columns of the lateral horns, which then project through the anterior roots to the paraspinal sympathetic chain *(dashed line)*. The impulse is propagated peripherally at that spinal level and also travels both cephalad and caudad in the sympathetic chain, exiting at multiple thoracic and lumbar levels *(dashed line)* and resulting in sympathetic hyperactivity. (From Crosby E, St. Jean B, Reid D, Elliot RD. Obstetric anaesthesia and analgesia in chronic spinal cord injured women. Can J Anaesth 1992; 39:487-94.)

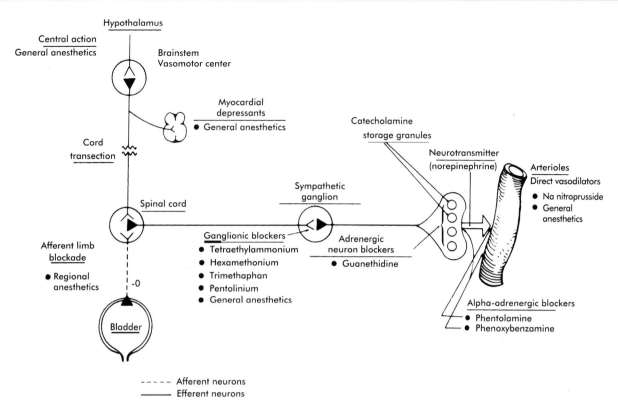

FIGURE 48-2. Sites of action of the agents used for control of the hypertension of autonomic hyperreflexia. (From Schonwald G, Fish KJ, Perkash I. Cardiovascular complications during anesthesia in chronic spinal cord injured patients. Anesthesiology 1981; 55:550-8.)

cesarean delivery rate was 47% for women with a lesion above T5 and 26% for women with a lesion below this level.[44] Preterm delivery occurred in 19% of patients.

Anesthetic Management

Women with a lesion at or above T6 are at risk for autonomic hyperreflexia. This syndrome can be distinguished from other causes of intrapartum hypertension by the occurrence of cyclic hypertension (i.e., blood pressure increases during contractions and decreases between contractions).[45]

Administration of regional anesthesia is the most common method for the prevention or treatment of autonomic hyperreflexia during labor and delivery. Spinal anesthesia has effectively controlled blood pressure in paraplegic patients undergoing general surgical procedures.[46-48] Some anesthesiologists have criticized the use of spinal anesthesia in paraplegic patients; they contend that distortion of the vertebral column makes it more difficult to predict and control the level of anesthesia. However, published data do not lend support to this argument.[46-48] If spinal anesthesia is chosen, it seems appropriate to insert a catheter and use a continuous technique.

Most obstetric anesthesiologists prefer the use of epidural analgesia for the prevention or treatment of autonomic hyperreflexia during labor and delivery. Case reports have noted the successful epidural administration of 0.25% or 0.5% bupivacaine or the administration of combined spinal-epidural (CSE) anesthesia for this purpose.[49-51] Baraka[45] reported the successful epidural administration of meperidine, an opioid with local anesthetic qualities. Abouleish et al.[52] noted that epidural fentanyl alone did not effectively treat the hypertension of autonomic hyperreflexia but that the addition of 0.25% bupivacaine resulted in a decrease in blood

<table>
<tr><td colspan="2">Box 48-1 MEDICAL COMPLICATIONS OF SPINAL CORD INJURY AGGRAVATED BY PREGNANCY</td></tr>
</table>

PULMONARY
- Decreased respiratory reserve
- Atelectasis and pneumonia
- Impaired cough

HEMATOLOGIC
- Anemia
- Deep vein thrombosis
- Thromboembolic phenomena

UROGENITAL
- Chronic urinary tract infections
- Urinary tract calculi
- Proteinuria
- Renal insufficiency

DERMATOLOGIC
- Decubitus ulcers

CARDIOVASCULAR
- Hypertension
- Autonomic hyperreflexia

From Crosby E, St. Jean B, Reid D, Elliot RD. Obstetric anaesthesia and analgesia in chronic spinal cord-injured women. Can J Anaesth 1992; 39:489.

pressure to baseline levels. In one case, the use of 3 mg of epidural morphine (followed by epidural administration of 0.25% bupivacaine during more advanced labor) was effective in the treatment of autonomic hyperreflexia.[53] Maehama et al.[54] reported the successful use of magnesium sulfate for management of autonomic hyperreflexia during labor.

The anesthesiologist must remember that the typical epidural test dose will not identify unintentional subarachnoid injection. Therapeutic doses of a local anesthetic agent should be administered cautiously. The cephalad sensory level can be fully assessed only if it is more cephalad than the level of the spinal cord lesion. Alternatively, a partial assessment can be performed by evaluating segmental reflexes below the level of the lesion. For example, the anesthesiologist can lightly stroke each side of the abdomen above and below the umbilicus. The anesthesiologist looks for contraction of the abdominal muscles and deviation of the umbilicus toward the stimulus. Reflexes will be absent below the level of the block.

Patients with spinal cord injury often have low baseline blood pressures and some degree of hemodynamic instability. Some anesthesiologists recommend the use of an intraarterial catheter for the continuous assessment of blood pressure.[47-51] Alternative means of treating autonomic hyperreflexia should be available if regional anesthesia is not successful (see Figure 48-2).

If cesarean delivery is necessary, I prefer to give epidural anesthesia with 2% lidocaine and 1:200,000 epinephrine. Severe respiratory insufficiency or technical difficulties with regional anesthesia may necessitate the use of general anesthesia.[55] If general anesthesia is required, a depolarizing muscle relaxant such as succinylcholine should not be given during the period of denervation injury. By a conservative definition, this period begins 24 hours after the injury and lasts for 1 year. The use of succinylcholine during this period of denervation injury may result in severe hyperkalemia.[56] Rather, a nondepolarizing muscle relaxant should be used to facilitate laryngoscopy and intubation.

MYASTHENIA GRAVIS

Myasthenia gravis is an autoimmune disorder characterized by episodes of muscle weakness that are made worse by activity. Its prevalence is approximately 40 to 80 per million. In women the onset peaks between 20 and 30 years of age.[57] In this age group the ratio of affected females to males is 3 to 1.

This disease has been classified according to severity as follows[57]:
- I: Ocular myasthenia
- IIA: Mild generalized myasthenia with slow progression, no crises, drug responsive
- IIB: Moderate generalized myasthenia with severe skeletal and bulbar involvement, no crises, inadequate drug response
- III: Acute, rapidly progressive myasthenia with respiratory crises and poor drug response; high mortality
- IV: Late severe myasthenia, progressive over 2 years from class I to II

Myasthenia gravis results from abnormal autoimmune regulation that leads to the production of antibodies against the nicotinic acetylcholine receptor on the neuromuscular endplate of skeletal muscle. This results in receptor destruction as well as antibody-induced blockade of the remaining acetylcholine receptors.[58] Smooth and cardiac muscle are not affected.

Thymic hyperplasia is common, and thymic tumors occur in approximately 10% of patients. There is an association between myasthenia gravis and other autoimmune disorders such as rheumatoid arthritis and polymyositis. In general, an early age of onset and a long duration of purely ocular myasthenia are good prognostic signs.

Medical Management

Treatment includes thymectomy, administration of anticholinesterase medications and/or immunosuppressive agents, and plasmapheresis. Thymectomy helps approximately 96% of patients; 46% of these develop complete remission, and 50% are asymptomatic or improve with therapy.[59] Thymectomy seems to exert a favorable influence on the outcome of pregnancy. One study noted decreased maternal and perinatal morbidity as well as less frequent clinical exacerbations in patients who had undergone thymectomy.[60]

Anticholinesterase drugs, which inhibit the breakdown of acetylcholine, are the mainstay of therapy. Edrophonium is administered as a diagnostic test; decreased muscle weakness within minutes after an intravenous dose of 10 mg confirms the diagnosis of myasthenia. Physostigmine crosses the blood-brain barrier and is not used for chronic therapy. Neostigmine and pyridostigmine are quaternary ammonium compounds that do not cross the blood-brain barrier. These drugs may be administered orally or intravenously. In general, pyridostigmine is preferred because it has less severe muscarinic side effects.[61]

Corticosteroids and azathioprine have been used with some success. Plasmapheresis can be especially helpful for patients in crisis. One study noted that preoperative plasmapheresis resulted in less need for mechanical ventilation and less time in the intensive care unit postoperatively.[62]

Myasthenia can present with two types of crises. A **cholinergic crisis** results from an excess of the muscarinic effects of anticholinesterase medication combined with a poor response to anticholinesterase therapy. In contrast, a **myasthenic crisis** results from a worsening of the disease. These two crises can be distinguished by the administration of edrophonium; the symptoms will not improve if a cholinergic crisis is present. An improvement indicates the need for a higher dose of anticholinesterase medication.

Many drugs can cause a worsening of myasthenic symptoms. These patients are extremely sensitive to drugs that can potentiate muscle weakness.[63] These agents include neuromuscular blocking agents, quinidine, propranolol, aminoglycoside antibiotics, and tocolytic agents such as magnesium sulfate,[64,65] terbutaline, and ritodrine.[66] One case report noted worsened symptoms after the maternal administration of betamethasone.[66]

Obstetric Management

The course of myasthenia during pregnancy varies. In general, approximately one third of patients improve, one third worsen, and one third show no change.[67] Approximately 30% of patients experience a relapse postpartum.

Myasthenia results in an increase in pregnancy wastage, preterm labor, and maternal mortality and morbidity.[67,68] Plauché[67] noted that maternal mortality is approximately 40 per 1000 live births, and perinatal mortality is approximately 68 per 1000 births.

During pregnancy, maternal physiologic changes may require altered doses of anticholinesterase drugs. Anticholinesterase agents are quaternary ammonium compounds with minimal placental transfer. Each patient should be monitored carefully for progressive respiratory compromise secondary to diaphragmatic elevation during pregnancy. Aggressive therapy of myasthenic crises is essential. Anticholinesterase drugs have known oxytocic effects[68]; thus uterine activity should be moni-

tored during the administration of these drugs. Vital capacity can be measured to monitor fatigue during labor.[69] During labor, intravenous administration of an anticholinesterase drug may be needed. The treatment of the myasthenic parturient with preeclampsia is problematic. The use of magnesium sulfate for seizure prophylaxis may be associated with a significant increase in muscle weakness and may be contraindicated.[70]

The uterus consists of smooth muscle; therefore myasthenia gravis should not affect the first stage of labor. The second stage of labor also requires the use of striated muscle; therefore forceps delivery may be required.

Maternal antibodies to the acetylcholine receptor are transferred across the placenta. Neonatal myasthenia gravis occurs in approximately 16% of infants of mothers with myasthenia gravis.[67] Alpha-fetoprotein blocks the binding of the antibody to the acetylcholine receptor.[71] The rapid decrease in postpartum alpha-fetoprotein concentrations may be responsible for the onset of transient neonatal myasthenia. The infant presents with symptoms of myasthenia (feeding problems, hypotonia, and respiratory difficulty) within the first 4 days of life.[72] Anticholinesterase therapy may be required. The symptoms abate as the antibodies are metabolized, and resolution occurs within 2 to 4 weeks.

Anesthetic Management

Each patient should undergo early antepartum consultation with an anesthesiologist. This evaluation should include an assessment of the degree of bulbar and respiratory involvement. Pulmonary function testing should be performed in patients with evidence of respiratory compromise.

Patients with some degree of respiratory compromise may be more susceptible to the respiratory depression associated with opioids. Thus opioids should be used cautiously, if at all. Regional anesthesia allows prevention of the respiratory depression associated with opioids, and it is the preferred method of analgesia during labor and vaginal delivery.[69,73] Plasma cholinesterase activity is decreased in a patient who is taking an anticholinesterase drug. Ester local anesthetic agents may have a prolonged half-life, and patients may be at risk for local anesthetic toxicity. Therefore an amide local anesthetic agent should be given for epidural anesthesia. Because the dose of local anesthetic agent used for spinal anesthesia is small, the anesthesiologist can safely give either an ester or an amide local anesthetic agent. D'Angelo and Gerancher[73] reported the administration of CSE analgesia for labor and spontaneous vaginal delivery in a patient with severe myasthenia gravis. The CSE technique offers the advantages of effective analgesia with minimal motor block, but the intrathecal opioid component is associated with some risk of respiratory depression.

For cesarean delivery, regional anesthesia is preferred unless the patient has a significant degree of bulbar involvement or respiratory compromise.[74] In these cases, a high level of anesthesia may impair respiratory function. It seems prudent to secure the airway before surgery in patients with severe bulbar involvement or respiratory compromise.

Sodium thiopental, ketamine, and propofol have been used successfully for the induction of general anesthesia in patients with myasthenia gravis.[70,75,76] Muscle relaxants have an unpredictable effect in these patients. In general, muscles affected by the disease are more sensitive to depolarizing agents, and non-affected muscles are more resistant.[77] Succinylcholine may not be metabolized rapidly by patients who are taking an anticholinesterase agent.

Myasthenic patients are extremely sensitive to nondepolarizing muscle relaxants. If a nondepolarizing muscle relaxant must be given, the anesthesiologist should administer an agent with a short half-life (e.g., rocuronium, atracurium, vecuronium).[59] Volatile halogenated agents potentiate muscle relaxation. Neuromuscular blockade should be continually monitored with a nerve stimulator, and small doses of neostigmine may be given cautiously for the reversal of neuromuscular blockade.

After delivery, fluid shifts and a decreased alpha-fetoprotein concentration may necessitate an adjustment of the dose of anticholinesterase drug. Some patients who receive general anesthesia require postoperative ventilation. Earlier studies identified four factors that suggest an increased risk of postoperative ventilation in the nonobstetric patient: (1) duration of myasthenia greater than 6 years, (2) history of chronic respiratory disease, (3) pyridostigmine dose greater than 750 mg per day, and (4) vital capacity less than 2.9 L.[78] However, more recent work has failed to validate these factors and has identified a different list of factors that predict an increased risk of postoperative ventilation: (1) female gender, (2) $FEF_{25-75\%}$ less than 3.3 L/sec and less than 85% of that predicted, (3) FVC less than 2.6 L/sec and less than 78% of that predicted, and (4) $MEF_{50\%}$ less than 3.9 L/sec and less than 80% of that predicted.[79]

EPILEPSY

Epilepsy is a condition in which the patient experiences one of a variety of forms of recurrent seizure activity in the absence of metabolic disorders or acute brain disease. Box 48-2 lists a classification scheme for seizure disorders.[80]

Medical Management

A variety of anticonvulsant drugs are used for seizure therapy (Table 48-2).[81] It is preferable to treat a patient with a single agent if possible. The dose is adjusted to keep the serum level within the therapeutic range.

Prognosis for medical control of seizures is good for patients with generalized seizure disorders; 5-year remissions occur in 70% of patients, and 50% of these patients are able to discontinue their medications.[82] Patients with simple

---

Box 48-2   CLASSIFICATION OF SEIZURES

Generalized seizures—bilateral and symmetric, without local onset
- Tonic-clonic (grand mal) seizures
- Absence seizures (petit mal)
  1. Simple—loss of consciousness only
  2. Complex—with movements

Partial (focal) seizures—have a focal origin
- Simple—typically without loss of consciousness
  1. Motor
  2. Sensory
  3. Autonomic
  4. Psychic
- Complex—typically with impaired consciousness (includes temporal lobe epilepsy)
- Partial seizures with secondary generalization

From Commission on Classification and Terminology of the International League Against Epilepsy. Proposal for revised clinical electroencephalographic classification of epileptic seizures. Epilepsia 1981; 22:489-501.

partial seizures also have a good prognosis; as many as 92% of patients are in remission by 8 years.[83] Complex partial seizures (e.g., temporal lobe epilepsy) are more difficult to control.[84]

Interaction with Pregnancy

Approximately 0.5% of all parturients have a chronic seizure disorder.[85] Pregnancy exerts a variable effect on the frequency of seizures. Approximately one third of epileptic women experience an increase in seizure frequency during pregnancy, and approximately one half experience no change.[86]

A variety of etiologies have been proposed for the increase in seizure frequency in some pregnant women. Increased estrogen concentrations lower the seizure threshold.[87] Increased sodium and water retention, alkalosis secondary to hyperventilation, sleep deprivation, and increased stress and anxiety also have been suggested as mechanisms.[88] Anticonvulsant drug levels often decrease during pregnancy, often despite the administration of an increased dose.[85] Decreased plasma protein binding and increased drug clearance help explain the increased dose requirements during pregnancy.[89,90]

Maternal seizures can have devastating consequences. Hypoxia and acidosis that occur during a generalized seizure can result in fetal distress or intrauterine fetal death.[91] During the past three decades the overall risk of certain obstetric complications in epileptic women has declined. Nonetheless, some studies suggest that epileptic women have a twofold increase in the incidence of preeclampsia, preterm labor, and placental abnormalities.[92]

Infants of mothers with epilepsy are approximately twice as likely to have adverse pregnancy outcomes, including intrauterine fetal death, cesarean section, neonatal and perinatal death, low birth weight and abnormal development.[92] The risk of congenital malformations is approximately 4% to 6%.[92] Malformations have been associated with all currently used therapeutic modalities; those most often seen include cleft lip and palate, and cardiac, neural tube, and urogenital defects. Animal studies suggest that newer agents such as felbamate and gabapentin have less teratogenic effect in animals, but adequate human studies have not been performed.[93]

Infants of mothers on chronic anticonvulsant therapy are at risk for a deficiency in vitamin K-dependent clotting factors. These infants may have a coagulation defect even when

TABLE 48-2	ANTICONVULSANT DRUGS USED FOR EPILEPSY DURING PREGNANCY					
				Types of seizures*		
Drug	Dose	Side effects	Toxicity	Tonic-clonic	Absence	Complex partial
Phenytoin (Dilantin)	Average: 400 mg/day Range: 300-1200 mg/day Therapeutic level: 10-20 µg/mL	Ataxia, drowsiness, gum hyperplasia, hypertrichosis, nystagmus	Rash, serum sickness, pseudolymphoma, Stevens-Johnson syndrome, lupus erythematosus, macrocytic anemia, rare hepatic or marrow toxicity, cerebellar degeneration, peripheral neuropathy	+	−	+
Phenobarbital	Average: 120 mg/day Range: 30-210 mg/day Therapeutic level: 10-35 µg/mL	Drowsiness, ataxia, nystagmus	Rash, possible teratogenicity	+	−	+
Primidone (Mysoline)	Average: 1000 mg/day Range: 500-2000 mg/day Therapeutic level: 4-12 µg/mL	Drowsiness, nausea, ataxia, nystagmus (tachyphylaxis typical)	Rash, adenopathy, lupus erythematosus, macrocytic anemia, arthritis, edema	+	−	+
Carbamazepine (Tegretol)	Average: 600 mg/day Range: 200-1200 mg/day Therapeutic level: 4-8 µg/mL	Drowsiness, dizziness, blurred vision, ataxia, gastrointestinal disturbance	Blood dyscrasia (rare)	+	−	+
Ethosuximide (Zarontin)	Average: 1000 mg/day Range: 500-2000 mg/day Therapeutic level: 40-100 µg/mL	Nausea, abdominal pain, drowsiness, personality change, headache	Rash, nephropathy, marrow depression	−	+	−
Clonazepam	Average: 3 mg/day Range: 1.5-20 mg/day Therapeutic level: 0.01-0.07 µg/mL	Drowsiness, dizziness, ataxia	Coma	+	+	+

*A plus sign denotes that the drug is useful in the indicated form of seizure, and a minus sign indicates that it is not.
From Dalessio DJ. Current concepts: Seizure disorders and pregnancy. N Engl J Med 1985; 312:561.

there is no clinical evidence of abnormal maternal coagulation. Anticonvulsant agents that are enzyme inducing (e.g., phenytoin, phenobarbital, carbamazepine) are most likely to cause this problem. Affected infants are at risk for neonatal hemorrhage and respond to vitamin K (1 mg) given intramuscularly at birth. Some physicians also believe that women receiving chronic anticonvulsant therapy should receive vitamin K during the final month of pregnancy.[94] However, recent data suggest that antenatal maternal administration of vitamin K may not reduce the risk of neonatal bleeding.[95]

Anesthetic Management

Serum levels of anticonvulsant drugs should be checked to ensure therapeutic levels. If the patient experiences a seizure during labor, airway protection and support of ventilation are essential. Small doses of a benzodiazepine or sodium thiopental stop most seizures. Fetal bradycardia may necessitate immediate delivery.

There is no contraindication to the administration of regional anesthesia in these patients. In a retrospective review of 100 epileptic obstetric patients, 19 received general anesthesia, 48 received spinal anesthesia, 21 received epidural or caudal anesthesia, and 12 received pudendal block.[96] Of the five women who had a postpartum seizure, four had received spinal anesthesia and one had received general anesthesia with enflurane. No seizures occurred in patients who received epidural or caudal anesthesia. The authors speculated that alterations in CSF dynamics may have predisposed these patients to postpartum seizures. Merrell and Koch[97] suggested that epidural anesthesia may have an anticonvulsant effect in preeclamptic women.

If general anesthesia is necessary, it seems prudent to avoid drugs such as ketamine, enflurane, and meperidine, which may lower the seizure threshold.[88,98] Sevoflurane has a stronger epileptogenic property than isoflurane, but coadministration of nitrous oxide and hyperventilation both counteract this property.[99] Low doses of propofol also have been shown to cause activation of the electrocorticogram in epileptic patients, but at higher doses burst suppression was induced.[100] Induction of general anesthesia can be performed with sodium thiopental and succinylcholine, and the anesthesia may be maintained with a mixture of oxygen, nitrous oxide, and isoflurane. One study noted that some patients who receive phenytoin are resistant to vecuronium but not to atracurium.[101] Some physicians recommend the avoidance of meperidine for postoperative analgesia because of one report of myoclonic seizures in several patients who had received meperidine.[88]

MYOTONIA AND MYOTONIC DYSTROPHY

Myotonia is the term used to describe prolonged contraction of certain muscles after stimulation, followed by a delay in relaxation.[102] Myotonic dystrophy is the most common myotonic disorder. It has a prevalence of 5 per 100,000 populations.[103] This disorder is inherited in an autosomal dominant pattern, and the gene is known to be located on chromosome 19.[104] Specific muscles become dystrophic or wasted; typically those muscles include the hand, facial, masseter, and pretibial muscles. The disorder is slowly progressive, and symptoms may not become apparent until the second or third decade.[102] There is a wide range in the severity of the disease. Over time continual deterioration occurs, with gradual involvement of pharyngeal and laryngeal muscles, proximal limb muscles, and the diaphragm. Uterine smooth muscle is affected, and cardiac conduction abnormalities often are present. Patients typically succumb to either pulmonary or cardiac failure.

Congenital myotonic dystrophy is a severe form of myotonic dystrophy that presents early in infancy with hypotonia and feeding difficulties.[105] Myotonia becomes apparent during the first few years of life. In most cases the mother has myotonic dystrophy.

Myotonia congenita is a milder familial disorder that is characterized by myotonia of the skeletal muscles; multisystem involvement does not occur.[106] Unlike with myotonic dystrophy, cardiac abnormalities are not present. Smooth muscles are never affected. In some cases, muscle hypertrophy rather than wasting occurs. This disorder can be compatible with long life.

Drugs such as quinine and procainamide are most commonly used to relieve myotonic symptoms.[105,106] Corticosteroids, phenytoin, and tocainide also have been prescribed.

Obstetric Management

In patients with myotonic dystrophy, symptoms of weakness and myotonia remain unchanged or worsen during pregnancy. Antepartum evaluation should include pulmonary function testing to evaluate the severity of restrictive lung disease caused by muscle wasting. Antepartum evaluation also should include an electrocardiogram (ECG), which may demonstrate conduction abnormalities.

There is an increased risk of spontaneous abortion and preterm labor in patients with myotonic dystrophy.[107] Sholl et al.[108] reported that ritodrine tocolysis may provoke symptoms of myotonia.

Muscle weakness may result in a prolonged second stage of labor and an increased incidence of instrumental delivery.[107] Uterine involvement may result in uterine atony and an increased risk of obstetric hemorrhage.[109,110] The neonate may present with respiratory distress if affected by congenital myotonic dystrophy.

Patients with myotonia congenita also have been reported to have temporary worsening of symptoms during pregnancy.[111] Obstetric problems have not been described, most likely because this disease involves skeletal muscle only; uterine smooth muscle is not affected in patients with myotonia congenita.

Anesthetic Management

Patients with myotonic disorders may be especially sensitive to the respiratory depressant effects of opioid analgesics and general anesthesia.[112] All sedatives should be used with caution; in some cases, opioids or sedatives may precipitate apnea. Thus regional anesthesia is preferred for labor and vaginal or cesarean delivery. However, myotonia is an intrinsic muscle disorder that is not relieved by spinal or epidural anesthesia.[113] Only local infiltration with a local anesthetic agent relieves the myotonia. Cold is a known trigger of myotonia; thus the patient should be kept warm. Shivering, which often accompanies labor and delivery, also may provoke myotonia. Therefore some anesthesiologists recommend simultaneous intrathecal or epidural administration of an opioid such as sufentanil.[114] Patients with myotonic dystrophy have a high incidence of pulmonary complications after general anesthesia.[115]

If general anesthesia is required, depolarizing agents such as succinylcholine should be avoided because fasciculations may trigger myotonia,[116] which may make ventilation and intubation difficult. These patients seem to have a normal response to nondepolarizing muscle relaxants. However, careful neuromuscular monitoring is essential, particularly in those with significant muscle weakness. Patients receiving quinine may require a decreased dose of a nondepolarizing muscle relaxant.[117] Although myotonic dystrophy has not been associated with an increased risk for malignant hyperthermia (MH), some cases of MH have been reported in patients with myotonia congenita.[118] Both spinal and epidural anesthesia have been used successfully in patients with myotonic dystrophy.[114,119,120]

MUSCULAR DYSTROPHY

This group of disorders is characterized by a progressive degeneration of skeletal muscle with intact innervation.[121] Research regarding the subsarcolemmal muscle fiber protein dystrophin has led to a reclassification of these disorders. Analysis of dystrophin quality and quantity can be used diagnostically both before and during pregnancy and in some cases can identify carriers.

Duchenne and Becker muscular dystrophies are transmitted as X-linked recessive disorders. These disorders occur almost exclusively in males and are not discussed here. The most common muscular dystrophies that affect females include fascioscapulohumeral dystrophy and limb-girdle dystrophies.

Fascioscapulohumeral dystrophy is an autosomal dominant, slowly progressive disorder that primarily involves the muscles of the shoulders and face.[121] Over time the pelvic and pretibial muscles may be affected. Infrequently, cardiac tachycardia and arrhythmias have been reported.

Limb-girdle dystrophies involve a slow degeneration of the shoulder and pelvic muscles.[121] The inheritance pattern and severity are variable. Cardiac conduction disorders occur in some patients.

Obstetric Management

These dystrophinopathies have varied manifestations, and the classification of these disorders is defined by DNA and dystrophin analysis. Management should focus on the individual patient's symptoms and severity of disease. If significant weakness is present, pulmonary function testing should be obtained to assess the extent of restrictive disease. An antepartum ECG should be considered. Severe pelvic wasting may necessitate instrumental vaginal delivery. Pregnant women with muscular dystrophies do not seem to have an increased incidence of adverse pregnancy outcomes, except for an increased incidence of operative delivery.[122]

Anesthetic Management

Regional anesthesia is preferred for labor and vaginal or cesarean delivery. Severe disease may result in both airway abnormalities and spinal deformities, which may complicate the administration of either general or regional anesthesia.[123] These patients are at risk for developing a hypermetabolic syndrome similar to MH when they are exposed to succinylcholine and/or a volatile halogenated anesthetic agent. The mechanism for this response is not well defined but may

be related to the ability of these agents to exacerbate the instability and permeability of the dystrophin-deficient muscle membranes.[124-126] Thus triggering agents should be avoided in patients with muscular dystrophy who require general anesthesia. In general, these patients have a normal response to nondepolarizing muscle relaxants, but careful neuromuscular monitoring is needed, especially in patients with severe muscle wasting.

THE PHAKOMATOSES (CONGENITAL ECTODERMOSES)

In this category of disorder, cutaneous abnormalities are associated with progressive "quasineoplastic" disorders.[127] This group of disorders includes neurofibromatosis, tuberous sclerosis, and cutaneous angiomatoses with CNS abnormalities.

Neurofibromatosis

Neurofibromatosis represents the excessive proliferation of neural crest elements such as Schwann cells, melanocytes, and fibroblasts. Clinical manifestations include hyperpigmented lesions (café-au-lait spots) accompanied by a variety of cutaneous and subcutaneous tumors. The incidence is approximately 1 per 3000. Half of these cases are sporadic, and half are transmitted in an autosomal dominant fashion. The range of severity and progression is large, and the neurologic symptoms depend on the location of the tumors. Tumors that involve the optic or acoustic nerves, other intracranial tumors, and paraspinal neurofibromas are a cause of concern. Some patients require surgical excision of the tumors. There also is an increased risk of pheochromocytoma in these patients.[128]

OBSTETRIC MANAGEMENT

Pregnancy may exacerbate the disease and cause an increase in tumor growth.[129] Regression occurs after delivery. Neurofibromatosis has been associated with a poor perinatal outcome.[130] However, a more recent review of 247 pregnancies did not confirm the increased incidence of preeclampsia, preterm delivery, intrauterine growth restriction, and perinatal mortality reported previously.[131] The cesarean delivery rate in this group was 36%.

ANESTHETIC MANAGEMENT

The anesthesiologist should thoroughly assess the patient's current symptoms and known lesions and should give special attention to the airway because neck and laryngeal tumors are common.[132]

Regional anesthesia can be given for labor and vaginal or cesarean delivery in most patients. However, severe kyphoscoliosis caused by the presence of paraspinal tumors may complicate the administration of regional anesthesia in some patients. Patients may have asymptomatic paraspinal or intracranial tumors. For this reason, some authors have opined that regional anesthesia should be administered only after careful clinical and radiographic evaluations have been performed.[133]

If general anesthesia is required, muscle relaxants should be used cautiously, given the conflicting reports of dose response in these patients. Both increased and decreased sensitivity to succinylcholine, as well as an increased sensitivity to nondepolarizing agents, have been reported.[134-136] However, a recent study noted minimal alteration in dose response, and

the authors recommended no alteration in the dose of either succinylcholine or nondepolarizing muscle relaxants in these patients.[134]

Tuberous Sclerosis

Tuberous sclerosis is a phakomatosis characterized by epilepsy, mental retardation, and adenoma sebaceum. The brain shows abnormal growth of glial cells in hamartomas called *tubers*.[127] Hamartomatous tumors can occur in multiple organs, including the heart, kidneys, liver, and lungs. The inheritance pattern is autosomal dominant with a variable expression, and the disease is slowly progressive.

OBSTETRIC AND ANESTHETIC MANAGEMENT

There are few reports of pregnancy in women with tuberous sclerosis. The obstetrician and anesthesiologist should know the locations of lesions in an individual patient. Hemorrhage into the tumors, renal failure, and hypertension may complicate pregnancy.[137] Renal involvement seems to represent an important prognostic factor during pregnancy, and spontaneous rupture of a renal angiomyolipoma has been reported.[138] Although published reports have included several patients who required cesarean delivery, the authors made no specific mention of anesthetic management or complications.[137,138]

Cutaneous Angiomatosis with CNS Abnormalities

This group of phakomatoses consists of disorders in which a cutaneous vascular anomaly is accompanied by CNS abnormalities (Table 48-3).[139] There are few reports of pregnancy in patients with these disorders. Patients may present with neurologic problems related to hemangiomas of the CNS.

TABLE 48-3	CUTANEOUS ANGIOMATOSES WITH CNS ABNORMALITIES
Name	**Pathology and symptoms**
Sturge-Weber	Encephalotrigeminal angiomatosis (port wine nevus) with cerebral calcification and seizures
Klippel-Trenaunay-Weber	Dermatomal hemangiomas Spinal vascular malformations Limb hypertrophy
Epidermal nevus syndrome	Linear nevus with ipsilateral cerebral malformations
Rendu-Osler-Weber	Diffuse telangiectasias in skin and organs
Louis Bar	Ataxia and telangiectasias Diffuse CNS abnormalities Decreased levels of IgA Recurrent pulmonary infections
von Hippel-Lindau	Hemangioblastoma of cerebellum and retina Ataxia
Fabry	Deficiency of d-galactosides leading to progressive blood vessel, renal, and nerve cell accumulation of ceramide trihexoside

From Adams RD, Victor M, Ropper AH. Principles of Neurology, 6th ed. New York, McGraw-Hill 1997:1018-9.

Cesarean delivery with epidural anesthesia has been reported in a patient with spinal hemangiomas.[140]

LANDRY–GUILLAIN-BARRÉ SYNDROME

Acute idiopathic polyneuritis, also known as *Landry–Guillain-Barré syndrome,* is an inflammatory demyelinating illness with a reported incidence of approximately 1 case per 100,000 persons per year.[141] In 60% of patients a viral illness precedes neurologic symptoms by 1 to 3 weeks. Cases also have occurred after the administration of antirabies and influenza vaccines.

Patients present with weakness that first involves the limbs, followed by involvement of the trunk, neck, and facial muscles. Loss of reflexes, total motor paralysis, and respiratory failure can occur. Sensory loss typically is not detectable. Symptoms peak at 2 to 3 weeks. The majority of patients recover completely; approximately 10% have severe residual disability. Approximately 3% of patients do not survive.[141]

Nerve conduction studies show a slowing of conduction. Pathologic changes include lymphoid cellular infiltration and areas of demyelination that most likely result from a cell-mediated immunologic reaction against peripheral nerves. Autonomic nervous system involvement and dysfunction may occur.

The treatment is largely supportive and may include mechanical ventilatory support. Plasmapheresis reduces the duration of illness if it is instituted during the evolution phase, and this therapeutic modality has been used safely during pregnancy.[142,143]

Obstetric Management

The incidence of this syndrome seems to be lower in pregnant women than in nonpregnant women. Using data from several nationwide registries, Jiang et al.[144] found that the age-adjusted relative risk of Guillain-Barré syndrome seems to be lower during pregnancy and then increases during the 3 months after delivery. In severe cases the risk of preterm labor is increased, and neurologic deterioration may occur after delivery.[145] Termination of pregnancy does not appear advantageous for the course of the disease; indications for induction of labor include autonomic dysfunction. Instrumental vaginal delivery may be necessary.[145]

Anesthetic Management

Anesthetic management depends upon the status of the patient at the time of delivery. Case reports have documented the successful use of both epidural and CSE anesthesia.[18,146,147] However, some authors have expressed concern about the use of epidural anesthesia in these patients. Steiner et al.[148] implicated epidural anesthesia as a trigger of Guillain-Barré syndrome in four patients. These authors did not establish a cause-and-effect relationship, and I believe that epidural anesthesia is appropriate for women with a history of Guillain-Barré syndrome.

If general anesthesia is necessary, succinylcholine most likely should be avoided because of the risk of hyperkalemia in patients with acute muscle wasting.

The parturient who presents with a history of remote Guillain-Barré syndrome may have persistent diminished respiratory reserve, even in the absence of obvious residual disability.[149] Pulmonary evaluation should be considered before the administration of anesthesia. Approximately 5% of

patients relapse, and a small number of these develop a chronic disorder. However, there are no data that link relapse with any particular anesthetic technique.[141]

POLIO

Poliomyelitis is a disease caused by a picornavirus that is transmitted by means of the fecal-oral route. Most cases are asymptomatic or accompanied by only mild systemic symptoms. More severe symptoms and nervous system involvement occur in approximately 1% of patients.[150] Motor neurons in the cerebral cortex, brainstem, and spinal cord are affected. Asymmetric flaccid paralysis develops over several days. Bulbar paralysis is more common in young adults. The CSF findings are consistent with viral meningitis. Recovery occurs 3 to 4 months after onset, but residual deficits often persist.

A slowly progressive syndrome called **postpoliomyelitis muscular atrophy** may develop as many as 40 years after the acute illness. Klingman et al.[151] speculated that the increased functional demands are too great for the surviving neurons, and that these demands result in the late death of additional motor neurons. Others believe that this syndrome results from a reactivation of the initial viral infection.[152]

Obstetric Management

Currently, polio is a cause for concern only in countries with ineffective vaccination programs. If the parturient should require vaccination during pregnancy, oral polio vaccine does not appear to have harmful effects on fetal development.[153]

A history of previous poliomyelitis will affect labor and delivery only if residual deficits have resulted in pelvic asymmetry or an inability to push effectively during the second stage of labor.[154]

Anesthetic Management

Some physicians have feared that administration of regional anesthesia might cause reactivation of the virus and postpoliomyelitis muscular atrophy in patients with a history of poliomyelitis. Crawford et al.[18] reported the successful use of epidural analgesia with no adverse complications in patients with a history of polio. We currently provide regional anesthesia for labor and delivery in patients with a previous history of poliomyelitis.

BRAIN NEOPLASMS

Intracranial neoplasms vary in histology, clinical presentation, and prognosis (Table 48-4).[155] The yearly incidence of primary brain neoplasms is approximately 15 per 100,000.

Gliomas are the most common intracranial neoplasms. They account for approximately 45% of all intracranial tumors.[155] These tumors are derived from anaplasia of astrocytes. This category includes glioblastoma multiforme, astrocytoma, ependymoma, medulloblastoma, and oligodendrocytoma. These tumors vary in invasive potential. Glioblastoma multiforme is the most lethal. Oligodendrocytomas seem to have a better prognosis.

Meningiomas account for 15% of all brain tumors.[155] These benign tumors originate from the dura mater or arachnoid. Surgery typically is curative.

Pituitary adenomas are relatively common and have been found in 20% of pituitary glands postmortem.[155] Only a fraction of these tumors cause symptoms. Thus pituitary adenomas account for only 7% of brain tumors detected clinically. Because of their location, these tumors may cause visual field deficits. Tumors may secrete prolactin, growth hormone, or ACTH. Hypothalamic compression may result in diabetes insipidus. Bromocriptine often provides effective medical therapy for prolactin-secreting adenomas. Radiation and surgery also represent effective therapy, and the prognosis is generally good.

Schwannomas, also called **neurinomas,** account for 7% of all brain tumors. These lesions originate in the Schwann cells surrounding the nerve.[155] Clinical presentation depends on the location of the tumor. Acoustic neuromas result when the eighth nerve is involved; these lesions often are seen in patients with neurofibromatosis. The treatment is surgical excision.

Metastatic carcinomas account for 6% of all brain neoplasms.[155] Prognosis and therapy depend on the tumor of origin.

All brain tumors may share several pathophysiologic features. Neurologic deficits can result from mass effect, even if the tumor is benign. Tumor enlargement also may result in increased intracranial pressure (ICP). Brain edema is a prominent feature of cerebral neoplasms; it may result from a combination of vasogenic and cytotoxic mechanisms.

The potential for herniation must be considered in any patient with a mass lesion. The brain is divided into three basic compartments. The falx cerebri separates the cerebrum into right and left halves, and the tentorium isolates the cerebellum. High pressure from a mass can cause shifts from one compartment to another with devastating effects.

Obstetric Management

The incidence of primary brain tumors first presenting in pregnancy does not appear to be greater than that in aged-matched, nonpregnant women.[156] Approximately 5% to 20% of patients with **choriocarcinoma** have brain metastases at the time of diagnosis.[157] Patients with primary brain tumors have an increased incidence of spontaneous abortion, possibly because of hormonal factors.[158]

Although pregnancy does not affect the incidence of brain tumors, some of these lesions appear to grow faster during pregnancy. Visual field defects from pituitary adenomas worsen as a result of tumor enlargement during pregnancy. Symptoms may improve during the postpartum period.[159] Edema and the increased blood volume of vascular tumors

TABLE 48-4 INTRACRANIAL TUMORS

Type of intracranial tumor	% Occurrence
Glioma	45
Meningioma	15
Pituitary adenoma	7
Schwannoma	7
Metastatic carcinoma	6
Miscellaneous (e.g., craniopharyngioma, dermoid, epidermoid, pinealoma)	20
TOTAL	100

From Adams RD, Victor M, Ropper AH. Principles of Neurology, 6th ed. New York, McGraw-Hill 1997:642-94.

may account for some of these observations.[160] Hormonal effects also may play a role because estrogen and progesterone receptors are present in meningiomas and some gliomas.[160]

Management during pregnancy depends on the nature of the tumor. Surgery for benign tumors such as meningiomas can be delayed until the postpartum period. Women with more aggressive, malignant tumors or with tumors causing seizures or severe visual impairment may require surgery during pregnancy. Some women may opt for surgery after elective abortion.

In the normal parturient, CSF pressure may increase significantly with painful uterine contractions.[161] In patients with an intracranial mass lesion, this could result in an increased risk of herniation. The location and size of the tumor needs to be assessed in each individual case so that an appropriate plan can be designed. In general, either a pain-free second stage (with instrumental vaginal delivery to avoid pushing) or cesarean delivery may be appropriate.[162]

Anesthetic Management

Anesthetic considerations for surgery during pregnancy are discussed in Chapter 16. There may be some conflict between maternal and fetal interests in the patient with increased ICP. Hyperventilation often is used to decrease ICP; however, hyperventilation and hypocapnia may adversely affect utero-placental perfusion. Fetal heart rate (FHR) should be monitored during surgery when possible. The administration of mannitol can result in fetal hypovolemia in laboratory animals; it seems reasonable to use furosemide as a first-line diuretic.[163]

The patient with a less aggressive tumor may delay definitive therapy until after delivery. The choice of anesthesia for labor and vaginal delivery is controversial. Epidural anesthesia prevents the increase in ICP that can result with pushing during the second stage of labor.[164] However, there is concern that unintentional dural puncture might result in herniation in women with increased ICP. There are several published reports of the successful use of epidural anesthesia for labor and vaginal delivery in women with an intracranial neoplasm.[164,165] Spinal anesthesia for emergency cesarean delivery in a patient with a glioblastoma also has been reported.[166] A recent case report described a parturient with an occult brain tumor who had fatal transtentorial brain herniation following unintentional dural puncture during attempted placement of an epidural catheter.[167]

Many anesthesiologists favor general anesthesia for cesarean section.[168] The risks of increased ICP and a full stomach must be weighed. The induction may include administration of sodium thiopental and a short-acting nondepolarizing agent. Most anesthesiologists avoid succinylcholine in patients with increased ICP. A combination of isoflurane, nitrous oxide, and low-dose fentanyl is a commonly used technique for maintenance of anesthesia.

BENIGN INTRACRANIAL HYPERTENSION

Benign intracranial hypertension, also known as *pseudotumor cerebri*, is defined as an increase in ICP without a demonstrable etiology. Four criteria have been described: (1) CSF pressure above 200 mm H_2O, (2) normal CSF composition, (3) no alteration in the state of consciousness, and (4) absence of focal intracranial lesions.[169] The disorder most often occurs in obese women of childbearing age; this suggests that hormonal

factors may play a role in the pathophysiology. The majority of patients present with headache; in some cases, visual symptoms occur. Over time the disorder generally improves, but there is a small risk of recurrence.

Traditional therapy has included serial lumbar punctures and the administration of a carbonic anhydrase inhibitor and/or corticosteroid. These therapeutic modalities vary in efficacy. Lumboperitoneal shunting may be required in severe cases with visual symptoms. Weight loss seems to improve the condition.

Interaction with Pregnancy

Symptoms of benign intracranial hypertension worsen during pregnancy in 50% of cases.[170] Surgical management with shunt placement has resulted in clinical improvement and normal perinatal outcome in pregnant women with severe symptoms.[171] Otherwise, symptoms typically improve after delivery. This disorder does not seem to adversely affect maternal and perinatal outcomes.[172]

Anesthetic Management

Deliberate lumbar puncture represents a common form of treatment for this disorder. Cerebellar tonsillar herniation does not occur because of the uniform, global increase in ICP. Paruchuri et al.[173] noted that there are only two published cases of cerebellar tonsillar herniation after diagnostic lumbar puncture in patients with this disorder. Both patients had presented with severe headache, neck pain exacerbated by movement, and focal neurologic deficits. In the absence of these signs and symptoms, the anesthesiologist can safely give regional anesthesia for labor and vaginal or cesarean delivery.[169,174]

Some anesthesiologists recommend the administration of general anesthesia for cesarean section for patients with a lumboperitoneal shunt.[169] They contend that local anesthetic agent that reaches the subarachnoid space may escape into the peritoneum, and that therefore it might be difficult to achieve adequate anesthesia. Moreover, the performance of regional anesthesia may result in trauma to the shunt catheter. However, Bédard et al.[175] reported the successful administration of epidural anesthesia in a preeclamptic patient with a lumboperitoneal shunt for the treatment of benign intracranial hypertension. Preoperative radiographic examination may help the anesthesiologist avoid needle placement near the catheter, although such imaging was not used in this case. Epidural anesthesia also has been used successfully in patients with ventriculoperitoneal and ventriculoatrial shunts.[176,177]

MATERNAL HYDROCEPHALUS WITH SHUNT

Hydrocephalus results from a variety of etiologies. The most common include intracranial hemorrhage in preterm infants, fetal and neonatal infections, the Arnold-Chiari malformation, aqueductal stenosis, and the Dandy-Walker syndrome.[178] The Arnold-Chiari malformation includes extension of a portion of cerebellar tissue into the cervical canal, with progressive hydrocephalus. The Dandy-Walker syndrome results from failure of development of the midline of the cerebellum, with resultant hydrocephalus of the fourth ventricle.

Ventriculoatrial or ventriculoperitoneal shunt catheters are placed for the treatment of many of these disorders. Because of advances in neonatal and neurosurgical care,

hydrocephalic women with CSF shunt catheters currently are reaching childbearing age in increasing numbers.

Obstetric Management

Obstetric management depends on the presence of other medical and neurologic conditions. In general, hydrocephalus does not increase the incidence of obstetric complications.[179] However, neurologic complications may occur in as many as 76% of pregnant women with a preexisting shunt.[180] These complications include severe headache, shunt obstruction, and increased ICP. Most symptoms resolve postpartum.

The mother with neurologic stability can undergo labor and vaginal delivery. Elective cesarean delivery is recommended only if the symptoms are severe or result in neurologic instability.[180]

Anesthetic Management

Anesthetic management may depend on the location of the shunt. There has been concern that some of the local anesthetic agent entering the CSF may escape into the atrium or peritoneum and result in inadequate analgesia. However, epidural anesthesia has been used in patients with lumboperitoneal, ventriculoatrial, and ventriculoperitoneal shunts.[175-177] Because of the risk of shunt infection, some physicians recommend the administration of a prophylactic antibiotic regimen similar to that used for the prophylaxis of bacterial endocarditis.

SUBARACHNOID HEMORRHAGE

Spontaneous subarachnoid hemorrhage occurs with an incidence of 1 to 5 per 10,000 pregnancies.[181] Whether pregnancy itself is a risk factor is controversial.[181] Aneurysms and arteriovenous malformations are the most common causes in women of childbearing age (Figure 48-3).[182] Box 48-3 lists a variety of less common etiologies. The prognosis is very serious, regardless of the etiology. Maternal mortality ranges from 13% to 35% after aneurysm rupture and from 8% to 28% after rupture of an arteriovenous malformation.[181]

Holcomb and Petrie[183] concluded that cerebral aneurysms and arteriovenous malformations present in approximately equal proportions during pregnancy. Dias and Sekhar[184] reviewed 154 published cases of intracranial subarachnoid hemorrhage during pregnancy. They noted that aneurysms were responsible for intracranial hemorrhage in 77% of the patients, and arteriovenous malformations were responsible in the remaining 23%.

Most authors have reported a progressive increase in the incidence of aneurysm bleeding throughout gestation, increasing in parallel with the physiologic increase in blood volume.[181,184] Re-hemorrhage during the same pregnancy occurs in approximately half of patients with an aneurysm hemorrhage.[181] Because of the risk of re-hemorrhage, a pregnant patient with a history of aneurysm bleeding who is deemed operable generally is referred for surgical clipping. Surgical management of aneurysms during pregnancy has been associated with significantly lower maternal and fetal mortality in affected patients.[184] Once a curative surgical procedure has been performed, it is unnecessary to treat this patient any differently during labor and delivery, when compared with a patient without an aneurysm. If an aneurysm is found incidentally during pregnancy and has not bled, management should be based on the specific clinical situation, including aneurysm size and location. Two cases of successful endovascular treatment of ruptured intracranial aneurysms in parturients have been reported; this approach avoids the need for craniotomy.[185]

Bleeding from arteriovenous malformations has been reported by some authors to occur with equal frequency throughout the course of pregnancy and by others to occur more frequently with advancing gestational age.[181,184,186] Whether pregnancy increases the risk of bleeding from an arteriovenous malformation is controversial.[187] Arteriovenous malformations have been reported to have a 25% chance of rebleeding during the same pregnancy.[181,186] The data regarding surgical management during pregnancy varies, with some authors noting that surgery does not significantly affect maternal or fetal mortality.[184]

Obstetric Management

If the lesion has been cured surgically, the patient requires no special care during labor and delivery. For an untreated aneurysm or arteriovenous malformation, hemodynamic stress during labor and delivery should be minimized. Current data do not demonstrate a definite advantage of cesarean delivery over assisted vaginal delivery.[181,183,184] For vaginal delivery, epidural anesthesia and the use of low

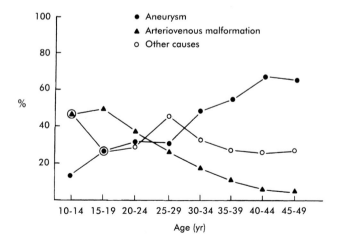

FIGURE 48-3. Relative probability of major causes of subarachnoid hemorrhage for women by age. (From Donaldson JO. Neurology of Pregnancy, 2nd ed. London, WB Saunders 1989:139.)

Box 48-3 OTHER CAUSES OF SPONTANEOUS SUBARACHNOID HEMORRHAGE DURING PREGNANCY

Hematologic disorders
   Anticoagulant therapy
   Placental abruption with disseminated intravascular coagulation
Mycotic aneurysm from subacute bacterial endocarditis
Vasculitis (e.g., lupus erythematosus)
Metastatic choriocarcinoma
Eclampsia
   Early—hypertensive intracerebral hemorrhage
   Late—cerebral infarction and multiple petechial hemorrhages
Postpartum cerebral phlebothrombosis
Rupture of spinal cord arteriovenous malformation
Ectopic endometriosis

From Donaldson JO. Neurology of Pregnancy, 2nd ed. London, WB Saunders, 1989: 140.

forceps may be performed to shorten the second stage of labor and attenuate fluctuations in blood pressure. The decision regarding method of delivery should be based on the individual patient and her pregnancy history.

Anesthetic Management

If the parturient has undergone surgical repair of either an aneurysm or arteriovenous malformation, anesthetic management need not differ from that of other obstetric patients. Those with untreated lesions should be managed to maintain hemodynamic stability and avoid hypertension. Regional anesthesia is generally preferred.[188-191] If vaginal delivery is planned, epidural or CSE anesthesia should be considered. For cesarean delivery, either epidural or spinal anesthesia can be used. Some anesthesiologists contend that epidural anesthesia provides greater hemodynamic stability and is thus preferred for cesarean delivery.[189]

In some cases, the neurosurgeon may ligate or excise the vascular lesion *during* pregnancy, *before* delivery.[192] There are several published cases of neurovascular intracranial surgery during pregnancy.[193-195] The anesthesiologist should consider the principles of anesthetic management for pregnant women undergoing nonobstetric surgery (see Chapter 16). In addition, it is critical to maintain stable blood pressure during induction of anesthesia, laryngoscopy, and intubation. The patient should receive adequate sedation before and after arrival in the operating room. Placement of an intraarterial catheter is mandatory. The anesthesiologist may attenuate the hypertensive response to laryngoscopy and intubation by administration of intravenous esmolol, labetalol, lidocaine, nitroglycerin, or nitroprusside. An assistant should maintain cricoid pressure during induction of anesthesia.

Succinylcholine can be used for intubation. It seems prudent to give a defasciculating dose of a nondepolarizing muscle relaxant before the administration of succinylcholine in these patients. Regardless of the choice of muscle relaxant, it is critical that laryngoscopy and intubation not be performed until the patient is anesthetized adequately. The risks of hypertension and intracranial bleeding as well as the risk of aspiration should be considered during induction of anesthesia.

The anesthesiologist may maintain anesthesia with nitrous oxide and modest doses of isoflurane and an opioid. Aggressive maternal hyperventilation may result in decreased uterine blood flow. However, the anesthesiologist may use modest hyperventilation (e.g., $PaCO_2$ of 28 to 30 mm Hg) as needed to reduce maternal ICP. The anesthesiologist should maintain left uterine displacement in patients who are beyond 20 weeks' gestation. Intraoperative FHR monitoring allows the anesthesiologist to assess the fetal response to maternal general anesthesia and hyperventilation. At the Brigham and Women's Hospital, we use intraoperative FHR monitoring beginning at 24 weeks' gestation. Typically an obstetric nurse monitors the FHR tracing during surgery and requests obstetric consultation if it is needed. An adverse change in the FHR tracing should prompt the anesthesiologist to ensure adequate maternal oxygenation, ventilation, and perfusion.

Use of deliberate hypotension may compromise uteroplacental perfusion. However, several authors have reported the safe use of deliberate hypotension during neurovascular intracranial surgery in pregnant women.[193-195] There is no consensus regarding a safe level of hypotension in these patients. There also is no consensus on the ideal method for achieving deliberate hypotension in pregnant women. Prolonged administration of large doses of nitroprusside may result in fetal cyanide toxicity.[196] Short-term administration of nitroprusside seems safe.[197,198] Intraoperative FHR monitoring allows the anesthesiologist to assess the FHR response to deliberate hypotension. Endovascular treatment under general anesthesia avoids the need for craniotomy and deliberate hypotension.[185]

In some cases, the obstetrician and neurosurgeon may perform a *combined* procedure (e.g., a cesarean section followed by ligation or excision of the neurovascular lesion).[199-202] Principles of anesthetic management are similar to those described for intracranial neurovascular surgery during pregnancy.

Rarely, anesthesiologists may provide care for pregnant women who are receiving **extended somatic support** after brain death. Powner and Bernstein[202] recently reviewed 11 reports of 10 cases of brain death during pregnancy, wherein somatic support was provided until successful delivery. Intracranial hemorrhage was the cause of maternal brain death in 6 of the 10 patients. The longest period of support was 107 days, from 15 to 32 weeks' gestation. All 10 infants survived. The authors concluded that preservation of uteroplacental blood flow is the most important priority during extended somatic support, but they acknowledged that this goal is difficult to achieve because of hemodynamic instability, the high prevalence of infection, and other adverse consequences (e.g., diabetes insipidus) of brain death.

CORTICAL VEIN THROMBOSIS

Cerebral venous thrombosis is associated with dehydration, polycythemia, leukemia, and infection of the face or sinuses.[203] Thromboses commonly involve the cavernous sinus, lateral sinus, sagittal sinus, or cortical veins. Primary cortical vein thrombosis is the type most often seen in the parturient. The incidence of cerebral venous thrombosis in the parturient has been estimated to be approximately 8.9 cases per 100,000 deliveries, and is strongly associated with cesarean delivery.[204] Most cases occur within the second and third weeks postpartum.[205] The etiology is unclear. Pregnancy may predispose patients to this condition because of at least two factors.[206,207] First, traumatic damage to the endothelial lining of vessels may occur during the second stage of labor. Second, pregnancy is a hypercoagulable state.

Affected patients may present with headache, nausea and vomiting, and blurred vision. In severe cases, lateralizing neurologic signs, lethargy, and seizures may occur. Care should be taken to differentiate cortical vein thrombosis from postdural puncture headache (PDPH). In general, the headache with cortical vein thrombosis is more diffuse in location and its intensity does not vary with position.[206,207] Diagnosis can be confirmed by MRI or angiography. Treatment includes anticonvulsant and anticoagulation therapy, provided that there is no evidence of intracranial hematoma or subarachnoid hemorrhage. In some cases, residual neurologic deficit and seizures may persist. One study noted that approximately 80% of parturients with this condition had a good outcome, compared with 58% of nonobstetric patients.[208]

Obstetric and Anesthetic Management

Cortical vein thrombosis rarely occurs before delivery. Neurologic instability with maternal and fetal deterioration

may necessitate urgent delivery. Maternal anticoagulation contraindicates the administration of regional anesthesia. The anesthesiologist should avoid systemic hypotension, which may reduce cerebral perfusion pressure and blood flow to injured areas already subjected to marginal perfusion. If the patient has an asymmetric cerebral hematoma, dural puncture may precipitate herniation of the brainstem. Thus it seems preferable to give general anesthesia for cesarean section, with special attention to the treatment of increased ICP.

MOTOR NEURON DISORDERS

Motor neuron diseases include a group of disorders that are characterized by progressive muscular weakness and atrophy. These disorders may affect motor function only, or they also may result in sensory deficits. There are few data on the course of these disorders in pregnant women. This discussion focuses on three of these disorders: amyotrophic lateral sclerosis and primary spinal muscular atrophy, which are pure motor neuron disorders, and peroneal muscular atrophy, which includes both motor and sensory degeneration. Currently there is no cure for any of these degenerative disorders.

Amyotrophic Lateral Sclerosis

Amyotrophic lateral sclerosis has an annual incidence of approximately 1 per 100,000.[209] This disease involves progressive degeneration of anterior horn cells with progressive atrophic weakness and hyperreflexia. Patients typically succumb to respiratory failure within 6 years.

This disease is more often seen in patients older than 50 years of age, but there are reports of this disorder in pregnant women.[210] Physicians should assess and frequently monitor the parturient's degree of respiratory compromise during pregnancy and throughout the peripartum period. Epidural anesthesia has been used in these patients without evidence of worsened neurologic function postoperatively.[211,212] If general anesthesia is required, these patients may be sensitive to the effects of nondepolarizing muscle relaxants.[213]

Spinal Muscular Atrophy

Primary spinal muscular atrophy is a disorder that also involves degeneration of anterior horn cells. However, these patients tend to be younger than those afflicted with amyotrophic lateral sclerosis, and this disorder progresses more slowly. Some types of this disorder are hereditary. This disease tends to involve mainly the spinal cord, without involvement of the corticospinal tract.

Spinal muscular atrophy is associated with an increased incidence of preterm labor.[214] One series noted that pregnancy was associated with an exacerbation of muscle weakness in 8 of 12 patients.[214] Epidural and spinal anesthesia have been used successfully in these patients.[215,216]

Peroneal Muscular Atrophy

Peroneal muscular atrophy, also known as *Charcot-Marie-Tooth disease,* typically is inherited as an autosomal dominant trait.[217] This disorder involves a progressive sensory and motor degeneration of peripheral nerves and roots. The peroneal nerve is affected early. The disorder progresses to involve all the nerves and muscles of the legs and finally the hands. Paresthesias typically are present.

At least one report has suggested that peroneal muscular atrophy worsens during pregnancy, perhaps because of fluid retention and edema around the nerve.[218] This disorder occasionally causes respiratory embarrassment. Thus physicians should assess the patient's respiratory function during pregnancy. Epidural anesthesia has been used.[219] One case report suggested that these patients have a normal response to nondepolarizing muscle relaxants.[220]

ISOLATED MONONEUROPATHIES DURING PREGNANCY

Pregnancy is associated with an increased incidence of several specific mononeuropathies: Bell's palsy, carpal tunnel syndrome, and meralgia paresthetica.

Bell's Palsy

Bell's palsy is a syndrome of acute onset that involves paralysis of the facial nerve. The incidence during pregnancy is approximately 188 per 100,000 per exposure-year, which is approximately 10 times higher than expected in nonpregnant patients.[221] Some studies suggested an association with preeclampsia, perhaps on the basis of increased interstitial edema.[222]

The prognosis for recovery is good, especially if the initial paralysis is partial.[223] Patients may benefit from a short course of prednisone.

Dorsey and Camann[224] retrospectively reviewed 36 cases of Bell's palsy associated with pregnancy; 25 women developed symptoms during the third trimester, and the remaining 11 developed symptoms during the first week postpartum. Of the 36 women, 27 received spinal or epidural anesthesia. The authors concluded that "regional anesthesia during labor and delivery may be safe in patients with pregnancy-associated Bell's palsy." They suggested that "the appropriate anesthetic for a given patient may be chosen without concern for the co-existing Bell's palsy."

Carpal Tunnel Syndrome

Carpal tunnel syndrome results from compression of the median nerve in the flexor retinaculum at the wrist. Patients typically report paresthesias and weakness in the median nerve distribution. Symptoms are worse on awakening. Patients may be treated with splinting. Severe symptoms may require surgery. Most cases resolve spontaneously within the first 2 months postpartum.[225]

Meralgia Paresthetica

Meralgia paresthetica is a syndrome that involves compression of the lateral femoral cutaneous nerve. Obesity and the exaggerated lordosis of pregnancy can stretch the nerve.[226] Patients report paresthesia in the lateral thigh, typically beginning after the first trimester. Symptoms typically resolve within 3 months of delivery.[227]

KEY POINTS

- **Symptoms of multiple sclerosis may worsen postpartum, regardless of the anesthetic technique that is used. However, the long-term prognosis of this disease most likely is unaffected by pregnancy.**
- **Multiple sclerosis does not contraindicate the use of regional anesthesia.**
- **Continuous epidural anesthesia is the method of choice for the prevention or treatment of autonomic hyperreflexia during labor and delivery in patients with spinal cord injury.**
- **Patients with myasthenia gravis require close surveillance during labor. Increasing muscle weakness may require an adjustment in the dosage of the anticholinesterase drug. Severe respiratory involvement may preclude the use of regional anesthesia for cesarean delivery.**
- **The anesthesiologist should avoid succinylcholine in patients with myotonic dystrophy because fasciculations can trigger myotonia.**
- **Regional anesthesia does not appear to precipitate the onset of postpoliomyelitis muscular atrophy.**
- **The parturient with an untreated intracranial aneurysm or arteriovenous malformation should be treated to maintain hemodynamic stability; epidural anesthesia should be considered during labor and delivery.**
- **There is an increased incidence of Bell's palsy, carpal tunnel syndrome, and meralgia paresthetica during pregnancy. Symptoms typically resolve during the first few weeks postpartum.**

REFERENCES

1. Kurland LT. The frequency and geographic distribution of multiple sclerosis as indicated by mortality statistics and morbidity surveys in the United States and Canada. Am J Hyg 1952; 55:457-81.
2. Kurtzke JF. Patterns of neurologic involvement in multiple sclerosis. Neurology 1989; 39:1235-8.
3. McDonald WI. The mystery of the origin of multiple sclerosis. J Neurol Neurosurg Psychiatr 1986; 49:113-23.
4. Johnson KP. The historical development of interferons as multiple sclerosis therapies. J Mol Med 1997; 75:89-94.
5. Durelli L, Isoardo G. High-dose intravenous immunoglobulin treatment of multiple sclerosis. Neurol Sci. 2002 Apr;23 Suppl 1:S39-48.
6. Watson CW. Effect of lowering of body temperature on the symptoms and signs of multiple sclerosis. N Engl J Med 1959; 261:1253-9.
7. Mueller B, Zhang J, Chritchlow C. Birth outcomes and need for hospitalization after delivery among women with multiple sclerosis. Am J Obstet Gynecol 2002; 186:446-52.
8. Damek DM, Shuster E. Pregnancy and multiple sclerosis. Mayo Clin Proc 1997; 72:977-89.
9. Confavreux C, Hutchinson M, Hours MM, et al. Rate of pregnancy-related relapse in multiple sclerosis. N Engl J Med 1998; 339:285-91.
10. Whitaker JN. Effects of pregnancy and delivery on disease activity in multiple sclerosis. (editorial). N Engl J Med 1998; 339:339-40.
11. Roullet E, Verdier-Taillefer MH, Amarenco P, et al. Pregnancy and multiple sclerosis: A longitudinal study of 125 remittent patients. J Neurol Neurosurg Psych 1993; 56:1062-5.
12. Baskett PJ, Armstrong, R. Anaesthetic problems in multiple sclerosis. Anaesthesia 1970; 25:397-401.
13. Bamford C, Sibley W, Laguna J. Anesthesia in multiple sclerosis. Can J Neurol Sci 1978; 5:41-4.
14. Tui C, Preiss AL, Barcham I, Nevin MI. Local nervous tissue changes following spinal anesthesia in experimental animals. J Pharmacol Exp Ther 1944; 81:209-17.
15. Shapira K. Is lumbar puncture harmful in multiple sclerosis? J Neurol Neurosurg Psychiatr 1959; 22:238.
16. Stenuit J, Marchand P. Les sequells de rachi-anaesthesie. Acta Neurol Psychiatr Belg 1968; 68:626-35.
17. Warren TM, Datta S, Ostheimer GW. Lumbar epidural anesthesia in a patient with multiple sclerosis. Anesth Analg 1982; 61:1022-3.
18. Crawford JS, James FM, Nolte H, et al. Regional analgesia for patients with chronic neurologic disease and similar conditions. Anaesthesia 1981; 36:821.
19. Bader AM, Hunt CO, Datta S, et al. Anesthesia for the obstetric patient with multiple sclerosis. J Clin Anesth 1988; 1:21-4.
20. Leigh J, Fearnley SJ, Lupprian KG. Intrathecal diamorphine during laparatomy in a patient with advanced multiple sclerosis. Anaesthesia 1990; 43:640-2.
21. Donaldson JO. Neurology of Pregnancy, 2nd ed. London, WB Saunders, 1989:217.
22. Stein G, Morton J, Marsh A, et al. Headaches after childbirth. Acta Neurol Scand 1984; 69:74-9.
23. Safra MJ, Oakley GP. Association between cleft lip with or without cleft palate and prenatal exposure to diazepam. Lancet 1975; ii:478-80.
24. Nulman I, Rovet J, Stewart DE, et al. Neurodevelopment of children exposed in utero to antidepressant drugs. N Engl J Med 1997; 336: 258-62.
25. Paulson GW. Headaches in women, including women who are pregnant. Am J Obstet Gynecol 1995; 173:1734-41.
26. Stewart WF, Shechter A, Rasmussen BK. Migraine prevalence: A review of population based studies. Neurology 1994; 44(suppl 4):S17-23.
27. Somerville BW. The influence of progesterone and estradiol upon migraine. Headache 1972; 12:93-102.
28. Silberstein SD. Migraine and pregnancy. Neurol Clin 1997; 15:209-31.
29. Chen TC, Leviton A. Headache recurrence in pregnant women with migraine. Headache 1994; 34:107-10.
30. Davis ME, Adair FL, Pearl S. The present status of oxytocics in obstetrics. JAMA 1936; 107:261-7.
31. Fox AW, Chambers CD, Anderson PO, et al. Evidence-based assessment of pregnancy outcome after sumatriptan exposure. Headache 2002; 42:8-15.
32. Marcoux S, Berube S, Brisson J, Fabia J. History of migraine and risk of pregnancy-induced hypertension. Epidemiology 1992; 3:53-6.
33. Rosene KA, Featherstone HJ, Benedetti TJ. Cerebral ischemia associated with parenteral terbutaline use in pregnant migraine patients. Am J Obstet Gynecol 1982; 143:405-7.
34. Kalsbeek WD, McLaurin RL, Harris BS, Miller JD. National head and spinal cord injury survey: Major findings. J Neurosurg 1980; 52:S19-31.
35. Donaldson JO. Neurology of Pregnancy, 2nd ed. London, WB Saunders, 1989:11.
36. Adams RD, Victor M, Ropper AH. Principles of Neurology, 6th ed. New York, McGraw-Hill, 1997:1227-36.
37. Kuhn RA. Functional capacity of the isolated human spinal cord. Brain 1950; 73:1-51.
38. Marshall J. Observations on reflex changes in the lower limbs in spastic paraplegia in man. Brain 1954; 77:290-304.
39. Kurnick NB. Autonomic hyperreflexia and its control in patients with spinal cord lesions. Ann Intern Med 1956; 44:678-86.
40. Crosby E, St. Jean B, Reid D, Elliot RD. Obstetric anaesthesia and analgesia in chronic spinal cord-injured women. Can J Anaesth 1992; 39:487-94.
41. Schonwald G, Fish KJ, Perkash I. Cardiovascular complications during anesthesia in chronic spinal cord injured patients. Anesthesiology 1981; 55:550-8.
42. Catanzarite VA, Ferguson JE, Weinstein C, Belton SR. Preterm labor in the quadriplegic parturient. Am J Perinatol 1986; 3:115-8.
43. Greenspoon JS, Paul RH. Paraplegia and quadriplegia: Special considerations during pregnancy and labor and delivery. Am J Obstet Gynecol 1986; 155:738-41.
44. Westgren N, Hultling C, Levi R, Westgren M. Pregnancy and delivery in women with a traumatic spinal cord injury in Sweden, 1980-1991. Obstet Gynecol 1993; 81:926-30.
45. Baraka A. Epidural meperidine for control of autonomic hyperreflexia in a paraplegic parturient. Anesthesiology 1985; 62:688-90.
46. Lambert DH, Deane RS, Mazuzan JE. Anesthesia and the control of blood pressure in patients with spinal cord injury. Anesth Analg 1982; 61:344-8.
47. Hambly PR, Martin B. Anaesthesia for chronic spinal cord lesions. Anaesthesia 1998; 53:273-89.

48. Thorn-Alquist AM. Prevention of hypertensive crises in patients with high spinal lesions during cystoscopy and lithotripsy. Acta Anaesthesiol Scan (suppl) 1975; 57:79-82.

49. Stirt JA, Marco A, Conklin KA. Obstetric anesthesia for a quadriplegic patient with autonomic hyperreflexia. Anesthesiology 1979; 51:560-2.

50. Agostoni M, Giorgi E, Beccaria P, et al. Combined spinal-epidural anaesthesia for caesarean section in a paraplegic woman: Difficulty in obtaining the expected level of block. Eur J Anaesth 2000; 17:329-31.

51. Kobayashi A, Mizobe T, Tojo H, Hashimoto S. Autonomic hyperreflexia during labour. Can J Anaesth 1995; 42:1134-6.

52. Abouleish EI, Hanley ES, Palmer SM. Can epidural fentanyl control autonomic hyperreflexia in a quadriplegic parturient? Anesth Analg 1989; 68:523-6.

53. Pauzner D, Wolman I, Niv D, David MP. Epidural morphine-bupivacaine combination for the control of autonomic hyperreflexia during labor. Gynecol Obstet Invest 1994; 37:215-6.

54. Maehama T, Izena H, Kanazawa K. Management of autonomic hyper-reflexia with magnesium sulfate during labor in a woman with spinal cord injury. Am J Obstet Gynecol 2000; 183:492-3.

55. Ahmed AB, Bogod DG. Anesthetic management of a quadriplegic patient with severe respiratory insufficiency undergoing cesarean section. Anaesthesia 1996; 51:1043-5.

56. Stone WA, Beach TP, Hamelberg W. Succinylcholine: Danger in the spinal-cord injured patient. Anesthesiology 1970; 32:168-9.

57. Adams RD, Victor M, Ropper AH. Principles of Neurology, 6th ed. New York, McGraw-Hill, 1997:1459-71.

58. Richman DP, Agius MA. Acquired myasthenia gravis: Immunopathology. Neurol Clin 1994; 12:273-84.

59. Baraka A. Anaesthesia and myasthenia gravis. Can J Anaesth 1992; 39:476-86.

60. Eden RD, Gall SA. Myasthenia gravis and pregnancy: A reappraisal of thymectomy. Obstet Gynecol 1983; 62:328-33.

61. Donaldson JO. Neurology of Pregnancy, 2nd ed. London, WB Saunders, 1989:66.

62. d'Empaire G, Hoaglin DC, Perlo VP, Pontoppidan H. Effect of prethymectomy plasma exchange on postoperative respiratory function in myasthenia gravis. J Thorac Cardiovasc Surg 1985; 89:592-6.

63. Barrons RW. Drug-induced neuromuscular blockade and myasthenia gravis. Pharmacotherapy 1997; 17:1220-32.

64. Cohen BA, London RS, Goldstein PJ. Myasthenia gravis and preeclampsia. Obstet Gynecol 1976; 48(suppl):35-7S.

65. Bashuk RG, Krendal DA. Myasthenia gravis presenting as weakness after magnesium administration. Muscle Nerve 1990; 13:708-12.

66. Catanzarite VA, McHargue AM, Sandberg EC, Dyson DC. Respiratory arrest during therapy for premature labor in a patient with myasthenia gravis. Obstet Gynecol 1984; 654:819-22.

67. Plauché WC. Myasthenia gravis in mothers and their newborns. Clin Obstet Gynecol 1991; 34:82-99.

68. McNall PG, Jafarnia MR. Management of myasthenia gravis in the obstetrical patient. Am J Obstet Gynecol 1965; 92:518-25.

69. Rolbin WH, Levinson G, Shnider SM, Wright RG. Anesthetic considerations for myasthenia gravis and pregnancy. Anesth Analg 1978; 57:441-7.

70. Benshushan A, Rojansky N, Weinstein D. Myasthenia gravis and preeclampsia. Isr J Med Sci 1994; 30:229-33.

71. Hatada Y, Munemura M, Matsuo I, et al. Myasthenia crises in the puerperium: The possible importance of alpha-fetoprotein. Case Report. Br J Obstet Gynaecol 1987; 94:480-2.

72. Namba T, Brown SB, Grob D. Neonatal myasthenia gravis: Report of two cases and a review of the literature. Pediatrics 1970; 45:488-504.

73. D'Angelo R, Gerancher JC. Combined spinal and epidural analgesia in a parturient with severe myasthenia gravis. Reg Anesth Pain Med 1998; 23:201-3.

74. Mitchell PJ, Bebbington M. Myasthenia gravis in pregnancy. Obstet Gynecol 1992; 80:178-81.

75. Riegler R, Lischka A, Neumark J. Problems of anesthesia for cesarean section in myasthenia gravis. Anaesthesist 1983; 32:403-6.

76. O'Flaherty D, Pennant JH, Rao K, Giesecke AH. Total intravenous anesthesia with propofol for transternal thymectomy in myasthenia gravis. J Clin Anesth 1992; 4:241-4.

77. Foldes FF, McNall PG. Myasthenia gravis: A guide for anesthesiologists. Anesthesiology 1962; 23:837-72.

78. Leventhal SR, Orkin FK, Hirsh RA. Prediction of the need for postoperative mechanical ventilation in myasthenia gravis. Anesthesiology 1980; 53:26-30.

79. Naguib M, el Dawlatly A, Ashour M, Bamgboye EA. Multivariate determinants of the need for postoperative ventilation in myasthenia gravis. Can J Anaesth 1996; 43:1006-13.

80. Commission on Classification and Terminology of the International League Against Epilepsy. Proposal for revised clinical and electroencephalographic classification of epileptic seizures. Epilepsia 1981; 22:489-501.

81. Dalessio DJ. Current concepts: Seizure disorders and pregnancy. N Engl J Med 1985; 312:559-63.

82. Annegers JF, Hauser WA, Elveback LR. Remission of seizures and relapse in patients with epilepsy. Epilepsia 1979; 20:729-37.

83. Elwes RD, Johnson AL, Shorvon SD, Reynolds EH. The prognosis for seizure control in newly diagnosed epilepsy. N Engl J Med 1984; 311:944-7.

84. Schmidt D. Prognosis of chronic epilepsy with complex partial seizures. J Neurol Neurosurg Psychiatr 1984; 47:1274-8.

85. Rutherford JM, Rubin PC. Management of epilepsy in pregnancy: Therapeutic aspects. Br J Hosp Med 1996; 55:620-2.

86. Schmidt D, Canger R, Avanzini G, et al. Change of seizure frequency in pregnant epileptic women. J Neurol Neurosurg Psychiatr 1983; 46:751-5.

87. Ramsay RE. Effect of hormones on seizure activity during pregnancy. J Clin Neurophysiol 1987; 4:23-5.

88. Yerby MS. Pregnancy and epilepsy. Epilepsia 1991; 32(S6):S51-9.

89. Nau H, Kuhnz W, Egger HJ, et al. Anticonvulsants during pregnancy and lactation: Transplacental, maternal and neonatal pharmacokinetics. Clin Pharmacokinet 1982; 7:508-43.

90. Perucca E, Crema A. Plasma protein binding of drugs in pregnancy. Clin Pharmacokinet 1981; 7:336-52.

91. Higgens TA, Comerford JB. Epilepsy in pregnancy. J Ir Med Assoc 1974; 67:317-20.

92. Lowe SA. Drugs in pregnancy: Anticonvulsants and drugs for neurological disease. Best Practice and Research in Clinical Obstetrics and Gynaecology 2001; 15:863-76.

93. Morrell MJ. The new antiepileptic drugs and women: Efficacy, reproductive health, pregnancy, and fetal outcome. Epilepsia 1996; 37:34-44.

94. Cornelissen M, Steegers-Theunissen R, Kollée L, et al. Supplementation of vitamin K in pregnant women receiving anticonvulsant therapy prevents neonatal vitamin K deficiency. Am J Obstet Gynecol 1993; 168:884-8.

95. Kaaja E, Kaaja R, Ratila R, Hiilesmaa V. Enzyme-inducing antiepileptic drugs in pregnancy and the risk of bleeding in the neonate. Neurology 2002; 58:549-53.

96. Aravapalli R, Abouleish E, Aldrete JA. Anesthetic implications in the parturient epileptic patient. Anesth Analg 1988; 67:S266.

97. Merrell DA, Koch MA. Epidural anaesthesia as an anticonvulsant in the management of hypertension and the eclamptic patient in labour. S Afr Med J 1980; 58:875-7.

98. Modica PA, Tempelhoff R, White PF. Pro- and anticonvulsant effect of anesthetics. Anesth Analg 1990; 70:303-15.

99. Iijima T, Nakamura Z, Iwao Y, Sankawa H. The epileptogenic properties of the volatile anesthetics sevoflurane and isoflurane in patients with epilepsy. Anesth Analg 2000; 91:989-95.

100. Smith M, Smith SJ, Scott CA, Harkness WF. Activation of the electrocorticogram by propofol during surgery for epilepsy. Br J Anaesth 1996; 76:499-502.

101. Ornstein E, Matteo RS, Schwartz AE, et al. The effect of phenytoin on the magnitude and duration of neuromuscular block following atracurium or vecuronium. Anesthesiology 1987; 67:191-6.

102. Adams RD, Victor M, Ropper AH. Principles of Neurology, 6th ed. New York, McGraw-Hill, 1997:1392.

103. Stoelting RK, Dierdorf SF. Anesthesia and Co-existing Disease, 3rd ed. New York, Churchill Livingstone Inc., 1993:437-8.

104. Shaw DJ, Brook JD, Meredith AL, et al. Gene mapping and chromosome 19. J Med Genet 1986; 23:2-10.

105. Adams RD, Victor M, Ropper AH. Principles of Neurology, 6th ed. New York, McGraw-Hill, 1997:1423-6.

106. Adams RD, Victor M, Ropper AH. Principles of Neurology, 6th ed. New York, McGraw-Hill, 1997:1476-80.

107. Shore RN, MacLachlan TB. Pregnancy with myotonic dystrophy: Course complications and management. Obstet Gynecol 1971; 38:448-54.

108. Sholl JS, Hughey MJ, Hirschmann RA. Myotonic muscular dystrophy associated with ritodrine tocolysis. Am J Obstet Gynecol 1985; 151:83-6.

109. Arulkumaran S, Rauff M, Ingemarsson I, et al. Uterine activity in myotonic dystrophy. Br J Obstet Gynaecol 1986; 93:634-6.

110. Blumgart CH, Hughes DG, Redfern N. Obstetric anaesthesia in dystrophia myotonica. Anaesthesia 1990; 45:26-9.

111. Gilchrist JM. Muscle disease in the pregnant woman. In Devinsky O, Feldman E, Hainline B, editors. Neurologic Complications of Pregnancy. (Vol. 64 of Advances in Neurology). New York, Raven Press, 1994:196.

112. Russell SH, Hirsch NP. Anaesthesia and Myotonia. Br J Anaesth 1994; 72:210-6.
113. Donaldson JO. Neurology of Pregnancy, 2nd ed. London, WB Saunders, 1989:75.
114. Camann WR, Johnson MD. Anesthetic management of a parturient with myotonia dystrophica: A case report. Reg Anesth 1990; 15:41-3.
115. Mathicu J, Allard P, Gobeil G, et al. Anesthetic and surgical complications in 219 cases of myotonic dystrophy. Neurology 1997; 49:1646-50.
116. Paterson IS. Generalized myotonia following suxamethonium: Case report. Br J Anaesth 1962; 34:340-2.
117. Hook R, Anderson EF, Noto P. Anesthetic management of a parturient with myotonia atrophica. Anesthesiology 1975; 43:689-92.
118. Brownell KW. Malignant hyperthermia: Relationship to other diseases. Br J Anaesth 1988; 60:303-8.
119. Campbell AN, Thompson N. Anaesthesia for caesarean section in a patient with myotonic dystrophy receiving warfarin therapy. Can J Anaesth 1995; 42:409-14.
120. Cherng YG, Wang YP, Liu CC, et al. Combined spinal and epidural anesthesia for abdominal hysterectomy in a patient with myotonic dystrophy. Reg Anesth 1994; 19:69-72.
121. Adams RD, Victor M, Ropper AH. Principles of Neurology, 6th ed. New York, McGraw-Hill, 1997:1414-31.
122. Rudnik-Shoneborn S, Glauner B, Rohng D, Zerres K. Obstetric aspects in women with fascioscapulohumeral muscular dystrophy, limb girdle muscular dystrophy, and congenital myopathies. Arch Neurol 1997; 54:888-94.
123. Pash MP, Balaton J, Eagle C. Anaesthetic management of a parturient with severe muscular dystrophy, lumbar lordosis and a difficult airway. Can J Anaesth 1996; 43:959-63.
124. Gronert GA, Fowler W, Cardinet GH, et al. Absence of malignant hyperthermia contractures in Becker-Duchenne dystrophy at age 2. Muscle Nerve 1992; 15:52-6.
125. Allen GC. Malignant hyperthermia susceptibility. Anesthesiol Clin North Am 1994; 12:513-35.
126. Denborough, Michael. Malignant hyperthermia. Lancet 1998; 352: 1131-36.
127. Adams RD, Victor M, Ropper AH. Principles of Neurology, 6th ed. New York, McGraw-Hill, 1997:1010-20.
128. Joffe D, Robbins R, Benjamin A. Caesarean section and phaeochromocytoma resection in a patient with Von Hippel Lindau disease. Can J Anaesth 1993; 40:870-4.
129. Ginsburg DS, Hernandez E, Johnson JW. Sarcoma complicating Von Recklinghausen's disease in pregnancy. Obstet Gynecol 1981; 58:385-7.
130. Sharma JB, Gulati N, Malik S. Maternal and perinatal complications in neurofibromatosis during pregnancy. Int J Gynaecol Obstet 1991; 34:221-7.
131. Dugoff L, Sujansky E. Neurofibromatosis type 1 and pregnancy. Am J Med Genet 1996; 66:7-10.
132. Hirsch NP, Murphy A, Radcliffe J. Neurofibromatosis: Clinical presentations and anesthetic implications. Br J Anaesth 2001; 86:555-64.
133. Dounas M, Mercier F, Lhuissier C, Benhamou D. Epidural analgesia for labour in a parturient with neurofibromatosis. Can J Anaesth 1995; 42:420-4.
134. Richardson MG, Setty GK, Rawoof SA. Responses to nondepolarizing neuromuscular blockers and succinylcholine in von Recklinghausen neurofibromatosis. Anesth Analg 1996; 82:382-5.
135. Mittershciffthaler G, Maurhard U, Huter O, Brezinka C. Prolonged action of vecuroneum in neurofibromatosis. Anaesteziol Reanimatol 1989; 14:175-8.
136. Naguib M, Al-Rajeh SM, Abdulatif M, Ababtin WA. The response of a patient with Von Recklinghausen's disease to succinylcholine and atracurium. Middle East J Anesthesiol 1988; 9:429-34.
137. Petrikovsky BM, Vintzileos AM, Cassidy SB, Egan JF. Tuberous sclerosis in pregnancy. Am J Perinatol 1990; 7:133-5.
138. Forsnes EV, Eggleston MK, Burtman M. Placental abruption and spontaneous rupture of renal angiomyolipoma in a pregnant woman with tuberous sclerosis. Ob Gyn 1996; 88:725.
139. Adams RD, Victor M, Ropper AH. Principles of Neurology, 6th ed. New York, McGraw-Hill, 1997:1018.
140. Ogasawara KK, Ogasawara EM, Hirata G. Pregnancy complicated by Von Hippel-Lindau disease. Obstet Gynecol 1995; 85:829-31.
141. Adams RD, Victor M, Ropper AH. Principles of Neurology, 6th ed. New York, McGraw-Hill, 1997:1312-8.
142. Guillain-Barré Study Group. Plasmapheresis and acute Guillain-Barré syndrome. Neurology 1985; 35:1096-104.
143. Gautier PE, Hantson P, Vekemans NC, et al. Intensive care management of Guillain-Barré syndrome during pregnancy. Intensive Care Med 1990; 16:460-2.

144. Jiang GX, de Pedro-Cuestra J, Strigard K, et al. Pregnancy and Guillain-Barré syndrome: A nationwide register cohort study. Neuroepidemiology 1996; 15:192-200.
145. Rockel A, Wissel J, Rolfs A. Guillain-Barré syndrome in pregnancy: An indication for caesarean section? J Perinat Med 1994; 122:393-8.
146. McGrady EM. Management of labour and delivery in a patient with Guillain-Barré syndrome. Anaesthesia 1987; 42:899.
147. Vassiliev DV, Nystrom EU, Leicht CH. Combined spinal and epidural anesthesia for labor and cesarean delivery in a patient with Guillain-Barré syndrome. Reg Anesth Pain Med. 2001; 26:174-6.
148. Steiner I, Argov Z, Cahan C, Abramsky O. Guillain-Barré syndrome after epidural anesthesia: Direct nerve root damage may trigger disease. Neurology 1985; 35:1473-5.
149. Sibert K, Sladen RN. Impaired ventilatory capacity after recovery from Guillain-Barré syndrome. J Clin Anesth 1994; 6:133-8.
150. Adams RD, Victor M, Ropper AH. Principles of Neurology, 6th ed. New York, McGraw-Hill, 1997:764-7.
151. Klingman J, Chui H, Corgiat M, Perry J. Functional recovery: A major risk factor for the development of postpoliomyelitis muscular dystrophy. Arch Neurol 1988; 45:645-7.
152. Sharief MK, Hentges R, Chiardi M. Intrathecal immune response in patients with the post-polio syndrome. N Engl J Med 1991; 325:749-55.
153. Harjulehto-Mervaala T, Avo T, Hiilesmaa VK, et al. Oral polio vaccination during pregnancy: Fetal development and perinatal outcome. Clin Infect Dis 1994; 18:414-20.
154. Daw E, Chandler G. Pregnancy following poliomyelitis. Postgrad Med J 1976; 52:492-6.
155. Adams RD, Victor M, Ropper AH. Principles of Neurology, 6th ed. New York, McGraw-Hill, 1997:642-96.
156. Roelvink NC, Kamphorst W, van Alphen HA, Rao BR. Pregnancy-related primary brain and spinal tumors. Arch Neurol 1987; 44: 209-15.
157. DeAngelis LM. Central nervous system neoplasms in pregnancy. In Devinsky O, Feldman E, Hainline B, editors. Neurologic Complications of Pregnancy. (Vol. 64 of Advances in Neurology). New York, Raven Press, 1994:139-52.
158. Choi NW, Schuman LM, Gullen WH. Epidemiology of primary central nervous system neoplasms. II. Case-control study. Am J Epidemiol 1970; 91:467-85.
159. Enoksson P, Lunberg N, Sjostedt S, et al. Influence of pregnancy on visual fields in suprasellar tumors. Acta Psychiatr Neurol Scand 1961; 36:524-38.
160. Isla A, Alvarez F, Gonzalez A, et al. Brain tumor and pregnancy. Obstet Gynecol 1997; 89:19-23.
161. Marx GF, Zemaitis MT, Orkin LR. Cerebrospinal fluid pressures during labor and obstetrical anesthesia. Anesthesiology 1961; 22:348-54.
162. Finfer SR. Management of labour and delivery in patients with intracranial neoplasms. Br J Anaesth 1991; 67:784-7.
163. Bruns PD, Linder RO, Drose VE, Battaglia F. The placental transfer of water from fetus to mother following the intravenous infusion of hypertonic mannitol to the maternal rabbit. Am J Obstet Gynecol 1963; 86:160-7.
164. Kepes ER, Andrews IC, Radnay PA, et al. Conduct of anesthesia for delivery with grossly raised cerebrospinal fluid pressure. N Y State J Med 1972; 72:1155-6.
165. Goroszeniuk T, Howard RS, Wright JT. The management of labour using continuous lumbar epidural analgesia in a patient with malignant cerebral tumour. Anaesthesia 1986; 41:1128-9.
166. Atanassoff PG, Alon E, Weiss B, et al. Spinal anaesthesia for caesarean section in a parturient with brain neoplasm. Can J Anaesth 1994; 41:163-4.
167. Su TM, Lan CM, Yang LC, et al. Brain tumor presenting with fatal herniation following delivery under epidural anesthesia. Anesthesiology 2002; 96:508-9.
168. Chang L, Looi-Lyons L, Bartosik L, Tindal S. Anesthesia for cesarean section in two patients with brain tumours. Can J Anaesth. 1999; 46: 61-5.
169. Bedson Cr, Platt F. Benign intracranial hypertension and anesthesia for cesarean section. Internat J Obst Anesth 1999; 8:288-90.
170. Koontz WL, Herbert WNP, Cefalo RC. Pseudotumor cerebri in pregnancy. Obstet Gynecol 1983; 62:324-7.
171. Shapiro S, Yee R, Brown H. Surgical management of pseudotumor cerebri in pregnancy: Case report. Neurosurgery 1995; 37:829-31.
172. Digre KB, Varner MW, Corbett JJ. Pseudotumor cerebri and pregnancy. Neurology 1984; 34:721-9.
173. Paruchuri SRA, Lawlor M, Kleinhomer K, et al. Risk of cerebellar tonsillar herniation after diagnostic lumbar puncture in pseudotumor cerebri (abstract). Reg Anesth 1993; 18(suppl):99.

174. Palop R, Choed-Amphai E, Miller R. Epidural anesthesia for delivery complicated by benign intracranial hypertension. Anesthesiology 1979; 50:159-60.

175. Bédard JM, Richardson MG, Wissler RN. Epidural anesthesia in a parturient with a lumboperitoneal shunt. Anesthesiology 1999; 90:621-3.

176. Kaul B, Vallejo MC, Ramanathan S, et al. Accidental spinal analgesia in the presence of a lumboperitoneal shunt in an obese parturient receiving enoxaparin therapy. Anesth Analg 2002; 95:441-3,

177. Littleford JA, Brockhurst NJ, Bernstein EP, Georgoussis SE. Obstetrical anesthesia for a parturient with a ventriculoperitoneal shunt and third ventriculostomy. Can J Anaesth 1999; 46:1057-63.

178. Adams RD, Victor M, Ropper AH. Principles of Neurology, 6th ed. New York, McGraw-Hill, 1997:1003-6.

179. Bradley NK, Liakos AM, McAllister JP, et al. Maternal shunt dependency: implications for obstetric care, neurosurgical management, and pregnancy outcomes and a review of selected literature. Neurosurgery 1998; 43:448-60.

180. Wisoff JH, Kratzert KJ, Handwerker SM, et al. Pregnancy in patients with cerebrospinal fluid shunts: Report of a series and review of the literature. Neurosurgery 1991; 29:827-31.

181. Wilterdink JL, Feldman E. Cerebral hemorrhage. In Devinsky O, Feldman E, Hainline B, editors. Neurologic Complications of Pregnancy. (Vol. 64 of Advances in Neurology). New York, Raven Press, 1994:13-23.

182. Donaldson JO. Neurology of Pregnancy, 2nd ed. London, WB Saunders, 1989: 137-40.

183. Holcomb WL, Petrie RH. Cerebrovascular emergencies in pregnancy. Clin Obstet Gynecol 1990; 33:467-72.

184. Dias MS, Sekhar LN. Intracranial hemorrhage from aneurysms and arteriovenous malformations during pregnancy and the peurperium. Neurosurgery 1990; 27:855-66.

185. Piotin M, de Souza Filho CBA, Kothimbakam R, Moret J. Endovascular treatment of acutely ruptured intracranial aneurysms in pregnancy. Am J Obstet Gynecol 2001; 185:1261-2.

186. Sadasivan B, Malik G, Lee C, Ausman JI. Vascular malformations and pregnancy. Surg Neurol 1990; 33:305-13.

187. Mas JL, Lamy C. Stroke in pregnancy and the puerperium. J Neurol. 1998; 245:305-13.

188. Hudspith NJ, Popham PA. The anaesthetic management of intracranial haemorrhage from arteriovenous malformations during pregnancy: Three cases. Internat J Obstet Anesth 1996; 5:189-93.

189. Viscomi CM, Wilson J, Bernstein I. Anesthetic management of a parturient with an incompletely resected cerebral arteriovenous malformation. Reg Anesth 1997; 22:192-7.

190. Sharma SK, Herrera ER, Sidawi JE, et al. The pregnant patient with an intracranial arteriovenous malformation: Cesarean or vaginal delivery using regional or general anesthesia? Reg Anesth 1995; 20:455-8.

191. Anaesthesia for caesarean section in a patient with an intracranial arteriovenous malformation. Anaesth Intens Care 1999; 27:66-8.

192. Stoodley MA, Macdonald RL, Weir BK. Pregnancy and intracranial aneurysms. Neurosurg Clin N Am 1998; 9:549-56.

193. Donchin Y, Amirav B, Sahar A, Yarkoni S. Sodium nitroprusside for aneurysm surgery in pregnancy. Br J Anaesth 1978; 50:849-51.

194. Dhamee MS, Goh M. Deliberate hypotension for clipping of cerebral aneurysm during pregnancy. Anesthesiol Rev 1985; 12:20-2.

195. Newman B, Lam AM. Induced hypotension for clipping of a cerebral aneurysm during pregnancy: A case report and brief review. Anesth Analg 1986; 65:675-8.

196. Naulty J, Cefalo RC, Lewis PE. Fetal toxicity of nitroprusside in the pregnant ewe. Am J Obstet Gynecol 1981; 139: 708-11.

197. Ellis SC, Wheeler AS, James FM, et al. Fetal and maternal effects of sodium nitroprusside used to counteract hypertension in gravid ewes. Am J Obstet Gynecol 1982; 143:766-70.

198. Nelson SH, Suresh MS. Comparison of nitroprusside and hydralazine in isolated uterine arteries from pregnant and nonpregnant patients. Anesthesiology 1988; 68:541-7.

199. Conklin KA, Herr G, Funy D. Anaesthesia for cesarean section and cerebral aneurysm clipping. Can Anaesth Soc J 1984; 31:451-4.

200. Lennon RL, Sundt TM, Gronert GA. Combined cesarean section and clipping of intracerebral aneurysm. Anesthesiology 1984; 60:240-2.

201. Whitburn RH, Laishley RS, Jewkes DA. Anaesthesia for simultaneous caesarean section and clipping of intracerebral aneurysm. Br J Anaesth 1990; 64:642-5.

202. Powner DJ, Bernstein IM. Extended somatic support for pregnant women after brain death. Crit Care Med 2003; 31:1241-9.

203. Donaldson JO. Neurology of Pregnancy, 2nd ed. London, WB Saunders, 1989:160.

204. Lanska DJ, Kryscio RJ. Peripartum stroke and intracranial venous thrombosis in the National Hospital Discharge Survey. Obstet Gynecol 1997; 89:413-8.

205. Donaldson JO. Stroke. Clin Obstet Gynecol 1981; 24:825-35.

206. Ravindran RS, Zandstra GC. Cerebral venous thrombosis versus post lumbar puncture headache. Anesthesiology 1989; 71:478-9.

207. Younker D, Jones MM, Adenwala J, et al. Maternal cortical vein thrombosis and the obstetric anesthesiologist. Anesth Analg 1986; 65:1007-12.

208. Cantu C, Barinagarrementeria F. Cerebral venous thrombosis associated with pregnancy and puerperium. Stroke 1993; 24:1880-4.

209. Adams RD, Victor M, Ropper AH. Principles of Neurology, 6th ed. New York, McGraw-Hill, 1997: 1090.

210. Jacka MJ, Sanderson F. Amyotrophic lateral sclerosis presenting during pregnancy. Anesth Analg 1998; 86:542-3.

211. Hara K, Sakura S, Saito Y, et al. Epidural anesthesia and pulmonary function in a patient with amyotrophic lateral sclerosis. Anesth Analg 1996; 83:878-9.

212. Kochi T, Oka T, Mizuguchi T. Epidural anesthesia for patients with amyotrophic lateral sclerosis. Anesth Analg 1989; 68:410-2.

213. Rosenbaum KJ, Neigh JL, Strobel GE. Sensitivity to nondepolarizing muscle relaxants in amyotrophic lateral sclerosis: Report of two cases. Anesthesiology 1971; 35:638-41.

214. Pugh CP, Healey SK, Crane JM, Young D. Successful pregnancy and spinal muscular atrophy. Obstet Gynecol 2000; 95:1034.

215. Weston LA, DiFazio C. Labor analgesia and anesthesia in a patient with spinal muscular atrophy and vocal cord paralysis. Reg Anesth 1996; 21:350-4.

216. Harris SJ, Moaz K. Cesarean section conducted under subarachnoid block in tow sisters with spinal muscular atrophy. Internat J Obstet Anesth 2002; 10:125-7.

217. Adams RD, Victor M, Ropper AH. Principles of Neurology, 6th ed. New York, McGraw-Hill, 1997:1343-5.

218. Rudnik-Schoneborn S, Rohrig D, Nicholson G, Zerres K. Pregnancy and delivery in Charcot-Marie-Tooth disease type 1. Neurology 1993; 43:2011-6.

219. Scull T, Weeks S. Epidural analgesia for labour in a patient with Charcot-Marie-Tooth disease. Can J Anaesth 1996; 43:1150-2.

220. Brian JE, Bayles GD, Quirk JG, Clark RB. Anesthetic management for cesarean section of a patient with Charcot-Marie-Tooth disease. Anesthesiology 1987; 66:410-2.

221. McGregor JA, Guberman A, Amer J, Goodlin R. Idiopathic facial nerve paralysis (Bell's palsy) in late pregnancy and the early puerperium. Obstet Gynecol 1987; 69:435-8.

222. Shmorgun D, Chan WS, Ray JG. Association between Bell's palsy in pregnancy and preeclampsia. QJM 2002; 95:359-62.

223. Adour KK. The bell tolls for decompression? N Engl J Med 1975; 292:748-50.

224. Dorsey DL, Camann WR. Obstetric anesthesia in patients with idiopathic facial paralysis (Bell's palsy): A 10-year survey. Anesth Analg 1993; 77:81-3.

225. Ekman-Ordeberg G, Salgeback S, Ordeberg G. Carpal tunnel syndrome in pregnancy: A prospective study. Acta Obstet Gynecol Scand 1987; 66:233-5.

226. VanDiver T, Camann W. Meralgia paresthetica in the parturient. Int J Obstet Anesth 1995; 4:109-12.

227. Massey EW. Mononeuropathies in pregnancy. Semin Neurol 1988; 8:193-6.

Chapter 49
Obesity

Robert D'Angelo, M.D. · David D. Dewan, M.D.

Various definitions exist for obesity (Table 49-1). Most commonly a person with a body mass index (BMI) of ≥ 30 kg/m^2 is considered obese. The incidence of overweight individuals is increasing in the general population at an alarming rate and is reaching epidemic proportions.[1] It has been estimated that obesity causes approximately 300,000 preventable deaths per year and may soon cause as much preventable disease and death as cigarette smoking.[2] The most recent data from the National Center for Health Statistics suggest that 54% of Americans are overweight and 21% are obese.[1] The increasing prevalence of obesity among nonpregnant patients extends to the pregnant population. At Wake Forest University, the percentage of patients who weighed more than 300 lb at the time of delivery increased from 0.18% in 1978 to 0.35% in 1989[3] and to 1.9% in 2002.

There is an increased incidence of hypertension, coronary artery disease, cerebrovascular disease, diabetes mellitus, gallbladder disease, and liver disease in obese, nonpregnant patients.[4,5] Unfortunately, pregnancy-associated weight gain affects the weight of women after pregnancy.[6] Fortunately, pregnancy primarily results in an accumulation of lower body fat, which confers less health risk than upper body fat.[7,8] Regardless of its etiology, however, morbid obesity is associated with a twofold to twelvefold increase in mortality.[4,9,10]

PHYSIOLOGIC CHANGES OF OBESITY

Pulmonary Changes

Excess body weight requires increased energy expenditure proportionate to the increase in body mass and surface area. Increased energy expenditure increases oxygen consumption and CO_2 production independent of the metabolic rate, which remains constant among obese patients. Oxygen consumption and CO_2 production double as weight doubles.[11] The obese patient's respiratory quotient resembles that of a patient with normal weight, and exercise studies of obese patients have revealed that oxygen consumption and CO_2 production are directly proportional to the work performed.[12] Minute ventilation obligatorily increases to meet demand, except in the 5% to 10% of patients with the pickwickian

syndrome, who display a decreased sensitivity to CO_2.[13] Unfortunately, obesity impairs the body's ability to meet these demands. Specifically, excess weight worsens pulmonary mechanics, alters lung volumes, and impairs oxygenation.

PULMONARY MECHANICS

Increased chest wall weight requires greater energy expenditure during ventilation to move the greater mass. Cullen and Formel[14] concluded that the oxygen cost of breathing rises proportionately with weight, except for those with coincidental pulmonary disease. In contrast, Sharp et al.[15] reported that respiratory work efficiency among obese patients falls when measured as a ratio of mechanical work divided by the oxygen cost of breathing. This implies a decreased efficiency of respiratory muscles in obese patients. The weight gain associated with pregnancy further increases the work of breathing in obese patients. Frequent shallow respirations may represent a more efficient breathing pattern than large tidal volumes in obese patients. Noble[16] documented an increase in tidal volume after weight loss by obese patients; this suggests that the obese patient conserves energy by decreasing tidal volume. This ventilatory pattern contrasts with the increased tidal volume that typically accompanies pregnancy. Nonetheless, most morbidly obese pregnant women have a Pa_{CO_2} that is normal for pregnancy. However, pulmonary reserve is decreased.

LUNG VOLUMES

Obesity alters lung volumes. Increased abdominal weight restricts diaphragmatic movement, especially in the supine or Trendelenburg position; this encourages smaller tidal volumes (Figure 49-1). Increased chest wall weight decreases the expansive tendency of the chest wall. Functional residual capacity (FRC) declines, and it may be less than closing capacity. This results in airway closure during tidal ventilation in morbidly obese patients. Similarly, expiratory reserve volume, vital capacity, inspiratory capacity, total lung capacity, and maximum minute ventilation all decrease in the morbidly obese patient. Although total compliance decreases, pulmonary compliance and airway resistance remain normal.[4]

TABLE 49-1	INDICES OF OBESITY AND THEIR PARAMETERS	
Index	**Definition**	**Values**
Overweight	20% > ideal	
Obesity	> 20% over ideal	
Morbid obesity	Ideal weight × 2	
Broca index	Ideal female weight	Ht (cm) − 105
Body mass (Quetelet) index	$\dfrac{Wt\,(kg)}{Ht\,(m)^2}$	Normal = 25, obese > 30
Ponderal index	$\dfrac{Ht\,(in)}{\sqrt[3]{Wt\,(lb)}}$	Obese < 11.6

From Dewan DM. The obese parturient. In James FM, Wheeler AS, Dewan DM, editors. Obstetric Anesthesia: The Complicated Patient, 2nd ed. Philadelphia, FA Davis, 1988:468.

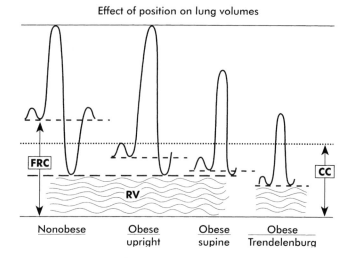

FIGURE 49-1. In obesity, decreased chest wall compliance results in a functional residual capacity *(FRC)* that decreases at the expense of expiratory reserve volume *(ERV)*. Closing capacity *(CC)* stays normal. (From Vaughan RW. Pulmonary and cardiovascular derangements in the obese patient. In Brown BR, editor. Anesthesia and the Obese Patient. Philadelphia, FA Davis, 1982:26.)

Pregnancy also alters lung volumes. In the nonobese pregnant patient, expiratory reserve volume and FRC decline approximately 20% to 25% by term. Eng et al.[17] examined a series of pregnant women whose estimated prepregnant weights ranged from 50% to 140% above normal and compared lung volumes during the third trimester and again at 2 months postpartum. With the exception of FRC, the lung volume changes resembled those that occur in nonobese pregnant women. However, FRC decreased less in obese pregnant women than in nonobese pregnant women, perhaps offering some protection from premature airway closure in the overweight gravida.

OXYGENATION

Pulmonary diffusion typically remains normal, except in some patients with massive obesity.[4] Decreased chest wall compliance and the greater weight of abdominal contents promote airway closure in the dependent portion of the lung. Ventilation preferentially occurs in the more compliant, nondependent portion of the lung. In contrast, pulmonary blood flow preferentially occurs in the dependent portion of the lung. This results in ventilation-perfusion mismatch and hypoxemia.[18] Barrera et al.[19] suggested that there is a relative hyperperfusion of poorly ventilated alveoli in obese patients.

Consistent with the positional deterioration of lung volumes, oxygenation worsens in the supine and Trendelenburg positions. Although oxygenation does not necessarily correlate linearly with weight,[20] massive weight loss improves PaO2 and expiratory reserve volume. Weight loss does not improve forced expiratory volume in 1 second, forced vital capacity, or maximum mid-expiratory flow.[21]

The increased ventilation and cardiac output that occur during pregnancy may confer some protection to obese women. Two studies noted maternal PaO2 measurements of approximately 85 to 86 mm Hg in obese pregnant women.[17,22] Although these measurements are less than those seen in normal pregnant women, they exceed those observed in morbidly obese, nonpregnant patients presenting for gastric bypass. Other physicians have argued that pregnancy does not improve oxygenation in obese patients.[23]

Cardiovascular Changes

Obesity increases blood volume and cardiac output. A weight increase from 70 to 170 kg results in a doubling of cardiac output and blood volume in nonpregnant patients.[24] The cardiac index remains normal. Increased cardiac output primarily results from increased stroke volume. The systemic arteriovenous oxygen difference remains normal.[25]

Pulmonary blood volume increases in proportion to the increase in cardiac output and total blood volume. Pulmonary hypertension can occur and may be position dependent. Paul et al.[26] observed an 11% increase in oxygen consumption and a 30% increase in pulmonary capillary wedge pressure (PCWP) when morbidly obese patients assumed the supine position. Hypoxemia, if present, causes increased pulmonary vascular resistance. Airway obstruction also may increase pulmonary artery pressure. Teeple and Ghia[27] noted a decline in PCWP from 38 to 5 mm Hg after endotracheal intubation and relief of airway obstruction in an obese patient.

Hypertension occurs more frequently among obese patients; a BMI of greater than 30 is associated with a threefold increase in the incidence of hypertension.[9] Obesity offers no protection against the consequences of hypertension.[28] Mabie et al.[29] described a subset of obese, hypertensive pregnant women with increased left ventricular mass, normal systolic function, and abnormal diastolic function. They suggested that these findings reflect volume overload in the presence of inadequate left ventricular relaxation. Primary therapy for these patients includes a reduction of the expanded blood volume through vigorous diuretic therapy.

A clear relationship exists between obesity and death from cardiovascular causes. Drenick et al.[10] demonstrated a twelvefold increase in mortality among obese patients between the ages of 25 and 34 years; cardiovascular disease was the most common cause of death. Tseuda et al.[30] reported two cases of cardiac arrest in morbidly obese patients who were placed supine. They speculated that sudden circulatory changes associated with positional change accounted for the sudden death in these patients. Drenick and Fisler[31] also reported cases of postoperative cardiac arrest in obese patients that were not explained at autopsy.

Messerli et al.[32] documented a thirtyfold increase in premature ventricular contractions in obese patients with

eccentric left ventricular hypertrophy (LVH) when compared with lean subjects. Although LVH occurs in response to increased work load, there is an association between increased left ventricular mass and increased weight, even after controlling for age and blood pressure, especially in patients with a BMI of greater than 30.[33] Among morbidly obese pregnant women, left atrial size, left ventricular thickness, interventricular septal thickness, and left ventricular mass increase and left ventricular function remain similar to that of nonobese women.[34] Alexander[25] concluded that excess epicardial fat is not a prominent feature in obese patients with cardiac enlargement. Fatty infiltration of the heart can occur, especially in the right ventricle and perhaps in the conduction system, but eccentric LVH is the major cause of increased heart size. Inadequate hypertrophy and chamber dilation predispose some patients to myocardial decompensation.[35]

Gastrointestinal Changes

Vaughan et al.[36] observed that 88% of obese, nonpregnant patients presenting for surgery had a gastric pH of less than 2.5, and 86% had a gastric volume that exceeded 25 mL. These findings resemble those in a population of healthy pregnant patients who presented for elective cesarean section.[37] It is unclear whether the combination of pregnancy and obesity further increases gastric volume and decreases gastric pH.

Hiatal hernia is more common in obese patients than in nonobese patients. However, it is unclear whether obesity worsens pregnancy-associated changes in lower esophageal sphincter tone.[38-42] Altogether, it seems likely that the morbidly obese patient is at increased risk for pulmonary aspiration of gastric contents.

Endocrine Changes

Diabetes mellitus occurs more frequently among obese patients. Kissebah et al.[7] suggested that decreased insulin sensitivity is associated with upper body obesity. Farmer et al.[43] identified a relative insulin insufficiency among obese women during pregnancy.

Coagulation Changes

Most studies suggest that the obese patient is at increased risk for deep vein thrombosis and pulmonary thromboembolism,[44,45] although this is a matter of some dispute.[46] It is likely but unproved that obesity increases the risks of deep vein thrombosis and pulmonary thromboembolism associated with pregnancy.

INTERACTION WITH PREGNANCY

The median weight gain during pregnancy in the United States is 30.5 lb.[47] The incidence of morbid obesity among obstetric patients varies according to the definition used. Approximately 26% of pregnant women weigh more than 200 lb, 8% weigh more than 250 lb, and 2% weigh more than 300 lb.[48,49] At Wake Forest University, 1.9% of our pregnant patients weighed more than 300 lb in 2002.

Obstetricians have long believed that obesity adversely affects pregnancy outcome. In 1968, Tracy and Miller[50] reported that a pregnant weight exceeding 250 lb during any part of pregnancy increased the likelihood of complicating medical disease, obstetric complications, and operative delivery. Other studies have evaluated the effect of obesity on obstetric outcome. Unfortunately, these studies have not used a uniform definition of obesity during pregnancy.[52-54] A variety of definitions have been used to define obesity, including the following: (1) the weight-to-height ratio, (2) a prepregnant BMI greater than 29, (3) a weight of 90 kg *at any time* during pregnancy, (4) a greater than 20% increase in weight during pregnancy, and (5) a weight of greater than 200 lb during pregnancy. The optimal definition of obesity during pregnancy is unclear.

Obesity is associated with an increased risk of chronic hypertension, pregnancy-induced hypertension (PIH), and diabetes mellitus during pregnancy.[51,55-57] In our series of morbidly obese patients at Wake Forest University, we observed a fourteenfold increase in the incidence of chronic hypertension (28% versus 2%) among patients whose weight exceeded 300 lb at the time of delivery when compared with a control group of nonobese patients.[3] The greater risk of chronic hypertension may result in part from the fact that obese patients typically are older than nonobese patients.

Obesity results in a less marked increase in the incidence of PIH.[51,55,57] In our series, we observed a 16% incidence of preeclampsia among women whose weight exceeded 300 lb at the time of delivery, versus a 10% incidence of preeclampsia among a control group of nonobese patients.[3]

The diabetogenic state that accompanies pregnancy places the morbidly obese woman at high risk for insulin-dependent diabetes mellitus during pregnancy. Obesity results in a twofold to eightfold increase in the incidence of diabetes mellitus during pregnancy.[56,57]

Most important, obesity increases the risk of death during pregnancy.[58-62] Kaunitz et al.[59] suggested that advanced age and an increased incidence of hypertension, diabetes, thromboembolic disease, and infection are factors that increase the risk of maternal death among obese women. Likewise, several studies[61,62] have noted that obesity increases the likelihood of maternal death during anesthesia.

Progress of Labor and Method of Delivery

Increased BMI, increased prepregnancy weight, and excessive maternal weight gain increase the risk of cesarean section.[55-57,63] However, the reasons for the increased incidence of cesarean section among obese patients are unclear. Some obstetricians contend that abnormal presentation, fetal macrosomia, and prolonged labor are predisposing factors associated with the increased incidence of cesarean section among obese women. Some studies have suggested that abnormal presentation and multiple gestation are more common in obese patients than in nonobese patients.[50,64] However, neither Johnson et al.[51] nor Hood and Dewan[3] observed a higher incidence of malpresentation in obese pregnant women.

Hypertension and diabetes often prompt elective induction of labor, which may increase the risk of cesarean section. Garbaciak et al.[56] reviewed the records of 9667 patients who were subdivided into four weight categories: underweight, normal weight, overweight, and morbidly obese. As weight increased, the frequency of antenatal medical complications—including hypertension, PIH, and diabetes—also increased. The presence of medical complications increased the cesarean section rate for normal weight and obese patients but not for morbidly obese patients. This study suggests that factors other than medical complications account for the increased cesarean section rate among obese women.

Some,[63,65] but not all,[64] studies suggest that obese patients are at increased risk for abnormal labor. Some studies[39,56,63] have noted an increased incidence of meconium-stained amniotic fluid, umbilical cord accidents, and late fetal heart rate (FHR) decelerations during labor in obese patients. It seems unlikely that an increased incidence of fetal distress accounts for the increased incidence of cesarean section among obese patients. In our series of morbidly obese patients, the indications for cesarean section were remarkably similar for both normal weight and morbidly obese patients, with the exception of the diagnosis of failed induction. Likewise, the incidence of cesarean section for failure-to-progress was much higher in the morbidly obese group than in the control group, although the difference was not statistically significant. The frequent diagnosis of dystocia is consistent with the decreased incidence of preterm delivery and low birth weight (LBW) infants and the increased incidence of fetal macrosomia and post-term gestation in obese women in other studies.[23,55,56,63,64]

Maternal diabetes and obesity may independently increase the likelihood of fetal macrosomia.[24] Weight gain during pregnancy also may affect the risk of fetal macrosomia,[63] and some physicians have suggested that weight gain *during* pregnancy is more likely to increase the incidence of cesarean section than absolute weight *before* pregnancy. Bianco et al.[66] suggested that restricting maternal weight gain to less than 25 lb decreases the risk of delivering a large for gestational age (LGA) infant and improves neonatal outcome.[66] Others have not confirmed that excess maternal weight gain increases the risk of fetal macrosomia.[51] Abrams and Parker[55] noted that maternal weight gain significantly increased newborn birth weight for underweight, ideal weight, and moderately overweight women but not for women whose prepregnancy weights were greater than 135% of ideal.[67] These investigators and others have suggested that recommendations for a minimum weight gain for the morbidly obese woman are unnecessary. Crane et al.[52] have speculated that prepregnancy weight loss should decrease the cesarean delivery rate, and they suggested counseling to encourage preconception weight loss. Finally, Klebanoff et al.[68] noted that a maternal birth weight of more than 8 lb was second only to maternal weight during pregnancy as a predictor for fetal macrosomia. In summary, the morbidly obese patient, with or without diabetes and with or without excessive weight gain, is at increased risk for fetal macrosomia.[57]

Although it seems clear that fetal macrosomia increases the likelihood of cesarean section, Johnson et al.[51] observed an increased incidence of cesarean section among obese patients even when patients with hypertension, diabetes, and macrosomic infants were excluded from analysis. Bell et al.[69] concluded that obesity is an *independent* risk factor for cesarean section; they demonstrated a twofold increase in the incidence of cesarean section among patients with a BMI of 40 kg/m^2; each additional 10 kg/m^2 increase in BMI was associated with an additional increase in the likelihood of cesarean section.

Medicolegal considerations may increase the likelihood of cesarean section in obese patients.[64] For example, obstetricians may perform cesarean section to avoid the risk of shoulder dystocia during vaginal delivery. Others have suggested that soft tissue dystocia increases the risk of cesarean section in obese patients. In a discussion of infertility among obese patients, Prough and Askel[70] speculated that perineal fat and intrapelvic fat deposits near the sigmoid colon and lateral pelvic sidewalls may alter the shape of the vaginal canal.

Garbaciak et al.[56] also speculated that the increase in maternal pelvic soft tissue could narrow the birth canal.

Some physicians have suggested an increased likelihood of excessive blood loss during cesarean section in obese patients.[51] Prolonged, difficult surgery may be responsible for this observation. However, in our series, we did *not* observe increased blood loss during cesarean section among patients who weighed more than 300 lb.[3]

Perinatal Outcome

Obese women are at decreased risk for preterm delivery and delivery of a LBW infant.[51] Higher prepregnancy maternal weight increases the risk of late fetal death, although it protects against the delivery of a small-for-gestational-age (SGA) infant.[71] Infants of obese women also may have an increased risk of neural tube defects and other congenital malformations.[72]

Fetal macrosomia may predispose obese women to trauma at delivery[47] and increase the likelihood of shoulder dystocia during vaginal delivery.[56,63] Johnson et al.[63] noted an association between fetal macrosomia and an increased incidence of shoulder dystocia in patients weighing more than 250 lb. Perlow et al.[57] observed an increased frequency of neonatal intensive care unit admissions among the infants of obese women. Although Rahaman et al.[73] observed a tenfold increase in perinatal mortality among obese parturients, other investigators have not observed an increased incidence of neonatal depression or perinatal mortality among obese patients.[63,64] In our series, we observed no neonatal deaths among women who weighed more than 300 lb at delivery, despite the fact that 47% of those patients had antenatal complications.[3]

ANESTHETIC MANAGEMENT

Preanesthetic Assessment

The high incidence of coincidental medical disease among obese pregnant women necessitates an early, careful preanesthetic assessment. When concerns exist, a pulse oximeter may be used to assess the adequacy of maternal oxygenation. When questions exist regarding maternal ventilation, an arterial blood gas measurement is invaluable. The presence of preeclampsia necessitates the assessment of the platelet count. At Wake Forest University, we do not perform other coagulation tests unless there is clinical evidence of either coagulopathy or rapid deterioration of the patient.[74]

Unless the length of the sphygmomanometer cuff exceeds the circumference of the arm by 20%, systolic and diastolic blood pressure measurements may overestimate true maternal blood pressure. The use of an appropriate size of blood pressure cuff and an automatic blood pressure measurement device often obviate the need for intraarterial monitoring. However, the anesthesiologist may place an intraarterial catheter in patients with chronic hypertension or preeclampsia and in those who require frequent arterial blood gas measurements during and after cesarean section.

The anesthesiologist should anticipate the need for needles longer than those used for the administration of spinal and epidural anesthesia in patients of normal weight.[22,75] Fortunately, only a minority of obese patients require an epidural needle of extra length. In some cases, however, the hub of the epidural needle indents the skin, and successful catheter placement requires that a second individual pass the

catheter while the primary anesthetist maintains needle position. In contrast, spinal needles with extra length are often required when performing spinal anesthesia in obese patients.

Appropriately sized labor beds, transportation gurneys, and operating tables are imperative. Although there are reports of obese patients who required two operating tables, standard operating tables are typically rated to support a patient weight as high as 500 lb. However, in one case at Wake Forest University, the foot of the operating table collapsed during movement of the patient into the lithotomy position. This experience emphasizes the importance of having a sufficient number of personnel to assist with patient transport. Many patients are transported to the operating room after administration of epidural anesthesia for labor, and these patients typically are unable to help move themselves from the labor bed to the operating table.

Labor and Vaginal Delivery

Intravenous access must be established early during labor. It is difficult to establish intravenous access in some obese patients. However, the increased concentrations of steroid hormones during pregnancy cause venodilation, which may lessen the technical challenge. Rarely, central venous cannulation is the only available route.

Options for analgesia are identical to those for the lean patient. Although some obese women may not require analgesia or anesthesia for labor and spontaneous vaginal delivery,[64] obesity does not affect the severity of labor pain,[76] and most obese women desire analgesia during labor and vaginal delivery.

The potential for neonatal depression complicates the administration of systemic opioids during labor. For delivery, pudendal nerve block may be more difficult technically in obese patients. Inhalation analgesia (e.g., nitrous oxide) remains useful in some patients. However, nitrous oxide has limited efficacy, and it is unavailable in many birthing rooms. Further, inhalation analgesia entails the risk of loss of consciousness, which may precipitate disaster in an obese patient with a difficult airway. Finally, given the increased risk of fetal macrosomia and shoulder dystocia in obese patients, satisfactory anesthesia may be necessary to facilitate an atraumatic vaginal delivery.

Lumbar epidural analgesia is an excellent choice for labor and vaginal delivery in obese parturients. Epidural analgesia reduces oxygen consumption and attenuates the increase in cardiac output that occurs during labor and delivery. In our series, administration of epidural analgesia did not affect the likelihood of vaginal delivery in patients who weighed more than 300 lb when compared with similar patients who did not receive epidural analgesia during labor.[3] The use of epidural analgesia during labor allows the anesthesiologist to provide profound anesthesia for operative vaginal delivery. Likewise, the anesthesiologist may extend epidural anesthesia for cesarean section if necessary.

Buckley et al.[75] reported a 20% incidence of failed epidural analgesia in morbidly obese patients. They reported one patient with an inadequate block and 10 patients in whom they were unable to identify the epidural space. Our experience at Wake Forest University suggests that anesthesiologists can achieve a high rate of success with epidural analgesia. We achieved a 94% success rate in patients who weighed more than 300 lb at the time of delivery; this rate did not differ significantly from the 98% rate of success in a control group of nonobese parturients. However, the obese patients required more attempts to identify the epidural space, and a larger number of obese patients required placement of a second or third catheter.[3]

The increased depth of the epidural space among obese patients contributes to the high failure rate of epidural analgesia by increasing the rate of failure to identify the epidural space and also by increasing the incidence of unilateral blockade. Narang and Linter[77] observed that an increased depth of the epidural space exaggerates minor directional errors and increases the likelihood of identifying a lateral portion of the epidural space. Although ultrasonographic guidance has been suggested as a method to facilitate identification of the epidural space,[78] the applicability of this technique on a busy obstetric service is questionable. Use of the sitting position facilitates identification of the midline of the spinal column, and this often facilitates successful identification of either the subarachnoid or epidural space. Further, the distance from the skin to the epidural space is less when the patient is sitting.[79] When patients move from the sitting to the lateral position, the increase in skin-to-epidural space distance increases the likelihood of catheter displacement if the catheter is secured before the change in patient position.[80] The risk of unintentional catheter dislodgement is reduced if the patient assumes the lateral position before the anesthesiologist secures the epidural catheter with tape.

Ideally, epidural analgesia during labor should provide excellent pain relief with little motor block. It is especially important to minimize motor block during labor in obese parturients; otherwise, nursing care and patient transport are problematic. At Wake Forest University, we have relied on epidural administration of a dilute solution of bupivacaine. The addition of an opioid to the bupivacaine solution allows a further reduction in the concentration of the local anesthetic agent. Douglas et al.[81] used a continuous epidural infusion of bupivacaine and fentanyl to provide analgesia in a morbidly obese parturient whose pregnancy was complicated by angina, insulin-dependent diabetes mellitus, hypertension, asthma, and benign intracranial hypertension.

Unfortunately, the administration of both a local anesthetic and an opioid may mask the malposition of an epidural catheter. The administration of opioid by *any* route provides some pain relief. Given the technical difficulties associated with identification of the epidural space in an obese parturient, the anesthesiologist may be reluctant to remove a catheter that is believed to be positioned correctly because the patient experiences some pain relief. If the patient subsequently requires cesarean section, administration of large doses of a local anesthetic agent through a malpositioned catheter may result in inadequate anesthesia for surgery. In contrast, administering a local anesthetic agent alone to establish epidural analgesia during labor will only produce substantial pain relief if the catheter is positioned correctly within the epidural space. The presence of satisfactory epidural analgesia should be documented before the anesthesiologist adds opioid to the local anesthetic solution for an obese patient. The block should be bilateral and *near perfect*. Otherwise, the catheter should be removed and another one should be placed. In our series, the administration of a local anesthetic agent through the first catheter resulted in successful analgesia in only 50% of the obese patients, compared with 95% of the control patients. Careful evaluation of the epidural block and early replacement of malpositioned catheters were largely responsible for our ultimate success, which was documented

by the fact that only 1 of 55 cesarean sections attempted with epidural anesthesia required conversion to general anesthesia for patient discomfort.[3]

In cases of unintentional dural puncture, continuous spinal analgesia represents an alternative technique for providing labor analgesia.[82] Like continuous epidural analgesia, continuous spinal analgesia may be extended for emergency cesarean section. It is unclear whether morbid obesity affects the incidence of postdural puncture headache. However, the routine use of continuous spinal analgesia is not recommended because of the risk that providers may mistakenly give a larger (epidural) dose of local anesthetic through the spinal catheter. In this scenario the potential for a high spinal block in the uncontrolled setting of the labor suite could lead to a catastrophic loss of the airway.

There is little information regarding the efficacy and side effects of combined spinal-epidural (CSE) analgesia for morbidly obese parturients. However, because 10 μg of intrathecal sufentanil may increase end-tidal PCO_2 by as much as 13 mm Hg in normal-weight pregnant patients, the anesthesiologist should carefully consider the risk of respiratory depression in obese parturients.[83] Further, because of the potential for failed epidural analgesia after successful spinal analgesia, as well as the increased likelihood of cesarean section for dystocia, CSE analgesia is *not* the preferred technique for obese patients at Wake Forest University. We prefer early confirmation of the efficacy of epidural analgesia. Delayed recognition of failed epidural analgesia is a significant shortcoming of CSE analgesia.

Cesarean Section

In our series, 42 (48%) of 87 women who weighed more than 300 lb and who underwent a trial of labor subsequently underwent cesarean section.[3] Among nonobese patients, cesarean section is associated with an increased risk of maternal mortality,[84] and performance of emergency cesarean section further increases that risk.[85] Obesity increases the risk of anesthesia-related maternal death during cesarean section.[61-63] Among morbidly obese patients, cesarean section also increases the risk of maternal morbidity, and it may be associated with risk to the fetus.[86]

In addition, it may be difficult to position the patient appropriately and safely. The protuberant abdomen may shift remarkably when the patient is tilted toward the left. Thus the patient must be secured to the operating table before she is tilted leftward. However, it is important to initiate left uterine displacement immediately thereafter. Tseuda et al.[30] reported two obese patients who experienced acute cardiovascular collapse after placement in the supine position.

The anesthesia care team also may be asked to participate in cephalad retraction of the large panniculus. On occasion we have been asked to secure tethered retractors either to the ether screen or to another stable object. Both the obstetrician and the anesthesiologist must remain cognizant of the risk of hypotension and fetal compromise during cephalad retraction of the panniculus in a morbidly obese patient. Hodgkinson and Husain[86] reported the details of cesarean section performed in eight patients who weighed between 150 and 204 kg. Intraoperative fetal death occurred in one patient who received epidural anesthesia for cesarean section. This apparently was the result of a prolonged episode of hypotension associated with cephalad retraction of a large panniculus.

A careful, thorough airway assessment is essential. Large breasts, the increased anteroposterior diameter of the chest, airway edema, and decreased chin-to-chest distance all increase the likelihood of difficult laryngoscopy and failed intubation in obstetric patients.[87] Obesity exaggerates many of the anatomic changes of pregnancy. Increased fat in the neck and shoulders makes it more difficult to position the patient appropriately for intubation. Further, the fat pads on the back of the shoulders often restrict the range of motion of the neck, and this increases the likelihood of difficulty during mask ventilation, laryngoscopy, and intubation. However, Safar et al.[88] noted that extension of the neck increases upper airway obstruction during the administration of general anesthesia in obese patients.

Difficult mask ventilation often is accompanied by gastric distention with air, which increases the risk of regurgitation and pulmonary aspiration of gastric contents. Obesity often impairs accurate identification of the cricoid ring; thus it may be difficult for the assistant to apply cricoid pressure correctly during rapid-sequence induction of general anesthesia. Finally, in cases of failed intubation, obesity increases the likelihood of unsuccessful transtracheal jet ventilation. Although it is relatively easy to perform a cricothyrotomy in a thin individual, it is not as easy in an obese patient.

Obese pregnant patients require aggressive pharmacologic aspiration prophylaxis. A total of 30 mL of 0.3 M solution of sodium citrate effectively increases gastric pH within 5 minutes.[89] Administration of an H_2-receptor antagonist and metoclopramide provide additional protection,[90] but metoclopramide may be less effective in the presence of preexisting anticholinergic or opioid therapy.[91] The anesthesiologist must be aware that the patient remains at risk for aspiration at the end of surgery. Unfortunately, the efficacy of sodium citrate wanes after 60 minutes.[37]

SPINAL ANESTHESIA

In 1961, Catenacci et al.[92] reported their experience with the administration of anesthesia to 1000 patients who weighed more than 200 lb, who were less than 5 feet 6 inches tall, and who underwent nonobstetric surgery. Some 225 patients received spinal anesthesia; 36% of these patients experienced hypotension, and three patients suffered an unexplained cardiac arrest. Among those three patients, two had a combined spinal-general anesthetic technique. Nonetheless, this series underscores the hazards of spinal anesthesia in obese patients. Concerns regarding the use of spinal anesthesia in obese patients include technical difficulties and the potential for an exaggerated spread of anesthesia.

Spinal anesthesia is technically feasible in most morbidly obese parturients, although a spinal needle with extra length may be required. There is a variable distribution of fat among obese patients. In some obese patients, performance of spinal or epidural anesthesia is no more difficult than in nonobese patients. Blass[22] successfully performed spinal anesthesia in 25 morbidly obese patients in whom standard epidural needles were of insufficient length to reach the epidural space. Jacobs et al.[93] successfully performed continuous spinal anesthesia in a patient who weighed more than 500 lb. Sicuranza and Tisdall[94] reported the successful administration of spinal anesthesia in 16 patients who weighed more than 114 kg.

Many anesthesiologists worry that obesity may result in an unpredictable, exaggerated spread of the local anesthetic agent during administration of either spinal or epidural anesthesia. Hormonal and mechanical factors may be responsible

for the decreased local anesthetic dose requirement in pregnant women. Obesity may cause compression of the vena cava, which increases the flow of blood through the epidural venous plexus and reduces the cerebrospinal volume of the subarachnoid space. Magnetic resonance imaging (MRI) has confirmed that obese patients have reduced CSF volume.[95] A separate study using MRI demonstrated an inverse correlation between block height and lumbar CSF volume.[96] Therefore, lower CSF volumes in obese patients may increase the risk of a high spinal block. Pregnancy-induced engorgement of the epidural veins and inward movement of soft tissue through the intervertebral foramina (resulting from increased abdominal pressure) may be responsible for the reduced CSF volume in obese parturients.[95] Further, Greene[97] has suggested that the large buttocks often present in obese patients place the vertebral column in a Trendelenburg position and may result in an exaggerated spread of anesthesia. Others have performed studies that suggest that the maximal spread of anesthesia does not correlate with weight or BMI.[98,99] Norris[99] administered hyperbaric bupivacaine 12 mg intrathecally and found no correlation between height, weight, BMI, and the spread of spinal anesthesia. However, McCulloch and Littlewood[100] administered 4 mL of 0.5% bupivacaine to a group of obese patients. They identified a correlation between the spread of anesthesia and the degree of obesity. They suggested that obesity increases the likelihood of high spinal anesthesia. In summary, although the preponderance of evidence suggests little correlation between patient weight and the spread of anesthesia, the consequences of extensive blockade dictate caution when selecting single-shot spinal anesthesia for an obese patient with a difficult airway.

Loss of thoracic motor function may be problematic in the morbidly obese patient. Spinal anesthesia results in a more profound thoracic motor blockade than does epidural anesthesia. In theory, a profound thoracic motor blockade might adversely affect oxygenation and ventilation of the obese parturient. However, Blass[22] observed that spinal anesthesia was associated with only a slight decrease in maternal PaO_2 after the administration of spinal anesthesia in a group of pregnant women who weighed between 250 and 500 lb. Further, these PaO_2 measurements were higher than in unanesthetized nonpregnant patients. Moreover, Pitkanen[98] noted a decreased peak expiratory flow rate but no change in arterial blood gas measurements after the administration of spinal anesthesia.

When the choice of anesthesia for cesarean section is being considered, the anesthesiologist must consider the potential for prolonged surgery in obese patients. Johnson et al.[51] noted that the duration of cesarean section exceeded 2 hours in 55% of women who weighed more than 250 lb. In contrast, the mean ± SD operative time was 77 ± 31 minutes in our series.[3] Clearly, the duration of surgery may extend beyond the duration of single-shot spinal anesthesia. Intraoperative induction of general anesthesia is undesirable and perhaps hazardous. Continuous spinal anesthesia represents an alternative to single-shot spinal anesthesia.[82,93]

EPIDURAL ANESTHESIA

It often is easier to identify the epidural space with a large-gauge epidural needle than it is to identify the subarachnoid space with a small-gauge spinal needle. Epidural anesthesia offers other advantages, including the following: (1) the ability to titrate the dose of local anesthetic agent, (2) a decreased incidence of hypotension, and (3) a decreased potential for excess motor blockade.

At least two studies have suggested that obesity affects the spread of epidural anesthesia.[101,102] Hodgkinson and Husain[102] administered 20 mL of 0.75% bupivacaine epidurally at the L3 to L4 interspace during a period of 40 seconds. Patients remained horizontal for 40 minutes after drug injection. When the BMI exceeded 28, no patient required additional local anesthetic to achieve surgical anesthesia. Although the sensory level reached C5 in some patients, no patient required positive-pressure ventilation, and hypotension occurred in only 12% of the patients. The height of the block was proportional to BMI and weight but not height. Subsequently, Hodgkinson and Husain[101] again administered 20 mL of 0.75% bupivacaine epidurally at the L3 to L4 interspace. In this series, half of the patients remained sitting for 5 minutes after injection of the local anesthetic. The sitting position decreased the cephalad spread of anesthesia in those patients whose BMI exceeded 30. In contrast, the sitting position did not affect the spread of anesthesia in lean patients. Of course, bolus epidural injection of 20 mL of a local anesthetic agent is *unacceptable* in contemporary obstetric anesthesia practice. Incremental injection of local anesthetic most likely lessens the effect of obesity on the spread of epidural anesthesia. Neither patient position nor obesity affects the height of sensory block when 12 mL of 0.25% bupivacaine is administered for epidural analgesia during labor.[103]

Maitra et al.[104] administered continuous epidural anesthesia during cesarean section in a 182-kg parturient. They used a 26-gauge spinal needle to identify the spinous processes before attempting to advance the epidural needle. The anesthetic was complicated by an inability to safely tilt the patient to maintain left uterine displacement; thus the authors manually displaced the uterus leftward. Despite an incision-to-delivery interval of 12 minutes, maternal and neonatal outcome were excellent. Likewise, Neuman et al.[105] successfully used epidural anesthesia to facilitate the placement of a metal rod through the large panniculus of a 430-kg man with pickwickian syndrome. In this case, the physicians wanted to retract the panniculus upward before the administration of general anesthesia. This avoided the hemodynamic consequences of cephalad retraction of the panniculus.[86]

In our series of morbidly obese patients who received epidural anesthesia for cesarean section, we observed that these patients tolerated a high sensory level of anesthesia remarkably well.[3] In cases in which the sensory level exceeded the desired level, slight flexion of the operating table lessened patient complaints without adversely affecting the difficulty of surgery, and none of our patients experienced significant respiratory distress during surgery.

Placement of an epidural catheter facilitates the epidural administration of opioid and local anesthetic for postoperative analgesia. Further, there is evidence that epidural administration of bupivacaine decreases the risk of deep vein thrombosis after total hip replacement.[106] Thus some physicians have suggested that epidural anesthesia may decrease the risk of thromboembolic complications in parturients. However, this is an unproved advantage in obstetric patients.

GENERAL ANESTHESIA

Endotracheal intubation is essential, but it may be difficult or impossible with standard techniques. There is an association between obesity and a short neck, and both of these factors predispose patients to difficult tracheal intubation.[107] Buckley et al.[75] reported 9 difficult intubations among 68 morbidly obese, nonpregnant patients; an additional 4 patients

underwent elective awake intubations. In our series, the incidence of difficult intubation was 33% among morbidly obese patients who received general anesthesia for cesarean section.[3] One difficult intubation occurred in a patient who had undergone successful intubation during a previous cesarean section. Clearly, the history of a previous successful intubation does not guarantee the same result during a subsequent procedure. Lee et al.[108] reported their experience with difficult intubation in 284 morbidly obese patients who underwent gastric bypass surgery. The incidence of difficult intubation was 2.4% among patients whose weight was 1.5 to 1.75 times the ideal, but the incidence of difficult intubation tripled to 7.3% among those patients whose weight was 1.75 to 2 times the ideal.

The potential for failed intubation and difficult mask ventilation underscores the need for an additional pair of experienced hands during the administration of general anesthesia in the obese patient. The primary anesthetist fatigues rapidly while attempting mask ventilation of an obese patient. Further, the jaw-thrust maneuver may require the use of both hands, and a second person must be available to provide positive-pressure ventilation and cricoid pressure. The prepared anesthesiologist also has a short-handled laryngoscope, assorted laryngoscope blades, a variety of endotracheal tubes, and equipment for performing percutaneous cricothyrotomy and transtracheal ventilation immediately available.

Awake intubation, by either direct visualization or fiberoptic laryngoscopy, provides an alternative method of securing the airway. Successful awake intubation also has been performed with the Bullard laryngoscope in a morbidly obese parturient.[109] However, awake intubation poses challenges. Catecholamine release and blood pressure elevation during awake procedures may exacerbate existing hypertension and adversely affect uterine blood flow.[110] Further, some patients may require urgent administration of general anesthesia because of maternal hemorrhage or fetal distress. In these cases, it is difficult to perform awake laryngoscopy and intubation successfully unless the anesthesiologist has adequate time to prepare the patient's airway. However, the mother should not be endangered to deliver a distressed fetus. Specifically, the anesthesiologist should not proceed with rapid-sequence induction of general anesthesia if intubation is expected to be difficult.

In emergency situations (e.g., urgent cesarean section) wherein endotracheal intubation (via direct laryngoscopy) is anticipated to be difficult or impossible, continuous spinal anesthesia may be considered as an alternative to an awake intubation. The local anesthetic agent can be administered incrementally through the spinal catheter to safely achieve the desired sensory level. In this situation, we typically use 0.5% hypobaric bupivacaine and administer an initial 1-mL (5-mg) dose followed by 0.5-mL boluses every 5 minutes until the desired sensory level is achieved. A continuous spinal catheter minimizes the risk of catastrophic loss of the airway. Alternatively, an elective surgical airway can be considered.

When preanesthetic assessment does not suggest that intubation will be difficult, the anesthesiologist may proceed with rapid-sequence induction of general anesthesia if it is indicated. Administration of general anesthesia begins with effective pulmonary denitrogenation. During apnea, pregnant women become hypoxemic more rapidly than do nonpregnant patients.[111] Similarly, during apnea, obese patients become hypoxemic more rapidly than do nonobese patients.[112,113] Therefore adequate denitrogenation is essential

before the administration of general anesthesia. Although we demonstrated that four maximal inspirations of 100% oxygen within 30 seconds provided benefit similar to that provided by 3 minutes of tidal ventilation with 100% oxygen before rapid-sequence induction of general anesthesia for cesarean section,[114] a separate study demonstrated a more rapid onset of hypoxemia in patients who had four maximal inspirations of 100% oxygen when compared with similar patients who had 3 minutes of tidal ventilation with 100% oxygen.[115] Goldberg et al.[116] evaluated the use of these two techniques in morbidly obese nonpregnant patients undergoing gastric bypass surgery. The two techniques provided similar increases in Pao_2, but patients who used the 3-minute technique developed a slight retention of CO_2. The authors speculated that a blunted ventilatory response to CO_2 contributed to the increase in $Paco_2$. (In contrast, other studies suggest that obese patients have a normal ventilatory response to CO_2.[13]) It seems reasonable to let circumstances dictate the selected method of denitrogenation. When the 3-minute tidal ventilation technique is selected, the anesthesiologist should encourage the patient to take some deep breaths. The four-breath method of denitrogenation should be reserved for emergencies.

Obesity alters the distribution of and response to anesthetic drugs. An increased volume of distribution prolongs the elimination half-life of thiopental in obese patients.[117] The clinical significance of these findings in obstetric patients is unclear. Kumar et al.[118] observed similar times to opening of the eyes after the administration of methohexital and Althesin in obese patients. They suggested that the choice of intravenous agent is relatively unimportant in the absence of complicating medical disease. Ketamine is an excellent induction agent in nonobese patients; to our knowledge, no study has specifically evaluated the use of ketamine in obese pregnant women. The choice of drug and dose remains a matter of judgment. If the anesthesiologist chooses to give thiopental, administration of less than 4 mg/kg may increase the risk of maternal awareness, hypertension, and decreased uterine blood flow during light anesthesia. Administration of a larger dose may be associated with delayed arousal in the event of failed intubation. At Wake Forest University, we typically administer 4 mg/kg (up to a maximum dose of 500 mg) of thiopental during induction of general anesthesia in obese parturients.

Succinylcholine remains the muscle relaxant of choice for rapid-sequence induction. As with thiopental, the ideal dose is unclear. Adequate relaxation is essential; the anesthesiologist should not attempt laryngoscopy and intubation in the presence of incomplete muscle relaxation. Some anesthesiologists worry that administration of a large dose of succinylcholine delays the return of spontaneous ventilation in cases of failed intubation. Bentley et al.[119] observed increased pseudocholinesterase activity in obese, nonpregnant patients. They recommended that anesthesiologists administer succinylcholine "on the basis of total rather than lean body weight in adult patients." At our institution, we give at least 1.0 to 1.5 mg/kg (up to a maximum dose of 200 mg) of succinylcholine during rapid-sequence induction of general anesthesia in obese patients.

After intubation, the anesthesiologist should continue to monitor neuromuscular blockade during surgery. Cesarean section is technically difficult in the morbidly obese patient. Adequate muscle relaxation is essential. However, technical problems may mimic inadequate muscle relaxation. Morbidly obese patients most likely have a normal response to nonde-

polarizing muscle relaxants. However, Weinstein et al.[120] observed a prolonged duration of action after administration of vecuronium in obese patients. They speculated that impaired hepatic clearance may have contributed to the prolonged duration of neuromuscular blockade. In contrast, administration of atracurium (which does not require hepatic metabolism) is associated with a normal duration of action in obese patients. The time required to reverse atracurium-induced neuromuscular blockade is not affected by total body weight or BMI.[121]

No evidence suggests that obesity alters minimum alveolar concentration (MAC) for inhalation agents in pregnant women. However, obesity does affect blood-gas partition coefficients. The blood-gas partition coefficient for enflurane decreases from 2.03 ± 0.02 to 1.76 ± 0.03, whereas the reverse phenomenon occurs with halothane.[122] These changes most likely are clinically insignificant.

In theory, increased body fat serves as a reservoir for inhalation and intravenous agents. Likewise, the body fat reservoir could increase the threat of biotransformation of the volatile halogenated agents, which would increase the risk of organ toxicity. Bentley et al.[123] reported increased serum fluoride and bromide concentrations after 2 hours of halothane anesthesia in obese patients when compared with concentrations in nonobese patients. Rice and Fish[124] suggested that obese patients might be at risk for fluoride-induced nephrotoxicity after prolonged administration of enflurane; this might be a concern in an obese patient with severe preeclampsia and abnormal renal function. Fortunately, cesarean section is a relatively brief procedure, even in an obese patient. Nonetheless, isoflurane most likely is a better choice than halothane or enflurane because of its decreased biotransformation in morbidly obese patients.[125,126] Some anesthesiologists have suggested that the newer volatile halogenated agents (i.e., desflurane, sevoflurane) might reduce the time to extubation, when compared to isoflurane, in obese patients.[127,128] However, administration of sevoflurane is associated with higher serum inorganic fluoride concentrations in obese patients than in nonobese patients.[129]

The choice of supplemental anesthetic agents most likely is of limited significance. Cork et al.[130] evaluated outcome in 67 morbidly obese patients who were randomized to receive nitrous oxide in oxygen, combined with either fentanyl, enflurane, or halothane. Although patients in the fentanyl group opened their eyes on command sooner, the time to extubation did not differ significantly from that in patients who received enflurane or halothane. There was no difference among groups in other measures of outcome. The authors concluded that there was "little to commend one general anesthetic technique over another in morbidly obese patients."[130]

High concentrations of a volatile halogenated agent increase the likelihood of neonatal depression, uterine atony, and maternal blood loss. In contrast, a low concentration of a volatile agent increases the risk of maternal awareness, catecholamine release, hypertension, and decreased uterine blood flow. Most anesthesiologists administer nitrous oxide to nonobese pregnant patients to allow administration of a decreased concentration of a volatile halogenated agent. However, morbidly obese patients may require administration of a higher inspired concentration of oxygen. The anesthesiologist may be unable to give as high a concentration of nitrous oxide as would be given to a nonobese patient. Administration of general anesthesia results in decreased

FRC. Further, the supine and Trendelenburg positions may further decrease the FRC and increase the likelihood of intraoperative hypoxemia. Vaughan and Wise[131] observed that 77% of obese patients had a PaO_2 of less than 80 mm Hg while breathing 40% oxygen during surgery. Techniques that may improve intraoperative oxygenation include (1) use of a large tidal volume, (2) administration of positive end-expiratory pressure (PEEP), and (3) elevation of the panniculus.[132] Salem et al.[133] questioned the wisdom of using a large tidal volume and PEEP in obese patients. They observed improved oxygenation after the discontinuation of PEEP. Eriksen et al.[134] compared increasing tidal volume by 35% versus the effectiveness of PEEP. Although both techniques increased maternal PaO_2, neither technique increased oxygen delivery. PEEP may increase maternal PaO_2, but it may decrease cardiac output and oxygen delivery.[135] Decreased cardiac output results in decreased uterine blood flow, which may result in fetal compromise in a case of a prolonged induction-to-delivery interval. Nonetheless, it is imperative to maintain adequate maternal oxygenation.

Finally, airway obstruction may increase PCWP and precipitate cardiovascular decompensation. Thus it is important to avoid airway obstruction during induction of anesthesia and emergence from anesthesia.

POSTOPERATIVE COMPLICATIONS

Obstetricians have long feared an increased risk of maternal morbidity after cesarean section in obese patients. In our series, major postpartum complications occurred only in those patients who delivered by cesarean section.[3] Wolfe et al.[136] evaluated measures of morbidity in 100 obese women who underwent cesarean section. Prolonged surgery and increased operative blood loss were associated with an increased risk of postoperative morbidity. Neither the type of skin incision nor the anesthetic technique affected the incidence of postoperative morbidity. However, postoperative hypoxemia is more severe in obese patients than in nonobese patients.[137] Performance of a vertical abdominal incision increases the risk of postoperative hypoxemia.[138,139] Administration of supplemental oxygen and the use of the semirecumbent position offer some protection from postoperative hypoxemia.[140,141] Finally, obese patients are at increased risk for other postoperative pulmonary complications (e.g., atelectasis, pneumonia).[142] Preoperative pulmonary function may be the best predictor of postoperative pulmonary complications in obese patients.[75] Further, administration of general anesthesia may increase the risk of postoperative pulmonary complications in obese patients.

Postoperative Analgesia

Adequate pain control after cesarean section may improve maternal outcome. Intramuscular administration of an opioid results in variable, unpredictable absorption of the drug, especially in the morbidly obese patient. Intravenous administration of an opioid provides a more consistent result. Some physicians have suggested the use of patient-controlled analgesia in obese patients.[143] Physicians and nurses must be aware of the risk of respiratory depression, which poses a greater hazard in the obese patient than in the lean patient. Intravenously administered sufentanil is eliminated slowly in obese patients, and the anesthesiologist should consider a reduction in the maintenance dose in these patients.[144]

Thoracic epidural anesthesia decreases oxygen consumption and left ventricular stroke work.[145] Gelman et al.[145] documented decreased oxygen consumption, arterial-venous oxygen difference, and left ventricular stroke work during administration of thoracic epidural anesthesia in morbidly obese patients. Rawal et al.[146] observed that epidural administration of morphine resulted in earlier ambulation, fewer pulmonary complications, and shorter hospitalization when compared with intramuscular administration of morphine in morbidly obese patients who had undergone abdominal surgery. The role of intraspinal opioids in patients with pickwickian syndrome is unclear. Pellecchia et al.[147] reported the successful administration of epidural morphine in a nonpregnant patient with obstructive sleep apnea. However, Lamarche et al.[148] reported one case of respiratory arrest that occurred after epidural opioid administration in a nonpregnant patient with sleep apnea syndrome.

KEY POINTS

- Medical disease (e.g., hypertension, diabetes mellitus) complicates obstetric and anesthetic management of the morbidly obese parturient.
- The obese parturient is at increased risk for fetal macrosomia, shoulder dystocia, and cesarean section.
- Dystocia is the most common indication for emergency cesarean section. As many as 50% of morbidly obese parturients who undergo a trial of labor require cesarean section.
- Obesity increases the risk for anesthesia-related maternal mortality. Airway complications represent the most common cause of anesthesia-related maternal mortality.
- The anesthesiologist should perform a careful, thorough assessment of the airway in every obese parturient. The anesthesiologist should not proceed with rapid-sequence induction of general anesthesia when a difficult airway is anticipated.
- Early administration of epidural analgesia is advised in obese patients who undergo a trial of labor. Anesthesiologists should critically evaluate the quality of the epidural block, and they should replace a catheter that does not result in excellent analgesia.
- Regional anesthesia is feasible in morbidly obese patients who require cesarean section. However, the potential for prolonged surgery suggests that continuous epidural anesthesia is a better choice than single-shot spinal anesthesia.
- Continuous spinal anesthesia may be considered in cases of unintentional dural puncture or in emergency situations (e.g., urgent cesarean section) wherein difficult/impossible intubation is anticipated.

REFERENCES

1. Mokdad AH, Ford ES, Bowman BA, et al. Prevalence of obesity, diabetes, and obesity-related health risk factors, 2001. JAMA 2003; 289:76-9.
2. Allison DB, Fontaine KR, Manson JE, et al. Annual deaths attributable to obesity in the United States. JAMA 1999; 282:1530-8.
3. Hood DD, Dewan DM. Anesthesia and obstetric outcome in morbidly obese parturients. Anesthesiology 1993; 79:1210-8.
4. Bray GA. Complications of obesity. Ann Intern Med 1985; 103:1052-62.
5. Manson JE, Colditz GA, Stampfer MJ, et al. A perspective study of obesity and risk of coronary heart disease in women. N Engl J Med 1990; 322:882-9.
6. Smith D, Lewis CE, Caveny JL, et al. Longitudinal changes in adiposity associated with pregnancy. The CARDIA study. JAMA 1994; 271: 1747-51.
7. Kissebah A, Bydelingum N, Murray R, et al. Relation of body height and fat distribution to metabolic complications of obesity. J Clin Endocrinol Metab 1982; 54:254-60.
8. Kreisberg RA. Clues to disease from location of body fat. Contemp Obstet Gynecol 1987:130-44.
9. Malcolm R, Von JM, O'Neil PM, et al. Update on the management of obesity. South Med J 1988; 81:632-9.
10. Drenick E, Gurunanjappa B, Seltzer F, Johnson DG. Excessive mortality and causes of death in morbidly obese men. JAMA 1980; 243:443-5.
11. Dempsey JA, Reddan W, Rankin J, et al. Alveolar arterial gas exchange during muscle work in obesity. J Appl Physiol 1966; 21:1807-14.
12. Dempsey JA, Reddan W, Balke B, et al. Work capacity determinants and physiologic costs of weight support work in obesity. J Appl Physiol 1966; 21:1815-20.
13. Lourenco RV. Diaphragm activity in obesity. J Clin Invest 1969; 48:1609-14.
14. Cullen JH, Formel PF. The respiratory defects in extreme obesity. Am J Med 1962; 32:525-31.
15. Sharp JT, Henry JP, Sweany SK, et al. Effect of mass loading the respiratory system in man. J Appl Physiol 1965; 19:959-66.
16. Noble AB. The problem of obesity in anesthesia for abdominal surgery. Can Anesth Soc J 1962; 9:6-14.
17. Eng M, Butler J, Bonica JJ. Respiratory function in pregnant obese women. Am J Obstet Gynecol 1975; 123:241-5.
18. Vaughan R. Anesthetic management of a morbidly obese patient. 1987 Review Course Lecture, International Anesthesia Research Society Meeting, Lake Buena Vista, Fla, Mar 14, 1987.
19. Barrera F, Reidenberg MM, Winters WL, Hungspreugs S. Ventilation-perfusion relationships in the obese patient. J Appl Physiol 1969; 26:420-6.
20. Lee JJ, Larsen RH, Buckley JJ, Roberts RB. Pulmonary function and its correlation to the degree of obesity of 294 patients. Anesthesiol Rev 1981; 8:28-32.
21. Vaughan RW, Cork RE, Hollander D. The effect of massive weight loss on arterial oxygenation and pulmonary function tests. Anesthesiology 1981; 54:325-8.
22. Blass NH. Regional anesthesia in the morbidly obese patient. Reg Anesth 1979; 4:20-2.
23. Gould SF, Makowski EL. Obesity in pregnancy. Perinatol Neonatol 1981; May/June:49-59.
24. Alexander JK, Dennis DW, Smith WG, et al. Blood volume, cardiac output and distribution of systemic blood flow in extreme obesity. Cardiovasc Res Center Bull 1962; 1:39-44.
25. Alexander JK. The cardiomyopathy of obesity. Prog Cardiovasc Dis 1985; 27:325-34.
26. Paul B, Hoyt J, Boutros A. Cardiovascular and respiratory changes in response to change of position in the very obese. Anesthesiology 1976; 45:73-8.
27. Teeple E, Ghia JN. An elevated pulmonary wedge pressure resulting from an upper respiratory obstruction in an obese patient. Anesthesiology 1983; 59:66-8.
28. Bloom E, Reed D, Yano K, MacKlean C. Does obesity protect hypertensives against cardiovascular disease? JAMA 1986; 256:2972-6.
29. Mabie WC, Ratts TE, Ramanathan KB, Sibai BM. Circulatory congestion in obese hypertensive women: A subset of pulmonary edema in pregnancy. Obstet Gynecol 1988; 72:553-8.
30. Tseuda K, Debrand M, Zeok S, et al. Obesity supine sudden death syndrome: Report of two morbidly obese patients. Anesth Analg 1979; 58:345-7.
31. Drenick EJ, Fisler JS. Sudden cardiac arrest in morbidly obese surgical patients unexplained after autopsy. Am J Surg 1988; 155:720-6.
32. Messerli FH, Nunez BD, Ventura HO, Snyder DW. Overweight and sudden death: Increased ventricular ectopy in cardiopathy of obesity. Arch Intern Med 1987; 147:1725-8.

33. Lauer MS, Anderson KM, Kannel WB, Levy D. The impact of obesity on left ventricular mass and geometry. JAMA 1991; 266:231-6.

34. Veille JC, Hanson R. Obesity, pregnancy, and left ventricular functioning during the third trimester. Am J Obstet Gynecol 1994; 171:980-3.

35. Ford LE. Heart size. Circ Res 1976; 39:297-303.

36. Vaughan RW, Bauer S, Wise L. Volume and pH of gastric juice in obese patients. Anesthesiology 1975; 43:686-9.

37. Dewan DM, Floyd HM, Thistlewood JM, et al. Sodium citrate pretreatment in elective cesarean section patients. Anesth Analg 1985; 64:34-7.

38. Van Thiel D, Gavaler J, Joshi S, et al. Heartburn and pregnancy. Gastroenterology 1972; 72:666-8.

39. Ulmsten U, Sundstrom G. Esophageal manometry in pregnant and nonpregnant women. Am J Obstet Gynecol 1978; 132:260-4.

40. Brock-Utne J, Dow T, Dimopoulos G, et al. Gastric and lower oesophageal sphincter (LOS) pressures in early pregnancy. Br J Anaesth 1981; 53:381-4.

41. Van Thiel D, Wald A. Evidence refuting a role for increased abdominal pressure in the pathogenesis of heartburn associated with pregnancy. Am J Obstet Gynecol 1981; 140:420-2.

42. O'Brien TF. Lower esophageal sphincter pressure (LESP) and esophageal function in obese humans. J Clin Gastroenterol 1980; 2:145-8.

43. Farmer G, Hamilton-Nicol D, Southerland HW, et al. The ranges of insulin response and glucose tolerance in lean, normal, and obese women during pregnancy. Am J Obstet Gynecol 1992; 167:772-7.

44. Postlewait RW, Johnson WD. Complications following surgery for duodenal ulcer in obese patients. Arch Surg 1972; 105:438-40.

45. Sikorski JM, Hampson WG, Staddon GE. The natural history and etiology of deep vein thrombophlebitis after total hip replacement. J Bone Joint Surg 1981; 63B:171-7.

46. Kernstein MD, McSwain NE, O'Connell RC, et al. Obesity: Is it really a risk factor in thrombophlebitis? South Med J 1987; 80:1236-8.

47. Martin JA, Hamilton BE, Ventura SJ, et al. Births: Final Data for 2001. National Vital Statistics Reports. Hyattsville, MD; National Center for Health Statistics. 2002; Vol. 51, No. 2.

48. Ehrenberg HM, Dierker L, Milluzzi C, Mercer BM. Prevalence of maternal obesity in an urban center. Am J Obstet Gynecol 2002; 187:1189-93.

49. Lu GC, Rouse DJ, DuBard M, et al. The effect of the increasing prevalence of maternal obesity on perinatal morbidity. Am J Obstet Gynecol 2001; 185:845-9.

50. Tracy TA, Miller GL. Obstetric problems of the massively obese. Obstet Gynecol 1968; 33:204-8.

51. Johnson SR, Kolberg BH, Varner MW, Railsback LD. Maternal obesity in pregnancy. Surg Gynecol Obstet 1987; 164:431-7.

52. Crane S, Wojtowyca M, Dye T, et al. Association between pre-pregnancy obesity and the risk of cesarean delivery. Obstet Gynecol 1997; 89:213-16.

53. Wolfe HM, Zador IE, Gross TL, et al. The clinical utility of body mass index in pregnancy. Am J Obstet Gynecol 1991; 164:1306-10.

54. Keys A, Fidanze F, Karbonen M, et al. Indices of relative weight in obesity. J Chronic Dis 1972; 25:329-43.

55. Abrams BE, Parker J. Overweight and pregnancy complications. Int J Obesity 1988; 12:293-303.

56. Garbaciak JA, Richter M, Miller S, et al. Maternal weight in pregnancy complications. Obstet Gynecol 1985; 152:238-45.

57. Perlow JH, Morgan MM, Montgomery D, et al. Perinatal outcome in pregnancy complicated by massive obesity. Am J Obstet Gynecol 1992; 167:958-62.

58. Maeder EC, Barno A, Mecklenburg F. Obesity: A maternal high risk factor. Obstet Gynecol 1975; 45:669-71.

59. Kaunitz A, Hughes J, Grimes D, et al. Causes of maternal mortality in the United States. Obstet Gynecol 1985; 65:605-12.

60. Rochat RW, Koonin LM, Atrash A, Jewett JF, and the Maternal Mortality Collaborative. Maternal mortality in the United States: Report from the maternal mortality collaborative. Obstet Gynecol 1988; 72:91-7.

61. May WJ, Greiss FC. Maternal mortality in North Carolina: A four year experience. Am J Obstet Gynecol 1989; 161:555-61.

62. Endler GC, Mariona FG, Solol RJ, Stevenson LB. Anesthesia-related mortality in Michigan 1972-1984. Am J Obstet Gynecol 1988; 159:187-93.

63. Johnson JW, Longmate JA, Frentzen B. Excessive maternal weight and pregnancy outcome. Am J Obstet Gynecol 1992; 167:353-72.

64. Peckham CH, Christianson RE. The relationship between pre-pregnancy weight and certain obstetric factors. Am J Obstet Gynecol 1971; 111:1-7.

65. Kerr MG. The problem of the overweight patient in pregnancy. J Obstet Gynaecol Br Commonw 1962; 69:988-95.

66. Bianco A, Smilen S, Davis Y, et al. Pregnancy outcome and weight gain recommendations for the morbidly obese woman. Obstet Gynecol 1998; 91:97-102.

67. Abrams BF, Laros RK. Prepregnancy weight, weight gain and birth weight. Am J Obstet Gynecol 1986; 154:502-9.

68. Klebanoff MA, Mills JL, Berendes HW. Mother's birth weight as a predictor of macrosomia. Am J Obstet Gynecol 1985; 153:253-7.

69. Bell E, Hartle H, Mayer D, et al. BMI predicts cesarean section in multicenter prospective cohort study (abstract). Anesthesiology 2001; 94:A81.

70. Prough SG, Askel S. Overweight, endocrine function, and infertility. Obesity Endocrinol Contemp Obstet Gynecol 1987; 63-78.

71. Cnattingius S, Bergstrom R, Lipworth L, Kramer, M. Prepregnancy weight and the risk of adverse pregnancy outcomes. N Engl J Med 1998; 338:147-52.

72. Waller DK, Mills JL, Simpson JL, et al. Are obese women at higher risk for producing malformed offspring? Am J Obstet Gynecol 1994; 170:514-48.

73. Rahaman J, Narayansingh GV, Roopnarinesing S. Fetal outcome among obese parturients. Int J Gynecol Obstet 1990; 31:227-30.

74. Leduc L, Wheeler J, Kirshon B, et al. Coagulation profile in severe preeclampsia. Obstet Gynecol 1992; 1:14-8.

75. Buckley FP, Robinson NB, Simonowitz DA, Dellinger ED. Anaesthesia in the morbidly obese: A comparison of anaesthetic and analgesic regimens for upper abdominal surgery. Anaesthesia 1983; 38:840-51.

76. Ranta P, Jouppila P, Spalding M, Jouppila R. The effect of maternal obesity and labour and labour pain. Anaesthesia 1995; 50:322-6.

77. Narang VPS, Linter SPK. Failure of extradural blockade in obstetrics: A new hypothesis. Br J Anaesth 1988; 60:402-4.

78. Wallace DH, Currie JM, Gilstrap LC, Santos R. Indirect sonographic guidance for epidural anesthesia in obese pregnant patients. Reg Anesth 1992; 17:233-6.

79. Hamza J, Mohammed S, Benhamou D, Cohen S. Paturient's posture during epidural puncture affects the distance from skin to epidural space. J Clin Anesth 1995; 7:1-4.

80. Hamilton C, Riley E, Cohen S. Changes in the position of epidural catheters associated with patient movement. Anesthesiology 1997; 86:778-84.

81. Douglas MJ, Flanagan ML, McMorland GH. Anaesthetic management of a complex morbidly obese parturient. Can J Anaesth 1991; 38:900-3.

82. Bell ED. Decreased incidence of post dural puncture headache in morbidly obese parturients following continuous spinal using 17 gauge tuohy needle.(abstract) Anesthesiology 1997; 87:A886.

83. Norris M, Ryan C, Fogel S, et al. Intrathecal sufentanil increases end-tidal CO_2 in laboring women (abstract). Anesthesiology 1997; 87:A885.

84. Hood DD, Dewan DM. Obstetric anesthesia. In Brown DL, editor. Risk and Outcome in Anesthesia. Philadelphia, JB Lippincott, 1992:356-413.

85. Moldin P, Hokegard K, Nielsen T. Cesarean section and maternal mortality in Sweden, 1973-1979. Acta Obstet Gynecol Scand 1984; 63:7-11.

86. Hodgkinson R, Husain FJ. Caesarean section associated with gross obesity. Br J Anaesth 1980; 52:919-23.

87. Samsoon GL, Young JR. Difficult tracheal intubation: A retrospective study. Anaesthesia 1987; 42:487-90.

88. Safar P, Escarraga LH, Chang F. Upper airway obstruction in the unconscious patient. J Appl Physiol 1959; 14:760-4.

89. O'Sullivan GM, Bullingham RE. Noninvasive assessment by radiotelemetry of antacid effect during labor. Anesth Analg 1985; 64: 95-100.

90. Goldberg ME, Norris MC, Larinjani GE, et al. The effects of atropine, metoclopramide and cimetidine on gastric contents in the morbidly obese population. Anesthesiol Rev 1989; 16:30-4.

91. Schmidt J, Jorgensen B. The effect of metoclopramide on gastric contents after preoperative ingestion of sodium citrate. Anesth Analg 1984; 63:841-3.

92. Catenacci AJ, Anderson JD, Boersma D. Anesthetic hazards of obesity. JAMA 1961; 175:657-65.

93. Jacobs LL, Berger HC, Fierro FE. Obesity and continuous spinal anesthesia: Case report. Anesth Analg 1963; 42:547-9.

94. Sicuranza BJ, Tisdall LH. Cesarean section in the massively obese. J Reprod Med 1975; 14:10-1.

95. Hogan Q, Prost R, Kulier A, et al. Magnetic resonance imaging of cerebrospinal fluid volume and the influence of body habitus and abdominal pressure. Anesthesiology 1996; 84:1341-9.

96. Carpenter RL, Hogan QH, Lui SS, et al. Lumbosacral cerebrospinal fluid volume is the primary determinant of sensory block extent and duration during spinal anesthesia. Anesthesiology 1998; 89:923-4.

97. Greene NM. Distribution of local anesthetics within the subarachnoid space. Anesth Analg 1985; 64:715-30.

98. Pitkanen MT. Body mass and spread of spinal anesthesia with bupivacaine. Anesth Analg 1987; 66:127-31.

99. Norris MC. Height, weight and spread of subarachnoid hyperbaric bupivacaine in the term parturient. Anesth Analg 1988; 67:555-8.

100. McCulloch WJD, Littlewood DG. Influence of obesity on spinal anesthesia with isobaric 0.5% bupivacaine. Br J Anesth 1986; 58:610-4.

101. Hodgkinson R, Husain FJ. Obesity, gravity and the spread of epidural anesthesia. Anesth Analg 1981; 60:421-4.

102. Hodgkinson R, Husain FJ. Obesity and the cephalad spread of analgesia following epidural administration of bupivacaine for cesarean section. Anesth Analg 1980; 59:89-92.

103. Milligan KR, Cramp P, Schatz L, et al. The effect of patient position and obesity on the spread of epidural analgesia. Int J Obstet Anesth 1993; 2:134-6.

104. Maitra AM, Palmer SK, Bachhuber SR, Abram SE. Continuous epidural anesthesia for cesarean section in a patient with morbid obesity. Anesth Analg 1979; 58:348-9.

105. Neuman GG, Baldwin CC, Petrini AJ, et al. Perioperative management of 430 kg (946 pound) patient with pickwickian syndrome. Anesth Analg 1986; 65:985-7.

106. Henny CP, Odoom JA, Cate HT, et al. Effects of extradural bupivacaine on the haemostatic system. Br J Anaesth 1986; 58:301-5.

107. Rocke DA, Murray WB, Rout CC, Gouws E. Relative risk analysis of factors associated with difficult intubation in obstetric anesthesia. Anesthesiology 1992; 77:67-73.

108. Lee JJ, Larson RH, Buckley JJ, Roberts RB. Airway maintenance in the morbidly obese. Anesthesiol Rev 1980; 7:33-6.

109. Cohn A, Hart R, McGraw S, Blass NH. The Bullard laryngoscope for emergency airway management in a morbidly obese parturient. Anesth Analg 1995;81:872-3.

110. Shnider S, Wright R, Levinson G, et al. Uterine blood flow and plasma norepinephrine changes during maternal stress in the pregnant ewe. Anesthesiology 1979; 50:524-7.

111. Byrne F, Oduro-Dominah A, Kipling R. The effect of pregnancy and pulmonary nitrogen washout. Anaesthesia 1987; 42:148-50.

112. Berthoud M, Peacock J, Reilly C. Effectiveness of preoxygenation in morbidly obese patients. Br J Anaesth 1991; 67:464-6.

113. Jense HG. Anesthesia Patient Safety Foundation Newsletter. December 1988:31.

114. Norris MC, Dewan DM. Preoxygenation for cesarean section: A comparison of two techniques. Anesthesiology 1985; 62:827-9.

115. Gambee M, Hetzka R, Fisher D. Preoxygenation techniques: Comparison of three minutes and four breaths. Anesth Analg 1987; 66:468-79.

116. Goldberg ME, Norris MC, Ghassem EL, et al. Preoxygenation in the morbidly obese: A comparison of two techniques. Anesth Analg 1989; 68:520-2.

117. Jung G, Mayersohn M, Perrier D, et al. Thiopental disposition in lean and obese patients undergoing surgery. Anesthesiology 1982; 56:269-74.

118. Kumar B, Harvey J, Cooper GM. Does obesity effect recovery? A study using intravenous methohexatol and althesin for short procedures. Anaesthesia 1983; 38:968-71.

119. Bentley JB, Borel JD, Vaughn RW, Gandolfi AJ. Weight, psuedocholinesterase activity, and succinylcholine requirement. Anesthesiology 1982; 57:48-9.

120. Weinstein JA, Matteo RS, Ornstein E, et al. Pharmacodynamics of vecuronium and atracurium in the obese surgical patient. Anesth Analg 1988; 67:1149-53.

121. Kirkegaard-Nielsen H, Lindholm P, Peterson HS, Severinsen I. Antagonism of atracurium-induced block in obese patients. Can J Anaesth 1998; 45:39-41.

122. Borel JD, Bentley JB, Vaughn RW, Gandolfi AJ. Enflurane blood gas solubility: Influence of weight and hemoglobin. Anesth Analg 1982; 61:1006-9.

123. Bentley JB, Vaughn RW, Gandolfi J, Cork RC. Halothane biotransformation in obese and nonobese patients. Anesthesiology 1982; 57:94-7.

124. Rice SH, Fish KJ. Anesthetic metabolism and renal functions in obese and nonobese Fischer 344 rats following enflurane or isoflurane. Anesthesiology 1986; 65:28-34.

125. Carpenter RL, Eger EC, Johnson BH, et al. The extent of metabolism of inhaled anesthetics in humans. Anesthesiology 1986; 65:201-5.

126. Strube PJ, Hulands GH, Halsey MJ. Serum fluoride levels in morbidly obese patients: Enflurane compared with isoflurane anaesthesia. Anaesthesia 1987; 42:685-9.

127. Torri G, Casati A, Comotti L, et al. Wash-in and wash-out curves of sevoflurane and isoflurane in morbidly obese patients. Minerva Anestesiol 2002; 68:523-7.

128. Juvin P, Vadam C, Malek L, et al. Postoperative recovery after desflurane, propofol, or isoflurane anesthesia amoun morbidly obese patients: a prospective, randomized study. Anesth Analg 2000; 91:714-9.

129. Higuchi H, Satoh T, Arimura S, et al. Serum inorganic fluoride levels in mildly obese patients during and after sevoflurane anesthesia. Anesth Analg 1993; 77:1018-21.

130. Cork RC, Vaughn RW, Bentley JB. General anesthesia for morbidly obese patients: An examination of postoperative outcomes. Anesthesiology 1981; 54:310-3.

131. Vaughan RW, Wise L. Intraoperative arterial oxygenation of obese patients. Ann Surg 1976; 84:35-42.

132. Wyner J, Brodsky JB, Merrell RC. Massive obesity and arterial oxygenation. Anesth Analg 1981; 60:691-3.

133. Salem MR, Dalal F, Zygmunt M, et al. Does PEEP improve intraoperative arterial oxygenation in grossly obese patients? Anesthesiology 1978; 48:280-1.

134. Eriksen J, Andersen J, Rasmusen J, Sorensen B. Effects of ventilation with large tidal volumes or positive end expiratory pressure on cardiorespiratory function in the anesthetized obese patients. Acta Anesthesiol Scand 1978; 22:241-7.

135. Santesson J. Oxygen transport in venous admixture in the extremely obese: Influence of anesthesia in artificial ventilation with and without positive end expiratory pressure. Acta Anaesthesiol Scand 1976; 20:387-94.

136. Wolfe HM, Gross TL, Sokol RJ, et al. Determinants of morbidity in obese women delivered by cesarean section. Obstet Gynecol 1988; 71:691-6.

137. Vaughan RW, Engelhart RC, Wise L. Postoperative hypoxemia in obese patients. Ann Surg 1974; 180:877-82.

138. Vaughan RW, Wise L. Choice of abdominal operative incision in obese patients: A study using blood gas measurements. Ann Surg 1975; 181:829-35.

139. Vaughan RW, Engelhart RC, Wise L. Postoperative alveolar-arterial oxygen tension difference: Relation to operative incision in obese patients. Anesth Analg 1975; 54:433-7.

140. Vaughan RW, Wise L. Postoperative arterial blood gas measurements: Effect of position on gas exchange. Ann Surg 1975; 182:705-9.

141. Vaughan RW, Bauer S, Wise L. Effect of position (semi-recumbent versus supine) on postoperative oxygenation in markedly obese. Anesth Analg 1976; 55:37-41.

142. Mircea N, Constantinescu C, Jianu E, et al. Risk of pulmonary complications in surgical patients. Resuscitation 1982; 10:33-41.

143. Levin A, Klein S, Brolin R, Pitchford D. Patient controlled analgesia for morbidly obese patient: An effective modality if used correctly (letter). Anesthesiology 1992; 76:857-8.

144. Schwartz AE, Matteo RS, Ornstein E, et al. Pharmacokinetics of sufentanil in obese patients. Anesth Analg 1991; 73:790-3.

145. Gelman S, Laws H, Potzick J, et al. Thoracic epidural versus balanced anesthesia in morbid obesity: Intraoperative and postoperative hemodynamic study. Anesth Analg 1980; 59:902-8.

146. Rawal N, Sjostrand U, Christoffersson E, et al. Comparison of intramuscular and epidural morphine for postoperative analgesia in the grossly obese: Influence of postoperative ambulation and pulmonary function. Anesth Analg 1984; 63:583-92.

147. Pellecchia DJ, Bretz KA, Barnette RE. Postoperative pain control by means of epidural narcotics in a patient with obstructive sleep apnea. Anesth Analg 1987; 66:280-2.

148. Lamarche Y, Martin R, Reiher J, Blaise G. Sleep apnea syndrome and epidural morphine. Can Anaesth Soc J 1986; 33:231-3.

Chapter 50
Renal Disease

Robert W. Reid, M.D.

"Children of women with renal disease used to be born dangerously or not at all—not at all if their doctors had their way."[1] This statement describes early experiences with maternal renal disease and pregnancy outcome. It remains true that renal disease, either preexisting or occurring during gestation, may impair maternal and fetal health. Experience and investigations during the last two decades have significantly improved the outcome for pregnant women with renal disease.[2]

It is helpful to review the renal physiologic changes that occur during normal pregnancy to understand and evaluate coexisting renal disorders. Early in gestation, increased vascular volume leads to renal enlargement. Hormonal changes result in dilation of the renal pelvis and ureters; dilation often is accompanied by decreased ureteral peristalsis. Dilated uterine and ovarian veins and the gravid uterus may obstruct ureter drainage at the pelvic brim. Together, these changes predispose pregnant women to vesicoureteric reflux and ascending infection. Alterations in glomerular hemodynamics and tubular function also occur. Increased cardiac output and decreased intrarenal vascular resistance cause an 80% increase in renal blood flow and a 50% increase in glomerular filtration rate (GFR) during pregnancy. These changes are somewhat less pronounced near term. Because of the increased GFR, a serum creatinine concentration greater than 0.8 mg/dL and a blood urea nitrogen (BUN) concentration greater than 13 mg/dL (which are normal values for the nonpregnant patient) suggest renal insufficiency in the pregnant patient. Tubular sodium reabsorption and osmoregulation are reset, allowing a "physiologic hypervolemia" during gestation. Modest proteinuria also occurs during pregnancy (e.g., up to 300 mg in 24 hours).[3]

Urinary tract infections (see Chapter 36) and hypertensive disorders of pregnancy (see Chapter 44) are discussed elsewhere in this text.

RENAL PARENCHYMAL DISEASE

Definition and Pathophysiology

Two general groups of disorders, **glomerulopathies** and **tubulointerstitial disease,** are considered under the rubric of renal parenchymal syndromes. Glomerulopathies are further subdivided into disorders that involve inflammatory or necrotizing lesions—the **nephritic syndromes**—and disorders that involve abnormal permeability to protein and other macromolecules—the **nephrotic syndromes**. More than 20 specific glomerulopathies exist. The nomenclature for these glomerulopathies is confusing, and specific diseases are not discussed in detail here.

Tubulointerstitial diseases include disorders characterized by abnormal tubular function. They result in abnormal urine composition and concentration but are not characterized by decreased GFR until late in the disease course. These diseases include interstitial nephritis, renal cystic disease, renal neoplasia, and functional tubular defects.

Patients with renal parenchymal disorders may remain asymptomatic for years, and they may exhibit only proteinuria and microscopic hematuria, with little if any evidence of reduced renal function. Spontaneous recovery or improvement with treatment occurs with many glomerulopathies. However, other patients exhibit progressive nephropathy, hypertension, and renal insufficiency. Approximately 120,000 patients in the United States have chronic renal failure; two thirds of these cases result from glomerulopathy, and one third result from tubulointerstitial disease.

Diagnosis

Women with preexisting disease may choose to become pregnant without the counsel of their nephrologist. When such patients become pregnant, the obstetrician and nephrologist seek to define the degree of renal involvement. Serial blood

pressure measurements are obtained to define the severity of hypertension and the efficacy of current antihypertensive therapy. Creatinine clearance and the degree of proteinuria should be determined. Urinalysis yields information regarding the presence of renal casts and the presence of bacteriuria. The determination of serum creatinine and BUN concentrations defines the extent of renal insufficiency. A serum creatinine concentration greater than 0.8 mg/dL, although normal in the nonpregnant woman, may represent significant renal insufficiency during pregnancy. The obstetrician may first detect renal dysfunction through routine prenatal screening tests. If proteinuria, hematuria, or azotemia is detected, a complete biochemical evaluation should be performed.

Both preeclampsia and renal disease may present with hypertension, proteinuria, and edema. The distinction between the two disorders often is unclear, especially after 20 weeks' gestation. Fisher et al.[4] evaluated 176 renal biopsies obtained from hypertensive women immediately postpartum, most of whom had a clinical diagnosis of preeclampsia. The clinicopathologic correlation was poor. Histologic evidence of preeclampsia (e.g., glomerular endotheliosis without hypercellularity) was present in only 65% of these hypertensive women. Primary renal disease was present in 20% and hypertensive nephrosclerosis in 11%. Nulliparous women (84%) were more likely to have a correct diagnosis of preeclampsia than parous women (38%).

Renal tissue biopsy often is used to establish a diagnosis in nonpregnant patients. Chen et al.[5] reported a series of 15 percutaneous renal biopsies performed in 15 pregnant women with onset of renal dysfunction of unknown cause during pregnancy. All patients underwent biopsy before 30 weeks' gestation. No biopsy-related complications occurred except in one patient who experienced gross hematuria. Histologic results provided useful clinical guidance that facilitated successful fetal outcome in 14 of the pregnancies. In contrast, Kuller et al.[6] reviewed 18 renal biopsies performed during pregnancy ($n = 15$) or in the immediate postpartum period ($n = 3$). In this series, renal hematoma was identified in 7 (39%) patients, and 2 (11%) patients required blood transfusion following the biopsy. Four intrauterine fetal deaths occurred, although none was a direct result of the biopsy. Because renal biopsy exposes the parturient to potential complications, many maternal-fetal medicine (MFM) physicians recommend biopsy only when sudden deterioration in renal function or symptomatic nephrotic syndrome occurs before 32 weeks' gestation, when definitive diagnosis may guide appropriate treatment. Beyond 32 weeks' gestation, MFM physicians typically prefer to delay biopsy until the postpartum period.

Effect of Pregnancy

The extent to which pregnancy affects preexisting renal disease depends upon the degree of renal insufficiency before pregnancy. Among women with mild antenatal renal insufficiency, pregnancy does not substantially alter the natural course of renal disease. In contrast, pregnant women with moderate or severe antenatal renal insufficiency often experience deterioration of renal function and exacerbation of hypertension. Katz et al.[7] studied the outcome of 121 pregnancies in 89 women with mild renal insufficiency (i.e., serum creatinine concentration less than 1.4 mg/dL). Hypertension complicated 23% of these pregnancies, and renal function decreased during 16% of these pregnancies, most often in those women with diffuse glomerulonephritis. However, the decrease in renal function was modest, and renal function returned to baseline after delivery. Only five (6%) women progressed to end-stage renal failure, and this occurred as many as 8 years after pregnancy. Jungers et al.[8] evaluated the effect of pregnancy on renal function among 360 women with primary glomerulonephritis. During the study period, 171 of the women became pregnant, and 189 women did not become pregnant. All study subjects had normal renal function at the time of entry into this study; and all of the patients who became pregnant had normal renal function at conception. In this case-control study, pregnancy was not identified as a risk factor for progression to end-stage renal failure.

In contrast, Jones and Hayslett[9] analyzed the outcome of 82 pregnancies in 67 women with preexisting moderate or severe renal insufficiency (i.e., serum creatinine greater than 1.4 mg/dL before pregnancy or at the first antepartum visit). The mean ± SD serum creatinine concentration increased from 1.9 ± 0.8 mg/dL in early pregnancy to 2.5 ± 1.3 mg/dL in the third trimester. The prevalence of hypertension rose from 28% at baseline to 48% during late pregnancy. Pregnancy-related loss of maternal renal function occurred in 43% of cases. A woman with a serum creatinine concentration that exceeds 2.0 mg/dL who becomes pregnant has a one-in-three chance of developing dialysis-dependent end-stage renal disease during or shortly after pregnancy.[10]

The pathophysiology by which pregnancy exacerbates renal disease is unknown. One hypothesis is that increased glomerular perfusion, which normally accompanies pregnancy, paradoxically causes further injury to the kidneys in patients with preexisting impairment of function. However, this hypothesis is unsupported by published data, which reveal no evidence of hyperfiltration (i.e., an initial decline in serum creatinine concentration) during early pregnancy in patients with renal disease. Epstein[10] outlined an alternative hypothesis in which preexisting renal disease may induce a cascade of platelet aggregation, microvascular fibrin thrombus formation, and endothelial dysfunction that leads to microvascular injury in the already tenuous kidneys.

Effect on the Fetus

The incidence of obstetric complications also is proportionate to the extent of preexisting maternal renal disease. Among parturients with mild antenatal renal insufficiency, the rate of preterm delivery is 20% and the rate of intrauterine growth restriction (IUGR) is 24%.[7] When the mother has moderate-to-severe preexisting renal insufficiency, these rates increase to 59% and 37%, respectively.[9] However, the fetal survival rate remains high in both populations—89% and 93%, respectively.

Alexopoulos et al.[11] described the outcome of 24 pregnancies in 17 women with biopsy-proven glomerular disease. All but two patients had normal renal function at the onset of pregnancy. The fetal survival rate was 75%. There were six preterm deliveries, three newborns that were small for gestational age (SGA), one stillbirth, and five elective abortions. Impaired renal function at conception portended worse fetal outcome.

Medical and Obstetric Management

During pregnancy, the nephrologist and the obstetrician monitor maternal renal function, blood pressure, and fetal development at frequent intervals. Monthly determination of serum creatinine concentration, creatinine clearance, and proteinuria

allows the recognition of renal deterioration. Some glomeru-lopathies respond to corticosteroids, and this management should be continued during pregnancy. Rapid deterioration of renal function that occurs before 32 weeks' gestation may require renal biopsy to exclude rapidly progressive glomeru-lopathies that require treatment. Antihypertensive therapy should be instituted (see Chapter 44). Recombinant human erythropoietin improves maternal anemia during pregnancy.[12] Protein restriction places the fetus at risk for IUGR and is not utilized. Deterioration of maternal renal function, the onset of preeclampsia, or evidence of fetal compromise may necessitate preterm delivery.

Hemodialysis and Chronic Ambulatory Peritoneal Dialysis

When renal disease has progressed to end-stage renal failure (i.e., the GFR is less than 5 mL/min), fertility is suppressed and conception and pregnancy are rare. Less than 10% of pre-menopausal dialysis patients have regular menses. Luteinizing hormone and follicle-stimulating hormone concentrations assume an anovulatory pattern, which causes 40% of affected women to be amenorrheic. Half of all female dialysis patients exhibit hyperprolactinemia because of reduced clearance and hypothalamic disturbances.[13] The European Dialysis and Transplant Association[14] reported only 16 pregnancies among 13,000 women of childbearing age who were undergoing dial-ysis. Toma et al.[15] surveyed 2504 dialysis units in Japan and reported 172 pregnancies among 38,889 women who were undergoing dialysis.

Two modalities of dialysis exist—extracorporeal hemodial-ysis and intracorporeal peritoneal dialysis. **Hemodialysis** is complicated by (1) the need for vascular access, (2) cardio-vascular instability, (3) large fluid and electrolyte shifts, (4) the need for anticoagulation of the extracorporeal circuit, and (5) the risk of hepatitis. Hypotension may compromise utero-placental perfusion and cause fetal distress. Even when hypotension and major fluid shifts are avoided, Doppler examination of uterine and umbilical artery flow during hemodialysis suggests the occurrence of a redistribution of arterial flow away from the uteroplacental vascular bed.[16] Fetal heart rate (FHR) monitoring is recommended during dialysis.[17,18] Rapid removal of maternal solutes and decreased oncotic pressure with attendant free-water diffusion into the amniotic cavity may lead to polyhydramnios.[18] Hemodynamic consequences are minimized by more frequent but shorter dialysis runs. **Chronic ambulatory peritoneal dialysis** allows less hemodynamic trespass, a more stable fetal environment, and the freedom to dialyze at home.[19] Complications of this modality include peritonitis and catheter difficulties.

Published reports have noted a wide range of successful outcomes in dialysis-dependent pregnant women, regardless of the modality of dialysis.[15,18-20] In the survey by Toma et al.,[15] 90 (52%) of the 172 pregnancies in women undergo-ing chronic hemodialysis were successful.

Maternal complications include anemia, hypertension, and malnutrition. Fetal complications include IUGR, fetal death, and preterm labor. BUN levels are kept below 80 mg/dL predialysis and 30 mg/dL postdialysis.[21] At birth, neonatal azotemia is similar to that of the mother. Although these infants often have low 1-minute Apgar scores, they typ-ically respond to resuscitative efforts and are vigorous at 5 minutes. The long-term effects of intrauterine azotemia on newborn cognitive development are unknown.[18]

Patients undergoing hemodialysis have a high prevalence of viral hepatitis, an increased frequency of active tuberculosis, and an increased frequency of infection with vancomycin-resistant enterococci, human immunodeficiency virus (HIV), and methicillin-resistant *Staphylococcus aureus* (MRSA). A 1995 survey of 2647 chronic hemodialysis centers in the United States revealed that 76% of these centers reuse dispos-able dialyzers.[22] The prevalence of hepatitis C virus (HCV) antibody was 10% among patients and 2% among staff at these hemodialysis centers. With increased surveillance for HCV and with the decline in the reuse of dialysis equipment, these infection risks are likely to decline. In 2002, Harmankaya et al.[23] presented encouraging data from a single hemodialysis unit. This group used dedicated, isolated dialysis machines for HCV-seropositive patients. Only 8 (4.8%) of 168 patients showed HCV seroconversion during an 8-year observation period. Four of these patients became HCV seropositive after they had undergone hemodialysis in other dialysis centers on holiday, and two of the patients had undergone blood transfu-sion within the 6 months preceding seroconversion.

Anesthetic Management

Anesthetic management is influenced by the extent of renal dysfunction and hypertension. The parturient with stable renal disease, mild-to-moderate renal insufficiency, well-controlled hypertension, and euvolemia requires minimal special con-sideration. In contrast, the dialysis patient with end-stage renal failure presents many anesthetic challenges (Box 50-1). Poorly controlled hypertension leads to left ventricular hyper-trophy and dysfunction. Symptoms of cardiovascular com-promise should prompt echocardiography to evaluate ventricular function. Uremic pericarditis, cardiomyopathy, and accelerated atherosclerosis rarely are seen until advanced uremia has been present for several years.

REGIONAL ANESTHESIA

Uremic toxins cause functional platelet defects and a pro-longed bleeding time. These defects are reversed by dialysis. Thrombocytopenia also may occur as a result of an increased peripheral destruction of platelets.

Uremic patients may be hypervolemic or hypovolemic, depending on the time that has elapsed since their last dialysis. Hypovolemia and autonomic neuropathy may lead to profound hypotension during the initiation of sympathetic blockade. This risk may be minimized through proper prehydration and slow induction of epidural anesthesia.[24] Before the administration of regional anesthesia, preexisting peripheral neuropathy should be documented for medicolegal purposes.

There are reports of systemic local anesthetic toxicity after bupivacaine brachial plexus blockade in patients with chronic renal failure.[25,26] However, Rice et al.[27] found no significant difference in the pharmacokinetic profile of bupivacaine after brachial plexus blockade in a group of uremic patients when compared with patients with normal renal function. There are no published data regarding the pharmacokinetics of epidu-rally administered local anesthetic agents in patients with chronic renal failure. Orko et al.[28] administered spinal anes-thesia with 0.75% bupivacaine to 20 nonpregnant patients with chronic renal failure and 20 control patients. Maximal segmental anesthesia occurred more rapidly in the patients with renal disease (21 versus 35 minutes). Further, the extent of sensory blockade was two segments higher in the patients with renal disease.

Box 50-1 CHRONIC RENAL FAILURE: ABNORMALITIES THAT MAY AFFECT ANESTHETIC MANAGEMENT

CARDIOVASCULAR

- Hypertension
- Fluid overload
- Ventricular hypertrophy
- Accelerated atherosclerosis
- Uremic pericarditis
- Uremic cardiomyopathy

PULMONARY

- Increased risk of difficult airway
- Recurrent pulmonary infections

METABOLIC AND ENDOCRINE

- Hyperkalemia
- Metabolic acidosis
- Hyponatremia
- Hypocalcemia
- Hypermagnesemia
- Decreased protein binding of drugs
- Hypoglycemia

HEMATOLOGIC

- Anemia
- Platelet dysfunction
- Decreased coagulation factors
- Leukocyte dysfunction

NEUROLOGIC

- Autonomic neuropathy
- Mental status changes
- Peripheral neuropathy
- "Restless leg" syndrome
- Seizure disorder

GASTROINTESTINAL

- Delayed gastric emptying
- Increased gastric acidity
- Hepatic venous congestion
- Hepatitis (viral or drug)
- Malnutrition

GENERAL ANESTHESIA

Patients with chronic uremia exhibit delayed gastric emptying and hyperacidity, which increases the risk of aspiration pneumonitis. In addition to sodium citrate, the anesthesiologist also should give an H_2-receptor antagonist and metoclopramide when time allows. Recommended single doses for patients with renal failure are ranitidine 50 mg, cimetidine 300 mg, and metoclopramide 10 mg intravenously. Weir and Chung[29] suggested that patients with chronic renal failure present greater intubation problems than normal patients; however, an objective analysis of airway difficulty has not been performed in this population.

Patients with chronic renal failure frequently have normochromic, normocytic anemia secondary to impaired erythropoietin production, chronic gastrointestinal bleeding, and vitamin deficiency. Typically this is well tolerated and does not require transfusion, unless excessive surgical bleeding occurs. Intravascular volume must be assessed before the induction of anesthesia. Central venous pressure monitoring should be considered when the hemodynamic condition is unclear. An intraarterial catheter also may aid the management of the parturient with poorly controlled hypertension. Hemodialysis fistulae should be padded carefully to prevent thrombosis in both the operating and recovery rooms. Blood pressure cuffs should not be placed on these extremities.

Thiopental and propofol exhibit normal volume of distribution and elimination in patients with renal failure. However, decreased albumin binding of thiopental allows an increased concentration of free drug.[30] Protein binding of propofol is unaffected by renal failure.[31] Uremia increases blood-brain barrier permeability to many drugs.[32] These changes may warrant a small decrease in the dose of thiopental or propofol for induction. The serum potassium concentration should be determined before the induction of anesthesia. If the potassium concentration is greater than 5.5 mEq/L, dialysis should be performed before an elective procedure. Succinylcholine will cause a 0.5 to 0.7 mEq/L increase in potassium concentration, which is similar to the increment that occurs in patients without renal disease.[33] If the patient is already hyperkalemic, this mild elevation may be sufficient to precipitate cardiac arrhythmias. Plasma cholinesterase concentrations are normal, even after dialysis.[34]

After delivery, neuromuscular blockade can be maintained with atracurium, which undergoes Hofmann nonenzymatic degradation and nonspecific esterase metabolism. Cisatracurium represents a good alternative neuromuscular blocker for patients with renal disease. Cisatracurium undergoes Hofmann degradation, but it undergoes little (if any) nonspecific esterase hydrolysis. Unlike atracurium, cisatracurium does not cause histamine release. The duration of action of atracurium or cisatracurium is *not* prolonged in patients with renal failure. Magnesium-containing antacids may lead to hypermagnesemia, which potentiates neuromuscular blockade.[35] Although anticholinesterase agents undergo renal elimination and have a prolonged duration in patients with renal insufficiency, the volume of distribution remains the same and standard doses are used for the reversal of neuromuscular blockade.

ACUTE RENAL FAILURE

Definition and Epidemiology

Acute renal failure (ARF) is an uncommon but serious complication of pregnancy. Rapid deterioration of renal function leads to an accumulation of fluid and nitrogenous waste products with impaired electrolyte regulation. In the mid-twentieth century, nearly a quarter of all cases of ARF were obstetric. Fortunately, during the last four decades, the incidence of ARF in developed countries has fallen significantly.[36,37] From 1958 to 1994, Stratta et al.[36] observed a steady decline in the incidence of ARF from 1 in 3000 to 1 in 18,000 pregnancies. With respect to all ARF cases, the proportion related to pregnancy fell from 43% to 0.5%. This progress has resulted from improved obstetric care and fewer septic abortions.

Pathophysiology and Diagnosis

ARF is suggested by a sharp elevation in the plasma creatinine (greater than 0.8 mg/dL) and BUN (greater than 13 mg/dL) concentrations. In complete renal failure, the serum creatinine concentration rises at the rate of 0.5 to 1.0 mg/dL/day. Urine output typically falls to less than 400 mL/day (oliguria), but some patients may be nonoliguric. Frank anuria is rare.[38] ARF is subdivided according to underlying etiology (i.e., prerenal, postrenal, intrarenal causes) (Box 50-2). The inciting

Box 50-2 CAUSES OF ACUTE RENAL FAILURE DURING PREGNANCY

PRERENAL

Hyperemesis gravidarum
Uterine hemorrhage
Heart failure

POSTRENAL

Urolithiasis
Ureteral obstruction by the gravid uterus

INTRARENAL

Acute tubular necrosis
Septic abortion
Amniotic fluid embolism
Drug-induced acute interstitial nephritis
Acute glomerulonephritis
Bilateral renal cortical necrosis
Acute pyelonephritis
Preeclampsia/eclampsia
HELLP syndrome
Acute fatty liver of pregnancy
Idiopathic postpartum renal failure

---

disorders vary among countries.[36,37,39-47] In those countries where access to elective abortion is restricted, septic abortion is the leading cause of pregnancy-related ARF. In other countries, severe preeclampsia-eclampsia, acute pyelonephritis of pregnancy, and bilateral renal cortical necrosis are the most common underlying disorders.

PRERENAL CAUSES

The most common prerenal causes of ARF—hyperemesis gravidarum[48] and obstetric hemorrhage—lead to hypovolemia and inadequate renal perfusion. Urinary indices show urinary osmolality greater than 500 mOsm/kg water, urine sodium less than 20 mEq/L, fractional sodium excretion less than 1%, and a urinary:plasma creatinine ratio greater than 40.[38] Concealed uterine hemorrhage from placental abruption may remain unrecognized until hypotension and renal failure ensue.[49] Women with preeclampsia may be more likely to develop ARF after hemorrhage because of preexisting intravascular contraction, prostacyclin deficiency, hyperreactivity to catecholamines, and coexisting coagulation disturbances.[45]

POSTRENAL CAUSES

The postrenal causes of ARF include nephrolithiasis and ureteral obstruction by the gravid uterus.[50,51] The latter complication is more likely in those parturients with polyhydramnios or multiple gestation.[52] Preexisting ureteral dilation and impaired peristalsis increase the risk of obstructive uropathy during pregnancy. Flank pain and decreased urine output during late gestation should alert the clinician to this possibility. Courban et al.[53] reported an unusual case of obstructive uropathy leading to ARF in a parturient with multiple uterine leiomyomas.

INTRARENAL CAUSES

Once prerenal and postrenal causes of ARF have been excluded, intrarenal processes remain. In general, oliguric intrarenal ARF is not easily reversed and must run its course. Causes include acute tubular necrosis, interstitial nephritis, and acute glomerulonephritis, as well as a few causes unique to pregnancy. These latter causes include renal cortical necrosis, acute pyelonephritis, severe preeclampsia-eclampsia, acute fatty liver of pregnancy, and idiopathic postpartum renal failure. A thorough history, review of medications, and urinalysis typically help determine the specific initiating factor.

Acute tubular necrosis results from nephrotoxic drugs, amniotic fluid embolism, rhabdomyolysis, intrauterine fetal death, and prolonged renal ischemia secondary to hemorrhage or septic shock. Urinalysis reveals dirty brown epithelial cell casts and coarse granular casts. Urinary indices show urine osmolality less than 350 mOsm/kg water, urine sodium greater than 40 mEq/L, fractional sodium excretion greater than 1%, and a urinary:plasma creatinine ratio less than 20.[38]

Acute interstitial nephritis is caused by nonsteroidal anti-inflammatory drugs (NSAIDs) and various antibiotics. These patients typically have fever, rash, eosinophilia, and urine eosinophils.

Acute glomerulonephritis is rare during pregnancy. It is suggested by hematuria, red cell casts, and proteinuria. Urinary indices of acute glomerulonephritis are similar to those of prerenal ARF.

Bilateral renal cortical necrosis, which rarely is observed in the nonobstetric patient, is responsible for 10% to 38% of cases of obstetric ARF.[46,49,54-56] It may occur during both early and late pregnancy. Placental abruption is the most common precipitating event. The pathogenesis of this disorder is unclear but may involve renal hypoperfusion or endothelial damage by endotoxin imposed on the normal hypercoagulable state of pregnancy. A single dose of endotoxin may precipitate bilateral renal cortical necrosis in pregnant animals, which has led some investigators to view this disorder as a clinical analog of the experimental Sanarelli-Shwartzman reaction.[45] Extensive microthrombi are found within the glomeruli and renal arterioles. Diagnosis is made by selective renal arteriography, which reveals an absent or patchy cortex. Renal biopsy also may be performed in the absence of active coagulopathy.[49]

Acute pyelonephritis is one of the most common infectious complications of pregnancy (see Chapter 36). Although acute pyelonephritis rarely leads to ARF in the nongravid patient, it accounts for 5% of cases of ARF among parturients.[57] The reason for this increased susceptibility is unclear. Whalley et al.[58] noted that acute pyelonephritis causes a marked reduction of GFR in pregnant women. In contrast, pyelonephritis causes little reduction in GFR in nonpregnant patients. The kidney may be more sensitive to bacterial endotoxins during pregnancy.

Severe preeclampsia-eclampsia has been blamed for 20% of the cases of obstetric ARF.[57,59] However, many cases of renal dysfunction and failure may only mimic preeclampsia and actually may result from other factors.[4] Other causes of ARF should be considered before explaining renal failure on the basis of preeclampsia.

Sibai and Ramadan[60] reported 32 cases of ARF associated with **HELLP syndrome** (Hemolysis, Elevated Liver enzymes, and Low Platelets). The majority of patients had a derangement of multiple organ systems and other obstetric complications (e.g., placental abruption, intrauterine fetal death, disseminated intravascular coagulation [DIC], postpartum hemorrhage, sepsis). Renal histology reveals thrombotic microangiopathy and acute tubular necrosis, suggesting pathogenesis of acute renal failure associated with HELLP syndrome.[61] In the Sibai and Ramadan[60] report, a total of 4 (13%) parturients died, and 10 (31%) required dialysis. The

perinatal mortality rate was 34%, and 72% of deliveries occurred preterm. Of interest, Flynn et al.[62] reported the successful use of cadaveric kidneys procured from a parturient who died following HELLP syndrome and ARF. Both recipients had acceptable graft function 2 years following transplantation.

Acute fatty liver of pregnancy (reversible peripartum liver failure)—a rare but life-threatening disorder of pregnancy—is associated with a 60% to 100% incidence of ARF. Specific clinical features of acute fatty liver of pregnancy are discussed in Chapter 45.

The syndrome of **idiopathic postpartum renal failure** was initially described by Robson et al.[63] in 1968. Subsequently, approximately 200 cases have been reported. This syndrome is characterized by ARF, microangiopathic hemolytic anemia, and thrombocytopenia occurring 2 days to 10 weeks after an uncomplicated delivery. It appears closely related to the hemolytic uremic syndrome. Idiopathic postpartum renal failure typically is preceded by an upper respiratory or gastrointestinal viral syndrome that rapidly progresses to ARF. The use of ethinyl estradiol as a contraceptive also may be causally related to this syndrome.[64] Spontaneous bleeding, congestive heart failure, hypertension, and seizures have been reported.[65,66] Some investigators believe that this syndrome represents a clinical analog to the generalized Shwartzman reaction, a condition induced in laboratory animals by two successive injections of endotoxin, which results in factor XII activation, thrombin generation, and fibrin deposition. Others consider the platelet deposition to be the primary event that leads to microvascular thrombi.[64] Management includes plasma infusion and antiplatelet therapy. The role of heparin therapy is controversial. The mortality rate among these patients is high. In a review of 67 patients,[67] 31 (46%) died, 8 (12%) required chronic dialysis or renal transplantation, 10 (15%) had residual renal impairment, and only 13 (19%) had complete recovery. In another review of 25 patients,[65] 8 (32%) parturients survived, 1 (4%) recovered normal renal function, 4 (16%) recovered with moderate chronic renal impairment, and 3 (12%) required long-term hemodialysis. Marcovici and Marzano[68] described the clinical course of a parturient who developed postpartum renal failure and acute pancreatitis. These authors cautioned that diuretics should be cautiously administered because they may increase the risk of pancreatitis.

Effect on the Mother and Fetus

Maternal mortality from ARF ranges from none to 34%.[36] This prognosis is better than that for ARF in the nonobstetric population because most obstetric patients are otherwise young and healthy. Stratta et al.[36] reported 84 cases of pregnancy-related ARF; 6% required hemodialysis. Although maternal prognosis has improved significantly in developed countries, mortality remains high (16%) among inner-city populations.[69] The prognosis for the fetus is worse than that for the mother, and more than 40% of these pregnancies end in fetal death.[42,56,70,71]

Medical and Obstetric Management

Management is directed toward rapid recognition of the underlying abnormality. Reversible disorders such as hypovolemia, concealed uterine hemorrhage, urinary tract infection, ureteral obstruction, and drug-induced ARF must be excluded. The urine-to-plasma osmolality ratio is a useful laboratory test to identify reversible prerenal causes. Intravascular volume should be optimized. Electrolytes and acid-base status should be monitored carefully. Hypertension must be managed aggressively. Many obstetric causes of ARF also may cause DIC; therefore, coagulation abnormalities should be excluded.[36]

Because urea and other metabolic products cross the placenta, hemodialysis or peritoneal dialysis should be directed toward maintaining the postdialysis BUN concentration at or below 30 mg/dL. Fluid shifts during hemodialysis should be minimized by short but frequent periods of dialysis. If the fetus is mature, delivery should be accomplished when the maternal condition is stabilized. The pediatrician must be alerted to the presence of high fetal BUN levels, which may lead to an osmotic diuresis and neonatal dehydration. Ertuk et al.[51] reported the first known delivery of a healthy infant during a hemodialysis session.

Anesthetic Management

The anesthesiologist should work with the obstetrician and nephrologist to optimize the maternal condition before the induction of labor or performance of cesarean section. Evaluation of maternal intravascular volume may require central venous or pulmonary artery pressure monitoring.[72] The level of azotemia, electrolyte balance, and hematologic status should be assessed. If the BUN level is greater than 80 mg/dL or the serum potassium is greater than 5.5 mEq/L, dialysis should be performed before elective vaginal or cesarean delivery. Regional anesthesia may be administered in the absence of coagulopathy, thrombocytopenia, or hypovolemia. Occult uterine hemorrhage should be excluded. Epidural anesthesia is preferred over spinal anesthesia when the intravascular volume status is in question because the level of sympathetic blockade may be established more slowly while appropriate volumes of intravenous fluid are administered. Normal saline without potassium should be administered. As the sympathetic blockade dissipates, the mother should be monitored for evidence of volume overload and pulmonary edema.

General anesthesia may be required for urgent cesarean delivery or in those patients with coagulopathy or hemorrhage. If a subclavian venous catheter was recently placed for hemodialysis access, pneumothorax should be excluded before the use of positive-pressure ventilation.

RENAL TRANSPLANTATION

Fewer than 1 in 800 women of childbearing age receiving chronic dialysis for renal failure become pregnant.[14] However, successful renal transplantation improves the fertility rate to more than 1 in 50. Since 1963, when Murray et al.[73] reported the first pregnancy after renal transplantation, many of these women have completed successful pregnancies.

Renal Hyperfiltration

When the transplant kidney is removed from a donor and is transplanted into an anephric recipient, it undergoes a process of hyperfiltration. This is a maladaptive response that, in the short term, attempts to bring the GFR toward the rate of a binephric system. In the long term, this hyperfiltration may lead to glomerular sclerosis and loss of renal function if it is associated with increased glomerular or capillary pressure.[74,75] In normal pregnancy, the GFR increases by 30% to 50% during the first and second trimesters and subsequently decreases somewhat during the third trimester. Theoretically,

this additional hyperfiltration of pregnancy predisposes the patient to a loss of renal function.

Baylis et al.[76,77] allayed many of these concerns by demonstrating that gestational hyperfiltration is not associated with increased glomerular pressure because of matching afferent and efferent arteriolar vasodilation. They produced hyperfiltration in rodent kidneys by performing uninephrectomy, maintaining the animals on a high-protein diet, and subjecting the animals to five consecutive pregnancies. They observed no functional impairment or renal histologic changes in this animal model. In addition, they demonstrated that glomerular pressure is lower in female rats than in male rats 10 months after uninephrectomy. Hakim et al.[78] have shown a similar gender advantage in humans after uninephrectomy.

Effect of Pregnancy on the Renal Allograft

Attempts to evaluate the impact of pregnancy on renal allograft function and survival are limited by the inability to randomize transplant patients to pregnancy or no pregnancy. Davison[79] surveyed 2309 pregnancies in 1594 women. Forty percent of the pregnancies did not progress beyond the first trimester (the spontaneous abortion rate was 13% and the elective abortion rate was 27%). The pregnancies that progressed beyond the first trimester were complicated by IUGR (25%), preterm delivery (50%), and hypertension and/or preeclampsia (30%). In most women, allograft function was enhanced during early pregnancy and deteriorated briefly during late pregnancy. Only 15% of the parturients experienced persistent renal impairment.[79]

Sturgiss and Davison[80] performed a case-control study of 36 renal transplant recipients: 18 became pregnant and 18 did not. Groups were matched according to age, early rejection episodes, primary renal function, time since transplant, and extent of histocompatibility. The authors noted no significant difference between the two groups in plasma creatinine concentration, GFR, mean arterial blood pressure, or the number who suffered graft loss or chronic rejection over a mean follow-up period of 12 years (Table 50-1).

Crowe et al.[81] reviewed 33 pregnancies in 29 renal transplant recipients. Mean serum creatinine concentrations and creatinine clearance remained stable throughout pregnancy and 1 year postpartum. However, mean urinary protein increased from 0.45 g/24 hr at onset of pregnancy to 1.11 g/24 hr at delivery. The proteinuria returned to baseline by 3 months postpartum. Little et al.[82] reported a series of 29 pregnancies among 19 women following renal transplantation. These pregnancies resulted in 23 (79%) live births. There was no change in renal allograft function during pregnancy. However, a mild elevation in serum creatinine concentration occurred during the early postpartum period. Renal allograft failure occurred in three (16%) women. Miniero et al.[83] reviewed 56 pregnancies in 42 women following renal transplantation. These women were maintained with cyclosporine, azathioprine, corticosteroids, and/or tacrolimus before and during gestation. The mean interval between transplantation and conception was 62 months (range of 12 to 180 months). Complications arose during pregnancy in 16 (44%) of 36 term pregnancies. Allograft rejection occurred in four (11%) cases; two (6%) of these rejections were irreversible.

Mehanty et al.[84] proposed an intriguing hypothesis, namely that mothers receiving renal allografts from offspring would have a better graft survival compared with either fathers receiving allografts from offspring or mothers receiv-

	TABLE 50-1	EFFECT OF PREGNANCY ON LONG-TERM FUNCTION OF RENAL ALLOGRAFTS*	
		Pregnant group (n = 18)	**Nonpregnant control group (n = 18)**
Plasma creatinine (mg/dL)		1.26 ± 0.83 (19% increase)	1.44 ± 0.59 (8% increase)
Glomerular filtration rate (mL/min)		58 ± 29 (18% decrease)	56 ± 32 (7% decrease)
Mean arterial pressure (mm Hg)		96 ± 12 (1% decrease)	101 ± 9 (5% increase)
Graft loss or chronic rejection		2 (11%)	2 (11%)

*Percentage increase or decrease represents change from initial assessment to end of follow-up. No statistically significant differences were noted.
From Sturgiss SN, Davison JM. Effect of pregnancy on long-term function of renal allografts. Am J Kidney Dis 1992; 19:167-72.

ing allografts from non-offspring. Fetal cells and DNA have been detected in maternal blood for decades after normal pregnancy and delivery. These investigators suggested that this microchimerism of fetal cells might induce tolerance and improve renal allograft survival in offspring donor to maternal recipient combinations. However, an initial study failed to support this hypothesis.

Effect on the Fetus

Although intercurrent pregnancy seems to have minimal impact on maternal health or allograft survival, fetal outcome is less favorable. Of the 56 pregnancies presented by Miniero et al.,[83] the obstetric outcome included 20 (36%) abortions and 20 (36%) preterm deliveries. All infants delivered before term exhibited significant IUGR. The Toronto Renal Transplant Program[85] reviewed 44 consecutive pregnancies in 26 women following renal transplantation. Of these, 12 (27%) pregnancies ended with abortion or intrauterine death and 32 (73%) pregnancies resulted in live-born infants. The mean infant weight in this group was 2540 g versus 3590 g in a control group. In Singapore, Tan et al.[86] reported abortion or stillbirth among 13 (31%) of 42 pregnancies following renal transplantation. The remaining successful pregnancies were complicated by preterm delivery (45%) and IUGR (86%). Toma et al.[15] surveyed 194 pregnancies in renal transplant recipients. Spontaneous or elective abortion occurred in 28 (14%) of these gestations, and successful delivery of surviving infants occurred in 159 (82%). The National Transplantation Pregnancy Registry[87] reported 53 (11%) fetal deaths in 461 pregnancies following renal transplantation.

Most posttransplantation protocols include a primary immunosuppressant (cyclosporine or tacrolimus) and one or two adjunctive agents (azathioprine, mycophenolate mofetil, sirolimus, and/or corticosteroids).[88] Despite transplacental exposure to these immunosuppressive drugs, congenital anomalies and other adverse effects are infrequent.[86,89-91] Kainz et al.[92] reported the outcome of 100 pregnancies in 84 women treated with tacrolimus following solid organ transplantation (27% kidney and 66% liver). Of 68 resulting live births, 4 (6%) neonates presented with a malformation of varied nature. Intrauterine exposure to cyclosporine impairs T-, B-, and NK-cell development and function in neonates. This effect, as well as depressed levels of serum immunoglobulin, persist during

the first year of life.[93] This places the infant at risk for suboptimal immunologic response following administration of classical vaccines, and for adverse effects following administration of live, attenuated vaccines. Delayed vaccination (until after 6 months of life) is recommended for infants exposed to immunosuppressant agents in utero.

Transplant recipients may become infected with cytomegalovirus (CMV) at the time of transplantation, or they may experience reactivation secondary to immunosuppression. Active CMV infection during pregnancy is associated with congenital anomalies (e.g., cerebral cysts, microcephaly, mental retardation). In addition, active neonatal CMV infection may lead to serious illness or death.

Following renal transplantation, residual impaired renal function may lead to false-positive biochemical screening for trisomy-21. Karidas et al.[94] demonstrated a significant correlation between free beta-human chorionic gonadotrophin (beta-hCG) and serum urea and creatinine concentrations. Similar alterations in alpha-fetoprotein (AFP) levels were not observed. In this setting, the double-marker biochemical test may be interpreted inaccurately. In patients with altered serum urea and creatinine concentrations, first-trimester nuchal translucency measurement, in combination with second-trimester ultrasonography, may be a more useful screening technique (see Chapter 6).

Medical and Obstetric Management

Discontinuation of immunosuppressive therapy, even years after transplantation, may lead to acute rejection. Thus, the immunosuppressive regimen must be continued during pregnancy unless toxicity results. Cyclosporine requirements increase during pregnancy, most likely because of enhanced metabolism.[95] The pregnant patient must be intensively monitored for any evidence of acute or chronic allograft rejection, infection, ureteral and renal artery obstruction, impaired renal function, hypertension, fluid volume disturbances, and/or anemia. Recombinant human erythropoietin has been used safely, and has successfully improved anemia in a few pregnant transplant recipients.[96,97]

Initial laboratory studies include (1) complete blood count, (2) renal function tests, (3) determination of serum electrolytes and glucose, and (4) viral serology for CMV, hepatitis B virus (HBV), hepatitis C virus (HCV), and HIV. Serial ultrasonography allows the recognition of fetal anomalies and the evaluation of fetal growth.

Cultures of the lower genital tract should be obtained in women with lesions that suggest herpes simplex virus (HSV) infection. A patient who presents with labor and evidence of active genital HSV infection should undergo cesarean section (see Chapter 36).

Vaginal examinations are minimized and always performed in a strict aseptic manner. The renal allograft typically is implanted in the extraperitoneal iliac fossa and does not impair vaginal delivery. Prophylactic antibiotics and stress-dose corticosteroids are indicated in patients who undergo cesarean section.

Anesthetic Management

In the absence of renal dysfunction or hypertension, anesthetic management is similar to that in the normal parturient. Strict aseptic technique is maintained during the placement of intravascular catheters and the performance of regional anesthetic techniques. Sowter et al.[98] reported an epidural abscess that occurred 23 days after epidural anesthesia in a nonpregnant patient receiving corticosteroid therapy for rheumatoid arthritis. Nevertheless, this complication is exceedingly rare, and immunosuppression itself should not be considered a contraindication to administration of epidural or spinal anesthesia, in the absence of systemic infection.

UROLITHIASIS

Definition and Epidemiology

Urolithiasis is characterized by the abnormal formation of calculi within the renal calyces or pelvis. Calculi may lodge within the ureters or bladder. Most stones are of the calcium oxalate (70%) or calcium phosphate (10%) type. The disorder affects 1% to 5% of the general population, but it is more common in the southeastern "stone belt" and mountainous regions. Symptomatic urolithiasis occurs during 1 in 240 to 1 in 3300 pregnancies[99,100] and is more common among Caucasians than African-Americans. Because pregnancy does not affect the rate of urolithiasis, this incidence approximates that observed among nonpregnant young women during a 9-month period.

Pathophysiology

The presence of urolithiasis presumes an underlying physiologic abnormality that leads to persistent supersaturation of the particular minerals involved. Supersaturation may occur secondary to acidic urine, oliguria, or an increased excretion of the stone constituents. During pregnancy, an elevated plasma 1,25-dihydroxyvitamin D level causes increased intestinal absorption of calcium, net mobilization of calcium from bone, and a state of absorptive hypercalciuria.[101] Ultimately, these changes provide calcium for the fetal skeleton. The fact that parturients rarely suffer from urolithiasis implies the occurrence of other physiologic changes during pregnancy that offset this stone-forming tendency. Calcium stone inhibitors such as citrate, magnesium, and glycoprotein are excreted in the urine to a greater extent during pregnancy.[102]

Diagnosis

Urolithiasis most commonly presents during the second or third trimester. Only 20% of affected pregnant women recount a prior history of renal calculi.[100] More than 80% of cases of gestational urolithiasis are diagnosed in parous women, which may reflect the increased incidence of this disease with advanced age.[103] Among 72 cases of urolithiasis reported by Lewis et al.,[99] 60% were right-sided, 36% were left-sided, and 4% were bilateral.

The diagnosis of urolithiasis during pregnancy may be confusing because it must be differentiated from ectopic pregnancy, preterm labor, appendicitis, pyelonephritis, and benign hematuria of pregnancy. A history of previous urolithiasis, recurrent urinary tract infections, or urologic surgery is suggestive. Symptoms include flank and abdominal pain, urgency, dysuria, nausea, and fever. Examination reveals costovertebral tenderness, abdominal tenderness, pyuria, and hematuria. Urolithiasis must be considered in a parturient with pyelonephritis who remains febrile or has continued bacteriuria despite 48 hours of parenteral antibiotics.

The initial imaging modality for the evaluation of urolithiasis during pregnancy is transabdominal ultrasonography.

This technology has evolved so that most cases of gestational urolithiasis may be diagnosed confidently without exposing the fetus to ionizing radiation. Specifically, color Doppler ultrasonography allows the identification of ureteral jets during pregnancy, and the asymmetry or absence of these jets indicates the presence of urinary calculi.[104-106] Vaginal ultrasonography may augment suboptimal transabdominal imaging. However, 40% of calculi are missed when the urinary tract is imaged with ultrasonography alone.[100]

If urinary calculi are not successfully visualized with ultrasonography, and if clinical suspicion for urolithiasis remains high, limited intravenous pyelography may be utilized.[100,102] Fetal radiation exposure during excretory urography is less than 1.5 rad. Exposure to 5 to 10 rads during the embryogenic period confers a 1% to 3% increase in the risk of congenital anomalies.[107] Of greater concern is the risk for childhood malignancies following radiation exposure in utero. Harvey et al.[108] studied 32,000 twins born in Connecticut from 1930 to 1969 (a time when twin gestations were diagnosed with limited abdominal radiography). The average radiation dose imposed on these fetuses was 1 rad (range of 0.16 to 4 rads). These children subsequently were found to have a 1.6-fold increase in the relative risk for leukemia and a 3.2-fold increase in the relative risk for childhood malignancies. These risks must be considered when selecting urologic imaging techniques. Magnetic resonance urography, with strongly T2-weighted sequences, also may show the site and type of obstruction without exposing the fetus to ionizing radiation.[105]

Effect of Pregnancy

In an effort to determine any effect of pregnancy on the natural history of urolithiasis, Coe et al.[109] reviewed the records of 58 pregnancies in women with the preexisting diagnosis of urolithiasis. The stone recurrence rate in this group was 0.49 stones per patient-year. This was not significantly different from the rate of 0.44 stones per patient-year in the general population.[110] These authors concluded that pregnancy does not alter the activity or severity of stone disease.

Effect on the Mother and Fetus

Urolithiasis seems to have minimal impact on the progress of gestation. Lewis et al.[99] observed that premature rupture of membranes occurred in 7% of patients with urolithiasis versus 3% in a control population. Obstetric outcome was otherwise similar to that of parturients without urolithiasis. Most often preterm labor resolves after passage or removal of the stone. Honoré[111] suggested that there is an increased incidence of renal stones among women who have a spontaneous abortion. He hypothesized that abnormalities of calcium hemostasis may lead to myometrial hyperirritability or abnormal hormonal secretion by the corpus luteum and/or placenta. Rare cases of ureteral rupture[112] and obstructed labor caused by a vesicular calculus[113,114] have been reported.

Urologic and Obstetric Management

During pregnancy, 70% of calculi pass spontaneously with conservative management (e.g., hydration, antibiotics if the patient is febrile, bed rest, analgesia).[99] Urologic intervention is indicated in the presence of persistent pyelonephritis, deterioration of renal function, massive hydronephrosis, persistent pain, or sepsis. Ureteral stent placement with ureteroscopy and ultrasonographic guidance is required in 29% of affected pregnant women, and percutaneous nephrostomy is required in 3% of patients.[99] Open ureterolithotomy or nephrectomy is required infrequently. Holmium:yttrium-aluminum-garnet (YAG) laser lithotripsy, using state of the art ureteroscopes, is an emerging technique for stone management in pregnancy.[115] Extracorporeal lithotripsy is not approved for use during pregnancy.[116]

Women with a history of urolithiasis should increase their intake of fluids. Calcium supplementation through prenatal vitamins should be avoided in women with recurrent urolithiasis. Medical management of stone disease may have untoward fetal effects. Thiazides are associated with fetal hyponatremia, hypoglycemia, and thrombocytopenia.[117] Although D-penicillamine, which is used to treat cystinuric urolithiasis, has been associated with congenital connective tissue defects,[118] some physicians consider this risk to be overstated if a low-methionine diet is avoided.[119] Adverse effects from xanthine oxidase inhibitors are unknown.[120]

Primary hyperparathyroidism should be considered when the parturient presents with (1) urolithiasis with or without pancreatitis, (2) hyperemesis beyond the first trimester, (3) a history of recurrent spontaneous abortion or intrauterine fetal death, (4) neonatal hypocalcemia or tetany, or (5) a total serum calcium concentration greater than 10.1 mg/dL during the second trimester or 8.8 mg/dL during the third trimester.[121,122]

Anesthetic Management

The ureters receive sensory innervation through the renal, ovarian, and hypogastric plexuses (T11 to L1 spinal segments). During conservative management of urolithiasis, epidural analgesia provides the patient with significant pain relief and facilitates the passage of the calculus, possibly through decreased ureteral spasm.[123-125] Ready and Johnson[123] reported the use of epidural analgesia in a patient with severe renal colic at 23 weeks' gestation. Analgesia that was maintained for 16 hours allowed the passage of the stone. Regional analgesia allows the anesthesiologist to avoid systemic opioids, which impair normal peristalsis in ureteric smooth muscle. Improved maternal pain control also may decrease endogenous catecholamine release and improve uteroplacental blood flow.

> **KEY POINTS**
>
> - **Pregnant women with moderate or severe renal insufficiency are at increased risk for deterioration of renal function, exacerbation of hypertension, and other obstetric complications. However, the rate of fetal survival is high.**
> - **Pregnancy does not affect the long-term survival of a renal allograft.**
> - **Immunosuppressive therapy must be continued during pregnancy in the patient with a renal transplant. The anesthesiologist should maintain strict aseptic technique during the placement of intravascular catheters and the performance of regional anesthetic techniques.**
> - **Epidural analgesia may facilitate the spontaneous passage of renal calculi.**

REFERENCES

1. Anonymous. Pregnancy and renal disease. Lancet 1975; 2:801-2.
2. Lindheimer MD, Davison JM, Katz AI. The kidney and hypertension in pregnancy: Twenty exciting years. Semin Nephrol 2001; 21:173-89.
3. Davison JM. Kidney function in pregnant women. Am J Kidney Dis 1987; 9:248-52.
4. Fisher KA, Luger A, Spargo BH, Lindheimer MD. Hypertension in pregnancy: clinical-pathological correlations and remote prognosis. Medicine (Baltimore) 1981; 60:267-76.
5. Chen HH, Lin HC, Yeh JC, Chen CP. Renal biopsy in pregnancies complicated by undetermined renal disease. Acta Obstet Gynecol Scand 2001; 80:888-93.
6. Kuller JA, D'Andrea NM, McMahon MJ. Renal biopsy and pregnancy. Am J Obstet Gynecol 2001; 184:1093-6.
7. Katz AI, Davison JM, Hayslett JP, et al. Pregnancy in women with kidney disease. Kidney Int 1980; 18:192-206.
8. Jungers P, Houillier P, Forget D, et al. Influence of pregnancy on the course of primary chronic glomerulonephritis. Lancet 1995; 346:1122-4.
9. Jones DC, Hayslett JP. Outcome of pregnancy in women with moderate or severe renal insufficiency. N Engl J Med 1996; 335:226-32.
10. Epstein FH. Pregnancy and renal disease. N Engl J Med 1996; 335:277-8.
11. Alexopoulos E, Bili H, Tampakoudis P, et al. Outcome of pregnancy in women with glomerular diseases. Ren Fail 1996; 18:121-9.
12. McGregor E, Stewart G, Junor BJ, Rodger RS. Successful use of recombinant human erythropoietin in pregnancy. Nephrol Dial Transplant 1991; 6:292-3.
13. Lim VS. Reproductive function in patients with renal insufficiency. Am J Kidney Dis 1987; 9:363-7.
14. Anonymous. Successful pregnancies in women treated by dialysis and kidney transplantation. Report from the Registration Committee of the European Dialysis and Transplant Association. Br J Obstet Gynaecol 1980; 87:839-45.
15. Toma H, Tanabe K, Tokumoto T, et al. Pregnancy in women receiving renal dialysis or transplantation in Japan: a nationwide survey. Nephrol Dial Transplant 1999; 14:1511-6.
16. Krakow D, Castro LC, Schwieger J. Effect of hemodialysis on uterine and umbilical artery Doppler flow velocity waveforms. Am J Obstet Gynecol 1994; 170:1386-8.
17. Nageotte MP, Grundy HO. Pregnancy outcome in women requiring chronic hemodialysis. Obstet Gynecol 1988; 72:456-9.
18. Hou S. Pregnancy in women requiring dialysis for renal failure. Am J Kidney Dis 1987; 9:368-73.
19. Jakobi P, Ohel G, Szylman P, et al. Continuous ambulatory peritoneal dialysis as the primary approach in the management of severe renal insufficiency in pregnancy. Obstet Gynecol 1992; 79:808-10.
20. Luciani G, Bossola M, Tazza L, et al. Pregnancy during chronic hemodialysis: a single dialysis-unit experience with five cases. Ren Fail 2002; 24:853-62.
21. Asrat T, Nageotte MP. Renal failure in pregnancy. Semin Perinatol 1990; 14:59-67.
22. Tokars JI, Miller ER, Alter MJ, Arduino MJ. National surveillance of dialysis associated diseases in the United States, 1995. ASAIO J 1998; 44:98-107.
23. Harmankaya O, Cetin B, Obek A, Seber E. Low prevalence of hepatitis C virus infection in hemodialysis units: Effect of isolation? Ren Fail 2002; 24:639-44.
24. Tighe KE, Smith ID, Bogod DG. Caesarean section in chronic renal failure. Eur J Anaesthesiol 1995; 12:185-7.
25. Gould DB, Aldrete JA. Bupivacaine cardiotoxicity in a patient with renal failure. Acta Anaesthesiol Scand 1983; 27:18-21.
26. Lucas LF, Tsueda K. Cardiovascular depression after brachial plexus block in two diabetic patients with renal failure. Anesthesiology 1990; 73:1032-5.
27. Rice AS, Pither CE, Tucker GT. Plasma concentrations of bupivacaine after supraclavicular brachial plexus blockade in patients with chronic renal failure. Anaesthesia 1991; 46:354-7.
28. Orko R, Pitkanen M, Rosenberg PH. Subarachnoid anaesthesia with 0.75% bupivacaine in patients with chronic renal failure. Br J Anaesth 1986; 58:605-9.
29. Weir PH, Chung FF. Anaesthesia for patients with chronic renal disease. Can Anaesth Soc J 1984; 31:468-81.
30. Ghoneim MM, Pandya H. Plasma protein binding of thiopental in patients with impaired renal or hepatic function. Anesthesiology 1975; 42:545-9.
31. Costela JL, Jimenez R, Calvo R, et al. Serum protein binding of propofol in patients with renal failure or hepatic cirrhosis. Acta Anaesthesiol Scand 1996; 40:741-5.
32. Freeman RB, Sheff MF, Haher JF, Schreiner GE. The blood-cerebrospinal fluid barrier in uremia. Ann Intern Med 1962; 56:233-40.
33. Miller RD, Way WL, Hamilton WK, Layzer RB. Succinylcholine-induced hyperkalemia in patients with renal failure? Anesthesiology 1972; 36:138-41.
34. Ryan DW. Preoperative serum cholinesterase concentration in chronic renal failure. Clinical experience of suxamethonium in 81 patients undergoing renal transplant. Br J Anaesth 1977; 49:945-9.
35. Ghoneim MM, Long JP. The interaction between magnesium and other neuromuscular blocking agents. Anesthesiology 1970; 32:23-7.
36. Stratta P, Besso L, Canavese C, et al. Is pregnancy-related acute renal failure a disappearing clinical entity? Ren Fail 1996; 18:575-84.
37. Selcuk NY, Tonbul HZ, San A, Odabas AR. Changes in frequency and etiology of acute renal failure in pregnancy (1980-1997). Ren Fail 1998; 20:513-7.
38. Mitch WE. Acute renal failure. In: Goldman L, Bennett JC, eds. Cecil Textbook of Medicine. Philadelphia: WB Saunders, 2000:567-71.
39. Diaz JH, De Gordon G, Hernandez L, Medina R. [Acute kidney insufficiency of obstetric origin. Experience at the Santo Tomas Hospital (1966-1981)]. Rev Med Panama 1990; 15:35-41.
40. Turney JH, Ellis CM, Parsons FM. Obstetric acute renal failure 1956-1987. Br J Obstet Gynaecol 1989; 96:679-87.
41. Zewdu W. Acute renal failure in Addis Abeba, Ethiopia: a prospective study of 136 patients. Ethiop Med J 1994; 32:79-87.
42. Randeree IG, Czarnocki A, Moodley J, et al. Acute renal failure in pregnancy in South Africa. Ren Fail 1995; 17:147-53.
43. Bamgboye EL, Mabayoje MO, Odutola TA, Mabadeje AF. Acute renal failure at the Lagos University Teaching Hospital: a 10-year review. Ren Fail 1993; 15:77-80.
44. Chugh KS, Singhal PC, Kher VK, et al. Spectrum of acute cortical necrosis in Indian patients. Am J Med Sci 1983; 286:10-20.
45. Grunfeld JP, Pertuiset N. Acute renal failure in pregnancy: 1987. Am J Kidney Dis 1987; 9:359-62.
46. Prakash J, Tripathi K, Pandey LK, et al. Renal cortical necrosis in pregnancy-related acute renal failure. J Indian Med Assoc 1996; 94:227-9.
47. Utas C, Yalçindag C, Taskapan H, et al. Acute renal failure in Central Anatolia. Nephrol Dial Transplant 2000; 15:152-5.
48. Hill JB, Yost NP, Wendel GD. Acute renal failure in association with severe hyperemesis gravidarum. Obstet Gynecol 2002; 100:1119-21.
49. Krane NK. Acute renal failure in pregnancy. Arch Intern Med 1988; 148:2347-57.
50. Khanna N, Nguyen H. Reversible acute renal failure in association with bilateral ureteral obstruction and hydronephrosis in pregnancy. Am J Obstet Gynecol 2001; 184:239-40.
51. Ertürk S, Akar H, Uçkuyu A, et al. Delivery of healthy infant during hemodialysis session. J Nephrol 2000; 13:75-7.
52. Homans DC, Blake GD, Harrington JT, Cetrulo CL. Acute renal failure caused by ureteral obstruction by a gravid uterus. JAMA 1981; 246:1230-1.
53. Courban D, Blank S, Harris MA, et al. Acute renal failure in the first trimester resulting from uterine leiomyomas. Am J Obstet Gynecol 1997; 177:472-3.
54. Chugh KS, Jha V, Sakhuja V, Joshi K. Acute renal cortical necrosis—a study of 113 patients. Ren Fail 1994; 16:37-47.
55. Seedat YK, Grant W, Chetty S. Bilateral renal cortical necrosis: a report of 2 cases. S Afr Med J 1976; 50:933-6.
56. Ventura JE, Villa M, Mizraji R, Ferreiros R. Acute renal failure in pregnancy. Ren Fail 1997; 19:217-20.
57. Grunfeld JP, Ganeval D, Bournerias F. Acute renal failure in pregnancy. Kidney Int 1980; 18:179-91.
58. Whalley PJ, Cunningham FG, Martin FG. Transient renal dysfunction associated with acute pyelonephritis of pregnancy. Obstet Gynecol 1975; 46:174-7.
59. Stratta P, Canavese C, Dogliani M, et al. Pregnancy-related acute renal failure. Clin Nephrol 1989; 32:14-20.
60. Sibai BM, Ramadan MK. Acute renal failure in pregnancies complicated by hemolysis, elevated liver enzymes, and low platelets. Am J Obstet Gynecol 1993; 168:1682-7; (discussion 1687-90).
61. Abraham KA, Kennelly M, Dorman AM, Walshe JJ. Pathogenesis of acute renal failure associated with the HELLP syndrome: A case report and review of the literature. Eur J Obstet Gynecol Reprod Biol 2003; 108:99-102.
62. Flynn MF, Power RE, Murphy DM, et al. Successful transplantation of kidneys from a donor with HELLP syndrome-related death. Transpl Int 2001; 14:108-10.
63. Robson JS, Martin AM, Ruckley V, Macdonald MK. Irreversible postpartum renal failure. A new syndrome. Q J Med 1968; 37:423-35.
64. Hayslett JP. Current concepts. Postpartum renal failure. N Engl J Med 1985; 312:1556-9.

65. Sun NC, Johnson WJ, Sung DT, Woods JE. Idiopathic postpartum renal failure: review and case report of a successful renal transplantation. Mayo Clin Proc 1975; 50:395-401.
66. Segonds A, Louradour N, Suc JM, Orfila C. Postpartum hemolytic uremic syndrome: a study of three cases with a review of the literature. Clin Nephrol 1979; 12:229-42.
67. Li PK, Lai FM, Tam JS, Lai KN. Acute renal failure due to postpartum haemolytic uraemic syndrome. Aust N Z J Obstet Gynaecol 1988; 28:228-30.
68. Marcovici I, Marzano D. Pregnancy-induced hypertension complicated by postpartum renal failure and pancreatitis: A case report. Am J Perinatol 2002; 19:177-9.
69. Nzerue CM, Hewan Lowe K, Nwawka C. Acute renal failure in pregnancy: A review of clinical outcomes at an inner-city hospital from 1986-1996. J Natl Med Assoc 1998; 90:486-90.
70. Naqvi R, Akhtar F, Ahmed E, et al. Acute renal failure of obstetrical origin during 1994 at one center. Ren Fail 1996; 18:681-3.
71. Lindheimer MD, Katz AI, Ganeval D, Grünfeld JP. Acute renal failure in pregnancy. In: Brenner BM, Lazarus JM, eds. Acute Renal Failure. New York: Churchill Livingstone, 1988:597-620.
72. Gilbert WM, Towner DR, Field NT, Anthony J. The safety and utility of pulmonary artery catheterization in severe preeclampsia and eclampsia. Am J Obstet Gynecol 2000; 182:1397-403.
73. Murray JE, Reid DE, Harrison JH, Merrill JP. Successful pregnancies after human renal transplantation. N Engl J Med 1963; 269:341-3.
74. Hostetter TH, Olson JL, Rennke HG, et al. Hyperfiltration in remnant nephrons: a potentially adverse response to renal ablation. Am J Physiol 1981; 241:F85-93.
75. Terasaki PI, Koyama H, Cecka JM, Gjertson DW. The hyperfiltration hypothesis in human renal transplantation. Transplantation 1994; 57:1450-4.
76. Baylis C, Wilson CB. Sex and the single kidney. Am J Kidney Dis 1989; 13:290-8.
77. Baylis C, Reckelhoff JF. Renal hemodynamics in normal and hypertensive pregnancy: lessons from micropuncture. Am J Kidney Dis 1991; 17:98-104.
78. Hakim RM, Goldszer RC, Brenner BM. Hypertension and proteinuria: long-term sequelae of uninephrectomy in humans. Kidney Int 1984; 25:930-6.
79. Davison JM. Dialysis, transplantation, and pregnancy. Am J Kidney Dis 1991; 17:127-32.
80. Sturgiss SN, Davison JM. Effect of pregnancy on long-term function of renal allografts. Am J Kidney Dis 1992; 19:167-72.
81. Crowe AV, Rustom R, Gradden C, et al. Pregnancy does not adversely affect renal transplant function. QJM 1999; 92:631-5.
82. Little MA, Abraham KA, Kavanagh J, et al. Pregnancy in Irish renal transplant recipients in the cyclosporine era. Ir J Med Sci 2000; 169: 19-21.
83. Miniero R, Tardivo I, Curtoni ES, et al. Pregnancy after renal transplantation in Italian patients: Focus on fetal outcome. J Nephrol 2002; 15:626-32.
84. Mahanty HD, Cherikh WS, Chang GJ, et al. Influence of pretransplant pregnancy on survival of renal allografts from living donors. Transplantation 2001; 72:228-32.
85. Sgro MD, Barozzino T, Mirghani HM, et al. Pregnancy outcome post renal transplantation. Teratology 2002; 65:5-9.
86. Tan PK, Tan AS, Tan HK, et al. Pregnancy after renal transplantation: experience in Singapore General Hospital. Ann Acad Med Singapore 2002; 31:285-9.
87. Armenti VT, Coscia LA, McGrory CH, Moritz MJ. National Transplantation Pregnancy Registry: Update on pregnancy and renal transplantation. Nephrol News Issues 1998; 12:19-23.
88. Gaston RS. Maintenance immunosuppression in the renal transplant recipient: An overview. Am J Kidney Dis 2001; 38:S25-35.
89. Bar J, Stahl B, Hod M, et al. Is immunosuppression therapy in renal allograft recipients teratogenic? A single-center experience. Am J Med Genet 2003; 116A:31-6.
90. Scott JR, Branch DW, Holman J. Autoimmune and pregnancy complications in the daughter of a kidney transplant patient. Transplantation 2002; 73:815-6.
91. Willis FR, Findlay CA, Gorrie MJ, et al. Children of renal transplant recipient mothers. J Paediatr Child Health 2000; 36:230-5.
92. Kainz A, Harabacz I, Cowlrick IS, et al. Review of the course and outcome of 100 pregnancies in 84 women treated with tacrolimus. Transplantation 2000; 70:1718-21.
93. Schen FP, Stallone G, Schena A, et al. Pregnancy in renal transplantation: immunologic evaluation of neonates from mothers with transplanted kidney. Transpl Immunol 2002; 9:161-4.
94. Karidas CN, Michailidis GD, Spencer K, Economides DL. Biochemical screening for Down syndrome in pregnancies following renal transplantation. Prenat Diagn 2002; 22:226-30.
95. Biesenbach G, Zazgornik J, Kaiser W, et al. Cyclosporin requirement during pregnancy in renal transplant recipients. Nephrol Dial Transplant 1989; 4:667-9.
96. Al Shohaib S. Erythropoietin therapy in a pregnant post-renal transplant patient. Nephron 1999; 81:81-3.
97. Thorp M, Pulliam J. Use of recombinant erythropoietin in a pregnant renal transplant recipient. Am J Nephrol 1998; 18:448-51.
98. Sowter MC, Burgess NA, Woodsford PV, Lewis MH. Delayed presentation of an extradural abscess complicating thoracic extradural analgesia. Br J Anaesth 1992; 68:103-5.
99. Lewis DF, Robichaux AG, Jaekle RK, et al. Urolithiasis in pregnancy: Diagnosis, management and pregnancy outcome. J Reprod Med 2003; 48:28-32.
100. Butler EL, Cox SM, Eberts EG, Cunningham FG. Symptomatic nephrolithiasis complicating pregnancy. Obstet Gynecol 2000; 96:753-6.
101. Gertner JM, Coustan DR, Kliger AS, et al. Pregnancy as state of physiologic absorptive hypercalciuria. Am J Med 1986; 81:451-6.
102. Loughlin KR, Ker LA. The current management of urolithiasis during pregnancy. Urol Clin North Am 2002; 29:701-4.
103. Horowitz E, Schmidt JD. Renal calculi in pregnancy. Clin Obstet Gynecol 1985; 28:324-38.
104. Burke BJ, Washowich TL. Ureteral jets in normal second- and third-trimester pregnancy. J Clin Ultrasound 1998; 26:423-6.
105. Grenier N, Pariente JL, Trillaud H, et al. Dilatation of the collecting system during pregnancy: physiologic vs obstructive dilatation. Eur Radiol 2000; 10:271-9.
106. Asrat T, Roossin MC, Miller EI. Ultrasonographic detection of ureteral jets in normal pregnancy. Am J Obstet Gynecol 1998; 178:1194-8.
107. Swartz HM, Reichling BA. Hazards of radiation exposure for pregnant women. JAMA 1978; 239:1907-8.
108. Harvey EB, Boice JD, Honeyman M, Flannery JT. Prenatal x-ray exposure and childhood cancer in twins. N Engl J Med 1985; 312:541-5.
109. Coe FL, Parks JH, Lindheimer MD. Nephrolithiasis during pregnancy. N Engl J Med 1978; 298:324-6.
110. Coe FL, Keck J, Norton ER. The natural history of calcium urolithiasis. JAMA 1977; 238:1519-23.
111. Honoré LH. The increased incidence of renal stones in women with spontaneous abortion: a retrospective study. Am J Obstet Gynecol 1980; 137:145-6.
112. Eaton A, Martin PC. Ruptured ureter in pregnancy: A unique case? Br J Urol 1981; 53:78-9.
113. Drago JR, Rohner TJ, Chez RA. Management of urinary calculi in pregnancy. Urology 1982; 20:578-81.
114. Armon PJ. Obstructed labour due to a vesical calculus. Br Med J 1977; 2:498.
115. Watterson JD, Girvan AR, Beiko DT, et al. Ureteroscopy and holmium:YAG laser lithotripsy: an emerging definitive management strategy for symptomatic ureteral calculi in pregnancy. Urology 2002; 60:383-7.
116. Streem SB. Contemporary clinical practice of shock wave lithotripsy: a reevaluation of contraindications. J Urol 1997; 157:1197-203.
117. Gray MJ. Use and abuse of thiazides in pregnancy. Clin Obstet Gynecol 1968; 11:568-78.
118. Mjolnerod OK, Dommerud SA, Rasmussen K, Gjeruldsen ST. Congenital connective-tissue defect probably due to D-penicillamine treatment in pregnancy. Lancet 1971; 1:673-5.
119. Gregory MC, Mansell MA. Pregnancy and cystinuria. Lancet 1983; 2:1158-60.
120. Maikranz P, Coe FL, Parks J, Lindheimer MD. Nephrolithiasis in pregnancy. Am J Kidney Dis 1987; 9:354-8.
121. Carella MJ, Gossain VV. Hyperparathyroidism and pregnancy: case report and review. J Gen Intern Med 1992; 7:448-53.
122. Schnatz PF, Curry SL. Primary hyperparathyroidism in pregnancy: Evidence-based management. Obstet Gynecol Surv 2002; 57:365-76.
123. Ready LB, Johnson ES. Epidural block for treatment of renal colic during pregnancy. Can Anaesth Soc J 1981; 28:77-9.
124. Romagnoli A. Letter: Continuous epidural block in the treatment of impacted ureteric stones. Can Med Assoc J 1973; 109:968.
125. Lloyd JW, Carrie LES. A method of treating renal colic. Proc R Soc Med 1965; 58:634-9.

Chapter 51
Respiratory Disease

Karen S. Lindeman, M.D.

ASTHMA

Definition

Asthma is defined by the presence of the following three characteristic findings: (1) reversible airway obstruction, (2) airway inflammation, and (3) airway hyperresponsiveness.[1] **Airway obstruction** produces the clinical manifestations of wheezing, cough, and dyspnea. **Airway inflammation** modulates the course of asthma by independently producing airway obstruction and enhancing airway responsiveness. **Airway hyperresponsiveness** is marked by exaggerated responses to a wide variety of bronchoconstrictor stimuli, including histamine, methacholine, prostaglandin $F_{2-alpha}$, hypoosmotic solutions, and cold air.[2]

Epidemiology

Asthma is an increasingly common problem among young, otherwise healthy women of childbearing age. Morbidity and mortality rates from this disease have increased during the last two decades. The prevalence of asthma increased 29% between 1980 and 1987, and hospitalization discharge rates increased threefold.[3] The reasons underlying these increases are unknown.

Asthma complicates pregnancy in approximately 6% of women.[4,5] However, the actual prevalence may be higher because at least 10% of the population suffers from nonspecific airway hyperresponsiveness that characterizes asthma. The prevalence of asthma is 12% among pregnant women in Australia.[6]

Pathophysiology

The underlying defect that produces the clinical syndrome of asthma is unknown. The most important potential mecha-

nisms include (1) an enhancement of contractility or an impairment of relaxation of airway smooth muscle, (2) a neural imbalance, (3) airway inflammation, and (4) changes in the function of airway epithelium.

AIRWAY SMOOTH MUSCLE

Contraction of airway smooth muscle is thought to be the most important factor in producing acute airway obstruction. For many years, an enhancement of airway smooth muscle responsiveness to contractile agonists was assumed to be a major mechanism of asthma. To test this hypothesis, investigators attempted to correlate airway responsiveness in vivo and in vitro in human subjects[7-11] and in the Basenji-greyhound dog model of asthma.[12] These studies did not demonstrate a significant correlation between the airway response to histamine or cholinergic agonists in vivo and airway smooth muscle contraction in vitro. Some studies actually demonstrated a negative correlation between the responses in vivo and in vitro,[11,12] suggesting that diminished responsiveness may represent a chronic adaptive response of airway smooth muscle.

Instead of an enhancement in responsiveness to contractile stimuli, a reduction in responsiveness to relaxant stimuli may contribute to airway obstruction. One study demonstrated impaired relaxant responses to isoproterenol in airway smooth muscle from human asthmatic subjects when compared with the responsiveness of airway smooth muscle from controls.[13] Other evidence substantiates the presence of impaired airway relaxation in asthmatic subjects in vivo.[14] Although the mechanism for this effect is poorly understood, a reduction in airway sensitivity to beta-adrenergic agonists could contribute to airway hyperresponsiveness by altering the balance between constricting and dilating influences.

NEURAL COMPONENTS

A balance between constricting and dilating influences also exists with respect to the autonomic nervous system. A shift in this balance, with an increase in constricting influences, may be a mechanism of asthma.

The parasympathetic nervous system provides the dominant constrictor input to the airways (Figure 51-1). Efferent cholinergic fibers travel in the vagus nerve to synapse in ganglia within the airway wall.[15] Postganglionic fibers release acetylcholine to activate muscarinic receptors and stimulate airway smooth muscle contraction. A negative feedback system limits acetylcholine release from nerve terminals. Muscarinic autoreceptors, or receptors on the nerve ending,[16] also are activated by acetylcholine and inhibit further release of acetylcholine from the nerve terminal.

The importance of exaggerated cholinergic efferent activity in the pathogenesis of airway hyperreactivity has been debated extensively. The relatively limited efficacy of anticholinergic agents in relieving clinical bronchospasm, as well as growing evidence supporting other mechanisms, suggests that this pathway has a limited role in the pathophysiology of asthma. However, this mechanism appears to be very important in the perioperative management of asthmatic subjects. Reflex stimulation of airway smooth muscle by placement of an endotracheal tube represents one of the most important causes of bronchospasm in the perioperative period.

An alternative mechanism by which the parasympathetic nervous system may contribute to airway hyperresponsiveness is through dysfunction of the muscarinic autoreceptors. Dysfunction of these receptors allows increased postganglionic release of acetylcholine after reflex stimulation.[17] This mechanism is well established in a guinea pig model of viral infection[18] and may explain the airway hyperresponsiveness that occurs for several weeks after an upper respiratory tract infection.[19] The role of this mechanism in the pathophysiology of clinical asthma is unclear.

The sympathetic nervous system primarily acts to decrease airway tone. In contrast to the parasympathetic nervous system, sympathetic innervation of airway smooth muscle in human subjects is either sparse or absent.[20] Circulating catecholamines activate beta-adrenoceptors in airway smooth muscle and provide the primary sympathetic efferent input to human airways. Because airways of normal human subjects do not become hyperresponsive after beta-adrenergic blockade,[21] it is unlikely that impaired catecholamine secretion contributes significantly to the pathogenesis of asthma.

The alpha-adrenergic system is thought to play a relatively minor role in determining the state of airway responsiveness. Although alpha-adrenoceptors are present in human airways,[22] the protective effects of alpha-adrenergic antagonists have been disappointing and can be attributed to other properties such as antihistamine activity.

In addition to cholinergic and adrenergic input, a third neural system—the nonadrenergic, noncholinergic (NANC) system—provides efferent nerves to the airways. Both constricting[23] and dilating[24] pathways have been identified. Nitric oxide serves as the inhibitory NANC neurotransmitter in human airways.[25] Potentially, a relative increase in constricting influences or a decrease in dilating influences in the NANC system could contribute to asthma. However, one study demonstrated no deficit in NANC inhibitory pathways in asthmatic subjects.[26] Although the role of the NANC system remains under investigation, current evidence does not support the idea that an imbalance of the NANC system is a major mechanism of asthma.

AIRWAY INFLAMMATION

Airway inflammation appears to serve primarily as a modulating influence in asthma. Inflammation is certainly present in some but not all asthmatic subjects.[27] The process of inflammation involves the occurrence of airway wall edema and infiltration of the mucosa by a variety of inflammatory cells, including neutrophils, mast cells, helper T lymphocytes, macrophages, and eosinophils.[28] These cells produce and release mediators of inflammation, including histamine, leukotrienes, platelet activating factor, prostaglandins, thromboxanes, cytokines, serotonin, and nitric oxide.[28] Mediators can modulate airway responsiveness by stimulating airway smooth muscle contraction,[2] directing migration of inflammatory cells,[30] modifying neural control of the airways,[31] increasing mucosal permeability,[32] or disrupting airway epithelium.[33] In addition, airway inflammation can reduce airway diameter to produce obstruction and can alter airway geometry to enhance responsiveness.[34] The overall importance of inflammation in asthma is unclear. Although inflammation appears to modulate the course of asthma, other factors certainly contribute to the pathogenesis.

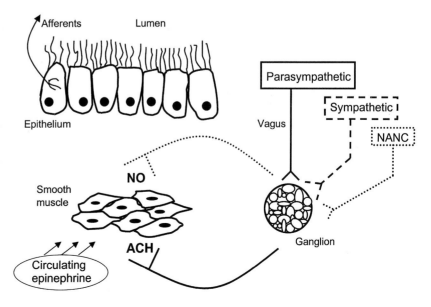

FIGURE 51-1. Neural control of the airway. Parasympathetic, sympathetic, and nonadrenergic, noncholinergic *(NANC)* efferents innervate ganglia within the airway wall. Postganglionic cholinergic efferents release acetylcholine *(ACH)* to constrict airway smooth muscle. Postganglionic NANC efferents release nitric oxide *(NO)* to relax airway smooth muscle. Circulating epinephrine relaxes the airway. Afferents from the airway originate in the epithelium.

AIRWAY EPITHELIUM

The epithelium provides a barrier to protect the subepithelial layers against stimuli that could provoke bronchospasm. Airways of asthmatic subjects demonstrate areas of epithelial destruction,[35] which might increase exposure to constrictor stimuli and enhance airway responsiveness.

In recent years it has become apparent that the epithelium not only has a barrier function but also plays an active role in the maintenance of airway tone. The epithelium produces constricting and dilating factors.[36,37] An alteration in the balance between these factors could alter airway responsiveness. In addition, the epithelium produces enzymes that are important in the metabolism of some constricting agents, such as neuropeptides.[38] Loss of the epithelium could reduce the quantities of these enzymes and potentiate the effects of constricting neuropeptides. The relative importance of these alterations in epithelial function in the pathogenesis of asthma is unknown.

Diagnosis

MEDICAL HISTORY

The classic symptoms of asthma include wheezing, cough, dyspnea, and chest tightness. A patient's medical history also should include information about the pattern and severity of the symptoms, precipitating and aggravating factors, and the duration and course of these symptoms.

PHYSICAL EXAMINATION

Physical examination is directed to the respiratory tract. Auscultation of the chest may reveal wheezing and a prolonged phase of expiration.

LABORATORY STUDIES

Laboratory studies that aid in the diagnosis of asthma depend on findings from the medical history and physical examination. In general, pulmonary function tests are useful to document the severity and establish the reversibility of obstruction (Box 51-1). In the absence of additional findings, other tests are not as useful in establishing the diagnosis of asthma. Bronchoprovocation tests (with agents such as methacholine or histamine) are used when the history and physical examination strongly suggest the presence of asthma but spirometry fails to reveal airway obstruction.

Interaction with Pregnancy

EFFECTS OF PREGNANCY ON ASTHMA

The overall course of asthma has been reported to improve, worsen, or remain the same during pregnancy.[39-42] The variable course of asthma in these studies may reflect differences in the severity of the populations studied because patients with more

---

severe symptoms are more likely to worsen during pregnancy.[40,42] Another reason for the variation in these studies is the variation in the methods of assessing the severity of asthma. Most studies used either clinical symptoms or requirements for pharmacologic therapy as indicators of the course of the disease. These measures do not correlate with objective measures of airway obstruction.[43] Juniper et al.[44] measured methacholine sensitivity before, during, and after pregnancy. Reductions in sensitivity to methacholine occurred during the second and third trimesters when compared with preconception or postpartum measurements (Figure 51-2). Although these findings suggest a reduction in airway hyperresponsiveness during pregnancy, the limited study population (16 subjects) makes extrapolation of the data to the general population uncertain.

Exacerbations of asthma rarely occur during labor and delivery. In one study, the incidence of symptoms during labor was only 10%,[40] and when these symptoms did occur, treatment was either minimal or not required. However, acute exacerbations of asthma are far more likely to occur after cesarean section than after vaginal delivery (41% and 4%, respectively).[45]

A number of mechanisms may be responsible for the changes in the clinical course of asthma during pregnancy (Box 51-2). An increase in the progesterone level is thought to be one mechanism that improves asthma during pregnancy. Progesterone relaxes smooth muscle in the uterus and gastrointestinal tract, and may or may not have similar effects on airway smooth muscle. However, evidence from clinical

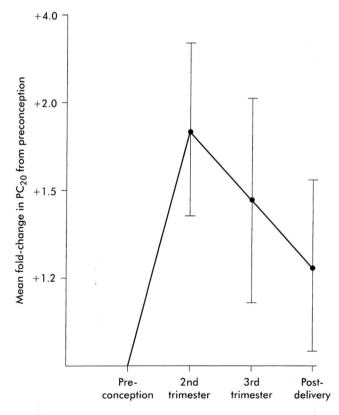

FIGURE 51-2. Airway responsiveness before, during, and after pregnancy expressed as fold change in PC_{20} (dose of methacholine needed to reduce FEV_1 by 20%) when compared with values before conception. ($n = 16$; $P = 0.033$ for the effect of pregnancy on airway responsiveness.) (From Juniper EF, Daniel EE, Roberts RS, et al. Improvement in airway responsiveness and asthma severity during pregnancy. Am Rev Respir Dis 1989; 140:924-31.)

Box 51-1 PULMONARY FUNCTION TESTS IN PATIENTS WITH ASTHMA
Forced vital capacity (FVC) is the volume of gas exhaled after maximal inspiration. • May be reduced in asthma. Forced expiratory volume in 1 second (FEV_1) is the volume exhaled in the first second after maximal inspiration. • May be reduced in asthma. $FEV_1/FVC < 0.75$ in asthma

studies does not support a central role for progesterone in attenuating airway hyperresponsiveness. Juniper et al.[44] detected no strong association between methacholine responsiveness and progesterone levels during pregnancy. In nonpregnant asthmatic patients, neither histamine[46] nor methacholine[47] responsiveness changed during the normal menstrual cycle, although progesterone levels fluctuated markedly. These data suggest that hormonal changes do not affect airway smooth muscle in the same manner as uterine or gastrointestinal smooth muscle. Alternatively, measurements of histamine and methacholine responsiveness may reflect factors other than smooth muscle contractility. In either case, mechanisms underlying the improvement in symptoms of asthma during pregnancy appear to involve factors other than hormonal effects on airway smooth muscle.

EFFECTS OF ASTHMA ON THE PARTURIENT AND FETUS

Several investigators have questioned whether maternal asthma adversely affects perinatal outcome. Studies have reported an increased incidence of preeclampsia,[39] cesarean delivery,[45] low birth weight (LBW) infants,[48] preterm labor,[49] antepartum and postpartum hemorrhage,[50] and perinatal mortality.[51] One study noted that diabetes mellitus was more common among severe asthmatic patients taking corticosteroids.[48] The risk of these adverse outcomes may be higher in patients with severe[48,51] or poorly controlled[52] asthma and in patients who are steroid dependent.[48] When asthma was carefully managed by a pulmonary physician, the risk of adverse outcomes was not increased significantly.[53] The importance of adequate control of asthma and the prevention of recurring episodes of status asthmaticus during pregnancy have been emphasized,[39,40,52] but no controlled studies have documented improved perinatal outcome. A recent multicenter, prospective, observational cohort study[54] noted that asthma was not associated with a significant increase in preterm delivery or other adverse perinatal outcomes other than a discharge diagnosis of neonatal sepsis. This study confirmed earlier observations that the cesarean delivery rate is increased among women with moderate or severe asthma.[54]

Potential mechanisms of increased perinatal morbidity and mortality in patients with uncontrolled asthma include hypoxemia and hypocapnia, which occur during acute exacerbations. Maternal hypocapnia (which may produce uterine vasoconstriction) and hypoxemia diminish fetal oxygen delivery. In addition, asthma-associated inflammatory mediators seem to impair placental function,[55] perhaps via their adverse effects on placental vascular function.[56]

Box 51-2 FACTORS THAT MAY IMPROVE OR WORSEN ASTHMA DURING PREGNANCY

IMPROVE

- Progesterone-induced relaxation of airway smooth muscle
- Increased production of bronchodilating prostaglandins
- Increased circulating cortisol

WORSEN

- Decreased sensitivity to beta-adrenergic agonists
- Increased production of bronchoconstricting prostaglandins
- Reduced sensitivity to circulating cortisol because of binding of steroid hormones (e.g., progesterone) to cortisol receptors

---

Medical Management

Pharmacologic therapy of asthma during pregnancy is directed toward avoiding acute exacerbations and episodes of status asthmaticus. Ideally, management should begin before conception. Although general principles typically dictate that unnecessary medication should be avoided during pregnancy, studies investigating the effects of asthma on perinatal outcome suggest that the risks of uncontrolled asthma are significantly higher. Medications that are currently used to treat asthma fall into two general categories—bronchodilators and antiinflammatory agents. These agents generally are safe for the fetus. The prophylactic use of antibiotics is unnecessary.

BRONCHODILATORS

Beta-adrenergic agonists exert beneficial effects in patients with asthma by activating beta$_2$-adrenergic receptors, which mediate a number of processes (Box 51-3). Short-acting beta-adrenergic agonists represent the most effective therapy for acute exacerbations of asthma.[57-59]

Daily use of long-acting beta-adrenergic agonists is thought to improve the control of asthma and reduce airway hyperresponsiveness, but the mechanism has not been clearly defined. Clinical trials documenting the safety of regular use of long-acting beta-adrenergic agonists have allayed previously held concerns. Despite well-maintained baseline bronchodilation, some patients develop a tolerance to the protective effect of a beta-adrenergic agonist in attenuating the response to a constrictor stimulus.[60] Although regular use of beta-adrenergic agonists in asthma may be beneficial in conjunction with other forms of therapy, these agents do not appear to provide optimal control of asthma when used alone. Conversely, no compelling evidence requires that beta-adrenergic agonists be discontinued after conception or that their use be reserved for treatment of an acute exacerbation.

Routes of administration include aerosol, oral, and parenteral. The aerosol route generally is preferred during pregnancy because high concentrations of the medication can be delivered directly to the site of activity in the airways. The aerosol route minimizes maternal systemic effects and potential fetal risk.

A limited number of human studies have investigated the fetal safety of chronic administration of a beta-adrenergic agonist. In one study of 259 asthmatic parturients, the use of an inhaled beta$_2$-adrenergic agonist was not associated with congenital malformations or an increased incidence of intrauterine growth restriction, preterm delivery, or perinatal mortality.[61] In addition, the fact that these agents have been used for many years without reports of teratogenicity suggests that their use should not be restricted because of fetal concerns. Optimal control of maternal symptoms of asthma appears to be more important for the fetus than any potential detrimental effects of beta-adrenergic agonists.

Methylxanthines (e.g., theophylline, aminophylline) have been used for many years in the chronic treatment of

---

Box 51-3 MECHANISMS OF BENEFICIAL EFFECTS OF BETA-ADRENERGIC AGONISTS IN ASTHMA

- Direct airway smooth muscle relaxation
- Enhanced mucociliary transport
- Decreased airway edema
- Inhibition of cholinergic neurotransmission

asthma. Although their mechanism of action is controversial, relaxation of airway smooth muscle is the most prominent effect. The ability of these agents to inhibit intracellular phosphodiesterase and increase concentrations of cyclic adenosine monophosphate (cAMP) is not the mechanism of bronchodilation because these effects do not occur at clinically relevant concentrations in vivo.[62]

Methylxanthines have been used for many years in pregnant asthmatic subjects without reported detrimental effects on the fetus.[63] Serum concentrations of these agents should be monitored carefully, especially in the third trimester, when theophylline clearance decreases.[64]

The addition of a methylxanthine to a regimen that already includes a beta-adrenergic agonist may not confer additional benefit,[65] perhaps because a major mechanism of the acute effects of methylxanthines is the release of catecholamines.[66] These agents typically are reserved for patients who respond poorly to other forms of therapy.

Bronchodilation with **anticholinergic agents** occurs through the blockade of muscarinic receptors on airway smooth muscle. Anticholinergic agents alone are not as effective as beta-adrenergic agonists.[67] Perhaps the limited efficacy of these agents results from the increase in acetylcholine release that results from the blockade of inhibitory autoreceptors on cholinergic nerves. However, unlike methylxanthines, anticholinergic agents enhance bronchodilation when they are combined with beta-adrenergic agonists.[67]

Although atropine was used in the past, the introduction of **quaternary compounds (e.g., ipratropium bromide)** allows aerosol delivery of a higher concentration of an anticholinergic agent to the lungs with less systemic absorption[67,68] and reduced concentrations in the fetus. Human data on potential teratogenicity are lacking, but ipratropium bromide is not associated with teratogenicity in animal studies.[69]

ANTIINFLAMMATORY AGENTS

Proposed mechanisms of **corticosteroid** action include (1) decreases in cellular infiltration and mediator release, (2) decreases in airway permeability, and (3) up-regulation of the beta-adrenergic system.[70] Unlike bronchodilators, these agents not only reduce airway sensitivity to a constrictor stimulus[71] but also decrease the maximal degree of airway narrowing,[72] which may predict the severity of an acute asthmatic episode.

The use of **inhaled corticosteroids** has gained popularity. This route of administration is effective and may limit fetal side effects. Effects of systemic and inhaled corticosteroids on the fetus are controversial. Neither systemic nor inhaled corticosteroids have been documented to increase the risk of congenital malformations in humans. Although some earlier studies documented an increased incidence of preterm and LBW infants in steroid-dependent mothers,[48,73] these studies did not distinguish between severe, poorly controlled disease and effects of the pharmacologic agent. When these factors were controlled, corticosteroid use during pregnancy was not associated with increased perinatal risk.[74]

Corticosteroids may increase perinatal morbidity by exacerbating maternal glucose intolerance, especially in women who also are treated with a beta-adrenergic agonist.[75] Thus careful monitoring of maternal glucose is indicated in asthmatic women who are treated with a corticosteroid during pregnancy. However, because of the efficacy of corticosteroids in controlling severe asthma during pregnancy,[76] these agents should not be withheld from the medical regimen.

Some authors have recommended that steroid-dependent asthmatic women receive large doses of parenteral steroids during labor to prevent complications related to adrenal suppression.[63,77,78] The scientific basis for this recommendation is questionable. Although physiologic glucocorticoid replacement reduced hemodynamic instability and mortality in adrenalectomized primates that underwent surgery, supraphysiologic doses provided no additional benefit.[79] There is little information regarding the benefit of steroid replacement therapy during labor. To my knowledge, there are no published clinical studies that have compared hemodynamic responses and morbidity in steroid-treated versus untreated patients during labor and delivery. Administration of physiologic doses of corticosteroids during labor and delivery seems warranted, but the benefit of supraphysiologic doses of steroids in the peripartum management of asthmatic women is unclear. The potential for adrenal insufficiency in infants of mothers taking corticosteroids appears to be very low.[78] This risk may be low because of the widespread use of either prednisone or prednisolone. In the mother, prednisone is converted rapidly to prednisolone, which crosses the placenta to a very limited extent.

Cromolyn sodium and **nedocromil sodium** belong to a class of drugs that are thought to reduce inflammation and mediator release primarily by stabilizing mast cells and perhaps other cells as well. Nedocromil also may prevent the release of constricting neuropeptides from sensory nerve terminals after exposure to an irritant stimulus.[80]

Cromolyn and nedocromil are administered as aerosols. Clinical experience suggests that their effects on the fetus are minimal, but placental transfer has not been evaluated. Although neither animal nor human studies have reported an increased risk of teratogenicity with cromolyn sodium, the number of studies is limited.[63] Because there is even less information regarding the fetal effects of nedocromil sodium, inhaled cromolyn sodium is preferred. Only a subset of asthmatic subjects respond to cromolyn, but the limited information regarding fetal effects does not support the need to discontinue cromolyn during pregnancy in those patients who respond.

Based on the observation that leukotrienes are released into the airways by immune cells and contribute to the inflammatory process, newer forms of antiinflammatory therapy include **leukotriene receptor antagonists** and **leukotriene synthesis inhibitors**.[81] There is no information regarding the safety of these agents during human pregnancy.

Obstetric Management

Three aspects of obstetric management of the asthmatic parturient may differ from that of the normal patient: (1) induction of labor, (2) management of postpartum hemorrhage, and (3) treatment of hypertension.

For induction of labor, prostaglandins should be administered cautiously in women with asthma. Prostaglandin $F_{2\text{-alpha}}$ constricts airways in vivo[2,82] and in vitro.[83] Airways of asthmatic subjects demonstrate an increased sensitivity to prostaglandin $F_{2\text{-alpha}}$, and its use to induce labor is associated with bronchospasm.[84] Prostaglandin E_2 dilates airways in vitro,[83] but aerosols can provoke bronchoconstriction in asthmatic subjects in vivo,[82] most likely through an irritant effect. Because of the known risk of bronchospasm after exposure to prostaglandin $F_{2\text{-alpha}}$ and the possible risk after exposure to prostaglandin E_2, alternative methods of induction of labor

are preferred in asthmatic women. Likewise, asthma represents a relative contraindication to the administration of 15-methyl prostaglandin $F_{2\text{-alpha}}$ (carboprost, Hemabate) for the treatment of postpartum hemorrhage.

The use of ergot alkaloids to treat postpartum hemorrhage in asthmatic women has been questioned.[63] Although controlled studies have not been performed, ergot alkaloids have been associated with episodes of acute bronchospasm,[85-87] either on the basis of their tryptaminergic actions or their ability to activate alpha$_1$-adrenergic receptors on airway smooth muscle. Oxytocin, which does not seem to affect airway tone, is the preferred ecbolic agent in asthmatic patients.

Beta-adrenergic receptor antagonists are used to treat hypertension in some pregnant women. In asthmatic patients, these agents may provoke bronchospasm,[88,89] possibly by blocking the bronchodilating properties of circulating epinephrine. Other antihypertensive agents (e.g., hydralazine, sodium nitroprusside, trimethaphan) do not seem to enhance airway responsiveness.

Anesthetic Management

PREOPERATIVE ASSESSMENT

During the preoperative evaluation, the anesthesiologist should assess the severity of the disease and whether an acute asthmatic episode is present. The medical history should include information about symptoms of wheezing, dyspnea, and cough. Further information should include the frequency and severity of symptoms, the course of these symptoms during pregnancy, and the date of the most recent exacerbation. Patients who suffer frequent, severe attacks are at increased risk for morbidity in the peripartum period.

Physical examination should focus on the pulmonary system. Chest auscultation may reveal wheezing, with or without a prolonged expiratory phase. However, wheezing may not be audible if air movement is markedly reduced. Additional signs of an acute exacerbation of asthma include tachypnea, an exaggerated (greater than 20 mm Hg) pulsus paradoxus, and the use of accessory respiratory muscles.

In a stable asthmatic parturient, laboratory tests add little to anesthetic management. However, if an acute exacerbation is suspected, chest radiographic examination, arterial blood gas measurements, and pulmonary function tests may assist with diagnosis and therapy. **Chest radiographic examination** helps diagnose precipitating or complicating conditions such as pneumonia, pneumothorax, and heart failure. During an episode of acute asthma, **arterial blood gas measurements** often reveal hypoxemia and respiratory alkalosis. After a prolonged, severe episode, arterial carbon dioxide tension rises as a result of fatigue. **Spirometry** measures the volume of gas exhaled over time (Box 51-1). The most convenient indirect measurement for assessing airway obstruction during labor is the **peak expiratory flow rate,** which can be measured at the bedside with a Wright peak-flow meter.[90]

MANAGEMENT DURING LABOR AND VAGINAL DELIVERY

The goals of analgesia for labor and delivery in asthmatic women include (1) provision of pain relief, (2) a reduction in the stimulus to hyperpnea, and (3) prevention or relief of maternal stress. It is especially important to prevent hyperpnea and stress in women who describe asthmatic episodes triggered by exercise or stress. These goals should be accomplished with minimal sedation, minimal paralysis of the muscles of respiration, and minimal depression of the fetus. Possible analgesic regimens include systemic opioids, paracervical block, pudendal nerve block, lumbar sympathetic block, and epidural or spinal analgesia using local anesthetic agents, opioids, or both.

Systemic opioids may provide reasonable pain relief and reduce the stimulus to hyperpnea, especially during the first stage of labor. In theory, opioids reduce the risk of bronchospasm in asthmatic subjects. Opiate receptors are thought to be present in the respiratory tract[91] and to inhibit the release of excitatory neuropeptides. The ability of moderate doses of morphine to attenuate bronchoconstriction in response to aerosolized capsaicin[92] (which causes a release of neuropeptides) suggests that opioids may inhibit bronchoconstriction resulting from stimulation of afferent sensory fibers. The clinical relevance of these findings has not been determined. Conversely, opioids may increase the risk of bronchospasm by releasing histamine. Although high doses of morphine are associated with increased plasma levels of histamine,[93] no controlled studies have documented an increased incidence of bronchospasm in asthmatic subjects. High doses of these agents are not desirable in subjects with active wheezing because of the risks of maternal and neonatal respiratory depression (see Chapter 20).

Paracervical and **pudendal nerve block** performed by an obstetrician are reasonable choices for analgesia during the first and second stages of labor, respectively. These techniques provide analgesia without sedation or paralysis of the respiratory muscles. The problems with these techniques in asthmatic women are similar to those in normal patients (see Chapter 22).

Lumbar sympathetic block also provides pain relief without sedation and motor block during the first stage of labor. Unfortunately, this technique requires special skills. Moreover, this block has a limited duration, and it does not provide analgesia or anesthesia for the second stage of labor (see Chapter 22).

Intrathecal and **epidural opioid** techniques are useful during the first stage of labor (see Chapter 21). The advantage of the absence of motor block in an asthmatic subject should be weighed against the risk of respiratory depression.

Advantages of the use of local anesthetic agents for **lumbar epidural analgesia** in asthmatic patients include continuous pain relief and a reduction in the stimulus to hyperventilation. These goals typically are achieved without maternal sedation or neonatal depression. Unlike other analgesic techniques, continuous lumbar epidural analgesia adds a margin of safety by providing the opportunity to extend the sensory block for cesarean section. This allows the anesthesiologist to avoid some of the risks of general endotracheal anesthesia. The most significant disadvantage of epidural local anesthetics in an asthmatic subject is the risk of a high thoracic motor block and respiratory insufficiency. Maintenance of a sensory level at the tenth thoracic dermatome minimizes this risk. In addition, the use of a dilute concentration of bupivacaine combined with a modest dose of fentanyl is safe for the fetus and produces satisfactory analgesia with less motor block than bupivacaine alone.[94]

MANAGEMENT DURING CESAREAN SECTION

The choice between regional anesthesia and general anesthesia for cesarean section depends on obstetric considerations and the respiratory status of the parturient. Because the presence of an endotracheal tube is the factor most closely associated with bronchospasm during the perioperative period,[95] techniques that avoid endotracheal intubation during light anesthesia minimize the risk of bronchospasm.

The most significant advantage of regional anesthesia in the asthmatic patient is that this technique obviates the necessity for endotracheal intubation. Regional anesthesia is associated with a lower incidence of bronchospasm in asthmatic subjects than general anesthesia.[95] Stable asthmatic patients can undergo either spinal anesthesia or epidural anesthesia. In unstable asthmatic patients who require the use of accessory muscles of respiration, regional anesthesia may not be appropriate because of impaired ventilatory capacity in the presence of a high thoracic motor block.

The adrenal medulla receives innervation from preganglionic sympathetic fibers arising from the sixth thoracic to the second lumbar spinal segment.[96] Some physicians have postulated that regional anesthesia and the ensuing sympathectomy could precipitate or potentiate bronchospasm during cesarean section in asthmatic subjects by reducing the adrenal output of epinephrine.[97] This possibility seems remote for several reasons. First, this hypothesis implies that an increase in circulating catecholamines decreases sensitivity of the airways to constricting stimuli. In fact, the severity of histamine-induced bronchoconstriction does not correlate with plasma catecholamine concentrations in asthmatic patients.[98] Second, epinephrine concentrations do not decrease during nonobstetric surgery performed under regional anesthesia with high thoracic sensory levels.[99,100] Third, the possibility that regional anesthesia may prevent increases in circulating epinephrine that are required to compensate for stress-induced bronchospasm does not appear to be valid. Bronchoconstriction does not stimulate epinephrine secretion in human asthmatic subjects.[101] These findings suggest that although basal levels of circulating epinephrine may play a significant role in the maintenance of airway tone, large increases do not afford a great degree of additional protection against intraoperative bronchospasm. Thus regional anesthesia (with a high thoracic sensory level) is appropriate for cesarean section in stable asthmatic subjects.

General anesthesia for asthmatic subjects undergoing cesarean section requires a balance between the competing considerations of aspiration and intraoperative bronchospasm. The high risk of aspiration mandates endotracheal intubation, but airway instrumentation provides the greatest stimulus for bronchospasm in the perioperative period.[95]

Most commonly, the options for endotracheal intubation include awake intubation or rapid-sequence induction, although mask induction of general anesthesia with sevoflurane has been described in a parturient in status asthmaticus.[102] Pretreatment with an aerosolized beta-adrenergic agonist, by its direct effects on airway smooth muscle, may reduce the risk of bronchospasm before endotracheal intubation. Indications for awake intubation in asthmatic subjects are similar to those for normal patients, but the additional risk of bronchospasm should be considered. The benefits of topical local anesthetics and airway nerve blocks should be weighed against a possible increase in the risk of aspiration from the loss of protective airway reflexes. Rapid-sequence induction for cesarean section is most often accomplished using either **thiopental** or **ketamine.** In an animal model of airway hyperresponsiveness, ketamine affords greater protection against reflex-mediated bronchoconstriction than thiopental,[103] most likely on the basis of its sympathomimetic properties. Alternatively, **propofol** provides better protection against bronchospasm associated with endotracheal intubation in asthmatic patients than does thiopental.[104] The mechanism for this effect is unknown but does not appear to result from the direct effects of propofol on airway smooth muscle.[105]

No controlled studies have compared the airway response to endotracheal intubation after induction with either ketamine or propofol, but propofol may be a better choice when stimulation of the sympathetic nervous system is not a desired outcome. **Lidocaine,** which also attenuates airway reflexes, may provide additional benefit. The intravenous route of administration is preferred; aerosol administration can provoke an increase in lung resistance in animals with airway hyperresponsiveness.[106]

In *nonasthmatic* parturients, maintenance of anesthesia typically includes administration of a low concentration of a volatile halogenated agent, with or without nitrous oxide, before delivery of the infant. After delivery, maintenance of anesthesia typically includes nitrous oxide and an intravenous opioid, with or without a low concentration of a volatile halogenated agent. In *asthmatic* parturients, the **volatile halogenated agents** are considered the agents of choice for the maintenance of anesthesia. These agents produce a dose-dependent reduction in airway responsiveness[107] through direct effects on airway smooth muscle,[108-113] inhibition of airway reflexes, and effects on airway epithelium.[110,113,114]

A high concentration of a volatile halogenated agent produces salutary effects on the airways, but it also increases the risk of hemorrhage during cesarean section. Halothane, enflurane, and isoflurane relax uterine smooth muscle in a dose-dependent fashion.[115] Alternatively, nitrous oxide, an intravenous opioid, and a low concentration of a volatile agent may be given. Although halothane and isoflurane are approximately equipotent bronchodilators at high concentrations (e.g., 1.7 minimal alveolar concentration [MAC]), halothane produces greater bronchodilation than isoflurane at lower concentrations (0.6 or 1.1 MAC), and may therefore be preferred for anesthesia during cesarean section.[116] A recent study[117] noted that sevoflurane (1.1 MAC) decreased respiratory system resistance as much or more than did an equipotent concentration of isoflurane or halothane in nonasthmatic human subjects with mild-to-moderate chronic lung disease; however, a comparative study of lower concentrations of these three agents has not been performed. The authors suggested that "sevoflurane may be a worthwhile alternative to the traditional choice of halothane as an adjunct to prevent and manage intraoperative bronchospasm."[117]

A bronchodilator can be added if bronchospasm occurs. The potential disadvantage of this technique is that the most effective bronchodilators (i.e., the beta-adrenergic agonists) also relax uterine smooth muscle. The administration of a beta-adrenergic agonist by aerosol delivers a relatively greater dose of drug to the airways and minimizes uterine relaxation.

Emergence from general anesthesia, like induction, requires a balance between reducing the risk of aspiration and reducing the risk of bronchospasm. Extubation of the trachea when the patient is awake minimizes the risk of aspiration, but the endotracheal tube may stimulate reflexes and precipitate bronchospasm as the depth of anesthesia is reduced. If bronchospasm occurs during emergence, bronchodilators can be administered. For refractory bronchospasm, continued mechanical ventilation in an intensive care unit may be required.

CIGARETTE SMOKING

Epidemiology

Cigarette smoking is a significant, preventable cause of maternal morbidity and perinatal morbidity and mortality. Approximately 80% of women who smoke continue to do so during pregnancy.[118]

Pathophysiology

Cigarette smoke is composed of a large number of separate components that produce a variety of biologic effects. Nonrespiratory effects of cigarette smoking are described in Chapter 52.

The primary respiratory effects of cigarette smoking include alterations in small airway function, increased mucus secretion, and impairment of ciliary transport.[119] The precise mechanisms for these effects are unknown. Smoking also is associated with an increase in nonspecific airway reactivity,[120] possibly on the basis of epithelial damage or altered airway geometry from increased mucus secretion. These changes lead to a marked increase in the incidence of postoperative pulmonary complications.[119]

Interaction with Pregnancy

Few studies have documented the respiratory effects of cigarette smoking during pregnancy. In one study, reductions in forced expiratory flow rates suggested that cigarette smoking increases maternal small airway resistance when compared with that in nonsmokers.[121] These and other abnormalities were similar to the changes in airway function observed in nonpregnant smokers. Although further studies are warranted, other respiratory effects of cigarette smoking in pregnant women are likely to be similar to those effects in nonpregnant women.

Cigarette smoking affects pregnancy in a number of ways. Among these, it reduces the risk of preeclampsia[122] and increases the risks of ectopic pregnancy[123] and placenta previa.[124] Further details regarding adverse maternal and fetal effects are described in Chapter 52.

Medical Management

Cessation of smoking is the preferred form of medical management. Smoking cessation programs are effective in pregnant women.[125] Nonpharmacologic methods are preferred to pharmacologic methods (e.g., nicotine patches) because of insufficient safety information for the latter.[126] Das et al.[127] demonstrated that smoking cessation before or during early pregnancy resulted in prompt improvement in maternal airway function. Former smokers had lung function measurements similar to those of nonsmokers. Further, the mean birth weight of babies born to ex-smokers was similar to that of babies born to nonsmokers and was significantly greater than that of babies born to pregnant women who continued to smoke. Smoking cessation reduces perioperative complications in the setting of nonobstetric surgery,[119] but there are no data on the effects of smoking cessation shortly before labor and delivery.

Anesthetic Management

Endotracheal intubation increases the risk of bronchospasm in smokers.[128] For vaginal delivery, any of the analgesic techniques described earlier are acceptable. For cesarean delivery, regional anesthesia achieves the goal of avoiding airway instrumentation and is therefore preferable to general anesthesia, although no controlled studies have documented differences in peripartum morbidity. If general anesthesia is required, the methods for reducing the risk of intraoperative bronchospasm described earlier may be considered. During induction of general anesthesia in smokers, the formulation of propofol containing sulfite results in greater respiratory resistance after endotracheal intubation than the formulation containing ethylenediaminetetraacetic acid (EDTA).[129] The clinical significance of this observation is unknown. One study noted that desflurane failed to reduce respiratory resistance after endotracheal intubation in smokers.[130] Therefore, desflurane may be less desirable than other agents (e.g., sevoflurane) for maintenance of general anesthesia in smokers.

CYSTIC FIBROSIS

Epidemiology

Cystic fibrosis is a lethal genetic disorder that is transmitted as an autosomal recessive trait. The disease occurs in approximately 1 in 2500 live Caucasian births.[131,132] Because of improvements in diagnosis and therapy, an increasing number of women with cystic fibrosis survive to reproductive age. The number of pregnancies reported to a national cystic fibrosis registry doubled between 1986 and 1990 from 52 to 111.[131]

Pathophysiology

Clinical features of cystic fibrosis result from abnormalities of epithelial tissues, especially in the respiratory, digestive, and reproductive tracts. The underlying mechanism is thought to be a defect in cAMP-mediated activation of chloride (Cl^-) conductance in the epithelium.[133,134] Normal epithelial cells secrete Cl^- in response to increased intracellular cAMP. In cystic fibrosis, a genetic mutation makes epithelial cells unable to alter Cl^- permeability in response to changes in cAMP.[133,134] The gene responsible for cystic fibrosis is located on chromosome 7 and encodes a protein known as the *cystic fibrosis transmembrane regulator (CFTR)*.[135,136] The CFTR is a Cl^- channel,[137,138] which also regulates the activity of other Cl^- channels.[139] Transfer of the coding region of normal CFTR DNA to cystic fibrosis cells restores the ability of these cells to secrete Cl^- in response to increased intracellular cAMP.[140,141]

In the lungs, abnormalities of electrolyte transport alter the composition of airway secretions. Inflammation, with infiltration of polymorphonuclear leukocytes, also contributes to changes in airway secretions.[142] Large numbers of disintegrating neutrophils release DNA in quantities sufficient to overwhelm the ability of deoxyribonuclease I (DNAse I), an endogenously released enzyme, to digest extracellular DNA. Undigested DNA increases the viscosity of airway secretions, which causes obstruction of small airways and reduced lung volumes. The ensuing ventilation-perfusion inequalities produce arterial hypoxemia. Some patients manifest hyperreactive airways. Spontaneous pneumothorax often occurs. Chronic airway obstruction and impaired mucus clearance increase the frequency of pulmonary infection. Most patients become colonized or infected with *Pseudomonas aeruginosa*. Eventually, tissue damage leads to bronchiectasis and pulmonary insufficiency. Chronic hypoxemia and lung destruction may produce pulmonary hypertension and cor pulmonale. Nonrespiratory manifestations of cystic fibrosis include pancreatic exocrine insufficiency, intestinal obstruction, and infertility.

Diagnosis

Clinical criteria for the diagnosis of cystic fibrosis include (1) the presence of chronic obstructive lung disease and colonization with *Pseudomonas aeruginosa* before age 20, (2) exocrine pancreatic insufficiency, and (3) a family history of cystic

fibrosis. Laboratory measurements of sweat Cl^- concentrations greater than 60 mEq/L assist with the diagnosis. Chest radiographic examination often demonstrates hyperinflation, and arterial blood gas measurements may show hypoxemia. Pulmonary function tests are useful to assess the severity of the disease. With serial measurements, the clinician should look for evidence of an increased residual volume and reduced FEV_1.[143]

Interaction with Pregnancy

EFFECT OF PREGNANCY ON CYSTIC FIBROSIS

Several factors may contribute to the deterioration of pulmonary function during pregnancy in patients with cystic fibrosis. These factors include (1) increased airway responsiveness and obstruction (as can occur in patients with asthma), (2) increased work of breathing, and (3) cardiovascular changes such as congestive heart failure and pulmonary hypertension associated with the increased blood volume of pregnancy.

Deterioration of pulmonary status is related to the severity of the disease before pregnancy. Canny et al.[144] noted that patients with mild cystic fibrosis had very little deterioration of pulmonary function. Edenborough et al.[145] noted that women with the poorest pulmonary function before pregnancy showed the greatest deterioration during pregnancy and had the greatest mortality. In a study that included a control group of nonpregnant women with cystic fibrosis, FEV_1 decreased similarly in both control and pregnant subjects for as many as 21 months postpartum, but few patients in either group suffered from severe cystic fibrosis.[146] A small study suggested that pregnancy does not appear to have long-term effects on the course of cystic fibrosis,[147] but larger studies are needed.

EFFECT ON CYSTIC FIBROSIS ON PREGNANCY

In patients with severe cystic fibrosis, perinatal complications are increased in the presence of poor maternal pulmonary function.[145,148] The mechanisms are thought to include chronic hypoxemia and poor maternal nutrition. However, the infant survival rate is higher than might be expected.[149] Canny et al.[144] observed that perinatal outcome was better in cystic fibrosis patients who manifested only mild pulmonary dysfunction.

Medical Management

Respiratory management of cystic fibrosis is primarily symptomatic.[150] Patients with large volumes of mucus production undergo postural drainage. Bronchodilators may help those patients who manifest a reversible component of airway obstruction. Continuous antibiotic therapy (e.g., nebulized tobramycin) has been advocated to reduce the incidence of recurrent pulmonary infection during pregnancy,[151] but indications for the use of this therapy and the effects on the fetus have not been defined. Continuous oxygen therapy may benefit patients with hypoxemia and cor pulmonale.

Other forms of therapy include (1) aerosolized human deoxyribonuclease I to reduce the viscosity of lung secretions, (2) lung transplantation,[152,153] and (3) gene therapy.[154] Current approaches to gene therapy include the transfer of the normal CFTR gene to the airway epithelium using viral carriers or nonviral carriers such as liposomes.[155] Other approaches include the use of a CFTR-channel opener to enhance Cl^- flux through existing channels, delivery of normal CFTR protein to the airways, and activation of non-CFTR Cl^- channels.[155]

Obstetric Management

Because of the influence of pregravid maternal health on pregnancy outcome, the primary obstetric issue centers on the advisability of pregnancy in patients with cystic fibrosis. Criteria for the termination of pregnancy are not clearly defined. Genetic counseling regarding the risks of cystic fibrosis in the offspring is another important component of obstetric management.

Anesthetic Management

Considerations regarding anesthetic management focus primarily on the pulmonary system. Because of the high incidence of hypoxemia in patients with cystic fibrosis, the continuous monitoring of maternal oxygen saturation guides oxygen therapy.

The goals of pain relief during labor are to provide adequate analgesia and prevent maternal hyperventilation while avoiding high thoracic motor block and respiratory depression. High thoracic motor block may impair the parturient's ability to cough and eliminate thick secretions. Hyperventilation increases the work of breathing and may cause decompensation in patients with severe pulmonary dysfunction. For pain relief, parenteral opioid analgesia may worsen pulmonary function by depressing respiratory drive and inhibiting cough. Intrathecal opioids have been used successfully[156] but patients should be monitored carefully for respiratory depression. Continuous lumbar epidural analgesia, with a sensory block maintained at the level of the tenth thoracic dermatome, can provide excellent pain relief and reduce the stimulus for hyperventilation with minimal motor block of the thorax. A dilute solution of bupivacaine, with or without an opioid, provides sensory analgesia with minimal motor block and is especially useful in this setting.[157,158]

Cesarean section necessitates the choice between general anesthesia and regional anesthetic techniques. Among patients with cystic fibrosis, no studies have documented differences in outcome between those receiving general or regional anesthesia. Regional anesthesia offers the advantage of avoiding endotracheal intubation, which may be associated with bronchospasm or obstruction of the endotracheal tube with secretions. Regional anesthesia also avoids positive-pressure ventilation, which may enlarge a preexisting pneumothorax. The primary consideration regarding regional anesthesia during cesarean section is to avoid a high thoracic motor block, which may impair ventilation and the ability to cough. Methods for reducing this risk include the use of a continuous catheter technique, which allows titration of the local anesthetic agent to achieve the desired sensory level, and the use of the lowest concentration of local anesthetic (with or without an opioid) that provides surgical anesthesia. Using this approach, Bose et al.[159] reported successful administration of epidural anesthesia—with a sensory level as high as T_6—in a patient suffering from respiratory failure associated with cystic fibrosis.

For general anesthesia, techniques to reduce the risk of bronchospasm during endotracheal intubation may be warranted. Additional considerations include (1) humidification of gases to prevent inspissation of mucus, (2) frequent suctioning, and (3) use of ventilator settings that allow an appropriately long expiratory phase to prevent air trapping. It may be prudent to avoid nitrous oxide because of the possibility of pneumothorax. These patients should be allowed to awaken fully before extubation. Chest physiotherapy may be required in the immediate postoperative period.

RESPIRATORY FAILURE

Epidemiology

Respiratory failure accounts for a significant proportion of maternal deaths.[160] The prevalence of respiratory failure during pregnancy is not known. A large number of these patients have adult respiratory distress syndrome (ARDS). The incidence of ARDS during pregnancy is approximately 1 in 3000 deliveries.[161]

Pathophysiology

The pathophysiology of respiratory failure depends on the underlying disorder. ARDS results from a group of predisposing conditions, but a common final pathway leads to similar manifestations. Damage to the alveolar and capillary membranes initiates a cascade of events leading to fluid transudation that often is accompanied by pulmonary venoconstriction. Direct injury to the alveolar and capillary membranes can result from pulmonary aspiration of gastric contents and perhaps oxygen toxicity. Indirect toxicity can result from humoral and cellular mechanisms.[162] Some experimental models suggest that endogenously released nitric oxide may serve as a mediator of lung injury,[163,164] although in other models nitric oxide serves a protective role by producing vasodilation.[165,166]

Transudation of fluid leads to atelectasis, airway obstruction, and altered ventilation-perfusion relationships. Both physiologic dead space and shunt fractions are increased.

Diagnosis

A variety of disorders can cause acute respiratory failure during pregnancy (Box 51-4). Specific diagnostic criteria depend on the disorder.

The diagnosis of ARDS depends on the exclusion of other disorders. Prominent characteristics of ARDS include arterial hypoxemia, radiographic evidence of pulmonary infiltrates, and reduced lung compliance in the setting of a recognized predisposing condition.[167]

Interaction with Pregnancy

Pregnancy is not known to alter the course of respiratory failure. Maternal mortality is approximately 50%,[161] which is similar to the rate in nonpregnant patients.[167]

The most significant effect of respiratory failure on pregnancy is a reduction in oxygen delivery to the fetus. This reduction results most commonly from maternal arterial hypoxemia or maternal hypotension, which often accompanies respiratory failure. Hypotension may result from associated underlying conditions and elevated mean airway pressures during mechanical ventilation. High rates of perinatal complications have been reported,[168] and preterm delivery is often required.[169]

Medical Management

Therapeutic strategies for managing respiratory failure during pregnancy do not differ significantly from those for nonpregnant patients. The primary goals of medical management are as follows: (1) eliminate predisposing condi-

---

> **Box 51-4 ETIOLOGY OF RESPIRATORY FAILURE DURING PREGNANCY**
>
> **ADULT RESPIRATORY DISTRESS SYNDROME (ARDS)**
> - Infection
>   - Bacterial or viral pneumonia
>   - Endometritis
>   - Pyelonephritis
>   - Sepsis
> - Preeclampsia
> - Hemorrhage
>   - Multiple transfusions
>   - Disseminated intravascular coagulation
> - Aspiration of gastric contents
> - Embolism
> - Drugs
>   - Salicylates
>   - Opioids
>
> **PULMONARY EMBOLISM**
> - Thromboembolism
> - Amniotic fluid embolism
> - Venous air embolism
>
> **CYSTIC FIBROSIS**
>
> **PULMONARY EDEMA**
> - Beta-adrenergic receptor agonists (e.g., ritodrine, terbutaline)
> - Cardiogenic

---

tions, (2) limit fluid transudation, and (3) maintain maternal oxygen delivery. Fluid restriction and diuretics help limit fluid transudation, although this therapy must be used cautiously when the underlying cause of respiratory failure is associated with intravascular fluid depletion. Methods of maintaining oxygen delivery include (1) administration of an increased inspired concentration of oxygen, (2) use of mechanical ventilation, (3) administration of bronchodilators, and (4) administration of pharmacologic agents to support the circulation. In recent years, several investigators have attempted to improve oxygen delivery by the administration of inhaled **nitric oxide** in patients with ARDS. Nitric oxide relaxes smooth muscle. Rapid inactivation of nitric oxide by binding to hemoglobin in the circulation allows inhaled nitric oxide to produce pulmonary vasodilation without systemic vascular effects. Selective pulmonary vasodilation in well-ventilated areas of the lung presumably would improve oxygen delivery. In a recently published randomized trial, Dellinger et al.[170] showed modest improvements in the oxygenation of patients with ARDS who were treated with inhaled nitric oxide, although mortality was not reduced. There are several anecdotal reports of the use of inhaled nitric oxide during pregnancy,[171-175] including one report of its use to improve oxygenation in a pregnant woman with fulminant pulmonary failure due to varicella pneumonia.[172]

Pneumothorax is a frequent complication of mechanical ventilation. For circulatory support, agents with both alpha- and beta-adrenergic activity are more likely to restore or protect uterine blood flow than selective alpha-adrenergic agonists.

PROCAINAMIDE

Obstetricians have given procainamide to the mother for transplacental cardioversion of a fetal tachyarrhythmia.[183] Rapid administration of procainamide can result in hypotension and widening of the QRS complex. A lupus-like syndrome occurs in some patients. Thus this drug is not considered a first-line antiarrhythmic drug during pregnancy.

BETA-ADRENERGIC RECEPTOR ANTAGONISTS

Propranolol, atenolol, and metoprolol have been widely used during pregnancy for a variety of indications, including hypertension, mitral stenosis, HOCM, and control of heart rate with both atrial and ventricular tachyarrhythmias. Labetalol has become a popular choice for the treatment of hypertension in women with preeclampsia. These medications readily cross the placenta. There have been reports of IUGR, fetal bradycardia, and neonatal hypoglycemia during maternal use of a beta-adrenergic receptor antagonist.[184] The incidence of these effects is low. However, the obstetrician and anesthesiologist should be aware of the potential for acute fetal bradycardia during or after intravenous administration of a beta-adrenergic receptor antagonist.[106-110] Esmolol rapidly crosses the placenta but is eliminated rapidly from the plasma of both maternal and fetal sheep.[106] Eisenach and Castro[107] observed that prolonged maternal administration of esmolol resulted in fetal hypoxemia in gravid ewes. It is unclear whether short-term maternal administration of esmolol adversely affects the human fetus. The FHR should be monitored during and after intravenous administration of a beta-adrenergic receptor antagonist such as esmolol.

CALCIUM-ENTRY BLOCKING AGENTS

There is limited published experience with the use of verapamil as an antiarrhythmic agent during pregnancy. Verapamil may be administered intravenously to suppress an acute maternal tachyarrhythmia.[185] However, intravenous administration of verapamil may result in hypotension, and maternal blood pressure should be monitored carefully.

Verapamil crosses the placenta to a limited degree. Murad et al.[186] noted that fetal blood concentrations were 35% to 45% of maternal blood concentrations. However, these levels are sufficient to produce a marked slowing of atrioventricular conduction in the fetus.[187]

Another calcium-entry blocking agent (nicardipine) has been used for the treatment of hypertension in women with severe preeclampsia.[188]

LIDOCAINE

Lidocaine has been used for the treatment of ectopic ventricular arrhythmias during pregnancy.[182] The patient should be monitored for evidence of local anesthetic toxicity (e.g., somnolence, tinnitus, dysgeusia, convulsions). Fetal acidosis, if present, may result in the phenomenon of ion trapping, with unexpectedly high fetal blood concentrations of lidocaine.

PHENYTOIN

This medication is used for the treatment of digitalis toxicity or refractory ventricular arrhythmias.[182] More often, phenytoin is administered as an anticonvulsant agent in women with a seizure disorder. These women are at risk for fetal malformations (i.e., the fetal hydantoin syndrome)[189] (see Chapter 13). Its use should be limited to the acute management of digitalis-induced arrhythmias that are unresponsive to alternative treatment.

AMIODARONE

This medication has been used to treat refractory maternal atrial and ventricular arrhythmias[190,191] and also for the treatment of fetal tachyarrthmias.[192] Initial reports suggested that amiodarone is safe during pregnancy. However, subsequent reports have noted a high incidence of adverse fetal effects (e.g., IUGR, preterm delivery, fetal hypothyroidism).[193,194] Amiodarone contains iodine, and chronic use presents a large load of iodine to both maternal and fetal tissues. The exposure to iodine is the proposed mechanism for the high incidence of hypothyroidism in adults using this medication, and it presumably has the same effect on the fetus.[193,195] At present, amiodarone is not often used in pregnant women except when refractory arrhythmias are unresponsive to other agents.[196]

ADENOSINE

Adenosine is a purine nucleoside that modulates conduction through the atrioventricular node.[197] The primary indication for adenosine is paroxysmal supraventricular tachycardia, which is the most common arrhythmia in pregnant women.[182] Adenosine has several features that make it attractive for use during pregnancy. The onset of action is rapid, and the duration of action is brief. Side effects (e.g., hypotension, dizziness, flushing, dyspnea) are common, but they are transient and minor.[197]

Several authors have described the safe and effective use of adenosine in pregnant women.[198,199] Afridi et al.[199] described the use of adenosine to treat hemodynamically significant supraventricular tachycardia associated with Wolff-Parkinson-White syndrome at 7 months of gestation. In that case, concomitant fetal bradycardia resolved when adenosine converted the maternal tachyarrhythmia to a normal sinus rhythm.

Caution should be exercised when using adenosine. Narrow-complex supraventricular rhythms respond well to adenosine, but if atrial fibrillation or flutter is present, conduction through an accessory tract may be enhanced and the rhythm disturbance may actually worsen.

Treatment of Congenital Heart Block and Bradyarrhythmias

Congenital complete heart block is a rare syndrome. There are published cases of asymptomatic women with this syndrome who underwent uncomplicated pregnancy and delivery.[200] Nonetheless, if congenital heart block is recognized in a pregnant woman, cardiology evaluation is warranted to determine whether placement of a pacemaker (either temporary or permanent) is indicated. In general, a pacemaker is indicated if the patient is symptomatic or in the presence of either a prolonged Q-T interval or left atrial enlargement. Women with permanent pacemakers for symptomatic bradyarrhythmias have had successful pregnancies and deliveries.[201] Pacemakers can be inserted by electrocardiographic or echocardiographic guidance to avoid fetal exposure to ionizing radiation.[202] During labor, the use of epidural anesthesia is recommended to minimize maternal expulsive efforts (which might cause a reflex slowing of heart rate) and to facilitate a painless instrumental vaginal delivery.

Prolonged Q-T Syndrome and Ventricular Tachycardia

Ventricular tachycardia may be associated with drugs, electrolyte abnormalities, and eclampsia. Idiopathic ventricular

tachycardia usually results from an abnormality of the right ventricular septum. Prolonged Q-T syndromes increase the risk for *torsades de pointes* and cardiac arrest during pregnancy.

Lidocaine is the preferred therapeutic agent, and procainamide is an alternative agent. Women who are hemodynamically unstable require immediate cardioversion.[203]

A beta-adrenergic receptor antagonist is used prophylactically in patients with a history of idiopathic ventricular tachycardia. Procainamide and sotalol are second-line medications, and amiodarone is reserved for the most refractory cases. Episodes of syncopal ventricular tachycardia or ventricular fibrillation justify the placement of an AICD.[203] Good pregnancy outcomes have been reported in women who had the device implanted during the second or third trimester or prior to pregnancy.[204,205]

Cardioversion

Ogburn et al.[206] have described the safe use of electrical cardioversion during pregnancy. The use of electrical cardioversion should be limited to patients with tachyarrhythmias who are unresponsive to medical therapy or to those with hemodynamic instability. An H_2-receptor antagonist and a clear oral antacid should be administered before cardioversion. (We avoid administration of metoclopramide in these patients because there is some evidence that it exacerbates tachycardia and tachyarrhythmias.[207]) The risk of pulmonary aspiration of gastric contents should be weighed against the risk of general anesthesia with endotracheal intubation. The judicious use of sedation rather than full general anesthesia and endotracheal intubation is usually preferred in this setting. A benzodiazepine, a barbiturate, or propofol can provide satisfactory sedation and amnesia. Women with severe hemodynamic instability may not tolerate the administration of *any* dose of a sedative drug. The FHR should be monitored because transient FHR abnormalities (and rarely, sustained fetal bradycardia) may occur during/after cardioversion.[208,209]

DISEASES OF THE AORTA

Marfan Syndrome

Marfan syndrome is a hereditary disorder of collagen and elastin. Patients with Marfan syndrome have long, slender extremities, joint laxity, and many other musculoskeletal abnormalities. In addition to MVP, patients with Marfan syndrome develop dilation of the ascending aorta, which may progress to a dissecting aneurysm, aortic incompetence, and rupture of the aorta. If aortic root involvement is noted, management should be directed toward strict blood pressure control and minimization of shear stress within the aorta.

Pyeritz[210] reviewed 32 women affected by Marfan syndrome who became pregnant; 16 died and 4 survived acute aortic dissection. Most of the women who suffered an aortic complication in association with pregnancy had preexisting aortic regurgitation, aortic root dilation, or other severe cardiovascular problems. Women with Marfan syndrome and minimal cardiovascular disease may tolerate pregnancy quite well. Nonetheless, these patients should be watched carefully for symptoms of aortic dissection.[211] Moreover, serial echocardiography may be misleading in the diagnosis of aortic dissection.[212]

Some evidence suggests that Marfan syndrome is associated with cervical incompetence, abnormal placentation, and postpartum hemorrhage.[213]

Aortic Dissection

There is an increased incidence of aortic dissection during pregnancy.[214] One half of all cases of aortic rupture in women less than 40 years of age are associated with pregnancy.[215] Some physicians have suggested that the cardiovascular changes of pregnancy (e.g., increased blood volume, cardiac output, stroke volume, and heart rate) impose significant stress on the wall of the aorta. Women with inherited connective tissue disorders (e.g., Marfan syndrome, Ehlers-Danlos disorder) are at increased risk. Other risk factors include systemic hypertension and a congenitally bicuspid aortic valve.[215] Konishi et al.[216] reviewed 51 cases of dissecting aneurysm of the aorta and its branches during pregnancy and the puerperium. Approximately 6% of cases occurred during the first trimester, 10% during the second trimester, and 51% during the third trimester. Approximately 14% of cases occurred during labor, and the remaining 20% of cases occurred during the puerperium.

PATHOPHYSIOLOGY

With aortic dissection, blood moves through a tear in the aortic intima and separates the intima from the adventitia. Most dissections extend distally, but proximal propagation can occur. A false lumen results, which can reconnect with the true lumen anywhere along the course of the dissection. Rupture of the aorta typically is fatal. It occurs most frequently in the pericardial space and left pleural cavity and produces both pericardial tamponade and hemothorax.[214]

The most common point of origin is within the ascending aorta within a few centimeters of the aortic valve. The second most common location is within the descending thoracic aorta just distal to the origin of the left subclavian artery. Debakey et al.[217] have identified three types of aortic dissection (Figure 40-4). A type I dissection extends beyond the ascending aorta into the descending aorta. A type II dissection is confined to the ascending aorta. Type III dissections originate in the descending thoracic aorta. A type III-A dissection remains above the diaphragm, and a type III-B dissection extends below the diaphragm. Type I and type II dissections may be complicated by aortic insufficiency, pericardial tamponade, dissection (or obstruction) of major branches of the aortic arch, compression of a mainstem bronchus, and laryngeal nerve compression.

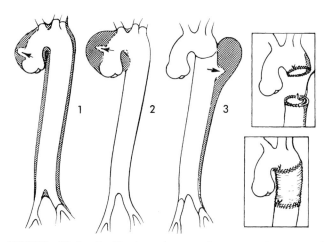

FIGURE 40-4. Classification of aortic dissections. (Courtesy of Dr. Lawrence H. Cohn, Boston.)

DIAGNOSIS

Prompt medical and surgical management increases the likelihood of survival in pregnant women with aortic dissection. Aortic dissection should be included in the differential diagnosis whenever a woman complains of severe chest or back pain during pregnancy or the puerperium. Other clinical symptoms and signs include shortness of breath, syncope, tachycardia, and an ischemic extremity. Dyspnea may be the result of pain or direct compression of a large airway by an expanding aneurysm. Differential blood pressure in the arms or differential pulses in the lower extremities may be noted.

Kao et al.[218] reported the case of a 23-year-old woman who received epidural anesthesia for delivery and subsequently complained of severe lower thoracic back pain that radiated to her right leg. Before the anesthetist could be consulted, the patient suffered a grand mal seizure and had a cardiorespiratory arrest.

Chest radiographic examination may reveal a widening mediastinum or hemothorax. Aortography establishes the definitive diagnosis. Magnetic resonance imaging is a useful technique for the evaluation of aortic disease because it avoids radiation exposure while providing excellent imaging of the aorta.[219]

MANAGEMENT

Pregnancy may affect the choice between medical and surgical therapy.[220] In almost all cases in which aortic dissection is suspected, aggressive control of blood pressure with a vasodilator agent is essential. The use of a beta-adrenergic receptor antagonist decreases the force of ventricular ejection, which decreases shear stress against the aortic wall. Management should include placement of an intraarterial catheter and measurement of CVP. Intravenous opioids are important for minimizing pain; this helps decrease forces that can extend the dissection.

The patient in extremis (with acute aortic insufficiency, tamponade, extensive distal dissection, and CNS ischemia) needs immediate surgery as a life-saving, resuscitative measure. In contrast, the patient with a known, small, controlled aortic dissection may undergo labor and delivery with dense epidural anesthesia. Maternal expulsive efforts should be avoided during the second stage of labor. Patients should receive medical therapy as discussed, with the decision to continue medical therapy or proceed to surgery based on the details of each particular patient. To date, no established guidelines exist to determine the optimal course of management in the acute yet stable case of aortic dissection during pregnancy.

INFECTIVE ENDOCARDITIS

Infective endocarditis is an ominous condition that imposes a formidable burden on the cardiovascular demands of pregnancy. Fortunately, it is a rare event during pregnancy. One report suggested that infective endocarditis occurs in approximately 1 in 8000 deliveries.[221] However, another study, which included an extensive review of the published literature in English and selected European journals, found only 124 cases during a 40-year period before 1986.[222] Among those cases, the maternal mortality rate was 29% and the fetal mortality rate was 23%.

The incidence of infective endocarditis in the obstetric population appears to be declining; this may be attributable to (1) a decreasing prevalence of rheumatic heart disease, (2) more pervasive use of aseptic technique during obstetric procedures, (3) more aggressive treatment of obstetric infections, and (4) a lower incidence of illegal abortion. However, intravenous drug abuse has emerged as a major cause of infective endocarditis in women of childbearing age.[223]

Pathophysiology

Infective endocarditis is defined as the invasion and colonization of the cardiac valves, endocardium, and congenital or prosthetic cardiac tissue by an infectious pathogen. Colonization results in the development of friable vegetations, which may produce emboli, hemodynamic compromise, and a fulminant clinical course. Although infective endocarditis typically occurs in association with a preexisting cardiac lesion (which provides a roughened surface for bacterial growth), structurally normal hearts also may be affected.[224] Risk factors for the infection of *preexisting cardiac lesions* include dental and urologic procedures, prolonged intravenous therapy, and intravenous drug abuse. Risk factors for the infection of *normal cardiac tissue* include prolonged intravenous therapy and intravenous drug abuse, infection of an arteriovenous shunt, and renal dialysis.[224]

Blood-borne bacteria that adhere to damaged or normal endocardial surfaces may lead to the formation of vegetations. Virtually any pathogen can cause endocarditis. Pathogens reported during pregnancy include *Streptococcus viridans*,[225] group B streptococcus,[226] *Staphylococcus aureus*,[224] *Neisseria gonorrhoeae*,[227] *Chlamydia trachomati*,[228] enterococcus,[229] *Salmonella enteritidis*,[230] *Mycobacterium fortuitum*,[231] and *Listeria monocytogenes*.[232]

Seaworth and Durack[222] found that streptococci caused the majority of cases (74%) of infective endocarditis that followed obstetric and gynecologic procedures. *Streptococcus viridans* was the predominant pathogen, and enterococci and group B streptococci were uncommon, except after abortion.[222] Women who are immunosuppressed or immunodeficient (e.g., those who have AIDS) are susceptible to uncommon and less-virulent pathogens.

Diagnosis

Prompt diagnosis and aggressive antibiotic therapy improve the clinical outcome. Infective endocarditis can be divided into two groups: subacute and acute. **Subacute endocarditis** is characterized by a slow, insidious onset of fever, weakness, malaise, and unexplained embolic phenomena. Blood cultures are positive in 90% of these cases. Murmurs typically result from the underlying cardiac lesion. Systemic embolism may develop at any time, giving rise to splinter hemorrhages and mucosal petechiae. Septic abscesses can lead to atrioventricular nodal dysfunction, conduction block, and arrhythmias. Other manifestations include splenomegaly and immune complex nephritis secondary to antigen-antibody complex deposition on the glomerular basement membrane. The latter complication may result in renal failure. The major causes of death include congestive heart failure, embolic cerebral infarction, arrhythmias, and renal failure.

Acute infective endocarditis is heralded by an abrupt onset of symptoms, including high fevers, shaking chills, and early onset of embolic phenomena. Skin and mucosal petechiae may occur. Murmurs occur in two thirds of patients with vegetations on the left side of the heart. Cardiac decompensation appears early. Cardiovascular function may worsen suddenly with erosion of a valve or

rupture of the chordae tendineae. Aortic ring abscesses may produce conduction disturbances or ventricular septal defects. The ECG may be normal or may demonstrate arrhythmias or conduction disturbances. Echocardiography helps localize valvular vegetations and also may reveal valvular incompetence or left ventricular failure. The major causes of death in this group are congestive heart failure, arrhythmias, uncontrolled sepsis, septic emboli, and mycotic aneurysm formation with rupture.

Medical and Surgical Management

The medical management of pregnant women is essentially identical to that for nonpregnant patients.[223] The identity of the pathogen and the laboratory determination of organism sensitivity dictate the choice of antibiotic therapy. Patients should receive a minimum of 4 to 6 weeks of parenteral antibiotic therapy. Complications such as congestive heart failure and arrhythmias are managed as outlined previously.

Indications for surgical intervention include fungal endocarditis, acquired conduction defects, progressive heart failure, acute hemodynamic deterioration, systemic embolization, and persistent sepsis. Bataskov et al.[227] reviewed 44 obstetric cases of infective endocarditis that required surgery. The operative mortality rate was 30%.

Obstetric and Anesthetic Management

Obstetric management may include the performance of early instrumental vaginal delivery to minimize maternal expulsive efforts during the second stage of labor.

Anesthetic management is dictated by the clinical presentation. Patients with evidence of cardiac decompensation require invasive hemodynamic monitoring. Controversy exists regarding the use of regional anesthesia in patients with systemic infection. It seems prudent to avoid regional anesthesia in patients with sepsis or acute infective endocarditis. However, in a patient with a recent history of infective endocarditis, administration of regional anesthesia can be considered, provided the patient is afebrile, culture negative, and hemodynamically stable.

Antibiotic Prophylaxis

Controversy remains regarding the indications for antibiotic prophylaxis. From a public health perspective, the indiscriminate use of antibiotics may promote the emergence of bacterial strains that are virulent and resistant to currently available antibiotics. Further, antibiotics may cause severe maternal allergic reactions and fetal toxicity (see Chapter 13).

Patients at high risk for endocarditis (e.g., surgically constructed systemic-pulmonary shunts or conduits, prosthetic valves, rheumatic heart disease, history of endocarditis) should receive antibiotic prophylaxis before undergoing operative procedures that produce bacteremia.[113,116] Controversy remains regarding the prophylactic use of antibiotics for uncomplicated labor and vaginal delivery.[5,116] Many obstetricians administer prophylactic antibiotics at the start of labor and for 24 hours after delivery. Prophylaxis typically consists of intravenous ampicillin and gentamicin. Vancomycin may be substituted for penicillin in patients who are allergic to penicillin.[116] An alternative regimen for low-risk patients consists of only two doses of amoxicillin (Table 40-2).

Antibiotic prophylaxis is not recommended for elective cesarean section, if labor has not yet begun and the membranes are intact.

TABLE 40-2	PROPHYLACTIC ANTIBIOTIC REGIMENS FOR GENITOURINARY/GASTROINTESTINAL PROCEDURES
Drug	**Dosage regimen**
Standard regimen Ampicillin, gentamicin, and amoxicillin	Intravenous or intramuscular administration of ampicillin 2.0 g, plus gentamicin 1.5 mg/kg (not to exceed 80 mg) 30 min before the procedure; followed by amoxicillin 1.5 g orally, 6 hr after the initial dose; alternatively, the parenteral regimen may be repeated once, 8 hr after the initial dose
Ampicillin-, amoxicillin-, penicillin-allergic patient regimen Vancomycin and gentamicin	Intravenous administration of vancomycin 1.0 g over 1 hr, plus intravenous or intramuscular administration of gentamicin 1.5 mg/kg (not to exceed 80 mg) 1 hr before the procedure; may be repeated once, 8 hr after the initial dose
Alternative low-risk patient regimen Amoxicillin	2.0 g orally 1 hr before procedure; then 1.5 g 6 hr after the initial dose

From Dajani AS, Taubert KA, Wilson W, et al. Prevention of bacterial endocarditis: Recommendations of the American Heart Association. JAMA 1997; 277:1794-1801.

KEY POINTS

- Heart disease is the primary medical cause of nonobstetric maternal mortality.
- Increasing numbers of women with congenital cardiac lesions are now reaching childbearing age and becoming pregnant. Therefore, anesthesiologists will encounter these women with increasing frequency.
- Pulmonary artery catheterization rarely is necessary in pregnant women with most forms of congenital heart disease, including Eisenmenger syndrome.
- Intrathecal administration of a lipophilic opioid represents an excellent choice of intrapartum analgesia for women who may not tolerate decreased SVR and decreased venous return.
- Recent reports suggest that few, if any, cardiac lesions represent an absolute contraindication to the use of epidural anesthesia, assuming that the induction of anesthesia proceeds slowly and the potentially adverse hemodynamic changes are corrected promptly. Single-shot spinal anesthesia can produce circulatory collapse in parturients with severe aortic stenosis, primary pulmonary hypertension, and Eisenmenger syndrome.
- The treatment of arrhythmias during pregnancy is similar to that for nonpregnant women.
- When CPR is required during pregnancy, the standard ACLS protocol should be used. Successful CPR during pregnancy requires the avoidance of aortocaval compression. Early evacuation of the uterus may facilitate both maternal and fetal survival.

REFERENCES

1. Tan J, de Swiet M. Prevalence of heart disease diagnosed de novo in pregnancy in a West London population. Br J Obstet Gynaecol 1998; 105:1185-8.
2. Sullivan JM, Ramanathan KB. Management of medical problems in pregnancy: a severe cardiac disease. N Engl J Med 1985; 313:304-9.
3. McFaul PB, Dornan JC, Lamki H, Boyce D. Pregnancy complicated by maternal heart disease. A review of 519 women. Br J Obstet Gynaecol 1988; 95:861-7.
4. Hess DB, Hess WL. Cardiovascular disease and pregnancy. Obstet Gynecol Clin North Am 1992; 19:679-92.
5. American College of Obstetrics and Gynecology. Cardiac Disease in Pregnancy. ACOG Technical Bulletin No. 168, 1992.
6. Siu SC, Colman JM. Heart disease and pregnancy. Heart (British Cardiac Society) 2001; 85:710-5.
7. Black S, Cuchiara RF, Nishimura RA, Michenfelder JD. Parameters affecting the occurrence of paradoxical air embolism. Anesthesiology 1989; 71:235-41.
8. Saidi AS, Bezold LI, Altman CA, et al. Outcome of pregnancy following intervention for coarctation of the aorta. Am J Cardiol 1998; 82:786-8.
9. Deal K, Wooley CF. Coarctation of the aorta and pregnancy. Ann Intern Med 1973; 78:708-13.
10. Perloff JK. Pregnancy and heart disease. In Braunwald E, editor. Heart Disease. Philadelphia, WB Saunders, 1988:1855-6.
11. Manullang TR, Chun K, Egan TD. The use of remifentanil for cesarean section in a parturient with recurrent aortic coarctation. Can J Anaesth 2000; 47:454-9.
12. Eisenmenger V. Die Angeborenen Defecte der Kammerscheidewand des Herzens. Z Klin Med 1897; 32:1-29.
13. Shime J, Mocarski EJM, Hastings D, et al. Congenital heart disease in pregnancy: Short and long term implications. Am J Obstet Gynecol 1989; 156:313-22.
14. Gleicher R, Midwall J, Hochberger D. Eisenmenger's syndrome and pregnancy. Obstet Gynecol Surv 1979; 34:721-41
15. Su NY, Lin SM, Hsen SS, et al. Anesthetic management of parturients with Eisenmenger's syndrome: Report of two cases. Acta Anaesthesiol Sin 2001; 39:139-44.
16. Mangano DT. Anesthesia for the pregnant cardiac patient. In Shnider SM, Levinson G, editors. Anesthesia for Obstetrics, 3rd ed. Baltimore, Williams & Wilkins, 1993:485-523.
17. Pollack KL, Chestnut DH, Wenstrom KD. Anesthetic management of a parturient with Eisenmenger's syndrome. Anesth Analg 1990; 70:212-4.
18. Spinnato JA, Kraynack BJ, Cooper MW. Eisenmenger's syndrome in pregnancy: Epidural analgesia for elective cesarean section. N Engl J Med 1981; 304:1215-7.
19. Goodwin TM, Gherman RB, Hameed A, Elkayam U. Favorable response of Eisenmenger syndrome to inhaled nitric oxide during pregnancy. Am J Obstet Gynecol 1999; 180: 64-7.
20. Lust KM, Bouts RJ, Dooris M, Wilson J. Management of labor in Eisenmenger syndrome with inhaled nitric oxide. Am J Obstet Gynecol 1999; 181:419-23.
21. Decoene C, Bourzoufi K, Moreau D, et al. Use of inhaled nitric oxide for emergency cesarean section in a woman with unexpected primary pulmonary hypertension. Can J Anaesth 2001; 48:584-7.
22. Panetta C, Schiller N. Evidence of patent ductus arteriosus and right-to-left shunt by finger pulse oximetry and Doppler signals of agitated saline in abdominal aorta. Am Soc Echo 1999; 12:763-5.
23. Schwalbe SS, Deshmukh SM, Marx GF. Use of pulmonary artery catheterization in parturients with Eisenmenger's syndrome. Anesth Analg 1990; 71:442-3.
24. Rosenthal E, Nelson-Piercy C. Value of inhaled nitric oxide in Eisenmenger syndrome during pregnancy (letter). Am J Obstet Gynecol 2000; 183:781-2.
25. Owen MD, Poss MJ, Dean LJ, Harper MA. Prolonged intravenous remifentanil infusion for labor analgesia. Anesth Analg 2002; 94:918-9.
26. Head BB, Owen J, Vincent RD, et al. A randomized trial of intrapartum analgesia in women with severe preeclampsia. Obstet Gynecol 2002; 99:452-7.
27. Ghai B, Mohan V, Khetarpal M, Malhotra N. Epidural anesthesia for cesarean section in a patient with Eisenmenger's syndrome. Internat J Obstet Anesth 2002; 11:44-7.
28. Cole PJ, Cross MH, Dresner M. Incremental spinal anaesthesia for elective Caesarean section in a patient with Eisenmenger's syndrome. Br J Anaesth 2001; 86:723-6.
29. Fuster V, Steele PM, Edwards WD, et al. Primary pulmonary hypertension: Natural history and the importance of thrombosis. Circulation 1984; 70:580-7.
30. Weiss BM, Zemp L, Seifert B, Hess OM. Outcome of pulmonary vascular disease in pregnancy: A systematic overview from 1978 through 1996. J Am Coll Cardiol 1998; 31:1650-7.
31. Khan MJ, Bhatt SB, Kryc JJ. Anesthetic considerations for parturients with primary pulmonary hypertension: Review of the literature and clinical presentation. Internat J Obstet Anesth 1996; 5:36-42.
32. Weeks SK, Smith JB. Obstetric anaesthesia in patients with primary pulmonary hypertension (editorial). Can J Anaesth 1991; 38:814-6.
33. O'Hare R, McLoughlin C, Milligan K, et al. Anaesthesia for caesarean section in the presence of severe primary pulmonary hypertension. Br J Anaesth 1998; 81:790-2.
34. Palmer CM, DiNardo JA, Hays RL, Van Maren GA. Use of transesophageal echocardiography for delivery of a parturient with severe pulmonary hypertension. Internat J Obstet Anesth 2002; 11:48-51.
35. Monnery L, Nanson J, Charlton G. Primary pulmonary hypertension in pregnancy: A role for novel vasodilators. Br J Anaesth 2001; 87:295-8.
36. Lam GK, Stafford RE, Thorp J, et al. Inhaled nitric oxide for primary pulmonary hypertension in pregnancy. Obstet Gynecol 2001; 98:895-8.
37. Easterling TR, Ralph DD, Schmucker BC. Pulmonary hypertension in pregnancy: treatment with pulmonary vasodilators. Obstet Gynecol 1999; 93: 494-8.
38. Rubin LJ, Badesch DB, Barst RJ, et al. Bosentan therapy for pulmonary arterial hypertension. N Engl J Med 2002; 346:896-903.
39. Channick RN, Simonneau G, Sitbon O, et al. Effects of the dual endothelin-receptor antagonist bosentan in patients with pulmonary hypertension: A randomised placebo-controlled study. Lancet 2001; 358:1119-23.
40. Stewart R, Tuazon D, Olson G, Duarte AG. Pregnancy and primary pulmonary hypertension : Successful outcome with epoprostenol therapy. Chest 2001; 119:973-5.

41. Robinson DE, Leicht CH. Epidural analgesia with low-dose bupivacaine and fentanyl for labor and delivery in a parturient with severe pulmonary hypertension. Anesthesiology 1988; 65:285-8.

42. Smedstad KG, Cramb R, Morison DH. Primary pulmonary hypertension: A series of eight cases. Can J Anaesth 1994; 41:502-12.

43. Breen TW, Janzen JA. Pulmonary hypertension and cardiomyopathy: Anaesthetic management for caesarean section. Can J Anaesth 1991; 38:895-9.

44. Cohen Y, Rudick V. Caesarean section in a parturient with severe pulmonary hypertension. Epidural ropivacaine or continuous spinal anaesthesia (letter). Acta Anaesthesiol Scand 2002; 46:620-22.

45. Autore C, Conte MR, Piccininno M, et al. Risk associated with pregnancy in hypertrophic cardiomyopathy. J Am Coll Cardiol 2002; 40:1864-9.

46. Fairley CJ, Clarke JT. Use of esmolol in a parturient with hypertrophic obstructive cardiomyopathy. Br J Anaesth 1995; 75:801-4.

47. Piacenza JM, Kirkorian G, Audra PH, Mellier G. Hypertrophic cardiomyopathy and pregnancy. Eur J Obstet Gynecol Reprod Biol 1998; 80:17-23.

48. Paix B, Cyna A, Belperio P, Simmons S. Epidural analgesia for labour and delivery in a parturient with congenital hypertrophic obstructive cardiomyopathy. Anaesth Intensive Care 1999; 27:59-62.

49. Boccio RV, Chung JH, Harrison DM. Anesthetic management of cesarean section in a patient with idiopathic hypertrophic subaortic stenosis. Anesthesiology 1986; 65:633-65.

50. Haering JM, Comunale ME, Parker RA, et al. Cardiac risk of noncardiac surgery in patients with asymmetric septal hypertrophy. Anesthesiology 1996; 85:254-9.

51. Wadsworth R, Greer R, MacDonald JMS, Vohra A. The use of remifentanil during general anaesthesia for cesarean delivery in two patients with severe heart dysfunction. Internat J Obstet Anesth 2002; 11:38-43.

52. American Heart Association. Silent Epidemic: The Truth about Women and Heart Disease. Dallas, the Association, 1989: 1-17.

53. Ginz B. Myocardial infarction in pregnancy. J Obstet Gynaecol Br Commonw 1952; 63:381-90.

54. Badui E, Enciso R. Acute myocardial infarction during pregnancy and puerperium: A review. Angiology 1996; 47:739-56.

55. Roth A, Elkayam U. Acute myocardial infarction associated with pregnancy. Ann Intern Med 1996; 125:751-62.

56. American College of Obstetricians and Gynecologists. Committee on Obstetrics: Maternal and Fetal Medicine. Cocaine in Pregnancy. ACOG Committee Opinion No. 114, 1992.

57. Caruth JE, Mirvis SB, Brogan DR, Wenger NK. The electrocardiogram in normal pregnancy. Am Heart J 1981; 102:1075-8.

58. National Council on Radiation Protection and Measurements: Medical radiation exposure of pregnant and potentially pregnant women. Washington, DC, 1977.

59. Meltzer RS, Serrvys PW, McGhie, J. Cardiac catheterization under echocardiographic control in a pregnant woman. Am J Med 1981; 71:481-4.

60. Shotan A, Gottlieb S, Goldbourt U, et al. Prognosis of patients with a recurrent acute myocardial infarction before and in the reperfusion era: A national study. Am Heart J 2001; 141:478-84.

61. Ascarelli MH, Grider AR, Hsu HW. Acute myocardial infarction during pregnancy managed with immediate percutaneous transluminal coronary angioplasty. Obstet Gynecol 1996; 88:655-7.

62. Webber MD, Halligan RE, Schumacher JA. Acute infarction, intracoronary thrombolysis, and primary PTCA in pregnancy. Cathet Cardiovasc Diagn 1997; 42:38-43.

63. Sanchez-Ramos L, Chami YG, Bass TA, et al. Myocardial infarction during pregnancy: Management with transluminal coronary angioplasty and metallic intracoronary stents. Am J Obstet Gynecol 1994; 171:1392-3.

64. Garry D, Leikin E, Fleisher AG, Tejawi N. Acute myocardial infarction in pregnancy with subsequent medical and surgical management. Obstet Gynecol 1996; 87:802-4.

65. Schumacher B, Belfort MA, Card RJ. Successful treatment of acute myocardial infarction during pregnancy with tissue plasminogen activator. Am J Obstet Gynecol 1997; 176:716-9.

66. Frenkel Y, Barkai G, Reisin L, et al. Pregnancy after myocardial infarction: Are we playing safe? Obstet Gynecol 1991; 77:822-5.

67. Listo M, Bjorkenheim G. Myocardial infarction during delivery. Acta Obstet Gynecol Scand 1966; 45:268-78.

68. Mabie WC, Anderson GD, Addington MB, et al. The benefit of cesarean section in acute myocardial infarction complicated by premature labor. Obstet Gynecol 1988; 71:503-6.

69. Rao TKL, Jacobs KH, El-Etr AA. Reinfarction following anesthesia in patients with myocardial infarction. Anesthesiology 1983; 59:499-505.

70. Cohen WR, Steinman T, Pastner B. Acute myocardial infarction in a pregnant woman at term. JAMA 1983; 250:2179-81.

71. Aglio LS, Johnson MD. Anaesthetic management of myocardial infarction in a parturient. Br J Anaesth 1990; 65:258-61.

72. Soderlin MK, Purhonen S, Haring P, et al. Myocardial infarction in a parturient. Anaesthesia 1994; 49:870-72.

73. Bonow RO, Carabello B, de Leon AC, et al. ACC/AHA Guidelines for the management of patients with valvular heart disease, executive summary: A report of the American College of Cardiology/American Heart Association Task Force on Practice Guidelines (Committee on Management of Patients With Valvular Heart Disease). J Heart Valve Dis 1998; 7: 672-707.

74. Bonow RO, Carabello B, de Leon AC, et al. Guidelines for the management of patients with valvular heart disease, executive summary: A report of the American College of Cardiology/American Heart Association Task Force on Practice Guidelines (Committee on Management of Patients with Valvular Heart Disease). Circulation 1998; 98:1949-84.

75. Gohlke-Barwolf C, Acar J, Oakley C, et al. [Recommendations for prevention of thromboembolism in heart valve diseases. Working Group on Valvular Heart Disease, European Society of Cardiology]. Zeitschrift fur Kardiologie 1995; 84:1018-32.

76. Roberts WC. The congenitally bicuspid aortic valve. Am J Cardiol 1970; 26:72-8.

77. Lao TT, Sermer M, MaGee L, et al. Congenital aortic stenosis and pregnancy-A reappraisal. Am J Obstet Gynecol 1993; 169:540-5.

78. Hustead ST, Quick A, Gibbs HR, et al. "Pseudo-critical" aortic stenosis during pregnancy: Role for Doppler assessment of aortic valve area. Am Heart J 1989; 1383-5.

79. Arias F, Pineda J. Aortic stenosis and pregnancy. J Reprod Med 1978; 4:229-32.

80. Bhargava B, Agarwal R, Yadav R, et al. Percutaneous balloon aortic valvuloplasty during pregnancy: Use of the Inoue balloon and the physiologic antegrade approach. Cathet Cardiovasc Diagn 1998; 45:422-5.

81. Easterling TR, Chadwick HS, Otto CM, Benedetti TJ. Aortic stenosis in pregnancy. Obstet Gynecol 1988; 72:113-8.

82. Brian JE, Seifen AB, Clark RB, et al. Aortic stenosis, cesarean delivery, and epidural anesthesia. J Clin Anesth 1993; 5:154-7.

83. Pittard A, Vucevic M. Regional anaesthesia with a subarachnoid microcatheter for caesarean section in a parturient with aortic stenosis. Anaesthesia 1998; 53:169-73.

84. Redfern N, Bower S, Bullock RE, Hull CJ. Alfentanil for caesarean section complicated by severe aortic stenosis. Br J Anaesth 1987; 59: 1309-12.

85. Kan RE, Hughes SC, Rosen MA, et al. Intravenous remifentanil: Placental transfer, maternal and neonatal effects. Anesthesiology 1998; 88:1467-74.

86. McCarroll CP, Paxton LD, Elliott P, Wilson DB. Use of remifentanil in a patient with peripartum cardiomyopathy requiring Caesarean section. Br J Anaesth 2001; 86:135-8.

87. Scott H, Bateman C, Price M. The use of remifentanil in general anaesthesia for caesarean section in a patient with mitral valve disease. Anaesthesia 1998; 53:695-7.

88. Paulus DA, Layon AJ, Mayfield WR, et al. Intrauterine pregnancy and aortic valve replacement. J Clin Anesth 1995; 7:338-46.

89. Tzankis G, Morse DS. Cesarean section and reoperative aortic valve replacement in a 38-week parturient. J Cardiothor Vasc Anesth 1996; 10:516-8.

90. Naidoo DP, Desai DK, Moodley J. Maternal deaths due to pre-existing cardiac disease. Cardiovasc J South Afr 2002; 13:17-20.

91. Stollerman GH. Rheumatic and heritable connective tissue diseases of the cardiovascular system. In Braunwald E, editor. Heart Disease. Philadelphia, WB Saunders, 1988:1710.

92. Rokey R, Hsu HW, Moise KJ, et al. Inaccurate noninvasive mitral valve area calculation during pregnancy. Obstet Gynecol 1994; 84:950-5.

93. Braunwald E. Valvular heart disease. In Braunwald E, editor. Heart Disease, 4th ed. WB Saunders, Philadelphia, 1992:1011.

94. Al Kasab SM, Sabag T, Al Zeibag M. Beta adrenergic blockade in the management of pregnant women with mitral stenosis. Am J Obstet Gynecol 1990; 165:37-40.

95. Vosloo S, Reichart B. The feasibility of closed mitral valvotomy in pregnancy. J Thorac Cardiovasc Vasc Surg 1987; 93:675-9.

96. Baron F, Zottoli E, Hill WC. Percutaneous balloon mitral valvuloplasty during a twin gestation. South Med J 2002; 95:358-9.

97. Uygur D, Beksac MS. Mitral balloon valvuloplasty during pregnancy in developing countries. Europ J Obstet, Gynecol Reprod Biol 2001; 96:226-8.

98. de Souza JAM, Martinez EE, Ambrose JA, et al. Percutaneous balloon mitral valvuloplasty in comparison with open mitral valve commissuro-

tomy for mitral stenosis during pregnancy. J Am Coll Cardiol 2001; 37:900-3.

99. Lee CH, Chow WH, Kwok OH. Percutaneous balloon mitral valvuloplasty during pregnancy: Long-term follow-up of infant growth and development. Hong Kong Med J 2001; 7:85-8.

100. Mangione JA, Lourenco RM, dos Santos ES, et al. Long-term follow-up of pregnant women after percutaneous mitral valvuloplasty. Catheterization Cardiovas Intervent 2000; 50:413-7.

101. Elkayam U. Pregnancy and Cardiovascular Disease, in Heart Disease: A Textbook of Cardiovascular Medicine. Braunwald E, editor. WB Saunders Company 2001; 2172-2191.

102. Hameed A, Karaalp IS, Tummala PP, et al. The effect of valvular heart disease on maternal and fetal outcome of pregnancy. J Am Coll Cardiol 2001; 37:893-9.

103. Naidoo DP, Moodley J. Management of the critically ill cardiac patient. Best Prac Res Clin Obstet Gynaecol 2001; 15:523-44.

104. Clark SL, Phelan JP, Greenspoon J, et al. Labor and delivery in the presence of mitral stenosis: Central hemodynamic observations. Am J Obstet Gynecol 1985; 152:984-8.

105. Hemmings GT, Whalley DG, O'Connor PJ, et al. Invasive monitoring and anaesthetic management of a parturient with mitral stenosis. Can J Anaesth 1987; 34:182-5.

106. Östman PL, Chestnut DH, Robillard JE, et al. Transplacental passage and hemodynamic effects of esmolol in the gravid ewe. Anesthesiology 1988; 69:738-41.

107. Eisenach JC, Castro MI. Maternally administered esmolol produces fetal a-adrenergic blockade and hypoxemia in sheep. Anesthesiology 1989; 71:718-22.

108. Larson CP, Shuer LM, Cohen SE. Maternally administered esmolol decreases fetal as well as maternal heart rate. J Clin Anesth 1990; 2: 427-9.

109. Losasso TJ, Muzzi DA, Cucchiara RF. Response of fetal heart rate to maternal administration of esmolol. Anesthesiology 1991; 74:782-4.

110. Ducey JP, Knape KG. Maternal esmolol administration resulting in fetal distress and cesarean section in a term pregnancy. Anesthesiology 1992; 77:829-32.

111. Cohn LH. Surgery for mitral regurgitation. JAMA 1988; 260:2883-7.

112. Oakley CM. Valvular disease in pregnancy. Curr Opin Cardiol 1996; 11:155-9.

113. Shapiro EP, Trimble EL, Robinson JC, et al. Safety of labor and delivery in women with mitral valve prolapse. Am J Cardiol 1985; 56:806-7.

114. Savage DD, Garrison RJ, Devereux RB, et al. Mitral valve prolapse in the general population. 1. Epidemiologic features: The Framingham Study. Am Heart J 1983; 106:571-6.

115. Shapiro EP, Trimble EL, Robinson JC, et al. Safety of labor and delivery in women with mitral valve prolapse. Am J Cardiol 1985; 56:806-7.

116. Dajani AS, Taubert KA, Wilson W, et al. Prevention of bacterial endocarditis: Recommendations of the American Heart Association. JAMA 1997; 277:1794-801.

117. Lee CN, Wu CC, Lin PY, et al. Pregnancy following cardiac valve replacement. Obstet Gynecol 1994; 83:353-6.

118. Elkayam U. Pregnancy through a prosthetic heart valve. J Am Coll Cardiol 1999; 33:1642-5.

119. Iturbe-Alessio I, Inescio M, Mutchinik O. Risks of anticoagulant therapy in pregnant women with artificial heart valves. N Engl J Med 1986; 315:1390-4.

120. Dalen E, Hirsh J (co-chairs). American College of Chest Physicians and the National Heart, Lung, and Blood Institute National Conference of Antithrombotic Therapy. Chest 1986; 89(suppl 2):1-106S.

121. Cooley DA, Chapman DW. Mitral commissurotomy during pregnancy. JAMA 1952; 150:1113-5.

122. Leyse R, Ofstum M, Dillard DH, Merendino KA. Congenital aortic stenosis in pregnancy, corrected by extracorporeal circulation. JAMA 1961; 176:1109-12.

123. Weiss BM, von Segesser LK, Alon E, et al. Outcome of cardiovascular surgery and pregnancy: A systematic review of the period 1984-1996. Am J Obstet Gynecol 1998; 179:1643-53.

124. Parry AJ, Westaby S. Cardiopulmonary bypass during pregnancy. Ann Thorac Surg 1996; 61:1865-9.

125. Yun EM, Royak A, Liu X, et al. The effects of cardiopulmonary bypass on uterine blood flow. Anesthesiology 1997; 87:A876.

126. Farmakides G, Schulman H, Mohtashemi M, et al. Uterine-umbilical velocimetry in open-heart surgery. Am J Obstet Gynecol 1987; 156:1221-2.

127. Khandelwal M, Rasanen J, Ludormirski A, et al. Evaluation of fetal and uterine hemodynamics during maternal cardiopulmonary bypass. Obstet Gynecol 1996; 88:667-71.

128. Burke AB, Hur D, Bolan JC, et al. Sinusoidal fetal heart rate pattern during cardiopulmonary bypass. Am J Obstet Gynecol 1990; 163:17-8.

129. Strickland RA, Oliver WC, Chantigian RC, et al. Anesthesia, cardiopulmonary bypass and the pregnant patient. Mayo Clin Proc 1991; 66: 411-29.

130. Mora CT, Grunewald KE. Reoperative aortic and mitral prosthetic valve replacement in the third trimester of pregnancy. J Cardiothorac Anesth 1987; 1:313-7.

131. Martin MC, Pernoll ML, Boruszak AN, et al. Cesarean section while on cardiac bypass: Report of a case. Obstet Gynecol 1987; 57:414-55.

132. Lamarra M, Azzu AA, Kulatilake NP. Cardiopulmonary bypass in the early puerperium: Possible new role for aprotinin. Ann Thorac Surg 1992; 54:361-3.

133. Nunley WC, Kolp LA, Dabinett LN, et al. Subsequent fertility in women who undergo cardiac surgery. Am J Obstet Gynecol 1989; 161:573-6.

134. Pearson GD, Veille JC, Rahimtoola S, et al. Peripartum cardiomyopathy: National Heart, Lung, and Blood Institute and Office of Rare Diseases (National Institutes of Health) Workshop Recommendations and Review. JAMA 2000; 283:1183-8.

135. Mehta NJ, Mehta RN, Khan IA. Peripartum cardiomyopathy: Clinical and therapeutic aspects. Angiology 2001; 52:759-62.

136. Brown B, Asaeda G. Prehospital rounds. Hypertension after having a baby. Emerg Med Serv 2002; 31:74-5.

137. Yagoro A, Tada H, Hidaka Y, et al. Postpartum onset of acute heart failure possibly due to postpartum autoimmune myocarditis. A report of three cases. J Int Med 1999; 245:199-203.

138. Irey NS, Norris HJ. Intimal vascular lesions associated with female reproductive steroids. Arch Pathol 1973; 96:227-34.

139. Adesonya CO, Anjorin FI, Sada IA, et al. Atrial natriuretic peptide, aldosterone, and plasma renin activity in peripartum heart failure. Br Heart J 1991; 65:152-4.

140. Sanderson JE, Adesanaya CO, Anjorin FI, Parry EH. Maternal cardiomyopathy of pregnancy: Heart failure due to volume overload? Am Heart J 1979; 97:613-21.

141. Felker GM, Jaeger CJ, Klodas E, et al. Myocarditis and long-term survival in peripartum cardiomyopathy. Am Heart J 2000; 140:785-91.

142. Aziz TM, Burgess MI, Acladious NN, et al. Heart transplantation for peripartum cardiomyopathy: A report of three cases and a literature review. Cardiovas Surg 1999; 7:565-7.

143. Elkayam U, Tummala PP, Rao K, et al. Maternal and fetal outcomes of subsequent pregnancies in women with peripartum cardiomyopathy. New Engl J Med 2001; 344:1567-71.

144. Futterman LG, Lemberg L. Peripartum cardiomyopathy: an ominous complication of pregnancy. Am J Crit Care 2000; 9:362-6.

145. Carlson KM, Browning JE, Eggleston MK, Gherman RB. Peripartum cardiomyopathy presenting as lower extremity arterial thromboembolism. A case report. J Reprod Med 2000; 45:351-3.

146. Bozkurt B, Villanueva FS, Holubkov R, et al. Intravenous immune globulin in the therapy of peripartum cardiomyopathy. J Am Coll Cardiol 1999; 34:177-80.

147. McIndoe AK, Hammond EJ, Babington R. Peripartum cardiomyopathy presenting as a cardiac arrest at induction of anesthesia for emergency cesarean section. Br J Anaesth 1995; 75:97-101.

148. McCarroll CP, Paxton LD, Elliott P, Wilson DB. Use of remifentanil in a patient with peripartum cardiomyopathy requiring caesarean section. Br J Anaesth 2001; 86:135-8.

149. George LM, Gatt SP, Lowe S. Peripartum cardiomyopathy: Four case histories and a commentary on anesthetic management. Anaesth Intens Care 1997; 25:292-6.

150. Hosenpud JD, Bennett LE, Keck BM, et al. The registry of the international society for heart and lung transplantation: Fourteenth official report. J Heart Lung Transplant 1997; 16:691-712.

151. Scott JR, Wagoner LE, Olsen SL, et al. Pregnancy in heart transplant recipients: Management and outcome. Obstet Gynecol 1993; 82:324-7.

152. Kossoy LR, Herbert CM, Wentz AC. Management of heart transplant recipients: Guidelines for the obstetrician-gynecologist. Am J Obstet Gynecol 1988; 159:490-9.

153. Morini A, Spina V, Aleandri V, et al. Pregnancy after heart transplant: Update and case report. Human Reprod 1998; 13:749-57.

154. Troche V, Ville Y, Fernandez H. Pregnancy after heart or heart-lung transplantation: A series of 10 pregnancies. Br J Obstet Gynaecol 1998; 105:454-8.

155. Kim KM, Sukhani R, Slogoff S, Tomich PG. Central hemodynamic changes associated with pregnancy in a long-term cardiac transplant recipient. Am J Obstet Gynecol 1996; 174:1651-3.

156. Eskandar M, Gader S, Ong BY. Two successful vaginal deliveries in a heart transplant recipient. Obstet Gynecol 1996; 87:880.

157. Yusuf S, Theodoropoulos S, Mathias CJ, et al. Increased sensitivity of the denervated transplanted human heart to isoprenaline both before and after β-adrenergic blockade. Circulation 1987; 75:696-704.

158. Camann WR, Goldman GA, Johnson MD, et al. Cesarean delivery in a patient with a transplanted heart. Anesthesiology 1989; 71: 618-20.

159. Branch KR, Wagoner LE, McGrory CH, et al. Risks of subsequent pregnancies on mother and newborn in female heart transplant recipients. J Heart Lung Transplant 1998; 17:698-702.

160. Eskandar M, Gader S, Ong BY. Two successful vaginal deliveries in a heart transplant recipient. Obstet Gynecol 1996; 88:880.

161. Rigg CD, Bythell VE, Bryson MR, et al. Caesarean section in patients with heart-lung transplants: A report of three cases and review. Internat J Obstet Anesth 2000; 9:125-132.

162. Rees GAD, Willis BA. Resuscitation in late pregnancy. Anaesthesia 1988; 43:347-9.

163. Goodwin APL, Pearce AJ. The human wedge: A maneuver to relieve aortocaval compression during resuscitation in pregnancy. Anaesthesia 1992; 47:433-4.

164. American Heart Association. Guidelines for cardiopulmonary resuscitation and emergency cardiac care: Special resuscitation situations. JAMA 1992; 268:2242-50.

165. Parker J, Balis N, Chester S, Adey D. Cardiopulmonary arrest in pregnancy: Successful resuscitation of mother and infant following immediate caesarean section in labour ward. Aust NZ J Obstet Gynaecol 1996; 36:207-10.

166. Cardosi RJ, Porter KB. Cesarean delivery of twins during maternal cardiopulmonary arrest. Obstet Gynecol 1998; 92:695-7.

167. Marx GF. Cardiopulmonary resuscitation of late pregnant women. Anesthesiology 1982; 56:156.

168. Kloeck W, Cummins RO, Chamberlain D, et al. Special resuscitation situations: An advisory statement from the International Liaison Committee on Resuscitation. Circulation 1997; 95:2196-210.

169. Finegold H, Darwich A, Romeo R, et al. Successful resuscitation after maternal cardiac arrest by immediate cesarean section in the labor room (letter). Anesthesiology 2002; 96:1278.

170. Baraka A, Kawkabani N, Haroun-Bizri S. Hemodynamic deterioration after cardiopulmonary bypass during pregnancy: Resuscitation by postoperative emergency cesarean section. J Cardiothor Vasc Anesth 2000; 14: 314-5.

171. American Heart Association. Textbook of Advanced Cardiac Life Support, 2nd ed, Dallas, The American Heart Association, 1994: 10-17.

172. Esposito BA, Grossi EA, Coppa G, et al. Successful treatment of postpartum shock caused by amniotic fluid embolism with cardiopulmonary bypass and pulmonary artery thromboembolectomy. Obstet Gynecol 1990; 8:572-4.

173. Lee RV, Rodgers BD, White LM, Harvey RC. Cardiopulmonary resuscitation of pregnant women. Am J Med 1986; 81:311-8.

174. Lopez-Zeno JA, Carlo WA, O'Grady JP, Fanaroff AA. Infant survival following delayed postmortem cesarean delivery. Obstet Gynecol 1990; 76:991-2.

175. Litwin MS, Loughlin KR, Benson CB, et al. Placenta percreta involving the urinary bladder. Br J Urol 1989; 64:283-6.

176. Long WB, Rosenblum S, Grady P. Successful resuscitation of bupivacaine-induced cardiac arrest using cardiopulmonary bypass. Anesth Analg 1989; 69:403-6.

177. Splinter WM, Dwane PD, Wigle RD, McGrath MJ. Clinical reports: Anaesthetic management of emergency caesarean section followed by pulmonary embolectomy. Can J Anaesth 1989; 36:689-92.

178. Shotan A, Ostrzega E, Mehra A, et al. Incidence of arrhythmias in normal pregnancy and relation to palpitations, dizziness, and syncope. Am J Cardiol 1997; 79:1061-4.

179. Lee SH, Chen SA, Wu TJ, et al. Effects of pregnancy on first onset and symptoms of paroxysmal supraventricular tachycardia. Am J Cardiol 1995; 76:675-8.

180. Dominguez A, Iturralde P, Hermosillo AG, et al. Successful radiofrequency ablation of an accessory pathway during pregnancy. Pacing Clin Electrophysiol 1999; 22:131-4.

181. Sherman JL, Locke RV. Transplacental neonatal digitalis intoxication. Am J Cardiol 1960; 6:834-7.

182. Rotmensch HH, Rotmensch S, Elkayam U. Management of cardiac arrhythmias during pregnancy. Drugs 1987; 33:623-33.

183. Dumesic DA, Silverman NH, Tobias S, Golbus MS. Transplacental cardioversion of fetal supraventricular tachycardia with procainamide. N Engl J Med 1982; 307:1128-31.

184. Pruyn SC, Phelan JP, Buchanan GC. Long-term propranolol therapy in pregnancy: Maternal and fetal outcome. Am J Obstet Gynecol 1979; 135:485-589.

185. Klein V, Repke JT. Supraventricular tachycardia in pregnancy: Cardioversion with verapamil. Obstet Gynecol 1984; 63: 165-85.

186. Murad SHN, Tabsh KMA, Conklin KA, et al. Verapamil: Placental transfer and effects on maternal and fetal hemodynamics and atrioventricular conduction in the pregnant ewe. Anesthesiology 1985; 62:49-53.

187. Wolff F, Brueker KH, Schlensker KH, Bolte A. Prenatal diagnosis and therapy of fetal heart rate anomalies: With a contribution on the placental transfer of verapamil. J Perinatol Med 1980; 8:203-8.

188. Seki H, Takeda S, Kinoshita K. Long-term treatment with nicardipine for severe pre-eclampsia. Internat J Gynaecol Obstet 2002; 76:135-41.

189. Hanson JW, Myranthopoulos NC, Harvey MAS, Smith DW. Risks of offspring of women treated with hydantoin anticonvulsant and emphasis of fetal hydantoin syndrome. J Pediatr 1976; 89:662-8.

190. Rey E, Bachrach LK, Buttow GN. Effects of amiodarone during pregnancy. Can Med Assoc J 1987; 136:959-60.

191. Foster CJ, Love HG. Amiodarone in pregnancy: Case report and review of the literature. Int J Cardiol 1988; 20:307-16.

192. Arnoux P, Seyral P, Llurens M. Amiodarone and digoxin for refractory fetal tachycardia. Am J Cardiol 1987; 59:166-7.

193. Laurent M, Betremieux P, Biron Y, Lellelloco A. Neonatal hypothyroidism after treatment with amiodarone during pregnancy. Am J Cardiol 1987; 60:142.

194. Widerhorn J, Bhandari AK, Bughi S, et al. Fetal and neonatal adverse effects profile of amiodarone treatment during pregnancy. Am Heart J 1991; 122:1162-6.

195. Nadamanee K, Piwonka RW, Singh BN, Hershman J. Amiodarone and thyroid function. Prog Cardiovasc Dis 1989; 6:427-37.

196. Schleich JM, Cilly FBD, Laurent MC, Almange C. Early prenatal management of a fetal ventricular tachycardia treated in utero by amiodarone with long term follow-up. Prenat Diagn 2000; 20:449-52.

197. Belardinelli L, Linden J, Berne RM. The cardiac effects of adenosine. Prog Cardiovasc Dis 1989; 6:73-97.

198. Mason BA, Ricci-Goodman J, Koos BJ. Adenosine in the treatment of maternal paroxysmal supraventricular tachycardia. Obstet Gynecol 1992; 80:478-80.

199. Afridi I, Moise KJ, Rokey R. Termination of supraventricular tachycardia with intravenous adenosine in a pregnant woman with Wolff-Parkinson-White syndrome. Obstet Gynecol 1992; 80:481-3.

200. Dalvi BV, Chaudhuri A, Kulkarni HL, Kale PA. Therapeutic guidelines for congenital complete heart block presenting in pregnancy. Obstet Gynecol 1992; 79:802-4.

201. Jaffe R, Gruber A, Fejgin M, et al. Pregnancy with an artificial pacemaker. Obstet Gynecol Surv 1987; 42:137-9.

202. Gudal M, Kervancioglo C, Oral D, et al. Permanent pacemaker implantation in a pregnant woman with the guidance of ECG and two-dimensional echocardiography. PACE 1987; 10:543-5.

203. Trappe HJ, Pfitzner P. [Cardiac arrhythmias in pregnancy]. Zeitschrift fur Kardiologie 2001; 90:36-44.

204. Bonini W, Botto GL, Broffoni T, Dondina C. Pregnancy with an ICD and a documented ICD discharge. Europace 2000; 2:87-90.

205. Olufolabi AJ, Charlton GA, Allen SA, et al. Use of implantable cardioverter defibrillator and anti-arrhythmic agents in a parturient. Br J Anaesth 2002; 89:652-5.

206. Ogburn PL, Schmidt G, Liinman J, Cefalo RC. Paroxysmal tachycardia and cardioversion during pregnancy. J Reprod Med 1983; 27:359-62.

207. Bevacqua BK. Supraventricular tachycardia associated with postpartum metoclopramide administration. Anesthesiology 1988; 68:124-5.

208. Chow T, Galvin J, McGovern B. Antiarrhythmic drug therapy in pregnancy and lactation. Am J Cardiol 1998; 82:58-62I.

209. Barnes EJ, Eben F, Patterson D. Direct current cardioversion during pregnancy should be performed with facilities available for fetal monitoring and emergency caesarean section. BJOG 2002; 109:1406-7.

210. Pyeritz RE. Maternal and fetal complications of pregnancy in the Marfan syndrome. Am J Med 1981; 71:784-90.

211. Tritapepe L, Voci P, Pinto G, et al. Anesthesia for cesarean section in a Marfan patient with recurrent aortic dissection. Can J Anaesth 1996; 43:1153-5.

212. Rosenblum NG, Grossman AR, Gabbe SG, et al. Failure of serial echocardiographic studies to predict aortic dissection in a pregnant patient with Marfan syndrome. Am J Obstet Gynecol 1983; 146:470-1.

213. Paternoster DM, Santarossa C, Vettore N, et al. Obstetric complications in Marfan's syndrome pregnancy. Minerva Ginecologica 1998; 50:441-3.

214. Pedowitz P, Perrell A. Aneurysms complicated by pregnancy. Am J Obstet Gynecol 1957; 73:720-35.

215. Tobis JM. Aortic dissection in pregnancy. In Elkayam U, Gleicher N, editors. Cardiac Problems in Pregnancy. New York, Alan R Liss, 1982:161-5.

216. Konishi T, Tatsuta N, Kumada K, et al. Dissecting aneurysm during pregnancy and the puerperium. Jpn Circ J 1980; 44:726.

217. Debakey ME, Henly WS, Cooley DA, et al. Surgical management of dissecting aneurysms of the aorta. J Thorac Cardiovasc Surg 1965; 49:130-49.

218. Kao YJ, Zavisca FG, Tellez JM, et al. Backache after extradural anaesthesia in the postpartum period: Dissection of thoracic aorta. Br J Anaesth 1991; 67:335-8.

219. Cigarroa JE, Isselbacher EM, DeSanctis RW, Eagle KA. Diagnostic imaging in the evaluation of suspected aortic dissection: Old standards and new directions. N Engl J Med 1993; 328:35-43.

220. Crawford ES, Palamara AE, Saleh SA, Roehm JOF. Aortic aneurysm: Current status of surgical treatment. Surg Clin North Am 1979; 59: 597-636.

221. Henry DM, Cotton DB. Bacterial endocarditis in pregnancy associated with septic renal embolization. South Med J 1985; 78:355-6.

222. Seaworth BJ, Durack DT. Infective endocarditis in obstetric and gynecologic practice. Am J Obstet Gynecol 1986; 154:180-8.

223. Cox SM, Leveno KJ. Pregnancy complicated by bacterial endocarditis. Clin Obstet Gynecol 1989; 32:48-53.

224. Weinstein L. Infective endocarditis. In Braunwald E, editor. Heart Disease, 3rd ed. Philadelphia, WB Saunders, 1988:1100.

225. O'Donnell D, Gillmer DJ, Mitha AS. Aortic and mitral valve replacement for bacterial endocarditis in pregnancy: A case report. S Afr Med J 1983; 64:1074.

226. Gallagher PG, Watanakunakorn C. Group B streptococcal endocarditis: Report of seven cases and review of the literature, 1962-1985. Rev Infect Dis 1986; 8:175-88.

227. Bataskov KL, Hariharan S, Horowitz MD, et al. Gonococcal endocarditis complicating pregnancy: A case report and literature review. Obstet Gynecol 1991; 78:494-5.

228. Vander Bel-Kahn JM, Watanakunakorn C, Menefee MG, et al. Chlamydia trachomatis endocarditis. Am Heart J 1978; 95: 627-36.

229. Mandell GL, Kaye D, Levison ME, Hook EW. Enterococcal endocarditis: An analysis of 38 patients observed at the New York Hospital-Cornell Medical Center. Arch Intern Med 1970; 2:258-64.

230. Gill GV. Endocarditis caused by Salmonella enteritidis. Br Heart J 1979; 42:353-4.

231. Alvarez-Elcoro S, Mateos-Mora M, Zajarias A. Mycobacterium fortuitum endocarditis after mitral valve replacement with a bovine prosthesis. South Med J 1985; 78:865-6.

232. Holshouser CA, Ansbacher R, McNitt T, Steele R. Bacterial endocarditis due to Listeria monocytogenes in a pregnant diabetic. Obstet Gynecol 1978; 51(suppl):9-10S.

Chapter 41
Endocrine Disorders

Richard N. Wissler, M.D., Ph.D.

DIABETES MELLITUS

Definition and Epidemiology

Diabetes mellitus (DM) is a common metabolic disorder, with a prevalence of 2.6% to 4.5% in the general adult population in the United States.[1,2] DM results from either a decrease in insulin secretion (type 1) or a resistance to insulin in target tissues (type 2). *Insulin-dependent diabetes mellitus* (IDDM) and *non-insulin-dependent diabetes mellitus* (NIDDM) are relatively synonymous terms for type 1 and type 2 DM, respectively. Currently, type 1 and type 2 DM are the preferred designations.[3] A combination of genetic and environmental factors contributes to both types of DM.[3] However, type 1 is primarily an autoimmune disorder, and type 2 occurs primarily in obese individuals. Type 2 DM accounts for 90% to 95% of the cases of DM in the United States. Gestational DM refers to DM or glucose intolerance that is first diagnosed during pregnancy. Gestational DM occurs in approximately 4% of pregnancies in the United States.[3]

Pathophysiology

Insulin is a peptide hormone secreted by the beta cells of the islets of Langerhans in the pancreas. Box 41-1 lists the factors that influence insulin secretion.[4,5] Insulin binds to specific cell-surface receptors in its target tissues, which include liver, skeletal muscle, and fat. The intracellular effects of insulin are mediated by means of tyrosine kinase in the beta-subunit of the receptor through a cascade of distal protein kinase-mediated phosphorylations.[6,7] Normal hepatic glucose metabolism represents a balance between the effects of insulin and several "counterregulatory" hormones (e.g., glucagon, cortisol, epinephrine, growth hormone).[8] This control system for glucose homeostasis normally permits rapid adjustments in glucose metabolism in the fed and fasted states. Insulin is also an important anabolic regulator of lipid and amino acid metabolism (Figure 41-1). The insulin deficiency (absolute or relative) that is associated with DM results in abnormalities in the metabolism of carbohydrates, lipids, and amino acids.

Acute and chronic complications occur in patients with DM (Box 41-2). The three major acute complications are diabetic ketoacidosis, hyperosmolar hyperglycemic nonketotic coma, and hypoglycemia.[9] **Diabetic ketoacidosis (DKA)** occurs almost exclusively in patients with type 1 DM. DKA may develop with the typical dose of insulin in the event of a new source of insulin resistance (e.g., infection, trauma, stress), or it may occur as a result of failure to administer the usual dose of insulin. DKA results from decreased uptake of glucose by insulin-responsive tissues (e.g., liver, skeletal muscle) and increased use of free fatty acids as a hepatic energy source. The lack of insulin favors lipolysis, beta-oxidation of free fatty acids in the liver, and hepatic formation of acetoacetate and beta-hydroxybutyrate from the excess acetyl-CoA generated by fatty acid oxidation.[10] These biochemical events result in metabolic acidosis, hyperglycemia, and dehydration secondary to an osmotic diuresis. Signs and symptoms of DKA include nausea, vomiting, weakness, tachypnea, hypotension, tachycardia, stupor, and acetone on the breath.[9] The diagnosis of DKA depends on the laboratory findings of hyperglycemia, ketosis, and acidosis. The traditional method for the diagnosis of ketonemia is the nitroprusside reaction, which detects acetoacetate but not the more plentiful beta-hydroxybutyrate. Recently developed enzymatic assays may allow routine clinical quantitation of blood levels of beta-hydroxybutyrate.[11]

Hyperosmolar hyperglycemic nonketotic coma (HHNC) occurs predominantly in patients with type 2 DM. The precipitating medical event typically is of a more serious nature than that of DKA.[9] The laboratory findings in HHNC are hyperglycemia (often more than 600 mg/dL), hyperosmolarity (greater than 310 mOsm), and moderate azotemia (serum blood urea nitrogen [BUN] of 70 to 90 mg/dL), without ketonemia or significant acidosis.[10] The absence of significant ketosis in HHNC may indicate an inhibition of lipolysis by hyperosmolarity[12] or low levels of insulin.[13]

Hypoglycemia is a continuing health threat in diabetic patients, especially those who receive insulin therapy. Symptomatic awareness of hypoglycemia and counterregulatory responses may be inadequate in some diabetic patients

Box 41-1 FACTORS THAT INFLUENCE INSULIN SECRETION

PHYSIOLOGIC

STIMULATION

- Glucose
- Amino acids
- Gastrointestinal peptide hormones (e.g., gastric inhibitory polypeptide)
- Ketone bodies (e.g., in starvation)
- Glucagon
- Parasympathetic stimulation
- Beta-adrenergic stimulation

INHIBITION

- Somatostatin
- Sympathetic stimulation (splanchnic nerve)
- Alpha-adrenergic stimulation

PHARMACOLOGIC AND EXPERIMENTAL

STIMULATION

- Cyclic AMP
- Theophylline
- Sulfonylureas
- Salicylates

INHIBITION

- Deoxyglucose
- Mannoheptulose
- Diazoxide
- Prostaglandins
- Diphenylhydantoin
- Beta-cell poisons
  - Alloxan
  - Streptozotocin

From West JB, editor. Best and Taylor's Physiological Basis of Medical Practice, 12th ed. Baltimore, Williams & Wilkins, 1991:757.

Box 41-2 MAJOR COMPLICATIONS OF DIABETES MELLITUS

ACUTE

Diabetic ketoacidosis (DKA)
Hyperosmolar hyperglycemic nonketotic coma (HHNC)
Hypoglycemia

CHRONIC

MACROVASCULAR (ATHEROSCLEROSIS)

- Coronary
- Cerebrovascular
- Peripheral vascular

MICROVASCULAR

- Retinopathy
- Nephropathy

NEUROPATHY

- Autonomic
- Somatic

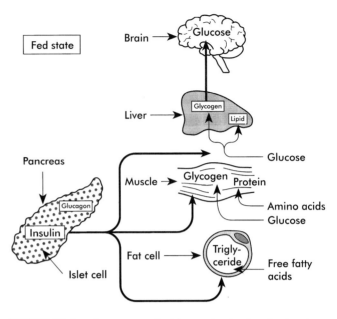

FIGURE 41-1. Substrate use in the fed state, showing the role of insulin in the promotion of fuel storage. (From Kitabachi AE, Murphy MB. Diabetic ketoacidosis and hyperosmolar hyperglycemic nonketotic coma. Med Clin North Am 1988; 72:1545-63.)

decreased caloric intake.[16] In one study, two diabetic pregnant patients (who were receiving insulin therapy) became hypoglycemic while fasting before cesarean section. Deliberate, inappropriate self-administration of insulin or an oral hypoglycemic agent can lead to factitious hypoglycemia.[17]

In general, the prevalence of chronic complications increases with the duration of DM.[18] The Diabetes Control and Complications Trial, a randomized multicenter study of patients with type 1 DM, demonstrated a positive relationship between tight glucose control and a lowered incidence or rate of progression of **retinopathy, nephropathy,** and **neuropathy.**[19] In a similar study of patients with type 2 DM—the UK Prospective Diabetes Study (UKPDS)—intensive glucose control lowered the incidence of microvascular complications but not mortality or macrovascular complications.[20] In contrast to glycemic control, antihypertensive therapy reduced the incidence of macrovascular complications and mortality in patients with both type 2 DM and chronic hypertension.[20] DM may affect **cardiovascular function** as a result of coronary atherosclerosis and autonomic neuropathy. In addition, DM may cause a cardiomyopathy by means of direct alterations in myocardial carbohydrate and lipid metabolism.[21]

Clinical Presentation and Diagnosis

The current diagnostic criteria for DM in nonpregnant patients are shown in Box 41-3.[3]

Gestational DM is associated with (1) advanced maternal age, (2) obesity, (3) a family history of DM, and (4) a history of prior stillbirth, neonatal death, or fetal malformation or macrosomia. Unfortunately, the clinical sensitivity of the medical history in detecting gestational DM is only 50%.[22] Three different forms of oral glucose tolerance tests (OGTTs) are used to diagnose gestational DM. The World Health Organization does not distinguish between pregnant and nonpregnant patients, and it recommends the 75-g, 2-hour OGTT (see Box 41-3). Others have recommended a 50-g, 1-hour OGTT in pregnant patients (with a cut-off plasma

with an autonomic neuropathy.[14] Beta-adrenergic receptor blocking agents should be avoided in diabetic patients for the same reason.[15] Hypoglycemia results from an imbalance between insulin or oral hypoglycemic agents and available metabolic fuels. In hospitalized patients with DM, major risk factors for hypoglycemia include renal insufficiency and

glucose concentration of 140 mg/dL) as a screening test for DM at 24 to 28 weeks' gestation.[23,24] Patients with a positive screen subsequently undergo a 100-g, 3-hour OGTT (Table 41-1).

Two areas of controversy exist regarding diagnostic testing for gestational DM. First, should a screening test be applied universally or used only in high-risk patients?[25-27] For example, women at low risk for gestational DM include those under 25 years of age with normal body weight and a negative family history for DM, who are not members of an ethnic/racial group with a high prevalence of DM (e.g., Hispanic, African-American, American Indian, and South or East Asian). Second, which diagnostic thresholds should be used in the 3-hour OGTT? The American Diabetes Association (ADA) has proposed diagnostic thresholds lower than those advocated by the National Diabetes Data Group (Table 41-1).[24] (The ADA criteria were formerly known as the criteria of Carpenter and Coustan.) Several studies suggest a health benefit associated with the use of the lower diagnostic thresholds.[28,29] However, some investigators are reluctant to endorse either threshold without consideration of cost-effectiveness.[25,30]

Glycosylated hemoglobin (GHb) measurements are used as time-integrated estimates of glycemic control, but not as a diagnostic test for DM. The normal range for hemoglobin A_{1C} in nondiabetic pregnant women is 4.1% to 5.9%.[31]

Interaction with Pregnancy

HOW DOES PREGNANCY AFFECT DIABETES MELLITUS?

Pregnancy is characterized by a progressive peripheral resistance to insulin at the receptor and postreceptor levels in the second and third trimesters (Figure 41-2).[32-34] The presumed mechanism involves an increase in counterregulatory hormones (e.g., placental lactogen, placental growth hormone,

---

Box 41-3 CRITERIA FOR THE DIAGNOSIS OF DIABETES MELLITUS (DM)

1. Symptoms of DM plus casual plasma glucose concentration ≥ 200 mg/dL. Casual is defined as any time of day without regard to time since last meal. The classic symptoms of DM include polyuria, polydipsia, and unexplained weight loss.

   or

2. Fasting plasma glucose (FPG) ≥ 126 mg/dL. Fasting is defined as no caloric intake for at least 8 hours.

   or

3. Two-hour postload plasma glucose (2hPG) ≥ 200 mg/dL during an oral glucose tolerance test (OGTT). This test should be performed as described by the World Health Organization, using a glucose load containing the equivalent of 75 g of anhydrous glucose dissolved in water.

- In the absence of unequivocal hyperglycemia with acute metabolic decompensation, these criteria should be confirmed by repeat testing on a different day.
- The third measurement (OGTT) is not recommended for routine clinical use.
- Normal fasting glucose = FPG < 110 mg/dL.
- Normal glucose tolerance = 2hPG < 140 mg/dL.
- Impaired fasting glucose = FPG ≥ 110 and < 126 mg/dL.
- Impaired glucose tolerance = 2hPG ≥ 140 and < 200 mg/dL.

From American Diabetes Association Expert Committee on the Diagnosis and Classification of Diabetes Mellitus. Report of the Expert Committee on the Diagnosis and Classification of Diabetes Mellitus. Diabetes Care 1997; 20:1183-97.

TABLE 41-1 ORAL GLUCOSE TOLERANCE TEST CRITERIA FOR THE DIAGNOSIS OF GESTATIONAL DIABETES MELLITUS*

| | Plasma glucose (mg/dL) | |
Hour	National Diabetes Data Group	American Diabetes Association
0	105	95
1	190	180
2	165	155
3	145	140

*100-g oral glucose dose. If any two measurements exceed the criteria, gestational diabetes mellitus is diagnosed. Note: mg/dL of glucose may be converted to mmol/L by multiplying by 0.0555.
From Jovanovic L, Pettitt DJ. Gestational diabetes mellitus. JAMA 2001; 286:2516-8.

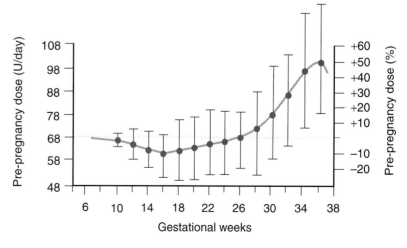

FIGURE 41-2. Insulin requirements in euglycemic women with type 1 diabetes mellitus during pregnancy. (From Crombach G, Siebolds M, Mies R. Insulin use in pregnancy: Clinical pharmacokinetic considerations. Clin Pharmacokinet 1993; 24:89-100.)

cortisol, progesterone) during pregnancy. The change in placental lactogen is a plausible mechanism, given that a graph of serum levels during pregnancy is similar in shape to that shown for insulin requirements in pregnant women with type 1 DM (Figure 41-2),[35] and placental lactogen has growth hormone-like activity. The insulin resistance of pregnancy may facilitate the provision of maternal glucose and amino acids for the fetus.[35]

Gestational DM develops when a patient cannot mount a sufficient compensatory insulin response during pregnancy. In some patients, gestational DM can be viewed as a preclinical state of glucose intolerance that is not detectable before pregnancy. After delivery most patients return to normal glucose tolerance but remain at increased risk for DM (predominantly type 2) in later life.[36,37] The recurrence rate for gestational DM in a subsequent pregnancy is 52% to 68%.[38,39]

In patients with pregestational DM, the therapeutic doses of insulin progressively increase during pregnancy because of peripheral insulin resistance.[40] At term, the daily insulin requirement typically is approximately 1.0 insulin units/kg, compared with 0.7 units/kg before pregnancy, although variations among individuals occur.[40] During late pregnancy in normal patients, basal and glucose-stimulated plasma insulin levels are twice the postpartum measurements.[41] These changes reflect pregnancy-related increases in pancreatic islet cell mass and glucose sensitivity, probably related to the net effect of competing progesterone and lactogenic hormone stimuli in the endocrine pancreas.[42,43] Near term, maternal overnight insulin requirements may *decrease,* presumably as a result of "siphoning of maternal fuels" by the growing fetus during the overnight maternal fast.[44,45]

Endogenous plasma insulin concentrations during labor and delivery in nondiabetic parturients differ from exogenous insulin requirements in laboring diabetic women. In nondiabetic parturients, the plasma glucose concentration is only one of many factors that affect endogenous insulin secretion. In nondiabetic parturients, glucose production and utilization markedly increase during painful labor, compared with postpartum measurements.[46] Plasma insulin concentrations remain unchanged except for a brief increase during the third stage of labor and immediately postpartum.[46,47] These observations suggest that glucose use during labor is largely independent of insulin. The pattern of plasma insulin concentrations in nondiabetic patients is similar with and without analgesia (e.g., nitrous oxide, meperidine).[47]

In patients with type 1 DM, insulin requirements decrease with the onset of the first stage of labor.[48] These patients may require no additional insulin during the first stage, although insulin requirements are modified by (1) the level of metabolic control before labor, (2) the residual effect of prior doses of subcutaneous insulin, and (3) the glucose infusion rate.[48-50] Insulin requirements increase during the second stage of labor, but the mechanism for this change is unknown.[48,49] The use of epidural analgesia or oxytocin does not affect exogenous insulin requirements during the first and second stages of labor.[48] After delivery (either vaginal or cesarean), insulin requirements in patients with type 1 DM decrease markedly for at least several days, although there is significant variability among individuals (Figure 41-3).[34,51,52] Presumably, the decreased insulin requirement results from the loss of counterregulatory hormones produced by the placenta. Pituitary growth hormone responses to hypoglycemia are blunted in late pregnancy, and this may contribute to impaired counterregulatory responses during the postpartum period.[53] Moreover, one case report suggested that endogenous insulin secretion may be temporarily restored during the peripartum period in patients with type 1 DM, perhaps as a result of the suppressive effect of pregnancy on autoimmunity.[54] The change in counterregulatory influences at the time of delivery may unmask a previously silent insulinoma.[55] The insulin requirements gradually return to prepregnancy levels within several weeks of delivery in patients with type 1 DM.[45]

Before the discovery of insulin in 1921, pregnancies were rare in diabetic patients. Subsequently, insulin therapy improved maternal outcome, but fetal and neonatal morbidity and mortality remained high. Insulin therapy resulted in the increased survival of patients with severe DM, which allowed these patients to reach childbearing age and become pregnant.[56] Despite improved obstetric and medical care, maternal mortality remains 10 times higher in diabetic patients than in nondiabetic patients.[57]

In 1949, Dr. Priscilla White[58] proposed a classification system of DM during pregnancy that was based on 439 consecutive cases. Physicians caring for pregnant diabetic patients

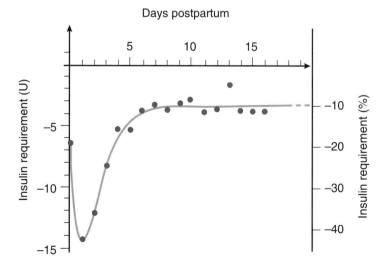

FIGURE 41-3. Insulin requirements in the postportum period. (From Crombach G, Siebolds M, Mies R. Insulin use in pregnancy: Clinical pharmacokinetic considerations. Clin Pharmacokinet 1993; 24:89-100.)

should be familiar with the White system, which has endured with some modifications (Table 41-2). White developed this system to emphasize the relationship among the duration of type 1 DM, vascular complications of type 1 DM, and poor fetal outcome.[59] In the 1950s, fetal survival rates were as follows: class A, 100%; class B, 67%; class C, 48%; class D, 32%, and class F, 3%.[59]

DKA occurs in 8% to 9% of diabetic pregnancies.[57,60] As is true for nonpregnant patients, DKA during pregnancy occurs almost exclusively in patients with type 1 DM. However, one case report described an episode of DKA in a patient with gestational DM and subsequent normal glucose tolerance in the nonpregnant state.[61] DKA results in a perinatal mortality rate as high as 30% to 70%, although outcome may have improved in recent years.[60,62] The increased risk of DKA during pregnancy reflects the metabolic adaptations of pregnancy, including peripheral insulin resistance.[34]

During pregnancy, DKA occurs most commonly during the second and third trimesters.[63] It is associated with the following factors: (1) beta-adrenergic agonist therapy, (2) emesis, (3) decreased caloric intake, (4) poor medical management, and (5) patient noncompliance.[64,65] Infection is another risk factor for DKA, and pregnant patients with pregestational type 1 DM have an infection rate 3.2 times higher than that in nondiabetic pregnant patients.[66] DKA may be the first clinical sign of type 1 DM during pregnancy.[62,67] Both the beta-adrenergic agonists (used to treat preterm labor) and the glucocorticoids (used to accelerate fetal lung maturity) have counterregulatory pharmacologic effects that oppose the action of insulin. Beta-adrenergic tocolytic therapy, with or without concurrent glucocorticoid therapy, can precipitate DKA during pregnancy.[68-70] Beta-adrenergic receptor stimulation worsens glucose intolerance by stimulating glucagon secretion.[71] Beta-adrenergic agents may exert this effect through *any* route of administration.[70-72] Beta-adrenergic agonists may be well tolerated in pregnant patients with DM, provided that increased insulin requirements are anticipated and doses are adjusted in response to frequent blood glucose monitoring.[67,70]

Several case reports have described fetal heart rate (FHR) patterns that are consistent with fetal distress during episodes of maternal DKA.[73-75] FHR responses normalized and preterm uterine contractions stopped after appropriate medical management of maternal DKA. The mechanism of fetal distress during DKA is unclear but may be related to changes in uterine blood flow. In a study of human uterine blood flow during cesarean section, Blechner et al.[76] demonstrated that acute maternal metabolic acidosis decreases uterine blood flow. In pregnant ewes, uterine arterial infusion of beta-hydroxybutyrate decreased uterine blood flow and fetal P_{O_2} by 12% and 26%, respectively.[77] A single human case report demonstrated reversible fetal blood flow redistribution during an episode of maternal DKA, based on Doppler pulsatility indices of the umbilical and middle cerebral arteries.[78]

Raziel et al.[79] reported a single case of **HHNC** during pregnancy. No conclusion can be drawn concerning HHNC and pregnancy, except that their simultaneous occurrence is rare.

Hypoglycemia is a significant health risk during pregnancy for patients with pregestational type 1 DM. Episodes of severe hypoglycemia occur during pregnancy in 33% to 71% of these patients.[80-82] This rate is approximately 3 to 15 times greater than that for similar groups of nonpregnant patients with type 1 DM,[80,81] and 73% of the episodes of severe hypoglycemia occur before 16 weeks' gestation.[82] In one study, patients with pregestational type 2 DM or gestational DM who required insulin therapy during pregnancy experienced no episodes of severe hypoglycemia.[81] The risk of hypoglycemia during pregnancy in patients with type 1 DM is increased with tight glucose control.[80,82,83] This mirrors the clinical experience in nonpregnant patients with type 1 DM, in which tight insulin therapy results in a threefold increase in the incidence of severe hypoglycemia.[84] Counterregulatory hormone responses to hypoglycemia are impaired after intensive insulin therapy in both pregnant and nonpregnant patients with type 1 DM.[85-87] Two small series of patients suggest that acute mild-to-moderate maternal hypoglycemia is not associated with acute alterations in fetal well-being in pregnant patients with type 1 DM.[85,88] Episodes of severe hypoglycemia before pregnancy are associated with an increased incidence of hypoglycemia during pregnancy.[82]

Airaksinen et al.[89] observed that pregnant patients with both type 1 DM and autonomic neuropathy were not more likely to develop severe hypoglycemia than those without autonomic neuropathy. However, this study evaluated relatively small groups of patients and may have lacked the statistical power to demonstrate differences among groups.

The relationship between pregnancy and the development of macrovascular complications of DM is largely unknown. Patients with pregestational type 1 DM have higher systolic and diastolic blood pressures during pregnancy and are three times more likely to have **pregnancy-induced hypertension (PIH)** than nondiabetic controls.[90,91] In women with pregestational type 1 DM, the risk of preeclampsia is increased with increased severity of diabetes (White classification), and proteinuria early in pregnancy is associated with an increased risk of adverse outcome.[92] **Myocardial infarction** occurs during diabetic pregnancies, but it is a rare complication.[93] The effect of PIH on the progression of **atherosclerotic disease** in diabetic patients is unclear.

Pregnancy may accelerate the development of **proliferative retinopathy,** a microvascular complication of DM. The following factors may affect the progression of diabetic retinopathy during pregnancy: (1) hypertension, (2) hyperglycemia,

TABLE 41-2	MODIFIED WHITE CLASSIFICATION OF DIABETES MELLITUS DURING PREGNANCY			
Class	Age of onset of diabetes (years)	Duration of diabetes (years)	Vascular disease	Insulin required
Gestational diabetes				
A₁	Any	Any	−	−
A₂	Any	Any	−	+
Pregestational diabetes				
B	>20	<10	−	+
C	10-19 or	10-19	−	+
D*	<10 or	>20	+	+
F	Any	Any	+	+
R	Any	Any	+	+
T	Any	Any	+	+
H	Any	Any	+	+

*Vascular disease in D is hypertension or benign retinopathy.
F, Nephropathy; *R*, proliferative retinopathy; *T*, status-post renal transplant; *H*, ischemic heart disease.
From Landon MB, Gabbe SG. Diabetes mellitus and pregnancy. Obstet Gynecol Clin North Am 1992; 19:633-54.

(3) duration of diabetes, and (4) the extent of baseline retinal disease.[94,95] The onset of strict glycemic control may *transiently* exacerbate diabetic retinopathy in pregnant or non-pregnant patients with type 1 DM. The Diabetes Control and Complications Trial[19] demonstrated that strict glycemic control is justified in nonpregnant patients. Long-term evaluation revealed that patients with strict glycemic control had less progression of diabetic retinopathy than patients who received conventional therapy.[19] Controversy remains regarding the affect of a rapid-acting human insulin analog (lispro) on the development or progression of diabetic retinopathy during pregnancy.[96,97]

In contrast to diabetic retinopathy, pregnancy does not accelerate the progression of **diabetic nephropathy.**[98,99] It is unclear whether pregnancy accelerates the progression of **somatic** or **autonomic neuropathy** in diabetic patients.

HOW DOES DIABETES MELLITUS AFFECT THE MOTHER AND FETUS?

Both pregestational and gestational DM are associated with an increased incidence of PIH, polyhydramnios, and cesarean section.[57,101-105] The incidence of **cesarean section** is increased threefold to tenfold in women with pregestational DM, and the incidence is increased 1.5 times in women with gestational DM.[57,102,103,105] Attempted vaginal birth after cesarean section in patients with gestational DM is associated with higher rates of operative vaginal delivery and repeat cesarean section compared with nondiabetic controls.[100] Pregestational DM but not gestational DM is associated with a twofold to threefold increase in the incidence of **preterm labor and delivery.**[101-103,106] Not all cases of preterm delivery result from preterm labor. In some cases, the obstetrician may effect preterm delivery for maternal or fetal indications.

Box 41-4 lists the fetal complications of maternal DM during pregnancy. **Fetal macrosomia** is a well-known complica-

---

Box 41-4 FETAL COMPLICATIONS OF MATERNAL DIABETES MELLITUS

DURING PREGNANCY AND THE PUERPERIUM

CHRONIC

Macrosomia/large for gestational age
- Shoulder dystocia
- Birth injury/trauma

Structural malformations[116]
- CNS: anencephaly, encephalocele, meningomyelocele, spina bifida, holoprosencephaly
- Cardiac: transposition of great vessels, ventricular septal defect, situs inversus, single ventricle, hypoplastic left ventricle
- Skeletal: caudal regression
- Renal: agenesis, multicystic dysplasia
- Gastrointestinal: anal/rectal atresia, small left colon
- Pulmonary: hypoplasia

ACUTE

Intrauterine/neonatal death
Neonatal respiratory distress syndrome
Neonatal hypoglycemia
Neonatal hyperbilirubinemia

AFTER PREGNANCY

Glucose intolerance
Possible impairment of cognitive development

---

tion of maternal DM. Most studies suggest that pregestational and gestational DM result in an increased incidence of fetal macrosomia.[101,102,107-111] Depending on the definition of macrosomia (4000 g versus 4500 g), pregestational DM results in fetal macrosomia in 9% to 25% of cases, which represents a fourfold to sixfold increase when compared with nondiabetic controls.[107-111] When a birth weight exceeds the 90th percentile for gestational age and gender, the neonate is considered large for gestational age (LGA). In one study of patients with pregestational DM, 38% of the newborns were LGA, and the overall rate of shoulder dystocia was 12%.[112]

Macrosomia results in an increased risk of **shoulder dystocia** and **birth trauma** at vaginal delivery.[104,110,111] However, some studies suggest that women with gestational DM are not at increased risk for shoulder dystocia when compared with nondiabetic controls.[102,103] Other risk factors for fetal macrosomia include maternal obesity and postterm delivery.[108] The use of intensive insulin therapy may reduce the risk of birth trauma in women with pregestational DM, despite the fact that these women deliver babies with an average birth weight 400 g higher than that in nondiabetic controls.[111]

Several potential mechanisms have been suggested for the development of fetal macrosomia in diabetic pregnancies. Maternal hyperglycemia results in fetal hyperglycemia, which results in reactive fetal hyperinsulinemia and an anabolic response in the fetus.[113] Moreover, maternal-to-fetal transplacental transfer of insulin has been demonstrated in humans with pregestational DM. This process most likely is facilitated by the presence of maternal antiinsulin antibodies. A weak but significant correlation exists between antibody titer and fetal macrosomia.[114] Shoulder dystocia may reflect the excessive growth of the fetal trunk (relative to the fetal head) in response to insulin.[115]

Women with pregestational DM are at increased risk for **fetal anomalies** (see Box 41-4). The incidence of major anomalies in these patients is 6% to 18%, which is 7 to 10 times higher than that in nondiabetic controls.[57,107,109,116,117] Overall, cardiovascular anomalies are most common, followed by anomalies of the central nervous system (CNS).[117,118] The caudal regression syndrome is uncommon, but it is 200 times more likely in diabetic than in nondiabetic pregnancies.[118] The incidence of major congenital anomalies in infants of women with gestational DM is 3% to 8%, which is less than that in infants of women with pregestational DM.[103,109,119] However, one study showed a relative risk of 20.6 for cardiovascular anomalies in patients with gestational DM who required insulin therapy when compared with nondiabetic controls.[117]

The following metabolic factors may be involved in the development of fetal structural malformations in diabetic pregnancies: (1) hyperglycemia, (2) hypoglycemia, (3) hyperketonemia, (4) somatomedin inhibitors, and (5) zinc deficiency.[116,120] The proposed mechanisms for the development of anomalies include (1) yolk sac failure, (2) reduced intracellular myoinositol, (3) arachidonic acid deficiency, and (4) oxygen-free radicals. Most fetal structural malformations that occur during diabetic pregnancies likely have a multifactorial etiology.[120] However, hyperglycemia during the period of critical organogenesis before the seventh week postconception is probably the single strongest etiologic factor in diabetic pregnant women.[116]

Studies have suggested that patient education and the initiation of strict glycemic control during the preconception period may decrease the rate of major congenital anomalies from 10% to 1% in patients with pregestational DM.[121-124]

The latter figure is equal to the baseline risk of major structural malformations in the general population. Strict glycemic control that is initiated during the preconception period increases the incidence of maternal hypoglycemic episodes. These studies suggest that hypoglycemia is not a significant factor in the etiology of human malformations because the rate of anomalies decreased tenfold despite hypoglycemic episodes.[121,122] Strict glycemic control before conception also has been associated with a threefold decrease in the incidence of spontaneous abortion in patients with pregestational DM.[125] Dicker et al.[126] observed normal induced ovulation, in vitro fertilization, and early embryonic development in a small series of infertile patients with pregestational DM who attended a preconception diabetes clinic. Unfortunately, only 36% of women with known pregestational DM receive appropriate medical care before conception.[116]

During the 1950s to 1970s, the **perinatal mortality rate** in patients with pregestational DM was 15% to 18%.[57,101] Subsequent studies noted a decrease in the perinatal mortality rate to 2%, which is similar to that in nondiabetic controls.[101,103,107] In contrast, another study noted a perinatal mortality rate of 8%, which was three times greater than that in nondiabetic controls.[112] When the entire population is considered, it is likely that the perinatal mortality rate remains higher in patients with pregestational DM than in nondiabetic controls. The perinatal mortality rate for patients with gestational DM is intermediate between the rate for those with pregestational diabetes and the rate for nondiabetic controls.[101,103,112]

Historically, **intrauterine fetal death** was responsible for approximately 40% of the perinatal deaths in pregnant patients with DM; 68% of the stillbirths occurred between 36 and 40 weeks' gestation.[58,60,112] In contemporary reports, the ratio of intrauterine to neonatal deaths in diabetic pregnancies has varied from 0 to 1.0.[60,112] Fetal macrosomia is a risk factor for intrauterine fetal demise in diabetic and nondiabetic pregnancies.[110] Recurrent episodes of intrauterine hypoxia may be a feature of diabetic pregnancies that end in stillbirth; episodes of hypoxia may reflect reduced uteroplacental blood flow and changes in fetal carbohydrate metabolism.[127] In recent years, **congenital anomalies** have emerged as the leading cause of perinatal mortality in diabetic pregnancies.[101,116,122] This likely reflects improved obstetric care during pregnancy, despite the lack of adequate glycemic control before conception.

Two series that included patients who delivered between 1950 and 1979 demonstrated an incidence of **neonatal respiratory distress syndrome (RDS)** in diabetic pregnancies that was 6 to 23 times that of nondiabetic controls.[57,128] Respiratory distress is more common among newborns who are delivered preterm and among those who are delivered by cesarean section without labor. When Robert et al.[128] controlled their data for these two confounding variables, neonatal RDS remained at a 5.6 times greater incidence among women with pregestational DM. More recent studies of patients with both pregestational and gestational DM have not demonstrated a significant difference in neonatal RDS between diabetic and nondiabetic pregnancies.[103,109,129,130]

The level of glycemic control during pregnancy affects the amniotic fluid phospholipid profile. Therefore poorly controlled diabetic pregnancies may have a higher incidence of "immature amniotic fluid fetal lung profiles" at 34 to 38 weeks' gestation, without an increase in the rate of clinical RDS.[130] In current obstetric practice, amniotic fluid analysis for phosphatidylglycerol (PG) is not performed in nondiabetic or well-controlled diabetic pregnancies at or beyond 38 weeks' gestation because of the low risk of neonatal RDS.[131] Measurement of PG in amniotic fluid is recommended when gestational age is uncertain, or when maternal diabetes is poorly controlled.

Neonatal hypoglycemia occurs in 5% to 12% of cases of pregestational and gestational DM.[103,107,109] This represents a sixfold to sixteenfold increased risk of neonatal hypoglycemia when compared with nondiabetic controls.[103,109] Neonatal hypoglycemia is presumed to result from the sustained fetal hyperinsulinemia that develops in response to chronic intrauterine hyperglycemia. Clinical studies have demonstrated increased fetal insulin levels and exaggerated fetal insulin responses to acute maternal hyperglycemia in diabetic pregnancies.[132,133] An acute increase in maternal glucose concentration, as might occur if a dextrose-containing solution were used for intravenous hydration before administration of regional anesthesia, can lead to reactive neonatal hypoglycemia, even in nondiabetic patients.[134]

There is a twofold to fivefold increase in the incidence of **neonatal hyperbilirubinemia** in patients with pregestational and gestational DM when compared with nondiabetic controls.[103,109] Both the etiology and the clinical significance are unknown, although one study noted the absence of long-term morbidity.[103]

DM develops more frequently in the offspring of diabetic mothers, most likely as a result of a combination of genetic and intrauterine environmental factors. Despite the well-known association of IDDM with HLA markers, studies of monozygotic human twins have suggested that genetic factors have a greater role in the etiology of type 2 DM than type 1 DM (100% versus 20% to 50% concordance, respectively).[135] In addition, fathers with type 1 DM are five times more likely than mothers with the same disease to have a child with type 1 DM. The intrauterine environment affects the development of glucose intolerance in the offspring.[135-137] In laboratory animals, the intrauterine diabetogenic influence can be demonstrated for at least three generations and represents a nongenetic mode of metabolic inheritance.[137] One animal study suggested that insulin secretion abnormalities in the offspring of diabetic pregnancies may represent a defect in sympathetic regulation of the pancreas as opposed to intrinsic pancreatic disease.[138]

Some investigators have suggested that **cognitive development** may be impaired in the children of diabetic mothers, although this is a matter of some dispute.[136]

Obstetric Management

In the management of **pregestational DM** during pregnancy, the first goal is to optimize glycemic control before conception. Early, strict glycemic control is the best way to prevent fetal structural malformations in patients with pregestational DM.[116,122] Determination of GHb concentrations may help the physician determine the adequacy of preconceptional glycemic control. Ultrasonography performed by an experienced examiner at 24 weeks' gestation has a positive predictive value of 90% and a negative predictive value of 97% in the diagnosis of major malformations.[139]

Contemporary obstetric management includes an emphasis on strict maternal glycemic control. During pregnancy, the patient should frequently determine the capillary blood glucose concentration by means of fingerstick and the use of a

reflectance meter.[41,140] These determinations permit timely adjustments in diet and insulin therapy. In general, insulin requirements progressively increase during the second and third trimesters. Both maternal and perinatal outcomes seem to improve when maternal glycemic control approaches that observed in normal pregnancies. Opinions vary regarding the optimum target glucose concentration in patients with pregestational DM. However, a fasting blood glucose concentration of 60 to 95 mg/dL seems appropriate. Of course, strict glycemic control results in an increased risk of maternal hypoglycemia.

Therapeutic insulin is available in several forms. Initially, insulin was isolated as a natural product from domestic animals (e.g., cattle, pigs). In the past 20 years, synthetic human insulin has become commercially available. Human insulin has largely replaced beef and pork insulin in human medicine, with an expected decrease in immune reactions among human recipients.[141,142]

The goal of insulin therapy is to provide plasma insulin concentrations that lead to tight glucose control without hypoglycemia. This goal is facilitated by having several insulin preparations with different subcutaneous absorption rates[142] (Table 41-3). Regular insulin can be administered by the intravenous or subcutaneous route. Regular insulin administered intravenously has a half-life of approximately 4 minutes.[143] The other native insulins listed in Table 41-3 (i.e., neutral protamine Hagedorn [NPH], lente, ultralente) represent chemical complexes of regular insulin with protamine or zinc, and subcutaneous administration of these insulins is associated with a delayed absorption and onset of action. An alternative therapeutic strategy is to administer a rapid-acting insulin by the subcutaneous route, using a continuous programmable pump.[144]

Human insulin therapy has been revolutionized over the past decade by the development of insulin analogs.[145-148] These molecules represent specific amino acid substitutions in portions of the human insulin protein not involved in receptor binding. Insulin analogs currently in clinical use include the short-acting and long-acting classes. Insulin **lispro** has reversal of amino acids at positions 28 and 29 on the B chain. Insulin **aspart** has aspartic acid instead of proline

in position 28 on the B chain. Insulin **glargine** has glycine instead of asparagine at position 21 of the A chain, and two arginines added to the C-terminus of the B chain. Lispro and aspart are rapid acting, with an onset and offset (when given subcutaneously) more physiologic than regular insulin. Glargine is relatively insoluble at neutral pH in the subcutaneous space. Compared with ultralente insulin, subcutaneous glargine has a sustained release without an initial peak of activity. It is likely that additional insulin analogs (e.g., fatty acid-activated insulins) will be introduced into clinical practice in the future.

Lispro, aspart, and glargine have all been used safely in human pregnancy. However, controversy continues regarding insulin lispro and a possible association with progression of diabetic retinopathy during pregnancy.[96,97] There is no evidence for significant variations in subcutaneous insulin uptake during pregnancy. However, studies have demonstrated variations in subcutaneous insulin uptake within and between nonpregnant individuals. The significant factors contributing to these variations include the preparation of insulin, injection site, injection concentration, injection volume, depth of subcutaneous injection, accuracy of intended dose, exercise, and environmental temperature.[141,149] Because insulin requirements decrease abruptly at delivery, it is important to verify the times, doses, insulin preparations, and routes of administration in the 24 hours before delivery to avoid maternal postpartum hypoglycemia.

The management of DKA is similar in pregnant and nonpregnant patients and includes the following therapeutic components: (1) intravenous hydration, (2) intravenous insulin, (3) treatment of the underlying cause of DKA, (4) careful monitoring of serum glucose and electrolytes, and (5) restriction of bicarbonate therapy to cases of extreme acidosis.[74,150,151] In addition, left uterine displacement should be maintained, and supplemental oxygen should be administered. Initial management of the critically ill mother should focus on the effective management of DKA. Fetal distress should resolve with appropriate medical management.[74-76]

In cases of gestational DM, the first goal is to make the diagnosis. In the United States, many obstetricians practice universal screening for gestational DM at 24 to 28 weeks' gestation.[152] Diet and exercise represent the initial therapeutic approaches for glycemic control in patients with gestational DM. Insulin therapy is started if the fasting glucose exceeds a threshold of 80 to 105 mg/dL.[40,127,153-155] In general, oral hypoglycemic agents are not used during pregnancy. These agents cross the placenta, and there is concern that they may result in fetal hyperinsulinemia and may be teratogenic. Recent clinical data with oral agents are encouraging but need to be confirmed.[25,156]

The timing of delivery represents an important decision in the management of diabetic pregnancies. White[58] noted, "Our problem must [be] . . . to prevent premature delivery of the infant of the diabetic mother prior to the period of its viability . . . and, secondly, the termination of the pregnancy at the point of viability and before the dreaded late intrauterine accident can occur." Typically a nonstress test is performed twice weekly in patients with pregestational DM, beginning at 32 weeks' gestation.[40,157] A nonreactive nonstress test should prompt the performance of a contraction stress test or fetal biophysical profile (see Chapter 6). Some maternal-fetal medicine specialists have advocated the use of Doppler umbilical artery flow velocimetry in diabetic pregnancies, but the efficacy of this modality remains unclear.[118,158] Risk factors for

TABLE 41-3	PHARMACOKINETICS OF HUMAN INSULIN, ADMINISTERED BY THE SUBCUTANEOUS ROUTE, IN NONPREGNANT HUMANS[144-147]		
Insulin Preparations	**Onset (hr)**	**Peak (hr)**	**Duration (hr)**
Short-Acting Class			
• Regular	0.5-1	2-4	4-8
• Lispro*	0.25	1	2-4
• Aspart*	0.25	1	2-4
Intermediate Class			
• NPH	1-4	6-10	12-20
• Lente	2-4	6-12	12-20
Long-Acting Class			
• Ultralente	3-5	10-16	18-24
• Glargine*	2	None	24

*Insulin analogs

abnormal fetal testing in diabetic pregnancies include maternal nephropathy, hypertension, and poor glycemic control.[159] No consensus exists regarding antepartum testing in women with well-controlled gestational DM.[25] Patients with poorly controlled gestational DM probably should have antepartum fetal surveillance similar to patients with pregestational DM.[25,160]

In the presence of reassuring fetal testing, delivery can be delayed until after 38 weeks' gestation.[40,157] If fetal testing is abnormal and amniotic fluid analysis indicates fetal pulmonary maturity, the fetus should be delivered as soon as possible. If fetal testing is abnormal but amniotic fluid analysis suggests that the fetal lungs are immature, the timing of delivery is more problematic.

The decision regarding the method of delivery requires consideration of several factors (e.g., estimated fetal weight, fetal condition, cervical dilation and effacement, previous obstetric history). The obstetrician is more likely to choose elective cesarean section in the diabetic parturient with evidence of fetal macrosomia.

Anesthetic Management

Few studies exist of the anesthetic management of pregnant patients with DM. In general, clinical decisions in these patients must be guided by logical extensions of studies of nonpregnant diabetic patients and nondiabetic pregnant patients.

The preanesthetic evaluation of the patient with DM should include a history and physical examination that focuses on the identification of the acute and chronic complications of DM (Box 41-2).[161] There are no published data on the relationship between the complications of DM and responses to anesthetic agents or anesthetic outcomes in pregnant patients. In a study of nonpregnant diabetic patients, preoperative evidence of **autonomic cardiovascular dysfunction** was predictive of the need for a vasopressor during general anesthesia.[162] With the potential for hypotension during regional anesthesia, noninvasive testing of autonomic function may be useful in obstetric patients with pregestational DM. For example, in nonpregnant diabetic patients the corrected QT interval on the electrocardiogram (ECG) correlates with the severity of autonomic neuropathy.[163] Patients with evidence of autonomic dysfunction may benefit from more frequent blood pressure determinations and more vigorous intravenous hydration before and during the administration of regional anesthesia. **Gastroparesis** is a manifestation of autonomic neuropathy in diabetic patients.[164] The nondiabetic pregnant patient is already at risk for gastric regurgitation and pulmonary aspiration (see Chapter 30). In patients with pregestational DM, I recommend the preanesthetic administration of metoclopramide (10 mg intravenously) to minimize the risk of aspiration secondary to diabetic gastroparesis. In nonpregnant diabetic patients, autonomic neuropathy is associated with a decreased cough reflex threshold and an increased incidence of obstructive sleep apnea.[165,166]

Several studies have examined the maternal, fetal, and neonatal effects of **regional anesthesia** for cesarean section in patients with pregestational DM.[167-170] Datta and Brown[167] observed that spinal anesthesia was associated with a slight but significant decrease in umbilical cord blood pH at delivery in patients with pregestational DM when compared with similar patients who received general anesthesia for cesarean section. Subsequently, these investigators noted an associa-

tion between fetal acidosis and peripartum maternal hypotension in patients with pregestational DM who received epidural anesthesia for cesarean section.[168] In both of these studies, acute maternal hyperglycemia (secondary to intravenous hydration with 5% dextrose before administration of regional anesthesia) was a potentially confounding factor.[167,168] A single case involving placental blood flow measurements in a diabetic patient who received spinal anesthesia for cesarean section is not interpretable because of other confounding factors.[171]

Neonatal acidosis does not occur during **spinal** or **epidural anesthesia** for cesarean section in diabetic parturients provided that (1) maternal glycemic control is satisfactory, (2) the patient receives aggressive preanesthetic volume expansion with a non-dextrose–containing balanced salt solution, and (3) hypotension is treated aggressively with ephedrine.[169,170] Because some diabetic parturients have chronic uteroplacental insufficiency, epidural anesthesia may be preferable to spinal anesthesia because the former results in a slower onset of sympathetic blockade. However, no clinical studies have directly addressed this issue in pregnant diabetic women.

Thalme and Engstrom[172] demonstrated normal umbilical artery pH measurements after the administration of **general anesthesia** in a small series of patients with pregestational DM.

No studies have compared the relative maternal safety of general versus regional anesthesia in pregnant diabetic patients. Gabbe et al.[173] reported one maternal death in a series of 261 pregnant women with gestational DM. This maternal death followed the induction of epidural anesthesia.

After administration of epidural anesthesia for cesarean section, Ramanathan et al.[170] observed an increased incidence of neonatal hypoglycemia in patients with pregestational DM when compared with nondiabetic controls (35% versus 7%). In this study, maternal glycemic control was fair (mean fasting plasma glucose level of 127 mg/dL), a non-dextrose–containing solution was used for intravenous hydration, and intravenous insulin therapy was adjusted based on frequent blood glucose determinations. This study illustrates the neonate's vulnerability to hypoglycemia after a diabetic pregnancy, despite meticulous anesthesia care at the time of delivery.

Maternal insulin requirements increase progressively during the second and third trimesters of pregnancy.[34] They decrease with the onset of labor, increase again during the second stage of labor, and decrease markedly during the early postpartum period.[48,49] Intravenous insulin therapy is the most flexible method of treatment during these rapid changes in physiologic insulin requirements. The absorption of subcutaneous insulin is unpredictable. Subcutaneous insulin therapy may increase the risk of maternal hypoglycemia, especially during the postpartum period.[49] Moreover, strict glycemic control in pregnant patients with type 1 DM increases the risk of maternal hypoglycemia as a result of impaired counterregulatory hormone responses. Intravenous glucose and insulin infusions during the peripartum period should be titrated to maintain a maternal blood glucose concentration of 70 to 90 mg/dL. During active labor, the glucose requirement is 2.5 mg/kg/min or more.[40,46] In nonpregnant patients with DM, many perioperative strategies have been proposed for metabolic control.[174-176] No convincing evidence suggests that one clinical strategy for perioperative diabetic control is superior in terms of patient outcome. Frequent blood glucose measurements (e.g., at 30- to 60-minute intervals), followed

by appropriate adjustment of glucose and insulin infusions, represent the cornerstone of optimal perioperative care in patients with DM.

Plasma concentrations of catecholamines (e.g., epinephrine, norepinephrine) increase during painful labor in nondiabetic women. The administration of either epidural or spinal anesthesia attenuates this physiologic response.[177,178] Catecholamines are counterregulatory hormones that oppose the activity of insulin.[8] In theory, the increased plasma concentrations of catecholamines should cause an increase in insulin requirements during the first stage of labor. However, insulin requirements remain low throughout the first stage of labor.[48] One study noted that the administration of epidural anesthesia does not affect insulin and glucose requirements during the first stage of labor.[48] Unfortunately, this study did not describe any details of epidural anesthesia, and it did not describe the methods of pain relief in the group of women who did not receive epidural anesthesia. There are no published data on the interaction between regional anesthesia and maternal plasma concentrations of catecholamines in diabetic pregnant women. There is one case report of symptomatic hypoglycemia following initiation of labor analgesia with a combined spinal-epidural technique in a patient with stable gestational DM.[179] However, others have questioned the general applicability of this case.[180]

There are no published data on the effects of DM on the pharmacokinetics and pharmacodynamics of anesthetic agents in pregnant women. In nonpregnant patients, DM is associated with a delayed onset of muscle relaxation with tubocurarine.[181] Bromage[182] described anecdotal evidence of reduced local anesthetic dose requirements during the administration of epidural anesthesia in a group of presumably nonpregnant diabetic patients. However, a pharmacokinetic study did not support the assertion of altered epidural vascular uptake of lidocaine in diabetic patients. In this study, peak plasma concentrations of lidocaine were similar after the administration of epidural anesthesia in nonpregnant patients with and without type 2 DM.[183]

Clinical studies have not directly addressed whether DM is a risk factor for anesthetic complications in pregnant patients. Perioperative peripheral nerve injuries have been described after the administration of anesthesia in nonpregnant diabetic patients. These nerve palsies may represent either unrecognized preanesthetic neurologic deficits or a propensity for nerve injury because of latent peripheral nerve disease.[184,185] Diabetic animals are more prone than controls to develop peripheral nerve injury after perineural infiltration with lidocaine, and the morphologic patterns suggest an ischemic mechanism.[186] It is important to perform a brief neurologic history and physical examination as part of the preanesthetic evaluation of all patients, especially those with DM (see Chapter 33. In addition, the anesthesiologist should ensure proper perioperative positioning and padding of the extremities during the administration of anesthesia in diabetic patients.

The diabetic "stiff-joint" syndrome has been described as a cause of difficult direct laryngoscopy and intubation in patients with DM.[187,188] This syndrome occurs in patients with long-standing type 1 DM and is associated with nonfamilial short stature, joint contractures, and tight skin.[189] Limited movement of the atlantooccipital joint may result in difficult direct laryngoscopy and intubation. During the preanesthetic evaluation of patients with DM, the anesthesiologist may screen for the stiff-joint syndrome by looking for the "prayer

sign" (Figure 41-4). Other investigators have suggested phalangeal visualization on an ink print of the palm (i.e., the palm print index) as an alternative screen for difficult intubation.[190] The anesthetic management of diabetic patients with suspected stiff-joint syndrome is controversial. Some authors recommend preanesthetic flexion-extension radiographic studies of the cervical spine, followed by awake intubation in affected patients.[188] Others have expressed doubt regarding the clinical significance of this syndrome and the reported frequency of airway management problems.[191,192] The term *diabetic scleredema* is synonymous with the stiff-joint syndrome. There is one case report of a pregnant patient with pregestational DM and diabetic scleredema who experienced an anterior spinal artery syndrome after the administration of epidural anesthesia for cesarean section.[193] The authors suggested that spinal cord vascular compression resulted from a combination of (1) preexisting microvascular disease, (2) an epidural space that was stiff because of connective tissue disease, and (3) administration of a large volume (e.g., 35 mL) of the local anesthetic agent. In patients with a history and physical examination that suggest diabetic stiff-joint syndrome, the anesthesiologist should consider two potential problems: (1) difficult direct laryngoscopy and intubation, and (2) a noncompliant epidural space.

Infection is an important cause of morbidity in pregnant women with pregestational DM.[63] There are no published data regarding the incidence of CNS infection after the administration of regional anesthesia in pregnant diabetic patients. Goucke and Graziotti[194] reported a case of epidural abscess after the epidural injection of local anesthetic and a corticosteroid in a nonpregnant patient with type 2 DM. DM

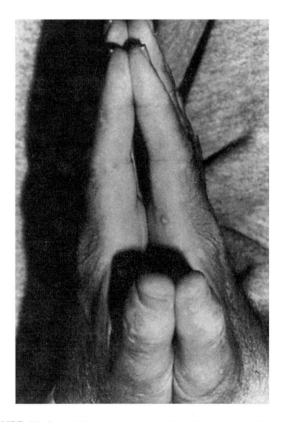

FIGURE 41-4. Inability to approximate the palmar surfaces of the phalangeal joints (prayer sign) despite maximal effort, secondary to diabetic stiff-joint syndrome. (From Hogan K, Rusy D, Springman SR. Difficult laryngoscopy and diabetes mellitus. Anesth Analg 1988; 67:1162-5.)

is a risk factor for the occurrence of spontaneous epidural abscess in nonpregnant patients. Strict aseptic technique should be used during the administration of regional anesthesia in all patients, especially those with DM.

THYROID DISORDERS

Thyroid Hormone Physiology

The follicular cells of the thyroid gland sequester iodine and synthesize thyroglobulin, an iodinated precursor protein. Thyroglobulin is secreted into the lumen of the microscopic thyroid follicles before it undergoes reuptake, proteolysis, and transport back through the follicular cells.[195,196] This process results in the systemic release of the thyroid hormones: thyroxine (T_4) and 3,5,3′ triiodothyronine (T_3). Reverse T_3 (3,3′,5′ triiodothyronine) is a structural variant with much less physiologic potency in most target organs.[197]

Thyroid hormone synthesis and release are controlled primarily by a trophic hormone from the pituitary—thyroid-stimulating hormone (TSH)—and the supply of iodine. The thyroid hormones normally participate in a negative feedback loop that regulates TSH secretion (Figure 41-5). This feedback loop includes the regulation of thyrotropin releasing hormone (TRH) production in the hypothalamus as well as a direct action on the pituitary.[198,199] The ratio of thyroid secretion rates for T_4 and T_3 is approximately 10:1 in normal nonpregnant humans.[200-202] This ratio may be altered by disease.[203]

The thyroid hormones are highly protein bound in the blood. In euthyroid nonpregnant humans, the normal total serum concentrations of T_4 and T_3 are 50 to 150 nmol/L and 1.4 to 3.2 nmol/L, respectively.[204-206] The unbound or free fractions of T_4 and T_3 are 0.03% and 0.3%, respectively.[207] Similar proportions of T_4 and T_3 are distributed among the three major plasma proteins that bind thyroid hormones: (1) thyroxine-binding globulin (TBG) (70% to 80%), (2) thyroxine-binding prealbumin or transthyretin (10% to 20%), and (3) albumin (10% to 15%).[208,209] The serum concentration of unbound or free T_4 typically is the major determinant of thyroid hormone activity in target tissues.[210] Thyroid hormones are temporarily inert while they are bound to plasma proteins. Changes in the concentrations of thyroxine-binding proteins can occur during various physiologic states (e.g., pregnancy) and disease processes. Thyroid hormone action does not change as long as the concentration of free T_4 remains constant, despite fluctuations in the total concentration of T_4.

Thyroid hormone is an endocrine regulator in many target organs, including the liver, kidneys, skeletal and cardiac muscles, brain, pituitary, and placenta.[211] The defined physiologic effects of thyroid hormones are mediated by regulation of specific gene products. These effects include (1) somatic and nervous system development, (2) calorigenesis, (3) augmented skeletal and cardiac muscle performance, (4) intermediary metabolism, and (5) feedback control.[212]

In the target tissues, the molecular actions of T_4 begin with the enzymatic deiodination of T_4 to T_3. Iodothyronine deiodinase is widely distributed in the body and occurs in at least two molecular forms.[213,214] Only 20% of the daily T_3 production is secreted by the thyroid gland; the remainder is formed by peripheral deiodination.[200] Next, T_3 enters the nuclei of target cells by diffusion or transport and binds to specific thyroid hormone receptors. These protein receptors have separate domains that bind to either T_3 or specific DNA sequences known as *thyroid-responsive elements*.[215] In the absence of T_3, native thyroid hormone receptors bind to DNA and exert a baseline negative effect on thyroid-responsive elements. When T_3 binds to its receptor, this negative effect is reversed and the transcription of specific gene products is enhanced.[212,215] The thyroid hormone receptor belongs to a family of structurally related, intracellular ligand-binding proteins.[216] Variations in the number and types of thyroid hormone receptors, as well as receptor linkage to development- or tissue-specific genomic expressions, provide additional levels of physiologic control and vulnerability to disease processes.[212,215,217]

Figure 41-6 demonstrates the specific sites in thyroid hormone synthesis that are affected by medications. Drugs also may affect (1) the concentrations of binding proteins, (2) deiodinase activity, and (3) peripheral uptake of thyroid hormones.[208-210,218]

In most cases, two tasks are associated with the laboratory evaluation of thyroid function. First, the serum concentration of free T_4 can be directly measured or indirectly calculated. Second, the serum concentration of TSH is measured to assess the negative feedback loop that controls the thyroid gland. The TSH concentration is judged as appropriate or inappropriate in the context of the serum concentration of free T_4. All laboratory tests have a better predictive value when they are used in groups of patients that are likely to have a given

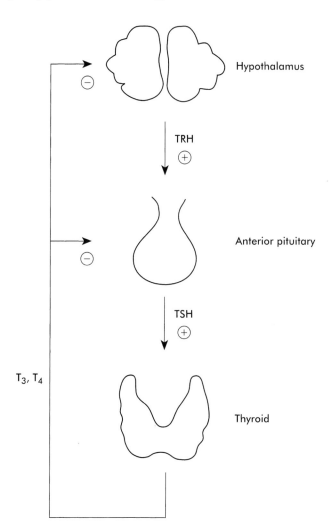

FIGURE 41-5. Normal feedback control of thyroid hormone secretion. (From Davies PH, Franklyn JA. The effects of drugs on tests of thyroid function. Eur J Clin Pharmacol 1991; 40:439-51.)

disorder.[219] Thyroid function tests are most useful in patients with a clinical presentation that suggests thyroid dysfunction.

During normal human pregnancy, the serum concentration of TBG steadily increases until it reaches a plateau at 20 weeks' gestation, when it is 50% greater than the nonpregnant level.[204] The increased concentration of TBG results from a prolonged half-life (not increased synthesis) during pregnancy.[209] The normal pregnant woman is euthyroid because the serum concentrations of free T_4 and T_3 are in the normal (or low-normal) range for nonpregnant humans.[204] However, the increased concentration of TBG means that the total serum concentrations of T_4 and T_3 during pregnancy are at or above the upper limit of normal for nonpregnant women.[204,220]

Human chorionic gonadotropin (hCG) is a placental protein that shares some structural features with TSH. The serum concentrations of TSH and hCG have an inverse relationship during normal human pregnancy.[204] This reflects the mild TSH-like activity that results from increased plasma concentrations of hCG during early pregnancy.[221,222] In addition, one study suggested that TSH may inhibit hCG synthesis in the placenta.[223]

Maternal iodine availability is decreased during pregnancy because of increased fetal uptake and increased maternal renal clearance.[223,224] In geographic areas with marginal iodine supplies, this may predispose the mother to goiter unless she has a dietary iodine supplement.[204,225,226]

Hyperthyroidism

DEFINITION AND EPIDEMIOLOGY

Hyperthyroidism is defined as an abnormal increase in the serum concentration of unbound or free thyroid hormones. The prevalence of hyperthyroidism in the general population is 0.2% to 1.9%, with a female to male ratio of 10:1.[227,228] Box 41-5 lists the various etiologies of hyperthyroidism. Graves' disease is responsible for 70% to 90% of the cases of hyperthyroidism.[229] Thyroiditis and the combined category of toxic adenoma and toxic multinodular goiter each account for approximately 5% of cases. There are multiple levels of interaction between the thyroid and reproductive endocrine systems in women, with specific implications for patients with hyperthyroidism and hypothyroidism.[230]

Box 41-5 ETIOLOGIES OF HYPERTHYROIDISM

ABNORMAL THYROID STIMULATOR

- Graves' disease
- Gestational trophoblastic neoplasia
- TSH-secreting pituitary tumor

INTRINSIC THYROID AUTONOMY

- Toxic adenoma
- Toxic multinodular goiter

INFLAMMATORY DISEASE (E.G., SUBACUTE THYROIDITIS)

EXTRINSIC HORMONE SOURCE

- Ectopic thyroid tissue
- Thyroid hormone ingestion

From Houston MS, Hay ID. Practical management of hyperthyroidism. Am Fam Physician 1990; 41:909-16.

PATHOPHYSIOLOGY

Graves' disease is an autoimmune thyroid disease.[221] The etiology of Graves' disease most likely is multifactorial and includes both **environmental** (e.g., stress, hormones) and **genetic** influences. Several autoantibodies against thyroid tissue have been described in Graves' disease. Autoantibodies directed against the TSH receptor in the thyroid gland may augment or inhibit TSH action, depending on their binding specificities. (These antibodies are called **thyroid receptor antibodies [TRAbs]**.) Therefore the binding specificities of TRAbs in the blood of each patient with Graves' disease affect the net thyroid-stimulating activity. Autoantibodies against thyroid peroxidase, the sodium-iodine cotransporter, and thyroglobulin also have been described in patients with Graves' disease.

Among untreated patients with Graves' disease, approximately 20% undergo spontaneous remission.[231] However, the prognosis for an individual patient cannot be predicted based on clinical or laboratory examinations.[216]

CLINICAL PRESENTATION AND DIAGNOSIS

Hyperthyroidism presents clinically as a physiologic state dominated by an increased metabolic rate. A hyperthyroid symptom scale has been developed based on 10 clinical factors: nervousness, sweating, heat intolerance, hyperactivity, tremor, weakness, hyperdynamic precordium, diarrhea, appetite, and degree of incapacitation.[218] This symptom scale has been useful in following the clinical course of patients with Graves' disease. Exophthalmus or infiltrative ophthalmopathy is clinically apparent in the majority of patients with Graves' disease.[231-233] However, other physical signs may occur at low frequency in affected patients: pretibial myxedema or dermopathy (1% to 2%) and nail changes or acropachy (less than 1%). The pathogenesis of infiltrative ophthalmopathy in Graves' disease remains unclear. On a descriptive basis, the primary orbital abnormality is enlargement of the extraocular muscles, which is accompanied by chronic inflammation.[233]

Hyperthyroidism stimulates the cardiovascular system beyond the demands of the underlying increased metabolic rate, resulting in a "hyperkinetic circulatory state."[234,235] Myocardial contractility, heart rate, stroke volume, and ventricular size all increase, and peripheral vascular resistance decreases in skin and muscle. Thyroid hormones can affect the ratio of alpha- and beta-adrenergic receptors in the heart.[235] A cardiomyopathy can be demonstrated during exercise in hyperthyroid patients that is independent of beta-adrenergic receptors and is reversible with normalization of thyroid function.[236] Elderly patients with hyperthyroidism are especially prone to develop atrial fibrillation.[235]

The diagnosis of hyperthyroidism depends by definition on the documentation of an increase in the serum concentration of unbound or free T_4. The more common forms of hyperthyroidism (e.g., Graves' disease, toxic adenoma, toxic multinodular goiter) may be differentiated from the less common forms by a radioiodine uptake study.[237] The identification of TSH-receptor autoantibodies may have some role in distinguishing Graves' disease from toxic adenoma or multinodular goiter.[231]

INTERACTION WITH PREGNANCY

Normal human pregnancy is a euthyroid state, with normal serum concentrations of unbound or free T_4 despite increased serum concentrations of TBG and total T_4.

Hyperthyroidism during pregnancy results from a distribution of etiologies that is similar to that in nonpregnant patients (Box 41-5). Graves' disease is the predominant cause of hyperthyroidism during pregnancy. The prevalence of hyperthyroidism during pregnancy is 0.2%, which is lower than the prevalence in the general population.[227,228,238-240] This may reflect a beneficial effect of the immunotolerance of pregnancy on autoimmune disorders such as Graves' disease.[231,239] Also, human pregnancy is associated with a change in the specificity of TSH receptor antibody activity from stimulatory to blocking activity.[241]

Gestational trophoblastic neoplasms frequently are associated with elevated serum hCG concentrations. High concentrations of hCG may possess significant thyroid-stimulating bioactivity because of the structural homology between hCG and TSH.[221,222] Transient hyperthyroidism during pregnancy has been reported in association with hyperemesis gravidarum.[242] Hyperthyroidism and hyperemesis gravidarum may be parallel disease processes, with elevated hCG as a shared mechanism.[242] Hyperthyroidism rarely may result from two coincident disease processes (e.g., Graves' disease and struma ovarii) in either pregnant or nonpregnant patients.[243]

Thyroid nodules occur in 4% to 7% of adults. Pregnancy is associated with an increase in number and size of thyroid nodules.[244] Pregnancy most likely does not affect the development or progress of thyroid carcinoma, although this remains a matter of some dispute.[245,246] The evaluation of thyroid nodules that present during pregnancy should include (1) measurement of serum TSH and free T_4 concentrations, (2) ultrasonographic examination (to differentiate cystic versus solid lesions), and (3) fine-needle aspiration or percutaneous needle biopsy. Malignant lesions can be treated surgically during pregnancy. Radioactive iodine therapy may be delayed until the postpartum period.[245]

MEDICAL AND SURGICAL MANAGEMENT

In nonpregnant patients, the current therapies for Graves' disease include radioactive iodine, antithyroid medications, and surgery.[237,247-249]

Radioactive iodine is administered orally as ^{131}I, in variable doses (i.e., 10 to 75 mCi).[248] All forms of iodine are sequestered by the thyroid gland, and ^{131}I exerts a therapeutic effect in Graves' disease primarily by means of the local emission of beta radiation. Hypothyroidism develops after a therapeutic dose of radioactive iodine in most patients with Graves' disease. This necessitates careful follow-up and long-term thyroid hormone replacement therapy.[247] In nonpregnant patients, the long-term health risks of radioactive iodine therapy are minimal.[248] Pregnancy represents a contraindication to radioactive iodine therapy because all forms of iodine readily cross the placenta to the fetus. Current recommendations are to delay pregnancy for 4 to 6 months after radioactive iodine therapy, although ^{131}I has a half-life of only 8 days.[248]

Propylthiouracil and **methimazole** are the antithyroid medications used to treat Graves' disease.[237,247] These drugs interfere with the incorporation of iodine into thyroglobulin and with subsequent coupling reactions in the thyroid gland (Figure 41-6). In addition, propylthiouracil inhibits iodothyronine deiodinase in peripheral tissues. These medications may be prescribed alone or at higher doses in combination with thyroxine, the latter known as "block and replace" therapy.[239] Typical oral doses are 5 to 15 mg two times daily for

methimazole and 100 to 150 mg three times daily for propylthiouracil.[237] The long-term clinical strategy is to adjust the dose downward as tolerated. Some patients with Graves' disease experience remission after the administration of an antithyroid medication.[247] The major complication of antithyroid medications is asymptomatic agranulocytosis (0.03% to 0.5%), which typically occurs within 3 months of starting therapy.[237,247] If treatment with antithyroid medications is unsatisfactory, the nonpregnant patient may receive radioactive iodine.

Surgical therapy of Graves' disease typically is reserved for those patients who cannot or will not undergo treatment with radioactive iodine or antithyroid medications. The opinions on surgical intervention vary widely.[237,247,249] In most cases, the preferred surgical procedure is a subtotal thyroidectomy, with preservation of a 4- to 10-g thyroid remnant.[249] Perioperative complications of thyroid surgery include (1) unilateral or bilateral vocal cord paralysis secondary to laryngeal nerve injury, (2) wound hematoma, (3) pneumothorax, (4) hypoparathyroidism, and (5) thyroid storm.[249,250]

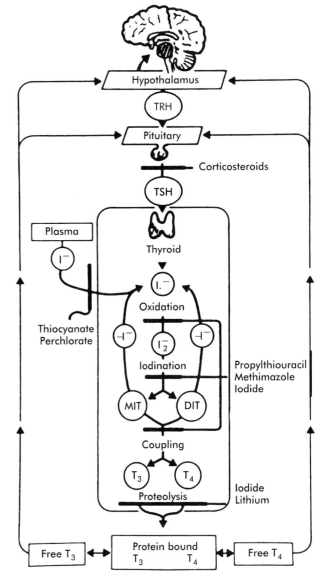

FIGURE 41-6. Effects of antithyroid medications on thyroid hormone synthesis and activity. (From Stehling LC. Anesthetic management of the patient with hyperthyroidism. Anesthesiology 1974; 41:585-95.)

Hypocalcemia secondary to acute hypoparathyroidism may present as laryngospasm during the postoperative period.[250]

Adjunctive therapies for hyperthyroidism include iodine, radiocontrast agents, lithium, and glucocorticoids (Figure 41-6).[237,247] Beta-adrenergic receptor antagonists also have been used to decrease the cardiovascular responses to increased concentrations of thyroid hormones.[247]

Thyroid Storm

Thyroid storm is a life-threatening exacerbation or decompensation of a preexisting hyperthyroid state.[251-256] Thyroid storm is a clinical diagnosis based on the following signs and symptoms: (1) fever, (2) mental and emotional disturbances, (3) tachycardia, (4) tachypnea, (5) diaphoresis, and (6) diarrhea. Without treatment, thyroid storm may progress to coma, multiorgan system failure, and death. The mortality rate approached 100% in earlier series, but improved therapy has decreased mortality to less than 20%.[254]

In most cases, thyroid storm is associated with a precipitating event in a patient with untreated or incompletely treated hyperthyroidism (Box 41-6). Historically, the precipitating events reflect the common serious medical illnesses of a given era.[251-253] In the past, cases of thyroid storm were categorized as "medical" or "surgical" depending on whether the exacerbation occurred during the perioperative period. With improved perioperative management, the incidence of *surgical* thyroid storm has decreased markedly, and this terminology rarely is used in contemporary medical practice.

In the past, 2% to 7% of patients hospitalized for hyperthyroidism experienced thyroid storm.[251-253] The current incidence of thyroid storm in hyperthyroid patients is difficult to determine.

The mechanism for the development of thyroid storm is unknown. Based on the clinical presentation and the known precipitating events, one hypothesis is that thyroid storm is caused by increased thyroid hormone and catecholamine secretion. Limited data suggest that total serum concentrations of T_4 and T_3 do not increase during thyroid storm in hyperthyroid patients,[257] although one case report suggests otherwise.[258] Alternatively, the precipitating event in thyroid storm may augment thyroid hormone action by increasing the circulating free fraction of thyroid hormones. This hypothesis is supported by data that demonstrate increased serum concentrations of free T_4 during thyroid storm as well as observations of changes in thyroid hormone binding during fever or systemic illness.[259]

Catecholamine secretion also may play a role in the development of thyroid storm. In hyperthyroid patients without thyroid storm, the endogenous secretion of epinephrine and norepinephrine is normal, as are the cardiovascular responses to exogenous epinephrine and isoproterenol.[260-262] These parameters have not been measured during episodes of thyroid storm. However, the symptoms of thyroid storm respond well to medications that block the synthesis or receptor binding of beta-adrenergic agents.[253,255,256] The role of the sympathetic nervous system in thyroid storm is supported by historical observations that spinal anesthesia to the fourth thoracic dermatome level is therapeutic.[263] It is unclear whether baseline catecholamine secretion is permissive for thyroid storm or whether a surge of catecholamines is necessary to trigger this condition.

Box 41-7 outlines the treatment of thyroid storm. Several points merit discussion. Glucocorticoid supplementation is described as a general supportive measure because of the relative deficiency of endogenous glucocorticoid production in patients with hyperthyroidism.[264,265] Glucocorticoids also inhibit both thyroid hormone production and the peripheral conversion of T_4 to T_3.[234] Propylthiouracil and methimazole decrease thyroid hormone production, but only propylthiouracil inhibits the peripheral conversion of T_4 to T_3. In addition to the relief of many symptoms of hyperthyroidism, propranolol inhibits the peripheral conversion of T_4 to T_3. This latter property of propranolol is not related to its beta-adrenergic receptor blocking activity and is not shared by most other beta-blockers.[266-268] Because of its dual action,

---

Box 41-6 EVENTS ASSOCIATED WITH PRECIPITATION OF THYROID STORM

Surgery	Stroke
Childbirth	Infection
Trauma	Diabetic ketoacidosis
Iodinated contrast agents	Hypoglycemia
[131]I treatment	Congestive heart failure
Emotional stress	Bowel infarction
Pulmonary embolism	

From Roth RN, McAuliffe MJ. Hyperthyroidism and thyroid storm. Emerg Med Clin North Am 1989; 7:873-83.

Box 41-7 TREATMENT OF THYROID STORM[252-256]

Prevention
General supportive measures
- Cooling blanket and ice
- Chlorpromazine (25 to 50 mg IV) or meperidine (25 to 50 mg IV) to diminish shivering
- Intravenous hydration
- Glucose and electrolyte replacement
- Oxygen
- Glucocorticoids: dexamethasone (2 to 4 mg IV) or hydrocortisone (100 to 300 mg IV)
- B-complex multivitamins

Reduction of synthesis and secretion of thyroid hormones
- Antithyroid medications: propylthiouracil (600 to 1000 mg orally per day) or methimazole (60 to 100 mg orally or rectally per day)
- Iodine: sodium iodide (1 g IV or Lugol's solution 30 drops orally) or supersaturated potassium iodide solution (SSKI 3 drops orally)
- Glucocorticoids

Reduction of peripheral conversion of thyroxine (T_4) to 3,5,3'-triiodothyronine (T_3)
- Propylthiouracil
- Glucocorticoids
- Radiographic contrast agents
  - Iopanoic acid (Telepaque) 3 g orally
  - Sodium ipodate (Oragrafin) 1 g orally
- Propranolol

Decrease in the metabolic effects of thyroid hormones
- Beta-adrenergic blocking agents
  - Propranolol
  - Esmolol
- Reserpine
- Guanethidine

Other therapeutic maneuvers
- Plasma exchange
- Dantrolene

Diagnosis and treatment of the underlying illness that precipitated thyroid storm.

propranolol is the beta-adrenergic receptor antagonist of choice in cases of thyroid storm. Esmolol also has been used successfully during the treatment of thyroid storm.[269-272] Esmolol is preferred in patients with a sensitivity to nonspecific beta-adrenergic receptor blockade (e.g., asthma). Moreover, patients with significant cardiomyopathy from hyperthyroidism may be very sensitive to beta-adrenergic receptor blockade.[236,273-274] In these patients, esmolol is advantageous because the dose may be titrated to the desired effect.[275] The drug's short half-life allows a rapid reversal of effect if needed.

Thyroid storm is an acute hypermetabolic state that may be difficult to distinguish clinically from malignant hyperthermia. Rhabdomyolysis is one of the few features of malignant hyperthermia that has not been reported in thyroid storm.[276] Three cases of thyroid storm that were treated with dantrolene have been reported.[277-279] Two patients survived, but the third succumbed to multiorgan system failure that antedated the dantrolene therapy. In another case, a patient with known Graves' disease undergoing subtotal thyroidectomy had an intraoperative hypermetabolic crisis that was initially diagnosed and treated as thyroid storm. Based on subsequent blood gas analysis, the correct diagnosis of malignant hyperthermia was made and the patient successfully treated with dantrolene.[280] Plasma exchange is another unusual but efficacious therapeutic option in cases of thyroid storm.[281]

In summary, treatment of thyroid storm includes general supportive measures plus the administration of glucocorticoids, propylthiouracil, sodium iodide, and propranolol. Some authorities recommend delaying iodine treatment until 1 hour after the administration of propylthiouracil to avoid increased iodine use by the thyroid gland.[254-256]

Preoperative Preparation

The risk of thyroid storm during the perioperative period can be minimized by appropriate preparation of the hyperthyroid patient. The majority of cases of perioperative thyroid storm involve thyroid surgery. The preoperative therapeutic goals are to inhibit thyroid hormone synthesis and secretion in patients with preexisting hyperthyroidism and to decrease the vascularity of the thyroid gland. The four main therapies used in preoperative preparation are administration of (1) an antithyroid medication (primarily propylthiouracil), (2) a beta-adrenergic receptor antagonist, (3) a glucocorticoid, and (4) iodine.[234,282,283] Iodine inhibits thyroid hormone secretion more effectively in hyperthyroid patients than in euthyroid patients because the latter are capable of mounting a compensatory TSH response as serum T_4 levels decrease.[284]

In some patients, beta-adrenergic receptor blockade alone may be sufficient to prevent perioperative thyroid storm.[285] However, thyroid storm has been reported after preoperative preparation with propranolol alone.[286-288] In some of these cases, the patients most likely did not receive effective beta-adrenergic receptor blockade. A 25% reduction in exercise-induced heart rate is a better indication of adequate beta-adrenergic receptor blockade than a change in the resting heart rate.[283] One advantage of beta-adrenergic receptor antagonists over antithyroid medications is the decreased time typically required for preoperative preparation (i.e., 2 weeks versus 6 to 8 weeks, respectively).[285] Several investigators have recommended preoperative preparation with a beta-adrenergic receptor antagonist, with the addition of iodine beginning 10 days before surgery.[283,289,290] The use of beta-adrenergic receptor antagonists entails a risk of hypoglycemia in hyperthyroid patients because these patients have reduced hepatic glucose reserves and because beta-adrenergic receptor blockade results in a pharmacologic blunting of sympathetic responses.[283]

No prospective, randomized studies have compared the efficacy of various methods of preoperative preparation of hyperthyroid patients. A reasonable clinical approach includes the use of multiple therapeutic agents (e.g., a beta-adrenergic receptor antagonist, iodine, and a glucocorticoid), with the doses titrated to the clinical response of each patient. These clinical parameters may include exercise-induced heart rate, fine tremor, weight gain, and recovery of muscle strength.[234,283] Baeza et al.[291] described a preoperative regimen for hyperthyroid patients that included oral betamethasone, propranolol, and iopanoic acid (Telepaque). Iopanoic acid is therapeutic in patients with hyperthyroidism because its metabolism results in the release of iodide; it also inhibits the peripheral conversion of T_4 to T_3.[292]

Elective surgery should not proceed without adequate preoperative preparation of hyperthyroid patients. In cases of emergency surgery, physicians should invoke the therapies discussed for the treatment of thyroid storm (Box 41-7).

Medical and Surgical Management During Pregnancy

All of the therapeutic options used in nonpregnant hyperthyroid patients should be efficacious in pregnant patients. However, the fetal effects of several of these therapies require a modification of the treatment of hyperthyroidism during pregnancy.

Radioactive iodine is contraindicated during pregnancy because iodine readily crosses the placenta to the fetus. The fetal effects of inadvertent maternal administration of ^{131}I vary with gestational age.[236] After 10 weeks' gestation, the fetal thyroid gland can sequester iodine, and ^{131}I may destroy or significantly damage the gland. Before 10 weeks' gestation, the risk to the fetus is less well defined and most likely approximates that of a low-level dose of radiation during early development.[224]

The mainstays of therapy for hyperthyroidism during pregnancy are the antithyroid medications propylthiouracil and methimazole.[223,224,279,280] These medications cross the placenta much more easily than the maternal thyroid hormones. Therefore maternal administration of an antithyroid medication may induce fetal hypothyroidism and goiter. Propylthiouracil and methimazole have similar efficacy in the treatment of hyperthyroidism during pregnancy.[281] In the past, propylthiouracil has been used more frequently than methimazole in pregnancy. This pattern of therapy was based on the perception that methimazole crossed the placenta more easily than propylthiouracil, and that methimazole was occasionally associated with a congenital scalp defect. Both of these concerns have been resolved favorably by recent data.[237,238,240,294] During pregnancy, treatment with propylthioural usually begins with an oral dose of 100 to 150 mg three times daily or methimazole 5 to 15 mg twice daily. Subsequently the dose is titrated downward to minimize the fetal effects. A pregnant patient is often maintained on a total daily dose of less than 100 mg of propylthiouracil. In a group of patients who were known to have Graves' disease and who were maintained on methimazole before pregnancy, administration of T_4 (100 µg/day) without methimazole beginning at 20 weeks' gestation resulted in a sixfold reduction in the postpartum rate of recurrent hyperthyroidism.[295] This effect was correlated with a

retained placental tissue. Initiating treatment with a low dose of nitroglycerin may relax the uterus sufficiently while minimizing potential complications (e.g., hypotension).

V. Anesthetic Choices for Cesarean Delivery

The literature suggests that spinal, epidural or CSE anesthetic techniques can be used effectively for cesarean delivery. When compared to regional techniques, the literature indicates that general anesthetics can be administered with shorter induction-to-delivery times. The literature is insufficient to determine the relative risk of maternal death associated with general anesthesia compared to other anesthetic techniques. However, the literature suggests that a greater number of maternal deaths occur when general anesthesia is administered. The literature indicates that a larger proportion of neonates in the general anesthesia groups, compared to those in the regional anesthesia groups, are assigned Apgar scores of less than 7 at 1 and 5 minutes. However, few studies have utilized randomized comparisons of general versus regional anesthesia, resulting in potential selection bias in the reporting of outcomes.

The literature suggests that maternal side effects associated with regional techniques may include hypotension, nausea, vomiting, pruritus and postdural puncture headache. The literature is insufficient to examine the comparative merits of various regional anesthetic techniques.

The Consultants agree that regional anesthesia can be administered with fewer maternal and neonatal complications and improved maternal satisfaction when compared to general anesthesia. The Consultants are equivocal about the possibility of increased maternal complications when comparing spinal or epidural anesthesia with CSE techniques. They agree that neonatal complications are not increased with CSE techniques.

Recommendations: The decision to use a particular anesthetic technique should be individualized based on several factors. These include anesthetic, obstetric and/or fetal risk factors (e.g., elective versus emergency) and the preferences of the patient and anesthesiologist. Resources for the treatment of potential complications (e.g., airway management, inadequate analgesia, hypotension, pruritus, nausea) should be available.

VI. Postpartum Tubal Ligation

There is insufficient literature to evaluate the comparative benefits of local, spinal, epidural or general anesthesia for postpartum tubal ligation. Both the Task Force and Consultants agree that epidural, spinal and general anesthesia can be effectively provided without affecting maternal complications. Neither the Task Force nor the Consultants agree that local anesthetic techniques provide effective anesthesia, and they are equivocal regarding the impact of local anesthesia on maternal complications. Although the literature is insufficient, the Task Force and Consultants agree that a postpartum tubal ligation can be performed safely within 8 hours of delivery in many patients.

Recommendations: Evaluation of the patient for postpartum tubal ligation should include assessment of hemodynamic status (e.g., blood loss) and consideration of anesthetic risks. The patient planning to have an elective postpartum tubal ligation within 8 hours of delivery should have no oral intake of solid foods during labor, and postpartum until the time of surgery. Both the timing of the procedure and the decision to use a particular anesthetic technique (i.e., regional versus general) should be individualized, based on anesthetic and/or obstetric risk factors and patient preferences. The anesthesiologist should be aware that an epidural catheter placed for labor may be more likely to fail with longer post-delivery time intervals. If a postpartum tubal ligation is to be done before the patient is discharged from the hospital, the procedure should not be attempted at a time when it might compromise other aspects of patient care in the labor and delivery area.

VII. Management of Complications

1. RESOURCES FOR MANAGEMENT OF HEMORRHAGIC EMERGENCIES

The literature suggests that the availability of resources for hemorrhagic emergencies is associated with reduced maternal complications. The Task Force and Consultants agree that the availability of resources for managing hemorrhagic emergencies is associated with reduced maternal, fetal and neonatal complications.

Recommendations: Institutions providing obstetric care should have resources available to manage hemorrhagic emergencies (Table 1). In an emergency, the use of type-specific or O-negative blood is acceptable in the parturient.

2. EQUIPMENT FOR MANAGEMENT OF AIRWAY EMERGENCIES

The literature suggests, and the Task Force and Consultants agree that the availability of equipment for the management of airway emergencies is associated with reduced maternal complications.

Recommendations: Labor and delivery units should have equipment and personnel readily available to manage airway emergencies. Basic airway management equipment should be immediately available during the initial provision of regional analgesia (Table 2). In addition, portable equipment for difficult airway management should be readily available in the operative area of labor and delivery units (Table 3).

3. CENTRAL INVASIVE HEMODYNAMIC MONITORING

There is insufficient literature to indicate whether pulmonary artery catheterization is associated with improved maternal, fetal or neonatal outcomes in patients with pregnancy-related hypertensive disorders. The literature is silent regarding the management of obstetric patients with central venous catheterization alone. The literature suggests that pulmonary artery catheterization has been used safely in obstetric patients; however, the literature is insufficient to examine specific obstetric outcomes. The Task Force and Consultants agree that it is not necessary to use central invasive hemodynamic monitoring routinely for parturients with severe preeclampsia.

Recommendations: The decision to perform invasive hemodynamic monitoring should be individualized and based on clinical indications that include the patient's medical history and cardiovascular risk factors. The Task Force recognizes that not all practitioners have access to resources for utilization of central venous or pulmonary artery catheters in obstetric units.

TABLE 1	SUGGESTED RESOURCES FOR OBSTETRIC HEMORRHAGIC EMERGENCIES*

1. Large bore iv catheters
2. Fluid warmer
3. Forced air body warmer
4. Availability of blood bank resources
5. Equipment for infusing iv fluids and/or blood products rapidly. Examples include (but are not limited to) hand squeezed fluid chambers, hand inflated pressure bags, and automatic infusion devices.

*The items listed represent suggestions. The items should be customized to meet the specific needs, preferences, and skills of the practitioner and health-care facility.

TABLE 2	SUGGESTED RESOURCES FOR AIRWAY MANAGEMENT DURING INITIAL PROVISION OF REGIONAL ANESTHESIA*

1. Laryngoscope and assorted blades
2. Endotracheal tubes, with stylets
3. Oxygen source
4. Suction source with tubing and catheters
5. Self-inflating bag and mask for positive pressure ventilation
6. Medications for blood pressure support, muscle relaxation, and hypnosis

*The items listed represent suggestions. The items should be customized to meet the specific needs, preferences, and skills of the practitioner and health-care facility.

TABLE 3	SUGGESTED CONTENTS OF A PORTABLE UNIT FOR DIFFICULT AIRWAY MANAGEMENT FOR CESAREAN SECTION ROOMS*

1. Rigid laryngoscope blades and handles of alternate design and size from those routinely used†
2. Endotracheal tubes of assorted size
3. Laryngeal mask airways of assorted sizes
4. At least one device suitable for emergency nonsurgical airway ventilation. Examples include (but are not limited to) retrograde intubation equipment, a hollow jet ventilation stylet or cricothyrotomy kit with or without a transtracheal jet ventilator, and the esophageal-tracheal combitube.
5. Endotracheal tube guides. Examples include (but are not limited to) semirigid stylets with or without a hollow core for jet ventilation, light wands, and forceps designed to manipulate the distal portion of the endotracheal tube.
6. Equipment suitable for emergency surgical airway access
7. Topical anesthetics and vasoconstrictors

*The items listed represent suggestions. The items should be customized to meet the specific needs, preferences, and skills of the practitioner and health-care facility.
†The Task Force believes fiberoptic intubation equipment should be readily available.
Adapted from Practice guidelines for management of the difficult airway: A report by the American Society of Anesthesiologists Task Force on Management of the Difficult Airway. Anesthesiology 1993; 78:599-602.

4. CARDIOPULMONARY RESUSCITATION

The literature is insufficient to evaluate the efficacy of CPR in the obstetric patient during labor and delivery. The Task Force is supportive of the immediate availability of basic and advanced life-support equipment in the operative area of labor and delivery units.

Recommendations: Basic and advanced life-support equipment should be immediately available in the operative area of labor and delivery units. If cardiac arrest occurs during labor and delivery, standard resuscitative measures and procedures, including left uterine displacement, should be taken. In cases of cardiac arrest, the American Heart Association has stated the following: "Several authors now recommend that the decision to perform a perimortem cesarean section should be made rapidly, with delivery effected within 4 to 5 minutes of the arrest."[3]

REFERENCES

1. Guidelines for Perinatal Care, 4th ed. American Academy of Pediatrics and American College of Obstetricians and Gynecologists, 1997, pp 100-102.
2. American Society of Anesthesiologists: Position on monitored anesthesia care, ASA Standards, Guidelines and Statements. Park Ridge, IL, American Society for Anesthesiologists, October 1997, pp 20-21.
3. Guidelines for cardiopulmonary resuscitation and emergency cardiac care: recommendations of the 1992 national conference. JAMA 1992; 268:2249.

Appendix C

American Society of Anesthesiologists Optimal Goals for Anesthesia Care in Obstetrics[*]

This joint statement from the American Society of Anesthesiologists (ASA) and the American College of Obstetricians and Gynecologists (ACOG) has been designed to address issues of concern to both specialties. Good obstetric care requires the availability of qualified personnel and equipment to administer general or regional anesthesia both electively and emergently. The extent and degree to which anesthesia services are available varies widely among hospitals. However, for any hospital providing obstetric care, certain optimal anesthesia goals should be sought. These include:

I. Availability of a licensed practitioner who is credentialed to administer an appropriate anesthetic whenever necessary. For many women, regional anesthesia (epidural, spinal or combined spinal-epidural) will be the most appropriate anesthetic.

II. Availability of a licensed practitioner who is credentialed to maintain support of vital functions in any obstetric emergency.

III. Availability of anesthesia and surgical personnel to permit the start of a cesarean delivery within 30 minutes of the decision to perform the procedure; in cases of VBAC, appropriate facilities and personnel, including obstetric anesthesia, nursing personnel, and a physician capable of monitoring labor and performing cesarean delivery, immediately available during active labor to perform emergency cesarean delivery (ACOG 1999). The definition of immediate availability of personnel and facilities remains a local decision, based on each institution's available resources and geographic location.

IV. Appointment of a qualified anesthesiologist to be responsible for all anesthetics administered. There are obstetric units where obstetricians or obstetrician-supervised nurse anesthetists administer anesthetics. The administration of general or regional anesthesia requires both medical judgment and technical skills. Thus, a physician with privileges in anesthesiology should be readily available.

Persons administering or supervising obstetric anesthesia should be qualified to manage the infrequent but occasionally life-threatening complications of major regional anesthesia such as respiratory and cardiovascular failure, toxic local anesthetic convulsions, or vomiting and aspiration. Mastering and retaining the skills and knowledge necessary to manage these complications require adequate training and frequent application.

To ensure the safest and most effective anesthesia for obstetric patients, the director of anesthesia services, with the approval of the medical staff, should develop and enforce written policies regarding provision of obstetric anesthesia. These include:

I. Availability of a qualified physician with obstetrical privileges to perform operative vaginal or cesarean delivery during administration of anesthesia. Regional and/or general anesthesia should not be administered until the patient has been examined and the fetal status and progress of labor evaluated by a qualified individual. A physician with obstetrical privileges who has knowledge of the maternal and fetal status and the progress of labor, and who approves the initiation of labor anesthesia, should be readily available to deal with any obstetric complications that may arise.

II. Availability of equipment, facilities, and support personnel equal to that provided in the surgical suite. This should include the availability of a properly equipped and staffed recovery room capable of receiving and caring for all patients recovering from major regional or general anesthesia. Birthing facilities, when used for analgesia or anesthesia, must be appropriately equipped to provide safe anesthetic care during labor and delivery or post-anesthesia recovery care.

Personnel other than the surgical team should be immediately available to assume responsibility for resuscitation of the depressed newborn. The surgeon and anesthesiologist are responsible for the mother and may not be able to leave her care for the newborn even when a regional anesthetic is functioning adequately. Individuals qualified to perform neonatal resuscitation should demonstrate:

A. Proficiency in rapid and accurate evaluation of the newborn condition including Apgar scoring.

B. Knowledge of the pathogenesis of a depressed newborn (acidosis, drugs, hypovolemia, trauma, anomalies and infection), as well as specific indications for resuscitation.

C. Proficiency in newborn airway management, laryngoscopy, endotracheal intubations, suctioning of airways, artificial ventilation, cardiac massage and maintenance of thermal stability.

In larger maternity units and those functioning as high-risk centers, 24-hour in-house anesthesia, obstetric and neonatal specialists are usually necessary. Preferably, the obstetric anesthesia services should be directed by an anesthesiologist with special training or experience in obstetric anesthesia. These units will also frequently require the availability of more sophisticated monitoring equipment and specially trained nursing personnel.

A survey jointly sponsored by the ASA and ACOG found that many hospitals in the United States have not yet achieved the above goals. Deficiencies were most evident in smaller delivery units. Some small delivery units are necessary because of geographic considerations. Currently, approximately 50 percent of hospitals providing obstetric care have fewer than 500 deliveries per year. Providing comprehensive care for obstetric patients in these small units is extremely inefficient, not cost-effective and frequently impossible. Thus, the following recommendations are made:

1. Whenever possible, small units should consolidate.

2. When geographic factors require the existence of smaller units, these units should be part of a well-established regional perinatal system.

---

[*]Approved by House of Delegates on October 28, 2000.

The availability of the appropriate personnel to assist in the management of a variety of obstetric problems is a necessary feature of good obstetric care. The presence of a pediatrician or other trained physician at a high-risk cesarean delivery to care for the newborn or the availability of an anesthesiologist during active labor and delivery when vaginal birth after cesarean delivery (VBAC) is attempted, and at a breech or twin delivery are examples. Frequently, these professionals spend a considerable amount of time standing by for the possibility that their services may be needed emergently but may ultimately not be required to perform the tasks for which they are present. Reasonable compensation for these standby services is justifiable and necessary.

A variety of other mechanisms have been suggested to increase the availability and quality of anesthesia services in obstetrics. Improved hospital design to place labor and delivery suites closer to the operating rooms would allow for more efficient supervision of nurse anesthetists. Anesthesia equipment in the labor and delivery area must be comparable to that in the operating room.

Finally, good interpersonal relations between obstetricians and anesthesiologists are important. Joint meetings between the two departments should be encouraged. Anesthesiologists should recognize the special needs and concerns of the obstetrician and obstetricians should recognize the anesthesiologist as a consultant in the management of pain and life-support measures. Both should recognize the need to provide high quality care for all patients.

REFERENCE

American College of Obstetricians and Gynecologists. Vaginal birth after previous cesarean delivery. ACOG Practice Bulletin. Washington, DC: ACOG, 1999.

BIBLIOGRAPHY

Committee on Perinatal Health, Toward Improving the Outcome of Pregnancy: The 90s and Beyond. White Plains, New York: March of Dimes Birth Defects Foundation, 1993.

Index

KEY POINTS

- **Patients with asthma, infection, respiratory failure, or cystic fibrosis and patients who smoke cigarettes may have reversible airway obstruction.**
- **In patients with airway hyperresponsiveness, endotracheal intubation provides one of the most significant stimuli for bronchospasm during the perioperative period.**
- **Inhaled beta$_2$-adrenergic agonists are the most effective therapy for perioperative bronchospasm.**
- **Most bronchodilators also produce uterine relaxation. However, administration by aerosol should minimize the effects on uterine tone.**
- **Regional anesthesia often is the anesthetic technique of choice in patients with respiratory disease because endotracheal intubation is not required.**
- **Techniques of regional anesthesia should be modified to reduce the likelihood of a high thoracic motor block in patients with significant respiratory disease.**

Obstetric Management

Because the benefits of delivery on the course of respiratory failure have not been documented, the indications for induction of labor or cesarean section in this setting are not well defined. Tomlinson et al.[176] retrospectively reviewed outcome for 10 pregnant patients who required intubation and mechanical ventilation for respiratory compromise. The maternal inspired oxygen requirements decreased an average of 28% by 24 hours after delivery, but positive end-expiratory pressure requirements did not change. The authors concluded that delivery did not result in uniform improvement in maternal respiratory function, and that obstetricians should exercise caution in making a decision to perform elective delivery in patients with respiratory failure.

Vaginal delivery is possible during mechanical ventilation,[161,170,177,178] but many affected women undergo cesarean section for standard obstetric indications.[161]

Anesthetic Management

The anesthetic management of patients with respiratory failure requires appropriate medical management. During labor, analgesia for mechanically ventilated patients can be provided by intravenous opioids, which often are used for sedation during mechanical ventilation. Regional anesthetic techniques provide epidural analgesia without the neonatal respiratory depression that is associated with high doses of opioids. The use of regional anesthetic techniques in patients with respiratory failure depends on underlying conditions and ongoing therapy. The anesthesiologist should give attention to the intravascular volume, the adequacy of coagulation, and the presence of infection.

In mechanically ventilated patients, general anesthesia often is the most convenient choice for cesarean section. Aside from the issues of medical management discussed previously, the techniques and pharmacologic agents do not differ substantially from those used in patients without respiratory failure.

REFERENCES

1. Expert Panel Report. Definition and diagnosis. Executive Summary: Guidelines for the Diagnosis and Management of Asthma. Bethesda, MD, Public Health Service, National Institutes of Health, US Government Printing Office, DHHS Publication No. 1991:91-3042A.

2. Boushey HA, Holtzman MJ, Sheller FR, Nadel JA. Bronchial hyperreactivity. Am Rev Respir Dis 1980; 121:389-414.

3. Expert Panel Report. Guidelines for the Diagnosis and Management of Asthma. Bethesda, MD, Public Health Service, National Institutes of Health, US Government Printing Office, DHHS Publication No. 1991:91-3042.

4. National Asthma Education Program. Report of the Working Group on Asthma and Pregnancy. Executive summary: Management of Asthma During Pregnancy. Bethesda, MD, US Government Printing Office, DHHS Publication No. 93-3279A.

5. Alexander S, Dodds L, Armson BA. Perinatal outcomes in women with asthma during pregnancy. Obstet Gynecol 1998; 92:435-40.

6. Kurinczuk JJ, Parsons DE, Dawes V, Burton PR 1999. The relationship between asthma and smoking during pregnancy. Women Health 29:31-47.

7. Vincenc KS, Black JL, Yan K, et al. Comparison of in vivo and in vitro responses to histamine in human airways. Am Rev Respir Dis 1983; 128:875-9.

8. Armour CL, Lazar NM, Schellenberg RR, et al. A comparison of in vivo and in vitro human airway reactivity to histamine. Am Rev Respir Dis 1984; 129:907-10.

9. Roberts JA, Raeburn D, Rodger IW, Thomson NC. Comparison of in vivo airway responsiveness and in vitro smooth muscle sensitivity to methacholine in man. Thorax 1984; 39:837-43.

10. Roberts JA, Rodger IW, Thomson NC. Airway responsiveness to histamine in man: Effect of atropine on in vivo and in vitro comparison. Thorax 1985; 40:261-7.

11. Goldie R, Spina D, Henry PJ, et al. In vitro responsiveness of human asthmatic bronchus to carbachol, histamine, β-adrenoceptor agonists and theophylline. Br J Clin Pharmacol 1986; 22:669-76.

12. Downes H, Austin DR, Parks CM, Hirshman CA. Comparison of drug responses in vivo and in vitro in airways of dogs with and without airway hyperresponsiveness. J Pharmacol Exp Ther 1986; 237:214-9.

13. Cerrina J, Ladurine MR, Labat C, et al. Comparison of human bronchial muscle responses to histamine in vivo with histamine and isoproterenol agonists in vitro. Am Rev Respir Dis 1986; 134:57-61.

14. Skloot G, Permutt S, Togias A. Airway hyperresponsiveness in asthma: A problem of limited smooth muscle relaxation with inspiration. J Clin Invest 1995; 96:2393-2403.

15. Richardson JB. State of the art: Nerve supply to the lungs. Am Rev Respir Dis 1979; 19:785-802.

16. Starke K, Gothert M, Kilbinger H. Modulation of neurotransmitter release by presynaptic autoreceptors. Physiol Rev 1989; 69:865-989.

17. Barnes PJ. Muscarinic autoreceptors in the airways: Their possible role in airway disease. Chest 1989; 96:1220-1.

18. Fryer AD, Jacoby DB. Parainfluenza virus infection damages inhibitory M$_2$ muscarinic receptors on pulmonary parasympathetic nerves in the guinea pig. Br J Pharmacol 1991; 109:267-71.

19. Empey DW, Laitinen LA, Jacobs L, et al. Mechanisms of bronchial hyperreactivity in normal subjects following upper respiratory tract infection. Am Rev Respir Dis 1976; 113:131-9.

20. Nadel JA, Barnes PJ. Autonomic regulation of the airways. Ann Rev Med 1984; 35:451-567.

21. Tattersfield AE, Leaver DG, Pride NB. Effects of beta-adrenergic blockade and stimulation on normal human airways. J Appl Physiol 1973; 35:613-9.

22. Spina D, Rigby PJ, Paterson JW, Goldie RG. α$_1$-Adrenoceptor function and autoradiographic distribution in human asthmatic lung. Br J Pharmacol 1989; 97:701-8.

23. Andersson RGG, Grundstrom N. The excitatory non-cholinergic, non-adrenergic nervous system of the guinea-pig airways. Eur J Respir Dis 1983; 64:141-57.

24. Richardson JB. Nonadrenergic inhibitory innervation of the lung. Lung 1981; 159:315-22.

25. Belvisi MG, Stretto CD, Barnes PJ. Nitric oxide is the endogenous neurotransmitter of bronchodilator nerves in human airways. Eur J Pharmacol 1992; 210:221-2.

26. Lammers J-W, Minette P, McCusker M, et al. Capsaicin-induced bronchodilation in asthmatic patients: Role of non-adrenergic inhibitory system. J Appl Physiol 1989; 98:325-30.

27. Hogg JC, James AL, Para PD. Evidence for inflammation in asthma. Am Rev Respir Dis 1991; 143:S39-42.

28. Tattersfield AE, Knox AJ, Britton JR, et al. Asthma. Lancet 2000; 360:1313-22.

29. Barnes PJ. NO or no NO in asthma? Thorax 1996; 51:218-20.

30. Lee TH, Lane SJ. The role of macrophages in the mechanisms of airway inflammation in asthma. Am Rev Respir Dis 1992; 145:S27-30.

31. Black JL. Control of human airway smooth muscle. Am Rev Respir Dis 1991; 143:S11-2.

32. Schwartz LB. Cellular inflammation in asthma: Neutral proteases of mast cells. Am Rev Respir Dis 1992; 145:S18-21.

33. Nadel JA. Biologic effects of mast cell enzymes. Am Rev Respir Dis 1992; 145:S37-41.

34. Moreno RH, Hogg JC, Pare PD. Mechanisms of airway narrowing. Am Rev Respir Dis 1986; 133:1171-80.

35. Laitinen LA, Heino M, Laitinen A, et al. Damage of the airway epithelium and bronchial reactivity in patients with asthma. Am Rev Respir Dis 1985; 131:599-606.

36. Flavahan NA, Aarhus LL, Rimele TJ, Vanhoutte PM. Respiratory epithelium inhibits bronchial smooth muscle tone. J Appl Physiol 1985; 58:834-8.

37. Frossard N, Muller F. Epithelial modulation of tracheal smooth muscle responses to antigenic stimulation. J Appl Physiol 1986; 61:1449-56.

38. Johnson AR, Ashton J, Schulz W, Erdos EG. Neutral metalloendopeptidase in human lung tissue and cultured cells. Am Rev Respir Dis 1985; 132:564-8.

39. Stenius-Aarniala B, Piirila P, Teramo K. Asthma and pregnancy: A prospective study of 198 pregnancies. Thorax 1988; 43:12-8.

40. Schatz M, Harden K, Forsythe A, et al. The course of asthma during pregnancy, postpartum, and with successive pregnancies: A prospective analysis. J Allergy Clin Immunol 1988; 81:509-16.

41. White RJ, Coutts II, Gibbs CJ, MacIntyre C. A prospective study of asthma during pregnancy and the puerperium. Resp Med 1989; 83:103-6.

42. Kircher S, Schatz M, Long L. Variables affecting asthma course during pregnancy. Ann Allergy Asthma Immunol 2002;89:463-466.

43. Teeter JG, Bleecker ER. Relationship between airway obstruction and respiratory symptoms in adult asthmatics. Chest 1998; 113:272-7.

44. Juniper EF, Daniel EE, Roberts RS, et al. Improvement in airway responsiveness and asthma severity during pregnancy. Am Rev Respir Dis 1989; 140:924-31.

45. Mabie WC, Barton JR, Wasserstrum N, Sibai BM. Clinical observations on asthma in pregnancy. J Mat Fet Med 1992; 1:45-50.

46. Weinmann GG, Zacur H, Fish JE. Absence of changes in airway responsiveness during the menstrual cycle. J Allergy Clin Immunol 1987; 79:634-8.

47. Juniper EF, Kline PA, Roberts RS, et al. Airway responsiveness to methacholine during the natural menstrual cycle and the effect of oral contraceptives. Am Rev Respir Dis 1987; 135:1039-42.

48. Perlow JH, Montgomery D, Morgan MA, et al. Severity of asthma and perinatal outcome. Am J Obstet Gynecol 1992; 167:963-7.

49. Liu S, Wen SW, Demissie K, et al. Maternal asthma and pregnancy outcomes. A retrospective cohort study. Am J Obstet Gynecol 2001; 184:90-6.

50. Alexander S, Dodds L, Armson BA. Perinatal outcomes in women with asthma during pregnancy. Obstet Gynecol 1998; 92:435-40.

51. Gordon M, Niswander KR, Berendes H, Kantor AG. Fetal morbidity following potentially anoxigenic obstetric conditions. VII. Bronchial asthma. Am J Obstet Gynecol 1970; 106:421-39.

52. McColgin SW, Glee L, Brian BA. Pulmonary disorders complicating pregnancy. Obstet Gynecol Clin North Am 1992; 19:697-717.

53. Schatz M, Zeiger RS, Hoffman CP, et al. Perinatal outcomes in the pregnancies of asthmatic women: A prospective controlled analysis. Am J Respir Crit Care Med 1995; 151:1170-4.

54. Dombrowski MP, Schatz M, Wise R, et al, for the National Institute of Child Health and Human Development Maternal-Fetal Medicine Units Network and the National Heart, Lung, and Blood Institute. Asthma during pregnancy. Obstet Gynecol 2004; 103:5-12.

55. Murphy VE, Zakar T, Smith R, et al. Reduced β-hydroxysteroid dehydrogenase type 2 activity is associated with decreased birth weight centile in pregnancies complicated by asthma. J Clin Endocrinol Metab 2002; 87:1660-8.

56. Clifton VL, Giles WB, Smith R, et al. Alterations of placental vascular function in asthmatic pregnancies. Am J Respir Crit Care Med 2001; 164:546-53.

57. Twentyman OP, Higenbottam TW. β-Agonists can be used safely and beneficially in asthma. Resp Med 1992; 86:471-6.

58. Pauwels RA, Lofdahl CG, Postma DS, et al. Effect of inhaled formoterol and budesonide on exacerbations of asthma. N Engl J Med 1997; 337:1405-11.

59. O'Byrne PM, Barnes PJ, Rodriguez-Roisin R, et al. Low dose inhaled budesonide and formoterol in mild persistent asthma. Am J Respir Crit Care Med 1998; 164:1392-7.

60. Cheung D, Timmers MC, Zwinderman AH, et al. Long-term effects of a long-acting β2-adrenoceptor agonist, salmeterol, on airway hyperresponsiveness in patients with mild asthma. N Engl J Med 1992; 327:1198-203.

61. Schatz M, Zeiger RS, Harden K, et al. The safety of inhaled beta-agonist bronchodilators during pregnancy. J Allergy Clin Immunol 1988; 82:686-95.

62. Bukowsky M, Nakatsu K, Hunt PW. Theophylline reassessed. Ann Intern Med 1984; 101:63-73.

63. Schatz M. Asthma during pregnancy: Interrelationships and management. Ann Allergy 1992; 68:123-37.

64. Carter BL, Driscoll CF, Smith GD. Theophylline clearance during pregnancy. Obstet Gynecol 1986; 68:555-9.

65. Littenberg G. Aminophylline treatment in severe, acute asthma. JAMA 1988; 259:1678-84.

66. Tobias JD, Kubos KL, Hirshman CA. Aminophylline does not attenuate histamine-induced airway constriction during halothane anesthesia. Anesthesiology 1989; 71:723-9.

67. Rebuck AS, Chapman KR, Abboud R, et al. Nebulized anticholinergic and sympathomimetic treatment of asthma and chronic obstructive airways disease in the emergency room. Am J Med 1987; 82:59-64.

68. Gross NJ, Skorodin MD. Anticholinergic antimuscarinic bronchodilators. Am Rev Respir Dis 1984; 129:856-70.

69. Barsky ER. Asthma and pregnancy. Postgrad Med 1991; 89:125-32.

70. Barnes PJ. Effect of corticosteroids on airway hyperresponsiveness. Am Rev Respir Dis 1990; 141:70-6.

71. Dutoit JI, Salome CM, Woolcock AJ. Inhaled corticosteroids reduce the severity of bronchial hyperresponsiveness in asthma but oral theophylline does not. Am Rev Respir Dis 1987; 136:1174-8.

72. Bel EH, Timmers MC, Zwinderman AH, et al. The effect of inhaled corticosteroids on the maximal degree of airway narrowing to methacholine in asthmatic subjects. Am Rev Respir Dis 1991; 143:109-13.

73. Fitzsimons R, Greenberger PA, Patterson R. Outcome of pregnancy in women requiring corticosteroids for severe asthma. J Allergy Clin Immunol 1986; 78:349-53.

74. Schatz M, Zeiger RS, Harden K, et al. The safety of asthma and allergy medications during pregnancy. J Allergy Clin Immunol 1997; 100:301-6.

75. Bernstein IM, Catallano PM. Ketoacidosis in pregnancy associated with parenteral administration of terbutaline and betamethasone. J Reprod Med 1990; 35:818-20.

76. Wendel PJ, Ramin SM, Barrett-Hamm C, et al. Asthma treatment in pregnancy: A randomized controlled study. Am J Obstet Gynecol 1996; 175:150-4.

77. Greenberger PA. Asthma during pregnancy. J Asthma 1990; 27:341-7.

78. Chung KF, Barnes PJ. Treatment of asthma. Br Med J 1987; 294:103-5.

79. Udelsman R, Ramp J, Gallucci WT. Adaptation during surgical stress: A reevaluation of the role of glucocorticoids. J Clin Invest 1986; 77:1377-81.

80. Verleden GM, Belvisi MG, Stretton CD, Barnes PJ. Nedocromil sodium modulates nonadrenergic, noncholinergic bronchoconstrictor nerves in guinea pig airways in vitro. Am Rev Respir Dis 1991; 143:114-8.

81. Horwitz RJ, McGill KA, Busse WW. The role of leukotriene modifiers in the treatment of asthma. Am J Respir Crit Care Med 1998; 157:1363-71.

82. Mathe AA, Hedquist P. Effect of prostaglandins F_{2a} and E_2 on airway conductance in healthy subjects and asthmatic patients. Am Rev Respir Dis 1975; 111:313-20.

83. Sweatman WFP, Collier HOJ. Effects of prostaglandins on human bronchial muscle. Nature 1968; 217:69.

84. Fishburne JI, Brenner WE, Braaksma JT, et al. Bronchospasm complicating intravenous prostaglandin F_{2a} for therapeutic abortion. Obstet Gynecol 1972; 39:892-6.

85. Louie S, Krzanowski JJ, Lockey RF. Effect of ergometrine on airway smooth muscle contractile responses. Clin Allergy 1985; 15:173-8.

86. Seller WFS, Long DR. Bronchospasm following ergometrine. Anaesthesia 1979; 34:909.

87. Crawford J. Bronchospasm following ergometrine. Anesthesia 1980; 35:397-8.

88. Barnes PJ. State of the art: Neural control of human airways in health and disease. Am Rev Respir Dis 1986; 134:1289-314.

89. Leff AR. Endogenous regulation of bronchomotor tone. Am Rev Respir Dis 1988; 137:1198-216.

90. Wright BM, McKerrow CB. Maximum forced expiratory flow rate as a measure of ventilatory capacity. Br Med J 1959; 2:1041-51.

91. Belvisi MG, Rogers DF, Barnes PJ. Neurogenic plasma extravasation: Inhibition by morphine in guinea pig airways in vivo. J Appl Physiol 1989; 66:268-72.

92. Fuller RW, Karlsson J-A, Choudry NB, Pride NB. Effect of inhaled and systemic opiates on responses to inhaled capsaicin in humans. J Appl Physiol 1988; 65:1125-30.

93. Rosow CE, Moss J, Philbin DM, et al. Histamine release during morphine and fentanyl anesthesia. Anesthesiology 1982; 56:93-6.

94. Chestnut DH, Owen CL, Bates JN, et al. Continuous epidural infusion analgesia during labor: A randomized, double-blind comparison of 0.0625% bupivacaine/0.0002% fentanyl versus 0.125% bupivacaine. Anesthesiology 1988; 68:754-9.

95. Shnider SM, Papper EM. Anesthesia for the asthmatic patient. Anesthesiology 1961; 22:886-92.

96. Bonica JJ. Autonomic innervation of the viscera in relation to nerve block. Anesthesiology 1968; 29:793-813.

97. Mallampati SR. Bronchospasm during spinal anesthesia. Anesth Analg 1981; 60:838-40.

98. Barnes PT, Ind PW, Brown MJ. Plasma histamine and catecholamines in stable asthmatic subject. Clin Sci 1982; 62:661-5.

99. Pflug AE, Halter JB. Effect of spinal anesthesia on adrenergic tone and the neuroendocrine responses to surgical stress in humans. Anesthesiology 1981; 55:120-6.

100. Shimosato S, Etsten BE. The role of the venous system in cardiocirculatory dynamics spinal and epidural anesthesia in man. Anesthesiology 1969; 30:619-28.

101. Sands MF, Douglas FL, Green J, et al. Homeostatic regulation of bronchomotor tone by sympathetic activation during bronchoconstriction in normal and asthmatic humans. Am Rev Respir Dis 1985; 131:993-8.

102. Que JC, Lusaya VO. Sevoflurane induction for emergency cesarean section in a parturient in status asthmaticus. Anesthesiology 1999; 90:1475-6.

103. Hirshman CA, Downes H, Farbood A, Bergman NA. Ketamine block of bronchospasm in experimental canine asthma. Br J Anaesth 1979; 51:713-8.

104. Pizov R, Brown RH, Weiss YS, et al. Wheezing during induction of general anesthesia in patients with and without asthma. Anesthesiology 1995; 82:1111-6.

105. Mehr EH, Lindeman KS. Effects of halothane, propofol, and thiopental on peripheral airway reactivity. Anesthesiology 1993; 79:290-8.

106. Downes H, Hirshman CA. Lidocaine aerosols do not prevent allergic bronchoconstriction. Anesth Analg 1981; 60:29-31.

107. Vettermann J, Beck KC, Lindahl SHE, et al. Actions of enflurane, isoflurane, vecuronium, atracurium, and pancuronium on pulmonary resistance in dogs. Anesthesiology 1988; 69:688-95.

108. Korenaga S, Takeda K, Ito Y. Differential effects of halothane on airway nerves and muscle. Anesthesiology 1984; 60:309-18.

109. Wiklund CU, Lim S, Lindsten J. Relaxation by sevoflurane, desflurane and halothane in the isolated guinea-pig trachea via inhibition of cholinergic neurotransmission. Br J Anaesth 1999; 83:422-9.

110. Brichant J-F, Gunst SJ, Warner DO, Rehder K. Halothane, enflurane, and isoflurane depress the peripheral vagal motor pathway in isolated canine tracheal smooth muscle. Anesthesiology 1991; 74:325-32.

111. Sayiner A, Lorenz RR, Warner DO, Rehder K. Bronchodilation by halothane is not modulated by airway epithelium. Anesthesiology 1991; 75:75-81.

112. Mercier FJ, Naline E, Bardou M, et al. Relaxation of proximal and distal isolated human bronchi by halothane, isoflurane and desflurane. Eur Respir J 2002; 20:286-92.

113. Warner DO, Brichant J-F, Rehder K. Direct and neurally mediated effects of halothane on pulmonary resistance in vivo. Anesthesiology 1990; 72:1057-63.

114. Park KW, Dai HB, Lowenstein E, et al. Epithelial dependence of the bronchodilatory effect of sevoflurane and desflurane in rat distal bronchi. Anesth Analg 1998; 86:646-51.

115. Laszlo A, Buljubasic N, Zsolnai B, et al. Interactive effects of volatile anesthetics, verapamil, and ryanodine on contractility and calcium homeostasis of isolated pregnant rat myometrium. Am J Obstet Gynecol 1992; 167:804-10.

116. Brown RH, Zerhouni EA, Hirshman CA. Comparison of low concentrations of halothane and isoflurane as bronchodilators. Anesthesiology 1993; 78:1097-1101.

117. Rooke A, Choi JH, Bishop MJ. The effect of isoflurane, halothane, sevoflurane, and thiopental/nitrous oxide on respiratory system resistance after tracheal intubation. Anesthesiology 1997; 86:1294-9.

118. Prager K, Malin H, Spiegler D, et al. Smoking and drinking behavior before and during pregnancy of married mothers of liveborn infants and stillborn infants. Pub Health Rep 1984; 99:117-27.

119. Pearce AC, Jones RM. Smoking and anesthesia: Preoperative abstinence and perioperative morbidity. Anesthesiology 1984; 61:576-84.

120. Gerrard JW, Cockcroft DW, Mink JT, et al. Increased nonspecific bronchial reactivity in cigarette smokers with normal lung function. Am Rev Respir Dis 1980; 122:577-81.

121. Das TK, Moutquin JM, Parent JG. Effect of cigarette smoking on maternal airway function during pregnancy. Am J Obstet Gynecol 1991; 165:675-9.

122. Marcoux S, Brisson J, Fabia J. The effect of cigarette smoking on the risk of preeclampsia and gestational hypertension. Am J Epidemiol 1989; 130:950-7.

123. Phillips RS, Tuomala RE, Feldblum PJ, et al. The effect of cigarette smoking, Chlamydia trachomatous infection, and vaginal douching on ectopic pregnancy. Obstet Gynecol 1992; 79:85-90.

124. Williams MA, Mittendorf R, Lieberman E, et al. Cigarette smoking during pregnancy in relation to placenta previa. Am J Obstet Gynecol 1991; 165:28-32.

125. Doman-Mullen P, Ramirez G, Groff JY. A meta-analysis of randomized trials of prenatal smoking cessation interventions. Am J Obstet Gynecol 1994; 171:1328-34.

126. American College of Obstetricians and Gynecologists. Smoking cessation during pregnancy. ACOG Educational Bulletin No. 260, Washington, D.C., 2000.

127. Das TK, Moutquin J-M, Lindsay C, et al. Effects of smoking cessation on maternal airway function and birth weight. Obstet Gynecol 1998; 92:201-5.

128. Kim SE, Bishop MJ. Endotracheal intubation but not laryngeal mask airway insertion, produces reversible bronchoconstriction. Anesthesiology 1999; 90:391-4.

129. Rieschke P, LaFleur BJ, Janicki PK. Effects of EDTA- and sulfite containing formulations of propofol on respiratory system resistance after tracheal intubation in smokers. Anesthesiology 2003; 98:323-8.

130. Goff MJ, Arain SR, Ficke DJ. Absence of bronchodilation during desflurane anesthesia. Anesthesiology 2000; 93:404-8.

131. Kotloff RM, FitzSimmons SC, Fiel SB. Fertility and pregnancy in patients with cystic fibrosis. Clin Chest Med 1992; 13:623-35.

132. Collins FS. Cystic fibrosis: Molecular biology and therapeutic implications. Science 1992; 256:774-9.

133. Hwang TC, Lu L, Zeitlin PL, et al. Cl− channels in cystic fibrosis: Lack of activation by protein kinase C and cAMP-dependent protein kinase. Science 1989; 244:1351-3.

134. Li M, McCann JD, Liedtke CM, et al. Cyclic AMP-dependent protein kinase opens chloride channels in normal but not cystic fibrosis airway epithelium. Nature 1988; 331:358-60.

135. Riordan JR, Rommens JM, Kerem BS, et al. Identification of the cystic fibrosis gene: Cloning and characterization of complementary DNA. Science 1989; 245:1066-73.

136. Rommens JM, Iannuzzi MC, Kerem BS, et al. Identification of the cystic fibrosis gene: Chromosome walking and jumping. Science 1989; 245:1059-65.

137. Anderson MP, Rich DP, Gregory RJ, et al. Generation of cAMP-activated chloride currents by expression of CFTR. Science 1991; 251:679-82.

138. Bear CE, Duguay F, Naismith AL, et al. Cl− channel activity in Xenopus oocytes expressing the cystic fibrosis gene. J Biol Chem 1991; 266:19142-5.

139. Egan M, Flott T, Afione S, et al. Defective regulation of outwardly rectifying Cl− channels by protein kinase A corrected by insertion of CFTR. Nature 1992; 358:581-4.

140. Drumm ML, Pope HA, Cliff WH, et al. Correction of the cystic fibrosis defect in vitro by retrovirus-mediated gene transfer. Cell 1990; 62:1227-33.

141. Rich DP, Anderson MP, Gregory RJ, et al. Expression of cystic fibrosis transmembrane conductance regulator corrects defective chloride channel regulation in cystic fibrosis airway epithelial cells. Nature 1990; 347:358-63.

142. Konstan MW, Hilliard KA, Norvell TM, Berger M. Bronchoalveolar lavage findings in cystic fibrosis patients with stable, clinically mild lung disease suggest ongoing infection and inflammation. Am J Respir Crit Care Med 1994; 150:448-54.

143. Kerem E, Reisman J, Corey M, et al. Prediction of mortality in patients with cystic fibrosis. N Engl J Med 1992; 326:1187-91.

144. Canny GJ, Corey M, Livingston RA, et al. Pregnancy and cystic fibrosis. Obstet Gynecol 1991; 77:850-3.

145. Edenborough FP, Stableforth DE, Webb AK, et al. Outcomes of pregnancy in women with cystic fibrosis. Thorax 1995; 50:170-4.

146. Frangolias DD, Nakielna EM, Wilcox PG. Pregnancy and cystic fibrosis: A case-controlled study. Chest 1997; 111:963-9.

147. Gilljam M, Antoniou M, Shin J, et al. Pregnancy in cystic fibrosis: Fetal and maternal outcome. Chest 2000; 118:85-91.

148. Odegaard I, Stry-Pedersen B, Hallberg K, et al. Maternal and fetal morbidity in pregnancies of Norwegian and Swedish women with cystic fibrosis. Acta Obstet Gynecol Scand 2002; 81:698-705.

149. Edenborough FP, MacKenzie WE, Stableforth DE. The outcome of 72 pregnancies in 55 women with cystic fibrosis in the United Kingdom 1977-96. BJOG 2000; 107: 254-61.

150. Ramsey BW. Management of pulmonary disease in patients with cystic fibrosis. N Engl J Med 1996; 335:179-88.

151. Valenzuela GJ, Comunale FL, Davison BH, et al. Clinical management of patients with cystic fibrosis and pulmonary insufficiency. Am J Obstet Gynecol 1988; 159:1181-3.

152. Hubbard RC, McElvaney NG, Birrer P, et al. A preliminary study of aerosolized recombinant human deoxyribonuclease I in the treatment of cystic fibrosis. N Engl J Med 1992; 326:812-5.

153. Shennib H, Adoumie R, Noirclerc M. Current status of lung transplantation for cystic fibrosis. Arch Intern Med 1992; 152:1585-8.

154. Rosenfeld MA, Collins FS. Gene therapy for cystic fibrosis. Chest 1996; 109:241-52.

155. Ackerman MJ, Clapham DE. Ion channels: Basic science and clinical disease. N Engl J Med 1997; 336:1575-86.

156. Hyde NH, Harrison DM. Intrathecal morphine in a parturient with cystic fibrosis. Anesth Analg 1986; 65:1357-8.

157. Howell PR, Kent N, Douglas MJ. Anaesthesia for the parturient with cystic fibrosis. Internat J Obstet Anesth 1993; 2:152-8.

158. Deshpande S. Epidural analgesia for vaginal delivery in a patient with cystic fibrosis following double lung transplantation. Internat J Obstet Anesth 1998; 7:42-5.

159. Bose D, Yentis M, Fauvel NJ. Caesarean section in a parturient with respiratory failure caused by cystic fibrosis. Anaesthesia 1997; 52:576-85.

160. Kaunitz AM, Hughes JM, Grimes DA, et al. Causes of maternal mortality in the United States. Obstet Gynecol 1985; 65:605-12.

161. Mabie WC, Barton JR, Sibai BM. Adult respiratory distress syndrome in pregnancy. Am J Obstet Gynecol 1992; 167:950-7.

162. Malik AB, Selig WM, Burhop KE. Cellular and humoral mediators of pulmonary edema. Lung 1985; 163:193-219.

163. Cruz MS, Moxley MA, Corbett JA, Longmore WJ. Inhibition of nitric oxide synthase attenuates NNMU-induced alveolar injury in vivo. Am J Physiol 1997; 273:L1167-73.

164. Kengatharen KM, De Kimpe SJ, Thiemermann C. Role of nitric oxide in the circulatory failure and organ injury in a rodent model of gram-positive shock. Br J Pharmacol 1996; 119:1411-21.

165. Pheng LH, Francoeur C, Denis M. The involvement of nitric oxide in a mouse model of adult respiratory distress syndrome. Inflammation 1995; 19:599-610.

166. Terada LS, Mahr NN, Jackobson ED. Nitric oxide decreases lung injury after intestinal ischemia. J Appl Physiol 1996; 81:2456-60.

167. Nunn JF. Applied Respiratory Physiology. London, Butterworths, 1987:450-9.

168. Catanzarite V, Willms D, Wong D, et al. Acute respiratory distress syndrome in pregnancy and the puerperium: Causes, courses and outcomes. Obstet Gynecol 2001; 97: 760-4

169. Jenkins TM, Troiano NH, Graves CR, et al. Mechanical ventilation in an obstetric population: Characteristics and delivery rates. Am J Obstet Gynecol 2003; 188: 549-52.

170. Dellinger RP, Zimmerman JL, Taylor RW, et al. Effects of inhaled nitric oxide in patients with acute respiratory distress syndrome: Results of a randomized phase II trial. Crit Care Med 1998; 26:15-23.

171. Goodwin TM, Gherman RB, Hameed A, Elkayam U. Favorable response of Eisenmenger syndrome to inhaled nitric oxide during pregnancy. Am J Obstet Gynecol 1999; 180:64-7.

172. Bugge JF, Tanbo T. Nitric oxide in the treatment of fulminant pulmonary failure in a young pregnant woman with varicella pneumonia. Eur J Anaesthesiol 2000; 17:269-72.

173. Lam GK, Stafford RE, Thorp J, et al. Inhaled nitric oxide for primary pulmonary hypertension in pregnancy. Obstet Gynecol 2001; 98: 895-8.

174. Monnery L, Nanson J, Charlton G. Primary pulmonary hypertension in pregnancy: A role for novel vasodilators. Br J Anaesth 2001; 87: 295-8.

175. Decoene C, Bourzoufi K, Moreau D, et al. Use of inhaled nitric oxide for emergency cesarean section in a woman with unexpected primary pulmonary hypertension. Can J Anesth 2001; 48:584-7.

176. Tomlinson MW, Caruthers TJ, Whitty JE, Gonik B. Does delivery improve maternal condition in the respiratory-compromised gravida? Obstet Gynecol 1998; 91:108-11.

177. Sosin D, Krasnow J, Moawad A, Hall JB. Successful spontaneous vaginal delivery during mechanical ventilatory support of the adult respiratory distress syndrome. Obstet Gynecol 1986; 68:19-23S.

178. Jenkins TM, Troiano NH, Graves CR, et al. Mechanical ventilation in an obstetric population: Characteristics and delivery rates. Am J Obstet Gynecol 2003; 188:549-52.

Chapter 52

Substance Abuse

David J. Birnbach, M.D.

Substance abuse is the ninth leading cause of death in the United States. Anesthesiologists world-wide can expect to encounter patients who are victims of this problem. Substance abuse is associated with various diseases and an increased risk of early death. Pregnant women who are victims of substance abuse may also be victims of violence and are at increased risk for sexually transmitted disease.[1]

For the years 1996 to 1998, the National Household Survey on Drug Abuse noted that 6.4% of nonpregnant women of childbearing age and 2.8% of pregnant women reported that they used illicit drugs. Over half of pregnant women who used illicit drugs also used cigarettes and alcohol. The authors estimated that during the first trimester, 202,000 pregnancies were exposed to illicit drugs, 1,203,000 pregnancies were exposed to cigarettes, and 823,000 pregnancies were exposed to alcohol.[1]

Anesthesiologists must be sensitive to the potential for pregnant women to be victims of drug abuse, and they must be aware of the problems and complications that may arise in these patients.[2]

COCAINE

Epidemiology

Cocaine (benzoylmethylecgonine, $C_{17}H_{21}NO_4$) is an alkaloid derived from the *Erythroxylon coca* plant.[3] Attitudes toward cocaine have changed dramatically since this drug was introduced to Western medicine in 1884 as the first local anesthetic.[4] Until the Pure Food and Drug Act was passed in 1906, cocaine was thought to have only beneficial properties and was added to many substances including Coca Cola.[5] After the Harrison Narcotic Act was passed in 1914, the use of cocaine began to decline in the United States. However, there were differing opinions regarding the risks associated with cocaine use.

As recently as 1980, the authors of a chapter in the *Comprehensive Textbook of Psychiatry* stated, "Used no more than 2 or 3 times a week, cocaine creates no serious problems."[6]

This belief changed in the early 1980s with the introduction of crack, an inexpensive alkaloidal cocaine that can be smoked. This form of cocaine currently is widely used in the United States.[7] In 1985, it was estimated that 30 million Americans had used cocaine and that more than 5 million Americans were using this drug regularly.[8] Experts on the subject of drug abuse estimate that the current use of cocaine far exceeds these earlier estimates that more than 30% of young adults in the United States having tried cocaine before the age of 30.[9] Medical examiners estimate that 30% of drug-related deaths involve cocaine.[2]

Before 1985, cocaine was used most often by affluent males. The demographics of cocaine use have changed. A cross section of the American population, including women of reproductive age, currently abuse this drug.[10] Evidence suggests that there is an increasing incidence of cocaine abuse during pregnancy[11,12] and that this has resulted in a variety of maternal and perinatal complications.[13] In addition, sexually transmitted diseases are more common among crack-cocaine users,[14] and breast-fed infants may be exposed to significant amounts of cocaine.[15]

Pathophysiology

Cocaine's pharmacologic effects are mediated by alterations in the activity of the neurotransmitters norepinephrine, dopamine, and serotonin. The euphoric effects of cocaine are believed to be mediated by a prolongation of dopamine's activity in the limbic system and cortex.[16,17] Studies that have used positron emission tomography (PET) suggest that cocaine's central nervous system (CNS) effects are related to both its affinity for the dopamine transporter and its fast pharmacokinetics.[18] Volkow et al.[18] hypothesized that periodic and frequent stimulation of the dopaminergic system secondary to the chronic use of cocaine favors activation of a circuit that involves the orbitofrontal cortex, cingulate gyrus, thalamus, and striatum. This circuit is abnormal in cocaine abusers, and its activation is thought to perpetuate the compulsive addiction to this drug.

The life-threatening effects of cocaine (e.g., vasoconstriction, hypertension, cardiac abnormalities) occur predominantly as a result of an accumulation of catecholamines. Hypotheses that explain the cocaine-induced accumulation of norepinephrine include (1) prevention of presynaptic reuptake and deactivation of norepinephrine, (2) blockade of catecholamine-binding mechanisms, and (3) stimulation of the sympathoadrenal axis.[19,20] Recent studies have found that the hypertension that occurs with inhalation of cocaine in nonanesthetized individuals is caused by a tremendous increase in cardiac output coincident with direct sympathetic stimulation; the increase in blood pressure activates the arterial baroreceptors, which results in reflex suppression of postganglionic sympathetic nerve activity.[2]

Cocaine affects all major organ systems and often causes life-threatening complications (Box 52-1).[21-40] Of special interest to the anesthesiologist is the risk of myocardial ischemia and infarction. An all-too-common emergency-room scenario is the diagnosis of myocardial ischemia in a young cocaine-

---

Box 52-1 LIFE-THREATENING MATERNAL COMPLICATIONS OF COCAINE ABUSE

CARDIOVASCULAR[21-28,39]
• Myocardial ischemia and infarction
• Hypertension
• Malignant arrhythmias
• Asystole
• Aortic rupture

PULMONARY[29,30]
• Aspiration
• Bronchospasm
• Pneumothorax
• Pneumomediastinum

CENTRAL NERVOUS SYSTEM[31,32]
• Convulsions
• Cerebrovascular accident
• Intracerebral hemorrhage
• Subarachnoid hemorrhage

RENAL[33,34]
• Renal failure

GASTROINTESTINAL[35]
• Bowel ischemia

HEPATIC[36,37]
• Hepatic failure
• Hepatic rupture

HEMATOLOGIC[38]
• Thrombocytopenia
• Disseminated intravascular coagulation

---

abusing patient who would otherwise not be at risk for cardiovascular disease. Potential mechanisms for cocaine-induced myocardial ischemia and depression include coronary artery vasospasm or thrombus, cardiomyopathy, and direct myocardial depression (Figure 52-1).[21-24] Cocaine smokers are also at risk for pulmonary edema.[40] Cardiovascular complications of cocaine abuse are not necessarily dose dependent. A recent study showed that chronic exposure to cocaine does not affect clearance of a bolus dose of cocaine in sheep.[41] Morbidity and mortality may occur during recreational use of small doses of cocaine in people without preexisting cardiac disease. It has been suggested that pregnancy results in an increased sensitivity to the cardiovascular effects of cocaine.[28]

Diagnosis

It is desirable but often difficult for the obstetrician to identify cocaine abuse during early pregnancy. A majority of pregnant cocaine addicts deny drug use when they are interviewed by physicians.[42] Therefore, physical examination and toxicology testing may be necessary to confirm the diagnosis.[43] Given the high frequency of concomitant opioid abuse in cocaine abusing parturients, anyone suspected of cocaine abuse should be tested for other illicit substances. There is an increased likelihood of maternal drug abuse in pregnant women who present with no prenatal care. Box 52-2 lists some of the signs and symptoms of cocaine abuse. Box 52-3 lists the differential diagnoses of hypertension during pregnancy. Physicians should consider the possibility of cocaine use in hypertensive pregnant women. Indeed, patients with cocaine intoxication may present with the classic triad of preeclampsia (i.e., hypertension, proteinuria, edema).[44]

Most often, the diagnosis of cocaine abuse is confirmed by means of urine toxicology. Current methods of urine toxicology include gas chromatography, mass spectrometry, and radioimmunoassay. Unfortunately, many of the currently available tests are performed in the hospital laboratory or at an outside laboratory, and often results are unavailable until several days after delivery of the newborn. A method that allows physicians to test the urine instantly is the OnTrak Abuscreen (Roche, Branchburg, NJ) assay for metabolites of cocaine. Cocaine is degraded into water-soluble metabolites (i.e., benzoylecgonine, ecgonine methyl ester) by (1) plasma cholinesterase, (2) other esterases in both plasma and liver, and (3) nonenzymatic hydrolysis.[45] The OnTrak latex agglutination inhibition test for benzoylecgonine provides a result within 4 minutes, which allows the perinatal team to make appropriate clinical decisions regarding the care of the patient. We evaluated the use of this test in a study of 85 women at risk for cocaine abuse in New York City.[46] We observed that the rapid test had a 100% sensitivity and 100% specificity when compared with standard hospital laboratory tests. The major differences between the OnTrak test and the laboratory tests were that the OnTrak method was less expensive and the result was available in 4 minutes rather than in 24 to 48 hours. Two of the cocaine-positive patients were admitted with a diagnosis of severe preeclampsia. Use of the OnTrak test allowed us to make the appropriate diagnosis, and the hypertension in these patients resolved after the administration of labetalol. This method allowed the obstetricians to avoid unnecessary preterm delivery of these patients.[47]

Urine testing remains positive for 24 to 72 hours after cocaine use, depending on the degree of use. Because of differences in metabolism, infant toxicology testing may

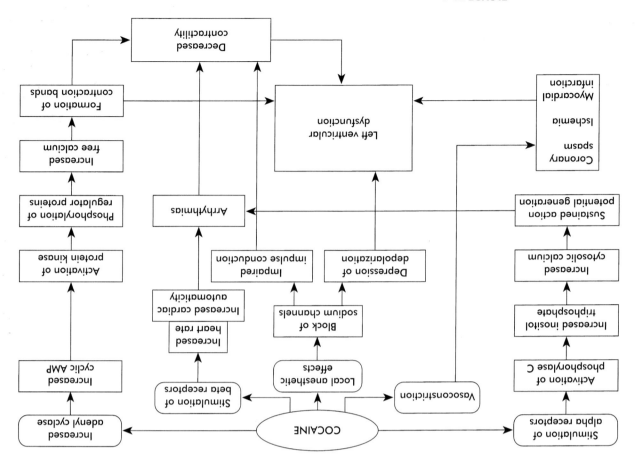

FIGURE 52-1. Mechanisms of cocaine-induced myocardial depression and dysfunction.

remain positive for several days after the maternal urine test becomes negative.[48] Recent studies have evaluated the use of newborn meconium and maternal hair for the detection of cocaine abuse and have found that these methods can greatly improve the detection of cocaine use in pregnant patients.[49,50]

Interaction with Pregnancy

Cocaine use during pregnancy is fraught with danger. This danger is exaggerated by the misconceptions that cocaine may be used safely, does not cross the placenta, and allows for easier and faster childbirth. Comprehensive prenatal care and patient education are of critical importance in the struggle to reduce the use of cocaine during pregnancy.

Woods and Plessinger[28] demonstrated that pregnancy enhances the cardiovascular toxicity of cocaine in gravid ewes. Cocaine and its breakdown products have a high water and lipid solubility as well as a low molecular weight. Thus cocaine freely crosses the placenta and produces direct effects on the fetus.[51] Indirect effects also occur. Maternal vasoconstriction causes decreased uteroplacental blood flow, uteroplacental insufficiency, and decreased fetal oxygenation.[52] Cocaine abuse is associated with an increased risk of placental abruption, premature rupture of the membranes, meconium-stained amniotic fluid, low birth weight (LBW), and congenital anomalies.[53] Chazotte et al.[54] evaluated fetal heart rate (FHR) tracings from fetuses exposed to cocaine in utero. They noted no specific, characteristic patterns, but they

observed a decrease in long-term variability and an increase in the frequency of uterine contractions. Evidence currently suggests that cocaine may have direct effects on several biochemical processes in the placenta.[55] For example, the function of the human placental serotonin transporter may be severely impaired by the maternal use of cocaine during pregnancy.[56] Cocaine may also have direct effects on the fetal vasculature, and a recent study suggested that perinatal cocaine exposure may affect neonatal cardiac function.[57] Although the effects of maternal cocaine abuse are thought to be cumulative, erratic use of cocaine during pregnancy may result in perinatal complications as severe as those that occur with daily use.[58] Box 52-4 summarizes the fetal and neonatal effects of maternal cocaine abuse.

Obstetric Management

The American College of Obstetrics and Gynecology (ACOG)[70] has made several recommendations regarding the management of pregnant patients who use cocaine:

1. The obstetrician should obtain a drug history during the first prenatal visit, and the patient should be warned about the dangers of drug use during pregnancy.
2. A woman who acknowledges use of cocaine should be counseled and offered support to aid in her abstinence.
3. The obstetrician should consider periodic urine testing in order to encourage and reinforce continual abstinence.
4. The obstetrician should consider testing the mother, neonate, or both in cases of unexpected preterm labor,

Box 52-2 SIGNS AND SYMPTOMS OF COCAINE ABUSE

Hypertension/tachycardia
Convulsions
Hyperreflexia
Tremors
Hyperpyrexia
Acidosis
Emotional lability
Dilated pupils

Box 52-3 DIFFERENTIAL DIAGNOSIS OF HYPERTENSION DURING PREGNANCY

Drug abuse
Preeclampsia/eclampsia
Chronic hypertension
Pain/noxious stimulation
Hypoxia/hypercarbia
Pheochromocytoma
Malignant hyperthermia
Opioid/alcohol withdrawal

Box 52-4 FETAL AND NEONATAL EFFECTS OF MATERNAL COCAINE ABUSE

Increased incidence of spontaneous abortion[59]
Increased incidence of preterm labor and premature rupture of membranes[60]
Increased incidence of placental abruption[61]
Decreased uteroplacental perfusion[62]
Increased incidence of fetal distress[46]
Fetal tachycardia/hypertension[62]
Increased incidence of congenital malformations[51,63-65]
Neonatal central nervous system irritability[59,66]
Perinatal cerebral infarction[67]
Intrauterine fetal death[68]
Neonatal myocardial infarction[69]

unexplained fetal growth restriction, or in women with placental abruption and no history of chronic hypertension.

5. Some states consider in utero drug exposure to be a form of child abuse or neglect under the law. Some states require that physicians report positive drug tests in pregnant women or their newborns to the states' child protection agency.[71,72]

6. When a maternal test is positive for cocaine metabolites, the neonatologist or pediatrician should be advised of the infant's exposure in utero.

Anesthetic Management

After a physician has determined that a patient is using cocaine, the anesthesiologist must decide whether the patient is an appropriate candidate for regional or general anesthesia. In some cases of severe fetal "distress," the anesthesiologist is asked to provide anesthesia for emergency cesarean section, regardless of the mother's hemodynamic status. We have had success with the administration of regional anesthesia in a large population of pregnant women who were abusing cocaine, and we have observed that life-threatening events are more common during general anesthesia than during regional anesthesia in these women. During administration of general anesthesia, the most frequently encountered problems are severe hypertension and arrhythmias after induction, laryngoscopy, and intubation.[73]

Regional anesthesia is not without risk, for several reasons. First, these patients are at risk for platelet abnormalities.[38] If regional anesthesia is selected, the anesthesiologist should ascertain that the patient has an acceptable platelet count. Second, these patients are at an increased risk for hypotension during regional anesthesia. We observed a greater decrease in maternal blood pressure in cocaine-positive patients than in cocaine-negative patients who received epidural anesthesia for cesarean section.[74] Third, ephedrine may not be an effective vasopressor in the patient with depleted catecholamine stores. Thus the anesthesiologist should prepare a dilute solution of phenylephrine and should plan to use phenylephrine if ephedrine does not effectively treat hypotension.[75] Fourth, cocaine addicts often complain of pain despite an adequate level of spinal or epidural anesthesia during cesarean section. Thus these patients may require opioid supplementation during surgery. Possible explanations include an abnormal affect among cocaine addicts, the anesthesiologist's desire to sedate patients who abuse drugs, and most likely, a central effect of cocaine, which may cause an abnormality of endorphins. Changes in both mu- and kappa-opioid receptor densities have been identified in regions with abundant dopaminergic terminals after binge patterns of cocaine administration.[76] The binding of opioid receptors by specific receptor-selective ligands has also been reported.[77] Of interest, a recent study demonstrated that intrathecal sufentanil 10 μg produced intrapartum analgesia of similar quality but shorter duration in laboring women who had abused cocaine than in parturients who had not abused cocaine.[78]

If general anesthesia is chosen, the anesthesiologist should be prepared to treat hypertension, arrhythmias, and myocardial ischemia.[79] Vertommen et al.[80] evaluated the administration of hydralazine for the treatment of cocaine-induced hypertension in gravid ewes. Intravenous administration of cocaine increased maternal mean arterial pressure (MAP) by approximately 30% and decreased uterine blood flow (UBF) by approximately 25% to 40%. Hydralazine successfully restored maternal MAP toward baseline, but it also resulted in profound maternal tachycardia and failed to restore UBF. The maternal heart rate increased by approximately 120% after the administration of hydralazine. Subsequently, Hughes et al.[81] performed a similar study to evaluate the use of labetalol for treatment of cocaine-induced hypertension in gravid ewes. Labetalol rapidly decreased maternal MAP toward baseline, but it did not restore UBF. Unlike hydralazine, labetalol did not increase maternal heart rate; rather, labetalol decreased maternal heart rate to baseline. The authors concluded that "labetalol may be preferable to hydralazine for treatment of the acutely cocaine-intoxicated parturient."[81]

In my practice, we treat severe hypertension secondary to cocaine abuse by giving labetalol plus nitroglycerin before the induction of general anesthesia. However, Hollander[82] has suggested that labetalol should not be used in cocaine-abusing patients because labetalol's antagonism of beta-adrenergic receptors is greater than its effect on alpha receptors. Cocaine abuse represents a relative contraindication to the use of propranolol because beta-adrenergic blockade may cause unopposed alpha-adrenergic receptor stimulation and exacerbated hypertension.[83] In addition, beta blockade has been reported to enhance cocaine-induced coronary vasoconstriction.[84] Güeret et al.[85] have suggested the use of benzodiazepines in patients with cocaine toxicity. Published evidence suggests that calcium-entry blocking agents may *not* be effective in preventing or treating cocaine toxicity.[86]

If possible, the anesthesiologist should avoid administering drugs that sensitize the myocardium to catecholamines (e.g., halothane) and those that release catecholamines or cause tachycardia (e.g., ketamine, atropine).[87,88] General anesthetic agents should be titrated carefully in these patients. The minimum alveolar concentration (MAC) for general anesthetic agents may be decreased in *chronic* cocaine addicts as a result of the depletion of catecholamines. In contrast, *acute* use of cocaine may result in increased concentrations of catecholamines, which may indicate a need for increased doses of anesthetic drugs (i.e., increased MAC). Cocaine use may also alter the response to succinylcholine.[89]

Table 52-1 outlines therapy for cocaine intoxication.

Cocaine addicts often abuse other drugs; they may combine cocaine with marijuana, alcohol, amphetamines, or heroin.[90-92] For example, cocaine mixed with alcohol attenuates the excitatory effects of cocaine in dogs.[93] Another common street drug is speedball, which is a combination of heroin and cocaine.[94] Patients may unknowingly mix drugs because street cocaine is often "cut" with multiple compounds, which may cause toxic cardiovascular and neurologic complications. Therefore, if single-drug abuse is suspected, the anesthesiologist should be prepared to encounter and treat the effects of multiple drugs. Cocaine toxicity is often seen many hours after the ingestion of cocaine. Therefore, patients should be considered at risk for cocaine-related complications even if the cocaine use occurred more than 24 hours earlier.[95]

AMPHETAMINES

Amphetamines are the third most widely abused class of drugs in the United States.[96] While cocaine is a coastal and urban drug, amphetamines and methamphetamines prevail in middle and western states, finding favor with workers engaged in prolonged shifts and repetitive tasks.[2] The amphetamines are a group of sympathomimetic drugs that cause profound CNS stimulation. These drugs are abused individually and with other drugs such as cocaine and heroin. Acute ingestion of an amphetamine causes catecholamine release from adrenergic nerve terminals and inhibition of catecholamine uptake. Signs and symptoms of amphetamine abuse resemble those of cocaine abuse and include hypertension, tachycardia, agitation, confusion, arrhythmias, dilated pupils, hyperreflexia, and fever.[97] The combination of hypertension, proteinuria, and fever, convulsions resulting from amphetamine abuse has been mistaken for eclampsia.[98] In addition, amphetamines cause

anorexia, which may lead to poor maternal nutrition and fetal intrauterine growth restriction (IUGR).[31]

Interaction with Pregnancy

In the 1950s and 1960s, some obstetricians supported the antenatal use of amphetamines to help with weight control. Several studies found no association between the use of amphetamines and congenital abnormalities.[99,100] Others have reported an increased incidence of congenital heart disease and neurologic abnormalities among these infants.[101,102] However, there is little doubt that the illicit use of amphetamines is associated with IUGR, preterm labor and delivery, placental abruption, fetal "distress," and an increased risk of perinatal mortality.[103,104]

Anesthetic Management

Amphetamine abuse may cause maternal or fetal instability that necessitates emergency cesarean section. The anesthesiologist must be aware of hypertension and arrhythmias after induction of general anesthesia, laryngoscopy, and endotracheal intubation. **Acute ingestion of amphetamines** increases dose requirements for general anesthetic agents.[105,106] It seems prudent to avoid agents that sensitize the myocardium to catecholamines; thus, isoflurane seems preferable to halothane. In contrast, **chronic ingestion of amphetamines** may decrease the MAC of volatile halogenated agents.[105] Elliott and Rees[107] noted that "chronic ingestion of amphetamine depletes the neurones of catecholamines, impairs the response to sympathomimetics and obtunds the stress response."[7] They noted that it may be difficult to differentiate between acute and chronic ingestion in a patient and suggested the use of invasive hemodynamic monitoring in patients with a history of amphetamine ingestion. Regional anesthesia may be used, but epidural or spinal anesthesia may precipitate severe hypotension, and the response to pressor agents is unpredictable. There are two published cases of cardiac arrest during epidural[108] and general[109] anesthesia for cesarean section in women who chronically abused amphetamines. Geerlings[110] has suggested that there is a high incidence of psychosis associated with the chronic use of amphetamines. Such behavior may complicate the management of obstetric patients who receive regional anesthesia.

ECSTASY

Ecstasy (3,4-methylenedioxymethamphetamine, or MDMA) and its derivatives MDA (Adam) and MDEA (Eve) have both stimulant and hallucinogenic properties. Ecstasy increases 5-hydroxytryptamine (5-HT or serotonin) levels, and, to a lesser extent, dopamine levels by stimulating release and inhibiting uptake.[111] High doses of ecstasy may have neurotoxic effects on central serotonergic systems.[112] Selective impairment of neuropsychological performance associated with regular ecstasy use is not reversed by prolonged abstinence in animals.[112] This is consistent with evidence that ecstasy has potent, selective neurotoxic effects on brain serotonergic systems in humans.[113] Also, former users report higher levels of depression than matched controls.[114] The average ecstasy user is Caucasian, is younger, and has more unplanned pregnancies than nonusers. She is more likely to smoke cigarettes, drink alcohol, and have episodes of binge drinking during pregnancy. Illicit drugs such as cocaine,

TABLE 52-1	THERAPY FOR COCAINE INTOXICATION
Symptom	**Therapy**
Hypertension/tachycardia	Nitroglycerin, labetalol, ± benzodiazepine[82]
Convulsions	Benzodiazepine/control airway
Tremors/central nervous system agitation	Benzodiazepine
Angina	Intravenous nitroglycerin ± labetalol[90]
Arrhythmias	Sodium bicarbonate,[86] lidocaine[91]

marijuana, methamphetamine, ketamine, gamma-hydroxy-butyrate, and psilocybin are often used with ecstasy. Over one third of pregnant ecstasy users report psychiatric/emotional problems such as clinical depression and/or anxiety.[115] Use of ecstasy may increase the risk of congenital cardiovascular and musculoskeletal anomalies.[116]

Reports of fatal toxicity are common. Serious morbidity and mortality have occurred from fulminant hyperthermia, cardiac arrhythmias, disseminated intravascular coagulation (DIC), rhabdomyolysis, acute renal failure, and hepatic toxic-ity. Hydration, electrolyte replacement, maintenance of urine output, cooling, anti-arrhythmia therapy, and management of anxiety are all essential goals of treatment. One report described the successful use of dantrolene for treatment of the hypermetabolic state (i.e., hyperthermia, tachycardia) in a case of massive overdose of ecstasy.[117]

OPIOIDS

The spectrum of opioid abuse includes morphine, heroin, meperidine, methadone, and fentanyl. Although there appears to be a decreased incidence of opioid abuse among pregnant women in the United States, opioid abuse continues to be a frequent problem in inner-city hospitals. It has been estimated that 250,000 women in the United States are intra-venous drug abusers, and 90% of these women are of child-bearing age.[118] An upsurge in the prevalence of opioid abuse may be related to cocaine abuse because heroin is used to ameliorate some of the effects of cocaine.[119] It has been esti-mated that more than 300,000 infants are exposed to opioids in utero.[120]

Perinatal opioid abuse is associated with a multitude of maternal and fetal sequelae. Many of the problems associated with intravenous drug abuse result from drug preparation and injection techniques, not from the opioid itself. Heroin sold on the street is routinely cut with a high proportion of adulterants such as talc and cornstarch.[121] These substances often cause more damage than the heroin itself. (For example, the injection of talc-diluted heroin causes talcosis.) Because the intravenous drug abuser does not use sterile technique when mixing or injecting the illicit drug, infectious sequelae are common. When sclerosis of the peripheral veins occurs, the intravenous drug abuser typically injects drugs into a cen-tral vein. The injection of illicit drugs into the internal jugu-lar, subclavian, and femoral veins is a major cause of morbidity and mortality. Pneumothorax, pneumomedi-astinum, hemothorax, thrombophlebitis, endocarditis, and embolic phenomena may occur.[122] Other maternal complica-tions of intravenous drug abuse include sexually transmitted disease, human immunodeficiency virus (HIV) infection and acquired immunodeficiency syndrome (AIDS), hepatitis, endocarditis, and other cardiovascular, pulmonary, and renal abnormalities.[123-125]

Although all drug-abusing patients tend to deny drug use to physicians, intravenous drug dependency is easier to recognize than cocaine abuse. Physicians must consider the diagnosis in women with track marks, thrombotic and sclerosed veins, sub-cutaneous abscesses or scarring, bizarre behavior, a history of drug-associated diseases, or an absence of prenatal care.

Interaction with Pregnancy

Fetal effects of maternal intravenous drug abuse include IUGR and fetal jeopardy. These problems most likely result

from several factors that include (1) a direct opioid effect on the fetus, (2) maternal use of multiple drugs, (3) poor mater-nal nutrition, (4) infection, and (5) opioid withdrawal.[126]

Many pregnant opioid addicts are given methadone to decrease the maternal risk of intravenous drug use. Infants born to mothers taking methadone weigh more than infants of mothers who abuse heroin. However, methadone is associ-ated with multiple fetal and neonatal problems including severe newborn withdrawal, neurobehavioral depression, and an increased incidence of perinatal mortality.[127,128] A recent study demonstrated that the maternal methadone dose does not correlate with neonatal withdrawal. The authors con-cluded that "maternal benefits of effective methadone dosing are not offset by neonatal harm."[128]

Drozdick et al.[129] recently reported a study of methadone trough levels in pregnant women addicted to heroin. The authors observed that the mean methadone serum trough level in asymptomatic pregnant women was approximately 0.3 mg/L, and they concluded that trough levels of 0.24 mg/L or greater should be adequate to prevent withdrawal symp-toms in pregnant women. The daily dose of methadone needed to achieve these levels typically is between 50 and 150 mg, but some patients may need a higher dose during the third trimester.[129]

A recent study found that electroacupuncture may also have a place in the treatment of morphine withdrawal.[130] Some physicians have suggested use of a naltrexone mainte-nance program for pregnant women with a recurrent pattern of heroin abuse. Early evidence suggests no obvious risk to the mother or developing fetus.[131]

Anesthetic Management

Physicians need to recognize maternal opioid overdose and maternal withdrawal. Overdose may even occur in a hospital-ized patient when visitors bring the patient a supply of drugs or when the patient has concealed drugs in her possessions or body. Overdose is characterized by coma, miosis, and respira-tory depression. Withdrawal occurs approximately 12 hours after the last opioid dose. Symptoms may include yawning, lacrimation, rhinorrhea, diarrhea, dehydration, fever, and sweating. Clonidine and methadone have been advocated for the treatment of opioid withdrawal.[132] To prevent withdrawal, the physician caring for an opioid addict should calculate the patient's typical daily opioid dose and administer that base-line amount, irrespective of additional considerations of acute pain relief.[133] Pain during labor or after surgery may require administration of an even larger dose of opioid.

The anesthesiologist often is involved in the care of preg-nant women who abuse drugs intravenously, for at least three reasons. First, intravenous access is limited and diffi-cult, and the obstetrician may request that the anesthesiolo-gist establish central venous access. Second, provision of intrapartum analgesia is often problematic. Third, these patients may require emergency cesarean section for nonre-assuring FHR status. The cause of fetal jeopardy is multifac-torial, but opioid withdrawal may cause fetal hypoxia and must be avoided.

If the mother receives opioids during labor to prevent withdrawal, the newborn may present with respiratory depression. Neonatal resuscitation should include active assis-tance of ventilation but not administration of naloxone. Naloxone may precipitate acute neonatal withdrawal syn-drome. Symptoms of neonatal withdrawal include irritability, poor feeding, hypertonicity, diarrhea, apnea, and autonomic dysfunction.[134]

Regional anesthetic techniques are advantageous for the opioid addict, provided that there are no contraindications such as coagulopathy, sepsis, or infection at the site of the block. Epidural anesthesia may be continued for pain relief after cesarean section; this allows physicians to provide analgesia without opioids. There appears to be an increasing incidence of spinal epidural abscess and disc space infection among intravenous drug abusers.[135] These spinal/epidural infections have occurred in drug abusers who did not receive regional anesthesia. Unfortunately, if an opioid addict develops spinal/epidural infection after the administration of regional anesthesia, the anesthesiologist undoubtedly will be blamed. Thus neurologic assessment should be undertaken before initiation of the block. Asymptomatic HIV infection, which is a major problem in these patients, does not contraindicate regional anesthesia.[136] The anesthesiologist may give opioids intravenously or intraspinally to relieve pain, but agonist-antagonist drugs via any route must be avoided because they may precipitate acute withdrawal.[137]

Despite the use of large doses of local anesthetic, regional anesthesia may provide inadequate pain relief in some opioid abusers.[138] It appears that the drug abuser may tolerate less pain than a normal patient. One explanation is that these patients have a decreased production of endogenous opioid peptides. Regardless of the cause, it is often necessary to provide intravenous opioid supplementation of regional anesthesia in the opioid addict.

General anesthesia may become necessary in these patients for multiple reasons (e.g., coagulopathy, sepsis, hemodynamic instability, combative behavior, patient refusal). Many of these patients have abnormal liver function. Therefore, drugs that are hepatotoxic or largely detoxified in the liver should be used with caution. Intravenous induction of anesthesia is typically smooth. Provided that the patient's physiologic opioid requirements are met, cross tolerance is not a problem during the maintenance of anesthesia.[133]

There may be some efficacy in the intraoperative and/or postoperative administration of a parenteral nonsteroidal antiinflammatory drug (NSAID) (e.g., ketorolac).[139] In addition, patient-controlled analgesia can be used safely and effectively in patients with a history of substance abuse.[140,141] In recovering addicts, the use of multimodal therapy with regional anesthesia and an NSAID may obviate the need for opioids. It has been suggested that the lack of adequate pain control is a major cause of relapse among addicts.[2]

MARIJUANA

Marijuana, a naturally occurring substance that is smoked for its hallucinogenic properties, is the most commonly used illicit drug among women of childbearing age. A survey of drug abuse noted that 56% of women 18 to 25 years of age acknowledged using marijuana.[142] It has been estimated that the incidence of marijuana use during pregnancy ranges from 10% to 27%.[134]

Interaction with Pregnancy

Marijuana may alter the pituitary release of trophic hormones and placental production of estrogen and progesterone, which may have an adverse effect on fertility and pregnancy.[143] Laryngospasm, bronchoconstriction, and increased carbon monoxide concentrations also may occur.[2,144] In addition, frequent and regular use of cannabis throughout pregnancy may be associated with small decrements in birth weight.[145]

The active ingredient in marijuana is delta-9-tetrahydro-cannabinol (THC); it is a highly lipid-soluble substance that accumulates in fatty tissues and freely crosses the placenta. Many women who use marijuana also use alcohol and nicotine. Thus it has been difficult to identify the specific effects of marijuana on the fetus. Investigators have used sophisticated statistical methods to separate the effects of these agents and currently have sufficient information to identify fetal complications of maternal marijuana use. Specifically, it appears that marijuana use results in decreased uteroplacental perfusion and impaired fetal growth.[146]

Anesthetic Management

As with cocaine abuse, tachycardia is common after marijuana use.[147] The anesthesiologist should entertain the possibility of drug abuse when determining the cause of unexplained intraoperative tachycardia. Marijuana-induced tachycardia can be treated with beta-adrenergic receptor blockade. The anesthesiologist should avoid giving anesthetic agents that cause tachycardia to patients with a known history of recent marijuana abuse. Thus the anesthesiologist most likely should avoid intravenous administration of ketamine, atropine, and pancuronium. It also seems prudent to avoid the addition of epinephrine to a solution of local anesthetic.

Chronic marijuana use may lead to lethargy, irritability, and respiratory tract infections.[148] Marijuana also may cause myocardial depression. During general anesthesia, marijuana and the volatile halogenated agents may have an additive effect and may result in cardiovascular depression.[149]

ETHANOL

It has been estimated that more than 15 million Americans have an alcohol problem, and 8% to 11% of women of child-bearing age are problem drinkers or alcoholics.[150] A recent study estimated that 15% of pregnant women in the United States consume alcohol, and 3.5% consume alcohol frequently.[151]

Interaction with Pregnancy

Alcohol is a known teratogen, and its use during pregnancy is associated with the fetal alcohol syndrome and alcohol-related neurodevelopmental disorder (ARND). Fetal alcohol syndrome was first described in France in 1968.[152] Subsequently, more than 800 clinical and research reports on fetal alcohol syndrome have been published.[153] Although the incidence of fetal alcohol syndrome varies based on location and diagnostic criteria, it is clear that fetal alcohol exposure continues to be a serious problem. For example, it has been estimated that the combined rate of fetal alcohol syndrome and ARND in Seattle is at least 9.1 per 1000 live births.[154]

Fetal alcohol syndrome is characterized by a spectrum of symptoms including a characteristic appearance, growth restriction, and mental retardation (Box 52-5).[152] Although severe manifestations are seen after the consumption of at least four to five drinks per day, minor manifestations (including neurobehavioral deficits) have been reported in the infants of mothers who abused lesser amounts of alcohol.

No safe level of intake has been established for pregnant women, although the American Council on Science and Health has recommended that pregnant women consume no more than two drinks daily.[155] Because a safe level of intake has not been determined, abstinence is the safest course during pregnancy and for women who plan to become pregnant.[156] Some investigators have suggested that heavy paternal alcohol abuse produces the fetal alcohol syndrome, but the evidence of paternal involvement in this disease is inconclusive.[157]

Multiple mechanisms for the teratogenic effects of maternal alcohol ingestion have been postulated. It has been suggested that acetaldehyde, a metabolic by-product of ethanol, may be toxic to the fetus and placenta.[156,157] Other possible mechanisms include abnormal protein synthesis, poor dietary intake, abnormal intestinal absorption, vitamin deficiencies, and genetic predisposition.

Anesthetic Management

Alcohol abuse can present with a multitude of medical problems including cardiac arrhythmias, cardiomyopathy, gastritis, pancreatitis, cirrhosis, psychosis, neuropathy, and coagulopathy. When evaluating a patient who may have an alcohol problem, the anesthesiologist should give special attention to a review of the cardiac, hematologic, neurologic, and hepatic systems. The anesthesiologist also should obtain a thorough history of alcohol intake including the time and quantity of last consumption. The anesthesiologist should also remember that patients who abuse alcohol often abuse other drugs.

Occasionally, an acutely intoxicated pregnant woman presents to the labor and delivery suite. Risks of acute alcohol intoxication include maternal pulmonary aspiration of gastric

---

contents and fetal "distress." If a parturient appears to be intoxicated, the blood alcohol concentration should be determined and a urine sample should be subjected to a toxicology screen. Kurth et al.[158] demonstrated that ethylcocaine, which is formed when alcohol is ingested with cocaine, is a very potent cerebral vasoconstrictor. This suggests that concurrent use of ethanol and cocaine may be especially hazardous.

Table 52-2 lists the anesthetic implications of alcohol abuse. Regional anesthesia is preferred in the absence of coagulopathy or severe neuropathy. It is prudent to document the presence or absence of peripheral neuropathy before the administration of regional anesthesia. Regional anesthesia allows the anesthesiologist to avoid the problems associated with the administration of general anesthesia in the alcoholic patient.

VAPOR SNIFFING

Recreational inhalation of toluene-based solvents has been reported during pregnancy and has been associated with an increased incidence of IUGR, preterm labor, and perinatal death.[159] Maternal manifestations of solvent abuse include renal tubular acidosis, electrolyte abnormalities, and cardiac arrhythmias. Optimal management of these patients requires early recognition of the problem. Although it is not possible to link a specific birth defect or developmental problem to prenatal exposure to a specific chemical, it is clear that inhalant abuse and its associated lifestyle place both the mother and the child at risk.[160] Kuczkowski[161] recently described the anesthetic management for emergency cesarean section in a parturient with solvent-related respiratory depression and fetal bradycardia.

CIGARETTE SMOKING

Great strides have been made in educating the public regarding the health risks associated with cigarette smoking, and

---

Box 52-5 SIGNS AND SYMPTOMS OF FETAL ALCOHOL SYNDROME

CRANIOFACIAL ABNORMALITIES
- Abnormalities of the eyes, mouth, ears, and maxilla

CNS ABNORMALITIES
- Irritability
- Retardation
- Hypotonia

CARDIAC ABNORMALITIES
- Atrial septal defect
- Ventricular septal defect
- Tetralogy of Fallot

UROLOGIC ABNORMALITIES
- Renal defects
- Hypospadius

MUSCULOSKELETAL ABNORMALITIES
- Hernias
- Scoliosis
- Pectus excavatum
- Pectus carinatum
- Abnormal joint movements

CUTANEOUS
- Hemangiomas

TABLE 52-2 SEQUELAE OF ALCOHOL ABUSE AND ANESTHETIC IMPLICATIONS

Sequelae	Anesthetic Implications
Cardiomyopathy	Increased risk of myocardial depression during general anesthesia
Increased gastric acid	Increased risk of pulmonary aspiration of gastric contents
Cross-tolerance with barbiturates	Increased induction dose of sodium thiopental required except when the patient is acutely intoxicated
Decreased albumin concentration	Increased sensitivity to many drugs as a result of decreased protein binding
Coagulopathy	Possible contraindication to the administration of regional anesthesia
Esophageal varices	Increased risk of bleeding with passage of a nasogastric tube, esophageal stethoscope, temperature probe, and suction catheter
Ascites	Abnormalities of intravascular volume and electrolytes
Liver disease	Decreased pseudocholinesterase activity and abnormal response to drugs that undergo hepatic metabolism
Electrolyte abnormalities	Prolonged activity of muscle relaxants

there has been a decline in the use of cigarettes among young Americans. However, cigarettes are an inexpensive, legal substance abused by millions of young Americans.

Interaction with Pregnancy

Cigarette smoking is a preventable cause of both maternal morbidity and perinatal morbidity and mortality. Unfortunately, more than 25% of pregnant women smoke during pregnancy.[162,163] Sloan et al.[163] anonymously collected urine samples from 181 women who presented to the University of Missouri Clinics for obstetric care and who resided in communities of less than 25,000 people. Of the 181 specimens, 83 (46%) contained nicotine, and 17 (9.4%) contained marijuana.

Approximately 80% of women who smoke continue to do so during pregnancy.[162] Heavy smokers are less likely to quit smoking during pregnancy than are light smokers; this is most likely because of their greater dependence on nicotine.

Cigarette smoke is composed of more than 1000 components, many of which affect the respiratory, cardiovascular, and immune systems. Nicotine and carbon monoxide are the two components of cigarette smoke that are the most harmful for the cardiovascular system. These substances adversely affect the health of the mother and fetus. The affinity of hemoglobin for carbon monoxide is greater than 200 times its affinity for oxygen; therefore, the inhalation of carbon monoxide produces significant levels of carboxyhemoglobin.[164] The presence of carboxyhemoglobin decreases the amount of hemoglobin that can combine with oxygen. Therefore, carboxyhemoglobinemia decreases the oxygen content of the blood. It also produces a left shift of the maternal oxyhemoglobin dissociation curve; this causes an increased affinity of hemoglobin for oxygen. The net effect is a decrease in the delivery of oxygen to both the mother and the fetus.

Nicotine worsens the insult to the fetus. Nicotine decreases uteroplacental perfusion and may produce fetal hypoxia.[165,166] Clark and Irion[166] observed that intravenous administration of nicotine increased uterine vascular resistance and decreased UBF in gravid ewes. Morrow et al.[167] used Doppler ultrasonography to evaluate uterine and umbilical blood flow velocity after cigarette smoking by pregnant women. They observed that cigarette smoking was associated with increased maternal heart rate and blood pressure. Cigarette smoking resulted in no change in the uterine artery systolic/diastolic velocity ratio. However, smoking was associated with an increase in FHR and in the umbilical artery systolic/diastolic velocity ratio, which suggested an increase in umbilical artery vascular resistance. These investigators concluded the following:[167]

Cigarette causes considerable changes in the feto-placental circulation that are similar to those seen in fetal growth retardation and are indicative of increased placental vascular resistance. These alterations in fetal blood flow may impair the oxygen exchange across the placenta, and in some cases, may adversely affect perinatal outcome.

Cigarette smoking causes changes in the placenta including hypertrophy, a decrease in vasculosyncytial membranes, cytotrophoblastic cell proliferation, focal syncytial necrosis, decreased pinocytosis, and thickening of the trophoblastic basement membrane.[168]

Cigarette smoking during pregnancy increases the risk of spontaneous abortion, preterm delivery, and low birth weight (LBW). The incidence of LBW in infants increases in proportion to the number of cigarettes smoked.[169] There appears to be an adverse interaction among cigarette smoking, maternal age, and parity. Chattingius et al.[170] noted that *older* smokers are at especially high risk for the delivery of small-for-gestational-age (SGA) infants, and *parous* smokers are at an especially high risk for preterm delivery and delivery of LBW infants. Other neonatal problems associated with cigarette smoking include sleep disturbances, feeding difficulties, sudden infant death syndrome (SIDS), learning disorders, and childhood cancers.[171,172]

Some physicians have suggested that nicotine replacement therapy should be used in women who have difficulty discontinuing the use of cigarettes during pregnancy.[173,174] Although nicotine is harmful to the fetus, transdermal nicotine therapy allows the patient to receive nicotine without exposure to the many other toxic chemicals that are found in cigarette smoke. Further, smoking delivers more nicotine at a more rapid rate and results in more intense cardiovascular and CNS stimulation than transdermal nicotine.[173]

Anesthetic Management

Respiratory consequences of cigarette smoking include an increase in mucus secretion, a decrease in mucociliary transport, and narrowing of the small airways.[175] Thus postoperative respiratory morbidity is the major risk associated with general anesthesia in patients who smoke cigarettes. Approximately 4 to 6 weeks of abstinence from cigarette smoking are required to allow a decrease in the risk of postoperative respiratory morbidity as compared to the nonsmoker. However, any period of abstinence improves the patient's readiness for anesthesia and surgery. After 48 hours of abstinence, carboxyhemoglobin concentrations fall toward those of nonsmokers. Decreased carboxyhemoglobin concentrations result in increased maternal oxygen content and delivery. In addition, a few days of abstinence may greatly improve mucociliary transport, and 1 to 2 weeks of abstinence result in a significant reduction in sputum volume.

Cigarette smoking also impairs the immune response. Further, cigarette smoking causes an induction of hepatic enzyme activity which may alter the metabolism of drugs such as theophylline, warfarin, and propranolol.[176,177] Miller[178] studied the effect of cigarette smoking on drug metabolism and found that diazepam and chlordiazepoxide produced greater drowsiness in nonsmokers and less drowsiness in heavy smokers. He concluded that "substances in cigarette smoke induce liver microsomal enzymes which increase the metabolism of these drugs."

CAFFEINE

Caffeine clearly is not an illicit substance, and perhaps a discussion of caffeine should not be included in a chapter on the subject of substance abuse. However, both patients and physicians have a significant interest in the implications of caffeine consumption during pregnancy. Caffeine is ingested daily in one of its many forms by a majority of the American population. Almost 80% of pregnant women have some form of daily ingestion of caffeine.[179] Caffeine, a methylxanthine, is an active ingredient in coffee (29 to 176 mg/cup), tea (8 to 107 mg/cup), cocoa (5 to 10 mg/cup), cola beverages (32 to 65 mg/12 oz), and solid milk chocolate (6 mg/oz).[179,180]

Abrupt discontinuation of the regular daily intake of caffeine may precipitate symptoms of caffeine withdrawal. Caffeine withdrawal may present as headache, muscle pains, or anxiety.[181,182] Silverman et al.[182] studied 62 normal adults with a history of low-to-moderate daily intake of caffeine; the mean daily dose of caffeine was 235 mg, or approximately 2.5 cups of coffee per day. The abrupt discontinuation of caffeine resulted in moderate or severe headache in 52% of the subjects. Further, 8% of the subjects had evidence of anxiety, and 11% had evidence of depression.

Interaction with Pregnancy

Caffeine is readily absorbed from the gastrointestinal tract, and it rapidly crosses the placenta. This results in fetal blood and tissue concentrations that are similar to maternal concentrations.[183,184] In 1980, the Food and Drug Administration (FDA) advised pregnant women to avoid all caffeine-containing foods or to use them sparingly.[185] Early studies had suggested that caffeine has an adverse effect during pregnancy, but most of these studies were performed in animals, and the implications of these findings for human beings were unclear. Human studies were flawed by the confounding effect of cigarette smoking. Linn et al.[186] evaluated the effects of coffee consumption in more than 12,400 women; they controlled for smoking, other habits, demographic characteristics, and medical history. They observed no association between coffee consumption and adverse outcomes of pregnancy, including preterm delivery and LBW infants. Similarly, Mills et al.[187] controlled for other risk factors in a multicenter study; the authors found no evidence that moderate caffeine use increased the risk of spontaneous abortion, IUGR, or microcephaly.

However, caffeine ingestion during pregnancy is not without risk. At least three cases of fetal arrhythmias caused by excessive maternal intake of caffeine have been reported.[188] These fetal arrhythmias occurred in utero and continued postpartum until they resolved spontaneously. They were not associated with any maternal arrhythmias or hemodynamic instability. The enzyme responsible for metabolizing caffeine is absent until several days after birth.[189]

Anesthetic Management

Withdrawal symptoms may present during labor, or they may occur in the patient who is fasting before or after cesarean section. There is a significant relationship between daily caffeine intake before surgery and postoperative headache.[190] Thus the anesthesiologist should consider caffeine withdrawal as a potential cause of postpartum headache, especially when the headache does not vary with a change in posture.

KEY POINTS

- Cocaine abuse remains a major public health problem, and the anesthesiologist should question all pregnant women about illicit drug use.
- The majority of women who abuse drugs *deny* drug use. If drug abuse is suspected, the patient should be tested.
- Rapid tests for urine metabolites of cocaine are available, inexpensive, and accurate.
- Drug abuse should be considered in the differential diagnosis for pregnant patients with severe hypertension, placental abruption, and/or no prenatal care.

- Cocaine abuse represents a relative contraindication to the use of propranolol because beta-adrenergic receptor blockade may cause unopposed alpha-adrenergic receptor stimulation and an exacerbation of hypertension.
- Opioid addicts must receive their daily dose of opioid to prevent symptoms of withdrawal.
- The anesthesiologist should not give an opioid antagonist or a mixed agonist-antagonist to a pregnant woman who is known or suspected to be an opioid addict.
- Physicians may safely use patient-controlled analgesia for postoperative pain management in opioid addicts.
- Nonsteroidal antiinflammatory drugs may also facilitate the provision of postoperative analgesia.
- Postoperative headache may be a manifestation of caffeine withdrawal.

REFERENCES

1. Ebrahim S, Gfroerer J. Pregnancy-related substance use in the United States during 1996-1998. Obstet Gynecol 2003; 101: 374-9.
2. Steadman JL, Birnbach DJ. Patients on party drugs undergoing anesthesia. Curr Opin Anaesthesiol 2003; 16:147-52.
3. Cregler K, Mark H. Medical complications of cocaine abuse. N Engl J Med 1986; 315:1495-500.
4. Freud S. On the general effects of cocaine (1885). Drug Depend 1970; 5:15-7.
5. Beattie GF. Soft drink flavours: Their history and characteristics. Perfumery and Essential Oil Record. 1956; 47:437-42.
6. Grinspoon L, Bakalar JB. Drug dependence: Non-narcotic agents. In Kaplan HI, Freedman AM, Sadock BJ, editors. Comprehensive Textbook of Psychiatry, vol 2. Baltimore, Williams & Wilkins, 1980:1621.
7. Hatsukami DK, Fischman MW. Crack cocaine and cocaine hydrochloride: Are the differences myth or reality? JAMA 1996; 276:1580-8.
8. Abelson H, Miller J. A decade of trends in cocaine use in the household population. Natl Inst Health Monograph Series 1985; 61:35-49.
9. Groerer SC, Brodsky MC. Frequent cocaine users and their use of treatment. Am J Public Health 1993; 83:1149-54.
10. Washton AM, Gold MS. Recent trends in cocaine abuse: A view from the national hotline, "800-Cocaine." Adv Alcohol Subst Abuse 1986; 6:31-47.
11. Neerhof MG, MacGregor SN, Retzky SS, Sullivan TP. Cocaine abuse during pregnancy: Peripartum prevalence and perinatal outcome. Am J Obstet Gynecol 1989; 161:633-8.
12. Kain ZN, Rimar S, Barash PG. Cocaine abuse in the parturient and effects on the fetus and neonate. Anesth Analg 1993; 77:835-45.
13. Rozenak D, Diamant YZ, Yaffe H, et al. Cocaine: Maternal use during pregnancy and its effect on the fetus and the infant. Obstet Gynecol Survey 1990; 45:348-59.
14. Sharpe TT. Sex-for-crack-cocaine exchange, poor black women, and pregnancy. Qual Health Res 2001; 11:612-30.
15. Winecker RE, Goldberger BA, Tebbett IR, et al. Detection of cocaine and its metabolites in breast milk. J Forensic Sci 2001; 46: 1221-3.
16. Gold MS, Washton AM, Dackis CA. Cocaine abuse: Neurochemistry, phenomenology, and treatment. Natl Inst Drug Abuse Res Monogr 1985; 61:130-50.
17. Sprauve ME. Substance abuse and HIV in pregnancy. Clin Obstet Gynecol 1996; 39:316-32.
18. Volkow ND, Ding YS, Fowler JS, Wang GJ. Cocaine addiction: Hypothesis derived from imaging studies with PET. J Addictive Dis 1996; 15:55-71.
19. Pitts DK, Marwah J. Autonomic actions of cocaine. Can J Physiol Pharmacol 1989; 67:1168-76.
20. Chiueh CC, Kopin IJ. Centrally mediated release by cocaine of endogenous epinephrine and norepinephrine from the sympathoadrenal medullary system of unanesthetized rats. J Pharmacol Exp Ther 1978; 205:148-54.
21. Kloner RA, Hale S, Alker K, Rezkalla S. The effects of acute and chronic cocaine use on the heart. Circulation 1992; 85: 407-19.
22. Nahas GG, Trouve R, Manger WM. Cocaine catecholamines and cardiac toxicity. Acta Anaesthesiol Scand 1990; 34:77-81.

23. Billman GE. Mechanisms responsible for the cardiotoxic effects of cocaine. FASEB J 1990; 4:2469-75.
24. Fraker TD, Temesy-Armos PN, Brewster PS, Wilkerson RD. Mechanism of cocaine-induced myocardial depression in dogs. Circulation 1990; 81:1012-6.
25. Liu SS, Forrester RM, Murphy GS, et al. Anaesthetic management of a parturient with myocardial infarction related to cocaine use. Can J Anaesth 1992; 39:858-61.
26. Chao CR. Cardiovascular effects of cocaine during pregnancy. Sem Perinatol 1996; 20:107-14.
27. Burkett G, Yasin SY, Palow D, et al. Patterns of cocaine binging: Effect on pregnancy. Am J Obstet Gynecol 1994; 171:372-8.
28. Woods Jr JR, Plessinger MA. Pregnancy increases cardiovascular toxicity to cocaine. Am J Obstet Gynecol 1990; 162:529-34.
29. Tashkin DP, Khalsa M, Gorelick D, et al. Pulmonary status of habitual cocaine smokers. Am Rev Respir Sys 1992; 145:92-100.
30. Bernasko JW, Brown G, Mitchell JL, Matseoane SL. Spontaneous pneumothorax following cocaine use in pregnancy. Am J Emerg Med 1997; 15:107.
31. King JC. Substance abuse in pregnancy. A bigger problem than you think. Postgrad Med 1997; 102:135-50.
32. Levine SR, Brust JCM, Futrell N, et al. Cerebrovascular complications of the use of the "crack" form of alkaloidal cocaine. N Engl J Med 1990; 323:699-704.
33. Lampley EC, Williams S, Myers SA. Cocaine-associated rhabdomyolysis causing renal failure in pregnancy. Obstet Gynecol 1996; 87:804-6.
34. Merigan KS, Roberts JR. Cocaine intoxication: Hyperpyrexia, rhabdomyolysis and acute renal failure. Clin Toxicol 1987; 25:135-48.
35. Nalbandian H, Sheth N, Dietrich R, Georgiou J. Intestinal ischemia caused by cocaine ingestion: Report of two cases. Surgery 1985; 97:374-6.
36. Moen MD, Caliendo MJ, Marshall W, Uhler ML. Hepatic rupture in pregnancy associated with cocaine use. Obstet Gynecol 1993; 82:687-9.
37. Kloss MW, Rosen GM, Rauckman EJ. Cocaine-mediated hepatotoxicity: A critical review. Biochem Pharmacol 1984; 33:169-73.
38. Orser B. Thrombocytopenia and cocaine abuse. Anesthesiology 1991; 74:195-6.
39. Livingston JC, Mabie BC, Ramanathan J. Crack cocaine, myocardial infarction, and troponin I levels at the time of cesarean delivery. Anesth Analg 2000; 91:913-5.
40. Hutter CM. Cocaine and pulmonary oedema. Anaesthesia 2003; 58: 285-6.
41. Burchfield DJ, Tebbett IR, Anderson KJ. Elimination of cocaine by pregnant sheep following single or multiple exposures. Toxicol Sci 2001; 63:157-9.
42. Knisely JS, Spear ER, Green DJ, et al. Substance abuse patterns in pregnant women. NIDA Res Monogr 1991; 108:280-1.
43. Spence MR, Williams R, DiGregorio GJ, et al. The relationship between recent cocaine use and pregnancy outcome. Obstet Gynecol 1991; 78:326-9.
44. Towers CV, Pircon RA, Nageotte MP, et al. Cocaine intoxication presenting as preeclampsia and eclampsia. Obstet Gynecol 1993; 81:545-7.
45. Stewart DJ, Inaba T, Lucassen M, et al. Cocaine metabolism: Cocaine and norcocaine hydrolysis by liver and serum esterases. Clin Pharmacol Ther 1979; 25:464-8.
46. Birnbach DJ, Stein DJ, Grunebaum A, et al. Cocaine screening of parturients without prenatal care: An evaluation of a rapid screening assay. Anesth Analg 1997; 84:76-9.
47. Birnbach DJ, Stein DJ, Grunebaum A. An instant approach to the differential diagnosis between preeclampsia and cocaine abuse (abstract). Am J Obstet Gynecol 1993; 168:A429.
48. Chasnof IJ, Lewis DE, Griffith DR, Willey S. Cocaine and pregnancy: Clinical and toxicological implications for the neonate. Clin Chem 1989; 35:1276-8.
49. Kline J, Ng SK, Schittini M, et al. Cocaine use during pregnancy: Sensitive detection by hair assay. Am J Public Health 1997; 87:352-8.
50. Oyler J, Darwin WD, et al. Cocaine disposition in meconium from newborns of cocaine-abusing mothers and urine of adult drug users. J Anal Toxicol 1996; 20:453-62.
51. Bingol N, Fuchs M, Diaz V, et al. Teratogenicity of cocaine in humans. J Pediatr 1987; 110:93-6.
52. Moore TR, Sorg J, Miller L, et al. Hemodynamic effects of intravenous cocaine on the pregnant ewe and fetus. Am J Obstet Gynecol 1986; 155:883-8.
53. Little BB, Ramin SM, et al. Peripartum cocaine use and adverse pregnancy outcome. Am J Human Biol 1999; 11:598-602.
54. Chazotte C, Forman L, Gandhi J. Heart rate patterns in fetuses exposed to cocaine. Obstet Gynecol 1991; 78:323-5.
55. Ganapathy V, Ramamoorthy S, Leibach FH. Transport and metabolism of monoamines in the human placenta. Trophoblast Res 1993; 7:35-51.

56. Prasad PD, Leibach FH, Mahesh VB, Ganapathy V. Human placenta as a target organ for cocaine action: Interaction of cocaine with the placental serotonin transporter. Placenta 1994; 15:267-78.
57. Sun LS, Takuma S, Lui R, Homma S. The effect of maternal cocaine exposure on neonatal rat cardiac function. Anesth Analg 2003; 97:878-82.
58. Burkett G, Yasin SY, Palow D, et al. Patterns of cocaine binging: Effect on pregnancy. Am J Obstet Gynecol 1994; 171:372-8.
59. Chasnof IJ, Burns WJ, Schnoll SH, Burns KA. Cocaine use in pregnancy. N Engl J Med 1985; 313:666-9.
60. Dinsmoor MJ, Irons SJ, Christmas JT. Preterm rupture of membranes associated with recent cocaine use. Am J Obstet Gynecol 1994; 171:305-9.
61. Acker D, Sachs BP, Tracey KJ, Wise WE. Abruptio placentae associated with cocaine use. Am J Obstet Gynecol 1983; 146:220-1.
62. Woods JR, Plessinger MA, Clark KE. Effect of cocaine on uterine blood flow and fetal oxygenation. JAMA 1987; 257:957-61.
63. Jasnosx KM, Hermansen MC, Snider C, Sang K. Congenital complete absence of the diaphragm: A rare variant of congenital diaphragmatic hernia. Am J Perinatol 1994; 11:340-3.
64. Fantel AG, MacPhail BJ. The teratogenicity of cocaine. Teratology 1982; 26:17-9.
65. Chavez GF, Mulinare J, Cordero JF. Maternal cocaine use during early pregnancy as a risk factor for congenital urogenital anomalies. JAMA 1989; 262:795-8.
66. Little BB, Snell LM, Klein VR, Gilstrap LC. Cocaine abuse during pregnancy: Maternal and fetal implications. Obstet Gynecol 1989; 73:157-60.
67. Chasnoff IJ, Bussey ME, Savich R, Stack CM. Perinatal cerebral infarction and maternal cocaine use. J Pediatr 1986; 108:456-9.
68. Martinez A, Larrabee K, Monga M. Cocaine is associated with intrauterine fetal death in women with suspected preterm labor. Am J Perinatol 1996; 13:163-6.
69. Bulbul ZR, Rosenthal DN, Kleinman CS. Myocardial infarction in the perinatal period secondary to maternal cocaine abuse. Arch Pediatr Adolesc Med 1994; 148:1092-6.
70. American College of Obstetrics and Gynecology Committee on Obstetrics: Maternal and Fetal Medicine. Cocaine in Pregnancy. ACOG Committee Opinion No. 114, Washington, D.C., September 1992.
71. Firestone D. Woman is convicted of killing her fetus by smoking cocaine. New York Times (Print) 2001; May 18: A12.
72. Frierson RL, Binkley MW. Prosecution of illicit drug use during pregnancy: Crystal Ferguson v. City of Charleston. J Am Acad Psychiatry Law 2001; 29:469-73.
73. Birnbach DJ, Stein DJ, Thomas K, et al. Cocaine abuse in the parturient: What are the anesthetic implications (abstract)? Anesthesiology 1993; 79:A988.
74. Birnbach DJ, Grunebaum A, Collins E, Cohen A. The effect of cocaine on epidural anesthesia (abstract). Am J Obstet Gynecol 1991; 164:400S.
75. Birnbach DJ, Stein DJ, Danzer BI, et al. Ephedrine resistance in the cocaine-positive parturient. Prevalence and treatment (abstract). Anesthesiology 1996; 85:A892.
76. Kreek MJ. Cocaine, dopamine and the endogenous opioid system. J Addictive Dis 1996; 15:73-96.
77. Unterwald EM, Horne-King J, Kreek MJ. Chronic cocaine alters brain mu opioid receptors. Brain Res 1992; 584:314-8.
78. Ross VH, Moore CH, Pan PH, et al. Reduced duration of intrathecal sufentanil analgesia in laboring cocaine users. Anesth Analg 2003; 97: 1504-8.
79. Boylan JF, Cheng DC, Sandler AN, et al. Cocaine toxicity and isoflurane anesthesia: Hemodynamic, myocardial metabolic, and regional blood flow effects in swine. J Cardiothoracic Vasc Anesth 1996; 10:772-7.
80. Vertommen JD, Hughes SC, Rosen MA, et al. Hydralazine does not restore uterine blood flow during cocaine-induced hypertension in the pregnant ewe. Anesthesiology 1992; 76:580-7.
81. Hughes SC, Vertommen JD, Rosen MA, et al. Cocaine induced hypertension in the ewe and response to treatment with labetalol (abstract). Anesthesiology 1991; A1075.
82. Hollander JE. The management of cocaine-associated myocardial ischemia. N Engl J Med 1995; 333:1267-71.
83. Ramoska E, Sacchetti A. Propranolol induced hypertension in the treatment of cocaine intoxication. Ann Emerg Med 1985; 14:1112-3.
84. Lange RA, Cigarroa RG, Flores ED, et al. Potentiation of cocaine-induced coronary vasoconstriction by beta-adrenergic blockade. Ann Int Med 1990; 112:897-903.
85. Guerot E, Sanchez O, Diehl JL, Fagon JY. Acute complications in cocaine users. Ann Med Interne (Paris) 2002; 153 (3 suppl): 1527-31.
86. Williams RG, Kavanagh KM, Teo KK. Pathophysiology and treatment of cocaine toxicity: Implications for the heart and cardiovascular system. Can J Cardiol 1996; 12:1295-301.

87. Murphy JL. Hypertension and pulmonary oedema associated with ket-amine administration in a patient with a history of substance abuse. Can J Anaesth 1993; 40:160-4.
88. Fleming JA, Byck R, Barash PG. Pharmacology and therapeutic applica-tions of cocaine. Anesthesiology 1990; 73:518-31.
89. Jatlow P, Van Dyke C, et al. Cocaine and succinylcholine sensitivity: A new caution. Anesth Analg 1979; 58:235-8.
90. Hollander JE, Hoffman RS, Gennis P, et al. Nitroglycerin in the treat-ment of cocaine associated chest pain: Clinical safety and efficacy. J Toxicol Clin Toxicol 1994; 32:243-56.
91. Shih RD, Hollander JE, Burstein JL, et al. Clinical safety of lidocaine in patients with cocaine-associated myocardial infarction. Ann Emerg Med 1995; 26:702-6.
92. Birnbach DJ, Browne IM, Kim A, et al. Identification of polysubstance abuse in the parturient. British Journal of Anaesthesia 2001; 87:488-90.
93. Mehta MC, Jain AC, Billie M. Effects of cocaine and alcohol alone and in combination on cardiovascular performance in dogs. Am J Med Sci 2002; 324:76-83.
94. Samuels SS, Schwalbe SS, Marx GF. Speedballs: A new cause of intraoper-ative tachycardia and hypertension. Anesth Analg 1991; 72:397-8.
95. Schindler CW, Tella SR, Erzouki HK, Goldberg SR. Pharmacological mechanisms in cocaine's cardiovascular effects. Drug Alcohol Depend 1995; 37:183-91.
96. Fischer SP, Healzer JM, Brock-Utne J. General anaesthesia in a patient on long-term amphetamine therapy: is there cause for con-cern? Anesth Analg 2000; 91:758-9.
97. Ong BH. Hazards to health: Dextroamphetamine poisoning. N Engl J Med 1962; 266:1321-2.
98. Elliot RH, Rees GB. Amphetamine ingestion presenting as eclampsia. Can J Anaesth 1990; 37:130-3.
99. Nora JJ, McNamara DG, Fraser FC. Dextroamphetamine sulphate and human malformations. Lancet 1967; 1:570-1.
100. Kalter H, Warkany J. Congenital malformations. N Engl J Med 1983; 308:491-7.
101. Nelson NM, Forfar JO. Associations between drugs administered during pregnancy and congenital anomalies of the fetus. Br Med J 1971; 1:523-7.
102. Oro AS, Dixon SD. Perinatal cocaine and methamphetamine exposure: Maternal and neonatal correlates. J Pediatr 1987; 111:571-8.
103. Eriksson M, Larsson G, Windbladh B, Zetterström R. The influence of amphetamine addiction on pregnancy and the newborn infant. Acta Paediatr Scand 1978; 67:95-9.
104. Little BB, Snell LM, Gilstrap LC. Methamphetamine abuse during preg-nancy: Outcome and fetal effects. Obstet Gynecol 1988; 72:541-4.
105. Johnston RR, Way WL, Miller RD. Alteration of anesthetic requirement by amphetamine. Anesthesiology 1972; 36:357-63.
106. Michel R, Adams AP. Acute amphetamine abuse: Problems during gen-eral anaesthesia for neurosurgery. Anaesthesia 1979; 34:1016-9.
107. Elliot RH, Rees GB. Amphetamine ingestion presenting as eclampsia. Can J Anaesth 1990; 37:130-3.
108. Samuels SI, Maze A, Albright A. Cardiac arrest during cesarean section in a chronic amphetamine abuser. Anesth Analg 1979; 58:528-30.
109. Smith DS, Gutsche BB. Amphetamine abuse and obstetrical anesthesia. Anesth Analg 1980; 59:710-1.
110. Gerrings PJ. Social and psychiatric factors in amphetamine users. Psychiatr Neurol Neurochir 1972; 75:219-24.
111. Lingford-Hughes A, Nutt D. Neurobiology of addiction and implica-tions for treatment. Br J Psych 2003; 182:97-100.
112. Gouzoulis-Mayfrank E, Daumann J, Tuchtenhagen F, et al. Impaired performance in drug free users of recreational ecstasy (MDMA). J Neurol Neurosurg Psych 2000; 68:719-25.
113. Morgan M, McFie L, Fleetwood H, Robinson JA. Ecstasy (MDMA): Are the psychological problems associated with its use reversed by pro-longed abstinence? Psychopharmacol 2002; 159:294-303.
114. Machines N, Handley SL, Harding GFA. Former chronic methylene-dioxymethamphetamine (MDMA or ecstasy) users report mild depres-sive symptoms. J Psychopharmacol 2001; 15:181-6.
115. Ho E, Karim-Tabesh L, Koren G. Characteristics of pregnant women who use ecstasy (3,4-methylenedioxymethamphetamine). Neurotoxicol Teratol 2001; 23:561-7.
116. McElhatton PR, Bateman DN, Evans C, et al. Congenital anomalies after prenatal ecstasy exposure. The Lancet 1999; 354:1441-2.
117. Singarajah C, Lavies NG. An overdose of ecstasy: A role for dantrolene. Anaesthesia 1992; 47:686-7.
118. Hoegerman G, Schnoll S. Narcotic use in pregnancy. Clin Perinatol 1991; 18:51-76.
119. Blanche F, Galea J. Cocaine trends and other drug trends in New York City, 1986-1994. J Addict Dis 1996; 15:1-12.
120. Spravve ME. Substance abuse and HIV in pregnancy. Clin Obstet Gynecol 1996; 39:316-32.
121. Gross EM. Autopsy findings in drug addicts. Pathol Ann 1978; 13:35-67.
122. Lewis JW, Groux N, Elliot JP, et al. Complications of attempted central venous injections performed by drug abusers. Chest 1980; 4:613-7.
123. Giuffrida JG, Bizzarri DV, Saure AC, et al. Anesthetic management of drug abusers. Anesth Analg 1970; 49:272-8.
124. Kliman L. Drug dependence and pregnancy: Antenatal and intrapartum problems. Anaesth Intensive Care 1990; 18:358-60.
125. Rodriguez EM, Mofenson LM, Chang BH, et al. Association of maternal drug use during pregnancy with maternal HIV culture positivity and perinatal HIV transmission. AIDS 1996; 10:273-82.
126. Naeye RL, Blanc W, LeBlanc W, Khatamee MA. Fetal complications of maternal heroin addiction: Abnormal growth, infections and episodes of stress. J Pediatr 1973; 83:1055-61.
127. Lee CC, Chiang CN. Maternal-fetal transfer of abused substances: Pharmacokinetic and pharmacodynamic data. Nat Inst Drug Abuse Res Monogr 1985; 60:110-47.
128. Berghella V, Lim PJ, Hill MK, et al. Maternal methadone dose and neonatal withdrawal. Am J Obstet Gynecol 2003; 189:312-7.
129. Drozdick J, Berghella V, Hill M, Kaltenbach K. Methadone trough levels in pregnancy. Am J Obstet Gynecol 2002; 187:1184-8.
130. Yu X, Cui J, Yu J. Tachycardia ameliorated by electroacupuncture in morphine withdrawal rats. Zhongguo Zhong Xi Yi Jie He Za Zhi 2000; 5:353-5.
131. Hulse GK, O'Neill G, Pereira C, Brewer C. Obstetric and neonatal out-comes associated with maternal naltrexone exposure. Aust N Z J Obstet Gynecol 2001; 41:424-8.
132. Gold MS, Pottash AL, Extein I, Kleiber HD. Clonidine in acute opiate withdrawal. N Engl J Med 1980; 302:1421-2.
133. Wood PR, Soni N. Anaesthesia and substance abuse. Anaesthesia 1989; 44:672-80.
134. Bell TG, Lau K. Perinatal and neonatal issues of substance abuse. Pediatr Clin North Am 1995; 42:261-75.
135. Koppel BS, Tuchman AJ, Mangiardi JR, et al. Epidural spinal infection in intravenous drug abusers. Arch Neurol 1988; 45:1331-7.
136. Hughes SC, Dailey PA, Landers D, et al. Parturients infected with human immunodeficiency virus and regional anesthesia: Clinical and immunologic response. Anesthesiology 1995; 82:32-7.
137. Weintraub SJ, Naulty JS. Acute abstinence syndrome after epidural injection of butorphanol. Anesth Analg 1985; 64:452-3.
138. Scheutz F. Drug addicts and local anaesthesia: Effectivity and general side effects. Scand J Dental Res 1982; 90:99-305.
139. Pavy TJG, Paech MJ, Evans SF. The effect of intravenous ketorolac on opioid requirement and pain after cesarean delivery. Anesth Analg 2001; 92:1010-4.
140. Boyle RK. Intra- and postoperative anaesthetic management of an opi-ate addict undergoing caesarean section. Anaesth Intensive Care 1991; 19:276-9.
141. Stacey BR, Brody MC, Burke DF. Patients with a substance abuse history can effectively use PCA (abstract). Anesthesiology 1990; 73:A759.
142. Day NL, Richardson GA. Prenatal marijuana use: Epidemiology, methodologic issues, and infant outcome. Clin Perinatol 1991; 18:77-91.
143. Smith CG, Asch RH. Drug abuse and reproduction. Fertil Steril 1987; 48:355-73.
144. Wu TC, Tashkin DP, Djahed B, Rose JE. Pulmonary hazards of smoking marijuana as compared with tobacco. N Engl J Med 1988; 318:347-51.
145. Fergusson DM, Horwood J, Northstone K, ALSPAC Study Team. Maternal use of cannabis and pregnancy outcome. BJOG 2002; 109:21-7.
146. Zuckerman B, Frank DA, Hingson R, et al. Effects of maternal mari-juana and cocaine use on fetal growth. N Engl J Med 1989; 320:762-8.
147. Beaconsfield P, Ginsburg J, Rainsford R. Marijuana smoking: Cardiovascular effects in man and possible mechanisms. N Engl J Med 1972; 287:202-12.
148. Wheeler SF. Substance abuse during pregnancy. Primary Care 1993; 20:191-207.
149. Stoelting RK, Martz RC, Gartner J, et al. Effects of delta 9-tetrahydro-cannabinol on halothane MAC in dogs. Anesthesiology 1973; 38:521-4.
150. Pietrantoni M, Knuppel RA. Alcohol use in pregnancy. Clin Perinatol 1991; 18:93-111.
151. Ebrahim SH, Luman ET, Floyd RL, et al. Alcohol consumption by preg-nant women in the United States during 1988-1995. Obstet Gynecol 1998; 92:187-92.
152. Lemoine P, Harrousseau H, Borteyru JP. Les enfants de parents alcooliques: Anomalies observees. A propos de 127 cas. Quest Med 1968; 25:477-82.
153. Abel EL. Alcohol and the fetus: Is zero the only option? Lancet 1983; 1:682-3.

154. Sampson PD, Streissguth AP, Bookstein FL, et al. Incidence of fetal alcohol syndrome and prevalence of alcohol-related neurodevelopmental disorder. Teratology 1997; 56:317-26.

155. American Council on Science and Health. Alcohol use during pregnancy. Nutrition Today 1982; 17:29-32.

156. Council on Scientific Affairs, American Medical Association. Fetal effects of maternal alcohol use. JAMA 1983; 249:2517-21.

157. Shepard TH. Catalog of Teratogenic Agents, 6th ed. Baltimore, Johns Hopkins University Press, 1989.

158. Kurth CD, Monitto CL, Albuquerque ML, et al. Effect of cocaine and cocaine metabolites on the cerebral microvasculature in piglets (abstract). Anesthesiology 1992; 77:A1039.

159. Wilkins-Haug L, Gabow PA. Toluene abuse during pregnancy: Obstetric complications and perinatal outcomes. Obstet Gynecol 1991; 77:504-9.

160. Jones HE, Balster RL. Inhalant abuse in pregnancy. Obstet Gynecol Clin North Am 1998; 25:153-67.

161. Kuczkowski KM. Solvents in pregnancy: An emerging problem in obstetrics and obstetric anaesthesia (letter). Anaesthesia 2003; 58:1036-7.

162. Prager K, Malin H, Spiegler D, et al. Smoking and drinking behavior before and during pregnancy of married mothers of live-born infants and stillborn infants. Pub Health Rep 1984; 99:117-27.

163. Sloan LB, Gay JW, Snyder SW, Bales WR. Substance abuse during pregnancy in a rural population. Obstet Gynecol 1992; 79:245-8.

164. Rodkey FL, O'Neal JD, Collison HA. Oxygen and carbon monoxide equilibria of human adult hemoglobin at atmospheric and elevated pressure. Blood 1969; 33: 57-65.

165. Philipp K, Pateisky N, Endler M. Effects of smoking on uteroplacental blood flow. Gynecol Obstet Invest 1984; 17:179-82.

166. Clark KE, Irion GL. Fetal hemodynamic response to maternal intravenous nicotine administration. Am J Obstet Gynecol 1992; 167:1624-31.

167. Morrow RJ, Ritchie JW, Bull SB. Maternal cigarette smoking: The effects on umbilical and uterine blood flow velocity. Am J Obstet Gynecol 1988; 159:1069-71.

168. Van der Veen F, Fox H. The effects of cigarette smoking on the human placenta: A light and electron microscopic study. Placenta 1982; 3:243-56.

169. Surgeon General. The health consequences of smoking for women. A report of the Surgeon General 1983. Washington, DC, US Government Printing Office, 1983:191-249.

170. Cnattingius S, Forman MR, Berendes HW, et al. Effect of age, parity, and smoking on pregnancy outcome: A population-based study. Am J Obstet Gynecol 1993; 168:16-21.

171. Stjernfeldt M, Berglund K, Lindssten J, Luduigsson J. Maternal smoking during pregnancy and risk of childhood cancer. Lancet 1986; 1:1350-2.

172. Kistin N, Handler A, Davis F, Ferre C. Cocaine and cigarettes: A comparison of risks. Paediatr Perinat Epidemiol 1996; 10:269-78.

173. Benowitz NL. Nicotine replacement therapy during pregnancy. JAMA 1991; 266:3174-7.

174. American College of Obstetricians and Gynecologists. Smoking and Reproductive Health. ACOG Technical Bulletin No. 180, Washington, D.C., May 1993.

175. Pearce AC, Jones RM. Smoking and anaesthesia: Preoperative abstinence and perioperative morbidity. Anesthesiology 1984; 61:576-84.

176. Becket AH, Triggs EJ. Enzyme induction in man caused by smoking. Nature 1967; 216:587.

177. Jusco WJ. Role of tobacco smoking in pharmacokinetics. J Pharmacokinet Biopharm 1978; 6:7-39.

178. Miller RR. Effect of smoking on drug action. Clin Pharm Ther 1977; 22:749-56.

179. Srisuphan W, Bracken MB. Caffeine consumption during pregnancy and association with late spontaneous abortion. Am J Obstet Gynecol 1986; 154:14-20.

180. Bunker ML, McWilliams M. Caffeine content of common beverages. J Am Diet Assoc 1979; 74:28-30.

181. Stringer KA, Watson WA. Caffeine withdrawal symptoms (letter). Am J Emerg Med 1987; 5:469.

182. Silverman K, Evans SM, Strain EC, Griffiths RR. Withdrawal syndrome after the double-blind cessation of caffeine consumption. N Engl J Med 1992; 327:1109-14.

183. Soyka LF. Effects of methylxanthines on the fetus. Clin Perinatol 1979; 6:37-51.

184. Goldstein A, Warren R. Passage of caffeine into human gonadal and fetal tissue. Biochem Pharmacol 1962; 17:166-8.

185. Goyan JE. Food and Drug Administration News Release No. P80-36, September 4, 1980.

186. Linn S, Schoenbaum SC, Monson RR, et al. No association between coffee consumption and adverse outcomes of pregnancy. N Engl J Med 1982; 306:141-5.

187. Mills JL, Holmes LB, Aarons JH, et al. Moderate caffeine use and the risk of spontaneous abortion and intrauterine growth retardation. JAMA 1993; 269:593-7.

188. Oei SG, Vosters RPL, Van der Hagen NLJ. Fetal arrhythmias caused by excessive intake of caffeine by pregnant women. Br Med J 1989; 298:568-9.

189. Weathersbee PS, Lodge JR. Caffeine: Its direct and indirect influence on reproduction. J Reprod Med 1977; 19:55-63.

190. Fennelly M, Galletly DC, Purdie GI. Is caffeine withdrawal the mechanism of postoperative headache? Anesth Analg 1991; 72:449-53.

Chapter 53

Trauma

B. Wycke Baker, M.D.

EPIDEMIOLOGY

Public health officials define trauma as a disease process.[2] Trauma especially threatens specific segments of the population (i.e., children, teenagers, young adults). Trauma occurs with seasonal and geographic variation; it is most prevalent during the summer and in urban areas. Risk factors include physical conditions (e.g., fatigue, intoxication) and environmental conditions (e.g., heavy traffic, bad weather). Frequent etiologies include motor vehicle accidents (MVAs), violent assaults, and fire. Most MVAs occur within 25 miles of home and account for more than half (i.e., approximately 50,000) of trauma-related deaths each year in the United States.[3]

Trauma is the leading cause of death for people under 45 years of age in the United States. Deaths resulting from trauma continue to increase at the alarming rate of more than 1% per year.[1] In many cases, trauma can be prevented. Current debate over national health system reform emphasizes the importance of preventive medicine and the allocation of resources to promote health maintenance and safety consciousness. Unfortunately, public safety measures (e.g., motorcycle helmets, automobile passenger restraints) often meet social and political resistance, and limited funding exists to investigate methods of injury prevention. As therapy for other medical and obstetric conditions improves, trauma may account for a greater percentage of the maternal and perinatal mortality rates.

The continuum of trauma care begins with basic life support in the field, progresses to specialized treatment at a regional referral center, and extends to comprehensive rehabilitation services after hospitalization. Anesthesiologists play a critical role throughout this process; they perform life-saving resuscitation, provide perioperative management, and offer ongoing consultation.

Management of a pregnant trauma patient requires the anesthesiologist to consider the unique changes in anatomy and physiology that occur during pregnancy. The location and pathophysiology of maternal injuries may differ from those that occur in nonpregnant patients. Potential disruptions in uteroplacental perfusion and the possibility of direct fetal injury place the fetus at risk for compromise.

Women of childbearing age are included among the population at greatest risk for trauma. Trauma occurs during approximately 5% to 10% of all pregnancies and ranks first among nonobstetric causes of maternal death.[4] The leading causes of trauma during pregnancy include MVAs, falls, violent assaults, suicides, and burn injuries. Falls may result from an unstable gait during pregnancy. Pregnant women also may be at increased risk for falling during physical activity and exercise.

Violence against pregnant women occurs with alarming frequency. Gazamarian et al.[5] reviewed 13 studies, published between 1963 and 1995, that examined the prevalence of violence against pregnant women. They observed that the prevalence of violence during pregnancy was 0.9% to 20.1%, and that two patterns of violence could be discerned. In the first pattern, "violence is a chronic problem for women who experience violence periodically or regularly; in the other pattern, violence is acute among women who had not experienced violence previously."[5] Further, they concluded that "violence may be a more common problem for pregnant women than preeclampsia, gestational diabetes, and placenta previa." Violent assaults often involve blunt trauma, penetrating trauma, or both, to the pregnant woman's abdomen. Despite recent efforts to prevent domestic violence, physical abuse frequently recurs during subsequent pregnancies. Gazamarian et al.[5] and others have urged the development and implementation of appropriate screening programs for women at risk for violence during pregnancy.

The incidence of trauma increases with each trimester of pregnancy. Approximately 8% of injuries occur during the first trimester, 40% of injuries during the second trimester, and 52% during the third trimester.[6] Rothenberger et al.[7] found that head injury and hemorrhagic shock account for most maternal deaths that result from trauma during pregnancy. In a retrospective study of pregnant women involved in MVAs in rural California, Crosby and Costiloe[8] found that maternal death was the most frequent cause of fetal death. More recently, Weiss et al.[3] noted that MVAs were the leading cause of fetal death even when maternal survival occurred. Fetal and perinatal death rates often exceed maternal death rates after penetrating abdominal trauma. For example, penetrating abdominal trauma during pregnancy causes maternal death in less than 5% of cases, but it results in direct fetal injury in 59% to 80% of cases. Perinatal death occurs in 41% to 71% of these cases. In contrast, limited published data suggest that the incidence, severity, and outcome of maternal burn injuries do not differ from those in the nonpregnant population and that fetal survival typically accompanies maternal survival.[10,11]

PATHOPHYSIOLOGY

Because trauma frequently causes hemorrhage and impairs respiratory function, hypoperfusion and hypoxia might be expected to emerge as predominant pathophysiologic processes. In fact, the pathophysiology of trauma during pregnancy is complex. Injuries can affect nearly all organ systems.

Like other diseases, trauma produces direct and indirect effects. For example, **direct tissue injury** from penetrating trauma, blunt trauma, or burns may trigger **indirect tissue injury** from shock, disseminated intravascular coagulation (DIC), and adult respiratory distress syndrome (ARDS).

Hemodynamic Changes

Pregnancy increases the mother's total blood volume and produces a number of hemodynamic changes, including *increased* cardiac output and heart rate, and *decreased* systemic vascular resistance (SVR). Some women also experience a decline in blood pressure. These changes may complicate the evaluation of intravascular volume, the assessment of blood loss, and the diagnosis of hypovolemic shock. In nonpregnant patients, signs of hypovolemic shock typically occur when hemorrhage results in the loss of a critical percentage (i.e., 20% or more) of total blood volume.[12] Griess[13] observed that a 30% to 35% decrease in maternal blood volume over 30 minutes produced no significant change in maternal blood pressure in gravid ewes. Pregnant women may be expected to have an improved tolerance to hemorrhage because of the 45% increase in total blood volume that occurs during pregnancy. Pregnant women who exhibit signs of hypovolemic shock may have lost a significantly greater percentage (40% or more) of total blood volume than nonpregnant patients.

Maternal hemodynamic measurements may not accurately reflect the status of the uteroplacental circulation. In contrast to the blood flow to other vital organs, there is little if any autoregulation of uterine blood flow. Uteroplacental perfusion is very sensitive to maternal hemodynamic changes. Griess[13] noted that uterine blood flow decreased by 10% to 20%—but maternal blood pressure did not change—in response to a rapid 30% to 35% decrease in maternal blood volume. Even when maternal hemodynamic measurements appear normal, uterine blood flow and fetal condition may be compromised.

Hematologic Changes

The dilutional anemia of pregnancy may complicate the assessment of intravascular volume and the assessment of blood loss in trauma victims. White blood cell counts often increase during pregnancy; the demargination of peripheral leukocytes accounts for this physiologic leukocytosis of pregnancy. Elevated counts do not necessarily signal infection in pregnant trauma victims.

Coagulation Changes

Pregnancy represents a state of accelerated but compensated intravascular coagulation, which is advantageous and disadvantageous for the trauma victim. Increased concentrations of coagulation factors may enhance hemostasis after trauma. However, pregnant patients are at increased risk for thromboembolic complications during periods of immobilization. DIC is a potential complication of severe trauma, placental abruption, or both. Massive transfusion may result in dilutional coagulopathy.

Acid-Base Changes

Buffering capacity during pregnancy is diminished by metabolic compensation for the respiratory alkalosis and by a physiologic decrease in hemoglobin concentration. As a result, pregnant trauma patients rapidly develop metabolic acidosis during periods of hypoperfusion and hypoxia.

Anatomic Changes

During the first trimester of pregnancy, the bony pelvis protects the uterus, and the fluid-filled amniotic sac protects the fetus from direct injury. Fort and Hartlin[14] reviewed 240 cases of trauma during early pregnancy and found no increase in fetal loss between pregnant victims of noncatastrophic trauma and pregnant controls. In contrast, *severe* abdominal trauma exposes the mother and fetus to distinct injuries during pregnancy. Pelvic fractures associated with blunt trauma to the lower abdomen may cause significant occult hemorrhage, which results in part from the increased tissue perfusion that is present as early as the first trimester. Urinary tract injuries occur in 10% to 15% of pelvic fractures. Compression of the bladder between the gravid uterus and pelvis increases the risk of bladder rupture. Pelvic fractures, hypovolemic shock, sepsis, and excessive exposure to ionizing radiation may cause first-trimester fetal loss.

During the second trimester, the pregnant uterus ascends out of the pelvis and displaces abdominal viscera cephalad. During this time, the anatomic pattern of injury is more variable. Cephalad displacement of the bowel may increase the risk of intestinal injury from penetrating trauma to the upper abdomen. Cephalad displacement of the bowel may also obscure the signs and symptoms of peritonitis. The gravid uterus may shield other structures (e.g., stomach, pancreas, mesentery, diaphragm) from injury. Hemorrhage into the retroperitoneal space occurs more often and may be more severe in pregnant than in nonpregnant patients.

Pearlman and Viano[15] reported the development of a pregnant crash-test dummy that they used to evaluate current passenger restraint systems. The crash-test dummy was designed to simulate a pregnant woman at 28 weeks' gestation. The investigators concluded that the current shoulder harness-lap belt combination resulted in the least transmission of force to the maternal abdomen and the least acceleration of the fetal head in simulated frontal collisions. This was true only when the lap belt was worn as low as possible on the abdomen, and when the shoulder harness was placed to the left of the uterus, between the breasts, and over the midportion of the clavicle. Other positions of the lap belt and shoulder harness resulted in a significantly increased transmission of force to the maternal abdomen, greater acceleration of the fetal head, or both. Further, the statistical evaluation of outcome. The following scoring systems provide an assessment of the severity of injury: (1) **anatomic injury scales** rely on physical examination and diagnostic procedure findings (e.g., Injury Severity Score); (2) **physiologic injury scales** (e.g., Champion Trauma Score, Glasgow Coma Scale) rely on assessment of physiologic responses and function; and (3) **combination injury scales** (e.g., Modified Injury Severity Scale) include key elements of anatomic and physiologic scales.[21-24] The Glasgow Coma Scale is the most widely used physiologic scoring system (Table 53-1). Injury scales help anesthesiologists and other medical personnel organize emergency care.

Regionalization of trauma and obstetric referral centers facilitates delivery of the specialized care that is required by pregnant trauma patients. However, smaller hospitals can and should establish procedures for the rapid mobilization of resources for emergency cases. Box 53-1 lists some of the resources that are required for the management of obstetric emergencies. Ideally, these resources should be kept together and readily available in an easily accessible central location. It is especially important that large amounts (i.e., four to eight units) of low-antibody-titer, type O, Rh-negative packed red blood cells are readily available for rapid administration to the trauma victim.

Airway Management

Airway evaluation and management is the first priority during initial resuscitation, and it is the anesthesiologist's primary responsibility. In pregnant trauma victims it is preferable to conduct airway management in a safe anesthetizing location (e.g., the operating room), which facilitates immediate access to a complete array of airway and monitoring equipment. The anatomic and physiologic changes of pregnancy (e.g., mucosal edema, increased oxygen consumption, decreased functional residual capacity) increase the difficulty and

TABLE 53-1 GLASGOW COMA SCALE

Response	Score
Eye opening	
Spontaneous	4
To voice	3
To pain	2
None	1
Verbal response	
Oriented	5
Confused	4
Inappropriate words	3
Incomprehensible words	2
None	1
Motor response	
Obeys commands	6
Purposeful movements (pain)	5
Withdraws (pain)	4
Flexion (pain)	3
Extension (pain)	2
None	1

Total Glasgow Coma Scale score = (I + II + III).
From Teasdale G, Jennett B. Assessment of coma and impaired consciousness: A practical scale. Lancet 1974; 2:81-4.

investigators observed that deployment of an airbag against a crash-test dummy wearing the lap belt and shoulder harness was associated with a small increase in force transmitted to the maternal abdomen and a modest increase in fetal head injury criteria. However, when the crash-test dummy was *unbelted*, airbag deployment resulted in a substantial increase in force transmitted to the maternal abdomen, as well as a substantial increase in fetal head injury criteria. The authors concluded that "use of the 3-point restraint system appears to reduce the likelihood of injury in this model." They emphasized the importance of the proper use of existing passenger restraint systems. Sims et al.[16] reported three cases of pregnant women (33 to 39 weeks' gestation) involved in MVAs in which the driver-side airbag deployed. None of these women or their fetuses sustained any injuries attributable to the airbag deployment.

A recent study of 322,704 singleton live births in Utah between 1992 and 1999 noted that pregnant women who did not wear their seatbelts during an MVA were twice as likely to experience excessive maternal bleeding—and nearly three times more likely to have a fetal death—than belted women involved in an MVA. The authors concluded that "wearing a seatbelt in a motor vehicle crash during pregnancy is a useful and effective intervention for reducing the risk of adverse pregnancy outcomes."[17]

OBSTETRIC COMPLICATIONS

Trauma to the pregnant uterus threatens both the fetus and the mother. Myometrial injury may cause the release of arachidonic acid and prostaglandins, which may precipitate **preterm labor**. Moreover, **premature rupture of membranes (PROM)** may occur, which increases the risk of infection and preterm labor. Severe abdominal trauma may cause **uterine rupture**, which occurs in 0.6% of all injuries during pregnancy.[18] Although it occurs infrequently, uterine rupture may be life threatening; maternal mortality rates approach 10%, and fetal mortality rates approach 100%. Penetrating uterine trauma often results in **fetal injury**. Case reports include descriptions of isolated injuries to the fetal membranes, umbilical cord, and placenta as well as direct fetal injuries. Fetal skull fracture and intracranial hemorrhage may occur in cases of blunt trauma during late pregnancy, after the fetal head has entered the pelvis.

Placental abruption complicates 1% to 5% of minor injuries and 20% to 50% of major injuries. Except for maternal death, placental abruption is the most frequent cause of fetal death after trauma. Even nonseriously injured pregnant women are at increased risk for placental abruption.[19] An acute decrease in transplacental gas exchange may lead to life-threatening fetal hypoxia and acidosis. Placental abruption also may cause overt or occult maternal hemorrhage and coagulopathy.

MANAGEMENT

Two principles guide the clinical management of trauma during pregnancy. First, guidelines for advanced life support apply to pregnant and nonpregnant patients; the "ABCs" of resuscitation" remain unaltered.[20] Second, maternal resuscitation is the most effective method of fetal resuscitation.

Logistic Considerations

Determination of the severity of injuries guides prehospital triage, directs clinical management, and provides data for the decrease the safety margin of airway management. Trauma can produce a wide range of airway-management problems, including facial fractures and cervical spine injuries. Some patients require the simplest airway maintenance maneuvers (e.g., administration of supplemental oxygen, suctioning, jaw thrust). **Tracheal intubation** is required if injuries result in any one of the following: (1) airway obstruction (2) compromised protective laryngeal reflexes and decreased ability to clear blood and secretions from the airway, (3) decreased adequacy of ventilatory efforts, or (4) hypoxemia despite administration of supplemental oxygen. Severe cases may require cricothyrotomy or tracheostomy. Early consultation with an otolaryngologist should be obtained if airway examination suggests that tracheal intubation may be difficult or impossible. In emergency circumstances, cricothyrotomy or tracheostomy may be difficult.

Respiratory failure is the most frequent cause of death when neck injuries involve the cervical spinal cord.[25] Airway management of patients with cervical spine injuries requires skill and attention. Flexion, extension, or rotation of the head and neck may worsen injuries. Until lateral cervical spine and odontoid view radiographs have excluded serious cervical spine injuries, I prefer techniques of **awake tracheal intubation** to avoid movement of the head and neck, reduce the risk of aspiration, and permit neurologic examination after intubation. Helpful measures that may decrease the risk of further neurologic injury include application of a cervical collar to maintain the head and neck in a neutral position and placement of the patient on a rigid backboard to immobilize the spine. Orotracheal intubation may be difficult in this position. In patients who are breathing spontaneously, the first choice is to perform fiberoptic nasotracheal intubation while the patient is awake. If technical problems (e.g., blood in the airway) interfere with fiberoptic visualization or if injuries (e.g., basilar skull fracture with cerebrospinal fluid [CSF] rhinorrhea) preclude nasotracheal intubation, other techniques (e.g., retrograde oral intubation while the patient is awake) should be considered.

Based on favorable outcome in nonpregnant trauma patients, many anesthesiologists and emergency medicine physicians consider rapid-sequence induction with cricoid pressure and orotracheal intubation a safe, effective method of airway control.[26] In uncooperative or combative patients, awake tracheal intubation may require too much time and may increase the risk of further neurologic injury. In selected cases, rapid-sequence induction may be safer than awake tracheal intubation, provided that physical examination reveals

---

Box 53-1 RESOURCES REQUIRED TO MANAGE OBSTETRIC EMERGENCIES

- Anesthesia machine and ventilator
- Standard airway and tracheal intubation equipment, including a fiberoptic bronchoscope, light source, cricothyrotomy set, jet ventilator, and tracheostomy tray
- Anesthesia drug cart
- Cart with all resuscitation drugs and a defibrillator
- Noninvasive and invasive monitoring equipment
- Electronic fetal monitor and ultrasonography equipment
- Primed infusion sets and pressure transducers
- An intravenous fluid warming cabinet
- Surgical packs
- A neonatal warmer and resuscitation equipment
- Four to eight units of low-antibody-titer, type O, Rh-negative packed red blood cells

---

acceptable conditions for orotracheal intubation. In these cases, the following precautions are recommended: (1) pharmacologic aspiration prophylaxis, if time and conditions allow; (2) denitrogenation before rapid-sequence induction of anesthesia; (3) application of cricoid pressure by an assistant; (4) application of neutral axial traction by a second assistant; and (5) minimal movement of the head and neck during laryngoscopy and orotracheal intubation.

Hemodynamic Resuscitation

Beginning with transport from the field and continuing throughout the hospital course, it is essential to avoid aortocaval compression in patients beyond 18 to 20 weeks' gestation. In these patients, the gravid uterus should be displaced away from the inferior vena cava and abdominal aorta at all times. In most cases, placing the patient in the lateral decubitus position relieves aortocaval compression. Alternatively, a folded blanket or wedge may be placed beneath the right hip, or the backboard or table may be tilted to the left. In some circumstances, it may be necessary to manually displace the uterus leftward.

The upper extremities provide the best sites for initial venous access. Two large-bore peripheral venous catheters may be placed to obtain blood samples for laboratory analyses (Box 53-2). In cases of hypovolemic shock, large-bore access to the central venous circulation permits more rapid volume resuscitation. I use the Seldinger technique to insert an 8.5-Fr central venous catheter into the internal jugular vein, the subclavian vein, or both, and rapidly infuse warmed (glucose-free) balanced salt solution. If hemorrhage is life threatening, low-antibody-titer, type O, Rh-negative packed red blood cells are transfused until type-specific or cross-matched blood is available.

Maternal hypotension may require vasopressor treatment. In my judgment, ephedrine is the vasopressor of choice for the treatment of modest hypotension in pregnant patients. Severe maternal hypotension may not respond to ephedrine. In such cases, either phenylephrine or epinephrine can be used.

It is preferable to place a radial intraarterial catheter as soon as possible to measure arterial blood pressure and facilitate the collection of arterial blood samples. Beat-to-beat monitoring of arterial blood pressure and heart rate, quantitative assessment of urine output, and frequent determination of blood gas tensions and acid-base status guide the initial resuscitation. Later, pulmonary artery catheterization with direct measurement of cardiac filling pressures, cardiac output, and SVR may guide postresuscitation management. The femoral vessels provide quick and easy vascular access during the resuscitation of nonpregnant patients.[27] In

---

Box 53-2 INITIAL LABORATORY ANALYSES FOR THE TRAUMA VICTIM

- Blood type, Rh status, and crossmatch
- Complete blood count
- Platelet count
- Prothrombin time
- Partial thromboplastin time
- Fibrinogen concentration
- Liver function tests
- Serum electrolyte levels
- Serum amylase levels
- Serum toxicology screen

contrast, catheterization of the femoral vessels may be difficult and dangerous in pregnant patients. Femoral catheters also increase the risk of thromboembolism and sepsis. In general, all vascular catheters inserted during the initial resuscitation of trauma patients should be removed and replaced within 24 hours.

Head Injury

Head trauma is the most frequent injury among MVA victims. During pregnancy, it is a leading cause of maternal death after trauma.[28] Increased intracranial pressure (ICP) frequently accompanies serious head injuries. Treatment of increased ICP includes (1) **physiologic methods** (e.g., mechanical hyperventilation, change in posture), (2) **pharmacologic methods** (e.g., hyperosmotic agents, diuretics, corticosteroids, barbiturates), and (3) **surgical methods** (e.g., ventriculostomy, craniotomy for decompression).

The following measures help promote cerebral venous drainage and help lower ICP: (1) elevating the head 30 to 45 degrees, (2) minimizing flexion or rotation of the head, and (3) avoiding catheterization of the internal and external jugular veins. Mechanical hyperventilation (i.e., $PaCO_2$ between 25 and 30 mm Hg) rapidly lowers ICP. The beneficial effect of hyperventilation diminishes after several hours, and a further decrease in $PaCO_2$ (i.e., less than 25 mm Hg) does not appear to provide additional therapeutic benefit. The hyperosmotic agent mannitol (0.25 to 1.0 g/kg intravenously over 20 minutes) transiently increases plasma osmolality, produces an osmotic gradient across the intact blood-brain barrier, and results in movement of fluid out of the brain. If the blood-brain barrier is not intact, mannitol may pass into the brain and worsen cerebral edema. In such cases, furosemide (1 mg/kg) may be safer than mannitol, and it may decrease the ICP more effectively. Furosemide decreases CSF formation and intravascular volume.

The usefulness of corticosteroids for treating head injury and an increased ICP is unclear. Corticosteroids (e.g., dexamethasone, 0.25 mg/kg every 6 hours) may decrease the formation of CSF and cerebral edema. Barbiturates decrease the ICP by decreasing cerebral blood flow and metabolism. Thiopental (1 to 3 mg/kg intravenous bolus) rapidly decreases the ICP for as long as 10 minutes. Pentobarbital (3 to 5 mg/kg loading dose; 2 mg/kg/hr continuous intravenous infusion) produces a more sustained decrease in the ICP.

Some methods of decreasing the maternal ICP may have deleterious effects on the fetus. Mechanical hyperventilation may limit gas exchange between the mother and the fetus in two ways: (1) it can significantly decrease the uterine blood flow by decreasing maternal cardiac output and blood pressure, and (2) in theory, it can decrease transplacental oxygen delivery by causing maternal respiratory alkalosis, which shifts the maternal oxyhemoglobin dissociation curve to the left.[29] Mannitol and furosemide therapy also may adversely affect the fetus. Both agents cross the placenta and can increase fetal urine output. Concern exists about the potential adverse effects of increased fetal plasma osmolality and decreased fetal intravascular volume.[30,31]

Despite these risks, prompt treatment of increased ICP during maternal resuscitation may be life saving for the mother and the fetus. The possibility of favorable maternal neurologic outcome justifies the temporary fetal risks of treatment. The fetal heart rate (FHR) is continuously monitored during efforts to decrease the maternal ICP. Careful, incre-

mental adjustments of maternal ventilation typically allow the achievement of a $PaCO_2$ that decreases ICP without producing abnormalities in the FHR tracing. Pulmonary artery catheterization allows the measurement of cardiac filling pressures, cardiac output, and SVR, which guides mannitol and furosemide therapy and facilitates the maintenance of maternal hemodynamic stability during acute treatment. Placement of a ventriculostomy catheter to drain CSF may help control the maternal ICP and may decrease fetal risk by decreasing requirements for hyperventilation, mannitol, and furosemide. Finally, prompt surgical intervention to correct the underlying problem (e.g., evacuation of a subdural or epidural hematoma) should optimize maternal and fetal outcome after head injury.

Diagnostic Procedures

The pregnant trauma patient often requires a radiologic skeletal survey, and she may require special radiologic procedures to diagnose injuries. In 1977, the National Council of Radiation Protection and Measurements described the risks of radiologic procedures during pregnancy.[32] The fetus appears to be most vulnerable to the nonlethal effects of radiation between 2 and 15 weeks' gestation. Abdominal and pelvic computed tomography (CT) scans expose the fetus to 5 to 10 rads.[33] These doses are unlikely to significantly increase the risks of mutagenesis, teratogenesis, and childhood cancer. Of course, physicians should eliminate unnecessary radiation exposure. When possible, a lead shield should be placed over the maternal pelvis and lower abdomen to decrease fetal radiation exposure.

Diagnostic peritoneal lavage is useful in cases of suspected intraabdominal injury.[34] After the first trimester, closed diagnostic peritoneal lavage (performed by means of needle paracentesis) may be less accurate and more dangerous than open diagnostic peritoneal lavage performed through a small supraumbilical incision. Based on findings during diagnostic peritoneal lavage, the mother may require laparotomy (Box 53-3).

Obstetric Management

Placental abruption may be a consequence of trauma during pregnancy.[19,35,36] Maternal signs and symptoms may include abdominal pain, uterine tenderness, uterine contractions, and vaginal bleeding. A recent study suggested that, among pregnant trauma victims, an admission white blood cell count > 20,000/mm³ may signal an increased risk of placental abruption.[37]

Electronic FHR monitoring may reveal fetal tachycardia or late FHR decelerations. Electronic FHR monitoring should begin as soon as possible because placental abruption typically manifests shortly after injury. Most clinicians agree that FHR monitoring should continue at least 4 hours because of concerns about delayed placental abruption. Electronic FHR monitoring should continue beyond 4 hours if one of the

Box 53-3 CRITERIA FOR POSITIVE DIAGNOSTIC PERITONEAL LAVAGE

- Red blood cell count greater than 20,000/mm³
- White blood cell count greater than 500/mm³
- Amylase level greater than 175 Somogyi units
- Presence of bile, bacteria, or intestinal contents in the lavage fluid

following situations is present: (1) placental abruption is sus-pected, (2) uterine activity is frequent, (3) rupture of mem-branes has occurred, (4) FHR abnormalities are present, or (5) maternal condition is critical. Additional testing may include ultrasonography, the nonstress test (NST), the con-traction stress test (CST), or the fetal biophysical profile. Ultrasonography helps establish fetal viability, determine ges-tational age, locate and assess the placenta, and estimate amniotic fluid volume. Ultrasonography does not consis-tently allow the identification of placental abruption. The obstetrician may perform a fetal biophysical profile (which includes ultrasonography and an NST) to assess fetal condi-tion after trauma (see Chapter 6).

Cesarean delivery may be necessary during laparotomy to improve surgical access to maternal injuries or to save a viable but compromised fetus. In particular, penetrating abdominal trauma that results in uterine and fetal injury may necessitate cesarean delivery. If such a delivery is anticipated, neonatol-ogy and pediatric surgery teams should be alerted.

Fetomaternal hemorrhage may occur after trauma during pregnancy, especially when injury to the uteroplacental circu-lation permits fetal red blood cells to enter the maternal cir-culation.[36,38] Fetomaternal hemorrhage occurs four to five times more often in pregnant trauma patients than in unin-jured pregnant women. In cases of abdominal trauma, uterine tenderness should increase the index of suspicion of fetoma-ternal hemorrhage. This type of hemorrhage occurs most often in patients with anterior uterine implantation sites. Fetomaternal hemorrhage may cause Rh isosensitization in the Rh-negative mother. Severe hemorrhage may result in fetal hypoxia or death. Surviving infants may have anemia.

The Kleihauer-Betke acid-elution assay helps detect and quantitate the volume of fetomaternal hemorrhage. In this assay, an acid phosphate buffer added to a sample of maternal venous blood elutes adult hemoglobin from maternal red blood cells but does not elute fetal hemoglobin from fetal red blood cells. After treatment with the acid phosphate buffer, the red blood cells subsequently are stained. Maternal red blood cells appear as "ghost" cells; in contrast, red blood cells that contain fetal hemoglobin have a dark stain. The obstetrician and pathologist can estimate the volume of feto-maternal hemorrhage by determining the fetal-to-maternal red blood cell ratio and the total maternal blood volume. Detection of fetomaternal hemorrhage is important in Rh-negative women because Rh(D)-immune globulin should be administered to prevent maternal Rh isosensitization. Sequential Kleihauer-Betke assays help detect ongoing feto-maternal hemorrhage. It may be necessary to administer more than one dose of Rh(D)-immune globulin to some Rh-negative pregnant women who are victims of trauma.

Perimortem Cesarean Delivery

When cardiac arrest occurs in a pregnant woman, standard resuscitation guidelines apply without modification. Although the success rate of cardiopulmonary resuscitation (CPR) in pregnant patients is unknown, data from nonpreg-nant patients indicate that initiation of CPR as soon as pos-sible after cardiac arrest increases the survival rate.[39] During effective CPR, cardiac output is approximately 30% of nor-mal values and depends on the efficacy of external chest compressions. Placing the patient supine on a firm, flat sur-face provides optimal resuscitation conditions for nonpreg-nant patients but exacerbates aortocaval compression in pregnant patients. Left lateral tilt or manual left uterine dis-placement may relieve aortocaval compression but may interfere with effective external chest compression and resuscitation efforts.

Cesarean delivery may facilitate maternal resuscitation by relieving aortocaval compression, increasing venous return to the heart, and increasing cardiac output during CPR.[40] When standard resuscitation efforts fail to restore maternal circula-tion, it may be difficult to make a decision to perform an immediate cesarean delivery. Factors to consider include the following: (1) the cause of maternal cardiac arrest, (2) the time interval since maternal cardiac arrest, (3) the probability of maternal survival, (4) the gestational age, (5) the probabil-ity of neonatal survival, and (6) the availability of personnel to care for the mother and neonate.[41] Katz et al.[42] have stated, "Unequivocally, if a pregnant woman suffers a cardiopul-monary arrest from any cause during the third trimester, a perimortem cesarean section should be performed." They have advocated the "4-minute rule," which states that peri-mortem cesarean delivery should begin within 4 minutes of cardiac arrest and that the fetus should be delivered within 5 minutes of maternal cardiac arrest. Performance of peri-mortem cesarean delivery within 4 to 5 minutes of maternal cardiac arrest increases the likelihood of maternal and neona-tal survival (Figure 53-1). In addition, case reports of infant survival after more than 20 minutes of maternal cardiac arrest support the performance of a perimortem cesarean delivery in any case of maternal cardiac arrest beyond 24 weeks' gestation when there is evidence of fetal cardiac activity.[43-48]

Anesthetic Management

Anesthetic management of pregnant trauma patients incor-porates the principles of anesthesia for trauma patients with those for pregnant patients undergoing nonobstetric surgery (Box 53-4). Resuscitation initiated during the preoperative period also may dominate the intraoperative course. Although hypovolemia precludes the administration of the typical doses of anesthetic agents, young patients may experience intraop-erative awareness during paralysis and light anesthesia, even when hypotension is severe. I administer a reduced dose of an induction agent (e.g., thiopental, etomidate) in hypo-volemic patients who require rapid-sequence induction of general anesthesia. Ketamine is unique among anesthetic agents because its sympathomimetic qualities result in car-diovascular stimulation. It is often used in trauma patients, but it causes myocardial depression in patients with severe hypovolemia and may increase ICP in patients with head injuries. Large doses (greater than 2 mg/kg) may increase uterine tone and decrease uteroplacental perfusion.[49,50] Small doses are less likely to adversely affect the uteropla-cental circulation.

Many anesthesiologists believe that balanced anesthetic techniques are superior to inhalation anesthetic techniques for the maintenance of hemodynamic stability during trauma surgery. In unstable patients, small doses of amnestic agents (e.g., midazolam, scopolamine) and small doses of an opioid (e.g., fentanyl) can be titrated until the patient's hemody-namic status permits the use of a volatile halogenated anes-thetic agent. The volatile halogenated agents provide distinct advantages in pregnant patients because they are easily titrated, minimize the risk of intraoperative awareness, decrease uterine activity by relaxing uterine smooth muscle, and may protect or restore uterine blood flow during noxious stimulation by decreasing plasma concentrations of catecholamines.[51] I prefer isoflurane because it has less effect on perfusion pressure in patients with hypovolemia than other volatile halogenated agents.[52] I avoid using nitrous oxide because it limits the inspired oxygen fraction and because it can expand air-filled cavities (e.g., pneumothorax).

Electronic FHR monitoring may help guide intraoperative anesthetic and obstetric management. During the administration of general anesthesia, decreased FHR variability reflects the transplacental transfer of anesthetic agents and is not necessarily a cause of concern. However, sustained fetal tachycardia or bradycardia or recurrent FHR decelerations suggest fetal compromise. FHR abnormalities may signal the need to (1) optimize maternal oxygenation, ventilation, and acid-base status; (2) expand maternal blood volume; (3) increase maternal perfusion pressure by administration of a vasopressor; (4) increase maternal oxygen-carrying capacity by transfusion of red blood cells; or (5) relieve aortocaval compression by increasing left uterine displacement or repositioning surgical retractors. An obstetric nurse or an obstetrician should be present to monitor the FHR and uterine activity, and an obstetrician should be immediately available to perform cesarean delivery of a viable fetus in case severe fetal distress occurs during surgery.

Uterine activity should be monitored during and after surgery. This facilitates the early diagnosis of preterm labor, which may be treated with a tocolytic agent such as terbutaline or magnesium sulfate (see Chapter 34).

ARDS may complicate the postresuscitation course. It is unclear whether the physiologic changes of pregnancy increase the risk of ARDS or whether its causes occur more frequently during pregnancy (Box 53-5).[53] In high-risk cases, I continue mechanical ventilation and monitor the patient for signs of ARDS after resuscitation.

Provision of care for the trauma patient may expose the anesthesiologist and other medical personnel to professional hazards. The treatment of trauma patients most likely

increases the risks of exposure to hepatitis and the human immunodeficiency virus (HIV). Strict adherence to universal precautions decreases the risk of infection.[54,55] Provision of care for the trauma victim also exposes physicians to medicolegal liability. Accidental injuries, unplanned surgery, and the lack of established physician-patient relationships contribute to the risk of litigation.[56] It is important to communicate with patients and family members in a direct, concerned, and timely manner and to complete medical documents in a thorough, legible, and timely fashion.

Box 53-4 PRINCIPLES OF ANESTHETIC MANAGEMENT OF PREGNANT TRAUMA PATIENTS

• Optimization of gas exchange
• Restoration of blood volume and tissue perfusion
• Protection of the brain and spinal cord
• Maintenance of uteroplacental circulation and fetal oxygenation
• Prevention of maternal awareness
• Detection of unrecognized injuries
• Correction of coagulopathy
• Maintenance of normothermia
• Avoidance of teratogenic drugs during the first trimester
• Prevention of preterm labor

Box 53-5 RISK FACTORS FOR ADULT RESPIRATORY DISTRESS SYNDROME IN PREGNANT TRAUMA PATIENTS

• Hypovolemic shock
• Massive transfusion
• Placental abruption
• Intrauterine fetal death
• Sepsis
• Tocolytic therapy

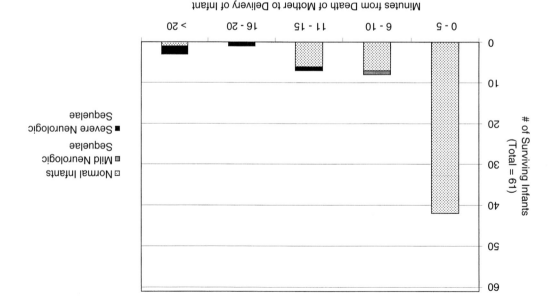

FIGURE 53-1. Infant survival after perimortem cesarean section, 1900-1985. A total of 61 infant survivals was reported. The true incidence of survival cannot be determined because the total number of perimortem cesarean deliveries is not known. The likelihood of infant survival is greatest when delivery takes place within 5 minutes of maternal cardiac arrest. Nevertheless, some infants delivered more than 20 minutes after maternal cardiac arrest have survived. (Data obtained from Katz VL, Dotters DJ, Droegemueller W. Infant survival following perimortem. Obstet Gynecol 1986; 68:555.)

KEY POINTS

- Trauma occurs in 5% to 10% of all pregnancies and ranks first among nonobstetric causes of maternal mortality.

- Head injuries and hemorrhagic shock account for most maternal deaths secondary to trauma.

- Maternal death and placental abruption are the most frequent causes of fetal death secondary to trauma.

- Hospitals should establish procedures to mobilize resources for emergency cases. It is especially important that hospitals establish procedures that facilitate the provision of large amounts of blood to the obstetric unit.

- Maternal resuscitation is the most effective method of fetal resuscitation.

- When cardiac arrest occurs in a pregnant woman, standard resuscitation guidelines apply without modification.

- The "4-minute rule" states that perimortem cesarean delivery should begin within 4 minutes of maternal cardiac arrest and that the fetus should be delivered within 5 minutes of maternal cardiac arrest.

- Electronic FHR monitoring helps guide anesthetic and obstetric management during maternal resuscitation, surgery, and postoperative management.

REFERENCES

1. American College of Surgeons Committee on Trauma. Advanced Trauma Life Support Student Manual. Chicago, American College of Surgeons, 1989.
2. Martinez R. Injury control: A primer for physicians. Ann Emerg Med 1990; 19: 97-101.
3. National Safety Council. Accident facts. Chicago, National Safety Council, 1987.
4. Pearlman MA, Tintinalli JE, Lorenz RP. A prospective controlled study of outcome after trauma during pregnancy. Am J Obstet Gynecol 1990; 162:1502-10.
5. Gazmararian JA, Lazorick S, Spitz AM, et al. Prevalence of violence against pregnant women. JAMA 1996; 275:1915-20.
6. Buchsbaum HJ. Penetrating injury of the abdomen. In Buchsbaum HJ, editor. Trauma in Pregnancy. Philadelphia, WB Saunders, 1979: 82-100.
7. Rothenberger D, Quattlebaum FW, Perry JF, et al. Blunt maternal trauma: A review of 103 cases. J Trauma 1978; 18:173-9.
8. Crosby WM, Costiloe JP. Safety of lap-belt restraint for pregnant victims of automobile collisions. N Engl J Med 1971; 284:632-6.
9. Weiss HB, Songer TJ, Fabio A. Fetal deaths related to maternal injury. JAMA 2001; 286:1863-8.
10. Deitch EA, Rightmire DA, Clothier J, Blass N. Management of burns in pregnant women. Surg Gynecol Obstet 1985; 161:1-4.
11. Smith BK, Rayburn WF, Feller I. Burns and pregnancy. Clin Perinatol 1983; 10:383-6.
12. Mattox KL, Bickell W, Pepe PE, et al. Prospective MAST study in 911 patients. J Trauma 1989; 29:8-11.
13. Greiss FC. Uterine vascular responses to hemorrhage during pregnancy. Obstet Gynecol 1966; 77:569-72.
14. Fort HT, Harbin RS. Pregnancy outcome after noncatastrophic maternal trauma during pregnancy." Obstet Gynecol 1970; 35:912-5.
15. Pearlman MD, Viano D. Automobile crash simulation with the first pregnant crash test dummy. Am J Obstet Gynecol 1996; 175:977-981.
16. Sims CJ, Boardman CH, Fuller SJ. Airbag deployment following a motor vehicle accident in pregnancy. Obstet Gynecol 1996; 88:726.
17. Hyde LK, Cook LJ, Olson LM, et al. Effect of motor vehicle crashes on adverse fetal outcomes. Obstet Gynecol 2003; 102:279-86.
18. Fries MH, Hankins GDV. Motor vehicle accidents associated with minimal maternal trauma but subsequent fetal demise. Ann Emerg Med 1989; 18:301-4.
19. Schiff MA, Holt VL, Daling JR. Maternal and infant outcomes after injury during pregnancy in Washington State from 1989 to 1997. J Trauma 2002; 53:939-45.
20. American College of Obstetricians and Gynecologists. Trauma During Pregnancy. ACOG Technical Bulletin No. 161. Washington, DC, 1991.
21. Baker SP, O'Neill B, Haddon W, et al. The injury severity score: A method for describing patients with multiple injuries and evaluating emergency care. J Trauma 1974; 14:187-90.
22. Champion HR, Sacco WJ, Carrazzo AJ, et al. Trauma score. Crit Care Med 1981; 9:672-5.
23. Teasdale G, Jennett B. Assessment of coma and impaired consciousness: A practical scale. Lancet 1974; 2:81-4.
24. Walker ML, Storrs BB, Mayer T. Factors affecting outcomes in the pediatric patient with multiple trauma. Child Brain 1984; 11:387-90.
25. Hastings RH, Marks JD. Airway management for trauma patients with potential cervical spine injuries. Anesth Analg 1991; 73:471-82.
26. Ballen J. Neuromuscular blockade in the emergency department. J Emerg Med 1987; 5:225-8.
27. Wax PM, Talan DA. Vascular access. In Callaham ML, editor. Current Practice of Emergency Medicine. Philadelphia, BC Decker, 1991:63-7.
28. Luce JM. Medical management of head injury (a review). Chest 1986; 89:864-72.
29. Levinson G, Shnider SM, deLorimier AA, et al. Effects of maternal hyperventilation on uterine blood flow and fetal oxygenation and acid-base status. Anesthesiology 1974; 40:340-7.
30. Bruns PD, Linder RO, Drose VE, Battaglia F. The placental transfer of water from fetus to mother following the intravenous infusion of hypertonic mannitol to the maternal rabbit. Am J Obstet Gynecol 1963; 86:160-7.
31. Witter FR, King TM, Blake DA. Adverse effects of cardiovascular drug therapy on the fetus and neonate. Obstet Gynecol 1981; 58:1005.
32. National Council on Radiation Protection and Measurements. Medical radiation exposure of pregnant women. NCRPM Report No. 54. Washington, DC, NCRPM, 1977.
33. Wagner LK, Archer BR, Zeck OF. Conceptus dose from two state-of-the-art CT scanners. Radiology 1986; 159:787-92.
34. Esposito TJ, Gens DR, Smith LG, Scorpio R. Evaluation of blunt abdominal trauma occurring during pregnancy. J Trauma 1989; 29:1628-32.
35. Pearlman MD, Tintinalli JE, Lorenz RP. Blunt trauma during pregnancy. N Engl J Med 1990; 323:1609-13.
36. Pak LL, Reece EA, Chan L. Is adverse pregnancy outcome predictable after blunt abdominal trauma? Am J Obstet Gynecol 1998; 179:1140-4.
37. Shah S, Miller PR, Meredith JW, Chang MC. Elevated admission white blood cell count in pregnant trauma patients: An indicator of ongoing placental abruption. J Am Surg 2002; 68:644-7.
38. Rose PG, Strohm PL, Zuspan FP. Fetomaternal hemorrhage following trauma. Am J Obstet Gynecol 1985; 153:844-7.
39. Swenson RD, Weaver WD, Niskanen RA, et al. Hemodynamics in humans during conventional and experimental methods of cardiopulmonary resuscitation. Circulation 1988; 78:630-3.
40. Strong TH, Lowe RA. Perimortem cesarean section. Am J Emerg Med 1989; 7:489-94.
41. Satin AJ, Hankins GDV. Cardiopulmonary resuscitation in late pregnancy. In Clark SL, Cotton DB, Hankins GDV, Phelan JP, editors. Critical Care Obstetrics, 2nd ed. Boston, Blackwell Scientific Publications, 1991:579.
42. Katz VL, Dotters DJ, Droegemueller W. Perimortem cesarean delivery. Obstet Gynecol 1986; 68:571-6.
43. Lopez-Zeno JA, Carlo WA, Fanaroff AA. Infant survival following delayed postmortem cesarean delivery. Obstet Gynecol 1990; 7:991-2.
44. Awwad JT, Azar GB, Aouad AT, et al. Postmortem cesarean section following maternal blast injury: Case report. J Trauma 1994; 36:260-1.
45. Chen HF, Lee CN, Huang GD, et al. Delayed maternal death after perimortem cesarean section. Acta Obstet Gynecol Scand 1994; 73:839-41.
46. Kaiser RT. Air embolism death in a pregnant woman secondary to oromortem cesarean section. Acad Emerg Med 1994; 1:555-8.
47. Lanoix R, Akkapeddi V, Goldfeder B. Perimortem cesarean section: Case reports and recommendations. Acad Emerg Med 1995; 2:1063-7.
48. LeSher AR, O'Connor RE. Cesarean section in a severely traumatized patient. Del Med J 1992; 64:619-22.
49. Seyde WC, Longnecker DE. Anesthetic influences on regional hemodynamics in normal and hemorrhaged rats. Anesthesiology 1984; 61:686-92.
50. Craft JB, Coaldrake LA, Yonekura JL, et al. Ketamine, catecholamines, and uterine tone in pregnant ewes. Am J Obstet Gynecol 1983; 146:429-34.

51. Shnider SM, Wright RG, Levinson G, et al. Plasma norepinephrine and uterine blood flow changes during endotracheal intubation and general anesthesia in the pregnant ewe (abstract). Anesthesiology 1978; 48:A115.

52. Horan BF, Prys-Roberts C, Roberts JG, et al. Haemodynamic responses to isoflurane anesthesia and hypovolemia in the dog, and their modification by propranolol. Br J Anaesth 1977; 49:1179-86.

53. Andersen HF, Lynch JP, Johnson TRB. Adult respiratory distress syndrome in obstetrics and gynecology. Obstet Gynecol 1980; 55:291-4.

54. Kelen GD. Human immunodeficiency virus (HIV-1) and the emergency department: Risks and risk protection for health care providers. Ann Emerg Med 1990; 19:242-5.

55. Centers for Disease Control. Guidelines for prevention of transmission of human immunodeficiency virus and hepatitis B virus to health-care and public-safety workers. MMWR 1989; 38:S-6.

56. Gild WM, Bennett JA. Medicolegal risks. In Brown DL, editor. Risk and Outcome in Anesthesia. Philadelphia, JB Lippincott, 1992:561-72.

Appendix A

American Society of Anesthesiologists Guidelines for Regional Anesthesia in Obstetrics*

These guidelines apply to the use of regional anesthesia or analgesia in which local anesthetics are administered to the parturient during labor and delivery. They are intended to encourage quality patient care but cannot guarantee any specific patient outcome. Because the availability of anesthesia resources may vary, members are responsible for interpreting and establishing the guidelines for their own institutions and practices. These guidelines are subject to revision from time to time as warranted by the evolution of technology and practice.

GUIDELINE I

REGIONAL ANESTHESIA SHOULD BE INITIATED AND MAINTAINED ONLY IN LOCATIONS IN WHICH APPROPRIATE RESUSCITATION EQUIPMENT AND DRUGS ARE IMMEDIATELY AVAILABLE TO MANAGE PROCEDURALLY RELATED PROBLEMS.

Resuscitation equipment should include, but is not limited to: sources of oxygen and suction, equipment to maintain an airway and perform endotracheal intubation, a means to provide positive pressure ventilation, and drugs and equipment for cardiopulmonary resuscitation.

GUIDELINE II

REGIONAL ANESTHESIA SHOULD BE INITIATED BY A PHYSICIAN WITH APPROPRIATE PRIVILEGES AND MAINTAINED BY OR UNDER THE MEDICAL DIRECTION[1] OF SUCH AN INDIVIDUAL.

Physicians should be approved through the institutional credentialing process to initiate and direct the maintenance of obstetric anesthesia and to manage procedurally related complications.

GUIDELINE III

REGIONAL ANESTHESIA SHOULD NOT BE ADMINISTERED UNTIL: (1) THE PATIENT HAS BEEN EXAMINED BY A QUALIFIED INDIVIDUAL[2]; AND (2) A PHYSICIAN WITH OBSTETRICAL PRIVILEGES TO PERFORM OPERATIVE VAGINAL OR CESAREAN DELIVERY, WHO HAS KNOWLEDGE OF THE MATERNAL AND FETAL STATUS AND THE PROGRESS OF LABOR AND WHO APPROVES THE INITIATION OF LABOR ANESTHESIA, IS READILY AVAILABLE TO SUPERVISE THE LABOR AND MANAGE ANY OBSTETRIC COMPLICATIONS THAT MAY ARISE.

Under circumstances defined by department protocol, qualified personnel may perform the initial pelvic examination. The physician responsible for the patient's obstetrical care should be informed of her status so that a decision can be made regarding present risk and further management.[2]

GUIDELINE IV

AN INTRAVENOUS INFUSION SHOULD BE ESTABLISHED BEFORE THE INITIATION OF REGIONAL ANESTHESIA AND MAINTAINED THROUGHOUT THE DURATION OF THE REGIONAL ANESTHETIC.

GUIDELINE V

REGIONAL ANESTHESIA FOR LABOR AND/OR VAGINAL DELIVERY REQUIRES THAT THE PARTURIENT'S VITAL SIGNS AND THE FETAL HEART RATE BE MONITORED AND DOCUMENTED BY A QUALIFIED INDIVIDUAL. ADDITIONAL MONITORING APPROPRIATE TO THE CLINICAL CONDITION OF THE PARTURIENT AND THE FETUS SHOULD BE EMPLOYED WHEN INDICATED. WHEN EXTENSIVE REGIONAL BLOCKADE IS ADMINISTERED FOR COMPLICATED VAGINAL DELIVERY, THE STANDARDS FOR BASIC ANESTHETIC MONITORING[3] SHOULD BE APPLIED.

GUIDELINE VI

REGIONAL ANESTHESIA FOR CESAREAN DELIVERY REQUIRES THAT THE STANDARDS FOR BASIC ANESTHETIC MONITORING[3] BE APPLIED AND THAT A PHYSICIAN WITH PRIVILEGES IN OBSTETRICS BE IMMEDIATELY AVAILABLE.

GUIDELINE VII

QUALIFIED PERSONNEL, OTHER THAN THE ANESTHESIOLOGIST ATTENDING THE MOTHER, SHOULD BE IMMEDIATELY AVAILABLE TO ASSUME RESPONSIBILITY FOR RESUSCITATION OF THE NEWBORN.[3]

The primary responsibility of the anesthesiologist is to provide care to the mother. If the anesthesiologist is also requested to provide brief assistance in the care of the newborn, the benefit to the child must be compared to the risk to the mother.

GUIDELINE VIII

A PHYSICIAN WITH APPROPRIATE PRIVILEGES SHOULD REMAIN READILY AVAILABLE DURING THE REGIONAL

*Approved by House of Delegates on October 12, 1988 and last amended on October 18, 2000.

[1]The Anesthesia Care Team (Approved by ASA House of Delegates 10/26/82 and last amended 10/25/95).

[2]Guidelines for Perinatal Care (American Academy of Pediatrics and American College of Obstetricians and Gynecologists, 1988).

[3]Standards for Basic Anesthetic Monitoring (Approved by ASA House of Delegates 10/21/86 and last amended 10/21/98).

ANESTHETIC TO MANAGE ANESTHETIC COMPLICATIONS UNTIL THE PATIENT'S POSTANESTHESIA CONDITION IS SATISFACTORY AND STABLE.

GUIDELINE IX

ALL PATIENTS RECOVERING FROM REGIONAL ANESTHESIA SHOULD RECEIVE APPROPRIATE POSTANESTHESIA CARE. FOLLOWING CESAREAN DELIVERY AND/OR EXTENSIVE REGIONAL BLOCKADE, THE STANDARDS FOR POSTANESTHESIA CARE[4] SHOULD BE APPLIED.

1. A postanesthesia care unit (PACU) should be available to receive patients. The design, equipment and staffing should meet requirements of the facility's accrediting and licensing bodies.
2. When a site other than the PACU is used, equivalent postanesthesia care should be provided.

GUIDELINE X

THERE SHOULD BE A POLICY TO ASSURE THE AVAILABILITY IN THE FACILITY OF A PHYSICIAN TO MANAGE COMPLICATIONS AND TO PROVIDE CARDIOPULMONARY RESUSCITATION FOR PATIENTS RECEIVING POSTANESTHESIA CARE.

---

[4]Standards for Postanesthesia Care (Approved by ASA House of Delegates 10/12/88 and last amended 10/19/94).

Appendix B

Practice Guidelines for Obstetrical Anesthesia: A Report by the American Society of Anesthesiologists Task Force on Obstetrical Anesthesia*

PRACTICE guidelines are systematically developed recommendations that assist the practitioner and patient in making decisions about health care. These recommendations may be adopted, modified, or rejected according to clinical needs and constraints.

Practice guidelines are not intended as standards of absolute requirements. The use of practice guidelines cannot guarantee any specific outcome. Practice guidelines are subject to periodic revision as warranted by the evolution of medical knowledge, technology, and practice. The guidelines provide basic recommendations that are supported by analysis of the current literature and by a synthesis of expert opinion, open forum commentary, and clinical feasibility data (Appendix).

A. PURPOSES OF THE GUIDELINES FOR OBSTETRICAL ANESTHESIA

The purposes of these Guidelines are to enhance the quality of anesthesia care for obstetric patients, reduce the incidence and severity of anesthesia-related complications, and increase patient satisfaction.

B. FOCUS

The Guidelines focus on the anesthetic management of pregnant patients during labor, non-operative delivery, operative delivery, and selected aspects of postpartum care. The intended patient population includes, but is not limited to, intrapartum and postpartum patients with uncomplicated pregnancies or with common obstetric problems. The Guidelines do not apply to patients undergoing surgery during pregnancy, gynecological patients or parturients with chronic medical disease (e.g., severe heart, renal or neurological disease).

*From Anesthesiology 1999, 90:600–11. © 1999 American Society of Anesthesiologists, Inc. Lippincott Williams & Wilkins, Philadelphia.

Developed by the Task Force on Obstetrical Anesthesia: Joy L. Hawkins, M.D. (Chair), Denver, Colorado; James F. Arens, M.D. Galveston, Texas; Brenda A. Bucklin, M.D., Omaha, Nebraska; Robert A. Caplan, M.D., Seattle, Washington; David H. Chestnut, M.D., Birmingham, Alabama; Richard T. Connis, Ph.D., Woodinville, Washington; Patricia A. Dailey, M.D., Hillsborough, California; Larry C. Gilstrap, M.D., Houston, Texas; Stephen C. Grice, M.D., Alpharetta, Georgia; Nancy E. Oriol, M.D., Boston, Massachusetts; Kathryn J. Zuspan, M.D., Edina, Minnesota.

Submitted for publication October 29, 1998. Accepted for publication October 29, 1998. Supported by the American Society of Anesthesiologists, under the direction of James F. Arens, M.D. Chairman of the Ad Hoc Committee on Practice Parameters. Approved by the House of Delegates, October 21, 1998. Effective date January 1, 1999. The methods and analyses used to develop these guidelines are described in Anesthesiology 1999; 90:600–11. A list of the articles used to develop these guidelines is available by writing to the American Society of Anesthesiologists.

Address reprint requests to American Society of Anesthesiologists: 520 North Northwest Highway, Park Ridge, IL 60068-2573.

Key words: Anesthesia cesarean section; analgesia labor and delivery.

C. APPLICATION

The Guidelines are intended for use by anesthesiologists. They also may serve as a resource for other anesthesia providers and health care professionals who advise or care for patients who will receive anesthesia care during labor, delivery and the immediate postpartum period.

D. TASK FORCE MEMBERS AND CONSULTANTS

The ASA appointed a Task Force of 11 members to review the published evidence and obtain consultant opinion from a representative body of anesthesiologists and obstetricians. The Task Force members consisted of anesthesiologists in both private and academic practices from various geographic areas of the United States.

The Task Force met its objective in a five-step process. First, original published research studies relevant to these issues were reviewed and analyzed. Second, Consultants from various geographic areas of the United States who practice or work in various settings (e.g., academic and private practice) were asked to participate in opinion surveys and review and comment on drafts of the Guidelines. Third, the Task Force held two open forums at major national meetings to solicit input from attendees on its draft recommendations. Fourth, all available information was used by the Task Force in developing the Guideline recommendations. Finally, the Consultants were surveyed to assess their opinions on the feasibility of implementing the Guidelines.

E. AVAILABILITY AND STRENGTH OF EVIDENCE

Evidence-based guidelines are developed by a rigorous analytic process. To assist the reader, the Guidelines make use of several descriptive terms that are easier to understand than the technical terms and data that are used in the actual analyses. These descriptive terms are defined below.

The following terms describe the availability of scientific evidence in the literature.

Insufficient: There are too few published studies to investigate a relationship between a clinical intervention and clinical outcome.

Inconclusive: Published studies are available, but they cannot be used to assess the relationship between a clinical intervention and a clinical outcome because the studies either do not meet predefined criteria for content as defined in the "Focus of the Guidelines," or do not meet research design or analytic standards.

Silent: There are no available studies in the literature that address a relationship of interest.

The following terms describe the strength of scientific data.

Supportive: There is sufficient quantitative information from adequately designed studies to describe a statistically significant relationship ($P < 0.01$) between a clinical intervention and a clinical outcome, using the technique of meta-analysis.

Suggestive: There is enough information from case reports and descriptive studies to provide a directional assessment of the relationship between a clinical intervention and a clinical outcome. This type of qualitative information does not permit a statistical assessment of significance.

Equivocal: Qualitative data have not provided a clear direction for clinical outcomes related to a clinical intervention and (1) there is insufficient quantitative information or (2) aggregated comparative studies have found no quantitatively significant differences among groups or conditions.

The following terms describe survey responses from Consultants for any specified issue. Responses are weighted as agree = +1, undecided = 0 or disagree = −1.

Agree: The average weighted responses must be equal to or greater than +0.30 (on a scale of −1 to 1) to indicate agreement.

Equivocal: The average weighted responses must be between −0.30 and +0.30 (on a scale of −1 to 1) to indicate an equivocal response.

Disagree: The average weighted responses must be equal to or less than −0.30 (on a scale of −1 to 1) to indicate disagreement.

GUIDELINES

I. Perianesthetic Evaluation

1. HISTORY AND PHYSICAL EXAMINATION

The literature is silent regarding the relationship between anesthesia-related obstetric outcomes and the performance of a focused history and physical examination. However, there are suggestive data that a patient's medical history and/or findings from a physical exam may be related to anesthetic outcomes. The Consultants and Task Force agree that a focused history and physical examination may be associated with reduced maternal, fetal and neonatal complications. The Task Force agrees that the obstetric patient benefits from communication between the anesthesiologist and the obstetrician.

Recommendations

The anesthesiologist should do a focused history and physical examination when consulted to deliver anesthesia care. This should include a maternal health history, an anesthesia-related obstetric history, an airway examination, and a baseline blood pressure measurement. When a regional anesthetic is planned, the back should be examined. Recognition of significant anesthetic risk factors should encourage consultation with the obstetrician.

2. INTRAPARTUM PLATELET COUNT

A platelet count may indicate the severity of a patient's pregnancy-induced hypertension. However, the literature is insufficient to assess the predictive value of a platelet count for anesthesia-related complications in either uncomplicated parturients or those with pregnancy-induced hypertension. The Consultants and Task Force both agree that a routine platelet count in the healthy parturient is not neces-

sary. However, in the patient with pregnancy-induced hypertension, the Consultants and Task Force both agree that the use of a platelet count may reduce the risk of anesthesia-related complications.

Recommendations

A specific platelet count predictive of regional anesthetic complications has not been determined. The anesthesiologist's decision to order or require a platelet count should be individualized and based upon a patient's history, physical examination and clinical signs of a coagulopathy.

3. BLOOD TYPE AND SCREEN

The literature is silent regarding whether obtaining a blood type and screen is associated with fewer maternal anesthetic complications. The Consultants and Task Force are equivocal regarding the routine use of a blood type and screen to reduce the risk of anesthesia-related complications.

Recommendations

The anesthesiologist's decision to order or require a blood type and screen or cross-match should be individualized and based on anticipated hemorrhagic complications (e.g., placenta previa in a patient with previous uterine surgery).

4. PERIANESTHETIC RECORDING OF THE FETAL HEART RATE

The literature suggests that analgesic/anesthetic agents may influence the fetal heart rate pattern. There is insufficient literature to demonstrate that perianesthetic recording of the fetal heart rate prevents fetal complications. However, both the Task Force and Consultants agree that perianesthetic recording of the fetal heart rate reduces fetal and neonatal complications.

Recommendations

The fetal heart rate should be monitored by a qualified individual before and after administration of regional analgesia for labor. The Task Force recognizes that continuous electronic recording of the fetal heart rate may not be necessary in every clinical setting[1] and may not be possible during placement of a regional anesthetic.

II. Fasting in the Obstetric Patient

1. CLEAR LIQUIDS

Published evidence is insufficient regarding the relationship between fasting times for clear liquids and the risk of emesis/reflux or pulmonary aspiration during labor. The Task Force and Consultants agree that oral intake of clear liquids during labor improves maternal comfort and satisfaction. The Task Force and Consultants are equivocal whether oral intake of clear liquids increases maternal risk of pulmonary aspiration.

Recommendations

The oral intake of modest amounts of clear liquids may be allowed for uncomplicated laboring patients. Examples of clear liquids include, but are not limited to, water, fruit juices without pulp, carbonated beverages, clear tea, and black coffee. The volume of liquid ingested is less important than the type of liquid ingested. However, patients with additional risk factors of aspiration (e.g., morbid obesity, diabetes, difficult airway), or patients at increased risk for operative delivery (e.g., nonreassuring fetal heart rate pattern) may have further restrictions of oral intake, determined on a case-by-case basis.

2. SOLIDS

A specific fasting time for solids that is predictive of maternal anesthetic complications has not been determined. There is insufficient published evidence to address the safety of *any* particular fasting period for solids for obstetric patients. The Consultants agree that a fasting period of 8 hours or more is preferable for uncomplicated parturients undergoing *elective* cesarean delivery. The Task Force recognizes that in laboring patients the timing of delivery is uncertain; therefore compliance with a predetermined fasting period is not always possible. The Task Force supports a fasting period of at least 6 hours before elective cesarean delivery.

Recommendations

Solid foods should be avoided in laboring patients. The patient undergoing elective cesarean delivery should undergo a fasting period for solids consistent with the hospital's policy for nonobstetric patients undergoing elective surgery. Both the amount and type of food ingested must be considered when determining the timing of surgery.

III. Anesthesia Care for Labor and Vaginal Delivery

A. OVERVIEW OF RECOMMENDATIONS

Anesthesia care is not necessary for all women for labor and/or delivery. For women who request pain relief for labor and/or delivery, there are many effective analgesic techniques available. Maternal request represents sufficient justification for pain relief, but the selected analgesia technique depends on the medical status of the patient, the progress of the labor, and the resources of the facility. When sufficient resources (e.g., anesthesia and nursing staff) are available, epidural catheter techniques should be one of the analgesic options offered. The primary goal is to provide adequate maternal analgesia with as little motor block as possible when regional analgesia is used for uncomplicated labor and/or vaginal delivery. This can be achieved by the administration of local anesthetic at low concentrations. The concentration of the local anesthetic may be further reduced by the addition of narcotics and still provide adequate analgesia.

B. SPECIFIC RECOMMENDATIONS

1. Epidural Anesthetics

a. Epidural Local Anesthetics. The literature supports the use of single-bolus epidural local anesthetics for providing greater quality of analgesia compared to parenteral opioids. However, the literature indicates a reduced incidence of spontaneous vaginal delivery associated with single-bolus epidural local anesthetics. The literature is insufficient to indicate causation. Compared to *single-injection spinal opioids* the literature is equivocal regarding the analgesic efficacy of single-bolus epidural local anesthetics. The literature suggests that epidural local anesthetics compared to spinal opioids are associated with a lower incidence of pruritus. The literature is insufficient to compare the incidence of other side-effects.

b. Addition of Opioids to Epidural Local Anesthetics. The literature supports the use of epidural local anesthetics when compared with *equal* concentrations of

epidural local anesthetics without opioids for providing greater quality and duration of analgesia. The former is associated with reduced motor block and an increased likelihood of spontaneous delivery, possibly as a result of a reduced total dose of local anesthetic administered over time.*

The literature is equivocal regarding the analgesic efficacy of *low* concentrations of epidural local anesthetics with opioids compared to *higher* concentrations of epidural local anesthetics without opioids. The literature indicates that low concentrations of epidural local anesthetics with opioids compared to higher concentrations of epidural local anesthetics are associated with reduced motor block.

No differences in the incidence of nausea, hypotension, duration of labor, or neonatal outcomes are found when epidural local anesthetics with opioids were compared to epidural local anesthetics without opioids. However, the literature indicates that the addition of opioids to epidural local anesthetics results in a higher incidence of pruritus. The literature is insufficient to determine the effects of epidural local anesthetics with opioids on other maternal outcomes (e.g., respiratory depression, urinary retention).

The Task Force and majority of Consultants are supportive of the case-by-case selection of an analgesic technique for labor. The subgroup of Consultants reporting a preferred technique, when all choices are available, selected an epidural local anesthetic technique. When a low concentration of epidural local anesthetic is used, the Consultants and Task Force agree that the addition of an opioid(s) improves analgesia and maternal satisfaction without increasing fetal or neonatal complications.

Recommendations: The selected analgesic/anesthetic technique should reflect patient needs and preferences, practitioner preferences or skills, and available resources. When an epidural local anesthetic is selected for labor and delivery, the addition of an opioid may allow the use of a lower concentration of local anesthetic and prolong the duration of analgesia. Appropriate resources for the treatment of complications related to epidural local anesthetics (e.g., hypotension, systemic toxicity, high spinal anesthesia) should be available. If opioids are added, treatments for related complications (e.g., pruritus, nausea, respiratory depression) should be available.

c. Continuous Infusion Epidural Techniques (CIE). The literature indicates that effective analgesia can be maintained with a low concentration of local anesthetic with an epidural infusion technique. In addition, when an opioid is added to a local anesthetic infusion, an even lower concentration of local anesthetic provides effective analgesia. For example, comparable analgesia is found, with a reduced incidence of motor block, using bupivacaine concentrations of *less than* 0.125% with an opioid compared to bupivacaine concentrations equal to 0.125% without an opioid.† No comparative differences are noted for incidence of instrumental delivery.

The literature is equivocal regarding the relationship between different local anesthetic infusion regimens and the incidence of nausea or neonatal outcome. However, the liter-

---

*No meta-analytic differences in the likelihood of spontaneous delivery were found when studies using morphine or meperidine were added to studies using only fentanyl or sufentanil.

†References to bupivacaine are included for illustrative purposes only, and because bupivacaine is the most extensively studied local anesthetic for CIE. The Task Force recognizes that other local anesthetic agents are equally appropriate for CIE.

ature suggests that local anesthetic infusions with opioids are associated with a higher incidence of pruritus.

The Task Force and Consultants agree that infusions using low concentrations of local anesthetics with or without opioids provide equivalent analgesia, reduced motor block, and improved maternal satisfaction when compared to higher concentrations of local anesthetic.

Recommendations: Adequate analgesia for uncompli-cated labor and delivery should be provided with the second-ary goal of producing as little motor block as possible. The lowest concentration of local anesthetic infusion that provides adequate maternal analgesia and satisfaction should be used. For example, an infusion concentration of bupivacaine equal to or greater than 0.25% is unnecessary for labor analgesia for most patients. The addition of an opioid(s) to a low concen-tration of local anesthetic may improve analgesia and mini-mize motor block. Resources for the treatment of potential complications should be available.

2. Spinal Opioids with or without Local Anesthetics

The literature suggests that spinal opioids with or without local anesthetics provide effective labor analgesia without sig-nificantly altering the incidence of neonatal complications. There is insufficient literature to compare spinal opioids with parenteral opioids. However, the Consultants and Task Force agree that spinal opioids provide improved maternal analge-sia as compared to parenteral opioids.

The literature is equivocal regarding analgesic efficacy of spinal opioids compared to epidural local anesthetics. The Consultants and Task Force agree that spinal opioids pro-vide equivalent analgesia compared to epidural local anes-thetics. The Task Force agrees that the rapid onset of analgesia provided by single-injection spinal techniques may be advantageous for selected patients (e.g., those in advanced labor).

Recommendations: Spinal opioids with or without local anesthetics may be used to provide effective, although time-limited, analgesia for labor. Resources for the treatment of potential complications (e.g., pruritus, nausea, hypotension, respiratory depression) should be available.

3. Combined Spinal-Epidural Techniques

Although the literature suggests that combined spinal-epidural techniques (CSE) provide effective analgesia, the lit-erature is insufficient to evaluate the analgesic efficacy of CSE compared to epidural local anesthetics. The literature indi-cates that use of CSE techniques with or without opioids results in a higher incidence of pruritus and nausea. The Task Force and Consultants are equivocal regarding improved analgesia or maternal benefit of CSE versus epidural techniques. Although the literature is insufficient to evaluate fetal and neonatal out-comes of CSE techniques, the Task Force and Consultants agree that CSE does not increase the risk of fetal or neonatal complications.

Recommendations: Combined spinal-epidural tech-niques may be used to provide rapid and effective analgesia for labor. Resources for the treatment of potential complica-tions (e.g., pruritus, nausea, hypotension, respiratory depres-sion) should be available.

4. Regional Analgesia and Progress of Labor

There is insufficient literature to indicate whether timing of analgesia related to cervical dilation affects labor and deliv-ery outcomes. Both the Task Force and Consultants agree that cervical dilation at the time of epidural analgesia administra-tion does not impact the outcome of labor.

The literature indicates that epidural analgesia may be used in a trial of labor for previous cesarean section patients with-out adversely affecting the incidence of vaginal delivery. However, randomized comparisons of epidural versus other specific anesthetic techniques were not found, and compari-son groups were often confounded.

Recommendations: Cervical dilation is not a reliable means of determining when regional analgesia should be ini-tiated. Regional analgesia should be administered on an indi-vidualized basis.

5. Monitored or Stand-by Anesthesia Care for Complicated Vaginal Delivery

Monitored anesthesia care refers to instances in which an anesthesiologist has been called upon to provide specific anes-thesia services to a particular patient undergoing a planned procedure.[2] For these Guidelines, stand-by anesthesia care refers to the availability of the anesthesiologist in the facility, in the event of obstetric complications. The literature is silent regarding the subject of monitored or stand-by anesthesia care in obstetrics. However, the Task Force and Consultants agree that monitored or stand-by anesthesia care for compli-cated vaginal delivery reduces maternal, fetal, and neonatal complications.

Recommendations: Either monitored or stand-by anes-thesia care, determined on a case-by-case basis for compli-cated vaginal delivery (e.g., breech presentation, twins, and trial of instrumental delivery), should be made available when requested by the obstetrician.

IV. Removal of Retained Placenta

1. ANESTHETIC CHOICES

The literature is insufficient to indicate whether a particular type of anesthetic is more effective than another for removal of retained placenta. The literature is also insufficient to assess the relationship between a particular type of anesthetic and maternal complications. The Task Force and Consultants agree that spinal or epidural anesthesia (i.e., regional anesthe-sia) is associated with reduced maternal complications and improved satisfaction when compared to general anesthesia or sedation/analgesia. The Task Force recognizes that circum-stances may occur when general anesthesia or sedation/anal-gesia may be the more appropriate anesthetic choice (e.g., significant hemorrhage).

Recommendations: Regional anesthesia, general endo-tracheal anesthesia, or sedation/analgesia may be used for removal of retained placenta. Hemodynamic status should be assessed before giving regional anesthesia to a parturient who has experienced significant bleeding. In cases involving signif-icant maternal hemorrhage, a general anesthetic may be preferable to initiating regional anesthesia. Sedation/analgesia should be titrated carefully due to the potential risk of pul-monary aspiration in the recently delivered parturient with an unprotected airway.

2. NITROGLYCERIN FOR UTERINE RELAXATION

The literature suggests and the Consultants agree that the administration of nitroglycerin is effective for uterine relaxation during removal of retained placental tissue.

Recommendations: Nitroglycerin is an alternative to terbutaline sulfate or general endotracheal anesthesia with halogenated agents for uterine relaxation during removal of